Foye's Principles of Medicinal Chemistry

FIFTH EDITION

Foye's Principles of Medicinal Chemistry

Fifth Edition

David A. Williams, Ph.D.

Professor of Chemistry
Massachusetts College of Pharmacy and Health Sciences
Boston, Massachusetts

Thomas L. Lemke, Ph.D.

Associate Dean for Professional Programs and
Professor of Medicinal Chemistry
College of Pharmacy
University of Houston
Houston, Texas

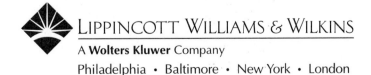

LIPPINCOTT WILLIAMS & WILKINS

A **Wolters Kluwer** Company

Philadelphia • Baltimore • New York • London
Buenos Aires • Hong Kong • Sydney • Tokyo

Editor: David Troy
Managing Editor: Matt Hauber
Marketing Manager: Anne Smith
Production Editor: Christina Remsberg
Designer: Armen Kojoyian
Compositor: Graphic World
Printer: Quebecor World-Dubuque

Library of Congress Cataloging-in-Publication Data
Williams, David A., 1938-
    Foye's principles of medicinal chemistry/David A. Williams, Thomas L. Lemke.—5th ed.
        p.   cm.
    Includes index.
    ISBN 0-683-30737-1
        1. Pharmaceutical chemistry. I. Title: Principles of medicinal chemistry. II. Lemke, Thomas L. III. Title.

RS403 .P75 2002
    616.07'56–dc21   2001050327

02 03 04 05
1 2 3 4 5 6 7 8 9 10

Preface

As defined by IUPAC, medicinal chemistry is a chemistry-based discipline, involving aspects of biological, medical and pharmaceutical sciences. It is concerned with the invention, discovery, design, identification and preparation of biologically active compounds, the study of their metabolism, the interpretation of their mode of action at the molecular level and the construction of structure-activity relationships (SAR), the relationship between chemical structure and pharmacological activity for a series of compounds.

As we begin a new century, we look back 30 years to the first edition of *Foye's Principles of Medicinal Chemistry* and then back 50 years to the first edition of Wilson and Gisvold's textbook, *Organic Chemistry in Pharmacy* (later renamed *Textbook of Organic Medicinal and Pharmaceutical Chemistry*), and can examine how the teaching of medicinal chemistry has evolved over the last half of the previous century. Fifty years ago the approach to teaching drug classification was based on chemical functional groups; in the 1970's it was the relationship between chemical structure and pharmacological activity for a series of compounds, and today, it is the integration of these principles with pharmacology and therapeutics into a single multi-semester course called pharmacodynamics, pharmacotherapeutics, or another similar name. Drug discovery and development maintains its role in traditional drug therapy, but its application to pharmacogenomics may well become the treatment modality of the future. The scope of knowledge in organic chemistry, biochemistry, pharmacology, and therapeutics allows scientists to make generalizations connecting the physico-chemical properties of small organic molecules and peptides to the receptor and biochemical properties of living systems. As a consequence, these generalizations, validated by repetitive examples, emerge in time as principles of drug discovery and drug mechanisms, principles that describe the structural relationships between diverse organic molecules and the biomolecular functions that predict their mechanisms toward controlling diseases.

The organizational approach we have taken in this textbook builds from the principles of drug discovery, physico-chemical properties of drug molecules, and ADMET (absorption-distribution-metabolism-excretion-toxicity), to their integration into therapeutic substances. Our challenge has been to provide a comprehensive description of drug discovery and pharmacodynamic agents in an introductory textbook. To address the increasing emphasis in U.S. pharmacy schools to integrating medicinal chemistry with pharmacology and clinical pharmacy and the creation of one-semester principle courses, we have organized the book into three parts: Part I: Principles of Drug Discovery; Part II: Pharmacodynamic Agents (with further subdivision into drugs affecting different systems of the body); and Part III: Recent Advances in Drug Discovery. Part I is designed for the one-semester course in principles of drug discovery, and Parts II and III for an integrated course or courses in pharmacodynamics/pharmacotherapeutics.

New features to this textbook include an overview of the drug development process from the perspective of an industrial research scientist (Michael Williams), an overview of drug receptors (David Triggle), case studies to supplement many of the pharmacodynamic chapters (Drs. Roche and Zito), additional new chapters, text boxes that explore special-interest topics or chapter-related topics, and selected readings and up-to-date references to encourage further exploration. In addition, a companion web page at http://connection.lww.com/pharmacy provides both a Student Resource Center, which contains the answers to the cases in the book and supplemental cases and study material, and a Faculty Resource Center, which contains the answers to the supplemental cases and a section for chapter updates.

We are both medicinal chemists, and our approaches to editing this fifth edition of *Foye's Principles of Medicinal Chemistry* are influenced by our respective academic backgrounds. We believe that our collaboration on this textbook represents a melding of our perspectives that will provide new dimensions of appreciation and understanding for all students. In editing this multi-authored book we have tried to ensure a more-or-less consistent style in the organization of the respective chapters.

We are indebted to our knowledgeable contributors, for without them this book would not exist; to Vickie Roche and Sandy Zito for creating the case studies; to our respective Deans, Department Chairs, and senior administrators for allowing us the time and facilities to complete this book; and to colleagues at our respective institutions who carefully reviewed portions of the chapter manuscripts and case studies for accuracy.

We gratefully acknowledge many other people who assisted and encouraged us in writing and editing this fifth edition of *Foye's Principles*. These include the managing editor Matt Hauber for his tactfulness in keeping us on schedule, the other editorial staff at LWW, and Donna Balado, who recruited us to this monumental task. We owe a very special ***thank you*** to our devoted wives for their understanding and sacrifices over the past several years.

With the publication of this fifth edition of this book, we celebrate and commemorate the contributions of William O. Foye whose vision founded this textbook. We also commemorate the contributions of Charles Wilson and Ole Gisvold, who founded the first textbook in pharmaceutical and medicinal chemistry and introduced many of us to the world of medicinal chemistry, and the contributions of research mentors who influenced our teachings in medicinal chemistry, William O Foye, Edward Smissman, and Philip S. Portoghese.

David A. Williams PhD
Professor of Chemistry
Massachusetts College of Pharmacy
   and Health Sciences
Boston, Massachusetts

Thomas L. Lemke PhD
Professor of Medicinal Chemistry
University of Houston
College of Pharmacy
Houston, Texas

INTRODUCTION TO MEDICINAL CHEMISTRY CASE STUDIES

We are pleased to introduce the student (and faculty) users of *Foye's Principles of Medicinal Chemistry* textbook to our medicinal chemistry case studies, one of which is contained at the end of most of the chapters in this book. (Answers to the case studies and additional cases are available in the Student Resource Center of the *Foye's Principles of Medicinal Chemistry* website, http://connection.lww.com/pharmacy.) This preface is written to explain their scope and purpose, and help those who are unfamiliar with our technique of illustrating the therapeutic relevance of chemistry get the most out of the exercise.

Like the more familiar therapeutic case studies, medicinal chemistry case studies are clinical scenarios that present a patient in need of a pharmacist's expert intervention. The learner, in the role of the pharmacist, evaluates the patient's clinical and personal situation and makes a drug product selection from a limited number of therapeutic choices. However, in a medicinal chemistry case study, only the structures of the potential therapeutic candidates are given. To make their professional recommendation, students must conduct a thorough analysis of *key structure activity relationships (SAR)* in order to predict such things as relative potency, receptor selectivity, and duration of action and potential for adverse reactions, and then apply the knowledge gained to meet the patient's therapeutic needs.

The therapeutic choices we offer in each case have been carefully selected to allow students to thoroughly review the therapeutically relevant chemistry of the classes of drugs used to treat a particular disease. By working thoughtfully and scientifically through the cases, students will not only master chemical concepts and principles and reinforce basic SAR, but also learn how to actively use their unique knowledge of drug chemistry when thinking critically about patient care. This skill will be invaluable to you when, as a practitioner, you are faced with a full gamut of therapeutic options to analyze in order to ensure the best therapeutic outcomes for your patients.

In short, here's what we hope you will gain by working our cases.

- Mastery of the important concepts needed to be successful in the medicinal chemistry component of your pharmacy curriculum;
- An understanding of the relevance of drug chemistry to pharmacological action and therapeutic utility, and the ability to discriminate between therapeutic options based on that understanding;
- An enhanced ability to think critically and scientifically about drug use decisions;
- A commitment to caring about the impact of your professional decisions on your patients' quality of life;
- An appreciation of your unique role as the chemist of the health care team.

We hope you find these case studies both challenging and enjoyable, and encourage you to use them as a springboard to more in-depth discussions with your faculty about the role of chemistry in rational therapeutic decision-making.

Victoria Roche
S. William Zito
11/02/01

Contributors

Ali R. Banijamali, Ph.D.
Senior Research Scientist
Uniroyal Chemical Company
Crompton Corporation
Middlebury, Connecticut

Eric Billings, Ph.D.
Director, NHLBI Bioinfermatics Care Facility
National Institutes of Health
Bethesda, Maryland

Raymond G. Booth, Ph.D.
Department of Medicinal Chemistry
School of Pharmacy
University of North Carolina
Chapel Hill, North Carolina

Ronald F. Borne, Ph.D.
Professor of Medicinal Chemistry
School of Pharmacy
The University of Mississippi
University, Mississippi

Robert W. Brueggemeir, Ph.D.
Professor, Medicinal Chemistry
College of Pharmacy
The Ohio State University
Columbus, Ohio

Patrick S. Callery, Ph.D.
Professor of Medicinal Chemistry
Department of Basic Pharmaceutical Sciences
West Virginia University
Morgantown, West Virginia

Alice M. Clark, Ph.D.
National Center for Natural Products Research
    and Department of Pharmacognosy
School of Pharmacy
The University of Mississippi
University, Mississippi

James T. Dalton, Ph.D.
Associate Professor of Pharmaceutics
College of Pharmacy
The Ohio State University
Columbus, Ohio

Malgorzata Dukat, Ph.D.
Associate Professor
Virginia Commonwealth University
School of Pharmacy
Richmond, Virginia

E. Kim Fifer, Ph.D.
Professor of Medicinal Chemistry
College of Pharmacy
University of Arkansas for Medical Sciences
Little Rock, Arkansas

William O. Foye, Ph.D., D.Sc (Hon)
Sawyer Professor of Pharmaceutical Sciences Emeritus
Massachusetts College of Pharmacy and Health Sciences
Boston, Massachusetts

David S. Fries, Ph.D.
T.J. Long School of Pharmacy
University of the Pacific
Stockton, California

Peter M. Gannett, Ph.D.
Basic Pharmaceutical Sciences
School of Pharmacy
West Virginia University
Morgantown, West Virginia

Richard A. Glennon, Ph.D.
School of Pharmacy
Virginia Commonwealth University
Richmond, Virginia

Robert K. Griffith, Ph.D.
School of Pharmacy
West Virginia University
Morgantown, West Virginia

Marc W. Harrold, Ph.D., R.Ph.
Associate Professor of Medicinal Chemistry
School of Pharmacy
Duquesne University
Pittsburg, Pennsylvania

Sunil S. Jambhekar, Ph.D.
Associate Professor of Industrial Pharmacy/Pharmaceutics
Massachusetts College of Pharmacy/HS
Boston, Massachusetts

David A. Johnson, Ph.D.
Department of Pharmacology-Toxicology
Duquesne University
Pittsburgh, Pennsylvania

V. Craig Jordan, Ph.D., D.Sc., M.D. (Hon)
Diana, Princess of Wales Professor of Cancer Research
Northwestern University Medical School
Chicago, Illinois

Stephen G. Kerr, Ph.D.
Massachussets College of Pharmacy and Health Sciences
Boston, Massachusetts

James J. Knittel, Ph.D.
Associate Professor of Medicinal Chemistry
College of Pharmacy
University of Cincinnati
Cincinnati, Ohio

Danny L. Lattin, Ph.D.
Dean
College of Pharmacy
South Dakota State University
Brookings, South Dakota

Barbara W. LeDuc, Ph.D.
Assistant Professor of Pharmacology
Massachussets College of Pharmacy and Health Sciences
Boston, Massachusetts

Thomas L. Lemke, Ph.D.
Associate Dean for Professional Programs and Professor
  of Medicinal Chemistry
College of Pharmacy
University of Houston
Houston, Texas

Matthias C. Lu, Ph.D.
Professor of Medicinal Chemistry
College of Pharmacy
University of Illinois at Chicago
Chicago, Illinois

Timothy J. Maher, Ph.D.
Professor of Pharmacology
Massachusetts College of Pharmacy and Health Sciences
Boston, Massachusetts

Ahmed S. Mehanna, Ph.D.
Department of Pharmaceutical Sciences
Massachusetts College of Pharmacy and Health Sciences
Boston, Massachusetts

Duane D. Miller, Ph.D.
Professor and Chairman
Department of Pharmaceutical Sciences
College of Pharmacy
University of Tennessee
Memphis, Tennessee

Lester A. Mitscher, Ph.D.
Kansas University Distinguished Professor
  of Medicinal Chemistry
School of Pharmacy
University of Kansas
Lawrence, Kansas

Michael Mokotoff, Ph.D.
Professor of Pharmaceutical Sciences
School of Pharmacy
University of Pittsburgh
Pittsburgh, Pennsylvania

Wendel Nelson, Ph.D.
School of Pharmacy
University of Washington
Seattle, Washington

John L. Neumeyer, Ph.D.
Matthews Distinguished Professor (Emeritus)
Harvard Medical School/McLean Hospital
Belmont, Massachusetts

Robert B. Palmer, Ph.D.
Assistant Professor
Medicinal Chemistry and Toxicology
University of New Mexico
Albuquerque, New Mexico

Douglas J. Pisano, Ph.D., RPh
Dean
School of Pharmacy—Worcester
Massachusets College of Pharmacy and Health Sciences
Boston, Massachusetts

Gary O. Rankin, Ph.D.
Professor and Chair
Department of Pharmacology
Joan C. Edwards School of Medicine
Marshall University
Huntington, West Virginia

Ronald E. Reid, Ph.D.
Professor of Pharmaceutical Chemistry
Faculty of Pharmaceutical Sciences
University of British Columbia
Vancouver, British Columbia, Canada

Victoria Roche, Ph.D.
School of Pharmacy and Allied Health Professions
Creighton University
Omaha, Nebraska

Manohar Sethi, Ph.D.
Associate Professor
School of Pharmacy
College of Pharmacy, Nursing, and Health Sciences
Howard University
Washington, DC

Robert D. Sindelar, Ph.D.
Department of Medicinal Chemistry
School of Pharmacy
The University of Mississippi
University, Mississippi

William Soine, Ph.D.
Department of Pharmaceutical Sciences
Virginia Commonwealth University
Richmond, Virginia

Marilyn K. Speedie, Ph.D.
Dean and Professor
College of Pharmacy
University of Minnesota
Minneapolis, Minnesota

Timothy S. Tracy, Ph.D.
Department of Basic Pharmaceutical Sciences
School of Pharmacy
West Virginia University
Morgantown, West Virginia

David J. Triggle, Ph.D.
University Distinguished Professor
School of Pharmacy and Pharmaceutical Sciences
University at Buffalo
State University of New York
Buffalo, New York

Robert A. Wiley, Ph.D.
College of Pharmacy
University of Iowa
Iowa City, Iowa

David A. Williams, Ph.D.
Associate Dean of Graduate Studies
Massachusetts College of Pharmacy and Health Sciences
Boston, Massachusetts

Michael Williams, Ph.D., D.Sc.
Department of Molecular Pharmacology
   and Biological Chemistry
Northwestern University School of Medicine
Chicago, Illinois

Robin M. Zavod, Ph.D.
Associate Professor of Pharmaceutical Sciences
Chicago College of Pharmacy
Midwestern University
Downers Grove, Illinois

S. William Zito, Ph.D.
College of Pharmacy and Allied Health Professions
St. John's University
Jamaica, New York

Contents

Introduction

Origins of Medicinal Chemistry

WILLIAM O. FOYE

In the so-called prescientific era, natural products having a history as folk remedies were in use, but little of the drug therapy of today is based on these remedies. Some of the natural products that are used today, either as extracts or derivatives, were often used originally for other purposes, such as arrow poisons, part of religious or other rituals, or even cosmetics. Examples of such products include opium, belladonna, cinchona bark, ergot, curare, nutmeg, calabar bean, foxglove, and squill. Many drugs originally used as folk remedies, on the other hand, have been abandoned. The following account points out some of the discoveries, accidents, and investigations that led to the present methods of searching for drugs. A comprehensive review of drug discoveries, with dates, names of investigators, and indications of times of isolation, synthesis, and pharmacology is given by Alfred Burger in the 4th edition, Part I, of Burger's Medicinal Chemistry, published in 1980. This includes over 1300 references; references are therefore not duplicated here.

EARLY INVESTIGATIONS OF NATURAL PRODUCTS

Before the development of chemistry as a science, drugs that had been used were either natural organic products or inorganic materials. Herbals and pharmacopeias listed plants that had been in use for thousands of years and resulted from efforts by various societies that had been made in the search to find cures for the various ills and diseases encountered and recognized. One of the first herbals was published in Basel in 1470 by Bartholomeus Anglicus, an English professor of theology in Paris, and the first pharmacopeia in the West was the *Nuovo Receptario Composito* published in Venice in 1498 by the College of Physicians. The First London Pharmacopeia was published in 1618. Among the earliest recorded uses of plant medicinals were those of the herb called "ma huang," a species of *Ephedra* used medicinally in China for over 5000 years, and one called "ch'ang shang" in China (2735 B.C.), later identified as *Dichroa febrifuga*. The use of squill as a cardiac tonic was recorded in the Ebers Papyrus (Egypt, ~ 1500 B.C.). The medical knowledge of the Greeks is known from the writings of Galen (129–199 A.D.), especially from his "On the Art of Healing," which relied on mixtures of herbs. Herbal medicine perhaps reached its greatest use in Europe during the seventeenth century, but gradually declined as physicians rejected the authoritarianism of the past in favor of experimentalism.

The Swiss physician, Paracelsus (1493–1541), made the first recorded challenge to the use of herbs, and urged the alchemists of his era to use their knowledge for developing chemical medicines, primarily from minerals. He also attempted to find the healing essence in pharmaceutical preparations, either organic or inorganic. His thinking was well ahead of its time, for the first active principle was not extracted from a plant until the beginning of the 19th century.

With the gradual decline of the magic and superstition that had accompanied the use of substances believed to have medicinal properties, physicians began to look for evidence of effectiveness in their preparations. Towards the end of the 18th century, serious doubt had arisen regarding the medicinal effects of most plant preparations, and the only remedies believed to have any value were cinchona bark for malaria and ipecacuanha for dysentery (both having come from the New World), and opium and belladonna, both plant extracts whose use had been revived.

English physicians had also experimented with the use of Priestley's "fixed air," or carbon dioxide, and Lavoisier's "dephlogisticated air," or oxygen. Carbonated drinks were administered with the hope of dissolving kidney stones, and oxygen was administered for resuscitation. Further experimentation with gases failed to elicit new remedies, although the euphoriant properties of both nitrous oxide and ether were discovered. Although Henry Hickman in England published a pamphlet recommending that some gases could be used to render surgical patients unconscious, it was not until the 1840s that Long and Wells in the United States showed that ether and nitrous oxide could be used as anesthetics for surgery.

Chemical experimentation in the late eighteenth and early nineteenth centuries led ultimately to its use in the discovery of new drugs. Antoine Fourcroy in Paris was able to analyze the content of mineral waters, believed to have medicinal value, and later examined solids and fluids in the human body. An associate, Vauquelin, assumed responsibility for medicinal analysis following the decision of the revolutionary Convention in 1793 to suppress academic and professional bodies formerly under the influence of the monarchy. He became the first director of the Ecole Supérieure de Pharmacie, and encouraged the association of chemistry with pharmacy in the developing curriculum. He also encouraged faculty members and their students to attempt the extraction of active principles from plants, and develop chemical assays for them.

1

Opium was among the first plant drugs to be investigated by the method of plant analysis introduced by Fourcroy. Opium had been mentioned in the Egyptian Ebers Papyrus and also by Homer in the Iliad, so its properties were known by the eighth century B.C. In 1803, Derosne, a Parisian pharmacist, devised an assay for opium in which he had isolated a crystalline salt. Later, Serturner, an Austrian apothecary, followed Derosne's work and showed that the narcotic principle of opium had an alkali-like character and could form salts with acids. Most previous plant extracts had been acidic in nature. He published his findings on the alkaline nature of the opium narcotic principle in 1817. Serturner's article was translated by Gay-Lussac, who pointed out the importance of the discovery of an organic alkaline constituent, and predicted that other organic alkaline materials would be found in plants. He proposed that the names of these materials should end in the suffix "ine." This was the first attempt to standardize the nomenclature of organic materials; he also changed Serturner's "morphium" to "morphine." Later, in 1818, the German chemist Meissner introduced the term "alkaloid" for the alkaline extracts of plants.

Antoine Fourcroy, the son of an apothecary, was one of the first to apply chemistry to pharmacy and medicine. He instituted the use of specific reagents to determine the presence of minerals, and analyzed various barks, looking for substitutes for cinchona bark. This work was regarded as a model for plant analysis, and encouraged others to examine cinchona and opium.

Thomas Anderson, professor of chemistry at the University of Glasgow, determined the composition of codeine, a mildly analgesic opium alkaloid. In 1853, an assistant, Henry How, conceived the idea that functional groups in natural products might be modified by chemical reagents. Among his experiments, he heated morphine with methyl iodide, hoping to convert the alkaloid to codeine. He obtained, however, a new substance which he identified as the quaternary salt of morphine. Later, the professor of chemistry at the University of Edinburgh, Arthur Crum Brown, prepared the same compound, along with quaternary ammonium salts of other alkaloids, for pharmacological examination by Thomas Fraser, professor of materia medica. This became one of the first attempts to correlate chemical structure with biological activity. He found that the quaternary salts of strychnine, brucine, thebaine, codeine, morphine, nicotine, atropine, and coniine all had curare-like paralyzing activity. This demonstrated that the quaternary ammonium function conferred curariform activity.

The work of Brown and Fraser stimulated Alder Wright, lecturer in chemistry at St. Mary's Hospital Medical School in London to treat morphine and codeine with organic acids. Among the products was diacetylmorphine, which was tested by F.M. Pierce in 1874. In 1887, Ralph Stockman, colleague of Thomas Fraser, and David Dott, a pharmacist, established that the ethyl ether of morphine was almost identical to the methyl ether (codeine) in pharmacological tests. These findings were not exploited, but von Mering in Germany persuaded the drug manufacturer, E. Merck of Darmstadt, to market the ethyl ether. It was introduced as Dionin in 1898, the first commercially available semisynthetic morphine derivative. It was promoted as a cough sedative in preference to codeine or other opiates.

In 1898, Heinrich Dreser of Friedrich Bayer and Company introduced diacetylmorphine as a safer pain reliever than morphine. It was described as a "heroic drug," was given the proprietary name of heroin, and it quickly became popular throughout the world. Four years passed before its addictive properties were recognized. Laws were later passed by governments to restrict its use.

Joseph Pelletier, an assistant professor at the Ecole Supérieure de Pharmacie, isolated the emetic principle from ipecacuanha root in 1817, in collaboration with a physiologist, Francois Magendie. The root had been used as an emetic by natives of Brazil and Peru mainly for dysentery. Pelletier and Magendie named the principle emetine. In the search for other plant alkaline materials, Pelletier and a student, Joseph Caventou, examined species of the *Strychnos* family, potent plant poisons. They succeeded in isolating both strychnine and brucine from these plants from research started in 1818. In 1820, they isolated quinine from cinchona bark, which had been introduced into Europe two centuries earlier from Ecuador as a cure for malaria. Since it was first described by an Augustinian monk, who had lived in Peru, it became known as "Jesuit's bark." It also became known as the English Remedy, when its use became publicized by an apprentice to an apothecary in Cambridge, Robert Talbor, following some toxic incidents and disputes over its efficacy. Talbor's preparation consisted of large doses of the powdered bark infused in wine. The Swedish botanist Linnaeus was able to classify the family of trees from which the barks were obtained as Cinchona, following collection of samples by Charles-Marie de la Condamine.

Following their isolation of quinine, Pelletier and Caventou urged medical practitioners to study the pure plant principles. Francois Magendie utilized animal tests and then treated patients with quinine, thus setting the present course of drug development. He also included it in his Formulaire of 1821, and knowledge of the efficacy of quinine became widespread. His method also provided some assurance that drugs would henceforth be of unchanging constitution. Pelletier and Caventou then started the manufacture of quinine on a large scale, and by 1826 they were producing 3600 kg of quinine sulfate yearly. Manufacturers in Germany followed suit when the details of the Pelletier and Caventou process for obtaining quinine from cinchona bark were published. The pharmaceutical industry thus became established, and pure, active drug principles gradually became available.

DEVELOPMENTS LEADING TO VARIOUS MEDICINAL CLASSES OF DRUGS
Anesthetics

The first use of synthetic organic chemicals for interference with life processes occurred when nitrous oxide, ether, and chloroform were introduced for anesthesia during the 1840s. Horace Wells, a dentist in Hartford, Connecticut administered nitrous oxide during a tooth removal in 1844 with no indication of pain by the patient. Crawford Long, a Georgia physician, had employed ether as an anesthetic for excising a growth on a patient's neck in 1842, but did not report his success until 1849. William Morton, a dentist, gave the first successful public demonstration of surgical anesthesia at the Massachusetts General Hospital in 1846, using ether and a recently designed inhaler. Chloroform had been used for "frolic partys," as had ether and nitrous oxide, and William Lawrence demonstrated its effectiveness as an anesthetic at St. Bartholomew's Hospital in London. In Paris, Pierre Fluorens tested both chloroform and ethyl chloride as anesthetics on animals.

Hypnotics and Analgesics

Early efforts to find synthetic drugs were consequently concentrated on anesthetics and hypnotics and eventually analgesics. Opium had been employed to kill pain and cause sleep from early but unrecorded times. Sydenham, the noted seventeenth century physician and founder of the clinical method, remarked that "without opium I would not care to practice medicine." Morphine was isolated from opium by Serturner in 1805, and was the first plant alkaloid to be isolated in relatively pure form. It was later found to have cough-suppressing properties.

Chloral hydrate appeared in 1869 from the laboratory of Rudolf Buchheim, who held the first ever university chair in pharmacology, at Dorpat in Estonia. Chloral hydrate was used on the mistaken assumption that it would liberate chloroform in the blood. It was not until 1948 that chloral was found to be metabolized to trichloroethanol, providing confirmation of Josef von Mering's contention of seventy years earlier. Paraldehyde was found to have hypnotic properties in 1883 in Milan, but this was already known to liberate acetaldehyde in the body. Acetaldehyde had been studied earlier in Paris, but caused marked bronchial irritation. Von Mering found that tertiary alcohols, principally tertiary amyl alcohol, were useful hypnotics in 1885. Urethane was introduced at the same time, but was then classified as a respiratory stimulant, and became the active ingredient of smelling salts. Sulphonal was found to be hypnotic by two professors at Freiburg in 1887. It was marketed by a dyestuffs manufacturer, F. Bayer and Co., and became the company's first profitable pharmaceutical.

Von Mering, on the assumption that a structure having a carbon atom carrying two ethyl groups would have hypnotic properties, investigated diethyl acetyl urea. This proved to be as potent as sulphonal. Further research led to 5,5-diethylbarbituric acid. Barbituric acid itself had been synthesized by Adolph von Baeyer in 1864. Although the diethyl derivative had been synthesized 20 years earlier, von Mering established that it was a useful hypnotic.

Antipyretics

Salicylic acid was introduced by Carl Buss in Switzerland as a possible cure for typhoid fever. It was found to be an effective antipyretic, and Buss published his findings in 1875. Because of its unpalatability, attempts were made to improve the drug. Professor von Nencki, also in Switzerland, combined salicylic acid with phenol to form the ester which he named salol (1883). This had poor solubility, but did provide some benefit for fevers. Since the compound was found to be hydrolyzed in the small intestine, the concept of the "salol principle" became known. This was an early example of a drug known to release controlled amounts of an active agent.

Large doses of salicylic acid were being used in the 1890s to control rheumatism, but the doses were unpleasant to take. Felix Hoffman of the Bayer laboratories found acetylsalicylic acid in the literature; it had been synthesized by von Gerhardt in 1853. Animal tests were encouraging, and it was released for clinical trial in Halle and Berlin in 1898. Results were published the following year, and the compound was found as effective as salicylic acid without the unpleasant side effects. The Bayer Company marketed the compound as an antipyretic, later as an antirheumatic, and it became the most widely used drug worldwide in the 20th century. It was given the proprietary name of Aspirin, derived from "a" for acetyl, and "spirin" from the name of the plant from which salicylic acid was first obtained, *Spirea ulmaria*. Aspirin also had disadvantages; ulceration in the stomach was caused by lumps of the undissolved tablets lodging against the stomach wall. Allowing the tablets to disintegrate before being swallowed provided a remedy, but the use of soluble calcium aspirin, recommended in Germany in 1913, was also an improvement. Ultimately, dispersible and effervescent formulations became more widely used.

Another antipyretic, Antipyrin or phenazone, was synthesized by Ludwig Knorr in 1884 with the mistaken assumption that he was preparing a portion of the quinine molecule. By the time it reached the market, manufactured by the Hoechst Dyeworks, Knorr had found that it was a pyrazolone derivative. Phenazone was the most widely used drug of its time, until replaced by aspirin. It is now known to cause agranulocytosis, a serious blood condition. It was also found to be a cure for headache, for which use all subsequent antipyretics were routinely considered. Pyramidon, or amidopyrine, was also marketed by Hoechst, following testing at Strasbourg University in 1896. It also became a best selling drug in Europe until it was found to cause agranulocytosis.

Another antipyretic was discovered at Strasbourg. In the attempt to rid patients with intestinal worms using naphthalene, Professor Kussmaul's assistants found no cure for the parasites but did find a potent antipyresis. It happened that the pharmacy in Strasbourg had supplied them with acetanilide instead of naphthalene. The compound was given the name Antifebrin. Acetanilide was cheaper to manufacture than the other antipyretics, and was used for many years, despite the fact that it inactivated hemoglobin, a condition known as methemoglobinemia.

The methoxy and ethoxy derivatives of acetanilide were synthesized at the dye works of F. Bayer and Company, under the direction of Carl Duisberg. They were tested at Freiburg University by Professor Kast, who found the ethyl ether was less toxic than acetanilide. It was marketed as phenacetin, and remained a popular antipyretic for about 90 years, until kidney damage was found in chronic users.

Other attempts were made to find an antipyretic superior to phenacetin. Von Mering collaborated with the Bayer Company (1893) in a clinical trial of paracetamol (P-hydroxy-acetanilide), which it was postulated to be a metabolite of phenacetin by Trefuel and Hinsberg in 1894. Von Mering found it to be an effective antipyretic and analgesic, but believed it also had a tendency to produce methemoglobinemia, which may have been due to contamination with P-aminophenol. Paracetamol was reinvestigated half a century later by Lester and Greenberg at Yale University, who showed that it was indeed a metabolite of phenacetin in humans. It was marketed by the Sterling-Winthrop Company in 1953, with the trade name of Panadol (acetaminophen). It was promoted as being safer than aspirin, particularly in children and those adults with ulcers. It was later found to cause liver damage from overdosage, however.

During the same era, of the late 1800s, some of the antipyretics were found to have antirheumatic effects. In 1874, salicin, the active principle from willow bark, was used to treat a patient with rheumatic fever. Later, the Dundee physician, Thomas MacLagan, reported his results on treating around 100 patients, claiming successful palliative effects. von Nencki, in Basel, had shown in 1870 that salicin was converted in the body to salicylic acid. This was tried on rheumatic fever patients with similar success. Others confirmed the value of salicylic acid for alleviating the effects of rheumatic fever.

Other antipyretics introduced in the 1880s were examined for antirheumatic effects. Phenazone was recommended in 1885 for its ability to ease joint pain. Acetanilide, phenazone, and amidopyrine were all used for years for rheumatic conditions. Amidopyrine, however, increased the risk of agranulocytosis. Attempts to avoid this problem resulted eventually in the derivative, phenylbutazone (Butazolidin), which was marketed in 1952. This drug still had the potential for causing agranulocytosis as well as aplastic anemia. Its metabolite, oxy-phenbutazone, was also used, but had the same serious side effects. Safer derivatives, azapropazone and feprazone were developed later.

Local Anesthetics

Local anesthetics were also developed during this fruitful period for drug discovery. A Viennese ophthalmologist, Carl Koller, had experimented with several hypnotics and analgesics for local anesthesia of the eye, and found one when his friend Sigmund Freud suggested that they attempt to establish how South American Indians allayed fatigue by chewing leaves of the coca bush. Cocaine had been isolated from the plant by Albert Niemann at Gottingen University in 1860, but was considered only a mild stimulant comparable to caffeine. Finding that cocaine numbed the tongue, Koller realized that he had found a local anesthetic. Animal tests at Vienna General Hospital revealed that it was effective in anesthetizing the eye. Koller and Dr. Gaertner at the hospital carried out tests on their own eyes, finding good local anesthesia with little irritation. A paper on Koller's findings was presented in Heidelberg in 1884, and within a month cocaine was being used in Europe and the United States.

By 1887, toxic effects of cocaine, associated with systemic cocaine circulation, and its addictive property were causing concern. Modifications in the structure (Albert Einhorn had proposed an incorrect structure in 1892) led to the synthesis of alpha- and beta-Eucaine by Georg Merling, working in Emil Fischer's laboratory in Berlin. These modified agents were nonaddictive but still irritating. Richard Willstätter, working in Einhorn's laboratory in Munich, determined the structures of both cocaine and atropine in 1898, and succeeded in synthesizing cocaine three years later.

Analogs of and portions of the cocaine molecule were then investigated, leading to synthesis of orthocaine by Einhorn in 1896 and benzocaine by Ritsert in 1902. Ernest Fourneau at Poulenc Freres in France developed Stovaine (amylocaine) which allowed the formation of non-irritating water-soluble salts by having an aliphatic amino group in the side chain. Heinrich Braun developed Novocaine (procaine) by combining elements of Einhorn's compound and adrenaline. It was the dominant local anesthetic for nearly half a century. Further research led to the introduction of Nupercaine (dibucaine) by Karl Miescher of Ciba in Switzerland, which became useful as a spinal anesthetic because of its long duration of action.

Holger Erdtman at Stockholm University started a long investigation for improved local anesthetics, and his assistant Nils Löfgren synthesized Xylocaine (lidocaine). It was marketed by Astra in 1948, and it became the most widely used local anesthetic for the rest of the century. Various modifications were developed giving longer acting anesthetics of which Marcain (bupivacaine) produced nerve blocks for up to eight hours. It became widely used for continuous epidural anesthesia in child birth.

Antiseptics

The concept of antiseptics was realized in 1750 by a military surgeon, Sir John Pringle, who had held the chair of moral philosophy at Edinburgh prior to military service. He examined the effects of various salts on preserving beef. This was the earliest attempt to compare the preservative properties of antiseptics, a term which he first used. Other experiments followed, in the attempt to find agents for wound disinfection. Various chlorine-based formulations were used, the most effective being chloride of lime. Ignaz Semmelweis, in Vienna, published data in 1861 showing a marked decline in mortality rate from puerperal fever when physicians first washed their hands in chloride of lime solution.

The antiseptic properties of coal tar were recognized in 1815, but a useful formulation, emulsified coal tar, was not found until 1859 by a Bayonne pharmacist. Friedlieb Runge, a chemist, had separated an acidic fraction from coal tar, in the 1830's, and named it carbolic acid. He found that it preserved both animal tissue and wood. The chemical constitution of carbolic acid was determined in 1841 by Laurent, who called it "acide phénique." It was later named phenol. Jules Lemaire published a book, "De l'Acide Phénique" in 1863, advocating the use of carbolic acid in surgery. But it was the publications of Joseph Lister at the University of Glasgow that established the effectiveness of phenol in surgery by halting the growth of bacteria that the recent research of Pasteur had shown to be the causative factor in infections.

Attempts to find antiseptics that could be used internally led to the trials of sulfocarbolic acid, salicylic acid, guaiacol, guaiacolsulfonic acid, and creosote from beechwood. Of greater significance was the synthesis by Albert Einhorn of diethylaminoacetylguaiacol hydrochloride (Guaiasonol), which was the first drug to be made water-soluble by incorporation of an aliphatic amine that could form a soluble salt. When Robert Koch found a method of growing bacteria in culture, in 1881, a rational search for chemotherapeutic agents could begin. Testing of the available antiseptics showed that mercuric chloride was the only agent that appeared to be sporicidal. Although this agent was not effective against all infectious organisms known, the experimental procedure developed by Koch served as the basis for the development of chemotherapy. Methyl violet also revealed limited success when used as internal antiseptic, so the idea of a universally effective internal antiseptic was regarded as futile.

A new possibility for infectious disease therapy became known during the early 1880s. In 1881, Louis Pasteur found that aging cultures of the cholera-causing organism had lost their ability to infect chickens. When the same chickens were later injected with fresh, virulent cultures of the organism, they were found to have developed an immunity to cholera. Pasteur correctly surmised that this was the result of their prior exposure to attenuated cultures, and later remarked that "chance favors the prepared mind." Thus, the science of immunology was born by a serendipitous discovery.

Following Koch's demonstration of the apparent sporicidal activity of mercurous chloride, and the unpleasant aspects of inorganic mercurials in humans, organic mercurials were developed. Mercury benzoate, carbolate, and salicylate were introduced in the late 1880s. These were quite insoluble in water, but were formulated in pills or in ointments, since they were absorbed transdermally. Solubilizing groups were then added to aromatic compounds, which resulted in a number of useful mercurials, including the sulfonic acid salts of phenol mercuric acid (Arterol), Afridol, merbaphen, mercurophen, mercurochrome, nitromersal, thiomersal, and phenylmercuric acetate and nitrate. Some of these agents are still in use, particularly as pharmaceutical preservatives.

Cardiac Stimulants

Use of a folklore remedy, foxglove, for treatment of dropsy by William Withering in 1775 led to the discovery that its primary function was as a cardiac stimulant. The plant, *Digitalis purpurea*, was then used as the powdered leaf. It was not until 1827, however, that Richard Bright was able to distinguish between dropsy due to kidney disease and that from heart failure. By 1890, the U.S. Dispensatory (16th Ed.) indicated that digitalis should be used solely in heart disease. Only in the early 1900s was a proper understanding of the effects of digitalis on the heart attained, due primarily to the introduction of the polygraph in 1902 by James Mackenzie, and of the electrocardiograph by William Einthoven a year later. Correct indication for the use of digitalis then became apparent for atrial fibrillation in which the heart beats become weak and irregular, and for certain forms of heart failure in sinus rhythm.

Attempts to isolate an active principle from digitalis were made in the 1820s, stimulated by the offering of a prize for isolation of a pure principle by the Société de Pharmacie in Paris. The award was won in 1841 by E. Homolle and T. Quevenne, chief pharmacist at the Hôspital de la Charité in Paris, for isolation of an active, crystalline material, probably consisting mainly of digitoxin. Other products were obtained later by other investigators: digitaline crystallisée by Nativelle in 1869, and digitoxin by Schmiedeberg in 1875. The former became known as digitalin, but was much less potent than digitoxin. These isolates were by then known as glycosides.

It took almost a half century before Adolf Windaus at Göttingen University established the correct structure for digitoxin (1928) and for digitalin (1929). Sydney Smith of Burroughs Wellcome and Company isolated and separated the glycosides of *Digitalis purpurea* and obtained a new one named digoxin. This is used more widely than either powdered digitalis leaves or digitoxin since it does not bind as strongly to proteins and permits both a more rapid build up to a therapeutic concentration and more rapid clearance from the body. Ouabain, a glycoside isolated by Arnaud in 1888 from the ouabain tree in East Africa, was found to be more easily crystallized than the digitalis glycosides and also provided a more rapid onset of action. This was also found to be present in an arrow poison used by the Somalis, and also found in arrow poisons prepared from the seeds of *Strophanthus gratus* and other varieties of *Strophanthus*. Arthur Stoll also isolated a crystalline cardiotonic glycoside from squill, the bulb of the sea onion (*Urginea maritima*) in 1933. Its structure was similar to that of the digitalis glycosides. This plant had been used by both the ancient Egyptians and Greeks. Its principal action was a reflex expectorant effect, with emesis caused by larger doses.

Antianginal Drugs

With the clinical application of the sphygmograph, pioneered by Thomas Brunton in 1867 at the Edinburgh Royal Infirmary, it became possible to measure rise in blood pressure. This accompanied attacks of angina pectoris. Brunton followed the usual practice by removing blood from the patient, and he became convinced that the relief of pain was due to lowering of arterial pressure. This led him to the use of amyl nitrite, already known to lower blood pressure in animals. Amyl nitrite had been synthesized in 1844 by Balard at the Sorbonne, but had also been found to cause severe headaches and was not presumed as a remedy for angina. Bernard Richardson showed that amyl nitrite caused dilation of the capillaries, and Arthur Gamgee demonstrated that dilation of blood vessels led to a drop in blood pressure.

Brunton experimented with other nitrites and found similar effects. He also examined nitroglycerin, which became available following Alfred Nobel's discovery of its use as an explosive. Other physicians adopted nitroglycerin, and William Murrell reported his use of nitroglycerin in Lancet in 1878, once a proper dosage had been determined. After the drug had been in use for some time, it was realized that it relaxed smooth muscle generally. A search for other compounds that might have this property was done by measuring their ability to dilate pieces of coronary artery. This led ultimately to finding activity among substitutes for papaverine, analogs of methadone, and local anesthetics based on the lidocaine structure. It is now known that some of these compounds with coronary dilating ability also have the ability to act as calcium antagonists.

Antiarrhythmic Drugs

The first discovery of an antiarrhythmic drug was made by a patient. Karl Wenckebach, a Dutch cardiologist, told a patient that there was nothing that could relieve attacks of atrial fibrillation. The patient disagreed, and returned the next day with a normal pulse. He had taken quinine. It had been known for sometime that quinine had a depressant action on the heart, but had not been used for

cardiac irregularities. Wenckebach tried quinine on other patients, but in only a few cases was the trial successful. He mentioned this in his book on cardiac arrhythmias, published in 1914. Four years later, W. Frey reported in a Viennese medical journal that quinidine was the most effective of the four principal cinchona alkaloids in controlling atrial arrhythmias. Use of quinidine became established by the early 1920s.

Use of local anesthetics in surgery was first done by Frederick Mantz of Cleveland, who was looking for drugs which could be applied directly to the heart to prevent arrhythmias during surgery. He found procaine to be highly effective, being superior to cocaine or piperocaine. He made his discovery known in 1936. Procaine, however, was rapidly metabolized by esterases in the blood, and also had side-effects on the central nervous system. A procaine analog resistant to esterases was found in procainamide, which also had much less effect on the central nervous system.

Early Developments in Infectious Disease Drugs
Antiprotozoal Drugs

Following his experiments with dyes to stain bacteria, Paul Ehrlich found that methylene blue stained nerve fibers. It was given to patients with a variety of neuritic and arthritic conditions and found to relieve pain, but it also damaged the kidney if used continuously. Ehrlich also knew that it stained the plasmodia that caused malaria, and had it administered to two patients in Berlin suffering from malaria. Both patients recovered from the disease, but the dye was ineffective against the more severe forms of the disease in the tropics. This cure of a mild form of malaria, however, was the first successful use of a synthetic drug against a specific infectious disease (1891).

Ehrlich did not continue work with methylene blue, primarily because there was no method for infecting animals with malaria to test potential drugs. However, in 1902 Laveran and Mesnil at the Pasteur Institute were able to infect mice and rats with two varieties of trypanosomes, causative organism for sleeping sickness. In collaboration with E. Nocard of the Pasteur Institute, Paul Ehrlich began his investigation of trypanocides. He was assisted by Dr. Shiga, sent to Ehrlich's laboratory by the head of the Tokyo Institute for Infectious Diseases, and Professor Kitasato, who had worked with Ehrlich previously. Arsenicals were found to be ineffective against trypanosomes, but benzopurpurin dyes showed promise. To increase the poor solubility of the dyes, sulfonic acid groups were introduced. This research resulted ultimately in the effective dyes Trypan Blue, and Afridol Violet. These dyes were obtained from first the Cassella Company and later from F. Bayer and Company. Use of a urea linkage in the compounds to interrupt conjugation removed the color, since the previous dyes caused coloration of the skin of patients. By 1917 more than a thousand naphthalene ureas had been tested, and the most effective was Bayer 205 or Germanin, later given the name suramin.

The structure of suramin was not revealed in the Bayer patent. Ernest Fourneau, head of the medicinal chemistry laboratory of the Pasteur Institute, deduced the structure by synthesizing a number of compounds based on intermediate naphthalene sulfonic acids which had appeared in Bayer patents. By 1924, he had the structure of a compound giving identical trypanocidal properties to those of suramin. This was published and given the name of moranyl (Fourneau 309). Since the structure had not previously been published, Bayer could not claim infringement of its patent. After this, disclosure of structures became standard practice in pharmaceutical patents.

Suramin remains one of the principal drugs for prevention and treatment of some forms of trypanosomiasis. Because of the sulfonic acid functions (six of them are included in suramin), the compound cannot enter the central nervous system, and so cannot be used in the later stages of sleeping sickness. The method of discovery of this agent, however, gave great stimulus to the development of chemotherapy. Within twelve years of its discovery, Bayer researchers had developed the first synthetic antimalarials and several other agents. The diamidines, of which pentamidine is a principal drug for trypanosomiasis, was developed by the same procedure of synthesis and testing of compounds against diseases of infected laboratory animals.

Arsenicals. A report on the medicinal effects of arsenic was published by Thomas Fowler in 1786. Potassium arsenite had been used previously to treat malaria in Hungary, but Fowler made his own preparation, which became known as Fowler's Solution. It was used throughout the nineteenth century as an alternative to quinine. There was also some evidence that arsenic preparations had beneficial effects in syphilis, and David Livingstone, the medical missionary who explored much of Central Africa, recommended arsenicals for alleviation of sleeping sickness.

Sir David Bruce showed in 1894 that protozoa were present in the blood of animals with sleeping sickness, and that Fowler's Solution temporarily eliminated the protozoa from the blood of infected cattle. The protozoa were later described as *Trypanosoma brucei*. Alphonse Laveran at the Pasteur Institute in 1902 found a method of infecting mice with trypanosomes, and found that Fowler's Solution caused a rapid, but temporary, disappearance of the protozoa from the blood of the infected mice. Less toxic arsenicals were sought, first by August Michaelis at Karlsruhe and Rostock, and then by Professor Ludwig Darmstadter in Charlottenburg. One of these, called Atoxyl (*P*-aminophenylarsonic acid), was sent to Ehrlich, who tested it against isolated cultures of trypanosomes and found it inactive. In 1905, however, Wolferstan Thomas of the Liverpool School of Hygiene and Tropical Medicine described the success of Atoxyl in treatment of animals experimentally infected with trypanosomes.

Robert Koch was asked by the German Sleeping Sickness Commission to evaluate the effect of Atoxyl on human populations in East Africa. He found that the necessary dose in humans for removing trypanosomes, by constant medication for six months, also presented a risk of blindness by damage to the optic nerve. Ehrlich decided to prepare analogs of Atoxyl, and found that the structure proposed by Bechamp was incorrect. Reaction with nitrous acid gave a diazonium salt, showing that the compound was not an anilide but the arsonic acid. This made a much wider range of analogs possible.

With financial support by the widow of the Frankfurt banker George Speyer, as well as by John D. Rockefeller in the U.S., a chemotherapy institute was built for Ehrlich and called the George Speyer-Haus. It was opened in 1906. Ehrlich described the principle guiding the design of new chemotherapeutic agents by the Latin phrase "corpora non agunt nisi fixata," meaning that organisms are not killed unless the chemotherapeutic agent had a high affinity for them. Ehrlich also devised the concept of therapeutic index, determined by measuring both the curative and lethal doses of therapeutic agents. He was influenced as well by the ideas on the existence of drug receptors proposed by John Langley, a Cambridge physiologist. Ehrlich then advanced the hypothesis that the parasitic action of arsenicals was due to their binding to receptors on the surface of the parasites. He was in hopes that the chemotherapeutic agents would bind only to receptors in the parasites and not those of the patient.

The isolation of the organism that caused syphilis was reported in Berlin in 1905 by Schaudinn and Hoffmann. Hoffmann asked for samples of Ehrlich's compounds for testing on syphilitic patients in his clinic in Bonn. Several other investigators also received samples of Ehrlich's compounds. In 1909 Ehrlich was joined by Sacachiro Hata, who had developed a method of infecting rabbits with syphilis while working at the Kitasato Institute in Tokyo. He tested the arsenicals prepared by Ehrlich's chemist, Alfred Bertheim, and found that the 606th compound prepared had good curative properties in rabbits infected with syphilis. Ehrlich arranged for the Hoechst Farbwerke to patent the compound. The compound was tested in humans with syphilis by Professor Alt of Uchtspringe and Professor Schreiber of Magdeburg. The compound was found to be a cure for syphilis. Results were announced at the Congress for Internal Medicine at Weisbaden in 1910, and Ehrlich received requests from numerous physicians for samples of the compound. Between April and December 1910, sixty-five thousand vials of "606" were supplied, while a plant for its production was being installed by Hoechst. The compound was marketed under the proprietary name of Salvarsan, later being given the approved name of arsphenamine. Its chemical name was 3-amino-4-hydroxyarsenobenzene, but it was known to the public as

"606" or Ehrlich-Hata "606." It had to be treated with dilute alkali prior to injection, to give a water-soluble but rather unstable salt. A more stable salt was obtained with neoarsphenamine, which included a sodium sulfoxylate function on the amino group, and required only the addition of water prior to injection, which was preferred by the physicians. The finding of a cure for syphilis with "606" represents the discovery of the first major chemotherapeutic agent, and has given Ehrlich the title of "the founder of chemotherapy." His concepts leading to this development are still the basis for much of chemotherapeutic research.

Arsphenamine and neoarsphenamine were difficult to manufacture, because of side reactions and difficulty of purification. In both Britain and France and later in the United States, during the First World War, difficulties were experienced in the drugs. The German patent on these compounds was then abrogated by the governments of these countries, and licences were issued to drug companies for their manufacture. With careful checking of individual batches of the compounds, reasonably pure drugs were produced. The French Military Medical Services administered over 94,000 injections of arsphenamine without a fatality, which also illustrates the extent of the spread of syphilis at the time. This experience of manufacturing a synthetic drug stimulated the growth of British, French, and American pharmaceutical industries.

By the end of the war, Jacobs and Heidelberger of the Rockefeller Institute had synthesized an analog of atoxyl called tryparsamide (N-(carbamoylmethyl analog of arsanilic acid), which was more effective than any other arsenical against trypanosomiasis. The Rockefeller Foundation patented the compound, but issued licenses free of charge to manufacturers who wished to market the drug. This was a fitting outcome for John D. Rockefeller's early support of Ehrlich's research and a tribute to Rockefeller's vision and generosity. It was also an appropriate conclusion to Ehrlich's research on atoxyl. Ehrlich had believed that arsonic acids caused neurotoxicity, leading to blindness. Fourneau, however believed this toxicity was due to impurities. He synthesized a number of phenylarsonic acids of which acetarsol proved to be a relatively safe antisyphilitic as well as amoebicide. It was manufactured by Poulenc Frères.

Thousands of arsenicals were synthesized in Europe and America during the 1920s and 1930s. During the First World War, W. Lee Lewis of the U.S. Chemical Warfare Service prepared a highly vesicant arsenical now known as Lewisite. Its deleterious effects were produced by absorption through the skin and hydrolysis to an arsenite. Fear that it might be used by the enemy during the Second World War led British scientists to search for an antidote. Professor Rudolph Peters of the biochemistry department at Oxford found that arsenite reacted with two adjacent thiol groups present in the pyruvate oxidase system. The

discovery that this reaction could be competitively inhibited by simple molecules containing two adjacent thiol groups resulted in the preparation of the effective antidote dimercaprol (BAL, or British Anti-Lewisite). This could be applied to the skin as an ointment, or be injected. This episode constitutes one of the earliest examples of rational drug design. Dimercaprol is still used as an antidote for poisoning by arsenic, mercury, lead, and other metals that react with the thiol groups of the pyruvate oxidase system.

Antimonials. Nicole and Mesnil at the Pasteur Institute followed up Laveran's finding of the value of Fowler's Solution in mice infected with trypanosomiasis by showing that intravenous injections of tarter emetic (antimony potassium tartrate) gave similar results. Cattle were later cured of trypanosomiasis with tartar emetic, but in doses too toxic for human use. Vianna, a Brazilian physician, injected tartar emetic in patients having a disease caused by a then unknown organism, later named *Leishmania braziliensis*, with favorable results (1912). Leishmaniasis now refers to a group of tropical diseases caused by protozoa first detected in 1900 by William Leishman. It is one of the most widespread of all communicable diseases, and its most common form, kala-azar, affects millions of children in tropical areas. Without treatment, the mortality rate from this disease is around 90%; with antimonial chemotherapy, the mortality rate is reduced to around 10%. Few chemotherapies have saved as many lives.

In Khartoum in 1918, J.B. Christopherson found that tartar emetic acted against schistosomiasis, a parasitic disease caused by a trematode worm which is transmitted by freshwater snails. Because of its toxicity and irritancy on injection, tartar emetic (the potassium salt) was gradually replaced by the more water soluble antimony sodium tartrate. Many antimonials, often of complex and uncharacterized polymeric structure, have been synthesized. Several of the best-known antimonials were prepared in the 1920s by E. Schmidt of the von Heyden Chemical Works in Germany and tested by Uhlenhuth at the University of Freiburg. One of these, stibophen, was marketed under the name of Fouadin, apparently to impress King Fouad of Egypt, where schistosomiasis is a major health problem. Sodium stibogluconate was later synthesized by Schmidt and tested at the I.G. Farben laboratories. It remains an important drug for cutaneous leishmaniasis.

Antimalarials

Lack of a suitable method of infecting laboratory animals with malaria prevented Ehrlich and others from finding cures for malaria. In 1924, however, W. Roehl at Bayer's Chemotherapeutic Institute developed a technique for screening potential antimalarials in canaries. Compounds that appeared promising were then tested in patients suffering from the paralysis and insanity of the later stages of syphilis were infected with malaria parasites. This procedure was first tried by Professor Wagner-Juaregg in Vienna.

Research on quinoline derivatives at Bayer under W. Schulemann started with modifications of methylene blue, first investigated by Ehrlich. Substitution of a diethylaminoethyl side-chain on methylene blue by Roehl gave an effective compound with a low therapeutic index. To avoid having a dye as a base for potential antimalarials, quinoline derivatives were investigated. With this side-chain substituted on the amino group of 8-aminoquinoline, the resulting compound cured infected canaries. Hundreds, if not thousands, of compounds were synthesized and tested by a small group of Bayer researchers. A promising 6-methoxy quinoline derivative was found to be curative in infected syphilitic patients and later patients with naturally acquired malaria. Clinical trials throughout the world followed, and the compound was successful. It was marketed as Plasmoquine and given the name pamaquin. Its structure was disclosed in 1928. Combination of pamaquin with quinine eliminated the parasites from both the blood and liver stages of the disease, producing outright cures.

Aminoacridines were synthesized by Mietzsch and Mauss at Bayer and tested by W. Kikuth, after the death of Roehl. More than 12,000 compounds were examined, the most effective being Atebrin, later given the approved name of mepacrine (quinacrine in the U.S.). This compound killed parasites in the erythrocytic phase of malaria. With the approach of World War II, it became apparent to both Britain and the U.S. that loss of the East Indies would result in the loss of quinine. By September, 1939, production of mepacrine at I.C.I. in the U.K. had reached pilot-plant stage, but full-scale production followed shortly. In the U.S., the Winthrop Chemical Co., which had been set up after World War I by I.G. Farben to distribute Bayer pharmaceuticals, was seized by the Custodian of Enemy Property and sold to Sterling Drug, Inc. After the Japanese moved into the East Indies and cut off the supply of quinine, the newly organized Sterling-Winthrop Co. was called upon to supply large quantities of quinacrine. The company sublicensed 11 American manufacturers to produce the drug, and by 1944 millions of quinacrine tablets had been made. This effort, along with that to produce large amounts of penicillin, provided the impetus for the U.S. to become the world's largest producer of pharmaceuticals.

During their North African campaign, German troops were supplied with another antimalarial, sontoquine (Resochin), which was a quinoline derivative. This provoked the search for quinoline antimalarials at Sterling-Winthrop, and led to the discovery of chloroquine by Surrey and Hammer. This compound caused fewer side effects than quinacrine, and in addition did not color the skin yellow. Another antimalarial discovered at Parke-Davis was amodiaquine, a substituted 4-aminoquinoline. Both of these compounds were superior to quinacrine and quinine. The antimalarial program at Columbia University under Elderfield

produced primaquine, an 8-aminoquinoline superior to amodiaquine for eradication of tertian malaria caused by *Plasmodium vivax*. It remained the most effective antimalarial for this type of malaria for the next 40 years, or until resistance to most antimalarials became a problem.

British antimalarial researchers investigated sulfonamides, particularly those containing pyrimidine, during the war. The most effective of compounds of this type was Sulphamethazine, synthesized by Francis Rose of I.C.I. Other research groups examined compounds of about 40 chemical classes, and from this effort was found the biguanides, of which chloroguanide (proguanil) was the most effective antimalarial. Clinical trials at the Liverpool School of Tropical Medicine showed it to be effective against the erythrocytic phase of malaria. It was marketed under the name of Paludrine.

In 1949, George Hitchings, of the New York laboratory of Burroughs Wellcome, noticed the structural analogy of one of their antifolic acid drugs to proguanil and tested it against malaria parasites. This gave encouraging results, and synthesis of a large series of derivatives led to discovery of pyrimethamine (Daraprine). It was tested in London at the Wellcome Laboratories of Tropical Medicine, and has been widely used as an alternative to proguanil.

Schistosomicidal Drugs

I.G. Farben initiated research on remedies for schistosomiasis in 1936. Kikuth and Goennert devised a screening method for testing compounds against *Schistosoma mansoni*. Their large number of antimalarial candidates provided active compounds, among them, the Miracils, of which Miracil D was an acceptable orally active remedy. It was given the name of lucanthone. Mauss and his colleagues at I.G. Farben also produced the mirasans, which were active in mice, but not in man. They served as the starting point for investigations in the Pfizer laboratories in Sandwich, England, which led to the discovery of oxamniquine (mansil). This was tested in patients in Brazil infected with *S. mansoni*, and cured 90% of them. It had poor activity, however, against *Schistosoma haematobium*, the prevalent schistosomal disease in Africa and the Middle East.

It was believed that lucanthone was converted metabolically to an active form. All attempts to identify the metabolite failed until Archer at Sterling Winthrop found that the metabolite was a hydroxy derivative, which was named hycanthone. Its greater potency allowed a smaller quantity, within water solubility limits, to be given by intramuscular injection. It has had widespread use against *S. mansoni*. This represents an early case, similar to that of finding sulfanilamide from prontosil, where a metabolite was found more effective than a drug in use.

CONCLUSION

The discoveries described in this short history form the basis for many of the later successes in drug development, including discoveries adequately described in following chapters and are not therefore recounted here. Most, if not all, of these earlier discoveries would be described today as empirical, or fortuitous, and a number of them were plainly accidental. Despite the relative lack of knowledge of the basic substances on which we now know drugs act, and prior to the marvelous advances in drug discovery methods in the last half of the twentieth century, these early discoveries represent an amazing amount of insight, accurate guesswork, and, of course, determination, by those accomplishing the research and led to the broad range of drug substances known before the age of more highly organized research in the 1900s. These "early" researchers deserve our gratitude and admiration, and the role of the human imagination in drug research should not be forgotten.

SUGGESTED READINGS

A. Albert, "Selective Toxicity, The Physico-chemical Basis of Therapy," 7th ed., New York, Methuen, 1984.

C. Hansch, P.G., Sammes, and J.B. Taylor, "Comprehensive Medicinal Chemistry," Vols.1–6, Oxford, Pergamon Press, 1990.

J. Nogrady, "Medicinal Chemistry, A Biochemical Approach," New York, Oxford University Press, 1985.

M.L. Podolsky, "Cures Out of Chaos," Williston, VT., Harwood Academic, 1998.

B.G. Reuben and H.A. Wittcoff, "Pharmaceutical Chemicals in Perspective," New York, John Wiley & Sons, 1989.

S.M. Roberts and B.J. Price, "Medicinal Chemistry, The Role of Organic Chemistry in Drug Research," New York, Academic Press, 1985.

W. Sneador, "Drug Discovery: The Evolution of Modern Medicines," New York, John Wiley & Sons, 1985.

M.E. Wolff, "Burger's Medicinal Chemistry and Drug Discovery," Vols. 1–5, New York, Wiley-Interscience, 1995–1997.

PART I

Principles of Drug Discovery

Overview: Drug Design and Development: A Perspective

MICHAEL WILLIAMS

INTRODUCTION

Without question, the drugs produced by the ethical pharmaceutical industry over the past century have irrevocably changed the fabric of society improving both the individual quality of life and life expectancy. Bacterial infections, polio, smallpox, tuberculosis and related diseases, and gastric ulcers that were once life threatening have, to a very major extent, become minor public health concerns although the emergence of bacterial resistance due to the overuse of antibiotics has begun to reverse this trend (1).

The increase in life expectancy resulting from drug therapy has also resulted in a shift in population demographics toward a more healthy, elderly population. As a consequence, diseases like cancer and neurodegenerative, degenerative and autoimmune diseases have become increasingly prevalent, resulting in an increase in health care needs and a greater consumption of the gross national product in providing health care. Drug regimens for birth control (2), compounds for erectile dysfunction (3) and new treatments for incontinence (4) are drugs that improve individual life choices and the quality of life. Similarly, HIV protease and reverse transcriptase inhibitors for the treatment of HIV infections in the space of a few years have changed a disease with a fatal prognosis to a potentially chronic one (5). Cancer is also being viewed as a potentially chronic, rather than fatal, disease with the potential for newer, non-cytotoxic approaches that include inhibition of the angiogenic events supporting tumor growth and proliferation (6).

Despite progress to date, as the ethical pharmaceutical industry enters the 21st century, there remains an increasing need for novel, innovative therapeutic agents not only in areas that are historically well served like anti-infectives (1), but also for the myriad of diseases associated with aging for which there are generally no effective medications but considerable demand.

Publication of draft sequences of the human genome (64,65) during the course of preparation of this chapter has added an additional dimension to the drug discovery process. While it was assumed that the human genome would be greater than the 10,000–25,000 genes found in *Drosophilia*; the finding that only 35,000 or so genes comprise the human genome has shifted the focus to identifying new drug targets from the genome to the proteome, those proteins, simple and complex, that are expressed by the genome (66).

Historical Evolution of the Pharmaceutical Industry

The ethical pharmaceutical industry originated in Japan in the 1600s with the establishment of Takeda in 1637. However, the modern era of drug discovery has its roots in the European and U.S. fine chemical industries of the 19th century (7,8). Apothecaries selling various herbal medicines and metals evolved over time into larger organizations, selling both ethical and patent medicines, based on technical improvements in drug manufacture from natural product sources. The U.S. industry was established near Philadelphia in the 1800s where emerging mechanization coupled with needs related to the U.S. Civil War, primarily in the area of analgesic alkaloids like morphine, led to the establishment of companies like Squibb, Parke-Davis and Eli Lilly. In England, Allen and Hanbury and May and Baker also marketed alkaloids while in Germany and Switzerland, Merck, Bayer, Schering, Roche, Ciba, Geigy and Sandoz subserved a similar role. Changes in pricing in the dyestuffs industry in the 1880s led several chemical companies to establish synthetic research efforts resulting in compounds like the antipyretic alkaloid, pyramidon (Hoechst). Research efforts focused in the area of immunology at Hoechst (in association with Ehrlich, Koch, and Behring) and at Wellcome in the U.K. (in association with Dale). The introduction of the non-steroidal anti-inflammatory drug (NSAID) aspirin as an antipyretic in 1889 led to the establishment of a legacy within the pharmaceutical industry (19) that survives to this day with the recent introduction of selective COX-2 inhibitors (10).

By the start of World War I in 1914, European pharmaceutical companies had established U.S. operations worth nearly a billion dollars. With the U.S. entry into the war in 1917, the Trading with the Enemy Act resulted in trust status for U.S. subsidiaries of German companies, eventually leading to the sale of these assets. Bayer's aspirin trademark was sold to Sterling, and only returned to Bayer in 1995 with the closure of Sterling Winthrop Pharmaceuticals, Eastman Kodak's ill conceived foray into pharmaceuticals. E. Merck's U.S. operation was the genesis of Merck, Sharp, and Dohme and subsequently Merck Research Laboratories, while Schering AG's U.S. assets evolved into Schering-Plough. The curtailment of the German pharmaceutical industry's U.S. presence resulted in an expansion of the Swiss industry as well as the subsequent formation of I.G. Farben in Germany. During the war, Sandoz, Ciba, and Geigy had a virtual monopoly on the supply of dyestuffs to the Allies, the profits from which permitted their expansion into pharmaceuticals. The French industry was established in the early 1900s with Poulenc which has sequentially become, Rhone Poulenc, Rhone Poulenc Rorer and, following a recent merger with Hoechst Marion Roussel, Aventis.

Despite positive interactions between German academia and industry in the late 1800s, in the U.S., industrial scientists were specifically excluded from membership of the American Society of Pharmacology and Experimental Therapeutics (ASPET) until 1941. Swann (11) has ascribed this to the training of American pharmacologists abroad who returned with the German concept of *Wissenschaft*— the "moral imperative of studying things for themselves— not their immediate utilities"—being well entrenched. However, academic scientists like R. Adams with Abbott and A.N. Richards with Merck followed the example of Ehrlich, Koch, and Behring's association with Hoechst and that of Dale with the Wellcome Research Laboratories in the U.K., playing an important role in the evolution of the U.S. pharmaceutical industry and its commitment to basic research. This continuing recognition of the fundamental importance of research resulted in Merck, Abbott, Upjohn, Lilly, Squibb, and Parke-Davis establishing viable biomedical research organizations during the 1920s that continue, in one form or another, to this day.

The development of antibiotics heralded the next growth phase of the pharmaceutical industry. Sulfa drugs were replaced by penicillin 13 years after Fleming's discovery in 1929. A co-operative effort in the U.S. led to other antibiotics like aureomycin (Lederle), chloromycetin (Parke-Davis) and teramycin (Pfizer) leading to further industry growth and increasing the global presence of companies like Glaxo, Beecham, and Boots from the U.K., Schering, Hoechst, and Bayer from Germany, Ciba, Geigy, Sandoz, and Roche from Switzerland, and Pfizer, Merck, Lederle, and Parke-Davis from the U.S. In the U.K., Burroughs Wellcome, Glaxo, British Drug Houses, May and Baker, and Boots had emerged as major entities in the industry by 1942.

The French and Belgian pharmaceutical industries attained prominence in the 1950s with the discovery of the psychotropic drugs like chlorpromazine (Rhone-Poulenc) and haloperidol (Janssen) that replaced controversial surgical techniques like prefrontal lobotomy for the treatment of the mentally ill (7,12). From the 1950s through the early 1970s, the industry continued to grow despite the thalidomide teratogenicity disaster in the early 1960s that led to the Kefauver-Harris Amendments to the U.S. FD & C Act of 1938 (13). Innovative research efforts within the U.S. industry increased in the mid 1970s with the recruitment of members of the U.S. National Academy of Sciences (e.g., P. Cuatrecasas (Burroughs Wellcome), P.R. Vagelos (Merck), P. Needleman (Monsanto)) as heads of internal research activities. This coincided with a greater molecular focus in the drug discovery process and the transition from the core techniques of biochemistry and molecular pharmacology to those of molecular biology and genomics. Concomitant with these changes came other paradigm shifts that markedly impacted both the culture and the business environment of the ethical pharmaceutical industry.

Drug Discovery Dynamics

A major change in the drug discovery process in the past quarter century has been the "biotechnology revolution" which has irrevocably altered the funding of the process, the technologies used to identify new compounds, and the cultural approach. While initially a description of the science encompassed in the techniques of molecular biology (14), the "biotechnology revolution" soon became associated with a new trend in biomedical research, with funds to start up "biotech" companies to exploit novel academic research discoveries for commercial gain being provided by venture capitalists, primarily in the U.S. In 1997, approximately 1150 biotechnology companies employed 300,000 individuals and generated $12 billion in revenues (15) approximately equal to that of Merck. Among the early biotech companies founded in the mid 1980s were Genentech, Genex, Genetic Systems, Cetus, Genetics Institute, and Amgen (15). Of these Genentech and Genetics Institute are now subsidiaries of Roche Biosciences and American Home Products, respectively while Amgen, Genzyme, Chiron, and Biogen have emerged as major pharmaceutical companies. The remainder have disappeared. The establishment of biotech companies also led to a long overdue entrepreneurial rejuvenation of the pharmaceutical industry based drug discovery process (16), and a shift of much of the innovative research base in the industry from "big pharma" to the smaller, more aggressive and highly focused, flexible and less bureaucratic "biotech" organizations. However, more recently, with a more realistic appreciation of the risks and time associated with the drug development process, venture capital interest in funding biotech has waned (17). Despite many new enabling, time and cost efficient technologies (e.g., genomics, combinatorial chemistry, high throughput screening), it still takes upwards of a decade or more to move a compound through the clinical trial process with an 80–90% risk of failure. The advent of Internet companies like Netscape and Amazon.com that offer almost immediate financial returns has further decreased venture capital interest in funding the biotech industry.

Another major paradigm shift in pharmaceutical R&D resulted from federal and insurance company pressures to contain health care costs and to control escalating drug costs (18,19). While only 4–7% of the total health care dollar in the U.S. is spent on prescription drugs, the cost to the individual for drugs in some instances approached a very tangible 30% in out of pocket expenses due to reimbursement structure. This focused considerable attention on the pharmaceutical industry which led the industry to focus various outreach programs to the public to increase the awareness of the benefits and cost effectiveness of drugs. Nonetheless, the momentum in containing health care costs resulted in the industry moving from an oligopoly to an oligopsony (18) and has resulted in highly restricted drug formularies. Increased costs for drug development, estimated at $359 million in 1991, at $627 million in 1995 and a projected $1.36 billion in 2000, have forced greater efficiencies in the industry (20–23) with considerable consolidation and the continued outsourcing of higher risk, early drug discovery efforts to venture capital funded biotech companies and clinical trials to clinical research organizations. The balance between the need for continued investment in innovative drug research and the economic constraints imposed by health care cost containment has raised the hurdle on what is deemed an appropriate return on investment for a drug in terms of break-even and peak sales (24). Thus a compound with peak sales of $400 million, which was thought to be an attractive investment in the 1980s, may now be a marginal product. It should be noted however that projecting sales is very much a crystal ball exercise with many unknowns. The projections for the recent launch (1999) of the selective COX-2 inhibitor, celecoxib were initially modest based on concerns about competition with generic NSAIDs. First year sales are anticipated to be in excess of $1.5 billion. In contrast, Pfizer's orally active phosophodiesterase 5 inhibitor, sildenafil (Viagra) for erectile dysfunction, which was launched in 1998, was at that time, the most successful new drug launch with projected sales of $5 billion or more. Due to its cardiovascular side effects that contraindicate its use in angina patients taking nitrates, sales of Viagra flattened considerably with first year sales reaching only $800 million.

Drug discovery and development has been the focus of the activities of many management consulting organization studies. One of these (21) focused attention on the required productivity in the R&D activities of major pharmaceutical companies to maintain profitability. This essentially took the number of innovative new drugs required to maintain growth rates and compared the likelihood of these being produced with present research and development investment and concluded that there were significant shortfalls between the two at almost all pharmaceutical companies. Suggested solutions were increased productivity without increasing R&D resources, new research strategies involving a balance between internal research and external alliances and improved integration of enabling technologies and their management under the rubric of improved information management (25). While more specific, these recommendations were highly reminiscent of those made by Weisbach and Moos some four years earlier (16).

An alternative or perhaps complimentary approach to improved productivity is consolidation. The first major consolidation in the pharmaceutical industry occurred in the early 1970s with the formation of Ciba-Geigy (26). Subsequent significant mergers/acquisitions were Monsanto and Searle (1985), Squibb and Bristol-Myers (1989), SmithKline Beckman and Beecham (1989), Parke-Davis and Warner-Lambert (Warner-Lambert), Roche Biosciences and Syntex (1994), Roche Biosciences and Genentech (1993/1999), Hoechst and Marion Merrill Dow (1995), Pharmacia and Upjohn (1995), Glaxo and Burroughs Wellcome (Glaxo-Wellcome) (1995), Astra and Fisons (1995), Parke Davis and Agouron (1999), Sugen and Pharmacia-Upjohn (1999). Interestingly, acquisition or consolidation appear to attain their own momentum. Thus Ciba Geigy mergered with Sandoz in 1996 to form Novartis, Astra with Zeneca in 1999 to form AstraZeneca and Hoechst Marion Roussel with Rhone Poulenc Rorer to form Aventis in 1999, Glaxo-Wellcome with SmithKline Beecham to form GlaxoSmithKline in 2000, Warner-Lambert/Parke-Davis with Pfizer in 2000, and Monsanto with Pharmacia-Upjohn to form Pharmacia in 2000. As the 20th century draws to a conclusion, further consolidations are anticipated to occur between a number of other large pharmaceutical companies that have already merged with an expectation of there being only 5–10 global pharmaceutical companies by the first decade of the 21st century. Similar consolidations have occurred in the energy (Amoco and BP), automobile (DaimlerChrysler), and entertainment (Polygram, MCA, and Universal Studios) industries. Consolidation has also occurred in the biotech industry with Agouron acquiring Alanex, Arris and Sequana merging to form Axys, which was acquired by the genomics company, Celera, and Elan Pharmaceuticals acquiring Athena and Neurex.

THE R&D PROCESS
Background

As already noted, the process involved in the identification of new compounds for the treatment of human disease is a prolonged, expensive and unpredictable endeavor with a high risk of failure, generally agreed to be in the region of 80%. In addition to the costs of bringing a drug to market, the time spent in moving it from the discovery process to the pharmacist's shelf can take from 8–14 years depending on the complexity of the clinical trials, the expertise, focus and risk orientation of the sponsoring company, and the length of the regulatory review process. As a result, many major pharmaceutical companies have yearly R&D budgets in the range of $2–5 billion per year (21,22).

While new technologies like genomics and combinatorial chemistry have had a major impact in identifying new targets and in enhancing compound synthesis and evaluation thus facilitating lead compound selection, the critical steps that occur beyond these initial stages, compound optimization, functional testing, animal model testing, metabolism, formulation, and pharmacokinetics have only recently become the focus of innovative science approaches. Compound optimization has however remained a relatively consistent activity over the past decade. In the early days of the biotechnology industry, the success in basic molecular biology research led to excessively optimistic statements by entrepreneurs that the R&D process could be cut short and consequently be made less expensive. This näiveté explains the spate (1993–1998) of failed clinical trials that have impacted the fortunes (and in some cases existence) of companies like Synergen, Regeneron, Celltech, Xoma, Cortech, Cephalon, British Biotech, and Centocor (15). Unfortunately, the drug development process remains the same whether the lead compound was prepared by traditional synthetic organic chemistry techniques or recombinant DNA technology.

The emphasis on resource efficiency has also focused on improving the time and cost of the clinical trials procedure. While a relatively standardized group of activities when compared to the discovery process (27), strategies designed to focus on niche markets (28) or on organizational dynamics (29,30) have the potential to produce cost savings and reduce the risk of clinical trials to the extent that this can be done.

R&D Strategies

Success in drug discovery is dependent on the ability to identify novel, patentable compounds known colloquially as New Chemical Entities (NCEs), that have the potential to treat a disease in a safe and efficacious manner. While enabling technology platforms like genomics and combinatorial chemistry contribute significantly to this process, a proprietary NCE position is absolutely essential to ensure marketing exclusively and to justify the investment in the R&D process, making medicinal chemistry a core element of the drug discovery process.

Drug discovery can be divided into four distinct steps: target identification and selection, target optimization, lead identification, and lead optimization. Superimposed on these scientific steps are the more intangible, yet critical processes that relate to the activities and integration of the individual scientist involved in drug R&D who represents a wide diversity of technical specialties, experiences, and cultural and ethnic backgrounds all of which must be melded into a team effort to advance drug discovery activities (31,32). To this end project management processes, company organization(s) and culture, resourcing practices, prioritization, and decision making (25,33) are critical factors for success. The best technologies will not lead to the most optimal outcomes in a dysfunctional cultural setting or when priorities and objective and consistent criteria for decision making are not part of the cultural norm. And as the greatest commercial opportunities are likely to occur in those therapeutic areas where unmet medical need and risk are both high, the effective use of innovative and well managed scientific approaches will continue to be a major factor in ensuring success for the future.

SCIENTIFIC ASPECTS OF DRUG DISCOVERY
Target Identification and Selection

The selection of a research target is based on a number of factors hopefully including the therapeutic franchise area of the company (34), evolving scientific knowledge, unmet medical need, the level of competition, perceived commercial opportunity, a serendipitous lead from high throughput screening, and the innovation of the drug discovery groups. For a biotech company, the project is, in essence, the *raison d'etre* of the company and a failure that can be absorbed in a larger organization with multiple opportunities can often mean the difference between life and death for a biotech company.

In a therapeutic area like hypertension, the R&D process is sufficiently well established to make drug discovery a relatively predictable process. An NCE that reduces blood pressure in the spontaneously hypertensive rat (SHR) model, unless it desensitizes its molecular target upon chronic administration or has a poor pharmacokinetic profile, will be active in humans. In other disease states e.g., Alzheimer's Disease (AD), rheumatoid arthritis (RA), and cancer, the knowledge related to the molecular events underlying disease pathophysiology is limited, making drug discovery and development in these areas complex and unpredictable. Thus the clinical trial, through the critical Phase II "go/no go" decision (see below) is a continuum of the research project, the evaluation of the compound in humans being the ultimate proof of principle of the hypothesis testing process. In terminating innovative, high risk research projects before definitive data is available that is relevant to the original hypothesis, there is a considerable danger of missing opportunities and "reinventing the wheel" as researchers at other companies pursue the self same targets. However well conceived, well planned, and well funded, four out of five research projects fail to reach a level of commercial interest because of the nature of the "cutting edge" research that innovative biomedical research routinely entails.

There has been an explosion in the identification of new targets over the last decade as many novel receptor and enzyme genes have been cloned and expressed from human genomic libraries using the techniques of molecular biology. This process has been accelerated with the various human genome initiatives (35–38). However, the patenting of these potential drug targets and limitations on their use in screening has resulted in yet another paradigm shift in industrial biomedical research where biological targets are no longer in the public domain. This has been a subject of considerable debate with concerns as to the negative impact of patenting on research activity (39) and led one observer to suggest (40) that the current trend in gene patenting would probably have allowed Newton to patent gravity.

In addition to issues related to the freedom to use a particular gene, the identification of the function of a newly identified gene is a major challenge as is its selection as a target for compound screening (41). Genomic targets for drug discovery can be identified using one of two techniques, expression profiling or positional cloning. The former initially involves the comparison of cDNAs derived from "normal" and diseased tissues using techniques like subtractive hybridization or differential display to identify genes that differ between the two. The source of the cDNAs can be from normal and diseased human tissues, cultured cells, or from experimental manipulation in animal models e.g., middle cerebral artery occlusion in rats as a model of cerebral ischemia. Often as many as a thousand genes or more can be found to differ between two reference cDNA libraries necessitating further criteria for the selection of those genes thought to be of primary interest. Additional analyses can be performed to pinpoint genes of particular relevance such as looking at multiple sources of diseased tissue (e.g., more than one geographical locale) to ensure that the genes identified are relevant to the disease rather than being unique to a familial population. Expression profiling of the genes in different tissues, e.g., brain, kidney, skin etc. can also aid in selecting candidate genes, and when using animal models. A time course to follow the appearance of gene differences can also be useful in selecting genes that are of primary interest. DNA microarrays provide yet another technique for assessing gene expression patterns to identify candidates. Advances in protein sequencing and analysis has given rise to a new approach to expression profiling termed proteomics, which examines differences in tissue samples at the protein level.

Positional cloning or polymorphism association involves gene mapping in combination with population genetics to identify those genes candidates involved in human diseases from the 100,000 genes thought to be present in the human genome. Traditionally, disease causing as distinct from disease associated genes have been sought in familial cohorts or isolated communities. For instance, the gene for asthma has reportedly been identified in a population of approximately a thousand individuals who show a propensity for asthma on the island of Tristan da Cuhna. Unfortunately, this gene may only relate to the disease inherited in that particular population and may not translate to identifying the gene(s) involved in sporadic asthma in a broader population. An alternative approach akin to the null hypothesis in experimental design is to obtain samples from patients diagnosed with the disease that can then be genotyped using largely automated processes to identify SNPs (single nucleotide polymorphisms). By examining a large number of diverse individuals from different populations affected with a disease and an equally diverse group of normals, the frequency of occurrence of an SNP can then be statistically associated with a given disease state without necessarily invoking an *a priori* approach. Techniques like linkage disequilbrium can then be used to identify the association between different SNPs and the disease state. Since many disease states are polygenomic e.g., involve more than one gene variant as well as predisposing environmental factors, it is important that the identification of disease associated genes is done using the maximum amount of data with the maximum rigor. As a hypothetical example, using limited patient source material in the search for the gene for a given disease may result in the generation of information that is hopefully disease associated or,

equally possibly, may identify genes that while important to the individual are either familial or disease related rather than disease causing.

Once a candidate gene has been objectively associated with a given disease to the extent that currently available information can provide, the challenge is then to identify its function both in order to understand the molecular pathophysiology of the disease and also to initiate a drug discovery program. The function of a gene can be theoretically determined using a functional genomics approach. Function can be ascribed by searching for structural homologies for a novel gene product and other, known proteins using genomic databases or by searching protein partners using 2-hybrid approaches (67). Simple organisms like *C. Elegans,* the zebra fish and *Aplysia californica* can be used to study related gene products, e.g., proteins of unknown function to see what role they play in the life of these relatively simple organisms and extrapolate these functions to humans. Modification of the mouse genome to produce knock-outs (ablation of a gene) and over expression of a particular gene (transgenics) can also be used to attempt to define function. These approaches are very labor- and time-intensive, however, and sometimes provide limited information. Knocking out a particular gene can lead to an embryo that is unable to survive or, alternatively, given the system redundancy necessary for survival, a particular gene defect can be overridden at the embryonic stage by compensatory physiological mechanisms. An alternative approach is to ablate gene products on an acute basis in the adult animal by utilizing antisense oligonucleotides. Newer transgenic techniques involve turning on genes when the animal reaches adulthood thus avoiding the compensatory mechanism that can emerge during embryogenesis

The factors required for the selection of an identified genomic product as a drug discovery target are complex. Obviously the degree of comfort with the identification of the target based on triangulation with a number of clinical and genomic databases is paramount as is the fit with the therapeutic franchise of a particular company. Once the degree of risk has been established, the accessibility of the target with available technologies, diagnostics, and pharmacogenomics (42) must then be ascertained. The latter refers to the use of genomic typing to determine which patients will respond favorably to a medication and those at risk for adverse effects based on their genetic makeup. For instance, if a compound shows side effects due to an unusual cytochrome P450 metabolism in a subsection of the general population, individuals with this response can be screened for and excluded from early clinical trials.

Target Optimization

Once a drug discovery target has been identified and validated for a given disease it needs to be available in an appropriate setting and in sufficient amounts to study its characteristics in terms of interactions with new compounds, e.g., ligand site topology and functional effects. At the very least a native or recombinant source of the target should be available to facilitate high throughput screening. Transient transfection can be used but is often complicated by variations in the amount of protein expressed which can confound the functional assessment of the activity of new compounds (43). In addition, a functional readout of receptor activation or enzyme activity should be available in order to readily discern between the activity of agonist and antagonist ligands. Ideally, sufficient quantities of a target protein should also be available to conduct X-ray crystallographic, computer-assisted molecule design (CAMD) and nuclear magnetic resonance (NMR) studies to aid in the design of new compounds with optimal properties (44,45).

Lead Identification

Once a target has been selected, the next step is the identification of novel compounds that interact with it with high potency, efficacy, and selectivity. *Affinity* refers to the ability of a new compound to bind tightly to its target and is measured in molar units. A typical high affinity ligand for a receptor will have an affinity measured in terms of competition for a radioligand that is selective for a specific receptor in isolated tissues, cell lines, or tissue homogenates, with an experimental ligand. The concentration of the latter that is required to inhibit binding of the radioligand by 50% (IC_{50} value) or an affinity constant (Ki) can be used to assess the interaction of a ligand with its target. Typically the IC_{50} or Ki value is in the nanomolar (10^{-9}M) range range. *Efficacy* refers to the ability of a ligand to elicit an effect on its target that can be measured in terms of a biochemical or physiologic response. For a receptor, a ligand may be an agonist, mimicking the effects of the endogenous ligand or an antagonist, which blocks the effects of the endogenous ligand (Chapter 4). By definition, a full agonist has an efficacy of 100% (unity = 1.0) while an antagonist has an efficacy of 0% (zero = 0). A partial agonist can have efficacy between 0 and 100% while a full agonist may have a response greater than 100% due to a higher intrinsic efficacy that may reflect the degree of coupling to the effector mechanism in different tissues. When such coupling is especially efficient, only a small percentage of the receptors on that tissue need be activated to elicit a full response. Thus it is not uncommon to find compounds that are specific for one receptor in terms of binding affinity that have substantially functional activity at other receptors for which they have lower affinity but are highly and efficiently coupled to effector systems.

By definition, a partial agonist is also a partial antagonist. Selectivity refers to the ability of a compound to recognize its target without interacting with other, related drug targets, e.g., G protein-coupled receptor family at similar concentrations which may lead to unwanted side effect liabilities. The structure activity relationship (SAR) for a novel series of compounds can be derived either by radioligand binding assays or functional assays involving biochemical responses (e.g., cyclic nucleotide production) or gene reporter systems (e.g., melanotroph responses, luciferin-luciferase linked light emitting reporter assays or calcium sensitive dyes). The availability of binding assays for over 100 different classes of receptors and enzymes can be used to derive a binding profile for a given ligand that will establish its specificity for binding to one target among a number of receptors or enzymes. The degree of selectivity required for a new ligand is an iterative process. Ideally a compound selectivity index of 100 to a 1000 or more is ideal but in some instances 50- to 100-fold can provide sufficient selectivity to derive a good therapeutic index.

Compound Sources

New compounds originate from natural product sources (46–48) (Chapter 1) or by synthetic effort (49,50) (Chapters 2 and 5). Chemical modification of a known pharmacophore series to derive an SAR represents the major means by which NCEs are developed. Such pharmacophores are usually the endogenous hormone or transmitter for the target enzyme or receptor (51). A 'lead' reported in the patent literature as possessing an interesting or unusual pharmacologic profile or a novel pharmacophore discovered by the targeted screening of a compound library or natural product sources can be an attractive target for initiating a research program.

Modern medicinal chemistry approaches can be complimented by various physical techniques in the area of structural biology.

Targeted High Throughput Screening

While a novel compound can be developed from a competitor's structure based on information available in patents or from a natural product, another approach to generating new leads is by serendipitously evaluating (or screening) compound sources and sample collections (52,53). By definition, high throughput screening (HTS) is a random process even though in targeted screening, the focus is on a defined molecular target. Screening is very much less precise than the synthetic approach in that many thousands of compounds are evaluated at a fixed concentration to derive a "yes or no" answer in terms of activity at a given target. Many hundreds of thousands of compounds can be evaluated per month. In the past decade, with the development of 96, 384, and 1536-well microtiter plates, the screening of compound libraries consisting of 300,000–400,000 samples that took up to 6 months to methodically work through can now be evaluated in a matter of weeks. HTS using radioligand binding assays provides information on the ability of the ligand to recognize its target—its affinity. Any active leads then have to be assessed in functional assays to determine whether the compounds are agonists or antagonists. More recently, the use of transfected receptors in various cell lines in combination with fluorescent calcium sensing dyes and fluorescent imaging plate readers (FLIPR) has allowed compound affinity and efficacy to be measured in real time.

HTS screening has obviously increased the need for continuous supplies of huge numbers of compounds. These are sourced from chemical libraries within and between pharmaceutical and chemical companies, from academia, especially in the previous Eastern Bloc countries, from natural product sources, or can be produced via combinatorial chemistry techniques. Using the latter approach, chemical libraries representing large number of oligonucleotides, carbohydrates, peptide/protein molecules can be made using nucleoside, sugar, and amino acid building blocks. Using 100 interchangeable building blocks, each with a molecular weight of 150, potentially results in the synthesis of 100 million tetrameric or 10 billion pentameric NCEs (49). While it is unlikely that combinatorial chemistry will replace the more traditional methods of lead identification, it has significantly accelerated the process of compound production especially in terms of using parallel synthesis techniques where limited numbers of compounds can be rapidly made.

Natural Product Sources

The discovery of important NCEs like the CCK_1 receptor antagonist, asperlicin, the immunosupressants, cyclosporin and FK 506, the various cholesterol lowering acids, and the nicotinic analgesic, epibatidine have focused the opportunities in natural product evaluation from the traditional realm of microbiology, anti-infectives, and anticancer agents to other therapeutic areas. Natural product sources include plants, microbes, marine flora and fauna, and arachnid and amphibian sources (46–48) (Chapter 1).

Lead Optimization

A molecule that is targeted as a potential drug has many required attributes. In addition to potency, efficacy, and selectivity a compound must be bioavailable and chemically and metabolically stabile. The intrinsic physicochemical properties governing these properties are not well understood and inevitably, the optimization of a novel lead can be loosely compared with that of a water bed, where adjusting the properties of one part can affect those in another. Very often, the optimal compound is a necessary compromise of these various attributes. For instance, one may accept a compound with less potency than another if it has an improved pharmacokinetic profile or a better selectivity for its target site.

Focused Synthetic Effort

Traditional synthetic medicinal chemistry approaches are highly focused and iterative in real time. Newly synthesized compounds are immediately evaluated for activity and selectivity so that this information can be used to aid in the design of subsequent compounds. The average cost of creating a single NCE in this manner is around $7500 due to the "hand-crafted" nature of the serial synthesis process. At this point, the complexity of the synthetic process, compound yield and cost of goods are less important than being able to make novel compounds in sufficient quantities for initial biological testing.

Bioavailability

Bioavailability of a compound is dependent on a number of factors that include solubility, the ability to cross biologic barriers including the gastrointestinal tract and the blood brain barrier by either passive or active diffusion processes, plasma protein binding, susceptibility to enzymatic modification (e.g., glucuronidation), and excretion properties (Chapter 7). NCEs that are highly potent and selective in vitro lack significant in vivo activity because they are unable to reach their sites of action. This may be due to a lack of absorption, first pass metabolism in the liver, or permeability limitations such as the blood-brain barrier. The potential of a compound as a drug candidate is therefore limited unless alternative formulations or derivatives (e.g., prodrugs) can overcome these obstacles. The less ionized a compound, the better it is absorbed and the more readily it can pass biological membrane barriers. Many of the physiochemical factors affecting bioavailability are poorly understood such that there are few hard and fast structure activity rules that can be applied across a chemical series with any degree of reasonable predictability. Oral bioavailability (F) is the fraction of the ingested dose of a compound that is available to the systemic circulation and is the product of the amount absorbed and that which avoids first pass metabolism. To assess an F value requires a dosing regimen and analytical techniques to measure nanogram quantities of the parent compound and potential metabolites in the plasma. Efforts are ongoing to use in vitro surrogate systems, e.g., Caco-2 cells to select compounds for in vivo evaluation (54). In transitioning from preclinical models of compound activity to the clinical situation, the plasma level of an NCE required for efficacy (ng/ml) rather than the absolute dose (mg/kg) is a useful predictor for establishing dosing regimens since it more accurately reflects the exposure of the target site to the compound and thus avoids interspecies variabilities in absorption and metabolism.

Empirically, the log of the octanol:water partition coefficient, logP has been used to predict the absorption potential of new compounds with a value of 0–3 representing an optimal window for absorption. LogP predictions do not hold well for peptides and the molecular weight of a compound has been used as an alternative predictor for absorption, the lower the molecular weight, the better the absorption profile (55).

Once the functional activity of an NCE has been established at its molecular target, it is important that the in vitro selectivity be reassessed in appropriate systems. Many different types of receptors employ G-protein linked and cyclic nucleotide pathways. Thus while a compound may be identified as selectively active at one receptor from its binding profile, there is always the possibility that it may alter second messenger production by more than one

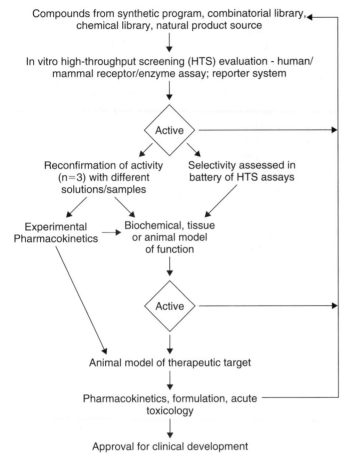

Fig. I.1. Flowchart for evaluation of new chemical entities.

receptor-mediated mechanism in a functional system. The use of appropriate antagonists or agonists can help clarify this situation

The evaluation of new chemical entities (NCEs) for activity at either receptors or enzymes generally occurs in a hierarchical manner predicated on knowledge and experience in a given area of research and exemplified in the Figure I.1 flow chart. Until the 1970s, drug discovery efforts were directed at largely empirical tissue or animal models that indirectly measured receptor function. This "black box" approach was unable to delineate those factors responsible for the efficacy of a given compound from those eliciting toxicity. The basis for a concentration ratio between these two events, the therapeutic index, was poorly understood, and the search for active entities free from major side effects was difficult to accomplish both conceptually and in practice. Modern drug discovery is based on the concept that receptor and enzyme subtypes exist and can be selectively targeted using novel ligands to elicit selective therapeutic responses free from the side effects associated with activation of other receptor subtypes of the same class. To some extent, the increased focus on the molecular basis of drug action has increased the understanding of those properties of a compound that are beneficial. However, many efficacious compounds produce their effects by interactions

with a unique set of targets which can complicate on overly reductionistic approach to the drug discovery process.

Compound evaluation progresses from in vitro selectivity and molecular target activity, to functional efficacy and selectivity, to activity in disease-predictive models. As a compound moves through this process, the criteria for interest become increasingly more stringent. Since there are three main attributes of a compound—efficacy, selectivity/toxicity, and bioavailability, an iterative process occurs with an NCE being modified to improve bioavailability. This sometimes results in a decrease in efficacy. The flow chart can then be used in a flexible manner to "rebalance" the attributes of an NCE.

Therapeutic Models

Animal models remain an important link between the molecular characterization of an NCE and its transition to the clinical setting. Beyond the SHR (spontaneously hypertensive rat), there are very few predictable animal models of human disease states; for instance, to our knowledge there is no such thing as a depressed rat although there are models like the behavioral despair where an experimental state of depression is induced and where many compounds shown to be antidepressants in humans have efficacy (56). Such surrogate models aid in selecting compounds and doses for clinical evaluation. For example, anti-inflammatory agents can be assessed by their ability to reduce the pain response associated with an injection of carageenin into the forepaw. Transgenic models of human diseases are also being developed that may prove useful in providing preclinical data for the initiation of clinical trials (57).

Sometimes therapeutic models can be complimented by the use of human tissues (blood or samples from surgical procedures or cadavers) or cloned and expressed human receptors or enzymes to assess NCE activity. This represents an important facet of the compound evaluation process. In the area of inflammation, human blood cells can be used to study complement, cytokine, leukotriene, and prostacyclin receptor function. NCEs identified in this manner also undergo evaluation in animal models relevant to the targeted disease state to validate the mechanistic hypothesis and to provide information relevant to biological activity and bioavailability in the species used for toxicology. This situation is paradoxical in that an NCE designed to have activity and selectivity at the human target may behave very differently in lower species adding an additional layer of complexity to the characterization of a compound of interest.

PRECLINICAL DEVELOPMENT
Absorption, Distribution, Metabolism, and Excretion (ADME)

In assessing NCE activity in vivo there is usually a correlation between drug efficacy and the plasma concentration of either the parent compound and/or its active metabolites. The interaction of these processes control the plasma concentration of the drug. Analysis of the time course of plasma drug concentration changes (pharmacokinetics) (Chapter 7) can contribute important insights into the ADME process that is essential to the new drug application package (IND). A temporal relationship can then be established between efficacy and drug levels and the metabolites formed and their elimination (Chapter 8) (58). Once this has been established, taking into account different drug vehicles, doses, species differences, routes of administration, and dosing regimens, ADME studies can be used to both design and monitor clinical trials thus reducing much in the way of trial and error in using biologic efficacy as the only readout.

Toxicological Safety Evaluation

Once a compound has evolved to lead status, its safety has to be evaluated in suitable in vitro and in vivo models (59). A compound is initially evaluated for mutagenicity in vitro in various cell culture models that assess effects on bacterial and mammalian cell replication. The Ames test, (bacterial mutagenicity) is usually one of the first toxicological test procedures carried out on a new compound series as is the mouse micronucleus test. Following such in vitro testing, an NCE is then evaluated in a short, rising dose study in two mammalian species (one non-rodent) to identify doses at which signs of toxicity are observed. Initial in vivo toxicologic testing is for 7, 14, or 28 days depending on the anticipated exposure to humans in initial clinical trials. While these time periods are subchronic, 7 day dosing provides sufficient safety data to expose subjects to a single dose and 14 and 28 days, sufficient for a rising, multiple dose study. For clinical studies of 2 weeks in duration, rodent toxicity studies of 2–4 weeks are required; for 2–4 week human trials, animal studies should be 1 month in duration. For clinical trials of 1–3 months, 3 month toxicity is required. The amount of planning, compound synthesis, and tissue assessment required for an in vivo toxicologic evaluation can take from 3–6 months for subacute toxicology. Chronic toxicity studies require 6–12 months of exposure. From these studies, a No Adverse Event Level (NOAEL) can be determined.

An NCE in clinical trials will also be evaluated over a 2 year period for reproductive effects, teratogenicity and immunologic and behavioral toxicity both in adult mammals and their offspring. In life carcinogenicity studies expose mice and rats to an investigational compound for more than two years.

CLINICAL DEVELOPMENT

Clinical development is divided into four distinct elements preceded by the filing of a Notice of Claimed Investigational Exemption for a New Drug—the IND in the U.S., the Clinical Trial Exemption (CTX) or Clinical Trial Certificate (CTC) outside the U.S., to the FDA (Food and Drug Administration) in the U.S., EMEA (European Medications Evaluation Agency) in the EU or their equivalents in Japan. The IND or CTX documents the preclinical safety and efficacy studies performed on an NCE and is not formally approved by either agency. Instead, the agencies have 30 days to review the IND or CTX and if no issues are raised, the sponsoring company can then proceed with human studies.

Differences in regulatory requirements in the U.S., Europe, and Japan have led to the formation of an International Conference on Harmonization of Technical Requirements (ICH) for registration of Pharmaceuticals for Human Use, whose stated role is to eliminate redundancy and duplication in the procedures for registering NCEs.

The four phases of clinical trials are (60):

Phase I: First-time exposure to humans to measure tolerance and safety in healthy volunteers. Rising dose studies are done with the NCE to determine the maximum tolerated dose (MTD) via the expected route of administration. Pharmacokinetic and bioavailability studies are also carried out at this time and may include multiple dosing regimens in preparation for the Phase II trials. Depending on the targeted disease, patients may also be included in the Phase I trials to more accurately reflect the targeted population, e.g., geriatric patients or to avoid exposing normal, healthy subjects to cytotoxic drugs for use in cancer patients. Drug tolerance may also vary between healthy volunteers and patients. For instance, schizophrenics tolerate doses of the antipsychotic, haloperidol that are 200-times higher than that tolerated by normal volunteers (60).

Phase II: Initial clinical investigation for treatment efficacy, these studies continue evaluation of the safety of a new compound. Phase II is colloquially divided into 'a' and 'b' stages, the former a limited trial to ascertain some degree of efficacy followed by Phase IIb, a more broad range (and expensive) trial involving a larger number of patients (100–300). During Phase II trials, biochemical or physiologic indices of drug efficacy are routinely sought as objective endpoints of drug action where possible. Later, clinical trials are usually conducted on a "double-blind" basis rather than "open." In double blind studies, neither the patient nor those involved in providing health care have knowledge of whether a placebo, a vehicle formulation identical to that used for the active principle of the NCE but lacking the NCE, or the drug is being given. This can rule out psychological aspects of drug treatment especially when evaluating CNS drugs. In those instances where there is no known treatment for a disease, it is ethical, as laid down in the revised (1975) Declaration of Helsinki, in order to prove efficacy, that the control group remains untreated. Placebo therapy can often appear to be effective and this can confound results from open studies that are usually carried out without a code and in some instances without an adequate control group. The phrase 'breaking the code' refers to the identification of which treatment a patient has received. A Phase IIa "signal"—the first indication of efficacy in the targeted population, is a major "go/no go" milestone in the clinical development of an NCE.

Regulatory agencies frequently require, in addition to a placebo arm, a comparative or positive control arm with a known drug (if available) to both validate the trial and to demonstrate that the NCE has comparable or superior efficacy and an equivalent or superior safety profile. If the positive control arm, say fluoxetine for an antidepressant, ibuprofen for an antiinflammatory, or ciprofloxocin for an antibiotic fails to show efficacy then the whole trial can be considered a failure.

Phase III—Pivotal clinical trials require full-scale evaluation of treatment in several different medical or regional centers. The design is to compare the new drug with known treatments and with placebo in controlled blinded trials. The dosage used in this stage is critical as Phase III data are those upon which regulatory decisions are made and that support the labeling and subsequent marketing of the compound. The number of patients involved in this portion of compound development can be several hundred to three thousand. Phase III studies also include an assessment of potential drug interactions.

Once sufficient data have been accumulated from a Phase III trial (which can take from 2–8 years), a company may then file a New Drug Application (NDA) to the FDA in the U.S. or a Product License Application (PLA) in the EU to request approval to market the NCE as a drug. The NDA or PLA is many thousands of pages in length containing efficacy data as a basis for the claimed indications as well as safety information and a summary of the risks and benefits for the agent. Once the FDA receives an NDA, it is given a priority for review based on therapeutic gain: Type A, important; Type B, modest; and Type C, little or none. The FDA has 180 days to complete an NDA review and issue an action letter that determines whether the NDA is approved, approvable requiring minor modifications or unapprovable having major deficiencies.

Phase IV—Postmarketing surveillance—this portion of the clinical trials occurs after the drug is approved and undertakes the monitoring of adverse effects and additional long term, large-scale studies of drug efficacy. In addition, Phase IV trials can be used to monitor both additional indications for a new drug for a subsequent NDA as well as gathering information to assess the pharmacoeconomics for the introduction of a new treatment modality. Such information can be used to convince health care payers that the use of a new drug offers significant benefit over existing therapy (surgery or other drugs) to the extent that there are savings in either the initial or long term as reflected in time for patient recovery and quality of life.

Many pharmaceutical companies have established clinical research units at major research hospitals across the world to facilitate the monitoring of compound development. In addition, several companies are accelerating compound evaluation in man by the use of Exploratory Clinical Research Units, small Phase I units that are geared to take novel, mechanism based compounds that have undergone toxicology to FDA standards into limited human evaluations to assess efficacy and proof of principle. Such units are especially important when a compound is developed preclinically on the basis of a novel mechanism of action which requires hypothesis testing in humans without the expense of full clinical evaluation. The FDA and ICH continue to examine ways to expedite the clinical trial process (61).

a) Line organization

b) Project team

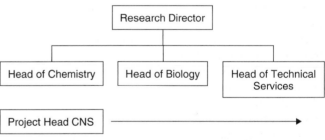

c) Matrix organization

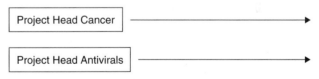

Fig. I.2. Organizational structures for drug discovery.

Organizational Aspects of Drug R&D

Once a drug target has been identified, a project team will need to be established and adequately resourced (31). The nature of this process and the technical makeup of the team is highly dependent on the structure of an organization as well as the individuals involved (30,33,62).

In established companies projects will be either **matrix,** established across therapeutic disciplines organized in a line management, technological manner (Figure I.2) or **dedicated,** where each project will have its own complement of the needed disciplines. Biotechnology companies will by necessity of size, function in the dedicated project team mode.

The size and makeup of a project team is highly dependent on the stage of the project (63). Thus, at an early stage, when the concept of a biological target is being validated, the project has a greater need for biological resources with little need for chemistry. Such a project stage has been termed **initiatory** (I). The complexity of the validation process depends on the type of target. If working with a traditional biological target, e.g., a new receptor or an inducible enzyme or a cloned and expressed target, the challenge will be to use the available test procedures and any known chemical leads to test the hypothesis. If genomically derived proteins represent the target of a program, there will be an additional need to establish the function of a protein associated with a given disease state. This can be a daunting undertaking, highly dependent on serendipity. Once data is available to validate the approach, the project moves into a **planning** (P) stage. This involves the development and implementation of appropriate screens and their integration into high throughput screens. Simultaneously, a small medicinal chemistry effort would be put in place to modify known pharmacophores and generate leads. With the identification of novel structures, the project would move to the **realized** (R) stage where full scale, critical mass chemistry, biology, pharmacokinetic, and animal testing resources are put in place. The final stage of a project is the **mature** (M) stage where compounds are in clinical testing and information is being fed back to the project team to improve the properties of second generation compounds known colloquially as "back-ups" or "follow-ons."

The flow chart (Figure I.1) is a proven tactical approach to effectively running a project. Providing a vehicle to objectively set criteria for compound selection and subsequent characterization thus permitting prioritization of the project team activities and providing clear guidelines for decision making. Project team effectiveness is dependent both on the quality of the science and the vision and commitment of the leader and the individual members of the team (31).

REFERENCES

1. Binder S, Levitt AM, Sacks JJ, Hughes JM. Emerging infectious diseases: public health issues for the 21st Century. Science 1999, 284:1311–1313.
2. Asbell B. The Pill. New York, Random House, 1995.
3. Cartledge J, Eardley I. Viagra and beyond. Curr Opin CPNS Invest. Drugs 1999,1:240,–247.
4. O'Brien J, Austin M, Sethi P, et al. Urinary incontinence: prevalence, need for treatment, and effectiveness of intervention by nurse. B Med J 1991,202:1308–1312.
5. Palella, FJ, Delaney, KM, Moroman AC, et al. Declining morbidity and mortality among patients with advanced human immunodeficiency virus infection. N Engl J Med 1998,338:853-860.
6. Fearon ER. Human cancer syndromes: clues to the origin and nature of cancer. Science 1997,278:1043–1050.
7. Sneader WJ. Drug Discovery. The Evolution of Modern Medicines. Chichester, U.K., John Wiley, 1997.
8. Liebenau J. Evolution of the pharmaceutical industry. Comp Med Chem 1990,1:81–98.
9. Mann CC, Plummer ML. The Aspirin Wars. New York, Knopf, 1991.
10. Vane JR, Bakhle YS, Botting RM. Cyclooxygenases 1 and 2. Ann Rev Pharmacol Toxicol 1998,38:97–120.
11. Swann JP. Academic Scientists and the Pharmaceutical Industry. New York, Johns Hopkins University Press, 1988.
12. Youngson R, Schott I. Medical Blunders. London, Robinson, 1996.
13. Drayer JI, Burns JP. From discovery to market: the development of pharmaceuticals. In: Wolff, ME, ed. Burger's Medicinal Chemistry and Drug Discovery, 5th Ed. Volume 1. Principles and Practice. Wiley, New York, 1995, pp. 251–300.
14. Williams M, Giordano T, Elder RA, Reiser HJ, Neil GL. Biotechnology in the drug discovery process: strategic and management issues. Med Res Rev 1993,13:399–448.
15. Dibner MD. Biotechnology and pharmaceuticals. 10 years later. BioPhar, September, 1997,24–29.
16. Weisbach JA, Moos WH. Diagnosing the decline of major pharmaceutical research laboratories: a prescription for drug companies. Drug Dev Res 1995,34:243–259.
17. Sapienza, AM, Williams M. Biotechnology, E-business and Darwin. Reflections on the industry in the Internet Age. IDrugs, 1999,2:971–973.
18. Thompson WL. Research investments in a managed-care, cost-containment oligopsony. Ann Rep Med Chem 1995,30:339–345.
19. DiMasi J, Hansen RW, Grabowski HG, et al. Research and development costs for new drugs by therapeutic category. PharmacoEcon 1995,7:52–169.
20. Arlington S. Accelerating drug discovery: creating the right environment. Drug Disc Today 1997,2:547–553.
21. Banerjee PK, Rosofsky M. Drug discovery: the quest for innovation and productivity. Scrip Magazine, November, 1997,35–38.
22. Carr G. The alchemists. A survey of the pharmaceutical industry. Economist February 21, 1998,3–18.
23. Regalado A, Drug development's preclinical bottleneck. Windhover's Review of Emerging Medical Ventures, December, 1997.
24. Drews J, Ryser S. Pharmaceutical innovation between scientific opportunities and economic constraints. Drug Disc Today 1997,2:365–36-72.
25. Vrettos N, Steiner M. Unleashing managerial advantage in pharmaceutical research and development. Drugs Made In Germany 1999,42:13–19.
26. deStevens G. Conflicts and resolutions. Med Res Rev 1995,15:261–275.
27. Spilker B. Multinational Pharmaceutical Companies: Principles and Practices. New York, Raven, 1994.
28. Jorgensen SI, Jensen I, Edwards M. Surviving as a niche player in the pharmaceutical industry: reflections from the field. Drug Dev Res 1993,30:112–120.
29. Boyatzias RE, Esteves MB, Spencer LM. Entrepreneurial innovation in pharmaceutical research and development. Human Resource Planning 1992,15:15–29.
30. Sapienza AM. Creating Technology Strategies. How To Build Competitive Biomedical R&D. New York, Wiley-Liss, 1997.
31. Williams M, Stork, D. Setting up the R&D team. In Hampton JJ, AMA Management Handbook. AMACOM, New York, 1994,7–25.
32. Sapienza AM. Managing Scientists. New York, Wiley, 1995.
33. Roussel PA, Saad KN, Erickson T. Third Generation R & D. Managing the Link to Corporate Strategy. Boston, MA, Harvard Business School Press, 1991.
34. Borisy A, Kalustain J. Drug franchises, In Vivo. The Business and Medicine Report. October, 1998, pp. 1–6.
35. Guyer S, Collins FS. How is the Human Genome Project doing, and what have we learned so far? Proc Natl Acad Sci USA 1995, 92:10841–10848.
36. Poste G. The case for genomic patenting. Nature 1995,378:534–536.
37. Drews G. Genomic sciences and the medicine of tomorrow. Nature Biotech 1996,14:1517–1518.

38. Scangos G. Drug discovery in the postgenomic era. Nature Biotech 1997,15:1220–1221.
39. Kiley, R. Patent on random complementary DNA fragments? Science 1993,257:915–918.
40. Davison F. Gene patenting. Nature 1996,379:111.
41. Williams M. Genomics, Proteomics and Gnomics. Curr Opin Invest Drugs 2001,2:437–439.
42. Marshall A. Getting the right drug into the right patient. Nature Biotech 15, 1249–1254.
43. Kenakin TP The classification of seven transmembrane receptors in recombinant expression systems. Pharmacological Rev 1996,48:413–465.
44. Greer J, Baldwin JJ, Erickson J, et al. Application of the three-dimensional structures of protein target molecules in structure-based drug design. J Med Chem 1994,37: 1035–1051.
45. Blundell T. Structure-based drug design. Nature 1996,384: Supplement 23–26.
46. Joyce C. Earthly Goods. Medicine Hunting in the Rain Forest. Little, Brown, Boston, 1994.
47. Daly JW. The chemistry of poisons in amphibian skin. Proc Natl Acad Sci USA 1995,92:9–13.
48. Sato A. The search for new drugs from marine organisms. J Toxicol Toxin Rev, 1996,15:171–198.
49. Gordon EM, Kerwin Jr. JF. Combinatorial Chemistry and Molecular Diversity in Drug Discovery. Wiley, New York, 1998.
50. Triggle DJ Chemical Diversity. Current Protocols Pharmacol. Wiley, New York, 1998, 9.0.1–9.0.18
51. Black JW Drugs from emasculated hormones: the principle of synoptic antagonism. Science 1989,245:486–492.
52. Hodgson J. Pharmaceutical screening: from off-the-wall to off-the-shelf. Biotechnology 1993,11:683–688.
53. Kenny BA, Bushfield M, Parry-Smith DJ, et al. The application of high throughput screening to novel lead discovery. Prog Drug Res 1998,41:246–269.
54. Artursson P. Epithelial transport of drugs in cell culture. I: A model for studying the passive diffusion of drugs over intestinal absorptive (Caco-2) cells. J Pharm Sci 1990,79: 476–482.
55. Navia MA, Chaturvedi PR. Design principles for orally bioavailable drugs. Drug Disc Today 1996,1:179–189.
56. Porsolt RD, Brossard G, Roux S. Models of affective illness: behavioral despair test in rodents, Current Protocols Pharmacol. Wiley, New York, 1998, 5.8.1–5.8.7.
57. Wilson JM Animal models of human disease for gene therapy. J Clin Invest 1996,97:1138–1141.
58. Rowland M, Tozer TN. Clinical Pharmacokinetics: Concepts and Applications, 3rd Ed. Philadelphia, Lea and Febiger, 1995.
59. Dorato MA, Buckley LA. Toxicology in the drug discovery and development process. Current Protocols Pharmacol. Wiley, New York, 1998, 10.3.1–10.3.30.
60. Cutler NR, Sramek JJ, Kurtz NM, et al. Accelerating CNS Drug Development, Wiley, Chichester, U.K., 1998.
61. Kessler DA, Feiden KL. Faster evaluation of vital drugs. Sci Amer 1995,272(3):48–55
62. Stork DA. Not all differences are created equal: not all should be managed the same: the diversity challenge in pharmaceutical R & D. Drug Dev Res 1998,43:174–181.
63. Williams M. Strategies for drug discovery. NIDA Research Monograph 1993,132:1–22.
64. International Human Genome Sequencing Consortium; Initial sequencing and analysis of the human genome. Nature 2001, 409:860–921.
65. Venter JC, Adams MD, Meyers EW, et al. The sequence of the human genome. Science 2001,291:1304–1351.
66. Williams M, Coyle JT, Shaikh S and Decker MW (2001). Same brain, new century. Challenges in CNS drug discovery in the postgenomic, proteomic era. Ann Rep Med Chem. 36:1–10.
67. Legrain P, Wojcik J, Gauthier J-M. Protein-protein interaction maps: a lead towards cellular functions. Trends Genetics 2001, 17:346–352.

1. Natural Products

ALICE CLARK

INTRODUCTION
History

Natural products have been a major source of drugs for centuries. With more than 25% of the pharmaceuticals in use today derived from natural products, interest in natural products research remains strong. This can be attributed to several factors, including unmet therapeutic needs that drive new drug discovery, the remarkable diversity of both chemical structures and biological activities of naturally occurring secondary metabolites, the utility of bioactive natural products as biochemical and molecular probes, the development of novel and sensitive techniques to detect biologically active natural products, improved techniques to isolate, purify, and structurally characterize these active constituents, advances in solving the demand for bulk supply of complex natural products, and the success of herbal remedies in the global marketplace. Enormous opportunities exist for multidisciplinary research that joins the forces of pharmacognosy and natural products chemistry, molecular and cellular biology, medicinal and analytical chemistry, biochemistry, pharmacology, and pharmaceutics to exploit the vast diversity of chemical structures and biological activities of natural products.

Prior to the early-mid 20th century, the use of natural products was limited principally to crude plant preparations and was based largely on empirical observation, i.e., an observed effect was the justification for continued use of a preparation. Little was known or understood regarding the chemistry of the plants that were being used. The early observations regarding the use of plants to control illness and injury were recorded as the various materia medica of the traditional and folkloric remedies in various cultures. These included, for example, the writings of Dioscorides in the first century A.D. (De Materia Medica), of Galen in the 2nd century, and the existing Chinese Materia Medica.

The 'renaissance' of natural products chemistry came with decades of research devoted to the isolation and structural characterization of chemical constituents of plants (and later, microorganisms), often absent any knowledge of (or interest in) the biological effects of such constituents. Following an era of purely "phytochemical" investigation came a period in which the biological effects of pure natural products and the important and pivotal role of natural products in understanding pharmacological and cellular processes were recognized. For example, the isolation and structure determination of morphine from *Papaver somniferum,* the isolation of the cardiac glycosides from *Digitalis* species, and the isolation of other CNS active alkaloids from a variety of plants and microbes all contributed to understanding human physiology and laid the foundation for modern medicinal chemistry and pharmacology.

The current state of the science brings a different perspective that incorporates an increasing understanding of cellular biochemistry, molecular biology, and genomics to the process of discovering biologically active natural products. Additionally, advances in techniques, such as miniaturization of bioassays and coupling of chromatographic and spectroscopic techniques, has dramatically changed the process itself, in essence creating a subdiscipline that deals with issues related to the rapid biologic evaluation of large numbers of samples that range from purified single chemical entities to complex mixtures and extracts (high throughput screening).

What is in store for the future? Clearly, the process of natural products drug discovery will continue to evolve, and the role of natural products in drug discovery and development will likely continue or even increase. Additionally, the public interest in botanicals and the growing recognition of the utility of botanicals by healthcare professionals continues to increase. For these reasons, the impact of this discipline on pharmacy education, research, and practice will continue to be important.

Important Principles

It is important to understand the definition of certain terms that will be used frequently throughout our discussion of natural products discovery. These terms are defined in Table 1.1 In some ways the discovery and development of natural product-derived drugs is very similar to the design of synthetic drugs, yet in other ways these processes are very different. For example, both must rely on biological assays of some kind in order to identify promising lead compounds for further development. The most fundamental difference between natural products as a source of new drugs, and design and synthesis as a source of new drugs is, in fact, simply the origination of the compound.

In the search for novel bioactive natural products with promising therapeutic potential, the approach determines outcome. One must ask "What is the goal of the discovery process?" Is it to discover a novel compound (a completely new and different chemical structure) that also possesses a new biological activity or mechanism of action, or is it acceptable to discover a known compound, or another variation of a known chemotype, with a new or novel biologi-

Table 1.1. Definitions of Natural Product Terms

Term	Definition
Pharmacognosy	Study of all aspects of biologically active natural products and/or their derivatives, and encompasses the chemistry of all living organisms (plants, microbes, animals).
Natural product	Single chemical compound that occurs naturally. This term is typically used to refer to an organic compound of limited distribution in nature (often called secondary metabolites).
Dereplication	Process of determining whether an observed biological effect of an extract or specimen is due to a known substance.
Bioassay-directed fractionation	Process of isolating active constituents from some type of biomass (plants, microbes, marine invertebrates, etc.) using a decision tree that is dictated solely by bioactivity.
Phytochemistry	Isolation of substances from plants without regard to biological activity (i.e., compound-driven).
Biodiversity prospecting	Process of collecting or surveying of a large set of flora (or fauna) for purpose of biological evaluation and isolation of lead compounds (1).
High-throughput screening (HTS)	"Process by which large numbers of compounds can be tested, in an automated fashion, for activity as inhibitors (antagonists) or activators (agonists) of a particular biological target such as cell-surface receptors or a metabolic enzyme" (2).
Lead compound	Compound that has a desirable biological activity with therapeutic relevance, but typically has some shortcoming that is likely to be overcome through the development of analogs (which may be designed and produced via a range of activities from the 'conventional' medicinal chemistry approach to combinatorial chemistry and combinatorial biosynthesis).
Biosynthesis	Process an organism uses to synthesize a chemical constituent.
Semi-synthesis	Synthetic modification of a natural product.
Combinatorial biosynthesis (biocombinatorial synthesis)	"Process of generating novel molecules from natural products by the genetic engineering of biosynthetic pathways in microorganisms" (3,4).

cal activity or mechanism? It is also possible to discover a novel compound that has a known biological activity or mechanism of action. The goal will dictate the approach, and the approach will control the outcome.

In the best case scenario, completely novel chemicals with previously unknown, but potentially therapeutically useful biological activities will be discovered. In this context, it is important to recognize the role of natural products as lead compounds. This has been the case in several disease states, where natural products were the first useful drugs for a specific disease (for example, the statins for cholesterol lowering and cyclosporin for immunosuppression).

APPROACHES TO DISCOVERING AND DEVELOPING NATURAL PRODUCTS AS POTENTIAL NEW DRUGS

The process of drug discovery from natural sources is rooted in the discipline of pharmacognosy, which has a significant interdisciplinary nature. Everything ranging from strategies for collecting natural product source material to meeting mass supply demands must be carefully considered in the process of natural products drug discovery. Failure to adequately address any of the steps in the process could result in failure to achieve the objective of identifying potential new drug candidates. The process

Table 1.2. Steps Necessary for Drug Development of Chemicals from Natural Sources

Sourcing, sample acquisition, processing, and storage of specimens
Evaluating biological activities of samples
Identifying the biologically active natural product(s) in active samples
Selecting and optimizing lead compounds for further development

consists of a number of concurrent and interactive activities, which are shown in Table 1.2.

One of the consistent challenges for the natural product chemist who aims to identify natural product-derived pharmaceuticals is the issue of how best to determine desirable biological activity. In the beginning, this was largely a trial and error process, i.e., through empirical observation it was determined which plant and animal products were effective for a variety of ailments. Through the years this process gave way to an equally random, but more scientifically validated process known as "screening." It is in this area that much of the debate regarding how best to discover a potential new drug rages. There are those who believe the best approach is "biodiversity prospecting" wherein one samples a broad array of plant, microbial, and animal species, searching for compounds with a predefined set of desirable biological activities. The goal is to survey as much specimen diversity as is possible. Current estimations of the number of species of plants that inhabit our planet range from 300,000 to 500,000, and only a very small percentage have been minimally evaluated. Although it is an important and appropriate undertaking, it would take many years of systematic, concerted effort to evaluate all the Earth's plants for a specific biological activity, and this is clearly not achievable in our lifetime!

Another approach to natural product drug discovery is to utilize the impressive quantity and quality of information derived by indigenous cultures that have used plant and animal products to control disease and injury. This discipline, referred to as ethnobotany, or ethnopharmacology, is a mix of sociology, medicine, anthropology and botany, and can provide very useful information to guide the natural products chemist in the search for new therapeutic agents. It is likely that most of the herbal remedies on the market today have derived from such ethnobotanical information. Supporters of this approach argue that it is unlikely that cultures would have continued to use a material for decades, or even centuries, if it failed to be effective. Given that much of this information is passed from generation to generation through oral history only, there is a sense of urgency to record and validate the knowledge of the "shaman" before the information is forever lost. On the other hand, there are some cultures that have carefully recorded, in written form, the information regarding the use of natural substances to treat illness and injury. The Chinese "Materia Medica" is a centuries-old treatise that documents in impressive detail the classification, description, preparation, and uses of thousands of medicinal plants. Likewise, the Ayurvedic system is similar in its level of detail and documentation of plants used in traditional medicine in India.

Much debate has also centered around the most appropriate manner of evaluation of natural products for desirable activities. Prior to the 70s and 80s, when major advancements in molecular biology were made, the discovery of a novel drug other than an antimicrobial relied largely on the use of animal models. However, in the 80s, with major advancements in molecular biology, there was a trend toward the utilization of receptor- or enzyme-based assay systems (sometimes referred to as mechanism-based assays) that measure very specific and selective activities. This has led to the development of a subdiscipline of drug discovery dedicated to the rapid evaluation of large numbers of pure compounds and natural product extracts for very specific biological activities, usually based on interactions with selected enzymes or receptors. This approach, known as high throughput screening (HTS), relies heavily on robotics and automation and has revolutionized the ability to routinely evaluate tens of thousands of samples. New assays using a specific target enzyme or receptor are rapidly developed and adapted for high throughput screening, making it possible to screen very large libraries of compounds in a very short time. These advancements have led to "turnover" of assays about every six months in industry, wherein a new assay is developed, the entire library of samples is evaluated, another new assay developed, the library screened again, and so on. While this approach clearly has a major role in the future of drug discovery, we should be reminded of two important points. First, the identification of a potential new target for drug discovery must come from somewhere, and this is usually from an understanding of the basic biology of the target system or from an understanding of the mechanism of action of a novel biologically active compound. Most of the latter have been derived from natural products discovered in assay systems that are not mechanism based (i.e., whole cell assays vs. enzymatic or receptor assays). The downside of the high throughput mechanism-based screening is that it selects only for activity by a specific mechanism, and activity via another mechanism may be missed. While

this is obviously important and useful, it does, nevertheless, restrict the search. Thus, it is critical to recognize the importance of identifying prototype biologically active compounds that are novel not only structurally, but mechanistically as well. A second point to keep in mind is that the need to penetrate a cell or to reach a particular tissue is never circumvented. Thus, there are those who also argue that, given the ultimate goal of using the drug in a whole animal system complete with complicated cellular and tissue barriers, compounds should be sought that are active in whole cell systems. Clearly, there is a need and a role for both approaches, and when taken in concert and coordinated to complement one another, the likelihood of identifying useful new drugs is substantially increased.

Finally, an area of much concern in the past, particularly from an industrial viewpoint, is the concern regarding a reliable and sufficient supply of natural product-derived drugs. This, indeed, has been perceived as an almost insurmountable problem in a few cases of compounds from plant or marine sources. It is difficult to know, however, whether there has ever been a really good drug candidate that was abandoned for the singular reason that supply was a major concern. Clearly, when the source is a cultivable terrestrial or aquatic microorganism (such as bacteria, fungi, or algae), the challenges are significantly more manageable, and this fact probably largely accounts for the greater focus on fermentation chemistry in industrial natural products discovery efforts. Nevertheless, there are a sufficient number of examples of plant-derived natural products that are used clinically without structural alteration to suggest that the concerns regarding supply should not be overriding, that is, if a drug is useful enough, the challenge of adequate supply will be addressed. One approach that has been quite successful is the development of simpler semisynthetic or synthetic analogs that are designed to incorporate the necessary pharmacophore of the more complex natural product and improve its pharmaceutical properties such as pharmacokinetics, compatibility, stability, etc. In these cases, the natural product serves as a prototype lead compound for the design and development of second generation agents with simpler, synthetically accessible structures and improved characteristics. In such cases, it is unlikely that large quantities of the original prototype natural product are required for mass production of the drug; however, this may occur if the improved agent is a semisynthetic derivative that uses a natural product as starting material, and issues related to supply are still important. A second approach has been to determine the genetic and environmental factors that influence the production of the critical secondary metabolite, and to couple this information with improved recovery techniques. A third, largely theoretical, approach to overcoming the supply issue is the use of tissue culture. While in principle this approach is quite appealing, thus far the production of important plant-derived drugs by tissue culture has met with limited success (5).

Regardless of the variations that may be undertaken in approaching natural products drug discovery, the process necessarily involves acquiring source materials, evaluating those materials for desirable biological activities, identifying the active constituent(s), optimizing lead compounds and developing drug candidates. A discussion of each of these processes is provided below.

Strategies and Approaches for Sourcing, Processing, and Archiving Natural Products for Drug Discovery

The goal of sourcing and sample acquisition is to obtain the maximum chemodiversity and therapeutically useful biological activity within the minimum number of collected samples. The goal of sample handling and preparation is to remove nuisance compounds that may interfere with bioassays in a nonspecific manner, to prepare the samples to be compatible with existing (and future) bioassays, and to store both the collected, unprocessed material and the processed samples in a manner that is easily retrievable and maximizes stability. Thus, the key decisions related to sourcing and sampling preparation are: what strategies to employ (including what sources on which to focus, i.e., plant, marine, microbial, insect, etc.), what quantity of specimen to collect, how to appropriately access and acquire specimens, how to store and process the collected samples, and how to handle and store the processed sample (usually extracts).

Sources of Natural Products

A number of strategies may be developed to select and acquire sources of natural products that are most likely to yield desirable compounds. Some strategies in use today include utilizing ethnobotanical and folklore information on medicinal plant use by specific cultures, exploring the relationship of genetic biodiversity and environmental factors to chemodiversity and specific biological activities, examining the chemical ecology of plants and animals, focusing on plants, microbes, or animals that exist in unusual habitats, investigating whether different plant parts and ages of plants are more likely to produce novel bioactive natural products, and biodiversity prospecting. An important primary consideration in any natural products drug discovery program, and particularly those relying on ethnobotanical or bioprospecting strategies, is the fact that the greatest biodiversity occurs in the tropical regions and the greatest ethnobotanical knowledge exists within various cultures that do not use "Western medicine," both of which often occur in developing countries. Access to the genetic property of developing countries is a complicated and sensitive matter that requires careful thought and attention to the concerns of all involved. All collections should be done as collaborative efforts with careful attention to issues of ownership of intellectual property, laws governing access to biodiversity, and political, social, and economic factors.

Initial sample size may vary, but certainly with recent advances in technology related to bioassays, isolation, dereplication, and structure elucidation, much smaller initial sample sizes are required than in the past. Initial sample size notwithstanding, attention must be given to the likelihood that additional quantities of source material will be required for promising specimens, necessitating the ability to re-collect the same specimen with confidence that similar results will be obtained with re-collected material. Once samples are acquired, voucher specimens (or type cultures, or other appropriate authenticated source material) must be maintained according to standard accepted methods and the collected specimens must be extracted or otherwise processed to prepare samples for biological evaluation. Recent developments that affect sourcing strategies include decreased access to plants and marine life, especially in developing countries. Developments that contribute to a greater range of specimens being collected and evaluated include a growing body of literature on methods to isolate, cultivate, and identify unusual microbes (slow-growing, nonabundant soil organisms, marine microbes, endophytes, etc.) and methods to collect and identify unusual marine invertebrates (Closed Circuit Underwater Breathing Apparatus, remote submersibles collecting from extreme environs, increasing taxonomic knowledge). In addition, the automation and miniaturization of extraction and bioassay techniques allows for collection of much smaller initial sample sizes, affording the opportunity to collect and evaluate specimens that were previously not accessible or sufficiently abundant. Also, improved geopositioning systems and abilities to dereplicate and structurally characterize relatively minor components (discussed later) also contribute to a diminishing demand for large initial sample sizes for screening.

There are three sources of natural products: plants, microorganisms, and animals, and there are advantages and disadvantages, opportunities and challenges associated with exploring each of these.

Plants.   There are significant advantages and opportunities associated with accessing plants as a source of new drugs; there are also substantial disadvantages and challenges. Fortunately, the chemical and biological diversity of plants drives the balance in favor of advantages and opportunities, and mandates that challenges and disadvantages be addressed and overcome. Several other authors have provided excellent reviews detailing some of these benefits and concerns (1, 6–10). One of the principal advantages of plants as a source of new pharmaceuticals is that the secondary metabolism of plants appears to have evolved over centuries to retain biochemical features that guarantee chemical diversity. However, as pointed out by others (11), this does not necessarily guarantee that biological activity (especially therapeutically useful activity for humans) will also exist. In other words, just because there is chemical diversity does not mean there will be useful therapeutic activity. Nevertheless, the fact that natural products are a source of new and varied chemical templates is an important advantage of searching plants for new chemotypes. Another important advantage of plants as a source of new drugs is that they have, as others have noted, "been carrying out combinatorial chemistry for centuries" (12), and have retained those biochemical features that may also contribute to "self defense." Chemical ecology (co-habitation and protection from surrounding organisms) likely accounts for many of the secondary metabolites produced by plants, and can be an important and useful strategy for identifying new leads for drug development.

There are two major challenges associated with searching for new drugs from plants: (a) identifying plants that likely produce new or novel natural products with potent and potentially useful bioactivity; and (b) identifying and isolating from the biomass of the plant those natural products that are new compounds or novel chemotypes with potentially useful bioactivity. In addition to these challenges are the problems of initial access to the plant material, especially from foreign countries, as well as the follow-up access and use of plant material, if necessary, to solve bulk supply issues. One of the most important problems that remains in this area, and one that represents a significant opportunity for research, is the development of rational, testable strategies for identifying "high hit ratio" plants. Reproducibility (or lack thereof) in re-collected material is also a significant concern, particularly as it relates to bulk supply. Whether due to seasonal variations, different plant parts or age of the plants, or other reasons, it is an obvious challenge that is a major driving force for the development of synthetic routes to important natural products. There must be an assurance of the ability to produce large quantities of a promising new drug candidate, by reisolation from the source plant, by tissue culture, or by synthesis (total or semisynthesis).

Microorganisms. As a source of new natural product drugs, microorganisms have the distinct advantage that, assuming a stable stock culture can be maintained, bulk supply is less of a concern, although there are problems on the front end, such as the increased challenge of dereplication (especially for soil organisms), the difficulties of establishing initial cultivation conditions (especially for marine microbes), and maintenance of stable cultures. An increasingly important advantage (in addition to scale-up capacity) of microbes is the potential for modification of natural biosynthetic pathways through combinatorial biosynthesis. Also, there remain many unexplored sources of microbes, such as marine aquatic microorganisms, organisms from extreme environs, and endophytes. Recent developments in methods to isolate, cultivate, and identify unusual microbes will undoubtedly contribute to the increased exploration of the chemistry of these organisms in the future.

Animals. It could be reasonably argued that one advantage of animals as a source of bioactive natural products is that they have likely developed chemical defenses to protect against other animal predators; thus there may be a greater likelihood of obtaining pharmacologically active compounds from them. Additionally, they have been minimally examined as a source of new drugs. Recent significant discoveries have propelled this source into the mainstream of natural products research. One such discovery was made by Daly and coworkers (13,14), who identified epibatidine from the South American tree frog, *Epipedobates tricolor.* While the toxicity of this compound probably precludes its development as a therapeutic agent, it has led to extensive studies to identify inhibitors of nicotinic receptors as analgesics. Also, the elegant work of Oliviera and coworkers (15) on the isolation and characterization of the cone snail venoms illustrates the combinatorial chemistry capacity of this animal. Organisms from the marine environment, particularly sponges and other invertebrates, are also recognized as an important source of potential new drugs (16,17).

Handling, Processing, and Storing Collected Specimens

One of the major concerns in natural products discovery is how (or even whether) to extract the biomass in order to maximize the recovery of truly interesting secondary metabolites while minimizing the presence of "nuisance compounds" that may account for non-specific false-positives in many biological assays. Thus, the goal of sample preparation is to select for positives and remove "nuisance" compounds, and to prepare the sample to be compatible with existing (and future) bioassays, storage, and retrieval. The key decisions are whether the biomass should be extracted, and if so, how it should be extracted. For plant samples, additional considerations include whether to extract fresh vs. dried, or ground vs. unground biomass. For microbes, what conditions should be used for initial cultivation is also a consideration. In the past, most biomass, whether plant or microbial, was extracted, usually with organic solvents. Consequently, mostly low molecular weight lipophilic compounds were obtained. Significant advancements have been made in the area of separations chemistry (18), including the use of supercritical fluids for extraction, various chromatographic techniques, and purification of water soluble natural products, and these provide new avenues for consideration in sample preparation that will be consistent with follow-up larger scale isolation (discussed later).

Both qualitative and quantitative differences may exist in the chemical profiles of fresh vs. dried plant material. Also, it has been reported that some secondary metabolites are sequestered in specific plant organs, eliminating the need for conventional grinding and extraction to recover interesting secondary metabolites (19). Much more work is needed to determine the impact of various methods of sample preparation on the overall objectives of detecting novel bioactive natural products in plant biomass.

Evaluating Natural Products for Potentially Therapeutic Biological Effects

The core foundation of every drug discovery program is the approach to the detection of desirable biological activities. The goal of biological evaluation is to identify compounds with selective and specific biological effects on contemporary and relevant disease targets, and to effectively predict in vivo efficacy, toxicity and pharmacokinetics. Typically, a tier of assays may be established (2), beginning with a primary assay that has a relatively high throughput capacity and is designed to detect samples with the most promise for yielding interesting compounds, followed by secondary assays to corroborate, quantify, and define specific activities, and tertiary assays designed to assess the clinical potential of promising compounds (usually animal models). The primary assay is usually designed to "screen" out the vast majority of samples with low to moderate activity or with non-selective activity. Prior to major advances in molecular biology, molecular pharmacology, and genomics, most assays for the discovery of new drugs were based on identifying compounds that effected an observable response in animals, or, for antibiotics, that inhibited the growth of the target pathogens. While this had the advantage of detecting those agents active in whole cell or whole animal systems, it was very laborious, expensive, and often impractical. With the advent of molecular biology techniques, primary assays are now typically mechanism-based, molecular target-specific bioassays. These are usually developed as high throughput screens, designed to screen large libraries of samples. It is important to recognize that specific challenges are associated with screening natural product extracts (as opposed to pure compounds or mixtures of compounds, such as might be produced through combinatorial synthesis). In particular, natural product extracts typically are colored, insoluble and consist of numerous compounds that may interact (synergistic and antagonistic), may result in false positives, and present significant challenges in assay sensitivity. Secondary assays are usually designed to corroborate and quantitate the activity observed in the primary assay, to establish the spectrum of activity, to provide insight into the mode of action, and to predict in vivo pharmaceutical properties. Important criteria for determining the relative importance of a lead compound usually include evidence to suggest it acts by a novel mechanism of action and evidence that it possesses desirable pharmaceutical properties. Claeson and Bohlin have provided an excellent overview of some of these challenges in designing bioassays specifically for natural products screening (2).

Key decisions in designing, utilizing and interpreting the results of biological assays include the selection of the target (therapeutic, systemic, cellular, molecular), establishing a threshold for "active," determining whether high throughput screening is necessary and appropriate for each assay, and, an important and consistently difficult problem, designing in vitro bioassays that will correlate with, and effectively predict in vivo outcomes. Advances in functional vs. affinity genomics and the use of transgenic systems, along with miniaturization and automation of biological assay techniques, have revolutionized the biological evaluation of all products, natural and synthetic. Additionally, the use of molecular biology techniques, such as incorporation of luciferase reporter genes into cell lines, and advances in instrumentation that allow the use of sensitive luminescent and colorimetric assays has provided a means of coupling bioassays with chromatographic and spectroscopic techniques, in some cases allowing on-line bioassay capability.

Identifying the Biologically Active Natural Product

One of the major challenges in natural product drug discovery is determining which of a number of approximately equally active samples to pursue for further study, usually for isolation and structure elucidation of the active constituent(s). This is best accomplished through a system of prioritization coupled with the process known as dereplication. Since isolation and structure elucidation may be among the most laborious, time-consuming, and expensive steps in natural product drug discovery, much attention is given to developing reliable methods of dereplication. The goal of dereplication is to select, for follow-up isolation and structure elucidation, only extracts that are likely to yield novel chemotypes, i.e., to "de-select" compounds with known activity profiles or structures. One of the best ways to achieve dereplication is to access unique sources, so that there is a greater assurance of obtaining novel chemotypes. Also, advances in coupling spectroscopic and chromatographic techniques can provide rapid and reliable structural information on small quantities of material, thus facilitating dereplication (20). Judicious use of the literature is a critical aspect of successful dereplication.

It is also important to prioritize samples for further study. Priority assignment may be based on a combination of factors, including biological activity profile, the results of literature searches that indicate minimal previous work on a specimen, and the availability of sufficient biomass for larger scale fractionation. Typically, once a priority position is assigned to a given sample, bioassay-directed fractionation is carried out to isolate pure active constituents. Recent developments that have affected the ability to isolate minor active constituents include the use of supercritical fluid chromatography, capillary electrophoresis, countercurrent chromatography, centrifugal partition chromatography, and spin columns, among others.

Structural characterization of isolated active compounds is accomplished most often using state-of-the-art spectroscopic techniques such as high field nuclear magnetic resonance spectroscopy (NMR), mass spectroscopy, and various methods to determine absolute and relative stereochemistry, especially X-ray crystallography.

Selecting and Optimizing Lead Compounds

New compounds that show promising therapeutic potential based on biological activity are subject to further studies aimed at developing a promising pharmaceutical candidate for preclinical studies and clinical trials. These studies involve medicinal chemistry to accomplish total synthesis, analog synthesis for structure-activity relationship studies, molecular modeling and computer aided drug design, and analytical and physical chemistry to establish the pharmaceutical properties of the compound. Studies to understand and predict pharmacokinetics, efficacy and toxicity in appropriate models, drug delivery and formulations, and metabolism, are all aimed at identifying the most suitable candidate for preclinical and clinical development. In particular, there is a growing utilization of in vitro model systems (e.g., microbial, tissue culture) to predict in vivo characteristics of new drug candidates. These topics are covered extensively in other chapters and will not be addressed in detail here.

DRUG DEVELOPMENT—NATURAL PRODUCTS

Once a drug candidate has been selected for development, there are essentially no differences between a natural product-derived new drug candidate and a synthetically-derived/designed new drug candidate in terms of the process of further development. The most notable difference, and a pressing concern, is the issue of assuring sufficient quantities are available for preclinical and clinical studies, and, ultimately, for commercial use. As noted earlier, for plant-derived compounds, the options for meeting bulk supply are through synthesis or semi-synthesis, re-isolation of wild or cultivated plant material, or by tissue culture scale-up. Of these, synthesis and isolation from plant material have been the most consistent in providing large quantities of specific plant-derived compounds. For microbes (especially terrestrial organisms), cultivation and large scale fermentation have been very successful. However, there remain many challenges to the bulk production of exciting new drug development candidates obtained from other sources, including plants and marine organisms. Various strategies are being investigated to meet these challenges, and include tissue culture of plants and aquaculture of marine invertebrates.

SELECTED EXAMPLES OF NATURAL PRODUCT-DERIVED DRUGS

Although the use of plant and animal products to control disease has been well documented for centuries, the biochemical basis for observed efficacies did not come under careful scientific scrutiny until the 18th and 19th centuries, particularly in the early to mid 1800s when a number of important, pharmacologically active natural products such as the cardiac glycosides and a variety of bioactive alkaloids (e.g., morphine, atropine, reserpine, and physostigmine) were discovered. Many of these biologically active natural products became important not only for their use directly as therapeutic agents or as prototype lead compounds for new drug development, but also as biochemical probes to unravel the principles of human pharmacology, a role for natural products which continues today (21). Shu (22) has provided an outstanding, comprehensive review of the role of natural products in drug development from the industry perspective.

Cardiovascular Drugs

The positive benefits of extracts of *Digitalis purpurea* (Foxglove) and *D. lanata* were recognized long before the active constituents were isolated and characterized structurally. The cardiac glycosides, which include digoxin, digitoxin, and deslanoside, exert a powerful and selective positive inotropic action on the cardiac muscle. Digoxin is still produced by mass cultivation and extraction of a strain of foxglove (*Digitalis purpurea*) that has been selected for maximum production of the bioactive glycosides (23). In addition to the cardiac glycosides, a number of naturally-occurring alkaloids are important drugs in the control of various cardiovascular conditions. For example, quinidine, isolated from the bark of the Cinchona tree, is an important anti-arrhythmic drug, and was also one of the earliest and most well-known examples of the critical role of chirality in drug action. Its diastereoisomer, quinine, has virtually no cardiac activity, but was recognized as one of the first anti-infective agents due to its efficacy against malaria. The discovery of the pharmacologic effects of components of the venom of the pit viper (*Bothrops jararaca*) ultimately led to the discovery of the role of angiotensin converting enzyme (ACE) in hypertension (24–26), and ACE inhibitors now constitute an important class of drugs that has had a major role in the management of cardiovascular disease (27). Other important naturally-occurring alkaloids active as cardiovascular drugs include reserpine, once one of the most useful antihypertensive agents known, and papaverine, a non-narcotic peripheral vasodilator. In addition, theophylline, a xanthine alkaloid, is an important bronchodilator used to control asthma in children. Ergotamine, an Ergot alkaloid obtained from a fungus that infects rye grass, is an important central vasoconstrictor that is used therapeutically to treat migraine headaches. One relatively recent addition to this class of drugs is the dopamine D_2 receptor agonist, cabergoline, launched in Belgium in 1993 as an antiprolactin. This drug is also being evaluated as a potential therapy for Parkinson's disease and as an anticancer agent for the treatment of breast cancer (28).

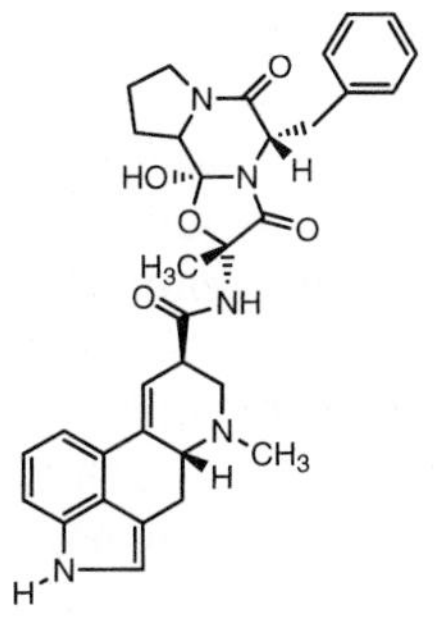

Ergotamine

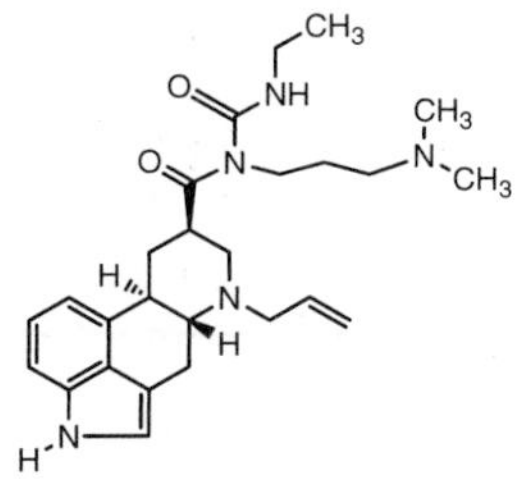

Cabergoline

to the development and introduction of nabilone (30), an effective anti-emetic that is widely used.

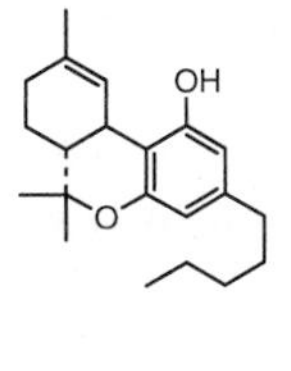

THC

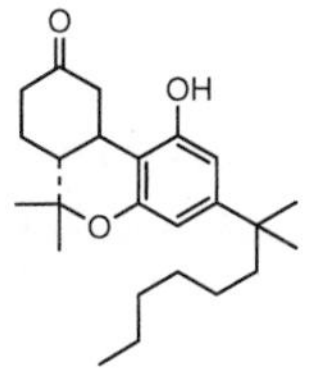

Nabilone

CNS Drugs

One of the most cited examples of important natural product-derived drugs is the neuromuscular blocker, d-tubocurarine, derived from the South American plant curare, which was used by South American Indians as an arrow poison (23). Tubocurarine led to the development of decamethonium, which, although structurally dissimilar to tubocurarine, was synthesized nevertheless based on the presumption at the time that tubocurarine contained two quaternary nitrogens (29). Likewise, the synthetic local anesthetics such as procaine and benzocaine were synthesized to mimic the nerve blocking activity of cocaine, a natural alkaloid obtained from the leaves of *Coca eroxylum*, but without the adverse side effects that have led to the abuse of cocaine. (23). The opium alkaloids, codeine and

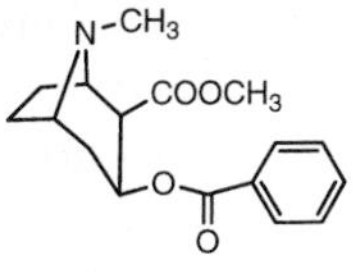

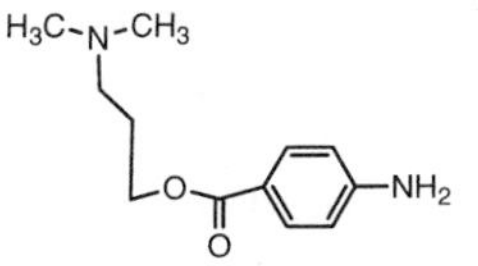

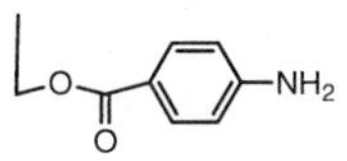

Recently, the recognition of the possibility that a number of vastly different CNS and peripheral nervous system diseases may be therapeutically controlled by selective nicotinic acetylcholine receptor (nAChR) agonists has opened a new area of drug design based on the nicotine molecule. Disorders such as Alzheimer's disease, Tourette's syndrome, Parkinson's disease, as well as other cognitive and attention disorders may ultimately be more effectively treated if agonists specific for certain subtypes of nAChRs can be discovered or designed. The characterization and understanding of these receptors was based largely on studies using agonists or antagonists, most of which are natural products, such as acetylcholine, arecoline, anabasine, lobeline, and methyllycaconitine. Recently, reports that the nicotine analog epibatidine, which was isolated from the skin of poisonous frogs, exhibits exceptional analgesic activity and is a very potent nAChR agonist have led to a num-

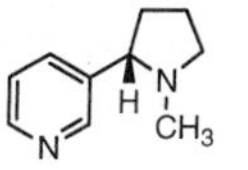

Cocaine

Procaine

Benzocaine

Nicotine

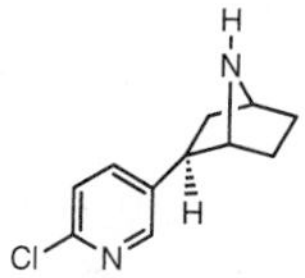

Epibatidine

morphine, served as models for the synthesis of naloxone, an important analog used to treat and diagnose opiate addicts (30), and also led to the discovery of the endogenous opioids, enkephalins and endorphins. Similarly, delta-9-tetrahydrocannabinol (THC), the component of *Cannabis sativa* responsible for the CNS effects seen with marijuana use, has also been found to reduce nausea associated with cancer chemotherapy. As a result, efforts to design semisynthetic or synthetic agents that mimic the desirable anti-emetic effects, while reducing the CNS effects of THC, led

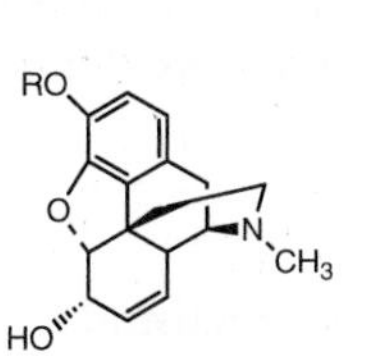

ber of synthetic studies on this molecule, including the synthesis of both pure enantiomers and the remarkable discovery that each enantiomer is very active (31).

Both physostigmine, a naturally-occurring alkaloid, and neostigmine, a synthetic analog of physostigmine, are important acetylcholinesterase inhibitors. Another acetylcholinesterase inhibitor, galanthamine, which is an alkaloid that occurs in the bulbs of daffodils, is currently being investigated as a possible therapy for cognitive impairment in Alzheimer's disease (32).

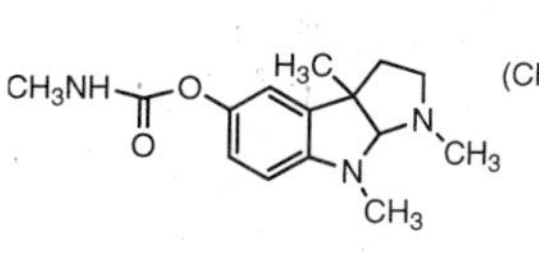

Morphine, R = H
Codeine, R = CH$_3$

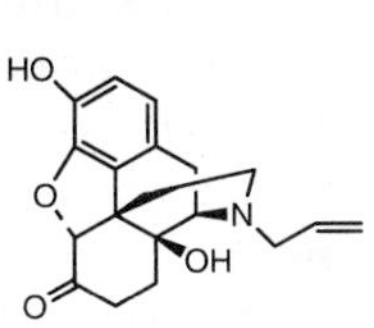

Naloxone

Physostigmine

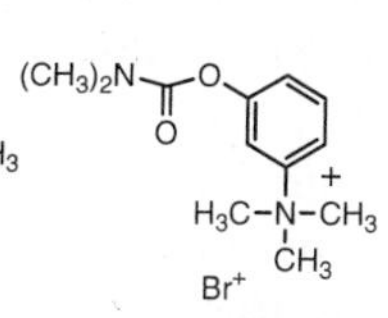

Neostigmine

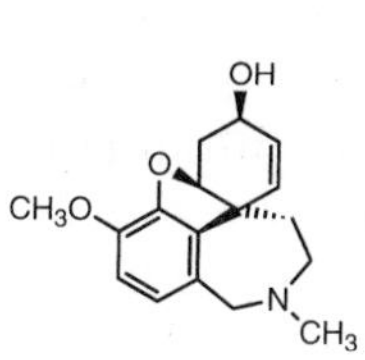

Galanthamine

Anti-infectives

There can be no argument that the antibiotics are among the most important classes of therapeutic agents and have had enormous impact on both life expectancy and quality of life. With the discovery of the natural penicillins as secondary metabolites of species of the fungus *Penicillium,* the course of medical history was dramatically changed and the antibiotic era was introduced. Antibiotics are, by definition, natural products or derivatives of natural products. During the course of some 50 years that followed Alexander Fleming's observations of the antibiotic effect of *Penicillium* toward *Staphylococcus,* and the subsequent isolation and characterization of the active constituent, penicillin N, by Howard Florey and Ernst Chain, hundreds of antibiotics have been isolated from scores of microorganisms (33). It is not unusual for two or three new antibiotics to be launched each year. Not only do these antibiotics serve as important drugs, but explorations into the mechanisms by which these natural products exert their action have led to an understanding of the biology of the target pathogens that would not likely have been possible without these important biochemical probes. Coupled with advances in molecular biology, significant advances in identifying new specific molecular targets in the pathogens are also being made.

The discovery of important anti-infectives is not limited to antibacterial or antifungal antibiotics from microbial sources. Long before the discovery of penicillin, native Amerindians knew that the bark of the South American "fever tree" *Cinchona succiruba,* was effective in controlling malaria (23). Quinine was ultimately identified as the active antimalarial constituent of the *Cinchona* bark. When the natural source of quinine was threatened during World Wars I & II, massive programs to synthesize multitudes of quinoline derivatives based on the quinine prototype ensued. From this intensive effort emerged the two drugs that remained the therapeutic standards for the treatment of malaria until the past decade: primaquine and chloroquine.

Quinine   Primaquine   Chloroquine

Today, new important anti-infectives are being discovered from microbial, plant, and animal sources. For example, the antimalarial agent artemisinin was isolated from the Chinese medicinal plant, *Artemisia annua.* Commonly known as Qinghaosu, this herbal remedy had been used in China for centuries for the treatment of malaria. In 1972, the active constituent was isolated and identified

as the sesquiterpene endoperoxide artemisinin. This compound, in addition to having a structure very different from any of the previously known antimalarial agents (i.e., quinolines), also exhibited antimalarial and pharmacologic profiles very different from the clinically useful agents. Specifically, with activity against strains of the parasite that had become resistant to conventional chloroquine therapy and the ability, due to its lipophilic structure, to cross the blood brain barrier, it was particularly effective for the deadly cerebral malaria. For this reason, several major programs were undertaken to produce artemisinin derivatives with more desirable pharmaceuti-

Artemisinin   Artemether

cal properties, and much has been published on synthetic and semisynthetic studies, microbial transformations, biological evaluations, mechanism of action studies, and pharmacologic profiles of artemisinin and related analogs (34–36). From these studies has emerged artemether, a derivative that is currently approved for the treatment of malaria in much of the world.

Another important class of anti-infective natural products to be introduced for human use in recent years are the avermectins, polyketide derived macrolides that were originally isolated from several species of *Streptomyces* (37). The major drug of this class, ivermectin, was originally developed to treat and control nematodes and para-

Ivermectin

sites of livestock. In recent years, however, ivermectin's potential for the treatment of human disease has also been realized, and it is now used to treat onchocerciasis (river blindness) (38,39), a disease that afflicts 40 million people worldwide (40).

Anticancer

Another therapeutic area where natural products have had a major impact on longevity and quality of life is in the chemotherapy of cancer. In fact, most of the major anticancer drugs are natural products from plants or microorganisms (41). Examples include such important anticancer drugs as bleomycin, doxorubicin, daunorubicin, vincristine, vinblastine, mitomycin, streptozocin, irinotecan (a camptothecin derivative), and etoposide and teniposide (podophyllotoxin derivatives).

The observation that fractions of the rosey periwinkle, *Catharanthus rosea,* produced severe leukopenia in rats led Gordon Svoboda and his coworkers at Eli Lilly to isolate and develop the two major anticancer drugs vincristine and vinblastine. These two complex, dimeric indole-indoline alkaloids are important therapies for the treatment of acute childhood leukemia (vincristine), Hodgkin's disease (vinblastine) and metastatic testicular tumors (vinblastine), and continue to be manufactured today by mass cultivation and processing of the natural source (23).

Over 40 years ago, the National Cancer Institute initiated a program to explore natural sources for potential new anticancer agents. Although this program went through periods of low productivity and little support, the discovery of one of the most exciting new drugs in recent history, paclitaxel, was a direct result of this effort. This compound as well as most other anticancer drugs, was dis-

Paclitaxel

covered using a system of screening large numbers of extracts of plants, microorganisms, and more recently, marine organisms, for inhibition of cancer cells grown in culture. A comprehensive account of the discovery and development of paclitaxel was recently published by the two pioneering natural product chemists who discovered this compound, Monroe Wall and Mansukh Wani (42). Although it took 15 years for the true benefit of paclitaxel to be fully realized, it was approved for the treatment of ovarian cancer in 1992 and for breast cancer in 1993, and is a rare example of the clinical use of the unaltered plant-derived natural product. Studies on the mechanism of anticancer action by paclitaxel revealed that it acted by a unique and novel mechanism, blocking depolymerization of microtubules (43). This led the way to the discovery of two new structurally unrelated classes of natural products that act by this same mechanism: the epitholones (44) and the discodermolides (45).

Another important plant-derived anticancer natural product isolated and identified by Wall and Wani is camptothecin, an alkaloid from the Chinese tree *Camptotheca*

acuminata Descne (46) that inhibits topoisomerase I. Irinotecan and topotecan as semisynthetic derivatives of camptothecin, were introduced in the U.S. in 1996 for the treatment of lung, ovarian, and colorectal cancers.

Camptothecin   Irinotecan

Topotecan

Two other important natural product-derived drugs that are part of the cancer chemotherapeutic arsenal are etoposide and teniposide (47). *Podophyllum peltatum,* used for years as a folk remedy, is the source of podophyllin, a crude resin used topically to treat condylomata acuminata. Podophyllin contains, among other things, the lignin podophyllotoxin. Studies directed at preparing a water soluble derivative of podophyllotoxin ultimately led to the discovery of a minor, but very active, constituent of the podophyllin resin, 4'-desmethoxy-1-epipodophyllotoxin glucoside (48). The ability to produce this minor, naturally occurring compound by semisynthetic modification of the more abundant podophyllotoxin was a breakthrough that allowed the preparation and evaluation of a number of analogs, some of which had extraordinary activity. Two of these analogs, etoposide and teniposide were introduced as anticancer drugs in 1983 and 1992, respectively. These compounds act by a mechanism (inhibition of topoisomerase II) that is different from that of podophyllotoxin (spindle poison), illustrating that structural similarity alone is not always a reliable predictor of similar biological effect.

A growing number of potential new drugs are being discovered from marine sources. The marine natural products dolostatin 10 and bryostatin 1 are two of the leading drug candidates among marine natural products that have advanced to clinical trials. Dolostatin 10, isolated from a sea hare, inhibits microtubule assembly and binds to tubulin at the vinblastine site (49). Bryostatin 1 is a protein kinase C partial agonist and was isolated from a marine bryozoan (49,50). Intensive efforts are underway to identify ecologically friendly, cost-effective means of producing these potentially important new anticancer agents.

Podophyllotoxin   Etoposide   Teniposide

Another example of the importance of natural product drug discovery and development to advances in the chemotherapy of cancer is the growing body of evidence

Dolostatin 10   Bryostatin 1

that the retinoids, derived from vitamin A (retinol), may have potential utility in the treatment of cancer. Although several retinoids are already used clinically (e.g., all-trans-retinoic acid [tretinoin], 13-cis-retinoic acid [isotretinoin] for acne and the synthetic analog, etretinate for severe psoriasis), it has recently been recognized that these compounds (and others such as fenretinide) may have significant potential in cancer chemotherapy. Although each of these drugs suffers from significant side effects that diminish its utility, it has been shown that the retinoids exert both their therapeutic and adverse effects through activation of retinoid receptors, for which there are several subtypes (51,52). This data, when coupled with synthetic ac-

Etretinate

Retinol: X = CH₂OH; Y = H
Tretinoin: X = COOH; Y = H
Isotretinoin: X = H; Y = COOH
Fenretinide: X = CONH- (ρ-hydroxyphenyl); Y = H

cessibility, suggest that synthetic retinoids based on the naturally occurring prototypes may be prepared that are more selective for specific receptor subtypes, thus offering the hope of separating the beneficial effects from the undesirable effects.

Cholesterol-Lowering Agents [Hypolipidemics]

Some of the most exciting natural products discovered in recent years are the cholesterol-lowering agents derived from fungi. These drugs act by inhibition of 3-hydroxy-3-methylglutaryl coenzyme A reductase (HMG-CoA reductase), an enzyme critical in the biosynthesis of cholesterol. The first of the HMG-CoA reductase inhibitors were isolated from *Penicillium* species (53,54). Compactin, from *P. brevicompactin,* was first reported as an antifungal agent (54). With the recognition of the mechanism of action of compactin came a search for other naturally occurring HMG-CoA reductase inhibitors that led to the discovery of lovastatin, a secondary metabolite of the fungus *Aspergillus terreus* (55). Although lovastatin was introduced on the market in 1989, many studies were undertaken to prepare improved synthetic analogs and led to the development of simvastatin (launched 1991), pravastatin (1991), and fluvastatin (1993).

Compactin: R₁ = R₂ = H   Pravastatin   Fluvastatin
Lovastatin: R₁ = H; R₂ = CH₃
Simvastatin: R₁ = R₂ = CH₃

Immunomodulators

The immunomodulator, cyclosporin, was originally isolated from a soil fungus, *Trichoderma polysporum* (56). This compound was a major breakthrough for organ transplantation, since it suppressed immunological rejection of the transplanted organ. Tacrolimus (FK-506), a secondary metabolite of *Streptomyces tsukubaensis,* was approved in 1994 for use as an immunosuppressant in organ transplantation.

FUTURE OF NATURAL PRODUCTS AND DRUG DISCOVERY

The importance of natural products in the future of drug discovery is clear: novel biologically active natural products will continue to serve as lead compounds for drug development and as biochemical probes for the discovery of pharmacologic and biochemical processes. There are a number of exciting developments occurring

Tacrolimus
(FK 506)

in the general arena of drug discovery for which natural products will play a central or peripheral role. Perhaps the most rapidly developing and exciting of these is the use of combinatorial chemistry, wherein a molecular scaffold is substituted in a random manner with a wide variety of substituents (57). Innovation and creativity regarding the molecular scaffolds will be substantially enhanced with the discovery of relatively simple, small molecular weight bioactive natural products. While combinatorial chemistry alone may provide completely new lead compounds, beginning a combinatorial approach with a nucleus that is already known to possess exciting biological activity (i.e., a bioactive natural product) should facilitate lead optimization and increase the likelihood of creating interesting drug candidates through this approach. In a similar vein, the "mixing" of genetic information encoding for specific secondary metabolites can produce "unnatural" natural products. This approach (combinatorial biosynthesis) has been used to produce, by biosynthetic manipulation, "hybrid" antibiotics possessing desirable properties of different naturally occurring compounds (58).

Finally, the use of bioactive natural products to probe the molecular and pharmacological processes of living organisms will continue with even greater sophistication, owing to the major advances being made in molecular biology. By coupling the technological capabilities to explore the inner workings of cells that molecular biology offers with the creativity and innovation of nature, in the form of a seemingly infinite supply of natural compounds with biological and chemical diversity, the future of natural product drug discovery is more promising than ever before. Clearly, the natural products discovered to date have played a vital role in improving the human condition, and this role will continue as long as there are unexplored sources of novel natural products.

REFERENCES

1. Soejarto DD. Biodiversity prospecting and benefit-sharing: perspectives from the field. J Ethnopharmacol 1996;51:1–15.
2. Claeson P, Bohlin L. Some aspects of bioassay methods in natural-product research aimed at drug lead discovery. Trends Biotech 1997;15:245–248.
3. Hutchinson CR. Drug Synthesis by Genetically Engineered Microorganisms. Biotechnology 1994;12:375–380.
4. Michels PC, Khmelnitsky YL, Dordick JS, et al. Combinatorial biocatalysis: a natural approach to drug discovery. Trends Biotech 1998;16:210–215.
5. Doernenburg H, Knoor D. Strategies for the improvement of secondary metabolite production in plant cell culture. Enzyme Microb Technol 1995;17:674–84.
6. Baker JT, Borris RP, Carte B, et al. Natural product drug discovery and development: new perspectives on international collaboration. J Nat Prod 1995; 58:1325–1357.
7. Elisabetsky E, Costa-Campos L. Medicinal Plant Genetic Resources and International Cooperation: the Brazilian Perspective. J Ethnopharmacol 1996;51:111–120.
8. Turner DM. Natural product source material use in the pharmaceutical industry: the Glaxo experience. J Ethnopharmacol 1996;51:39–44.
9. Boyd MR. The position of intellectual property rights in drug discovery and development from natural products. J Ethnopharmacol 1996;51:17–27.
10. Borris RP. Natural products research: perspectives from a major pharmaceutical company. J Ethnopharmacol 1996;51: 29–38.
11. Finn RD, Jones CG. Avenues of discovery in biopropsecting. Nature 1998;393:617.
12. Finn RD, Jones CG. In Romeo JT. et al., eds. Recent Advances in Phytochemistry. Plenum Press, 1996:295–312.
13. Spande TF, Hugo MG, Edwards MW, et al. Epibatidine: A novel (chloropyridyl)azabicycloheptane with potent analgesic activity from an Ecuadoran poison frog. J Am Chem Soc 1992;114: 3475–3478.
14. Daly JW. Thirty years of discovering arthropod alkaloids in amphibian skin. J Nat Prod 1996;61:162–172.
15. Oliviera BM, Hillyard DR, Marsh M, et al. Combinatorial peptide libraries in drug design: lessons from venomous cone snails. Trends Biotechnol 1995;13:422–426.
16. Cragg GM, Newman DJ, Weiss RB. Coral reefs, forests, and thermal vents: the worldwide exploration of nature for novel antitumor agents. Sem Oncol 1997;24:156–163.
17. Fenical W. New pharmaceuticals from marine organisms. Trends Biotech. 1997;15:339–341.
18. Cannell RJP. In Cannell RJP, ed. Natural products isolation. Totowa, NJ: Humana Press, 1998;1–51.
19. Duke SO, Canel C, Rimando AM, et al. Current and Potential Exploitation of Plant Glandular Trichome Productivity. In Advances in Botanical Research. New York: Academic Press, 2000; 31:37–67.
20. van Middlesworth F, Cannell RJP. Dereplication and Partial Identification of Natural Products. In Cannell RJP, ed. Natural Products Isolation. Totowa, New Jersey: Humana Press, 1998;279–327.
21. Clark AM. Natural products as a resource for new drugs. Pharm Res 1996;13:1133–1141.
22. Shu Y-Z. Recent Natural Products Based Drug Development: a pharmaceutical industry perspective. J Nat Prod 1998;61: 1053–1071.
23. Robbers JE, Speedie MK, Tyler VE, Pharmacognosy, 10th ed. Philadelphia: Lea & Febiger, 1996.
24. Ferreira SH. A bradykinin-potentiating factor (BPF) present in the venom of Bothrops jararaca. Brit J Pharmacol 1965;24: 163–169.
25. Ferreira SH, Greene LJ, Alabaster VA, et al. Activity of various fractions of bradykinin potentiating factor against angiotensin I converting eznyme. Nature 1970;225:379–380.
26. Ferreira SH, Bartelt DC, Greene LJ. Isolation of bradykinin-potentiating peptides from Bothrops jararaca. Biochem 1970;9: 2583–2593.

27. Jackson EK, Garrison JC. Renin and angiotensin. In Hardman JG, Limbird LE, Molinoff PB, et al, eds. The pharmacological basis of therapeutics. New York: McGraw-Hill, 1996;9: 733–758.

28. Cheng X-M. To market, to market 1993. In JA Bristol, ed. Annual Reports in Medicinal Chemistry. San Diego: Academic Press, 1994;29: 331–354.

29. Barlow RB, Ing HR. Curare-like action of polymethylene bisquaternary ammonium salts. Br J Pharmacol Chemother 1948; 3:298.

30. Hardeman JG, Limbird LE. Molinoff PB, et al, eds. The pharmacological basis of therapeutics, 9th ed. New York: McGraw-Hill, 1996.

31. McDonald IA, Cosford N, Vernier J-M. Nicotinic acetylcholine receptors: molecular biology, chemistry and pharmacology. In Bristol JA, ed. Annual reports in medicinal chemistry. New York: Academic Press, 1995;30:41–50.

32. Hieble JP, Ruffolo RR. Pharmacology of neuromuscular transmission. In Munson PL, Mueller RA, Breese GR, eds. Principles of pharmacology: basic concepts & clinical applications. New York: Chapman & Hall, 1995;145–159,1734.

33. Berdy J, ed. CRC Handbook of antibiotic compounds. Boca Raton: CRC Press, 1980.

34. Trigg PI. In Wagner H, Hikino H, Farnsworth NR, eds. Economic and medicinal plant research. London: Academic Press, 1989;3:19–55.

35. Wu Y-L, Li Y. Study on the chemistry of qinghaosu (artemisinin). Med Chem Res 1995;5:569–586.

36. Lee I-S, Hufford CD. Metabolism of antimalarial sesquiterpene lactones. Pharmac Ther 1990;48:345–355.

37. Davies, HG, Green RH. Avermectins and milbemycins. Nat Prod Repts 1986;3:87–121.

38. Awadzi K, Dadzie KY, Schulz-Key H, et al. The chemotherapy of onchocerciasis X. An assessment of four single dose treatment regimes of MK-933 (ivermectin) in human onchocerciasis. Ann Trop Med Parasitol 1985;79:63.

39. Greene BM, Taylor HR, Cupp EW, et al. Comparison of ivermectin and diethylcarbamazine in the treatment of onchocerciasis. New Engl J Med 1985;313:133–138.

40. Bradley SG, Marciano-Cabral F. Antiparasitic drugs. In Munson PL, Mueller RA, and Breese GR, eds. Principles of pharmacology: basic concepts & clinical applications. New York: Chapman & Hall, 1995;1437–1473.

41. Loo TL, Freireich EJ. Cancer chemotherapeutic drugs. In Munson PL, Mueller RA, Breese GR, eds., Principles of pharmacology: basic concepts & clinical applications. New York: Chapman & Hall, 1995;1475–1516.

42. Wall ME, Wani MC. Camptothecin and taxol: Discovery to clinic—Thirteenth Bruce F. Cain Memorial Award Lecture. Cancer Res 1995;55:753–760.

43. Schiff PB, Fant F, Horwitz SB. Promotion of microtubule assembly in vitro by taxol. Nature 1979;277:665–667.

44. Bollag DM, McQueney PA, Zhu J, et al. Epothilones, a new class of microtubule-stabilizing agents with taxol-like mechanism of action. Cancer Res 1995;55:2325–2333.

45. ter Haar E, Kowalski RJ, Hamel E, et al. Discodermolide, a cytotoxic marine agent that stabilizes microtubules more potently than taxol. Biochem 1996;35:243–250.

46. Wall ME, Wani MC, Cooke CE, et al. Plant antitumor agents. I. The isolation and structure of camptothecin, a novel alkaloidal leukemia and tumor inhibitor from Camptotheca acuminata. J Am Chem Soc 1966;88:388.

47. Stahelin H, von Wartburg A. The chemical and biological route from podophyllotoxin glucoside to etoposide: Ninth Bruce F. Cain Memorial Award Lecture. Cancer Research 1991;51:5–15.

48. Stahelin H, von Wartburg A. From podophyllotoxin glucoside to etoposide. In Jucker E, ed. Progress in drug research. Basel: Birkhauser-Verlag, 1989;33:169–266.

49. Pettit GR. Progress in the discovery of biosynthetic anticancer drugs. J Nat Prod 1996;59:812–821.

50. Pettit GR, Herald CL, Doubek DL, et al. Isolation and structure of bryostatin 1. J Am Chem Soc 1982;104:6846–6848.

51. Heyman RA, Mangelsdorf DJ, Dyck JA, et al. 9-cis retinoic acid is a high affinity ligand for the retinoid X receptor. Cell 1992; 68:397–406.

52. Allegretto EA, McClurg MR, Lazarchik SB, et al. Transactivation properties of retinoic acid and retinoid X receptors in mammalian cells and yeast. J Biol Chem 1993;268:26625–26633.

53. Gordon DJ, Rifkind BM. 3-Hydroxy-3-methylglutaryl coenzyme a (HMG-CoA) reductase inhibitors: a new class of cholesterol-lowering agents. Ann Int Med 1987;107:759–761.

54. Brown AG, Smale TC, King TJ, et al. Crystal and molecular structure of compactin, a new antifungal metabolite from Penicillium brevicompactum. J Chem Soc, Perkin Trans I 1976;1165–1170.

55. Alberts AW, Chen J, Kuron G, et al. A highly potent competitive inhibitor of hydroxymethylglutaryl-coenzyme A reductase and a cholesterol-lowering agent. Proc Natl Acad Sci USA 1980;77:3957–3961.

56. Ruegger A, Kuhn M, Lichti H, et al. Cyclosporin A, ein immunsuppressiv wirksamer Peptidmetabolit aus Trichoderma polysporum (Link ex Pers.) Rifai. Helv Chim Acta 1976;59:1075–1092.

57. Baum R. Combinatorial chemistry. Chem Eng News 1996;74:28.

58. Katz L, Donadio S. Polyketide synthesis: prospects for hybrid antibiotics. Annu Rev Microbiol 1993;47:875–912.

2. Drug Design and Relationship of Functional Groups to Pharmacologic Activity

JAMES KNITTEL AND ROBIN ZAVOD

Medicinal chemistry is the discipline concerned with determining the influence of chemical structure on biological activity. As such, it is therefore necessary for the medicinal chemist to understand not only the mechanism by which a drug exerts its effect, but also the physicochemical properties of the molecule. The term "physicochemical properties" refers to the influence of the organic functional groups present within a molecule on its acid/base properties, water solubility, partition coefficient, crystal structure, stereochemistry etc. All of these properties influence the absorption, distribution, metabolism and excretion (ADME) of the molecule. In order to design better medicinal agents the medicinal chemist needs to understand the relative contributions that each functional group makes to the overall physical chemical properties of the molecule. Studies of this type involve modification of the molecule in a systematic fashion and determination of how these changes affect biological activity. Such studies are referred to as studies of structure-activity relationships i.e., what structural features of the molecule contribute to, or take away from, the desired biological activity of the molecule of interest.

Because of the fundamental nature of its subject matter, this chapter includes numerous case studies throughout (as boxes) and at the end. In addition, a list of study questions at the end of—and unique to—this chapter provides further self-study material on the subject of drug design.

INTRODUCTION

Chemical compounds, usually derived from plants, have been used by humans for thousands of years to alleviate pain, diarrhea, infection and various other maladies. Until the 19th century these "remedies" were primarily crude preparations of plant material whose constituents were unknown and the nature of the active principal (if any) was also unknown. The revolution in synthetic organic chemistry during the 19th century produced a concerted effort toward identification of the structures of the active constituents of these naturally derived medicinals and synthesis of what were hoped to be more efficacious agents. By determining the molecular structures of the active components of these complex mixtures it was thought that a better understanding of how these components worked could be elucidated.

Relationship Between Molecular Structure and Biologic Activity

Early studies of the relationship between chemical structure and biologic activity were conducted by Crum-Brown and Fraser (1) in 1869. They showed that many compounds containing tertiary amine groups became muscle relaxants when converted to quaternary ammonium compounds. Compounds with widely differing pharmacological properties such as, strychnine (a convulsant), morphine (an analgesic), nicotine (deterrent, insecticide), and atropine (anticholinergic), all could be converted to muscle relaxants with properties similar to tubocurarine when methylated (Fig. 2.1). Crum-Brown and Fraser therefore concluded that muscle relaxant activity required a quaternary ammonium group within the chemical structure. This initial hypothesis was later disproven by the discovery of the natural neurotransmitter and activator of muscle contraction, acetylcholine (Fig. 2.2). Even though Crum-Brown and Fraser's initial hypothesis concerning chemical structure and muscle relaxation was proven to be incorrect, it demonstrated the concept that molecular structure does influence the biological activity of chemical compounds.

With the discovery by Crum-Brown and Fraser that quaternary ammonium groups could produce compounds with muscle relaxant properties scientists began looking

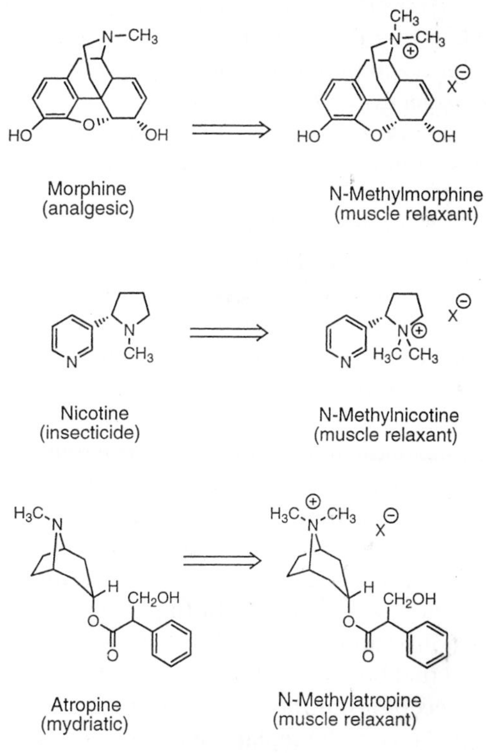

Morphine (analgesic) → N-Methylmorphine (muscle relaxant)

Nicotine (insecticide) → N-Methylnicotine (muscle relaxant)

Atropine (mydriatic) → N-Methylatropine (muscle relaxant)

Fig. 2.1. Effects of methylation on biologic activity.

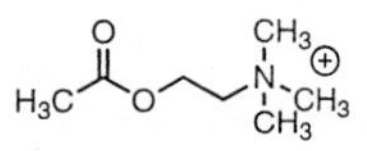

Fig. 2.2. Acetylcholine, a neurotransmitter and muscle relaxant.

for other organic functional groups that would produce specific biologic responses. The thinking at this period of time was that specific chemical groups, or nuclei (rings), were responsible for specific biologic effects. This lead to the postulate, which took some time to disprove, that "one chemical group gives one biological action." (2) Even after the discovery of acetylcholine by Loewi and Navrati (3) which effectively dispensed with Crum-Brown and Fraser's concept of all quaternary ammonium compounds being muscle relaxants, this was still considered dogma and took a long time to replace.

Selectivity of Drug Action and Drug Receptors

Though the structures of many drugs or xenobiotics were known at the turn of the century, or at least the composition of functional groups, it was still a mystery as to how these compounds exerted their effects. Utilizing his observations regarding the staining behavior of microorganisms, Ehrlich developed the concept of drug receptors (4). He postulated that certain "side chains" on the surfaces of cells were "complementary" to the dyes (or drug), thereby allowing the two substances to combine. In the case of antimicrobial compounds, this combining of the chemical to the "side chains" produced a toxic effect. This concept effectively was the first description of what later became know as the receptor hypothesis for explaining the biological action of chemical compounds. Ehrlich also discussed selectivity of drug action via the concept of a "magic bullet" for compounds that would eradicate disease states without producing undue harm to the organism being treated (i.e., the patient). This concept was later modified by Albert (5) and is generally referred to as "selective toxicity." Utilizing this concept Ehrlich developed organic arsenicals that were toxic to trypanosomes as a result of their irreversible reaction with mercapto groups present on vital proteins within the organism. The formation of As-S bonds resulted in death to the target organism. However, it was soon learned that these compounds were not only toxic to the target organism, but also to the host once certain blood levels of arsenic were achieved.

The "paradox" that resulted after the discovery of acetylcholine of how one chemical group can produce two different biologic effects, i.e., muscle relaxation and muscle contraction, was explained by Ing (6) using the actions of acetylcholine and tubocurarine as his examples. Ing hypothesized that both acetylcholine and tubocurarine act at the same receptor but that one molecule fits to the receptor in a more complementary manner and "activates" it, causing muscle contraction. Just how this activation occurs

was not elaborated upon. The larger molecule, tubocurarine, simple occupies part of the receptor and prevents acetylcholine, the smaller molecule, from occupying the receptor. With both molecules the quaternary ammonium functional group is a common structural feature and interacts with the same region of the receptor. If one closely examines the structures of other compounds that have opposing effects on the same pharmacologic system, this appears to be a common theme: Molecules that block the effects of natural neurotransmitters (antagonists) are generally larger in size than the native compound. Both compounds share common structural features, however, thus providing support to the concept that the structure of a molecule, its composition and arrangement of chemical functional groups, determines the type of pharmacologic effect that it possesses (i.e., structure-activity relationship). Thus, compounds that are muscle relaxants acting via the cholinergic nervous system will possess a quaternary ammonium or protonated tertiary ammonium group and will be larger than acetylcholine. Structure-activity relationships (SARs) are the underlying principle of medicinal chemistry. Similar molecules exert similar biological actions in a qualitative sense. A corollary to this is that structural elements (functional groups) within a molecule most often contribute in an additive manner to the physicochemical properties of a molecule and therefore its biological action. One need only peruse the structures of drug molecules in a particular pharmacologic class to become convinced of this (e.g., histamine H_1 antagonists; histamine H_2 antagonists; β-adrenergic antagonists; etc.). The objective of the medicinal chemist in his/her quest for better medicinal agents (drugs) is to discover what functional groups within a specific structure are important for its pharmacologic activity, and how can these groups be modified to produce more potent, selective and safer compounds.

An example of how different functional groups can yield compounds with similar physicochemical properties is shown with sulfanilamide antibiotics. In Figure 2.3 the structures of sulfanilamide and p-aminobenzoic acid (PABA) are shown. In 1940, Woods (7) demonstrated that PABA was capable of reversing the antibacterial action of sulfanilamide (and other sulfonamides antibacterials) and that both PABA and sulfanilamide had similar steric and electronic properties. Both compounds contain acidic func-

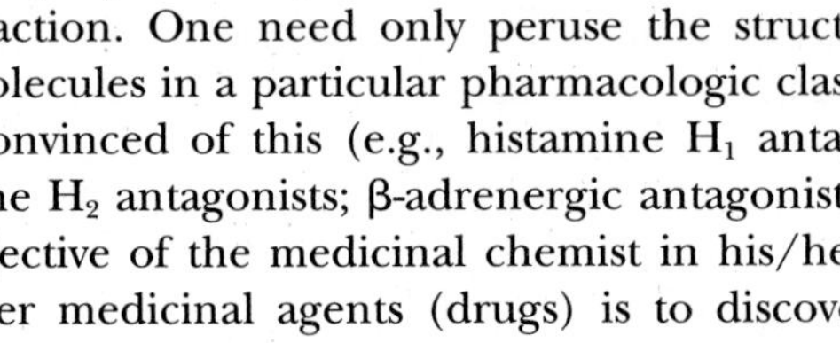

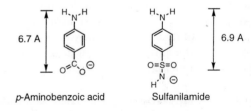

p-Aminobenzoic acid   Sulfanilamide

Fig. 2.3. Ionized forms of PABA and sulfanilamide. Comparison of distance between amine and ionized acids of each compound. Note how closely sulfanilamide resembles PABA.

tional groups with PABA containing an aromatic carboxylic acid and sulfanilamide an aromatic sulfonamide. When ionized at physiological pH both compounds have a similar electronic configuration and the distance between the ionized acid and the weakly basic amino group is also very similar. It should therefore be no surprise that sulfanilamide acts as an antagonist to PABA metabolism in bacteria.

PHYSICOCHEMICAL PROPERTIES OF DRUGS
Acid/Base Properties

The human body is composed of 70–75% water, which amounts to approximately 55 liters of water for a 160 lb (55 kg) individual. For an average drug molecule with a molecular weight of 200 g/mol and a dose of 20 mg this leads to a concentration of $\sim 2 \times 10^{-6}$ M solution. When considering the solution behavior of a drug within the body we are therefore dealing with a dilute solution. For dilute solutions the Brönsted-Lowry (8) acid/base theory is most appropriate for explaining and predicting acid/base behavior. This is a very important concept in medicinal chemistry since the acid/base properties of drug molecules directly affect absorption, excretion and compatibility with other drugs in solution. According to the Brönsted-Lowry Theory an acid is any substance capable of yielding a proton (H^+) and a base is any substance capable of accepting a proton. When an acid gives up a proton to a base it is converted to its *conjugate base*. Similarly, when a base accepts a proton it is converted to its *conjugate acid* form (Equations 2.1 and 2.2).

$$\text{Eq. 2.1} \quad \underset{\substack{\text{Acid} \\ \text{(acetic acid)}}}{CH_3COOH} + \underset{\substack{\text{Base} \\ \text{(water)}}}{H_2O} \rightleftharpoons \underset{\substack{\text{Conjugate} \\ \text{base} \\ \text{(acetate)}}}{CH_3COO^\ominus} + \underset{\substack{\text{Conjugate} \\ \text{acid} \\ \text{(hydronium)}}}{H_3O^\oplus}$$

$$\text{Eq. 2.2} \quad \underset{\substack{\text{Base} \\ \text{(methylamine)}}}{CH_3NH_2} + \underset{\substack{\text{Acid} \\ \text{(water)}}}{H_2O} \rightleftharpoons \underset{\substack{\text{Conjugate} \\ \text{Acid} \\ \text{(methylammonium)}}}{CH_3NH_3^\oplus} + \underset{\substack{\text{Conjugate} \\ \text{base} \\ \text{(hydroxide)}}}{^\ominus OH}$$

Note that when an acid loses its proton it is left with an extra pair of electrons that are no longer neutralized by the proton. This is the *ionized* form of the acid and is now very water soluble due to the charge. Since the acid has lost its proton it is often also referred to as having undergone dissociation. There are many different organic functional groups that behave as acids and these are listed in Table 2.1. It is important that the student learn to recognize these functional groups and their relative acid strengths. This will help the student to predict absorption, distribution, excretion and potential incompatibilities between drugs.

When a base is converted to its conjugate acid form it too becomes ionized. However, in this instance it becomes positively charged due to the presence of the extra proton. Most basic drugs are usually derived from primary, secondary and tertiary amines. Other organic functional groups that act as bases are shown in Table 2.2. Again the

student should familiarize himself with these functional groups and be able to readily recognize them by name and relative strengths.

Organic functional groups that are neither capable of giving up a proton, nor accepting a proton are considered to be neutral (or nonelectrolytes) with respect to their acid/base properties. Common functional groups of this type are shown in Table 2.3. In the case of quaternary ammonium compounds the molecule is not electrically neutral even though it is neither acidic nor basic. Additional reading on the acid/base behavior of the functional groups listed in Tables 2.1–2.3 can be found in Remington (9) and Lemke (10).

A molecule may contain multiple functional groups and therefore possess both acid and base properties. For example, ciprofloxacin (Fig. 2.4) a quinolone antibiotic, contains a secondary alkyl amine and a carboxylic acid. Depending upon the pH of the solution (or tissue) this molecule will either accept a proton, yield a proton or both. Thus it can be a base, acid or amphoteric (both acid and base) in its properties. Figure 2.5 shows the acid/base behavior of ciprofloxacin at two different locations of the gastro-intestinal tract. Note that at a given pH value (e.g., pH of 1.0–3.5) only one of the functional groups (the alkylamine) is ionized. In order to be able to make this prediction one has to understand the relative acid/base strength of acids and bases. Thus, one needs to be able to know which acid or base within a molecule containing multiple functional groups is the strongest and which is the weakest. The concept of pK_a not only indicates the relative acid/base strength of organic functional groups, but it also allows one to calculate, for a given pH, exactly how much of the molecule is in the ionized and unionized form.

Relative Acid Strength (pK_a)

Strong acids and bases completely dissociate or accept a proton in aqueous solution to produce their respective conjugate bases and acids. For example, mineral acids such as HCl or bases such as NaOH undergo complete dissociation in water with the equilibrium shifted completely to the right side as shown in equations 2.3 and 2.4:

$$\text{Eq. 2.3} \quad HCl + H_2O \longrightarrow Cl^\ominus + H_3O^\oplus$$

$$\text{Eq. 2.4} \quad NaOH + H_2O \longrightarrow Na^\oplus + OH^\ominus + H_2O$$

However, acids and bases of intermediate or weak strength incompletely dissociate or accept a proton and the equilibrium lies somewhere in between. The equilibrium is such that all possible species may exist. Note that in equations 2.3 and 2.4 water is acting as a base in one instance and as an acid in the other. Water is amphoteric, it may act as an acid or a base depending upon the conditions. Because we are always dealing with a dilute aqueous solution the strongest base that can be present is OH^- and the strongest acid H_3O^+. This is known as the leveling ef-

Table 2.1. Common Acidic Organic Functional Groups and Their Ionized (Conjugate Base) Forms

Acids	pKa			Conjugate Base
Phenol	9–11			Phenolate
Sulfonamide	9–10			Sulfonamidate
Imide	9–10			Imidate
Alkylthiol	10–11	R—SH	R—S$^{\ominus}$	Thiolate
Thiophenol	9–10			Thiophenolate
N-Arylsulfonamide	6–7			N-Arylsulfonamidate
Sulfonimide	5–6			Sulfonimidate
Alkylcarboxylic acid	5–6			Alkylcarboxylate
Arylcarboxylic acid	4–5			Arylcarboxylate
Sulfonic acid	0–1			Sulfonate

Acid strength usually increases as one moves down the table.

Table 2.2. Common Basic Organic Functional Groups and Their Ionized (Conjugate Acid) Forms

Base	pKa			Conjugate Acid
Arylamine	4–5			Arylammonium
Aromatic amine	5–6			Aromatic ammonium
Imine	3–4			Iminium
Alkylamines	10–11 / 9–10			Alkylammonium
Amidine	10–11			Amidinium
Guanidine	10–11			Guanidinium

Table 2.3. Common Organic Functional Groups That Are Considered Neutral Under Physiologic Conditions

R–CH₂–OH	Ether	Ester	Sulfonic acid ester
Alkyl alcohol			
Amide	Diarylamine	Nitrile	Quaternary ammonium
Amine oxide	Ketone & Aldehyde	Thioether	Sulfoxide Sulfone

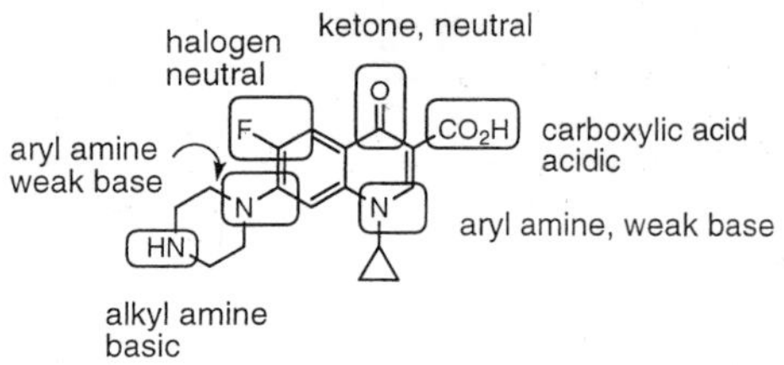

Fig. 2.4. Chemical structure of ciprofloxacin showing the various organic functional groups.

Stomach (pH 1.0 – 3.5)   Duodenum (pH ~4)

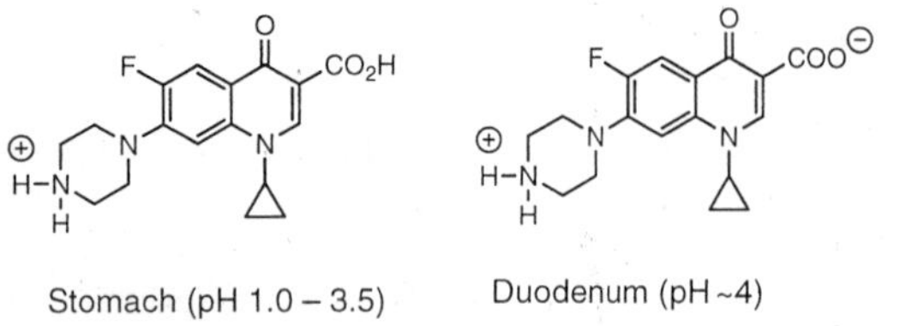

Fig. 2.5. Predominate forms of ciprofloxacin at two different locations within the gastrointestinal tract.

fect of water. Thus, some organic functional groups that are considered acids or bases with respect to their chemical reactivity do not behave as such under physiological conditions in aqueous solution. For example, alkyl alcohols such as ethyl alcohol, are not sufficiently acidic to undergo ionization to a significant extent in aqueous solution. Water is not sufficiently basic to remove the proton from the alcohol to form the ethoxide ion (Equation 2.5).

Eq. 2.5 $CH_3CH_2OH + H_2O \rightleftharpoons CH_3CH_2O + H_3O^{\oplus}$

Predicting the Degree of Ionization of a Molecule

From general principles it is possible to predict if a molecule is going to be ionized or unionized at a given pH simply by knowing if the functional groups present on the molecule are acid or basic. However, in order to be able to quantitatively predict the degree of ionization of a molecule one must know the pK_a values of the acid and basic functional groups present and the pH of the environment to which the compound will be exposed. The Henderson-Hassalbach equation (Equation 2.6) can be used to calculate the percent ionization of a compound at a given pH. This equation was used to calculate the major forms of ciprofloxacin in Figure 2.5.

Eq. 2.6 $pK_a = pH + \log \dfrac{[\text{acid form}]}{[\text{base form}]}$

The key to understanding the use of the Henderson-Hassalbach equation for calculating percent ionization is to realize that this equation relates a constant, pK_a, to the ratio of acid form to base form of the drug. Since pK_a is a constant for any given molecule, then the ratio of acid to base will determine the pH of the solution. Conversely, a given pH determines the ratio of acid to base. A sample calculation is shown in Figure 2.6 for the sedative hypnotic amobarbital.

When dealing with a base, the student must recognize that the conjugate acid form is the ionized form of the drug. Thus, as one should expect, a base behaves in a manner opposite to that of an acid. Figure 2.7 shows the calculated percent ionization for the decongestant

---

Absorption/Acid-Base Case

A long distance truck driver comes into the pharmacy complaining of seasonal allergies. He asks you to recommend an agent that will act as an antihistamine, but will not cause drowsiness. He regularly takes TUMs for indigestion because of the bad food that he eats while he is on the road.

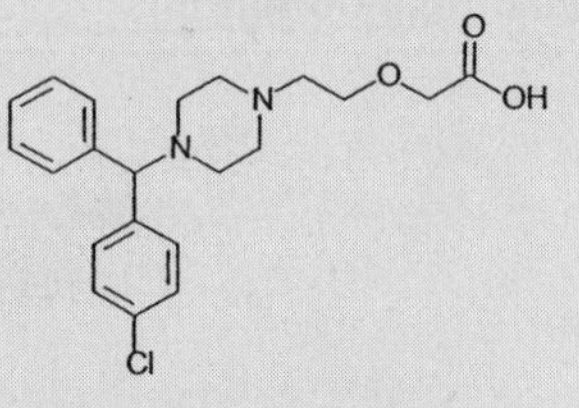

Cetirizine (Zyrtec) 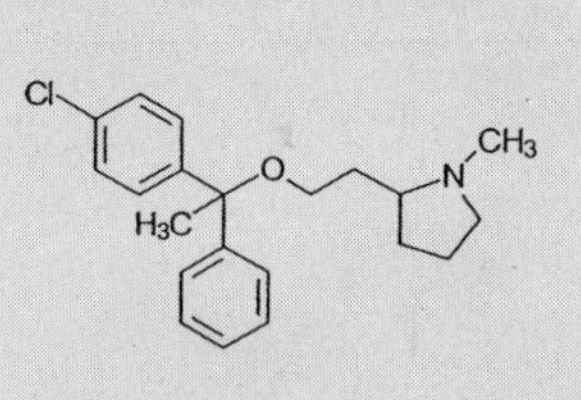   Clemastine (Tavist) 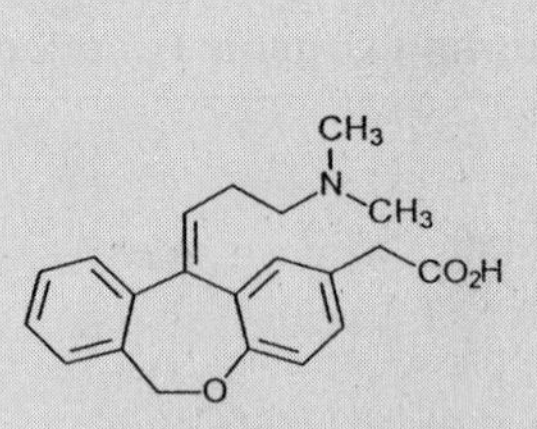   Olopatadine (Patanol)

1. Identify the functional groups present in Zyrtec and Tavist and evaluate the effect of each functional group on the ability of the drug to cross lipophilic membranes (e.g., blood brain barrier). Based on your assessment of each agent's ability to cross the blood brain barrier (and therefore potentially cause drowsiness), provide a rationale for whether the truck driver should be taking Zyrtec, or Tavist.
2. Patanol is sold as an aqueous solution of the hydrochloride salt. Modify the structure above to show the appropriate salt form of this agent. This agent is applied to the eye to relieve itching associated with allergies. Describe why this agent is soluble in water and what properties make it able to be absorbed into the membranes that surround the eye.
3. Consider the structural features of Zyrtec and Tavist. In which compartment will each of these two drugs be best absorbed? (stomach, pH = 1 or intestine, pH = 7.5).
4. TUMs neutralizes stomach acid (pH of stomach = 3.5). Based on your answer to question #3, determine whether the truck driver will get the full antihistaminergic effect if he takes his antihistamine at the same time as he takes his TUMs. Provide a rationale for your answer.

Acid Base Chemistry/Compatibility Cases

The IV technician in the hospital pharmacy gets an order for a patient that includes the two drugs drawn below. She is unsure if she can mix the two drugs together in the same IV bag and isn't sure how water-soluble either of the agents are.

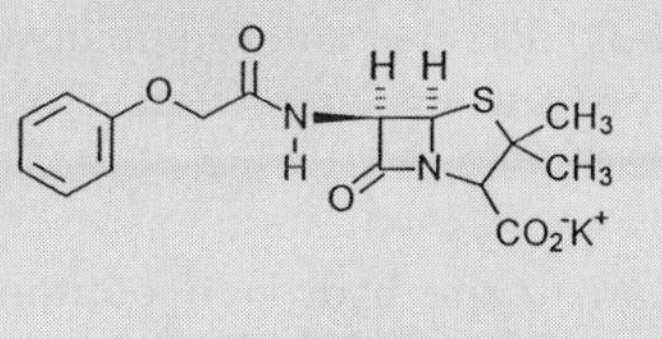

Penicillin V Potassium

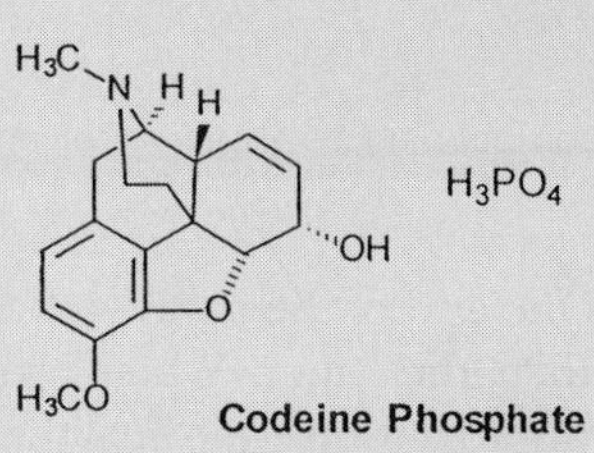

Codeine Phosphate

1. Penicillin V potassium is drawn in its salt form, whereas codeine phosphate is not. Modify the structure above to show the salt form of codeine phosphate. Determine the acid/base character of the functional groups in the two molecules drawn above, as well as the salt form of codeine phosphate.
2. As originally drawn above, which of these two agents is more water-soluble? Provide a rationale for your selection that includes appropriate structural properties. Is the salt form of codeine phosphate more or less water soluble than the free base form of the drug? Provide a rationale for your answer based on the structural properties of the salt form of codeine phosphate.
3. What is the chemical consequence of mixing aqueous solutions of each drug in the same IV bag? Provide a rationale that includes an acid/base assessment.

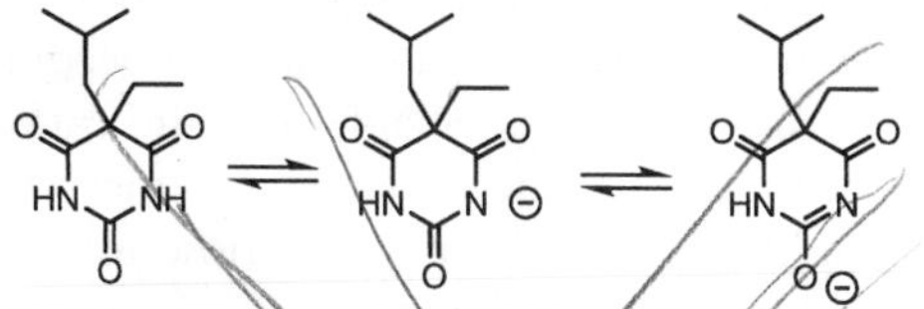

Acid form
pK$_a$ 8.0   Conjugate base

Question: At a pH of 7.4, what is the percent ionization of amobarbital?

Answer: $7.4 = 8.0 + \log \frac{[\text{acid}]}{[\text{base}]}$

$-0.6 = \log \frac{[\text{acid}]}{[\text{base}]}$

$10^{-0.6} = \frac{[\text{acid}]}{[\text{base}]} = \frac{0.25}{1}$

% acid form $= \frac{0.25 \times 100}{1.25} = 20\%$

Fig. 2.6. Calculation of % ionization of amobarbital. Calculation indicates that 20% of the molecules are in the acid (or protonated) form, leaving 80% in the conjugate base (ionized) form.

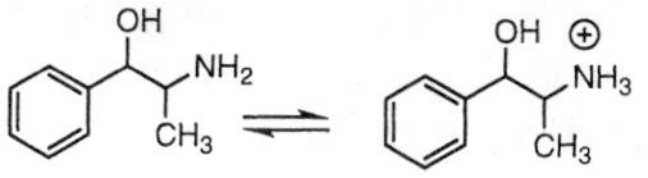

Base form   Conjugate acid form
pK$_a$ 9.4

Question: What is the percent ionization of phenylpropanolamine at pH 7.4?

Answer: $9.4 = 7.4 + \log \frac{[\text{acid}]}{[\text{base}]}$

$2.0 = \log \frac{[\text{acid}]}{[\text{base}]}$

$10^2 = \frac{[\text{acid}]}{[\text{base}]} = \frac{100}{1}$

% acid form $= \frac{100}{101} \times 100 = 99\%$

Fig. 2.7. Calculation of % ionization of phenylpropanolamine. Calculation indicates that 99% of the molecules are in the acid form which is the same as % ionization.

phenylpropanolamine. It is very important to recognize that for a base, the pK$_a$ refers to the conjugate acid or ionized form of the compound. To thoroughly comprehend this relationship, the student should calculate the percent ionization of an acid and a base at different pH values.

Water Solubility of Drugs

The solubility of a drug molecule in water greatly affects the routes of administration available and its absorption, distribution and elimination. Two key concepts to keep in mind when considering the water (or fat) solubility of a molecule are the hydrogen bond forming potential of the functional groups present in the molecule and the ionization of functional groups.

Hydrogen Bonds

Each functional group capable of donating or accepting a hydrogen bond will contribute to the overall water solubility of the compound. Hence, such functional groups will increase the hydrophilic (water loving) nature of the molecule. Conversely, functional groups that cannot form hydrogen bonds will not enhance hydrophilicity, and will actually contribute to the hydrophobicity (water hating) of the molecule. Hydrogen bonds are a special case of what are generally referred to as dipole-dipole bonds. Dipoles result from unequal sharing of electrons between atoms within a covalent bond. This unequal sharing of electrons results when two atoms involved in a covalent bond have significantly different electronegativities. As a result, partial ionic character develops between the two atoms, produc-

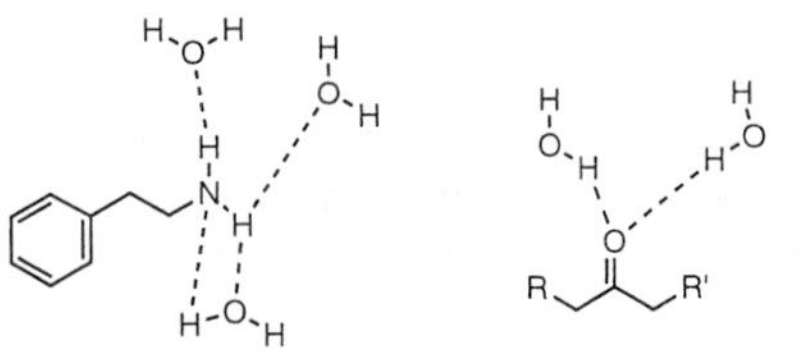

Fig. 2.8. Examples of hydrogen bonding between water and hypothetical drug molecules.

ing a permanent dipole: One end of the covalent bond has higher electron density than the other. When two molecules containing dipoles approach one another they align such that the negative end of one dipole is electrostatically attracted to the positive end of the other. When the positive end of the dipole is a hydrogen atom, this interaction is referred to as a *hydrogen bond* (or H-bond). Thus, for a hydrogen bond to occur at least one dipole must contain an electropositive hydrogen. The hydrogen atom must be involved in a covalent bond with an electronegative atom such as oxygen (O), nitrogen (N), sulfur (S) or selenium (Se). Of these four elements only O and N contribute significantly to the dipole and we will therefore only concern ourselves with the hydrogen bonding capability of OH and NH groups. This is only in reference to functional groups that "donate" hydrogen bonds.

Even though the energy involved for each hydrogen bond is small, 1–10 kcal/mol/bond, it is the additive nature of multiple hydrogen bonds that contributes to water solubility. We will see in Chapter 4 that this same bonding interaction is also important in drug-receptor interactions. Figure 2.8 shows several possible hydrogen bond types that may occur with different organic functional groups and water. As a general rule, the more hydrogen bonds that are possible,

Table 2.4. Common Organic Functional Groups and Their Hydrogen-Bonding Potential

Functional Groups	Number of Potential H-bonds
R—OH	3
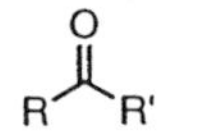 R—C(=O)—R'	2
R—NH$_2$	3
R—NH—R'	2
R—N(R')—R"	1
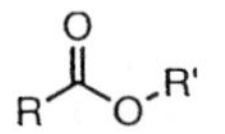 R—C(=O)—O—R'	2

the greater the water solubility of the molecule. Table 2.4 lists several common organic functional groups and the number of potential hydrogen bonds for each. This table does not take into account the possibility of *intramolecular* hydrogen bonds that could form. Each intramolecular hydrogen bond would decrease water solubility (and increase lipid solubility) since one less interaction with solvent occurs.

Ionization

In addition to the hydrogen bonding capability of a molecule, another type of bonding interaction plays an important role in determining water solubility: Ion-Dipole bonding. This type of bonding comes into play when one deals with organic salts. Ion-dipole bonds develop between either a cation or anion and a formal dipole such as water. A cation, having a deficiency in electron density, will be attracted to regions of high electron density. When dealing with water, this would be the two lone pairs of electrons associated with the oxygen atom. An anion will associate with regions of low electron density or the positive end of the dipole. In the case of water as solvent, this would be the hydrogen atoms (Fig. 2.9).

Not all organic salts are necessarily very water soluble. In order to associate with enough water molecules to become soluble, the salt must be highly dissociable; i.e., the cation and anion must be able to separate and each interact with water molecules. Highly dissociable salts are those formed from strong acids with strong bases, weak acids with strong bases and strong acids with weak bases. Strong acids are hydrochloric, sulfuric, nitric, perchloric and phosphoric acid. All other acids are considered to be weak. Sodium hydroxide and potassium hydroxide are considered to be strong bases, with all other bases classified as weak. Thus the salt of a carboxylic acid and alkylamine is a salt of a weak acid and weak base respectively, and therefore does not dissociate appreciable. This salt would not be very water soluble. Some examples of common organic salts used in pharmaceutical preparations are provided in Figure 2.10.

When dealing with the water solubility of ionized molecules one must also consider the possibility of intramolecular ionic bonding. Compounds with ionizable functional groups that produce opposite charges have the potential to interact with each other rather than water molecules. When this occurs such compounds often become very insoluble in water. A classic example is the amino acid tyrosine (Fig. 2.11). Tyrosine contains three very polar functional groups with two of these (the alkylamine and carboxylic acid) being capable of ionization, depending on the pH of the solution. The phenolic hy-

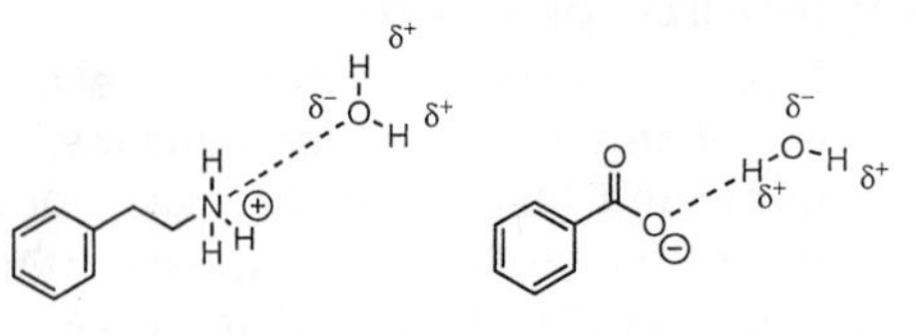

Fig. 2.9. Examples of ion-dipole bonds.

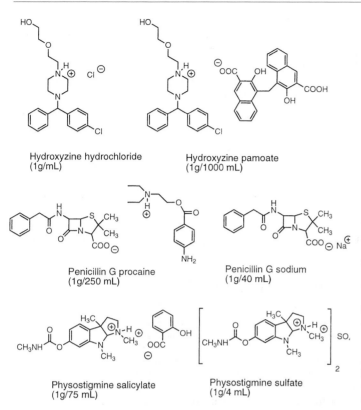

Hydroxyzine hydrochloride
(1g/mL)

Hydroxyzine pamoate
(1g/1000 mL)

Penicillin G procaine
(1g/250 mL)

Penicillin G sodium
(1g/40 mL)

Physostigmine salicylate
(1g/75 mL)

Physostigmine sulfate
(1g/4 mL)

Fig. 2.10. Water solubilities of different salt forms of selective drugs.

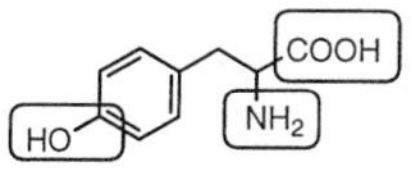

Fig. 2.11. Functional groups present in tyrosine, their hydrogen-bonding potential, and pK_a values.

droxyl is also ionizable, but it doesn't contribute under the conditions most often encountered in pharmaceutical formulations or physiologic conditions. Because of the presence of three very polar functional groups (two of them being ionizable) one would therefore expect tyrosine to be very soluble in water, yet its solubility is only 0.45 g/1000ml. Since the basic alkylamine (pK_a 9.1, for the conjugate acid) and the carboxylic acid (pKa 2.2) can react with one another a zwitterionic molecule is formed. The two charged groups are sufficiently close to allow a strong ion-ion bond to form, thereby keeping each of these groups from forming ion-dipole bonds with the surrounding water molecules. The lack of interaction of the ions with the water dipoles results in a molecule that is very insoluble (Fig. 2.12). Not all zwitterions or multiply charged molecules show this behavior. Only those containing ionized functional groups that are close enough to interact to form an ion-ion bond will be poorly soluble. The greater the separation between charges, the more highly water soluble the molecule will be.

Predicting Water Solubility: Empiric Approach

Lemke (10) has developed an empirical approach to predicting water solubility of molecules based upon the carbon solubilizing potential of several organic functional groups. If the solubilizing potential of the functional groups exceeds the total number of carbon atoms present, then the molecule is considered to be water soluble. Otherwise, it is insoluble. Functional groups that can interact either through intramolecular hydrogen bonds or ion-ion interactions will decrease the solubilizing potential of each group. It is difficult to quantitate how much such interactions will take away from water solubility, but recognizing these interactions will allow one to explain anomalous results.

Table 2.5 shows the water solubilizing potential for several organic functional groups common to many drugs. Since most drug molecules contain more than one functional group (i.e., are polyfunctional) the second column in the table will be used most often. A couple examples for predicting water solubility will be used to demonstrate Lemke's method. Anileridine (Fig. 2.13) is a narcotic analgesic containing three organic functional groups that contribute to water solubility: an aromatic amine (very weak base), a terti-

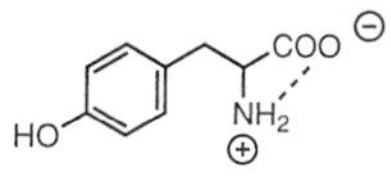

Fig. 2.12. Zwitterion form of tyrosine showing ion-ion bond.

Absorption/Binding Interactions Case

A 24-year-old male comes into the pharmacy and asks you for a recommendation for a treatment for the itching and burning he has recently noticed on both feet. He indicates that he would prefer a cream rather than a spray or a powder. Your recommendation to this patient is to use Lamisil, a very effective topical antifungal agent that is sold over the counter.

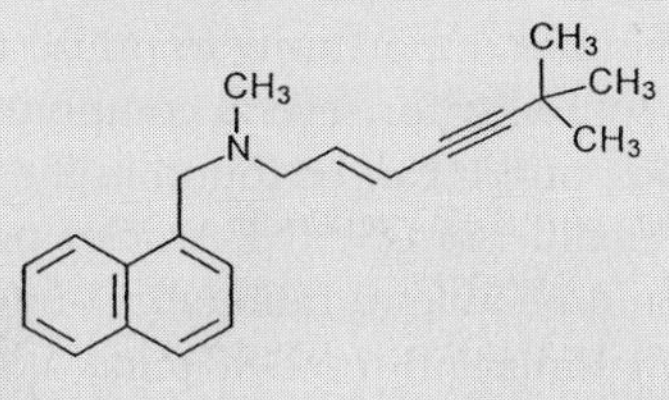

Terbinafine (Lamisil)

1. Identify the structural characteristics and the corresponding properties that make terbinafine an agent that can be utilized topically.
2. The biological target for drug action for terbinafine is squalene epoxidase. Consider each of the structural features of this antifungal agent and describe the type of interactions that the drug will have with the target for drug action. Which amino acids are likely to be present in the active site of this enzyme?

Binding Interactions

Each of these drug molecules interacts with a different biological target and elicits a unique pharmacologic response. For each of the three molecules, list the types of binding interactions that are possible with a target for drug action. For each type of binding interaction, provide one example of an amino acid that could participate in that interaction.

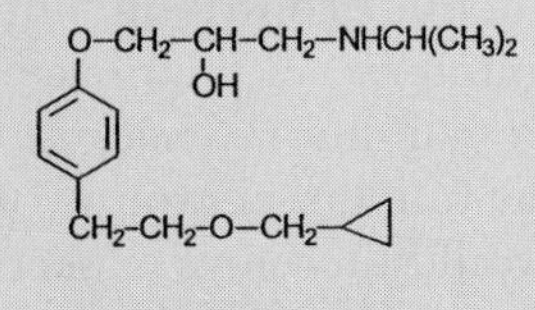

Betaxolol (Betoptic)

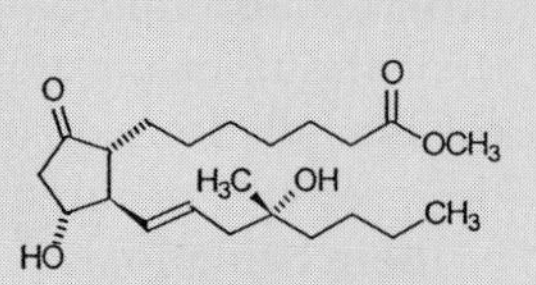

Misoprostol (Cytotec)

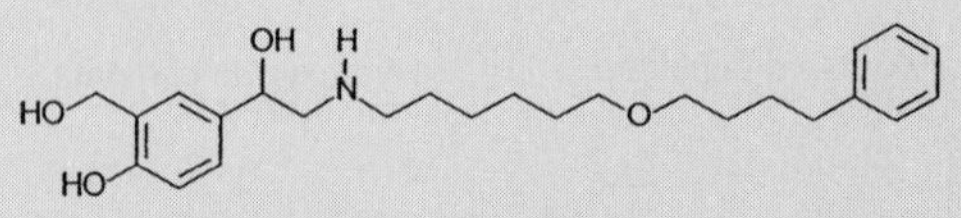

Salmeterol (Serevent)

Example: Binding Interaction: Van der Waals   Amino Acid: leucine

Table 2.5. Water-solubilizing Potential of Organic Functional Groups When Present in a Mono- or Polyfunctional Molecule

Functional Group	Monofunction Molecule	Polyfunctional Molecule
Alcohol	5 to 6 carbons	3 to 4 carbons
Phenol	6 to 7 carbons	3 to 4 carbons
Ether	4 to 5 carbons	2 carbons
Aldehyde	4 to 5 carbons	2 carbons
Ketone	5 to 6 carbons	2 carbons
Amine	6 to 7 carbons	3 carbons
Carboxylic acid	5 to 6 carbons	3 carbons
Ester	6 carbons	3 carbons
Amide	6 carbons	2 to 3 carbons
Urea, carbonate, carbamate		2 carbons

Water solubility is defined as >1% solubility (9).

ary alkylamine (weak base) and an ester (neutral). There are a total of 21 carbon atoms in the molecule with a solubilizing potential from the three functional groups of 9 carbon atoms. Since the solubilizing potential of the functional groups is less than the total number of carbons present, the prediction would be that anileridine is insoluble in water. This is indeed the case, for its solubility is reported in the U.S. Pharmacopeia (USP) as >1g/10,000ml or <0.01%. However, when the hydrochloride salt of anileridine is considered, not only do the three functional groups contribute a solubilizing potential of 9 carbons, but the positive charge of the alkylammonium also contributes to its ionization. Lemke estimates that each charge on a molecule (cationic

or anionic) contributes a solubilizing potential of 20–30 carbons. Thus, the solubilizing potential for these groups in anileridine hydrochloride is 29–39 carbons, which is more than the total number of carbon atoms in the molecule. The compound would therefore be soluble in water, and it is to the extent of 0.2g/ml or 20%. Problem 6 at the end of the chapter provides more opportunity to utilize this approach to predict water solubility for several compounds. Solubility data for these compounds can be found in the USP (USP 24 Approximate Solubilities of USP/NF Articles, pp 2299–2304). The student should be able to rationalize any discrepancies between his/her results and the USP data.

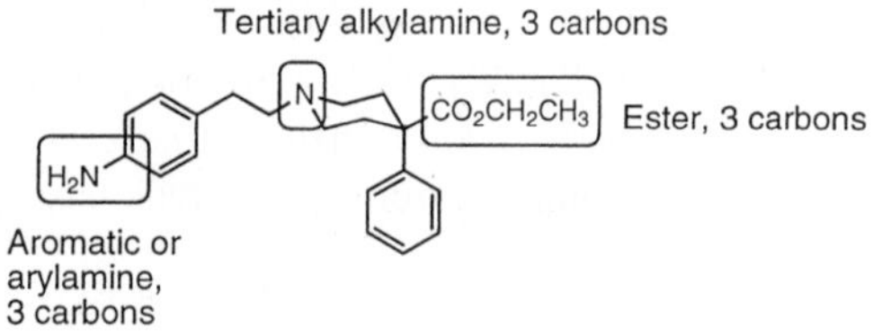

Predicting Water Solubility: Analytical Approach

Another method for predicting water solubility involves calculating an approximate logP, or log of the partition coefficient for a molecule. This approach is based on an approximation method developed by Cates (11) and discussed in Lemke (10). In this approach, one sums the hydrophobic or hydrophilic properties of each functional group present in the molecule. Before we can calculate logP values, we must first digress to a brief explanation of the concept of partition coefficient.

Tertiary alkylamine, 3 carbons

Ester, 3 carbons

Aromatic or arylamine, 3 carbons

Anileridine

Fig. 2.13. Identification of functional groups in anileridine.

Water/Lipid Solubility Case

When you look at any drug molecule there are a number of functional groups that are present that contribute to the properties of that drug molecule. Identify the types of functional groups present in each molecule and to which physical properties (water/lipid solubility) each contributes.

1. Structural Feature   Physical Property

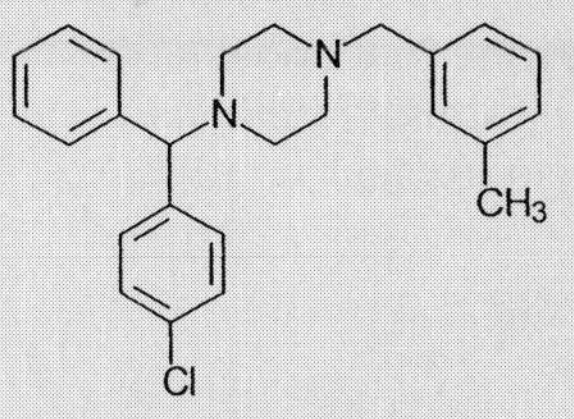

Meclizine
(Antivert)

2. Structural Feature   Physical Property

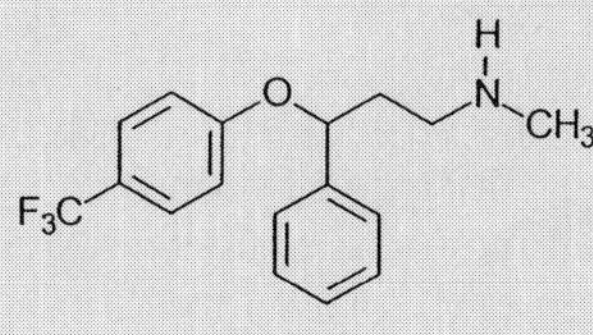

Fluoxetine
(Prozac)

3. Structural Feature   Physical Property

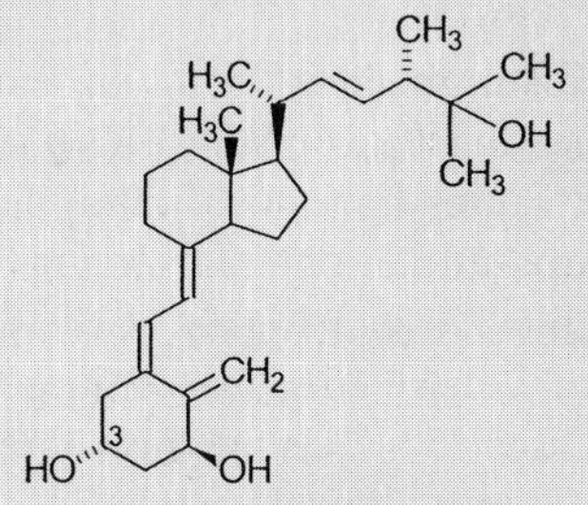

1, 25-dihydroxy Vit D₂

In its simplest form the partition coefficient, P, refers to the ratio of the concentrations of drug in octanol to that of water. Octanol is used to mimic the amphiphilic nature of lipid since it has a polar head group (primary alcohol) and a long hydrocarbon chain, or tail, such as that of fatty acids which make up part of a lipid membrane. Since P is logarithmically related to free energy (12) it is generally expressed as logP, and is therefore the sum of the hydrophobic and hydrophilic characteristics of the organic functional groups making up the structure of the molecule. Thus, logP is a measure of the solubility characteris-

tics of the entire molecule. Because each organic functional group contained within the molecule contributes to the overall hydrophobic/hydrophilic nature of the molecule, a hydrophobic/hydrophilic value (the hydrophobic

Eq. 2.7 $LogP = \Sigma\pi$ (fragments)

substituent constant, π) can be assigned to each organic functional group. Equation 2.7 defines this relationship.

When calculating logP from hydrophobic substituent constants the sum is usually referred to as $logP_{calc}$ or

Binding Interactions/Solubility Case

JK presents a prescription for her daughter (6 months old) for Donatussin Drops. She wants to know if this medication will have an effect on her daughter's alertness.

Components of Donatussin:
Phenylephrine (decongestant)
Chlorpheniramine (antihistamine)
Guaifenesin (expectorant)

Phenylephrine   Chlorpheniramine   Guaifenesin

1. Identify the structural features/functional groups of phenylephrine and guaifenesin that contribute to improved water solubility (medication given as drops). List the type(s) of interactions that these groups have with water and draw an example of these interactions (with appropriate labels) below.
2. Evaluate each of the three molecules and determine if each molecule contains any functional groups that will allow the drug to cross the blood brain barrier and have an effect on this child's alertness (create a list of relevant functional groups. for each molecule). Based on your evaluation, which agent is likely to have the most significant effect? Identify what property is necessary for these agents to cross this biological membrane.
3. Identify the binding interactions that chlorpheniramine and guaifenesin could have with their respective targets for drug action. Be sure to identify which functional groups will participate in each of these binding interactions.

ClogP to distinguish it from an experimentally determined value (logP$_{meas}$ or MlogP). Over the years extensive tables of π values have been compiled for organic functional groups and molecular fragments (see references 12–15). Table 2.6 is a highly abbreviated summary of π values from Lemke (10) based largely upon the manuscript by Cates (11). Using the values in this table, it is possible to obtain a fairly reasonable estimate of the water solubility of many organic compounds. As an example we

will once again use the narcotic analgesic anileridine to demonstrate the calculation of logP. This compound has a total of 21 carbon atoms, some aliphatic and some aromatic. We therefore need to separate these since aromatic carbon atoms, due to delocalized p orbitals for the sp² hybridized atoms, are more polar than aliphatic carbons. The compound also contains one tertiary alkylamine, one aromatic amine and an ester. Note that when dealing with esters and amides the oxygen, nitrogen and ester/amide carbon are counted in this π value. The remaining aliphatic carbons are then counted. Figure 2.14 summa-

Table 2.6. Hydrophilic-lipophilic Values (π V) for Organic Fragments (9)

Fragments	π Value
C (aliphatic)	+0.5
Phenyl	+2.0
Cl	+0.5
O$_2$NO	+0.2
IMHB	+0.65
S	0.0
O = C−O (carboxyl)	−0.7
O = C−N (amide, imide)	−0.7
O (hydroxyl, phenol, ether)	−1.0
N (amine)	−1.0
O$_2$N (aliphatic)	−0.85
O$_2$N (aromatic)	−0.28

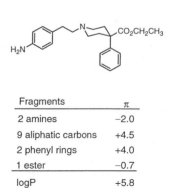

Fragments	π
2 amines	−2.0
9 aliphatic carbons	+4.5
2 phenyl rings	+4.0
1 ester	−0.7
logP	+5.8

Fig. 2.14. Calculation of logP for anileridine.

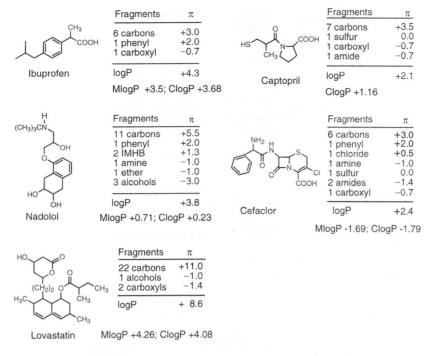

Fig. 2.15. ClogP calculations for selected compounds.

Questions We Can Now Answer About Any Drug Molecule

Based on your knowledge of acid/base chemistry, from where will this drug primarily be absorbed?
What is the solubility of the drug in the stomach, plasma, or in an aqueous IV?
What are the possible interactions that the drug could have with its respective target for drug action?
What is the compatibility of the drug if mixed with other drugs?
How should this drug be delivered? Is it stable in stomach acid?

rizes the logP calculation for anileridine. The calculation gives a ClogP value for anileridine of +5.8. Water solubility as defined by the USP is solubility of greater than 3.3%, which equates to an approximate logP of +0.5. Values less than +0.5 are therefore considered to be water soluble, and those greater than +0.5 are water insoluble. According to our calculation, anileridine would be predicted to be insoluble in water. This calculation agrees with the more empiric procedure discussed earlier. Other sample calculations are shown in Figure 2.15 and several problems are provided at the end of this chapter. In Figure 2.15, MlogP values (when available) and ClogP values obtained from the program MaclogP (16) are included for comparison purposes. Even though the π values used from Table 2.6 are not as extensive as those used in the computer program, there is good general agreement with most of these compounds with respect to their solubility (or insolubility) in water.

Predicting the percent ionization or water solubility of a molecule should not be viewed only as an exercise in arithmetic, but also as a way to understand the solution behavior of molecules, especially when dealing with admixtures and differences among molecules in their pharma-

cokinetics. The ionization state of a molecule not only influences its water solubility, but also its ability to traverse membranes and therefore its ability to be absorbed. Serum protein binding, and therefore the amount of free drug available for receptor binding, is also greatly influenced by the ionization state and the hydrophilic/hydrophobic nature of the molecule.

STEREOCHEMISTRY AND DRUG ACTION

The physicochemical properties of a drug molecule are not only dependent upon what functional groups are present in the molecule, but also the spatial arrangement of these groups. This becomes an especially important factor when a molecule is subjected to an asymmetric environment such as the human body. Since proteins and other biological macromolecules are asymmetric in nature, how a particular drug molecule interacts with these macromolecules is determined by the three-dimensional orientation of the organic functional groups present. If crucial functional groups are not occupying the proper spatial region surrounding the molecule, then productive bonding interactions with the biological macromolecule (or receptor) will not be possible, thereby potentially negating the desired pharmacologic effect. However, if these functional groups are in the proper three-dimensional orientation, the drug can produce a very strong interaction with its receptor. It is therefore very important for the medicinal chemist responsible for developing a new molecular entity for therapeutic use to understand not only what functional groups are responsible for the drug's activity, but also what three-dimensional orientation of these groups is also needed.

Enantiomers

Approximately one in every four drugs currently on the market can be considered to be a mixture. That is, these compounds are combinations of isomers. Yet for many of these compounds the biological activity may reside in only one isomer or at least predominate in one isomer. The majority of these isomeric mixtures are what are referred to as racemic mixtures (racemates). These are compounds, usually synthetic, that contain equal amounts of both possible enantiomers, or optical isomers. Enantiomers are isomers whose three-dimensional arrangement of atoms results in nonsuperimposable mirror images. These compounds have identical physical chemical properties except for their ability to rotate the plane of polarized light in opposite directions with equal magnitude. Enantiomers are also referred to as chiral compounds, antipodes or enantiomorphs. When introduced into an asymmetric, or chiral, environment, such as the human body, enantiomers will display different physical chemical properties producing significant differences in their pharmacokinetic and pharmacodynamic behavior. Such differences can result in adverse side effects or toxicity due to one of the isomers or the isomers may exhibit significant differences in absorption (especially active transport), serum protein binding and metabolism. With the latter one isomer may be converted into a toxic substance or may influence the metabolism of another drug. To further discuss the influence of stereochemistry on drug action, some of the basic concepts of stereochemistry need to be reviewed.

Stereochemical Definitions

Organic compounds can exist as isomers, compounds with the same number and kinds of atoms, but with different bonding arrangements. The arrangement of bonds within a molecule that provides it with a particular three-dimensional shape is referred to as the *configuration* of the molecule. Differences in configuration result in compounds with differing physicochemical properties such as solubility, melting point, or boiling point, just to name a few. For example, the empirical formula C_2H_6O can describe at least two different compounds: dimethyl ether (CH_3OCH_3) or ethyl alcohol (CH_3CH_2OH). The former has a boiling point of $-23.6°C$ (i.e., it is a gas), whereas the latter has a boiling point of $78.5°C$. Numerous other examples of isomers exist in which the empirical formula can describe two or more compounds with different physical and chemical properties (see problem 8 at the end of the chapter).

Diastereomers

Stereoisomers are compounds containing the same number and kinds of atoms, the same arrangement of bonds, but different three-dimensional structures i.e., they only differ in the three-dimensional arrangements of atoms in space. Stereoisomers are subdivided into two types: enantiomers and diastereoisomers. As indicated earlier, enantiomers are compounds whose three-dimensional arrangement of atoms is such that they are nonsuperimposable mirror images. Diastereoisomers are all stereoisomeric compounds that are not enantiomers. Thus, the term diastereoisomer includes compounds containing double bonds as well as ring systems. Unlike enantiomers, diastereoisomers exhibit different physical and chemical properties, including melting point, boiling point, solubility and chromatographic behavior. These differences in physical chemical properties allow for the separation of diastereoisomers from mixtures utilizing standard chemical separation techniques such as column chromatography or crystallization. Enantiomers cannot be separated using such techniques unless a chiral environment is provided or they are converted to diastereoisomers (e.g., salt formation with another enantiomer). Examples of enantiomers and diastereoisomers are provided in Figure 2.16.

Designation of Stereoisomers and Nomenclature

At first enantiomers were distinguished by their ability to rotate the plane of polarized light. Isomers rotating light to the right, or clockwise direction, were designated as dextrorotatory and this was indicated by a (+)-sign before the chemical name (e.g., (+)-amphetamine or dextroamphetamine). The opposite designation, levorotatory or (−)-, was given to compounds which rotated the plane of polarized light to the left or counterclockwise. The letters d- and l- were formerly used to indicate (+)- and (−)- respectively. A racemate (racemic mixture), i.e., a 1:1 mixture of enantiomers, is indicated by (±)-before the compound name. The student should be made aware that

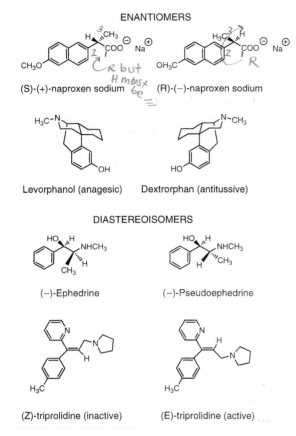

Fig. 2.16. Examples of stereoisomers.

this method of nomenclature is based upon a physical property of the molecule and does not provide any information concerning the *absolute configuration* or three-dimensional arrangement of atoms around the chiral center. Since the rotation of plane polarized light is a physical property, both the magnitude and direction of rotation can vary depending upon the conditions used. Thus, temperature, solvent and concentration of the substance are only three factors that need to be considered. A good example of this is the antibiotic chloramphenicol. There are

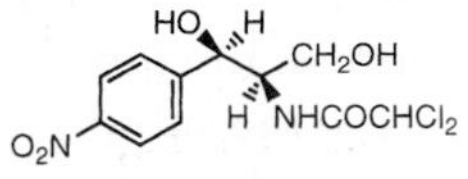

Chloramphenicol

two chiral centers in this molecule resulting in four possible stereoisomers. The isomer shown is dextrorotatory when its optical rotation is measured in ethanol, but levorotatory in ethyl acetate. It is obvious that the simple measurement of a physical property such as rotation of the plane of polarized light is not sufficient for the assignment of the absolute configuration of a molecule.

Fisher and Rosanoff in the late 19th century developed a system of nomenclature based upon the structure of glyceraldehyde (Fig. 2.17). Since there were no known methods for determining the absolute three dimensional arrangement of atoms in space at that time, the two isomers of glyceraldehyde were arbitrarily assigned the designation of D-(+)- and L-(−).

It wasn't until the 1950s that the absolute configurations were determined and it was found that Fisher had fortuitously guessed correctly. Assignments of configuration to other molecules were done based upon their relationship to D- or L-glyceraldehyde via synthesis irrespective of the observed direction of rotation of plane polarized light. Thus, via chemical degradation, it was possible to determine that (+)-glucose, (−)-2–deoxyribose and (−)-fructose had the same terminal configuration as D-(+)-glyceraldehyde and were therefore given the D-absolute configuration. Amino acids were assigned based upon their relationship to D-(+)- and L-(−)-serine (Fig. 2.17). Unfortunately, this system becomes very cumbersome with molecules containing more than one chiral center.

In 1956 Cahn, Ingold and Prelog devised a system of nomenclature for stereoisomers referred to as the Sequence Rule System (or CIP system). With this system, atoms attached to a chiral center are ranked according to their atomic number. Highest priority is given to the atom with highest atomic number and subsequent atoms are ranked accordingly from highest to lowest. When a decision cannot be made regarding priority, e.g., two atoms with the same atomic number attached to the chiral center, the process continues to the next atom until a decision can be made. The molecule is then viewed from the side opposite the lowest priority atom and the priority sequence from highest to lowest is determined. If the sequence is to the right, or clockwise, the chiral center is designated as the R absolute configuration. When the priority sequence is to the left, or counterclockwise, the designation is S. An example of this is seen in the neurotransmitter norepinephrine.

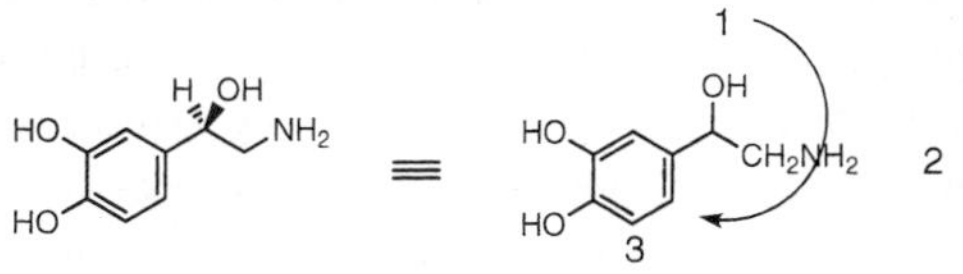

Norepinephrine   R

Degradation studies demonstrated that (−)-norepinephrine is related to D-(−)-mandelic acid and was therefore given the D-designation using the Fisher system. With the CIP system norepinephrine is assigned the R absolute configuration.

CHO   CHO
H——OH   HO——H
CH₂OH   CH₂OH

D-(+)-Glyceraldehyde   L-(−)-Glyceraldehyde

COOH   COOH
H——NH₂   H₂N——H
CH₂OH   CH₂OH

D-(+)-Serine   L-(−)-Serine

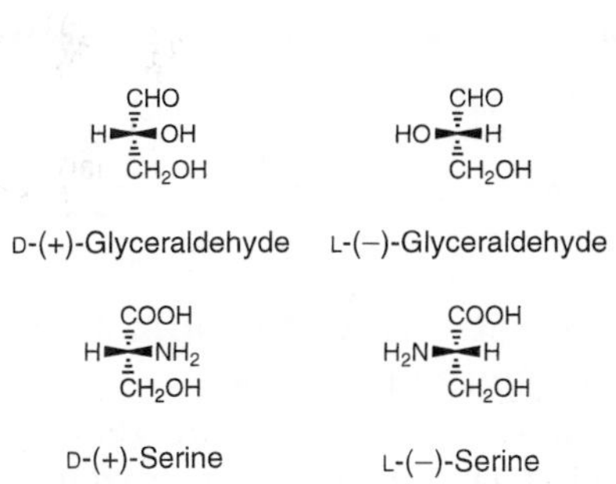

Fig. 2.17. Relationship of optical isomers of serine to D and L glyceraldehyde.

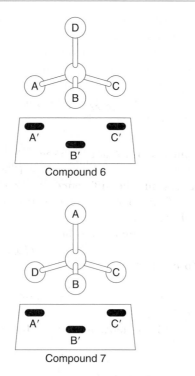

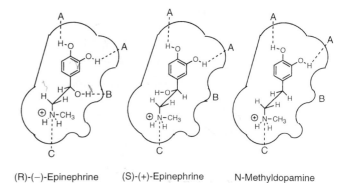

(R)-(−)-Epinephrine   (S)-(+)-Epinephrine   N-Methyldopamine

Fig. 2.19. Drug receptor interation of (R)- (−)-epinephrine, (S)-(+)-epinephrine, and N-methyldopamine.

Fig. 2.18. Optical isomers. Only in compound 6 do the functional groups A, B, and C align with the corresponding sites of binding on the asymmetric surface.

This was one of the earliest observations that enantiomers can exhibit differences in biological action. In 1933, Easson and Stedman (18) reasoned that differences in biological activity between enantiomers resulted from selective reactivity of one enantiomer with its receptor. They postulated that such interactions require a minimum of a three-point fit to the receptor. This is demonstrated in Figure 2.18 for two hypothetical enantiomers. In Figure 2.18, A, B, and C represent hypothetical functional groups that can interact with complementary sites on the hypothetical receptor surface, represented by A′, B′ and C′. Only one enantiomer is capable of attaining the correct orientation enabling all three functional groups to fit their respective sites on the receptor surface. The lack of achieving the same interactions with the other enantiomer explains its reduced biological activity since it is unable to properly fit the receptor and therefore cannot "trigger" the appropriate change in the receptor conformation. The Easson-Stedman Hypothesis states that the more potent enantiomer must be involved in a minimum of three intermolecular interactions with the receptor surface and the less potent enantiomer only interacts with two sites. This can be illustrated by looking at the differences in vasopressor activity of (R)-(−)-epinephrine, (S)-(+)-epinephrine and the achiral N-methyldopamine (Fig. 2.19). With (R)-(−)-epinephrine, the three points of interaction with the receptor site are the substituted aromatic ring, β-hydroxyl group and the protonated secondary ammonium group. All three functional groups interact with their com-

The student should note that the CIP system of nomenclature uses a set of arbitrary rules and therefore should be viewed as a system that keeps track of absolute configuration only. There are many instances where two molecules may have different absolute configurations as designated by the CIP system, but the same relative orientation of the functional groups relevant for biological activity. A case in point is the absolute configuration of the nonselective alpha-adrenogenic antagonist propranolol as compared to norepinephrine. Because of the ether oxygen, the priority sequence of the functional groups about the chiral center results in the assignment of the (S)-absolute configuration for the more active enantiomer of propranolol. However, close inspection of both (R)-norepinephrine and (S)-propranolol shows that the hydroxy group, basic amine and aromatic rings of both compounds occupy the same regions in 3D space.

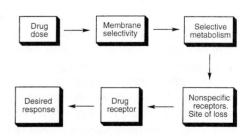

(R)-Norepinephrine   (S)-Propranolol

Stereochemistry and Biologic Activity
Easson-Stedman Hypothesis

In 1886 Piutti (17) reported different physiologic actions for the enantiomers of asparagine, with (+)-asparagine having a sweet taste and (−)-asparagine bland.

Fig. 2.20. Selective phases to which opitcal isomers may be subjected before biologic response.

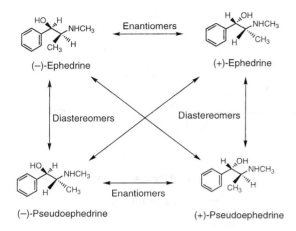

Fig. 2.21. Relationship between the diastereomers of ephedrine and pseudoephedrine.

plementary binding sites on the receptor surface producing the necessary interactions that stimulate the receptor. With (S)-(+)-epinephrine only two interactions are possible (the protonated secondary ammonium and the substituted aromatic ring). The β-hydroxyl group occupies the wrong region of space and therefore cannot interact properly with the receptor. N-methyldopamine can achieve the same interactions with the receptor as (S)-(+)-epinephrine and it is therefore not suprising that its vasopressor response is the same as (S)-(+)-epinephrine and less than (R)-(−)-epinephrine.

Not all stereoselectivity seen with enantiomers can be attributed to differences in reactivity at the receptor site. Differences in biological activity can also be due to differences in the ability of each enantiomer to reach the receptor site. Since the biological system encountered by the drug is asymmetric, each enantiomer may experience selective penetration of membranes, metabolism, absorption at sites of loss (e.g., adipose tissue) or excretion. Figure 2.20 shows the selective phases enantiomers may encounter prior to reaching the receptor. Not all of these processes may be encountered by a particular enantiomer, but such processes may provide enough of an influence to cause one enantiomer to produce a significantly better pharmacologic effect than the other. Conversely, such processes may also contribute to untoward effects of a particular enantiomer. The student must continually keep in mind that not all pharmacologic effects of a drug are necessarily beneficial to the patient and differences in pharmacologic action among stereoisomers provide excellent examples of this concept.

Diastereomers

As mentioned earlier, diastereoisomers are compounds that are non-superimposable, non-mirror image isomers. Such compounds can result from the presence of more than one chiral center in the molecule, double bonds or ring systems. These isomers have different physical and chemical properties and thus differences in biological ac-

tivity between such isomers can often be attributed to these properties.

Compounds containing more than one chiral center are probably the most common type of diastereoisomer used as drugs. The classic example of compounds of this type is the diastereoisomers ephedrine and pseudoephedrine (see Fig. 2.21). When a molecule contains two chiral centers there can be up to four possible stereoisomers consisting of two sets of enantiomeric pairs. For each enantiomeric pair there is inversion of both chiral centers, while the difference between diastereomers is inversion of only one chiral center (problem 9 at the end of the chapter helps illustrate this point). Figure 2.22 shows several examples of other compounds that contain two or more chiral centers and therefore are diastereoisomeric (problem 10 at the end of the chapter).

Restricted bond rotation due to carbon-carbon double bonds (alkenes or olefins) and similar systems such as C=N (imines) can produce stereoisomers. These are also referred to as geometric isomers, although they are more properly diastereoisomers. In compounds of this type substituents can be oriented on the same side or opposite sides of the double bond. The alkene 2–butene is a simple example of this.

cis or Z isomer   trans or E isomer

With 2-butene it is readily apparent that the methyl groups may be on the same side or opposite sides of the double bond. When they are on the same side the molecule is defined as the cis- or Z-isomer (from the German zusammen or "together"); when they are on opposite sides the designation is trans- or E- (from the German entgegen or "opposite"). With simple compounds such as 2-butene it is easy to determine which groups in the molecule are cis or trans to one another. However, this becomes more difficult to determine with more complex structures where it is less obvious which substituents should be referred to

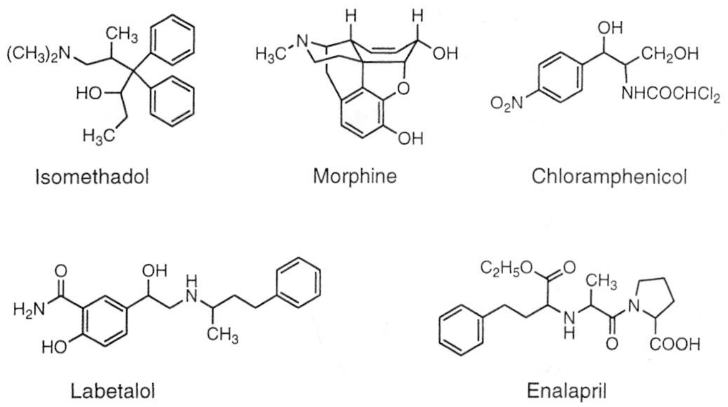

Isomethadol   Morphine   Chloramphenicol

Labetalol   Enalapril

Fig. 2.22. Examples of chiral drugs with two or more asymmetric centers.

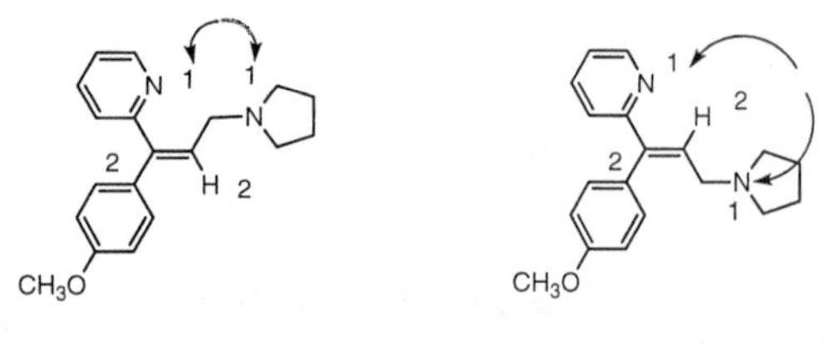

Fig. 2.23. Geometric isomers of triprolidine.

Decalin

trans-decalin

cis-decalin

when naming the compound. In 1968 Blackwood et al. (19) proposed a system for the assignment of "absolute" configuration with respect to double bonds. Using the CIP sequence rules, each of the two substituents attached to the carbon atoms comprising the double bond are assigned a priority of 1 or 2 depending upon the atomic number of the atom attached to the double bond. When two substituents of higher priority are on the same side of the double bond, this isomer is given the designation of cis or Z. When the substituents are on opposite sides, the designation is trans or E. The histamine H_1-receptor antagonist, triprolidine, (Fig. 2.23) is a good example for demonstrating how this nomenclature system works. The E-isomer of triprolidine is more active both in vitro and in vivo, indicating that the distance between the pyridine and pyrrolidine rings is critical for binding to the receptor.

Diastereoisomers (as well as enantiomers) can also be found in cyclic compounds. For example, the cyclic alkane 1,2-dimethylcyclohexane can exist as *cis/trans* diastereoisomers and the *trans* isomer can also exist as an enantiomeric pair. In Figure 2.24 each of the trans-enantiomorphs are depicted in the two possible chair conformations for the cyclohexane ring. Cyclohexane rings can exhibit significant conformational freedom that allows for the possibility of conformational isomers. Isomers of this type will be discussed in the next section. When two or more rings share a common bond (e.g., decalin) rotation around the bonds is even more restricted, preventing even ring "flipping" (conformationally rigid) from occurring thereby producing diastereoisomers and enantiomers.

In the case of the two-ring system of decalin, the rings can join together at the common bond either in the trans or cis configuration as shown. Steroids, a class of medicinally important compounds consisting of four fused rings (three cy-

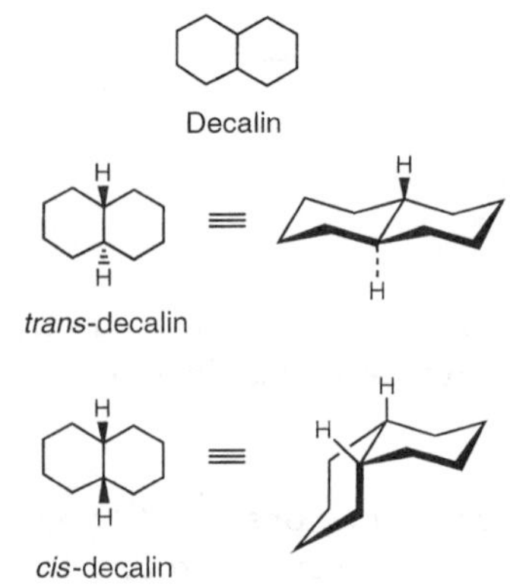

clohexane, 1 cyclopentane), exhibit significantly different biological activity when the first two cyclohexane rings are fused into different configurations referred to as the 5α or 5β-isomers (Fig. 2.25). The α-designation indicates that the substituent in the 5-position is below the "plane" of the ring system while the β-designation refers to the substituent being above this plane. What appears to be a very minor change in orientation for the substituent results in a very drastic change in the three-dimensional shape of the molecule and in its biological activity. Figure 2.25 shows the diastereoisomers 5α-cholestane and 5β-cholestane as examples. The chemistry and pharmacology of steroids will be discussed in more detail in Chapters 28 and 29.

Conformational Isomerism

With conformational isomerism we are dealing with a dynamic process, that is, isomerization takes place via rotation about one or more single bonds. Such bond rotation results in non-identical spatial arrangement of atoms in a molecule. Changes in spatial orientation of atoms due to bond rotation results in different *conformations* (or rotameters) whereas conversion of one enantiomer into another (or diastereoisomer) requires the breaking of bonds which has a much higher energy requirement than single bond rotation.

The neurotransmitter acetylcholine can be used to demonstrate the concept of conformational isomers.

Each single bond within this molecule is capable of undergoing rotation, and at room temperature such rotations

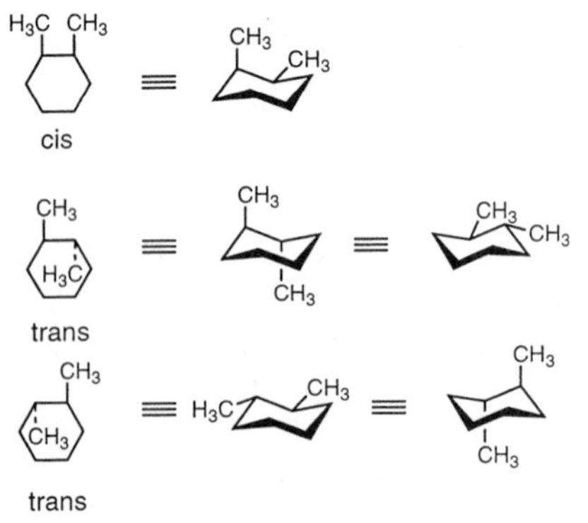

cis

trans

trans

Fig. 2.24. Diastereomers of 1,2-dimethylcyclohexane.

5α-Cholestane

5β-Cholestane

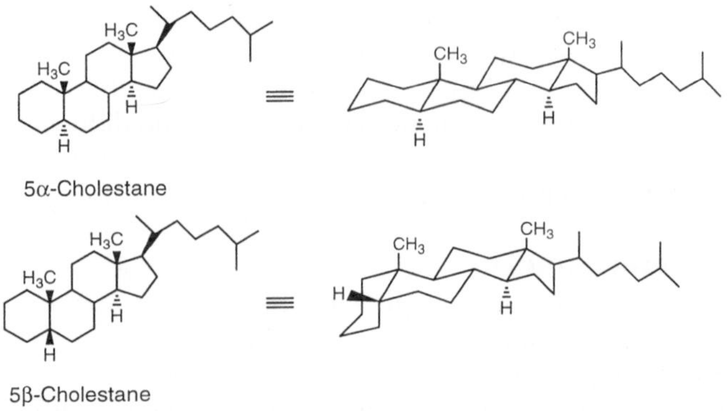

Fig. 2.25. The 5α and 5β conformations of the steriod nucleus cholestane.

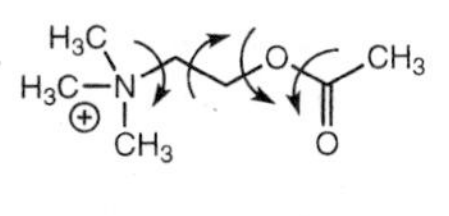

Acetylcholine

readily occur. Even though rotation around single bonds was shown by Kemp and Pitzer in 1936 (20) not to be free, but to have a energy barrier, this barrier is sufficiently low that at room temperature acetylcholine exists in many interconvertible conformations (see Chapter 10). Close observation reveals that rotation around the central C2–C3 bond produces the greatest spatial rearrangement of atoms than rotation around any other bond within the molecule. In fact, several rotatable bonds in acetylcholine produce redundant structures because all of the atoms attached to one end of some bonds are identical, resulting in no change in spatial arrangement of atoms (e.g., methyl groups). When viewed along the C2–C3 bond, acetylcholine can be depicted in the sawhorse or Newman projections as shown in Figure 2.26. When the ester and trimethylammonium group are 180° apart the molecule is said to be in the anti or staggered conformation (or anti or staggered rotamer). This conformation allows for maximum separation of the functional groups and is therefore considered to be the energetically most stable conformation. Other conformations are possibly more stable if factors other than steric interactions come into play; e.g., intramolecular hydrogen bonds. Rotation of one end of the C2–C3 bond by 120° or 240° results in the two gauche or skew conformations shown in Figure 2.26. These are considered to be less stable than the anti-conformer, although some studies suggest that an electrostatic attraction between the electron poor trimethylammonium and electron rich ester oxygen stabilizes this conformation. Rotation by 60°, 180° and 240° produce conformations where all of the atoms overlap or what are referred to as eclipsed conformations. These are the least stable conformers.

An interesting observation can be made with the two gauche conformers shown in Figure 2.26. These conformers are not distinct molecules and only exist for a transient period of time at room temperature. However, if these could be "frozen" into the conformations shown, they would be nonsuperimposable mirror images or enantiomers. Thus, a compound that is achiral, such as acetylcholine, can exhibit prochirality if certain conformational isomers can be formed. It is quite possible that such a situation could exist when acetylcholine binds to one of its receptors. Studies have suggested that the gauche conformation is the form that binds to the nicotinic receptor while the anti form (which is achiral) binds to the muscarinic receptor.

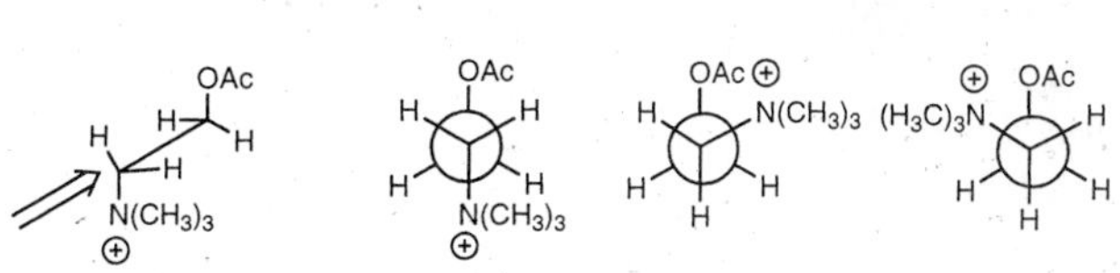

DRUG DESIGN: DISCOVERY AND STRUCTURAL MODIFICATION OF LEAD COMPOUNDS
Natural Product Screening

Perhaps the most difficult aspect of drug discovery for the medicinal chemist is that of lead discovery. Until the late 19th century the development of new chemical entities for medicinal purposes was primarily achieved through the use of natural products derived primarily from plant sources. As the colonial powers of Europe discovered new lands in the Western Hemisphere and colonized Asia, the Europeans learned of remedies derived from herbs for many ailments from the indigenous peoples of the newly discovered lands. Salicylic acid was isolated from the bark of willow trees after learning that Native Americans brewed the bark to treat inflammatory ailments. Further development of this lead compound by the Bayer Corporation of Germany resulted in acetylsalicylic acid or aspirin, the first non-steroidal anti-inflammatory agent. Teas obtained by brewing Cinchona bark were used by South American natives to treat chills and fever. Further study in Europe led to the isolation of quinine and quinidine, which were subsequently used to treat malaria and arrhythmias respectively. Following leads such as these chemists of the late 19th and early 20th centuries began to seek new medicinals from plant sources and to assay them for many types of pharmacologic actions. This approach to drug discovery is often referred to as natural product screening. With this approach compounds were isolated from natural sources based upon information obtained from indigenous peoples in many parts of the world. Until the mid-1970s this was one of the major approaches to obtaining new chemical entities as leads for new drugs. Unfortunately, this approach declined in favor of more rational approaches to drug design that developed during that period (see below). Recently, due to heightened awareness of the fragility of ecosystems on this planet, especially the rainforests, there has been a resurgence of screening products from plants before they become extinct. A new field of pharmacology, called ethnopharmacology, has emerged as a result. Ethnopharmacology is the term used to for the discipline of identifying potential natural product sources with medicinal products based upon native lore.

Compounds isolated from natural sources are usually tested in bioassays for the ailment that the plant material has been described to treat. Sometimes this may require several bioassays because the plant has been reported to be effective against several ailments. Often the treatment of different ailments requires different methods of preparation (e.g., brewing, chewing, direct application to wounds, etc.) or different parts of the same plant (e.g., roots, stem,

anti or staggered conformer

gauche or skew conformers

Fig. 2.26. Anti and gauche conformations of acetylcholine.

leaves, flowers, sap etc.). Each method of administration or part of the plant may involve different chemical compounds to produce the desired outcome. One can readily see that isolation of active constituents from plants that may be useful as medicinals is not a simple process and a number of variables are involved that may influence the amount of active compound or compounds that may influence the pharmacologic activity of the extract.

Random Screening of Synthetic Organic Compounds

This approach to discovering new chemical structures for a particular biological action began in the 1930s after the discovery of the sulfonamide class of antibacterials. Thousands of compounds and their synthetic intermediates were assayed in search of new structures that possessed antibacterial activity. All compounds available to the investigator (natural products, synthetic compounds), regardless of structure, were tested in the assays available at the time. This approach was also applied in the 1960s and 1970s in an effort to find agents that were effective against cancer. Some groups did not limit themselves to a particular biological activity, but tested compounds in a wide variety of assays. This approach was a precursor to what is now referred to as high throughput screening assays. This involves the bioassay of thousands of compounds in hundreds to thousands of bioassays simultaneously. This only became possible with the advent of computer controlled robotic systems for the assays and combinatorial chemistry techniques. These will be discussed further below.

What is crucial for random screening to be successful is a good bioassay system for the pharmacologic action of interest. Unfortunately, this means of lead discovery is very inefficient because no rational approach is taken to what compounds are to be tested to find new lead structures. Random screening eventually gave way to dedicated screening and rational design techniques.

Targeted Dedicated Screening and Rational Drug Design

This approach is more or less random in nature and involves greater knowledge of the therapeutic targets and some actual design based on physicochemical properties. Testing is usually with one or two models (e.g., specific receptor systems or enzymes) based on the therapeutic target. The design aspect often involves molecular modeling and the use of quantitative structure-activity relationships (QSAR) to better define the physicochemical properties that are crucial for biological activity. The drawback of these approaches is that they are better for developing a lead compound rather than discovery of the lead compound.

New Drug Discovery via Drug Metabolism Studies

New compounds have been "discovered" by investigating the metabolism of compounds that already are clinical candidates or, in rare instances, compounds that are already on the market. Metabolites of known compounds are isolated and then assayed for biological effects either on the same target system or a broader screen of several other target systems. The latter will be more useful if the metabolite being studied is a chemical structure that has been radically altered from the parent molecule through some unusual rearrangement reaction. More often the metabolite is not radically different from the parent molecule and therefore would be expected to have similar pharmacologic effects. The advantage is that a metabolite may possess better pharmacokinetic properties such as a longer duration of action, better absorption orally, or less toxicity with fewer side effects (e.g., terfenadine and its antihistaminic metabolite, fexofenadine). The sulfonamide antibacterial agents were discovered in this way. The azo dye prontosil was found to have antibacterial action in vitro only. It was soon discovered that this compound required reduction of the diazo group to produce 4-aminobenzene sulfonamide (Fig. 2.27) which was found to act as an antagonist to p-aminobenzoic acid, a crucial component in microbial metabolism.

New Drug Discovery via Observation of Side Effects

An astute clinician or pharmacologist may detect a side effect in a patient or animal model that could lead, upon further development, to a new therapeutic use for a particular chemical structure. Further development may even lead to an entirely new chemical class. This discovery of new lead compounds has occurred several times and will be discussed below.

One of the more interesting cases of drug development is that of the phenothiazine antipsychotics. These compounds can be traced back to the first histamine H_1-receptor antagonists developed in the 1930s. Bovet in 1937 (21) was the first to recognize that it should be possible to antagonize the effects of histamine and thereby treat allergic reactions. He tested compounds that were known to act on the autonomic nervous system and eventually discovered that benzodioxanes (Fig. 2.28) were capable of significant antagonism of the effects of histamine. In attempts to improve the antihist-

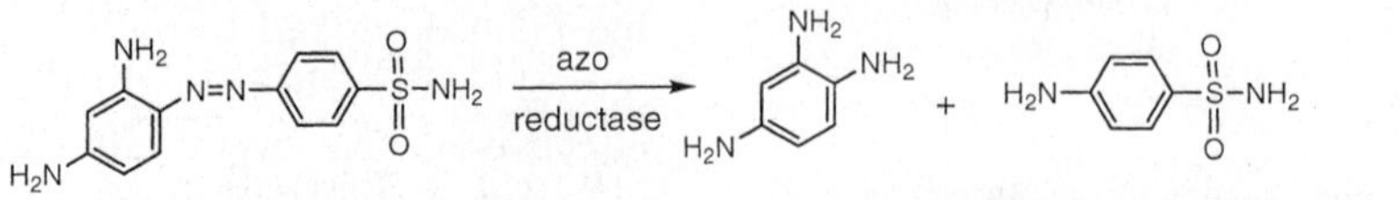

4-aminobenzenesulfonamide

Fig. 2.27. Metabolic conversion of prontosil to 4-aminobenzenesulfonamide.

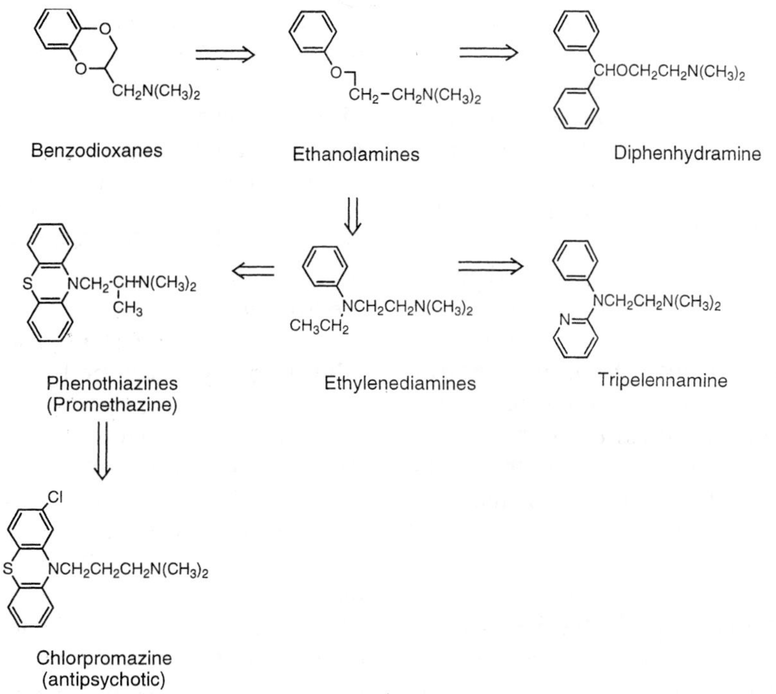

Fig. 2.28. Develpoment of phenothiazine-type antipsychotic drugs.

aminic action of the benzodioxanes it was discovered that ethanolamines also provided significant antihistaminic activity. Further development of this class ended up going in two directions. One approach led to the development of the diphenhydramine class of antihistamines and is represented by the first clinically useful H_1-receptor antagonist developed in the United States, diphenhydramine (Fig. 2.28). The other approach led to the ethylenediamine class represented by tripelennamine (Fig. 2.28).

Incorporation of the aromatic rings of the ethylenediamines into the tricyclic phenothiazine structure produced compounds (e.g., promethazine) with good antihistaminic action and relatively strong sedative properties. At first these compounds were found to not only be useful as antihistamines, but their very strong sedative properties lead to their use as potentiating agents for anesthesia (22). Further development to increase the sedative properties of the phenothiazines resulted in the development of chlorpromazine in 1950 (23).

Chlorpromazine was found to produce a tendency for sleep, but unlike the prior phenothiazines it also produced a disinterest in surroundings in patients and, with patients suffering psychiatric disorders, an ameliorative effect on the psychosis as well as relief of anxiety and agitation. These observations suggested that chlorpromazine had potential for the treatment of psychiatric disorders. Thus, what started out as attempts to improve antihistaminic activity, ultimately resulted in an entirely new class of chemical entity useful in an unrelated disorder (24).

Another example of how new chemical entities can be derived from compounds with unrelated biological effects

is that of the development of the K^+ channel agonist diazoxide (Fig. 2.29). This compound was developed as the result of the observation that the thiazide diuretics such as chlorothiazide not only had a diuretic component due to inhibition of sodium absorption in the distal convoluted tubule but also a direct effect on the renal vasculature. Structural modification to enhance this direct effect led to the development of diazoxide and related K^+ channel agonists for the treatment of hypertension.

REFINEMENT OF THE LEAD STRUCTURE
Determination of the Pharmacophore

Once a lead compound has been discovered for a particular therapeutic use, the next step is to determine the pharmacophore for this compound. The pharmacophore of a drug molecule is that portion of the molecule containing the essential organic functional groups that directly interact with the receptor active site and therefore confers upon the molecule the biologic activity of interest. Since drug receptor interactions are very specific, the pharmacophore may constitute a small portion of the molecule. It has been found on several occasions that what seem to be very complex molecules can often be reduced to simpler structures with retention of the desired biological action. A well known example of this is the narcotic analgesic morphine. Morphine is a tetracyclic compound with five chiral centers. Not only would simplification of the structure possibly provide molecules with fewer side effects, but a reduction in the number of chiral centers would also greatly simplify the synthesis of morphine derivatives and thereby decrease cost. Figure 2.30 shows

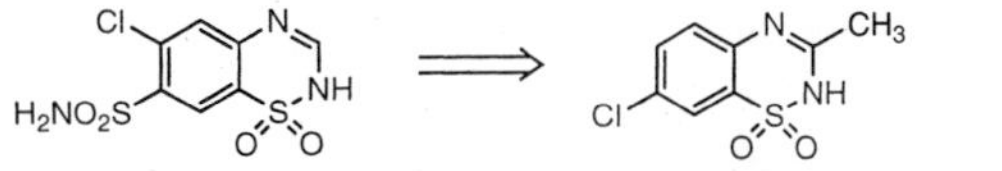

Fig. 2.29. Structural similarity of chlorothiazide, a diuretic, and diazoxide an antihypertensive that acts via opening of K⁺ channels.

how the morphine structure has been simplified in the search for compounds with fewer deleterious side effects such as respiratory depression and addiction potential. Within each class there are analogs that are less potent, equipotent and with potencies many times that of morphine. It can be readily seen from the figure that the pharmacophore of morphine must consist of a tertiary alkylamine that is at least four atoms away from an aromatic ring. A more detailed discussion of the chemistry and pharmacology of morphine can be found in Chapter 19.

Alterations in Alkyl Chains: Chain Length, Branching, Rings

Alterations in alkyl chains such as increasing or decreasing chain length, branching and changing ring size can have profound effects on the potency and pharmacologic activity of the molecule. Simply changing the length of an alkyl chain by one CH_2 unit or branching the chain will alter the lipophilic character of the molecule and therefore its absorption, distribution and excretion properties. If the alkyl chain is directly involved in the receptor interaction, then chain length and branching can alter the binding characteristics. Molecules that are conformationally flexible may become less flexible if branching is introduced at a key position of an alkyl chain. Changes in conformation will affect the spatial relationship of functional groups in the molecule, thereby influencing receptor binding. Changes as small as one CH_2 unit may seem trivial at first, but in many instances such small changes are important aspects in the design of analogs.

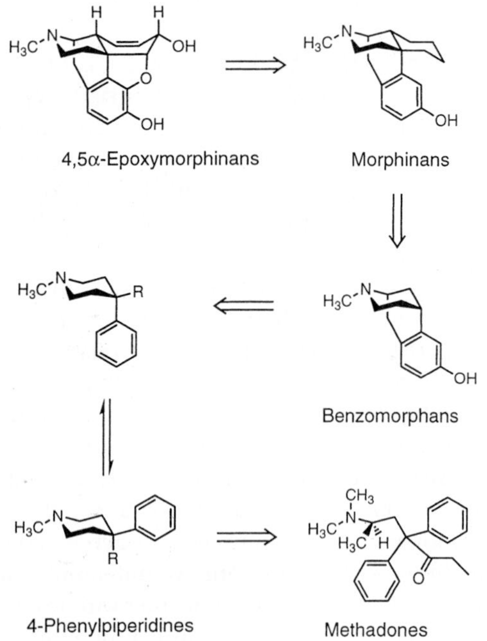

An example where simply increasing hydrocarbon chain length has significant effects not only on potency but also the agonist or antagonist action of a molecule is seen with a series of N-alkyl morphine analogs (Fig. 2.31). In this series, going from R = CH_3 (morphine) to R = $CH_2CH_2CH_3$ (N-propylnormorphine) produces a pronounced decrease in agonist activity and an increase in antagonist activity. When R = $CH_2CH_2CH_2CH_3$ (N-butylnormorphine) the compound is totally devoid of agonist or antagonist activity: i.e., the compound is inactive. However, further increases in chain length (R = $CH_2CH_2CH_2CH_2CH_3$ and R = $CH_2CH_2CH_2CH_2CH_2CH_3$) produce compounds with increasing potency as agonists. When R is β-phenylethyl the compound is a full agonist with a potency approximately 14× that of morphine (25,26).

Branching of alkyl chains can also produce drastic changes in potency and pharmacologic activity. If the mechanism of action is closely related to the lipophilicity of the molecule, then branching of a hydrocarbon chain will result in a less lipophilic compound and significantly altered biological effect. This decrease in lipophilicity as the result of hydrocarbon chain branching results from the chain becoming more compact and therefore produces less disruption of the H-bonding network of water. If the hydrocarbon chain is directly involved in receptor interactions, then branching can produce major changes in pharmacologic activity. For example, consider the phenothiazines promethazine and promazine:

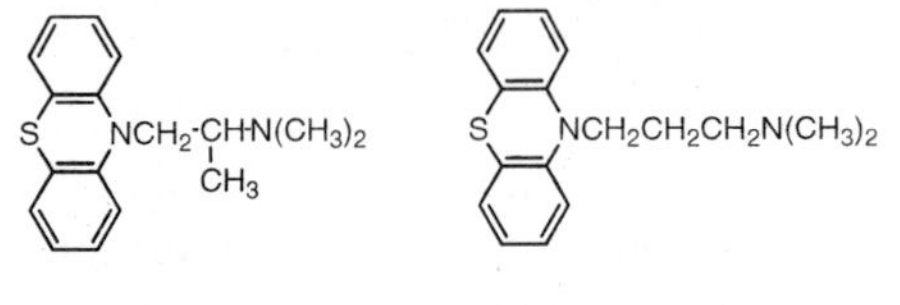

Promethazine   Promazine

The primary pharmacologic activity of promethazine is that of an antihistamine, whereas promazine is an antipsychotic. The only difference between the two is the alkylamine side chain. In the case of promethazine it contains a isopropylamine side chain while promazine has a n-propylamine. In this case the small change of one carbon atom from a branched to a linear hydrocarbon radically alters the pharmacologic activity.

Position isomers of substituents on aromatic rings may also possess different pharmacologic properties. Substituents on aromatic rings can alter the electron distribution throughout the ring which in turn can affect how the ring interacts with the receptor. Ring substituents may also influence the conformation of a flexible molecule, especially if they are located ortho to flexible side chains and

Fig. 2.30. Morphine pharmacophore and its relationship to analgesic derivatives.

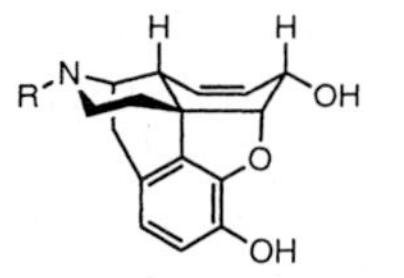

R	Pharmacologic activity
—CH$_3$	Analgesic (morphine)
—CH$_2$CH$_3$	Opioid agonist activity decreased
—CH$_2$CH$_2$CH$_3$	Opioid antagonist activity increased
—CH$_2$CH$_2$CH$_2$CH$_3$	Inactive as opioid agonist or antagonist
—CH$_2$CH$_2$CH$_2$CH$_2$CH$_3$ —CH$_2$CH$_2$CH$_2$CH$_2$CH$_2$CH$_3$	Opioid antagonist activity increased
—CH$_2$CH$_2$⬡	14X potency of morphine

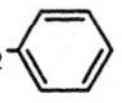

Fig. 2.31. Effect of alkyl chain length on activity of morphine.

can participate in steric or electronic intramolecular interactions (e.g., hydrogen, ion-dipole or ion-ion bonds). Ring substituents influence the conformations of adjacent substituents via steric interactions and may significantly affect receptor interactions. The observation that aromatic methoxy groups ortho to two other substituents take on a conformation perpendicular to the plane of the aromatic ring in hallucinogenic phenylalkylamines was used to explain the lack of hallucinogenic activity in these compounds (Fig. 2.32) by Knittel and Makriyannis (27).

FUNCTIONAL GROUP MODIFICATION: ISOSTERISM AND BIOISOSTERISM
Isosterism

When a lead compound is first discovered for a particular disease state, it often lacks the required potency and pharmacokinetic properties suitable for making it a viable clinical candidate. These may include undesirable side effects, physicochemical properties that limit bioavailability and adverse metabolic or excretion properties. These undesirable properties could be due to specific functional groups present in the molecule. The medicinal chemist therefore must modify the compound to reduce or elimi-

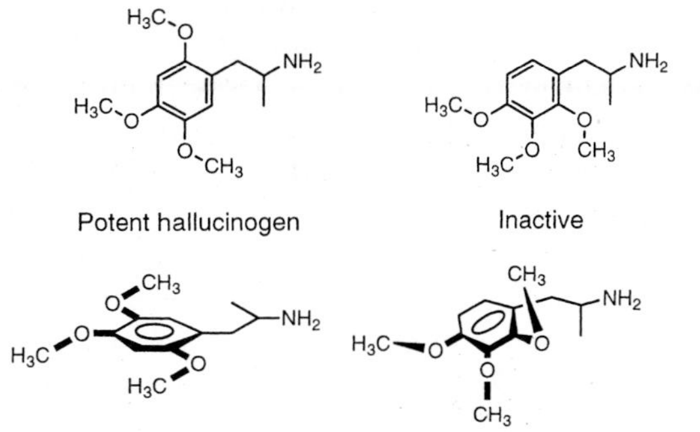

Fig. 2.32. Effect of positional isomers on structural conformation and biologic acitivity.

Table 2.7. Comparison of Physical Properties of N$_2$O and CO$_2$

Property	N$_2$O	CO$_2$
Viscosity at 20°C	148 × 10^{-6}	148 × 10^{-6}
Density of liquid at +10°C	0.856	0.858
Refractive index of liquid, D line 16°C	1.193	1.190
Dielectric constant of liquid at 0°C	1.593	1.582
Solubility in alcohol at 15°C	3.250	3.130

nate these undesirable features without losing the desired biological activity. Replacement or modification of functional groups with other groups having similar properties is known as isosteric or bioisosteric replacement.

In 1919, Langmuir first developed the concept of chemical isosterism to describe the similarities in physical properties among atoms, functional groups, radicals, and molecules (28,29). The similarities among atoms described by Langmuir primarily resulted from the fact that these atoms contained the same number of valence electrons and came from the same columns within the periodic table. This concept was limited to elements in adjacent rows and columns, inorganic molecules, ions and small organic molecules such as diazomethane and ketene. Table 2.7 shows a comparison of the physical properties of N$_2$O and CO$_2$ to illustrate Langmuir's concept.

To account for similarities between groups with the same number of valence electrons but different numbers of atoms, Grimm (30) developed his hydride displacement law. However, this is not a "law" in the strict sense, but more of an illustration of similar physical properties among closely related functional groups. Table 2.8 presents an example of hydride displacement. Descending diagonally from left to right in the table H atoms are progressively added to maintain the same number of valence electrons for each group of atoms within a column. Within each column the groups are considered to be "pseudoatoms" with respect to one another. Thus, NH$_2$ is considered to be isosteric to OH, etc. This early view of isosterism did not consider the actual location, motion, and resonance of electrons within the orbitals of these functional group replacements. Careful observation of this table reveals that some groups do share similar physical and chemical properties, but others have very different properties despite having the same number of valence electrons. For example, OH and NH$_2$ do share similar hydrogen bonding properties and should therefore be interchangeable if that is the only criterion necessary. But, the NH$_2$ group is basic whereas the OH is neutral. Hence, at

Table 2.8. Grimm's Hydride Displacement "Law"

C	N	O	F	Ne
	CH	NH	OH	FH
		CH$_2$	NH$_2$	OH$_2$
			CH$_3$	NH$_3$

physiological pH the NH₂ group would impart a positive charge to the molecule. If OH is being substituted by NH₂ the additional positive charge could have a significant effect on the overall physico-chemical properties of the molecule in which it is being introduced. The difference in physical chemical properties of the CH_3 group relative to the OH and NH₂ groups is even greater. In addition to basicity and acidity, this "law" fails to take into account other important physical chemical parameters such as electronegativity, polarizability, bond angles, size, shape of molecular orbitals, electron density, and partition coefficients which all contribute significantly to the overall physicochemical properties of a molecule.

Instead of considering only partial structures Hinsberg (31) applied the concept of isosterism to entire molecules. He developed the concept of "ring equivalents"; groups that can be exchanged for one another in aromatic ring systems without drastic changes in physical chemical properties relative to the parent structure. Benzene, thiophene and pyridine illustrate this concept (Fig. 2.33). A $-CH=CH-$ group in benzene is replaced by the divalent sulfur, $-S-$ in thiophene and a $-CH=$ is replaced by the trivalent $-N=$ to give pyridine. The physical properties of benzene and thiophene are very similar. For example, the boiling point of benzene is 81.1°C and that of thiophene is 84.4°C (at 760 mmHg). Pyridine, however, deviates with a boiling point of 115–116°C. Hinsberg therefore concluded that divalent sulfur (-S- or thioether) must resemble $-C=C-$ in shape and these groups were considered to be isosteric. Note that hydrogen atoms are ignored in this comparison. Today this isosteric relationship is seen in many drugs, e.g., H₁-receptor antagonists (Fig. 2.33).

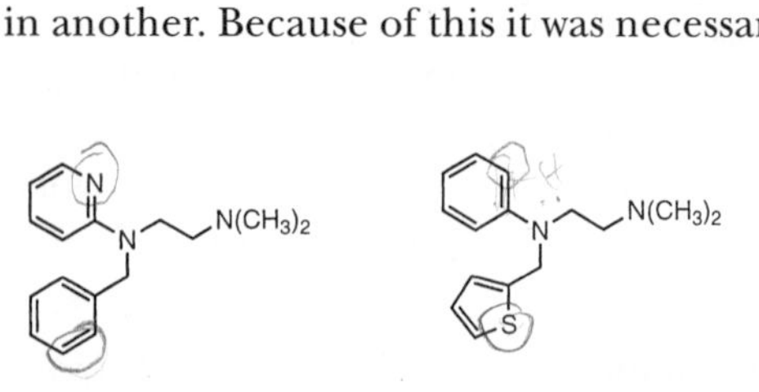

Bioisosterism

It is difficult to relate biological properties to physicochemical properties of individual atoms, functional groups or entire molecules because many physical and chemical parameters are involved simultaneously and are therefore difficult to quantitate. Simple relationships as described above often do not hold up across the many types of biological systems seen with medicinal agents. That is, what may work as an isosteric replacement in one biological system (or a given drug receptor) may not in another. Because of this it was necessary to introduce the term "bioisosterism" to describe functional groups related in structure and having similar biological effects. Friedman introduced the term bioisosterism and defined it as: "Bioisosteres are (functional) groups or molecules that have chemical and physical similarities producing broadly similar biological properties." (32) Recently Burger expanded this definition to take into account biochemical views of biological activity: "Bioisosteres are compounds or groups that possess near equal molecular shapes and volumes, approximately the same distribution of electrons, and which exhibit similar physical properties such as hydrophobicity. Bioisosteric compounds affect the same biochemically associated systems as agonist or antagonists and thereby produce biological properties that are related to each other." (33) The key point is that the same pharmacologic target is influenced by bioisoteres as agonists or antagonists. What may work as a bioisosteric group in one biological system (or receptor) may not have similar effects on another.

Classical and Nonclassical Bioisosteres

Bioisosteric groups can be subdivided into two categories: Classical and nonclassical bioisosteres. Functional groups that satisfy the original conditions of Langmuir and Grimm are referred to as classical bioisosteres. Nonclassical bioisosteres do not obey steric and electronic definitions of classical bioisoteres and do not necessarily have the same number of atoms as the substituent they replace. A wider set of compounds and functional groups are encompassed by nonclassical bioisoteres which produce, at the molecular level, qualitatively similar agonist or antagonist responses. In animals, many hormones, neurotransmitters etc. with very similar structures and biological actions can be classified as bioisosteres. An example would be the insulins isolated from various mammalian species. Even though these insulins may differ by several amino acid residues, they still produce the same biological effects. If this did not occur, the use of insulin to treat diabetes would have had to wait another 60 years for recombinant DNA technology to allow production of human insulin.

What may be a successful bioisosteric replacement for a given molecule interacting with a particular receptor in one instance, quite often has no effect or abolishes biological activity in another system. Thus, the use of bioisosteric replacement (classical or nonclassical) in drug design is highly dependent upon the biological system being investigated. No hard and fast rules exist to determine what bioisosteric replacement is going to work with a given molecule, although as the following tables and examples demonstrate, some generalizations have been possible. However, the medicinal chemist still must rely on experience and intuition in order to decide the best approach to be used when applying this strategy.

Tripelennamine   Methaphenilene

Fig. 2.33. Isosteric substitution of thiophene for benzene and benzene for pyridine.

Table 2.9. Classical Bioisosteres (Groups Within the Row Can Replace Each Other)

Monovalent bioisosteres
  F, H
  OH, NH
  F, OH, NH or CH$_3$ for H
  SH, OH
  Cl, Br, CF$_3$

Divalent bioisosteres
  $-C=S$, $-C=O$, $-C=NH$, $-C=C-$

Trivalent atoms or groups
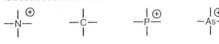

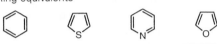

Tetrasubstituted atoms

$$-\overset{\underset{|}{|}}{N}\overset{\oplus}{} \quad -\overset{\underset{|}{|}}{C}- \quad -\overset{\underset{|}{|}}{P}\overset{\oplus}{} \quad -\overset{\underset{|}{|}}{As}-$$

Ring equivalents

Each category of bioisostere can be further subdivided as shown below, and examples are provided in Table 2.9:

  I. Classical Bioisosteres
    A. Monovalent atoms and groups
    B. Divalent atoms and groups
    C. Trivalent atoms and groups
    D. Tetrasubstituted atoms
    E. Ring equivalents
  II. Nonclassical Bioisosteres
    A. Exchangeable groups
    B. Rings versus noncyclic structure

Classical Bioisoteres

Substitution of hydrogen by fluorine is one of the most common monovalent isosteric replacements. Sterically hydrogen and fluorine are quite similar with their van der Waal's radii being 1.2 and 1.35 Å, respectively. Since fluorine is the most electronegative element in the periodic table, any differences in biological activity resulting from replacement of hydrogen with fluorine can be attributed to this property. A classical example of hydrogen replacement by fluorine is development of the antineoplastic agent 5-fluorouracil from uracil.

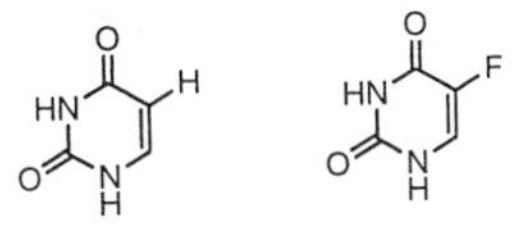

Another example is shown in Figure 2.34 where the chlorine of chlorothiazide has been replaced with

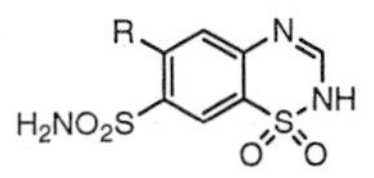

R =	Cl	Br	CF$_3$
σ	+0.23	+0.23	+0.54
π	+0.71	+0.86	+0.88
E_s	−0.97	−1.16	−2.40

Fig. 2.34. Isosteric replacement of Cl in thiazide diuretics. Comparison of physical chemical properties of the substituents.

bromine and a trifluoromethyl group. For each of the substitutions the electronic (σ, where σ^+ is electron withdrawing; σ^- electron donating) and hydrophobic (π) properties of each group are maintained relatively constant while the size of each group varies significantly as indicated by the Taft steric parameter (E_s).

Figure 2.35 shows an example of classical isosteric substitution of an amino for hydroxyl group in folic acid. The amino group is capable of mimicking the tautomeric forms of folic acid and providing the appropriate hydrogen bonds to the enzyme active site.

A tetravalent bioisosteric replacement study was done by Grisar et al. (33) with a series of α-tocopherol analogues (Fig. 2.36). α-Tocopherol has been shown to scavenge lipoperoxyl and superoxide radicals and to accumulate in heart tissue. This is thought to be part of its mechanism of action for reducing cardiac damage due to myocardial infarction. All of the bioisosteric analogues were found to produce similar biological activity.

Nonclassical Bioisoteres

As mentioned earlier, nonclassical bioisosteres are replacements of functional groups not defined by classical definitions. Some of these groups though mimic spatial arrangements, electronic properties or some other physicochemical property of the molecule or functional group crit-

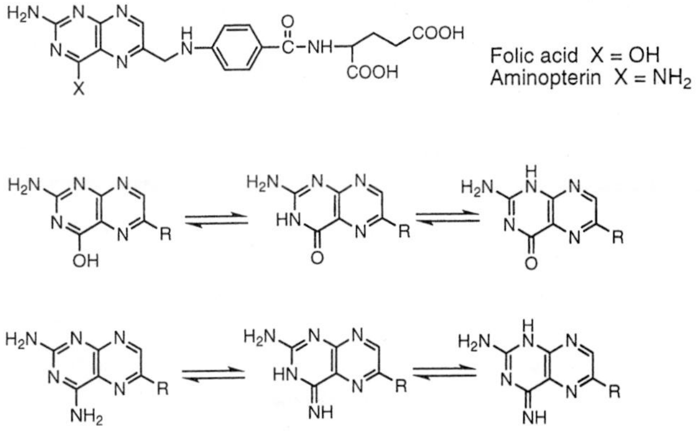

Folic acid X = OH
Aminopterin X = NH$_2$

Fig. 2.35. Isosteric replacement of OH by NH$_2$ in folic acid and possible tautomers of folic acid and aminopterin.

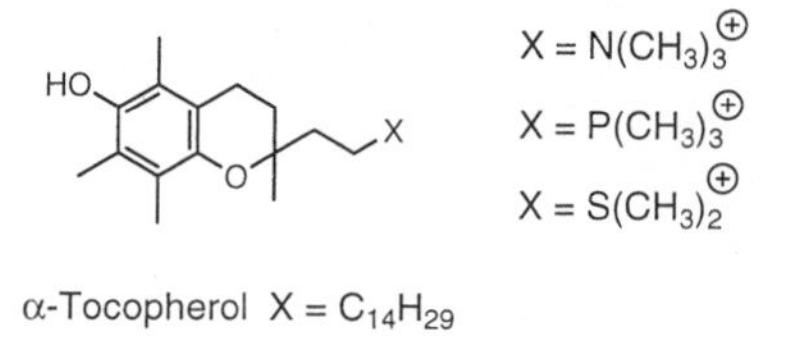

α-Tocopherol X = C₁₄H₂₉

X = N(CH₃)₃⊕
X = P(CH₃)₃⊕
X = S(CH₃)₂⊕

α-Tocopherol X = C₁₄H₂₉

Fig. 2.36. Tetravalent bioisoseres of α-tocopherol.

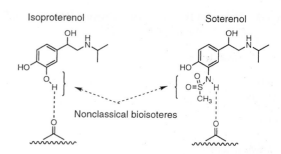

Fig. 2.38. Bioisosteric replacement of m-OH of isoproterenol with a sulfonamido group and similar hydrogen bonding capacity to a possible drug receptor.

ical for biological activity. One example is the use of a double bond to position essential functional groups into a particular spatial configuration critical for activity. This is shown with the naturally occurring hormone estradiol and the synthetic analog diethylstilbestrol in Figure 2.37. The trans isomer of diethylstilbestrol has approximately the same potency as estradiol while the cis isomer is only one-fourteenth as active. In the trans configuration the phenolic hydroxy groups mimic the correct orientation of the phenol and alcohol in estradiol (34,35). This is not possible with the cis isomer and more flexible analogs (Fig. 2.37) have little or no activity (36,37).

Another example of a nonclassical replacement is that of a sulfonamide group for a phenol in catecholamines (Fig. 2.38). With this example steric factors appear to have less influence on receptor binding than acidity and hydrogen bonding potential of the functional group on the aromatic ring. Both the phenolic hydroxyl of isoproterenol and the acidic proton of the arylsulfonamide have nearly the same pK_a values of approximately 10 (38). Both groups are weakly acidic and capable of losing a proton and interacting with the receptor as anions or participating as hydrogen bond donors at the receptor as shown in Figure 2.38). Since the replacement is not susceptible to metabolism by catechol O-methyltransferase, this replacement also has the added advantage of increasing the duration of action and making the compound orally active. Other examples of successful bioisosteric replacements are shown in Table 2.10 and a more detailed description of the role of biosisosterism can be found in the review by Patani and LaVoie (39).

SUMMARY

Medicinal chemistry involves the discovery of new chemical entities for the treatment of disease and the systematic study of the structure activity relationships of these compounds. Such studies provide the basis for development of better medicinal agents from lead compounds found via random screening, systematic screening and rational design. The role of the medicinal chemist is that of increasing the potency and duration of action of newly discovered compounds as well as decreasing adverse side effects. Without a thorough understanding of the physical chemical properties of the organic functional groups that comprise any given structure the task would be impossible.

For the pharmacist it is also important to understand the physical and chemical properties of the medicinal agents that he/she is dispensing. Not only will such knowledge help the practicing pharmacist to better understand the clinical properties of these compounds, but also to anticipate the properties of new agents that appear on the market. An understanding of the chemical properties of the molecule will allow the pharmacist to anticipate formulation problems (especially IV admixtures) as well as potential adverse interactions with other drugs as the result of serum protein binding and metabolism.

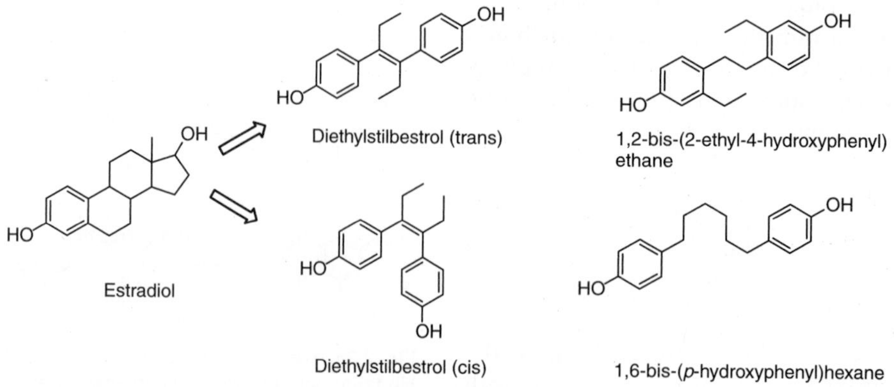

Diethylstilbestrol (trans)

1,2-bis-(2-ethyl-4-hydroxyphenyl) ethane

Estradiol

Diethylstilbestrol (cis)

1,6-bis-(p-hydroxyphenyl)hexane

Fig. 2.37. Noncyclic analogs of estradiol.

Table 2.10. Nonclassical Bioisosteric Replacements

Compound	Bioisosteric Replacement	Reference
		40
		41
		42
		43
		44
		45
		46

Problems

The following problems are provided for additional study:

1. Calculate the percent ionization of amobarbital at pH 2.0, 5.5 and 8.0. What trend is seen?

2. Calculate the percent ionization of phenyl-propanolamine at pH 2.0, 5.5 and 8.0. Compare these results with those obtained in Problem 1.

3. Calculate the percent ionization of sulfacetamide in the stomach, duodenum and ileum. Draw the structure of the predominate form of the drug in each tissue.

4. Referring to Figure 2.15, redraw each compound in its ionized form.

5. For the organic functional groups listed in Table 2.4, name each functional group and redraw them showing all potential hydrogen bonds with water.

6. Using the empiric method of Lemke, predict the water solubility for each of the following molecules. Note: Water solubility is defined as >1% solubility.

Aspirin	Carphenazine Maleate
Chlordiazepoxide	Codeine
Codeine Phosphate	Cyproheptadine Hydrochloride
Haloperidol	Phenytoin

7. Calculate the logP value for each of the following: Aspirin, Carphenazine, Codeine, Cyproheptadine, Haloperidol, Chlordiazepoxide, Phenytoin.

8. Using the Merck Index, find the chemical structures for the following empirical formulae. List as many physical chemical properties as possible for each compound and compare them within each group of isomers.

$C_4H_{10}O_2$ C_5H_8O
$C_5H_{11}O_2$ $C_7H_7NO_2$ $C_8H_8O_2$
$C_{12}H_{17}NO_3$
$C_{20}H_{30}O_2$

9. Using the Cahn-Ingold-Prelog rules, assign the absolute configuration to each chiral center of ephedrine and pseudoephedrine (Figure 2.21).

10. For the compounds shown in Figure 2.22 indicate, using an *, where the chiral centers are in each molecule.

11. Draw each possible stereoisomer for chloramphenicol and enalapril. Assign the absolute stereochemistry to each chiral center.

12. I. Draw the Newman projection along the CH_3-N bond of acetylcholine in the staggered conformation. Rotate the bond 120° and 240°. Are these rotameters conformational isomers? Explain why or why not.

     II. Repeat the above exercise with the N1–C2 bond of acetylcholine.

13. Draw the three most stable rotamers of norepinephrine. Of these rotamers, is there the possibility of an intramolecular interaction that would stabilize what would normally be considered to be an unstable rotameter? Explain.

CASE STUDY

Victoria F. Roche and S. William Zito

JO, a 57-year-old male executive, arrives at the pharmacy from his annual physical with refills for his blood pressure medications (Enalapril and Amlopidine) and a new prescription for Pepcid. He wants to know if he can take all three medications at the same time.

1. Complete the table below considering all three of the drug molecules.

Famotidine
(Pepcid)

Enalapril
(Vasotec)

Amlopidine
(Norvasc)

	Amine/Guanidine	Ketone	Carboxylic Acid	Amide
Which drug(s) contain this functional group?				
Hydrophobic or hydrophilic in character?				
Acidic, basic, or neutral as drawn				
Types of interactions possible with target for drug action				
Is this group a H-bond donor, H-bond acceptor, both or neither?				

2. Pepcid (famotidine; pKa = 10.5) is sold as a hydrochloride salt. Is the molecule as drawn acidic, basic or neutral? Given that Pepcid decreases the secretion of acid into the lumen of the stomach (stomach pH = 3.5 in presence of Pepcid), will Pepcid be ionized or unionized in the stomach?

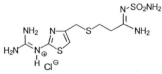

Famotidine hydrochloride

3. Considering the structural features of enalapril and amlodipine, determine the ionization state of each of these agents in the stomach (pH = 1) in the absence of Pepcid and in the presence of Pepcid (pH = 3.5). Use pKa = 9 for all aliphatic amines and pKa = 3 for all carboxylic acids.

4. Would you recommend that this patient take all three of these medications at the same time? Provide a brief rationale for your recommendation.

5. Enalapril is not administered as the active drug. It is readily hydrolyzed in the stomach to the active drug. Draw all of the products of hydrolysis.

CASE STUDY

Acid/Base Chemistry, Solubility and Absorption Case

Timoptic and Xalatan are agents that are used in the treatment of glaucoma. They are both dispensed as aqueous eye drops and the target for drug action for both drugs is a receptor in the eye.

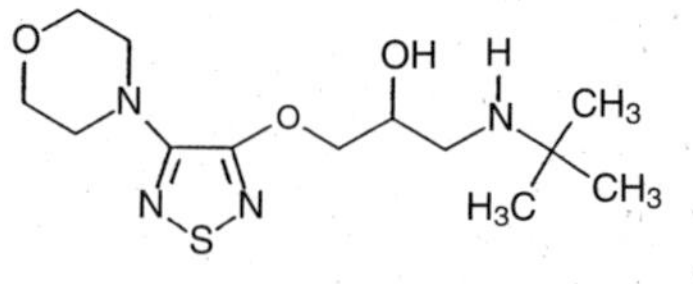

Timolol
(Timoptic)

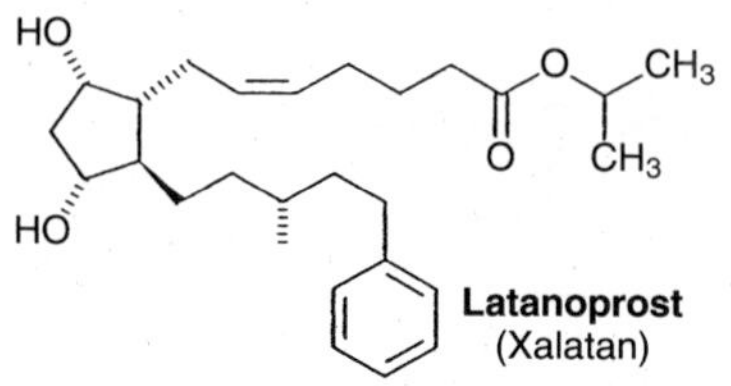

Latanoprost
(Xalatan)

1. *What is the acid/base character of Lantanoprost as drawn?*

   Circle One: ACID   BASE   NEUTRAL

2. *What is the acid/base character of Timolol as drawn?*

   Circle One: ACID   BASE   NEUTRAL

3. *Timolol is actually formulated as a water-soluble salt of maleic acid. Modify the structure below to show the salt form (ionized form) of timolol. Clearly identify the acid/base character of the salt form of this drug.*

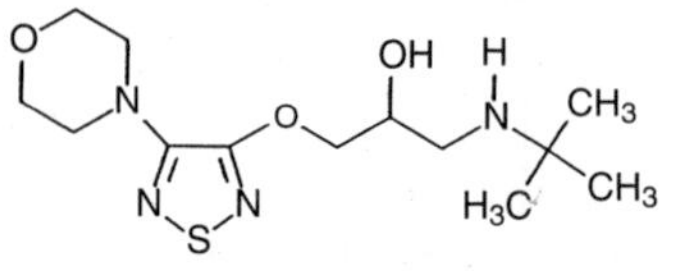

Timolol
(Timoptic)

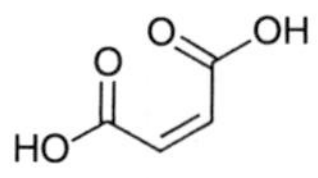

Maleic Acid

4. *Which of the functional groups in each of these drug molecules enhance the water solubility of these drugs?*

5. *Which of these two agents would you expect to be more hydrophobic and therefore more readily absorbed into the eye? Provide a structural rationale for your answer.*

6. *One of these agents is readily hydrolyzed and cannot be delivered orally. Which agent is unstable? Draw the products of hydrolysis.*

REFERENCES

1. Crum-Brown A, Fraser TR. Trans. Roy. Soc. Edinburgh 1869;25: 151.
2. Loewi O, Navrati E. Plugers Arch. Ges. Physiol. Menshen Tiere 1926;214: 689.
3. Ariëns EJ. A General Introduction to the Field of Drug Discovery. In: Ariëns EJ, ed. Drug Design, New York, Academic Press, 1971;1: 1–270.
4. Ehrlich P. In: Himmelweit F, ed. Collected Papers of Paul Ehrlich, London, Pergamon, 1957.
5. Albert A. The Long Search for Valid Structure-Action Relationships in Drugs. J. Med. Chem. 1982;25: 1–5.
6. Ing HR. Physiol. Rev. 1936;16: 527.
7. Woods DD. Br. J. Exp. Pathol. 1940;21: 74.
8. Piutti A. Compt. Red. 1886; 103: 134–138.
9. Shinkai JH, Gennaro AR. Organic Pharmaceutical Chemistry. In: Gennaro AR, ed. Remington's Pharmaceutical Sciences, Easton, Mack Publishing Company, 1990; 356–378.
10. Lemke TL. Review of Organic Functional Groups: Introduction to Medicinal Organic Chemistry. 3rd ed. Philadelphia: Lea & Febiger, 1992.
11. Cates, LA. Calculation of Drug Solubilities by Pharmacy Students. Amer. J. Pharm. Ed. 1981;45; 11–13.
12. Fujita T. The Extrathermodynamic Approach to Drug Design. In: Hansch C, ed. Comprehensive Medicinal Chemsitry, New York, Pergamon Press, 1990; 4: 497–560.
13. Tute MS. Principles and Practice of Hansch Analysis: A Guide to Structure-Activity Correlation for the Medicinal Chemist. In: Harper NJ, Simons AB, eds. Advances in Drug Research, London, Academic Press, 1971; 6: 1–77.
14. Hansch C, Leo A. Substituent Constants for Correlation Analysis in Chemistry and Biology. New York: John Wiley, 1979.
15. Hansch C, Leo A. Exploring QSAR: Hydrophobic, Electronic and Steric Constants, Washington, D.C.: American Chemical Society, 1995.
16. MacLogP v2.0.0, BioByte Corp., Claremont, CA
17. Pruitti A. Compt. Red. 1886; 103: 134–138.
18. Easson LH, Stedman E. Studies on the Relationship Between Chemical Constitution and Physiological Action. V. Molecular Dissymmetry and Physiological Activity. Biochem. J. 1933; 27: 1257.
19. Blackwood JE, Gladys CL, Loening KL, et al. J. Amer. Chem. Soc. 1968; 90: 509–510.
20. Kemp JD, Pitzer KS. Hindered Rotation of the Methyl Groups in Ethane. J. Chem. Phys. 1936; 4: 749.
21. Bovet D. C.R. Soc. Biol. (Paris). 1937; 124: 547.
22. Laboit H, et al. Presse Med. 1952; 60: 206.
23. Charpentier P, et al. C.R. Acad. Sci. (Paris). 1952; 325: 59.
24. Delay J, et al. Ann. Med. Psychol. (Paris). 1952; 110: 112.
25. McCawley EL, Hart ER, Marsh DF. J. Amer. Chem. Soc. 1941; 63: 314.
26. Clark RL, Pessolano AA, Weijlard J, et al. J. Amer. Chem. Soc. 1953; 75: 4964.
27. Knittel JJ, Makriyannis A. Studies on Phenethylamine Hallucinogens. 2. Conformations of Arylmethoxyl Groups Using 13C NMR. J. Med. Chem. 1981; 24: 906–909.
28. Langmuir I. J. Amer. Chem. Soc. 1919; 41: 868.
29. Langmuir I. J. Amer. Chem. Soc. 1919; 41: 1543.
30. Grimm HG. Z Elekrochemie. 1925; 31: 474.
31. Hinsberg O. J. Prakt. Chem. 1916; 93: 302.
32. Friedman HL. Symposium on Chemical-Biological Correlation. Natl. Acad. Sci. Natl. Res. Council, publ. No. 206, Washington, D.C., 1951, p. 295.
33. Burger A. Isosterism and Bioisosterism in Drug Design. Progress in Drug Research. 1991; 37: 288–371.
34. Grisar JM, Marciniak G, Bolkenius FN, et al. Cardioselective Ammonium, Phosphonium and Sulfonium Analogues of α-Tocopherol and Ascorbic Acid That Inhibit in Vitro and ex Vivo Lipid Peroxidation and Scavange Superoxide Radicals. J. Med. Chem. 1995; 38: 2880–2886.
35. Dodds EC, et al. Nature 1938; 141:247.
36. Walton E, Brownlee G. Nature 1943; 151; 305.
37. Blanchard EW, et al. Endocrinology. 1943; 32: 307.
38. Baker BR. J. Amer. Chem. Soc. 1943; 65: 1572.
39. Larsen AA, Gould WA, Roth HR, et al. Sulfonanilides. II. Analogs of Catecholamines. J. Med. Chem. 1967; 10: 462–472.
40. Patani GA, LaVoie EJ. Bioisosterism: A Rational Approach in Drug Design. Chem. Rev. 1996; 96: 3147–3176.
41. Watthey JWH, Desai M, Rutledge R, et al. J. Med. Chem. 1980; 23: 690.
42. Krause JL. Pharmacol. Res. Comm. 1983; 15: 119.
43. Macchia B, Balsamo A, Lapucci A, et al. Molecular Design, Synthesis and Anti-inflammatory Activity of a Series of β-Aminoxyproionic Acids. J. Med. Chem. 1990; 33: 1423–1430.
44. Street LJ, Baker R, Book T, et al. Synthesis and Biological Activity of 1,2,4-oxadiazole Derivatives: Highly Potent and Efficacious Agonists for Cortical Muscarinic Receptors. J. Med. Chem. 1990; 33: 2690–2697.
45. Wolff Me, Zanati G. J. Med. Chem. 1969; 12: 629.
46. Schaeffer HJ, et al. J. Pharm. Sci. 1964; 53: 1368.
47. Sawyer TK, Sanfilippo PJ, Hruby VJ, et al. 4-Norleucine, 7-D-phenylalanine-α-melanocyte-stimulating hormone: A Highly Potent α-Melanotropin with Ultralong Biological Activity. Proc. Natl. Acad. Sci. USA.1980; 77: 5754–5758.

3. Molecular Modeling and Drug Design

ERIC BILLINGS

INTRODUCTION

Historically, molecular modeling described software for the visualization of molecular structures. The ability to visualize molecules has proven to be such a convenient starting point for new software that the scope of molecular modeling has expanded dramatically. Over the past two decades, the term molecular modeling has expanded to include: visualizing two and three-dimensional structures; organizing many compounds and their properties into databases; providing tools for analyzing molecular properties; or simulating the behavior of molecules on an atomic level. The diverse molecular modeling packages have converged to offer a core of similar capabilities for manipulating molecules. They differ in their user interfaces and level of sophistication. Several have specialized functions for fields such as synthesis, toxicology, or structure determination using X-ray crystallography or NMR.

The first pharmaceutical successes in molecular modeling were in the 1980s as hundreds of X-ray crystallographic structures for drug leads and their target proteins became available. The expectations for molecular modeling were quite high based on these early successes of rational drug design and structural biology. It is perhaps not surprising that no single tool or technique can be a complete solution for drug development and molecular modeling has taken its place as another set of instruments for the elucidation of a drug's mechanism of action and in the design of the next, better therapeutic agent.

Molecular modeling is limited by the practical constraints of today's computers. If it were possible to build an infinitely fast computer a ligand's interaction with a large target could be computed with experimental accuracy or better. However, with today's computers, it is easy to pose a question that would take thousands of years to compute. Fortunately, there are many questions relevant to drug development that may be addressed today by selecting the right molecular modeling tool. Since computers double in speed every year and a half, computational tools continue to evolve as larger problems become tractable.

Studies undertaken with modern computational techniques may be organized along the three axes of molecular modeling (Figure 3.1). The first axis is simply the size of the system such as the number of atoms. The second axis is the accuracy, or resolution with which we wish to determine the result. The third axis is the time it takes for the event under study to occur. Since a finite amount of computer time exists, increasing the study along any one axis will force a trade-off along the other two.

To understand the first two axes, consider the preferred conformation of Penicillin-G (see Fig. 3.2), a typical β-lactam antibiotic. Since Penicillin-G is relatively small it's preferred conformation can be determined with high accuracy in a short amount of computer time. Expanding the system size of our study to include a series of β-lactams we might arrive at the limit of what we can compute in the time we're willing to wait. If we wanted to extend the system size further and examine the bound conformations of the β-lactam series to a β-lactamase (a system of roughly 50,000 atoms) we would have to reduce the accuracy to complete the calculations in a timely fashion. If the study were expanded still further to estimate the binding constant for each of 100,000 test compounds to the β-lactamase less accuracy would be possible. In this case, only a qualitative result with approximate ranking of the binding constants is currently possible.

The third axis of molecular modeling, the time it takes for an event to occur, poses several complications. For now, consider that a snapshot of the behavior of a system at one instant is fast and easy to compute.

However, catalysis, ligand binding and diffusion occur on the pico-, nano- and micro-second times scale. Simulating how a system evolves over these time scales adds up to millions or billions of snapshots to be computed and that can be prohibitive amount of computer time. Since a finite amount of computer time is available, studies of systems that evolve over time will require trade-offs in system size and accuracy. Events occurring over milli-seconds or more are currently beyond high-resolution techniques. Advanced computational chemistry methods have been developed to tackle many of the combinations of system size, accuracy and time scales. They are based on the principles of thermodynamics that capture the properties and behavior of molecules. That is, they approximate the free energy of the system mathematically and then derive the property or behavior of interest. These are combined with simulation, sampling and screening techniques to exam-

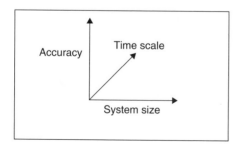

Fig. 3.1. Three axes of molecular modeling.

ine a compound's conformations or the effects of different functional groups.

There are several pitfalls to computational chemistry. Software packages are marketed to simplify our work by providing extensive default choices. It is relatively easy to construct a calculation using these defaults that is incapable of providing a meaningful result. It is the responsibility of the practitioner to determine the appropriate method for the quality of the result needed. A second pitfall is to over interpret the results. Little effort is made in most packages to provide error analysis. A good application of computational chemistry techniques ensures that a level of accuracy appropriate to the question is used and balances the amount of computer time necessary with the importance of the result. An appreciation of molecular modeling and its pitfalls requires an understanding of the fundamentals presented in this chapter.

This chapter is designed to encourage readers to use molecular modeling software and to appreciate its usefulness and pitfalls. It first reviews the visualization of molecules and their properties. This is easy and immediately useful. A review of the physical principles is provided to illustrate the mathematical basis underlying the subsequent computational techniques. The balance of the chapter is organized along the chemistry are introduced, followed by molecular mechanics and structure activity relationships. Techniques that allow an examination of events that evolve over time are then introduced including molecular dynamics and sampling. Sampling techniques approximate the effects of time and can be faster to compute. They include methods such as Monte Carlo techniques for ligand docking and other screening methods.

VISUALIZING MOLECULES AND THEIR PROPERTIES

Molecular modeling software enabled scientists to visualize the compounds they worked with as early as the 1970s. Although the early versions only displayed black and white pictures of the atoms within small compounds, it was a powerful tool for developing a mental model of a compound and its properties. Now, modern computers with specialized software allow scientists to literally step inside a room and view a virtual display of a biological system of interest. Interactive devices allow scientists to virtually "push" a ligand into its target's active site to develop a better understanding of its interaction. However, most molecular modeling is done with a stand-alone workstation or PC using commercial or freely available software. The fundamental approach to displaying molecules and their properties is the same for all molecular modeling software. This section reviews the mechanics of visualization and then several applications of interest.

Mechanics of Visualization

The graphic display of molecules and their properties is accomplished by dividing a complex display into small parts. The smallest parts of graphics are called primitives and consist of points, vectors and polygons.

Polygons are planar and have three or more sides. They are the building blocks for more complex surfaces. Within the graphics workstation or PC, they are individually assigned coordinates that define their shape and position. Molecular modeling software combines three primitives into "objects" such as atoms, bonds, or surfaces such as those depicting helices in proteins or a complex binding pocket. The final display observed may be built up of hundreds or thousands of objects that in turn represent thousands or millions of graphic primitives. Fortunately, a variety of software has already been developed with sophisticated interfaces that can insulate the user from the details of computer graphics. However, an appreciation of the mechanics of modeling makes learning their use and mastering their full power easier (Fig. 3.2).

A comfortable, intuitive user interface depends on the ability to create, modify and move several independent objects such as a ligand and its target. An abstract world containing the ligand and its target is built up of graphical primitives through a series of coordinate systems and transformations. First, the primitives necessary for the overall display are given individual coordinate systems. Points, vectors and polygons are defined to form specific shape (Figure 3.3). Second, these are transformed to the next level of object space to construct bonds and atoms. A transformation is a mathematical operation for changing the coordinates of all the vertices of primitives at once. Matrices are used to perform the individual transformations because computers are very efficient at performing them and they may be combined to reduce the overall work required. In the third operation, each molecule is defined by transforming the coordinates of its nuclei to their relative position within the molecule's object space. Changes to the atoms' relative positions, such as rotating atoms about a covalent bond, are accomplished within this "object space." Fourth, each of the molecules is transformed (rotated or translated) into a common "world" coordinate system. This transformation allows the individual molecules to be positioned relative to one another. Fifth, the transformation to "viewer" space is accomplished when the user selects which orientation of the overall system to look at. This transformation is what the user often defines when moving the displayed molecules with the mouse or dials. Sixth, the three-dimensional, transformed world coordinates are mapped to two-dimensional "display" coordinates. This transformation adds perspective so distant objects appear smaller or fainter to the user.

The display process may seem overly complicated with multiple coordinate systems and transformations. However, this approach has been developed for computers since the transformations are matrix operations that computer hardware can handle very efficiently. Since the

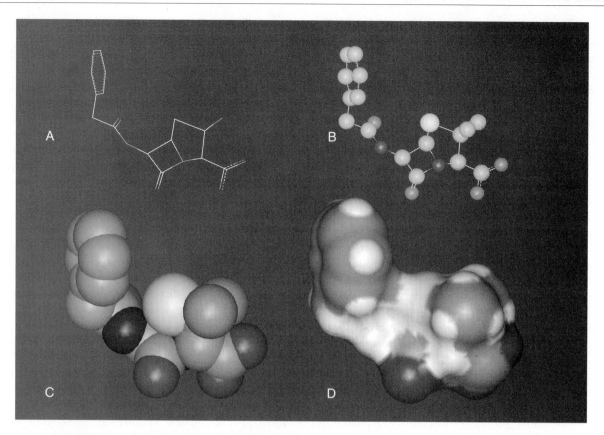

Fig. 3.2. Penicillin-G displayed with different levels of detail. Penicillin-G displayed using different representations (Clockwise from top left): (A) Stick display shows structure in a simple, nearly transparent form. (B) Ball and stick highlights atom placement and type. (C) CPK model shows the full van der Waals radii of the heavy atom. (D) The solvent accessible surface displays the surface of closest approach by other small molecules such as water. Coordinates for small molecules may be found on-line by searching a database to locate the compound of interest. The coordinates are often saved in a file format created for the Cambridge Crystal Database (1) or Brookhaven Protein Databank (2). Molecular modeling software will read in the atom types, labels and coordinates and prepare the data for display. These images are generated with Insight from Molecular Simulations, Incorporated.

transformations may be combined into a single operation, modern workstations can display systems and rotate them as quickly as the user can move the mouse or turn a dial. Since visualization is central to many areas of science and business, customized computer hardware has been specially developed to perform these operations quickly and efficiently. The interested reader may find several texts (3) on the subject of computer graphics.

Smooth motion of molecules on the display is accomplished when the computer generates enough discrete images to convince the human eye. The average person requires the motion to be broken into at least 30 images per second. High performance workstations have dedicated hardware called "geometry engines" specially designed to display large, complex systems fast enough to appear as smooth motion in real-time. Although desktop PCs have steadily increased in performance and can now display typical macromolecules, a high performance workstation is needed for real-time manipulation of a complex display such as a macromolecule, its surface and some associated properties.

In addition, modern workstations are able to generate a three-dimensional view of a complex display. The stereo-scopic effect (Fig 3.4) is achieved by presenting slightly different views to the left and right eye, mimicking our own binocular vision. This may be accomplished by displaying the images side by side or through the use of special glasses. Active LCD-type and passive polarized lenses (like those used at 3D movies) have been developed to improve the stereoscopic effect. Active glasses are synchronized with the display device that alternates between the display of the left and right eye images. When the left eye image is displayed the left eye lens is clear and the lens covering the right eye becomes opaque. Then, when the right eye image is displayed the left lens becomes opaque and the right eye lens becomes clear. The images are displayed more than 60 times per second so that each eye "sees" smooth motion.

Molecular Structures

The varieties of biological macromolecules targeted by therapeutic agents include proteins, nucleotides, and assemblies such as lipid bilayers or even highly specific compounds. Proteins and nucleotides frequently maintain a specific overall structure by first folding into local sub-domains. Diverse protein targets such as enzymes, genetic activating factors and membrane-bound receptors have common structural motifs that may be visualized to characterize the overall structure (Fig. 3.5.)

Proteins and nucleotides are a major focus in molecular modeling and a common vocabulary has been developed for describing their components and structures. The specific sequence of amino acid residues (or nucleotide bases) in the protein (or DNA or RNA) is termed the primary structure. The secondary structure is then defined as protein's local structure such as a stretch of 10 residues that form a helix. The tertiary structure is the overall arrangement of the secondary elements, such as group of helices. Quarternary structure is used to describe the interaction of the protein with its cofactors, substrates or other copies of itself that may assemble to form an active complex. The same terms are used to describe the structure of DNA and RNA even though they form different shapes.

Object space	Graphic primitives	points	vectors	polygons
Transformation	Build chemical entities			
Object space	Atoms, bonds, surfaces	atoms	bonds	surfaces
Transformation	Build chemical entities			
Object space	Molecules, surfaces			
Transformation	Set relative positions			
World space	All objects			
Transformation	Rotate, translate, zoom			
Viewer space	User's preferred view			
Transformation	Reduce 3D to 2D Add perspective			
Final 2D Display				

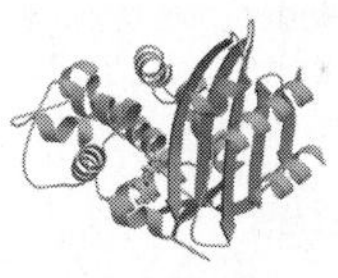

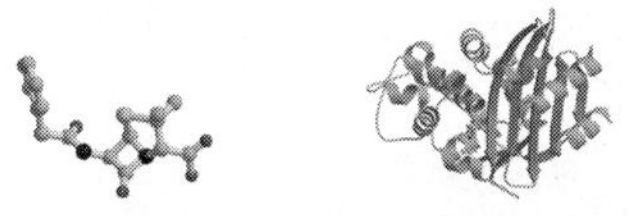

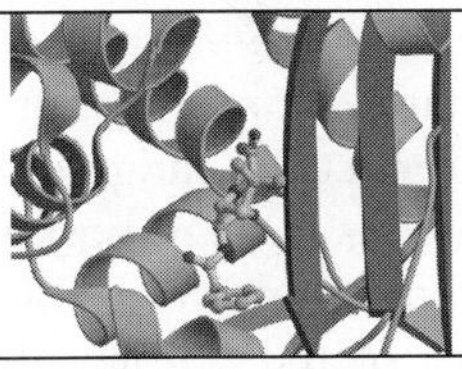

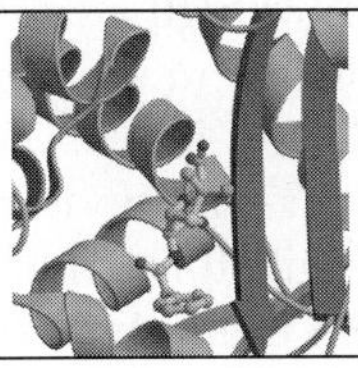

Fig. 3.3. Steps in Computer Graphics.

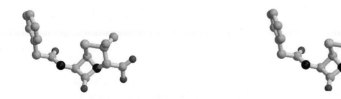
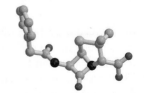

Fig. 3.4. Stereoscopic views of penicillin-G. A three-dimensional view of a molecule can be achieved by using two images. Three views of Penicillin-G are provided to illustrate different methods for stereo viewing. First, special viewers with mirrors may be placed over the page to direct different images to each eye to achieve a three-dimensional view. The "wall-eye" and "cross-eye" methods achieve the same result without the additional hardware. Try these two methods and then use the one that is most comfortable. For "wall-eye" viewing look between the left and center images and slowly focus the eyes further behind the paper until each eye is looking at its own image. Conversely, "cross-eye" viewing is accomplished by looking between the center and right images. Slowly cross the eyes until each eye is looking at its own image to achieve the three-dimensional view.

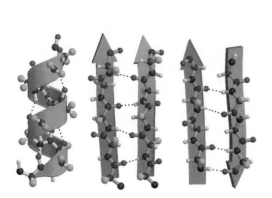

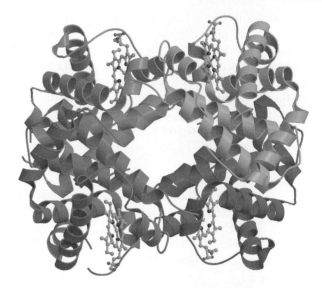

Fig. 3.5. *Visualizing macro-molecular structure. The secondary structural elements may be visualized using molecular modeling software. A typical α-helix; parallel β-sheet and antiparallel β-sheet are shown left to right. The hydrogen bonding patterns that stabilize each of these three motifs are shown with dashed lines. Secondary structural elements such as α-helices, β-strands and loops can be stylized to highlight their location within the overall tertiary structure. For example, the image of hemoglobin on the right shows the individual sub-units have the secondary structure of alpha helices. The relative position of the individual sub-units is the quaternary structure of hemoglobin. Hemoglobin's quaternary structure is a tetramer with four heme groups. These images were generated using freely available software called MolScript (4).*

Molecular Properties

Molecular modeling software offers several techniques beyond traditional graphs and tables of data. The properties of the molecules may be visualized in a number of ways. They may be mapped onto the surface of the molecule using colors to reflect the range of values of a property. For example, regions that are positively charged may be shown with different intensities of blue while negative regions are in shades of red. Other physical properties such as hydrophobicity could also be displayed. Non-physical properties such as how highly conserved the underlying residue is, or its similarity to another protein are often very informative as well. If a metric can be developed to characterize a property it may be displayed in three dimensions with the molecule for added insight.

Trypsin is an excellent example of the useful display of molecular properties (Figure 3.6). It is a serine protease that selectively cleaves the amide bond adjacent to a positively charged residue such as lysine or arginine. An evaluation of the electrostatics of its active site might provide some insight about its selectivity. A surface for the molecule was determined by computing the nearest approach of a water molecule to each atom. Some atoms are buried in the protein core and have no surface associated with them. Others are on the exterior of the protein and the solvent-accessible surfaces area for the individual atoms may be combined to construct a surface for the molecule. This molecular solvent-accessible surface (SAS) may then be colored, textured or modified to reflect the local value of a molecular property of interest.

The selectivity of trypsin is evident from the display of the electrostatic properties in its active site. The substrate protein lays in the groove extending from the lower left to the upper right. The catalytic serine is located just below the center of the image. The crystal structure included the protease-inhibitor, benzamidine, bound inside a negatively charged pocket adjacent to the serine. An amide bond is presented to the serine for hydrolysis when the R-group from the adjacent residue is positioned into the negatively charged pocket. The positively charged residues preferentially insert into the pocket that is now clearly negatively charged in the image. This selectively of this pocket for positively charged residues determines the specificity of trypsin.

BASIS OF COMPUTATIONAL CHEMISTRY

Molecular modeling provides a diverse set of computational techniques for analyzing both the form and function of molecules. In the previous section we examined how molecular modeling software can facilitate our understanding of the "form" of molecules by providing visualization tools. In this section, we will examine the computational tools used to understand and quantify the "function" of molecules. Accurate modeling of molecular behavior implies that the results reproduce experiment and establish trends that are in accord with the principles of thermodynamics. Successful tools have been implemented in several times by quantifying the specific interactions between molecules. A thorough appreciation for the basis of these tools in thermodynamics is the focus of this section.

The basis for molecular modeling and computational chemistry techniques is best understood within the framework of thermodynamics. The central aim of the various methods is to capture just enough of the chemistry of the system in an equation to be able to mathematically predict the behavior of some system of interest. If too much is included then the calculation takes too long or is intractable. If too little is included then the results may be incorrect or worse, misleading. Because energy plays such an important role in computational techniques a brief review of the basic tenets is appropriate. In this section we'll recap the underlying physics and the mathematical basis for many computational techniques.

A mathematical description of the energy of the system is the natural choice for many calculations. It embodies both the capacity of the system to do work and to respond to external forces. As an example, a peptide may respond to the electrostatic attraction of chymotrypsin by folding into its active site. The work of pepsin may be to hydrolyze the peptide bond. The energy of the system includes potential forms such as electrostatic attraction and the chemical energy stored in bonds. Kinetic forms of energy such as atomic vibration and electron motion are often included. Several successful and familiar forms of the expression for the energy are described in detail in the next section

ACCURACY AXIS: COMPUTING MOLECULAR BEHAVIOR

The use of an energetic description of the system has several advantages. First, the methods may be derived from experimental results. That is, the energy expressions may be calibrated with control systems before they are applied to some new system of interest. Second, the energy expression's level of detail may be systematically expanded to improve its accuracy. Conversely, it may be simplified to speed calculations for practical reasons. Third and perhaps most important, it allows the computational tools to be used in conjunction with established methods such as reaction rate theory and statistical mechanics.

Computational tools have theoretical and practical limits. It is possible to compute many properties and the evolution of a system, if its free energy may be computed and its initial conditions are known. The Heisenberg Uncertainty Principle places a theoretical limit on our knowledge of the initial position and momentum of all the particles. In a sense, computational methods differ in their level of approximations and each of these adds to errors. Chaos Theory, measurement and numerical errors place practical limits as well. However, with careful planning, their collective effects may be minimized and molecular modeling can be conducted within these limits with accurate results.

Free energy is a thermodynamic quantity that allows us to compare, quantitatively, the different possible configurations of a system. Free energy has two components, enthalpy and entropy. Enthalpy is a way of calculating the energy costs necessary to bring atoms together into one configuration. Entropy is a quantity that puts individual configurations into the perspective of all that are possible.

Enthalpy: A Numerical Snapshot of a Structure's Energy

The enthalpy of a system is the energy required to bring its components into a specific configuration. This may be written as:

$$H = U + PV$$

where H is the enthalpy, U is the internal energy of the system, P is the pressure and V is the volume. Consider a simple system consisting of a ball at the top of a hill (Figure 3.7). In freshman physics, we learned that the potential energy in this system is due to gravitation and is due to the attraction between the masses of the ball and the earth. The further the ball is from the center of mass of

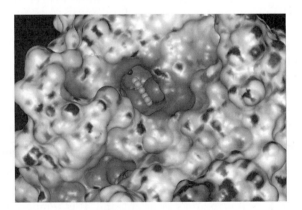
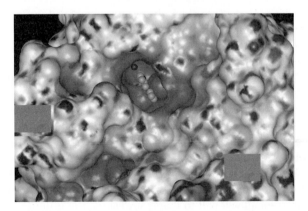

Fig. 3.6. Visualizing Molecular properties. The stereo image of the active site of trypsin was created using the molecular modeling software package Insight (5). Trypsin's three-dimensional structure was obtained from an X-ray crystallographic structure (6) downloaded from the Brookhaven Protein Databank (2). Hydrogen atoms were added using Insight to complete the valence requirements since X-ray structures do not typically include hydrogens. Next, a solvent-accessible surface was computed. The electrostatic potential in the vicinity of the protein was computed using a Poisson-Boltzmann (PB) calculation. PB calculations include an implicit model of counter-ion re-arrangement and the effects of the shape of the protein surface, providing a more accurate view. The surface was then colored in shades of red for negative regions, white for neutral and blue for positive regions.

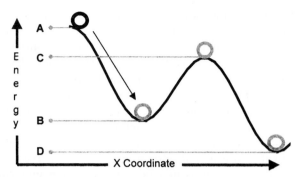

Fig. 3.7. Exploring energy landscapes. The figure depicts several important points on a one-dimensional potential energy surface including the Initial position (A), local minimum (B), transition state (C) and the global minimum (D). The independent X coordinate can represent any structural variable of interest including a position (as in our example of the ball on a hill), the dihedral angle of butane or a reaction coordinate, for example.

the earth, the greater the potential energy of the ball. Intuitively we know that the ball will roll down the hill due to the pull of gravity. In this instance, the internal energy of the system is the gravitational potential energy. In physical terms, the potential energy of the ball is greater when at the top of the hill (A) and would be lower if it were to roll down (to B). As the ball is accelerated down the hill, the potential energy due to gravitation is converted into the kinetic energy of the ball rolling down the slope. Several important concepts may be derived from this simple example.

First, only energy differences are meaningful. It is not necessary to know the absolute value of the energy at A in Figure 3.7 to know if the ball will roll down the hill. The important consideration is the slope, or the value at A relative to the surrounding points. The slope at any point may be used to determine the direction of the force acting on the ball, in this case to the right. This means the ball experiences a force in the direction that will reduce its energy. Mathematically this is expressed as

$$\Delta U / \Delta X = -\vec{F}$$

The ball will experience a force, $\vec{F}$, in the direction that will reduce its energy the most quickly, e.g., straight down the hill. This provides us with a mathematical tool for determining the preferred state of a system.

Second, a lower energy is more probable at equilibrium: A system will seek to minimize its energy by rearranging. The ball rolls down the hill from A to B (in Figure 3.7). If only the slope of the curve is used as a guide than the ball will roll to B and stop since the potential energy surface reaches a minimum there and moving beyond B would only increase its energy (positive slope). However, there is clearly a lower minimum at point D. Reaching or at least sampling the global minimum, D, is an important part of computational chemistry we will come back to.

Third, energy frequently and freely re-partitions between kinetic (movement) and potential forms. In this example, the ball rolls down the hill, converting the gravitational potential energy into kinetic energy. However, its enthalpy, H, remains constant since it is the sum of the potential and kinetic energy components plus any work done to the system. It is essentially an energetic snapshot of the system in one configuration at one point in time. For example, the energy required to assemble a molecule from infinitely separated atoms is an enthalpy called its heat of formation, ΔH_f. Since enthalpy is only a snapshot of one configuration, it is not enough to describe the complete behavior of a system. We must expand our analysis to include the effects of all configurations and this leads to an additional term called entropy.

Entropy: What are the Possibilities?

Entropy represents the tendency of a system to adopt all of its possible configurations. The energy components so far in this section have been enthalpies, a description of the energy necessary to bring the individual components into a specific state. However, many possible states are accessible to molecular systems. The occupation of states can be thought of in two ways. First, a molecule might adopt a particular configuration 40% of the time. Alternatively, in a large ensemble of these molecules, 40% might be in that configuration at any point in time. Entropy quantifies the tendency of an ensemble of molecules to adopt many configurations.

Consider the case of simplified butane. Lets assume that we are only interested in the energy associated with the rotation about the central dihedral angle of the system. Figure 3.8 depicts the excess potential energy for the rotation (a part of the enthalpy). The potential energy curve is for a single molecule and shows three minima: B and F are regional minima and D is the global minimum on the potential energy surface. We would expect to find that butane has adopted the cis configuration since it has the lowest energy. We can quantify this expectation by establishing a relationship between the energy of a state and the likelihood that it is occupied.

The probability that an individual state will be adopted can be related to the energy of the state. Specifically, the higher the energy of a given state, the less likely a molecule will be to adopt it. Maxwell Boltzmann established a proportionality between the probability, P, of a specific state, X, and its relative energy, ΔE:

$$P(X) \alpha\ e^{\frac{-\Delta E}{kT}}$$

where k is Boltzmann's constant and T is temperature. The term, ΔE, represents the difference in the energy compared to a reference state.

Formally, this relationship is true for systems that have arrived at equilibrium with a constant temperature and pressure. However, the essential feature is that many states are accessible and we can only determine the probability of a given state being occupied. In order to establish an exact probability, this equation must be normalized:

$$P(x) = e^{\frac{-\Delta E}{kT}} \Big/ \int e^{\frac{-\Delta E}{kT}}\, dx$$

where the denominator is an integral over all possible states. The denominator is often called the Partition Function. Figure 3.8 includes the probability of a given angle after normalization (gray line).

An experimental sample of 10^{20} butane molecules will have molecules in many of the accessible states. Examination of the probability of these states in Figure 3.8 reveals a few important concepts about the probability function. First, even though there is a single global minimum, not all molecules will adopt it. Second, small increases in the energy (relative to kT) dramatically reduce the probability of a state. A consequence of this is that the more low energy states there are, the larger the Partition Function. The final concept is perhaps the most important for understanding several of the approximations in computational chemistry. The probability of a state may NOT be determined by a calculation of that single, isolated state. It must include the effects of all the possible states of the dihedral angle so that the denominator may be determined. An exact result will require a calculation involving all possible states.

Entropy is the property of a system that quantifies its tendency to occupy all possible states. Entropy, S, is related to the number of locally accessible states. That is to say, the more states there are with a similar energy, the less likely any one state will be occupied. For example, the gauche minima (at B and F) increase the entropy of the system at low values of E. Consequently, at low values of E, the global minimum (at D in Figure 3.8) is less likely to be occupied. All three increase the entropy of the system at low values

of E because they are states with similar energies. More formally, under equilibrium conditions:

$$S = k \ln \omega(E)$$

where $\omega(E)$ is the density of states of the system for a given energy and volume. The density of states is a measure of the possible states that are accessible to a system with energy, E. $\omega(E)$ is formally defined in texts on Statistical Thermodynamics (7). Interested readers are encouraged to review these more detailed discussions.

We will find in the following sections that simple models of average interactions may sometimes be used to approximate entropic terms and save dramatic amounts of computer time. These approximations introduce inaccuracies that may be acceptable under certain conditions. Their use increases the range of questions that may be addressed with computational techniques, although at some risk.

Free Energy: Connecting to Experiment

Experiments usually measure a property of an ensemble of molecules and therefore represent an averaged value. The property is not measured for a single molecule but for experimental samples of nano to millimolar concentrations and nano- to milli-liter sizes. Thus, the property is averaged over 10^5 to 10^{17} molecules that occupy many different states. If an experiment were able to measure the dihedral angle of individual butane molecules, for example (see Figure 3.8), it would find that there were some molecules at nearly every possible angle (state). Many experiments measure a large ensemble of molecules under equilibrium conditions of temperature and pressure. The behavior of the system is not governed by the enthalpy or entropy alone but by the overall free energy of the system. The Gibbs free energy, G, is defined as:

$$G = H - TS$$

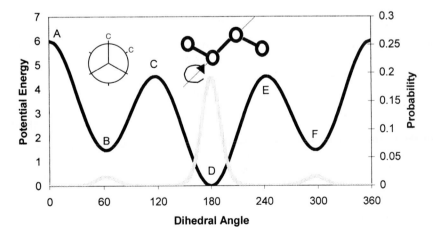

Fig. 3.8. Potential energy surface of a dihedral angle. Small molecules are comprised of bonded atoms and typically adopt the most favorable conformation. This one dimensional potential energy surface (Black line) represents the excess conformational energy for the dihedral angle formed by the four carbons in butane, for example. Butane has the trans (180°) configuration (D) as its favorable, low energy state. The cis (0°) position (A) is the relative maximum. The gauche (60° and 300°) positions (B, D) are local minima. The probability of a given state (gray line) is also shown.

where the Gibbs free energy is a conserved quantity under constant temperature and pressure conditions. Experimental data such as binding constants, reaction rates, diffusion rates etc. may frequently be used to determine the free energy and not the individual enthalpy and entropy.

Computational techniques are usually designed to approximate the free energy of the system. In the next section several computational methods are introduced which differ in their formulation of the (configurational) energy, E, of the system. All of the methods compute the energy, E, as a function of the coordinates and velocities of the atoms in the system, X^N. An expression for the free energy, G, may then be derived (8):

$$G = \langle E(X^N)\rangle - \frac{\langle E(X^N)\rangle^2}{2!kT} + \ldots$$

where <. . .> indicates an average over multiple states. This equation may be compared directly with the previous one. The first term estimates the enthalpy and the higher order terms approximate the entropy. Thus, we arrive at the important result that it is possible to use computational methods to compute the individual components of the free energy. Formally, this is an approximation of the Helmholtz free energy and differs by PV, where P is the pressure and V is the volume. However, computational methods frequently ignore this term since it is a constant for most studies.

NOTE: The concepts developed within this section are to illustrate the underlying physical chemistry of both experiment and computational methods. Thermodynamic principles are rigorously derived in more detailed texts on the subject of Statistical Thermodynamics. Although an effort has been made to point out where the development changed thermodynamic ensembles, important topics such as the momenta of the systems and differences between ensembles have been omitted for the sake of brevity. Interested readers are encouraged to pursue textbooks on the topic for a richer appreciation of statistical thermodynamics.

ACCURACY AXIS: COMPUTING MOLECULAR BEHAVIOR

The energy of a molecule is of great use in determining its behavior and properties. The mathematical form that describes the energy and momentum of the system is called a Hamiltonian. Several Hamiltonians have been developed to encapsulate the underlying chemistry of molecules at various levels of detail. In general, the more detailed the description the more accurate and generally useful the result. On the other hand, the more detailed the description the longer the calculation takes. For example, quantum-mechanical methods offer some of the most detailed and robust expressions for the energy. However, they are lengthy calculations for small systems (10 to 50 atoms) and completely intractable for larger ones. Thus, the available computing resources place a practical limit on our approaches. It is necessary, therefore, to balance the comprehensiveness of the Hamiltonian with the computing resources available. The trade-off is that the more complex and general the equation for the energy, the longer it will take to compute. To be effective, the Hamiltonian must contain terms necessary to reproduce the effect under study. For example, in order to study electron re-arrangement, the Hamiltonian must contain terms for electrons. Although this seems obvious, molecular modeling software packages often make it easy for the casual user to accept the default values, use the wrong tool and then report the misleading results with the same confidence as if it were calculated with the correct tool.

There are two general methods that we widely used in molecular modeling (Table 3.1). It is important to understand their foundations as well as their relative accuracy and generality. Quantum-mechanical methods use the Schrödinger equation to describe the nucleus and electrons and are the most rigorous method in use for describing the energy and include quantum effects explicitly. Molecular-mechanical methods treat molecules without atomic resolution. Atom-atom interactions are computed using an empirical equation that includes quantum effects implicitly.

Quantum Mechanics

Quantum mechanical methods offer the most detailed description of a molecule's chemical behavior. Several molecular properties are only accessible with these methods because they explicitly require a description of the molecule's electronic structure. One could reasonably argue that all properties are based on electronic structure and therefore all calculations should be based on these methods. However, the practical limitations of available computer time reduce the size of these studies to a few tens of atoms (with the most accurate methods). Quantum-mechanical calculations must be reserved for those questions that are of sufficient interest to justify the investment.

Quantum mechanical methods are usually based on the Schrödinger wave equation for the behavior of nuclei and electrons that was developed in 1926. It captured both the wave and particle nature of particles and consequently was the most detailed view of their behavior. Physicists were so enthused with its success that, three years after its introduction, the pre-eminent physicist P.A.M. Dirac was compelled to report:

Table 3.1. A Comparison of Methods for Computing Molecular Behavior

	Quantum Mechanics	Empirical Force Field
Basis	Schrödinger's Equation	Classical Hamiltonian
Smallest level of detail	Electrons, nuclei	Atoms
Parameterization	None	By atom type
Relative Computer time	10^8	10^4
Minimization, Dynamics	Yes	Yes
Includes bioavailability, metabolism, excretion	Impractical	Impractical

The underlying physical laws necessary for the mathematical theory of a large part of physics and the whole of chemistry are thus completely known, and the difficulty is only that the exact application of these laws leads to equations much too complicated to be soluble (9).

After 70 years of active research this is still a true statement. We can only find analytical solutions for the hydrogen atom and the H_2^+ molecule. The systems of interest in medicinal chemistry require special numerical methods that will be introduced shortly. Understanding and solving Schrödinger's equation is difficult at best. Fortunately, easy-to-use software has already been developed to find solutions. Keep in mind that the programs' goal is to find the solutions to Schrödinger's equation in order to describe the behavior of the molecules. To do this will require a description of the energy of the system and a description of how the electrons are distributed around the nuclei.

Schrödinger's equation may be written in a general way to describe all systems. It contains the potential (U) and kinetic (K) energy components of the total energy, E. It also contains a mathematical expression for the distribution of the electrons around the molecule, Ψ (pronounced "p-sigh"). In the case of the hydrogen atom, Ψ represents the familiar *s, p, d, f, . . .* orbitals and their complex shapes. For larger systems, Ψ describes even more complex geometries. The Schrödinger equation,

$$H\Psi = (U + K)\Psi = E\Psi$$

contains the Hamiltonian, H, which is shorthand notation for operations necessary to add up the total energy of the system. The Hamiltonian is an "operator," a mathematical construct which operates on the molecular orbital, Ψ, to determine the energy.

The hydrogen atom and molecule are the easiest examples for quantum mechanical methods. The hydrogen atom is comprised of a proton (P_1) and an electron (e_1). The dimensions of the atom are small enough and the energies large enough that the principles of relativity can have an effect on the results. Some reasonable assumptions must be made to simplify the calculation. If we omit a detailed analysis of the inner electrons and focus on the valence electrons in detail it is possible to simplify the terms in the Hamiltonian. One further assumption is that the movement of the nucleus is negligible compared to the electrons since they are 1800 times more massive. The result is the non-relativistic, time-independent form of the Hamiltonian:

$$H\Psi = \left(-\frac{1}{2}\nabla_1^2 + \frac{1}{R_1}\right)\Psi = E\Psi$$

where $-1/2\,\nabla_1^2$ represents the kinetic energy of the electron (including its ground state component) and $1/R_1$ is

the potential energy due to the electrostatic attraction between the proton and the electron in atomic units. R_1 is measured from the origin (O) of a convenient coordinate system.

The hydrogen molecule is a four-body problem and is a good example for the numerical methods in use today. All of the interactions between the two protons (P_1 and P_2) and two electrons (e_1 and e_2) must be represented in the Hamiltonian. In this case the Hamiltonian is:

$$H = -\frac{1}{2}\nabla_1^2 - \frac{1}{2}\nabla_2^2 + \frac{1}{R_1R_2} -$$

$$\frac{1}{R_1r_1} - \frac{1}{R_1r_2} - \frac{1}{R_2r_1} - \frac{1}{R_2r_2} + \frac{1}{r_1r_2}$$

Where the eight terms reflect the increased complexity of a many-body problem. The 1st and 4th terms, and the 2nd and 7th terms are the energies of the two isolated hydrogen atoms. The 3rd term is the interaction of the two protons. The 5th and 6th terms are the interaction of each proton with the electron of the other hydrogen atom. The 8th term is the interaction of the two electrons. The reader can imagine the proliferation of terms in a small drug with 25 atoms and 150 electrons.

The computation of electron-electron interactions quickly becomes the dominant component of quantum-mechanical calculations. The number of electron-electron interactions increases as n^2 where n is the number of electrons. However, the quantum nature of the calculation increases as n^4, since the probability of finding each electron in space is proportional to the square of the orbital. Consequently, much research has been done on ways to simplify the evaluation of electron-electron interactions. The method described below is based on *ab initio* methods which are derived "from the beginning" premises of quantum theory. Semi-empirical methods, such as MOPAC and AM1, substitute simple approximations for the majority of the electron-electron interactions. The semi-empirical methods are dramatically (100–1000 times) faster and are suitable for many applications. We will focus on the more general *ab initio* methods. The semi-empirical ones are simplifications worthy of further study for the interested reader (10).

Hartree-Fock methods are the most common approaches to *ab initio* calculations. Hartree and Fock simplified calculations by combining the electrons into an averaged field. This allowed the Hamiltonian to be calculated for each electron independently using a new term for its interaction with the overall electron cloud:

$$H_i = -\frac{1}{2}\nabla_1^2 - \frac{1}{R_1 r_1} - \frac{1}{R_2 r_1} + V$$

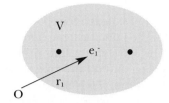

The averaged field, V, is due to the presence of all of the other electrons in the molecular orbitals. Thus, an electron interacts with one entity, the field V, rather than many other electrons. Once the individual electron's Hamiltonian is computed it may be combined with the other electrons to determine the overall energy and the molecular orbitals. The molecular orbitals are described using a set of mathematical functions called a basis set. Each set of basis functions is centered on an individual atom and may be combined with other basis functions to describe an extended orbital that may be occupied by electrons. An orbital is a linear combination of basis functions. The coefficients which define how much of a given basis function is part of each orbital are determined during the calculation.

The Hartree-Fock approximation requires an iterative approach to solve because the molecular orbitals are used to compute the averaged field, V, that in turn depends on the molecular orbitals. The initial molecular orbitals are educated guesses. They are used to compute the average field, V. This completes one iteration of the algorithm. The set of molecular orbitals is then varied slightly to see if an improved (lower energy) set may be located. If the new set is improved (i.e., has a lower energy) then it is used to compute a new V. The new V is then used to see if an improved set of orbitals may be found. This iterative procedure continues to refine the solution until a self-consistent field (SCF) has been determined. A self-consistent field means that the final set of molecular orbitals is the lowest energy consistent with the averaged field due to those orbitals. Since the Hartree-Fock method is a numerical solution it must have some convergence criteria for deciding when to terminate. The criteria are based on the set of orbitals, V and the energy E, which are monitored at each step. When the change in one of these three is less than some acceptable error the calculation stops.

The Hartree-Fock approximation simplifies the calculations but introduces systematic errors. The errors are due to the fact that electron movements may be correlated with other electrons. That is, the approximation suffers when the orbital of one electron selectively impacts a subset of the electrons that have been averaged in the field, V. Electron correlation methods have been developed to counter-act these effects. They are beyond the scope of this chapter but the reader will see methods such as MP2, CASS, CI and others cited in the literature. The literature in this field is often confusing due to the shorthand nota-

tions that describe the Hamiltonian (e.g., HF), the basis set (e.g., STO-3G) and the electron correlation method (e.g., MP2) used. A thorough review of basis sets and methods (11) should precede any detailed work.

The quantum-mechanical methods offer generality and accuracy. In theory, the methods may be applied to any element and molecule since no empirical parameters are necessary. In practice this is true with the caveat that heavier elements require substantially more computer resources. This method does not require the lengthy parameterization process that the empirical force field methods did. Therefore it may be applied to many systems almost immediately. The molecular orbitals and their energies are usually an intermediate solution to a quantum-mechanical calculation.

There are many properties of molecules that may be determined following a successful determination of the molecular orbitals and their occupancy. For example, dipole moments, magnetic susceptibility, chemical shielding, spin-spin coupling constants and electron affinities. Two calculations will provide proton and electron affinities as well as estimates of pK shifts. Several versions of *ab initio* methods are available. Commercial software packages with more sophisticated user interfaces are available such as Gaussian (12). Also, academic versions at low cost and with a variety of methods under development are also available such as GAMESS (13) and GAMESS-U.K. (14).

Molecular Mechanics

Molecular mechanics is based on simple empirical approximations of atomic and molecular interactions. The Hamiltonian in molecular mechanics classically describes the energy of the whole system as the sum of the inter- and intra-molecular interactions. Simply put, atoms are treated like a set of balls with springs connecting them. Additional terms are included to improve their geometry and to reproduce charge interactions. The energy of a molecular system is evaluated two atoms at a time without quantum mechanics. The molecular mechanics potential energy function (Figure 3.9) further breaks down the pair-wise interactions into non-bonded interactions and internal coordinates. The non-bonded terms include an electrostatic and van der Waals component. Atoms within one to three bonds are treated with internal coordinate terms. This type of potential energy function is sometimes referred to as an empirical force field because the energetic terms have simple form and parameters that are derived from experimental data and *ab initio* calculations.

The basic form of empirical force fields has been varied as part of efforts to improve their treatment of various biological systems. Extensive work has been done on the systematic improvement of the both the form and parameters used (15). However, this consensus form is common to AMBER (16) and CHARMM (17), two popular empirical force fields.

$$E = \frac{1}{2}k_r(r - r_0)^2 + \frac{1}{2}k_\theta(\theta - \theta_0)^2 + \sum k_{\phi i}(1 + \cos(n\phi + \delta)) + \frac{q_1 q_2}{rD} + e\left[\frac{r_{min}}{r_{ij}^{12}} - 2\frac{r_{min}}{r_{ij}^6}\right]$$

Fig. 3.9. Empirical Force Fields

Internal Coordinates

The bond and angle internal coordinates are treated like simple springs that keep them near their equilibrium bond length (r_0) and equilibrium bond angle (θ_0). The first two terms in the equation above use Hooke's Law to approximate the bond vibration:

$$E = \frac{1}{2}k_r(r - r_0)^2 + \frac{1}{2}k_\theta(\theta - \theta_0)^2$$

where k_r and k_θ are the bond and angle force constants. These two parameters are specific to the type atoms and the bond order (e.g., $-C-C-$, $-C = C-$, $-C-N$ etc.). The values for the parameters are derived from X-ray crystallographic structures and infrared spectra. The squared term in Hooke's Law results in both compression (negative displacement) and expansion (positive displacement) of the bond from its equilibrium value (r_0) increasing the energy. The bond term is symmetric about the equilibrium bond length and we know this is an approximation. It actually takes more energy to compress the bond than to stretch it. If necessary, we can use a Morse function that takes more time to compute but does a better job. In general, as long as the bond length is not too far from the equilibrium the approximation is a good one. The angle term uses a similar term to increase the energy when the bond angle deviates from its equilibrium value. The energy of the dihedral angles must be periodic since, for example, dihedral angles across single bonds are free to rotate. This term's potential energy surface is the same as the butane central dihedral angle (Figure 3.8) and is treated as a sum of cosine terms. The parameters for this term are adjusted to reproduce infrared and crystallographic data:

$$E = \sum k_{\phi i}(1 + \cos(n\phi + \delta))$$

where $k\phi$ is the dihedral force constant, n determines the periodicity of the term and δ adjusts phase for each term.

Non-Bonded Interactions

The non-bonded interactions, the electrostatic and van der Waal's terms, are applied to nearly all pairs of atoms. They are not computed for pairs of atoms treated by the internal coordinates since the bond, angle and dihedral terms provide a better approximation of their interaction. The non-bonded terms are usually smaller in magnitude individually but they can have a dominant effect because of the their large number. The number of atom pairs is $N(N-1)/2$, where N is the number of atoms in the system. A typical model of a protein (without solvent) might have 5,000 atoms with 25,000,000 atom-pair interactions and 15,000 internal coordinate terms to calculate. It is no surprise that the non-bonded interactions usually take more

than 90% of the computer time for a simulation. There are several methods for reducing the number of interactions that need to be calculated but each introduces artifacts. Recently, the Ewald method has gained general acceptance as a way to include all interactions within an acceptable amount of computation (18) using some mathematical cleverness and periodic boundary conditions.

Electrostatic interactions between atoms are calculated using Coulomb's Law. Each atom is assigned a charge to represent both formal charges and partial charges that arise due to unequal sharing of electrons. The partial charges are frequently derived from quantum mechanical calculations that are described in the next section. Although the form of Coulomb's Law is simple, it captures the underlying physics. The magnitude of the interaction is proportional to the atoms' charges (q_1 and q_2) and inversely proportional to their separation (r_{ij}) and the dielectric constant (D).

$$E = \frac{q_1 q_2}{rD}$$

The dielectric constant is a bulk property of the environment of the system. The dielectric of a vacuum is 1, which implies that there is no polarization of the environment. If a solvent, such as water or methanol, is explicitly included in the system than a dielectric of 1 is used since the orientation of the solvent molecules will polarize in the presence of the electric field. If water is the solvent, it is possible to use continuum models and reduce the amount of computation required. This does add artifacts to the simulation but they are fairly well characterized and the computation time is dramatically reduced.

The van der Waal term describes a more complex interaction between non-bonded atoms. At a large distance a net attraction exists between all (even neutral) atoms due to the concerted oscillation of their electrons. However, at close range the electrons and nuclei strongly repel each other. As a result, the van der Waal term has both a repulsive and an attractive component. Consequently, it uses the Lennard-Jones or 6–12 function in which r_{ij} is the distance between the atoms, r_{min} is the distance of minimum energy, and $-e$ is the minimum energy.

$$E = e\left[\frac{r_{min}}{r_{ij}^{12}} - 2\frac{r_{min}}{r_{ij}^6}\right]$$

The most widely used empirical force field methods include AMBER, CVFF and CHARMM. These empirical force fields have slightly different or additional terms to improve the energetic description of specific moieties (e.g., out of plane bending for benzene substituents). However, the basic form of the potential energy function is the same. The programs themselves are organized quite differently. The most popular commercial packages offer mature, sophisticated user interfaces with easier point-and-click interfaces for many functions. The academic versions typically offer more advanced features and methods that are under development. Their user interfaces are improving but lack robust point-and-click interfaces. Each offers advantages and disadvantages that must be considered before selecting one program and spending the time to learn it.

The advantages of empirical force field methods lie in their ability to treat thousands of atoms and direct connection with statistical thermodynamics. Many biological systems such as enzymes, structural proteins, DNA and their complexes are within the range of molecular mechanics. Scoring functions and simulations based on empirical force fields have successfully analyzed binding modes, folding mechanisms and allosteric effects. The simulations may be analyzed with statistical thermodynamic methods to estimate the free energy of binding or folding. Trajectories of atoms may be used to derive diffusion constants or to compare with NMR estimates of atomic motion. The flexibility of empirical force field methods must be balanced with the time required to develop parameters for a new system. Proteins, nucleotides and carbohydrates parameter sets continue to evolve but have been useful for more than 10 years. Novel lead compounds will often require parameterization to achieve meaningful results.

Comparison of Methods

A comparison of the two methods of molecular modeling is given in Table 3.2

TIME SCALE AXIS: SAMPLING AND SIMULATION

The time scale axis represents the ability to calculate the behavior of a system over time. Simulation represents our best efforts to reproduce the behavior of nature based on our understanding of thermodynamics and the mechanics of motion. Sampling is the process of selecting a few configurations of a system that estimate its overall motion. Care must be used in sampling to select configurations of sufficient quantity and diversity to be representative. Simulation studies, because of their basis in thermodynamics, are used phenomena that evolve over time. Both sampling and simulation may be used to study phenomena such as diffusion, correlation studies of active site interactions, energetic effects of mutations, reaction coordinates and ligand binding. For example, a ligand's interaction with its target may be studied by simulating its movement at its binding site and determining the critical interactions. The simulation may then be analyzed to extract thermodynamic properties such as the free energy of binding and the ligand's binding constant.

Table 3.2. Summary of Molecular Modeling Methodologies and their Capabilities

Use	Empirical Force Fields (Classical)	Quantum Mechanical	
		Semi-empirical	*Ab initio*
Geometry optimization	Yes	Yes	Yes
Molecular dynamics	Yes	Limited	No
Vibrational spectra	Yes	Yes	Yes
Thermodynamic values			
Heat of formation, ΔH	No	Yes	Yes
Relative ΔG of binding	Yes	No	No
Chemical reactivity			
Topology	Fixed	Variable	Variable
Transition states	No	Yes	Yes
Reaction coordinate	No	Yes	Yes
Force constants	No	Yes	Yes
Molecular properties			
Electrostatics	Yes	Yes	Yes
Hydrophobicity	Yes	No	No
Lipophilicity	Yes	No	No
Proton affinity	No	Yes	Yes
Electron affinity	No	Yes	Yes
Practical differences			
Tractable number of atoms	<50,000	<200	<50
Tractable number of compounds	1	1	1
Relative CPU time/iteration	10^4	10^6	10^8
Disk space requirements	5–5000MB	5–10MB	5–2000MB
Memory requirements (RAM)	5–100MB	5–100MB	5–1000MB
Popular programs	CHARMM	MOPAC	GAUSSIAN
	AMBER	AMPAC	GAMESS-UK
	Discover		CADPAC

The ability of computational tools to compute a particular property or geometry is listed for each of the theoretical methods. Estimates of the relative accuracy are general and are strongly dependent on the system under study. In some cases, additional work must be done to derive a property for a given method. For example, an empirical force field estimate of hydrophobicity could be computed by performing molecular dynamics with additional analysis of the trajectories of the atoms. *The large disk space requirement reflects the use of simple, fast linear free energy relationships for estimating the binding of a database containing hundreds of thousands of possible ligands.

An understanding of simulation is built upon two concepts that are used extensively in molecular modeling. The first is an appreciation for the large number of possible conformations molecules may have. For example, a protein backbone has two angles, ψ and ϕ, that may be used to describe its conformation. The shape of an entire protein backbone may be described by defining ψ and ϕ for each residue (assuming the amide bond is always trans). If we wish to consider the conformations for a pentapeptide in detail we might evaluate it in 30° increments of ψ and ϕ. Each of the 10 angles would have 360°/30° possibilities for a total of 12^{10} or approximately 62 billion possibilities! Even if 1000 conformations could be calculated per second, it would take nearly two years to complete the study. Clearly, studies must find more effective ways than brute force to sample the possible conformations. The challenge of sampling conformations is trying to ensure that we end up considering the most populated state, the global minimum.

The second important concept is energy minimization or geometry optimization. Thermodynamics tells us that only the low energy states are significantly occupied. A review of the potential energy surface of the dihedral angle of butane (Figure 3.8) shows three minima. A molecule is much more likely (according to the Boltzmann probability) to adopt one of the minimum energy conformations. Energy minimization is the process of evaluating the energy of any conformation and determining the nearest minima. It is possible to locate the most populated states using energy minimization.

The key to improved sampling will be combining an effective method for generating starting points with some amount of energy minimization. Diverse starting conformations will ensure a broad sampling of the potential energy surface and the conformations it represents. Energy minimization will reduce the time spent considering high-energy states by avoiding them during the search for the local minima. Since generation of starting conformations and energy minimization use computer time, a balance must be struck that optimizes the search for the low energy structures.

Energy Minimization

Energy minimization is the process of changing the geometry of a structure to reduce its energy. Lower energy states are of interest because molecules preferentially adopt them. Consequently, they are more indicative of molecular behavior than their high-energy neighbors. Empirical force field and quantum-mechanical methods are used for geometry optimization because they are able to compute a structure's energy and its derivatives as a function of its coordinates and velocities. It is possible to build a simple algorithm to move down the potential energy surface to lower energy structures if the energy function and its derivatives are known.

Geometry optimization is an iterative procedure of computing the energy of a structure and then making incremental changes to reduce the energy. As an example of geometry optimization recall the potential energy surface for the central dihedral of butane (Figure 3.8). The slope of the energy function gives us both a magnitude and a sign. If the current conformation has an angle (ϕ_i) of 330° then the slope is large and positive. While it is clear for this one-dimensional potential energy surface that there is only one local minimum at 300°, more complex surfaces require less obvious steps than simply moving to the minima. Consequently, energy minimization is implemented as an iterative procedure whereby the energy is evaluated and then atoms are moved a small step toward a lower energy. In the example of butane, the next angle would be

$$\phi_{i+1} = \phi_i - \Delta E(\phi) \times k$$

where k is a scale factor that determines how large a step along ϕ to take for a given slope. The negative sign before the slope implies a move "down" the potential energy surface toward a minimum. If the minimum is reached then the slope is zero (by definition) and no charges are made to the angle. The process is repeated until the energy changes are acceptably small or computer time is exhausted.

Energy minimization has been extensively studied and more expedient methods than this are generally used. However, this "Steepest Descent" method is robust and still in use. Other methods take advantage of the second derivative to improve the rate of convergence to the minimum. Still others use a combination of first and second derivatives to reduce the amount of time required to compute the second derivatives. In general, a robust method like Steepest Descent is used initially to reduce the highest energy interactions. This is followed by a more time-consuming method using some second derivatives that converges to the answer more efficiently.

Molecular Dynamics

One of the methods for simulating the behavior of a system is molecular dynamics. The dynamics of a system may be broken down into the movements of each of its atoms. If their velocities and the forces acting on them can be quantified then their movement may be calculated. The equations of motion of the atoms may be derived from the potential energy function and an observation by Isaac Newton:

$$\Delta E / \Delta X = -\vec{F} = -m\vec{a}$$

where ΔE is the change in the internal energy, F is the force vector, m is the mass of the atom and a is the acceleration. Newton realized that the acceleration of an object could be related to the forces applied to it. It is then possible to approximate the movement of an atom a short time into the future, Δt, using a Taylor expansion:

$$\vec{r}(t + \Delta t) = \vec{r}(t) + \vec{v}\Delta t + \vec{a}\frac{\Delta t^2}{2} + \ldots$$

This expression states that the position of an atom at some time in the future, $\vec{r}(t + \Delta t)$ may be found from its initial position ($\vec{r}$), velocity ($\vec{v}$) and acceleration ($\vec{a}$) The new position is now in terms of known quantities since molecular dynamics calculations keep track of atomic positions and velocities at each step.

This approach requires that we use a value of Δt that is small enough to correctly simulate the fastest atomic motions. The C-H bonds vibrate with a period of about 10^{-14} seconds. To simulate these motions, the time step must be roughly one-tenth of that, or 10^{-15} seconds. Simulations become unstable with values much larger than this one femtosecond time step. Simulations are unstable when forces are applied for a longer time interval (Δt) than they are really valid. For example, if the attractive force of a carbon acting on a hydrogen (in a C-H bond) is applied for too long a time interval, the hydrogen will have been repositioned too close to the carbon. During the next time step a very strong repulsive force will lead to the hydrogen being repositioned well beyond its typical bond length. This oscillatory process will continue until the energy of the bond is no longer conserved and the molecular dynamics software indicates an error condition.

Currently, a simulation of a system with up to 500,000 atoms is the limit of what is possible. However, a target enzyme, ligand, solvent and counter-ions are typically only 20–30,000 atoms. A complete study of such a system might require several weeks of computer time. There are several steps that are common to most simulations of this size.

1. Build the target protein model from an NMR or X-ray crystallographic structure.
2. Place the ligand into the putative binding site.
3. Add counter-ions and immerse this into a periodic box of water.
4. Perform an energy minimization to remove any high energy artifacts from the construction process.
5. Heat the system over 25 ps using molecular dynamics.
6. Allow the system to equilibrate so that the total energy and core structures have stabilized at the selected temperature (25ps–1 ns).
7. Begin the production phase of the study (250ps to 25 ns).

This molecular dynamics study may then be post-processed in several ways. First, the study may attempt to locate the lowest energy binding modes. In this case the trajectories of the atoms may be sampled at 1ps intervals and the resulting structures then subjected to energy minimization. The resulting structures could be ranked according to their energy and used to evaluate the expected binding mode. A second use would be to track the interatomic distances between residues of interest. A third use is to derive quantities such as the free energy of binding, correlation functions, diffusion constants or a potential of mean force. The full power of statistical thermodynamics may be applied to a simulation since the time averaged quantities may be used to approximate the free energy.

The basis of molecular dynamics in thermodynamic principles establishes it as our best attempt at reproducing molecular behavior. There are other methods of simulation besides molecular dynamics such as Langevin dynamics (19) that approximate Brownian dynamics with an implicit solvent model. There are other stochatic boundary condition models as well. (For an in-depth review please see 20). However, in each method, an effort is made to determine the trajectories and velocities of all atoms at each time step. Once achieved, the data may be used as a starting point for understanding the behavior of the system of interest.

Monte Carlo Sampling Method

An important sampling technique combines random selection and Boltzmann's probability theorem to explore a potential energy surface. The potential energy must be a function of the velocity of the particles, which is generally the case for empirical force field applications. The Metropolis Monte Carlo method (21) or Monte Carlo for short, is an example of a stochastic process. That is, it uses probabilistic methods as a tool to sample configurations accessible to the system. Random selection of configurations is an acceptable method for the generation of sample structures. In a search for the lowest energy structure, each random configuration receives an equal amount of computer time. High and low energy structures are treated the same and each configuration (X_i) is independent of the others. Each time a new structure with a lower energy is generated, it is adopted as the current, best structure (X_c). The Metropolis Monte Carlo method introduces a bias into the acceptance of the current structure that has two benefits.

The first advantage of Monte Carlo methods is that it allows a configuration to be evaluated based on its energy relative to the current configuration (X_c). This has the benefit of allowing local energy barriers to be traversed, improving the search of the local configuration space. The Metropolis Monte Carlo method introduces a bias based on the Boltzmann probability. Each time a new configuration (X_i) is generated, its energy $E(X_i)$ is compared to the energy of the current configuration, $E(X_c)$. If its energy is lower the new configuration is adopted. If the energy of X_i is higher, the probability of adopting the new configuration is determined from:

$$p = e^{\dfrac{-(E(Xi) - E(Xc))}{kT}}$$

The value of p is compared to a random number (between 0 and 1). If the probability, p, is greater than the random number, the new configuration is adopted.

The second advantage of Monte Carlo is that more computer time is spent searching in low energy regions. The extent of the changes in the configurations may be tied to the energy level so that when a low energy structure is located smaller changes in the configuration are attempted. This focuses the computer time on exploring local minima in the potential energy surface. At regular intervals larger changes in the conformation may be attempted to test for other regional minima.

SCREENING TECHNIQUES

Screening techniques are practical approaches to make sense of a less-than-complete description of the molecules in the system. They are necessary because of incomplete knowledge of the ligand; incomplete knowledge of the target; inaccuracies in computational methods; or limitations on the length of time available for computation. Selection of the right screening technique must balance the axes of molecular modeling to achieve an acceptable accuracy for the size of the system and the properties sought. The right screening technique is also dependent on the amount of experimental data available. Structural information such as an X-ray crystallographic or NMR 3D structure can significantly enhance the quality of the result. Numerous techniques have been developed to identify lead compounds and to rank order a set of congeners. They vary in their requirements for structural information about the compound and the target. They also vary from estimating binding for a database of 100,000 compounds simulation to a detailed analysis of a single compound to determine its mechanism of actin.

The techniques are similar to their attempt to improve their quality and generality by including as many of the principles of computational chemistry as possible. Scoring functions are generally based on simplified empirical force fields that include estimates of the enthalpy and perhaps an estimate of entropy. Parameters for the scoring functions are increasingly derived from quantum mechanical calculations for improving the overall accuracy. Sampling schemes are designed to explore as much of the relevant regions of conformation spaces as possible. In short, screening techniques attempt to incorporate as much of the thermodynamic underpinnings as possible and still get the study completed within an acceptable time frame.

Generating Test Compounds

Pharmaceutical companies treat the databases of compounds they have synthesized or purchased as a valued corporate asset. The databases may have up to 300,000 compounds and be supplemented by another database of virtual compounds that have been enumerated, geometry optimized but never synthesized. These compounds are then used in screening operations against targets they've identified. Programs such as CONCORD (22) are able to generate three-dimensional structures from two-dimensional descriptions using artificial intelligence and geometry optimization. Virtual combinatorial chemistry can generate thousands of compounds for analysis. Large sets of compound data, both experimental and virtual exists to use in screening efforts.

Screening Without a Target Structure

If no structural information is available about a target then only a subset of the available techniques may be applied. Two and three-dimensional QSAR techniques may be used. The activity or binding constants for a series of compounds may be used to estimate the role of different pharmacophores. The common elements of the compounds with high affinity are used to establish a two or three-dimensional map of their interaction sites. These descriptions may then be used for database searching and de novo ligand design methods. The flexibility of larger compounds is problematic since no single geometry is representative of all the different conformations. The DGEOM (23) program addresses the problem of generating possible conformations for a given compound. However, extensive computer time is requires to consider ligand flexibility. It is possible to convert a three-dimensional QSAR into a map of the cavity of the binding site. This may then be used for some of the screening methods for a simplified model of a target.

Homology modeling is a significant advancement in approximating the three-dimensional structure of a target. A homology model is based on the concept that proteins with high homology (40% or more) or high similarity (60% or more) will likely adopt a similar protein fold. Regions that are highly conserved are more likely to retain their three-dimensional shape. The primary sequence of the target of interest may be aligned with a protein whose X-ray crystallographic structure is known. Allowances for insertions and deletions may be made in the primary sequence. The binding site of the target of interest may then be approximated for modeling purposes. Software packages such as Homology (24) facilitate the process of homology modeling.

Screening Compounds to a Simplified Model of a Target

It is frequently necessary or of more interest to study the binding of thousands of compounds at low resolution than to study fewer compounds at high resolution. This is often the case when searching for lead compounds. The GRID approach (25) maps the binding site by superimposing a grid and calculating the electrostatics, hydrogen bonding sites or lipophilicity at each grid point. DOCK is a suite of programs that uses a similar approach (26) for scoring. DOCK provides other tools for scoring compounds, attempting alternate orientations and performing geometry optimization to include the flexibility of the ligand. A grid-based approach dramatically reduces the computer time. Each ligand's interaction is computed with the limited number of grid points and not all of the target's atoms.

Screening Compounds for Target with Known Structure

The three-dimensional structure is known for many pharmaceutical targets. To examine thousands of compounds, a low-resolution technique such as LUDI (27) uses rules to estimate the free energy of binding. LUDI interaction sites include hydrogen donors and acceptors, lipophilic-aliphatic and lipophilic-aromatic sites. A simple energy function avoids the use of an explicit calculation of all atom pairs. LUDI is typically re-parameterized for each target system to improve its performance. Once re-parameterized it is fast enough for interactive use with molecular modeling software.

An alternative to database screening is the de novo design of a compound to fit the binding site. Programs such as GROW (28) and LEGEND (29) use "seed" structures and add functional groups to optimize the use of possible binding sites. These tools have been most effective when used to support drug design efforts rather than to automate them.

Refining a Lead Compound with a Known Target

When a lead compound has been identified and the three dimensional structure of the target is known, computational techniques with higher accuracy may be warranted. Empirical force field or quantum-chemical methods may be used to study the interactions associated with binding in detail. The detailed mechanism of action may be more fully understood and aspects that are inaccessible experimentally may be worked out. A large array of computational techniques may be used to incrementally improve on a compound. Simulation is readily accomplished with explicit, all-atom models. Free energy perturbation studies may be used to predict binding constants in silico. Searches through a database of substituents may be executed to test effects on binding. Effects of mutations of the target may be examine. Quantum-chemical studies of reaction paths for suicide-inhibitors or substrate analogs are possible. Excellent reviews of computer-assisted drug design are available for the interested reader (30).

SUMMARY

Molecular modeling provides an array of valuable tools for drug design and analysis. Simple visualization of molecules and easy access to structural databases have become essential components on the desktop of the medicinal chemist. Commercial software continues to expand upon the core user interface. New algorithms from industry and academia are quickly incorporated into the high-end packages. Public domain packages are becoming more stable and offering functionality that rivals some of the commercial offerings. Computers continue to double in speed every year and a half while graphic displays become more sophisticated and intuitive. All of these elements make molecular modeling an integral part of drug design.

Molecular modeling continues to extend its role. Exciting new techniques, such as computational enzymology, and genomic and proteomic search engines promise to extend the range of molecular modeling tools. The quality of the methods is also improving as more computer power

facilitates greater sampling, longer simulations and improved statistics. Quantum-mechanical calculations are improving the quality of empirical force field parameters and speeding the development of new parameters. New parameters are under development for carbohydrate chemistry for adjuvant studies and lipid bilayer simulations. Drug design is a synthetic rather than a linear process. As new insights into molecular interactions appear, new methods must be developed and incorporated. The extensibility of computational chemistry will ensure that it will continue to have a vital role in visualizing and organizing our understanding of molecular interactions.

REFERENCES

1. Abola, E et al. Protein Databank. In: Allen, FH et al., ed. Crystallographic Databases-Information Content, Software Systems, Scientific Applications. Bonn/Cambridge/Chester: Data Commission of the International Union of Crystallography, 1987;107–132.
2. HM Berman, J. Westbrook, Z Feng, et al. The Protein Data Bank. Nucleic Acids Research, 28, pp. 2235–242 (2000).
3. Rogers, DF, Adams, JA, Mathematical Elements for Computer Graphics. Second Edition. New York: McGraw-Hill, Inc., 1990.
4. Kraulis, PJ MOLSCRIPT: A Program to Produce Both Detailed and Schematic Plots of Protein Structures. Journal of Applied Crystallography (1991) vol 24, pp. 946–950.
5. Insight 97, Molecular Simulations Incorporated, San Diego, CA.
6. Schroder, HK, Willassen, NP, Smalas, AO Structure of a Non-Psychrophilic Trypsin from a Cold-Adapted Fish Species. Acta Crystallogr., Sect. D, 1998; 54:780.
7. McQuarrie, DA, Statistical Mechanics. New York: Harper-Collins Publishers, 1976.
8. Beveridge, DL and DiCapua, FM Free Energy Via Molecular Simulation: Applications to Chemical and Biomolecular Systems. In: Annu. Rev. Biophys. Biophys. Chem. 1989; 18:431–492.
9. P.A.M. Dirac Proc. Roy. Soc. London 123, p. 714, 1929.
10. Stewart JJP Semi-empirical Molecular Orbital Methods. In: Lipkowitz KB, Boyd DB, eds. Reviews in Computational Chemistry. New York: VCH Publishers, Inc. 1990; 1.
11. Feller, D and Davidson, ER Basis Sets for Ab Initio Molecular Orbital Calculations and Intermolecular Interactions. In: Lipkowitz BK, Boyd DB, eds. Review in Computational Chemistry. New York: VCH Publishers, Inc. 1990; 1.
12. Gaussian 98 (Revision A.7), MJ Frisch, GW Trucks, HB Schlegel, et al. Gaussian, Inc., Pittsburgh PA, 1998.
13. MW Schmidt, KK Baldridge, JA Boatz, et al. J Comput. Chem. 1993:14, 1347–1363.
14. GAMESS-U.K. is a package of ab initio programs written by MF Guest, JH van Lenthe, J Kendrick, et al. with contributions from RD Amos, RJ Buenker, M Dupuis, et al. The package is derived from the original GAMESS code due to M Dupuis, D Spangler and J Wendoloski, NRCC Software Catalog. Vol. 1, Program No. QG01 (GAMESS), 1980.
15. Dinur, U and Hagler, AT New Approaches to Empirical Force Fields In: Lipkowitz KB, Boyd DB, eds. Reviews in Computational Chemistry. New York: VCH Publishers, Inc. 1990;2.
16. Weiner, SJ et al. J. Comp. Chem., 1986 7:230.
17. Brooks, BR et al. J. Comp. Chem., 1983 4:187.
18. Essman U et al. A smooth particle mesh Ewald method. J. Chem. Phys., 103(19), 8577.
19. Ermak DL, J. Chem. Phys. 1975 62:4189.

20. Allen MP, Tildesley DJ Computer Simulations of Liquids 1987 Oxford, U.K. Oxford University Press.

21. Metropolis N, Rosenbluth AW, Rosenbluth MN, et al. J. Chem. Phys. 1953; 21:1087–1092.

22. Rusinko III, A et al. University of Texas, Austin and Tripos Associates, St. Louis, MO 1988.

23. Blaney JM, Crippen GM, Dearing A, et al. JS QCE Bull. 1990 10:37.

24. Homology, San Diego, CA, Biosym Technologies, Inc.

25. Goodford PJ J. Med. Chem. 1985 28:849.

26. Kuntz, ID et al. J. Mol. Biol. 1982 161:269.

27. Böhm, J-J J. Comput. Aided Molec. Des. 1992 6:61.

28. Moon JB, Howe WJ Proteins: Struct. Funct. Genet. 1991 11:314.

29. Nishibata Y, Itai A Tetrahedron 1991 47:8985.

30. Martin YC, Willett, P Designing Bioactive Molecules: Three-Dimensional Techniques and Applications 1998 Washington, DC: American Chemical Society.

4. Receptors and Drug Action

TIMOTHY J. MAHER AND DAVID A. JOHNSON

INTRODUCTION

The human body is an example of a exquisitely designed, extremely complex machine that functions day-in and day-out to allow for the survival of the organism in response to a never-ending onslaught of external challenges. When one considers the enormous variety of environmental stressors that the body is continually subjected to, it is not surprising to anticipate the existence of a multitude of checks and balances associated with its physiological and biochemical systems. These systems, including endocrine, nervous, and enzymatic, typically function in concert to adapt to changing environmental conditions. While some systems are designed to respond quickly, i.e., within milliseconds, and for a short time, others are designed to act more slowly, but usually have significantly longer duration, i.e., months to years. Together these systems support the organism's survival. However, misfunctioning of the control of such systems often leads to disease and potentially the eventual demise of the individual.

The use of specific chemical compounds to treat disease dates back to early man. Many primitive cultures utilized plants and other natural sources in an attempt to mitigate the influences of evil spirits and other factors rooted in superstition, which were believed to be the foundations of such illnesses. Over the centuries a number of serendipitous observations involving the ability of largely botanical preparations to alter disease processes laid the foundation for the modern day more systematic approach to the discovery of medicinals for therapeutic use. The collaboration of chemical scientists and biological scientists continue this quest for the "magic bullet" to treat those diseases that challenge the individual's well-being.

HISTORICAL PERSPECTIVES

For years it had been known that some drugs were capable of producing their effects by acting at specific sites within the body. Claude Bernard was first to demonstrate this in the mid-1800s with his classical experiments involving curare (1). He showed that this neuromuscular blocking agent, which was used as an arrow poison by the South American natives, was capable of preventing skeletal muscle contraction following nerve stimulation, but was without effect when the muscle was stimulated directly. This work demonstrated for the first time a localized site of action for a drug and most importantly suggested that a gap or *synapse* existed between the nerve and the muscle. From these findings he also postulated that some chemical substance normally communicated the information between the nerve and the target tissue, in this case the muscle. These findings established the foundations for what is known today as *chemical neurotransmission*, a process frequently disrupted by diseases, and likewise the target of many therapeutic agents.

Investigations by J.N. Langley in the early 1900s established the initial foundations for the interaction of drugs with specific cellular components, later to be identified and termed receptors (2). Prior to this time many of the leading experts believed that most drugs acted non-selectively on virtually all of the cells in the body to produce their biological responses, a response resulting from their general physical characteristics, e.g., lipid solubility, and not related to specific structural features of the compound. Langley noted that compounds like pilocarpine, which act to mimic the parasympathetic division of the autonomic nervous system, were very selective and also extremely potent. Additionally, a compound like atropine, was capable of blocking in a rather selective fashion the effects of pilocarpine and parasympathetic nervous system stimulation. Importantly, he concluded that these two compounds interacted with the same component of the cell.

Paul Ehrlich, a noted microbiologist during the late 19th and early 20th centuries, is credited with coining the term *receptive substance* or *receptor* (3). His observations that various organic compounds appeared to produce their antimicrobial effects with a high degree of selectivity, led him to speculate that drugs produced their effects via binding to such a receptive substance. The interaction of the drug with the receptor was analogous to a "lock" and "key." Thus, certain organic compounds would fit properly into the receptor and activate it, leading to a high degree of specificity. While such a situation might be considered ideal for drug therapy, in actuality few drugs interact only with their intended receptors. The frequency of side effects not associated with a simple extension of their desired pharmacological actions, indicates that drug molecules can also combine with other receptors or non-receptor entities on or within cells to produce a host of other, and often undesirable, effects.

Some drugs produce their desired effects without interaction with a specific receptor. For instance, osmotic diuretics produce their pharmacologic effects simply by creating an osmotic gradient in the renal tubules, and thereby foster the elimination of water in the urine. This is purely the result of a physical characteristic of the drug.

Similarly, antacids produce their beneficial effects by chemically neutralizing the hydrochloric acid found in the gastrointestinal tract. No absorption of the drug is even required for its effects to be realized. Often, the failure of a drug to be absorbed and thus only act locally at the desired biological site constitutes a tremendous advantage regarding the safety of that compound. Unfortunately, from a practical standpoint, most pharmacologic agents require absorption following administration in order to reach the intended target, and thus side effects are typically a serious consideration.

More sophisticated mechanisms can also be involved in the non-receptor actions of therapeutic agents. For instance, the antineoplastic agent mechlorethamine, a nitrogen mustard, produces its beneficial (pharmacologic) and adverse (toxicologic) effects via interaction with many cellular components, in both cancerous and normal cells. Via its conversion to a highly reactive electrophilic ethyleniminium ion intermediate, this agent reacts with nucleophilic cellular components, such as amino, hydroxyl, sulfhydryl, phosphate, carboxyl and imidazole groups. In particular, by alkylating the N-7 position of guanine in DNA this agent produces miscoding (cytosine normally base pairs with guanine in DNA, however thymine now substitutes for cytosine) and the eventual death of the cell results (4). When one realizes that all replicating cells contain a N-7 nitrogen in guanine in their DNA, it is easy to see why mechlorethamine produces non-selective destruction of cells throughout the body. Thus, no specific receptor is involved in the actions of this class of pharmacologic agent.

AFFINITY—THE ROLE OF CHEMICAL BONDING

In the early 1900s A.V. Hill utilized nicotine and curare in isolated muscle preparations and noted the effects of temperature in his experiments (1). He concluded that the ability of a drug to produce an effect must result from specific chemical interactions between the drug and specific sites, and also noted that the effects of many drugs were reversible, since washing the isolated tissue oftentimes restored the sensitivity of the tissue to nerve stimulation. These studies set the foundation for our understandings of the chemical interactions between drugs and receptors.

When a drug interacts with a receptor there is believed to be a number of chemical attractive forces responsible for the initial interaction. Compounds that are attracted to a receptor macromolecule are said to have *affinity* for that receptor, and may be classified as *agonists* or *antagonists*. Additionally, compounds with affinity are also referred to as *ligands*. Agonists are those compounds that have affinity for the receptor and are also capable of producing a biological response as a result of its interaction with the receptor (5). As will be noted later, the ability to produce a response is referred to as *efficacy* or *intrinsic activity*. Drugs that are capa-

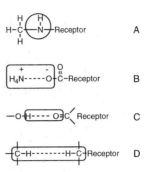

Fig. 4.1. Various drug-receptor bonds. A, covalent; B, ionic; C, hydrogen; D, hyrdophobic.

ble of interacting with the receptor but not activating it to produce a response are termed *antagonists*. This class of drug is said to have affinity, but lacks intrinsic activity. The affinity of a compound for a receptor is dependent upon its proper three-dimensional characteristics such as 1) its size, 2) stereochemical orientation of its functional groups, and 3) its physical and electrochemical properties such as ionic and dipole interactions.

Assuming that a compound has been distributed to the general vicinity of a receptor, a function of its physical characteristics, the binding of the drug to the receptor will initially depend upon the types of chemical bonds that can be established between the drug and its receptor. The overall strengths of these bonds will vary (Fig. 4.1), and will determine the degree of affinity between the drug and the receptor.

Covalent Bond

The strongest of bonds involved in drug-receptor interactions is the covalent bond where two atoms, one from the ligand and one from the receptor, share a pair of electrons. Because of the significant strength of the covalent bond, 50–150 kcal/mol, covalent bonding often results in a situation where the ligand is irreversibly bound by the receptor, and thus leads to the receptor's eventual destruction via endocytosis and chemical destruction. Full recovery of cellular function therefore requires the synthesis of new receptors.

An example of an irreversible covalent bond formation between drug and receptor involves the longlasting blockade of α-adrenoceptors by phenoxybenzamine (Chapter 11). Once phenoxybenzamine is converted to a highly reactive carbonium ion intermediate, this haloalkylamine can covalently link, via alkylation with amino, sulfhydryl or carboxyl groups at the α-adrenoceptor. The receptor is thus rendered irreversibly nonfunctional and eventually destroyed. The synthesis of new receptor requires a number of days, thus accounting for the extremely prolonged duration of the block associated with this agent. As will be discussed below, this property of phenoxybenzamine to irreversibly bind the α-adrenoceptor was critical for the demonstration of spare receptors (6,7). Since other receptors and cellular components also contain molecular groups that are likewise capable of interacting with the activated phenoxybenzamine intermediate, it is not surprising to find that receptors that mediate the actions of other neurotransmitters (e.g., acetylcholine, serotonin and histamine) are also subject to alkylation and blockade, demonstrating the lack of selectivity of phenoxybenzamine.

Another important example of a class of compounds that produces its effects via a covalent bond to its receptor are the organophosphate acetylcholinesterase inhibitors. Examples of such agents include the insecticides parathion and malathion, and the nerve gas agents sarin, soman and tabun. These compounds are capable of alkylating the active site of this enzyme that normally is responsible for metabolizing acetylcholine, the neurotransmitter found at the neuromuscular junction and within many sites of the autonomic and central nervous systems. Reaction of the enzyme with its normal substrate acetylcholine leads to a readily hydrolyzable acetylated enzyme, which rapidly regenerates the active enzyme. However, covalent bonding by the organophosphates results in phosphorylation of a serine within the active site of the enzyme, which is extremely stable and essentially irreversible. Recovery of enzymatic function in the tissue requires the synthesis of new enzyme molecules.

Ionic Bond

When two ions of opposite charge are attracted to each other through electrostatic forces, an ion bond is formed. The strength of this type of bond varies between 5–10 kcal/mol, and decreases proportionally to the square of the distance between the two atoms. The ability of a drug to bind to a receptor via ionic interactions therefore increases significantly as the drug molecule diffuses closer to the receptor. Additionally, the strength associated with the ionic bond is strong enough to support an initial transient interaction between the receptor and the drug, but unlike the covalent bond not so strong as to prevent dissociation of the complex.

The tendency of an atom to participate in ionic bonding is determined by its degree of electronegativity. Hydrogen as a standard, has an electronegativity value of 2.1 (Linus Pauling Units). Fluorine and chlorine atoms, and hydroxyl, sulfhydryl, and carboxyl groups form strong ionic bonds because of a stronger attraction for electrons than does hydrogen. On the other hand, alkyl groups do not participate in ionic bonds because of a weaker tendency to attract electrons than does hydrogen.

Hydrogen Bond

Hydrogen that is linked via a covalent bond to a strongly electronegative atom, such as oxygen, nitrogen or sulfur, develops a relative positive charge and will be attracted to another atom possessing a relative negative charge via what is termed hydrogen bonding. A water molecule which behaves as an electronic dipole (the hydrogens are relatively positive due to the attraction of electrons by the oxygen) can easily bond to other water molecule through hydrogen bonding. At 2–5 kcal/mol, a single hydrogen bond is relatively weak and would not be expected to support a drug-receptor interaction alone, but when multiple hydrogen bonds are formed between drugs and receptors, as is typically the case, a significant amount of stability is conferred upon the drug-receptor interaction. Thus, hydrogen bonding is most likely an essential requirement for many drug-receptor interactions.

Hydrophobic Interactions

Hydrophobic interactions between nonpolar organic molecules also can contribute to the binding forces that attract a ligand to its receptor. Theorists have suggested that in order for these forces to operate, a momentary dipolar structure needs to exist in order to allow for such association. This induced dipolar structure may occur as a result of a temporary imbalance of charge distribution within molecules. These forces are very weak (0.5–1 kcal/mol) and decrease proportionally to the seventh power of the interatomic distance. These bonds, also referred to as van der Waals' forces or London forces, require that the two nonpolar molecules come in close proximity to one another.

AFFINITY—THE ROLE OF CONFORMATION

Most therapeutically useful drugs bind only transiently to their intended receptor. The combination of a variety of

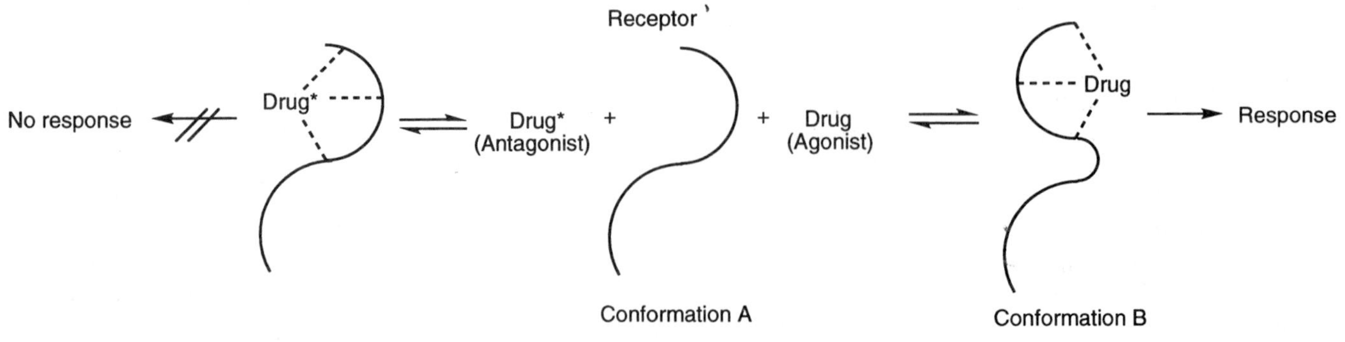

Fig. 4.2. Diagramatic representation of drug-induced fit theory, in which an agonist (drug) or antagonist (drug*) interacts with two different conformations of the receptor.

bonds including ionic, hydrogen and van der Waals' attractive forces can contribute to the binding of a drug to the receptor. The critical portion of the structure of the drug which is believed to bind to the receptor is termed the *pharmacophore*. Once the drug has bound, a biologic response may result (e.g., especially if an agonist). Following or in the process of binding to the receptor there may be a conformational change in the receptor that initiates the activation of the biologic response, and also changes the attractive environment between the drug and the receptor. This conformational change in the receptor may also allow for the dissociation of the drug-receptor complex. This simple explanation of the interaction of a drug with a receptor producing a biologic response is commonly referred to as *the occupancy theory*, and predicts that the response is directly related to the number of receptors bound by an agonist.

Another theory of drug-receptor interactions termed the *rate theory* suggests that the number of drug-receptor interactions per unit time determines the intensity of the response. Thus, drugs that associate with and then rapidly dissociate from the receptor, thus allowing other drug molecules to subsequently interact with the receptor, would be expected to produce the most robust responses. The *induced-fit theory* suggests that as the drug approaches the receptor a conformational change occurs in the receptor to allow for effective binding (Fig. 4.2). According to this theory the receptor does not normally exist in the proper conformation for drug binding. Following dissociation of the drug the receptor can then revert to its original configuration. In this theory an antagonist can induce a conformational change in the receptor, however the change is not the proper change required for a biologic response to be elicited. Combining the induced-fit and rate theories yields the *macromolecular pertubation theory* which suggests that two types of conformational changes exist, and that the rate of their existence determines the observed biologic response. Agonists produce the specific pertubation required for a biologic response, while antagonists produce a non-specific pertubation which fails to yield a biologic response. This theory can partially account for the activity of partial agonists. Finally, the *activation-aggregation theory* indicates that receptors are always in a dynamic equilibrium between active and inactive states. Agonists function by shifting the equilibrium toward the activated state, while antagonists prevent the activated state.

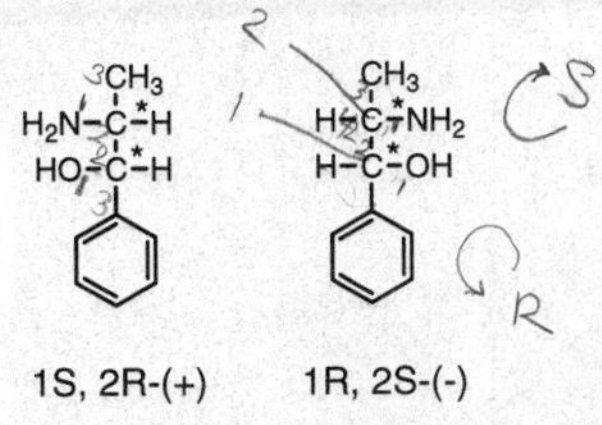

This theory can account for the activity of inverse agonists which produce neither a typical agonist response nor an antagonist response (i.e., blocking the receptor), but rather produce responses opposite to those of the agonist.

AFFINITY—THE ROLE OF STEREOCHEMISTRY

Very specific three-dimensional requirements must be satisfied for a compound to effectively act as an agonist. To elegantly demonstrate the specificity of a drug for its receptor, the unique three-dimensional characteristics of chiral compounds can be used as an example. As early as 1901 Pasteur noted the significance of asymmetric compounds in biological systems (8). Since that time, much has been learned from chiral compounds regarding three-dimensional binding requirements of receptors. For instance, although the individual *enantiomers* (non-superimposable mirror images) of norephedrine (2-amino-3-phenyl-1-propanol; Fig. 4.3) have identical molecular weights, melting points, lipid solubility and empirical formulae, these compounds have significantly different alpha adrenoceptor agonistic activities. The 1R,2S enantiomer (levo) is about 100 times more potent than the 1S,2R enantiomer (dextro) *in vivo* and *in vitro* (9,10). (Because there are two chiral centers, there is also another set of stereoisomers called diasteriomers, 1S,2S and 1R,2R that have an even different pharmacologic profile.) Thus, the greater efficacy of the 1R,2S enantiomer is most likely dependent upon its ability to bind and activate the receptor as a result of its preferential fit into the receptor.

Since labetalol, an adrenoceptor blocking agent structurally related to epinephrine, has two asymmetric centers, four diastereomers exist, Figure 4.4. The formulation available for use as a mixed α- and β-adrenoceptor blocker, contains equal amounts of each diastereomer. The R,R isomer accounts for much of the β-adrenoceptor blocking activity, while the S,R isomer has the greatest effect on α-adrenoceptors. The S,S isomer has some α-adrenoceptor blocking activity, but has no activity at β-adrenoceptors. The R,S isomer is essentially devoid of activity at both α- and β-adrenoceptors.

Many synthetically prepared therapeutic agents are a mixture of two enantiomers (racemates), with one enan-

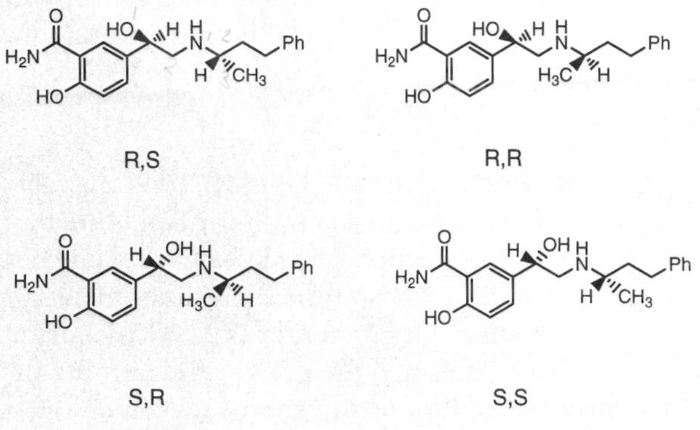

Fig. 4.3. Projection formulae of 2-amino-3-phenyl-1-propanol stereoisomers. From Maher TJ, Johnson DA. Drug Dev Res 1991; 24:149.

Fig. 4.4. Diastereomers of labetalol.

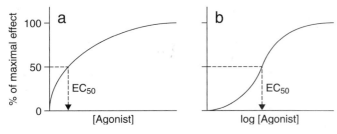

Fig 4.5. Plot of (a) dose or concentration and (b) log of the dose or concentration of a drug versus the effect produced.

tiomer termed the *eutomer* being largely responsible for the desired pharmacologic effect (11). The other enantiomer termed the *distomer* may be inactive, or even contribute more significantly to the toxicity of the therapeutic agent. Thus in the future, knowledge of chirality should play a significant role in the advances gained in receptor theory, as well as in therapeutics.

RECEPTOR BINDING AND DRUG DISCOVERY

The discovery of pharmacological agents by modern pharmaceutical companies and universities often involves the use of receptor-ligand binding techniques. Following the synthesis of a series of new chemically-related compounds, which may constitute hundreds to thousands of compounds, the determination of the desired biological activity used to be a rather daunting task. Prior to the advent of receptor-ligand binding techniques the initial screening of these compounds involved individually injecting each agent into experimental animals or incubating each agent with isolated tissues (e.g., intestine, heart, skeletal muscle), techniques that require a large investment of resources including personnel, time, animals and money. Nowadays receptor-ligand binding techniques are used to narrow large numbers of compounds down to those which display greatest affinity for a receptor, thereby significantly decreasing the time and cost associated with identifying "lead" compounds. However, one danger associated with such an initial screening approach is the failure to recognize potentially useful compounds that might require biotransformation prior to exerting a biological effect, such as a pro-drug. Additionally, it should be remembered that ligand binding based on the affinity of a drug for a receptor does not differentiate agonists from antagonists. Despite these potential pitfalls associated with receptor-ligand binding techniques, modern day drug discovery relies heavily upon these approaches.

DOSE-RESPONSE RELATIONSHIPS

A.J. Clark is generally given credit for being the first to apply the law of mass action principles to the concept of drug-receptor interactions, thus providing further evidence for dose-effect phenomenon (12). This concept as applied by Clark states that the greater the number of agonist molecules present at the site of the receptors, the greater will be the response, i.e., a direct relationship.

However, these principles of the law of mass action in receptor-drug interactions have been questioned. The law of mass action applies to compounds dissolved in fluids, that are allowed to diffuse freely. Now that much is known about the anchoring of most receptors to, or within, cell membranes where receptor-drug interactions are thought to occur, this environment would actually constitute a solid-liquid interface, and thus the law of mass action as applied to compounds dissolved in fluids where they are allowed to diffuse freely might not be completely applicable.

Equation 4.1 illustrates the interaction of a drug [D] with a receptor [R], which results in a drug-receptor complex [DR] and a biologic response. The interaction between most therapeutically useful drugs and its receptor is generally reversible.

Eq. 4.1 $$[D] + [R] \rightleftharpoons [D \sim R] \longrightarrow \text{Biologic Response}$$

Following administration of a drug one can monitor the biologic responses produced. Plotting the dose or concentration of the drug versus the effect produced (% response) yields a rectangular hyperbolic function as illustrated in Figure 4.5a. This type of function is mathematically difficult to accurately extrapolate quantitative information from due to the constantly changing slope of the curve. However, when the effect produced is plotted against the log of the drug concentration or dose administered, a sigmoidal function results, Figure 4.5b. This function possesses a relatively linear portion of the curve about its central point, thereby making quantitative extrapolations more accurate.

Dose-response curves are typically plotted to determine both quantitative and qualitative parameters of *potency* and *efficacy*. Potency is inversely related to the dose required to produce a given response (typically half-maximum), while efficacy is the ability of a drug to produce a full response (100% maximum). In Figure 4.6, Drug X is equally efficacious to Drug Y, but Drug X is more potent than Drug Y. That is to say, both Drug X and Y can produce a 100% response with Drug X reaching that response at a lower dose. Visual inspection of such dose-response curves allows for easy qualitative interpretations, e.g., in a series of curves, those positioned to the left are more potent than

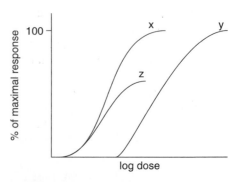

Fig 4.6. Dose–response relationship.

those positioned to the right. Additionally illustrated, in Figure 4.6, Drug Z is more potent than Drug Y, and Drug Z is equipotent to Drug X. However, comparisons of efficacy are visually apparent as the greater the maximum response (i.e., efficacy), the higher the maximum point on the dose-response curve. Thus, in Figure 4.6 Drugs X and Y are of equal efficacy, and of greater efficacy than Drug Z.

PRESYNAPTIC AND POSTSYNAPTIC RECEPTOR LOCATIONS

When an action potential arrives at the nerve cell's axon, a depolarization-induced exocytosis of neurotransmitter from its storage sites in the *presynaptic* terminal occurs. Through this process the action potential continues the flow of information to the target site, typically the *postsynaptic* cell. The neurotransmitter is believed to diffuse across the extracellular fluid filled space known as the synapse and interact with postsynaptic receptors. However, the released neurotransmitter may also be capable of interacting with presynaptic receptors located on the neurons that just released the neurotransmitter. The function of these receptors typically involve the regulation of nerve transmission, and are referred to as *autoreceptors* since the neurotransmitters that activate them function to control their own release.

An exquisite example of both receptor locations and the action of autoreceptors in the control of neurotransmission is observed in norepinephrine-containing postganglionic neurons of the sympathetic nervous system (Fig. 4.7) (13). Norepinephrine, which is capable of stimulating both α- and β-adrenoceptors, initially is released and is present in low concentration in the synapse. Low concentrations of this agent are capable of preferentially stimulating β-adrenoceptors located presynaptically, which function to increase the release of more neurotransmitter and thereby magnify the intended response. Additionally, the epinephrine released from the adrenal medulla during sympathetic stimulation is thought to also play an important role in facilitating neuronal norepinephrine release. This is an example of a positive feedback system which allows for a rapid rise in the concentration of the neurotransmitter, and thus the intended signal. Following this initial period of robust norepinephrine release, very high norepinephrine concentrations in the synaptic cleft result, which then is capable of stimulating other presynaptic autoreceptors, this time which terminate the additional release of neurotransmitter. This negative-feedback system allows for the signal to be terminated very quickly.

Together, the presynaptic facilitatory β-adrenoceptor-mediated mechanism and the presynaptic inhibitory α-adrenoceptor-mediated mechanism allow for a rapid, robust and well-controlled signal to be delivered. If one were to design a system that was to respond quickly to stressors, such as the sympathetic nervous system is believed to be designed to do, a system that turns on rapidly and can be

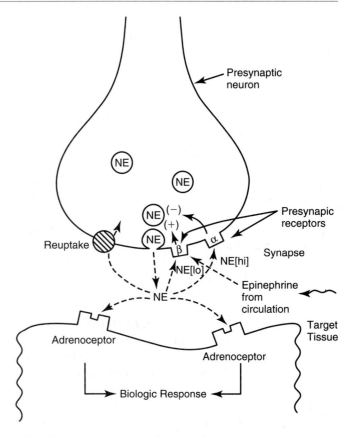

Fig. 4.7. Autoreceptor control of neurotransmission as observed in norepinephrine-containing postganglionic neurons of the sympathetic nervous system. NE, norepinephrine; NE[lo], low norepinephrine concentration; NE[hi], high norepinephrine concentration, α, alpha adrenoceptor; β, beta adrenoceptor; (−), inhibit; (+), stimulate.

terminated quickly would be ideal, and presumably of an evolutionary advantage. Additionally, many other neurotransmitter autoreceptors have been identified, for instance in the serotoninergic, dopaminergic and histaminergic transmitter systems. There are even examples whereby a neurotransmitter can interact with a presynaptic receptor to influence the release of a different neurotransmitter. For instance, norepinephrine released from neurons in the gastrointestinal tract can function to decrease acetylcholine release.

RECEPTORS AND THE BIOLOGIC RESPONSE
Signal Transduction

Signal transduction is the process by which receptor activation results in the modification of cellular structure and functions. The process of signal transduction serves several critical roles. First, it enables extracellular molecules to affect cellular function without entering the intracellular environment. This "long distance" communication is accomplished by the binding of an agonist to the receptor protein and stabilizing the receptor structure in an active conformation. The active receptor conformation can then facilitate the flow of ions through a membrane channel by the removal of steric or electronic hindrances (opening of channel gates). For those receptors which produce signals via activation of intracellular metabolic pathways, the active state or conformation changes the intracellular molecular environment in such a way as to activate, directly or indirectly, intracellular regulatory enzymes. Second, several different signals may affect one another by facilitating or inhibiting the activation of regulatory enzymatic proteins via common or opposing metabolic pathways. Thus, signal transduction mechanisms can interact in such a way as to yield an integrated response to multiple stimuli. Third, via the activation of enzymes and the production of second messengers (e.g., cyclic-AMP, DAG, IP_3), an initially weak signal can be amplified, and its duration prolonged, to produce a robust cellular response. This amplification can occur through several mechanisms. The kinetic time-frame for enzyme activation and the presence of key metabolites may be much longer than the time of receptor activation itself. Thus, a brief activation of a small number of receptors may result in a magnified response by the cell. Amplification can also occur via a molecular "cascade" where one initial signal can trigger a multitude of intracellular reactions which lead to an enhanced cellular response. Outcomes of signal transduction may include one or more of the following: 1) a change in cell membrane polarity in electrically excitable tissues such as nerves and muscles which then results in the facilitation or inhibition of an action potential, thus affecting the excitability of the tissue; 2) the activation of cytosolic metabolic cascades resulting in alterations in cellular morphology or function; and 3) gene activation leading to the synthesis of new proteins which may then modify cellular structures and physiology.

Ligand-gated Ion Channels

The most rapid cellular responses to receptor activation are mediated via ligand-gated ion channels (LGICs) (Fig. 4.8). The main component of this signal transduction pathway is a plasma membrane spanning protein composed of multiple peptide subunits, each of which contains four membrane spanning domains. The nicotinic acetylcholine receptor is perhaps the best characterized LGIC. The nicotinic receptor is composed of 5 distinct subunits, two α, and, depending on the receptor subtype,

various combinations of additional α, β, γ and δ subunits. The binding of an acetylcholine molecule to the binding site on each of two α subunits induces a conformational change in the receptor, opening a sodium selective ion channel through the center of the protein. The result is depolarization of the surrounding plasma membrane. Other neurotransmitter activated LGICs include GABA (γ-aminobutyric acid), glycine, glutamate and serotonin receptors. These receptors share a similar structural conformation and function to the nicotinic receptor, except for the specificity of the ligand binding site and selectivity of the channel for particular ions. The primary reason for the rapidity (milliseconds), of the cellular response with LGICs is that the transduction of the signal requires the activation of a single molecule. This transduction mechanism therefore, is especially well suited for physiologic processes necessitating an immediate response such as the stimulation of nerves and muscles.

G-protein Coupled Receptors

G-protein coupled receptors are a class of large membrane bound proteins, which share a well conserved structure, and transduce their signal via the activation of an intracellular guanine nucleotide binding protein (G-protein). This family of proteins has seven hydrophobic domains which span the plasma membrane and therefore is sometimes referred to as having a serpentine structure (Fig. 4.9). The extracellular region of the protein is composed of the amino terminus and several loops which comprise the ligand binding site. Smaller ligands tend to bind deep within the extracellular loops, close to the plasma membrane, while larger molecules have binding sites which are more superficial. The carboxy end of the receptor is located in the area of the protein which protrudes into the cytoplasm. The intracellular side of the receptor also includes the binding site for the G-protein which usually binds to the third loop between the sixth and seventh transmembrane regions of the protein. Close to the carboxy terminus are serine and threonine residues which are targets for ATP-dependent phosphorylation. Following prolonged activation, phosphorylation of these residues is hypothesized to occur via a negative feedback regulatory metabolic pathway which facilitates the binding of modulating molecules, that subsequently impair the coupling of G-proteins to the receptor. The result is receptor desensitization.

There are over 100 different G-protein coupled receptors which bind to a variety of ligands encompassing biogenic amines, such as acetylcholine, norepinephrine and serotonin; amino acid neurotransmitters such as glutamate and glycine, and peptide hormones such as angiotensin II and somatostatin. There are multiple G-protein coupled receptor types for a single ligand. The result is the possibility that a single ligand can activate a variety of transduction pathways and produce a multiplicity of cellular responses. Thus a receptor is defined not just by which ligand

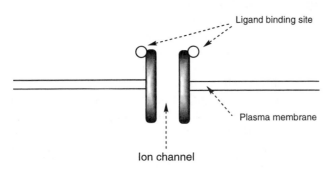

Fig. 4.8. Ligand-gated ion channel receptor.

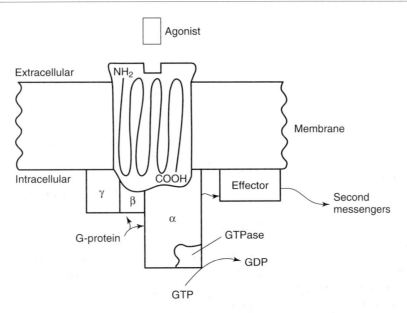

Fig. 4.9. G-protein coupled receptor. α, β, γ, correspond to G-protein subunits.

binds to it, but also by how the signal is transduced and the resulting physiologic response. As an example, there are at least nine different adrenergic receptor subtypes. Norepinephrine can bind to the β_1 receptor, which is coupled to a G-protein(designated G_s). Following receptor stimulation, there is activation of the enzyme adenylyl cyclase, thus leading ultimately to an increase in heart rate and force of contraction. Norepinephrine binding to α_1-receptors, on the other hand, results in the binding to a different G-protein (G_q), which activates the production of the second messengers inositol triphosphate (IP_3) and diacylglycerol (DAG), which then initiate a cascade of intracellular events leading to smooth muscle contraction. Therefore, a single ligand can induce a wide range of responses as a consequence of coupling to different G-proteins. Which G-protein is activated depends on factors such as the presence and availability of individual G-proteins within a particular cell type, kinetic issues such as the binding affinity of the G-protein for the receptor protein, and finally, the affinity of the activated G-protein subunits for signal transduction enzymes.

G-proteins. G-proteins are heterotrimeric in structure with the subunits (in decreasing size), designated as α, β, and γ. At least 13 types of G-proteins have been identified,

which are divided among four families, G_s, G_i, G_q, and G_{12}. Individual G-proteins transduce the receptor activation signal via one of a number of second messenger systems discussed below. The best understood second messenger systems associated with each G-protein family are summarized in Table 4.1.

It is the characteristics of the α subunit which determine the designation of the G-protein. Receptor activation leads to a conformational change in the associated G-protein; triggering the release of bound GDP from the α-subunit, which is then replaced by a molecule of GTP. With the binding of GTP, the α-subunit GTP complex dissociates from the αβ-subunits and binds to a particular target enzyme, resulting in its activation or inhibition. Within a short period of time the α-subunit catalyzes the dephosphorylation of the associated GTP molecule to GDP, resulting in the reassociation of the α-subunit with the αβ-subunits and thus the return of the G-protein to the inactivated state (Fig. 4.9). Variations on this scheme include the activation of proteins such as G-protein gated ion channels by dissociated αβ-subunits and the ability of receptor proteins to activate more than a single G-protein. The simultaneous activation of more than one type of G-protein coupled receptor results in the initiation of multiple signals which can then interact with one another (a phenomenon commonly referred to as cross talk). This interaction can be of several types: If both receptors utilize a common signal transduction pathway, the activation can result in an additive response by the cell. Conversely, if simultaneous receptor activation triggers opposing signal transduction pathways, then the outcome will be an attenuated cellular response. Other types of interactions may include the desensitization or activation of other receptor proteins or second messenger pathways. The final outcome of the activation of multiple signals is an integrated response by the cell.

Table 4.1. G-Protein Transducers and Second Messenger

G-Protein Transducer Family	Second Messenger System
G_s	Enhance adenylyl cyclase activity
G_i	Inhibit adenylyl cyclase activity
G_q	Stimulate phospholipase C activity
G_{12}	Modulate sodium/hydrogen ion exchanger

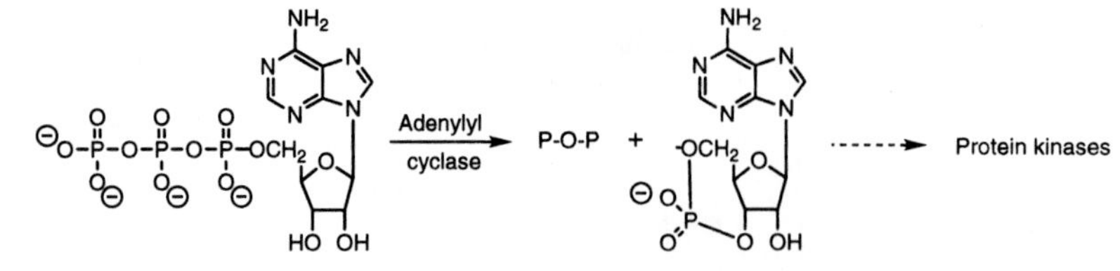

Fig. 4.10. Conversion of ATP to c-AMP catalyzed by adenylyl cyclase.

Second Messenger Pathways. As discussed above, in response to receptor activation, G-proteins activate plasma membrane bound enzymes which then trigger a metabolic cascade resulting in a cellular response. The products of these enzymatic actions are termed second messengers since they mobilize other enzymatic and structural proteins which then produce the cellular response. The enzymes which catalyze the synthesis of second messengers generally fall into two categories, those that convert the purine triphosphates ATP and GTP into their respective cyclic monophosphates, and enzymes which synthesize second messengers from plasma membrane phospholipids. The most thoroughly studied second messenger system is controlled by a family of 10 plasma membrane bound isoenzymes of adenylyl cyclase which catalyze the conversion of ATP to cyclic adenosine monophosphate (c-AMP) (Fig. 4.10). Adenylyl cyclase is activated by the G_s family of G-proteins and inhibited by G_i proteins. Following synthesis, c-AMP activates c-AMP-dependent protein kinases (PKAs) by triggering the dissociation of regulatory subunits from catalytic subunits. The catalytic subunits then activate other target proteins via phosphorylation, which then trigger the cellular response. The magnitude of the cellular response is proportional to the concentration of c-AMP. Degradation of c-AMP occurs via phosphodiesterases or by reducing c-AMP concentration via active transport out of the cell. The result is termination of the signal.

A similar, although less ubiquitous second messenger pathway is associated with guanylyl cyclase. Guanylyl cyclase is activated in response to catalytic receptors selective for ligands including atrial natriuretic factor and nitric oxide. When stimulated guanylyl cyclase then catalyzes the synthesis of c-GMP from GTP. Cyclic-GMP subsequently activates c-GMP-dependent protein kinases which then activate other proteins. The actions of c-GMP are terminated by enzymatic degradation of the second messenger or the dephosphorylation of substrates. One effect of this second messenger pathway is the relaxation of smooth muscle via the dephosphorylation of myosin light chains.

The generation of second messengers from plasma membrane phospholipids is mediated primarily by G-protein activation of phospholipase C. There are three families of phospholipase C (PLC), designated PLC-β, PLC-γ, and PLC-δ. Phospholipase C-β can be activated by the α-subunit of the G_q family of G-proteins or the βγ subunits of other G-proteins. PLC-γ is activated via tyrosine kinase receptors, however, the mechanism for PLC-δ is not yet understood. Upon activation, PLC hydrolyzes phosphatidyl inositol-4,5-bisphosphate to diacylglycerol (DAG) and inositol-1,4,5-triphosphate (IP_3) (Fig. 4.11). IP_3 is water soluble and diffuses into the cytoplasm where it triggers the release of calcium from intracellular stores. Intracellular calcium then binds to the protein calmodulin and also to protein kinase C (PKC), both of which then stimulate, via phosphorylation a broad range of enzymes and other proteins including specific kinases. The other product of PLC, DAG is lipid soluble and remains in the plasma membrane where it facilitates the activation of PKC by calcium. The signal is terminated via inactivation of IP_3 by dephosphorylation, while DAG is inactivated by phosphorylation to phosphatidic acid or deacetylation to fatty acids. The concentration of intracellular calcium is reduced by sequestration within cytoplasmic organelles or transport out of the cell. Activation of phospholipase D hydrolyzes phosphatidylcholine to phosphatidic acid which can then be metabolized to DAG via phosphatidate phosphohydro-

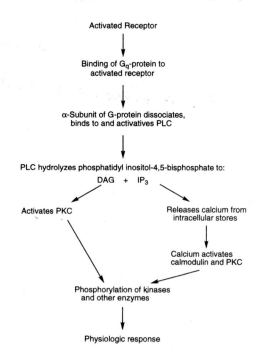

Fig 4.11. Phospholipase C second messanger cascade. DAG, diacylglycerol; IP_3, inositol-1,4,5-triphosphate; PLC, phospholipase C; PKC, protein kinase C.

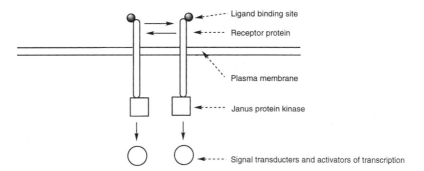

Fig. 4.12. Diagrammatic representation of an enzyme coupled receptor.

lase. This pathway prolongs the duration of elevated levels of DAG. Phospholipase A$_2$ is activated by increased concentrations of intracellular calcium and metabolizes phosphatidylcholine to arachidonic acid. Arachidonic acid then functions as a substrate for the synthesis of autocoids including prostaglandins, thromboxane A$_2$ and leukotrienes.

Catalytic Receptors

Catalytic receptors are a class of plasma membrane bound receptors which are characterized by a monomer with a ligand binding site in the extracellular domain, a single membrane spanning domain, and an intracellular domain with enzymatic activity. This family of receptors is activated predominately by peptide hormones such as insulin, epidermal growth factor, platelet derived growth factor and atrial natriuretic factor (ANF). The catalytic portion of the receptor functions as a protein kinase targeting primarily tyrosine residues, however, the receptor for ANF rather than having kinase activity, metabolizes GTP to c-GMP. Receptor activation occurs by ligand binding, which then triggers dimerization of receptor proteins via the cross phosphorylation of tyrosine residues. The dimeric protein is the active form of the catalytic receptor. One consequence of activation via dimerization is that the intracellular signal can be maintained even after the ligand has dissociated from the binding site. The phosphorylation of intracellular proteins by this receptor type results in effects such as the opening of ion channels, changes in cytoplasmic function, or the initiation of genomic expression.

Enzyme Coupled Receptors

Enzyme coupled receptors are similar in their function to catalytic receptors except rather than inherent catalytic activity, enzyme coupled receptors bind to separate enzymatic proteins (Fig. 4.12). This class of receptor binds cytokines including growth hormone, erythropoietin and interferon. Like catalytic receptors, enzyme coupled receptors are activated via dimerization following ligand binding. Kinase activity is accomplished by a separate non-covalently bound protein kinases of the Janus-kinase (JAK) family. Following dimerization, JAKs are activated and phosphorylate receptor tyrosine residues. The phosphorylated receptor then binds other molecules termed "signal transducers and activators of transcription" (STATS), which are phosphorylated by the JAKs and subsequently dissociate into the cytoplasm. The STATS then translocate to the nucleus where they initiate gene transcription.

Cytoplasmic Receptors

Cytoplasmic receptors differ from those described above in that they are not associated with the plasma membrane but are located within the cytoplasm (Fig. 4.13). Cytoplasmic receptors are composed of a single polypeptide with three functional domains. The amino terminal contains a binding site for a modulator protein termed heat shock protein-90 (HSP-90) which is associated with the receptor in the absence of agonist. In the middle of the receptor peptide is a binding site for DNA, and the carboxy terminus contains the ligand binding site. Cytoplasmic receptors are activated by lipid soluble ligands which passively diffuse through the plasma membrane. Agonists include nitric oxide, steroid hormones and vitamin D. Ligand binding activates the receptor by inducing the dissociation of HSP-90. The receptor then translocates to the nucleus and binds to a DNA response element which then initiates translation of the target gene. The response to this type of signal transduction is relatively slow, requiring 30 minutes to several hours following protein binding. Moreover, the duration of the response can last long after the concentration of the ligand has fallen to zero. The duration of the response is related to turnover rate of the synthesized protein, however, it may also be affected by a ligand with extremely high binding affinity, possibly resulting in prolonged receptor activation.

RECEPTOR SUBTYPES

Careful examination of the effects of a series of sympathomimetics by Ahlquist led him to postulate the existence of at least two types of adrenoceptors, which he termed α and β (21). Realizing that adrenoceptor agonists were capable of causing either relaxation or contraction of isolated smooth muscles, he noted that while a compound like norepinephrine had potent excitatory actions but

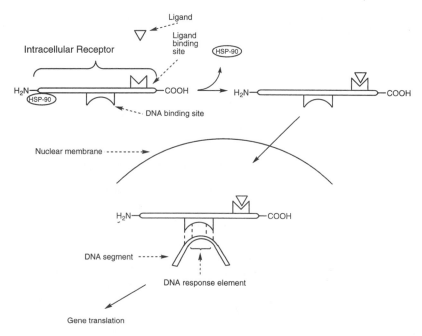

Fig. 4.13. Cytoplasmic receptor found within the cell. The receptor contains an attached heat shock protein-90 (HSP-90), a ligand binding site, and a DNA binding site.

weak inhibitory actions, another catecholamine, isoproterenol had potent inhibitory actions but weak excitatory actions. When a series of related compounds were tested for potency in various tissues, it was demonstrated that for the α-adrenoceptor the order of potency was: epinephrine $\geq$ norepinephrine $>>>$ isoproterenol, and for the β-adrenoceptor the order of potency was: isoproterenol $>$ epinephrine $\geq$ norepinephrine. Following the findings of Ahlquist, others utilized specific antagonists that had become available to further support this designation of receptor subtypes. Additionally, with the development of highly selective antagonists, the classification of receptors into subtypes has expanded at a tremendous rate (22). For example, the α-adrenoceptor noted above can be subclassed as α_{1A}, α_{1B}, α_{1C}, α_{1D} and α_{2A}, α_{2B} and α_{2C} based on cloning experiments, Table 4.2.

However, the therapeutic significance of such distinctions is not yet known due to a lack of selective agonists or antagonists. Some therapeutic distinction can be made

between α_1 and α_2 adrenoceptors in a general way in that α_1 vasoconstriction antagonism by prazosin, or central nervous system α_2 adrenoceptor stimulation by clonidine, both are useful in the treatment of hypertension. Similarly, β-adrenoceptor antagonists are available that antagonize β_1 adrenoceptors with some selectivity. Thus the use of metoprolol, a selective β_1 antagonist, is effective and relatively safe in hypertensive patients with compromised airway function, while the use of a non-selective (β_1 and β_2) antagonist such as propranolol would be clearly contraindicated in such a patient.

A summary of the most important receptor subtypes from a therapeutic standpoint is presented in Table 4.3. The reader should realize that this is a simplification of what is currently known about the various receptor subtypes. For instance, within the general category of serotonin receptors, at least 13 subtypes can be identified from cloning experiments. However, the lack of selective agonists and antagonists to characterize the pharmacology of

Table 4.2. Adrenoceptor Families

Receptor Type	Subtype	Transduction Mechanism	Tissue Function
α_1	1A	Activates $G_{q/11}$	Smooth muscle and myocardial contraction
α_1	1B	Activates $G_{q/11}$	Smooth muscle contraction
α_1	1D	Activates $G_{q/11}$	Smooth muscle contraction
α_2	2A	Activates $G_{i/o}$	Hypotension, sedation, analgesia, anesthesia
α_2	2B	Activates $G_{i/o}$	Vasoconstriction
α_2	2C	Activates $G_{i/o}$	Not established
β_1	—	Activates G_s	Increases heart rate and force of contraction
β_2	—	Activates G_s	Smooth muscle relaxation
β_3	—	Activates or inhibits adenylyl cyclase	Lipolysis, cardioinhibition

Table 4.3. Survey of Receptor Subtypes

Receptor Class	Subtype	Selective Agonist	Selective Antagonist	Effector	Cloned
Adrenoceptor	α_1	Phenylephrine	Prazosin	IP_3/DAG	Yes
	α_2	Clonidine	Yohimbine	↓cAMP	Yes
	β_1	Dobutamine	Atenolol	↑cAMP	Yes
	β_2	Terbutaline	Butoxamine	↑cAMP	Yes
Dopamine receptors	D_1	Fenoldopam	Dihydroxidine	↑cAMP	Yes
	D_2	Bromocriptine	(−) Sulpiride	↓cAMP	Yes
Excitatory amino acid receptor	NMDA	NMDA	D-AP5	↓Na^+/Ca^{++}	Yes
	AMPA	AMPA	CNQX	↑Na^+	Yes
	Kainate	Kainate	?	↑Na^+/K^+	Yes
GABA receptors	$GABA_A$	Muscimol	Bicuculline	↑Cl^-	Yes
	$GABA_B$	Baclofen	Saclofen	↓cAMP	Yes
Histamine receptor	H_1	2-(m-Fluorophenyl) Histamine	Mepyramine	IP3/DAG	Yes
	H_2	Dimapril	Ranitidine	↑cAMP	Yes
Muscarinic receptors	M_1	Oxotremorine	Pirenzepine	IP_3/DAG	Yes
	M_2	Oxotremorine	AF-DX116	↓cAMP	Yes
Nicotinic receptor	N_{muscle}	?	Decamethonium	↑Na^+/Ca^{++}	Yes
	$N_{neuronal}$	?	Hexamethonium	↑Na^+/Ca^{++}	Yes
Opioid receptor	Mu	Sufentanil	CTAP	↓cAMP	Yes
	Delta	[DAla²]deltorphin	Naltrindole	↓cAMP	Yes
	Kappa	Dynorphin	Nor-binaltorphimine	↓cAMP	Yes
Serotonin receptor (5-HT)	$5\text{-}HT_{1A}$	8-OH-DPAT	Spiperone	↓cAMP	Yes
	$5\text{-}HT_{2A}$	α-Methyl-5-HT	Ketanserin	IP_3/DAG	Yes

?, no known selective compounds available; cloned, receptor subtype has been cloned and the amino acid structure is known. Chemical abbreviations used: AF-DX116, 11-([2-{(di-ethylamino)methyl}-1-piperidinyl]acetyl)-5-11-dihydro-6H-pyridol[2,3-b] [1,4]benzodiazepine-6-one; AMPA, D,L-α-amino-3-hydroxy-5-methyl-4-isoxalone propionic acid; cAMP, cyclic adenosine 3′,5′-monophosphate; CNQX, 6-cyano-7-nitroquinoxaline-2,3-dione; CTAP, D-Phe-Cys-Tyr-DTrp-Arg-Thr-Pen-Thr-NH₂; DAG, diacyl glycerol; D-AP5, D-amino-5-phospho-nopentanoate; GABA, γ-aminobutyric acid; 5-HT, 5-hydroxytryptamine, serotonin; IP-3, inositol 1,4,5-triphosphate; NMDA, N-methyl-D-asparatate; 8-OH-DPAT, 8-hydroxy-2-(di-n-propylamino)tetralin.

each of these subtypes, has hindered our understanding of their individual functions and importance from a therapeutic standpoint. Our ability to eventually develop drugs that selectively manipulate such receptor subtypes has enormous therapeutic implications.

SPARE RECEPTORS

Biological systems often have built in safety factors to enhance the efficiency of receptor-stimulus coupling and thereby assure the desired neurotransmission. In many tissues containing α-adrenoceptors, in order to produce a maximum response, only a small percentage of the available receptors need be occupied. This depends on the particular tissue being studied and the agonist utilized. Occupancy of 100% of the available receptors is therefore not always required since *spare receptors* or *receptor reserve* are present. Studies utilizing phenoxybenzamine, which alkylates the α-adrenoceptor, and therefore irreversibly inactivates the receptor, indicate that only 5–10% of the available receptors need be activated to elicit a maximum response to a *full*, or *strong agonist* such as norepinephrine or phenylephrine (6,7,23). However, to obtain a maximum response to a *partial agonist* like ephedrine, nearly 100% of the receptors need to be occupied. The explanation behind this difference may involve a less than ideal receptor-drug interaction for partial agonists. A partial agonist may function as an antagonist if it interferes with the ability of a full agonist to bind to its receptor and produce a response. However, in the absence of a full agonist, the partial agonist only displays agonistic activity.

DYNAMIC NATURE OF RECEPTORS

As characteristic of most of the individual components of living systems, receptors are not static, rather they are constantly in a state of dynamic adaptation. One could envision these protein molecules floating within the fluid mosaic of the biological membrane awaiting interaction with normal physiological signals. The function of such receptors, once stimulated, involves attempts at correcting perturbations of the normal physiology of the cell or organism. This role in maintaining homeostasis within the organism requires constant adaptations to the changing environment. One approach of responding to such unpredictable challenges to homeostasis that appears to have developed in just about every species studied, involves the ability of receptors to change in response to such external assaults. Receptors are known to be able to decrease in actual number, or in their affinity for an agonist when stimulated at higher than normal frequencies. This alteration in the availability or functional capacity of a given receptor most likely constitutes an adaptive mechanism whereby the cell or organism is protected from agonist overload. For example, the chronic administration of a β-adrenoceptor agonist such as isoproterenol, is known to produce a *desensitization* of the β-adrenoceptors in the heart (24). During this period of overstimulation, the cell somehow recognizes the abnormal intensity of stimulation and initiates an adaptive change in the cell to protect its homeostasis. This is accomplished by a process of *down-regulation* of the receptor. As a general principle, the body will always attempt to maintain homeostasis, whether perturbed by environmental challenges, disease processes, or even the administration of drugs. Actually, the body sees the administration of drugs as a pertubation of homeostasis and usually attempts to overcome the effects of the drug by invoking receptor adaptations. However, oftentimes with appropriate dosing schedules drugs can be used with little observed receptor adaptation such that the desired pharmacologic effect continues to be observed.

In a similar fashion to the example described above, chronic administration of the β-adrenoceptor antagonist propranolol leads to a state of receptor *supersensitivity* or *up-regulation*. The cells within the tissue, such as the heart, sense an alteration in the normal rate of basal β-adrenoceptor stimulation, and thus respond by either increasing the number or affinity of the receptors for their natural agonists, norepinephrine and epinephrine. Additionally, an enhanced efficiency of the interaction between the receptor and its transducing systems may also account for a portion of the observed supersensitivity. The knowledge that such a receptor adaptation occurs has paramount practical therapeutic implications, since abrupt withdrawal of this class of agents may precipitate acute myocardial infarction, and thus this practice should be scrupulously avoided.

Some pathophysiologic states are characterized by perturbations in receptor dynamics. Prinzmetal's angina is thought to be characterized by an imbalance between vasodilatory β_2 adrenoceptor function and vasoconstrictor α_1 adrenoceptor function. In this disease state, the excessive alpha vasoconstriction of coronary arteries leads to myocardial ischemia and pain. The inadvertent use of a β-adrenoceptor antagonist, which is safely employed in typical angina pectoris to prevent β-adrenoceptor vasodilation, may leave unopposed the alpha vasoconstrictor influences and actually precipitate anginal pain. Thus, an understanding of the role receptors play in physiology, pathophysiology and pharmacology is essential for optimal therapeutic interventions.

FUTURE DIRECTIONS

Our understanding of the nature and role of receptors has increased tremendously since the early work of Langley and Ehrlich. Today with the advances made in the field of molecular biology, it is possible to clone individual receptor subtypes (see Table 4.3) and determine their function in cell culture. By modifying the amino acid structure at those sites believed to be involved in agonist binding, a better appreciation of the interaction of drugs currently available, and the rational design of those awaiting discovery, may be realized. Additionally, as we begin to be able to determine the structure of receptor subtypes through cloning techniques, we hopefully will better understand those disease processes that result from, or lead to, receptor adaptations or dysfunction.

REFERENCES

1. Leake CD. A Historical Account of Pharmacology in the 20th Century. Springfield, Charles C. Thomas, 1975.
2. Langley, JN. On the reaction of cells and nerve endings to certain poisons. J Physiol 1905;33:374.
3. Ehrlich, P. In: Himmelweit F, ed. Collected Papers of Paul Ehrlich. vol III , London: Pergammon, 1957.
4. Price CC. Chemistry of alkylation. In: Sartorelli AC and Johns DG, eds. Antineoplastic and Immunosuppressive Agents, Part II Handbuch der Experimentellen Pharmakologie, Vol. 38, Berlin, Springer-Verlag, 1975.
5. Nickerson M. Receptor occupancy and tissue response. Nature 1956;178:697.
6. Minneman KP, Abel PW. Relationship between alpha-1 adrenoceptor density and functional response of rat vas deferens. Studies with phenoxybenzamine. Naunyn Schmiedebergs Arch Pharmacol 1984;327:238–246.
7. Besse JC, Furchgott RF. Dissociation constants and relative efficacies of agonists acting on alpha adrenergic receptors in rabbit aorta. J Pharmacol Exp Ther 1976;197:66–78.
8. Pasteur L. On the assymetry of naturally occurring organic compounds, the foundations of stereochemistry. In: Richardson GM, ed. Memoirs by Pasteur, Van't Hoff Le Bel and Wislicenus. Stuttgart: Birkhauser, 1901.
9. Moya-Huff FA, Maher TJ. Beta-adrenoceptor influences on the alpha-1 and alpha-2 mediated vasoconstriction induced by phenylpropanolamine and its two component isomers in the pithed rat. J Pharm Pharmacol 1988;40:876–878.
10. Johnson DA, Maher TJ. Vasoactive properties of phenylpropanolamine and its enantiomers in isolated rat caudal artery. Drug Dev Res 1991;23:159–169.
11. Maher TJ, Johnson DA. Review of chirality and its importance in pharmacology. Drug Dev Res 1991;24:149–156.
12. Parascandola J, Clark AJ. Quantitative pharmacology and the receptor theory. Trends Pharmcol Sci 1982;4:421–423.
13. Starke K. Presynaptic alpha-autoreceptors. Rev Physiol Biochem Pharmacol 1987;107:73–146.
14. Brisson A, Unwin PNT. Quarternary structure of the acetylcholine receptor. Nature 1985;315:474–477.
15. Kemp JA, Leeson PD. The glycine site of the NMDA receptor—five years on. Trends Pharmacol Sci 1993;14:20–25.
16. Kobilka BK. Adrenergic receptors as models for G protein-coupled receptors. Annu Rev Neurosci 1992;15:87–114.
17. Gilman AG. G proteins: transducers of receptor-generated signals. Annu Rev Biochem 1987;56:615–649.
18. Berridge MJ. Inositol triphosphate and diacylglycerol: two interacting second messengers. Ann Rev Biochem 1987;56:159–193.
19. Chinkers M, Garbers DL, Chang MS, et al. A membrane form of guanylate cyclase is an atrial naturetic peptide receptor. Nature 1989; 338:78–83.
20. Evans RM. The steroid and thyroid hormone receptor superfamily. Science 1988;240:889–895.
21. Ahlquist RP. A study of the adrenotropic receptors. Am J Physiol 1948;153:586–600.
22. Minneman KP, Esbenshade TA. Alpha-1 adrenergic receptor subtypes. Annu Rev Pharmacol Toxicol 1994;34:117–133.
23. Furchgott RF. The use of beta-haloalkylamines in the differentiation of receptors and in the determination of dissociation constants of receptor-agonist complexes. In: Harper NJ, Simmonds AB, eds. Advances in Drug Research, Vol. 3 New York, Academic Press, 1966.
24. Tattersfield AE. Tolerance to beta-agonists. Bull Eur Physiopathol Respir 1985;21:1s-5s.

ADDITIONAL SUGGESTED READINGS

Ariens EJ. Affinity and intrinsic activity in the theory of competitive inhibition: problems and theory. Arch Int Pharmacodynam 1954;99:32–49.

Black JW, Leff P. Operational models of pharmacological agonists. Proc R Soc Lond [Biol.] 1983;220:141–162.

Bylund DB. Subtypes of alpha-1 and alpha-2 adrenergic receptors. FASEB J 1992;6:832–839.

Kebabian JW, Neumeyer JL. The RBI Handbook of Receptor Classification. Natick, MA, Research Biochemicals International, 1998.

Kenakin T. Pharmacologic Analysis of Drug-Receptor Interaction, 2nd Ed. New York, Raven, 1993.

Tallarida RJ, Jacobs LS. The Dose Response Relation in Pharmacology. New York, Springer-Verlag, 1979.

Trends In Pharmacological Sciences. 2000 Receptor & Ion Channel Nomenclature Supplement. Oxford, Elsevier Science Ltd, 2000.

5. Drug Design Through Enzyme Inhibition

STEPHEN KERR

INTRODUCTION

The concept of utilizing small molecules that specifically target one or more enzymatic systems present in the body is not new. Historically, compounds that were extracted from natural products have been used as medicinal agents (Chapter 1). Subsequently, they have been shown to have their therapeutic effect by targeting certain systemic enzymes (1). A classic example is the bark of the willow tree, known since ancient days to have antipyretic and analgesic effects. Its active ingredient, salicin, a glycoside, is metabolized in vivo to salicylic acid, which is a known inhibitor of cyclooxygenase, a key enzyme in the formation of prostaglandins which are mediators of pain and fever. Similarly, physostigmine, isolated from the West African Calabar bean was used as a treatment for glaucoma in the mid 1800s.

Physostigmine's mechanism of action was only later determined to be inhibition of acetylcholinesterase (1).

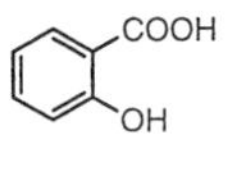

Salicylic acid 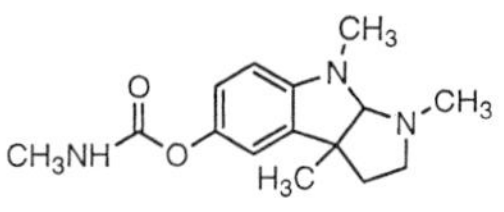   Physostigmine

Inhibition of acetylcholinesterase in the eye leads to improved drainage and thus a decrease in the intra ocular pressure giving relief to glaucoma patients. It was only in the 20th century when the concept of the "magic bullet" with selective toxicity, introduced by Ehrlich as a rational approach to chemotherapy (1), that the concept of rational design of enzyme inhibitors followed. The discovery in 1935 of the antibacterial activity of the azo dye, Prontosil, by Domagk (2), and the subsequent explanation in 1940 by Woods (3) of its metabolic reduction to sulfanilamide, an antimetabolite of p-aminobenzoic acid, finally paved the way for the rational design of enzyme inhibitors (Fig. 5.1). p-Aminobenzoic acid is an essential metabolite utilized in the bacterial synthesis of folic acid. Sulfanilamide, by its structural resemblance to p-

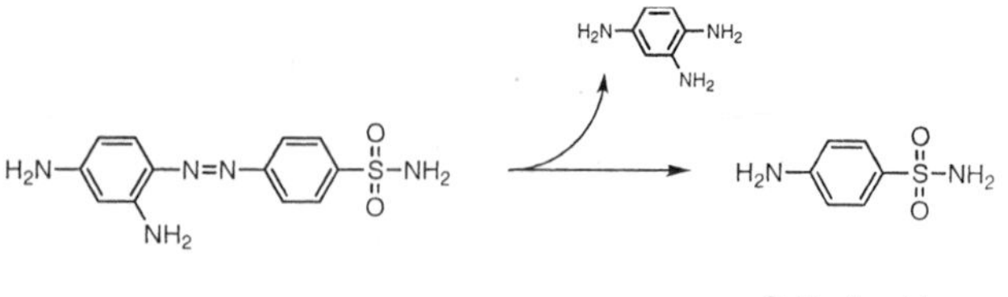

Prontosil   Sulfanilamide

Fig. 5.1. Metabolic reduction of prontosil to sulfanilamide.

100

aminobenzoic acid (see Chapter 2, Fig 2.3), competes for and selectively inhibits the bacterial enzyme, dihydropteroate synthase (Fig. 5.2). In the absence of dihydropteroic acid, the bacteria are unable to synthesize tetrahydrofolic acid, an essential cofactor in one-carbon transfers, involved in the de novo synthesis of purines and in the synthesis of thymidylate. This concept of designing drugs as antimetabolites, or structural analogs of essential metabolites became the hallmark for the development of enzyme inhibitors. This was especially important in cancer therapy during the early days of rational drug design (4). As mechanisms of enzymes became better understood, the inhibitor design strategy grew more sophisticated resulting in more potent and selective inhibitors being developed. Present day focus on drug design through enzyme inhibition makes use of the antimetabolite theory as well as detailed kinetic and mechanistic information on the enzymatic pathways. These strategies utilize sophisticated assays, enzyme crystal structures and active site environments, site directed mutagenesis experiments of catalytic residues of enzymes, and molecular docking experiments utilizing computers. It must be mentioned however, that in the drug design process, designing a potent inhibitor of an enzyme is only the first step in the long and difficult process of drug development (Principles of Drug Discovery). Other factors including pharmacokinetic profile of the inhibitor, toxicities and side effects, animal and preclinical studies must all be satisfactorily completed before the inhibitor can even enter clinical studies as a new drug candidate. Hence, even though there is an enormous amount of data on enzyme inhibitors only a selected few turn out to be marketable drugs. In succeeding paragraphs, general concepts of enzyme inhibitor and rational drug design will be discussed with selected examples.

GENERAL CONCEPTS OF ENZYME INHIBITION

The body is composed of thousands of different enzymes, many of them acting in concert in order to maintain homeostasis. While disease states may arise due to the malfunctioning of a particular enzyme, or the introduction of a foreign enzyme through infection by microorganisms, inhibiting a specific enzyme to alleviate a disease state is a challenging process. Most bodily functions occur through a cascade of enzymatic systems and it becomes extremely difficult to design a drug molecule that can selectively inhibit an enzyme and result in a therapeutic benefit. However, in order to address the

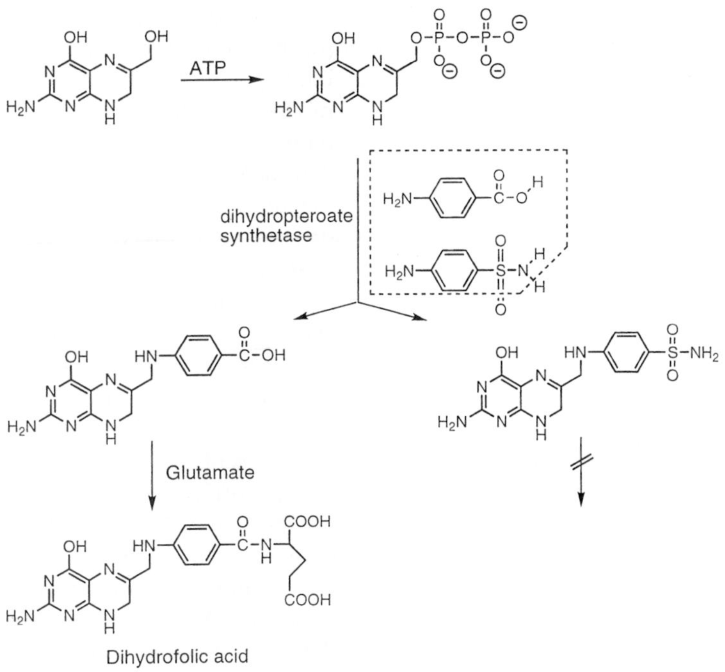

Fig. 5.2. Metabolic pathway leading to dihydrofolic acid and its inhibition by sulfanilamide. This figure shows the structural resemblance to *p*-aminobenzoic acid.

problem, the basic mechanism of enzyme action needs understanding. Once knowledge of a particular enzymatic pathway is determined and the mechanism and kinetics worked out, the challenge is then to design a suitable inhibitor that is selectively utilized by the enzyme causing its inhibition.

Enzymes (E) represent the best known chemical catalysts since they are uniquely designed to carry out specific chemical reactions in a highly efficient manner (5). They initially act by binding a substrate (S) to form an enzyme-substrate complex [E·S] which undergoes specific chemistry (catalysis) to give the enzyme-product complex [E·P] followed by dissociation of product (P) and free enzyme (E). Equation 5.1 represents a simplified version of this scenario, where K_d, is the enzyme-substrate dissociation constant and k_{cat} represents the rate constant for the cat-

Eq. 5.1 $$E + S \underset{}{\overset{K_d \text{ (or } K_m)}{\rightleftharpoons}} [E \cdot S] \overset{k_{cat}}{\rightleftharpoons} [E \cdot P] \rightleftharpoons E + P$$

alytic step (chemical modification step or slowest step in the overall pathway). If the binding step of E + S to form [E · S] is relatively fast as compared to the catalytic step, and one assumes steady-state conditions, then K_m, the Michaelis constant, (the substrate concentration at half maximum velocity [Vmax/2]), may be equated to the K_d (Eq. 5.2). The rate of the reaction can then be derived in terms of K_m and V_{max} (or $k_{cat} = V_{max}/[E]$). From the knowledge of the dissociation constant ($K_{m(d)}$) and the rate constant for catalysis (k_{cat}) it is then possible to compare inhibitors and the dissociation constant for the in-

hibitors, K_i, in relation to the natural substrates and the effect on the catalytic rates. These kinetic parameters, k_{cat} and $K_{m(d)}$ (or K_i) can then give an indication as to the affinity (K_i versus $K_{m(d)}$) and specificity (k_{cat}/K_i or

Eq. 5.2   Michaelis-Menten equation: $v = \dfrac{Vmax\,[S]}{Km + [S]}$

Lineweaver-Burk equation: $\dfrac{1}{v} = \dfrac{Km}{Vmax} \cdot \dfrac{1}{[S]} + \dfrac{1}{Vmax}$

$k_{cat}/K_{m(d)}$) of the inhibitor for a particular enzyme. Equation 5.3 represents the general scheme of reversible inhibition and Figure 5.3 illustrates graphically and mathematically the relationship of the velocity of the enzyme reaction to the substrate [S] and inhibitor [I] concentration as well as the kinetic parameters K_m, k_i and V_{max} (or $k_{cat} = V_{max}/[E]$).

Inhibition of enzymes may be broadly classified under two categories—reversible and irreversible inhibitors (Eq. 5.4). In the presence of inhibitor, the enzyme-substrate complex [E·S] is replaced by [E·I] which may block or retard the formation of product. In the presence of a reversible inhibitor, the enzyme is tied up and the reaction is retarded or stopped, however the enzyme can be subsequently regenerated from the enzyme-inhibitor complex, [E·I], to react again with substrate and produce product (see Eq. 5.3). On the other hand, irreversible inhibition implies that the enzyme can not be regenerated and the only way for catalysis to proceed would be if new molecules of the enzyme are generated from gene transcription and translation. Irreversible inhibition is commonly associated

Eq. 5.3(a)   Competitive Inhibition

$$E + S \xrightleftharpoons{K_m} [E \cdot S] \xrightleftharpoons{} E + P$$

$$E + I \xrightleftharpoons{K_i} [E \cdot I] \xrightarrow{\;/\!/\;} P$$

Eq. 5.3(b)   Noncompetitive Inhibition:

$$E + S \xrightleftharpoons{K_m} [E \cdot S] \searrow \; + I$$

$$[E \cdot S \cdot I]$$

$$E + I \xrightleftharpoons{K_i} [E \cdot I] \nearrow \; + S$$

Eq. 5.4 $E + I \xrightleftharpoons{K_i} [E \cdot I]$ (reversible inhibition)

$E + I \xrightarrow{K_i} [E - I]$ (irreversible inhibition)

with covalent bond formation between inhibitor and enzyme [E—I] which *cannot* be easily broken and is often defined as a time dependent loss of enzyme activity. Reversible inhibition on the other hand does not necessarily imply non-covalent bond formation. In many instances reversible inhibition can occur through covalent bond formation, but these bonds can be hydrolyzed to regenerate free enzyme and inhibitor. Thus for a reversible enzyme inhibitor there is no time dependent loss of activity and enzyme activity can always be recovered. There are instances when reversible inhibition tends to look kinetically like irreversible inhibition. This scenario results whenever there is a tight binding of a reversible inhibitor to the enzyme and consequently the dissociation of the enzyme from this enzyme-inhibitor complex is extremely slow. Kinetically it is extremely difficult to distinguish this type of inhibition from an irreversible inhibitor because over time the enzyme does tend to look like it loses its activity, and, for all practical purposes the enzyme behaves as if it were irreversibly tied up. In order to differentiate between tight binding reversible and irreversible inhibitors, one can dialyse the enzyme-inhibitor complex. In case of the reversible inhibitor, on dialysis, the inhibitor will be removed from the enzyme, resulting in recovery of the enzyme activity; however, this is not so with the irreversible one.

Reversible Enzyme Inhibition

Reversible enzyme inhibition may be classified under two main headings, competitive and non-competitive, with both following Michaelis-Menten kinetics. Competitive inhibition,

by definition, requires that the inhibitor competes with the substrate for binding to the enzyme at the active site and this binding is mutually exclusive. That is to say that if the inhibitor binds to the enzyme the substrate will not be able to bind and vice-versa. But, competitive inhibition also suggests that the inhibition can be reversed in the presence of saturating amounts of substrate, since in this case all enzyme active sites will be occupied by substrate displacing inhibitor. In contrast, non-competitive inhibition implies independent binding, i.e., both inhibitor and substrate may bind to the enzyme at different sites. Since binding of the inhibitor to the enzyme is at a site other than the active site, non-competitive inhibition can not be reversed by increasing the concentration of substrate. Graphing the kinetics of inhibition (Fig. 5.3), the Lineweaver-Burk plot of $\frac{1}{v}$ versus $1/[S]$ shows distinguishing characteristics between the two types of inhibition. In competitive inhibition, while there is no change in the maximum velocity of the reaction (V_{max}, the intercept on the Y-axis remains constant in presence of inhibitor), the slope of the curve (K_m/V_{max}) is different with the inhibitor present, and the K_m changes due to the presence of the competitive inhibitor (Fig. 5.3, competitive inhibition). In the case of non-competitive inhibition, only the V_{max} of the reaction decreases while the K_m remains unchanged (intercept on the X-axis unchanged with inhibitor, Fig. 5.3, non-competitive inhibition).

Most of the rationally designed and clinically useful reversible inhibitors are competitive inhibitors. These inhibitors generally bear some structural resemblance to the natural substrate of the enzyme. The design of such inhibitors would thus seem a logical and rational task which is uniquely suited to the medicinal chemist who can utilize the principles of bio-isosteric modification of natural enzyme substrates and metabolites, or modification of "lead" structures and structure activity relationships, to create selective and potent inhibitors. However, there are pitfalls in this endeavor since even the most rationally designed drug must still overcome transport and other cellular barriers before exerting its effects. In the case of the non-competitive inhibitors, the design is not as straightforward. These inhibitors can have widely differing structures which in many instances bear no resemblance to the natural substrate. In general, inhibitors of the non-competitive type have been primarily obtained through random screening of chemically novel molecules followed by further synthetic manipulation of the pharmacophore to optimize their inhibitory effects.

Examples of Reversible Inhibitors

The design of enzyme inhibitors has included random screening of synthetic chemical agents, natural products and combinatorial libraries followed by molecular optimization or structure activity relationships of so called "lead" structures as well as bio-isostere analogs of the enzyme substrates themselves. Drugs (e.g. finasteride) have also been developed for one indication but based on observed side-effects have lead to other uses.

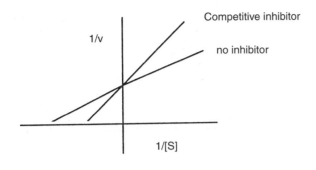

$$v = \frac{V_{max}}{1 + (K_m/[S])(1 + [I]/K_i)}$$

(K_m increases, V_{max} unchanged)

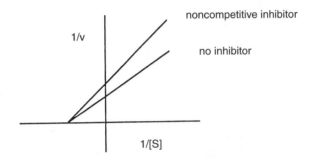

$$v = \frac{V_{max}/(1 + [I]/k_i)}{1 + (K_m/[S])}$$

(K_m unchanged, V_{max} decreases)

Fig. 5.3. Graphic representation of competitive and noncompetitive enzyme inhibition.

The rational approach in the design of enzyme inhibitors is greatly aided if the enzymatic reaction is characterized in terms of its kinetic mechanism. Such a characterization would include the knowledge of the kinetic parameters (rate constants and dissociation constants) of individual steps in the overall reaction pathway, as well as, the characterization of (any) intermediates involved in these individual steps. Examples of such "rational" inhibitors include both the reversible and irreversible inhibitors of enzymes.

Antimetabolites

Antimetabolites are agents that interfere with the functioning of an essential metabolite and are most often designed as structural analogs of the natural metabolite. As described earlier, the mechanism of action of sulfanilamide is that of a competitive inhibitor of *p*-aminobenzoic acid. However, in the case of the sulfanilamide the mechanism was only determined after the bacterial inhibitory action was noted. This is often the case when a drug is discovered to

Uses of Finasteride

Finasteride (Proscar) an inhibitor of steroid 5α-reductase, an enzyme involved in the catalytic reduction of testosterone to dihydrotestosterone, was originally developed as an agent to treat prostate hyperplasia. In addition to this original use, finasteride is presently also indicated as an agent (Propecia) to stimulate hair growth for treatment of male pattern baldness. This benefit was recognized as a useful side effect observed during clinical trials of finasteride as an anti-prostate agent.

have a certain therapeutic effect and later this effect is "rationalized" as being due to an enzyme inhibitory action (1). Other classic examples of a competitive inhibitor acting as an antimetabolite include a number of nucleoside analogs used as antiviral and anti-cancer agents. These agents again bear structural resemblance to natural nucleosides which in their triphosphate form are substrates for nucleic acid polymerases involved in the synthesis of nucleic acids. Nucleic acid polymerases catalyze the condensation of the free 3'-hydroxy-end of a nucleic acid with an incoming 5'-triphosphate derivative of a nucleoside (dNTP) resulting in a 3',5'-phospho-diester linkage. Hence, nucleoside analogs in order to compete with the natural substrate in the synthesis of nucleic acid must be converted intracellularly to their mono, di and finally triphosphate derivative before exerting their inhibitory effects on nucleic acid synthesis. Certain drug design strategies incorporate a "masked" phosphate group on the nucleoside, such that once absorbed they enter into the systemic circulation as the monophosphate (6). The majority of these analogs are designed such that they lack the 3'-hydroxy group and are dideoxy derivatives of the natural substrate. These analogs thus ensure that once they are incorporated into nucleic acid further extension of the nucleic acid is prevented due to the lack of a 3'-hydroxy group.

Inhibition of Human Immunodeficiency Virus-Reverse Transcriptase (HIV-RT)

Azidothymidine (AZT). The advent of AIDS stimulated a great interest in designing inhibitors against the essential viral polymerase—HIV-RT. AZT is a potent inhibitor of HIV-RT, the retroviral polymerase which catalyzes the for-

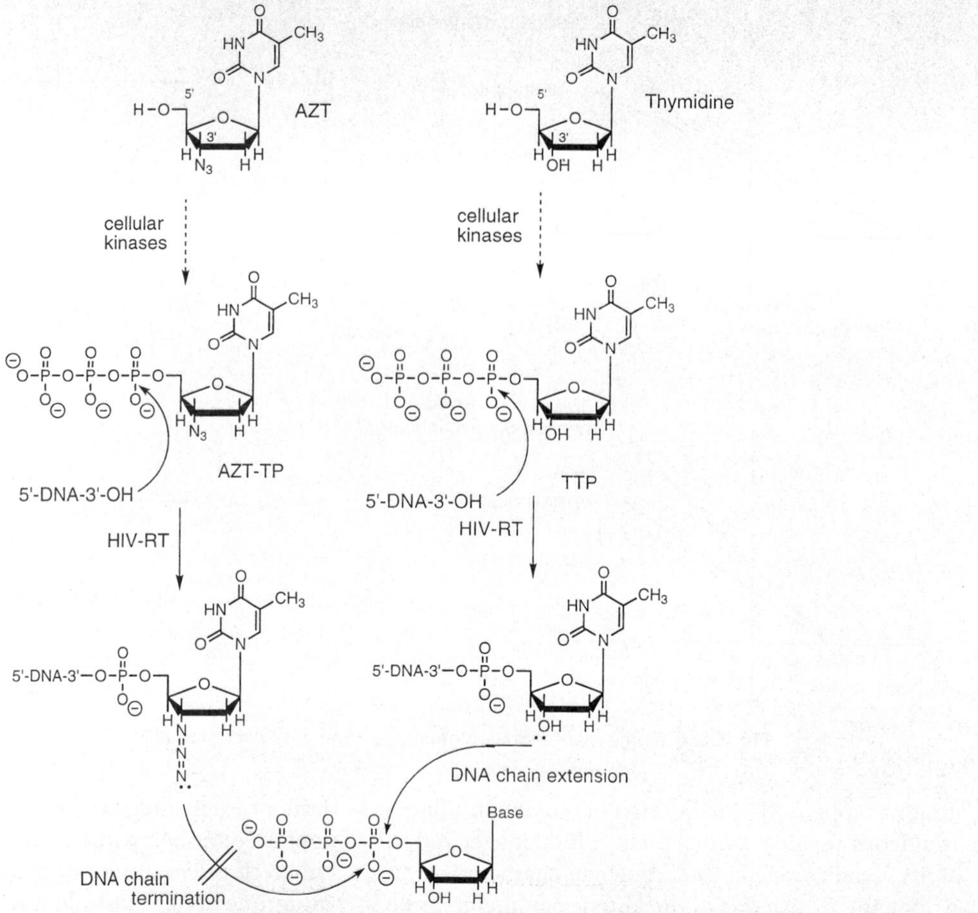

Fig. 5.4. Activation, incorporation, and chain-terminating action of AZT, a thymidine analog, as a reversible inhibitor of HIV-RT.

Historical Development of AZT

Interestingly, AZT was originally synthesized as an anti-cancer agent to inhibit cellular DNA synthesis but was found to be too toxic. Subsequently in the mid eighties during a random screening of nucleoside agents for potential inhibitory effects against HIV-RT, AZT was found to have selectivity for the HIV-RT (7). As such its effects on host cell polymerases result in its dose-limiting bone-marrow toxicity.

mation of proviral DNA from viral RNA. AZT is structurally similar to the natural nucleoside thymidine but has an azide group (-N$_3$) rather than a hydroxy group (-OH) at the 3'-position of the sugar, deoxyribose (Fig. 5.4). AZT is activated intra-cellularly to its triphosphate and competes with thymidine triphosphate for uptake by HIV-RT into DNA (8). Once incorporated, further chain extension of the DNA is prevented since there is no 3'-hydroxyl group to continue the DNA synthesis. In this fashion, AZT is an effective chain terminator of viral DNA synthesis.

Dideoxycytidine (ddC [Zalcitabine®]) and 3-Thiacytidine (3-TC [Lamivudine®]). 2,'3'-Dideoxycytidine is another antiretroviral agent used against HIV-RT. In this case ddC

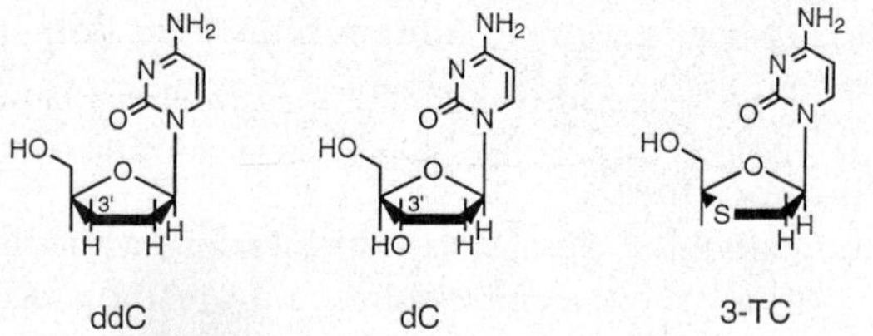

resembles the natural metabolite, deoxycytidine (dC), and as in the case of AZT, is a 3'-deoxy analog of dC where the 3'-OH group of deoxycytidine is replaced by a H-atom. Similarly, 3-TC is another anti-HIV agent which resembles dC. However, in this example, rather than replacing the 3'-hydroxyl functionality as in ddC, the 3'-carbon position of the sugar has been substituted by a sulfur (S) atom.

Nevirapine. An example of a potent non-competitive inhibitor of HIV-reverse transcriptase is the drug Nevirapine, a benzodiazepine analog (9), which is extremely tight-binding

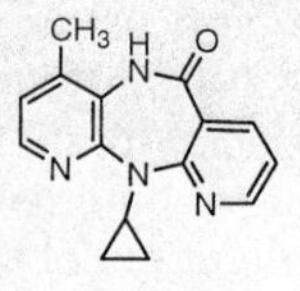

Nevirapine

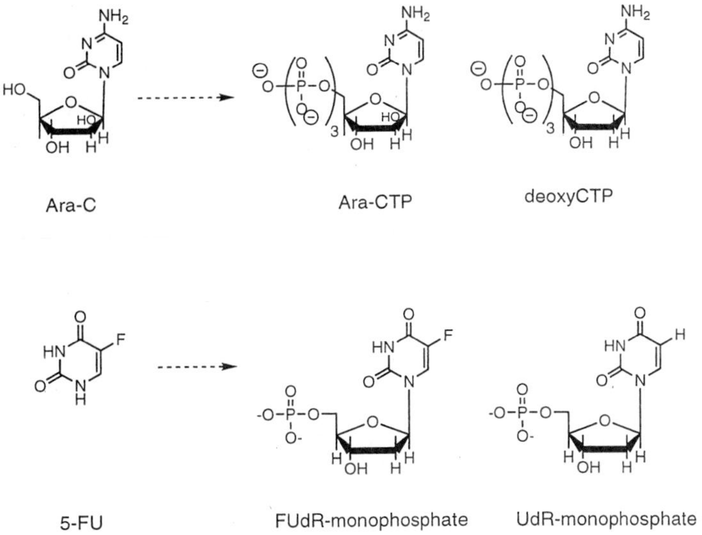

Fig. 5.5 Structures of pyrimidine antimetabolites used in cancer chemotherapy.

to the enzyme, having a K_i in the nanomolar range. As can be seen in the structure of nevirapine, the drug bears no resemblance to any of the natural nucleotide substrates and was discovered through a random screening program. X-ray crystallographic studies of HIV-RT complexed with nevirapine have shown it binding in a hydrophobic pocket present at a site adjacent and slightly overlapping the nucleotide binding site of HIV-RT (10). Kinetic studies with the enzyme have revealed an extremely slow binding rate for the drug, however, once bound, the polymerization rate for the reaction is effectively reduced (11).

A drawback for nevirapine however, is that the virus can develop resistance very rapidly, through mutation of the amino acid residues in the binding pocket (12), and thus its usefulness in limited to combination therapy with other anti-retroviral agents rather than single drug therapy.

Reversible Inhibitors Used in Cancer Therapy. The design of several anti-cancer agents have been based on the antimetabolite theory. Because cancer results in over-proliferation and uncontrolled cell growth, drugs designed against cancer have been based upon inhibiting DNA synthesis in the cell. Thus, these drugs have been targeted against those enzymes, including nucleic acid polymerases, thymidylate synthase and dihydrofolate reductase (DHFR) that play a role in DNA synthesis. Examples of drugs that have been designed against nucleic acid polymerases include cytosine arabinoside (Ara-C) and 5-fluorouracil (5-

FU) (Fig. 5.5). Cytosine arabinoside is first converted to its triphosphate and as such it functions as an antimetabolite of deoxycytidine triphosphate (deoxy CTP) to inhibit DNA polymerase. Ara-C, as can be seen from its structure, is the arabino isomer of cytidine. That is to say the 2'-hydroxyl functionality in ara-C is in the arabino configuration rather than the ribo configuration of cytidine. Because of this stereochemical change in the placement of the 2'-hydroxyl function, Ara-C tends to resemble deoxycytidine rather than cytidine. In this way, Ara-C inhibits DNA polymerases by competing with deoxycytidine. 5-FU is an analog of the pyrimidine base uracil where the H at the 5-position in uracil has been substituted by an isosteric fluorine (F) atom. This makes 5-FU look very similar to uracil. 5-FU, after conversion to 5-fluorodeoxyuridine monophosphate (FUdR-monophosphate, FdMP), is an inhibitor of thymidylate synthase, the enzyme involved in the de-novo synthesis of thymidylate. In this case the FdMP is an antimetabolite of deoxyuridine monophosphate (UdR-monophosphate, dUMP).

Methotrexate is a potent inhibitor of DHFR, the enzyme responsible for the reduction of folic acid to dihydro and tetrahydro folic acid, precursors to one-carbon donation in purine and pyrimidine de-novo synthesis. Methotrexate is an analog of folic acid where the 4-hydroxyl group (-OH) on the pteridine ring of folic acid has been replaced by an amino (-NH$_2$) functionality and the nitrogen atom at the 10-position is methylated (Fig. 5.6).

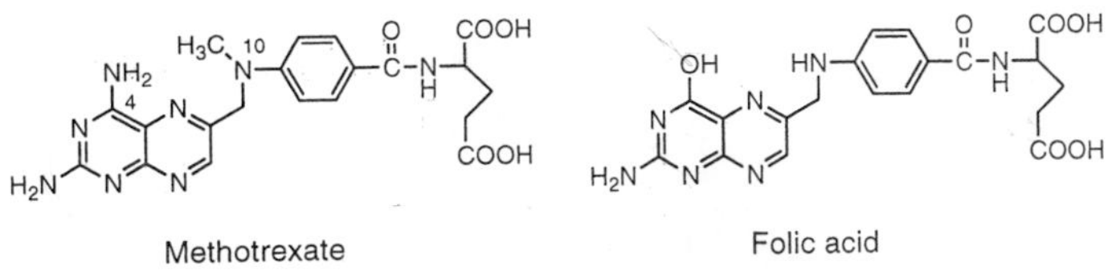

Fig. 5.6. Methotrexate the antimetabolite of folic acid.

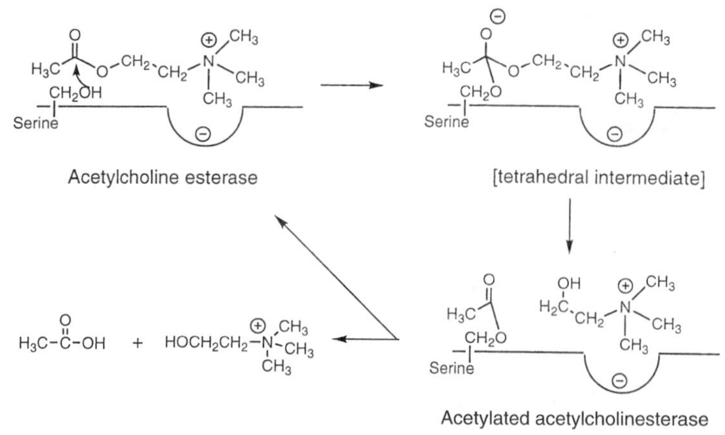

Fig. 5.7. Mechanism of hydrolysis of acetylcholine by acetylcholine esterase.

These substitutions led to methotrexate having an affinity for DHFR with orders of magnitude greater than that for the natural metabolite, folic acid, and allows it to be an extremely potent inhibitor.

Inhibition of Acetylcholinesterase

Acetylcholinesterase (AChE) is the enzyme that catalyzes the catabolism of the neurotransmitter acetylcholine to acetate and choline (Chapter 10). Thus, inhibition of AChE would lead to increased concentrations of acetylcholine and a prolonged action of the neurotransmitter. Inhibitors of AChE have found use in cases of myasthenia gravis, glaucoma and Alzheimer's disease. In order to appreciate the design of these inhibitors it is useful to first understand the mechanism of action of AChE. AChE has an anionic site which can bind the positively charged quaternary ammonium group of the choline functionality and an active esteratic site which contains a nucleophilic serine residue involved in the hydrolysis of the ester bond (Fig. 5.7). The mechanism involves the attack of the nucleophilic serine hydroxy group on the carbonyl group of acetylcholine to form a tetrahedral intermediate which breaks down resulting in the release of choline and an intermediate, acetylated serine which subsequently hydrolyses to release AChE.

Physostigmine has been used in the treatment of glaucoma. It is an alkaloid with a carbamate moiety which resembles the ester linkage of acetylcholine. Being an alkaloid it is protonated at physiological pH, and thus can bind to the anionic site of AChE. Following the mechanism of AChE the serine residue of the enzyme can attack the carbonyl group of physostigmine and in the process the serine is carbamylated (Fig. 5.8). This carbamyl serine intermediate is stable and subsequent hydrolysis by water occurs extremely slowly. The carbamylated enzyme is only slowly regenerated with a half-life of 38 min., more than seven orders of magnitude slower than that for the natural substrate, acetylcholine. This is an example of a reversible inhibitor which is involved in covalent bond formation with the enzyme which ultimately gets hydrolyzed.

Inhibitors of Angiotensin-Converting Enzyme

Angiotensin-converting enzyme (ACE) is a carboxypeptidase having a zinc ion as a cofactor and is involved in the renin-angiotensin cascade of blood pressure control (13). The design of the anti-hypertensive drug, captopril, a clinically important and potent reversible inhibitor of ACE is an example of one of the early endeavors and successes of a rationally designed enzyme inhibitor (14). The design of captopril was based on several factors. These included the knowledge that: a) ACE was similar in its enzymatic mechanism to carboxypeptidase A, except that ACE cleaved off a dipeptide, while carboxypeptidase A cleaves single amino acid residues from the carboxyl end of the protein; b) the discovery of L-benzylsuccinic acid as a potent inhibitor of carboxypeptidase A and, c) studies of a potent pentapeptide inhibitor of ACE, $BPP_{5\alpha}$ (Glu-Lys-Trp-Ala-Pro), from the venom of the Brazilian viper (*Bothrops jararaca*) that showed that the N-terminal peptide fragments including tetra, tri and the dipeptide fragment (Ala-Pro) of $BPP_{5\alpha}$ retained some inhibitory activity. Benzylsuccinic acid has been described as a bi-product inhibitor of carboxypeptidase A wherein its design was based on the combination of the products of the peptidase reaction; i.e., the two peptide fragments, one with a free carboxyl end which coordinates the zinc ion of the protease,

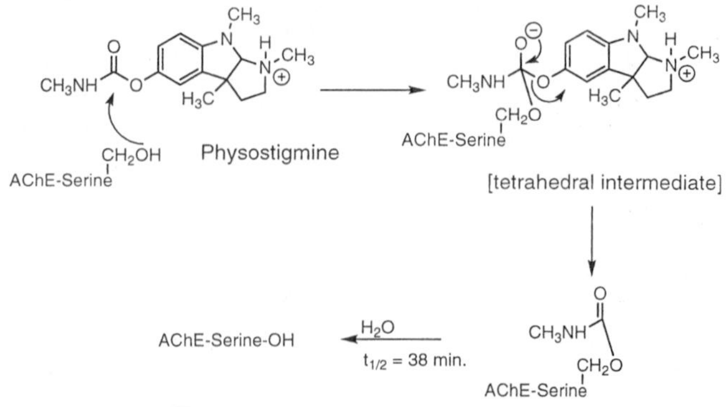

Fig. 5.8. Mechanism of inhibition of acetylcholine esterase by physostigmine.

the other with a free amino terminus (Fig. 5.9) (15). In the case of benzylsuccinic acid, the amino (-NH$_2$) functionality is replaced by the isosteric methylene (-CH$_2$-) group. Utilizing the above concepts, it was rationalized that succinyl-amino acids could similarly behave as a bi-product inhibitors of ACE. Starting with a succinyl-proline moiety, the structural activity developmental effort finally resulted in captopril with the substitution of the stronger zinc coordinating mercapto functionality in place of the carboxylic residue (of succinic acid) and a stereospecific R methyl group on the succinyl function to represent the methyl group on the natural L-Ala residue in Ala-Pro (the dipeptide fragment that had previously shown inhibitory activity). Captopril soon became highly successful in the clinic as an anti-hypertensive agent and in combination with diuretics has proved to be the treatment of choice in controlling hypertension.

Following on the heels of captopril was another byproduct ACE inhibitor, enalaprilat. Enalaprilat incorporated a phenylethyl moiety with the S-configuration, and made use of a hydrophobic binding pocket in ACE that was overlooked during the design of captopril (16). Recalling that the tripeptide fragment of BPP$_{5\alpha}$ (Trp-Ala-Pro) contained the aromatic tryptophan residue and showed weak inhibitory properties, suggested the benefit of an aromatic binding site. Substituting the tryptophan residue with a phenyl group allowed the design of enalaprilat which retained the carboxylic group as the coordinating ligand for zinc and resulted in a 20-fold increase in potency over captopril. Enalaprilat, a diacid, however was poorly absorbed

from the gastrointestinal tract and thus a prodrug ethyl ester of enalaprilat, enalapril was developed. Enalapril had superior pharmacokinetics to enalaprilat and was rapidly metabolized to the active drug.

Transition-State Analogs

Transition-state analogs are compounds that resemble the substrate portion of the hypothetical transition state of an enzymatic reaction. All chemical reactions progressing from substrate to product must cross an energy barrier and proceed through a transition state or activated high energy complex. This energy barrier is described as the activation energy. In the case of enzyme catalyzed reactions it is accepted that the enzyme reduces this energy barrier as compared to the non-enzyme catalyzed reaction. Factors contributing to this reduced energy barrier are several and include stabilization of the transition state and intermediate forms of the reaction during the course of transition from substrate to product, as well as, conformational effects of distortion of the substrate while traversing towards the product (5). It was Pauling who initially suggested in 1948 that compounds resembling the transition state of an enzyme catalyzed reaction would be effective inhibitors of the enzyme since the substrate transition state should have the greatest affinity for the enzyme (17). Wolfenden later proposed that thermodynamically it is possible to relate the hypothetical equilibrium dissociation constants between substrate and its transition state of an enzyme catalyzed reaction with that of the non-enzyme catalyzed one (18). Using such an analysis he showed that

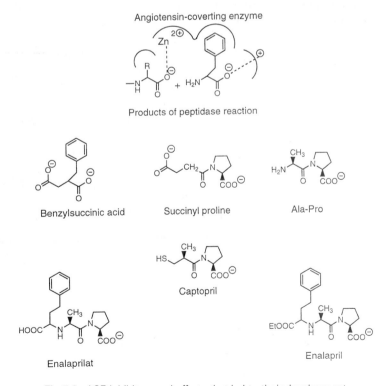

Fig 5.9. ACE inhibitors and efforts that led to their development.

the ratio of the hypothetical transition state dissociation constants of non-enzyme catalyzed reaction to that of the enzyme catalyzed one is equal to the ratio of the first order rate constants of formation of transition state for enzyme catalyzed reaction to non-catalyzed reaction. Since the ratio of the enzyme catalyzed rate constant to that of the non-catalyzed one ranges from 10^7 to 10^{10}, it follows then that the substrate transition state would bind the enzyme 10^7 to 10^{10}-fold more tightly than the substrate itself (19). Hence, transition-state analogs that resemble the substrate would be extremely tight binding compounds. In order to design a transition-state inhibitor knowledge of the enzyme chemistry and its mechanism is a basic requirement. It must be understood however, that these substrate transition states are by nature unstable transient species existing no more than a few pico seconds. Nevertheless experimental evidence has shown that even crudely designed transition-state inhibitors resembling the substrate are extremely potent inhibitors (19).

Transition-State Inhibitor of Adenosine Deaminase. Adenosine deaminase is the enzyme that hydrolyzes adenosine (or deoxyadenosine) to inosine (or deoxyinosine) and is important for purine metabolism. High levels of adenosine are toxic to B-cells of the immune system and can result in an immuno-compromised state. Also, people who lack the gene for adenosine deaminase have the genetic condition of SCID (severe combined immunodeficiency) and are extremely susceptible to opportunistic infections. Many cancer and anti-viral agents are also degraded by this enzyme and hence there is a role for the development of inhibitors of this enzyme (20). The mechanism proposed for adenosine deaminase is a nucleophilic

attack of water at the 6-position of the purine base to form a tetrahedral intermediate (Fig. 5.10). The transition state presumably resembles this intermediate.

In the course of the deaminase reaction the hybridization of the G-carbon changes from an sp^2 hybridized state to an sp^3 state. Subsequently, there is a loss of ammonia to give the product inosine. In order to develop a transition-state inhibitor for this enzyme, one would have to factor in this change in the hybridization of the substrate molecule and thus molecules having an sp^3-hybridized carbon at this position and resembling the substrate would potentially be candidates for transition-state inhibitors. The compound, 1,6-dihydro-6-hydroxymethylpurine has such geometry and its potent inhibitory properties of adenosine deaminase ($K_i < 1$ μM as compared to a K_m for adenosine of 31 μM) has been rationalized as being a transition-state inhibitor (21). Two compounds that nature has provided, coformycin and its deoxyribose analog, deoxycoformycin (Fig. 5.10), are extremely potent inhibitors of adenosine deaminase, ($K_i = 0.002$ nM). Both of these compounds contain a seven member ring structure which through its flexibility is presumed to resemble the hypothesized distorted sp^2–sp^3 transition state that forms during the addition of water to adenosine (22).

Irreversible Enzyme Inhibition

As previously described, irreversible enzyme inhibition is defined as "time dependent inactivation of the enzyme" which implies that the enzyme has in some way or form been permanently modified since it can no longer carry out its function. This modification is due to the result of a covalent bond being formed with the inhibitor and some amino acid residue present in the protein. Furthermore, this bond is extremely stable and for all practical purposes is not hydrolyzed to give back the enzyme in its original state or structure. In most examples of irreversible inhibition, a new enzyme must be generated through gene transcription and translation for the enzyme to continue its normal catalytic action. Basically, there are two types of irreversible enzyme inhibitors, the affinity labels or active site directed irreversible inhibitors and the mechanism based irreversible enzyme inactivators.

Affinity Labels and Active Site Directed Irreversible Inhibitors

The affinity labels are those chemical entities that are inherently reactive and can target any nucleophilic residue in the enzyme, especially those residing in and around the catalytic center of the protein. These agents generally resemble the substrate so that they may bind in the active site of the enzyme. In most examples, these agents also contain an electrophilic functional group, which includes groups such as: halo-methyl ketones (X-CH$_2$C=O, where X = halide), sulfonyl fluorides (SO$_2$F), nitrogen mustards ((ClCH$_2$CH$_2$)$_2$NH), diazoketones (COCHN$_2$) and other such reactive groups, that can "label" or alkylate a nucleophilic amino acid residue present in the enzyme. They

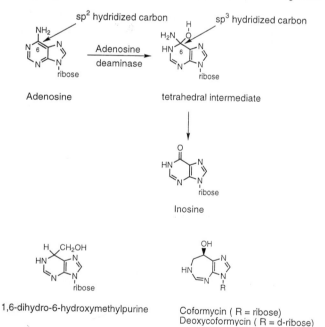

Fig. 5.10. Mechanism and transition-state inhibitors of adenosine deaminase.

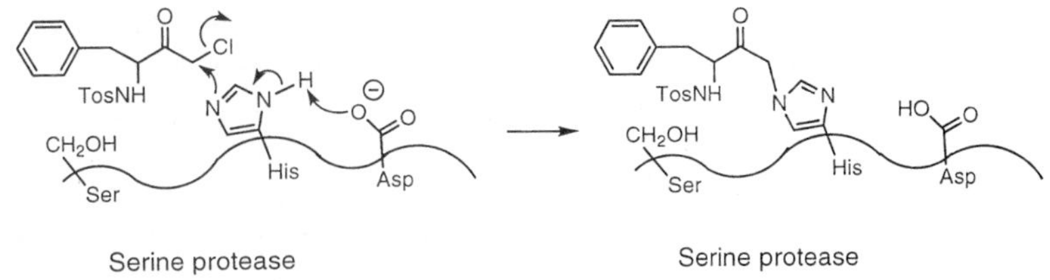

Fig. 5.11. Mechanism of affinity label of serine protease with TPCK.

generally tend to be indiscriminate in their action and have little therapeutic value since they are non-selective and thus inherently toxic. They have been used mainly as biochemical tools to probe active sites of enzyme so as to discern the types of amino acid residues present in and around the catalytic center of an enzyme. The classic example of an affinity label is TPCK (tosyl-phenylalanyl-chloromethyl-ketone), an irreversible inhibitor of the serine protease, chymotrypsin (17). Since TPCK resembles the amino acid phenylalanine, it can

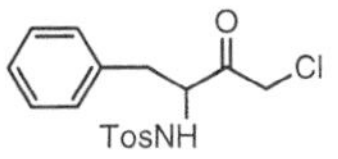

bind to the active site of the chymotrypsin whose selectivity is for such hydrophobic amino acid residues (Phe and Tyr). In the course of normal peptide hydrolysis, the reactive chloromethyl-ketone labels the nucleophilic histidine residue present as part of the catalytic triad (Ser-His-Asp) in the active site of the protease (Fig. 5.11). Another similarly designed affinity label is TLCK (tosyl-lysyl-chloromethyl-ketone) whose specificity is for the protease trypsin. Trypsin cleaves peptide bonds adjacent to the basic amino acids, lysine and arginine. It was found that TLCK was a specific inhibitor of trypsin but had no activity for chymotrypsin. On the other hand TPCK while extremely specific for chymotrypsin showed no activity for trypsin.

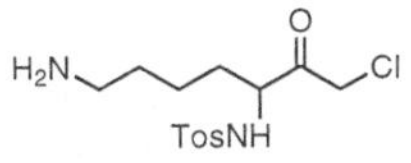

Because of the inherent reactivity and non-selectivity of these affinity labels and their limited utility in drug therapy,

the late B.R. Baker extended this concept to design inhibitors that would have greater selectivity and specificity and thus be potential drug candidates (23). He designed several analogues, termed active site directed irreversible inhibitors, targeted towards thymidylate synthase, a key enzyme involved in the de novo metabolism of thymidylate. These analogues contained a substrate binding region linked to a reactive group such as a halomethyl ketone by a tether whose chain length could be manipulated. The substrate portion of the analogue ensures both affinity and rapid binding to the enzyme active site. Once bound, areas in and around the binding site and on the surface of the enzyme could be probed for nucleophilic amino acid residues. By manipulating the length of the tether, ideal inhibitors could then be designed such that any suitably located, sufficiently nucleophilic amino acid residue, present on the surface of the enzyme could potentially be alkylated by the halomethyl ketone (Fig. 5.12). Once alkylated, the tether "bridges" the active site with the labeled amino acid residue thus "tying up" and preventing further catalysis by the enzyme.

Mechanism-Based Irreversible Enzyme Inactivators

Overview. The mechanism-based irreversible inhibitors have also been termed as "suicide substrates," "k_{cat} inhibitors," "Trojan horse inhibitors" or "latent alkylating agents." These inhibitors are inherently unreactive but upon normal catalytic processing by the enzyme, are activated into highly reactive moieties (24–26). These reactive

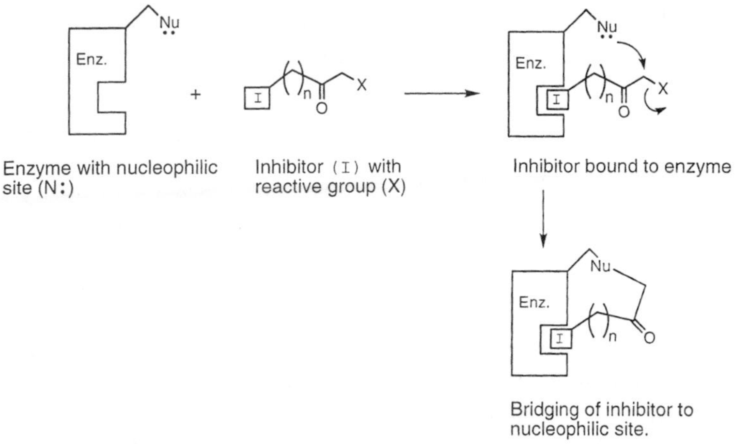

Fig. 5.12. Model showing Baker's (23) active site-directed irreversible inhibitors.

Eq. 5.5 $E + S \underset{K_i}{\overset{}{\rightleftharpoons}} [E \cdot S] \xrightarrow{k_{cat}} [E \cdot S^*] \xrightarrow{k_{inact}} [E-S]$

$\downarrow k_{diff}$

$E + S^* + Nu: \longrightarrow [Nu-S]$

functionalities can then irreversibly alkylate a nucleophilic amino acid residue or cofactor present in the enzyme and in essence, cause the enzyme's death ("suicide"). Basically, these inhibitors have a latent reactive functionality that only becomes apparent after binding and acted upon by the normal catalytic machinery of the enzyme. This type of inhibitor design differs from the preceding one in that these inhibitors have one more level of selectivity built in to them. The kinetic scheme for such inhibition is shown in Equation 5.5, where enzyme, E, binds with substrate (inhibitor) S to give an [E − S] complex with dissociation constant of K_i. Next the [E − S] complex is converted into a highly activated complex [E − S*] by the catalytic machinery (k_{cat}) of the enzyme, which can then go on to alkylate the enzyme, [E-S]. Note that it is possible for the reactive species [S*] to diffuse (dissociate) from the enzyme and react with some other target (nucleophilic species), i.e., the system is "leaky;" however, if this happens then the inhibitor can not be classified as a "true" suicide substrate because specificity is lost.

There are several requirements that need to be met by these inhibitors in order for them to be classified as suicide substrates. These include: inactivation should be time dependent (reaction should be irreversible); kinetics should be first-order; the enzyme should show saturation phenomenon; the substrate should be able to protect the enzyme; stoichiometry of the reaction should be 1:1 (one active site to one inhibitor).

Examples of Suicide Substrates. During the past three decades, besides the rational design of hundreds of molecules that have been synthesized and tested as suicide substrates, it has also come to light that nature, herself, has known about this mechanistic mode of enzyme inhibition and has provided us with several extremely potent mechanism-based suicide inactivators. Below are a few selected examples to demonstrate the mode of action of these inhibitors.

Halo Enol Lactones. Halo enol lactones are an example of suicide inhibitors for serine proteases. These analogs were developed by Katzenellenbogen and coworkers at the University of Illinois (27). Upon normal catalytic processing by the serine hydroxyl functionality, they give rise to a reactive halo-methyl ketone which subsequently alkylates a nearby nucleophilic residue on the enzyme (Fig. 5.13). Other suicide inactivators for the serine proteases have also been designed by various researchers (25).

Clauvulinic Acid. Clavulanic acid is a potent inhibitor of bacterial β-lactamase (28). This enzyme is a serine protease and can hydrolyze β-lactams such as the penicillin antibiotics. It is the principal enzyme responsible for penicillin resistant bacteria. Clavulanic acid itself is a β-lactam and if given in combination with penicillin, is preferentially taken up by β-lactamase and hydrolyzed. However in the process of hydrolysis, the molecule undergoes a cleavage leading to the formation of a "Michael acceptor," which subsequently alkylates a nucleophilic residue on the enzyme causing irreversible inhibition (Fig. 5.14). Such combinations of a β-lactamase inhibitor and a penicillin have resulted in clinically useful agents (clavulanic acid plus amoxicillin).

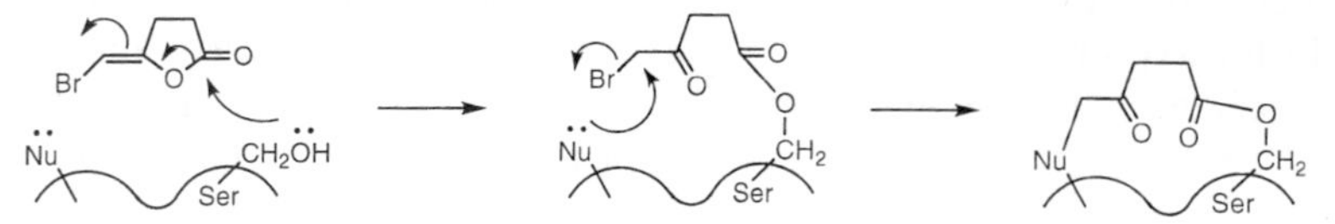

Fig. 5.13. Mechanism-based inhibition of serine proteases by Katzenellenbogen's halo enol lactone.

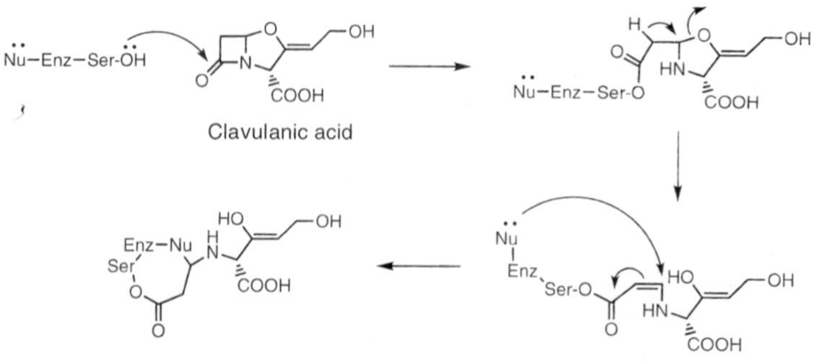

Fig. 5.14. Mechanism-based inhibition of β-lactamases by clavulinic acid.

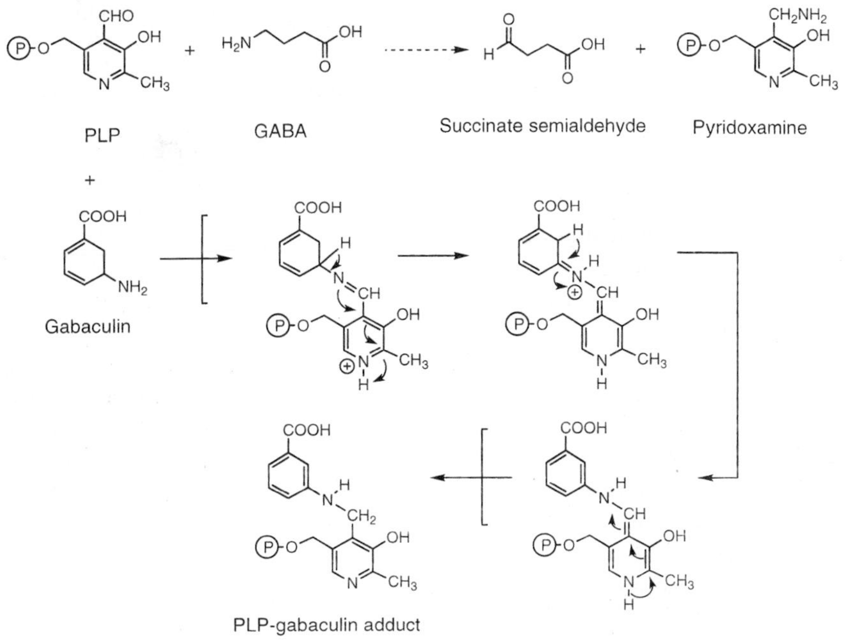

Fig. 5.15. Pyridoxal phosphate dependent GABA-Transaminase reaction and the mechanism of suicide inhibition by gabaculin.

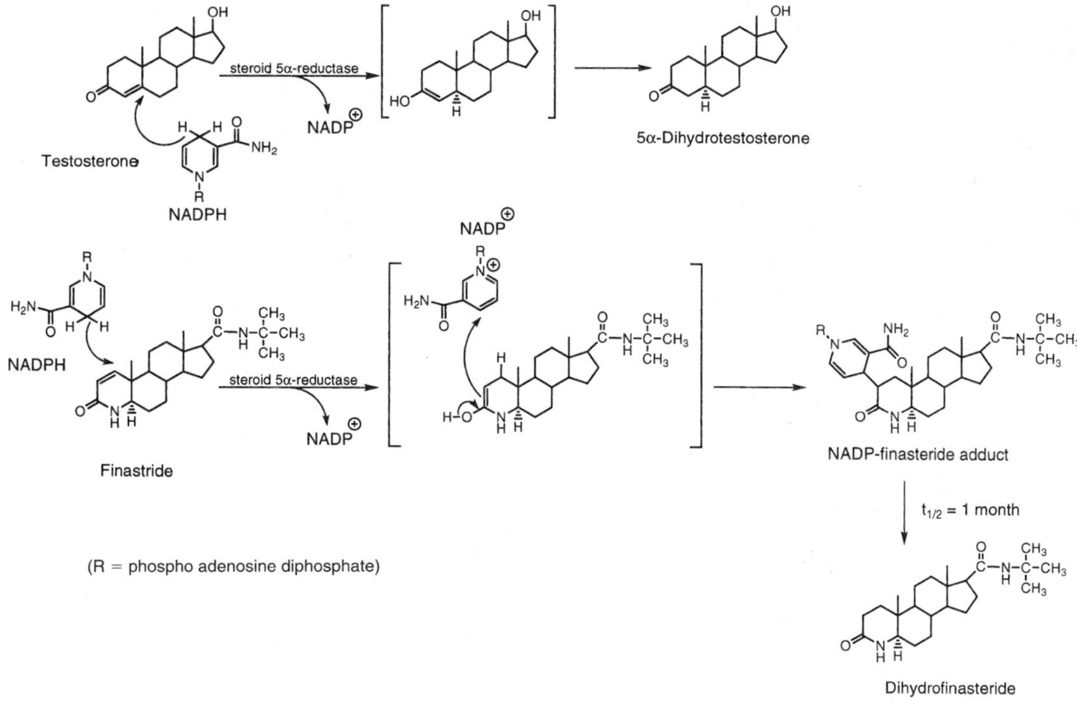

Fig. 5.16. Mechanism of steroid reductase reduction on finasteride and testosterone and the structure of hypothesized NADPH-dihydrofinasteride adduct (30).

Gabaculin. Gabaculin, a naturally occurring neurotoxin, is a potent mechanism-based inhibitor of the enzyme GABA-Transaminase (GABA-T) with an interesting mechanism of action (29). GABA-T is a pyridoxal phosphate (PLP) dependent enzyme involved in the catabolism (transamination, Fig. 5.15) of the excitatory neurotransmitter, GABA to succinate semialdehyde and pyridoxamine. As part of the normal catalytic mechanism of PLP dependent enzymes, the amino group of gabaculin first forms a Schiff base with the aldehyde of PLP (Fig. 5.15).

Next, this adduct undergoes an aromatization reaction resulting in an extremely stable covalent bond with the cofactor, PLP. Hence in this case, rather than an enzymatic nucleophilic residue being alkylated, the cofactor is "tied up" resulting in the inhibition.

Finasteride.   Finasteride is a clinically useful agent in the treatment of prostate hyperplasia and male pattern baldness. It is a potent inhibitor of human steroid-5α-reductase, the enzyme responsible for the reduction of testosterone to dihydrotestosterone (Fig. 5.16). The inhibitory action of finasteride has been attributed both to its similarity in structure to testosterone which allows it to bind to the enzyme and be reduced to dihydrofinasteride in place of testosterone as well as to its ability to act as a mechanism based inhibitor, where it can tie up the cofactor, NADPH by forming a covalent NADP-dihydrofinasteride adduct (Fig. 5.16). This adduct very slowly releases dihydrofinasteride with a half life of one month (30).

The above discussion has attempted to explain the essentials of drug design through enzyme inhibition with a few choice examples. The reader is referred to suggested reading material for more detailed explanations and insights into the rationale and design strategies of enzyme inhibitors. In conclusion, drug design by enzyme inhibition is a continually developing enterprise since there will always be the need to discover more selective and more potent inhibitors in an effort to increase the therapeutic benefit to patients. This chapter has tried to give a brief insight into this fascinating area of medicinal chemistry and the various types of enzyme inhibitors that can be rationally designed.

REFERENCES

1. Albert A. Selective toxicity—the physico-chemical basis of therapy. 7th ed. New York: Chapman & Hall, 1985.
2. Domagk G. Ein beitrag zur chemotherapie der bakteriellen infektionen. Dtsch Med Wochenschr 1935; 61: 250–253.
3. Woods DD. Relation of p-aminobenzoic acid to mechanism of action of sulphanilamide. Br J. Exp Pathol 1940; 21: 74–90.
4. Albert A. Selective toxicity—the physico-chemical basis of therapy. Chap. 9, 7th. ed. New York: Chapman & Hall, 1985.
5. Fersht A. Enzyme Structure and Mechanism. 2nd ed. New York: W.H. Freeman, 1985.
6. Sastry JK, Nehete PN, Khan S, et al. Membrane-permeable dideoxyuridine 5′-monophosphate analogue inhibits human immunodeficiency virus infection. Molecular Pharmacology 1992; 41: 441–445.
7. Mitsuya H, Weinhold KJ, Furman PA, et al. 3′-Azido-3′-deoxythymidine (BW A509U): an antiviral agent that inhibits the infectivity and cytopathic effect of human T-lymphotropic virus type III/lymphadenopathy-associated virus in vitro. Proc Natl Acad Sci(USA); 1985; 82:7096–7100.
8. Furman PA, Fyfe JA, St. Clair MH, et al. Phosphorylation of 3′-azido-3′-deoxythymidine and selective interaction of the 5′-triphosphate with human immunodeficiency virus reverse transcriptase. Proc Natl Acad Sci(USA); 1986; 83:8333–8337.
9. Grob PM, Wu JC, Cohen KA, et al. Nonnucleoside inhibitors of HIV-1 reverse transcriptase: nevirapine as a prototype drug. AIDS Res Hum Retrovir; 1992; 8:145–152.
10. Kohlstaedt LA, Wang J, Friedman JM, et al. Crystal structure at 3.5 A resolution of HIV-1 reverse transcriptase complexed with an inhibitor. Science; 1992; 256:1783–1790.
11. Spence RA, Kati WM, Anderson KS, et al. Mechanism of inhibition of HIV-1 reverse transcriptase by nonnucleoside inhibitors. Science. 1995; 267:988–993.
12. Mellors JW, Dutschman GE, Im GJ, et al. In vitro selection and molecular characterization of human immunodeficiency virus-1 resistant to non-nucleoside inhibitors of reverse transcriptase. Mol Pharmacol; 1992; 41:446–451.
13. Harrold M. Calcium Blockers; Angiotensin Converting Enzyme Inhibitors; Angiotensin Antagonists. In: Lemke T and Williams DA eds. Foyes Principles of Medicinal Chemistry. Chap. 23, 5th ed. Philadelphia: Williams & Wilkins, 2001.
14. Cushman DW, Cheung HS, Sabo EF, et al. Design of potent competitive inhibitors of angiotensin-converting enzyme. Carboxyalkanoyl and mercaptoalkanoyl amino acids. Biochemistry; 1977; 16: 5484–5491.
15. Byers LD, Wolfenden R. Binding of the by-product analog benzylsuccinic acid by carboxypeptidase A. Biochemistry; 1973;12: 2070–2078.
16. Patchett AA, Harris E, Tristram EW, et al. A new class of angiotensin-converting enzyme inhibitors. Nature 1980; 288: 280–283.
17. Walpole CSJ, Wrigglesworth R. In: Enzyme inhibitors in medicine; Natural Products Reports 1989; 63: 311–346.
18. Wolfenden R. Transition state analogues for enzyme catalysis. Nature 1969; 223:704–705.
19. Wolfenden R. Transition state analogues as potential affinity labeling agents. Methods Enzymol 1977; 46: 15–28.
20. Shannon WM, Schabel FM Jr. Antiviral agents as adjuncts in cancer chemotherapy. Pharmacol Therap 1980; 11:263–390.
21. Evans BE, Wolfenden RJ. A potential transition state analog for adenosine deaminase. J Am Chem Soc 1970; 92: 4751–4752.
22. Nakamura H, Koyama G, Iitaka Y, et al. Structure of Coformycin, an unusual nucleoside of microbial origin. J Am Chem Soc 1974; 96: 4327–4328.
23. Baker BR. Design of active site directed irreversible enzyme inhibitors. New York: Wiley, 1967.
24. Walsh C. Recent developments in suicide substrates and other active site-directed inactivating agents of specific target enzymes. Horiz Biochem Biophys 1977; 3: 36–81.
25. Abeless RH. Suicide enzyme inactivators. Chem Eng News 1983; 61 (38): 48–55.
26. Rando RR. Mechanism based irreversible enzyme inhibitors. Methods Enzymol 1977; 46: 28–41.
27. Kraft GA, Katzenellenbogen JA. Synthesis of halo enol lactones. Mechanism based inactivators of serine proteases. J Am Chem Soc 1981; 103: 5459–5466.
28. Charnas RL, Knowles JR. Inactivation of RTEM beta-lactamase from Escherichia coli by clavulanic acid and 9-deoxyclavulanic acid. Biochemistry 1981; 20: 3214–3219.
29. Rando RR. Mechanisms of naturally occurring irreversible enzyme inhibitors. Accts Chem Res 1975; 8: 281–288.
30. Bull HG, Garcia-Calvo M, Andersson S, et al. Mechanism-based inhibition of human steroid 5α-reductase by finasteride: enzyme-catalyzed formation of NADP-dihydrofinasteride, a potent bisubstrate analog inhibitor. J Am Chem Soc 1996; 118: 2359–2365.

SUGGESTED READING

Abeless RH. Suicide enzyme inactivators. Chem Eng News 1983; 61 (38): 48–55.

Albert A. Selective toxicity—the physico-chemical basis of therapy. 7th. ed. New York: Chapman & Hall, 1985.

Baker BR. Design of active site directed irreversible enzyme inhibitors. New York: Wiley, 1967.

Kalman TI, ed. Drug Action & Design-Mechanism Based Enzyme Inhibitors. New York: Elsevier Science, 1979.

Seiler N, Jung MJ, Kock-Weser J., eds. Enzyme-activated irreversible inhibitors. New York: Elsevier North Holland, 1978.

Silverman RB. The organic chemistry of drug design and drug action. New York: Academic Press, 1992

Smith JS, ed. Smith and Williams' Introduction to the principles of drug design and action. 3rd. ed. Amsterdam: Harwood Academic Press, 1998

Walpole CSJ, Wrigglesworth R. Enzyme inhibitors in medicine. Natural Products Reports; 1989; 63: 311–346.

Wolfenden R. Transition state analogues as potential affinity labeling agents. Methods. Enzymol 1977; 46: 15–28

6. Peptide and Protein Drugs

MICHAEL MOKOTOFF

INTRODUCTION

Living cells produce an impressive diversity of macromolecules (proteins, nucleic acids, polysaccharides) that serve as structural components, biocatalysts, hormones, receptors, or repositories of genetic information. These macromolecules are biopolymers constructed of monomer units or building blocks and for proteins the monomer units are α-amino acids. Proteins may contain substances other than α-amino acids, for example glycoproteins contain carbohydrates. However, the 3-dimensional structure and the biological properties of proteins are determined largely by the kinds of amino acids present, the order in which they are linked together in the polypeptide chain, and thus the spatial relationship of one α-amino acid to another.

Bacterial cells, plants, and animals contain a wide variety of peptides and proteins, consisting anywhere from 3 to 200 plus residues (each amino acid is considered a residue), many of which have profound biological activity. In humans, biological functions as diverse as growth, calcium metabolism, sexual reproduction, lactation, formation of glucocorticoid and mineralocorticoid steroids, production of thyroid hormones, water balance, induction or augmentation of uterine contraction during labor, erythropoiesis, glucose metabolism, etc. are known to be under the control of peptides and proteins. One should recognize that in humans proteins are also important as enzymes, structural components of various tissues, and are indispensable to receptor conformation. Therefore, it is not surprising that in today's medicine peptides and proteins continue to grow in popularity for their potential use in drug therapy.

The pharmaceutical industry is very much involved in the production of many of these important peptides and proteins by way of synthetic procedures as well as via biotechnology. Peptides of low to moderate molecular weight, peptide mimetics, and those containing pseudopeptide bonds or fraudulent amino acids will continue to be made by synthetic procedures rather than by biotechnology. This chapter will therefore discuss certain of the physical and chemical properties of peptides and proteins, the limitations to their use as medicinal agents, the methodology used in their synthesis, and modifications aimed to improve their stability and biological action. Having this background the chapter continues with a discussion of the importance of the peptide and protein hormones that are commercially available for diagnostic purposes or for the treatment of various disease states.

Where there are analogs of these hormones these too are discussed, particularly the chemical changes that were made and the implications of these changes to the overall biological action.

History

It may seem strange to the reader to think that just shortly before the end of the 19th century, it was not recognized that proteins consisted of peptide bonds between individual amino acids. It was not until the early 1900s that two individuals, Hofmeister (1) and Fischer (2), reported that the linkages between amino acids were indeed amide or peptide bonds. Due to the complexity of having multiple reactive functional groups present in the amino acids, each of which necessitated selective protection, there was no common method for the synthesis of peptides. In fact, it was not until 1932 when Bergmann and Zervas (3) developed a suitable blocking group for the α-amino function, the carbobenzoxy group (to be discussed later), that peptide synthesis began to come of age. The discovery in the 1940s of the peptide antibiotics as biologically important natural products, gave impetus for further refinements and advances in peptide synthesis. These events were then followed by such important milestones in peptide hormone discovery as the isolation, structure determination and synthesis of oxytocin by duVigneaud and co-workers (4,5,6) and the determination of the structure of insulin by Sanger (7). In the late 1960s and into the early 70s the isolation, identification and synthesis of several important hypothalamic hormones, e.g., thyrotropin-releasing hormone (TRH) (8, 9), luteinizing-hormone releasing factor (GnRH) (10), and growth hormone inhibiting factor (somatostatin) (11) was accomplished by two independent groups led by Drs. Guillemin and Schally.

It was these discoveries which served as incentives for further refinements in the synthesis of peptides, particularly such advances as the formation of the peptide bond via the coupling agent N,N'-dicyclohexylcarbodiimide (DCC) (12), the selective blocking of the α-amine functionality by the tert-butyloxycarbonyl (Boc) acid-sensitive group (13), and the 9-fluorenylmethyloxycarbonyl (Fmoc) base-sensitive blocking group (14). Probably, the crowning achievement in peptide synthesis was the report by Merrifield of his concept of a method in which peptides could be more rapidly synthesized by "growing" the peptides on solid support (15). His goals were to simplify and to accelerate peptide synthesis in a way that would make the preparation of long peptides practical and amenable to automation. These goals were realized in a few short years, and the syntheses of a wide variety of peptides and proteins have, and continue to appear in the literature (16, 17, 18).

As a measure of the importance of these historical events, it is significant that Nobel Prizes were awarded to those individuals most responsible for several of these advances. The following are quotes from the Nobel Prize Committee: Dr. DuVigneaud (Chemistry, 1955) "for his work on biochemically important sulphur compounds, especially for the first synthesis of a hormone"; Dr. Sanger (Chemistry, 1958) "for his work on the structure of proteins, especially that of insulin"; Drs. Guillemin and Schally (Medicine and Physiology, 1977, also with Dr. Yalow) for their work that "opened new vistas within biological and medical research far outside the border of their own spheres of interest"; Dr. Merrifield (Chemistry, 1984) for the development of a "simple and ingenious automated laboratory technique for rapidly synthesizing peptide chains in large quantities on a routine basis, called solid-phase peptide synthesis."

CHEMICAL AND PHYSICAL PROPERTIES OF PEPTIDES AND PROTEINS

The title of this chapter is "Peptide and Protein Drugs" therefore it is important to discuss the similarities and differences between peptides and proteins. Both are similar in that they are made up of repeating units, or residues, of α-amino acids that are linked together by peptide bonds, also known as amide bonds. Peptides in general are smaller in size, usually consisting of less than 50 residues (e.g., gonadotrophin-releasing hormone contains 10 residues and corticotrophin has 39 residues), and their three-dimensional structures are not always well defined. In contrast, proteins generally have very well defined three-dimensional structures and are considerably larger, consisting of over 50 residues (e.g., insulin has 51 residues and somatropin has 191 residues).

The Peptide Bond and Primary Structure of Peptides

A peptide is a compound that consists of at least two amino acids linked by an amide bond, an example of which is the tripeptide alanine-valine-glycine (Ala-Val-Gly) (Fig. 6.1). The properties of the peptide bonds that make up this tripeptide (framed in dotted lines), like other amide bonds, are controlled by the conjugation that exists between the lone-pair electrons on the nitrogen and the adjacent carbonyl group. The major consequence of this

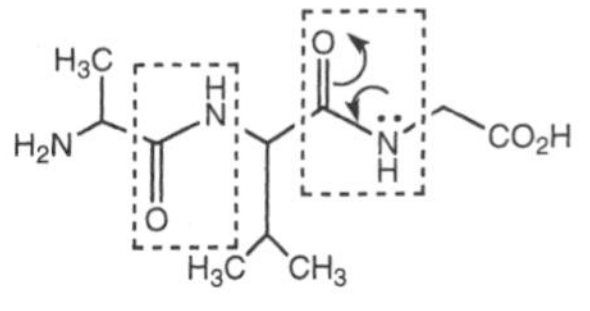

Fig. 6.1. A tripeptide, Ala-Val-Gly, indicating the planarity of the peptide bonds that are framed in dotted lines.

conjugation is that all peptide bonds are planar, as a result of the requirement that the nitrogen, carbon, and oxygen p-orbitals must lie in the same plane in order for the nitrogen lone-pair to conjugate with the carbonyl π-bond (19). It is this planarity and lack of free rotation about the C-N bond that causes the existence of two stable conformations, *cis* and *trans*, which is so important to the three-dimensional shape of peptides and proteins. However, in natural peptides and proteins, the peptide bond generally exists in the *trans*-form. The symbols for the natural, DNA encoded, amino acids found in human protein are shown in Table 6.1.

In the tripeptide shown in Figure 6.1, Ala-Val-Gly can be referred to as the primary structure of this peptide. That is to say, the primary structure of any peptide or protein is the number and sequence of the amino acids present (20). By convention, if the sequence is fully known, the peptide structures are written with the symbol for the α-amino, or N-terminal, residue at the left. This is followed in order with the symbols of all the other residues connected by hyphens, and terminating on the right with the symbol for the α-carboxy, C-terminal, residue. In the above example, Ala is the N-terminal residue and is understood, as written, to contain a free α-amino group, while Gly is the C-terminal residue and is understood, as written, to contain a free α-carboxylic acid. Several other conventions used in writing the primary structure of a peptide can be explained using the following model hexapeptide, Ac-Leu-Phe-Asp(OMe)-Lys(Ac)-Ser-Ile-NH$_2$. Ac-Leu is understood to mean that the α-amino group of the N-terminal amino acid is acetylated (Ac). When the symbol for an amino acid is followed in parentheses by an abbreviation, as is Asp(OMe) and Lys(Ac), this indicates that the side chain is protected by the group named in the parentheses; the Asp side chain carboxylic acid is protected as its methyl ester (OMe), and Lys side chain amino group is acetylated. Finally, the representation Ile-NH$_2$ is understood to indicate that the C-terminal residue does not exist as a free carboxyl but rather as its C-terminal amide, -CO-NH$_2$. Many important biologically active peptides actually exist as C-terminal amides, examples of which include gonadotropin-releasing hormone, oxytocin, and vasopressin.

Stereochemical Features of Amino Acids, Peptides and Proteins

Although there are some 300 different amino acids that occur in nature, only 20 of these are DNA encoded, all 20 of which are α-amino acids, and can be found in proteins from plants, animals and microbes. The structure and nomenclature for these 20 natural amino acids can be found in Table 6.1 (21). The amino acids in the table are not listed alphabetically; rather they are tabulated according to properties determined by their side-chain (R) functionality. Interestingly, 19 of the DNA encoded amino acids have the same stereochemistry and are chiral, while the 20th, Gly, is achiral because its side-chain group is H. The

Table 6.1. Twenty, DNA-encoded Amino Acids Found in Human Protein

Name[a]	R	pI[b]	Acidity/Basicity, Polarity[c]
Alanine, Ala, A	—CH₃	6.02	N, SNP
Glycine, Gly, G	—H	5.97	N, SP
Isoleucine, Ile, I	—CH(CH₃)—CH₂CH₃	6.02	N, LNP
Leucine, Leu, L	—CH₂—CH(CH₃)—CH₃	5.98	N, LNP
Valine, Val, V	—CH(CH₃)—CH₃	5.97	N, LNP
Aspartic acid, Asp, D	—CH₂-CO₂H	2.98	A, SP
Glutamic acid, Glu, E	—CH₂-CH₂-CO₂H	3.22	A, LP
Arginine, Arg, R	—(CH₂)₃—NH—C(=NH)—NH₂	10.76	B, LP
Lysine, Lys, K	—(CH₂)₄-NH₂	9.74	B, LP
Histidine, His, H	—CH₂-imidazole	7.59	WB, IP
Cysteine, Cys, C	—CH₂-SH	5.02	WA, SNP
Methionine, Met, M	—CH₂-CH₂—SCH₃	5.74	N, LNP
Serine, Ser, S	—CH₂-OH	5.68	N, SP
Threonine, Thr, T	—CH(OH)—CH₃	5.60	N, SNP
Tyrosine, Tyr, Y	—H₂C-C₆H₄-OH	5.67	N, IP
Asparagine, Asn, N	—CH₂—C(=O)—NH₂	5.41	N, SP
Glutamine, Gln, Q	—CH₂-CH₂—C(=O)—NH₂	5.65	N, LP
Phenylalanine, Phe, F	—H₂C-C₆H₅	5.48	N, LNP
Tryptophan, Trp, W	—CH₂-indole	5.89	N, IP

Proline, Pro, P with a pI = 6.30 is neutral, of intermediate polarity, and does not fit the general structure.

[a]Name of amino acid, 3-letter, 1-letter abbreviation.
[b]pI is the pH at which each amino acid is ionically balanced, carries no net charge, and exists entirely in its zwitterion form.
[c]Side-chains are acidic (A), weakly acidic (WA), basic (B), weakly basic (WB), or neutral (N); polarity is based on the size of the amino acid's side chain and degree of its polarization, small polar (SP), intermediate polar (IP), large polar (LP), small nonpolar (SNP), and large nonpolar (LNP).
Data from references 19–21.

19 chiral amino acids are all configurationally related to L-glyceraldehyde and therefore are still known as L-amino acids, albeit that this is an outdated nomenclature.

A more informative system for indicating the stereochemistry of chiral carbon uses the Cahn-Ingold-Prelog system, in which the four groups on an asymmetric carbon

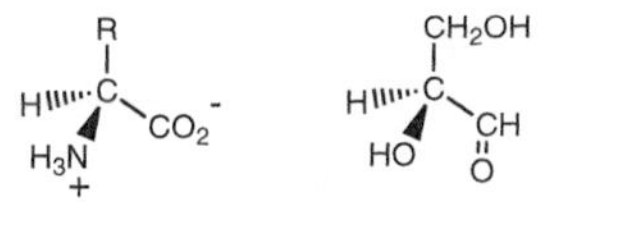

L-amino acid   L-Glyceraldehyde

are ranked according to a set of rules, the so-called *R/S* nomenclature (22). Using this nomenclature one can show that 18 of the 19 chiral, DNA encoded, amino acids are of the *S*-configuration, and only Cys is *R*. This is due to the sequencing rules (22) in which the side-chain CH_2SH (sulfur bonded to carbon) takes precedence over CO_2H (oxygen bonded to carbon). In addition, the side-chains of Ile and Thr each have an additional chiral center, and the DNA encoded forms exist as Ile (*S,S*) and Thr (*S,R*) (see Table 6.1).

Conformational Features of Peptides and Proteins

Previously, we defined the primary structure of a peptide or protein simply as its sequence, but it should be recognized that this only describes its linear, or one-dimensional, structure. If one wants to know more about a polypeptide or protein's three-dimensional shape it is necessary to have information about its *secondary* structure, or its well-defined conformation that is controlled by torsional angles (also called dihedral angles or rotations) and hydrogen-bonds. The *tertiary* structure, or well-defined folding, of a polypeptide or protein affords its biologically active, three-dimensional structure. Finally, some proteins can also exist in a *quaternary* structure, which occurs when two or more protein monomers (subunits) combine into a multisubunit protein.

Let's explore further the *secondary* structure of a polypeptide. The conformation of a peptide is very much dependent upon the spatial arrangement of the atoms that make up the bonds about each peptide residue of the backbone, which consists of repeating N-C_α-C units. These different conformations can vary by simple rota-

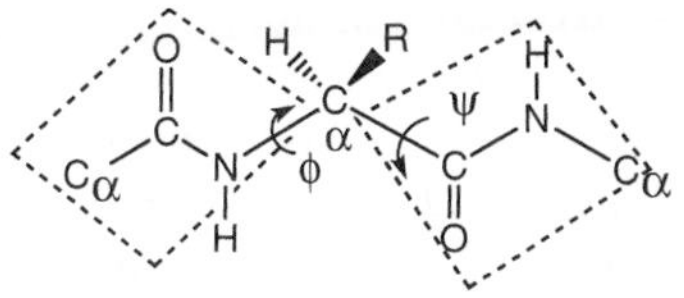

Fig. 6.2. Representation of a portion of a polypeptide backbone that indicates rotation about N-Cα (angle Φ, phi) and the Cα-C (angle Ψ, psi) bonds. Each Cα is a pivot point linking two adjacent planar peptide residues, as indicated by the dotted planes. The outer Cα's are shown devoid of substituents for ease of viewing.

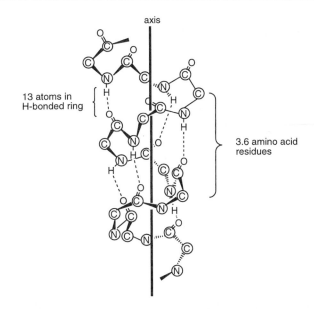

Fig. 6.3. Right-handed α-helix indicating H-bonds (dashed lines) that occur between each carbonyl oxygen and peptide N-H four residues removed; the ring formed by this H-bond contains 13 atoms. Adapted from reference 23.

tions without breaking a covalent bond or changing the chirality of atoms, in contrast to changing the configuration, which requires bond breaking. Consider Figure 6.2, which represents a section of a polypeptide chain containing two peptide units which can pivot about C_α, by rotation of the N-C_α and C_α-C bonds affording varying torsional angles ϕ (phi) and ψ (psi), respectively. As ϕ and ψ are rotated varying conformations are formed, many of which are forbidden by steric interference caused by both backbone and side-chain atoms from adjacent residues (19, 23).

Those structures that have allowed ϕ and ψ values are further stabilized by hydrogen bonds (H-bonds) formed between N-H····O=C of neighboring peptide bonds, giving rise to what are known as *secondary* structures. The most common polypeptide and protein *secondary* structures found in nature are the α-helix and the β-pleated sheet. The α-helix involving L-amino acids, first proposed by Pauling et al. in 1951 (24), is a right-handed spiral structure that is often found in fibrous and globular proteins, wherein the torsion angles ϕ and ψ are ideal for most residues. The α-helix has very definite and regular properties and is often referred to as a 3.6_{13} helix (19). A 3.6_{13} helix contains 3.6 residues per turn and forms an H-bonded ring of 13 atoms between every carbonyl O^1 and peptide H^{13}. This means that every carbonyl oxygen of residue *n* is bonded to the hydrogen on α-amino nitrogen *n* + 4 (Fig. 6.3). Although not shown in Figure 6.3, the side chains will project out from the helix and will not interfere with its stability (25).

In contrast to the α-helix, which has a coiled backbone, in the β-sheet conformation the polypeptide chain is nearly fully extended and two or more separate chains, or

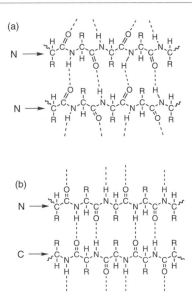

Fig. 6.4. Examples of (a) parallel and (b) antiparallel β-pleated sheets, shown with only two chains, that are held together by H-bonds (dashed lines). Note the difference in the H-bonds in the parallel (slanted and regularly spaced) and antiparallel (perpendicular with alternating wide and narrow spacing) sheets. Adapted from reference 23.

β-strands, can assemble side by side, wherein they are held together by H-bonds. The H-bonds are again between the carbonyl oxygen and the NH group of the backbone. The β-sheet can exist in two types, parallel and antiparallel, and in both cases the torsional angles φ and ψ are sterically favorable. In the former case the two stretches of polypeptide or protein are oriented in the same direction, whereas in the latter case the chains are oriented in opposite directions (see Fig. 6.4) (25). The β-sheet is not completely planar and if viewed along the backbone they resemble that of a pleated sheet. Furthermore, the side chains protrude on alternating sides of the β-sheet.

Other conformational changes that can occur in proteins, especially when they exist in relatively compact structures, is for the backbone to fold back on itself or to make a *turn*, that is, a site where the polypeptide chain reverses its overall direction. It is these reverse turns, for example β-turn or hairpin bend, which afford proteins with globular properties (26). A further discussion of turns is beyond the scope of this chapter, but the interested reader can find many good discussions of this topic in other sources (23, 25, 27).

When a protein which exists as an α-helix, β-sheet, or combination of both, folds into its biologically active globular shape it becomes compacted and takes on a three-dimensional shape or *tertiary* structure (21). In this case amino acid residues which might be far apart in the *primary* structure may wind up quite close to each other and this can be stabilized via noncovalent, usually hydrophobic, interactions. That is, *tertiary* structures are formed and stabilized because of hydrophobic interactions between the side chains of amino acid residues. In some globular

proteins several subunits can combine with a well-defined stoichiometry and symmetry, giving rise to what is known as the *quaternary* structure of the protein. A good example of this is hemoglobin, whose *quaternary* structure is a tetramer consisting of two α- and two β-chain subunits.

METABOLISM AND DRUG DELIVERY CONSEQUENCES

Peptides and proteins are metabolized quite extensively in the kidney, liver, and the gastrointestinal (GI) tract via the enzymatic hydrolysis of the peptide bond. Metabolism can also occur in nasal mucosa, the lung, and in blood. Because large proteins can assume complex *tertiary* structures, which thus better shields or "hides" internal peptide bonds, they are often metabolized slower, or less completely, than smaller proteins or polypeptides (28).

The enzymes involved in peptide bond hydrolysis, and thus the degradation of peptides and proteins, are known as peptidases and can be found in the blood, in the vascular bed, in the interstitial fluid, on cell membranes, and within cells. These enzymes include carboxypeptidases (cleaves C-terminal residues), dipeptidyl carboxypeptidases (cleaves dipeptides from the C-terminus), aminopeptidases (cleaves N-terminal residues), and amidases (cleaves internal peptide bonds). The oral administration of protein or peptide drugs generally results in very extensive metabolism within the GI tract, the loss of biologic activity, and little to no systemic absorption of the original drug. This is due to the prevalence of peptidases within the GI tract, wherein the protein or peptide drugs undergo first-pass metabolism. Even if these drugs are administered parenterally they still can undergo extensive metabolism because of their secretion across the intestinal mucosa and from hydrolyzing enzymes found in plasma and the vascular bed.

The fate of orally administered peptide drugs and the action of peptidases in their digestion occur as follows. As the peptide drugs enter the stomach, wherein the gastric juice has a pH of about 2, they are acted upon by pepsin, an enzyme secreted by the gastric mucosa. This enzyme is known as an endopeptidase, which means it can hydrolyze "internal" peptide bonds at the carbonyl side of aromatic (Tyr, Phe, Trp) and acidic (Asp, Glu) amino acid residues. From the stomach the contents continue on into the small intestine, the pH rises to about 7, and there the peptidases trypsin, chymotrypsin and elastase continue the digestion. These enzymes are endopeptidases secreted by the pancreas. Trypsin generally cleaves at the carbonyl side of basic (Lys, Arg) residues, chymotrypsin at aromatic (Tyr, Phe, Trp) residues, and elastase at small or sterically nonhindered (Ala, Gly, Ser) residues. Finally, the oligopeptides (peptides containing only a few residues) that are remaining after endopeptidase hydrolysis can be further acted upon by two exopeptidases, namely carboxypeptidase and aminopeptidase. An exopeptidase is one that cleaves at the termini of peptides. The net result is a thorough breakdown of peptides and proteins into single amino acids and smaller dipeptides and tripeptides. For the most part these enzymes are all specific for the natural amino acids of the L-configuration.

Chemical Methodology for Decreasing Proteolysis

Attempts to modify peptides in a way that makes them more resistant to the onslaught of peptidases, thereby enhancing the biologic activity and duration of action, has been pursued by peptide chemists. When metabolism studies indicate a predominant cleavage site, attempts can be made to replace that residue with another that retains the receptor-binding activity of the peptide while yielding enhanced resistance to peptidase activity. Often, this can be accomplished by replacing the offending L-residue with its enantiomer, the D-amino acid or another D-residue. Many peptidases are unable to cleave at peptide bonds consisting of a "fraudulent" D-amino acid, and peptides containing such changes can have enhanced biologic activity because of an increase in their half-life (29). Such successes have been documented, as will be discussed later with the superagonists of gonadotropin-releasing hormone. Also, the replacement of an L-amino acid with L-proline, or N-methylation of the amide nitrogen, offers the possibility of generating a peptide that is more resistant to enzymatic hydrolysis (29). The introduction of pseudo (ψ) peptide bonds (30) and the design of retro-inverso peptides (31) are two examples of strategies that can afford more peptidase-resistant peptides, topics which will be discussed later in this chapter.

Alternative Drug Delivery Methods for Peptides and Proteins

As one might imagine from the foregoing discussion, a major barrier to the use of peptides as clinically useful drugs has to do with their poor delivery properties. This is because proteolytic enzymes present at most routes of administration are able to quickly metabolize most peptides. Peptides and proteins are, for the most part, hydrophilic in nature and for this reason do not readily penetrate lipophilic biomembranes. Also, as discussed earlier, they have short biological half-lives because of rapid metabolism and clearance, all of which detracts from their efficient use in drug therapy. It is for these reasons that alternative drug delivery methods for peptides and proteins are an area of particular interest to the pharmaceutical industry.

To appreciate the problems of drug absorption via different routes, one only has to look at Table 6.2. This table compares the percent of dose that is absorbed for two important peptides, insulin and an analog of gonadotropin-releasing hormone, leuprolide, when administered by the oral, nasal, buccal, rectal, vaginal, and subcutaneous (SC) routes (32). Note the poor bioavailability when the drugs are administered orally. Several of the alternative routes of administration that have been, or are being, investigated

for the delivery of peptide and protein drugs include those shown in Table 6.2, as well as transdermal, parenteral (including SC), targeted, and pulmonary routes (33). While space does not allow a detailed discussion of each of these routes, the following generalities can be made.

A patient's least favorite method of drug administration is clearly the parenteral route, be it by intravenous (IV), intramuscular (IM), or SC injection. Besides the pain involved, it is a route that does not easily allow for self-administration, especially when the drug has to be given IM or IV. However, in emergency situations, when rapid onset of action is warranted, the IV route is preferred; the peptide drug can act very fast because it is placed directly into the blood stream and no absorption is involved. On the other hand, when a more sustained action is desired IM administration is preferred due to the ability to introduce larger volumes of fluid directly into skeletal muscle. The disadvantages of the IM route are pain after injection, possible degradation of the peptide at the injection site, slow absorption, and difficulty of self-injection. A SC injection of a peptide drug, which can be self-administered (e.g., insulin), affords a slower absorption rate when compared to the intramuscular route and is useful for long-term therapy, but there is decreased potency of the drug because of degradation and poor absorption (34). There has been some progress in improving parenteral dosage forms that allows for better patient compliance, e.g., biodegradable microspheres of poly(D,L-lactide-glycolide) for sustained release IM injection of leuprolide acetate for up to 6 months (35), or the administration of goserelin acetate dispersed in a matrix of D,L-lactic and glycolic acids copolymer. The latter is injected SC as a solid pellet the size of a grain of rice for use up to 3 months (see later discussions on these gonadotropin-releasing hormone analogs).

Interest in the delivery of peptide and protein drugs by the nasal route has been studied extensively because of, generally, a significant improvement in bioavailability over the oral route, and it is noninvasive. Although the nasal route avoids first-pass hepatic metabolism, there is still a significant degree of enzymatic degradation that occurs in the nasal mucosa, especially by aminopeptidases (36). Also, the higher molecular weight of peptides and proteins, coupled with their more hydrophilic properties,

Table 6.2. Dose of Insulin and Leuprolide Absorbed (%) Via Different Routes of Administration

Route	% Dose Absorbed	
	Insulin	Leuprolide
Oral	0.05	0.05
Nasal	30	2–3
Buccal	0.5	—
Rectal	2.5	8
Vaginal	18	38
Subcutaneous	80	65

Adapted from reference 32.

generally affords compounds with poor absorptive properties. Therefore, in order to obtain successful nasal delivery of peptides and proteins the coadministration of protease inhibitors and permeation enhancers is generally required (37, 38). Still, there are only a limited number of peptides, of mostly lower molecular weight, commercially available for nasal use, e.g., calcitonin, desmopressin, and nafarelin.

The delivery of peptide and protein drugs via the pulmonary route, that is, by inhalation therapy, has recently become an area of intense research interest to the biotechnology industry (33). This method is also noninvasive and allows the delivery of peptide and protein drugs to lung epithelium that is highly permeable and easily accessed via inhalation (39). That is not to say this methodology, which generally uses particles that are dry or liquid and delivers them with the use of dry-powder dispensers or liquid-aerosol generators, is not without problems (33). Problems such as protein stability, reproducible delivery devices, particle size, and bioavailability of the inhaled protein still need to be solved before pulmonary delivery gains greater acceptance. However, recent studies regarding the delivery of insulin by dry-powder inhalation have caused increased interest. In these Phase II studies the investigators have demonstrated that "inhaled insulin achieves the same blood glucose control traditionally obtained through several daily insulin injections" (40). Other aerosolized peptides and proteins that show no adverse effect on the lung, such as leuprolide acetate, interferon-α, heparin, and α-1 antitrypsin, are in various stages of development (40). A good treatise on inhalation therapy of peptide and protein drugs can be found in the book edited by Adjei and Gupta (41).

MAJOR METHODS OF PEPTIDE SYNTHESIS

Although there have been many advances in the chemistry of peptide synthesis, the problems that can occur during the large scale synthesis of even a medium size peptide, for example 20–35 residues, can be quite challenging and expensive, especially by the classical solution phase methodology. The alternative method of peptide synthesis, on solid-phase, has certainly grown in popularity and eliminated some of these problems, but is not without its own limitations. A description of these two methodologies, the synthesis of peptides in solution or by solid-phase, is described below.

Synthesis in Solution

The synthesis of peptides in solution, either by stepwise elongation or segment condensation, allows one to isolate the intermediates along the way and purify them to homogeneity. As a result of this the eventual final product is usually less contaminated with by-products and is easier to isolate in a homogeneous form. This method is also more amenable to the preparation of bulk quantities of peptides than is the solid-phase method. The trade off, however, is that the solution method is laborious and time consuming, especially as the size of the peptide grows wherein the problem of maintaining the peptide in solution becomes formidable. Also, when using the segment method there is always the danger of racemization occurring during the coupling of the segments. One of the more prolific laboratories that report outstanding achievements in the solution syntheses of complicated large peptides and proteins is that of Sakakibara in Japan (42).

Selective Protection of the α-Amino Group

In order to be able to form a peptide bond between two amino acids, e.g., Ala-Val, the nucleophilicity of the amino function in Ala must be removed. Thus only the amino group of Val is nucleophilic and only it can react with the activated carboxyl group (to be discussed below) of Ala. If this dipeptide is then to be elongated to a tripeptide, e.g., Gly-Ala-Val, the nucleophilicity of the Ala amine must be reinstated so that it now can react with an activated carboxyl group of Gly. The key then is to be able to easily protect and deprotect the amino functions of amino acids without inverting the chirality of the individual amino acids or disrupting any of the peptide bonds.

As previously mentioned the first group that fit these criteria was the carbobenzoxy (Cbz, Z) group discovered by Bergmann and Zervas (3) (Fig. 6.5). The advantages of the Cbz blocking group are that its amino acid derivatives are stable, crystalline and therefore commercially available for all of the natural amino acids. When the Cbz group is bound to the α-amine the resulting urethane functionality (RO_2C-NH-) imparts stability towards racemization (43). The Cbz group is stable to base but it can be removed by treatment with hydrogen bromide in glacial acetic acid (HBr/AcOH) or liquid hydrogen fluoride (HF). Both acidic catalysts promote acidolytic, not hydrolytic, cleavage resulting from protonation of the urethane carbonyl. In addition, the Cbz group is readily cleaved by catalytic hydrogenation in the presence of palladium (Pd/H_2), except in the presence of the sulfur containing amino acids, Cys and Met, in which the sulfur poisons the Pd catalyst. Conversely, the Cbz group is not useful for α-amino protection in solid phase peptide synthesis (SPPS) because the two acidolytic methods used in Cbz cleavage would

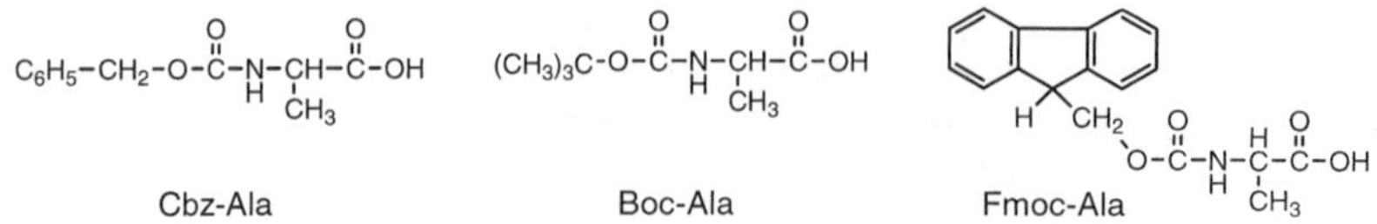

Fig. 6.5. Three urethane-type amino protecting groups, Cbz Boc, and Fmoc, shown attached to Ala.

also cleave the side chain blocking groups of the trifunctional amino acids. Also, Pd/H_2 cleavage is not useful in SPPS because Pd, being a solid, would contaminate the polymers used in SPPS. A further disadvantage of the Cbz group is that upon acidolytic cleavage benzyl cations can form and potentially alkylate the amino acids Trp and Met. Therefore, the addition of a scavenger agent (e.g., anisole) which can preferentially react with benzyl cations is usually added to the acid cleavage reagent.

The introduction of the Boc group (13) was a significant step forward as a protecting group for the α-amino function (Fig. 6.5). In addition to the advantages mentioned above for the Cbz group, including the urethane protection against racemization, the Boc group's ease of cleavage under milder acid conditions, such as trifluoroacetic acid (TFA), broadens its use in peptide synthesis, especially to that of SPPS. Furthermore, its resistance to cleavage by Pd/H_2 but sensitivity to TFA allows for differential blocking of trifunctional amino acids when using both Boc and Cbz groups. A disadvantage with the use of the Boc group, like with the Cbz group, is the possible formation of tert-butyl cations, which could alkylate the amino acids Trp and Met. Again, this can be minimized by the addition of a scavenger agent to the acidolytic cleavage reagent.

In the synthesis of peptides the repeated use of acid in the cleavage of the α-amino protecting group can cause variable amounts of unwanted side products to occur. In order to circumvent the need for repeated acidolytic cleavages, Carpino and Han (14) introduced the now popular Fmoc protecting group (Fig. 6.5). The main advantage of this urethane blocker is the fact that it is stable to acid but readily cleaved by organic base such as piperidine. It too, like Boc, is very useful in either solution or solid phase synthesis, and because it is base labile one can use various acid labile blocking groups for the side chains of the trifunctional amino acids. One disadvantage is that the commercially available Fmoc-amino acids are somewhat more expensive than the corresponding Boc- or Cbz-amino acids. Another disadvantage is that there can be some premature deblocking by the free amines, such as those found in amino acids or growing peptides, that are the nucleophilic components of the coupling reaction.

Selective Protection of the α-Carboxyl Group

In the solution synthesis of peptides by the stepwise elongation method (the addition of one amino acid at a time) or segment condensation method (the synthesis of several segments which are then joined to make the whole), the carboxyl function of the C-terminal residue must be blocked so that it does not partake in future coupling reactions. Clearly the easiest to prepare and least expensive of the groups protecting the α-carboxyl function is the methyl or ethyl ester. However, these esters are only cleaved by alkaline hydrolysis and that can lead to undesirable side reactions. Furthermore, these esters are not compatible with the conditions necessary to cleave the

Fmoc group, in that piperidine can react with these simple esters.

The benzyl (Bzl) ester is another widely used blocker for the carboxyl function and is easily prepared with inexpensive reagents. It is readily cleaved with liquid HF or by Pd/H_2. Alternatively, the Bzl ester is stable to TFA. Therein lies the reason why the Bzl ester is especially useful when Boc-amino acids are used; TFA cleaves the Boc group but not the Bzl ester, whereas Pd/H_2 can cleave the Bzl group but not the Boc group.

The tert-butyl (Bu^t) ester is easily prepared with inexpensive reagents, is cleavable with TFA and other acidolytic reagents (HF), yet it is stable to Pd/H_2. As a result it is a very popular blocking group because it is compatible with both Cbz— and Fmoc-amino acids. For example, the Cbz group can be cleaved via Pd/H_2 whereas the Bu^t ester is stable, while the converse is also true, the Bu^t ester can be cleaved with TFA and the Cbz group is stable. In the case of Fmoc-amino acids, the Bu^t ester is stable under the basic conditions needed to cleave the Fmoc group.

Selective Protection of Trifunctional Amino Acids

A trifunctional amino acid, as seen in Table 6.1, is one that has an additional functional group as part of its side-chain. For ease of discussion these can be divided into the following groups, as determined by their side-chain functionality: monoamino dicarboxylic acids (Asp, Glu); hydroxyl containing (Ser, Thr, Tyr); sulfur containing (Cys, Met); basic (Arg, His, Lys); weakly basic (Trp); neutral (Asn, Glu). In the discussion below it is important to recognize that the goal is selective protection of the side-chain functionality so that it does not participate in any chemistry during the assembly of the peptide, but instead undergoes cleavage at the end of the synthesis. That is, the side-chain protecting group should be stable to the conditions needed to cleave either the α-amino or α-carboxyl blocking groups during peptide chain elongation.

Irrespective of whether solution phase or SPPS is practiced, if Boc-amino acids are used with monoamino dicarboxylic acids then the side-chain carboxyl is usually protected as its Bzl ester. However, because of the potential for intramolecular succinimide formation with Asp(Bzl) peptides, the replacement of Bzl with a cyclohexyl (cHex) ester reduces this undesirable side reaction (43, 44). On the other hand, if Fmoc-amino acids are used then the side-chain carboxyl is usually protected as its Bu^t ester. Similarly, when using Boc-Ser and Boc-Thr the hydroxyl function is protected as the Bzl ether. However, in the case of Tyr the Bzl ether is not stable enough during the repeated TFA treatments needed to cleave the Boc group. Therefore, in the case of Boc-Tyr the preferred blocking group for the phenolic hydroxyl is the 2-bromo-carbobenzoxy (2Br-Z, $BrC_6H_4CH_2OCO$). When N$^\alpha$-Fmoc is used, the hydroxyl groups of Ser, Thr, and Tyr are usually protected by the Bu^t ether.

The amino acid Cys contains a free sulfhydryl (SH) function that is very nucleophilic and easily oxidized, thus it must be protected. A discussion of the several different blocking groups used to protect the sulfur is beyond the scope of this chapter, but the interested reader should consult those references whose main thrust is peptide synthesis (43, 45). The amino acid Met does not contain a free SH, but rather a methylthio ether, S-CH$_3$, and as such it is most often used unprotected. Some investigators prefer using Boc-Met protected as its sulfoxide, Boc-Met(O), in order to prevent alkylation of the sulfur and partial conversion to the sulfoxide during the synthesis. The sulfoxidation is most common during acidic cleavage of other blocking groups. The use of the sulfoxide would of course necessitate a reduction step at the end of the synthesis to convert Met(O) back to Met, which can be accomplished by the low/high HF cleavage procedure (46). When using Fmoc-Met the side-chain is unprotected.

Of the three basic amino acids, Arg, Lys and His, Arg is the most basic and is mainly used with the guanyl nitrogen (N^G) protected, even though at pH 9 the guanidino group (pKa 12.5) is virtually fully protonated. When N$^\alpha$-Boc is used, the preferred protection for N^G is the tosyl (Tos) group, which is cleavable with HF at the end of the synthesis. On the other hand, when N$^\alpha$-Fmoc is used one of the more popular N^G-blockers is the 2,2,5,7,8-pentamethyl-chroman-6-sulfonyl (Pmc) group, which like the Tos group is also of the sulfonyl type (see structure below). The presence of the aromatic methyls as well as the chroman oxygen imparts greater acidolytic lability, and the Pmc group is cleavable with TFA at the end of the synthesis. A more recent entry into N^G-protection is Fmoc-Arg(Pbf), where Pbf is 2,2,4,6,7-pentamethyldihydrobenzofuran-5-sulfonyl (below). The advantage of the Pbf group reportedly is a greater TFA lability when compared to its structural analog Pmc (47).

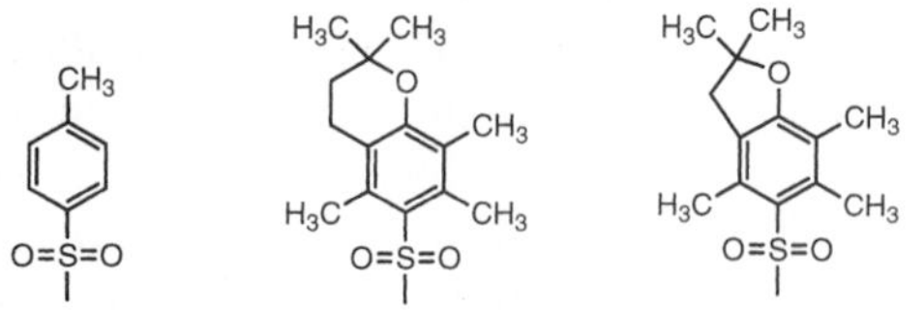

Tos   Pmc   Pbf

The side chain of basic amino acid Lys is usually protected with the 2-chloro-carbobenzoxy (2Cl-Z, ClC$_6$H$_4$CH$_2$OCO) group when using N$^\alpha$-Boc, because the presence of the 2-Cl increases the stability of the group to repeated treatments with TFA necessary for removing Boc groups. When N$^\alpha$-Fmoc protection is used the side-chain amine is simply protected with the Boc group. Finally, the least basic of the three, His, is always used with the imidazole ring protected, otherwise it is susceptible to racemization during activation of the carboxyl for peptide coupling. There are two different ring nitrogens in

the imidazole ring of His, namely N$^\pi$ and N$^\tau$. It is known that the N$^\pi$ electrons, which do not participate in the aromaticity of the imidazole ring, as do the N$^\tau$ electrons, are

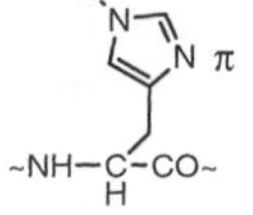

His residue

responsible for causing racemization (43). Therefore, two similar derivatives which block the π-N are the benzyloxy-methyl (Bom) and the *tert*-butyloxymethyl (Bum) groups, both of which are commercially available as Boc-His(N$^\pi$-Bom) and Fmoc-His(N$^\pi$-Bum). Whereas Boc-His(N$^\pi$-Bom) is widely used, Fmoc-His(N$^\pi$-Bum) is prepared by a multi-step procedure and is quite expensive. For the latter reason, when using Fmoc chemistry peptide chemists often use the less expensive Fmoc-His(N$^\tau$-Trt), where Trt is the triphenylmethyl (trityl) group. Although the Trt group is attached at the τ-nitrogen it still suppresses racemization because it is able to reduce the basicity of the imidazole ring and its steric bulk hinders racemization.

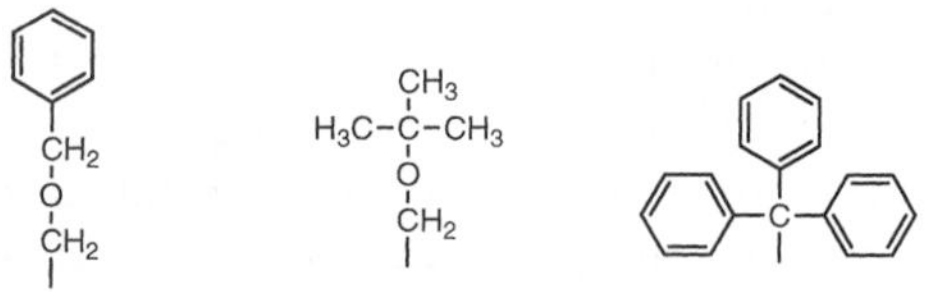

Bom   Bum   Trt

The aromatic, weakly basic and weakly nucleophilic Trp is susceptible to two side reactions, oxidation and alkylation of the indole ring by cations generated during acidolytic cleavages. Therefore, when using N$^\alpha$-Boc chemistry the formyl (For) group is often attached to the indole nitrogen, i.e., Boc-Trp(For). The formyl group is removable at the end of the synthesis by treatment with the low/high HF procedure (46). When using N$^\alpha$-Fmoc chemistry, peptide chemists have generally used Trp without side-chain protection. However, the use of Fmoc-Trp(Boc) has recently gained in popularity because it prevents sulfonation by-products that may occur during deprotection of peptides containing Pmc and Pbf protected Arg residues (48).

Finally, the neutral amino acids Asn and Gln can be used in peptide synthesis without side-chain protection, providing that the chemist is aware of the potential for dehydration of the carboxamide side-chain to a nitrile during peptide bond formation. This nitrile formation, which can occur with a variety of carboxyl activating reagents, is dramatically minimized by the addition of 1-hydroxybenzotriazole (HOBt) to the activating solution (43). During Fmoc chemistry with Asn and Gln, the use of the Trt side-chain blocking group has gained in popularity because it prevents nitrile formation as well as enhancing solubility in dimethylformamide, an organic solvent commonly used in peptide synthesis.

Major Methods of Peptide Bond Formation

To form a new peptide bond one must activate the α-carboxyl group of a suitably blocked amino acid so as to react it with the free α-amino group of another suitably blocked amino acid or growing peptide. The activation methodologies most often used can be divided into three main classes, 1) the carbodiimide coupling reagents, 2) the active esters, and 3) the phosphonium and uronium coupling reagents.

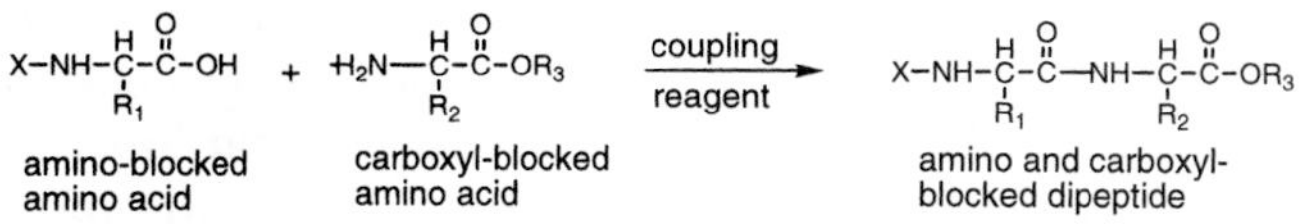

The reagent DCC (Fig. 6.6), which was previously discussed as one of the important discoveries that helped drive the field of peptide synthesis (12), is probably the most popular of the carbodiimide-type coupling reagents in use today. DCC can be considered to be a dehydrating agent inasmuch as it effects the removal of a molecule of water from the amino and carboxyl groups involved in the coupling. Details of the mechanism can be found elsewhere (49).

Some of the advantages of the carbodiimides are that they are inexpensive reagents, generally insensitive to moisture, and can effect rapid coupling. Two disadvantages are that quite extensive racemization can occur when coupling peptide segments, specifically the residue whose carboxyl is being activated, as well as nitrile formation of Asn and Gln residues, as discussed above. However, the addition of HOBt to carbodiimide couplings can very effectively minimize both of these disadvantages (49). Another annoying problem with the use of DCC, more so in SPPS than solution phase, is that its by-product, dicyclohexylurea (DCU) (below), is highly insoluble in most solvents used in peptide coupling. In SPPS, DCC is often replaced with diisopropylcarbodiimide (DIC) because its by-product, diisopropylurea (DIU) (below), is more soluble in the solvents used in this technique and does not contaminate the solid polymer phase.

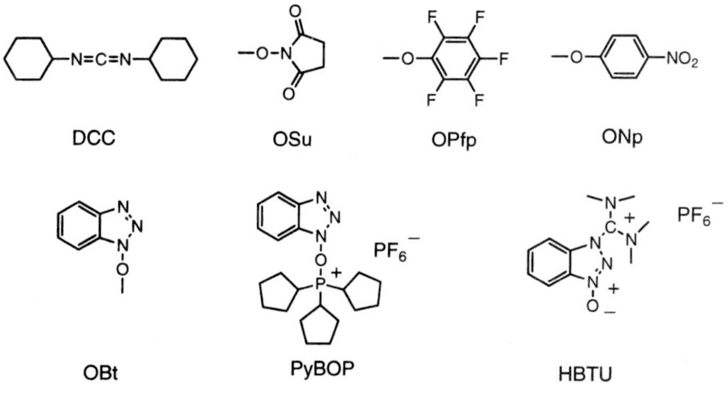

Fig 6.6. Structures of several of the reagents used in peptide bond formation.

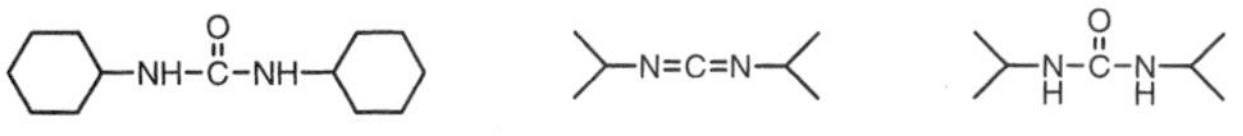

An active ester is a suitably protected amino acid whose carboxyl group has been esterified with a hydroxyl moiety that is easily eliminated upon attack of the carbonyl group by the nucleophilic amino component. When the hydroxyl moiety is a phenol it will contain either an electron withdrawing group (*para*-nitrophenol) or electronegative elements (pentafluorophenol), which affords a better leaving group. When using Boc-protected residues two popular active esters are the *para*-nitrophenol (ONp) and N-hydroxy-succinimde (OSu) esters (Fig. 6.6). When using Fmoc-protected residues the one active ester that is both commercially available and widely used is the pentafluorophenol (OPfp) ester (Fig. 6.6). Those derivatives that are commercially available are generally crystalline and reasonably stable. On the other hand, the 1-hydroxybenzotriazole (OBt) active ester (Fig. 6.6) is very popular with both Boc and Fmoc chemistries. However, the OBt-esters are not commercially available because they usually are neither isolable nor stable and have to be prepared *in situ* from a protected amino acid, HOBt, and a carbodiimide. Still this method finds wide use in both solution phase and SPPS.

More recently the use of phosphonium, for example benzotriazole-1-yl-oxy-tris-pyrrolidino phosphonium hexafluorophosphate (PyBOP) and uronium, for example 2-(1H-benzotriazole-1-yl)-1,1,3,3-tetramethyluronium hexafluorophosphate (HBTU), coupling reagents have gained wide use in effecting peptide bond formation, particularly in SPPS (Fig. 6.6). The structures of PyBOP and HBTU both incorporate an equivalent of HOBt and the final reactive Boc or Fmoc amino acid species is the corresponding OBt active ester (49).

Solid Phase Peptide Synthesis

Historically, the Merrifield strategy of SPPS, as originally published in 1963 (15), consisted of attaching the C-terminal amino acid of the peptide to be synthesized, N^α-Boc protected, to a solid polymer support via an ester linkage (50). This ester linkage was designed to be stable to all chemical conditions involved in the elongation of the peptide, but able to be cleaved from the polymer at the end of the synthesis without effecting the integrity of the final peptide. An additional requirement was that the side-chain protecting groups are stable during the synthesis but removable at the end, preferably at the same time that the final peptide was cleaved from the polymer. The original solid support used to attach the growing peptide was a chloromethylated polystyrene polymer (resin). Today, several newer and more versatile polymers are popular and have, for the most part, replaced the original resin. A scheme that illustrates Merrifield's concept of SPPS is shown in Figure 6.7.

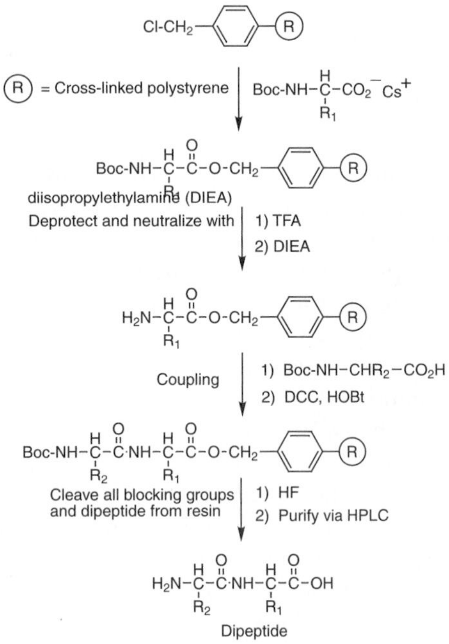

Fig. 6.7. Scheme based on Merrifield's methodology for Boc-based SPPS.

The following are several of the advantages that one can expect when using the technique of SPPS. The attachment of the growing polypeptide to an insoluble polymer allows soluble reagents and by-products to be readily removed by simple filtration and washing of the insoluble polypeptide-bound polymer. This reduces the loss of valuable peptide that occurs in solution phase peptide synthesis as a result of repeated isolation and purification of peptide intermediates. Another advantage is the ability to use excess soluble reagents, which are easily removed by filtration, in order to force reactions to completion and thereby achieve high yields. The most valuable advantage is the ability to automate all the operations of the polypeptide synthesis, thus drastically reducing time, labor, and cost involved in the synthesis. The disadvantages of SPPS are the inherent cost of using excess reagents and solvents in order to force the couplings to near completion and the actual purification of the final cleaved product can be difficult.

Boc Chemistry

The use of Boc-based SPPS for the synthesis of peptide acids necessitates that the peptide chains are linked to the resins as benzyl esters and that the side-chain protecting groups generally have a similar reactivity, so that these bonds are stable to repeated TFA cleavages of the N^α-Boc group. The need for a more stable benzyl ester linkage of the peptide to the Merrifield solid support culminated in the development of the phenylacetamidomethyl (PAM) resin. Similarly, the need to synthesize peptide C-terminal amides gave rise to the 4-methylbenzhydrylamine (MBHA) resin (51) (Fig. 6.8). Merrifield-, PAM- and MBHA-resins linked to all of the natural Boc-amino acids are commercially available.

Fmoc Chemistry

The growth in the use of N^α-Fmoc-based SPPS has been driven by the desire to avoid the repetitive acidolytic (TFA) treatment required in BOC-based SPPS and to evade the final HF cleavage needed to remove the peptide from its resin, as well as all blocking groups. The repetitive TFA and final HF treatments are often the cause of unwanted by-products. Fmoc-based SPPS allows the use of side-chain protection with *tert*-butyl-derived esters, ethers, and urethanes that are stable to the recurring mild secondary base (piperidine) treatment necessary to cleave the N^α-Fmoc group. All of the side-chain blockers can be cleaved, along with the peptide-to-resin linkage, via only one TFA treatment at the end of the synthesis. Problems encountered with Fmoc-based SPPS are the premature cleavage of the Fmoc group and the potential for by-products during cleavage of the peptide from its resin when Met and Trp are present. These problems and others are adequately addressed in several good reviews of this topic (52, 53).

Combinatorial Peptide Synthesis

Perhaps the reader can surmise from the above discourse on peptide synthesis that the preparation of a single peptide, its purification, and biologic testing is an arduous and time-consuming task. Therefore, building on Merrifield's SPPS methodology, investigators in the 1980s began developing methods for synthesizing large numbers of peptides simultaneously and screening them for biologic activity. These ideas, which have firmly taken root within the medicinal chemistry discipline and now expanded to small organic molecules, are collectively referred to as *combinatorial chemistry*, or the ability "to make a large number of chemical variants all at one time; to test them for bioactivity .... and then to isolate and identify the most promising compounds for further development" (54). This gives rise to a large number of compounds, or what is now referred to as a combinatorial library, of biologically screenable compounds.

The combinatorial method of peptide and small molecule construction can be accomplished by two general

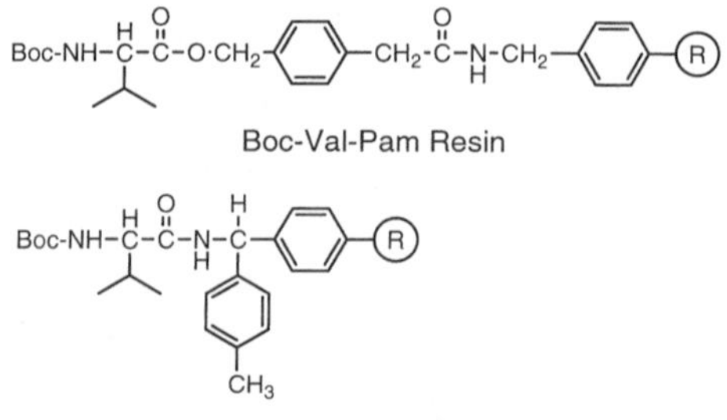

Fig. 6.8. Examples of Boc-Val attached to the phenylacetamidomethyl (PAM) resin and to the 4-methylbenzhydrylamine (MBHA) resin. The former is used to prepare peptides with a C-terminal carboxylic acid, whereas the latter is used for the preparation of peptide C-terminal amides.

methods, parallel synthesis or split-and-mix synthesis. Geysen and colleagues (55) were the first to introduce the parallel synthesis approach, wherein "all the products are assembled separately in their own reaction vessels," as in a single well of a microtiter plate (56). A typical plastic microtiter plate contains eight rows and 12 columns of small wells, thus 96 wells in which combinatorial parallel synthesis can take place. If, for example, each of the wells in the eight rows were pre-loaded with a different amino acid already attached to a polymeric support, then their SPPS coupling with a different blocked amino acid in each of the 12 columns would afford a 96-member library of dipeptides (Fig. 6.9). Of course, after removing unreacted chemicals and "reloading" each column with a different blocked amino acid, a 96-member library of tripeptides could be prepared, and so forth. After cleaving these dipeptides, tripeptides, or larger peptides, from the polymer the entire plate of 96 different compounds could be screened for biologic activity. If many microtiter plates

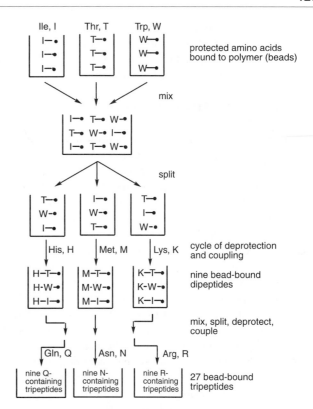

Fig. 6.10. Schematic representation of the split-and-mix technique.

were used, one could see how a large library of peptides could be constructed. Nowadays, robotic machines are used to carry out these repetitive steps and hundreds and thousands of compounds can be made in a day.

The split-and-mix technique, or "one-bead-one-compound," has been reviewed by Lam and co-workers (57) and was first developed by Furka and co-workers (58). In the parallel method each well contains only one peptide, whereas in the split-and-mix technique a single vessel may contain a mixture of closely related peptides. This occurs because the technique requires the repetition of three operations, a) a division into equal portions of the polymer upon which the peptide is growing, b) the coupling of each portion with a different amino acid, and c) the homogenous mixing of these portions (59) (Fig 6.10). By using the method outlined in Figure 6.10, wherein one starts with only three amino acids bound to a polymer, the number of peptides would triple after each coupling step, according to the formula 3^n. However, if all 20 of the natural amino acids were bound to a polymer one could generate 3,200,000 different peptides after only five couplings, according to the formula 20^n (59).

Each of the vessels are then evaluated for biologic activity and those with the most potent activity would be processed by a variety of techniques to determine which particular peptide(s) are responsible for the activity (56). An important difference between the split-and-mix technique and parallel synthesis is that the former method affords small quantities of a large number of peptides, whereas the latter method yields larger quantities of a smaller number of peptides (54).

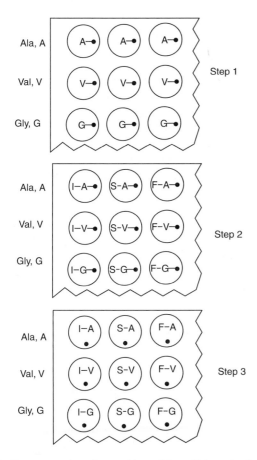

Fig. 6.9. Representation of a combinatorial parallel synthesis of a 96-member library of dipeptides in a typical plactic microtiter plate of eight rows and 12 columns; only the upper left three rows and three columns are shown. Step 1 shows three rows of wells containing three different amino acids that are already attached to a polymeric solid phase, as represented by the solid circles. In step 2 all eight rows are treated with the particular protected amino acids shown in each of the 12 columns, giving rise to 96 different polymer-bound dipeptides. In step 3, the dipepides are cleaved from the solid support in preparation for testing them for biologic activity.

A discussion of the many novel techniques and advances in combinatorial peptide synthesis is beyond the scope of this chapter and the interested reader may want to check several of the current reviews on this topic (60, 61, 62).

TOPOLOGICAL MODIFICATIONS OF PEPTIDES

In regards to biologically active peptides, a common assumption is that their activities depend on their three-dimensional structures. On the surface where contact between ligand and receptor occurs, the relative spatial arrangements of the side-chain groups on the peptide pharmacophore are critical for receptor recognition and probably determine, in many cases, the affinity, selectivity and activity of the peptide for a particular receptor protein. Therefore, side chain modifications of a given peptide may provide important insights into the conformational and topological requirements for its activity (63).

Alternatively, other structure-activity studies of peptides have involved modifications of the peptide backbone. In this regard there has been great interest in the replacement of some peptide bonds with pseudopeptide (ψ) bonds (30), because among other things it may modify the backbone conformation as well as limit enzymatic degradation, as briefly mentioned above. Still another fascinating topological modification that has shown promise in limiting enzymatic degradation, while retaining or enhancing biologic activity, is referred to as the retro-inverso modification (31), briefly mentioned above. Both of these modifications will now be discussed in more detail.

Peptides Containing Pseudopeptide (ψ) Bonds

The modification of the peptide backbone by replacement of the normal peptide bond, -CONH-, with an isosteric unit generally does not alter the overall dimensions of the peptide. A replacing unit is referred to as a pseudopeptide bond and any peptide analog containing a modified bond is referred to as a pseudopeptide. The symbol ψ was originally introduced (64) with specific reference to the sulfur-based CH_2S peptide bond replacement and later used for various CH_2S containing pseudopeptides. With an increase in peptide bond replacements the term has taken on a broader meaning and now is referred to by the symbols $\psi[\ ]$. The ψ refers to the absence of the peptide bond and the bracket, $[\ ]$, that is inserted between the named amino acid residues specifies the replacement structure for the peptide bond (30). For example, Ala$\psi[CH_2S]$Gly refers to the pseudopeptide $NH_2CH(CH_3)CH_2SCH_2CO_2H$. Several examples of the types of pseudopeptides that have been reported in the literature, as well as the nomenclature used to designate the replacement, are shown in Table 6.3. A useful reference for the synthesis of several pseudopeptide bonds is that reported by Spatola (65).

One pseudopeptide replacement that has been utilized more often than others, in attempts at modifying the pep-

Table 6.3.   Examples of Peptide Backbone Modifications

Unit-Replacing Peptide (-CONH-) Bond	Nomenclature Symbol
-CH$_2$S-	$\psi[CH_2S]$
-CONCH$_3$-	$\psi[CONCH_3]$
-COO-	$\psi[COO]$
-COS-	$\psi[COS]$
-COCH$_2$-	$\psi[COCH_2]$
-CSNH-	$\psi[CSNH]$
-CH$_2$NH-	$\psi[CH_2NH]$
-NHCO-	$\psi[NHCO]$
-CH$_2$CH$_2$-	$\psi[CH_2CH_2]$
-CHCH-	$\psi[CHCH]$
-CH$_2$CONH-	$\psi[CH_2CONH]$
-CONHO-	$\psi[CONHO]$
-CHOHCH$_2$NH-	$\psi[CHOHCH_2NH]$
-COCH$_2$NH-	$\psi[COCH_2NH]$
-CHOHNH-	$\psi[CHOHNH]$
-CHOHCH$_2$O-	$\psi[CHOHCH_2O]$
-CHOHCH$_2$-	$\psi[CHOHCH_2]$

tide backbone, is the $\psi[CH_2NH]$ unit (66). This unit has gained popularity because of its ready incorporation into peptides during conventional SPPS and it often affords receptor antagonists (67,68).

Retro-Inverso Peptides

Another approach that has been used to transform biologically active peptides with short half-lives, and therefore of little therapeutic use, into novel and more enzymatically stable analogs is that of the retro-inverso modification. This modification involves reversing one or more amide groups within the peptide backbone, which can be accomplished by using a correctly substituted gem-diaminoalkyl residue

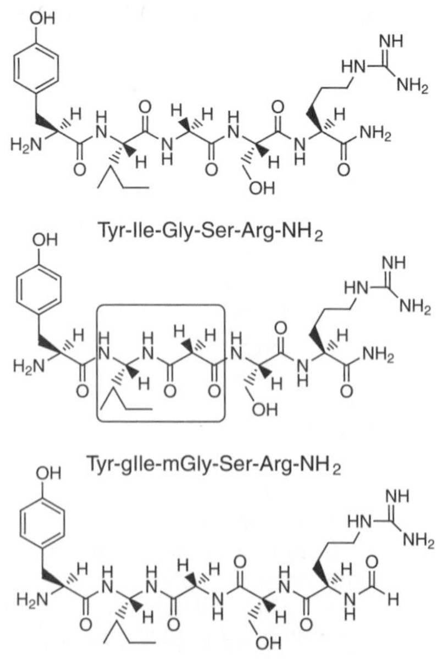

Tyr-Ile-Gly-Ser-Arg-NH$_2$

Tyr-gIle-mGly-Ser-Arg-NH$_2$

Fig. 6.11. A spatial representation of the antimetastatic peptide, Tyr-Ile-Gly-Ser-Arg-NH$_2$ (all L-configuration), and two types of partial retro-inverso analogs. The portion enclosed in the frame is the so-called "pairwise" modified segment (69). Adapted from reference 70.

(gXaa, wherein Xaa refers to the 3-letter notation for any amino acid, e.g., Val, Ala, and "g" indicates gem-diaminoalkyl) as the N-terminal residue and a substituted malonic acid residue (mXaa, "m" stands for malonic acid) as the C-terminal residue (31, 69). The aim of this topological approach is to devise analogs wherein a particular reversed peptide bond (NHCO) still maintains its planarity and the spatial orientation of the side chains is retained as close as possible to that of the original peptide. This necessitates that the chirality of amino acids placed between the gem-di-aminoalkyl and malonic acid residues must be reversed (rXaa, wherein "r" refers to a reversed direction of the peptide bond) (Fig. 6.11)(70). Retro-inverso analogs of several peptides, in particular partial retro-inverso analogs, have generally displayed enhanced enzymatic stability as well as increased bioavailability and potency (69). For the interested reader, Chorev and Goodman have published an article describing some of the more encouraging developments that have been reported with retro-inverso peptides (71).

COMMERCIALLY AVAILABLE PEPTIDE AND PROTEIN HORMONES AND ANALOGS WITH MEDICINAL USE

In the following sections we will introduce a wide variety of peptide and protein hormones, natural as well as their analogs, that are commercially available for the treatment of various diseases, or are used for diagnostic purposes. Several of these hormones are obtained synthetically, some from natural sources, while others are obtained via genetic engineering. These hormones are listed, for the most part, according to their endocrine organ of origin.

Hormones of Hypothalamic Origin

The hypothalamus, which is a relatively small organ that is located in the brain and responsible for thermoregulation, among other functions, is the secretory source of a number of peptide hormones that are transported to the pituitary gland situated immediately below it. These hormones regulate the synthesis of other peptide hormones produced by the anterior pituitary (adenohypophysis), and are thus called releasing hormones (RH) or releasing factors (RF), or inhibitory factors (IF), as the case may be. The release of these hypothalamic hormones is regulated via cholinergic and dopaminergic stimuli from higher brain centers, and their synthesis and release is controlled by feedback mechanisms from their target organs.

Thyrotropin-Releasing Hormone (TRH, Protirelin, Thypinone)

Physicochemical Properties. TRH was the first of the releasing factors to be identified and then synthesized. It consists of a tripeptide structure: pGlu-His-Pro-NH$_2$. The presence of three rings imparts some steric hindrance to the enzymatic hydrolysis of the two peptide bonds and affords partial oral activity, a rarity among peptide hormones (72). Still, the hormone is quickly inactivated *in vivo* and is only available for parenteral administration. It is active in picogram (10^{-12}) amounts and (upon pituitary gland receptor contact) it causes a many fold increase in the quantity of thyrotropin (thyroid stimulating hormone, TSH) released from this gland. TRH has been less successfully modified than other hypothalamic peptides and therefore there are no analogs that are commercially available.

Therapeutic Applications. Presently the use of TRH is as an adjunct diagnostic agent helpful in distinguishing between hypothalamic (tertiary) and pituitary (secondary) hypothyroidism. Primary hypothyroidism is a malfunction at the level of the thyroid gland. In the normal human, the IV administration of TRH is expected to cause a maximal secretion of TSH within 15–30 minutes. In the hypothyroid patient, the administration of TRH should cause the release of TSH if the defect is tertiary hypothyroidism, but no increase of TSH levels in a patient with secondary hypothyroidism.

Gonadotropin-Releasing Hormone (GnRH)

Physicochemical Properties. GnRH is a decapeptide (Fig. 6.12) that effects the release of the gonadotropins, luteinizing hormone (LH) and follicle stimulating hor-

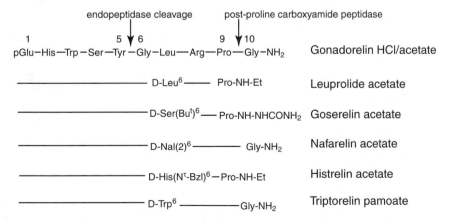

Fig. 6.12. GnRH based drugs that are commercially available. Leuprolide, goserelin, nafarelin, histrelin, and triptorelin are all superagonists, contain a D-amino acid in place of Gly^6, and three of the five are missing C-terminal Gly. The line indicates an identical sequence of amino acids.

mone (FSH), from the anterior pituitary gland, but not in equal amounts (FSH release is partially inhibited by the gonadal protein inhibin). Therefore, GnRH is intimately involved in the control of both male and female reproduction (Chapter 29). In contrast to what was found with TRH, medicinal chemists have capitalized on the relatively simple decapeptide structure of GnRH in that many analogs have been prepared as possible fertility and antifertility agents, several of which are commercially available, especially those which are referred to as superagonists. It is known that GnRH can be degraded by preferential enzymatic cleavage between Tyr^5-Gly^6 and Pro^9-Gly^{10} (73,74). Structure-activity relationship studies of GnRH analogs have shown that when Gly^6 is replaced with certain D-amino acids, as well as with changes in the peptide C-terminus, they generally experience a reduced attack by proteolytic enzymes, resulting in a longer-lasting action and, for that reason, are referred to as superagonists (75,76). Furthermore, when these D-amino acids at position 6 are hydrophobic the half-life is enhanced (77) (Fig. 6.12).

Physiologic Action of GnRH Agents. In physiological doses GnRH agonists are able to induce ovulation and spermatogenesis by increasing the levels of LH and FSH and as a result the sex-steroid levels, as does the normal hormone. However, in larger therapeutic doses GnRH agonists, especially the superagonists, block implantation of the fertilized egg, cause luteolysis of the corpus luteum, and thus act as postcoital contraceptive agents, although not an approved use. This "paradoxical" antifertility effect seen with the superagonists has been attributed to the fact that GnRH must be administered in a low dose, pulsatile manner in order for it to be therapeutically effective as a fertility agent. Natural GnRH release from the hypothalamus occurs in a pulsatile manner. When GnRH, or especially a superagonist, is administered in pharmacological doses each day, LH and FSH levels will initially rise but then will begin to fall after a few days because of target tissue desensitization/down-regulation of pituitary GnRH receptors. The continued use of these agents, in a non-pulsatile manner, will result in a drastic drop of the gonadal steroid levels to near castrate levels in both males and females, thereby giving rise to their use in such conditions as precocious puberty, endometriosis, and advanced metastatic breast and prostate carcinoma (78). It should be pointed out, however, that the GnRH superagonists typically take about 2 weeks to finally desensitize the GnRH receptors and during this time there is a transient rise in LH and FSH levels, which often results in an initial "flare-up" of the original symptoms. The following discussion concerns the medicinal chemistry of the commercially available products of GnRH and its analogs.

Specific Drugs

Gonadorelin HCl (Factrel). Gonadorelin hydrochloride (Fig. 6.12), administered by injection is used as a diagnostic agent to evaluate the ability of the anterior pituitary to produce the gonadotropins, LH and FSH. As such it finds use in evaluating abnormal gonadotropin regulation, as in precocious puberty and delayed puberty, or in differentiating between hypothalamic and pituitary gonadal antifertility.

Gonadorelin Acetate (Lutrepulse). Gonadorelin acetate, which is available as a powder for injection via the Lutrepulse Pump kit, is the identical synthetic decapeptide equivalent of human GnRH, but used as its acetate salt (Fig. 6.12). Gonadorelin acetate is intended to induce ovulation in women diagnosed with primary hypothalamic amenorrhea and is used to treat infertility caused by defective GnRH stimulation from the hypothalamus. The key here is that the natural hypothalamic production of GnRH occurs in a pulsatile manner, which ultimately causes pulsatile release, from the pituitary, of mainly LH and to a lesser extent FSH. The goal of the pulsatile administration of gonadorelin acetate is to approximate the natural hormone secretion pattern of the hypothalamus.

The Lutrepulse Pump delivers microgram quantities of gonadorelin acetate, via IV, in a pulsatile manner, over 7 consecutive days at a pulse period of 1 minute, every 90 minutes. After this period an ovarian ultrasound is usually performed to monitor the size of the developing follicle before refilling the pump. When the ovarian follicle reaches a target diameter, ovulation may be induced by an injection of human chorionic gonadotropin (hCG). This combination, if followed by unprotected sexual intercourse, is reportedly effective in permitting pregnancy to occur; multiple births can and do occur.

Leuprolide Acetate (Lupron, Viadur). Leuprolide acetate is a synthetic nonapeptide analog of GnRH that possesses greater potency than the natural hormone, is a superagonist, and is commercially available. Note that leuprolide acetate contains D-Leu and NH-Et in place of Gly^6 and Gly^{10}-NH_2, respectively (Fig. 6.12), both of which are substitutions that hinder enzymatic degradation. Leuprolide acetate is reportedly 15 times the potency of natural GnRH (78). When given continuously and in therapeutic doses, leuprolide acetate inhibits LH and FSH secretion by desensitizing/down-regulating the GnRH receptors, as discussed above. After an initial stimulation, chronic administration of leuprolide acetate results in the suppression of ovarian and testicular steroidogenesis. In premenopausal females, estrogens are reduced to postmenopausal levels, while in males, testosterone is reduced to castrate levels.

Leuprolide acetate is administered by injection daily or as depot injection monthly, every 3 or 4 months, as a palliative treatment in advanced prostatic carcinoma or as an alternative to orchiectomy or estrogen therapy. An implant version (Viadur) is also available for long-term palliative therapy; after implantation of the device into the upper arm, leuprolide acetate is continuously released over a 12-month period. Since dihydrotestosterone, a metabolite of testosterone, is able to stimulate the growth of prostate cancer, the ability of leuprolide acetate to bring testosterone to near castrate levels is why this drug finds use as a palliative in this advanced disease. The addition of a non-peptidyl antiandrogen, such as flutamide or bicalutamide, to the leuprolide acetate regimen prevents adrenal and testicular synthesized androgens from binding to or being taken up by target cancer tissue. This combination therapy can help with controlling the initial flare, is used in attempts to block all sources of androgen, and is usually referred to as maximal androgen blockade (MAB).

The FDA also approves the monthly and three monthly depot formulations for use in women diagnosed with endometriosis, but not for longer than 6 months because of the chance of developing osteoporosis. Endometriosis, a painful disorder of the female reproductive tract, occurs in women during their childbearing years. The disease involves the growth of endometrial tissue (which is normally shed monthly with menstruation) in areas outside the uterus, usually the pelvic region, where it swells and bleeds internally during the monthly menstrual cycle. The inability of the blood to leave the body leads to inflammation of the surrounding areas as well as the formation of scar tissue. Several of the symptoms of endometriosis are painful urination and bowel movements, severe menstrual cramps, pain during sexual intercourse, and possible infertility. Since estrogens stimulate the growth of endometrial tissue, the ability of this drug to drastically reduce estrogen levels suggests why leuprolide acetate is useful in treating endometriosis.

Central precocious puberty that is idiopathic, or gonadotropin dependent, can cause the development of secondary sexual characteristics before the age of 8 years in girls and 9 years in boys. Besides the psychologic and physiologic changes that can occur because of entering puberty too early, there is the risk of the child failing to reach his or her full adult height. Therefore, leuprolide acetate's ability to suppress LH and sex steroid levels (testosterone and estradiol) to prepubertal levels is the reason leuprolide acetate is approved for use in treating children with this disease. The use of this drug in a child with precocious puberty will slow or stop their secondary sexual development, slow linear growth and skeletal maturation, and in females it will effect a cessation of menstruation.

Uterine leiomyoma (fibroids), which is a benign neoplasm that is derived from smooth muscle, can cause excessive vaginal bleeding that may progress to anemia. Leuprolide acetate, concomitant with iron therapy, is used in treating anemia that arises from uterine leiomyoma. The decrease in the formation of the steroid sex hormones decreases fibroid and uterine volume that effects a relief of clinical symptoms (pelvic pain) and also stops the excessive bleeding, thus correcting the anemia problem.

Goserelin Acetate (Zoladex). Like leuprolide acetate, goserelin acetate is a synthetic nonapeptide analog of GnRH that possesses greater potency than the natural hormone, also is a superagonist, and is commercially available. Note that it contains D-Ser(Bu^t) and NH-NHCONH$_2$ in place of Gly^6 and Gly^{10}-NH$_2$, respectively (Fig. 6.12). That is, the C-terminal modification simply has a NH substituting for the CH$_2$ of Gly and like the C-terminal change in leuprolide acetate this inhibits enzymatic degradation of the peptide by the post-proline carboxyamide peptidase.

Goserelin acetate is available in the form of a solid pellet, about the size of a grain of rice, that is administered as a SC implant for the palliative treatment of advanced, metastatic breast cancer in either pre- or perimenopausal women, or similarly as a palliative in advanced prostatic cancer. Again, as mentioned above with leuprolide acetate, the rationale for this drug's use is its ability as a superagonist to bring the levels of estradiol or testosterone to near castrate levels, thus slowing the progression of breast or prostate carcinoma, respectively. Similar to leuprolide acetate, goserelin acetate is also approved for use in treating endometriosis for up to 6 months.

Goserelin acetate finds use, in combination with the antiandrogen flutamide, for shrinking prostate carcinoma prior to radiation therapy. The stipulation is that it be used in prostate carcinoma that has a Jewett staging of B2-C (locally confined to the prostate gland, one or both lobes may be involved, and seminal vesicles may be involved). The treatment should start 8 weeks before radiation treatment begins and be continued through the radiation treatment.

It has been reported that women who are to undergo hysterectomy for menorrhagia can benefit from prior treatment with goserelin acetate because the latter is able to induce endometrial thinning. This thinning of the endometrium improves the operating environment by causing less intrauterine bleeding, increased postoperative amenorrhea, and decreased dysmenorrhea following surgery (79). Therefore, this drug is approved for inducing endometrial thinning prior to hysterectomy for heavy menstrual bleeding.

Nafarelin Acetate (Synarel). Nafarelin acetate is a synthetic superagonist decapeptide analog of GnRH that possesses greater potency than the natural hormone, contains D-Nal(2)^6 [Nal = 3-(2-naphthyl)-Ala] in place of Gly^6, but the C-terminus, Gly^{10}-NH$_2$, is identical with natural GnRH (Fig. 6.12). This GnRH superagonist is available commercially as a 0.2% solution to be administered nasally for the relief of the signs and symptoms of endometriosis. It is a useful alternative for women with endometriosis who cannot tolerate danazol, a synthetic androgen also used for treating endometriosis, but which can produce androgenic/anabolic side effects, such as weight gain, edema, and undesirable changes in lipoprotein ratios. The observed side effects of nafarelin acetate are related to falling estrogen levels and include decreased libido, amenorrhea, hot flashes, and vaginal dryness. Estrogen of course is needed for the growth of endometrial tissue, thus decreased estrogen leads to shrinkage of errant endometrial tissue. When used consistently nafarelin acetate will inhibit ovulation and stop menstruation.

Nafarelin acetate, as the nasal solution, is also used in children, male and female, for the treatment of central precocious puberty. It will suppress LH and thus the estradiol or testosterone levels to prepubertal levels, thereby arresting early secondary sexual development, slowing linear growth and skeletal maturation, and menstruation stops in girls.

Histrelin Acetate (Supprelin). Histrelin acetate is another synthetic superagonist nonapeptide analog of GnRH that possesses greater potency than the natural hormone, contains D- His(N^τ-Bzl)^6 in place of Gly^6, and the C-terminus is identical with leuprolide acetate, namely NH-Et in place of Gly^{10}-NH$_2$ (Fig. 6.12). It is used to treat central, or idiopathic (unexplained), precocious puberty. It is meant to be administered by a parent as a daily injection to a child diagnosed with this disease. The drug, similar to those discussed above, will effect a return to normal hormone levels when given correctly. By following a consistent regimen of a single injection at the same time each day, puberty will be controlled and a repeat of the initial flare of symptoms when therapy was started can be avoided. Treatment can be discontinued when the child reaches the appropriate age for the normal start of puberty, about the age of 11–12 for girls and 12–13 for boys.

Triptorelin Pamoate (Trelstar Depot). Triptorelin pamoate is another synthetic superagonist decapeptide analog of GnRH that, like nafarelin acetate, contains only a single amino acid substitution in the natural hormone, namely D-Trp^6 for Gly^6 (Fig. 6.12). In the treatment of advanced prostrate cancer it is important to reduce serum testosterone levels to very low levels, typically to that which can be achieved by orchiectomy or estrogen therapy. When either of these two latter methods is unacceptable to the patient, an alternative approach is "chemical castration," which can be achieved by use of leuprolide or goserelin acetates, and now also triptorelin pamoate. This product is available for IM depot injection monthly, wherein serum concentration drops to a level generally seen in surgically castrated men.

Ganirelix Acetate (Antagon). Ganirelix acetate is an analog of GnRH with substitutions at residues 1, 2, 3, 6, 8 and 10. It is not a superagonist, but rather a synthetic decapeptide with high antagonist activity. Ganirelix acetate is the first GnRH antagonist to be marketed and it is approved for the suppression of LH surges, which

Ac-D-Ala(2-naphthyl)-D-Phe(p-Cl)-D-Ala(3-pyridyl)-Ser-Tyr-D
      H$_2$N-D-Ala-Pro—Lys—Leu—Lys
• 2 CH$_3$CO$_2$H   NH   NH
                        CH$_3$CH$_2$N=C   C=NCH$_2$CH$_3$
                        CH$_3$CH$_2$NH   NHCH$_2$CH$_3$

promotes ovulation, in women who are undergoing ovarian hyperstimulation fertility treatment. The goal of this drug is to significantly reduce the number of medication days necessary to suppress LH surges, thereby maintaining eggs in the ovaries. *In vitro* fertilization treatment cycles have historically been initiated via the administration of leuprolide acetate to suppress the premature release of LH. This inhibits ovulation so that the eggs remain available for retrieval by a fertility specialist. For this purpose leuprolide acetate is usually injected for as many as 26 days. Clinical studies have shown that ganirelix can shut down the LH surge and this can be accomplished in only 5 days of treatment. The suppression of LH is more pronounced than that of FSH, and the shorter treatment time minimizes unpleasant side effects such as hot flashes and headaches.

Cetrorelix Acetate (Cetrotide). Cetrorelix acetate is an analog of GnRH with amino acid substitutions at residues 1, 2, 3, 6,

Ac-D-Nal(2)-D-Phe(p-Cl)-D-Ala(3-pyridyl)-Ser-Tyr-D-Orn(carbamoyl)
                                        H$_2$N-D-Ala-Pro-Arg-Leu
          • Acetate

and 10. Each of these substitutions is a synthetic, non-DNA directed amino acid and, like ganirelix acetate above, imparts GnRH antagonist activity to cetrorelix acetate. This drug, like ganirelix acetate, is marketed for use in women undergoing assisted reproductive technology (ART) procedures wherein it is necessary to control their LH surge. This allows the follicles to develop to a size, as determined by ultrasound, that increases the success of timed insemination or in the retrieveal of oocytes that will improve the success rate of *in vitro* fertilization. Like ganirelix acetate, cetrorelix acetate has an advantage over GnRH agonists, such as leuprolide acetate, by reducing the fertility therapy cycle to days rather than weeks.

Somatostatin

Physiological Action. Somatostatin, a cyclic 14-peptide that was isolated by the Guillemin group (80) in 1973, is

S————————————————————S
Ala-Gly-Cys-Lys-Asn-Phe-Phe-Trp-Lys-Thr-Phe-Thr-Ser-Cys

probably the most thoroughly investigated and most important of the inhibitory factors produced by the hypothalamus. The principal activity of somatostatin, of hypothalamic origin, is inhibition of the release of growth hormone (GH) from the anterior pituitary. Too much GH, as in pituitary tumors, causes acromegaly, a form of giantism. On the other hand, too little GH leads to dwarfism. Somatostatin has also been identified in the pancreas and the gastrointestinal (GI) tract and besides inhibiting the secretion of both insulin and glucagon from the pancreas, somatostatin of GI origin inhibits the secretion of a variety of intestinal peptides, e.g., gastrin, secretin, pepsin, and renin. Unfortunately, the short half-life of somatostatin, less than 3 minutes, has precluded its use as a therapeutic agent. Many derivatives of somatostatin have been prepared in order to increase its duration of action or to enhance its selectivity of action. The culmination of these structure activity studies has been the development of octreotide acetate.

Synthetic Analogs

Octreotide Acetate (Sandostatin). Octreotide acetate, a long-acting octapeptide analog of somatostatin, has a half-life of about 1.5 hours. From pioneering work at the Salk Institute

$$
\begin{array}{c}
\text{S}\!\!-\!\!-\!\!-\!\!-\!\!-\!\!-\!\!-\!\!-\!\!-\!\!-\!\!-\!\!\text{S} \\
| \qquad\qquad\qquad\quad | \\
\text{D-Phe-Cys-Phe-D-Trp-Lys-Thr-Cys-Thr-ol}
\end{array}
$$

it was known that not all of the residues in somatostatin were necessary to elicit its full biologic activity (81), and from the Veber group (82) it was suggested that the essential fragment was the tetrapeptide Phe[7]-Trp-Lys-Thr[10]. These facts helped in designing the potent drug now known as octreotide acetate (83). This drug suppresses the secretion of gastroenteropancreatic peptides such as gastrin, vasoactive intestinal peptide (VIP), insulin, and glucagon, as well as pituitary GH. It is more potent than natural somatostatin in inhibiting glucagon, insulin and GH.

Octreotide acetate is used in the palliative treatment of patients with metastatic carcinoid tumors, which are tumors of the endocrine system, GI tract, and lung (gastroenteropancreatic). Carcinoid tumors secrete increasing amounts of vasoactive substances, including histamine, serotonin, bradykinin, and prostaglandins. Octreotide acetate inhibits or suppresses the release of these vasoactive substances and thus is useful in treating the severe diarrhea, facial flushing and wheezing episodes that accompany carcinoid tumors. In addition, it finds use in the palliative management of vasoactive intestinal polypeptide (VIP)-secreting tumors (VIPomas, usually pancreatic tumors). Patients with VIPomas suffer a profuse watery diarrhea syndrome and octreotide acetate decreases the release of damaging intestinal tumor cell secretions, promoting a reduction of hypokalemia by regulating electrolyte imbalances (84).

An excessive secretion of GH from the pituitary can cause the disorder known as acromegaly, which is characterized by a progressive enlargement of the head, face, hands, feet and thorax. Inasmuch as octreotide acetate is able to decrease the secretion of GH from the pituitary, it is used in treating patients with acromegaly who are unresponsive to prior pituitary radiation or surgery. In the treatment of acromegaly it is used because it reduces the blood levels of both GH and insulin-like growth factor-I (IGF-I) (85).

Indium In-111 Pentetreotide (OctreoScan). Somatostatin, and thus octreotide, receptors have a broad distribution not only in normal tissue but also in a wide variety of human tumors such as small cell lung cancers, brain tumors, malignant breast tumors, and pituitary and endocrine pancreatic tu-

mors (86). For this reason octreotide was constructed as a radionuclide-containing peptide by reacting the amino terminus with an active ester of diethylenetriaminepentaacetic acid (DTPA) to give DTPA-octreotide, and then chelating it with the radionuclide [111]In (87). This radiopharmaceutical is used as a diagnostic agent for the early detection and localization of small tumors and their metastases in the body, especially tumors that originate from neuroendocrine cells.

Growth Hormone-Releasing Factor (GRF)

Overview. Whereas somatostatin inhibits the release of pituitary GH, GRF is a positive effector in that it stimulates pituitary release of GH. GRF, a 44-residue-containing peptide, is found in the hypothalamus in only minute quantities. In fact, it was first elucidated in 1983, not from the hypothalamus but from human pancreatic tumors of acromegalic patients, and therefore was referred to as hp-GRF. However, hpGRF is identical to hypothalamic GRF. Growth hormone deficiency (GHD) in children can be treated with recombinant human GH or, as has been shown in earlier studies, with synthetic GRF (88). However, the fact that the biologic activity of GRF actually resides in the first 29 residues, beginning from the amino end, gave rise to the development of sermorelin acetate.

Sermorelin Acetate (Geref, Geref Diagnostic). Sermorelin acetate is a synthetic peptide containing the first 29 amino acid residues as found in human GRF and it finds use in treating children with idiopathic GHD and growth failure. As a diagnostic agent it is used to help elucidate the cause of a child's abnormal growth, that is, differentiating between hypothalamic or pituitary dysfunction. Sermorelin acetate is able to directly stimulate the pituitary to release GH. Many children with GHD have adequate reserves of GH, but the stimulus for its release is absent. Sermorelin acetate can help distinguish that child who lacks GH, or whose supply is inadequate, from one whose problem is at the hypothalamic level.

In a child whose growth deficiency has been diagnosed as due to inadequate secretion of natural GRF, and whose pituitary reserves of GH are intact, sermorelin acetate can trigger the release of GH so that it can be utilized for growth. The earlier that GHD can be diagnosed in a child the better, since early treatment affords a greater chance that the child will attain their maximum growth potential. An adequate amount of GH promotes nitrogen retention in the form of protein, stimulates lipolysis, increases the secretion of insulin, and perhaps enhances the production of insulin-like growth factor 1 (IGF-1), the latter of which augments several of the actions of follicle stimulating hormone (FSH). Therefore, it is not surprising that sermorelin acetate has two other approved orphan drug uses that depend upon the actions of enhanced amounts of GH: AIDS-associated catabolism and resulting weight loss, and as an adjunct to gonadotropin therapy in the anovulatory woman who fails to ovulate in response to adequate treatment with either clomiphene citrate or gonadotropin therapy alone.

Corticotropin-Releasing Hormone (Corticorelin, CRH), Corticorelin Ovine Triflutate (Acthrel)

The primary function of this hypothalamic 41-peptide is the regulation of the release of adrenocorticotropin hormone (ACTH) from the anterior pituitary gland, which then stimulates the release of hydrocortisone from the adrenal gland. The human peptide (hCRH) and the sequence found in sheep (oCRH) are both available by synthesis. ACTH deficiency in humans is usually associated with a pituitary disorder rather than a deficiency of CRH (89) and hCRH or oCRH can be used to distinguish between pituitary hypersecretion of ACTH (Cushing's disease) and ectopic ACTH secretion, both conditions of which cause a hypersecretion of hydrocortisone. In the case of ectopic ACTH secretion, the administration of CRH will elicit little to no response in the production of ACTH and hydrocortisone.

Synthetic oCRH, as its trifluoroacetate salt, is available for use as a diagnostic agent for patients with ACTH-dependent Cushing's syndrome, as described above. The ovine form of the peptide is used because of its longer half-life and somewhat greater potency when compared to the human sequence.

Hormones Originating in the Anterior Lobe of the Pituitary Gland

The pituitary, lying just below the hypothalamus, is a small gland that can be divided into an anterior and posterior lobe. This gland is responsible for the secretion of nine important peptide hormones, only two of which are released by the posterior gland. The anterior pituitary peptide hormones control the important functions of linear growth, reproduction, carbohydrate, fat and protein metabolism via hydrocortisone liberation, and the production of the thyroid hormones so important for regulating growth and energy metabolism.

Somatotropin (GH)

Somatotropin, or GH, is a protein containing 191 amino acids that is secreted by the anterior pituitary in response to the presence of GRF as secreted from the hypothalamus. The release of GH, as discussed above, is inhibited by somatostatin. Its primary function in the body is in promoting skeletal growth. When GH is absent in childhood, or if there is an inadequate supply, dwarfism results. Before 1985 children of short stature were sometimes treated with human GH (hGH) of pituitary origin, which was obtained from cadavers. However, the FDA approved hGH of natural origin was discontinued when several young adults, who had received hGH as children, died. Their deaths were attributed to contaminated hGH. The contaminant was an infective agent, a prion, that causes Creutzfeldt-Jakob disease (CJD), a rare and fatal neurodegenerative disease (90). Naturally occurring hGH has been replaced with material that is prepared by recombinant DNA procedures.

Somatrem (Protropin). Somatrem was the first hGH to be prepared by genetic engineering and it contains the identical human sequence of 191 amino acids plus an additional amino acid, Met, at the N-terminus. It is indicated for the long-term treatment of children who have growth failure due to GHD, and who still have open epiphyses, generally children with a bone age less than 12–13 years. Chronic renal failure in children is often accompanied with impeded growth, apparently as a result of abnormalities in the GH/IGF-1 axis (91). For the latter reason somatrem is approved for treating growth failure in children with chronic renal failure, and the drug should be administered until the time of renal transplantation.

Somatropin (Humatrope, Nutropin, Serostim, Genotropin, Norditropin). Somatropin, which is hGH that is also prepared by recombinant DNA procedures, contains exactly the same sequence of 191 amino acids as the natural hormone. Except for Serostim, these products are indicated for the long-term treatment of children who fail to grow because of inadequate secretion of the body's normal endogenous GH, and in treating growth problems associated with chronic renal failure. Even adults who are diagnosed with GHD, which could arise as a result of pituitary or hypothalamic disease, surgery, radiation therapy, or other reasons, can benefit from hGH replacement therapy via treatment with Somatropin. Turner's syndrome, a genetic disease in which there is a complete or partial absence of one of the two X-chromosomes in females, causes short stature as one of the many symptoms of this syndrome. Girls suffering from Turner's syndrome can benefit from the use of Somatropin during their growth years (92).

As previously indicated during the discussion of sermorelin acetate, hGH is a protein with anabolic properties and therefore promotes somatic growth. This anabolic property is the basis for the orphan drug uses of hGH: AIDS-associated catabolism or weight loss, cachexia due to AIDS, and use as an anabolic in severely burned patients (93).

Gonadotropins

Chemistry. The gonadotropins, FSH and LH, are large glycoproteins that are released by the anterior pituitary upon a signal from GnRH when it is secreted by the hypothalamus. Both FSH and LH consist of two non-covalently associated α- and β-subunits. The α-subunit, which contains 92 amino acid residues, is identical in both hormones, whereas the β-subunit consists of 121 residues in LH (94) and 111 in FSH (94) which are dissimilar. Thus, the β-subunit gives each hormone its specific function.

Physiologic Properties. LH and FSH are referred to as gonadotropins because they act on the female and male gonads, which effects the production of the sex steroids, estradiol and testosterone, respectively. In the female, FSH and LH act in concert in the regulation of ovarian function: egg maturation, ovulation, and transformation of the ruptured follicle to the corpus luteum. In males, spermatogenesis is dependent on these two hormones. Specifically, FSH in females enables the maturation of ovarian follicle cells and their secretion of estradiol, whereas in males it stimulates the maturation of sperm in the testes. On the other hand, LH promotes ovulation, formation of the corpus luteum and progesterone secretion in females, whereas in males it enables the secretion of testosterone from the testes.

According to the Research Initiatives Committee and the Public Communications Committee of The Endocrine Society, "infertility is the inability of a sexually active couple, who is not using any contraception, to achieve pregnancy in one year, the time in which 90% of couples succeed." In the case of male infertility, the quality and quantity of the sperm produced is involved. Female infertility can be due to several factors such as the inability to produce an egg, to ovulate, for fertilization to occur, and for the fertilized ovum to implant in the uterus. Several of the commercially available gonadotropins that can help in enhancing both male and female fertility are discussed below.

Menotropins (Pergonal, Humegon, Repronex). Human menopausal gonadotropins, or menotropins, is a natural product that is obtained from the urine of postmenopausal women and then biologically standardized (international units, IU) for FSH and LH activities, in an approximate ratio of 1:1 (available as 75 or 150 IU of LH and FSH). Menotropins is used in males with primary (hypothalamic) or secondary (pituitary) hypogonadism to stimulate spermatogenesis, providing they have previously been treated with human chorionic gonadotropin (hCG, a peptide hormone of placental origin that has activity very similar to LH, and which will be discussed later) to effect sufficient masculinization. In females, menotropins and hCG are given sequentially for the purposes of inducing ovulation in women who have difficulty ovulating because of either hypothalamic or pituitary hormonal dysfunction. The menotropins is given for 7–12 days, and after clinical evaluation (via ultrasound) indicates the presence of a mature follicle a single dose of hCG is given to simulate the typical LH surge that normally causes ovulation. Also, women can use the combination of menotropins and hCG to promote the development of multiple follicles when participating in an *in vitro* fertilization program requiring the recruitment of follicles.

Urofollitropin (Fertinex). Urofollitropin is a natural product that is also obtained from the urine of postmenopausal women and then highly purified so as to contain only FSH (reportedly minute amounts of LH are present). This product is used for its ability to stimulate follicle development and, as such, it is administered early in the follicular phase of women participating in an *in vitro* fertilization program, particularly the ovulating woman whose cause of infertility is due to a fallopian tube abnor-

mality. Therapy is continued daily until it is clinically demonstrated that the follicles are mature. If ovulation induction and pregnancy is the goal of the anovulatory woman then it is initiated by the administration of hCG.

This drug is also indicated for women whose infertility is caused by polycystic ovary syndrome (PCOS), which is generally observed clinically as enlarged, cystic ovaries containing relatively small follicles. Furthermore, these patients often develop hirsutism, their androgen and LH levels appear elevated while FSH levels are low, and the early exposure to these improper hormone levels may be causing the follicular atresia (95). Therefore urofollitropin, as an exogenous source of FSH, is useful in stimulating follicle maturation to preovulatory size, with little or no exposure of the follicles to additional LH (96). Again, when the follicles have matured to preovulatory size, ovulation is assisted by the administration of hCG. The couple is then advised to engage in sexual intercourse daily, beginning on the day prior to hCG administration and until ovulation has occurred.

Lately it has become desirable to have a non-natural source of pure FSH. It is believed that exposure to increased amounts of LH early in follicular development, as would be the case with menotropins, is detrimental to fertility. Also, urofollitropin is derived from menopausal urine and the demand for this product is outstripping the limited supply of this natural product (96). These problems are especially noteworthy in treating infertility in women with PCOS, and may be solved with the recent availability of two forms of recombinant FSH (r-FSH), which are discussed below.

Follitropin Alfa (Gonal-F). Follitropin alfa is a human FSH preparation of recombinant DNA origin. Since FSH is a glycoprotein, small alterations in the carbohydrate side chain attachments afford different isoforms, which thus results in different pharmacokinetic and pharmacodynamic properties. Follitropin alfa isoforms tend to be acidic and these acidic isoforms are metabolically cleared from the body at a slower rate (96). Because it is of recombinant origin, and not isolated from urine, it is free of any additional substances, such as urinary proteins and LH. It is marketed, like urofollitropin, for enhancing the development of multiple follicles that can then be induced to ovulate, via hCG administration, so that the oocytes can be collected for *in vitro* fertilization. It is also approved for use in anovulatory women, due to PCOS, who wish to become pregnant, wherein it can enhance follicle maturation prior to hCG use for final ovulation. Men can also benefit from therapy with follitropin alfa if their infertility is related to hypothalamic or pituitary hormonal dysfunction and not primary testicular failure; it induces spermatogenesis.

Follitropin Beta (Follistim). This is a human FSH preparation of recombinant DNA origin, which differs chemically from natural FSH and follitropin alfa only by slight variances in the composition of the carbohydrate side chains. In this case follitropin beta exists in isoforms that are higher in pH than follitropin alfa. These more basic isoforms of FSH reportedly have excellent receptor-binding activity and greater potency (96, 97). Follitropin beta is approved for the same uses as follitropin alfa.

Adrenocorticotropin Hormone (Corticotropin, ACTH, Acthar)

Chemistry. The anterior pituitary, under the influence of the hypothalamic peptide hormone CRH, releases ACTH, a single-chain peptide of 39 residues. It is derived from a much larger precursor protein known as pro-opiomelanocortin, the latter is the precursor of the melanocyte-stimulating hormones (MSH), the lipotropins, and other biologically active peptides (98). The sequence of 24 amino acid residues beginning from the amino terminus contains all of the biologic activity of the parent. The remaining 15 carboxy-terminal residues confers species specificity and enhances ACTH's stability towards proteolytic cleavage. Residues 1–24 are identical in humans, pigs, sheep, and beef, whereas the species differ only slightly from each other in the final 15 residues. Furthermore, the amino-terminal residues 1–13 in ACTH are identical with the full structure of α-MSH. Structure activity studies suggest that within the biologically active sequence 1–24, residues 6–10 (His-Phe-Arg-Trp-Gly) are responsible for the steroidogenic activity, while basic residues 15–18 (Lys-Lys-Arg-Arg) are responsible for binding to the ACTH receptor (98).

Physiologic Activity. The main action of ACTH is in regulating the function of the adrenal cortex. The adrenal cortex synthesizes and secretes hydrocortisone, aldosterone, and to a minor extent the testosterone precursors androstenedione and dehydroepiandrosterone. Angiotensin II and Na^+-K^+ levels mainly control the secretion of aldosterone, whereas ACTH is responsible for the regulation of the glucocorticoid hydrocortisone.

The hormone is usually obtained from the pituitaries of pigs and is available only in parenteral form. Primary adrenocortical insufficiency, Addison's disease, is due to adrenocortical hypofunction, whereas secondary adrenocortical insufficiency is due to inadequate ACTH secretion from the pituitary. The commercial use of ACTH is primarily reserved (cosyntropin is usually preferred) as an aid in the diagnosis of primary adrenocortical insufficiency or adrenocortical function, as determined by plasma cortisol concentrations prior to and following drug administration. Patients who have Addison's disease do not substantially increase plasma cortisol concentration after ACTH administration because the adrenal cortex is not functioning properly.

Cosyntropin (Cortrosyn). Cosyntropin is a synthetic polypeptide consisting of 1–24 amino acid residues of human ACTH, but which has the full biologic activity of its parent. Since it is of synthetic origin it is less allergenic than ACTH of natural origin. For this reason, cosyntropin is the preferred diagnostic agent to be used in the screening of patients suspected of having adrenocortical insufficiency. It acts rapidly on the adrenal cortex and thus it is possible to perform a 30-minute test of adrenal function in a physician's office or as an outpatient, by observing the plasma cortisol response. In this case of rapid screening, cosyntropin is administered parenterally after a control blood sample has been taken. A second blood sample is then taken exactly 30 minutes later and compared to the control cortisol level.

Hormones Released by the Posterior Lobe of the Pituitary Gland

As previously discussed, the pituitary gland is responsible for the secretion of nine important peptide hormones, only two of which are released by the posterior lobe. Actually, these two hormones, oxytocin and vasopressin, are synthesized in neurons originating in the hypothalamus and are transported to the posterior pituitary for storage until release is required.

$$\begin{array}{c} S\text{———————}S \\ | \qquad\qquad\qquad | \\ \text{Cys-Tyr-Ile-Gln-Asn-Cys-Pro-Leu-Gly-NH}_2 \end{array}$$

Oxytocin (Pitocin, Syntocinon)

Oxytocin is a 9-peptide, wherein six residues form a ring that is closed by a disulfide bridge. Oxytocin has uterotonic action, contracting the muscles of the uterus, and is sometimes used clinically to induce childbirth. It also has some activity in milk ejection (but not milk secretion, which is regulated by prolactin) in lactating women, but is no longer used for this purpose. Oxytocin effects the contraction of smooth muscle cells in the uterus, but studies have shown that the plasma concentration of oxytocin does not increase sharply during childbirth and therefore the role of oxytocin in the induction of labor is not fully known. Exogenous oxytocin, prepared synthetically, is used clinically to induce labor during childbirth, when medically necessary because of such problems as hypertension in the mother-to-be as a result of preeclampsia or eclampsia, Rh factor problems (erythroblastosis fetalis), and in a pregnancy that has exceeded 42 weeks. It also finds some use in promoting, post delivery, the expulsion of the placenta.

Vasopressin (Antidiuretic Hormone, ADH, Pitressin)

Overview. Human vasopressin (VP), or Arg-vasopressin, is chemically very similar to oxytocin and therefore is sometimes referred to as [Phe³, Arg⁸]oxytocin. The normal action of vasopressin in humans is the control of water reabsorption by the renal tubules, thus it is antidiuretic in action and often referred to as the antidiuretic hormone (ADH). When it is present in a concentration

$$S\text{————————}S$$
$$|\qquad\qquad\qquad\qquad |$$
Cys-Tyr-Phe-Gln-Asn-Cys-Pro-Arg-Gly-NH$_2$

$$S\text{————————}S$$
$$|\qquad\qquad\qquad\qquad |$$
Gly-Gly-Gly-Cys-Tyr-Phe-Gln-Asn-Cys-Pro-Lys-Gly-NH$_2$

higher than needed for antidiuretic action it causes a contraction of arterioles and capillaries and increases blood pressure, thereby its name vasopressin. An inadequate output of pituitary ADH can cause diabetes insipidus, which is characterized by the chronic excretion of large amounts of pale urine and results in dehydration and extreme thirst. Although vasopressin can be used for treating diabetes insipidus, the hormone has a short duration of action and is usually only reserved for emergency, rather than chronic, treatment of this disease.

Vasopressin Derivatives

Desmopressin Acetate (DDAVP, Stimate). Desmopressin, as its acetate salt, is a synthetic analog of VP in which the

$$H_2C\text{–}H_2C\text{–}\overset{\overset{\displaystyle O}{\|}}{C}\text{—Tyr-Phe-Gln-Asn-Cys-Pro-D-Arg-Gly-NH}_2$$
$$|\qquad\qquad\qquad\qquad\qquad\qquad |$$
$$S\text{————————————}S$$

N-terminal Cys is devoid of its α-amino function (1-Deamino) and where Arg^8 is present as its D-isomer (D-Arg^8), thus the commercial acronym, DDAVP. Apparently, the manipulation of the VP structure has increased its half-life, probably due to the presence of D-Arg and the absence of an N-terminal amine, such that desmopressin is available for oral, parenteral, or nasal use. It can be used by all three of these routes of administration to prevent or control polydipsia (excessive thirst), polyuria, and dehydration of patients with diabetes insipidus caused by a deficiency of VP. It has also been approved for the treatment of nocturnal enuresis (bed-wetting), which is thought to be the result of an absence of the normal nighttime rise in VP levels. Also, desmopressin is known to effect an increase in both plasma factor VIII (antihemophilic factor) and plasminogen activator. It therefore is approved by the FDA for use, parenterally and nasally, in reducing episodes of spontaneous or trauma-induced bleeding in patients with hemophilia A and Type I Von Willebrand's disease, but only if these patients demonstrate a plasma factor VIII activity that is above 5%. The commercial nasal product (Stimate) for treating patients with hemophilia A and Type I Von Willebrand's disease is 15 times stronger than the nasal form of desmopressin, which is used in treating diabetes insipidus.

Lypressin (Lys^8-VP, Diapid). Lypressin is porcine vasopressin and differs from the human hormone by the substitution of Lys for Arg at position 8. The commercial product is synthetically prepared and available in the form of a nasal spray for the treatment of diabetes insipidus. It is useful for patients who have become refractory to other forms of treatment.

Terlipressin (Glypressin). Terlipressin is a long acting analog of VP that was prepared by attaching a tripeptide unit to the N-terminus of Lys^8-VP. It is available as an orphan drug for the treatment of bleeding esophageal varices. Bleeding esophageal varices is a life threatening condition that occurs as a result of cirrhosis of the liver. In chronic liver cirrhosis, either due to excess alcohol consumption or from viral hepatitis, there is damage to the liver, scarring, and thus obstruction of blood flow coming from the stomach and intestines. This blockage of blood flow through the liver raises portal blood pressure and causes distension of veins along the walls of the esophagus thus creating varices (dilated veins) that are prone to ulceration, rupture, and massive bleeding (99). Terlipressin is able to lower portal pressure by reducing the blood that flows to the stomach and intestines, thereby decreasing the danger of bleeding from esophageal varices.

Hormone of Placental Origin

Overview. When the female monthly menstrual cycle is interrupted by pregnancy the placenta begins to release a hormone, human chorionic gonadotropin, whose function it is to maintain and prolong the life of the ovarian corpus luteum. The corpus luteum is important for the continued production, principally, of progesterone. Progesterone is especially important at this time because it prepares the uterus for pregnancy and helps in the maintenance of the placenta.

Human Chorionic Gonadotropin (hCG, A.P.L., Profasi HP, Pregnyl)

Placental hCG is a complex protein that consists of an α- and β subunit, of which the α-subunit has an identical sequence of 92 amino acid residues to that found in both LH and FSH, while the β subunit contains 145 amino acids and is responsible for its biologic specificity. The action of hCG very closely resembles that of LH, although hCG has a longer half-life, and also appears to have minimal FSH activity. It appears in the maternal bloodstream, and thus urine, shortly after conception when the fertilized ovum becomes implanted in the endometrium. As a result of this early release of hCG its detection in the urine forms the basis for the home pregnancy kits that have become so popular for the early prediction of pregnancy.

Because hCG, like LH, stimulates the production of testosterone by the testes it is used in young males (4–9 years) for treating prepubertal cryptorchidism, wherein it stimulates testicular descent, as well as for treating male hypogonadism. It also finds a use in treating infertility due to pituitary dysfunction, when used in combination with menotropins (as previously discussed) or clomiphene, to induce ovulation and pregnancy in anovulatory females. The commercial products are of natural origin, that is, the crude protein is obtained from the urine of pregnant women and then is purified.

Choriogonadotropin Alfa (Ovidrel)

Choriogonadotropin alfa is obtained by recombinant DNA technology and is biologically and chemically identical to hCG of natural origin. Presently it is approved, as above for hCG of urinary origin, for inducing ovulation in women with infertility due to anovulation. It also can be used in women participating in ART therapy, when they are properly pretreated with an agent that has desensitized the pituitary (e.g., a GnRH antagonist or superagonist), for the purpose of aiding in the final maturation of the eggs within the ovaries. A distinct advantage of this product is that it can be self-administered by the patient via SC injection.

Hormone Secretion Originating in the Parathyroid Gland

Overview

The parathyroid glands (four) exist in two pairs, one pair is embedded on the back surface of each of the two lobes of the thyroid gland. These very small glands are responsible for the secretion of parathyroid hormone (PTH), the result of which is an increase in the concentration of calcium ion (Ca^{2+}) in body fluids.

Parathyroid Hormone (PTH)

The Ca^{2+} concentration in body fluids is carefully regulated in humans and when it falls below normal levels the parathyroid glands secrete PTH. PTH is an 84-residue single-chain polypeptide that has a strong influence on the osteoclast cells of bone and results in these cells releasing some of their calcium into the bloodstream. At the same time it inhibits osteoblasts, thus reducing the rate of Ca^{2+} deposition in bone. Increased activity of the parathyroid, or hyperparathyroidism, results in the formation of too much parathyroid hormone and causes a potentially serious calcium imbalance. Calcitonin, to be discussed below, has an opposing action to that of PTH.

Teriparatide Acetate (Parathar)

Teriparatide is a synthetic polypeptide consisting of the first 34 amino acid residues from the N-terminal end of PTH and has been shown to contain all the structural requirements for full biologic activity. It is used parenterally as a diagnostic agent for patients presenting with hypocalcemia due to either hypoparathyroidism or pseudohypoparathyroidism. Hypoparathyroidism is relatively rare and usually is the result of operative removal or damage of the parathyroid glands during thyroid surgery. On the other hand, pseudohypoparathyroidism is not due to PTH deficiency but to target organ (bone and kidney) unresponsiveness to the hormone and is of genetic origin.

Hormone Secretion by the Parafollicular C Cells of the Thyroid Gland

Overview

The majority of the thyroid gland contains follicular cells responsible for the production of the thyroid hormones, however, there is another population of endocrine cells within the thyroid known as C (clear) cells, or parafollicular cells, which are responsible for producing the hormone calcitonin (CT). As previously mentioned, CT has an opposing action to that of PTH, which means it is responsible for decreasing the Ca^{2+} concentration in body fluids. It accomplishes this by inhibiting the activity of osteoclasts, thereby decreasing Ca^{2+} release from bone. The actual biosynthesis and release of CT is regulated by the concentration of Ca^{2+} in plasma, i.e., when it is high CT secretion increases.

Human Calcitonin (Cibacalcin) and Salmon Calcitonin (Calcimar, Miacalcin)

Calcitonin is a single-chain polypeptide consisting of 32 amino acid residues (Fig. 6.13). Calcitonins as obtained from different species are identical at 7 of the first 9 residues, contain Gly at position 28, and all terminate with Pro-NH_2. The C-terminal proline amide (Pro-NH_2) is very important for the biologic function of CT, as is the disulfide-bridge between Cys residues at positions 1 and 7. In contrast, the residues from 10 to 27 can be varied and seem to influence CT's potency as well as its duration of action; salmon CT differs from human CT at 16 amino acid residues.

Both species of CT are synthetically prepared and are commercially available, however salmon CT is generally preferred for medical uses because, on a weight basis, it is about 50 times as potent. Both human and salmon CT, in parenteral form, are approved for treating Paget's disease of

```
S————————————————————S
Cys–Ser–Asn–Leu–Ser–Thr–Cys–Val–Leu–Gly–Lys–Leu–Ser–Gln–Glu–Leu–His–Lys–Leu–Gln–
1               5                   10                  15                  20

Thr–Tyr–Pro–Arg–Thr–Asn–Thr–Gly–Ser–Gly–Thr–Pro-NH2     Salmon CT
                25                  30

S————————————————————S
Cys–Gly–Asn–Leu–Ser–Thr–Cys–Met–Leu–Gly–Thr–Tyr–Thr–Gln–Asp-Phe–Asn–Lys–Phe–His–
1               5                   10                  15                  20

Thr–Phe–Pro–Gln–Thr–Ala–Ile–Gly–Val–Gly–Ala–Pro-NH2     Human CT
                25                  30
```

Fig. 6.13. Primary structures of salmon and human calcitonin (CT).

bone, which is generally seen in older persons and involves increased bone resorption and the resulting softening of bones. However, only salmon CT is used in treating postmenopausal osteoporosis or hypercalcemia of malignancy (multiple myeloma or advanced breast carcinoma). Furthermore, only salmon CT (Miacalcin) is available in a nasal spray formulation for treating postmenopausal osteoporosis.

Hormones of Endocrine Pancreatic Origin

The exocrine pancreas consists mostly (about 99%) of gland cells known as pancreatic acini, which are responsible for secreting several digestive enzymes. The endocrine pancreas, or remaining 1% of the gland, consists of a group of cells known as pancreatic islets or islets of Langerhans. Each of these islets consists of four distinct cell types known as α, β, δ, and F cells (100). The α cells produce glucagon, the β cells produce insulin, the δ cells produce a peptide that is identical with somatostatin of hypothalamic origin, and the F cells produce a hormone known as pancreatic polypeptide, of which little is known. Insulin, glucagon, and somatostatin are essential in regulating carbohydrate, lipid, and amino acid metabolism. Insulin is responsible for promoting the storage of glucose as glycogen and effecting hypoglycemia, while glucagon mobilizes glucose from its glycogen stores and causes hyperglycemia. Whereas the primary action of somatostatin of hypothalamic origin is to inhibit the release of GH from the pituitary, pancreatic somatostatin suppresses the production of both insulin and glucagon. Inasmuch as Chapter 27 is devoted primarily to a discussion of insulin and oral hypoglycemic agents, in this chapter we will be brief in our coverage of glucagon and, especially, insulin.

Insulin

Overview. Three peptide hormones are essential in the regulation of carbohydrate, lipid, and amino acid metabolism: insulin, glucagon, and somatostatin. Somatostatin suppresses the production of both insulin and glucagon. Insulin encourages anabolism rather than catabolism because it promotes the synthesis of glycogen, proteins, and lipids. Therefore, a deficiency of insulin causes extreme changes in the entire metabolic pattern to occur. A lack of insulin leads to diabetes mellitus, which is characterized by elevated blood glucose levels, excess glucose in the urine, and failure to properly utilize carbohydrates and lipids. If untreated diabetes mellitus can be fatal, and even when treated there can be numerous circulatory and renal complications, and some metabolic abnormalities may lead to blindness (diabetic retinopathy). While insulin causes hypoglycemia, glucagon mobilizes glucose from its glycogen stores, and causes hyperglycemia.

Chemistry. Proinsulin, which is a single-chain of 86 amino acid residues, is enzymatically transformed into insulin within the β-cells. The conversion involves the cleavage of a connecting C-peptide, which contains between 30–35 residues, the number and sequence varying among different species; human C-peptide consists of 35 residues.

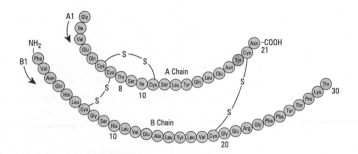

Fig. 6.14. Primary structure of human insulin chains A and B, including the inter-chain disulfide bonds A7-B7 and A20-B19 and intra-chain disulfide bond A6-A11.

The resulting human insulin consists of two peptide chains, designated A (having 21 residues) and B (having 30 residues), which are inter-chain connected by two disulfide bonds. Furthermore, the A-chain also contains an intra-chain disulfide bond between Cys[6] and Cys[11] (Fig. 6.14)

The primary sequences of insulin from several species are known and of these porcine insulin is the closest to that of humans. Their A-chains are identical and they differ only in their B-chains; Ala[30] (porcine) in place of Thr[30] (human). Human and bovine insulin differs in each chain; Ala[8] and Val[10] in the A-Chain (bovine) and Ala[30] in the B-chain (bovine). Commercial human insulin is produced biosynthetically, via rDNA technology, or semisynthetically by Thr[30] exchange for Ala[30] in insulin obtained from porcine sources. There also is a genetically engineered human insulin in which the order of the B-chain amino acids at positions 28 and 29 are reversed, specifically Lys[28] and Pro[29]. This is known as insulin lispro (Humalog) and its advantage is a more rapid onset and shorter duration of action than normal human insulin. Further details of the chemistry and formulations of the commercially available insulin products are discussed in Chapter 27.

Glucagon (GlucaGen Emergency Kit, GlucaGen Diagnostic Kit)

His-Ser-Gln-Gly-Thr-Phe-Thr-Ser-Asp-Tyr-Ser-Lys-Tyr-Leu-Asp-Ser-Arg ⌐
Thr-Asn-Met-Leu-Tyr-Gln-Val-Phe-Asp-Gln-Ala-Arg ⌐

Glucagon is a 29-amino acid straight-chain polypeptide of α-cell pancreatic origin. Glucagon triggers liver glycogenolysis and gluconeogenesis, thereby elevating glucose levels. The principal action of glucagon is, thus, the liver-mediated release into the blood of abnormally high concentrations of glucose, which causes hyperglycemia. This means that glucagon has an effect on blood glucose levels that is opposite to what occurs with insulin. In addition, glucagon has a relaxant effect on the GI tract and can also increase the force of the contraction of the heart muscle.

Glucagon from human, bovine and ovine sources are chemically identical. Therefore, glucagon as a powder for injection is obtained commercially from either beef or pork pancreas, wherein it is used in the treatment of severe hypoglycemic reactions in diabetic patients or during insulin shock therapy in psychiatric patients. In 1998 glucagon of rDNA origin became available and is being marketed for emergencies due to severe hypoglycemic reactions in diabetic patients and also, diagnostically, for use during radiologic examinations to temporarily inhibit GI tract movement.

OTHER BIOLOGICALLY SIGNIFICANT PEPTIDES AND PROTEINS

There are several other biologically significant peptides and proteins, as well as peptides and proteins not directly used in medicine. Table 6.4 summarizes some of the more interesting ones.

Table 6.4. Additional Significant Peptides and Proteins of Biological Interest, Several of Which Are Commercially Available

Name	Trade Name (if Applicable)	General Use or Action
Angiotensin II		Vasoconstricting 8-peptide involved in blood pressure regulation.
Atrial natriuretic peptide		28-peptide, vasodilator, that increases glomerular filtration and diuresis.
Bradykinin		9-peptide, produced in response to tissue damage, inflammation, viral infections, etc. Produces pain, increased vascular permeability, and the synthesis of prostaglandins.
Denileukin diftitox	Ontak	rDNA-derived fusion protein consisting of diphtheria toxin fragments A & B and interleukin-2. Used in treating cutaneous T-cell lymphoma.
Deslorelin	Somagard	GnRH superagonist used in treating central precocious puberty.
Epidermal growth factor (human)		rDNA-derived protein used in accelerating the regeneration of corneal epithelium and stromal tissue healing in non-healing corneal defects.
Insulin-like growth factor-I (human)		Protein of rDNA origin that has orphan drug status and is used in treating post-poliomyelitis syndrome.
Interferon alfa-2a	Roferon A	Protein of rDNA origin that has orphan drug status and is used for a number of malignancies: chronic myelogenous leukemia, renal-cell carcinoma, and AIDS-related Kaposi's sarcoma.
Interleukin-2	Teceleukin	Protein of rDNA origin that has orphan drug status and is used in treating renal-cell carcinoma and metastatic malignant melenoma.
Pentagastrin	Peptavlon	Synthetic 5-peptide analog of the C-terminal portion of gastrin. Used in diagnosing gastric secretory problems such as anacidity and hypersecretion and the diseases related to these problems.
Prolactin		Protein hormone structurally related to hGH. It is synthesized and released in a pulsatile manner from the anterior pituitary. Its principal site of action is the mammary gland, effecting breast growth during pregnancy and lactation. The hormone itself has no therapeutic value.
Relaxin		Polypeptide hormone secreted mainly by the corpus luteum during pregnancy. It facilitates the birth process by dilating the birth canal and relaxing the joint between the pubic bones. As an orphan drug it is used in treating progressive systemic sclerosis.
Secretin	Secretin Ferring Powder	27-peptide used in diagnosing pancreatic exocrine disease and gastrinoma (Zollinger-Ellison syndrome).
Thymopentin	Timunox	Synthetic 5-peptide consisting of residues 32-36 of thymopoietin, an immunologically active polypeptide. It is an immunomodulating investigational drug in treating asymptomatic HIV positive patients.
Vasoactive intestinal polypeptide		28-peptide that is structurally related to secretin and glucagon, among others. It has a diverse range of biological actions, including vasodilation and electrolyte secretion. It has orphan drug status for the treatment of acute esophageal food impaction.

CASE STUDY

Victoria F. Roche and S. William Zito

Mrs. H is a 31-year-old woman who has been married for 5 years. She has recently visited her gynecologist because of severe pelvic pain before and during her period. Lately, the pain has increased and is also occurring during sexual intercourse. She was diagnosed with endometriosis after a pelvic exam and laparoscopic observation of endometric lesions. The gynecologist wants to treat her with a Gonadotropin-Releasing Hormone (GnRH) superagonist. Which of the following peptide structures (1–4) would you recommend?

1. *Identify the therapeutic problem(s) where the pharmacist's intervention may benefit the patient.*

2. *Identify and prioritize the patient specific factors that must be considered to achieve the desired therapeutic outcomes.*

3. *Conduct a thorough and mechanistically oriented structure-activity analysis of all therapeutic alternatives provided in the case.*

4. *Evaluate the SAR findings against the patient specific factors and desired therapeutic outcomes and make a therapeutic decision.*

5. *Counsel your patient.*

$$\text{pGlu-His-Trp-Ser-Tyr-Gly-Leu-Arg-Pro-Gly-NH}_2$$
(1)

$$\text{pGlu-His-Trp-Ser-Tyr-D-Nal(2)-Leu-Arg-Pro-Gly-NH}_2$$
(2)

$$\text{pGlu-His-Trp-Ser-Tyr-Gly-Leu-Arg-Pro-NH}_2$$
(3)

$$\text{D-Phe-Cys-Phe-D-Trp-Lys-Thr-Cys-Thr-ol}$$
(4)

REFERENCES

1. Hofmeister F. Ergeb Physiol, Biol Chem Exp Pharmakol 1902;1:759–802.
2. Fischer E. Untersuchungen über aminosaüren, polypeptide, und proteine. Ber Dtsch Chem Ges 1906;39:530–610.
3. Bergmann M, Zervas L. A general process for the synthesis of peptides. Ber Dtsch Chem Ges1932;65:1192–1201.
4. Pierce JG, Gordon S, du Vigneaud V. Further distribution studies on the oxytocic hormone of the posterior lobe of the pituitary gland and the preparation of an active crystalline flavianate. J Biol Chem 1952;199:929–940.
5. du Vigneaud V, Ressler C, Trippett S. The sequence of amino acids in oxytocin, with a proposal for the structure of oxytocin. J Biol Chem 1953;205:949–957.
6. du Vigneaud V, Ressler C, Swan JM, et al. The synthesis of an octapeptide amide with the hormonal activity of oxytocin. J Am Chem Soc 1953;75:4879–4880.
7. Sanger F. A disulphide interchange reaction. Nature 1953; 171:1025–1026.
8. Burgus R, Dunn TF, Desiderio D, et al. Molecular structure of the hypothalamic hypophysiotropic TRF factor of ovine origin: mass spectrometry demonstration of the PCA-His-Pro-NH2 sequence. C R Acad Sci Paris 1969;269: 1870–1873.
9. Bøler J, Enzmann F, Folkers K, et al. The identity of chemical and hormonal properties of the thyrotropin releasing hormone and pyroglutamyl-histidyl-proline amide. Biochem Biophys Res Commun 1969;37:705–710.
10. Matsuo H, Baba Y, Nair RMG, et al. Structure of the porcine LH- and FSH-releasing hormone. I. The proposed amino acid sequence. Biochem Biophys Res Commun 1971;43:1334–1339.
11. Brazeau P, Vale W, Burgus R, et al. Hypothalamic polypeptide that inhibits the secretion of immunoreactive pituitary growth hormone. Science 1973;179:77–79.
12. Sheehan JC, Hess GP. A new method of forming peptide bonds. J Am Chem Soc 1955;77:1067–1068.
13. Carpino LA. Oxidative reactions of hydrazines. IV. Elimination of nitrogen from 1,1-disubstituted-2-arene sulfonyl hydrazides. J Am Chem Soc 1957;79:4427–4431.
14. Carpino LA, Han GY. The 9-fluorenylmethoxycarbonyl amino-protecting group. J Org Chem 1972;37:3404–3409.
15. Merrifield RB. Solid phase peptide synthesis, I: the synthesis of a tetrapeptide. J Am Chem Soc 1963;85:2149–2154.
16. Hernandez J-F, Bersch B, Pétillot Y, et al. Chemical synthesis and characterization of the epidermal growth factor-like module of human complement protease C1r. J Peptide Res 1997;49:221–231.
17. Hackeng TM, Dawson PE, Kent SBH, et al. Chemical synthesis of human protein S thrombin-sensitive module and first epidermal growth factor module. Biopolymers 1998;46:53–63.
18. Chen H, Pyluck AL, Janik M, et al. Peptides corresponding to the epidermal growth factor-like domain of mouse fertilin: synthesis and biological activity. Biopolymers 1998;47:299–307.
19. Bailey PD. An introduction to peptide chemistry. Chichester, UK: John Wiley & Sons, 1990.
20. Jakubke HD, Jeschkeit H. Amino acids, peptides and proteins. New York: John Wiley & Sons, 1977.
21. Doolittle RF. Proteins. Scientific Amer 1985;253:88–99.
22. Cahn RS, Ingold C, Prelog V. Specification of molecular chirality. Angew Chem Int Ed Engl 1966;5:385–415.
23. Horton HR, Moran LA, Ochs RS, et al. Principles of biochemistry. Englewood Cliffs: Neil Patterson Publishers/ Prentice Hall, 1993.
24. Pauling L, Corey RB, Branson HR. The structure of proteins: two hydrogen-bonded helical configurations of the polypeptide chain. Proc Natl Acad Sci USA 1951;37:205–211.
25. Creighton TE. Proteins: structures and molecular principles. New York: WH Freeman, 1983.
26. Chou K-C. Prediction of β-turns. J Peptide Res 1997; 49: 120–144.
27. Rose GD, Gierasch LM, Smith JA. Turns in peptides and proteins. In: Anfinsen CB, Edsall JT, Richards FM, eds. Advances in protein chemistry. Vol 37. Orlando: Academic Press, 1985.
28. Colburn WA. Peptide, peptoid, and protein pharmacokinetics/pharmacodynamics. In Garzone PD, Colburn WA, Mokotoff M, eds. Peptides, peptoids and proteins. Pharmacokinetics and pharmacodynamics, vol 3. Cincinnati: Harvey Whitney, 1991.
29. Alvares AP, Pratt WB. Pathways of drug metabolism. In: Pratt WB, Taylor P, eds. Principles of drug action. The basis of pharmacology. 3rd ed. New York: Churchill Livingstone, 1990.
30. Spatola AF. Peptide backbone modifications: a structure activity analysis of peptides containing amide bond surrogates, conformational constraints, and replacement. In: Weinstein B, ed. Chemistry and biochemistry of amino acids, peptides, and proteins. New York: Marcel Dekker, 1983.
31. Goodman M, Chorev M. On the concept of linear modified retro-peptide structures. Acc Chem Res 1979;12:1–7.
32. Lee VHL. Changing needs in drug delivery in the era of peptide and protein drugs. In: Lee VHL, ed. Peptide and protein drug delivery. New York: Marcel Dekker, 1991.
33. Pettit DK, Gombotz WR. The development of site-specific drug delivery systems for protein and peptide biopharmaceuticals. Trends Biotechnol 1998;16:343–349.
34. Banerjee PS, Hosny EA., Robinson JR. Parenteral delivery of peptide and protein drugs. In: Lee VHL, ed. Peptide and protein drug delivery. New York: Marcel Dekker, 1991.
35. Sanders LM. Controlled delivery systems for peptides. In: Lee VHL, ed. Peptide and protein drug delivery. New York: Marcel Dekker, 1991.
36. Sarkar MA. Drug metabolism in the nasal mucosa. Pharmaceutical Res 1992;9:1–9.
37. Su KSE. Nasal route of peptide and protein drug delivery. In: Lee VHL, ed. Peptide and protein drug delivery. New York: Marcel Dekker, 1991.
38. Sayani AP, Chien YW. Systemic delivery of peptides and proteins across absorptive mucosae. Crit Rev Ther Drug Carrier Syst 1996;13:85–184.
39. Edwards DA, Ben-Jebria A, Langer R. Recent advances in pulmonary drug delivery using large, porous inhaled particles. J Appl Physiol 1998;85:379–385.
40. Patton JS. Deep-lung delivery of proteins. Modern Drug Discovery 1998;Sept/Oct:19–28.
41. Adjei AL, Gupta PK, eds. Inhalation delivery of therapeutic peptides and proteins. New York: Marcel Dekker, 1997.
42. Nishio H, Inui T, Nishiuchi Y, et al. Chemical synthesis of dendrotoxin I: revision of the reported structure. J Peptide Res 1998;51:355–364.
43. Bodanszky M. Principles of peptide synthesis. 2nd ed. Berlin: Springer-Verlag, 1993.
44. Tam JP, Wong TW, Riemen MW, et al. Cyclohexyl ester as a new protecting group for aspartyl peptides to minimize aspartimide formation in acidic and basic treatments. Tetrahedron Lett 1979; 4033–4036.
45. Annis I, Hargittal B, Barany G. Disulfide bond formation in peptides. In: Fields GB, ed. Solid-phase peptide synthesis. Methods in enzymology. vol 289. New York: Academic Press, 1997.
46. Tam JP, Heath WF, Merrifield RB. S_N2 deprotection of synthetic peptides with a low concentration of hydrogen fluoride in dimethyl sulfide: evidence and application in peptide synthesis. J Am Chem Soc 1983;105:6442–6455.

47. Carpino LA, Shroff H, Triolo SA, et al. The 2,2,4,6,7-pentamethyldihydrobenzofuran-5-sulfonyl group (Pbf) as arginine side chain protectant. Tetrahedron Lett 1993;34:7829–7832.

48. White P. Fmoc-Trp(Boc)-OH: A new derivative for the synthesis of peptides containing tryptophan. In: Smith JA, Rivier JE, eds. Peptides: chemistry and biology (proceedings of the 12th american peptide symposium). Leiden: ESCOM, 1992.

49. Alberico F, Carpino LA. Coupling reagents and activation. In: Fields GB, ed. Solid-phase peptide synthesis. Methods in enzymology. vol 289. New York: Academic Press, 1997.

50. Merrifield B. Concept and early development of solid-phase peptide synthesis. In: Fields GB, ed. Solid-phase peptide synthesis. Methods in enzymology. vol 289. New York: Academic Press, 1997.

51. Mokotoff M. Current state of the art in the preparation of synthetic peptides. In Garzone PD, Colburn WA, Mokotoff M, eds. Peptides, peptoids and proteins. Pharmacokinetics and pharmacodynamics, vol 3. Cincinnati: Harvey Whitney, 1991.

52. Wellings DA, Atherton E. Standard Fmoc protocols. In: Fields GB, ed. Solid-phase peptide synthesis. Methods in enzymology. vol 289. New York: Academic Press, 1997.

53. Atherton E, Sheppard RC. Solid phase peptide synthesis. A practical approach. Oxford: IRL Press, 1989.

54. Borman S. Combinatorial chemists focus on small molecules, molecular recognition, and automation. C&EN 1996; February 12:29–54.

55. Geysen HM, Meloen RN, Barleling SJ. Use of peptide synthesis to probe viral antigens for epitopes to a resolution of a single amino acid. Proc Natl Acad Sci USA 1984;81:3998–4002.

56. Plunkett MJ, Ellman JA. Combinatorial chemistry and new drugs. Scientific American 1997;April:69–73.

57. Lam KS, Lebl M, Krchňák V. The "one-bead-one-compound" combinatorial library method. Chem Rev 1997;97:411–448.

58. Furka Á, Sebestyén F, Asgedom M, et al. General method for rapid synthesis of multicomponent peptide mixtures. Int J Peptide Protein Res 1991;37:487–493 .

59. Furka Á. Introduction to combinatorial chemistry. In: Advanced ChemTech Handbook of combinatorial & solid phase organic chemistry, 1999. Louisville: Advanced Chem Tech, Inc.

60. Obrecht D, Villalgordo JM. Solid-supported combinatorial and parallel synthesis of small-molecular-weight compound libraries. New York: Pergamon, 1998.

61. Cabilly S, ed. Combinatorial peptide library protocols. Totowa, NJ: Humana Press, 1998.

62. Miertus S, Fassina G, eds. Combinatorial chemistry and technology. Principles, methods, and applications. New York: Marcel Dekker, Inc., 1999.

63. Zhao M, Kleinman HK, Mokotoff M. Synthetic laminin-like peptides and pseudopeptides as potential antimetastatic agents. J Med Chem 1994;37:3383–3388.

64. Fok K-F, Yankeelov JA, Jr. Peptide-gap inhibitors: I. Competitive inhibition of aminopeptidase M by a hydrolytically resistant dipeptide analogue of glycylleucine. Biochem Biophys Res Commun 1977;114:273–278.

65. Spatola AF. Synthesis of pseudopeptides. In: Conn PM, ed. Methods in neurosciences. Vol 13. Neuropeptide analogs, conjugates, and fragments. San Diego: Academic Press, 1993.

66. Coy DH, Heinz-Erian P, Jiang NY, et al. Probing peptide backbone function in bombesin: a reduced peptide bond analogue with potent and specific receptor antagonist activity. J Biol Chem 1988; 263:5056–5060.

67. Coy DH, Hocart SJ, Sasaki Y. Solid phase reductive alkylation technique in analogue peptide-bond and side-chain modification. Tetrahedron 1988;44:835–841.

68. Mokotoff M, Ren K, Wong LK, et al. Synthesis and biological evaluation of novel potent antagonists of the bombesin/gastrin releasing peptide receptor. J Med Chem 1992;35:4696–4703.

69. Chorev M, Goodman M. A dozen years of retro-inverso peptidomimetics. Acc Chem Res 1993;26:266–273.

70. Zhao M, Kleinman HK, Mokotoff M. Synthesis and activity of partial retro-inverso analogs of the antimetastatic laminin-derived peptide, YIGSR-NH₂. J Peptide Res 1997;49:240–253.

71. Chorev M, Goodman M. Recent developments in retro peptides and proteins—an ongoing topochemical exploration. Trends Biotechnol 1995;13:438–445.

72. Nogrady T. Medicinal chemistry. A biochemical approach. 2nd ed. New York: Oxford University Press, 1988.

73. Barbieri RL, Friedman AJ. Gonadotropin releasing hormone analogs. New York: Elsevier, 1991.

74. Crowley WF Jr, Conn PM. Modes of action of GnRH and GnRH analogs. New York: Springer-Verlag, 1991.

75. Karten MJ, Rivier JE. Gonadotropin-releasing hormone analog design. Structure-function studies toward the development of agonists and antagonists: rationale and perspective. Endocrin Rev 1986;7:44–66.

76. Sealfon SC, Weinstein H, Millar RB. Molecular mechanisms of ligand interaction with the gonadotropin-releasing hormone receptor. Endocrin Rev 1997;18:180–205.

77. Coy DH, Vilchez-Martinez JA, Coy EJ, et al. Analogs of luteinizing hormone-releasing hormone with increased biological activity produced by D-amino acid substitutions in position 6. J Med Chem 1976;19:423–425.

78. Conn PM, Crowley WF Jr. Gonadotropin-releasing hormone and its analogs. In: Coggins CH, Hancock, EW, eds. Annual Rev Med, vol 45. Palo Alto: Annual Reviews, Inc, 1994.

79. Sowter MC, Singla AA, Lethaby A. The use of preoperative endometrial thinning agents before hysteroscopic surgery for menorrhagia (heavy menstrual bleeding) (Cochrane Review). In: The Cochrane Library, Issue 4, 1998. Oxford: Update Software.

80. Brazeau P, Vale W, Burgus R, et al. Hypothalamic polypeptide that inhibits the secretion of immunoreactive pituitary growth hormone. Science 1973;179:77–79.

81. Rivier J, Brazeau P, Vale W, et al. Somatostatin analogs. Relative importance of the disulfide bridge and of the Ala-Gly side chain for biological activity. J Med Chem 1975; 18:123–126.

82. Veber DF, Freidinger RM, Schwenk-Perlow D, et al. A potent cyclic hexapeptide analogue of somatostatin. Nature 1981; 292:55–58.

83. Bauer W, Briner U, Doepfner W, et al. SMS 201–995: A very potent and selective analogue of somatostatin with a prolonged action. Life Sci 1982;31:1133–1140.

84. Lamberts SWJ, van der Lely A-J, de Herdner WW, et al. Octreotide. New Eng J Med 1996;334:246–254.

85. Ezzat S, Snyder PJ, Young WF, et al. Octreotide treatment of acromegaly. A randomized, multicenter study. Ann Int Med 1992;117:711–718.

86. Bruns C, Stolz B, Albert R, et al. OctreoScan 111 for imaging somatostatin receptor-positive islet cell tumor in rat. Hormone Metab Res-Suppl 1993;27:5–11.

87. Bakker WH, Albert R, Bruns C, et al. [¹¹¹In-DTPA-D-Phe¹]-Octreotide, a potential radiopharmaceutical for imaging of somatostatin receptor-positive tumors: synthesis, radiolabeling and in vitro validation. Life Sci 1991;49:1583–1591.

88. Duck SC, Schwarz HP, Costin G, et al. Subcutaneous growth hormone-releasing hormone therapy in growth hormone-deficient children: first year of therapy. J Clin Endocrin Metab 1992;75:1115–1120.

89. Orth DN. Corticotropin-releasing hormone in humans. Endocrine Rev 1992;13:164–191.

90. Hintz RL. Untoward events in patients treated with growth hormone in the USA. Horm Res 1992;38:44–49 (Suppl).

91. Powell DR. Effects of renal failure on the growth hormone-insulin-like growth factor axis. J Pediatr 1997;131:S13–S16.

92. Rosenfeld RG, Frane J, Attie KM, et al. Six year results of a randomized prospective trial of human growth hormone and oxandrolone in Turner syndrome. J Pediatr 1992;121:49–55.

93. Clemmons DR, Underwood LE. Role of insulin-like growth factors and growth hormone in reversing catabolic states. Horm Res 1992;38:37–40.

94. Combarnous Y. Molecular basis of the specificity of binding of glycoprotein hormones to their receptors. Endocrine Rev 1992;13:670–691.

95. Homburg R, Giudice LC, Chang RJ. Polycystic ovary syndrome. Hum Reprod 1996; 11:465–466.

96. Prevost RR. Recombinant follicle-stimulating hormone: new biotechnology for infertility. Pharmacother 1998;18:1001–1010.

97. De Leeuw R, Mulders J, Voortman G, et al. Structure-function relationship of recombinant follicle stimulating hormone (Puregon). Molec Human Reprod 1996;2:361–369.

98. Imura H. Adrenocorticotropic hormone. In: DeGroot LJ, ed. Endocrinology. 3rd ed. Philadelphia: WB Saunders Co, 1995.

99. Law AW, Gales MA. Octreotide or vasopressin for bleeding esophageal varices. Ann Pharmacother 1997;31:237–238.

100. Martini FH. Fundamentals of anatomy and physiology. 4th ed. Upper Saddle River, NJ: Prentice Hall, 1998:621.

7. Physicochemical and Biopharmaceutical Properties of Drug Substances and Pharmacokinetics

SUNIL JAMBHEKAR

Introduction

Throughout its history, the pharmacy profession has been primarily concerned with the manner in which drugs produce their pharmacologic effects and the dosage forms through which drugs are administered. Since the early 20th century efforts have been directed to determining, understanding, and providing rational explanations of drug effects on biological systems but are limited only by our ability to correlate the observed physiologic events with a reasonable hypothesis or concept. Pharmacists, at one time, were closely involved in formulating a prescription written by a physician for a patient. Today most of the formulating is done by the pharmaceutical manufacturer.

Early descriptions of drug action were confined to their reference as tonic or toxic effects. This approach was followed by the concept of receptor theory, which for decades remained primarily an operational concept that was useful for discussing the new actions of drugs on a molecular level (1). However, research in receptor theories has provided evidence that the drug receptors do exist as distinct entities, and a limited success has been attained in the characterization of receptors (2,3).

An extension of the receptor theory of drug action is an increased emphasis on the importance of physicochemical properties of the drug and the relationship of such properties to the pharmacologic responses. Because these properties play an important role in determining biological action of pharmaceuticals, it is appropriate to refer to these properties as biopharmaceutical properties of drug substances. Examples of such properties include solubility, partition coefficients, diffusivity, degree of ionization, polymorphism, etc., which, in turn, are determined by the chemical structure and stereochemistry of drug substances.

A consideration of these biopharmaceutical properties is fundamental to discussing several important aspects of the overall effects. For a given chemical entity (drug), there will often be a difference in physiological availability and, presumably, in clinical responses. This is primarily because drug molecules must cross various biological membranes and interact with intercellular and intracellular fluids before reaching the elusive region called the "site of action." Under these conditions, the biopharmaceutical properties of the drug must contribute favorable to facilitate absorption and distribution processes to augment the drug concentration at various active sites. Furthermore, equally important is the fact that these biopharmaceutical properties of a drug must ensure a specific orientation on the receptor surface so that a sequence of events is initiated which leads to the observed pharmacological effects. Drug molecules deficient in the required biopharmaceutical properties, may generally display marginal pharmacologic action or be totally ineffective.

Biopharmaceutics may be defined as the study of the influence of formulation factors on the therapeutic activity of a drug product or dosage forms. It involves the study of the relationship between some of the physicochemical properties of a drug and the biological effects observed following the administration of a drug via various dosage forms or drug delivery systems. Almost any alteration in a drug delivery system is likely to alter the drug delivery rate and the amount of the drug delivered to the desired place in the body. This includes the chemical nature of the drug (ester, salts, complexes etc.), the particle size and surface area of the drug, the type of dosage forms (solution, suspension, capsule, tablet), and the excipients and processes used in the manufacturing of the drug delivery systems.

Drugs, via drug delivery systems, are most often administered to human subjects by the oral route. Compared to other routes of drug administration, especially the intravenous route, this route is unusually complex with respect to the physicochemical conditions existing at the absorption site. Therefore, before we discuss how the biopharmaceutical properties of a drug in a dosage form may affect the availability and the action of a drug, it is prudent for the reader to review the gastrointestinal physiology.

Gastrointestinal Physiology

Figure 7.1 schematically represents the gastrointestinal tract and some of the problems encountered in a consideration of drug absorption from the site following administration of a drug via dosage forms. The stomach may be divided into two main parts: a) the body of the stomach, and b) the pylorus. Histologically, these parts correspond to the pepsin and HCl secreting area and the mucus secreting area of the gastric mucosa, respectively. In the human, the stomach contents are usually in the pH range of 1 to 3.5, with pH 1–2.5 being the most common range. Furthermore, there is a diurnal cycle of gastric acidity in humans. During the night, stomach contents are usually more acidic i.e., pH is about 1.3, while, during the day, because of food consumption, the pH is less acidic. However, the recovery of stomach acidity occurs quite rapidly. The presence of protein, being amphoteric in nature, acts as an ex-

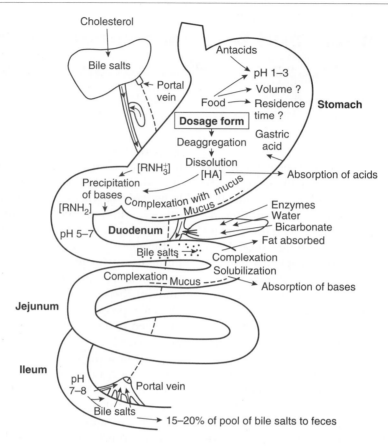

Fig. 7.1. Processes occurring along with drug absorption in the gastrointestinal tract, and the factors that affect drug absorption (4).

cellent buffer, and as digestion proceeds, the liberated amino acids increase the neutralizing capacity enormously.

The small intestine is divided anatomically into three sections: the duodenum, jejunum, and ileum. All three areas are involved in the digestion and absorption of food. The available absorbing area is increased by surface folds in the intestinal lining. The surface of these folds possess villi and microvilli (Fig. 7.2). The duodenal contents in the human are usually in the pH range of 5 to 7. There is a gradual decrease in acidity along the length of the gastrointestinal tract with the ultimate pH being 7 to 8 in the lower ileum. It has been estimated that approximately 8

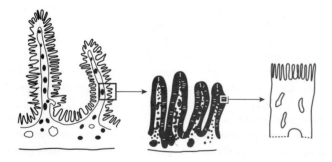

Fig. 7.2. The epithelium of the small intestine at different levels of magnification. From left to right: the intestinal villi and microvilli that constitute the brush border.

liters of fluid enters the upper intestine per day and approximately 7 liters of this arises from digestive juices and fluids, and about a liter from oral intake.

Over the entire length of the large and small intestine and the stomach is the brush border, consisting of a uniform coating (3 mm thick) of mucopolysaccharide. This coating layer serves to act as a mechanical barrier to bacteria or food particles.

When a dosage form containing a drug or drug molecules moves from the stomach through the pylorus into the duodenum, the dosage form encounters a rapidly changing environment with respect to pH. Furthermore, digestive juices secreted into the small bowel contain many enzymes not found in the gastric juices. Digestion and absorption of foodstuff occur simultaneously in the small intestine. Intestinal digestion is the terminal phase of preparing foodstuff for absorption and consists of two processes: 1) completion of the hydrolysis of large molecules to smaller ones which can be absorbed, and 2) brining the finished product of hydrolysis into an aqueous solution or emulsion.

Drug absorption, whether it be from the gastrointestinal tract or other sites, requires the passage of the drug in a molecular form across the barrier membrane. Most drugs are presented to the body as solid or semi-solid dosage forms, and the drug particles must first be released from these dosage forms. These drug particles must first

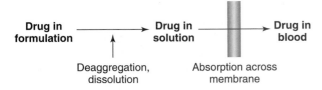

Fig. 7.3. Sequence of events in drug absorption from formulations.

dissolve, and if they possess the desirable biopharmaceutical properties, they will pass from a region of high concentration to a region of low concentration across the membrane into the blood or general circulation (Fig. 7.3).

A knowledge of biological membrane structure and its general properties is pivotal in understanding absorption processes and the role of the biopharmaceutical properties of drug substances.

Biological Membrane

The prevalent view is that the gastrointestinal membrane consists of a bimolecular lipoid layer covered on each side by protein with the lipid molecule oriented perpendicular to the cell surface (Fig. 7.4). The lipid layer is interrupted by small water filled pores which are approximately 4 angstroms in radius and a molecule having a radius of 4 angstroms or less may pass through the water filled pores. Thus, membranes have a specialized transport system to assist the passage of water soluble material and ions through the lipid interior, a process sometimes referred to as "convective absorption." The rate of permeation of such small molecules through the pore is affected

not only by the relative sizes of the holes and the molecules but also by the interaction between permeating molecules and the membrane. When permeation through the membrane occurs, the permeating substance is considered to have transferred from solution in the luminal aqueous phase to the lipid membrane phase, then to the aqueous phase on the other side of the membrane. Biological membranes differ from a polymeric membrane in that they are composed of small ampipathic molecules, phospholipid and cholesterol. The protein layer associated with membranes is hydrophobic in nature. Therefore, biological membranes have a hydrophilic exterior and hydrophobic interior. Cholesterol is a major component of most mammalian biological membranes, and its removal will render the membrane highly permeable. Cholesterol complexes with phospholipids and its presence reduces the permeability of the membrane to water, cations, glycerides, and glucose. The shape of the cholesterol molecule allows it to fit closely with the hydrocarbon chains of unsaturated fatty acids in the bilayer. It is the general opinion that the cholesterol makes the membrane more rigid. The flexibility of the biological membrane to reform and adapt to a changed environment is its important feature. The details of membrane structure are still widely debated, and a more recent membrane model is shown in Figure 7.4.

In addition to biopharmaceutical factors, several physiological factors may also affect the rate and extent of gastrointestinal absorption. These factors are as follows: properties of epithelial cells, segmental activity of the bowel, degree of vascularity, effective absorbing surface

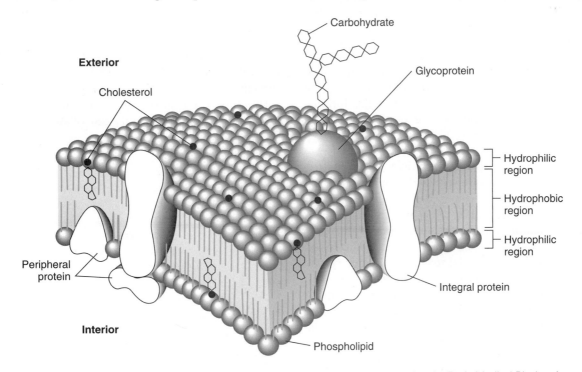

Fig. 7.4. Basic structure of an animal cell membrane. Reprinted with permission from Marks et al., eds. Basic Medical Biochemistry. Baltimore: Williams & Wilkins, 1996

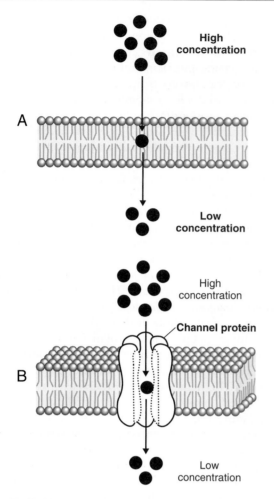

Fig. 7.5. A, Simple diffusion; **B,** membrane channels. Reprinted with permission from Marks et al., eds. Basic Medical Biochemistry. Baltimore, Williams & Wilkins, 1996.

area per unit length of gut, the surface and interfacial tensions, the electrolyte content and their concentration in luminal fluid, the enzymatic activity in the luminal contents, and gastric emptying rate of the drug from stomach.

Mechanisms of Drug Absorption

Drug transfer is often viewed as the movement of a drug molecule across a series of membranes and spaces Figure 7.5, a and b), which, in aggregate, serve as a macroscopic membrane. The cells and interstitial spaces lying between the gastric lumen and the capillary blood or structure between sinusoidal space and the bile canaliculi are examples. Each of the cellular membranes and spaces may impede drug transport to varying degrees and, therefore, any one of them can be a rate limiting step to the overall process of drug transport. This complexity of structure makes quantitative prediction of drug transport difficult. A qualitative description of the processes of drug transport across functional membranes are as follows:

Passive Diffusion

The transfer of most drugs across a biological membrane occurs by passive diffusion, a natural tendency for molecules to move from higher concentration to one of lower concentration. This movement of drug molecules is caused by the kinetic energy of the molecules. The rate of diffusion depends upon the magnitude of the concentration gradient (dC) across the membrane and can be represented by the following equation:

Eq. 7.1 $$-\frac{dC}{dt} = K^* dC = K(C_{abs} - C_b)$$

where $-dC/dt$ is the rate of diffusion across a membrane, K^* is a complex proportionality constant that includes the area of membrane, the thickness of the membrane, the partition coefficient of the drug molecule between the lipophilic membrane and the aqueous phase on each side of the membrane, and the diffusion coefficient of the drug.

The gastrointestinal absorption of a drug from an aqueous solution requires transfer from the lumen to the gut wall followed by penetration of the epithelial membrane by a drug molecule to the capillaries of the systemic circulation. Upon entering the blood, the drug distributes itself rapidly in the blood. Because of the volume differences at absorption and distribution sites, the drug concentration in blood (C_b) will be much lower than the concentration at the absorption site (C_{abs}). This concentration gradient is maintained throughout the absorption process, i.e., ($C_{abs}-C_b$). As a result, the concentration gradient, (dC in Equation 7.1), is approximately equal to C_{abs} and, hence, Equation 7.1 can be written as:

Eq. 7.2 $$-\frac{dC}{dt} = K^* C_1$$

Because absorption by passive diffusion is a first order process, the rate of absorption (dC/dt in Equation 7.2) is directly proportional to the concentration at the site of absorption (C_1). The greater the concentration of drug at the absorption site, the faster is the rate of absorption (Fig. 7.6).

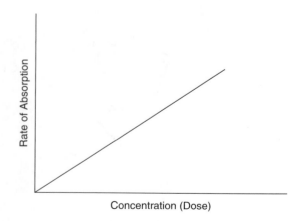

Fig. 7.6. Effect of drug concentration on the rate of absorption owing to passive diffusion.

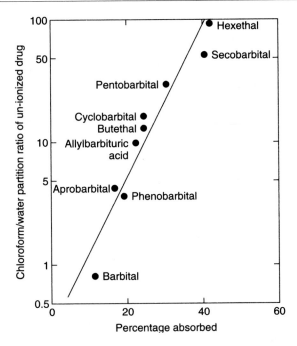

Fig. 7.7. Comparison between colonic absorption of barbiturates in the rat and lipid-to-water partition coefficient of the unionized form of the barbiturates. Reprinted from Ref. 5.

The percent of dose absorbed at any time, however, remains unchanged.

A major source of variation is membrane permeability, which depends on the lipophilicity of the drug molecule. This is often characterized by its partition between oil and water. The lipid solubility of a drug, therefore, is a very important physicochemical property governing the rate of transfer through a variety of biological membrane barriers. Figure 7.7 illustrates the role of partition coefficients in the drug absorption process and that there is a good correlation between the percentage of drug absorption and the partition coefficient of an un-ionized drug.

Carrier Mediated or Active Transport

Although most drugs are absorbed by passive diffusion, some drugs of therapeutic interest and some chemicals of nutritional values are absorbed by the action of transporter proteins i.e., a carrier mediated transport mechanism (Fig. 7.8). In this type of transport, membranes have a specialized role. The usual requirement for active transport is structural similarities between the drug and the substrate normally transported across the membrane. Active transport differs from passive diffusion in the following ways: 1) the transport of the drug occurs against a concentration gradient, 2) the transport mechanism can become saturated at high drug concentration, and 3) a specificity for a certain molecular structure may promote competition in the presence of a similarly structured compound. This, in turn, may decrease the absorption of a drug.

Active or facilitated absorption of a drug is usually explained by assuming that transporter proteins i.e., carriers in membranes are responsible for shuttling these solutes in mucosal or serosal direction. The number of apparent carriers in membranes, however, is limited. Therefore, the rate of transfer may be described by the following equation:

Eq. 7.3 $\text{Absorption rate} = \dfrac{dC}{dt} = \dfrac{V_{max}*C}{K_m + C}$

where, C is the solute concentration at the absorption site and V_{max} (the maximum theoretical transfer rate) and K_m (the concentration of drug at $\frac{1}{2} V_{max}$) are constants. In low doses or concentration, when $K_m \gg C$, reduces Equation 7.3 to

Eq. 7.4 $\dfrac{dC}{dt} = \dfrac{V_{max}}{K_m}*C = K*C$

Equation 7.4 indicates that the apparent first order kinetics is observed. Under these conditions there are sufficient number of carriers available so that a constant proportion of solute molecules presented to the membrane is

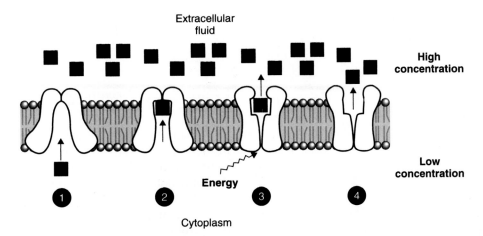

Fig. 7.8. Active transport. Reprinted with permission from Marks et al., eds. Basic Medical Biochemistry. Baltimore: Williams & Wilkins, 1996.

transported across. As the solute concentration increases, the number of free carriers is reduced and the proportion of solute molecules transferred across the membrane is reduced until a maximum absolute number saturation is reached. When $C >> K_m$, then:

Eq. 7.5   Absorption rate $= \dfrac{dC}{dt} = V_{max}$

Equation 7.5 indicates that a further increase in solute concentration will not result in any further increase in the rate of absorption (Fig. 7.9).

The capacity limited characteristics of carrier mediated processes suggest that the bioavailability of drugs absorbed in this manner should decrease with increasing doses. Therefore, the use of a large single oral dose of these drugs is irrational and, if larger daily doses are necessary, one should use divided doses. Examples of substances that are active transported include amino acids, methyldopa, 5-fluorouracil, penicillamine, and levodopa.

Convective Absorption

The absorption of small molecules, with molecular radii less than about 4 angstroms, through water filled pores of biological membrane, is referred to as convective absorption. The rate of absorption due to this mechanism is equated to the product of a sieving coefficient, the rate of fluid or water absorption and the concentration of solute in the luminal content. The sieving coefficient is indirectly related to the relative sizes of the pores and the molecules.

Ion-Pair Absorption

In 1967, Higuchi (6) suggested that highly ionized compounds, such as quaternary ammonium compounds, may possibly be absorbed by ion pair mechanism. In vitro, a relatively large organic anion can combine with

relatively large cation to form an ion pair which will cross a water-organic solvent interface and transfer to an organic phase.

The pH-Partition Hypothesis on Drug Absorption

Drug absorption is influenced by many physiological factors. Additionally, it also depends upon many physicochemical properties of the drug itself. Shore, Brodie, Hogben, Schanker, and Tocco (5,7–12) concluded from their research that most drugs are absorbed from the gastrointestinal tract by a process of passive diffusion of the un-ionized moiety across a lipid membrane. Furthermore, the dissociation constant, lipid solubility and the pH of the fluid at the absorption site determine the extent of absorption from a solution. The interrelationship among these parameters is known as the pH-partition theory. This theory provides a basic framework for the understanding of drug absorption from the gastrointestinal tract and drug transport across the biological membrane. The principle points of this theory are as follows:

1. The gastrointestinal and other biological membranes act like lipid barriers
2. The un-ionized form of the acidic or basic drug is preferentially absorbed
3. Most drugs are absorbed by passive diffusion
4. The rate of drug absorption and the amount of drug absorbed are related to its oil-water partition coefficient, the more lipophilic the drug, the faster is its absorption
5. Weak acidic and neutral drugs may be absorbed from the stomach but basic drugs are not.

When a drug is administered intravenously, it is immediately available to body fluids for distribution to the "site of action." However, all extravascular routes can influence the overall therapeutic activity of the drug, due primarily to its dissolution rate: a step necessary for a drug to be available in a solution form. When a drug is administered orally in a dosage form such as a tablet, capsule, suspension or intravenously, the rate of absorption across the biological membrane is frequently controlled by the slowest step in the following sequence:

Dosage form $\xrightarrow{\text{dissolution}}$ Drug in solution form

$\xrightarrow{\text{absorption}}$ Drug in general circulation

In many instances, the slowest step or rate limiting step in the sequence is the dissolution of the drug. When dissolution is the controlling step, any factors that affect the rate of dissolution must also influence the rate of absorption. This, in turn, affects the extent and duration of action. Several factors can influence the dissolution rate of drug from solid dosage forms and, therefore, the therapeutic activity. These factors include solubility of a drug,

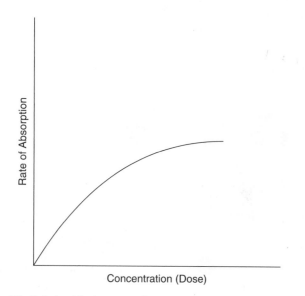

Fig. 7.9. Relationship between drug concentration and rate of absorption owing to active transport.

particle size and surface area of drug particles, crystalline and salt form of a drug and the rate of disintegration.

The absorption rate of drugs can also be affected by interaction or formation of complexes in the gastrointestinal tract. Generally, such complex formation reduces the concentration of free drug at the absorption site. Because the complexed drug is either slowly absorbed or not absorbed, the net effect is the reduction of concentration of drug at absorption site and slower rate of absorption.

Ionization and pH at Absorption Site

The fraction of the drug existing in its un-ionized form in a solution is a function of both the dissociation constant of a drug and the pH of the solution at the absorption site. The dissociation constant, for both weak acids and bases, is often expressed as pK_a (the negative logarithm of a dissociation constant, K_a). The Henderson-Hasselbach equation for the ionization of a weak acid, HA, is derived from the following equation:

Eq. 7.6 $$HA + H_2O \rightleftharpoons A^- + H_3O^+$$

We may express the equilibrium constant as follows:

Eq. 7.7 $$K_a = \frac{_aH_3O^+ \times _aA^-}{_aHA}$$

where, K_a is the equilibrium or dissociation constant and $_a$ is the activity coefficient. Assuming the activity coefficients approach unity in dilute solutions, the activity coefficient may be replaced by concentration terms and Equation 7.7 becomes:

Eq. 7.8 $$K_a = \frac{[H_3O^+][A^-]}{[HA]}$$

The negative logarithm of K_a is referred to as pK_a. Thus,

Eq. 7.9 $$pK_a = -\log K_a$$

Taking the logarithm of the expression for the dissociation constant of a weak acid in Equation 7.8 yields the following:

Eq. 7.10 $$-\log K_a = -\log [H_3O] - \log \frac{[A^-]}{[HA]}$$

where A^- is the ionized form of a weak acid and HA is the un-ionized form.

Eq. 7.11 $$pH - pK_a = \log \frac{[Ionized]}{[Un\text{-}ionized]}$$

Assuming α = fraction of ionized species and $1 - \alpha$ is the fraction remaining as the un-ionized form, Equation 7.11 can be written as:

Eq. 7.12 $$pH - pK_a = \log \frac{\alpha}{1 - \alpha}$$

or

Eq. 7.13 $$\frac{\alpha}{1 - \alpha} = \text{Antilog} (pH - pK_a)$$

From Equation 7.13, the fraction or percentage absorbable and nonabsorbable form of a weak acid can be

calculated, provided the pH condition at the site of administration is known. Analogously, the dissociation or basicity constant for a weak base is derived as follows:

Eq. 7.14 $$B + H_2O \leftrightarrow BH^+ + OH^-$$

The dissociation constant, K_b

Eq. 7.15 $$K_b = \frac{(_aOH)(_aBH)}{_aB} = \frac{[OH^-][BH]}{[B]}$$

Eq. 7.16 and $$pK_b = -\log K_b$$

The pK_a and pK_b values provide a convenient means of comparing the strength of weak acids and bases. The lower the pK_a, the stronger the acid; the lower the pK_b, the stronger the base. pK_a and pK_b values of conjugate acid-base pairs are linked by the expression:

Eq. 7.17 $$pK_a + pK_b = pK_w$$

where pK_w is the negative logarithm of dissociation constant of water. Taking the logarithm of Equation 7.15 and rearranging yields:

Eq. 7.18 $$-\log K_b = -\log [OH^-] - \log \frac{[BH^+]}{[B]}$$

Though the dissociation constant of a weak base is described by the term K_b, it is conventionally expressed in terms of K_a because of the relationship expressed in Equation 7.17.

Equation 7.18 can be written as:

Eq. 7.19 $$pH = pK_w - pK_b - \log \frac{[BH^+]}{[B]}$$

Since $pK_w - pK_b = pK_a$, Equation 7.19 takes the following form for a weak base. BH^+ is the ionized form and B is the unionized form:

Eq. 7.20 $$pK_a - pH = \log \frac{[Ionized]}{[Un\text{-}ionized]}$$

Again, assuming α = fraction of ionized species and $1 - \alpha$ is the fraction of un-ionized species, Equation 7.20 becomes:

Eq. 7.21 $$pK_a - pH = \log \frac{\alpha}{1 - \alpha}$$

or

Eq. 7.22 $$\frac{\alpha}{1 - \alpha} = \text{antilog} (pK_a - pH)$$

From Equation 7.22, one can calculate the fraction or percent of absorbable and nonabsorbable form of a weak base, given the pH condition at the site of drug absorption. Figure 7.10 shows the pK_a values of several drugs and the relative acid or base strength of these compounds.

The relationship between pH and pK_a and the extent of ionization is given by Equations 7.13 and 7.22 for weak acids and weak bases, respectively. Accordingly, most weak acidic drugs are predominantly in the un-ionized form at lower

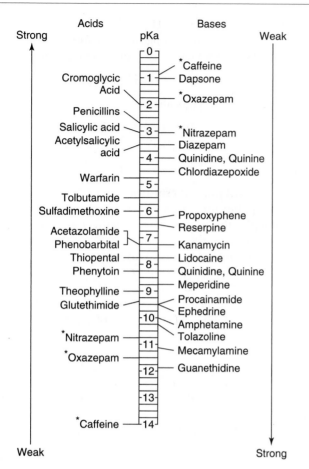

Fig. 7.10. pK$_a$ values of certain acidic and basic drugs. Drugs denoted with an asterisk are amphoteric (13).

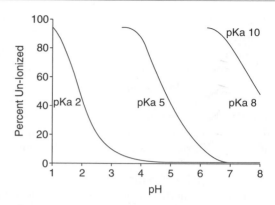

Fig. 7.11. For very weak acids, pK$_a$ values greater than 8.0 are predominantly un-ionized at all pH values between 1.0 and 8.0. Profound changes in the fraction un-ionized occur with pH for an acid with a pK$_a$ value that lies within the range of 2.0 to 8.0. Although the fraction un-ionized of even strong acids increases with hydrogen ion concentration, the absolute value remains low at most pH values shown (13).

Stronger bases such as guanethidine (pK$_a$ > 11) are ionized throughout the gastrointestinal tract and tend to be poorly absorbed.

The evidence of the importance of dissociation in drug absorption is found in the result of studies in which pH at the absorption site is changed (Tables 7.1 and 7.2). Table 7.2 clearly shows the decreased absorption of a weak acid at pH 8.0, compared to pH 1.0. On the other hand, an increase to pH 8.0 promotes the absorption of a weak base with practically nothing absorbed at pH 1.0. The data in Table 7.2 permits a comparison of intestinal absorption of acidic and basic drugs from buffered solutions ranging from pH 4.0 to 8.0. These results are in agreement with pH-partition hypothesis.

Lipid Solubility

Partition Coefficient. Some drugs may be poorly absorbed after oral administration even though they are available predominantly in the un-ionized form in the gastrointestinal tract. This is attributed to the low lipid

pH of the gastric fluid and may, therefore, be absorbed from the stomach as well as from intestine. Some very weak acidic drugs such as phenytoin and many barbiturates, whose pK$_a$ values are greater than 7.0 are essentially unionized at all pH values. Therefore, for these weak acidic drugs transport is more rapid and independent of pH, provided the un-ionized form is lipophilic or nonpolar. Furthermore, it is important to note that the fraction un-ionized changes dramatically only for weak acids with pK$_a$ values between 3 to 7. Therefore, for the weak acids a change in the rate of transport with pH is expected as shown in Figure 7.11.

Although the transport of weak acids with pK$_a$ values less than 3.0 should theoretically depend on pH, the fraction un-ionized is so low that transport across the gut membrane may be slow even under the most acidic conditions.

Most weak bases are poorly absorbed, if at all, in the stomach since they are present largely in the ionized form at low pH. Codeine, a weak base with pK$_a$ of about 8.0 will have about 1 in every million molecules in its un-ionized form at gastric pH of 1.0. Weakly basic drugs such as dapsone, diazepam and chlordiazepoxide are essentially unionized through the intestine. Strong bases, those with pK$_a$ values between 5 and 11, show pH dependent absorption.

Table 7.1. Comparison of Gastric Absorption of Acids and Bases at pH 1 and 8 in the Rat

	pK$_a$	Percent Absorbed at pH 1	Percent Absorbed at pH 8
Acids			
5-Sulfosalicylic acid	<2.0	0	0
5-Nitrosalicylic acid	2.3	52	16
Salicyclic acid	3.0	61	13
Thiopental	7.6	46	34
Bases			
Aniline	4.6	6	56
p-Toluidine	5.3	0	47
Quinine	8.4	0	18
Dextromethorphan	9.2	0	16

Table 7.2. Comparison of Intestinal Absorption of Acids and Bases in the Rat at Several pH Values (13)

		Percent Absorbed from Rat Intestine			
	pK$_a$	pH 4	pH 5	pH 7	pH 8
Acids					
5-Nitrosalicyclic acid	2.3	40	27	0	0
Salicyclic acid	3.0	64	35	30	10
Acetylsalicyclic acid	3.5	41	27	—	—
Benzoic acid	4.2	62	36	35	5
Bases					
Aniline	4.6	40	48	58	61
Amiopyrine	5.0	21	35	48	52
p-Toluidine	5.3	30	42	65	64
Quinine	8.4	9	11	41	54

solubility of the un-ionized molecule. A guide to lipid solubility or lipophilic nature of a drug is provided by a property called partition coefficient. This parameter, therefore, influences the transport and absorption processes of drugs, and is one of the most widely used properties in quantitative structure-activity relationships.

The movement of molecules from one phase to another is called partitioning. Drugs partition themselves between the aqueous phase and lipophilic membrane; preservative emulsions partition between the water and oil phases; antibiotics partition from body fluids to microorganisms; and drug and other adjuvants can partition into the plastic and rubber stoppers of containers. It is therefore important that this process is understood.

If two immiscible phases are placed adjacent to each other, one containing a solute soluble in both phases, the solute will distribute itself into two immiscible phases until equilibrium is attained and, therefore, no further transfer of solute occurs. At equilibrium, the chemical potential of the solute in one phase is equal to its chemical potential in the other phase. If we consider an aqueous (w) and an organic (o) phase, we write according to theory:

Eq. 7.24 $\qquad \mu^{\ominus}_w + RT \ln a_w = \mu^{\ominus}_o + RT \ln a_o$

where a represents the activity coefficient of a solute. Rearranging Equation 7.24 yields

Eq. 7.25 $\qquad \dfrac{\mu^{\ominus}_w - \mu^{\ominus}_o}{RT} = \ln \dfrac{a_w}{a_o}$

The term on the left side of Equation 7.25 is a constant at a given temperature and pressure. Therefore,

Eq. 7.26 $\qquad \dfrac{a_w}{a_o} = \text{constant or } \dfrac{a_o}{a_w} = \text{constant}$

These constants are the partition or distribution coefficients, P. If the solute under consideration forms an ideal solution in both phases or solvent, the activity coefficient can be replaced by the concentration term and Equation 7.26 becomes:

Eq. 7.27 $\qquad P = \dfrac{C_o}{C_w}$

Equation 7.27 is used conventionally to calculate the partition coefficient of a drug. In Equation 7.27, C_o, the concentration of drug in the organic or oil phase, is divided by the concentration in the aqueous phase. The greater the value of P, the higher the lipid solubility of the solute. It has been demonstrated for several systems that the partition coefficient can be approximated by the solubility of the solute in the organic phase divided by the solubility in the aqueous phase. Therefore, the partition coefficient is a measure of the relative affinities of the solute for an aqueous or non-aqueous or oil phase. The effect of lipid solubility and, hence, partition coefficient on the absorption of a series of barbituric acid derivatives is shown in Table 7.3.

It must be clearly understood that, though drugs with greater lipophilicity and, therefore, partition coefficient are better absorbed, it is imperative that drugs exhibit some degree or aqueous solubility. This is essential since the availability of the drug molecule in a solution form is a prerequisite for the drug absorption, and the biological fluids at the site of absorption are aqueous in nature. Therefore, from a practical view point, drugs must exhibit a balance between hydrophilicity and lipophilicity. This factor is always taken into account while a chemical modification is being considered as a way of improving the efficacy of a therapeutic agent.

The critical role of lipid solubility in drug absorption is a major guiding principle in the drug discovery and development process. Polar or hydrophilic molecules such as gentamicin, ceftrixine and streptokinase are poorly absorbed following oral administration and must therefore be administered parenterally. Lipid soluble drugs with favorable partition coefficients are generally well absorbed after oral administration. Very often, the selection of a compound with higher partition coefficient from a series of research compounds, provides improved pharmacologic activity. Occasionally the structure of an existing drug is modified to develop a similar pharmacologic activity with improved absorption. Chlortetracycline, which dif-

Table 7.3. Comparison of Barbiturate Absorption in Rat Colon and Partition Coefficient (Chloroform/Water) of Undissociated Drug

Barbiturate	Partition Coefficient	Percent Absorbed
Barbital	0.7	12
Apobarbital	4.9	17
Phenobarbital	4.8	20
Allylbarbital	10.5	23
Butethal	11.7	24
Cyclobarbital	13.9	24
Pentobarbital	28.0	30
Secobarbital	50.7	40
Hexethal	>100	44

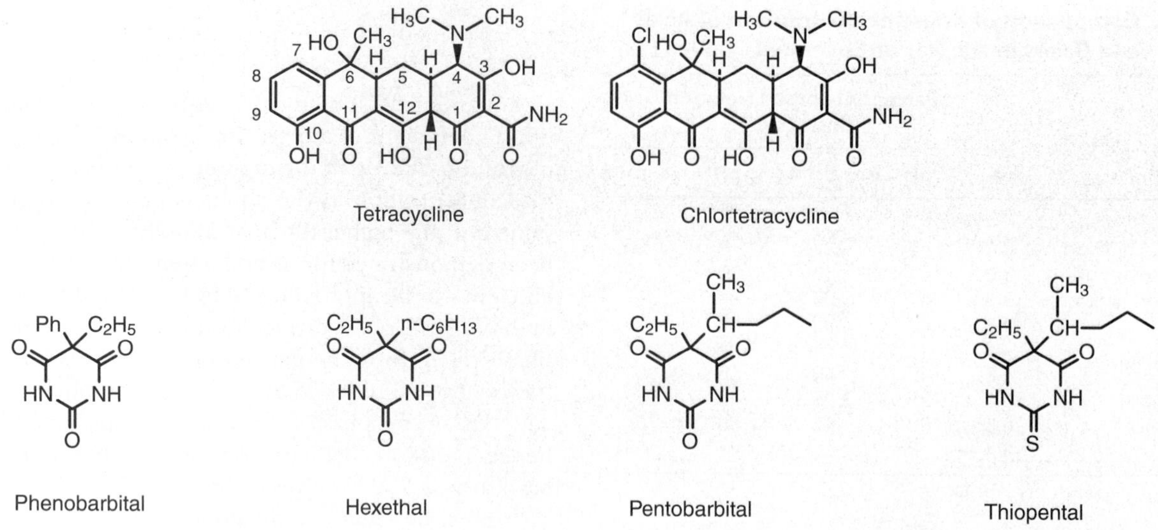

Tetracycline   Chlortetracycline

Phenobarbital   Hexethal   Pentobarbital   Thiopental

Fig. 7.12. Drug pairs in which chemical modification enhances lipophilicity.

fers from tetracycline by the substitution of a chlorine at C-7, substitution of a n-hexyl (Hexethal) for a phenyl ring in phenobarbital, or replacement of the 2-carbonyl of pentobarbital with a 2-thio group (thiopental) are examples of enhanced lipophilicity (Fig. 7.12).

It is important to note that even a minor molecular modification of a drug may promote the risk of also altering the efficacy and safety profile of a drug. For this reason, medicinal chemists prefer the development of a lipid soluble prodrug of a drug with poor oral absorption characteristics.

Prodrugs. Prodrugs are designed to improve permeability and oral absorption of the parent drug. They are more lipid soluble than the parent drug, and should be rapidly converted to the parent compound during absorption from the gut wall or the liver. Pivampicillin, a prodrug of ampicillin, is an ester and more lipid soluble, and therefore, more efficiently absorbed than the parent compound ampicillin (16).

The pH partition theory provides a basic framework for the understanding of drug absorption and is, sometimes, an oversimplification of a more complex process. For example, experimentally observed pH-absorption curves are less steep (Fig. 7.13) than that expected theoretically and are shifted to higher pH values for bases and lower pH values for acids.

This deviation, observed experimentally, is attributed by several investigators to factors such as limited absorption of ionized species of drugs, the presence of an unstirred diffusion layer adjacent to the cell membrane, and a difference between lumenal pH and cell membrane surface pH.

Absorption of Drugs from Solid Dosage Forms and Suspension

When a drug is administered orally via tablet, capsule or suspension as drug delivery systems, the rate of absorption is often controlled by how fast the drug particles dissolve in the fluid at the site of administration. Hence, dissolution rate is often the rate limiting (slowest) step in the following sequence:

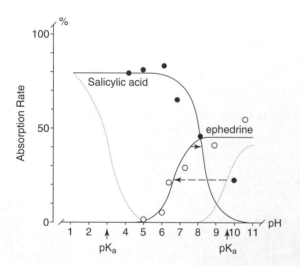

Fig. 7.13. Relationship between absorption rates of salicylic acid and ephedrine and bulk phase pH in the rat small intestine in vivo. *Dashed lines,* curves predicted by the pH-partition theory in the absence of an unstirred layer (17).

$$\boxed{\text{Solid drug}} \xrightarrow[\text{Step I}]{\text{Dissolution}} \boxed{\begin{array}{c}\text{Drug in}\\\text{Solution}\end{array}}$$

$$\xrightarrow[\text{Step II}]{\text{Absorption}} \boxed{\begin{array}{c}\text{Drug in Systemic}\\\text{Circulation}\end{array}}$$

When Step I or dissolution of the drug is controlling the rate of absorption, it is said to be dissolution rate limited.

Figure 7.14 describes the absorption of aspirin from solution and two different types of tablets.

It is clear from Figure 7.14 that aspirin absorption from solution is more rapid than from tablet formulations. This rapid absorption is an indication of the absorption being dissolution rate limited. A general relationship describing the dissolution of a drug was first reported by Noyes and Whitney (19). The equation derived by Noyes and Whitney states that:

Eq. 7.28 $$\frac{d_c}{d_t} = KS\,(C_s - C)$$

where d_c/d_t = the dissolution rate, K is a constant, S is the surface area of the dissolution solid, C_s is the equilibrium solubility of drug in the solvent, and C is the concentration of drug in the solvent at time t.

The constant K in Equation 7.28 has been shown to be equal to D/h, where D is the coefficient of the dissolving material of the drug and h is the thickness of the diffusion layer surrounding the dissolving solid particles. This diffusion layer is thin stationary film of a solution adjacent to the surface of a solid particle (Fig. 7.15) and is saturated with drug, i.e., drug concentration in the diffusion layer is equal to C_s, the equilibrium solubility. The term $(C_s - C)$ in Equation 7.28 represents the concentration gradient for the drug between the diffusion layer and the bulk solution. If dissolution is the rate limiting step in the absorption process, the term C in Equation 7.28 is negligible compared to C_s. Under this condition. Equation 7.28 is reduced to:

Eq. 7.29 $$\frac{dc}{dt} = \frac{DSC_s}{h}$$

Equation 7.29 describes a diffusion-controlled dissolution process. It is visualized that, when solid drug particles are introduced to the fluids at the absorption sites, the drug promptly saturates the diffusion layer (Fig. 7.15). This is followed by the diffusion of drug molecules from the dif-

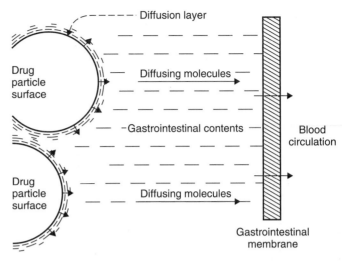

Fig. 7.15. Dissolution from a solid surface (4).

fusion layer into the bulk solution, which are instantly replaced in the diffusion layer by molecules from the solid crystal or particle. This is a continuous process. Even though it oversimplifies the dynamics of the dissolution process, Equation 7.29 is a qualitatively useful equation and clearly indicates the effects of some important factors on the dissolution, and therefore, the absorption rate of drugs. When dissolution is the rate limiting factor in the absorption, then bioavailability is affected. These factors are listed in Table 7.4.

The Noyes-Whitney equations (Equations 7.28 and 7.29) demonstrate that the equilibrium solubility (C_s) is one of the major factors determining the rate of dissolution. Changes in the characteristics of solvents, such as pH, affecting the solubility of the drug, affect its dissolution rate. Similarly, the use of a different salt or other physicochemical form of a drug, which have a solubility different from the parent drug, usually affects the dissolution rate. Increasing the surface area of a drug exposed to the dissolution medium, by reducing the particle size, usually increases the dissolution rate. In the discussion to follow, some of the more important factors affecting dissolution, and therefore absorption, are presented in greater detail.

Dissolution and pH: Solubility of Weak Acids and Bases

The solubility of weak acids and bases is a function of the pH of the medium. Therefore, differences in the dissolution rate are expected to occur in different regions of the gastrointestinal tract. The solubility of weak acid is obtained by:

Eq. 7.30 $$C_s = [HA] + [A^-]$$

where [HA] is the intrinsic solubility of the un-ionized acid, i.e., C_o, and $[A^-]$ is the concentration of its anion,

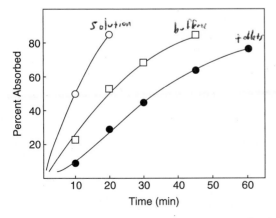

Fig. 7.14. Absorption of aspirin after oral administration of a 650-mg dose in solution (O), in buffered tablets (□), or in regular tablets (●) (18).

which can be expressed in terms of its dissociation constant, K_a, and C_o, i.e.,

Eq. 7.31
$$C_s = C_o + \frac{K_a C_o}{[H^+]}$$

Analogously, the solubility of a weak base is obtained by

Eq. 7.32
$$C_s = C_o + \frac{C_o [H^+]}{K_a}$$

By substituting Equations 7.31 and 7.32 into Equation 7.29 for the term C_s, the following dissolution rate equations are obtained:

For weak acids:

Eq. 7.33
$$\frac{dc}{dt} = \frac{K'(C_0 + K_a C_0)}{[H^+]}$$

or

Eq. 7.34
$$\frac{dc}{dt} = \frac{K' C_0 (1 + K_a)}{[H^+]}$$

and for a weak base:

Eq. 7.35
$$\frac{dc}{dt} = \frac{K' C_0 (1 + [H^+])}{K_a}$$

Equations 7.33 through 7.35 show that K′ is equal to DS/h. Equations 7.34 and 7.35 clearly suggest that the dissolution rate of weak bases decreases with increasing pH. Hence, the dissolution rate of weak bases is maximum in gastric fluid, but for weak acids it is at a minimum. Furthermore, the dissolution rate of weak acids increases as the solid drug particles move to the more alkaline regions of the gastrointestinal tract. Figure 7.16 illustrates the dissolution rates of weak acids as a function of pH (20).

The absorption of a salt of weak acid or base can be explained by using the following figure:

| Salt of Weak Acid or Base | Dissolution $\longrightarrow$ | Ionized form of Weak Acid or Base |

$$\begin{array}{c} K_1 \\ \longrightarrow \\ \longleftarrow \\ K_2 \end{array} \quad \boxed{\text{Un-ionized form of Weak Acid or Base}}$$

where K_1 and K_2 represent the rate constants associated with the formation of unionized and ionized species of a

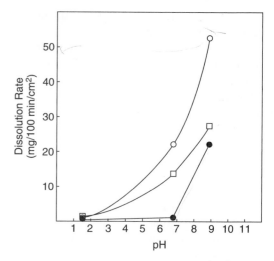

Fig. 7.16. pH-Dependent dissolution of salicylic acid (O), benzoic acid (□), and phenobarbital (●) (20).

compound, respectively. The ratio of these two rate constants represent the dissociation constant of a compound. The absorption of the unionized species of a molecule disturbs the equilibrium of the process. To regain the equilibrium, some of the ionized species, therefore, get converted into unionized species, which are then absorbed through the membrane. This process, being a continuous one, permits the absorption of the unionized species to take place. Therefore, a drug molecule will eventually be absorbed.

The relatively poor dissolution of weak acids at the pH of gastric fluid diminishes further the importance of the stomach as a drug absorption site. Although gastric absorption of weak acids may occur from solution, it is unlikely that much of the drug dissolves and is absorbed during the short residence time as solid dosage form in the stomach. A study by Ogata (21) proposed that the critical value of solubility that separates acid drugs from the absorption sites (stomach or intestine) is about 30 mg/mL in 0.1N HCl when 1 gram of drug is administered orally. The authors found that, if the solubility of a drug is less than 3 mg/mL, practically no absorption occurs in the stomach. Changes in the gastric pH also alter the solubility of certain drugs and may affect the dissolution and absorption rates. A patient with achlorhydria has a higher gastric

Table 7.4. How to Change Parameters of Dissolution Equation to Increase (+) or Decrease (−) Rate of Solution (4)

Equation Parameter	Comments	Effect on Rate of Solution
D (diffusion coefficient of drug)	May be decreased in presence of substances that increase viscosity of the medium	(−)
A (area exposed to solvent)	Increased by micronization and in "amorphous" drugs	(+)
δ (thickness of diffusion layer)	Decreased by increased agitation in gut or flask	(+)
c_s (solubility in diffusion layer)	That of weak electrolytes altered by change in pH, by use of appropriate drug salt or buffer ingredient	(−)(+)
c (concentration in bulk)	Decreased by intake of fluid in stomach, by removal of drug by partition or absorption	(+)

pH and absorbs aspirin more rapidly than a normal subject. On the other hand, similar differences were not observed with respect to the absorption rates of acetaminophen, a much weaker acid, whose solubility would be unaffected by changes in pH (22).

The relationships between dissolution rate and hydrogen ion concentration, described in Equations 7.34 and 7.35, are approximations and tend to overpredict the dissolution rate of weak acids in the small intestine and weak bases in the stomach. In reality, the hydrogen ion concentration $[H^+]$ of the bulk is not equal to the hydrogen ion concentration $[H^+]$ of the diffusion layer.

Salts

The dissolution rate of a particular salt is usually different from that of a parent compound. Sodium or potassium salts of weak acids dissolve more rapidly than the free acid. The same is true with HCl or other salts of weak bases. Table 7.5 illustrates the dissolution rate differences between some weak acids and their sodium salts.

The differences in the dissolution rates of salt and parent compound can be explained by taking into consideration the pH of the diffusion layer. At a given pH, regardless of salt or free acids/bases, a drug will have a fixed solubility. The classical dissolution equation predicts a slower dissolution of a salt of a drug and the concept of diffusion layer becomes useful.

For sodium or potassium salts of weak acids, the pH of the solution in a diffusion layer is greater than the pH of the diffusion layer for the corresponding weak acid. On the other hand, the pH of the solution in the diffusion layer for hydrochloride salts of weak bases is always smaller than the diffusion layer of the corresponding free base. Therefore, effective solubility and dissolution rate of soluble salts on drug absorption are available in the literature. The potassium salt of penicillin V yields higher peak plasma concentration of antibiotic than the corresponding free acid. (23) Sodium salts of barbiturates are reported by Anderson (24) to provide a rapid onset of sedation. Some salts have a lower

solubility and dissolution rate than their parent compounds. Examples include aluminum salts of weak acids and pamoate salts of weak bases. In these particular examples, insoluble films of either weak acids or pamoic acid appear to form in the dissolving solids, which further retards the dissolution rate.

Surface Area and Particle Size

A drug dissolves more rapidly when its surface area is increased. This is usually accomplished by reducing the particle size of a drug. Therefore, many poorly soluble and slowly dissolving drugs are currently marketed in micronized or microcrystalline form. The problems of low water solubility and particle size were not fully appreciated, but have resulted in reducing the therapeutic dose of some drugs without sacrificing therapeutic efficacy. For example, since the original marketing of spironolactone, its dose has been reduced from 500 mg to 25 mg as a result of a reformulation which includes micronization. A similar result has been obtained for grieseofulvin.

Summary

At one time, it was common to assume that the biologic response to a drug was simply a function of the intrinsic pharmacologic activity of the drug molecule. Today, while assessing the potency of most drugs, consideration is given to plasma drug concentration-response than dose response relationships. The concentration of a drug in the plasma is dependent on the rate and extent of absorption, which in turn is influenced by the physicochemical properties of drug substances. Drug absorption may markedly affect the onset and intensity of a biologic response of a drug. Clinically significant differences in the absorption of closely related drugs such as lincomycin and clindamycin, penicillin and pivampicillin, or secobarbital and sodium secobarbital are invariably due to significant differences in their physicochemical properties.

Dissolution is simply a process by which a solid substance goes into solution. The determination of dissolution rates of pharmaceutical substances from dosage forms does not predict their bioavailability or their in-vivo performance, but rather it indicates the potential availability of drug substance for absorption. Therefore, it is essential for pharmacists and pharmaceutical scientists to know and understand the importance of dissolution and its potential influence on the rate and extent of absorption and availability for drugs.

Factors affecting the dissolution rate of a drug from a dosage form can be related to the physicochemical properties of a drug, the formulation of a dosage form, and dissolution apparatus and test parameters.

The chapter has examined a few fundamental physicochemical properties of drugs, such as their solubility, particle size, partition coefficient, dissociation constant, and crystalline state, which affect the drug's dissolution rate and absorption. Although the magnitude and significance of these

Table 7.5. Dissolution Rate of Weak Acids and Their Sodium Salts (25)

Compound	pK$_a$	Dissolution Rate (mg/100 min/cm²)		
		0.1 N HCl pH 1.5	0.1 M Phosphate pH 6.8	0.1 M Borate pH 9.0
Benzoic acid	4.2	2.1	14	28
Sodium salt		980	1770	1600
Phenobarbital	7.4	0.24	1.2	22
Sodium salt		~200	820	1430
Salicylic acid	3.0	1.7	27	53
Sodium salt		1870	2500	2420
Sulfathiazole	7.3	<0.1	~0.5	8.5
Sodium salt		550	810	1300

factors must be determined individually for each drug product, the material presented here may serve as a guideline.

PHARMACOKINETICS
Introduction

The events following drug administration can be divided into two phases: a pharmacokinetic phase in which the ability to adjust a dose, alter the dosage form, and alter the frequency and the route of administration are related to drug concentration-time relationship in the body; and a pharmacodynamic phase in which the drug concentration at the sites of action is related to the magnitude of effect(s) produced. Once both of these phases have been defined for a drug, a dosage regimen for a drug can be established to achieve the optimum therapeutic goals in individual patients and in predicting what may happen when a dosage regimen is changed.

The sites into which drugs are routinely administered are broadly classified as intravascular and extravascular. The intravascular administration refers to the placement of a drug directly into blood, either intravenously or intra-arterially. And, since the drug is placed directly into blood, it is imperative that the drug be administered as a solution. The extravascular routes of administration include oral, intramuscular, sublingual, buccal, subcutaneous, dermal, rectal, and nasal routes. To enter the blood, a drug administered extravascularly must be absorbed from the site of administration. And, if a drug is administered through solid dosage forms such as tablets, capsules etc., then the drug must first dissolve at the site of administration. Therefore, the dissolution of a drug is essential prior to its absorption. On the other hand, no such absorption step is required when a drug is administered intravenously.

Pharmacokinetics is the scientific discipline that deals with mathematical description of biological processes affecting drugs and that is affected by drugs. And, in addition to signifying the relationship of ADME processes to the intensity and time course of pharmacologic effects of drugs pharmacokinetics describes the time course of a drug's absorption, distribution, metabolism and excretion (ADME) which takes place following the administration of a drug. It is therefore necessary to describe and analyze these processes and their effects in relation to their rates, rate constants or time course. A qualitative description of these processes is quite insufficient and seldom leads to adequate and accurate characterizations of the effects of drugs on the body and effects of the body on the drugs. Pharmacokinetics is a quantitative study whose purposes are:

1. To develop mathematical expressions that permits one to describe the temporal changes of the drug concentration;
2. To determine constraints that describe ADME processes succinctly;
3. To make predictions and extrapolations based on the mathematical expressions; and
4. To help establish dosage regimen which will result in improved drug utilization in patients.

At a fundamental level, pharmacokinetics is a tool useful to pharmacists and physicians to optimize the dosage regimen of drugs for individuals who may differ in their intrinsic response and their ability to absorb and eliminate drugs. Adjustment of dosage regimen to account for individual differences and disease states is, in essence, an exercise in clinical pharmacokinetics and clinical pharmacy practice.

A basic tenet of pharmacokinetics is that the magnitude of both the desired response and toxicity are functions of drug concentration in the blood. Furthermore, it is not only the efficacy of a drug at the site of action that determines the intensity and duration of its pharmacologic or therapeutic effects, but also the amount of a drug and the rate at which the drug gets to the site of action. The vital processes of the body may delay the transport of drug molecules across membranes, convert drug molecules into metabolites, and remove them from the body as metabolites and/or unchanged form. This, in turn, may result in therapeutic failure as a result of drug concentrations being too low or unacceptable toxicity as a consequence of too high a drug concentration. Between these limits of concentrations lies a region associated with therapeutic success. This region may be regarded as a therapeutic range or "therapeutic window." Each drug may possess its own "therapeutic window." And, since rarely can the drug concentration be measured at the site of drug action, the drug concentration is measured at alternative and more accessible sites such as plasma or serum and urine.

Figure 7.17 illustrates the concentration or therapeutic window for a drug. The terms MTC (minimum-toxic concentration) and MEC (minimum effective concentration) describe the limit of therapeutic range for a drug. If the administered dose of a drug produces the plasma concentration within this range, the drug will likely produce its therapeutic effect. The term onset of action is defined as the time at which the drug enters the therapeutic range (i.e., above the minimum effect con-

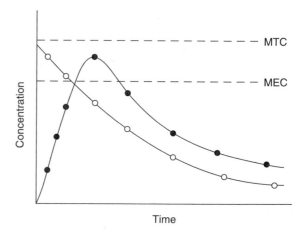

Fig. 7.17. Typical plasma concentration vs. time profile following the administration of a dose of a drug by intravascular (○) and extravascular routes (●).

centration), and when the plasma concentration of a drug falls below the therapeutic range is defined as the termination of action. The time span between the termination and the onset of action is described as the duration of action.

It is clear from Figure 7.17 and the definitions that an optimum dosage regimen might be defined as one that maintains the plasma concentration of a drug within the therapeutic range. Furthermore, it may be obvious from the discussion that the success of a drug in providing the desired drug concentration depends on factors such as how rapidly the drug reaches the general circulation from the site of administration, particularly following the oral and other extravascular routes, is the drug reaching the general circulation in sufficient amounts to provide plasma concentration within the therapeutic range, and the pharmacokinetic properties of a drug.

The purpose of this section in this chapter is to provide students a brief overview and the functional understanding of basic pharmacokinetics. Emphasis is placed upon how to carry out pharmacokinetic analysis of the data and how to use the pharmacokinetic parameters for predictive purposes. The mathematical equations presented in the chapter have been chosen because of their general utility for predicting the plasma concentrations following the administration of a drug by intra and extravascular routes. Furthermore, this chapter attempts to review and illustrate how the chemical modification of a drug through molecular modifications, may alter selected pharmacokinetic parameters of drugs and, therefore, possibly altering the pharmacologic response.

Compartmental Concepts

The most commonly employed approach to pharmacokinetic characterization of a drug is to depict the body as a system of compartments even though these compartments often do not have any apparent physiologic reality. These frequently used compartment models are illustrated in Figure 7.18.

The one compartment (I) assumes the body as a single homogenous unit (central compartment). The simplest model is particularly useful for pharmacokinetic analysis of plasma concentration and the urinary excretion data for drugs that are very rapidly distributed in the body. The two

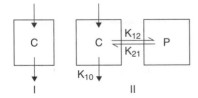

Fig. 7.18. Schematic representation of the one- (I) and the two- (II) compartment models commonly used in pharmacokinetics. The arrows represent transfer of a drug due to the first order process. The central compartment (plasma, highly perfused organs) is designated C, the peripheral (tissue) compartment is designated P.

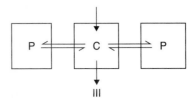

Fig. 7.19. Schematic representation of a three-compartment model commonly used in pharmacokinetics. The arrows represent transfer of a drug due to the first order process. The central compartment is designated C, the peripheral compartment is designated P.

compartments (II) consist of a central component, which includes the plasma and other highly perfused organs, connected to a peripheral or tissue compartment. Each compartment can be considered to include a group of tissues, fluids or parts of organs. A somewhat more complex model illustrated in Figure 7.19 is the three-compartment model (III), which consists of a central compartment connected to more than one peripheral compartment that differ in their relative accessibility to a drug. This model may be chosen if the data available warrants such a model.

The selection of a model depends much on the site and tissue being sampled, the frequency of sampling collection, and the ultimate goals of the study. The general operating rule in selecting a model for pharmacokinetic analysis of plasma concentration versus time data is to postulate the minimum number of compartments necessary to accurately describe the pharmacokinetics of a given drug. An approach to selecting the number of compartments should be parsimonious unless experimental evidence dictates that such parsimony may lead to errors in estimation of pharmacokinetic parameters of drugs and, therefore, the use of equations predicting blood levels of drugs.

Linear and Non-linear Pharmacokinetics

Linear Pharmacokinetics. Many processes in pharmacokinetics can be described accurately by a first order process. This means that the rate of a drug biotransformation, the rate of transfer of a drug between compartments, and the rate of absorption and elimination of drugs from the body are directly proportioned to the size of the dose administered. It is also true that passive diffusion is responsible for the transfer of a drug in the body and there is a directly proportional relationship between the administered dose and the resulting drug concentration in the body. This dose proportionality is often used as an indicator of linear pharmacokinetics. It is important, however, to recognize that the pharmacokinetic parameters such as the elimination half-life and the elimination rate constant are independent of the size of the dose administered. Therefore, linear pharmacokinetics is regarded as dose independent kinetics.

Non-linear Pharmacokinetics

The rate of elimination of a few drugs (i.e., ethanol, salicylate, phenytoin, etc.) by biotransformation and some other transfer processes involve protein carrier systems. These drugs are not removed from the body by a first order process, which means the rate of elimination is not proportional to the concentration of drug or the dose administered. In most of these cases, elimination follows zero order kinetics; the rate of change of drug concentration is independent of the drug concentration. A constant amount of a drug, rather than the constant percent of the remaining amount of drug is eliminated per unit time (i.e., mg/min or mcg.ml^{-1}.min^{-1}).

The most frequently reported reason for non-linear kinetics is that biotransformation and transfer processes require protein carrier systems. These systems are specific with respect to substrates that have finite capacities. The kinetics of these processes are often described by the Michaelis-Menten equation (Fig. 7.3–7.5).

This non-linear or dose dependent elimination kinetics may also be the result of effects other than the limited capacity of biotransformation or elimination processes. If a drug is partly reabsorbed from the renal tubules by a recycling process with limited capacity, then the elimination of large doses proceeds relatively more rapidly than the smaller doses. Similarly, lesser binding of drugs to plasma constituents or tissues at higher dosing may result in relatively more rapid drug elimination that is observed at lower drug concentrations.

There is evidence that some drug metabolites can inhibit their own formation. This process of product inhibition can also cause dose dependent effects, with large doses being eliminated relatively more slowly than the small doses. While the rate of decline of a drug concentration in the post distribution phase, at any given level of a drug in the body, will be independent of the dose in the case of simple Michaelis-Menten kinetics. In cases of product inhibition, this rate tends to decrease with increasing doses.

Intravascular Administration
Intravenous Bolus Administration and One-Compartment Model

Following the administration by intravenous injection, if a drug distributes very rapidly in the body, this confers upon the body the characteristics of a one-compartment model, and if the drug elimination from the body can be described by a first order process, then a plot of the logarithm of plasma drug concentration as a function of time yields a straight line as shown in Figure 7.20.

The equation responsible to describe plasma drug concentration against time is as follows:

Eq. 7.36 $\qquad C_p = (C_p)_0 \, e^{-Kt}$

where, C_p is the plasma drug concentration at time t, $(Cp)_0$ is the initial plasma drug concentration (i.e., t = 0) immediately after the injection, K is the first order elimination rate constant, and t represents time. Equation 7.37 can also be written as follows:

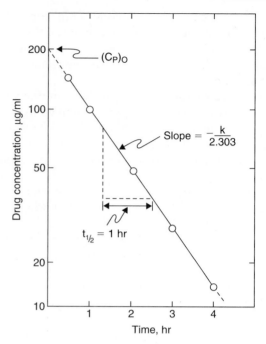

Fig. 7.20. Schematic representation of plasma concentration of drug in the body as a function of time following rapid intravenous injection.

Eq. 7.37 $\qquad \ln C_p = \ln(C_p)_0 - Kt$

or

Eq. 7.38 $\qquad \log C_p = \log(C_p)_0 - \dfrac{Kt}{2.303}$

The initial plasma drug concentration, $(Cp)_0$, may be obtained by extrapolation of the line (Fig. 7.20) to time = 0 or the y intercept of plasma drug concentration vs. time plot. Figure 7.20 shows that a plot of the log of plasma drug concentration vs. time will be linear under the stated condition.

Three primary factors determine the plasma concentration of the administered drug: 1) the route of administration, 2) the uptake of drug by body tissues, and 3) the elimination of the drug from the body. In the case of intravenous administration, since the drug is introduced directly into the blood, there is no delay due to the absence of the drug absorption process. The drug plasma level, however, depends on the dose size and the maximum plasma drug concentration occurs immediately after completion of the dose administration.

The Elimination Rate Constant and Half-life

The elimination rate constant, K, can be determined from the slope of the straight line as follows:

Eq. 7.39 $\qquad (\text{slope}) \times (2.303) = -K$

It is, however, much easier to determine the elimination rate constant by making use of the relationship:

Eq. 7.40 $\qquad K = \dfrac{0.693}{t_{1/2}}$

where, $t_{1/2}$ is the time required for any drug concentration to decrease by one half (i.e., 50%) and is also known as the biologic or the elimination half-life. The elimination half-life is a pharmacokinetic property of a drug and it is independent of the size of the administered dose, when the administered drug exhibits the characteristics of a first order process.

The elimination half-life ($t_{1/2}$) and the elimination rate constant (K) of a drug also play an important role in determining the plasma concentration of a drug at a given time. For instance, a drug with a short elimination half-life will be eliminated from the body much quicker than a drug with a longer elimination half-life. These two parameters of a drug, therefore, become important in maintaining the desired drug blood levels in the body. In essence these two parameters provide a quantifiable index of the presence of a drug in the body.

The process of drug elimination includes biotransformation and excretion and begins almost immediately when circulation of blood distributes some of the drug to organs capable of metabolizing the drug or excrete it from the body. Among the organs of drug elimination, the liver is the principal site of biotransformation and the kidney is primarily responsible for excretion of unchanged drugs and their metabolites. However, other organs may also participate in the elimination of selected drugs.

The consequence of biotransformation of the drug to metabolite depends on the pharmacologic activity of the individual metabolite(s). Metabolites may be active or completely inactive. Active metabolite(s) may be more or less potent than the parent drug and may exhibit similar or dissimilar action. The kinetics of distribution and elimination of metabolites may differ from those of the parent drug since each metabolite differs from the parent drug in its physicochemical properties as a result of functional group additions or changes.

The elimination rate constant (K) is the sum of the individual rate constants that characterize the elimination of a drug from the body and the form of metabolite or unchanged drug. Thus:

Eq. 7.41 $$K = K_u + K_m$$

where, K_u and K_m represent the first order rate constant associated with excretion and the form of metabolite or unchanged drug, respectively, removed from the blood.

The Apparent Volume of Distribution

This is a proportionality constant that relates the dose of drug (mg) and its concentration (C_p) in the body at a given time. This relationship is shown in Equation 7.42,

Eq. 7.42 $$(X)_t = V * (C_p)_t$$

where $(X)_t$ and $(C_p)_t$ are the dose of the drug and its plasma concentration, respectively, at a given time. The apparent volume of distribution (V) is determined by rearranging Equation 7.42 as follows:

Eq. 7.43 $$V = \frac{(X)_0}{(C_p)_0} = \frac{Dose}{(C_p)_0}$$

where X_0 is the administered dose of the drug and $(Cp)_0$ its initial plasma concentration.

The apparent volume of distribution (V) is usually a characteristic of a drug rather than the biological system. However, selected disease state and other factors that may influence the blood composition, total body fluid, and the permeability characteristic of tissue may bring about changes in the value of the apparent volume of distribution. In most situations, the apparent volume of distribution of a drug is independent of the drug concentration since doubling the amount of a drug in the body usually results in doubling of its plasma concentration (linear pharmacokinetics).

The magnitude of the apparent volume of distribution rarely corresponds to the plasma volume, extracellular volume or the volume of the body fluid. "V" may vary from a few liters (7 total liters) to several hundred liters in a human. The value of "V" for a drug depends upon its ability to penetrate into tissues in the body and the degree of binding of a drug to a plasma protein, among other factors. Because of differences in the magnitude of the apparent volume of distribution of a drug, a given dose of a drug with a relatively high volume of distribution will provide low initial drug concentrations and vice a versa (Eq. 7.42).

Clearance. One of the most important pharmacokinetic properties of a drug is clearance (Cl). In pharmacokinetic terms, clearance refers to the hypothetical volume of distribution from which the drug is entirely removed or cleared in unit time (ml/min). In other words, it is an index of drug elimination from the body. Clearance is a function of both the intrinsic ability of certain organs, such as kidneys and liver, to excrete or metabolize a drug and the blood flow rate to these organs. The concept of clearance can be illustrated by assuming the elimination in a single organ as depicted in Figure 7.21.

Under the conditions described in Figure 7.21 the venous concentration of drug (C_V) will always be less than the arterial concentration (C_A) because of the drug being eliminated or excreted during the passage of blood

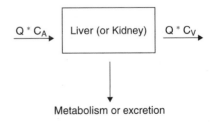

Fig. 7.21. Schematic representation of drug elimination by the liver (or kidney). Q * C_A is the rate at which the drug enters the liver (or kidney) and Q * C_V is the rate at which the drug leaves the liver (or kidney). The venous drug concentration C_V is less than the arterial drug concentration C_A.

through the organ. The rate at which the drug enters the organ is the product of blood flow rate (Q) and the arterial concentration (C_A). The rate at which the drug leaves the organ, on the other hand, is equal to the product of blood flow rate (Q) and venous concentration (C_v).

Eq. 7.44   The rate in = $Q * C_A$

Eq. 7.45   The rate out = $Q * C_V$

The difference between the rate in and rate out is the rate of elimination of a drug by the organ.

Eq. 7.46   Elimination rate = $Q(C_A - C_V)$

The dimensionless ratio of elimination rate to the rate at which a drug enters the organ ($Q * C_A$) is defined as the extraction ratio (ER) and is obtained as follows:

Eq. 7.47 $E_R = \dfrac{Q(C_A - C_V)}{Q * C_A} = \dfrac{(C_A - C_V)}{C_A}$

The extraction ratio (E_R) of a drug ranges from 0 to 1 depending on how well the organ eliminates or excretes the drug from the blood flowing through it. If an organ does not eliminate the drug, then $C_A = C_V$ and the extraction ratio is equal to zero (low extraction ratio). If, on the other hand, the organ avidly removes the drug so that $C_V \cong 0$, then the extraction ratio is equal to one (high extraction ratio). If liver is the organ responsible for metabolizing the drug then the extraction ratio may be described by using the notation, E_H.

Using the extraction ratio number (i.e., E_R or E_H), the drugs have been classified as having a low ($E_R < 0.3$), intermediate (E_R between 0.3 to 0.7) or high ($E_R > 0.7$) extraction ratio drugs. Table 7.6 lists the representative drugs with their hepatic or extraction ratios.

The influence of blood flow and intrinsic clearance of an organ on the clearance of a drug is determined by the extraction ratio of the drug.

The clearance of a drug may also be viewed as a proportionality constant relating the elimination rate of a drug to its plasma concentrations at a given time and is expressed as

Eq. 7.48 $(Cl) = \dfrac{\text{Rate of elimination}}{(\overline{C}_p)}$

where $(\overline{C}_p)$ is the average plasma concentration of a drug at a time that corresponds to the rate of elimination and follows from an earlier equation (Eq. 7.11) that:

Eq. 7.49 $(Cl) = Q * E_R$

where Q and E_R terms have been previously defined and since the drug elimination follows a first order process, clearance is independent of the drug concentrations or the dose administered.

The total body clearance (Cl) of a drug the from blood is equal to the ratio of the overall elimination rate to drug concentration (Eq. 7.48); where the overall elimination rate is comprised of the sum of the elimination processes occurring in all organs and the removal of a drug in all its forms. Therefore, the overall clearance (Cl_S) represents the renal clearance (i.e., unchanged form of a drug) and metabolic clearance (i.e., removal of a drug as metabolic by kidney). It is also very useful to keep in mind that the clearance can be expressed as the product of the apparent volume of distribution (V) and the elimination rate constant (K) for drugs that exhibit characteristics of one compartment model. Thus:

Eq. 7.50 $(Cl)_S = V * K$

Table 7.6. Hepatic and Renal Extraction Ratios of Selected Drugs and Metabolites (13)

		Low (<0.3)	Intermediate (0.3–0.7)	High (>0.7)
Hepatic[a] extraction		Carbamazepine Diazepam Digitoxin Indomethacin Phenobarbital Phenytoin Procainamide Salicylic Acid Theophylline Tolbutamide Valproic Acid Warfarin	Aspirin Quinidine Codeine Nortriptyline	Alprenolol Arabinosyl-cytosine Desipramine Doxepin Isoproterenol Lidocaine Meperidine Morphine Nitroglycerin Pentazocine Propoxyphene Propranolol
Renal[a] extraction		Atenolol Cefazolin Chlorpropamide Digoxin Furosemide Gentamicin Lithium Phenobarbital Sulfisoxazole Tetracycline	Cimetidine Cephalothin Procainamide (Some) Penicillins	(Many) Glucuronides Hippurates (Some) Penicillins (Many) Sulfates

[a]At least 30% of the drug is eliminated by this route.

Renal Clearance. Drug elimination occurs by renal excretion and an extra-renal pathway, usually hepatic metabolism. Renal clearance is defined as the proportionality constant between the urinary excretion rate and the plasma concentration:

Eq. 7.51
$$\left(\frac{dXu}{dt}\right)_{\bar{t}} = (Cl)_r * \bar{C}_p$$

where $\left(\dfrac{dXu}{dt}\right)_{\bar{t}}$ is the average urinary excretion rate (mg/hr); Cl_r is the renal clearance (ml/hr) and $\bar{C}_p$ is the plasma drug concentration. Equation 7.51, however, presents practical difficulty in measuring renal clearance since plasma drug concentration changes continually. This can be avoided by taking a modified approach. Equation 7.51 is rearranged, during a small time interval, (dt) to:

Eq. 7.52
$$(Xu)_t = (Cl)_r * C_p * dt$$

where ($C_p * dt$) corresponds to the area under the plasma concentration- time curve (AUC). The urine collection interval, dt, is composed of many such very small increments of time, and the amount of drug excreted in a collection interval is the sum of the drug amount excreted in each small time interval line. Then:

Eq. 7.53
$$(Cl)_r = \frac{\text{Total amount of drug excreted (i.e.,} (X_u)_\infty)}{(AUC)_0^\infty}$$

where $(X_u)_\infty$ is the total amount excreted in the urine and $(AUC)_0^\infty$ is the area under the plasma concentration time curve from t = 0 to t = ∞.

To account for all the administered drugs in the urine when the drug is administered intravenously is often not possible. This may be due to the excretion of some of the drug by an extra renal route, excretion of a metabolite by an extra-renal route, further biotransformation of primary metabolite into chemical forms that are not identified by the analytical method used or formation of unknown, and unidentified primary metabolites. If the metabolites can be identified in the urine then one can determine the metabolite clearance by using the following equation:

Eq. 7.53
$$(Cl)_m = \frac{\text{Total amount of drug excreted (i.e.,} (X_{mu})_\infty)}{(AUC)_0^\infty}$$

Hepatic Clearance. Although metabolism can take place in many organs, the liver frequently has the greater metabolic capacity and, therefore, has been most thoroughly studied. The most direct quantitative measure of the liver's ability to eliminate a drug is hepatic clearance, which includes biliary excretion clearance and hepatic metabolic clearance.

Eq. 7.55
$$(Cl)_H = Q_H * E_H$$

where Q_H is the sum of the hepatic portal and hepatic arterial blood flow rates, whose values are 1050 and 300 ml/min, respectively; E_H is the hepatic extraction ratio.

Under conditions of normal body functions, the pharmacokinetic behavior of most drugs can be established within reasonable limits and optimal dosage regimens can be designed using the observed values of the pharmacokinetic parameters of the drug. However, when the renal function is compromised as a consequence of acute or chronic renal diseases or patient's age, drugs that are eliminated predominantly through the kidneys are likely to be retained in the body for a longer duration and accumulate to the extent of providing toxic drug levels with repeated dosing. If the drug is converted to a metabolite, the accumulation of active metabolite may also lead to toxic effect and, though most metabolites are inactive, their accumulation with repeated dosing may produce toxic reactions by displacement of the parent drug from plasma protein and by inhibiting further drug metabolism.

Renal failure can result from a variety of pathological conditions. If renal impairment is rapid in onset and of short duration, then renal failure is described as acute. The primary cause of this may be prerenal i.e., acute congestive heart failure or, shock intrarenal i.e., acute tubule necrosis or, post renal i.e., hypercalcemia. The condition is generally reversible, however, complete restoration of renal function may take 6 to 12 months.

Chronic renal failure is almost always caused by intrinsic renal diseases and is characterized by slow, progressive development. Unlike the acute condition, chronic renal impairment is generally irreversible. The degree or loss of kidney functional capacity in the chronic condition is best described in terms of intact "nephron" hypothesis in which the diseased kidney is comprised of nephrons, which are essentially non-functional due to pathologic conditions, together with normal nephrons. Progressive renal impairment is the result of an increasing fraction of non-functional nephrons.

The prolonged and progressive nature of chronic renal failure is of particular concern in older patients who may require a variety of medications, both for their renal condition and other unrelated conditions. The inability of these patients to excrete drugs and drug metabolites adequately and the influence of their uremic conditions on the functions of other physiological systems require careful drug dosage adjustments to obtain accurate and adequate blood levels without increased toxicity.

Compounds (e.g., drugs) are cleared by kidneys due to passive filtration through the glomerulli or also by active secretion in the kidney tubule. Once in the nephrons, compounds may also be reabsorbed into the circulation. The glomerular filtration rate (GFR) can be measured by using any compound, which is filtered by glomerulli and not secreted and reabsorbed. Although exogenous compounds such as urea and insulin can be used for this purpose, the relative ease of using endogenous creatinine has made this the method of universal choice. In principle, the following equation determines the relationship between the creatine clearance (Cl_{cr}), the serum creatinine concentration (Cs_{cr}) and creatinine excretion rate $\left(\dfrac{dX_u}{dt}\right)_{\bar{t}*c_r}$

Eq. 7.56 $\qquad (Cl)_{cr} = \dfrac{(dXu/dt)_{\bar{t}cr}}{(C_s)_{cr}}$

Serum creatinine concentration is constant unless there is a change in the rate of production of creatinine in the body or creatinine clearance.

The creatinine clearance in normal kidneys is about 110–130 mL/min. This value declines with progressive renal impairment and drops to zero in severe renal impairment. Creatinine clearance values of 20–30 mL/min signify moderate renal impairment and values of less than 10mL/min signify several renal impairment. Creatinine is poorly secreted and not subject to tubular reabsorption and therefore its clearance is a useful measure of the glomerular filtration rate. Although creatinine clearance tells us about only one aspect of renal function (i.e., filtration), it is an excellent indicator for assessing the severity of renal impairment.

The extent to which decreased renal function influences drug elimination is a function of the percentage of circulating drug being cleared by the kidneys. From the literature, it is clear that the influence of renal impairment on the elimination half-life of a drug will be a direct function of the percentage of a drug cleared through the kidneys. If the elimination half-life of a drug, which is cleared essentially unchanged via the kidneys, is plotted against the endogenous creatinine clearance (Fig. 7.22), the result will be a hyperbola.

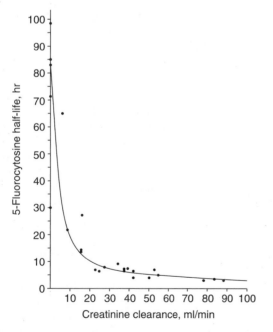

Fig. 7.22. Curvilinear relationship between the elimination half-life of 5-Fluorocytosine and renal function (creatinine clearance) (20).

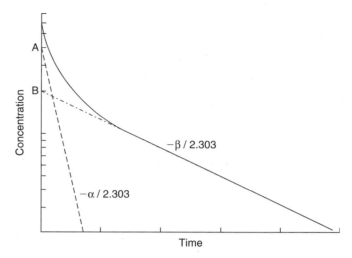

Fig. 7.23. Semi-logarithic plot of drug concentration in the plasma against time after the administration of a rapid intravenous injection when the body may be represented as a two compartment open model. The dashed line is obtained by "feathering" the curve.

Intravenous Bolus Administration: (Two-compartment Model)

Following the administration of a drug intravenously, it usually takes finite time before the distribution equilibrium is attained in the body. During this distribution phase, the drug concentration in the plasma will decline more rapidly than in the post-distribution phase as shown in Figure 7.23. There are three possible types of two compartment models. They differ in that the elimination of the drug occurs from the central compartment, peripheral compartment or both compartments. These three types of two-compartment models are, mathematically, indistinguishable on the basis of available concentration data. The type of a two-compartment model, illustrated in Figure 7.18, is most often used to describe the pharmacokinetics of drugs. It is assumed in this model that drug elimination from a two-compartment model occurs exclusively from the central compartment because the site of biotransformation and excretion i.e., liver and kidney are well-perfused with blood and, therefore, presumably rapidly accessible to drug in the systemic circulation. Whether or not this distribution phase is apparent will depend on the early collection of blood samples. A distribution phase may last for only a few minutes or for hours.

A semi-logarithmic plot of plasma drug concentration as a function of time (Fig. 7.23) after rapid intravenous injection of a drug can often be resolved into two linear components. This can be done graphically by employing the method of residual or "feathering" as shown in Figure 7.23 where the slopes of rapid and slow exponential are designated as (α) and (β), respectively. The intercepts on the concentration axis are designated A and B.

The entire plasma concentration time curve may be described by the following equation:

Eq. 7.57 $\qquad C_p = Ae^{-\alpha t} + Be^{-\beta t}$

where (α) and (β) are the first order distribution and disposition rate constants, respectively. A biexponential decline in the plasma drug concentration justifies, mathematically, the representation of the body as a two-compartment model.

The inter-compartmental rate constants (K_{21} and K_{12}) (Eqs. 7.58, 7.60) and the elimination rate constant (K_{10}) (Eq. 7.59) for the drug that exhibits the characteristics of a two-compartment model can be determined from the knowledge of (α), (β), A, and B (Fig. 7.23). This is achieved by employing the following equations:

Eq. 7.58
$$K_{21} = \frac{A\beta + B\alpha}{A + B}$$

where K_{21} is the rate constant associated with the transfer of a drug from compartment two to one (i.e., from the peripheral P to the central compartment C):

Eq. 7.59
$$K_{10} = \frac{\alpha * \beta}{K_{21}}$$

where K_{10} is the elimination rate constant of the drug.

Eq. 7.60
$$K_{12} = \alpha + \beta - (K_{21} + K_{10})$$

where K_{12} is the rate constant associated with the transfer of the drug from compartment one to two (i.e., from the central compartment C to the peripheral compartment P). Determination of these rate constants permits an assessment of the relative contribution of distribution and the elimination processes to the drug concentration versus time profile.

The transfer rate constant, K_{12}, is also required to calculate the amount of drug in the peripheral compartment (X_p) as a function of time after an intravenous administration:

Eq. 7.61
$$X_P = \frac{X_0 . K_{12}}{(\beta - \alpha)} (e^{-\alpha t} - e^{-\beta t})$$

where X_0 is the administered dose.

Extravascular Route of Administration

When a drug is administered by extravascular routes, absorption is a requisite for a drug to reach the general circulation. Absorption is defined here as a process of a drug proceeding from the site of administration to the site of measurement within the body, generally blood, plasma or serum. Figure 7.24 represents the passage of a drug through the GI tract into the general circulation.

When a drug is administered orally, there are several possible sites for drug loss. One such site is the gastrointestinal lumen, where the decomposition of a drug may occur. If it is assumed that the drug survives destruction in the gut lumen and is metabolized by enzymes as it passes through the membrane of the gastrointestinal tract then, though the drug leaves the site of administration, it is considered not to be absorbed systemically. Indeed, loss at any site in the gastrointestinal tract prior to reaching the site of measurement may contribute to decrease in the systemic absorption of the drug. The requirement for an orally administered drug to pass through the gastrointestinal tract makes the extent of absorption not always complete. The loss of a drug, as it passes for the first time through GI membrane and the lining, during absorption, is known as the first pass effect.

Figure 7.25 represents the time course of a drug and metabolite at each site in the body.

The rate or the change in the amount of drug in the body (dX/dt), following the administration of a drug by an extravascular route, is a function of both the absorption rate (K_aX_a) and the elimination rate (KX).

Eq. 7.62
$$\frac{dX}{dt} = K_aX_a - KX$$

where K_aX_a is the first order rate of absorption and KX is the first order elimination rate and K_a and K are the first order absorption and elimination rate constants, respectively.

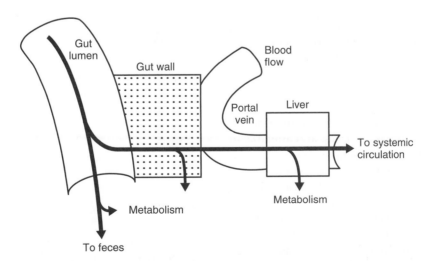

Fig. 7.24. After oral administration, a drug must pass sequentially through gut lumen, gut wall and then through the liver before reaching the general circulation. Metabolism may occur in the lumen before absorption, in the gut wall during the absorption or in the liver after absorption and before reaching the systemic circulation. Reprinted with permission from reference 13.

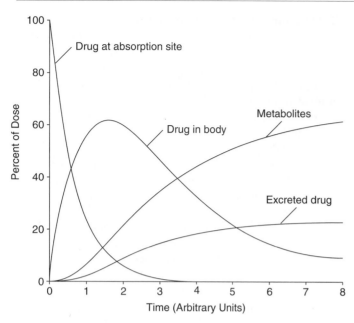

Fig. 7.25. Time course of a drug at each site following administration.

When the absorption rate is greater than the elimination rate (i.e., $K_aX_a > KX$), the amount of drug in the body and drug concentration in the plasma increases with the time. Conversely, when the amount of drug remaining at the absorption site (X_a) is sufficiently small the elimination rate exceeds the absorption rate (i.e., $KX > K_aX_a$) and, therefore, the amount of drug in the body and the drug concentration in the plasma decreases with time.

The maximum or peak plasma concentration, after drug administration, occurs at the moment when the absorption rate equals the elimination rate (i.e., $K_aX_a = KX$). The faster the drug is absorbed, the higher the maximum plasma concentration and the shorter the time required, following the administration of a dose, to observe the peak plasma concentration.

Integration of Equation 7.62 from $t = 0$ to $t = t$ and converting the amount to concentration, results in the following equation:

Eq. 7.63 $C_P = \dfrac{K_aF(X_a)_0}{V(K_a - K)}(e^{-Kt} - e^{-K_at})$

where $(Xa)_0$ is the administered dose and F is the fraction of the administered dose that is absorbed and available to reach the general circulation. Equation 7.63 is often used to determine plasma concentration after administration of a drug by an extravascular route when administered drug manifests the characteristics of a one-compartment model.

The absorption rate constant (K_a) of a drug is frequently larger than the elimination rate constant (K). Under such a condition, at some time after drug administration, the value of the term e^{-K_at} in Equation 7.63 approaches zero indicating that there is no more drug available for absorption, and Equation 7.63 simplifies to:

Eq. 7.64 $C_P = \dfrac{K_aF(X_a)_0}{V(K_a - K)}\left(e^{-Kt}\right)$

Eq. 7.65 $C_P = \text{Intercept}\left(e^{-Kt}\right)$

Eq. 7.66 $\log C_P = \log \text{Intercept} - \dfrac{Kt}{2.303}$

When the absorption is complete, the term X_aK_a disappears from the Equation 7.26 and the equation is reduced to:

Eq. 7.67 $-\dfrac{dX}{dt} = KX$

During the post-absorption phase, the decline in the plasma concentration with time follows first order kinetics. A typical plot of plasma concentration vs. time is shown in Figure 7.26.

The intercept of the extrapolated line (I*) is a complex function of absorption and elimination rate constants (K_a and K, respectively) as well as the dose or amount absorbed, $F.(X_a)_0$, and the apparent volume of distribution (V). It is, however, incorrect to assume that the intercept approximates the ratio of dose over the apparent volume of distribution unless the drug is rapidly and completely absorbed, which rarely occurs.

Importance of Absorption Rate. The influence of absorption on the drug concentration time profile is shown in Figure 7.27.

Administration of an equal dose of a drug in three different dosage forms or by three different extravascular routes or three different formations results in three times

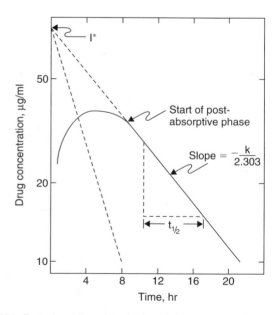

Fig. 7.26. Typical semilogarithmic plot of drug concentration vs. time profile in plasma following the administration of a drug by an extravascular route. The dashed line represents the "feathered line" used to obtain the absorption rate constant.

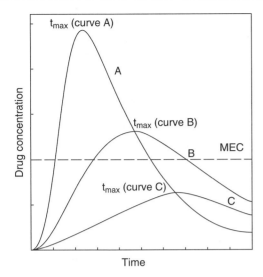

Fig. 7.27. A representation of the effects of drug concentration in the body at different absorption rate constants.

the drug in the plasma. The faster the drug is absorbed ($K_a \gg K$), the greater the peak plasma concentration and the shorter the time required to achieve peak plasma drug concentration.

Many drugs do not exhibit demonstrable pharmacologic effects or do not elicit a desired degree of pharmacologic response unless a minimum concentration is reached at the site of an action and, therefore, minimum therapeutic concentration in the plasma. Thus, the absorption rate of a drug may affect the clinical response if it fails to yield the minimum effective concentration (MEC). As evident in Figure 7.27, the more rapid is drug absorption, the faster is its onset of response (i.e., curve A). When the drug is absorbed rather slowly as curve C, the MEC level is just barely attained. The intensity of maximum pharmacologic effects is a function of the drug concentration. The data presented in Figure 7.27 suggests that the administered dose of a drug in curve A may produce a more intense response than observed in curves B and C.

The peak plasma drug concentration is always lower, following the administration of a drug by extravascular route, than its initial plasma concentration following the administration of an identical dose by intravenous solution. In the former, at peak time, some drugs may still remain at the absorption site and some have been eliminated while the entire dose is in the body immediately following the intravenous administration.

The delay between drug administration and a drug reaching general circulation may be of particular importance when a rapid onset of effect is desired. This delay is called lag time and can be anywhere between a few minutes to many hours. Lag time is generally attributed to the slow and poor absorption of the drug due to either slow disintegration and dissolution of the drug from the dosage form or due to slow removal of the coating material from coated tablets.

Determination of Peak Time (t_{max})

The determination of peak time (t_{max}) can be achieved by employing the following equation:

Eq. 7.68
$$t_{max} = \frac{\ln\left(\dfrac{Ka}{K}\right)}{(K_a - K)}$$

where t_{max} is the peak time and K_a and K are the first order absorption and elimination rate constants, respectively. Equation 7.68 shows that the peak time (t_{max}) is a function only of the relative magnitude of the absorption and the elimination rate constants. As the rate of absorption decreases (i.e., smaller K_a value), the peak time (t_{max}), will be higher as shown in Figure 7.27, progressing from curve C to curve A.

The rate of drug absorption varies when the extravascular route is changed, when a formulation of a drug is changed or when the dosage form is changed. These changes will be reflected in different peak times for the same dose of a drug. However, the peak time will be unaffected by a mere change in the size of the administered dose. In many disease states, the impairment in the renal function may affect the elimination rate constant thereby producing a change in the peak time.

Determination of Peak Plasma Concentrations (C_p)max

The peak (maximum) plasma drug concentration ($C_p)_{max}$ in the body occurs at time (t_{max}) which is described by substituting t_{max} for time (t) in Equation 7.63.

Eq. 7.69
$$(C_p)_{max} = \frac{K_a F(X_a)_0}{V(K_a - K)}\left(e^{-Kt_{max}} - e^{-K_a t_{max}}\right)$$

Equation 7.69 is further simplified into:

Eq. 7.70
$$(C_p)_{max} = \text{Intercept}\left(e^{-Kt_{max}} - e^{-K_a t_{max}}\right)$$

where the intercept of the plasma drug concentration verses time is equal to $\dfrac{K_a F(X_a)_0}{V(K_a - K)}$ as described earlier in the Equations 7.64 through 7.66. A much simpler expression can be obtained as follows. At peak time:

Eq. 7.71
$$e^{-K_a t_{max}} = \frac{K}{K_a} e^{-K_a t_{max}}$$

Substituting for $e^{-Kt_{max}}$ in Equation 7.69 yields:

Eq. 7.72
$$(C_p)_{max} = \frac{K_a F(X_a)_0}{V(K_a - K)}\left(\frac{K_a - K}{K_a}\right)(e^{-K_a t_{max}})$$

which upon the cancellation of terms, is readily simplified into:

Eq. 7.73
$$(C_p)_{max} = \frac{F(X_a)_0}{V}\left(e^{-K_a t_{max}}\right)$$

where F is the fraction of the dose absorbed; $(X_a)_0$ is the administered dose, V is the apparent volume of distribution; and K and t_{max} are elimination rate constants and peak time, respectively. Equation 7.73 suggests that the peak plasma concentration of a drug is a function of a dose entering the general circulation, the apparent volume of distribution, and the first order rate constants for absorption and elimination. Again, like absorption rate constant, the fraction of the administered dose reaching general circulation will depend upon the route of administration, the formulation, and the dosage form. These factors, therefore, will contribute to the peak plasma concentration of a drug.

Bioavailability

The bioavailability of a drug is defined as the rate and extent to which the administered dose of a drug reaches the general circulation. Generally, rapid and complete absorption of a drug is desirable if it is used for pain, allergy response, insomnia and other conditions when a quick onset of action is desired. As indicated earlier (Fig. 7.27), the more rapid is the absorption, the shorter is the onset of action and greater the intensity of a pharmacologic response.

The efficacy of a single dose is a function of both the rate and the extent of absorption. Therefore, in order for two dosage forms or two extravascular routes to be comparable with regard to the bioavailability following the administration of a drug, the absorption rate of a drug and the extent to which a drug reaches general circulation from each dosage form or extravascular route must be comparable.

The useful estimate of relative absorption rates of a drug from different products, through different routes of administration or different conditions (i.e., with or without food or in the presence of other drugs, etc.) can be made by comparing the magnitude of time of occurrence of peak concentration (t_{max}) and peak concentration (C_p)$_{max}$ and the area under the peak plasma concentration curve, $(AUC)_0^\infty$. The peak time and the peak plasma concentration can be determined by employing Equations 7.68 and 7.70 or 7.73, respectively, and the extent of absorption can be determined as follows.

Estimating the Extent of Absorption

The extent of absorption can be estimated by determining the total area under the plasma drug concentration verses time curve, $(AUC)_0^\infty$, or the total amount of an unchanged drug excreted in urine $(X_u)_\infty$ after the administration of a drug. The area under the plasma concentration versus time curve can be estimated by several methods such as a planimeter, an instrument for measuring the area of a plan figure and the cut and weight method, which weighs the paper of plasma concentration time curve. The weight is converted to weight per unit area. The most common methods, however, are the application of trapezoidal rule and equation, when possible. In a single dose study, we can not determine the area under the plasma concentration time curve, $(AUC)_0^\infty$, by the use of trapezoidal rule alone. In this case, a widely used practice is to determine (AUC) from t = 0 to t = t* (the last sam-

pling time) by means of trapezoidal rule and estimate the remaining area by employing the following equation:

Eq. 7.74 $$(AUC)_{t^*}^\infty = C_p^*/K$$

where $(AUC)_{t^*}^\infty$ is the area under the plasma concentration time from the last sampling time to time ∞, C_p^* is the last observed plasma concentration and K is the first order elimination rate constant. This area under the curve, $(AUC)_{t^*}^\infty$, will be added to the area under the curve obtained from t = 0 to t = t* to calculate the total area under the plasma concentration time curve.

Eq. 7.75 $$(AUC)_0^\infty = (AUC)_0^t{}^* + (AUC)_{t^*}^\infty$$

When an intravenous administration of a drug exhibits the characteristics of a one compartment model, the total area under the plasma concentration curve is estimated by employing the following equation:

Eq. 7.76 $$(AUC)_0^\infty = \frac{Dose}{V * K}$$

where VK is the systemic clearance of a drug.

Following the administration of a drug by an intravenous injection, if it is necessary to use a two-compartment model, the area under the plasma concentration time curve (AUC) from t = 0 to t = t* (the last sampling time) $(AUC)_0^\infty$ may be estimated by using trapezoidal rules, as mentioned earlier. And, the area under plasma concentration time curve (AUC) from t* to t = ∞ may be computed by using the following equation:

Eq. 7.77 $$(AUC)_{t^*}^\infty = C_p^*/\beta$$

where Cp* is the last observed plasma concentration and β is the first order disposition rate constant.

When a drug is administered by an extravascular route, one may use the following equation to determine the area under the plasma concentration time curve $(AUC)_0^\infty$.

Eq. 7.78 $$(AUC)_0^\infty = \frac{F * Dose}{V * K}$$

If it is desired to assess the relative extent of drug absorption from a product, a comparison of the total area under the plasma concentration from the product to that obtained for a reference drug standard is done. The reference standard may be an intravenous injection, an orally administered aqueous or water miscible solution or another product accepted as a standard.

When it is desired to assess the absolute bioavailability, the reference drug standard becomes an intravenous injection and when it is desired to judge the bioequivalence, the reference standard is an innovator product. If the area under the plasma drug concentration time, $(AUC)_0^\infty$, values are identical, following the administration of equal doses of a drug through a test product and the reference intravenous solution, we conclude that the drug from the test product is completely absorbed and not subject to presystemic metabolism.

Frequently, however, the standard is an innovator product or another established product. If the area under the plasma concentration time, $(AUC)_0^\infty$, values are identical, following the administration of equal doses of the test and the reference products, the conclusion is that the test product is completely bioavailable relative to the standard. It is essential to use the term relative to the standard since we do not know if the standard is completely absorbed or available. And, when two products produce comparable peak plasma drug concentrations and t_{max} and the reference standard is an innovator product, the products are judged to be bioequivalent.

By using the ratio of area under the plasma concentration time curve for extravascular to intravenous routes, one can determine the absolute bioavailability of a drug from a test product as follows:

$$\text{Eq. 7.79} \qquad F = \frac{(AUC)_0^\infty \text{ Oral}}{(AUC)_0^\infty \text{ I.V. Solution}}$$

where, F is the absolute bioavailability of a drug or the fraction of the administered dose that reaches the general circulation following the administration of equal dose of a drug. If the administered doses of a drug are different then the area under the plasma drug concentration time curve, $(AUC)_0^\infty$, estimates can be scaled approximately to permit comparison under identical conditions or equivalent doses, assuming of course, that the area under the plasma drug concentration time curve $(AUC)_0^\infty$ is directly proportioned to the administered dose.

The relative bioavailability (F_{rel}) of a drug from a test product may be determined by using the following expression.

$$\text{Eq. 7.80} \qquad F_{rel} = \frac{(AUC)_0^\infty \text{Test product}}{(AUC)_0^\infty \text{References standard}}$$

Equation 7.80 assumes that the doses administered from each product are identical, and if not, $(AUC)_0^\infty$ values should be scaled for the dose differences.

The determination of bioavailabilities from the urinary excretion of an unchanged drug, following the administration by intravenous solution, can be assessed by using the following equations:

$$\text{Eq. 7.81} \qquad (X_u)_\infty = \frac{(Dose) * K_u}{K}$$

where $(X_u)_\infty$ is the amount of drug excreted in unchanged form in the urine after the administration of a dose and K_u and K are the first order excretion and the elimination rate constants, respectively. On the other hand, for drugs administered by an extravascular route, the amount of an unchanged drug excreted in urine $(X_u)_\infty$ is obtained by:

$$\text{Eq. 7.82} \qquad (X_u)_\infty = \frac{F(Dose) * K_u}{K}$$

where F is the fraction of the administered dose that reaches the general circulation. Therefore, the bioavail-

ability of a drug following its extravascular administration can be expressed as:

$$\text{Eq. 7.83} \qquad F = \frac{(X_u)_\infty \text{ extravascular}}{(X_u)_\infty \text{ intravascular}}$$

To determine the assessment of relative bioavailability (F_{rel}), the Equation 7.83 becomes

$$\text{Eq. 7.84} \qquad F_{rel.} = \frac{(X_u)_\infty \text{ Test product}}{(X_u)_\infty \text{ Std. product}}$$

and Equations 7.83 and 7.84 are applicable under the condition that the administered doses are identical. The utility of these equations depends on how much of the drug is eliminated by urinary excretion, the sensitivity of the analytical procedure, and the variability in urinary output of the drug. Many drugs are extensively metabolized and little, if any, drug appears in an unchanged form in the urine. In such cases, the biovailability is estimated from the plasma concentration time data.

Following oral administration, a drug must pass sequentially from the gastrointestinal lumen, through the gut wall, and through the liver before reaching the general circulation (Fig. 7.24). Since the gut wall and liver are the sites of drug metabolism, a fraction of the amount of drug absorbed may be eliminated or metabolized before reaching the general circulation. Therefore, an oral dose of a drug may be completely absorbed yet incompletely available to reach the general circulation because of presystemic or first pass effect (metabolism) in the gut wall or liver. If such is the case then it will be reflected in the values of $(AUC)_0^\infty$ for the administered dose.

Criteria have been developed to identify and quantify the extent of presystemic metabolism and to indicate when it is occurring. The determination of presystemic metabolism requires only that the systemic availability of a drug is less than the fraction of the dose absorbed. The fraction absorbed may be determined from the urinary excretion of a drug and metabolite after oral administration of a drug relative to that after intravenous administration. Many drugs undergoing presystemic metabolism in humans have been identified on the basis of this type of information. Differentials between the gut wall and the liver, as the site of presystemic metabolism in humans are more difficult, though relatively easy in animals.

The liver is the most important site of presystemic elimination because of high levels of drug metabolizing enzymes, its ability to rapidly metabolize different types of drugs, and its unique anatomical location. The following are selected examples of drugs that are subject to considerable hepatic first pass metabolism: β blockers, propranolol and metoprolol; the analgesics, propoxyphene, meperidine and pentazocine; the antidepressants, imipramine and nortriptyline; and the antiarrhythmic, lidocaine.

Hepatic presystemic metabolism is most easily understood when liver is the sole organ of drug elimination. Under these conditions, the clearance of the drug, as determined following intravenous administration of the drug, is equal to:

$$\text{Eq. 7.85} \qquad (\text{Cl})_H = \frac{\text{Dose}}{(\text{AUC})_0^\infty}$$

Hepatic clearance, however, is also equal to:

$$\text{Eq. 7.86} \qquad (\text{Cl})_H = Q_H * E_H$$

where $(\text{Cl})_H$ is the hepatic clearance; Q_H is the hepatic blood flow rate; and E_H is the dimensionless hepatic extraction ratio of the drug. Hepatic blood flow rate (Q_H) has a mean range from about 1.1 to 1.8 liters/minute, with an average of about 1.5 liters/minute. Hepatic extraction ratio (E_H) of a drug may range from 0 to 1, depending on the liver's ability to metabolize the drug. The maximum hepatic clearance of a drug, excluding hepatic metabolism, is equal to hepatic blood flow; this occurs when $E_H = 1.0$ (i.e., hepatic extraction ratio). The fraction of a drug eliminated from portal blood (Fig. 7.24) during the absorption is given by the hepatic extraction ratio, E_H; the remainder of the drug (i.e., $1 - E_H$) escapes into the systemic circulation, and then is cleared from the circulation by the liver according to Equation 7.50.

If the fraction of the oral dose is absorbed and then subjected to hepatic presystemic metabolism, the area under the plasma concentration $(\text{AUC})_0^\infty$, following the oral administration of a drug is given by:

$$\text{Eq. 7.87} \qquad (\text{AUC})_0^\infty = \frac{F(X_a)_0(1 - E_H)}{Q_H * E_H}$$

Since $Q_H * E_H$ is equal to hepatic clearance (Eq. 7.86), which under these conditions, is given by the ratio of an intravenous dose to an area under the concentration time curve $(\text{AUC})_0^\infty{}_{\text{I.V.}}$. Equation 7.87 can be rewritten as:

$$\text{Eq. 7.88} \qquad \frac{(\text{AUC})_0^\infty \text{oral}}{(\text{AUC})_0^\infty \text{IV}} = \frac{F(X_a)_0(1 - E_H)}{(X_0)\ \text{IV}}$$

The ratio of $(\text{AUC})_0^\infty$ after oral and intravenous administration of equal doses of drugs is the systemic availability (i.e., fraction absorbed). If it is assumed that drug is completely absorbed (i.e., $F = 1$) then Equation 7.88 reduces to:

$$\text{Eq. 7.89} \qquad F = (1 - E_H)$$

Equation 7.89 shows that the systemic availability of the drug depends on the hepatic extraction ratio of the drug, and those drugs with low hepatic extraction ratios such as antipyrine, tolbutamide, and warfarin undergo little presystemic metabolism.

An estimate of hepatic extraction ratio (E_H) may be made from determination of the clearance of a drug following intravenous administration and comparing this value to the mean value of liver blood flow according to Equation 7.86, when rearranged:

$$\text{Eq. 7.90} \qquad E_H = \frac{(\text{Cl})_H}{Q_H}$$

The intravenous clearance of propranolol is about 1.05 liters/minute. Assuming that the average liver blood flow is about 1.5 liters/minute, we can determine the hepatic extraction for propranolol (E_H) is 0.7 and fraction absorbed (F) is 0.3. This means that, although propranolol is well absorbed, only 30% of the oral dose is available for systemic circulation.

This type of information, in conjunction with F (fraction absorbed) value, has been used to substantiate the predominantly hepatic presystemic elimination of several drugs including propranolol, lidocaine, pentazocine, etc. The plasma concentrations for pentazocine, following the oral administration of a 100 mg dose and an intravenous administration of a 30 mg dose, are shown in Figure 7.28. Figure 7.28 shows that, though the intravenous dose is smaller, this route of administration provides higher plasma concentration than an oral dose. The systemic availability (F) of pentazocine after oral administration was reported to be 11% to 32% with a mean of 18%. This low systemic availability is consistent with its high hepatic clearance (Cl_H).

Intravenous Infusion

If a drug is administered intravenously at a constant rate, its plasma concentration at any time will be provided by the following equation:

$$\text{Eq. 7.91} \qquad C_p = \frac{Q}{VK}(1 - e^{-Kt})$$

where Q is the constant infusion rate (dose/unit time).

The plasma drug concentration will rise (Fig. 7.29) with time after the start of an infusion and will slowly approach a constant level, at which the rate of elimination of the drug from the body equals the rate of infusion.

After the commencement of an infusion, it takes about 4.32 elimination half-lives of the drug for the plasma con-

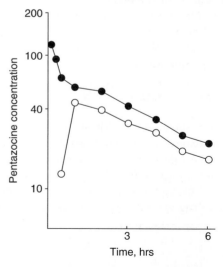

Fig. 7.28. Pentazocine concentration in plasma (ng/mL) after administration of 100 mg orally (○) or 30 mg intravenously (●) (26).

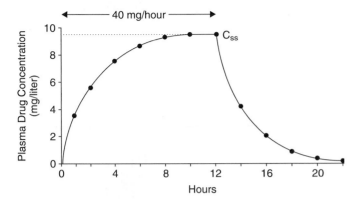

Fig. 7.29. Typical plasma concentration vs. time profile following the administration of a drug by intravenous infusion.

centration of the drug to be within 5% of the constant plateau level and 7 times the half-life for the concentration to be within 1% of the plateau level. The plateau or true steady state plasma concentration can be determined from Equation 7.91 by recognizing that the term (e^{-Kt}) approaches zero with increased time. Therefore:

Eq. 7.92 $$(C_p)_{ss} = \frac{Q}{VK}$$

where (C_p) is the true steady state plasma concentration; Q is the constant infusion rate, and VK is the systemic clearance of a drug. Equation 7.92 permits one to calculate the infusion rate necessary to attain and then maintain the desired steady state plasma concentration of a drug if the systemic clearance of the drug is available. Equation 7.92 also provides a convenient way to determine the apparent volume of distribution of a drug by means of intravenous infusion experiment if infusion rate (Q), the elimination rate constant (K), and the steady state plasma concentration $(C_p)_{ss}$ are known.

The decline of plasma concentration after the infusion is stopped can be calculated by employing the following equation:

Eq. 7.93 $$(C_p)_{t'} = (C_p)_T e^{-Kt'}$$

where $(C_p)_{t'}$ is the plasma concentration at (t') following the cessation of infusion; $(C_p)_T$ is the plasma concentration at a time the infusion is stopped.

Because the time required to reach the steady state plasma drug concentration $(C_p)_{ss}$ will be quite long for a drug with a long elimination half-life, the administration of an intravenous loading dose (D_L) is often desired and convenient to attain the desired drug concentration immediately and then maintain this concentration by the continuous infusion. The loading dose (D_L) required to attain the desired drug concentration is calculated as follows:

Eq. 7.94 $$D_L = (C_p)_{ss} \cdot V$$

Eq. 7.95 $$D_L = \frac{Q}{K}$$

Using Equation 7.92 or 7.95, one can determine the infusion rate (Q) needed to maintain the plasma concentration obtained by the administration of the loading dose (D_L).

Repetitive Drug Administration: (Multiple Dosing)

If a fixed intravenous dose of a drug is administered repeatedly at a constant time interval (τ), the plasma concentration of a drug at any time may be calculated by the following expression:

Eq. 7.96 $$(C_p)_t = \frac{X_0}{V}\left(\frac{1 - e^{-nK\tau}}{1 - e^{-K\tau}}\right)e^{-Kt}$$

where n is the number of doses that have been administered, t is the time between t = 0 and t = (τ); (τ) is dosing interval; X_0 is the dose administered; V is the apparent volume of distribution of the drug and K is the elimination rate constant. At the plateau, Equation 7.96 reduces to:

Eq. 7.97 $$(C_p)_\infty = \frac{X_0}{V}\left(\frac{e^{-Kt}}{1 - e^{-K\tau}}\right)$$

where $(C_p)_\infty$, is the steady state plasma concentration.

The maximum plasma concentration of a drug (Fig. 7.30) at the steady state, $(C_p)_\infty$ max, and its minimum plasma concentration at the steady state, $(C_p)_\infty$ min, can be determined by setting t = 0 and t = ∞, respectively. Equation 7.97 then becomes:

Eq. 7.98 $$(C_p)_\infty \text{max} = \frac{X_0}{V}\left(\frac{1}{1 - e^{-K\tau}}\right)$$

and

Eq. 7.99 $$(C_p)_\infty \text{min} = \frac{X_0}{V}\left(\frac{1}{1 - e^{-K\tau}}\right)e^{-K\tau}$$

When drugs are administered as repetitive doses (multiple doses), it is often of practical use to determine the "average" plasma concentration at the plateau or steady state, $(C_p)_{ss}$ "average." This is obtained by:

Eq. 7.100 $$(C_p)_{ss} \text{ "average"} = \frac{(X_0)}{VK\tau}$$

$(C_p)_{ss}$ "average" plasma concentration of the drug at the steady state; (τ) is the dosing interval; (X_0) is the administered dose, and VK is its systemic clearance. Equation 7.100 clearly indicates by knowing the apparent volume of distribution and the elimination rate constant, obtained from the administration of a single intravenous bolus dose, the "average" plasma concentration of a drug can be predicted for the intravenous bolus administration of a fixed dose (X_0) at a constant dosing interval (τ). Additionally, Equation 7.100 also clearly indicates that only the size of the dose (X_0) and the dosing interval (τ) may be adjusted to obtain the desired "average" steady state plasma drug concentration.

It is important to recognize that the "average" steady state plasma drug concentration, $(C_p)_{ss}$ "average," is neither the arithmatic or geometric mean of $(C_p)_{oo}$ max and $(C_p)_{oo}$ min, but rather the ratio of the area under the plasma concen-

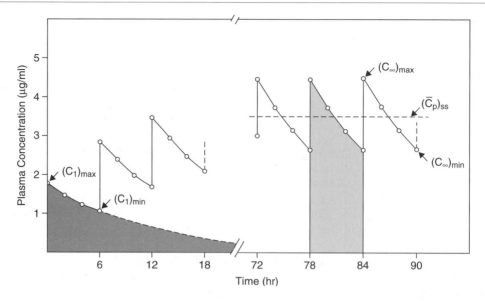

Fig. 7.30. Typical plasma concentration for a drug administered intravenously on a fixed dose and fixed dosing interval.

tration time curve during the dosing interval (τ) at the plateau over the dosing interval (τ). We know from Equation 7.76 that the ratio of a dose over systemic clearance (VK) equals the area under the plasma concentration time curve $(AUC)_0^\infty$. Therefore, substituting dose/clearance from Equation 7.76 into Equation 7.100 provides the following:

Eq. 7.101 $(C_p)_{ss} \text{ "average"} = \dfrac{(AUC)_0^\infty}{\tau}$

$(AUC)_0^\infty$ represents the area under the plasma drug concentration time curve following the administration of a single intravenous bolus dose.

When the drug is administered by oral route (Fig. 7.31), the mathematical expressions are more complicated than analogous equations for intravenous administration.

Eq. 7.102 $(C_p)_\infty = \dfrac{K_a F (X_a)_0}{V(K_a - K)} \left(\dfrac{e^{-Kt}}{1 - e^{-K\tau}} - \dfrac{e^{-K_a t}}{1 - e^{-K_a \tau}} \right)$

where $(Xa)_0$ is the dose administered; F is the fraction absorbed; K_a and K are the first order absorption and the elimination rate constants, respectively; V is the apparent volume of distribution; and t and τ are time and dosing intervals, respectively. Following the administration of each successive dose in the post absorption period, Equation 7.101 reduces to:

Eq. 7.103 $(C_p)_\infty \text{min} = \dfrac{K_a F (X_a)_0}{V(K_a - K)} \left(\dfrac{e^{-Kt}}{1 - e^{-K\tau}} \right)$

The "average" steady state plasma concentration of a drug when administered by an extravascular route can be obtained by employing the following equation:

Eq. 7.104 $(C_p)_{ss} \text{ "average"} = \dfrac{F(X_a)_0}{VK\tau}$

or by substituting Eq. 7.78 into Eq. 7.104, then

Eq. 7.105 $(C_p)_{ss} \text{ "average"} = \dfrac{(AUC)_0^\infty}{\tau}$

where F is the fraction absorbed or absolute bioavailability of a drug. Taking the ratio of Equations 7.104 and 7.100, following the attainment of the steady state condition, permits one to determine the bioavailability of a drug; of course, this assumes that the administered doses are identical.

Repeated administration of a fixed dose at a constant dosing interval (τ) produces a gradual increase of drug levels in the body until the steady state condition is attained. This increase is the result of drug accumulation (R) due to the sequential dosing of the drug. Therefore, predicting the degree of accumulation of a drug under defined conditions becomes important. Multiplying each side of Equation 7.100 by the apparent volume of distribution and divided by the administered dose, Equation 7.106 is obtained:

Eq. 7.106 $\dfrac{X_{ss} \text{ average}}{(X_0)} = \dfrac{1}{K\tau} = \dfrac{1.44 * t\frac{1}{2}}{\tau}$

where $\dfrac{X_{ss} \text{ average}}{X} = R = \text{Drug accumulated}$

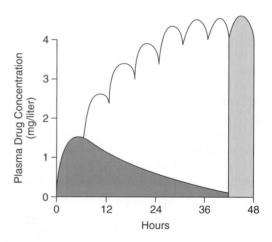

Fig. 7.31. Typical plasma concentration for a drug given orally on a fixed dose and fixed dosing interval.

where (X_{ss} "average" is the "average" amount of drug in the body at the steady state condition. The ratio of the "average" amount of a drug at its steady state and the administered dose is defined as drug accumulation (R). Equation 7.106 describes that the magnitude of drug accumulation is a function of the elimination half-life of a drug and the dosing interval chosen. For example, if a drug with an elimination half-life of 12 hours (i.e., K = 0.0577 hr^{-1}) is administered every 6 hours (τ), the ratio of $(X)_{ss}$ "average" over dose is 2.9. This means that repeated administration of a fixed dose of a drug in the body is about 2.9 times the amount administered in a single dose. It is also clear from Equation 7.106 that the drug accumulation ratio (R) is directly proportional to the elimination half-life of the drug ($t_{1/2}$), and inversely proportional to the dosing interval (τ); however, R is independent of the size of the administered dose.

Since considerable time may elapse before a steady state condition is attained as a result of repeated drug administration, it is often desirable to administer a large dose initially (i.e., initial loading dose, D_L) in order to achieve the desired drug levels immediately. Equation 7.36 which describes the time course of drug concentration after a single intravenous bolus dose may be written as:

Eq. 7.107
$$(C_p)_1 \min = \frac{X_0}{V} (e^{-K\tau})$$

where $(C_p)_1 \min$ is the drug concentration immediately prior to the administration of the second dose of the same size as the first one (i.e., the minimum concentration occurs at t = (τ) following the administration of the first dose). The minimum steady state plasma concentration, $(C_p)_{oo}$ is given by Equation 7.99. Thus, the ratio of $(C_p)_{oo} \min$ to $(C_p)_1 \min$ (i.e., Equation 7.99 and Equation 7.107) is another way to measure the drug accumulation (R). This ratio may be calculated by means of the expression:

Eq. 7.108
$$R = \frac{(C_p)_\infty \min}{(C_p)_1 \min} = \frac{1}{1 - e^{-K\tau}}$$

This ratio of minimum drug concentrations, numerically, is not equal to the ratio of "average" dose of a drug at steady state and the dose administered (Eq. 7.106).

If one wished to administer a loading dose (D_L) that produces the minimum concentration equal to $(C_p)_{oo} \min$:

Eq. 7.109
$$(C_p)_1 \min = (C_p)_\infty \min = \frac{D_L}{V} e^{-K\tau}$$

Dividing the Equation 7.99 by Equation 7.109 will result in:

Eq. 7.110
$$1 = \frac{D}{D_L(1 - e^{-K\tau})}$$

Equation 7.110, upon rearrangement, yields an expression to determine the loading dose (D_L):

Eq. 7.111
$$\frac{D_L}{D} = \frac{1}{(1 - e^{-K\tau})}$$

In Equations 7.110 and 7.111, D_L is the loading dose and D is the maintenance dose. Equation 7.111 permits the calculation of loading dose (D_L) for the chosen maintenance dose (D) and dosing interval (τ), and is applicable not only for the administration of a drug by intravenous bolus but also by the extravascular route. When a drug is administered by extravascular route, however, it is essential that each maintenance dose (D_L) be administered following the complete absorption of a drug from the previous dose. Conversely, Equation 7.111 also permits the determination of the maintenance dose (D) required to maintain the minimum drug level produced by the administration of the initial dose (D_L) for any chosen dosing interval (τ).

SUMMARY

From this discussion, the efficacy of a drug is not determined by its pharmacodynamic characteristics alone, but efficacy also depends to a large extent on the pharmacokinetic parameters of the drug since ADME processes control the rate and extent to which an administered dose of a drug reaches its site of action.

In light of a high degree of structural variability of drugs, multiplicity of kinetics and metabolite kinetics, the task of establishing a clear correlation between structured chemistry of substituents and their pharmacokinetic properties appear somewhat daunting. However, the pharmacokinetic fate of a drug molecule appears to be a consequence of its physical-chemical properties and may, therefore, to some extent, be predicted from its chemical structure.

Although medication in the formulation has received considerable attention, many of the alterations in the formulation may be considered as chemical changes. Most of what has been reported applies primarily to the gastrointestinal absorption of drugs and may be viewed as attempts to:

1. Maximize the rate of absorption by increasing dissolution rate (i.e., micronization, salt of acid or bases, amorphous form and metastable polymorph (etc.)
2. Decrease the loss of a drug due to its degradation in the stomach (i.e., acid, insoluble esters or salt and chemically stable derivatives of a drug)
3. Extend the duration of action by reducing the release rate of a drug from a dosage form such as timed release, depot forming injectable, macro crystals and slowly dissolving salts, and
4. Decrease the loss of a drug by reducing the complex formation.

These examples for enhancing gastrointestinal absorption represent the response to a particular problem with the parent compound and, therefore, may be viewed as "corrective" research. It is of considerable interest to see this aspect of research become "predictive and preventive" where pharmacokinetic parameters of drugs are required in the early phases of drug design to optimize the effectiveness of drugs.

An immediate problem facing those who would consider optimizing all factors of a drug is physically locating the receptor site and defining the ideal time course for the drug-receptor interaction, sustained effects, etc. An ideal drug molecule should reach the site of action, arrive rapidly in sufficient quantity, remain at the site of action for sufficient time, be excluded from other sites and be removed from the site, when appropriate. However, such an ideal drug molecule rarely exists and alternate available approaches are chosen to optimize the effectiveness of a drug. Furthermore, if there is a correlation between a biologic response and the blood levels of a drug in the biological fluid then the pharmacokinetic parameters will play an important role in influencing the biologic response since these parameters influence the magnitude of blood level of a drug in the body. While the task of examining the examples of drugs illustrating the connection between biologic response and pharmacokinetics study is not an easy one, the results do convey the important facts that:

1. Pharmacokinetic parameters influence the biological responses, which are critical in drug design and
2. Pharmacokinetic parameters can be modified by subtle structural change, which, in turn, may influence the blood level desired.

The ultimate goal is to design a drug molecule, which exhibits the desired pharmacologic effect as a result of the proper balance of ADME processes. Figure 7-32 illustrates how modification of a parent structure can influence the availability of a drug to the receptor site.

The following are some of the processes in Figure 7.32 that may be altered by changing a substituent group on the drug molecule:

I. Supply and loss:
   A) Rate of transfer from the dosage form.
   B) Binding of a drug in the depot and
   C) Stability of a drug in the depot.
II. Distribution in the body:
   A) Binding of a drug in the central and peripheral compartments.
   B) Apparent volume of distribution and
   C) Transfer of a drug to the receptor sites.
III. Drug-receptor interaction.

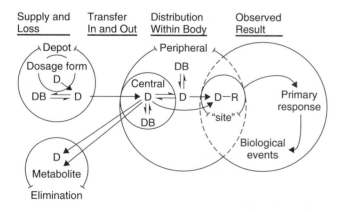

Fig. 7.32. Scheme illustrates how some of the processes can be altered by changing a substituent group on a drug molecule (27).

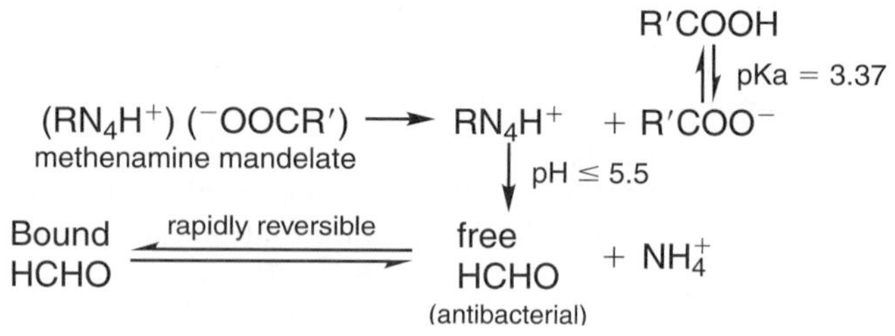

$$(RN_4H^+)(\,^-OOCR') \longrightarrow RN_4H^+ + R'COO^-$$

R'COOH, pKa = 3.37

pH ≤ 5.5

Bound HCHO ⇌ (rapidly reversible) free HCHO + NH_4^+

(antibacterial)

Fig. 7.33. Conversion of methenamine to formaldehyde in acidic pH.

Consider the following well-known example for the design of a urinary tract antieffective. The site of infection is the urinary tract. The example selected is the pro-drug, methenamine. In acidic pH, methenamine is converted to formaldehyde, which acts as an antibacterial agent (Fig. 7.33). Tablets of methenamine are often enteric coated to prevent conversion to formaldehyde in the stomach. Methenamine is cleared intact from the kidney into the urine where it is hydrolyzed to formaldehyde if the pH is less than 3.5. The rate of hydrolysis is controlled by the urinary pH.

The influence of structural effects on pharmacokinetic parameters can be illustrated by using the following examples. The steady state levels of the antibiotic, carbenicillin are known to be twice that of ampicillin. These higher blood levels of carbenicillin, following intravenous administration, have been attributed to its efficacy in the treatment of relatively resistant infections such as Pseudomonas. The reason for these differences in the higher steady state plasma concentration is the larger apparent volume of distribution for ampicillin since the elimination rate constants are similar. If all the factors were equal, one may argue that an increased value for the apparent volume of distribution is a clinical advantage since bacteria germinate more frequently in the tissue than in the blood. An antibiotic's effectiveness depends upon its penetration into tissues, particularly inflamed tissue. Thus, if plasma protein binding is equal for both antibiotics, the antibiotic with a larger volume of distribution would appear to be reaching the site of action with better efficacy, though this is by no means unequivocal. Therefore, the spectrum of research activity in the area of antibiotics would imply that the following goals for molecular modifications are generally pursued as: 1) increased tissue distribution, 2) longer half-life to maintain a higher blood level and decrease the frequency of dose administration, and 3) decreased binding capacity to foods and plasma protein, etc.

The author would like to acknowledge the assistance of Mr. Mukur Gupta in preparing this chapter.

REFERENCES
1. Ariens EJ. Intrinsic Activity: Partial Agonists and Partial Antagonists. J Cardiovasc Pharmacol 1983; 5: S8–S15.
2. Venter JC, Fraser CM. Mechanism of Action and Regulation. In: Kito S, Segawa T, Kuriyama K, ed. Neurotransmitter Receptors. New York. New York. Plenum Press, 1984.

3. Lefkowitz RJ, Stadel JM, Caron MG. Adenylate Cyclase-coupled Beta-adrenergic Receptors: Structure and Mechanisms of Activation and Desensitization. Ann Rev Biochem 1983; 52: 159–186.

4. Florence AT and Attwood D. Physiochemical Principles of Pharmacy; 2nd ed. New York. NY 10001. Chapman and Hall, 1988.

5. Schanker LS. J Pharmacol Exp Therap 1959; 126: 283–294.

6. Wagner JG. Biopharmaceutics and Relevant Pharmacokinetics, 1st ed. Hamilton, IL. The Hamilton Press, 1971.

7. Shore PA, Brodie BB, Hogben CAM. The Gastric Secretion of Drugs: A pH Partition Hypothesis. J Pharmacol Exp Therap 1957; 119: 361–369.

8. Hogben CAM, Tocco DJ, Brodie BB, et al. On the Mechanism of Intestinal Absorption of Drugs. J Pharmacol Exp Therap 1959; 125: 275–282.

9. Schanker LS. On the Mechanism of Absorption of Drugs from the Gastrointestinal Tract. J Med Pharm Chem 1960; 2: 343–359.

10. Schanker LS. Mechanism of Drug Absorption and Distribution. Ann Rev Pharmacol 1961; 1: 29–44.

11. Schanker LS. Passage of Drugs Across the Gastrointestinal Epithelium in Drugs and Membrane. In: Hogben CAM, ed. Proceedings of the First International Pharmacology Meeting vol 4. New York: The Macmillan Company, 1963.

12. Schanker LS. Physiological Transport of Drug. In: Harper NJ and Simons AB, ed. Advances in Drug Research; London: Academic Press, 1966.

13. Rowland M and Tozer T. Clinical Pharmacokinetics: Concepts and Application 2nd ed. Philadelphia: Lea and Febiger, 1989.

14. Schanker LS. Absorption of Drugs from the Rat Small Intestine. J Pharmacol Exp Therap 1958; 128: 81–87.

15. Zimmerman JJ, Feldman S. Physical-Chemical Properties and Biologic Activity. In: Foye WO, ed. Principles of Medicinal Chemistry, 3rd ed. Philadelphia: Lea and Febiger, 1988.

16. Foltz EL. Clinical Pharmacology of Pivampicillin. Antimicrob Agents Chemotherap 1970: 442–454.

17. Winne D. The Influence of Unstirred Layers on Intestinal Absorption In Intestinal Permeation Workshop Conference Hoechest vol 4. In: Kramer M and Lauterbach F, ed. Excerpta Medica International Congress series #391. Amsterdam-Oxford, 1977: 58–64.

18. Levy G, Leonard JR, Procknal JA. Development of In Vitro Dissolution Tests Which Correlate Quantitatively With Dissolution Rate Limited Absorption. J Pharm Sci 1965; 54: 1319–1325.

19. Noyes NA, Whitney WR. The Rate of Solution of Solid Substances in their own Solution. J Am Chem Soc 1897; 19: 930–942.

20. Gibaldi M. Biopharmaceutics and Clinical Pharmacokinetics. 4th ed. Philadelphia: Lea and Febiger, 1991.

21. Ogata H, Shibazoki T, Inoue T, et al. Studies on Dissolution Tests of Solid Dosage Forms. IV. Relation of Absorption Sites of Sulfonamides Administered Orally in Solid Dosage Forms to Their Solubilities and Dissolution Rates. Chem Pharm Bull 1979; 27: 1281–1286.

22. Pottage A, Nimmo J, Prescott LF. The Absorption of Aspirin and Paracetamol in Patients with Achlorhydria. J Pharm Pharmacol 1974; 26: 144.

23. Juncher H, Raaschou F. Solubility of Oral Preparation of Penicillin V. Antibiotic Med 1957; 4: 497.

24. Anderson KW. Oral Absorption of Quinalbarbitone and its Sodium Salt. Arch Int Pharmacodyn Therap 1964; 147: 171.

25. Nelson E. Comparative Dissolution Rates of Weak Acids and Their Sodium Salts. J Am Pharm Assoc (Sci. Ed.) 1958; 47: 297.

26. Ehrnebo M, Boreus L, Lonroth U. Bioavailability and First-Pass Metabolism of Oral Pentazocine in Man. Clin Pharmacol Therap 1977; 22, 888.

27. Notari R. Pharmacokinetics and Molecular Modification: Implications in Drug Design and Evaluation. J Pharm Sci 1973; 62 (6), 865–881.

SUGGESTED READINGS

Ganellin C, Roberts S. eds. Medicinal Chemistry: The role of organic chemistry in drug research. 2nd ed. New York: Academic Press, 1993.

Garrett E. Classical Pharmacokinetics to Frontiers. J Pharmacokin Biopharm 1973; 1 (5), 341–361.

Gibaldi M. Biopharmaceutics and Clinical Pharmacokinetics. 4th ed. Philadelphia: Lea and Febiger, 1991.

Gibaldi M, Perrier D. Pharmacokinetics, 2nd ed., Volume 15. Drugs and the Pharmaceutical Sciences. New York: Marcel Dekker, Inc., 1982.

Hug C. Pharmacokinetics of Drugs Administered Intravenously. Anesth. Analg 1978; 57, 704–723.

Rowland M, Tozer T. Clinical Pharmacokinetics: Concepts and Application. 3rd ed. Philadelphia: Lea and Febiger, 1994.

Taylor J, Kennewell P. Modern Medicinal Chemistry, Ellis Horwood Series in Pharmaceutical Technology. New York: Ellis Horwood, 1993.

Wagner J. A Modern View of Pharmacokinetics. J Pharmacokin Biopharm 1973; 1 (5), 363–401.

Wagner J. Do You Need a Pharmacokinetic Model, and, If So, Which One? J Pharmacokin Biopharm 1975; 3 (6), 457–478.

Welling P. Pharmacokinetics: Processes and Mathematics. Monograph 185. Washington DC: American Chemical Society, 1986.

Wermuth C, Koga N, Konig H, et al. Medicinal Chemistry for the 21st Century. IUPAC. Boston: Blackwell Scientific Publications, 1992.

8. Drug Metabolism

DAVID A. WILLIAMS

INTRODUCTION

Humans are exposed throughout their lifetime to a large variety of drugs and nonessential exogenous (foreign) compounds (collectively referred to as *xenobiotics*) that may pose health hazards. Drugs taken for therapeutic purposes as well as occupational or private exposure to the vapors of volatile chemicals or solvents pose possible health risks; smoking and drinking involve the absorption of large amounts of substances with potential adverse health effects. Furthermore, the ingestion of natural toxins in vegetables and fruits, pesticide residues in food, as well as carcinogenic pyrolysis products from fats and protein formed during the charbroiling of meat have to be considered. Most of these xenobiotics undergo enzymatic biotransformations by xenobiotic-metabolizing enzymes in the liver and extrahepatic tissues, and are eliminated by excretion as hydrophilic metabolites. In some cases, especially during oxidative metabolism, numerous chemical procarcinogens form reactive metabolites capable of covalent binding to biopolymers such as proteins or nucleic acids—critical components which can lead to mutagenicity, cytotoxicity, and carcinogenicity. Therefore, insight into the biotransformation and bioactivation of xenobiotics becomes an indisputable prerequisite for the assessment of drug safety and risk estimation of chemicals and drugs.

Detoxication and toxic effects of drugs and other xenobiotics have been studied extensively in various mammalian species. Frequently, differences in sensitivity to these toxic effects were observed and can now be attributed to genetic differences between species in the isoenzyme/isoforms of cytochrome P450 monooxygenases (CYP450). The level of expression of the CYP450 enzymes is regulated by genetics and a variety of endogenous factors such as hormones, gender, age, disease, and the presence of environmental factors such as inducing agents. Drugs were developed and prescribed under the old paradigm that "one dose fits all" which largely ignores the fact that humans (adults and children) are genetically and metabolically different, resulting in a variable response to drugs.

Drugs can no longer be regarded as chemically stable entities that elicit the desired pharmacologic response and then are excreted from the body. Drugs undergo a variety of chemical changes in humans by enzymes of the liver, intestine, kidney, lung, and other tissues, with subsequent alterations in the nature of their pharmacologic activity, duration of activity, and toxicity. Thus, the pharmacologic and toxicologic activity of a drug (or xenobiotic) is in many ways the consequence of its metabolism.

Drug therapy is becoming oriented more to controlling metabolic, genetic, and environmental illnesses (such as cardiovascular disease, mental illness, cancer, and diabetes) rather than to short-term therapy. In most of these cases, drug therapy lasts for months or even years and the problem of drug toxicity from long-term therapy has become increasingly important.

The practice of prescribing several drugs simultaneously is commonplace, thus an awareness of possible drug-drug interactions is essential to avoid catastrophic synergistic effects and chemical, enzymic, and pharmacokinetic interactions that may produce toxic side effects.

The study of xenobiotic metabolism has developed rapidly during the past few decades (1–3). These studies have been fundamental in the assessment of drug efficacy, safety, and the design of dosage regimens; in the development of food additives and the assessment of potential hazards of contaminants; in the evaluation of toxic chemicals; and in the development of pesticides and herbicides and their metabolic fate in insects, other animals, and plants. The metabolism of drugs and other xenobiotics is fundamental to many toxic processes such as carcinogenesis, teratogenesis, and tissue necrosis. Often, the same enzymes involved in drug metabolism also carry out the regulation and metabolism of endogenous substances. The inhibition and induction of these enzymes by drugs and xenobiotics may consequently have a profound effect on the normal processes of intermediary metabolism, such as tissue growth and development, hemopoiesis, calcification, and lipid metabolism.

Familiarity with the mechanisms of drug metabolism can often predict the consequences of drug-drug interactions, drug-food interactions and herbal-drug–drug interactions to explain a patient's adverse responses to drug regimens. Incorporating pharmacogenomics into the selection of drug regimens will change the way in which drugs are chosen for patients. Selection based on the patient's individual genetic makeup could eliminate the unpredictable response of drug treatment due to genetic polymorphisms that effects metabolism, clearance and tolerance. Pharmacogenomic testing to predict a patient's phenotype (i.e., poor metabolizer) and thus their ability to metabolize drugs will become commonplace in the future. Armed with such knowledge, improved selection of proper drug regimen and dose can be assured prior to beginning therapy.

The increased knowledge of drug metabolism, fed by the need for greater safety evaluation of drugs and chemicals, has resulted in a proliferation of publications and a series of monographs that present the current state of knowledge of foreign compound metabolism from biochemical and pharmacologic viewpoints (2–3).

PATHWAYS OF METABOLISM

Drugs, plant toxins, food additives, environmental chemicals, insecticides, and other chemicals foreign to the body undergo enzymic transformations that usually result in the loss of pharmacologic activity. The term detoxication describes the result of such metabolic changes. Although drug metabolism usually leads to detoxication, the processes of oxidation, reduction, glucuronidation, sulfation, and other enzyme-catalyzed reactions may lead to the formation of a metabolite having therapeutic or toxic effects. This process is often referred to as bioactivation. One of the earliest examples of bioactivation was the reduction of Prontosil to the antibacterial agent sulfanilamide. Other examples of drug metabolism leading to therapeutically active drugs include the hydroxylation of acetanilid to acetaminophen, and the N-demethylation of the antidepressant imipramine to desipramine and the anxiolytic diazepam to desmethyldiazepam. The insecticide parathion is desulfurized by both insects and mammals to paraoxon.

Most drugs and other xenobiotics are metabolized by enzymes normally associated with the metabolism of endogenous constituents, e.g., steroids and biogenic amines. The liver is the major site of drug metabolism, although other xenobiotic-metabolizing enzymes are found in nervous tissue, kidney, lung, plasma, and the gastrointestinal tract (digestive secretions, bacterial flora, and the intestinal wall).

Although hepatic metabolism continues to be the most important route of metabolism for xenobiotics and drugs, other biotransformation pathways play a significant role in the metabolism of these substances. Among the more active extrahepatic tissues capable of metabolizing drugs are the intestinal mucosa, kidney, and lung (see Extrahepatic Metabolism). The ability of the liver and extrahepatic tissues to metabolize substances to either pharmacologically inactive or bioactive metabolites before reaching systemic blood levels is called *first pass metabolism or the presystemic first pass effect.* Other metabolism reactions occurring in the gastrointestinal tract are associated with the bacterial and other microflora of the tract. The bacterial flora can affect metabolism through the: 1) production of toxic metabolites, 2) formation of carcinogens from inactive precursors, 3) detoxication, 4) exhibition of species differences in drug metabolism, 5) exhibition of individual differences in drug metabolism, 6) production of pharmacologically active metabolites from inactive precursors, and 7) production of metabolites not formed by animal tissues.

Phase 1 Reactions

The pathways of xenobiotic metabolism are divided into two major categories. Phase 1 reactions (biotransfor-mations) include oxidation, hydroxylation, reduction, and hydrolysis. In these enzymatic reactions, a new functional group is introduced into the substrate molecule, an existing functional group is modified, or a functional group or acceptor site for phase 2 transfer reactions is exposed, thus making the xenobiotic more polar and therefore more readily excreted.

Phase 2 Reactions

Phase 2 reactions (conjugation) are enzymatic syntheses whereby a functional group such as alcohol, phenol, amine, is masked by the addition of a new group, for example, acetyl, sulfate, glucuronic acid, or certain amino acids, which further increases the polarity of the drug or xenobiotic. Most substances undergo both phase 1 and phase 2 reactions, sequentially.

Those xenobiotics that are resistant to metabolizing enzymes or are already hydrophilic are excreted largely unchanged. This basic pattern of xenobiotic metabolism is common to all animal species, including man, but species may differ in details of the reaction and enzyme control.

Factors Affecting Metabolism

As indicated earlier, drug therapy is becoming oriented more to controlling metabolic, genetic, and environmental illnesses than to short-term therapy associated with infectious diseases. In most cases, drug therapy lasts for months or even years and the problems of drug-drug interactions and chronic toxicity from long-term drug therapy has become more serious. Therefore, a greater knowledge of drug metabolism is essential. Several factors influencing xenobiotic metabolism include:

1. **Genetic factors.** Individual differences in drug effectiveness (drug sensitivity or drug resistance), drug interactions and drug toxicity may depend on racial and ethnic characteristics with the population frequencies of the many polymorphic genes and the expression of the metabolizing enzymes. Pharmacogenetics focuses primarily on genetic polymorphisms (mutations) responsible for interindividual differences in drug metabolism and disposition (4). Genotype-phenotype correlation studies have validated that inherited mutations result in two or more distinct phenotypes causing very different responses following drug administration. The genes encoding for CYP2A6, CYP2C9, CYP2C19 and CYP2D6 are functionally polymorphic, therefore at least 30% of CYP450 dependent metabolism is performed by polymorphic enzymes. For example, mutations in the CYP2D6 gene, result in poor, intermediate, or ultra-rapid metabolizers of more than 30 cardiovascular and CNS drugs. Thus, each of these phenotypic subgroups experience different responses to drugs extensively metabolized by the CYP2D6 pathway ranging from severe toxicity to complete lack of efficacy. For example, ethnic specificity has been observed with the sensitivity of the Japanese and Chinese to ethanol as compared to the Caucasians; CYP2C19 polymorphism (affects about 20% Asians and 3% Caucasians) and the variable metabolism of

omeprazole (proton pump inhibitor) and antiseizure drugs; and the polymorphic paraoxonase (PON1) catalyzed hydrolysis of the neurotoxic organophosphates and of lipid peroxides (atherosclerosis) (see section on Genetic Polymorphism in this chapter).

Incorporating pharmacogenomics, the study of heritable traits affecting patient response to drug treatment, into drug therapy will alter the way in which drug regimens are chosen for patients based on their individual genetic makeup (4); thus, eliminating the unpredictable response of drug treatment due to genetic polymorphisms that effect metabolism, clearance and tolerance. Understanding how individuals are genetically predisposed to differences in metabolism risk may result in new classes of drugs that are metabolized by non-polymorphic CYP450 enzymes.

2. **Physiologic factors.** Age is a factor because the very young and the old have impaired metabolism. Hormones (including those induced by stress), sex differences, pregnancy, changes in the intestinal microflora, diseases (especially those involving the liver), and nutritional status can also influence drug and xenobiotic metabolism.

Because the liver is the principal site for xenobiotic and drug metabolism, liver disease can modify the pharmacokinetics of drugs metabolized by the liver (5,6). Several factors identified as major determinants of the metabolism of a drug in the diseased liver are the nature and extent of liver damage, hepatic blood flow, the drug involved, the dosage regimen, and the degree of participation of the liver in the pharmacokinetics of the drug. Liver disease affects the elimination half-life of some drugs but not of others, although all undergo hepatic biotransformation (Table 8.1). Some results have shown that the capacity for drug metabolism is impaired in chronic liver disease, which could lead to drug overdosage. Consequently, because of the unpredictability of drug effects in the presence of liver disorders, drug therapy under these circumstances is complex, and more than the usual caution is needed (6).

Table 8.1. The Effect of Liver Disease in Humans on the Elimination Half-Life of Various Drugs

Difference Reported	No Difference Reported
Acetaminophen*	Chlorpromazine
Amylbarbital	Dicoumarol
Carbenicillin	Phenytoin
Chloramphenicol	Phenylbutazone
Clindamycin	Salicylic Acid
Diazepam	Tobutamide
Hexobarbital	
Isoniazid	
Lidocaine	
Meperidine	
Meprobamate	
Pentobarbital	
Phenobarbital	
Prednisone	
Rifamycin	
Tolbutamide	
Theophylline	

*Drug for which clearance is disputable but may be increased.

Substances influencing drug and xenobiotic metabolism (other than enzyme inducers) include lipids, proteins, vitamins, and metals. Dietary lipid and protein deficiencies diminish microsomal drug metabolizing activity. Protein deficiency leads to a reduction in hepatic microsomal protein and lipid deficiency; oxidative metabolism is decreased because of an alteration in endoplasmic reticulum membrane permeability affecting electron transfer. In terms of toxicity, protein deficiency would increase the toxicity of drugs and xenobiotics by reducing their oxidative microsomal metabolism and clearance from the body.

3. **Pharmacodynamic factors.** Dose, frequency, and route of administration, plus tissue distribution and protein binding of the drug, affect its metabolism.

4. **Environmental factors.** Competition of ingested environmental substances with other drugs and xenobiotics for the metabolizing enzymes and poisoning of enzymes by toxic chemicals, such as carbon monoxide or pesticide synergists, alter metabolism. Induction of enzyme expression (the number of enzyme molecules increased but activity is constant) by other drugs and xenobiotics is another consideration.

Such factors may change not only the kinetics of an enzyme reaction, but also the whole pattern of metabolism, thereby altering the bioavailability, pharmacokinetics, pharmacologic activity or the toxicity of a xenobiotic. Species differences in response to xenobiotics must be considered in the extrapolation of pharmacologic and toxicologic data from experiments in animals to humans. The primary factors in these differences are probably the rate and pattern of drug and xenobiotic metabolism in the various species.

DRUG BIOTRANSFORMATION PATHWAY (PHASE 1)
Human Hepatic Cytochrome P450 Enzyme System
Introduction

Oxidation is probably the most common reaction in xenobiotic metabolism. This reaction is catalyzed by a group of membrane-bound monooxygenases found in the smooth endoplasmic reticulum of the liver and other extrahepatic tissues, called the cytochrome P450 monooxygenase enzyme system (7) (*the abbreviation CYP450 will be used for this enzyme system*). CYP450 has also been called a mixed-function oxidase (MFO) or microsomal hydroxylase. The tissue homogenate fraction containing the smooth endoplasmic reticulum is called the microsomal fraction. CYP450 functions as a multicomponent electron-transport system responsible for the oxidative metabolism of a variety of endogenous substrates (such as the steroids, fatty acids, prostaglandins, and bile acids), and exogenous substances (xenobiotics) including drugs, carcinogens, insecticides, plant toxins, environmental pollutants, and other foreign chemicals. Central to the functioning of this unique superfamily of heme proteins is a iron-protoporphyrin. The iron-protoporphyrin is coordinated to the

Table 8.2. Hydroxylation Mechanisms Catalyzed by CYP450

Aromatic hydroxylation

$$CH_3CO-N-C_6H_5 \xrightarrow{[OH]} CH_3CO-N-C_6H_4-OH$$
$$\quad\quad\quad\; H \quad\quad\quad\quad\quad\quad\quad\quad\quad H$$

Aliphatic hydroxylation

$$R-CH_3 \xrightarrow{[OH]} R-CH_2-OH$$

Deamination

$$R-CH(NH_2)-CH_3 \xrightarrow{[OH]} (R-C(OH)(NH_2)-CH_3) \longrightarrow R-CO-CH_3 + CH_2O$$

O-Dealkylation

$$R-O-CH_3 \xrightarrow{[OH]} (R-O-CH_2-OH) \longrightarrow R-OH + CH_2O$$

N-Dealkylation

$$R-N(CH_3)_2 \xrightarrow{[OH]} (R-N(CH_2OH)(CH_3)) \longrightarrow R-NH-CH_3 + CH_2O$$

$$R-NH-CH_3 \xrightarrow{[OH]} (R-NH-CH_2OH) \longrightarrow R-NH_2 + CH_2O$$

N-Oxidation

$$(CH_3)_3-N \xrightarrow{[OH]} ((CH_3)_3-NOH) \longrightarrow (CH_3)_3-NO + H^+$$

Sulfoxidation

$$R-S-R' \xrightarrow{[OH]} (R-\underset{OH}{S}-R') \longrightarrow R-\underset{O}{S}-R' + H^+$$

sulfur of cysteine and has the ability to form a complex with carbon monoxide, the result of which is a complex which has its major absorption band at 450 nm (thus the title of these metabolizing enzymes CYP450). CYP450 has an absolute requirement for NADPH (reduced form of nicotinamide adenine dinucleotide phosphate) and molecular oxygen (dioxygen). The rate at which various compounds are metabolized by this system depends on the species, strain, nutritional status, tissue, age, and pretreatment of the animals. The variety of reactions catalyzed by CYP450 include (Table 8.2): the oxidation of alkanes and aromatic compounds; the epoxidation of alkenes, polycyclic hydrocarbons, and halogenated benzenes; the dealkylation of secondary and tertiary amines and ethers; the deamination of amines; the conversion of amines to N-oxides, hydroxylamine, and nitroso derivatives, and dehalogenation of halogenated hydrocarbons. It also catalyzes the oxidative cleavage of organic thiophosphate esters, the sulfoxidation of some thioethers, the conversion of phosphothionates to the phosphate derivatives, and the reduction of azo and nitro compounds to primary aromatic amines.

The most important function of CYP450 is its ability to "activate" molecular oxygen (dioxygen), permitting the incorporation of one atom of oxygen into an organic sub-

strate molecule concomitant with the reduction of the other atom of oxygen to water. The introduction of a hydroxyl group into the hydrophobic substrate molecule provides a site for subsequent conjugation with hydrophilic compounds (Phase 2), thereby increasing the aqueous solubility of the product for its transport and excretion from the organism. This enzyme system not only catalyzes xenobiotic transformations in ways that usually lead to detoxication, but in some cases, in ways that lead to products having greater cytotoxic, mutagenic, or carcinogenic properties. A nonheme, microsomal flavoprotein monooxygenase is responsible for the oxidation of certain nitrogen and sulfur-containing organic compounds.

Components of CYP450

CYP450 consists of at least two protein components: a heme protein called cytochrome P450 and a flavoprotein called NADPH-CYP450 reductase containing both flavin mononucleotide (FMN) and flavin dinucleotide (FAD). CYP450 is the substrate- and oxygen-binding site of the enzyme system, whereas the reductase serves as an electron carrier, shuttling electrons from NADPH to CYP450. A third component essential for electron transport from NADPH to CYP450 is a phospholipid, phosphatidylcholine that facilitates the transfer of electrons from NADPH-CYP450 reductase to CYP450 (7). Although the phospholipid does not function in the system as an electron carrier, it has great influence upon the CYP450 monooxygenase system. The phospholipid makes up about 1/3 of the hepatic endoplasmic reticulum and contributes to a negatively charged environment at neutral pH.

Of the three components involved in microsomal oxidative xenobiotic metabolism, CYP450 is important because of its vital role in oxygen activation and substrate binding. CYP450 is an integral membrane protein deeply imbedded in the membrane matrix. The environment surrounding the enzyme is negatively charged at neutral pH due to the phospholipids. The electron components of CYP450 are located on the cytoplasmic side of the endoplasmic reticulum, and the hydrophobic active site towards the lumen of the endoplasmic reticulum (8). The active site of CYP450 consists of a hydrophobic substrate-binding domain in which is imbedded an iron protoporphyrin (heme) prosthetic group. This group is exactly like that of hemoglobin, peroxidase, and the b-type cytochromes. The iron in the iron-protoporphyrin is coordinated with four nitrogens via a tetradentate to the porphyrin ring. X-ray studies reveal that in the ferric state the two non-porphyrin ligands are water and cysteine (Fig. 8.1). The cysteine thiolate ligand (proximal) is present in all states of the enzyme and is absolutely essential for the formation of the reactive oxenoid intermediate. The sixth (distal) coordination position is occupied by an easily exchangeable ligand, most likely water, which is labile and easily exchanged for stronger ligands such as cyanide, amines, imidazoles, and pyridines. The ferrous form loses the water ligand com-

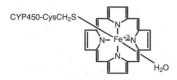

Fig. 8.1. Ferric heme thiolate catalytic center of CYP450. The porphyrin side chains are deleted for clarity.

pletely, leaving the sixth position open for binding ligands such as oxygen and carbon monoxide.

The vast array of xenobiotics presents a unique challenge to the human body to metabolize these lipophilic foreign compounds, and makes it impractical to have one enzyme for each compound or each class of compounds. Therefore, whereas most cellular functions are usually very specific, xenobiotic oxidation requires CYP450s with diverse substrate specificities and regioselectivities (multiple sites of oxidation). Several types of CYP450 enzymes can be found in a single species of animal. For example, the rat has more than 40 different CYP450 genes, each coding for a different version of the enzyme (isoform) that can metabolize almost any lipophilic compound to which they are exposed.

Classification of the CYP450 Multigene Family

Nebert classified the CYP450 supergene family on the basis of their structural (evolutionary) relationships (9). The CYP450 monooxygenases resulting from this supergene family have been subdivided into families with greater than 40% amino acid homology and subfamilies with greater than 55% homology (9). CYP450s are named using the root symbol CYP (CYtochrome P450), followed by an Arabic numeral designating the family member (CYP1, CYP2, CYP3, etc.), a letter denoting the subfamily (CYP1A, CYP2C, CYP2D, CYP2E), and another Arabic numeral representing the individual gene. Names of genes are written in italics. The nomenclature system is based solely on sequence similarity among the CYP450s and does not indicate the properties or function of individual P450s. Of the over 17 CYP450 isoforms that have been identified to date, the major isoforms responsible for drug metabolism in the liver are presented in Figure 8.2 (10). It

is quite evident that the CYP3A and CYP2C families are the isoforms most involved in the metabolism of clinically relevant drugs, and the CYP1A2 isoform is predominantly involved in the bioactivation of environmental substances.

CYP450s probably evolved initially for the regulation of endogenous substances, such as metabolizing cholesterol to maintain membrane integrity and for steroid biosynthesis and metabolism, rather than for metabolizing foreign compounds. The CYP450s are either involved in highly specific steroid hydroxylations located in the inner mitochondrial membrane or bound to the endoplasmic reticulum of the cell having broad substrate specificity. In evolutionary terms, CYP450s evolved from a common ancestor and only more recently (during the last 100 million years) have CYP450 genes taken on the role of producing enzymes for metabolizing a vast array of lipophilic foreign compounds. The emergence of the xenobiotic-CYP450 genes probably evolved from the steroidogenic CYP450s for enhancing animal survival by synthesizing new CYP450s for metabolizing plant toxins in the food chain. It is not surprising that animals and humans possess a large array of diverse CYP450 enzymes capable of handling a multitude of xenobiotics. Interindividual variation in the expression of xenobiotic-CYP450 genes (genetic polymorphism) or their inducibility may be associated with differences, for example, in individual susceptibility to cigarette smoke carcinogenesis. Certain CYP450 isoforms that clearly exhibit genetic polymorphism are known to metabolize and generally inactivate therapeutic agents. The extent of CYP450 polymorphisms in humans is being investigated to determine the risk or protection against cancer. Food mutagens are typically carcinogens in tissue, but they are activated by CYP1A2 in the liver and CYP3A. Specific forms of CYP450 in hepatic microsomes are regulated by hormones (e.g., CYP3A subfamily), and are induced or inhibited by drugs, food toxins, and other environmental xenobiotics (see the section on induction and inhibition of cytochrome P450 isoforms). Identification of a specific CYP450 isoform as the major form responsible for metabolism of a drug in humans permits reconciliation of its toxicity or other pharmacologic effects.

Substrate Specificity

No evidence exists that the active oxygenating species differ between CYP450s, suggesting the substrate specificities, substrate affinity, regioselectivity, and rates of reaction are probably a consequence of topographic features of the active site of apoproteins (7,8,11). Because a primary function of these enzymes is the metabolism of hydrophobic substrates, it is likely that hydrophobic forces are important in the binding of many substrates to the apoproteins. Nonspecific binding is consistent with the multiple substrate orientations in the active site necessary for the broad regioselectivities observed. A specific binding requirement would decrease the diversity of substrates. Some CYP450 isoforms have constrained binding sites and thus metabolize small

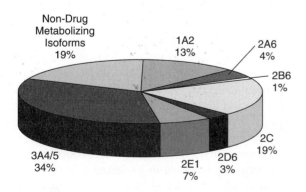

Fig. 8.2. Total human P450 isoforms expressed in the liver that metabolize drugs.

The Other CYP450 Isoforms

The other CYP450 isoforms catalyzing the oxidation of steroids, bile acids, fat-soluble vitamins and other endogenous substances include CYP4, arachidonic acid or fatty acid metabolism; CYP5, thromboxane A2 synthase converts arachidonic acid into thromboxane A2 which causes platelet aggregation; CYP7A, 7 α-hydroxylase catalyzes the rate-determining step in the biosynthesis of bile acids from cholesterol; CYP7B brain specific form of 7 α-hydroxylase catalyzing the synthesis of the neurosteroids, 7 α-hydroxy dehydroepiandrosterone and 7 α-hydroxy pregnenolone; CYP8A prostacyclin synthase catalyzes the synthesis of prostaglandin I₂ and the regulation of hemostasis that opposes CYP5; CYP8B, 12 α-hydroxylase in bile acid biosynthesis; CYP11A1, the first step in mitochondrial steroid biosynthesis that oxidatively cleaves the 17 side chain of cholesterol to pregnenolone, defects in this enzyme lead to a lack of glucocorticoids, feminization and hypertension; CYP11B1, a mitochondrial 11-beta hydroxylase that hydroxylates 11-deoxycortisol to hydrocortisone or 11-deoxycorticosterone to corticosterone; CYP11B2, mitochondrial aldosterone synthase that hydroxylates corticosterone at the 18 position to aldosterone; CYP17, 17-alpha hydroxylase and 17-20 lyase (two enzymes in one) are required for production of testosterone and estrogen (lack of this enzyme affects sexual development at puberty); CYP19, aromatase, catalyzes the aromatization of ring A of testosterone to estrogen (lack of this enzyme causes an estrogen deficiency and failure of females to develop at puberty); CYP21, C21 steroid hydroxylase (lack of this enzyme prevents cortisol synthesis, diverting excess 17-hydroxy progesterone into overproduction of testosterone biosynthesis); CYP24, mitochondrial 25–hydroxyvitamin D3 24-hydroxylase for the degradation/inactivation of vitamin D metabolites; CYP26A1, all-trans-retinoic acid hydroxylase, may be involved in terminating the retinoic acid signal and thus turning off a developmental switch.; CYP26B1, retinoic acid hydroxylase may hydroxylate the cis-retinoic acids not recognized by the CYP26A1; CYP26C retinoic acid hydroxylase function is not known; CYP27A1, 27-hydroxylase that oxidizes cholesterol 17-side chain as the first step in bile acid biosynthesis to the feedback inhibitors, cholic acid and chenodeoxycholic acid and also 25-hydroxylates vitamin D3; CYP27B1, mitochondrial vitamin D3 1-alpha hydroxylase activates vitamin D3; CYP27C1, unknown function; CYP39, 7 hydroxylase of 24-hydroxy cholesterol with unknown function; CYP46 cholesterol 24-hydroxylase with unknown function; CYP51, lanosterol 14-alpha demethylase, for converting lanosterol into cholesterol, inhibited by ketoconazole (Nelson, DR; www.drnelson.utmem.edu/cytochromeP450.html).

organic molecules (e.g., CYP2E1); CYP1A1/2 have planar binding sites and only metabolize aromatic planar compounds (i.e., polycyclic aromatic hydrocarbons [PAH]); CYP2D6 exhibits high affinities with specific apoprotein interactions (hydrogen bonds, ion-pair formation) for specific substrates such as lipophilic amines); and CYP3A4 has broader affinity for a variety of lipophilic substrates (m.w. range 200–1200). If the CYP450 isoforms are tightly membrane bound, substrate access to the active site would be limited to compounds that can diffuse through the membrane, whereas a different CYP450 isoform may be bound less tightly and will metabolize hydrophilic compounds.

In the past, the CYP450s were often referred to as having broad and overlapping specificities, but it became apparent that the broad substrate specificity is attributed to multiple isoenzymic forms of CYP450. The phenotype of an individual with respect to the forms and amounts of the individual CYP450s expressed in the liver can determine the rate and pathway of the metabolic clearance of a compound (see discussion on genetic polymorphism in this chapter). Significant differences exist between humans and animal species with respect to the catalytic activities and regulation of the expression of the hepatic drug metabolizing CYP450s. These differences often make it difficult to extrapolate to humans the results of CYP450–mediated metabolism studies performed experimentally in animal species. Caution is warranted in the extrapolation of rodent data to humans, because some isoforms are similar between species (e.g., CYP1A and CYP3A subfamilies),

whereas other subfamilies are different (e.g., CYP 2A, 2B, 2C, and 2D).

The unique and diverse characteristics of the CYP450 ensure that predicting the metabolism of xenobiotics will be difficult. To date, no crystal structure for a mammalian membrane-bound CYP450 isoform has been described.

Cytochrome P450 Isoforms Metabolizing Drugs/Xenobiotics (11,12)

Figure 8.3 shows the participation (%) of hepatic CYP450 isoforms in the metabolism of drugs and xenobiotics (10). Outstanding is the fact that more than 1/3 of all the drugs are metabolized by one isoform, CYP3A4, increasing the potential for drug-drug interactions. When two drugs are metabolized by the same isoform, only one drug can serve as a substrate at one time, increasing the likelihood of a drug-

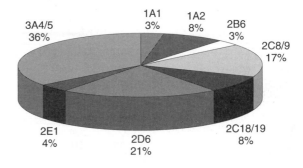

Fig. 8.3. Percent of clinically important drugs metabolized by human CYP450 isoforms.

Table 8.3. Some Substrates and Reaction Type for Human Subfamilies CYP1A2

Phenacetin (O-deethylation)
Acetaminophen (benzoquinone imine)
Theophylline (N1-and N3-demethylation)
Caffeine (N1- and N3-demethylation)
Imipramine (N-demethylation)
Estradiol (2- and 4-hydroxylation)
Antipyrine (N-demethylation)
Fluoroquinolones (3'-hydroxylation of piperazine ring)
Fluvoxamine

drug interaction especially if one drug has a lower therapeutic threshold.

Family 1

The CYP1A subfamily plays an integral role in the metabolism of two important classes of environmental carcinogens, polycyclic aromatic hydrocarbons (PAH) and aryl amines (Table 8.3) (13). The PAH are commonly present in the environment as a result of industrial combustion processes and in tobacco products. Several potent carcinogenic aryl amines result from the pyrolysis of amino acids in cooked meats and can cause colon cancer in rats. Environmental and genetic factors can alter the expression of this subfamily of these enzymes.

CYP1A1. CYP1A1 (also called aromatic hydrocarbon hydroxylase, AHH) is primarily expressed in extrahepatic tissues, small intestine, placenta, skin and lung, and also in the liver in response to the presence of CYP1A1 inducers such as PAH (i.e., in cigarette smoke, and the carcinogen 3-methylcholanthrene), α-naphthoflavone (a noncarcinogenic inducer related to dietary flavones), and indole-3-carbinol (found in Brussels sprouts and related vegetables). CYP1A1 metabolizes a range of PAH, including a large number of procarcinogens and promutagens. Diethylstilbestrol and 2-and 4-hydroxyestradiol (catecholestrogens) are oxidized by CYP1A1 to their quinone analogs, which are normally reduced to inactive metabolites (14). In the absence of a detoxifying reduction step, however, the quinones may accumulate and initiate carcinogenic processes or cell death by covalently damaging DNA or cel-

lular proteins. Interindividual variation in the inducible expression of CYP1A1 might be related to a genetic difference in aromatic hormone receptor (Ah) expression, which could explain differences in individual susceptibility to cigarette smoke-induced lung cancer. Therefore, genetic factors appear to be important in the expression of the CYP1A1 gene in humans and its involvement in human carcinogenesis. Women who smoke are at greater risk than men of developing lung cancer (adenocarcinoma) and chronic obstructive pulmonary diseases. The mechanism for the induction of the CYP1A1 gene begins with binding of the inducing agent(s) to a cytosolic receptor protein, the Ah receptor, which is translocated to the nucleus and binds to the DNA of the CYP1A1 gene, thus enhancing its rate of transcription. The presence of the Ah receptor in hepatic and intestinal tissues may have implications beyond xenobiotic metabolism and may play a role in the induction of other genes for the control of cellular growth and differentiation. On the other hand, CYP1A1 may metabolize procarcinogens to hydroxylated inactive compounds that are not mutagenic. The question of how the bowel protects itself from ingested compounds known to be activated by CYP1A1 (i.e., PAH) remains unanswered (13).

CYP1A2. CYP1A2 (also known as phenacetin O-deethylase, caffeine demethylase, or antipyrine N-demethylase) catalyzes the oxidation (and in some cases bioactivation) of aryl amines, nitrosamines, aromatic hydrocarbons, the bioactivation of promutagens and procarcinogens, caffeine, and other substances (Tables 8.3 and 8.4). It is expressed in the liver to the extent of 13% (range of up to 40×), intestine, and stomach, and is induced by smoking, polycyclic aromatic hydrocarbons, and isosafrole (a noncarcinogenic dietary compound). CYP1A2 is primarily responsible for the activation of the carcinogen aflatoxin B1 under ordinary conditions of human exposure and the pneumotoxin ipomeanol. The latter activation occurs in the liver and not in the lungs by CYP2F1 and CYP4B1 as previously thought. Evidence for polymorphism of this isoform has been reported, and it is likely that low CYP1A2 activity will be associated with altered susceptibility to the bioactivation of procarcinogens, promutagens, and

Table 8.4. Some Procarcinogens and Other Toxins Activated by Human Cytochrome P450s

CYP1A1	CYP1A2	CYP2E1	CYP3A4
Benzo[a]pyrene and other polycyclic aromatic hydrocarbons	4-Aminobiphenyl	Benzene	Aflatoxin B1
	2-Naphthylamine	Styrene	Aflatoxin G1
	2-Aminofluorene	Acrylonitrile	Estradiol
	2-Acetylaminofluorene	Vinylbromide	6-Aminochrysene
	2-Aminoanthracene	Trichlorethylene	Polycyclic hydrocarbon dihydrodiols
	Heteropolycyclic amines (2-aminoquinolines)	Carbon tetrachloride	
	Aflatoxin B1	Chloroform	
	Ipomeanol	Methylene chloride	
		N-nitrosodimethylamine	
		1,2-Dichloropropane	
		Ethyl carbamate	

Table 8.5. Some Substrates and Reaction Type for Human Subfamily CYP2C

CYP2C8	CYP2C9	CYP2C19
S-Warfarin (7-hydroxylation)	S-Warfarin (7-hydroxylation)	Omeprazole (hydroxylation)
Tolbutamide (methyl hydroxylation)	Tolbutamide (methyl hydroxylation)	(S)-Mephenytoin (4'-hydroxylation)
Retinoic acid	Retinoic acid	Diazepam (N-demethylation)
Retinol	Retinol	Proguanil (cyclization)
	Naproxen (O-demethylation)	Imipramine (N-demethylation)
	Ibuprofen (i-butyl hydroxylation)	Propranolol (side chain hydroxylation)
	Chlorpheniramine	(R)-mephenytoin (N-demethylation)
	Diclofenac (4'-hydroxylation)	Mephobarbital (side chain hydroxylation)
	Tienilic acid (thiophene ring hydroxylation)	Loratidine (descarbethoxyation)
	Δ-1 THC (7-hydroxylation)	
	Phenytoin (4-hydroxylation)	
	Hexobarbital (3'-hydroxylation)	
	(R)-Mephenytoin (4'-hydroxylation)	
	Testosterone (16a-hydroxylation)	
	Phenylbutazone (4-hydroxylation)	
	Sulfinpyrazone (aromatic hydroxylation)	
	Chloramphenicol	

other xenobiotics known to be substrates for this enzyme. The expression of the CYP1A2 gene in the stomach becomes an important issue for gastric carcinogenesis induced by smoking and the metabolic activation of the procarcinogens, aryl amines, to mutagens (13). Clinical studies have suggested that the N-demethylation of imipramine is greater in smokers than in nonsmokers.

Family 2

CYP2A6. CYP2A6 is the only member of this subfamily that is primarily expressed in the liver and may also be expressed in lung and nasal epithelium. It has a low level of hepatic expression and represents approximately 4% of the total hepatic CYP450 isoforms (Fig. 8.2). It catalyzes the 7-hydroxylation of coumarin (coumarin 7-hydroxylase), hydroxylation of aflatoxin B1, nicotine (C-oxidation to cotinine), naproxen, tacrine, clozapine, mexiletine, and cyclobenzaprine, as well as the bioactivation of nitrosamines, and procarcinogens. CYP2A6 exhibits polymorphism with an incidence of 2% in the Caucasian population. This population is characterized as poor metabolizers. Smokers with a defective CYP2A6 gene smoke fewer cigarettes, implicating a genetic factor in nicotine dependence.

CYP2B6. There is limited data on the CYP2B6 isoform and it represents less than 1% of the total hepatic CYP450 isoforms. Its level of expression is low and phenobarbital appears to induce its formation. The role of CYP2B6 in human drug metabolism is questionable, although cyclophosphamide, ifosfamide, bupropion, and nicotine are metabolized by this isoform.

CYP2C. The human CYP2C subfamily is the most complex family consisting of CYP2C8, CYP2C9, and CYP2C19, metabolizing about 25% of the clinically important drugs (Fig. 8.3) including (S)-warfarin, (S)-mephenytoin, and tolbutamide (Table 8.5). It represents approximately 20%

of the total CYP450 isoforms in the liver (Fig. 8.2). CYP2C8 is primarily expressed in extrahepatic tissues (kidney, adrenal, brain, uterus, breast, ovary and intestine) and metabolizes the tricyclic antidepressants, diazepam, and verapamil. Its level of expression is less than CYP2C9 and CYP2C19. CYP2C9 and CYP2C19 are found primarily in the liver and intestine. The expression of CYP2C19 in the liver is less than that for CYP2C9. CYP2C9 and CYP2C19 exhibit polymorphism (difference in the DNA sequence for the *CYP2C* gene) that changes the enzyme's ability to metabolize its substrates (i.e., poor metabolizer phenotype). Because of this genetic difference in expressing CYP2C isoforms, it is important to be aware of a person's race when prescribing drugs that are metabolized differently by different populations (see the section later in this chapter concerning genetic polymorphism). CYP2C9 is involved in tolbutamide methyl hydroxylation, and is a factor in the 4'-hydroxylation of phenytoin, 6/7–hydroxylation of S-warfarin, and (R)-mephenytoin. CYP2C19 ((S)-mephenytoin hydroxylase) is the isoform associated with the 4'-hydroxylation of (S)-mephenytoin. The CYP2C subfamily apparently is not inducible in humans.

CYP 2D6. CYP2D6 polymorphism is perhaps the most studied CYP450 (see section of polymorphism). This enzyme is responsible for at least 30 different drug oxidations representing about 21% of the clinically important drugs (Fig. 8.3). CYP2D6 is only 3% expressed in the liver and minimally in the intestine and it does not appear to be inducible (Fig. 8.2). Since there may be no other way to clear drugs metabolized by CYP2D6 from the system, poor metabolizers of CYP2D6 substrates may be at severe risk for adverse drug reactions or drug overdose. The metabolism of debrisoquine by CYP2D6 is one of the most studied examples of metabolic polymorphism, with its molecular basis of defective metabolism being well understood (Table 8.6) (see the section in this chapter on

Table 8.6. Some Substrates and Reaction Type for Human CYP2D6 Isoform

Cardiovascular Drugs
　　Debrisoquine (4-hydroxylation)
　　Quinidine (hydroxylation)
　　Flecainide (O-dealkylation)
　　Propafenone (4-hydroxylation)
　　Mexiletine (4-hydroxylation and methyl hydroxylation)
　　Guanoxan (6- and 7-hydroxylation)
　　Indoramin (6-hydroxylation)
　　Lidocaine (3-hydroxylation)
　　Encainide (N-demethylation, O-demethylation)
　　Captopril
β-Adrenergic Blockers
　　Propranolol (4'-hydroxylation)
　　Bifuralol (1'-hydroxylation)
　　Metoprolol (O-demethylation)
　　Timolol (O-dealkylation)
　　Alprenolol (4-hydroxylation)
Tricyclic Antidepressants
　　Amitriptyline (10-hydroxylation)
　　Clomipramine (hydroxylation)
　　Nortriptyline (10-hydroxylation)
　　Imipramine (2-hydroxylation)
SSRI
　　Fluoxetine(N-dealkylation)
　　Paroxetine
　　Venlafaxine
　　Nefazodone
　　Sertraline

Other Psychotropic Drugs
　　Clozapine (aromatic hydroxylation)
　　Methoxyphenamine (4-hydroxylation, N-demethylation)
　　Thioridazine (aromatic hydroxylation)
　　Perphenazine (aromatic hydroxylation)
　　Methoxyamphetamine (O-demethylation and b-oxidation)
Opioids
　　Codeine (O-demethylation)
　　Dextromethorphan (O-demethylation)
Antihistamine Drugs
　　Chlorpheniramine (N-demethylation, ring hydroxylation, deamination)
　　Clemastine
　　Diphenhydramine (N-demethylation, ring hydroxylation, cleavage ether bond)
　　Hydroxyzine (ring hydroxylation)
　　Promethazine (ring hydroxylation, S-oxidation, N-demethylation)
　　Tripelennamine
Miscellaneous Drugs
　　Perhexiline (4'-hydroxylation)
　　Phenformin (4-hydroxylation)
　　Sparteine (N-oxidation)
　　Tolterodine (2-hydroxylation)
　　Dolasetron (hydroxylation of indole ring)
　　Ondansetron (hydroylation of indole ring)
　　Tropisetron (hydroxylation of indole ring)

genetic polymorphism). This isoform metabolizes a wide variety of lipophilic amines and is probably the only CYP450 for which a charged or ion-pair interaction is important for substrate binding. It also appears to preferentially catalyze the hydroxylation of a single enantiomer (stereoselectivity) in the presence of enantiomeric mixtures. Quinidine is an inhibitor of CYP2D6 and concurrent administration with CYP2D6 substrates results in increased blood levels and toxicity for these substrates. If the pharmacologic action of the CYP2D6 substrate depends on the formation of active metabolites, quinidine inhibition results in a lack of a therapeutic response. The interaction of two substrates for CYP2D6 can prompt a number of clinical responses. For example, depending on which substrate has the greater affinity for CYP2D6, the first pass hepatic metabolism of the substrate (drug) with weaker affinity will be inhibited by a second substrate having greater affinity. The result of which will be a decrease and prolongation of elimination of the first substrate, leading to a higher plasma concentration and an increased potential for adverse toxicity.

CYP2E1. Few drugs are metabolized by CYP2E1 but it plays a major role in the metabolism of numerous halogenated hydrocarbons (including volatile general anesthetics) and a range of low-molecular weight organic compounds, including dimethyformamide, acetonitrile, acetone, ethanol, benzene, as well as in the activation of acetaminophen to its reactive metabolite, N-acetyl-*p*-benzoquinoneimine (Table 8.7) (15,16). CYP2E1 is of most interest because of the toxicity and carcinogenicity of it's metabolites. This isoform is expressed in the liver

Table 8.7. Some Substrates and Reaction Type for Human CYP2E1 Isoform

Acetaminophen (*p*-benzoquinone imine)
Styrene (epoxidation)
Theophylline (C-8 oxidation)
Disulfiram
Halogenated Hydrocarbons
　　Dehalogenation of chloroform, methylene chloride
General Anesthetics (fluorinated hydrocarbons)
　　Enflurane, Halothane, Methoxyflurane, Sevoflurane, Desflurane
Miscellaneous Organic Solvents
　　Ethanol (to acetaldehyde)
　　Glycerin
　　Dimethylformamide (N-demethylation)
　　Acetone
　　Diethylether
　　Benzene (hydroxylation)
　　Aniline (hydroxylation)
　　Acetonitrile (hydroxylation to cyanohydrin)
　　Pyridine (hydroxylation)

(7%), kidney, intestine, and lung, and is inducible by ethanol, isoniazid, 4-methylpyrazole and other chemicals (Tables 8.8 and 8.9). It is also known as microsomal ethanol oxidizing system (MEOS), benzene hydroxylase, or aniline hydroxylase. CYP2E1 is induced in alcoholics. There is a polymorphism associated with this isoform that is more common in Chinese people. This isoform also appears to be related to smoking induced cancer (c.f., CYP1A2). Most of the same compounds that induce CYP2E1 are also substrates for the enzyme. The induction of this enzyme in humans can cause enhanced susceptibility to the toxicity and carcinogenesis of CYP2E1 substrates. Some evidence shows interindividual variation in the in vitro liver expression of this isoform. Diabetes and dietary alterations (i.e., fasting, obesity) result in the induction of CYP2E1. Ketogenic diets (increased serum ketone levels), including those deficient in carbohydrates or high in fat, are known to enhance the metabolism of

halogenated hydrocarbons in rats (16). The mechanism of induction appears to be a combination of an increase in CYP2E1 transcription, m-RNA translation efficiency, and stabilization of CYP2E1 against proteolytic degradation. The induction of CYP2E1 resulting from ketosis (i.e., starvation, a high-fat diet, uncontrolled diabetes, obesity)

Table 8.8. Substrates and Reaction Type for Human CYP3A4 Isoform

Nifedipine, nicardipine, felodipine, etc. (aromatization)	Trazolam
Cyclosporin (N-demethylation and methyl oxidation)	Imipramine (N-demethylation)
Erythromycin (N-demethylation) and analogs	Clotrimazole
Midazolam (methyl hydroxylation)	"Azole" antifungals
Dihydroergotamine (proline hydroxylation)	Rifampin, rifabutin, and related compounds
Codeine (N-demethylation)	Glibenclamide
Diazepam (C-7-hydroxylation)	Valproic acid (hydroxylation and dehydrogenation)
Dextromethorphan (N-demethylation)	Theophylline (C-8 oxidation)
Dolasetron (N-oxide)	Carbamazepine (epoxidation)
Quinidine (N-oxidation and C-3 hydroxylation)	Tolterodine (N-demethylation)
Lidocaine (N-deethylation)	Steroids
Diltiazem (N-deethylation)	Testosterone (6β-hydroxylation)
Tamoxifen (N-demethylation)	Progesterone (6β-hydroxylation)
Lovastatin (6-hydroxylation)	Estradiol (2- and 4-hydroxylation)
Verapamil (N-demethylation)	17a-Ethynylestradiol (2- and 4-hydroxylation)
Δ^1 THC (6β-hydroxylation)	Norethisterone (2-hydroxylation)
Amiodarone (N-deethylation)	Hydrocortisone (6b-hydroxylation)
Cocaine (N-demethylation)	Prednisone (6b-hydroxylation)
Dapsone (N-oxidation)	Prednisolone (6b-hydroxylation)
Terfenadine (N-dealkylation, methyl hydroxylation)	Dexamethasone

Table 8.9. Some Substrates that Inhibit the CYP450 Isoforms

Acebutolol	2D6	Fluvoxamine	1A2, 2C19, 2C9,	Phenacetin	1A2
Amiodarone	2C9, 2D6, 3A4		2D6, 3A4	Phenylbutazone	2C9
Amitriptyline	2D6	Grapefruit (juice)	3A4,1A2	Pilocarpine	2A6
Atorovastatin	3A4	Glibdenclamide	3A4	Pindolol	2D6
Betaxolol	2D6	Haloperidol	2D6	Pravastatin	3A4, 2C9, 2D6
Bufuraolol	2D6	Ifosfamide	3A4	Propafenone	2D6
Caffeine	1A2	Indinavir	3A4	Propranolol	2D6
Cannabinoids	3A4	Isoniazid	1A2	Propofol	1A2, 2E1
Chlorpheniramine	2D6	Itraconazole	2C9, 3A4	Propoxyphene	3A4
Chlorpromazine	2D6	Ketoconazole	3A4, 2C19, 2D6, 1A2	Quinidine	2D6, 3A4
Cimetidine	1A2, 2C18, 2C9,	Ketoprofen	2C9	Ranitidine	2D6, 3A4
	2D6, 2E1, 3A4	Lansoprazole	1A2	Ritonavir	2A6, 2C19, 2C9,
Ciprofloxacin	1A2	Levofloxacin	1A2		2D6, 3A4
Citalopam	2D6	Lidocaine	1A2	Rivastatin	3A4
Clarithromycin	1A2, 3A4	Lomefloxacin	1A2	Saquinavir	3A4
Clemastine	3A4	Lomustine	2D6	Sertindole	2D6, 3A4
Clomipramine	2D6, 3A4	Lovastatin	3A4, 2C19, 2D6	Sertraline	2C19 ,2D6, 3A4
Clotrimazole	3A4	Metronidazole	2C9, 3A4	Simvastatin	3A4, 2C9, 2D6
Cyclosporine	3A4	Mexiletine	1A2	Sulfinpyrazone	2C9, 2C8, 3A4
Danazol	3A4	S-Mephenytoin	2C19	Sulfonamides	2C9
Desipramine	2D6	Mibefradil	3A4, 2D6	Tacrolimus	3A4
Diazepam	2C9, 2C19	Miconazole	3A4	Tamoxifen	3A4
Diclofenac	2C9	Midazolam	3A4	Thioridazine	2D6
Diltiazem	1A2, 3A4	Nefazodone	2D6	Tocainide	3A4
Disulfram	2C9, 2E1	Nifedipine	3A4	Tolbutamide	2C19, 2C9
Enoxacin	1A2	Nelfinavir	3A4	Topiramate	2C19
Erythromycin	1A2, 3A4	Nevirapine	3A4	Troglitazone	2C19, 2C9, 3A4
Felbamate	2C19	Nitrendipine	3A4	Troleandomycin	3A4
Felodipine	3A4	Norfloxacin	1A2, 2D6, 3A4	Venlafaxine	2D6, 3A4
Flecainide	2D6	Ofloxacin	1A2	Verapamil	3A4
Fluconazole	2C19 , 2C9, 3A4	Omeprazole	2C19, 2C9, 3A4	Vinblastine	2D6
Fluoxetine	2C19 , 3A4, 2D6	Orphenadrine	2B6	Vinorelbine	2D6
Fluphenazine	2D6	Paroxetine	2D6, 2C19	Warfarin	2C9
Flurbiprofen	2C9	Perhexiline	2D6	Zafirlukast	2C9, 3A4, 1A2
Fluvastatin	2C9, 2D6, 3A4	Perphenazine	2D6		

or exposure to alcoholic beverages or other xenobiotics may be detrimental to individuals simultaneously exposed to halogenated hydrocarbons (increased hepatotoxicity from halothane, chloroform). Chronic alcohol intake is known to enhance the hepatotoxicity of halogenated hydrocarbons. Testosterone appears to regulate CYP2E1 levels in the kidney and pituitary growth hormone for regulating hepatic levels of CYP2E1. Kidney damage from halocarbons was greater for male rats but not for female rats. This finding may have implications for sexual differences in the nephrotoxicity of CYP2E1 substrates in humans.

Family 3

CYP 3A4. The CYP3A subfamily includes the most abundantly expressed CYP450s in the human liver and intestine (extrahepatic metabolism), but only two forms have been characterized, CYP3A4 and CYP3A5. Approximately one third of the total CYP450 in the liver and two-thirds in the intestine, is CYP3A4. This isoform is responsible for the metabolism of more than one third of the clinically important drugs. CYP3A4 is expressed in the intestine, lung, placenta, kidney, uterus and brain and is glucocorticoid inducible. CYP3A7 is expressed only in fetal livers (approximately 50% of total fetal CYP450 enzymes), and little is known about its substrate specificity, except for the 16-hydroxylation of dehydroepiandrosterone- 3-sulfate, and its ability to hydroxylate allylic and benzylic carbons. The CYP3A4 subfamily metabolizes a range of clinically important drugs (Table 8.8) and is inhibited by a number of xenobiotics, including erythromycin (Table 8.9). It also appears to activate aflatoxin B1 and possibly benzo[a]pyrene metabolism. The interindividual differences reported for the metabolism of nifedipine, cyclosporin, triazolam, and midazolam are probably related to changes in induction and not to polymorphism. CYP3A binding is predominantly lipophilic (7). Drugs known to be substrates for CYP3A4 have a low and variable oral bioavailability that may be explained by prehepatic metabolism by a combination of intestinal CYP3A4 and P-glycoprotein in the enterocytes of the intestinal wall (for more discussion see the oral bioavailability section in this chapter). Therefore, it is the expression and function of the CYP3A4 that governs the rate and extent of metabolism of the substrates for the CYP3A subfamily. The induction of the CYP3A subfamily by phenobarbital in humans may be ultimately responsible for many of the well documented interactions between barbiturates and other drugs (11).

It is clear that no one animal model or combination of animal models reflects the metabolic capabilities of humans. By having a complete understanding of the factors (such as inducers, inhibitors, and effect of disease state) that alter the expression and activity of the enzyme responsible for the metabolism of a particular compound, and by a determination of responsible isoforms and patient phenotyping, it may be possible to predict drug interactions and metabolic clearance.

An alphabetical listing of the clinically important drugs and their CYP450 isoforms catalyzing their oxidative metabolism is presented in Table 8.10.

Catalytic Cycle of Cytochrome P450 — Steps of the Catalytic Cycle

The many variant CYP450 isoforms isolated show a remarkable uniformity for the catalytic mechanism (12,17). The current view illustrating the cyclic mechanism for the reduction and oxygenation of CYP450 as it interacts stepwise with substrate molecules, electron donors, and oxygen is shown in Figure 8.4 and can be summarized as follows (17):

Step a. The ferric CYP450 binds reversibly with a molecule of the substrate (RH) resulting in a complex analogous to an enzyme-substrate complex. The binding of the substrate facilitates the first one-electron reduction step.

Step b. The substrate complex of ferric-CYP450 undergoes reduction to a ferrous-CYP450 substrate complex by an electron originating from NADPH and transferred by the flavoprotein, NADPH-CYP450 reductase, from the $FNMH_2/FADH$ complex.

Step c. The reduced CYP450 complex readily binds dioxygen as the ferrous iron sixth ligand to form oxyCYP450 complex.

Step d. OxyCYP450 undergoes auto-oxidation to a superoxide anion.

Step e. The ferric superoxide anion undergoes further reduction by accepting a second electron from the flavoprotein (or possibly cytochrome b_5) to form the equivalent of a two-electron reduced complex, peroxyCYP450. The cycle can be aborted (uncoupled) from subsequent substrate hydroxylation at this step by xenobiotics that can cause the superoxide anion to disproportionate to hydrogen peroxide and dioxygen with regeneration of the starting point of the cycle, the ferric heme protein-substrate complex.

Step f. The ferric peroxyCYP450 complex undergoes heterolytic cleavage of peroxide anion to water and to a highly electrophilic perferryl oxenoid intermediate ($Fe^{5+}=O$) or a perferryl oxygen-cysteine-porphyrin resonance-stabilized complex. This perferryl oxygen species represents the catalytically active oxygenation species.

Step g. Abstraction of a hydrogen from the substrate by the perferryl oxygen species gives rise to a carbon-centered radical-perferric hydroxide pair, radical addition to a π-bond, or electron abstraction from a heteroatom to form a heteroatom-centered radical-cation perferryl intermediate.

Step h. Subsequent radical recombination (oxygen rebound) or electron-transfer (deprotonation) yields the hydroxylated product and the regeneration of the ferric cytochrome P450 enzyme complex.

Up to the final step the oxidizable substrate has been an inactive spectator in the chemical events of oxygen activation. None of the preceding oxygenated intermediates has been sufficiently reactive to abstract hydrogen from the substrate. The perferryl iron oxenoid complex (Step

Table 8.10. Drugs and the CYP450 Isoforms Catalyzing Their Metabolism

Acetaminophen	1A2, 2E1, 3A4	Estrogens	3A4	Nelfinavir	3A4
Alfentanil	3A4	Ethanol	2E1	Nevirapine	3A4
Alprazolam	3A4	Ethinyl estradiol	3A4	Nicardipine	3A4
Amiodarone	3A4	Ethosuximide	3A4	Nicotine	2A6, 2B6
Amitriptyline	1A2, 2C9, 2D6, 3A4	Etoposide	3A4	Nifedipine	3A4
		Felbamate	2E1, 3A4	Nimodipine	3A4
Amlodipine	3A4	Felodipine	3A4	Nisoldpine	3A4
Anastrozole	3A4	Fenfluramine	2D6	Nitrendipine	3A4
Artemether	3A4	Fentanyl	2D6, 3A4	Nortriptyline	1A2, 2D6
Artemisinin	2B6	Fexofenadine	3A4	Olanzapine	1A2
Astemizole	3A4	Finasteride	3A4	Omeprazole	2C19, 2C8, 3A4
Atorvastatin	3A4	Flecainide	2D6	Ondansetron	3A4, 2D6, 2E1
Benztropine	2D6	Fluconazole	3A4	Oral contraceptives	3A4
Bepridil	3A4	Fluoxetine	2D6, 3A4	Oxycodone	2D6
Bisoprolol	2D6	Fluphenazine	2D6	Oxybutynin	3A4
Bupropion	2B6	Flutamide	3A4	Paclitaxel	2C8, 3A4
Buspirone	3A4	Fluvoxamine	2D6	Paroxetine	2D6
Busulfan	3A4	Glimepiride	2C9	Perphenazine	2D6
Caffeine	1A2	Glyburide	3A4	Phenacetin	1A2
Cannabinoids	3A4	Granisetron	3A4	Phenformin	2D6
Carbamazepine	3A4	Halofantrine	3A4	Phenol	2E1
Carisoprodol	2C19	Haloperidol	3A4	Phenytoin	2C19, 2C9
Carvedilol	2C9, 2D6	Halothane	2E1	Pimozide	3A4
Cerivastatin	3A4	Hexobarbital	2C19, 2C9	Piroxicam	2C19, 2C9
Chloroquin	3A4, 2D6	Hydrocodone	2D6, 3A4	Pravastatin	3A4
Chlorpheniramine	2D6, 2C9, 2B1	Hydrocortisone	3A4, 2D6	Prednisone	3A4
Chlorpromazine	2D6, 3A4	Hydroxyzine	2D6	Progesterone	3A4
Chlorzoxazone	2E1	Ibuprofen	2C9	Proguanil	2C19
Cimetidine	3A4	Ifosfamide	2B6, 3A4	Propafenone	1A2, 2D6, 3A4
Cisapride	3A4	Imipramine	1A2, 2C19, 2C9, 2D6, 3A4	Propranolol	1A2, 2C19, 2D6
Clarithromycin	3A4			Quinidine	3A4
Clindamycin	3A4	Indinavir	3A4, 2D6	Quinine	3A4
Clemastine	2D6	Indomethacin	2C9	Repaglinide	3A4
Clomipramine	1A2, 2C19, 2D6, 3A4	Irinotecan	3A4	Retinoic acid	2C19, 2C8
		Isoflurane	2E1	Rifabutin	3A4
Clonazepam	3A4	Isoniazid	2E1	Rifampin	3A4
Clozapine	1A2, 2D6, 2A6	Isotretinoin (retinoids)	1A2, 2C8, 3A4	Riluzole	1A2
Cocaine	3A4	Isradipine	3A4	Risperidone	2D6, 3A4
Codeine	2D6, 3A4	Itraconazole	3A4	Ritonavir	1A2, 2A6, 2C19, 2C9, 2D6, 2E1, 3A4
Cyclobenzaprine	1A2, 2A6, 2D6, 3A4	Ketoconazole	3A4		
		Labetalol	2D6		
Cyclophosphamide	2B6, 3A4	Lansoprazole	2C19, 3A4	Ropivacaine	1A2, 2D6
Cyclosporine	3A4	Lidocaine	3A4	Salmeterol	3A4
Dapsone	2C9, 3A4	Loperamide	3A4	Saquinavir	3A4
Delavirdine	3A4, 2DS6	Lopinavir	3A4, 2D6	Selegiline	2D6
Desipramine	1A2, 2D6	Loratadine	2C19, 3A4, 2D6	Sertindole	2D6
Dexamethasone	3A4	Losartan	2C9, 3A4	Sertraline	2D6, 3A4
Dexfenfluramine	2D6	Lovastatin	3A4	Sevoflurane	2E1
Dextromethorphan	2D6, 3A4	Maprotiline	2D6	Sildenafil	2C9, 3A4
Diazepam	1A2, 2C19, 2C8, 3A4	Mefenamic acid	2C9	Simvastatin	3A4
		Mefloquine	3A4	Sulfentanil	3A4
Diclofenac	2C8/9	Meperidine	2D6	Sulfamethoxazole	2C9
Diphenhydramine	2D6	Mephenytoin	2C19	Tacrine	1A2, 2A6
Diltiazem	3A4	Mephobarbital	2C8	Tafenoquin	3A4, 2C9
Disopyramide	3A4	Methadone	1A2, 2D6	Tacrolimus	3A4
Divalproex sodium	2C19	Methamphetamine	2D6	Tamoxifen	1A2, 2A6, 2B6, 2D6, 2E1, 3A4
Docetaxel	3A4	Metoprolol	2D6		
Dolasetron	2D6, 3A4	Mexiletine	2D6, 2A6	Taxotere	3A4
Donepezil	2D6, 3A4	Mibefradil	3A4	Temazepam	3A4
Dorzolamide	2B1, 3A4, 2E1	Miconazole	3A4	Teniposide	3A4
Doxorubicin	3A4	Midazolam	3A4	Terfenadine	3A4
Doxylamine	2D6	Mifepristone	3A4	Testosterone	3A4
Dronabinol	2C9	Mirtazapine	1A2, 2C9, 2D6, 3A4	Theophylline	1A2, 2E1, 3A4
Enalapril	3A4			Thioridazine	2D6
Encainide	2D6	Morphine	2D6	Tiagabine	3A4
Enflurane	2E1	Naproxen	2C19, 2C9, 2A6	Timolol	2D6
Ergot Alkaloids	3A4	Navelbine	3A4	Tolbutamide	2C8, 2C9
Erythromycin	3A4	Nefazodone	3A4	Tolterodine	2D6, 3A4

continued

Table 8.10—*continued*

Tramadol	2D6	Tropisetron	2D6	Vinca alkaloids	3A4
Trazodone	2D6	Valproic acid	2C19	Vincristine	3A4
Torsemide	2C9	Venlafaxine	2D6, 3A4	R-Warfarin	1A2, 3A4
Tretinoin	3A4	S-Warfarin	2C19, 2C9	Zafirlukast	2C9
Triazolam	3A4	Yohimbine	2D6	Zileuton	1A2, 2C9, 3A4
Tripelennamine	2D6	Verapamil	3A4, 1A2, 2C9		
Troleandomycin	3A4	Vinblastine	3A4		

Oxygen Activation

Elemental oxygen (dioxgen) is a relatively unreactive form of oxygen which exists as an unpaired diradical in the triplet form. Alternatively, singlet oxygen is a form of dioxygen in which the diradical electrons are paired. In this form oxygen is too reactive for biological systems. Free oxygen atoms (oxenes), formed by splitting dioxgyen, are highly reactive, but are not known to exist in biochemical processes. The solution to the problem of a reactive form of oxygen lies in the suggestion that the reduction of dioxygen occurs to one of the reactive oxygen species (ROS) such as superoxide radical anion, peroxide, hydroxyl radical or oxygen atom.

$$O_2 + e^- \longrightarrow {:O\!=\!O}\cdot^{\ominus} \quad \text{Superoxide radical anion}$$

$$O_2 + 2e^- + 2H^+ \longrightarrow H_2O_2 \quad \text{Peroxide}$$

$$O_2 + 2e^- + 2H^+ \longrightarrow 2HO^- + H_2O \quad \text{Hydroxyl radical}$$

$$O_2 + 2e^- + 2H^+ \longrightarrow O + H_2O \quad \text{Oxygen atom}$$

Reactive oxygen species (ROS)

Any of these reactive oxygen species could oxidize an organic substrate with the net insertion of an oxygen atom. In each case, reductive reactions are required for activation of dioxygen to one of the ROS from electrons supplied by NADPH. The generation of a carbon-centered radical and a hydroxyl radical with triplet oxygen atom has been found to be relevant to a number of enzymatic and chemical reactions, involving oxenoids (oxygen rebound mechanism)(18). The function of CYP450 monooxygenases is usually the hydroxylation of a substrate. A reactive radical-like iron oxenoid intermediate is generated, reactive enough to split aliphatic C-H bonds, add to bonds α to heteroatoms or remove single electrons from heteroatoms. The mechanisms of cytochrome P450 are not fully understood and the reactive oxygen intermediate has not been isolated or even spectroscopically observed.

g), however, is a competent hydrogen abstractor, even for relatively inert terminal methyl groups on hydrocarbon chains. Evidence shows that the oxidant is selective in its choice of hydrogen atoms, balancing stability of the resulting carbon radical with stereochemical constraints. Because the inert aliphatic region of the substrate has been converted to a highly reactive radical, the process is described as substrate activation. Various studies have shown that the hydroxylation or alkene formation proceeds not by a direct one-step insertion of the oxygen atom, but by a two-step, two-electron process involving radical or cationic substrate intermediates with subsequent radical recombination (oxygen rebound) to products (Fig. 8.5) (18).

Despite considerable experimental evidence, the proposed mechanism and intermediates of monooxygenation of unsaturated substrates (alkenes, alkynes, aromatics) remains controversial (11,19). The proposed mechanism for the oxidation of π-bonds in alkenes involves a stepwise sequence of one-electron transfer between the radical complex and the perferryl oxygen intermediate ($[Fe^{5+}\!=\!O]$) (alkene oxidation Fig. 8.6). Following the initial formation of an unsaturated-P450 π-complex, the one-electron transfer yields either a π-complex or a radical σ-complex. These complexes can either collapse to the epoxide, undergo a 1,2-group migration to a carbonyl product (step b Fig. 8.6), or give a vinyl hydroxylated product (step c, Fig. 8.6). The presence of an oxygen radical in the porphyrin ring allows some substrate radicals to covalently bond through N-alkylation of a pyrrole nitrogen rather than to recombine with $(Fe\text{-}OH)^{3+}$. This deviation from the normal course of reaction explains the suicide inhibition exhibited by some xenobiotics, such as the oral contraceptives (20).

In the case of aromatic oxidations (Fig. 8.6), following the initial formation of an arene-P450 π-complex, one-

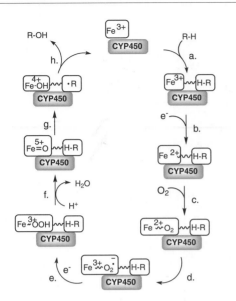

Fig. 8.4. Cyclic mechanism for CYP450. The substrate is RH and the valence state of the heme iron in CYP450 is indicated.

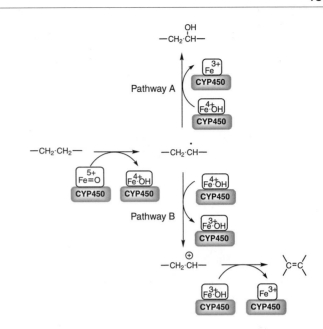

Fig. 8.5. Proposed mechanisms for the hydroxylation and dehydrogenation of alkanes.

electron transfer yields either a π-complex or a radical σ-complex. The radical σ-complex can collapse to the arene epoxide (step d Fig. 8.6) while the π-complex can proceed to an arene oxide or can undergo a NIH shift (1,2-group migration) to a phenolic product (step e Fig. 8.6). Arene oxides are highly unstable entities and rearrange (NIH shift) nonenzymatically to phenols or hydrolyzed enzymatically with epoxide hydrolase to 1,2-dihydrodiols (trans configuration) (step f Fig. 8.6), which are subsequently dehydrogenated to 1,2-diphenols. The oxidation of aromatic compounds can be highly specific to individual CYP450 isoforms, suggesting that substrate binding and orienta-

tion in the active site may dominate the mechanism of oxidative catalysis.

Heteroatom-containing substrates usually undergo hydroxylation adjacent (α) to the heteroatom, as compared to other positions. Reactions of this type include N-, O-, S-dealkylation, dehydrohalogenations, and oxidative deamination (dealkylation) reactions. Two mechanisms have been suggested (Fig. 8.7). One is the abstraction of a hydrogen atom from the carbon adjacent to the heteroatom, and the resultant carbon radical is stabilized by the het-

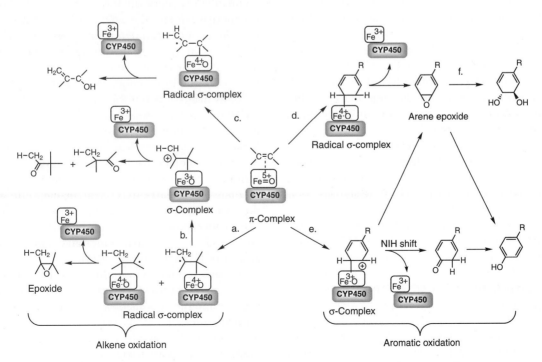

Fig. 8.6. Proposed mechanisms for oxidation of alkene and aromatic compounds.

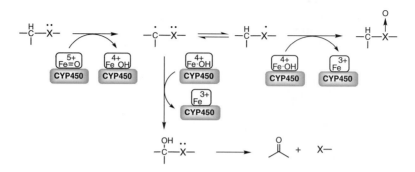

Fig. 8.7. Proposed mechanism for heteraotom-compound oxidation, dealkylation, and dehalogenation.

eroatom. Alternatively, abstraction of an electron from the heteroatom to form a heteroatom radical subsequently transfers a hydrogen atom from the more labile α-carbon to generate a carbon radical. Collapse of the carbon radical-perferric hydroxide radical pair hydroxylates the carbon adjacent to the heteroatom, generating an unstable geminal hydroxy heteroatom-substituted intermediate (e.g., carbinolamine, halohydrin, hemiacetal, hemiketal, or hemithioketal) that breaks down, releasing the heteroatom and forming a carbonyl compound (19).

Xenobiotics containing heteroatoms (N, S, P, and halogens) frequently are metabolized by heteroatom oxidation to its corresponding heteroatom oxide (tertiary amine to its N-oxide, sulfides to sulfoxides, phosphines to phosphine oxides). Heteroatom oxidation can also be attributed to a microsomal flavin-containing monooxygenase. As in the case for heteroatom α-hydroxylation, one electron oxidation of the heteroatom occurs as the first step to form the heteroatom cation perferric hydroxide radical intermediate, which collapses to generate the heteroatom oxide. This reaction is favored by the absence of α-hydrogens and stability of the heteroatom radical-cation (19).

All of the known oxidative reactions catalyzed by CYP450 monooxygenase can be described in the context of a mechanistic scheme involving the ability of a high valent iron oxenoid species to bring about the stepwise one-electron oxidation through the abstraction of hydrogen atoms, abstraction of electrons from heteroatoms, or the addition to π-bonds. A series of radical recombination reactions completes the oxidation process.

Induction and Inhibition of Cytochrome P450 isoforms
Induction

Many drugs, environmental chemicals, and other xenobiotics enhance the metabolism of themselves or of other co-ingested/inhaled compounds, thereby altering their pharmacologic and toxicologic effects (21,22). Prolonged administration of a drug or xenobiotic can lead to enhanced metabolism of a wide variety of other compounds. Enzyme induction is a dose-dependent phenomenon.

Drugs and xenobiotics exert this effect by inducing transcription of CYP450 mRNA and synthesis of xenobiotic-metabolizing enzymes in the smooth endoplasmic reticulum of the liver and other extrahepatic tissues (21). This phenomenon is called enzyme induction, and the term has been used to describe the process by which the rate of synthesis of an enzyme is increased relative to the rate of synthesis in the uninduced organism. In many older studies of mammalian systems, the term induction was inferred from the increase in enzyme activity, but the amount of enzyme protein had not been determined. Enzyme induction is important in interpreting the results of chronic toxicities, mutagenicities, or carcinogenesis and explaining certain unexpected drug interactions in patients.

Many drugs and xenobiotics stimulate the activity of the CYP450 isoforms, as shown in Table 8.11. These stimulators have nothing in common as far as their pharmacologic activity or chemical structures are concerned, but they are all metabolized by one or more of the CYP450 isoforms. Most are lipid soluble at physiologic pH. Polycyclic aromatic hydrocarbons (PAH) in cigarette smoke, xanthines and flavones in foods, halogenated hydrocarbons in insecticides, polychlorinated biphenyls, and food additives are but a few of the environmental chemicals that alter the activity of CYP450 enzymes (23).

Enzyme induction can alter the pharmacokinetics and pharmacodynamics of a drug with clinical implications for the therapeutic actions of a drug and increased potential for drug interactions. As a result of induction, a drug may be either metabolized more rapidly to metabolites that are more potent, more toxic, or less active than the parent

Table 8.11. Drugs that Induce the Expression of CYP450 Isoforms

Barbiturates	3A4, 2C9, 2C19, 2B6	4-Methylpyrazole	2E1
Carbamazepine	3A4, 2C9, 2D6	Omeprazole	1A1/2, 3A4
Charbroiled Meats	1A1/2	Phenobarbital	3A4, 2C, 2B6, 2D6, 1A2
Cigarette Smoke	1A1/2	Phenytoin	3A4, 1A2, 2B6, 2C8, 2C19, 2D6
Clotrimazole	1A1/2, 3A4	Primidone	3A4, 2C8, 1A2, 2B6
Ethanol	2E1	Psoralen	1A1/2
Erythromycin	3A4	Polycyclic aromatic hydrocarbons	1A1/2
Glucocorticoids (Dexamethasone, prednisone)	3A4, 2A6	Rifampin	2C8, 2C9,2C19, 3A4
Griseofulvin	3A4	Ritonavir	2D6
Isoniazid	2E1	St. Johns Wort	3A4
Lansoprazole	1A1/2, 3A4	Troglitazone	3A4
Mephenytoin	2B6	Topiramate	3A4

drug. Induction can also enhance the activation of procarcinogens or promutagens. Not all inducing agents enhance their own metabolism; e.g., phenytoin induces CYP3A4, but is hydroxylated by CYP2C9, which is constitutive. Some of the more common enzyme inducers of CYP450 subfamilies, which may also be substrates for the same CYP450 isoform, include phenobarbital (CYP2B6, CYP2C, and CYP3A4), rifampicin (CYP3A4), and cigarette smoke (CYP1A1/2) (see Table 8.9). The broad range of drugs metabolized by these CYP450 subfamilies (see Tables 8.3 to 8.7, and Table 8.10) and that are also affected by these enzyme inducers raises the issue of clinically significant drug interactions and their clinical implications. Examples of a clinical CYP450 drug interaction and a herbal drug-drug interaction include rifampin and oral contraceptives and St. John's Wort and oral contraceptives. Both induce the expression of CYP3A4, thereby reducing the serum levels of the oral contraceptive because of increased oxidative metabolism of the oral contraceptives by CYP3A4 to less active metabolites, increasing the risk for pregnancy. Drugs poorly metabolized by CYP450 enzymes are less affected by enzyme induction. Inducers of CYP450 isoforms also stimulate the oxidative metabolism or synthesis of endogenous substances, such as the hydroxylation of androgens, estrogens, progestational steroids (synthetic oral contraceptives), glucocorticoids, vitamin D, and bilirubin, decreasing their biologic activity. These enzyme inducers might also be implicated in deficiencies associated with these steroids. For example, the induction of C-2 hydroxylation of estradiol and synthetic estrogens by phenobarbital, dexamethasone, or cigarette smoking in women results in the increased formation of the principal and less active metabolite of these estrogenic substances, reducing their effectiveness (24). Thus, cigarette smoking in premenopausal women could result in an estrogen deficiency, increasing the risk of osteoporosis and early menopause. Postmenopausal women who smoke and take estrogen replacement therapy may lose the effectiveness of the estrogen.

In addition to enhancing metabolism of other drugs, many compounds, when chronically administered, stimulate their own metabolism, thereby decreasing their therapeutic activity and producing a state of apparent tolerance. This self-induction may explain some of the change in drug toxicity observed in prolonged treatment. The sedative action of phenobarbital, for example, becomes shorter with repeated doses and can be explained in part on the basis of increased metabolism.

The time course of induction varies with different inducing agents and different isoforms, except that CYP1A induction involves the Ah receptor. Increased transcription of CYP450 mRNA has been detected as early as 1 hour after the administration of phenobarbital, with maximum induction after 48 to 72 hours. After the administration of PAH, such as 3-methylcholanthrene and benzo[a]pyrene, maximum induction of CYP1A subfamily is reached within 24 hours. Less potent inducers of hepatic drug metabolism may take as long as 6 to 10 days to reach maximum induction (21). Exposure to a variety of xenobiotics may preferentially increase the hepatic content of specific forms of CYP450 (21,22). Therefore, the process of enzyme induction involves the adaptive increase in the content of specific enzymes in response to the enzyme-inducing agent. Other inducible metabolizing enzymes include UDP-glucuronosyl transferase and glutathione transferase.

Induction—Specific Inducers

Phenobarbital and Rifampin. Phenobarbital and rifampin are probably the enzyme inducers studied most extensively. These drugs could alter the pharmacokinetics and pharmacodynamics of many concurrently administered drugs listed in Tables 8.5 (CYP2C) and 8.8 (CYP3A4), raising the issue of clinically significant drug interactions.

Cigarette Smoke. Cigarette smoke has been shown to increase the hydrocarbon-inducible isoforms CYP1A1 and CYP1A2 in the lungs, liver, small intestine, and placenta of cigarette smokers. A decrease in the pharmacologic action and stimulation of the metabolism of several drugs is the end result. Cigarette smoking has been reported to lower the blood levels for theophylline, imipramine, estradiol, pentazocine, and propoxyphene; decrease urinary excretion of nicotine; and decrease drowsiness from chlorpromazine, diazepam, and chlordiazepoxide, although the plasma levels, half-life, or total clearance for diazepam are unchanged.

Dietary Substances.   A diet containing Brussels sprouts, cabbage, and cauliflower stimulated CYP450 activity in rat intestine (25). It was subsequently determined that indole derivatives (indole-3–carbinol) were responsible for the enzyme induction. Other examples of chemicals found naturally in foods that enhance metabolism in animals are flavones, safrole, eucalyptol, xanthines, β-ionone, and organic peroxides. Volatile oils in soft woods (e.g., cedar) have been shown to be enzyme inducers.

Alcohol.   Sober alcoholics show an increase in CYP2E1 enzyme activity, leading to more rapid clearance of drugs and xenobiotics that are substrates for this isoform from the body. As discussed previously, hepatic CYP2E1 oxidizes ethanol, and chronic ethanol intake increases the activity of CYP2E1 through enzyme induction (15). When intoxicated, alcoholics are more susceptible to the action of various drugs because of inhibition of drug metabolism due to excessive quantity of alcohol in the liver and an additive or synergistic effect in the central nervous system. The basis for this inhibition is unknown. Furthermore, moderate ethanol consumption reduces the clearance of some drugs, presumably because of competition between ethanol and the other drugs for hepatic biotransformation. The changes in drug metabolism in alcoholics can also be attributed to other factors, such as malnutrition, other drugs, and the trace chemicals that determine the flavor and odor of alcoholic beverages. Heavy drinkers metabolize phenobarbital, tolbutamide, and phenytoin more rapidly than nonalcoholics, which may be clinically important because of problems in adjusting drug therapy in alcoholics.

Inhibition

Another method of altering the in vivo effects of xenobiotics metabolized by CYP450s is through the use of inhibitors (see Table 8.9). The CYP450 inhibitors can be divided into three categories according to their mechanism of action: reversible inhibition, metabolite intermediate complexation of CYP450, or mechanism-based inactivation of CYP450 (22,26). The polysubstrate nature of CYP450 is responsible for the large number of documented interactions associated with the inhibition of drug oxidation and drug biotransformation.

Reversible Inhibition.   Reversible inhibition of CYP450 is the result of reversible interactions at the heme-iron

active center of CYP450, the lipophilic sites on the apoprotein, or both. The interaction occurs before the oxidation steps of the catalytic cycle, and their effects dissipate quickly when the inhibitor is discontinued. The most effective reversible inhibitors are those that interact strongly with both the apoprotein and the heme-iron. It is widely accepted that inhibition has an important impact on the oxidative metabolism and pharmacokinetics of drugs whose metabolism cosegregates with that of an inhibitor (see Tables 8.5 to 8.7, and Table 8.10) (26). Drugs interacting reversibly with CYP450 include the fluoroquinolone antimicrobials, cimetidine, the azole antifungals, quinidine (specific for CYP2D isoforms), and diltiazem. Cimetidine is the only H-2 antagonist that inhibits CYP450 by interacting directly with the CYP450 heme-iron through one of its imidazole ring nitrogen atoms. Cimetidine is not a universal inhibitor of CYP450 oxidative metabolism, but it does bind differentially to several CYP450 isoforms (Table 8.8). Cimetidine inhibits the oxidation of theophylline (CYP1A), chlordiazepoxide (CYP2C), diazepam (CYP2C), propranolol (CYP2C and CYP2D), warfarin (CYP2C), and antipyrine (CYP1A), but not that of ibuprofen (CYP2C), tolbutamide (CYP2C), mexiletine (CYP2D), 6-hydroxylation of steroids (CYP3A), and carbamazepine (CYP3A) (22). The imidazole-based azole antifungals are potent inhibitors of CYP3A and of the CYP450-mediated biosynthesis of endogenous steroid hormones. The azole antifungals exert their fungiostatic effects through inhibition of fungal P450, inhibiting the oxidative biosynthesis of lanosterol to ergosterol, thereby affecting the integrity and permeability of the fungal membranes.

CYP450 Complexation Inhibition.   Noninhibitory alkylamine drugs have the ability to undergo CYP450-mediated oxidation to nitrosoalkane metabolites (Fig. 8.8), which have a high affinity for forming a stable complex with the reduced (ferrous) heme intermediate for the CYP2B, CYP2C, and CYP3A subfamilies. This process is called metabolite intermediate complexation (26). Thus, CYP450 isoform is unavailable for further oxidation and synthesis of the new enzyme is required to restore CYP450 activity. The process relies on at least one cycle of the CYP450 catalytic cycle to generate the required heme intermediate. The macrolide antibiotics, troleandomycin, erythromycin, clarithromycin and their analogs are selective inhibitors of CYP3A4 that are capable of inducing the expression of hepatic and extrahepatic CYP3A4 mRNA and induction of their own biotransformation into nitrosoalkane metabolites. The clinical significance of this inhibition with CYP3A4 is the long-lived impairment of the metabolism of a large number of co-

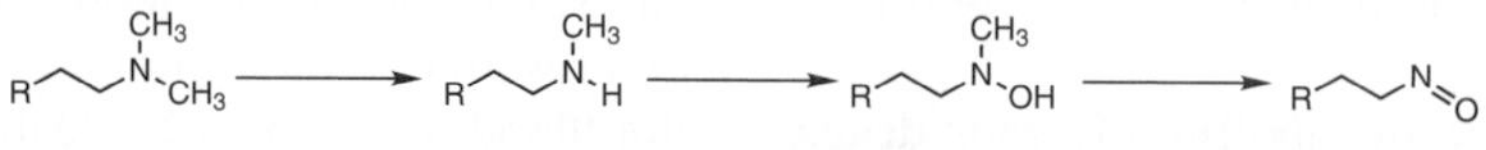

Fig. 8.8. Sequence of oxidation of dialkylamine to nitroso metabolite intermediate.

administered substrates for this isoform and the potential for drug-drug interactions and time-dependent non-linearities in their pharmacokinetics upon long term administration (see Table 8.9). For the macrolides to be so metabolized, they must possess an unhindered dimethylamino sugar and the whole compound must be lipophilic. Other alkylamine-based drugs demonstrating this type of inhibition include orphenadrine (antiparkinson drug), the antiprogestin, mifepristone (CYP3A), and SKF525A (the original CYP450 inhibitor). Methylenedioxyphenyl compounds (i.e., the insecticide synergist piperonyl butoxide and the flavoring agent isosafrole) generate metabolite intermediates that form stable complexes with both the ferric and ferrous state of CYP450.

Mechanism-based Inhibition. Certain drugs that are noninhibitory of CYP450 contain functional groups that, when oxidized by CYP450, generate metabolites that bind irreversibly to the enzyme. This process is called mechanism-based inhibition ("suicide inhibition") and requires at least one catalytic CYP450 cycle during or subsequent to the oxygen transfer step when the drug is activated to the inhibitory species. Alkenes and alkynes were the first functionalities found to inactivate CYP450 by generation of a radical intermediate that alkylates the heme structure (see the section on alkene and alkyne hydroxylation)(20,26). Iron is lost from the heme and abnormal N-alkylated porphyrins are produced. Drugs that are mechanism-based inhibitors of CYP450 include the 17 α-acetylenic estrogen, 17 α-ethynylestradiol, the 17 α-acetylenic progestin, norethindrone (norethisterone) and their radical intermediate that N-alkylates heme of CYP3A; chloramphenicol and its oxidative dechlorination to an acyl moiety that alkylates CYP450 apoprotein; cyclophosphamide (CYP3A) and its generation of acrolein and phosphoramide mustard; spironolactone and its 7-thio metabolite that alkylates heme; 8-methoxypsoralen (a furocoumarin) and its epoxide metabolite which alkylates the CYP450 apoprotein of CYP2A6, 21-halosteroids; halocarbons; and secobarbital. The selectivity of CYP450 isoform destruction by several of these inhibitors indicates the involvement of this isoform in its bioactivation of such drugs.

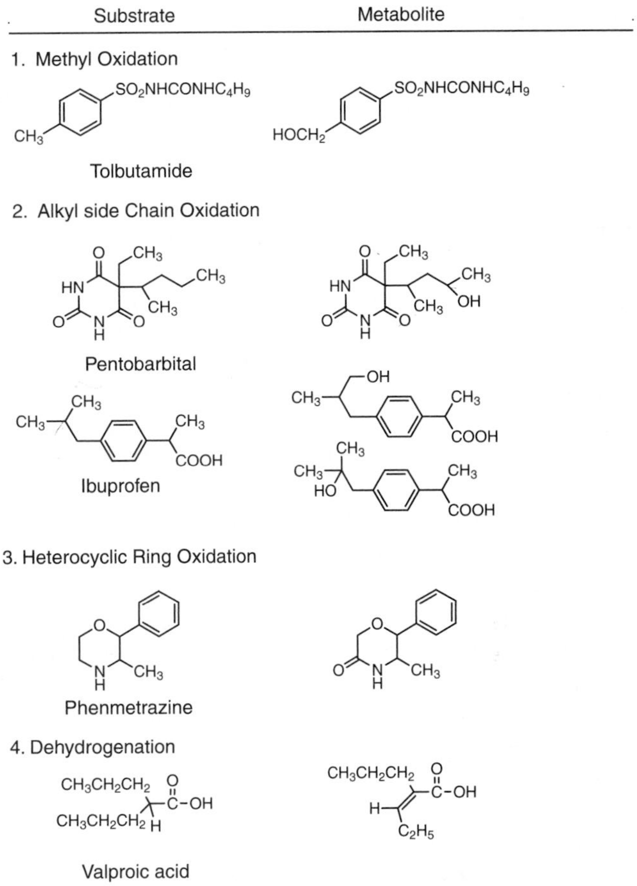

Oxidations Catalyzed by Cytochrome P450 Isoforms

Aliphatic and Alicyclic Hydroxylations. The accepted mechanism for the hydroxylation of alkane carbon-hydrogen bonds has previously been discussed (19) and is shown in Figure 8.5. The principal metabolic pathway for the methyl group is oxidation to the hydroxymethyl derivative followed by its nonmicrosomal oxidation to the carboxylic acid (e.g., tolbutamide, Fig. 8.9). On the other hand, some methyl groups are oxidized only to the hydroxymethyl derivative, without further oxidation to the acid. Where there are several equivalent methyl groups,

Fig. 8.9. Examples of phase 1 xenobiotic oxidative metabolism of aliphatic and alicyclic hydrocarbons catalyzed by CYP450.

usually only one is oxidized. For aromatic methyl groups, the para methyl is the most vulnerable.

Alkyl side chains are often hydroxylated on the terminal or the penultimate carbon atom (e.g., pentobarbital, Fig. 8.9). The isopropyl group is an interesting side chain which undergoes hydroxylation at the tertiary carbon and at either of the equivalent methyl groups (e.g., ibuprofen, Fig. 8.9). Hydroxylation of alkyl side chains attached to an aromatic ring does not follow the general rules for alkyl side chains, because the aromatic ring influences the position of hydroxylation. Generally, oxidation occurs preferentially on the benzylic methylene group and to a lesser extent at other positions on the side chain.

The methylene groups of an alicycle are readily hydroxylated, generally at the least hindered position, or at an activated position, e.g., α to a carbonyl (cyclohexanone); α to a double bond (cyclohexene); α to a phenyl ring (tetralin). The products of hydroxylation often show stereoisomerism. Nonaromatic heterocycles generally undergo oxidation at the carbon adjacent to the heteroatom (e.g., phenmetrazine, Fig. 8.9).

In addition to hydroxylation reactions, CYP450s can catalyze the dehydrogenation of an alkane to an alkene (olefin). The reaction is thought to involve the formation of a carbon radical, electron transfer to the perferryl complex of CYP450 giving a carbocation, and deprotonation to a dehydrogenated product alkene (see Fig. 8.5)(19). An example of the ability of CYP450 to function both as a dehydrogenase and monooxygenase has been demonstrated with the antiseizure valproic acid. While the major metabolic products in humans are β-oxidation and acyl glucuronidation, several alkenes are formed including (E)2-ene isomer (Fig. 8.9) (27). Presumably, the CYP3A subfamily catalyzes these reactions. The factors determining whether CYP450 catalyzes hydroxylation (oxygen rebound/recombination) or dehydrogenation (electron transfer) remains unknown, but hydroxylation is generally favored. In some instances, dehydrogenation may be the primary product, i.e., 6,7-dehydrogenation of testosterone.

Alkene and Alkyne Hydroxylation. The oxidation of alkenes yields primarily epoxides and a series of products derived from 1,2-migration (Fig. 8.6 and previous discussion). The stereochemical configuration of the alkene is retained during epoxidation. The epoxides can differ in reactivity. Those that are highly reactive either undergo pH catalyzed hydrolysis to excretable vicinal dihydrodiols or react covalently (alkylate) with macromolecules such as proteins or nucleic acids leading to tissue necrosis or carcinogenicity. Moreover, the ubiquitous epoxide hydrolase can catalyze the rapid hydrolysis of epoxides to nontoxic vicinal dihydrodiols. Several drugs (carbamazepine, cyproheptadine, and protriptyline), however, were found to form stable epoxides at the 10,11-position during biotransformation (Fig. 8.10). The fact that these epoxides could be detected in the urine indicates these oxides are not particularly reactive and should not readily react covalently with macromolecules.

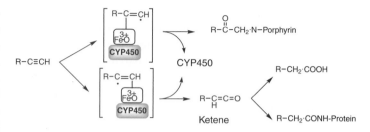

Fig. 8.11. Alkyne oxidation catalyzed by CYP450.

The epoxidation of terminal alkenes is accompanied by the mechanism-based ("suicide") N-alkylation of the heme-porphyrin ring. If the π-complex attaches to the alkene at the internal carbon, the terminal carbon of the double bond can irreversibly N-alkylate the pyrrole nitrogen of the porphyrin ring (20). The heme adduct formation is mostly observed with monosubstituted, unconjugated alkenes (i.e., 17α-ethylenic steroids and 4-ene metabolite of valproic acid).

In addition to the formation of epoxides, heme adducts, and hydroxylated products, carbonyl products are also created. These latter products result from the migration of atoms to adjacent carbons, 1,2-group migration. For example, during the CYP450 catalyzed oxidation of trichloroethylene, a 1,2-shift of chloride occurred to yield chloral (Fig. 8.10).

Like the alkenes, alkynes (acetylenes) are readily oxidized but usually faster. Depending on which of the two alkyne carbons are attacked, different products are obtained (20). If attachment of CYP450 occurs on the terminal alkyne carbon, a hydrogen atom migrates, forming a ketene intermediate that readily hydrolyzes with water to form an acid or that can alkylate nucleophilic protein side chains (i.e., lysinyl or cysteinyl) to form a protein adduct (Fig. 8.11). The effect of attaching the perferryl oxygen at the internal alkenyl carbon is N-alkylation of a pyrrole nitrogen in the porphyrin ring by the terminal acetylene carbon, with the formation of a keto heme adduct (Fig. 8.11). The latter mechanism has been proposed for the irreversible inactivation of CYP3A4 with 17 α-alkenyl steroids (i.e., 17 α-ethynylestradiol).

Aromatic Hydroxylation. The metabolic oxidation of aromatic carbon atoms by CYP450 depends on the isoform catalyzing the oxidation and the oxidation potential of the aromatic compound. The products usually are phenolic products and the position of hydroxylation can be influenced by the type of substituents on the ring according to the theories of aromatic electrophilic substitution (Fig. 8.6). For example, electron-donating substituents enhance *p*- and *o*-hydroxylation, whereas electron-withdrawing substituents reduce or prevent *m*-hydroxylation. Moreover, steric factors must also be considered, because oxidation usually occurs at the least hindered position. For monosubstituted benzene compounds, parahydroxylation usually predominates, with some ortho product being

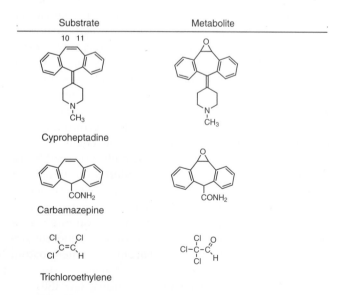

| Substrate | Metabolite |

Cyproheptadine

Carbamazepine

Trichloroethylene

Fig. 8.10. Examples of phase 1 xenobiotic oxidative metabolism of alkenes and alkynes catalyzed by CYP450.

formed (Fig. 8.12). When there is more than one phenyl ring, usually only one is hydroxylated (e.g., phenytoin).

The hydroxylation of aromatic compounds by CYP450 has traditionally been considered to be mediated by an arene oxide (epoxide) intermediate followed by the "NIH shift" as previously discussed (19) (Fig. 8.6). The formation of phenols and the isolation of urinary dihydrodiols, catechols, and glutathione conjugates (mercapturic acid derivatives) implicates arene oxides as intermediates in the metabolism of benzene and substituted benzenes in mammalian systems. The arene oxides are also susceptible to conjugation with glutathione to form premercapturic acids (see the section on glutathione conjugation).

The CYP1A2 and CYP3A subfamilies are important contributors to 2- and 4-hydroxylation of estradiol, and CYP3A4 for the 2-hydroxylation of the synthetic estrogens, for example, 17 α-ethynylestradiol (24). The principal metabolite (as much as 50%) for estradiol is 2-hydroxyestradiol, with 4-hydroxy and 16 α-hydroxyestradiol as the minor metabolites (Fig. 8.12). The 2-hydroxy metabolite of both estradiol and ethynylestradiol have limited or no estrogenic activity, whereas the C-4 and C-16 α-hydroxy metabolites have a potency similar to estradiol. In humans, 16 α-hydroxyestradiol is the major estrogen metabolite in pregnancy and in breast cancer. The metabolites 16 α-hydroxyestrone and 4-hydroxyestrone may be carcinogenic in specific cells because they are capable of damaging cellular proteins and DNA after their further activation to quinone intermediates.

Xenobiotic-metabolizing enzymes not only detoxify xenobiotics but also cause the formation of active intermediates (bioactivation), which in certain circumstances may elicit a diversity of toxicities, including mutagenesis, carcinogenesis, and hepatic necrosis (23). Some nucleophiles, in addition to

glutathione, such as other sulfhydryl compounds (most effective), alcohols, and phosphates, can react with arene oxides. Many of these nucleophiles are found in proteins and nucleic acids. The covalent binding of these bioactive epoxides to intracellular macromolecules provides a molecular basis for these toxic effects (see the discussion on toxicity from oxidative metabolism in this chapter).

N-Dealkylation, Oxidative Deamination and N-oxidation
N-Dealkylation. The dealkylation of secondary and tertiary amines to yield primary and secondary amines, respectively, is one of the most important and frequently encountered reactions in drug metabolism. The proposed mechanism for oxidative N-dealkylation involving α-hydrogen abstraction or an electron abstraction from the nitrogen by the perferryl oxygen has been previously discussed (19) (Fig. 8.7).

Typical N-substituents removed by oxidative dealkylation are methyl, ethyl, n-propyl, isopropyl, n-butyl, allyl, and benzyl. Usually, dealkylation occurs with the smaller alkyl group initially. Substituents that are more resistant to dealkylation include the tert-butyl (no α-hydrogen) and the cyclopropylmethyl. In general, tertiary amines are dealkylated to secondary amines faster than secondary amines are dealkylated to primary amines. This difference in rate has been correlated with lipid solubility. Appreciable amounts of secondary and primary amines therefore accumulate as metabolites that are more polar than the parent amine, thus slowing their rates of diffusion across membranes and reducing their accessibility to receptors. Frequently, these amine metabolites contribute to the pharmacologic activity of the parent substance (e.g., imipramine, Fig. 8.13) or produce unwanted side effects,

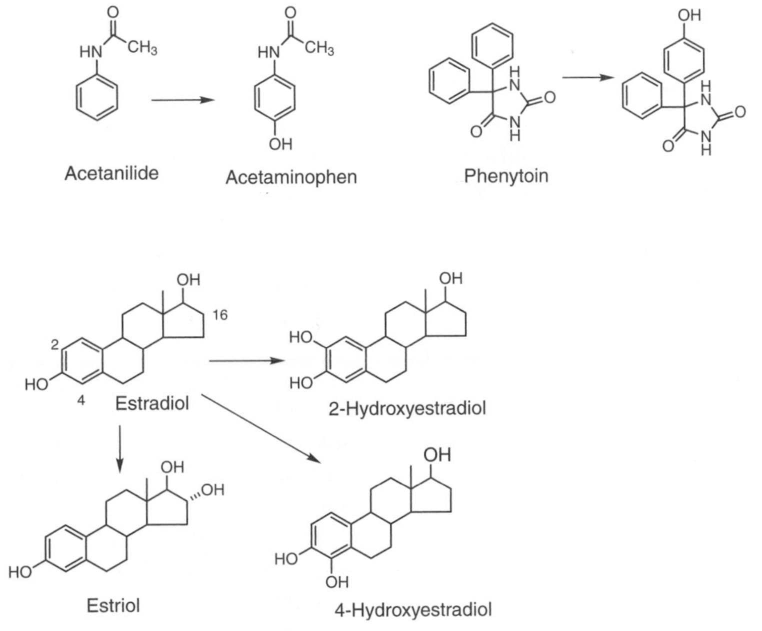

Acetanilide   Acetaminophen   Phenytoin

Estradiol   2-Hydroxyestradiol

Estriol   4-Hydroxyestradiol

Fig. 8.12. Examples of phase 1 xenobiotic oxidative metabolism of aryl compounds catalyzed by CYP450.

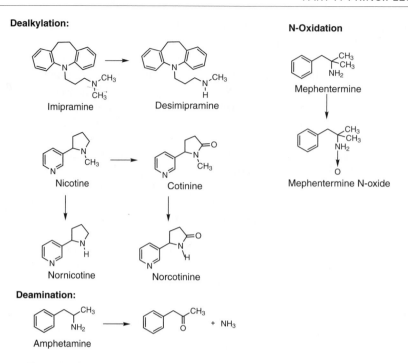

Fig. 8.13. Examples of phase 1 oxidation reactions catalyzed by CYP450.

such as hypertension, resulting from the N-dealkylation of N-isopropylmethoxamine to methoxamine. The design of an analogous drug without these unwanted drug metabolites can be achieved by proper choice of replacement substituents, for example, substituting the N-isopropyl group in N-isopropylmethoxamine with a tert-butyl (N-tert-butyl-methoxamine or butoxamine). N-dealkylation of substituted amides and aromatic amines occurs in a similar manner. N-substituted nonaromatic nitrogen heterocycles undergo oxidation on the α-carbon to a lactam (cotinine) as well as N-dealkylation (Nicotine to nornicotine, cotinine and norcotinine, Fig. 8.13).

Oxidative Deamination. The mechanism of oxidative deamination follows a pathway similar to that of N-dealkylation. Initially, oxidation to the imminium ion occurs, followed by decomposition to the carbonyl metabolite and ammonia. Oxidative deamination can occur with α-substituted amines, exemplified by amphetamine (Fig. 8.13). Disubstitution of the α-carbon inhibits deamination (e.g., phentermine). Some secondary and tertiary amines, and amines substituted with bulky groups, can undergo deamination directly, without N-dealkylation, for example, fenfluramine. Apparently, this behavior is associated with increased lipid solubility.

N-oxidation. In general, N-oxygenation of amines form stable N-oxides with tertiary amines and amides and hydroxylamines with primary and secondary amines when no α-protons are available (e.g., mephentermine, arylamines) (Fig. 8.13). Tertiary amines having a hydrogen(s) on the adjacent carbon, dealkylate via the N-oxide. Rearrangement of the N-

oxide to a carbinolamine, which subsequently collapses, gives rise to the secondary amine. The amine metabolites can be N-conjugated, increasing their excretion.

O- and S-Dealkylation. Oxidative O-dealkylation of ethers is a common metabolic reaction with a mechanism of dealkylation analogous to that of N-dealkylation; oxidation of the α-carbon and subsequent decomposition of the unstable hemiacetal to an alcohol (or phenol) and a carbonyl product (19). Thioethers are also dealkylated by the same mechanism to hemithioacetals.

$$Ar-O-CH_3 \longrightarrow Ar-O-\overset{\cdot\cdot}{\underset{}{C}}H_2^{\oplus} \longrightarrow Ar-O-CH_2OH \longrightarrow Ar-OH + CH_2O$$

The majority of ether groups in drug molecules are aromatic ethers, e.g., codeine, prazocin, and verapamil. For example, codeine is O-demethylated to morphine (Fig. 8.14). The rate of O-dealkylation is a function of chain length, i.e., increasing chain length or branching reduces the rate of dealkylation. Steric factors and ring substituents influence the rate of dealkylation, but are complicated by electronic effects. Some drug molecules contain more than one ether group, in which case, usually only one ether is dealkylated. The methylenedioxy group undergoes variable rates of dealkylation to the 1,2-diphenolic metabolite. Metabolism of such a group is also being capable of forming a stable complex with and inhibiting of CYP450.

Aliphatic and aromatic methyl thioethers undergo S-dealkylation to thiols and carbonyl compounds. For example, 6-methylthiopurine is demethylated to give the active anticancer drug, 6-mercaptopurine (Fig. 8.14). Other thioethers are oxidized to sulfoxides (see N- and S-oxidations).

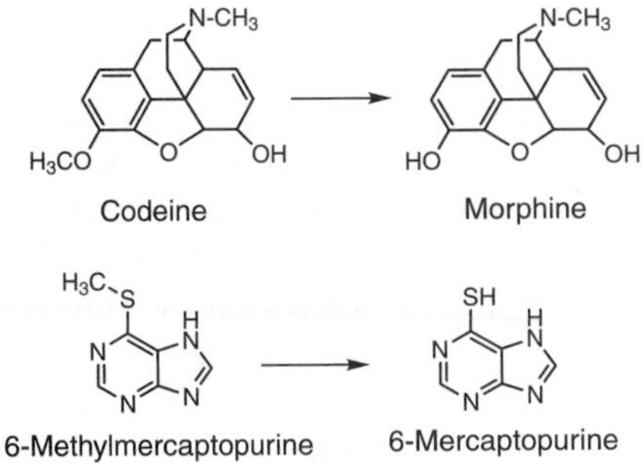

Fig. 8.14. Examples of phase 1 xenobiotic of O- and S-dealkylations catalyzed by CYP450.

Dehalogenation. Many halogenated hydrocarbons, such as insecticides, pesticides, general anesthetics, plasticizers, flame retardants, and commercial solvents, undergo a variety of different dehalogenation biotransformations (15,16). Because of our potential exposure to these halogenated compounds as drugs and environmental pollutants in air, soil, water, or food, it is important to understand the interactions between metabolism and toxicity. Some halogenated hydrocarbons form glutathione or mercapturic acid conjugates, whereas others undergo dehydrohalogenation and reductive dehalogenation catalyzed by CYP2E1. In many cases, reactive intermediates including radicals, anion, and cations are produced that may react with a variety of tissue molecules.

Halogenated hydrocarbons differ in their chemical reactivity as a result of the electron-withdrawing properties of the halogens on adjacent carbon atoms, resulting in the α-carbon developing electrophilic character. The halogen atoms also have the ability to stabilize α-carbon cations, free radicals, carbanions, and carbenes.

Oxidative dehydrohalogenation is a common metabolic pathway for many halogenated hydrocarbons (16,19). CYP450-catalyzed oxidation generates the transient *gem*-halohydrin (analogous to alkane hydroxylation) that can eliminate the hydrohalic acid to form carbonyl derivatives (aldehydes, ketones, acyl halides, and carbonyl halides) (Fig. 8.7). This reaction requires the presence of at least one halogen and one α-hydrogen. *Gem*-Trihalogenated hydrocarbons are more readily oxidized than are the gem-di-halogenated and monohalogenated compounds. The acyl halides and the carbonyl halides formed are reactive intermediates that can react either with water to form carboxylic acids or nonenzymatically with tissue molecules (with a potential for eliciting increased toxicity). Chloramphenicol ($RNHCOCHCl_2$) is biotransformed into an acyl halide ($RNHCOCOCl$) that selectively acylates the apoprotein of CYP450 (26).

An excellent example of oxidative dehydrohalogenation leading to significant hepato- and nephrotoxicity is seen with the fluorinated inhalation anesthetics (Fig. 8.15). The toxicity of halothane and the fluranes is related to their metabolism to either an acid chloride (or fluoride) or a trifluoroacetate intermediate (Chapter 14, Fig. 14.6). The CYP2E1 has been identified as the isoform catalyzing the biotransformation of the fluranes (16, 28, 29). The hydroxylated intermediate decomposes spontaneously to reactive intermediates, an acid chloride (or fluoride) or trifluoroacetate, which can either react with water to form halide anions and a fluorinated carboxylic acid, or bind covalently to tissue proteins producing an acylated protein. The acylated protein becomes a "hapten" stimulating an immune response and a hypersensitivity reaction. Halothane has received the most attention because of its ability to cause "halothane-associated" hepatitis. This immunologic reaction occurs after repeated exposure in surgical patients to tri-fluoroacetylate (TFA) protein. The patient is sensitized to future exposures of the volatile anesthetic. After subsequent exposure to a fluorinated anesthetic, the antigenic TFA-protein stimulates an immune response, producing halothane-like hepatitis. Because of the common metabolic pathway involving CYP2E1 for enflurane, isoflurane, desflurane, and methoxyflurane, halothane-exposed patients who have

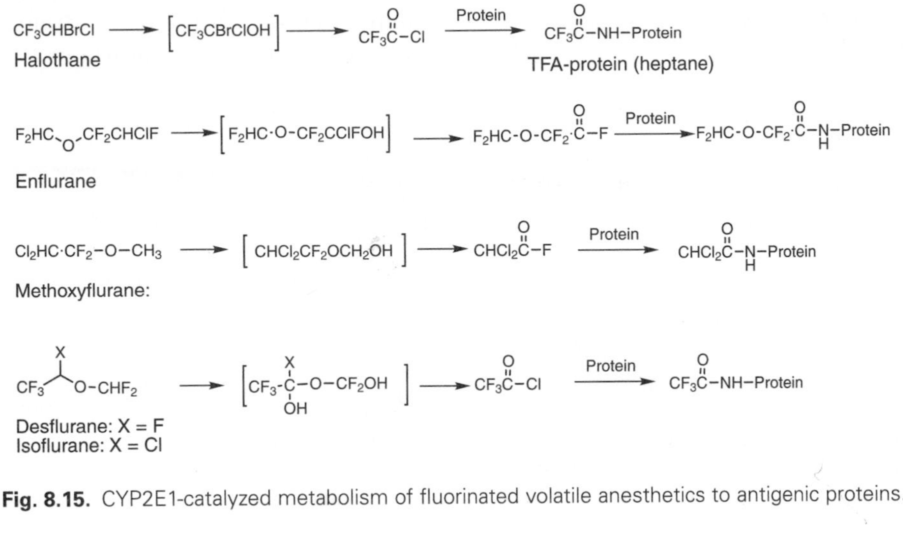

Fig. 8.15. CYP2E1-catalyzed metabolism of fluorinated volatile anesthetics to antigenic proteins.

halothane hepatitis can show cross-sensitization to one of the other fluranes, triggering an idiosyncratic hepatic necrosis. The formation of antigenic protein is related to the amount of CYP2E1 catalyzed metabolism for each agent; halothane (20 to 40%) > enflurane (2 to 8%) > isoflurane (0.2 to 1%) > desflurane (< 0.1%). Enough fluoride ion is generated from oxidative dehalogenation during flurane anesthesia to produce subclinical nephrotoxicity. Interestingly, female rats metabolize halothane more slowly than do males and are less susceptible than males to hepatotoxicity. For patients with pre-existing liver dysfunction, isoflurane or desflurane may be a better anesthetic choice.

In today's environment, most humans have been exposed to many CYP2E1 enzyme-inducing agents (including recreational, industrial, agricultural chemicals and alcohol), having an unknown effect on hepatic toxicity from volatile anesthetics. Enhanced activity for CYP2E1 has been observed in obesity, isoniazid therapy, ketogenic diets, and alcoholism.

Azo and Nitro Reduction. In addition to the oxidative systems, liver microsomes also contain enzyme systems that catalyze the reduction of azo and nitro compounds to primary amines. A number of azo compounds, such as Prontosil and sulfasalazine (Fig. 8.16), are converted to aromatic primary amines by azoreductase, an NADPH-dependent enzyme system in the liver microsomes. Evidence exists for participation of CYP450 in some reductions. Nitro compounds, for example, chloramphenicol and nitrobenzene, are reduced to aromatic primary amines by a nitroreductase, presumably through nitrosamine and hydroxylamine intermediates. These reductases are not solely responsible for the reduction of azo and nitro compounds; reduction by the bacterial flora in the anaerobic environment of the intestine may also occur.

N- and S-Oxidations Catalyzed by Flavin Monooxygenase

The major hepatic monooxygenase systems responsible for the oxidation of many drugs, carcinogens, pesticides, aromatic polycyclic hydrocarbons, and other xenobiotics containing nitrogen, sulfur, or phosphorus are CYP450 monooxygenase and microsomal flavin-containing monooxygenase (FMO) (30). The FMO exhibits broader substrate specificities than CYP450 monooxygenases and has a mechanism distinctly different from the CYP450 monooxygenase. Because oxygen activation occurs before substrate addition, any compound binding to 4 α-hydroperoxyflavin, the enzyme-bound monooxygenating FMO intermediate, is a potential substrate. Typically, FMO catalyzes oxygenation of the N and S heteroatoms ("soft nucleophiles") (Fig. 8.17) but not heteroatom dealkylation reactions. The products formed from FMO catalyzed oxidation are consistent with a direct two-electron oxidation of the heteroatom. Thus, FMO constitutes an alternative biotransformation pathway for N- and S-containing lipophilic xenobiotics. FMO is not normally inducible by phenobarbital nor affected by CYP450 inhibitors. With few exceptions, however, xenobiotic substrates for FMO are also substrates for the isoforms of CYP450 producing similar oxidation products. Which monooxygenase is responsible for the oxidation can be readily determined because FMO is thermally labile in the absence of NADPH, whereas CYP450 is stable.

Of the many nitrogen functional groups in xenobiotics, only secondary and tertiary acyclic, cyclic, and arylamines, hydroxylamines, and hydrazines are oxidized by FMO and excreted in the urine (Fig. 8.17). The tertiary amines form stable amine oxides, and secondary amines are sequentially oxidized to hydroxylamines, nitrones, and a complex mixture of products. Secondary N-alkylarylamines can be N-oxygenated to reactive N-hydroxylated metabolites that are responsible for the toxic, mutagenic, and carcinogenic activity of these aromatic amines. For example, the chemically unstable hydroxylamine intermediates of aromatic amines degrade into bladder carcinogens (see the discussion for this type of toxic mechanism under glucuronic acid conjugation in this chapter), and the hydroxamic acid intermediates of N-arylacetamides are bioactivated into liver carcinogens. Hepatic FMO, however, will not catalyze the oxidation of primary alkyl- or arylamines, except for the carcinogenic N-hydroxylated derivatives of 2-aminofluorene, 2-aminoanthracene, and other amino polycyclic aromatic hydrocarbons.

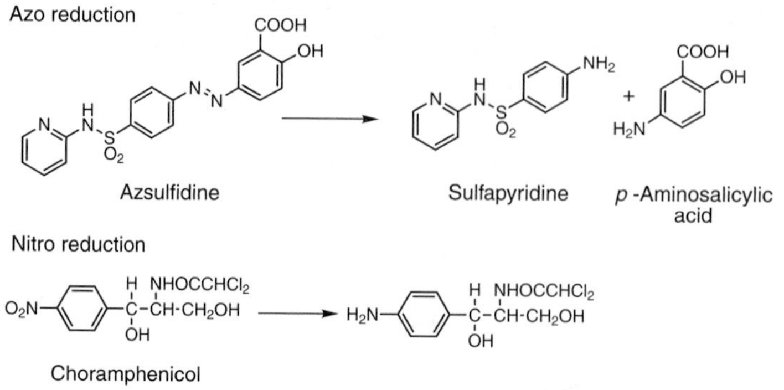

Fig. 8.16. CYP450 catalyzed reduction of azo and nitro compunds.

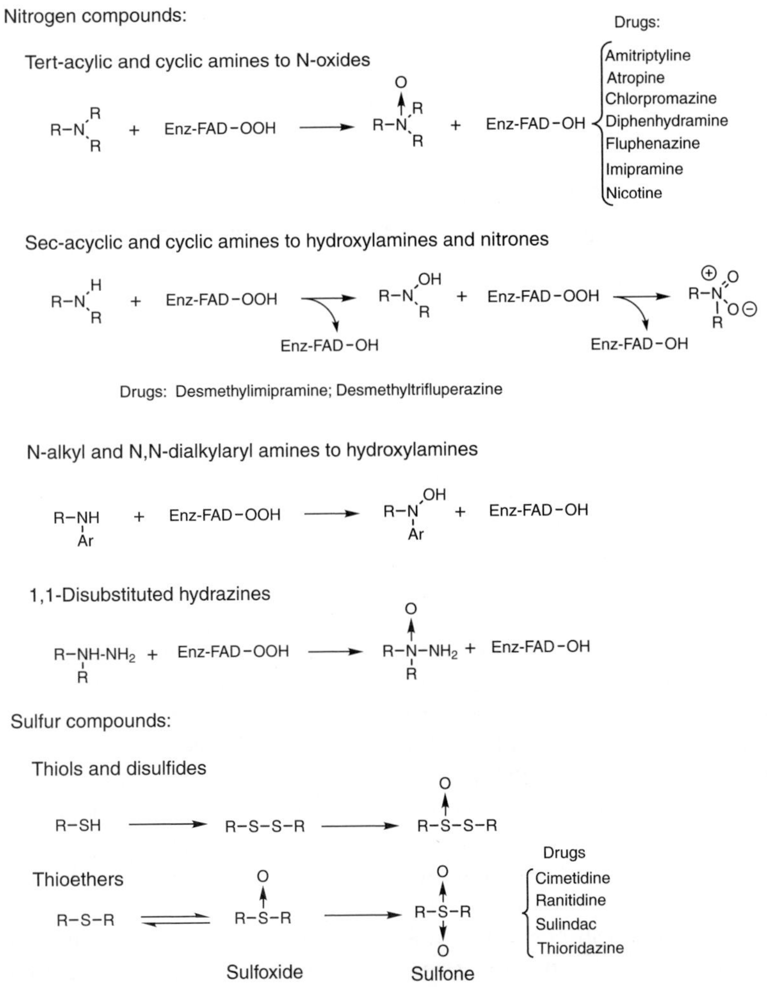

Nitrogen compounds:

Tert-acylic and cyclic amines to N-oxides

Drugs:
Amitriptyline
Atropine
Chlorpromazine
Diphenhydramine
Fluphenazine
Imipramine
Nicotine

Sec-acylic and cyclic amines to hydroxylamines and nitrones

Drugs: Desmethylimipramine; Desmethyltrifluperazine

N-alkyl and N,N-dialkylaryl amines to hydroxylamines

1,1-Disubstituted hydrazines

Sulfur compounds:

Thiols and disulfides

Thioethers

Drugs
Cimetidine
Ranitidine
Sulindac
Thioridazine

Sulfoxide   Sulfone

Fig. 8.17. Examples of flavin monoxygenase (FMO) oxidations.

S-Oxidation occurs almost exclusively by FMO (Fig. 8.17). Sulfides are oxidized to sulfoxides and to sulfones, thiols to disulfides, and thiocarbamates, mercaptopyrimidines, and mercaptoimidazoles (i.e., the antithyroid drug methimazole) via sulfenates (RSOH) to sulfinates (RSO$_2$H), all of which are eliminated in the urine.

FMO does not catalyze epoxidation reactions or hydroxylation at unactivated carbon atoms of xenobiotics. Primary aromatic amines and amides, aromatic heterocyclic amines and imines, and the aliphatic primary amine phentermine are N-oxidized by CYP450 to hydroxylamines. CYP450 oxidizes carbon disulfide to carbon dioxide and hydrogen sulfide and the antipsychotic phenothiazines to sulfoxides.

The major steps in the catalytic cycle for FMO are shown in Figure 8.18 (31). Like most of the other monooxygenases, FMO requires NADPH and oxygen as cosubstrates to catalyze the oxidation of the xenobiotic substrate. But unlike CYP450, the xenobiotic being oxidized does not need to be bound to the 4 α-hydroperoxyflavin intermediate (FAD-OOH) for oxygen activation to occur. Apparently, FMO is present within the cell in its enzyme-bound activated-hydroperoxide (Enz-FAD-OOH) state ready to oxidize any suitable lipophilic substrate that binds to it. FMO uses a nonradical, nucleophilic displacement type of mechanism binding dioxygen with a reduced flavin. The reactive oxygen intermediate is a reactive derivative of hydrogen peroxide, flavin-4 α-hydroperoxide (See insert in Fig. 8.18), which is reactive enough to successfully attack a lone electron pair on a heteroatom such as nitrogen or sulfur but not reactive enough to attack a typical C-H bond. These studies suggest the xenobiotic substrate (Sub.) interacts with the 4 α-hydroperoxyflavin form of FMO and is oxidized by oxygen transfer from Enz-FAD-OOH to form the oxidized product (Oxidized sub.). Neither the substrate nor the oxidized substrate is essential for any other steps in the cycle. Steps 2 to 5 simply regenerate the oxygenating agent Enz-FAD-OOH from Enz-FAD-OH, NADPH, oxygen, and a proton. Any compound readily crossing cell membranes by passive diffusion and penetrating to the FMO-bound hydroperoxyflavin intermediate is a potential substrate, thus explaining the broad substrate specificity exhibited for FMO. The fact that the xenobiotic substrate is not required for activation of the

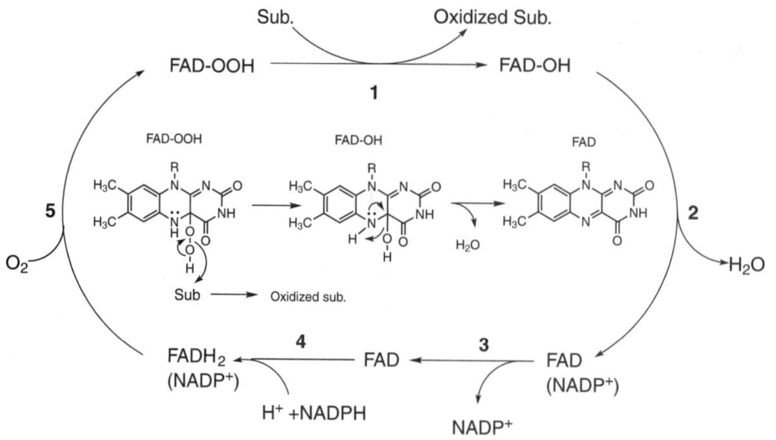

Fig. 8.18. FMO catalytic cycle. Oxygenated substrate is formed by nucleophilic attack of a substrate (Sub.) by the terminal oxygen of the enyme-bound hydroperoxyflavin (FAD-OOH) followed by heterolytic cleavage of the peroxide (1). The release of H_2O (2) or of $NADP^+$ (3) is rate limiting for reactions catalyzed by liver FMO. Reduction of flavin by NADPH (4) and addition of oxygen (5) complete the cycle by regeneration of the oxygenated FAD-OOH (34).

FMO-hydroperoxyflavin state distinguishes FMO from CYP450 monooxygenases, in which substrate binding initiates the CYP450 catalytic cycle and activation of oxygen to the perferryl oxygenating agent. It is not unusual for FMO oxidation products to undergo reduction to the parent xenobiotic, which can enter into repeated redox reactions called metabolic cycling.

Results of substrate specificity studies suggest that the number of ionic groups on endogenous substrate is an important factor enabling FMO to distinguish between xenobiotic and endogenous substrates, preventing the indiscriminate oxidation of physiologically important amine and sulfur compounds (32). Without exception, FMO readily catalyzes the oxidation of uncharged amines or sulfur compounds (in equilibrium with its respective monocation or monoanion; sulfur compounds, the charge is on sulfur atom). FMO will not catalyze the oxidation of dianions (e.g., thiamine pyrophosphate), dications (e.g., polyamines), dipolar ions (e.g., amino acids and peptides), or other polyionic compounds with one or more anionic groups (i.e., COO-) distal to the heteroatom (e.g., coenzyme A).

Unlike the CYP450 system, only three isoforms of hepatic FMO have been characterized in the adult human liver (33): minor form I (or FMO 1A1) which is the major form in fetal tissue; major form II (FMO 1D1); and form III, of which little is currently known. The substrate specificities for these isoforms have not been reported. The availability of different forms of FMO may be of clinical importance in the pharmacologic and toxicologic properties of FMO-dependent drug oxidations.

Peroxidases and Other Monooxygenases

Peroxidases are hemoproteins and perhaps are the most closely related enzymes to CYP450 monooxygenase (34). The normal course of peroxide (ROOH) catalyzed oxidation involves the formation of the $[FeO]^{+3}$ intermediate analogous to the perferryl complex in CYP450. It can per-

form heteroatom oxygenation and aromatization (oxidation) of 1,4-dihydropyridines (calcium channel blockers).

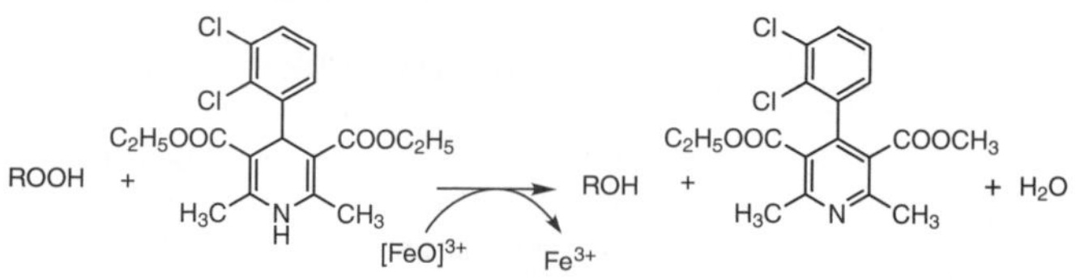

Other monooxygenases catalyzing oxidation reactions similar to CYP450 include dopamine β-monooxygenase, a mammalian copper containing enzyme catalyzing carbon hydroxylation, epoxidation, S-oxygenation, and N-dealkylation reactions, and non-heme iron-containing enzymes from bacteria and plants.

Nonmicrosomal Oxidations

In addition to the microsomal monooxygenases, other oxidases and dehydrogenases that catalyze oxidation reactions are present in the mitochondrial and soluble fractions of tissue homogenates.

Oxidation of Alcohols

Alcohol dehydrogenase is an NAD-specific enzyme located in the soluble fraction of tissue homogenates. It exhibits a broad specificity for alcohols; most primary alcohols are readily oxidized to their corresponding aldehydes. Some secondary alcohols are oxidized to the ketones, whereas other secondary and tertiary alcohols are excreted unchanged or as their conjugate metabolite. Some secondary alcohols show mixed activity because of steric factors and lack of affinity of the substrate for the enzyme.

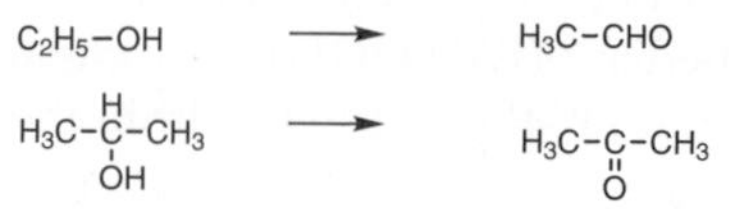

Oxidation by alcohol dehydrogenase is the principal pathway for ethanol metabolism, but the microsomal isoform CYP2E1 also plays a significant role in ethanol metabolism and tolerance. Apparently, two thirds of ingested ethanol is oxidized by alcohol dehydrogenase and the remainder by CYP2E1; during intoxication, however, ethanol induces the expression of CYP2E1. The induction of CYP2E1 contributes to the activation of some xenobiotics, increasing the vulnerability of the heavy drinker to anesthetic drugs, over-the-counter analgesics, prescription drugs, and chemical carcinogens. In turn, the excessive amounts of acetaldehyde generated causes hepatotoxicity, lipid peroxidation of membranes, formation of protein adducts, and other cellular changes.

Although the toxicity of methanol and ethylene glycol in humans has long been recognized, frequent reports of such toxicity are not surprising given the number of consumer products containing methanol and ethylene glycol (automotive antifreeze). Methanol (wood alcohol, methyl alcohol) is commonly used as a solvent in organic synthetic procedures, and is available to consumers in a variety of products ranging from solid fuels (Sterno), paint removers, solvent for "ditto" copy machines, motor fuels, antifreeze, and unintentional ingredient in alcoholic beverages. Oral methanol toxicity in humans is characterized by its rapid absorption from the gut followed by a latent period of many hours before metabolic acidosis (lowered blood pH and bicarbonate levels) and ocular toxicity is evident. The metabolic acidosis and blindness result from the excessive accumulation of formic acid and the inability of the hepatic tetrahydrofolate pathway to oxidize formate to carbon dioxide. The rate of elimination of methanol from the blood is relatively slow compared to ethanol, accounting for its long latency period. Its half-life ranges from 2 to 3 hours at low blood concentration to 27 hours at high blood concentration. Evidence supports the singular role of liver alcohol dehydrogenase in the metabolism of methanol to formaldehyde, although it is oxidized slowly by alcohol dehydrogenase (about one sixth the rate of ethanol). The demonstration that methanol is a substrate for alcohol dehydrogenase provides a rational basis for the use of ethanol in the treatment of methanol toxicity. Ethanol depresses the rate of methanol oxidation by acting as a competitive substrate for alcohol dehydrogenase, reducing the formation of formaldehyde. On the other hand, formaldehyde is not usually detected in the blood because of its rapid metabolism by aldehyde dehydrogenase to formate. Although human exposure to methanol vapor is less prevalent, methanol is rapidly absorbed through the skin or by inhalation and can result in methanol poisoning, depending on severity of exposure. Ethylene glycol is oxidized to hydroxyacealdehyde and glyoxal and subsequently to oxalate by aldehyde dehydrogenase. When eliminated into the urine, oxalate forms calcium oxalate crystals that can block the kidney tubules. 4-Methylpyrazole (Fomepizole) is an alcohol dehydrogenase inhibitor that is used as an antidote for the treatment of methanol or ethylene glycol poisoning.

Alcohol dehydrogenase also functions as a reductase when it catalyzes the reduction of an aldehyde or ketone to an alcohol. In addition, other NADP- or NAD-dependent dehydrogenases in the cytosol are capable of reducing a variety of ketones. Ketones are stable to further oxidation and consequently yield reduction products as major metabolites. Examples of reduction are chloral hydrate to trichloroethanol, naltrexone to 6-β-hydroxynaltrexol, methadone to α-methadol and dolasetron to dihydrodolasetron. These alcohol metabolites are all pharmacologically active.

Aldehyde Dehydrogenase

A NAD-specific aldehyde dehydrogenase catalyzes the oxidation of endogenous aldehydes, such as those produced by the oxidation of primary alcohols or the deamination of biogenic amines, and of exogenous aldehydes to the corresponding carboxylic acids. By inhibiting this enzyme, disulfuram (Antabuse) and metronidazole produce an unpleasant set of reactions (flushing, abdominal cramping, headache) when small amounts of alcohol are ingested. Antabuse is used therapeutically in controlling alcohol abuse. Aldehyde dehydrogenase deficiency exhibits significant polymorphic expression in Chinese.

$$H_3C-CHO \longrightarrow H_3C-COOH$$

Molybdenum Hydroxylases

Molybdenum hydroxylases are additional non-CYP450 enzymes capable of catalyzing the oxidation of drugs. The molybdenum hydroxylases, which include aldehyde oxidase, xanthine oxidase and xanthine dehydrogenase, are more commonly found in the cytosol of mammalian liver, and carry out the oxidation and detoxification of a number of structurally different azaheterocycles (35). The efficient oxidation of endogenous purine nucleosides suggests that their metabolism and detoxification might be an important physiological role for the molybdenum hydroxylases. Among the azaheterocycles metabolized are derivatives of pyridine, quinoline, pyrimidine, purine, quinazoline and pteridines. These hydroxylases generally oxidize the carbon α to the nitrogen of the azaheterocycle to oxo metabolites (also called lactams). The molybdenum hydroxylases contain a common electron transfer system in each subunit; one molybdenum atom, two Fe/S clusters and one flavin adenine dinucleotide molecule. The molybdenum hydroxylases catalyse their reactions differently than CYP450 and other hydroxylase enzymes, requiring water rather than molecular oxygen as the source of the oxygen atom incorporated into the metabolite, and with the concomitant reduction of molecular oxygen to superoxide (36). The active sites possess a catalytically labile $Mo^{V}-OH$ (or possibly $Mo^{VI}-OH_2$) group that is transferred to the substrate during the course of the hydroxylation reaction.

Aldehyde Oxidase. In addition to metabolizing some aldehydes, aldehyde oxidase also oxidizes a variety of azaheterocycles, but not thia- or oxaheterocycles. Of the various purine
nucleosides metabolized by aldehyde oxidase, the 2-hydroxy-
and 2-amino derivatives are more efficiently metabolized,
and for the N^9-substitutents, the typical order of preference
is the acyclic nucleosides (9-[(hydroxy-alkyloxy)methyl]-
purines) > 2′-deoxyribofuranosyl > ribofuranosyl > arabi-
nofuranosyl > H). The kinetic rate constants for purine
analogs revealed that the pyrimidine portion of the purine
ring system is more important for substrate affinity than the
imidazole portion. Aldehyde oxidase is inhibited by potassium cyanide and menadione (synthetic vitamin K).

Aldehyde oxidase metabolizes an assortment of azaheterocycles including the short-acting sedative-hypnotic drug,
zaleplon (a pyrazolo[1,5a] pyrimidine derivative) to its 5-
oxo metabolite; the anticancer drug thioguanine to 8-
oxothioguanine; the α2 adrenergic agonist brimonidine (a
pyrimidine derivative) to its 2-oxo-, 3-oxo- and 2,3-dioxo-
metabolites; quinine and quinidine to their 2-quinolone
metabolites; the pro-antiviral drug, famiclovir (a purine derivative) to its active 6-oxo metabolite (penciclovir); O^6-ben-
zylguanine to its 8-oxo metabolite (also formed primarily
from CYP3A4); the metabolism of the anticancer drug
DACA (an acridine-4-carboxamide derivative) to its 9-
acridone metabolite; the antiseizure drug, zonisamide (a
1,2-benzisoxazole derivative), is primarily metabolized by
reductive cleavage of the 1,2-benzisoxazole ring to 2-sul-
famoylacetylphenol. Although the azaheterocycles thiazole
and oxazole are not metabolized by aldehyde oxidase, their
carbocyclic analogs, benzothiazole, benzoxazole and 1,2-
benzisoxazole are metabolized. On the other hand, the heterocycles, benzothiophene and benzofuran, which do not
contain a nitrogen atom, are not metabolized by or inhibit
aldehyde oxidase.

The hepatotoxic and neurotoxic MPTP (1-methyl-4-
phenyl-1,2,3, 6-tetrahydropyridine) is metabolized by aldehyde oxidase to its non-toxic MP-2-pyridone metabolite
(MPTP lactam). Although S-cotinine is formed primarily
from S-nicotine in human smokers by CYP2A6, in vitro
studies suggest that aldehyde oxidase contributes to S-
nicotine metabolism by oxidizing the intermediate
metabolite (S-nicotine Δ-1′,5′-iminium ion) to S-coti-
nine.These results suggest that hepatic aldehyde oxidase is
a key detoxification enzyme for MPTP and S-nicotine.

Both aldehyde oxidase and xanthine oxidase contribute to the first-pass hepatic metabolism of orally administered methotrexate (a 2,4-diaminopteridine) to its 7-
hydroxymethotrexate metabolite.

Xanthine Oxidase and Xanthine Dehydrogenase. Xanthine oxidase and xanthine dehydrogenase represent different forms of the same gene product. Xanthine dehydrogenase and xanthine oxidase are interconvertable, thus these
two enzyme forms and their reactions are often referred to
as xanthine oxidoreductase. Xanthine oxidase is the rate-

limiting enzyme in purine catabolism of hypoxanthine to
uric acid via xanthine. Both xanthine oxidase and xanthine
dehydrogenase play important roles in the metabolism of a
number of purine anticancer drugs to their active and inactive metabolites. Although xanthine oxidase is strongly inhibited by the antigout drug, allopurinol, aldehyde oxidase
oxidizes it to oxypurinol. Only xanthine dehydrogenase requires NAD+ as an electron acceptor for the oxidation of
azaheterocycles. 6-Mercaptopurine is metabolized by xanthine oxidase to 6-mercaptouric acid.

6-Mercaptopurine   6-Mercaptouric acid

Oxidative Deamination of Amines

Monoamine oxidase (MAO) and diamine oxidase
(DAO) catalyze oxidative deamination of amines to the
aldehydes in the presence of oxygen. The aldehyde products can be metabolized further to the corresponding alcohol or acid by aldehyde oxidase or dehydrogenase.

Monoamine Oxidase (MAO). Monoamine oxidase is a
mitochondrial membrane flavin-containing enzyme that
catalyzes the oxidative deamination of monoamines according to the following equation:

$$R\text{-}CH_2\text{-}NH_2 \;+\; O_2 \;\longrightarrow\; [\,R\text{-}CH=NH\,] \;\longrightarrow\; R\text{-}CHO \;+\; NH_4^{\oplus}$$

Substrates for this enzyme include several monoamines,
secondary and tertiary amines in which the amine substrates are methyl groups. The amine must be attached to
an unsubstituted methylene group, and compounds having substitution at the α-carbon atom are poor substrates
for MAO, e.g., aniline, amphetamine, and ephedrine, but
are oxidized by the microsomal CYP450 enzymes rather
than by MAO (Fig. 8.13). For secondary and tertiary
amines, alkyl groups larger than a methyl and branched
alkyl groups, i.e., isopropyl, t-butyl, or β-phenylisopropyl,
inhibit MAO oxidation, but such substrates may function
as reversible inhibitors of MAO. Nonselective irreversible
inhibitors of MAO include hydrazides (phenelzine) and
tranylcypromine, and the MAO-B selective inhibitors pargyline and selegiline. Monoaminic oxidase is important in
regulating the metabolic degradation of catecholamines
and serotonin (5-HT) in neural tissues, and hepatic MAO
has a crucial defensive role in inactivating circulating
monoamines or those that originated in the gastrointestinal tract and were absorbed into the systemic circulation
(e.g., tyramine). Two types of MAO isolated are MAO-A
and MAO-B. They show dissimilar substrate preferences
and different sensitivities to inhibitors. MAO-A is found
mainly in peripheral adrenergic nerve terminals and
shows substrate preference for 5-hydroxytryptamine, norepinephrine, and epinephrine; MAO-B is found principally in platelets and shows selectivity for nonphenolic,

lipophilic β-phenethylamines. Common substrates to both MAO-A and MAO-B are dopamine, tyramine, and other monophenolic phenylethylamines.

MPTP (1-methyl-4-phenyl-1,2,3,6-tetrahydropyridine), a contaminant in the synthesis of reversed esters of meperidine, was discovered to be a highly selective neurotoxin for dopaminergic cells, producing parkinsonism (32). The neurotoxicity of MPTP is associated with cellular destruction in the substantia nigra along with severe reductions in the concentration of dopamine, norepinephrine, and serotonin. The remarkable neurotoxic action for MPTP involves a sequence of events beginning with the metabolic activation of MPTP to the toxic metabolite MPP$^+$ (1-methyl-4-phenylpyridinium ion) by MAO-B, specific uptake and accumulation of MPP$^+$ in the nigrostriatal dopaminergic neurons, and ending with the inhibition of oxidative phosphorylation (of NADH dehydrogenase in complex I). This inhibition results in mitochondrial injury depriving the sensitive nigrostriatal cells of oxidative phosphorylation with their eventual cell death (neurotoxic actions of MPP$^+$). MAO-B inhibitors (e.g., deprenyl) blocked this biotransformation.

MPTP   MPP$^+$

Diamines, such as $H_2N\text{-}(CH_2)_n\text{-}NH_2$, in which n is less than six, are not attacked and show little affinity for MAO. If the intermolecular distance between the amine groups is increased, the rate of oxidation by MAO increases. Evidently, the second amine group interferes with attachment of the amine to the enzyme.

Diamine Oxidase (DAO). Diamine oxidase attacks both diamines and histamine in much the same way MAO attacks monoamines, forming aldehydes. This enzyme is inhibited by carbonyl-blocking reagents and produces hydrogen peroxide, supporting the role of pyridoxal phosphate and the flavin prosthetic groups in the catalytic action of the enzyme. DAO is recovered in the supernatant after centrifugation and removal of particulate matter. It is present in kidneys, intestines, liver, lung, and nervous tissue. It limits the biologic effects of histamine and the polymethylene amines putrescine and cadaverine. It also attacks monoamines, but at a higher substrate concentration.

$H_2N\text{-}(CH_2)_4\text{-}NH_2$ $H_2N\text{-}(CH_2)_5\text{-}NH_2$

Putrescine   Cadaverine

Plasma amine oxidases are in blood plasma of mammals and include spermine oxidase, which deaminates spermine and other polyamines.

Miscellaneous Reductions

Disulfides (e.g., disulfiram), sulfoxides (e.g., dimethylsulfoxide), N-oxides, double bonds such as those in pro-

gestational steroids, and dehydroxylation of aromatic and aliphatic hydroxyl derivatives are examples of reductions occurring in microsomal or nonmicrosomal (usually cytosol enzymes) fractions.

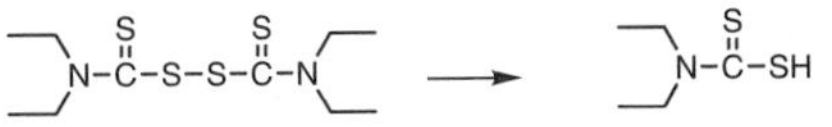

Disulfiram   Diethyldithiocarbamic acid

$CH_3SOCH_3 \longrightarrow CH_3SCH_3$

Dimethylsulfoxide   Dimethylsulfide

Various studies on the biotransformation of xenobiotic ketones have established that ketone reduction is an important metabolic pathway in mammalian tissue. Because carbonyl compounds are lipophilic and may be retained in tissues, their reduction to the hydrophilic alcohols and subsequent conjugation are critical to their elimination. Although ketone reductases may be closely related to the alcohol dehydrogenases, they have distinctly different properties and use NADPH as the cofactor. The metabolism of xenobiotic ketones to free alcohols or conjugated alcohols has been demonstrated for aromatic, aliphatic, alicyclic, and unsaturated ketones (e.g., naltrexone, naloxone, hydromorphone, and daunorubicin). The carbonyl reductases are distinguished by the stereospecificity of their alcohol metabolites.

β-Oxidation

Alkyl carboxylic acids, as their coenzyme A (CoA) thioesters, are metabolized by oxidation at the carbon β to the carboxylic carbon (β-oxidation). This pathway involves the oxidative cleavage of two carbon units at a time (as acetate), beginning at the carboxyl terminus and continuing until no more acetate units can be removed. The reaction is terminated when a branch (e.g., valproic acid) or aromatic group is encountered. The metabolism of even and odd phenylalkyl acids can serve as an example:

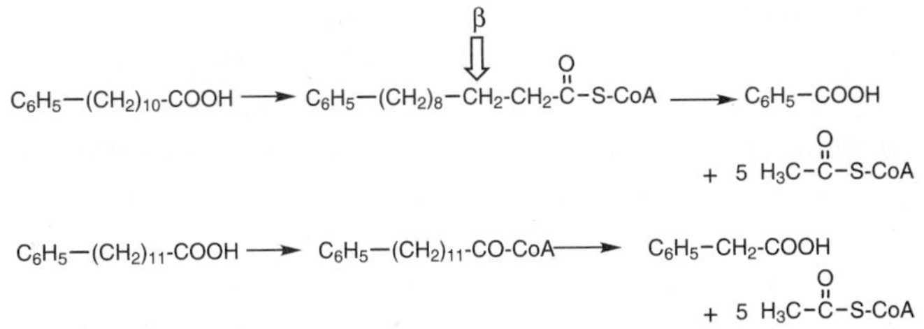

Hydrolysis

In general, esters and amides are hydrolyzed by enzymes in the blood, liver microsomes, kidneys, and other tissues. Esters and certain amides are hydrolyzed rapidly by a group of enzymes called carboxylesterases. The more lipophilic the amide, the more favorable it is as a substrate for this enzyme. In most cases, the hydrolysis of an ester or amide bond in a toxic substance results in bioinactivation to hydrophilic metabolites that are readily excreted. Some of these metabolites may yield conjugated metabolites (i.e., glucuronides). Carboxylesterases include cholinesterase (pseudocholinesterase), arylcarboxyesterases, liver microso-

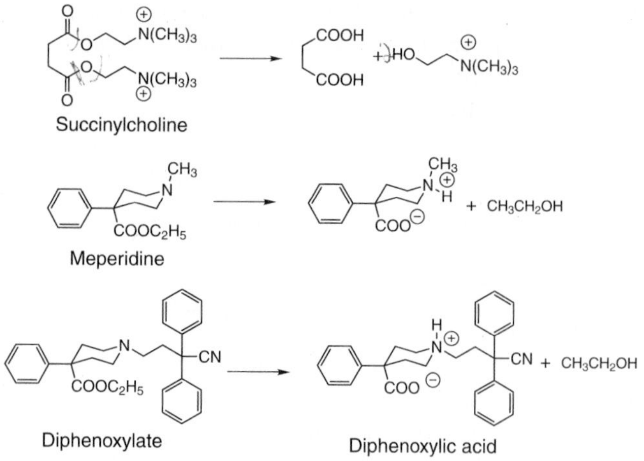

Fig. 8.19. Examples of hydrolysis reactions.

one of the major metabolites detected in human urine. Amide hydrolysis of phthalylsulfathiazole and succinylsulfathiazole by bacterial enzymes in the colon releases the antibacterial agent sulfathiazole.

Summary

In summary, phase 1 metabolic transformations introduce new and polar functional groups into the molecule, which may produce one or more of the following changes:

1. Decreased pharmacologic activity-*deactivation*
2. Increased pharmacologic activity-*activation*
3. Increased *toxicity-carcinogenesis, mutagenesis, cytotoxicity*
4. Altered pharmacologic activity

Drugs exhibiting increased activity or activity different from the parent drug generally undergo further metabolism and conjugation, resulting in deactivation and excretion of the inactive conjugates.

DRUG CONJUGATION PATHWAYS (PHASE 2)

Conjugation reactions represent probably the most important xenobiotic biotransformation reaction (36). Xenobiotics are usually lipophilic, well absorbed in blood, but slowly excreted in the urine. Only after conjugation (phase 2) reactions have added an ionic hydrophilic moiety, such as glucuronic acid, sulfate, or glycine to the xenobiotic, is water solubility increased and lipid solubility decreased enough to make urinary elimination possible. The major proportion of the administered drug dose is excreted as conjugates into the urine and bile. Conjugation reactions may be preceded by phase 1 reactions. For xenobiotics with a functional group available for conjugation, conjugation alone may be its fate.

Traditionally, the major conjugation reactions (glucuronidation and sulfation) were thought to terminate pharmacologic activity by transforming the parent drug or phase 1 metabolites into readily excreted ionic polar products. Moreover, these terminal metabolites would have no significant pharmacologic activity, i.e., poor cellular diffusion and affinity for the active drug's receptor. This long-established view changed, however, with the discovery that morphine 6-glucuronide has more analgesic activity than morphine in humans and minoxidil sulfate is the active metabolite for the antihypertensive minoxidil. For most xenobiotics, conjugation is a detoxification mechanism. Some compounds, however, form reactive intermediates that have been implicated in carcinogenesis, allergic reaction, and tissue damage.

Sequential conjugation for the same substance gives rise to multiple conjugated products (see P-aminosalicylic acid in Fig. 8.20). The xenobiotic can be a substrate for more than one metabolizing enzyme. For example, different conjugation pathways could compete for the same functional group. The outcome is an array of metabolites excreted in the urine or feces. The factors determining

mal carboxylesterases, and other unclassified liver carboxylesterases. Cholinesterase hydrolyzes choline-like esters (succinylcholine) and procaine, as well as acetylsalicylic acid. Genetic variant forms of cholinesterase have been identified in human serum (e.g., succinylcholine toxicity when administered as ganglionic blocker for muscle relaxation). Meperidine is hydrolyzed only by liver microsomal carboxylesterases (Fig. 8.19). Diphenoxylate is hydrolyzed to its active metabolite, diphenoxylic acid, within 1 hour (Fig. 8.19). Presumably, the peripheral pharmacologic action of diphenoxylate is attributed to zwitterionic diphenoxylic acid, which is readily eliminated in the urine.

A distinct type of esterase is the enzyme serum paraoxonase (PON1) which appears to act as an important guardian against the neurotoxicity of organophosphates and cellular damage from oxidized lipids in the LDL proteins (37). PON1 (A-esterase) is similar to arylesterase in that it catalyzes the hydrolysis of phenyl acetate and other aryl esters. Without PON1, the organophosphate is free to react with and irreversibly inhibit acetylcholinesterse (Chapter 10). PON1 also exhibits a substrate dependent polymorphism. Individuals susceptible to the toxic effects of organophosphates such as paraoxon and chlorpyrifos (Dursban) are deficient in this isoenzyme.

Esters that are sterically hindered are hydrolyzed more slowly and may appear unchanged in the urine. For example, approximately 50% of a dose of atropine appears unchanged in the urine of humans. The remainder appears to be unhydrolyzed biotransformed products.

As a rule, amides are more stable to esterase hydrolysis than are esters, and it is not surprising to find amides excreted largely unchanged. This fact has been exploited in developing the antiarrhythmic drug procainamide. Procaine is not useful because of its rapid esterase hydrolysis, but 60% of a dose of procainamide was recovered unchanged from the urine of humans, with the remainder mostly N-acetylprocainamide. On the other hand, the deacylated metabolite of indomethacin (a tertiary amide) is

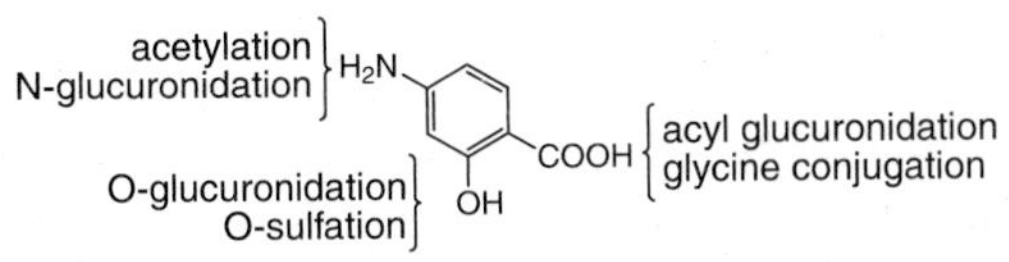

Fig. 8.20. Sequential conjugation pathways for *p*-aminosalicylic acid.

the outcome of this interplay include availability of cosubstrates, enzyme kinetics (V_{max}), substrate affinity (Km) for the metabolizing enzyme, and tissues. When a cosubstrate is low or depleted, the competing reactions can take over. The reactivity of the functional group determines all subsequent events. For example, major conjugation reactions at the phenolic hydroxyl groups are sulfation, ether glucuronidation, and methylation; for amine groups, acetylation, sulfation, glucuronidation; for carboxyl groups amino acid conjugation, ester glucuronidation.

Conjugation enzymes may show stereospecificity toward enantiomers when a racemic drug is administered. The metabolite pattern of the same drug administered orally and intravenously may be different because of presystemic intestinal conjugation. A current and in-depth review of the different phase 2 conjugations is available in reference 38.

Glucuronic Acid Conjugation

Glucuronide formation is probably the major and most common route for xenobiotic Phase 2 metabolism to water-soluble metabolites, and accounts for the major share of the conjugated metabolites found in the urine and bile (38). Its significance lies in the readily available supply of glucuronic acid in the liver and in the many functional groups forming glucuronide conjugates, e.g., phenols, alcohols, carboxylic acids, and amines.

Mechanism of Glucuronide Conjugation

The reaction involves the direct condensation of the xenobiotic (or its phase 1 product) with the activated form of glucuronic acid, uridine diphosphate glucuronic acid (UDPGA). The overall scheme of reactions is shown in Figure 8.21. The reaction between UDPGA and the acceptor compound is catalyzed by UDP-glucuronosyl transferases (UGT), a multigene family of isozymes located along the endoplasmic reticulum of liver, epithelial cells of the intestine and other extrahepatic tissues. Its unique location in the endoplasmic reticulum (ER) along with the CYP450 isoforms has important physiologic effects in the neutralization of reactive intermediates generated by the CYP450 isoforms and in controlling the levels of reactive metabolites present in these tissues.(Fig. 8.22). This cartoon depicts the spatial orientation and the interrelationship of the ER membrane-bound enzymes such as CYP450, UGTs and membrane-bound transporters (39). The transporters carry the UDPGA and xenobiotics (D) from the cytosol into the ER lumen, and transport the glucuronide metabolite from the ER lumen into the cytosol. The presence of the active site for UGT towards the ER lumen catalyzes the reaction between the substrate and UDPGA. The resultant glucuronide has the β-configuration about carbon 1 of glucuronic acid. With the attachment of the hydrophilic carbohydrate moiety containing an easily ionizable carboxyl group (pK_a 3-4), a lipid-soluble substance is converted into a conjugate that is poorly reabsorbed by the renal tubules from the urine and is excreted more readily into the urine or, in some cases, into the bile. Endogenous substances conjugated with glucuronic acid include steroids, bilirubin, and thyroxine. Not all glucuronides are excreted by the kidneys. Some are excreted into the intestinal tract with bile (enterohepatic cycling), where β-glucuronidase pres-

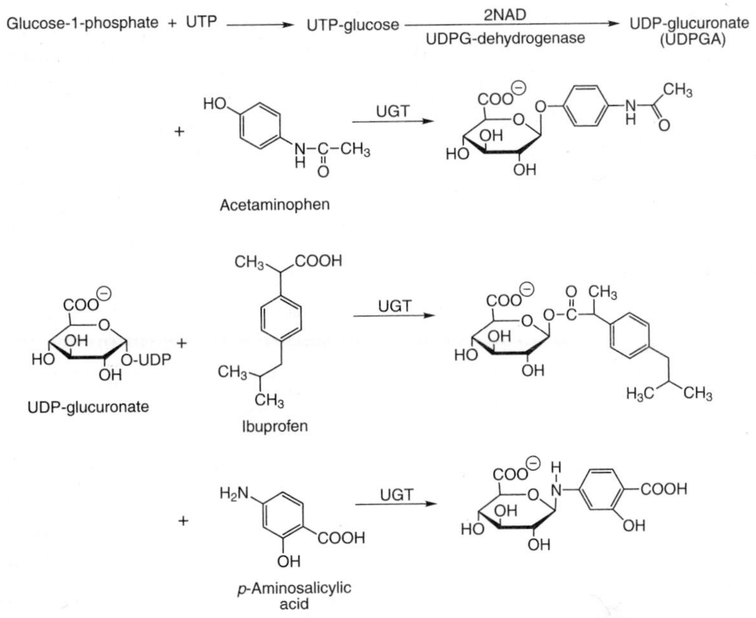

Fig. 8.21. Glucuronidation pathway catalyzed by UDP-glucuronosyl transferases (UGTSs).

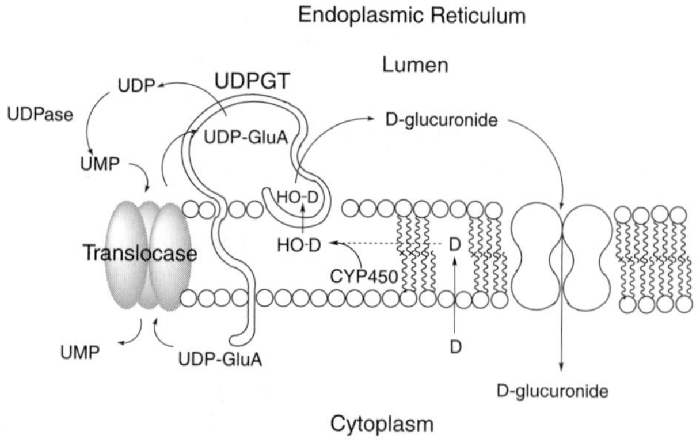

Fig. 8.22. Proposed topological model of UGT. A lipophilic drug (D) reaches the active site of CYP450 from the membrane or cytoplasm and is hydroxylated. The hydroxylated metabolite is transfered to UGT where glucuronidation occurs followed by release into the lumen and excretion from the cell. UDP-GluA is synthesized in the cytoplasm and transported via translocase (adapted from reference 62).

ent in the intestinal flora hydrolyzes the C^1-O-glucuronide back to the aglycone (xenobiotic or their metabolites) for reabsorption into the portal circulation.

UDP-glucuronosyl Transferase Families

The UGTs have been classfied into families according to similarities in amino acid sequences, analogous to the CYP450 family. The human UGT family is divided into two subfamilies, UGT1 and UGT2 (40). There is considerable overlap in substrate specificities between the two families. The human UGT1A1 isoform is primarily responsible for the glucuronidation of bilirubin, estradiol and other estrogenic steroids; UGT1A3 and UGT1A4 catalyze the glucuronidation of drugs with tertiary amines and hydroxylated xenobiotics; UGT1A6 exhibits limited substrate specificity for planar phenolic substances; UGT1A9 has a wide range of substrate specificity and can glucuronidate nonplanar phenols, plant substances such as anthraquinones and flavones, steroids and other phenolic drugs; and UGT1A10 glucuronidates mycophenolic acid an inhibitor of inosine monophosphate dehydrogenase. Human family 2 isoform UGT2B4 catalyzes the glucuronidation of the 6 α-hydroxyl group of bile acids; UGT2B7 is involved with the 3- and 6-glucuronidation of morphine and 6-glucuronidation of codeine; UGT2B11 glucuronidates a wide range of planar phenols, bulky alcohols and polyhydroxylated estradiol metabolites; and UGT2B15 catalyzes the glucuronidation of the 17 α-hydroxyl group of dihydrotestosterone and other steroidal compounds, and phenolphthalein. UGT1A isoforms are inducible with 3-methylcholanthrene and cigarette smoking, and UGT2B family is inducible by barbiturates.

UDP-glucuronosyl Transferase Distribution

The human liver has been established as the most important tissue for all routes of metabolism including glu-

curonidation. Studies have shown that the rate of glucuronidation is not uniform in the different sections of the liver; UGT1A6 content was greatest in the middle; UGT2B2 was uniformly distributed throughout the liver; UGT1A6 was also found in the bile duct epithelium and in the endothelium of the hepatic artery and portal vein. The UGTs expressed in the intestine include UGT1A1 (bilirubin glucuronidating isoform), UGT1A3, UGT1A4, UGT1A6, UGT1A8, UGT1A9 and UGT1A10. Substrate specificities of intestinal UGT isoforms are comparable to those in the liver. UGT isoforms in the intestine can glucuronidate orally administered drugs such as morphine, acetaminophen, alpha and beta adrenergic agonists and other phenolic phenethanolamines, and other dietary xenobiotics reducing their oral bioavailability (first pass metabolism). Although UGT isoforms are found in kidney, brain and lung, they are not uniformly distributed, with UGT1A6 being the isoform that is ubiquitous in extrahepatic tissue.

O, N, and S-Glucuronides

The xenobiotics forming glucuronides with alcohols and phenols are ether glucuronides; aromatic and some aliphatic carboxylic acids form ester (acyl) glucuronides; aromatic amines form N-glucuronides, and sulfhydryl compounds form S-glucuronides, both of which are more labile to acid than are the O-glucuronides (Fig. 8.21). Some tertiary amines (e.g., tripelennamine) have been reported to form quaternary ammonium N-glucuronides. Substances containing a 1,3-dicarbonyl structure, e.g., phenylbutazone, can undergo formation of C-glucuronides by direct conjugation without prior metabolism. The acidity of the methylene carbon of the 1,3-dicarbonyl group determines the degree of C-glucuronide formation.

Acyl Glucuronides

Drug-acyl glucuronides are reactive conjugates at physiologic pH. The acyl group of the C^1-acyl glucuronide can migrate via transesterification from the original C-1 position of the glucuronic acid to the C-2, C-3, or C-4 positions. The resulting positional isomers are not hydrolyzable by β-glucuronidase, giving the appearance of a new unknown conjugate(s). Under physiologic or weakly alkaline conditions, however, the C^1-acyl glucuronide can hydrolyze in the urine to the parent substance (aglycone) or undergo acyl migration to an acceptor macromolecule. The pH catalyzed migration of the acyl group from the drug C^1-O-acyl glucuronide to a protein or other cellular constituent occurs with the formation of a covalent bond to the protein (41). The acylated protein becomes a "hapten" and could stimulate an immune response against the drug, resulting in the expression of an hypersensitivity reaction, or other forms of immunotoxicity. A high incidence of anaphylactic reactions have been reported for several nonsteroidal anti-inflammatory drugs (NSAIDs, also known as NSAIAs) (benoxaprofen, zomepirac, indoprofen, alclofenac, ticrynafen, and ibufenac) that have been removed from the market. All of these NSAIDs are metabolized by humans to acyl glucuronides. Similar reactions have been reported for other NSAIDs including tolmetin, sulindac, ibuprofen, ketoprofen, and acetylsalicylic acid. The frequency of the immunotoxic response may be related to the stability of the acyl glucuronide, the chemical rate kinetics for the migration of the acyl group, and the concentration and stability/half-life of the antigenic protein. When the acyl glucuronide is the primary metabolite, patients with decreased renal function (i.e., elderly individuals) or when probenecid is coadministered, renal cycling of the unconjugated (aglycone) parent drug or metabolite is likely to occur, resulting in the plasma accumulation of the aglycone. The reduced elimination of the acyl glucuronide increases its hydrolysis back to the aglycone or the migration of the C^1-O-acyl group to an acceptor macromolecule.

Bioactivation and Toxic Glucuronides

Generally, glucuronides are biologically and chemically less reactive than their parent molecules, and are readily eliminated without interaction with intracellular substances. Some glucuronide conjugates, however, are more active than the parent drug (42). Morphine, for example, forms the 3-O- and 6-O-glucuronides in the intestine and in the liver. The 3-O-glucuronide is the primary glucuronide metabolite of morphine with a blood concentration 20 times morphine. Pharmacologically, it is an opiate antagonist. On the other hand, 6-O-glucuronide, with a blood concentration twice that of morphine, is a more potent μ-receptor agonist and 650× more analgesic than morphine in humans, whether administered orally or parentally. Thus, the analgesic effects of morphine are the result of a complex interaction of the drug and its two metabolites with the opiate receptor. Apparently, the 6-O-glucuronide can pass into the brain via an anion transport system.

Glucuronidation is also capable of promoting cellular injury (e.g., hepatotoxicity, carcinogenesis) by facilitating the formation of reactive electrophilic (electron-deficient) intermediates and their transport into target tissues (23). The induction of bladder carcinogenesis by aromatic amines may occur as the result of the glucuronidation of

N-hydroxylarylamine. These O-glucuronides become concentrated in the urine, where they are readily hydrolyzed by the acid pH of the urine back to the N-hydroxylarylamines. Elimination of water under these conditions leads to the formation of electrophilic arylnitrenium species. This reactive species can bind covalently with endogenous cellular constituents, e.g., nucleic acids and proteins, initiating carcinogenesis.

Sulfation and glucuronidation occur side by side, often competing for the same substrate (most commonly phenols, i.e., acetaminophen), and the balance between sulfation and glucuronidation is influenced by such factors as species, dose, availability of cosubstrates, and inhibition and induction of the respective transferases.

Sulfate Conjugation

Sulfate conjugation is an important reaction in the biotransformation of steroid hormones, catecholamine neurotransmitters, thyroxine, bile acids, phenolic drugs, and other xenobiotics (38). The major physiologic consequence of sulfate conjugation of a drug or xenobiotic is its increased aqueous solubility and excretion because the pKa of the sulfonate groups is about 1–2. The sulfate conjugates are almost totally ionized in physiologic solutions and possess a smaller volume of distribution than unconjugated steroids and drugs. However, in certain instances, sulfate conjugation can result in bioactivation to reactive electrophiles or therapeutically active conjugates (e.g., minoxidil sulfate). The cytosolic sulfotransferases are generally associated with the conjugation of phenolic steroids, neurotransmitters, and xenobiotics. The membrane bound sulfotransferases are localized in the Golgi apparatus of most cells and are responsible for the sulfation of glycosaminoglycans, glycoproteins, and the tyrosinyl group of peptides and protein, but are not generally associated with xenobiotic metabolism.

Mechanism of Sulfate Conjugation

A xenobiotic is sulfated by transfer of an active sulfate from 3'-phosphoadenosine-5'-phosphosulfate (PAPS) to the acceptor molecule, a cytosolic reaction catalyzed by a multigene sulfotransferases (Fig. 8.23); PAPS is formed enzymatically from ATP and inorganic sulfate. Sulfate

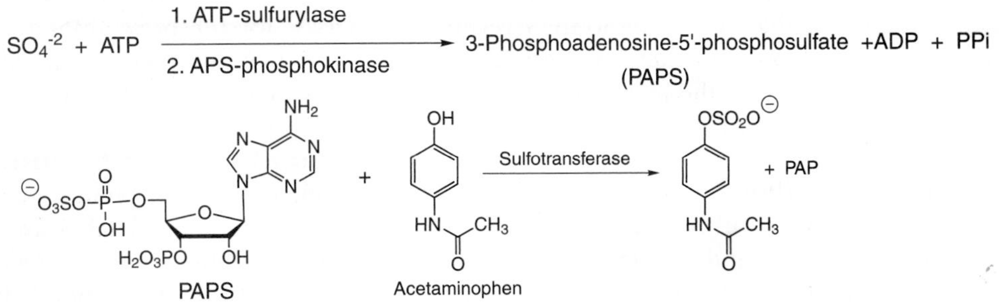

Fig. 8.23. Sulfation pathways.

conjugation is principally a reaction of phenols, and to a lesser extent of alcohols, to form highly ionic and polar sulfates (R-O-SO$_2$H). The availability of PAPS and its precursor inorganic sulfate determines the reaction rate. The total pool of sulfate is usually limited and can be readily exhausted. With increasing doses of a drug, conjugation with sulfate becomes a less predominant pathway. At high doses with a competing substrate (i.e., acetaminophen), glucuronidation usually predominates over that of sulfation, which prevails at low doses. Other precursors for sulfate include L-methionine and L-cysteine. When PAPS, inorganic sulfate, or the sulfur amino acids are low or depleted or when a substrate for sulfation is given in high doses, competing reactions with glucuronidation can take over. O-methylation is also a competing reaction for catecholamine.

Sulfotransferase Family

In humans, sulfotransferases are divided into two families, SULT1 and SULT2 (43). The isoforms SULT1A1, SULT1A2 and SULT1A3 catalyze the sulfation of many phenolic drugs, catecholamine, hormones, aromatic amines, and other xenobiotics (44). SULT1A1/2 (formerly known as phenol sulfotransferase-thermally stable) preferentially sulfates small planar phenols in the micromolar concentration range, estradiol and synthetic estrogens, phytoestrogens, acetaminophen, the N-oxide of minoxidil, N-hydroxyaromatic and heterocyclic amines; SULT1A3 (formerly known as phenol sulfotransferase-thermally labile) selectively sulfates the catecholamines dopamine, norepinephrine, and epinephrine, the N-oxide of minoxidil, thyroid hormones, but not estrogenic steroids and other hydroxy-steroids; SULT1B1 catalyzes the sulfation of the thyroid hormones; SULT1C1 is involved with the bioactivation of procarcinogens via sulfation; SULT1E1 (formerly known as estrogen sulfotransferase, EST) preferentially sulfates estradiol in the nanomolar range; SULT2A1 (formerly known as DHEA-ST or dehydroepiandrosterone sulfotransferase) conjugates DHEA, estradiol (micromolar range), the synthetic estrogens and other estrogen metabolites; and SULT2B1 (formerly known as hydroxysteroid sulfotransferase, HST) sulfates DHEA and pregnenolone.

Sulfate conjugation appears to be an important reaction in the transport and metabolism of steroids. Sulfation decreases the biologic activity of the steroid because the steroid sulfates are not capable of binding to their receptors; it provides for the transport of an inactive form of the steroid to its target tissue where the active steroid is regenerated by sulfatases at the target tissue.

Sulfotransferase Distribution

SULT1A families are abundantly expressed in the liver, small intestine, brain, kidneys, and platelets (43). For example, phenol is sulfated by a sulfotransferase in the liver, kidneys, and intestines, whereas steroids are sulfated only in the liver. The broad diversity of compounds sulfated in human tissues is due in part to the multi-isoforms of the cytosolic sulfotrasnferases and their overlapping substrate specificities. Sulfate conjugates are almost totally ionized and are therefore excreted mostly in the urine, but biliary elimination is common for steroids. On hydrolysis of biliary sulfate conjugates in the intestine by sulfatases, the parent drug (or xenobiotic) or its metabolites may be reabsorbed into the portal circulation for eventual elimination in the urine as a sulfate conjugate (enterohepatic cycling). The rate of sulfation appears to be age dependent, decreasing with age. An important site of sulfation, especially after oral administration, is the intestine. The result is a presystemic first pass effect, decreasing drug bioavailability for several drugs for which the primary route of conjugation is sulfation. Drugs such as isoproterenol, albuterol, steroid hormones, α-methyldopa, acetaminophen, and fenoldopam are affected. Competition for intestinal sulfation between coadministered substrates may influence their bioavailability with either an enhancement of or decrease in therapeutic effects. An example would be coadministration of acetaminophen and the oral contraceptive ethynylestradiol.

Bioactivation and Toxicity

As with glucuronidation, sulfation is a detoxication reaction, although sulfate conjugates have been reported to be pharmacologically active (e.g., minoxidil sulfate, dehydroepiandrosterone sulfate, and morphine 6-sulfate) or are converted into unstable sulfate conjugates that form reactive intermediates implicated in carcinogenesis and tissue damage. Sulfation of an alcohol generates a good leaving group and can be an activation process for alcohols to produce a reactive electrophilic species (23). However, N-sulfates, like the N-glucuronides, are capable of promoting cytotoxicity by facilitating the formation of reactive electrophilic intermediates. Sulfation of N-oxygenated aromatic amines is an activation process for some arylamines that can eliminate the sulfate to an electrophilic species capable of reacting with proteins or DNA, e.g., 2-acetylaminofluorene. N-sulfation of arylamines to arylsulfamic acids, R-NHSO$_3$H, is a minor pathway.

Stereoselectivity

SULT1A3 displays stereoselectivity in the sulfation of chiral phenolic phenethanolamines. This isoform may be partly responsible for the enantiomer specific metabolism observed for the beta adrenergic agonists. For example, the (+) enantiomers of terbutaline and isoproterenol and the (−) enantiomer of albuterol are selectively sulfated.

Conjugation with Amino Acids

Conjugation with amino acids is an important metabolic route in the metabolism of xenobiotic carboxylic acids prior to elimination (38). Glycine, the most common amino acid, forms water-soluble ionic conjugates with aromatic, arylaliphatic, and heterocyclic carboxylic acids. These amino acid conjugates are usually less toxic than

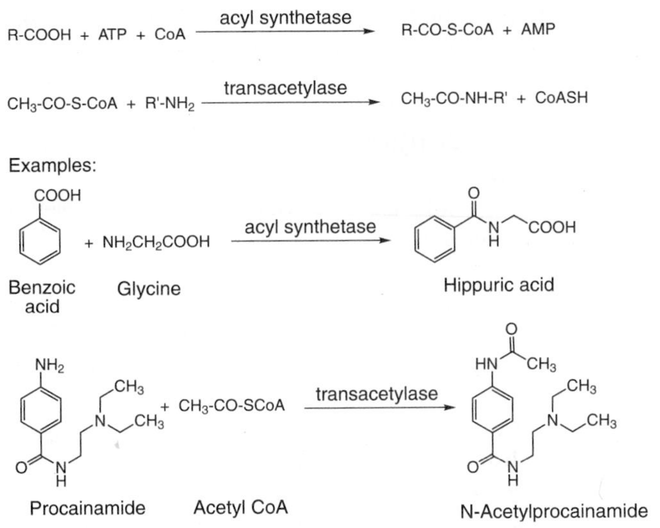

$$R\text{-COOH} + ATP + CoA \xrightarrow{\text{acyl synthetase}} R\text{-CO-S-CoA} + AMP$$

$$CH_3\text{-CO-S-CoA} + R'\text{-}NH_2 \xrightarrow{\text{transacetylase}} CH_3\text{-CO-NH-R'} + CoASH$$

Examples:

Benzoic acid + Glycine $\xrightarrow{\text{acyl synthetase}}$ Hippuric acid

Procainamide + Acetyl CoA $\xrightarrow{\text{transacetylase}}$ N-Acetylprocainamide

Fig. 8.24. Amino acid conjugation pathways of carboxylic acids with glycine and acetylation pathways.

their precursor acids and are excreted readily into the urine and bile. These reactions involve the formation of an amide or peptide bond between the xenobiotic carboxylic acid and the amino group of an amino acid, usually glycine. The xenobiotic must first be activated to its coenzyme A (CoA) thioester before reacting with the amino group (Fig. 8.24). The formation of the xenobiotic acyl CoA thioester is of critical importance in intermediary metabolism of lipids as well as intermediate and long chain fatty acids.

The major metabolic biotransformations for xenobiotic carboxylic acids include conjugation with either glucuronic acid or glycine. The metabolic fate of these carboxylic acids depends on the size and type of substituents adjacent to the carboxyl group. Most unbranched aliphatic acids are completely oxidized and do not usually form conjugates, although branched aliphatic and aryl-aliphatic acids are resistant to β-oxidation and form glycine or glucuronide conjugates. Interestingly, substitution of the α-carbon favors glucuronidation rather than glycine conjugation. Benzoic and heterocyclic aromatic

acids are principally conjugated with glycine. Glycine conjugation is preferred for xenobiotic carboxylic acids at low doses, and glucuronidation is preferred at high doses with broad substrate selectivity. In humans and some species of monkeys, glutamine forms a conjugate with phenylacetic acids and related arylacetic acids. Bile acids form conjugates with glycine and taurine by the action of enzymes in the microsomal fraction rather than in the mitochondria.

2-Arylpropionic acids ("profens") are a major group of nonsteroidal anti-inflammatory drugs (NSAIDs) that exist in two enantiomeric forms (41). The anti-inflammatory activity (inhibition of cyclooxygenase) for the NSAIDs resides with the S(+) enantiomer. The intriguing aspect for the metabolism of the NSAID is their unidirectional chiral inversion from the R(−) to the S(+) enantiomer (Fig. 8.25). The NSAID acyl CoA thioester is the critical intermediate for this chiral inversion of the 2-arylpropionic acids and the formation of the thioester is stereospecific for the pharmacologically inactive R-enantiomer (43). Racemic ibuprofen and related anti-inflammatory 2-arylpropionic acids (e.g., benoxaprofen, carprofen, cicliprofen, clidanac, fenoprofen, indoprofen, ketoprofen, loxoprofen, and naproxen) undergo in vivo metabolic inversion to the more active S-enantiomer via the formation, epimerization, and hydrolysis of their respective acyl CoA thioesters (45). The unidirectional R- to S-inversion of ibuprofen is attributed to the stereoselective thioester formation of (R)-ibuprofen CoA, and not to the stereoselectivity of either the epimerization or hydrolysis steps (46). S(+)-ibuprofen does not form its CoA thioester in vivo. Because the formation of 2-arylpropionyl CoA thioester is analogous to the activation and metabolism of medium and long chain fatty acids, it seems possible that conditions either elevating (e.g., diabetes or fasting) or depleting CoA may alter CoA thioester formation of the 2-arylpropionic acids and their in vivo metabolic inversion. Amino acid conjugation (i.e., CoA activation) is more sensitive to steric hindrance than is glucuronidation (e.g., arylacetic acids).

In contrast to the enhanced reactivity and toxicity of the various glucuronide, sulfate, acetyl and glutathione conjugates, amino acid conjugates have not proven toxic. It has been proposed that amino acid conjugation is a detoxication pathway for reactive acyl CoA thioesters.

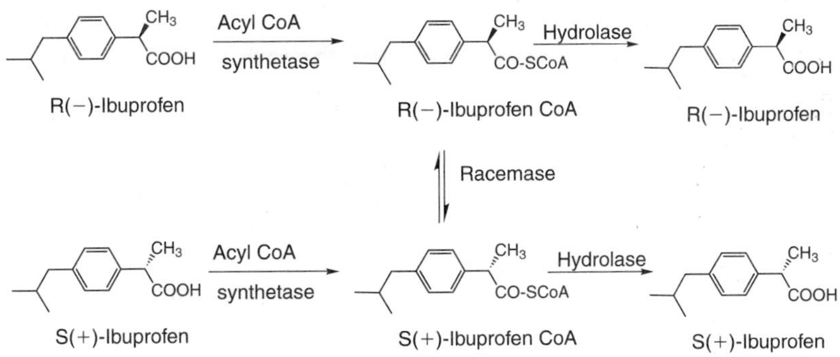

Fig. 8.25. Stereospecific inversion of R(−) to S(+)-ibuprofen.

Acetylation

Acetylation is principally a reaction of amino groups involving the transfer of acetyl CoA to primary aliphatic and aromatic amines, amino acids, hydrazines, or sulfonamide groups (38). The liver is the primary site of acetylation, although extrahepatic sites have been identified. Sulfonamides, being difunctional, can form either N^1 or N^4 acetyl derivatives, and, in some instances, the diacetylated derivative has been identified. Secondary amines are not acetylated. Acetylation may produce conjugates that retain the pharmacologic activity of the parent drug, e.g., N-acetylprocainamide (see Fig. 8.24).

The existence of genetic polymorphism in the rate of acetylation has important consequences in drug therapy and tumorigenicity of xenobiotics. Acetylation polymorphism has been associated with differences in human drug toxicity between the two acetylator phenotypes, slow and fast acetylators. Slow acetylators are more prone to drug-induced toxicities and accumulate higher blood concentrations of the unacetylated drug (e.g., hydralazine and procainamide-induced lupus erythematous, isoniazid-induced peripheral nerve damage, sulfasalazine-induced hematologic disorders) than rapid acetylators. Fast acetylators eliminate the drug more rapidly by conversion to its relatively nontoxic N-acetyl metabolite. For some drug substances, however, fast acetylators may pose a greater risk of liver toxicity than slow acetylators because they produce toxic metabolite(s) more rapidly, e.g., isoniazid forms the hepatotoxic monoacetylhydrazine metabolite. Thus, differences in acetylator phenotype can influence adverse drug reactions.

The possibility arises that genetic differences in acetylating capacity may confer differences in susceptibility to chemical carcinogenicity from arylamines. The tumorigenic activity of arylamines (1 in Fig. 8.26) may be the result of a complex series of sequential metabolic reactions commencing with N-acetylation (2 in Fig. 8.26), subsequent oxidation to arylhydroxamic acids (3 in Fig. 8.26) and metabolic transformation to acetoxyarylamines by N, O-acyltransferase (4 in Fig. 8.26). The acetoxyarylamine can eliminate the acetoxy group to form the reactive arylnitrenium ion (5 in Fig. 8.26) which is capable of covalently binding to nucleic acids and proteins, thus increasing the risk for development of bladder and liver tumors (47). The rapid acetylator phenotype is expected to form the acetoxyarylamine metabolite at a greater rate than the slow acetylator, and thereby presents a greater risk for the development of tumors than the slow acetylator.

Glutathione Conjugation and Mercapturic Acid Synthesis

Mercapturic acids are S-derivatives of N-acetylcysteine synthesized from glutathione (GSH) (36). It is generally accepted that most compounds metabolized to mercapturic acids first undergo conjugation with glutathione, catalyzed by the enzyme glutathione S-transferase (GST), a multigene isoenzyme family abundantly found in the soluble supernatant liver fractions. In humans, GSTs are divided into two isoforms, GSTM1 and GSTT1. The principal drug substrates for GSTM1 are the nitrosourea and mustard-type anticancer drugs. GSTT1 metabolizes small organic molecules such as solvents, halocarbons and electrophilic compounds (e.g., αβ-unsaturated carbonyl compounds). The reaction is depicted in Figure 8.27.

GST apparently increases the ionization of the thiol group of GSH, increasing its nucleophilicity toward electrophiles and conjugating with these potentially harmful electrophiles, thereby protecting other vital nucleophilic centers in the cell such as nucleic acids and proteins. Glutathione is also capable of reacting nonenzymatically with nucleophilic sites on neighboring macromolecules. Once conjugated with GSH, the electrophiles are usually excreted in the bile and urine.

A range of functional groups yields thioether conjugates of GSH, as well as products other than thioethers (Fig. 8.27). The nucleophilic attack by GSH occurs on electrophilic carbons with leaving groups such as halogen (alkyl, alkenyl, aryl, or aralkyl halides), sulfate (alkylmethanesulfonates), and nitro (alkyl nitrates) groups, ring opening of small ring ethers (epoxides, β-lactones, such as β-propiolactone), and the Michael-type addition to the activated β-carbon of an α,β-unsaturated carbonyl compound, such as acrolein. Organic nitrate esters (e.g., the coronary vasodilator nitroglycerin) undergo a dismutation reaction that results in the oxidation of GSH to GSSG (through formation of the labile S-nitrate conjugation product), and reduction of the nitrate ester to an alcohol and inorganic nitrite. The lack of substrate specificity gives argument to the fact that glutathione transferase has undergone adaptive changes to accommodate the variety of xenobiotics to which it is exposed. Usually, the conjugation of an electrophilic compound with GSH is a reaction of detoxication, but some carcinogens have been activated through conjugation with GSH (19).

The enzymatic conjugation of GSH with epoxides provides a mechanism of protecting the liver from injury caused by certain bioactivated intermediates (see the subsequent section on toxicity from oxidative metabolism). Not all epoxides are substrates for this enzyme, but the more chemically reactive epoxides appear to be better substrates. Important among the epoxides that are substrates for this enzyme are

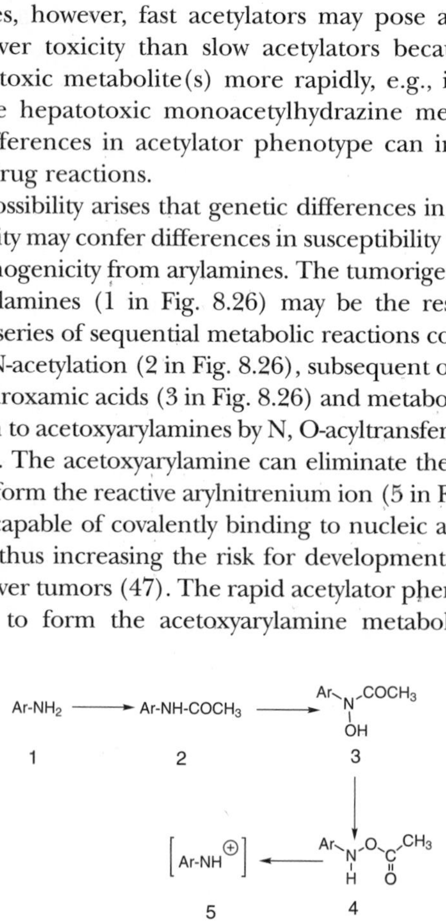

Fig. 8.26. Bioactivation of acetylated arylamines.

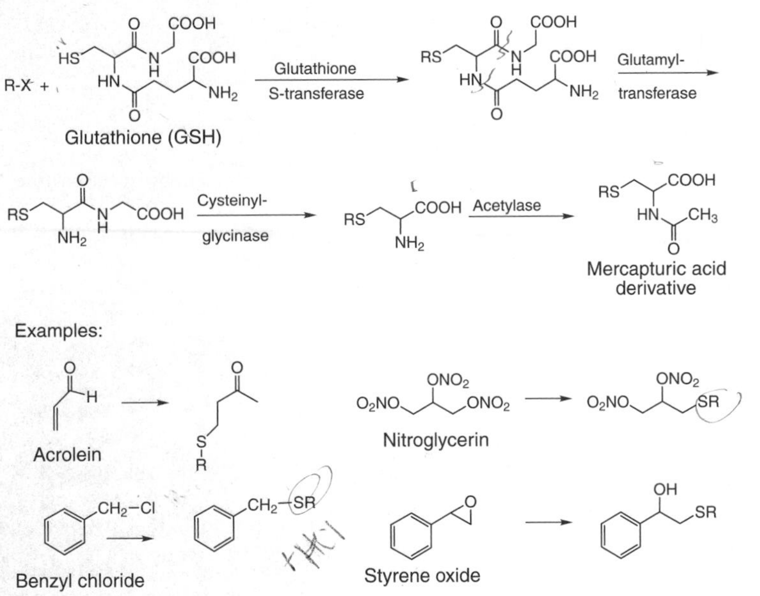

Fig. 8.27. Glutathione and mercapturic acid conjugation pathways.

those produced from halobenzenes and PAH through the action of CYP450 monooxygenase. Epoxide formation exemplifies bioactivation because the epoxides are reactive and potentially toxic, whereas their GSH conjugates are inactive. Conjugation of GSH with the epoxides of aryl hydrocarbons eventually results in the formation of hydroxymercapturic acids (premercapturic acids), which undergo acid-catalyzed dehydration to the mercapturic acids. The halobenzenes are usually conjugated in the para-position.

Monohalogenated, *gem*-dihalogenated, and vicinal dihalogenated alkanes undergo glutathione transferase-catalyzed conjugation reactions to produce S-substituted glutathione derivatives that are metabolically transformed into the more stable and less toxic mercapturic acids. This common route of metabolism occurs through nucleophilic displacement of a halide ion by the thiolate anion of glutathione (see the discussion on glutathione conjugation). The mutagenicity of the 1,2-dihaloethanes (e.g., the pesticide and fumigant, ethylene dibromide) has been attributed to GSH displacing bromide with the formation of the S-(2-haloethyl) glutathione, which subsequently rearranges to a reactive episulfonium ion electrophile that in turn alkylates a DNA. Many of the halogenated hydrocarbons exhibiting nephrotoxicity undergo the formation of similar S-substituted cysteine derivatives.

The mercapturic acid pathway appears to have evolved as a protective mechanism against xenobiotic-induced hepatotoxicity or carcinogenicity, serving to detoxify a large number of noxious substances that we inhale or ingest or that are produced daily in the human body. A correlation exists between the hepatotoxicity of acetaminophen and levels of GSH in the liver. The probable mechanism of toxicity that has emerged from animal studies is that acetaminophen is CYP1A2 and CYP2E1 oxidized to the N-acetyl-*p*-benzo-

quinonimine intermediate that conjugates with and depletes hepatic GSH levels (Fig. 8.28). This action allows the benzoquinonimine to bind covalently to tissue macromolecules. The mercapturic acid derivative of acetaminophen represents approximately 2% of the administered dose of acetaminophen. Thus, the possibility exists that those toxic metabolites that usually are detoxified by conjugating with GSH exhibit their hepatotoxicity (or perhaps carcinogenicity) because the liver has been depleted of GSH and is incapable of inactivating them. Pretreatment of animals with phenobarbital often hastens the depletion of GSH by increasing the formation of epoxides or other reactive intermediates.

Methylation

Methylation is a common biochemical reaction but appears to be of greater significance in the metabolism of endogenous compounds than for drugs and other foreign compounds (38). Methylation differs from other conjugation processes in that the O-methyl metabolites formed may in some cases have as great or greater pharmacologic activity and lipophilicity than the parent molecule (e.g., the conversion of norepinephrine to epinephrine). Methionine is involved in the methylation of endogenous and exogenous substrates because it transfers its methyl group via the activated intermediate S-adenosylmethionine (SAM) to the substrate under the influence of methyl transferases (Fig. 8.29). Methylation results principally in the formation of O-methylated, N-methylated, and S-methylated products.

O-Methylation

The process of O-methylation is catalyzed by the magnesium-dependent enzyme catechol-O-methyltransferase (COMT) transferring a methyl group to the meta- or less frequently to the paraphenolic-OH (regioselectivity) of cat-

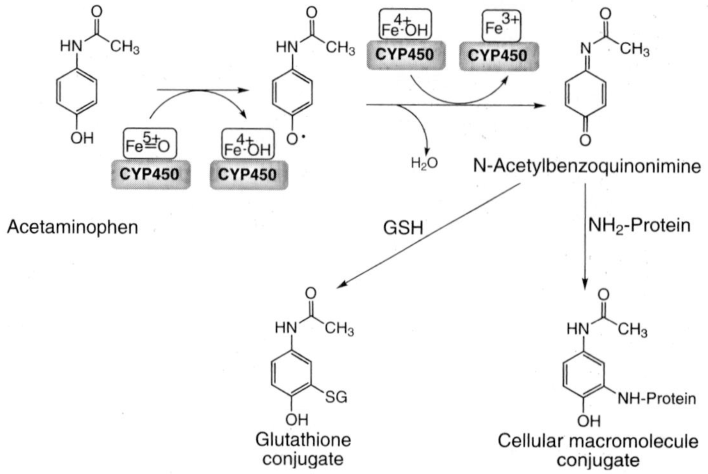

Fig. 8.28. Proposed mechanism for the CYP450-catalyzed oxidation of acetaminophen to its N-acetyl-*p*-benzoquinoneimine intermediate, which can further react with either glutathione (GSH) or cellular macromolecules (NH$_2$-Protein).

echolamines (e.g., norepinephrine), as well as their deaminated metabolites. It does not methylate monohydric or other dihydric phenols. The meta/para product ratio depends greatly on the type of substituent attached to the catechol ring. Substrates specific for COMT include the catecholamines: norepinephrine, epinephrine, and dopamine; catechol amino acids: L-DOPA and α-methyl-DOPA; and 2- and 4-hydroxyestradiol metabolites of estradiol. The enzyme is thought to function in the biologic inactivation of the adrenergic neurotransmitter norepinephrine as well as other endogenous and exogenous catechol-like substances. It is found in liver, kidneys, nervous tissue, and other tissues.

Hydroxyindole-O-methyltransferase, which O-methylates N-acetylserotonin, serotonin, and other hydroxyindoles, is found in the pineal gland and is involved in the formation of melatonin. This enzyme differs from COMT in that it does not methylate catecholamines and has no requirement for magnesium iron.

N-Methylation

The N-methylation of various amines is among several conjugate pathways for metabolizing amines. Specific N-methyltransferases catalyze the transfer of active methyl groups from SAM to the acceptor substance. Phenylethanolamine-N-methyltransferase (PNMT) methylates a number of endogenous and exogenous phenylethanolamines (e.g., normetanephrine, norepinephrine, and norephedrine) but does not methylate phenylethylamines. Histamine-N-methyl transferase specifically methylates histamine, producing the inactive metabolite N^1-methylhistamine. Amine-N-methyltransferase will N-methylate a variety of primary and secondary amines from a number of sources, including endogenous biogenic amines (serotonin, tryptamine, tyramine, and dopamine) and drugs (desmethylimipramine, amphetamine, and normorphine). Amine-N-methyl transferases seem to have a role in recycling N-demethylated drugs.

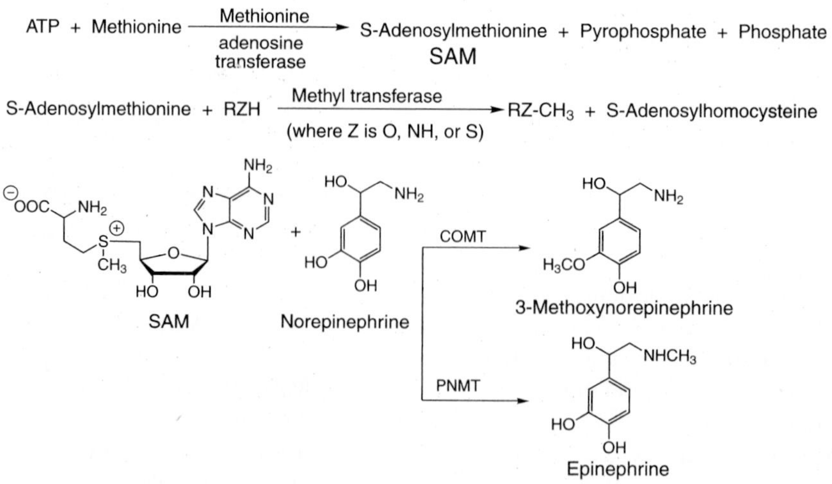

Fig. 8.29. Methylation pathways.

Thiol Methylation

Thiols are generally considered toxic, and the role of thiol S-methyl transferases is a non-oxidative detoxification pathway of these compounds (see the discussion of flavin-containing monooxygenases). The S-methylation of sulfhydryl compounds also involves a microsomal enzyme requiring SAM. Although a wide range of exogenous sulfhydryl compounds are S-methylated by this microsomal enzyme, none of the endogenous sulfhydryl compounds, e.g., cysteine and GSH, can function as substrates. S-methylation clearly represents a detoxication step for thiols. Dialkyldithiocarbamates (e.g., disulfiram) and the antithyroid drugs (e.g., 6-propyl-2-thiouracil), mercaptans, and hydrogen sulfide (from thioglycosides as natural constituents of foods, mineral sulfides in water, fermented beverages, and bacterial digestion) are S-methylated. Other drugs undergoing S-methylation include captopril, thiopurine, penicillamine, and 6-mercaptopurine.

Conjugation of Cyanide

The toxicity of hydrogen cyanide is the result of its ionization to cyanide ion in biologic tissues. It is a powerful metabolic inhibitor that arrests cellular respiration by inactivating cytochrome enzymes fundamental to the respiratory process, as well as combining with hemoglobin to form cyanomethemoglobin, which is incapable of transporting oxygen to tissues. With the wide prevalence of cyanoglycosides in plant materials, the ability to detoxify cyanide is a vital function of the liver, erythrocytes, and other tissues. Rhodanese, a mitochondrial enzyme in liver and other tissues, catalyzes the formation of thiocyanate from cyanide rapidly in the presence of thiosulfate and colloidal sulfur, but cysteine and GSH are poor sulfur donors. The detoxification of cyanide depends on the availability of a physiologic pool of thiosulfate, the origin of which is not known. A possible source for thiosulfate is the transamination of cysteine to β-mercaptopyruvate and transfer of the mercapto group by a sulfur transferase to sulfite producing thiosulfate. Depletion of this pool increases cyanide toxicity. In the presence of excess cyanide, however, minor pathways for cyanide metabolism may occur, including oxidation to cyanate (NCO^-), reaction with cobalamin (vitamin B_{12}) to form cyanocobalamin, and the formation of 2-iminothiazolidine-4-carboxylic acid from the nonenzymatic reaction between cystine and cyanide (48).

$$S_2O_3^{2-} + CN^- \longrightarrow CNS^- + SO_3^{2-}$$

ELIMINATION PATHWAYS

Most xenobiotics are lipid-soluble and are altered chemically by the metabolizing enzymes, usually into less toxic and more water-soluble substances, before being excreted into the urine (or bile in some cases). The formation of conjugates with sulfate, amino acids, and glucuronic acid is particularly effective in increasing the polarity of drug molecules. The principal route of excretion of drugs and their metabolites is in the urine. If drugs and other compounds foreign to the body were not metabolized in this manner, substances with a high lipid-water partition coefficient could be reabsorbed readily from the urine through the renal tubular membranes and into the plasma. Such substances would therefore continue to be recirculated and their pharmacologic or toxic effects would be prolonged. Very polar or highly ionized drug molecules are often excreted in the urine unchanged.

Urine

Tubular reabsorption is greatly reduced by conversion of a drug into a more polar substance with a lower partition coefficient. In general, the more resistance a drug is to the metabolizing enzymes, the greater is the therapeutic action and the smaller the dose needed to achieve a particular therapeutic goal.

Urine is not the only route for excreting drugs and their metabolites from the animal body. Other routes include bile, saliva, lungs, sweat, and milk. The bile has been recognized as a major route of excretion for many endogenous and exogenous compounds.

Enterohepatic Cycling of Drugs

The liver is the principal organ for the metabolism and eventual elimination of xenobiotics from the human body either in the urine or in the bile. Steroid hormones, bile acids, drugs and their respective conjugated metabolites when eliminated in the bile are available for reabsorption from the duodenal-intestinal tract into the portal circulation, undergoing the process of enterohepatic cycling (EHC) (49). Nearly all drugs are excreted in the bile, but only a few are concentrated in the bile. For example, the bile salts are so efficiently concentrated in the bile and reabsorbed from the GI tract that the entire body pool recycles several times per day. Therefore, enterohepatic cycling is responsible for the conservation of bile acids, steroid hormones, thyroid hormones and other endogenous substances. In humans, compounds excreted into the bile usually have a molecular weight greater than 500, whereas with rats, the critical molecular weight is 325. Consequently, biliary excretion is more common in the rat than in man. Compounds with a molecular weight between 300 and 500 are excreted in both urine and bile. Some compounds would not be expected to be excreted in the bile because of a molecular weight of less than 300 and a relatively nonpolar structure. Compounds excreted into bile are usually strongly polar substances that may be charged (anionic) (e.g., dyes) or uncharged (e.g., cardiac glycosides and steroid hormones). Biotransformation of this type of compound by means of phase 1 and phase 2 reactions would produce a conjugated metabolite, which is usually anionic, more polar, and has a molecular weight greater than that of the parent compound. They are most often present as their glucuronide conjugates, because glucuronidation adds 176 to the molecular weight of the parent compound.

Unchanged drug in the bile is either excreted with the feces, metabolized by the bacterial flora in the intestinal tract, or reabsorbed into the portal circulation.

Not unexpectedly, the bacterial intestinal flora plays a direct involvement in EHC and the recycling of drugs through the portal circulation (see Extraheptic metabolism). Conjugated drug and metabolites excreted via the bile may be hydrolyzed by enzymes of the bacterial flora releasing the parent drug, or its phase I metabolite, for reabsorption into the portal circulation (50). Among the numerous compounds metabolized in the enterohepatic circulation are the estrogenic and progestational steroids, digitoxin, indomethacin, diazepam, pentaerythritol tetranitrate, mercurials, arsenicals, and morphine. The oral ingestion of xenobiotics inhibiting the gut flora (i.e., non-absorbable antibiotics) can effect the pharmacokinetics of the initial drug.

The impact of EHC on the pharmacokinetics and pharmacodynamics of a drug depends on the importance of biliary excretion of the drug relative to renal clearance and on the efficiency of GI absorption. EHC becomes dominant when biliary excretion is the major clearance mechanism for the drug. Because the majority of the bile is stored in the gall bladder and released upon the ingestion of food, intermittent spikes in the plasma drug concentration is observed following re-entry of the drug from the bile via EHC. From a pharmacodynamic point of view, the net effect of EHC is to increase the duration of a drug in the body and to prolong its pharmacologic action.

Chronic treatment with the enzyme inducer, phenobarbital, enhances the biliary excretion of drug molecules and their metabolites by increasing liver size, bile flow, and more efficient transport into the bile. This behavior is not shared by all inducers of the CYP450 monooxygenases. The route of administration may also influence excretion pathways. Direct administration into the portal circulation might be expected to result in more biliary excretion than could be expected via the systemic route.

DRUG METABOLISM AND AGE

Approximately 20% of the population is over the age of 65 and is responsible for more than 40% of the national drug expenditures. People over 65 represent a significant portion of the population, that is the most medicated and accounts for more than 25% of all prescription drugs dispensed. The average elderly patient in a health care facility could receive as many as 10 medications daily, which results in the potential for a greater incidence of adverse drug reactions. The widespread use of medications in the elderly will increase the potential for an increased incidence of drug-related interactions. Not unexpectedly, these interactions will be related to changes in drug metabolism and clearance from the body (Table 8.12). The interpretation of the age-related alteration in drug response must consider the contributions of absorption, distribution, metabolism, and excretion (51). Drug therapy

Table 8.12. Effect of Age on the Clearance of Some Drugs

No Change	Decrease
Acetaminophen*	Acetaminophen*
Aspirin	Alprazolam
Diclofenac	Amitriptylene
Digitoxin	Carbenoxolone
Diphenhydramine	Chlordiazepoxide
Ethanol	Chlormethiazole
Flunitrazepam	Clobazam
Heparin	Desmethyldiazepam
Lormetazepam	Diazepam
Midazolam	Labetalol
Nitrazepam	Lidocaine
Oxazepam	Lorazepam
Phenytoin (±)	Morphine
Prazosin	Meperidine
Propylthiouracil	Nifedipine and other dihydropyridines
Temazepam	Norepinephrine
Thiopental (±)	Nortriptyline
Tolbutamide (±)	Phenytoin
Warfarin	Piroxicam
	Propranolol
	Quinidine
	Quinine
	Theophylline
	Verapamil

*Drug for which clearance is disputable but may actually be increased.

in the elderly is expected to become one of the more significant problems for clinical medicine. It has been well documented that the metabolism of many drugs and their elimination is impaired in the elderly.

Metabolism in the Elderly

The decline in drug metabolism because of old age is associated with physiological changes having pharmacokinetic implications affecting the steady-state plasma concentrations and renal clearance for the parent drug and its metabolites (52). Those changes relevant to the bioavailability of drugs in the elderly are decreases in hepatic blood flow, glomerular filtration rate, hepatic microsomal enzyme activity, plasma protein binding, and body mass. Because the rate of a drug's elimination from the blood through hepatic metabolism is determined by hepatic blood flow, protein binding and intrinsic clearance, a reduction in hepatic blood flow can lead to an increase in drug bioavailability and decreased clearance, with the symptoms of drug overdose and toxicity as the outcome. Drugs whose elimination is dependent upon hepatic blood flow have a high extraction ratio and undergo extensive first pass metabolism when administered orally. Available evidence suggests that age is associated with a reduction in first-pass metabolism of some but certainly not all drugs. Those orally administered drugs exhibiting a reduction in first pass metabolism in the elderly include the dihydropyridine calcium antagonists, chlormethiazole, diazepam, lorazepam, chlordiazepoxide, alprazolam, propranolol, verapamil, labetalol, theophylline, morphine, amitriptyline, nortriptyline. The bioavailability of drugs with low extraction ratios depends upon the percent of drug-protein binding and not upon first-pass hepatic metabolism. In as much as drug binding to plasma proteins is an important factor in the rate of drug metabolism, it appears not to be a significant factor in the elderly.

Age related changes in drug metabolism are a complicated interplay between the age-related physiological changes, genetics, environmental influences (diet and nutritional status, smoking and enzyme induction), concomitant diseases states, and drug intake. In most studies the elderly appear as responsive to drug metabolizing enzyme activity (Phase I and II) as young individuals. All of the common pathways of drug conjugation, including glucuronidation, sulfation and glycine conjugation are variably affected by aging. Given the number of factors that determine the rate of drug metabolism, it is not surprising that the effects of aging on drug elimination by metabolism has yielded variable results even for the same drug. Therefore, the bioavailability of a drug in the elderly and the potential for drug toxicity, is largely dependant upon its extraction ratio and mode of administration. The fact that drug elimination may be altered in old age, suggest that initial doses of metabolized drugs should be reduced in older patients and then modified according to the clinical response (52). A decrease in hepatic drug metabolism coupled with age-related alterations in clearance, volume of distribution, and receptor sensitivity can lead to prolonged plasma half-life and increased drug toxicity (Table 8.13).

Fetal Metabolism

The ability of the human fetus and placenta to metabolize xenobiotics is well established. A 1973 clinical study reported that women ingest an average of 10 drugs during pregnancy, not including anesthetics, intravenous fluids, vitamins, iron, nicotine, cosmetic products, artificial sweeteners, or exposure to environmental contaminants. The majority of these substances readily cross the placenta, thus exposing the fetus to a large number of xenobiotic agents. The knowledge of the effects of prenatal exposure to drugs, environmental pollutants (e.g., smoking), and other xenobiotics (e.g., ethanol) on the fetus has led to a de-

crease in the exposure to these substances during pregnancy. The human fetus is at special risk from these substances because of the presence of the CYP450 monooxygenase system, which is capable of metabolizing xenobiotics during the first part of gestation. Placentas of tobacco smokers have shown a significant increase in the rate of placental CYP450 monooxygenase activity (CYP1A subfamily). There is increasing concern for this type of enzyme activity because this enzyme system is known to catalyze the formation of reactive metabolites that are capable of covalently binding to macromolecules producing permanent effects (e.g., teratogenic, hepatotoxic, or carcinogenic) in the fetus and newborn. A more disturbing fact is that the other conjugation enzymes (i.e., glucuronosyl transferases, epoxide hydrase, glutathione transferase, sulfotransferase), which are important for the formation of phase 2 conjugates of these reactive metabolites, are found in low to negligible levels, increasing the exposure of the fetus to these potentially toxic metabolites.

Fetal drug metabolism functions either as a protective mechanism against environmental xenobiotics to transform active molecules into inactive molecules, or as a toxifying system when transforming innocuous substances into reactive molecules. The placenta is not a barrier for protecting the fetus from xenobiotics, but almost every drug present in the maternal circulation will cross the placenta and reach the fetus. However, for some drugs, the placental efflux transport-protein, P-glycoprotein (P-gp), (to be discussed later in this chapter) functions as a materno-fetal barrier, pumping drugs and P-gp substrates out of the fetal circulation back into the maternal circulation (53). Recent results demonstrate that the placental P-gp functions as a materno-fetal barrier to protect the fetus from exposure to potentially harmful teratogenic xenobiotics/drugs and endogenous substances that have been absorbed through the placenta. P-gp inhibitors should be carefully evaluated for their potential to increase fetal susceptibility to drug/chemical-induced teratogenesis. On the other hand, selective inhibition of P-gp could be used clinically to improve pharmacotherapy of the unborn child. Depending upon the pharmacologic activity of the parent substance or its metabolites, both fetal and adult maternal drug metabolism may be viewed as complimentary, yet contradictory. Because metabolites are generally more water soluble than the parent substance, when formed in the fetus, drug metabolites may be trapped and accumulate on the fetal side of the placenta. Such accumulation can result in drug-induced toxicities or developmental defects. However, the difference between fetal and adult metabolism can be used advantageously, and constitutes the rational for transplacental therapy; e.g., the administration of betamethasone several days before delivery can increase the production of surfactant in the fetal lung and prevent respiratory distress syndrome in the neonate.

The activity of CYP3A isoenzymes in the human fetal liver is similar to that seen in adult liver microsomes. The

Table 8.13. Examples of Drugs Exhibiting First-Pass Metabolism

Acetaminophen	Isoproterenol	Oxprenolol
Albuterol	Lidocaine	Pentazocine
Alprenolol	Meperidine	Propoxyphene
Aspirin	Methyltestosterone	Propranolol
Cyclosporin	Metoprolol	Salicylamide
Desmethylimipramine	Dihydropyridines	Terbutaline
Fluorouracil	(Nifedipine)	Verapami
Hydrocortisone	Nortriptyline	
Imipramine	Organic nitrates	

fetal activity for CYP3A7 isoenzyme is unusual as most other fetal isoenzymes of CYP450 exhibit 5–40% of the adult isoenzymes. Fetal and neonatal drug metabolizing enzyme activities may differ from those in the adult.

Neonatal Metabolism

From the day of birth, the neonate is exposed to drugs and other foreign compounds persisting from pregnancy as well as those transferred via breast milk. Fortunately, many of the drug-metabolizing enzymes operative in the neonate developed during the fetal period. The routine use of therapeutic agents during labor and delivery, and during pregnancy, is widespread, and consideration has to be given to the fact that potentially harmful metabolites can be generated by the fetus and newborn. Consequently, the use of drugs that are capable of forming reactive metabolic intermediates should be avoided during pregnancy, delivery, and the neonatal period. The activity of Phase 1 and 2 drug-metabolizing enzymes high at birth, decrease to normal levels with increasing age. There is evidence of increased activity of drug-metabolizing enzymes in liver microsomes of neonates resulting from treatment of the mother during the pregnancy with enzyme inducers (e.g., phenobarbital).

GENETIC POLYMORPHISM

The reality of drug therapy is that many drugs do not work in all patients. By current estimates the percentage of patients who will react favorably to a specific drug ranges from 20% to 80%. Drugs have been developed and dosage regimens prescribed under the old paradigm that "one dose fits all" which largely ignores the fact that humans are genetically different, resulting in interindividual differences in drug metabolism and disposition (4). It is widely accepted that genetic factors have an important impact on the oxidative metabolism and pharmacokinetics of drugs. Genotype-phenotype correlation studies (pharmacogenetics) have shown that inherited mutations in CYP450 genes (allelles) result in distinct phenotype-subgroups. For example, mutations in the CYP2D6 gene result in poor (PM), intermediate (or extensive, EM), and ultra-rapid (UM) metabolizers of CYP2D6 substrates (54) (Table 8.6). Each of these phenotypic subgroups experience different responses to drugs extensively metabolized by the CYP2D6 pathway, ranging from severe toxicity to complete lack of efficacy. Genetic studies confirm that "one dose does not fit all," leaving the question of why we would continue to develop and prescribe drugs under the old paradigm. As early as 1997, the FDA recognised that identifying genetic polymorphisms might allow for the safe dosing, marketing and approval of drugs that would otherwise not be approved and advised pharmaceutical companies to incorporate the knowledge of genetic polymorphisms into drug development (see insert). Importantly, pharmacogenomic testing (the study of heritable traits affecting patient response to drug treatment) can significantly increase the

---

FDA Advisory on Genetic Polymorphism

"When a genetic polymorphism affects an important metabolic route of elimination, large dosing adjustments may be necessary to achieve the safe and effective use of the drug ... indeed in some cases understanding how to adjust the dose to avoid toxicity may allow the marketing of a drug that would have an unacceptable level of toxicity were its toxicity unpredictable and unpreventable."

From FDA's *"Guidance of Industry, Drug Metabolism/Drug Interaction Studies in the Drug Development Process: Studies in Vitro"* April 1997.

---

likelihood of developing drug regimens that benefit most patients without severe adverse events.

Polymorphisms are expressed for a number of metabolizing enzymes, but the polymorphic CYP450 isoforms most important for drug metabolism include CYP2A6, CYP2C9, CYP2C19 and CYP2D6. These polymorphic isoforms give rise to phenotypic-subgroups in the population differing in their ability to perform clinically significant biotransformation reactions with obvious clinical ramifications (55). Metabolic polymorphism may have several consequences, e.g., when enzymes that metabolize drugs that are used either therapeutically or socially are deficient, adverse or toxic drug reactions may occur in these individuals. The discovery of genetic polymorphism resulted from the observation of increased frequency of adverse effects or no drug effects after normal doses of drugs to some patients, e.g., hyper-CNS response from the administration of the antihistamine, doxylamine or no analgesic response with codeine. Polymorphism is a difference in DNA sequence found at 1% or higher in a population and expressed as an amino acid substitution in the protein sequence of an enzyme, resulting in changes in its rate of activity (Vmax) or affinity (Km). Thus, mutant DNA sequences can lead to interindividual differences in drug metabolism. Furthermore, the polymorphisms do not occur with equivalent frequency in all racial or ethnic groups. Because of these differences, it is important to be aware of a person's race and ethnicity when drugs are given that are metabolized differently by different populations (54,56). Since there is no other way to adequately clear these drugs from the body, PM may be at greater risk for adverse drug reactions or toxic overdoses. The signs and symptoms of these overdoses are primarily extensions of the drug's common adverse effects or pharmacologic effects (Table 8.14) (56). The level of adverse reactions or overdosage depends very much on the overall contribution of the mutant isoform to the drug's metabolism. Perhaps the most interesting explanation for the various mutant isoforms is that they evolved as protective mechanisms against alkaloids and other substances common in the food chain for the different ethnicities. Although much effort has gone into finding polymorphisms of *CYP3A4* and *CYP1A2* genes, none have yet to be discovered.

Table 8.14. Impact of Human CYP450 Polymorphisms on Drug Treatment in Poor Metabolizers (65)

Polymorphic Enzyme	Decreased Clearance	Adverse Effects (Overdosage)	Reduced Activation of Prodrug
CYP2C9	S-Warfarin	Bleeding	Losartan
	Phenytoin	Ataxia	
	Losartan		
	Tolbutamide	Hypoglycemia	
	NSAIDs	GI bleeding?	
CYP2C19	Omeprazole		Proguanil
	Diazepam	Sedation	
CYP2D6	TC antidepressants	Cardiotoxicity	Tramadol
	SSRIs	Serotonin syndrome	Codeine
	Anti-arryhtmic drugs	Arrythmias	Ethylmorphine
	Perhexiline	Neuropathy	
	Haloperidol	Parkinsonism?	
	Perphenazine		
	Zuclopenthixol		
	S-mianserin		
	Tolterodine		
CYP2A6	Nicotine		

Occasionally, one derives benefit from an unusual CYP phenotype. For example, cure rates for peptic ulcer treated with omeprazole are substantially greater in individuals with defective CYP2C19, owing to the sustained high plasma levels achieved.

CYP2C9 and CYP2C19

CYP2C9 and CYP2C19 are the main isoforms for the metabolism of the antiseizure drug, phenytoin, and for the anticoagulant S-warfarin. Although CYP2C19 metabolizes fewer drugs than does CYP2D6, the drugs it does metabolize are clinically important (Table 8.5). In Caucasians, CYP2C19 deficit is found in the poor metabolizer (PM) phenotype which is only seen in 8–13% of the population; in 20–30% of the Asian population (11–23% Japanese and 5–37% in Chinese); up to 20% of the black African-American population; in 14–15% of the Saudi Arabians and Ethiopians; and up to 70% of the Pacific Islanders (54,56). The more common mutant allele in these individuals is CYP2C19*2 which expresses an inactive enzyme. The large interindividual variability observed in the therapeutic response to the antiseizure drug mephenytoin is attributed to CYP2C19 polymorphism which catalyzes the p-hydroxylation of its (S) stereoisomer (55). The R-enantiomer is N-demethylated by CYP2C8 with no difference in its metabolism between PM and extensive metabolizers (EM).

CYP2C9 is the primary isoform for the metabolism of the antiseizure drug, phenytoin, the anticoagulant S-warfarin and the hypoglycemic drug, tolbutamide. Other clinically important drugs are listed in Table 8.5. At least six different mutant CYP2C9 alleles have been identified; of these the two alleles primarily responsible for CYP2C9 deficiency are CYP2C9*2 and CYP2C9*3 and code for enzymes with reduced affinity for subtrates (54,56). However, a deficiency of this isoform is seen in 8–13% of Caucasians, 2–3% black African Americans and <1% of the Asians. PM indi-

viduals possessing this deficient isoform variant are ineffective in clearing (S)-warfarin (so much so that they may be fully anticoagulated on just 0.5mg of warfarin a day) and in the clearance of phenytoin, which has a potentially very toxic narrow therapeutic range. On the other hand, the prodrug losartan will be poorly activated and ineffective.

CYP2D6

CYP2D6 is of particular importance because it metabolizes a wide range of commonly prescribed drugs including antidepressants, antipsychotics, β-adrenergic blockers and antiarrythmics (Table 8.6). The CYP2D6 deficiency is a clinically important genetic variation of drug metabolism characterized by three phenotypes, the UM, the EM and the PM. The PM phenotype is inherited as an autosomal recessive trait with five out of 30 of the known CYP2D6 gene mutations leading to either zero expression or the expression of a nonfunctional enzyme (54). Approximately 12–20% of Caucasians express the CYP2D6*4 allele and <5% express the other CYP2D6 alleles; up to 34% of black African Americans express the CYP2D6*17 allele and <5% express the other CYP2D6 alleles; up to 50% of Chinese-Asians express the CYP2D6*10 allele and <5% express the other CYP2D6 alleles; these individuals are referred to as PM (54,56). Conversely, the 20–30% of Saudi Arabians and Ethiopians who express the CYP2D6*2XN allele are known as ultrafast metabolizers (UM) of CYP2D6 substrates because they express excess enzyme since they have multicopies of the gene (54). Inasmuch as CYP2D6 is not inducible, individuals of Ethiopian and Saudi Arabian descent have genetically developed a different strategy to cope with the (presumed) high load of alkaloids and other substances in their diet; thus the high expression of CYP2D6 using *multiple copies* of the gene. Those individuals deficient in CYP2D6 will be predisposed to adverse effects or drug toxicity from antidepressants or neuroleptics caused by inadequate metabolism or long half-lives, but will find the metabolism of prodrugs in these patients to be ineffective due to lack of activation, e.g., codeine which must be metabolized by O-demethylation to morphine. UM will require a dose much higher than normal to attain therapeutic drug plasma concentrations (e.g., a patient required a daily dose of about 300 mg nortryptyline in order to achieve therapeutic plasma levels) or where a lower dose for prodrugs that require metabolic activation. Individuals with PM phenotype are also characterized by loss of CYP2D6 stereoselectivity in hydroxylation reactions. It can be anticipated that large differences in steady-state concentration for CYP2D6 substrates will occur between individuals with the different phenotypes when they receive the same dose. Depending on the drug and reaction type, a 10- to 30-fold difference in blood concentrations may be observed in the PM phenotype debrisoquine polymorphism (57).

CYP2A6

CYP2A6 is of particular importance because it activates a number of procarcinogens to carcinogens and is the major isoform metabolizing nicotine to cotinine. Approximately 15% of Asians express the *CYP2A6*4del* allele and <2% Caucasians express the other *CYP2AD6*2* allele; both alleles express zero or a nonfunctional enzyme; these individuals are referred to as PM (54,56). A benefit from being a PM of CYP2A6 substrates might be the protection from some carcinogens and smoking, owing to the high plasma levels of nicotine achieved with fewer cigarettes.

Acetylation

Acetylation, a nonmicrosomal form of metabolism, also exhibits polymorphisms and was first demonstrated in the acetylation of isoniazid (see the section on acetylation). Several forms of acetyl transferase occur in humans. Some clinically used drugs undergoing polymorphic acetylation include isoniazid, procainamide, hydralazine, phenelzine, dapsone, caffeine, some benzodiazepines, and possibly the carcinogenic secondary N-alkylaryl amines (2-aminofluorene, benzidine, and 4-aminobiphenyl). Intestinal acetyl transferase appears not to be polymorphic (i.e., 5-aminosalicylic acid). The proportion of fast acetylation phenotype in Caucasians is about 30–45%, in the Oriental population, 80–90%, and in Canadian Eskimos, 100%. The incidence of drug-induced systemic lupus erythematosus from chronic procainamide therapy is more likely to appear with slow acetylators.

Other Polymorphic Metabolizing Enzymes

The polymorphism for CYP2E1 is expressed more in Chinese than Caucasians. CYP2E1 PM exhibit tolerance to alcohol and less toxicity from halohydrocarbon solvents.

The only FMO pathway exhibiting polymorphism is the genetic disease trimethylaminuria, in which individuals excrete diet-derived free trimethylamine in the urine. Usually, trimethylamine undergoes extensive FMO N-oxidation.

In human populations, serum paraoxonase (PON1) exhibits a substrate dependent polymorphism to the neurotoxic effects of organophosphates in those susceptible individuals that are deficient in PON1 (i.e., poor metabolizers) (37). PON1 catalyzes the hydrolysis of paraoxon, chlorpyrifos (Dursban) and other organophosphates.

Polymorphism has been associated with serum cholinesterases (particularly succinyl cholinesterase causing skeletal muscle paralysis), alcohol dehydrogenases, aldehyde dehydrogenases, epoxide hydrolase, and xanthine oxidase (55). Approximately 50% of the Oriental population lack aldehyde dehydrogenase, resulting in high levels of acetaldehyde following ethanol ingestion and causing the symptoms of nausea and flushing. People with genetic variants of cholinesterase respond abnormally to succinylcholine, procaine, and other related choline esters. The clinical consequence of reduced enzymic activity of cholinesterase is that succinylcholine and procaine are not hydrolyzed in the blood, resulting in prolongation of their respective pharmacologic activities.

A suggestion has been made that EM phenotypes may be more prone than PM phenotypes to develop cancers because they are better able to activate procarcinogens. Such interindividual variations may have a major influence in determining the risk of cancer. The activity of a particular CYP450 isoform may be a rationale for predicting the individual risk from exposure to carcinogenic compounds.

Our increasing knowledge of genetic polymorphism has contributed a great deal to our understanding of interindividual variation in the metabolism of drugs, how to change dose-regimens accordingly to minimize drug toxicity or to improve therapeutic efficacy. In humans, drugs not subject to polymorphic metabolism also exhibit substantial interindividual variation in their disposition, attributed to a great extent to environmental factors such as inducing agents, smoking, and alcohol ingestion.

ORAL BIOAVAILABILITY

Oral bioavailability (Chapter 7) is the fraction of the total dose of a drug that reaches the systemic circulation. The low oral bioavailability for a drug may be the result of disintegration and dissolution properties of the drug formulation, solubility of the drug molecule in the GI environment, membrane permeability, presystemic intestinal metabolism, hepatic first-pass metabolism, or susceptibility to membrane transporters such as P-glycoprotein efflux. Other routes of administration (e.g., subcutaneous, intravenous, inhalation, and nasal) for susceptible drugs have been investigated in an attempt to overcome the pronounced presystemic metabolism. The extent of first-pass metabolism depends upon the drug delivery system, since a formulation may increase or decrease the rate of dissolution, the residence time of a drug in the gastrointestinal tract, and the dose. The more prolonged the residence time, the greater is the efficiency of first-pass metabolism. The drug form and delivery system should yield optimal bioavailability and pharmacokinetic profiles resulting in a reproducible clinical response.

Studies are being performed to determine the effect of pre-systemic and hepatic first-pass metabolism on the toxicity and carcinogenicity of xenobiotics. For a nontherapeutic toxic substance, the existence of a first-pass effect is desirable because the liver can bioinactivate it, preventing its distribution to other parts of the body. On the other hand, first-pass metabolism may increase its toxicity by biotransforming the toxicant to a more toxic metabolite, which can re-enter the blood and exert its toxic effect.

Presystemic First Pass Metabolism

Although hepatic metabolism continues to be the most important route of metabolism for xenobiotics, the ability of the liver and intestine to metabolize substances to either pharmacologically inactive or bioactive metabolites before reaching systemic blood levels is called prehepatic or *presystemic first pass metabolism,* which results in the low systemic availability for susceptible drugs. Sulfation and glucuronidation are presystemic intestinal first pass metabolism major pathways in humans for acetaminophen, phenylephrine, terbutaline, albuterol, fenoterol, and isoproterenol.

The discovery that CYP3A4 is found in the mucosal enterocytes of the intestinal villi signifies its role as key determinant in the oral bioavailability of its numerous drug substrates (Table 8.8) (58). Drugs known to be substrates for CYP3A usually have a low and variable oral bioavailability that may be explained by presystemic first pass metabolism by the small intestine CYP450 isoforms. The concentration of functional intestinal CYP3A is influenced by genetic disposition, induction, and inhibition which determines to a great extent drug blood levels and therapeutic response. Xenobiotics when ingested orally can modify the activity of intestinal CYP3A enzymes by induction, inhibition, and stimulation. By modulation of the isoform pattern in the intestine, a xenobiotic could alter its own metabolism and that of others in a time- and dose-dependent manner. Its concentration in the intestine is comparable to that of the liver. The oral administration of dexamethasone induces the formation of CYP3A and erythromycin inhibits it. The glucocorticoid inducibility of CYP3A4 may also be a factor in differences of metabolism between males and females. Studies have suggested that intestinal CYP3A4 C-2 hydroxylation of estradiol contributed to the oxidative metabolism of endogenous estrogens circulating with the enterohepatic recycling pool (24). Norethisterone has a low oral bioavailability of 42% because of oxidative first pass metabolism (CYP3A), but levonorgestrel is completely available in women with no conjugated metabolites.

Several clinically relevant drug interactions between orally co-administered drugs and CYP3A4 can be explained by a modification of drug metabolism at the CYP450 level. If a drug has high presystemic elimination (low bioavailability) and is primarily metabolized by CYP3A4 then co-administration with a CYP3A4 inhibitor can be expected to alter the drug's pharmacokinetics by reducing its metabolism, thus increasing its plasma concentration. Drugs and some foods (e.g., grapefruit juice) that are known inhibitors, inducers, or substrates for intestinal CYP3A4 can potentially interact with the metabolism of a co-administered drug affecting its AUC and rate of clearance (Tables 8.9 and 8.11) (59). Inducers can reduce absorption and oral bioavailability, whereas these same factors are increased by inhibitors. For example, erythromycin can enhance the oral absorption of another drug by inhibiting its metabolism in the small intestine by CYP3A4. Prednisone, prednisolone, and methylprednisolone (but not dexamethasone), by virtue of being competitive substrates for CYP3A4, are competitive inhibitors of synthetic glucocorticoid metabolism. This is because a major metabolic pathway for synthetic glucocorticoids involves CYP3A4. In addition to co-administered drugs, metabolic interactions with exogenous CYP3A4 substrates secreted in the bile are possible. The poor oral bioavailability for cyclosporin is attributed to a combination of intestinal metabolism by CYP3A4 and efflux by P-glycoprotein (60).

Because the intestinal mucosa is enriched with glucuronosyltransferases, sulfotransferases, and glutathione transferases, presystemic first pass metabolism for orally administered drugs susceptible to these conjugation reactions results in their low oral bioavailability (47). Presystemic metabolism often exceeds liver metabolism for some drugs. For example, more than 80% of intravenously administered albuterol is excreted unchanged in urine with the balance as glucuronide conjugates, whereas when it is administered orally, less than 5% is systemically absorbed because of intestinal sulfation and glucuronidation. Presystemic metabolism is a major pathway in humans for most β-adrenergic agonists, e.g., glucuronides or sulfates for terbutaline, fenoterol, albuterol, and isoproterenol, morphine (3–O-glucuronide), acetaminophen (O-sulfate), and estradiol (3–O-sulfate). The bioavailability of orally administered estradiol or ethynylestradiol in females is about 50%, whereas mestranol (3-methoxy-ethynylestradiol) has greater bioavailability because it is not significantly conjugated. Levodopa has a low oral bioavailability because of its metabolism by intestinal L-aromatic amino acid decarboxylase. The activity of this enzyme depends on the percent bound of its cofactor pyridoxine (vitamin B_6). Tyramine, which occurs in fermented foods such as cheeses and red wines, ripe bananas, and yeast extracts, is metabolized by both MAO-A and MAO-B in the gut wall.

The extensive presystemic first pass sulfation of phenolic drugs, for example, can lead to increased bioavailability of other drugs by competing for the available sulfate pool, resulting in the possibility of drug toxicity (38). Concurrent oral administration of acetaminophen with ethynylestradiol resulted in a 48% increase in ethynylestradiol blood levels. Ascorbic acid, which is sulfated, also increases the bioavailability of concurrently administered ethynylestradiol. Sulfation and glucuronidation occur side by side, often competing for the same substrate, and the balance between sulfation and glucuronidation is influenced by several factors such as species, doses, availability of cosubstrates, inhibition, and induction of the respective transferases.

First Pass Metabolism

Several orally administered drugs are known to undergo liver first-pass metabolism during their transport to the systemic circulation from the gastrointestinal tract (e.g., metoprolol). Thus, the liver can remove substances from the blood after their absorption from the gastrointestinal tract, thereby preventing distribution to other parts of the body. This effect can seriously impair the bioavailability of an orally administered drug, reducing the amount of the drug that reaches the systemic circulation and ultimately its receptor to produce its pharmacologic effect. Drugs subject to first-pass metabolism are included in Table 8.10.

P-Glycoprotein

Another factor that must be considered in the oral bioavailability of many CYP3A4 substrates is intestinal P-glycoprotein (P-gp) (61).

Originally discovered as a transmembrane transporter-protein associated with the resistance (elimination) of anticancer drugs, P-gp can also play a role in how a drug is absorbed, distributed, metabolized and eliminated from the body (60,61). Considering its role as a transporter protein (efflux pump), it is logical that it should exhibit saturable (non-linear) kinetics. P-gp exhibits a broad specificity for a large number of substrates, inhibitors and inducers (Table 8.15). The common link between P-gp substrates is that most of the same compounds are also substrates for CYP3A4. The close physical location of P-gp and CYP3A4 in the endothelial cells of the intestinal mucosa allows these proteins to work in concert with each other to decrease drug plasma concentrations of CYP3A4 substrates, suggesting a complementary protective mechanism for these two proteins, forming a barrier to the absorption intestinal of CYP3A4 substrates. Hepatic and renal P-gp also appear to function in a complementary manner promoting the elimination of substrates into the bile and urine respectively. For example, if a drug is a substrate for intestinal P-gp, its oral absorption will be incomplete and while this same drug will be actively transported by the renal tubules into the urine, enhancing its elimination. On the other hand, inhibiting P-gp would be expected to improve the oral bioavailability of P-gp substrates, but if the inhibitor is also a substrate for CYP3A4, increased me-

Description of P-Glycoprotein

P-gp is a transmembrane ATP-dependent active transport protein that is strategically expressed in the luminal endothelial cells of organs associated with lipophilic xenobiotic absorption and distribution. For example, P-gp in the intestinal mucosa functions to move xenobiotics into the intestine to block their absorption into the portal circulation; P-gp in the endothelial cells of the brain functions as a blood-brain barrier to move substances out of the brain into systemic circulation; P-gp in the endothelial cells of the renal proximal tubules of the kidney and in the canicular membranes of hepatocytes functions to increase xenobiotic elimination into the urine and bile, respectively (62). P-gp is also expressed in the endothelial cells of adrenal cortex and medulla, of the testis and ovaries, of the peripheral nerves (functions as a blood-nerve barrier) and of the pancreas; in the epithelial cells of the placenta where it serves as the materno-fetal barrier for the fetus, and in the stem cells of the bone marrow. The particular localization of P-gp suggests that this transmembrane transporter-protein probably evolved as a protective mechanism against the absorption of xenobiotics to increase their transport out of these organs and tissues. It appears that the substrates, inhibitors or inducers are non-selective for various P-gps. P-gp should exhibit saturation/non-linear kinetics; at or near saturation concentrations, an increase in drug absorption can result in 2–3-fold increase in plasma drug concentration. P-gp activity is controlled by a variety of endogenous and environmental stimuli which evoke stress responses including cytotoxic agents, heat shock, irradiation, genotoxic stress, inflammation, inflammatory mediators, cytokines and growth factors.

tabolism (pre-systemic) would occur. Drugs with low oral bioavilability or high first-pass metabolism may be particulary susceptible to alterations in the transport kinetics of P-gp. Because P-gp exhibits saturation (non-linear) kinetics, drugs with low dosages can have their oral bioavailability enhanced by increasing its oral dosage thus saturating the P-gp pump. As with CYP3A4, there is significant interindividual variation (4–10 fold) in the intestinal expression of P-gp which could explain the variance observed in the pharmacokinetics for CYP3A4 substrates. The interactive nature of CYP3A4 and P-gp will be of importance in controlling and improving the oral bioavailability of CYP3A4 substrates and drug regimens. The presence of inhibitors of P-gp in grapefruit juice (such as 6,7-dihydroxybergamottin and other furanocoumarins) has confirmed that the inhibition of efflux transport of drugs as well as of drug metabolism by CYP3A4 could be an important cause of drug-grapefruit juice interaction (63).

In summary, oral bioavailability for xenobiotics is dependent upon a combination of factors including physical properties of the drugs and formulation, and biologic factors including metabolizing enzymes, membrane permeability, and the membrane efflux pump, P-gp.

Table 8.15. Some Substrates, Inhibitors and Inducers for P-glycoprotein

Substrate		Inhibitors		Foods
acetolol	lidocaine*	amiodarone*	lovastatin*	daidzein
amiodarone*	loperamide*	amitriptyline*	maprotiline	genistein
atorvastatin*	methotrexate	astemizole*	mefloquine*	grapefruit juice*
celiprolol	mibefradil	atorastatin*	mibefradil*	orange juice
cimetidine*	nadolol	carvedilol	midazolam*	isoflavones
ciprofloxacin	nelfinavir*	chlorpromazine*	mifepristone*	
colchicine	nicardipine*	clarithromycin*	nelfinavir*	**Inducers**
cyclosporin*	ondansetron*	cyclosporin*	nicardipine*	dexamethasone*
daunorubicin*	paclitaxel*	desipramine	nifedipine*	prazosin
debrisoquine	pravastatin*	dexverapamil*	nitrendipine*	progesterone*
dexamethasone*	quinidine*	diltiazem*	ofloxacin	quercetin
DHEA	quinolones	dipyridamole	prochlorperzine	rifampin
digoxin*	rantidine	disulfiram	progesterone*	St. John's Wort*
diltiazem*	rifampin*	doxepin	propanolol	
docetaxel*	ritonavir*	erythromycin*	propafenone*	
domperidone*	saquinaivr*	felodipine*	quinidine*	
doxorubicin*	tacrolilmus*	flupenthixol	quinine*	
enoxacin	taxol*	fluphenazine	reserpine	
erthromycin*	teniposide*	glibenclamide	rifampin*	
estradiol*	terfenadine*	haloperidol*	ritonavir*	
etoposide*	timolol	hydrocortisone*	saquinavir*	
fexofenadine*	verapamil*	imipramine*	tacrolimus*	
hydrocortisone*	vinblastine*	itraconazole*	testosterone*	
idarubicin	vincristine*	ivermectin	tamoxifen*	
indinavir*	vindesine*	ketoconazole*	trimipramine	
ivermectin		lidocaine*	verapamil*	

*CYP3A4 substrate, inhibitor or inducer.

EXTRAHEPATIC METABOLISM

Because the liver is the primary tissue for xenobiotic metabolism, it is not surprising that our understanding of mammalian CYP450 monooxygenase is based chiefly on hepatic studies. Although the tissue content of CYP450s is highest in the liver, CYP450 enzymes are ubiquitous and their role in extrahepatic tissues remains unclear. The CYP450 pattern in these tissues differs considerably from that in the human liver (64). In addition to liver tissue, CYP450 enzymes are found in lung, nasal epithelium, intestinal tract, kidney and adrenal tissues, and brain. It is possible that the expression of the polymorphic genes and induction of the isoforms in the extrahepatic tissues may affect activity of the CYP450 isoforms in the metabolism of drugs, endogenous steroids and xenobiotics. Therefore, characterization of CYP450, UGT, SULT and other polymorphic drug metabolizing enzymes in extrahepatic tissues is important to our overall understanding of the biologic importance of these families of isoforms to improved drug therapy, design of new drugs and dosages forms, toxicity, and carcinogenicity.

The mucosal surfaces of the gastrointestinal tract, the nasal passages, and lungs are major portals of entry for xenobiotics into the body and as such are continuously exposed to a variety of orally ingested or inhaled airborne xenobiotics including drugs, plant toxins, environmental pollutants, and other chemical substances. As a consequence of this exposure, these tissues represent a major target for necrosis, tumorigenesis, and other chemically induced toxicities. Many of these toxins and chemical car-

cinogens are relatively inert substances that must be bioactivated in order to exert their cytotoxicity and tumorigenicity. The epithelial cells of these tissues are capable of metabolizing a wide variety of exogenous and endogenous substances, and provide the principal and initial source of biotransformation for these xenobiotics during the absorptive phase. The consequences of such presystemic biotransformation is either a decrease in the amount of xenobiotic available for systemic absorption by facilitating the elimination of polar metabolites, or toxicification by activation to carcinogens, which may be one determinant of tissue susceptibility for the development of intestinal cancer. The risk of colon cancer may depend on dietary constituents that contain either procarcinogens or compounds modulating the response to carcinogens.

Intestinal Metabolism

Mounting evidence shows that many of the clinically relevant aspects of CYP450 may in fact occur at the level of the intestinal mucosa and could account for differences among patients in dosing requirements. The intestinal mucosa is enriched with CYP450 isoforms, glucuronosyl transferases, sulfotransferases and glutathione S-transferases making it particularly important for orally administered drugs susceptible to oxidation (58), glucuronidation or sulfation conjugation pathways (38), or glutathione conjugation pathways. The highest concentrations of CYP450s occur in the duodenum with a gradual tapering into the ileum. CYP2E, CYP3A, CYP2C8, CYP2C9, CYP2C19, and CYP2D6 have been identified in the human intestine. Therefore, intestinal CYP450 isoforms provide potential presystemic first pass metabolism of ingested xenobiotics affecting their oral bioavailability (e.g., hydroxylation of naloxone) or bioactivation of carcinogens or mutagens. It is not surprising that dietary factors can affect the intestinal CYP450 isoforms. For example, a two-day dietary exposure to cooked Brussels sprouts significantly decreased the 2 α-hydroxylation of testosterone, yet induced CYP1A2 activity for PAH. An 8 oz. glass of grapefruit juice inhibited the sulfoxidation metabolism of omeprazole (CYP3A4) but not its hydroxylation (CYP2C19), increasing its systemic blood concerntration. These types of interactions between a drug and a dietary inhibitor could result in a clincially significant drug interaction.

UGT isoforms in the intestine can glucuronidate orally administered drugs such as morphine, acetaminophen, alpha and beta adrenergic agonists and other phenolic phenethanolamines, and other dietary xenobiotics. This is a result of reduction in their oral bioavailability (increasing first pass metabolism), thus altering their pharmacokinetics and pharmacodynamics. The UGTs expressed in the intestine include UGT1A1 (bilirubin glucuronidating isoform), UGT1A3, UGT1A4, UGT1A6, UGT1A8, UGT1A9 and UGT1A10. Substrate specificities of intestinal UGT isoforms are comparable to those in the liver. Glucuronidase hydrolysis of biliary glucuronide conjugates in the intestine can contribute to enterohepatic cycling of the parent drug.

Likewise, the sulfotransferases in the small intestine can sulfate orally administered drugs and xenobiotics for which the primary route of conjugation is sulfation (such as isoproterenol, albuterol, steroid hormones, α-methyldopa, acetaminophen, fenoldopam) decreasing their oral bioavailability, thus altering their pharmacokinetics and pharmacodynamics. Competition for intestinal sulfation between coadministered substrates may influence their bioavailability with either an enhancement of or decrease in therapeutic effects. Sulfatase hydrolysis of biliary sulfate conjugates in the intestine can contribute to enterohepatic cycling of the parent drug.

The occurrence of intestinal CYP450 enzymes and bacterial enzymes in the microflora allows the metabolism of relatively stable environmental pollutants and food-derived xenobiotics (i.e., plants contain a variety of protoxins, promutagens, and procarcinogens) into mutagens and carcinogens (50). For example, cruciferous vegetables (Brussels sprouts, cabbage, broccoli, cauliflower, and spinach) are all rich in indole compounds (e.g., indole3-carbinol), which with regular and chronic ingestion are capable of inducing some intestinal CYP450s (CYP1A subfamily) and inhibiting others (CYP3A subfamily). It is likely these vegetables would also alter the metabolism of food-derived mutagens (e.g., heterocyclic amines produced during charbroiling of meat are CYP450 N-hydroxylated and become carcinogenic in a manner similar to aryl amines) and carcinogens.

The extent of a drug's metabolism in the small bowel and its role in clinically relevant drug interaction remain

to be evaluated and must be taken into account in oral pharmacokinetics analysis of future drug interaction studies. Clinically significant interaction will not always occur when a drug is combined with other isoform subfamily substrates. Oral co-administration of a drug with drugs interacting with its metabolism need not be avoided, but the blood concentration of the drug must be monitored closely and the dose should be adapted to avoid adverse drug reactions.

Intestinal Microflora

When drugs are orally ingested, or when there is considerable biliary excretion of a drug or its metabolites into the gastrointestinal tract such as with a parentally administered drug (enterohepatic cycling or recirculation), the intestinal bacterial microflora can have a role in drugs' metabolism. The microflora plays an important role in the enterohepatic recirculation of xenobiotics via their conjugated metabolites (e.g., digoxin, oral contraceptives norethisterone and ethynylestradiol, and chloramphenicol) and endogenous substances (steroid hormones, bile acids, folic acid and cholesterol), which re-enter the gut via the bile (50). Compounds eliminated in the bile are conjugated with glucuronic acid, glycine, sulfate, glutathione, and once secreted into the small intestine, the bacterial β-glucuronidase, sulfatase, nitroreductases, and various glycosidases catalyze the hydrolysis of the conjugates. The activity of orally administered conjugated estrogens, e.g., Premarin, involves the hydrolysis of the sulfate conjugates by sulfatases, releasing estrogens to be reabsorbed from the intestine into the portal circulation. The clinical use of oral antibiotics (e.g., erythromycin, penicillin, clindamycin, and aminoglycosides) has a profound effect on the gut microflora and the enzymes responsible for the hydrolysis of drug conjugates undergoing EHC. Bacterial reduction includes nitro reduction of nitroimidazole, azo reduction of azides (sulfasalazine to 5-aminosalicylic acid and sulfapyridine), and reduction of the sulfoxide to its sulfide. The sulfoxide of sulindac is reduced by both gut microflora and hepatic CYP450s. Other ways in which bacterial flora can affect metabolism are the following: (1) production of toxic metabolites, (2) formation of carcinogens from inactive precursors, (3) detoxication, (4) exhibition of species differences in drug metabolism, (5) exhibition of individual differences in drug metabolism, (6) production of pharmacologically active metabolites from inactive precursors, and (7) production of metabolites not formed by animal tissues. In contrast to the predominantly hepatic oxidative and conjugative metabolism of the liver, gut microflora is largely degradative, hydrolytic, and reductive, with a potential for both metabolic activation and detoxication of xenobiotics.

Lung Metabolism

Some of the hepatic xenobiotic biotransformation pathways are also operative in the lung (65). Because of the differences in organ sizes, the total content of the pulmonary xenobiotic-metabolizing enzyme systems is generally lower than in the liver, creating the impression of a minor role for the lung in xenobiotic elimination. CYP2E1 is the CYP450 isoform that is expressed in the lung to the greatest extent. The other CYP450s, FMO, epoxide hydrolase, and the phase 2 conjugation pathways, however, are comparable to those in the liver. Thus, the lungs may play a significant role in the metabolic elimination or activation of small molecular weight inhaled xenobiotics. When drugs are injected intravenously, intramuscularly, or subcutaneously, or after skin absorption, the drug initially enters the pulmonary circulation after which the lung becomes the organ of first pass metabolism for the drug. The blood levels and therapeutic response of the drug are influenced by genetic disposition, induction, and inhibition of the pulmonary metabolizing enzymes. By modulation of the CYP450 isoform pattern in the lung, a xenobiotic could alter its own metabolism and that of others in a time- and dose-dependent manner. Because of its position in the circulation, the lung provides a second pass metabolism for xenobiotics and their metabolites exiting from the liver, but it is also susceptible to the cytotoxicity or carcinogenicity of hepatic activated metabolites. Antihistamines, β-blockers, opioids, and tricyclic antidepressants are among the basic amines known to accumulate in the lungs as a result of their binding to surfactant phospholipids in lung tissue. The significance of this relationship to potential pneumotoxicity remains to be seen.

Nasal Metabolism

The nasal mucosa is recognized as a first line of defense for the lung against airborne xenobiotics because it is constantly exposed to the external environment (66). Drug metabolism in the nasal mucosa is an important consideration not only in drug delivery, but also for toxicologic implications because of xenobiotic metabolism of inhaled environmental pollutants or other volatile chemicals. CYP450 enzymes in the nasal epithelial cells can convert some of the airborne chemicals to reactive metabolites, increasing the risk of carcinogenesis in the nasopharynx and lung (e.g., nitrosamines in cigarette smoke). The most striking feature of the nasal epithelium is that CYP450 catalytic activity is higher than in any other extrahepatic tissue, including the liver. Nasal decongestants, essences, anesthetics, alcohols, nicotine, and cocaine have been shown to be metabolized in vitro by CYP450 enzymes from the nasal epithelium. The fact that the CYP450s in the nasal mucosa are active, first pass metabolism should be considered when delivering susceptible drugs to the nasal tissues. Flavin monooxygenases, carboxylesterases, aldehyde dehydrogenase, and other conjugation (phase 2) enzymes are also active in the nasal epithelium.

Metabolism in Other Tissues

The isoforms of CYP450s and their regulation in the brain are of interest in defining the possible involvement of CYP450s in central nervous system toxicity and carcinogenicity. The CYP450s present in the kidney and adrenal tissues include isoforms primarily involved in the hydroxylation of steroids, arachidonic acid, and 25-hydroxycholcalciferol.

STEREOCHEMICAL ASPECTS OF DRUG METABOLISM

In addition to the physicochemical factors that affect xenobiotic metabolism, stereochemical factors play an important role in the biotransformation of drugs. This involvement is not unexpected because the xenobiotic-metabolizing enzymes are also the same enzymes that metabolize certain endogenous substrates, which for the most part are chiral molecules. Most of these enzymes show stereoselectivity (but not stereospecificity), i.e., one stereoisomer enters into biotransformation pathways preferentially, but not exclusively. Metabolic stereochemical reactions can be categorized as follows: substrate stereoselectivity, when two enantiomers of a chiral substrate are metabolized at different rates; product stereoselectivity, in which a new chiral center is created in a symmetric molecule and one enantiomer is metabolized preferentially; substrate-product stereoselectivity, in which a new chiral center of a chiral molecule is metabolized preferentially to one of two possible diastereomers (67). An example of substrate stereoselectivity is the preferred decarboxylation of S-α-methyldopa to S-α-methyldopamine, with almost no reaction for R-α-methyldopa. The reduction of ketones to stereoisomeric alcohols and the hydroxylation of enantiotropic protons or phenyl rings by monooxygenases are examples of product stereoselectivity. For example, phenytoin undergoes aromatic *p*-hydroxylation of only one of its two phenyl rings to create a chiral center at C-5 of the hydantoin ring, methadone is reduced preferentially to its α-diastereometric alcohol, and naltrexone is reduced to its 6-β-alcohol. An example of substrate-product stereoselectivity is the reduction of the enantiomers of warfarin and the β-hydroxylation of S-α-methyldopamine to (1R:2S)-α-methylnorepinephrine, whereas R-α-methyldopamine is hydroxylated to only a negligible extent. In vivo studies of this type can often be confused by the further biotransformation of one stereoisomer, giving the false impression that only one stereoisomer was formed preferentially. Moreover, some compounds show stereoselective absorption, distribution, and excretion, which proves the importance of also performing in vitro studies. Although studies on the stereoselective biotransformation of drug molecules are not yet extensive, those that have been done indicate that stereochemical factors play an important role in drug metabolism and, in some cases, could account for the differences in pharmacologic activity and duration of action between enantiomers (see the discussion of chiral inversion of the NSAID).

TOXICITY FROM OXIDATIVE METABOLISM

The mechanism of toxicity for xenobiotics is generally accepted as resulting from bioactivation to reactive intermediates, which are responsible for toxic manifestations. Many of these metabolites have pharmacologic and toxicologic effects, some of which may differ from those of the parent drug. Many carcinogens elicit their biologic property through a covalent linkage to DNA. This process can lead to mutations and potentially to cancer. Most chemical carcinogens of concern are relatively inert and require activation by the xenobiotic-metabolizing enzymes before they can undergo reaction with DNA or proteins (cytotoxicity). There are many ways to bioactivate procarcinogens, promutagens, plant toxins, drugs, and other xenobiotics (23). Oxidative bioactivation reactions are by far the most studied and common. Conjugation reactions (phase 2), however, are also capable of activating these xenobiotics producing electrophiles, in which the conjugating derivative acts as a leaving group. These reactive intermediates are mostly electrophiles (electron-deficient substances), such as epoxides, quinones, or free radicals formed by the CYP450 monooxygenases and FMO. Reactive intermediates tend to be oxygenated in sterically hindered positions, making them nonacceptable substrates for subsequent detoxicating enzymes, such as epoxide hydrolase and glutathione S-transferases. Therefore, their principal fate is covalent linkage to intracellular macromolecules, including enzyme proteins and DNA. Experimental studies indicate that the CYP1A subfamily can oxygenate aromatic hydrocarbons (e.g., PAH) in sterically hindered positions, and activation by N-hydroxylation (e.g., aryl acetamides) appears to depend either on FMO or CYP450 isoforms. The formation of chemically reactive metabolites is important because they frequently cause a number of different toxicities, including tumorigenesis, mutagenesis, tissue necrosis, and hypersensitivity reactions.

Some toxic chemicals exert their toxic action by lethal injury or biologic autooxidation (lipid peroxidation).

Lethal injury involves the disruption of cellular energy metabolism by inhibition of oxidative phosphorylation (e.g., MPTP) or ATPase, resulting in disruption of subcellular organelles, cell death, and tissue necrosis. Because the early stages of lethal injury are reversible, complete recovery may occur. Autooxidation is the process whereby cellular components are irreversibly oxidized and damaged by free radicals or free-radical generating systems. This results in the oxidation and depletion of glutathione, various thiol enzymes, or lipid peroxidation which in turn leads to the disruption of cellular membranes, and to cell death, tissue necrosis, and the death of the organism. When cell death does not occur, nonlethal changes such as mutations and malignant transformations are likely.

Our understanding of these reactions was advanced by the studies of Gillette and co-workers (68). They proposed that the proportion of the dose that binds covalently to critical macromolecules could depend on the quantity of the reactive intermediate that forms.

A scheme illustrating the complexities of metabolically induced toxicity is shown in Figure 8.30. The figure represents chemical carcinogen metabolism, but it can be applied to other toxicities. Reactions that proceed via the open arrows eventually lead to neoplasia. Some carcinogens may form the "ultimate carcinogen" directly through CYP450 isoform metabolism; others, like the PAH (e.g., benzo[a]pyrene), appear to involve a minimum three-step reaction sequence forming an epoxide, then the diol, and perhaps a second epoxide group on another part of the molecule. Others form the N-hydroxy intermediate that requires transferase-catalyzed conjugation (e.g., O-glucuronide, O-sulfate) to form the "ultimate carcinogen." The quantity of "ultimate carcinogen" formed should relate directly to the proportion of the dose that binds or alkylates DNA.

The solid-arrow reaction sequences are intended to show detoxification mechanisms, which involve several

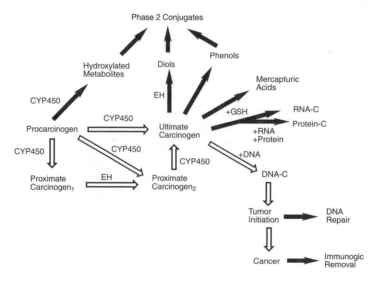

Fig. 8.30. Methylation pathways.

steps. First, the original chemical may form less active products (phenols, diols, mercapturic acids, and other conjugates). Second, the "ultimate carcinogen" may rearrange so as to be diverted from its reaction with DNA (or whatever is the critical macromolecule). Third, the covalently bound DNA may be repaired. Fourth, immunologic removal of the tumor cells may occur. Several mechanisms within this scheme could regulate the quantity of covalently bound carcinogen: (1) the activity of the rate-limiting enzyme, such as epoxide hydrolase, monooxygenase, or one of the transferases, could be involved; (2) the availability of co-substrates, e.g., glutathione, UDP-glucuronic acid, or PAPS, may be rate limiting; (3) specific monooxygenase activities for detoxification and activation must be considered; (4) availability of alternate reaction sites for the ultimate carcinogen, e.g., RNA and protein may be involved; (5) possible specific transport mechanisms that deliver either the procarcinogen or its ultimate carcinogen to selected molecular or subcellular sites.

Most lipid-soluble exogenous aromatic compounds and most compounds with olefinic unsaturation are metabolized in humans and in animals through epoxide formation. The importance of metabolically produced epoxides in mediating adverse biologic effects has aroused concern about clinically used drugs known to be metabolized to epoxides. Drugs possessing structural features prone to metabolic epoxidations are abundant. Metabolically produced epoxides have been reported for allobarbital, secobarbital, protriptyline, carbamazepine, cyproheptadine, and are implicated with 8-methoxypsoralen and other furanocoumarins (6,7-dihydroxybergamottin in grapefruit juice), phenytoin, phensuximide, phenobarbital, mephobarbital, lorazepam, and imipramine (62). The alarming biologic effects of some epoxides, however, do not imply that all epoxides have similar effects. Epoxides vary greatly in molecular geometry, stability, electrophilic reactivity, and relative activity as substrates for epoxide-transforming enzymes (e.g., epoxide hydrolase, glutathione S-transferase, and others).

Other studies have revealed toxic metabolites for isoniazid, acetaminophen, phenacetin, furosemide, and cephaloridine (69). Isoniazid is acetylated to its major metabolite acetylisoniazid, which is hydrolyzed to acetylhydrazine and isonicotinic acid (see Chapter 37). Acetylhydrazine is further metabolized by the CYP450 monooxygenase to an N-hydroxy intermediate that dehydrates into an acylating intermediate, which can then initiate the process that leads to hepatic necrosis. Acetaminophen is among the safest of all analgesics when taken in normal therapeutic doses, but it has been known to cause acute hepatic necrosis, sometimes fatal in both adults and children, when taken in excessive doses or after prolonged or repeated administration. The oxidation of acetaminophen to the chemically reactive N-acetyl-p-benzoquinoneimine, catalyzed by the isoforms CYP1A2 and 2E1, can either bind covalently with glutathione to form an inactive product, or with cellular macromolecules, initiating the processes

leading to hepatic necrosis (see Fig. 8.28). Furosemide, a frequently used diuretic drug, is reportedly a teratogen. When administered in large doses, it produces hepatic necrosis in mice. The hepatic toxicity apparently results from metabolic activation of the furan ring, possibly through an epoxide. Cephaloridine produces renal necrosis via metabolic activation of the thiophene ring in a manner similar to that described for furosemide. The concept that the pattern of metabolism can change with the dose accounts for the fact that some drugs may not be toxic unless a certain threshold dose is exceeded. For example, with acetaminophen and furosemide, no necrosis or covalent binding occurs until a dose of 100 mg/kg in animals is exceeded. Enzyme induction may enhance the formation of reactive intermediates and the severity of the tissue injury. Glutathione plays a protective role in the hepatic tissue injury produced by acetaminophen (see the section on glutathione conjugation), but not by furosemide. One method for preventing liver injury in the event of acetaminophen overdosage is the use of acetylcysteine, which traps the reactive metabolite similar to that with GSH.

The fact that numerous organic compounds that are essentially nontoxic as long as their structure is preserved can be converted into cytotoxic, teratogenic, mutagenic, or carcinogenic compounds by normal biotransformation pathways in animals and in humans is now well established (23). The "reactive intermediate" (an electrophile) process involves the reaction of an intermediate with cellular constituents, forming either nontoxic products or binding covalently with essential macromolecules, and initiating processes that eventually lead to the toxic effect. A better understanding of the mechanisms underlying these reactions may lead to more rational approaches to the development of nontoxic therapeutic drugs. For the present, it seems that new advances in drug therapy cannot occur without some risk of causing structural tissue lesions. Special attention to risk factors is required for drugs that will be used for long periods in the same patient.

N-nitrosamines ($R_2N-N=O$) have been implicated as mutagenic, carcinogenic, and teratogenic substances in animals, and have been suspected in some human cancers. Although they occur naturally in trace amounts, they can be formed by reaction of nitrite with secondary or tertiary amines. Among the amines to which people are exposed are drugs and agricultural chemicals. Some of these amines (e.g., methapyrilene, an antihistamine previously available in over-the-counter sleeping aids) have been shown to form N-nitroso compounds by reaction with nitrite and to be mutagenic with bacteria. These reactions can occur in food preserved with nitrite or in the stomach from dietary nitrites. Nitrosamines have to be activated metabolically before they can exert their carcinogenic or other toxic effects. One of the proposed mechanisms is hydroxylation of the α-carbon by CYP450 (similar to N-dealkylation) with subsequent N-dealkylation and spontaneous rearrangement to possible alkyl carbonium ions, which, in turn, can covalently bind to cellular macromolecules (19). Studies with dimethylnitrosamine have shown methylation to occur at the N-7 position in guanine as well as S-methylation of cysteine. The molecular basis of nitrosoamine-induced carcinogenesis or mutagenesis is not clearly understood at this time.

DRUG INTERACTIONS

Drug interactions represent a common clinical problem which has been compounded by the introduction of many new drugs and the expanded use of herbal medicines. Drug interactions occur when the efficacy or toxicity of a medication is changed by co-administration of another substance, drug, food (i.e., grapefruit) or herbal-product (70,71). Pharmacokinetic interactions often occur as a result of a change in drug metabolism. For example, CYP3A4 oxidizes a broad spectrum of drugs and its location in the small intestine and liver permits an effect on both presystemic and systemic drug disposition. Some interactions with CYP3A4 subtrates/inhibitors may also involve inhibition of P-gp. Other clinically important drug interactions resulting from the co-administration of CYP3A4 substrates or inhibitors include rhabdomyolysis with the co-administration of some 3-hydroxy-3-methylglutaryl-coenzyme A reductase inhibitors ("statins"); symptomatic hypotension with some dihydropyridine calcium antagonists; excessive sedation can result from benzodiazepine or non-benzodiazepine hypnosedatives; ataxia with carbamazepine; and ergotism with ergot alkaloids.

The clinical importance of any drug interaction depends on factors that are drug-, patient- and administration-related. Drugs with low oral bioavailability or high first pass metabolism are particularly susceptible to drug interactions as a result of co-administration of inhibitors that alter absorption, distribution and elimination. Generally, a doubling or more in plasma drug concentration has the potential for enhanced adverse or beneficial drug response. Less pronounced pharmacokinetic interactions may still be clinically important for drugs with a steep concentration-response relationship or narrow therapeutic index. In most cases, the extent of drug interaction varies markedly among individuals; this is likely to be dependent on interindividual differences in CYP450 content (polymorphism), pre-existing medical conditions and, possibly, age. Interactions may occur under single dose conditions or only at steady state. The pharmacodynamic consequences may or may not closely follow pharmacokinetic changes. Drug interactions may be most apparent when patients are stabilized on the affected drug and the CYP450 substrates or inhibitors are then added to the regimen (70). One reason for the increased incidence of drug interactions is the practice of simultaneously prescribing several potent drugs as well as ingesting nonprescription products and herbal products concurrently with potent prescribed medications.

An excellent example of a drug interaction that resulted in a life-threatening ventricular arrhythmia associated with QT prolongation (Torsades de pointes) occurred when CYP3A4 substrates or inhibitors were co-administered with terfenadine, astemizole, cisapride or pimozide. This potentially lethal drug interaction lead to the withdrawal of terfenadine and cisapride from clinical use, and the introduction of fexofenadine, the metabolite of terfenadine (Allegra) without this interaction (71).

Beneficial Drug Interactions

A beneficial drug interaction, for example, is the co-administration of a CYP3A4 inhibitor with cyclosporin which allows a reduction of the dosage and cost of the immunosuppressant. Certain HIV protease inhibitors, such as saquinavir, have a low oral bioavailability because of CYP3A4 metabolism. Its oral bioavailability can be profoundly increased by the addition of a low dose of a CYP3A4 inhibitor such as ritonavir. This concept of altering drug pharmacokinetics by adding a low subtherapeutic dose of a CYP3A4 inhibitor (ritonavir) to increase the oral bioavailability of another protease inhibitor, lopinavir (CYP3A4 substrate), led to the marketing of Kaletra, a new drug combination of lopinavir and ritinavir.

Grapefruit Juice

Grapefruit juice is a beverage often consumed at breakfast for its health benefits and to mask the taste of drugs or foods. However, unlike other citrus fruit juices, grapefruit juice can significantly increase the oral bioavailability of drugs primarily metabolized by intestinal CYP3A4 causing an elevation in their serum concentrations (Table 8.16). However, those drugs with high oral bioavailabilities greater than 60% (Table 8.16) are all likely safe to take with grapefruit juice as their high oral bioavailability leaves little room for elevation by grapefruit juice. The importance of the interaction appears to be influenced by individual patient susceptibility, type and amount of grapefruit juice and administration-related factors.

The mechanism by which grapefruit produces its effect is through inhibition of the enzymatic activity and decrease in the intestinal expression of CYP3A4. The P-gp eflux pump also transports many CYP3A4 substrates, and thus the pres-

Historical Significance of Grapefruit Juice

The discovery that grapefruit juice can markedly increase the oral drug bioavailability of CYP3A4 drugs was based on an unexpected observation from an interaction study between the dihydropyridine calcium channel antagonist, felodipine, and ethanol in which grapefruit juice was used to mask the taste of the ethanol. Subsequent investigations confirmed that grapefruit juice significantly increased the oral bioavailability of felodipine by reducing presystemic felodipine metabolism through selective inhibition of CYP3A4 expression in the intestinal wall.

Table 8.16. CYP3A4 Substrates and Interactions with Grapefruit Juice (59)

Drug	Interaction*	Drug	Interaction*
Calcium channel blockers		HMG-CoA reductase inhibitors	
Amlodipine	Y	Atorvastatin	Y
Felodipine	Y	Cerivastatin	Y?
Nifedipine	Y	Fluvastatin	N?
Nimodipine	Y	Lovastatin	Y
Nisoldipine	Y	Pravastatin	N?
Nitrendipine	Y	Simvastatin	Y
Pranidipine	Y		
		CNS Drugs	
Antiarrhythmics		Buspirone	Y
Diltiazem	N	Carbamazepine	Y
Verapamil	N	Diazepam	Y
Quinidine	N	Midazolam	Y
		Triazolam	Y
Antihistamines			
Ebastine	Y?	Immunosuppressants	
Loratidine	Y?	Cyclosporine	Y
		Tacrolimus	Y?
HIV protease inhibitors			
Indinavir	N?	Other	
Nelfinavir	N?	Methadone	Y
Ritonavir	N?	Sildenafil	Y
Saquinavir	Y		
Macrolides			
Clarithromycin	N		

*"Yes" and "No" indicate published evidence of the presence or absence of an interaction with grapefruit juice. "Yes?" and "No?" indicate expected findings based on available data. Those drugs with Y or Y? should not be consumed with grapefruit juice in an unsupervised manner.

ence of inhibitors of P-gp in grapefruit juice (such as 6',7'-dihydroxybergamottin and other furanocoumarins) could be a related factor for drug–grapefruit juice interactions (63). Numerous studies have shown that grapefruit juice acts on intestinal CYP3A4, not at the hepatic level.

Does the quantity of juice matter? The majority of the presystemic CYP3A4 inhibition is obtained following ingestion of 1 glass of grapefruit juice, however, 24 hours after ingestion of a glass of grapefruit juice, 30% of its effect is still present (59). The reduction in intestinal CYP3A4 concentration is rapid; a 47% decrease occurred in a healthy volunteer within 4 hours after consuming grapefruit juice. Daily ingestion of grapefruit juice results in a loss of CYP3A4 from the small intestine epithelium. Consumption of very large quantities of grapefruit juice (6–8 glasses per day) may lead to inhibition of hepatic CYP3A4.

The active constituents found in grapefruit juice responsible for its effects on CYP3A4 include flavonoids

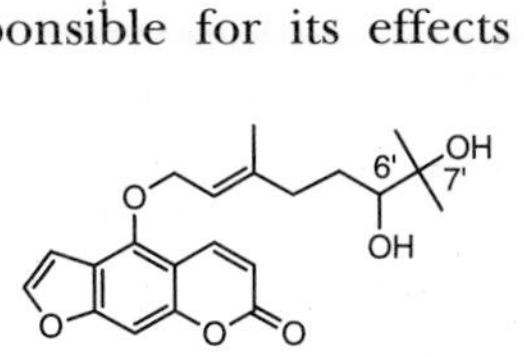

6',7'-Dihydroxybergamottin

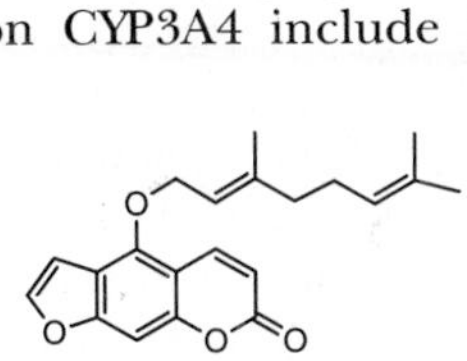

Bergamottin

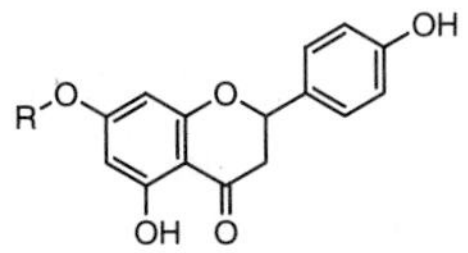

Naringin   R: rhamnose-glucoside-
Naringenin R: H-

(e.g., naringenin, naringin) and furanocoumarins (e.g., bergamottin, 6',7'-dihydroxybergamottin) (72). Of particular interest are the effects of naringin and 6',7'-dihydroxybergamottin, on the activity of intestinal CYP3A4. The majority of studies to date have used either freshly squeezed grapefruit juice, reconstituted frozen juice, commercial grapefruit juice, grapefruit segments, or grapefruit extract; all are capable of causing drug interactions with CYP3A4 substrates (blended grapefruit juices have not yet been investigated). The active constituents in grapefruit juice are present not just in the juice but also in the pulp, peel, and core of the fruit and are responsbile for its flavor. Bergamottin and 6',7'-dihydroxybergamottin have been found to be potent mechanism-based inhibitors of CYP3A4, and naringenin isomers are competitive inhibitors of CYP3A4 (72). Higher concentrations of 6',7'-dihydroxybergamottin and naringin are present in grapefruit segments. Thus, any therapeutic concern for a drug interaction with grapefruit juice should now be extended to include whole fruit and other products derived from the grapefruit peel. The difference in the in vitro CYP3A4 inhibition between grapefruit juice and orange juice is that orange juice contained no measurable amounts of 6',7'-dihydroxybergamottin.

If a patient has been taking medication with grapefruit juice for some time without ill effects, is it safe to continue to do so? Much of this unpredictability is due to the inconsistency of the juice concentrations and the sporadic manner in which grapefruit juice is consumed, suggesting that this approach may not be entirely safe (59). Given the unpredictability of the effect of grapefruit juice on the oral bioavailability the drugs in Table 8.16, patients should be advised to avoid this combination, thus preventing onset of potential adverse effects. Each patient's situation should be considered, and advice should be based on consumption history and the specific medications involved. The benefits of increased and controlled drug bioavailability by grapefruit juice may in the future be achieved through either standardizing the constituents or co-administration of the isolated active ingredients. This would then lead to a safe, effective, and cost-saving means to enhance the absorption of many therapeutic agents.

Drug pharmacokinetics can be altered by food through changes in drug solubility as well as the nutritional status of a patient. The fact that grapefruit juice can increase the bioavailability of certain drugs, by their reducing presystemic intestinal metabolism, has led to renewed interest in the area of "food-drug interactions" with particular interest on the effects of grapefruit constitutents. Specific natural occurring chemicals present in food have been associated with drug interactions. For example, severe hypertensive reactions have occurred when patients treated with MAO inhibitors have ingested cheeses and other foods rich in the biogenic amine tryramine.

P-glycoprotein

It is obvious from the earlier discussion regarding P-glycoprotein, that P-gp-mediated transport plays an important role in pharmacokinetic-mediated drug-drug interaction (60). Thus, inhibition of P-gp mediated transport could dramatically increase the systemic bioavailability of an otherwise poorly absorbed drug. Similar consequences could be expected with a reduction in renal or biliary clearances (e.g., digoxin). Numerous investigations with drugs such as digoxin, etoposide, cyclosporin, vinblastine, taxol, loperamide, domperidone, and ondansteron demonstrate that P-gp has an important role in determining the pharmacokinetics of substrate drugs (60). For example, if drug A is a substrate for both P-gp and *only* for CYP3A4, and a second drug B is added that is an inhibitor for both P-gp and CYP 3A4 (see Table 8.15), then the plasma drug concentration for unmetabolized drug A will be elevated with increased potential for drug interactions as adverse effects or for causing a drug overdose. If drug A is a substrate for multiple CYP isoforms, then drug A will be metabolized by these other isoforms, with minimal effect on plasma drug concentrations. On the other hand, if the second drug B is only an inhibitor for P-gp, then drug A will be subject to CYP3A4 metabolism, thus decreasing the plasma concentration for drug A to subtherapeutic levels. The effect of P-gp inhibition is to increase the oral bioavailability so that the later actions of CYP3A4 inhibition will be increased. One of the best examples is the interaction between digoxin and quinidine. Quinidine blocks P-gp in the intestinal muscosa and in the proximal renal tubule, thus

digoxin elimination into the intestine and urine is inhibited, increasing the plasma digoxin concentration to toxic levels. Another example is with loperamide. Loperamide is an opiate antidiarrheal that is normally kept out of the brain by the P-gp pump, however, inhibition of P-gp allows accumulation of loperamide in the brain leading to respiratory depression. The current relevant clinical data for drug interactions increasingly can be found on the World Wide Web.

Food-Drug Interactions

Besides interactions with drugs, interactions with naturally occurring compounds, present in food, may be important. For example, severe hypertensive reactions have occurred when patients treated with MAO inhibitors have ingested cheeses and other foods rich in the biogenic amine tyramine.

Herbal Drug-Drug Interactions

As the use of herbal medicines continues to increase, there is an increasing need to predict and avoid these potential adverse herbal-drug–drug interactions. Currently, nearly one in five adults taking prescription medicines are also taking at least one herbal medicine. The mechanisms for herbal-drug–drug interactions are similar to those for drug-drug interactions affecting the pharmacokinetics of the respective drug. Little is known regarding the pharmackinetics properties of many of the substances in herbal medicines. Therefore, the potential for herbal-drug–drug interactions has greatly increased. A commonly reported herbal-drug–drug interaction is between St. John's Wort and indinavir, a HIV protease inhibitor. St. John's Wort induces the metabolism of indinavir, a CYP3A4 substrate, leading to drug resistance and treatment failure. St. John's Wort decreases the absorption of digoxin apparently by inducing P-gp in the intestinal and renal endothelium increasing digoxin elimination in the intestine and urine, respectively. Licorice when taken with steroids can reduce their metabolism and elimination.

Miscellaneous Drug Interactions

The ability of drugs and other foreign substances to stimulate (induction) metabolism of other drugs has already been discussed. Phenobarbital, for example, stimulates metabolism of a variety of drugs, e.g., phenytoin and coumarin anticoagulants. Stimulation of bishydroxycoumarin metabolism can create a problem in a patient undergoing anticoagulant therapy. If phenobarbital administration is stopped, the rate of metabolism of the anticoagulant decreases, resulting in greater plasma concentrations for bishydroxycoumarin and enhanced anticoagulant activity, increasing possibility of hemorrhage. Serious side effects have resulted from this type of interaction.

These observations point out that combined therapy of a potent drug, e.g., bishydroxycoumarin, and a inducer of drug metabolism, e.g., phenobarbital, can create a hazardous situation if the enzyme inducer is withdrawn and therapy with the potent drug is continued without an appropriate decrease in dose.

Some drugs are competitive inhibitors of nonmicrosomal metabolic pathways. Serious reactions have been reported in patients treated with an MAO inhibitor, such as trancypromine or iproniazid, because they usually are sensitive to a subsequent dose of a sympathomimetic amine, e.g., amphetamine, or a tricyclic antidepressant, e.g., amitriptyline, which is metabolized by MAO.

Allopurinol, a xanthine oxidase inhibitor used for the treatment of gout, inhibits metabolism of 6-mercaptopurine and other drugs metabolized by this enzyme. A serious drug interaction results from the concurrent use of allopurinol for gout and 6-mercaptopurine to block the immune response from a tissue transplant or as antimetabolite in neoplastic diseases. In some cases, however, allopurinol is used in conjunction with 6-mercaptopurine to control the increase in uric acid elimination from 6-mercaptopurine metabolism. The patient should be supervised closely, because allopurinol, an inhibitor of purine metabolism, given in large doses, may have serious effects on bone marrow.

GENDER DIFFERENCES IN DRUG METABOLISM

The role of gender as a contributor to variability in xenobiotic metabolism is not clear, but increasing numbers of reports show differences in metabolism between men and women, raising the intriguing possibility that endogenous sex hormones, or hydrocortisone, or their synthetic equivalents may influence the activity of inducible CYP3A. For example, N-demethylation of erythromycin was significantly higher in females than males. Nevertheless, the N-demethylation was persistent throughout adulthood. In contrast, males exhibited unchanged N-demethylation values.

Gender-dependent differences of metabolic rates have been detected for some drugs. Side chain oxidation of propranolol was 50% faster in males than in females, but no differences between genders were noted in aromatic ring hydroxylation. N-demethylation of meperidine was depressed during pregnancy and for women taking oral contraceptives. Other examples of drugs cleared by oxidative drug metabolism more rapidly in men than in women included chlordiazepoxide and lidocaine. Diazepam, prednisolone, caffeine, and acetaminophen are metabolized slightly faster by women than by men. No gender differences have been observed in the clearance of phenytoin, nitrazepam, and trazodone, which interestingly are not substrates for the CYP3A subfamily. Gender differences in the rate of glucuronidation have been noted.

More investigation is warranted, and future pharmacokinetic studies examining the alteration in drug metabolism in one gender needs to be re-examined with respect to the other gender. Even in postmenopausal women, CYP3A function may be altered and influenced by the lack of estrogen or the presence of androgens.

MAJOR PATHWAYS OF METABOLISM

Table 8.10 contains an extensive list of commonly used drugs and the CYP450 isoforms which catalyze their metabolism. In addition, phase 1 and phase 2 metabolic pathways for some common drugs are listed in Table 8.17.

Table 8.17. Metabolic Pathways of Common Drugs

Drug	Pathway
Amphetamines	Deamination (followed by oxidation and reduction of the ketone formed) N-oxidation N-dealkylation Hydroxylation of the aromatic ring (aromatic oxidation) Hydroxylation of the β-carbon atom Conjugation with glucuronic acid of the phenol and alcohol products from the ketone formed by deamination
Barbiturates	Oxidation and complete removal of subtituents at carbon 5 N-dealkylation at N^1 and N^3 Desulfuration at carbon 2 (thiobarbiturates) Scission of the barbiturate ring at the 1:6 bond to give substituted malonylureas
Phenothiazines	N-dealkylation in the N^{10} side chain N-oxidation in the N^{10} side chain Oxidation of the heterocyclic S atom to sulfoxide or sulfone Hydroxylation of one or both aromatic rings Conjugation of phenolic metabolites with glucuronic acid or sulfate Scission of the N^{10} side chain

continued

Table 8.17—*continued*

Drug	Pathway
Sulfonamides	Acetylation at the N^4 amino group
	Conjugation with glucuronic acid or sulfate at the N^4 amino group
	Acetylation or conjugation with glucuronic acid at the N^1 amino group
	Hydroxylation and conjugation in the heterocyclic ring, R
Phenytoin	Hydroxylation of one aromatic ring
	Conjugation of phenolic products with glucuronic acid or sulfate
	Hydrolytic scission of the hydantoin ring at the bond between carbons 3 and 4 to give 5,5-diphenylhydantoic acid
Meperidine	Hydrolysis of ester to acid
	N-dealkylation
	Hydroxylatin of aromatic ring
	N-oxidation
	Both N-dealkylation and hydrolysis
	Conjugation of phenolic products
Pentazocine	Hydroxylation of terminal methyl groups of the alkenyl side chain to give cis and trans (major) alcohols
	Oxidation of hydroxymethyl product of the alkenyl side chain to carboxylic acids
	Reduction of alkenyl side chain and oxidation of terminal methyl group
Cocaine	Hydrolysis of methyl ester
	Hydrolysis of benzoate ester
	N-dealkylation
	Both hydrolysis and N-dealkylation
Phenmetrazine	Oxidation to lactam
	Aromatic hydroxylation
	N-oxidation
	Conjugation of phenolic products
Ephedrine	N-dealkylation
	Oxidative deamination
	Oxidation of deaminated product to benzoic acid
	Reduction of deaminated product to 1,2-diol
Propranolol	Aromatic hydroxylation at C—4'
	N-dealkylation
	Oxidative deamination
	Oxidation of deaminated product to naphthoxylactic acid
	Conjugation with glucuronic acid
	O-dealkylation
Indomethacin	O-demethylation
	N-deacylation of p-chlorobenzoyl group
	Both O-dealkylation and N-deacylation
	Conjugation of phenolic products with glucuronic acid
	Other conjugation products

Table 8.17—*continued*

Drug	Pathway
Diphenoxylate 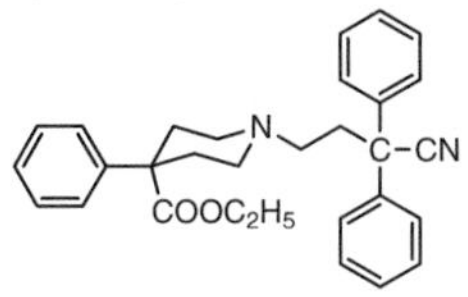	Hydrolysis of ester to acid Hydroxylation of one aromatic ring attached to the N-alkyl side chain
Diazepam 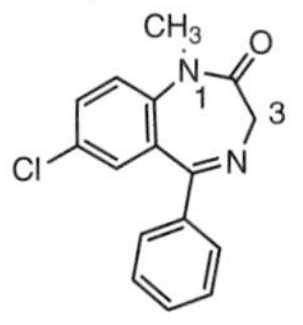	N-dealkylation at N1 Hydroxylation at carbon 3 Conjugation of phenolic products with glucuronic acid Both N-dealkylation of N1 and hydroxylation at carbon 3
Prostaglandins 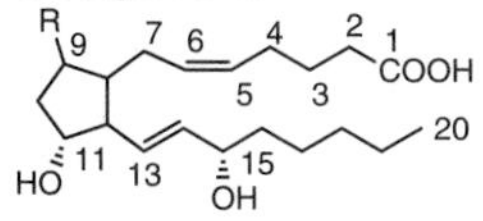	Reduction of double bonds at carbons 5 and 6, and 13 and 14 Oxidation of 15-hydroxyl to ketone β-Oxidation of carbons 1, 2, 3 and 4 ω-Oxidation of carbon 20 to acid
Cyproheptadine 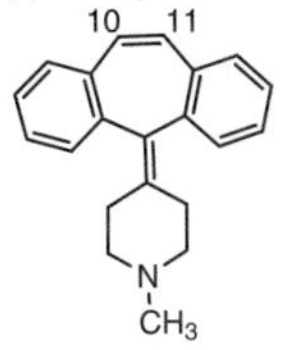	N-dealkylation 10,11-Epoxide formation Both N-dealkylation and 10,11-epoxidation
Hydralazine 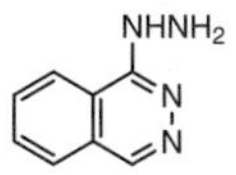	N-acetylation with cyclization to a methyl-s-triazolophthalazine N-formylation with cyclization to an s-triazolophthalazine Aromatic hydroxylation of benzene ring Oxidative loss of hydrazinyl group to 1-hydroxy Hydroxylation of methyl of methyl-s-triazolophthalazine Conjugation with glucuronic acid
Methadone 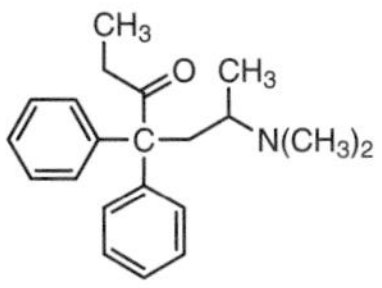	Reduction of ketone to hydroxyl Aromatic hydroxylation of one aromatic ring N-dealkylation of alcohol product N-dealkylation with cyclization to pyrrolidine
Lidocaine 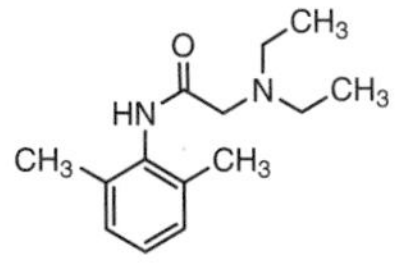	N-dealkylation Oxidative cyclization to a 4-imidazolidone N-oxidation of amide N Aromatic hydroxylation ortho to methyl Hydrolysis of amide
Imipramine 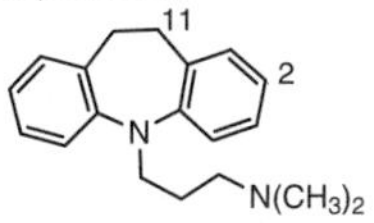	N-dealkylation Hydroxylation at C-11 Aromatic hydroxylation (C-2) N-oxidation Both N-dealkylation and hydroxylation
Cimetidine 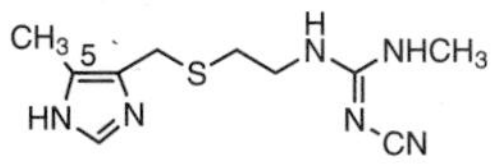	S-oxidation Hydroxylation of 5-methyl

continued

Table 8.17—*continued*

Drug	Pathway
Valproic acid $CH_3CH_2CH_2$ $CH_3CH_2CH_2$ $\rangle$—COOH	CoA thioester Dehydrogenation to (E) 2-ene Dehydrogenation to (E) 2,4-diene Dehydrogenation to 4-ene 3-Hydroxylation
Piroxicam	Pyridine 3′-hydroxylation Hydrolysis of amide Decarboxylation
Caffeine	N^3-demethylation N^1-demethylation N^7-demethylation to theophylline C-8 oxidation to uric acids Imidazole ring opened
Theophylline	N^3-demethylation N^1-demethylation C-8 oxidation to uric acids Imidazole ring opened 1-Me xanthine to 1-Me uric acid-xanthine oxidase
Nicotine	Pyrrolidine 5′-hydroxylation to continine Pyrrolidine N-oxidation (FMO) N-demethylation (nornicotine and norcotinine) Pyridine N-methylation 3′-Hydroxylation of cotinine
Ibuprofen	CoA thioester and epimerization of R− to S+ enantiomer Methyl hydroxylation to CH_2OH CH_2OH to COOH Acylglucuronide
Tamoxifen	N-demethylation 4′-Hydroxylation N-oxidation (FMO) 4-O-sulfate 4-O-glucuronide
Lovastatin	6′-Hydroxylation 3′-Side chain hydroxylation 3′-Hydroxylation β-oxidation of lactone O-glucuronides
Ciprofloxacin	Piperazine 3′-hydroxylation N-sulfation

Table 8.17—*continued*

Drug	Pathway
Labetalol	O-sulfate (major) O-glucuronide
Acetaminophen	O-glucuronide O-sulfate Oxidation to N-acetyl-p-benzoquinoneimine Conjugation of N-acetyl-*p*-benzoquinoneimine with glutathione
Tripelennamine	*p*-Hydroxylation Benzylic C-hydroxylation N-depyridinylation N-debenzylation
Felodipine	Aromatization Ester hydrolysis Methyl hydroxylation

REFERENCES

1. Williams RT. Detoxication Mechanisms 2nd ed. New York: J Wiley and Sons, 1959.
2. Drug Metabolism Reviews. New York: Marcel Dekker; Drug Metabolism and Disposition Baltimore: Lippincott Williams & Wilkins; Xenobiotica.London: Taylor and Francis.
3. Anders M. ed. Bioactivation of Foreign Compounds. New York: Academic Press, 1985; Caldwell J, Jakoby W. eds. Biological Basis of Detoxication. New York: Academic Press, 1983; Jakoby W. Ed. Enzymatic Basis of Detoxication Vol I and II. New York: Academic Press, 1980; Jakoby W, Bend JR, Caldwell J. eds. Metabolic Basis of Detoxication-Metabolism of Functional Groups. New York: Academic Press, 1982; Mulder GJ. ed. Conjugation Reactions in Drug Metabolism: An Integrated Approach. London: Taylor and Francis, 1990; Ortiz de Montellano PR. ed. Cytochrome P450: Structure Mechanism and Biochemistry. 2nd ed. New York: Plenum Press, 1995; Testa B, Jenner P. eds. Drug Metabolism: Chemical and Biochemical Aspects. New York: Marcel Dekker, 1976; Testa B, Jenner P. eds. Concepts in Drug Metabolism. New York: Marcel Dekker, 1981.
4. Murphy MP. Pharmacogenomics: A New Paradigm for Drug Development. Drug Discovery World. 2000; 1:23–32.
5. Wilkinson GR Schenker S. Drug disposition and liver disease. Drug Metab Rev 1975; 4: 139–175: McLean AJ Morgan DJ. Clinical Pharmacokinetics in Patients with Liver Disease. Clin Pharmacokinet 1991; 21: 42–69.
6. Rodighiero V. Effects of liver disease on pharmacokiunetics. An Update. Clin Pharmacokin. 1999; 37:399–443.
7. Groves JT, Han Y-Z. Models and Mechanisms of Cytochrome P450. In: Ortiz de Montellano PR. ed. Cytochrome P450: Structure Mechanism and Biochemistry. 2nd ed. New York: Plenum Press, 1995.
8. von Wachenfeldt C, Johnson EF. Structures of Eukaryotic Cytochrome P450 Enzymes. In: Ortiz de Montellano PR. ed. Cytochrome P450: Structure Mechanism and Biochemistry. 2nd ed. New York: Plenum Press, 1995.
9. Nebert DW, Nelson DR, Coon MJ, et al. The P450 superfamily: update on new sequences, gene mapping, and recommended nomenclature. DNA Cell Biol 1991; 10: 1; Gonzalez FJ, Gelboin HV. Human Cytochromes P450: Evolution and cDNA-Directed Expression. Environ Health Persp 1992; 98: 810–885.
10. Rendic S, DiCarlo FJ. Human Cytochrome P450 Enzymes: A Status Report Summarizing Their Reactions Substrates Inducers and Inhibitors. Drug Metab 1997; 29: 413–580.
11. Guengerich FP. Enzymatic Oxidation of Xenobiotic Chemicals. Crit Rev Biochem Mol Biol 1990; 25: 97–153; Wighton SA, Stevens JC The Human Hepatic Cytochromes P450 Involved in Drug Metabolism. Crit Rev Toxicol 1992; 22: 1–21.
12. Ortiz de Montellano PR. Oxygen Activation and Reactivity. In: Ortiz de Montellano PR ed. Cytochrome P450: Structure Mechanism and Biochemistry. 2nd ed. New York: Plenum Press, 1995.
13. Traber PG, McDonnell WM, Wang R. Expression and Regulation of Cytochrome P450I genes (CYP1A1 and CYP1A2) in the Rat Alimentary Tract. Biochim Biophys Acta 1992; 1171: 167–175.
14. Roy D, Bernhardt A, Strobel H, et al. Catalysis of the Oxidation of Steroid and Stilbene Estrogens to Estrogen Quinone Metabolites by the β-Naphthoflavone-Inducible Cytochrome P450 1A Family, Arch Biochem Biophys 1992; 296: 450–456.
15. Koop DR. Oxidative and Reductive Metabolism of Cytochrome P4502E1. FASEB J 1992; 6: 724–730.
16. Raucy JL, Kraner JC, Lasker JM. Bioactivation of Halogenated Hydrocarbons by Cytochrome P4502E1. Crit Rev Toxicol 1993; 23: 1–20.

17. White RE, Coon MJ. Oxygen Activation by Cytochrome P450. Ann Rev Biochem 1980; 49: 315–356; White RE. The Involvement of Free Radials in the Mechanisms of Monooxygenases Pharmacol Ther 1991; 49: 21–42.

18. Groves JT. Key Elements of the Chemistry of Cytochrome P450. The Oxygen Rebound Mechanism J Chem Educ 1985; 62: 928–31.

19. Guengerich FP, MacDonald TL. Chemical Mechanisms of Catalysis by Cytochromes P450: A Unified View Accts Chem Res 1984; 17: 9; Guengerich FP, MacDonald TL. Mechanisms of Cytochrome P450 Catalysis FASEB J 1990; 4:2453; Ortiz de Montellano PR. Cytochrome P-450 catalysis: radical intermediates and dehydrogenation reactions. Trends Pharmacol Sci 1989; 10: 354–9.

20. Ortiz de Montellano PR, Correia MA. Inhibition of Cytochrome P450 Enzymes In: Ortiz de Montellano PR. ed . Cytochrome P450 Structure Mechanism and Biochemistry. 2nd Ed. New York: Plenum Press 1995; Ortiz de Montellano PR. In: Alkenes and Alkynes. In: Anders M. ed. Bioactivation of Foreign Compounds New York: Academic Press 1985 pp. 121–155.

21. Whitlock JP, Denison MS. Induction of Cytochrome P450 Enzymes that Metabolize Xenobiotics. In: Ortiz de Montellano PR ed. Cytochrome P450: Structure Mechanism and Biochemistry. 2nd ed. New York: Plenum Press, 1995; Okey AB. Enzyme Induction in the Cytochrome P450 System. Pharmacol Ther 1990; 45: 241–298.

22. Barry M, Feely J. Enzyme Induction and Inhibition Pharmacol Ther 1992; 48: 71–94.

23. Guengerich FP. Metabolic Activation of Carcinogens. Pharmacol Ther 1992; 54: 17–61.

24. Martucci CP, Fishman J. P450 Enzymes of Estrogen Metabolism. Pharmacol Ther 1993; 57: 237–257.

25. Conney AH. Pantuck EJ, Kuntzman R, et al. Nutrition and chemical biotransformations in man. Clin Pharmacol Ther 1977; 22: 707–711.

26. Murray M, Reidy GF. Selectivity in the Inhibition of Mammalian Cytochromes P-450 by Chemical Agents. Pharmacol Rev 1990; 42: 85–101; Murray M. P450 Enzymes. Clin Pharmacokinet 1992; 23 132–146.

27. Ballie TA. Metabolism of Valproate to Hepatotoxic Intermediates. Pharm Weekbl [Sci] 1992; 14: 122–125.

28. Thummel KE, et al. Human Liver Microsomal Enflurane Defluorination Catalyzed by Cytochrome P-450 2E1. Drug Metab Dispos 1993; 21: 350–356.

29. Elliot RH, Strunun L. Hepatotoxity of Volatile Anesthetics. Br J Anaesth 1993; 70: 339–348.

30. Zeigler DM. Flavin-containing monooxygenases. Drug Metab Rev 1988; 19: 1–32.

31. Zeigler DM. Flavin-containing monooxygenases: enzymes adapted for multisubstrate specificity. Trends Pharmacol Sci 1990; 11:321–324.

32. Singer TP, Ramsay RR. Mechanism of Neurotoxicity of MPTP. FEBS Lett 1990; 274: 1–8.

33. Dolphin C, Shepard EA, et al. Cloning Primary Sequence and Chromosomal Mapping of a Human Flavin-Containing Monooxygenase. J Biol Chem 1991; 266: 12379–12385; Cashman JR, Wang Z, Yang L, Wighton SA. Stereo- and Regioselective N- and S- Oxidation of Tertiary Amines and Sulfides in the Presence of Adult Liver Microsomes. Drug Metab Dispos 1993; 21: 492–501.

34. Hollenberg PF. Mechanism of Cytochrome P450 and Peroxide Catalyzed Xenobiotic Metabolism FASEB J 1992; 6: 686–94; Marnett LJ, Kennedy TA. Comparison of the Peroxidase Activity of Hemoproteins and Cytochrome P450. In Ortiz de Montellano PR ed. Cytochrome P450 Structure Mechanism and Biochemistry. 2nd Ed. New York: Plenum Press 1995.

35. Hille R. Molybdenum enzymes. Essays Biochem 1999;34:125–37.

36. Beedham C. Molybdenum hydroxylases as drug-metabolizing enzymes. Drug Metab Rev 985;16:119–56; Beedham C. The role of non-P450 enzymes in drug oxidation. Pharm World Sci 1997;19:255–63.

37. Costa LG, Li WF, Richter RJ, et. al. The Role of Paraoxonase (PON1) in the detoxication of organophosphates and its human polymorphism. Chemico-Biological Reactions 1999; 119–120: 429–439.

38. Mulder GJ ed. Conjugation Reactions in Drug Metabolism: An Integrated Approach. New York: Taylor and Francis 1990.

39. Jansen PLM, Mulder PJ, Burchell B, et al. New Developments in Glucuronidation Research: Report of a Workshop on "Glucuronidation its role in health and disease." Hepatology 1992; 15:532–44.

40. Burchell B, Mcgurk K, Brierly CH, et al. UDP-glucuronosyltransferases. In: Guengerich FP. Ed. Comphrehensive Toxicology Vol. 3. New York: Pergamon Elsevier Science 1997.

41. Spahn-Langguth H, Benet LZ. Acylglucuronides Revisited; is the Glucuronidation Process a Toxification as well as a Detoxication Mechanism. Drug Metab Rev 1992; 24: 5–48.

42. Mulder GJ. Pharmacological Effects of Drug Conjugates: Is Morphine 6-Glucuronide an Exception. Trends Pharmacol Sci 1992; 13: 302–304.

43. Falani CN. Enzymology of human cytosolic sulfotransferases. FASEB J. 1997; 11:206–216.

44. Raftigianis RB, Wood TC, Weinshilboum RM. Human Phenolsulfotransferases SULT1A2 and SULT1A1. Biochem. Pharmacol. 1999; 58:605–616.

45. Caldwell J, Hutt AJ, Fournel-Gigleux S. The Metabolic Chiral Inversion and Dispositional Enantioselectivity of the 2-Arylpropionic Acids and Their Biological Activity. Biochem Pharmacol 1988; 37: 105–115.

46. Tracy TS, Wirthwein DP, Hall SD. Metabolic Inversion of (R)-Ibuprofen. Drug Metab Dispos 1993; 21: 114–119.

47. Nelson SD. Arylamines and Arylamide: Oxidation Mechanisms. In Anders M, ed. Bioactivation of Foreign Compounds. Academic Press: New York: 1985 pp. 349–375.

48. Ahmed AE, et al. Nitriles. In Anders M, ed. Bioactivation of Foreign Compounds. Academic Press. New York: 1985 pp. 485–489.

49. Dobrinska MR. Enterohepatic Circulation of Drugs. J Clin Pharmacol 1989; 29: 577–580.

50. Ilett KF, Tee LBG, Reeves PT, et al. Metabolism of Drugs and Other Xenobiotics in the Gut Lumen and Wall. Pharmacol Ther 1990; 46: 67–93.

51. Schmucker DL. Aging and Drug Dispostion: An Update. Pharmacol. Rev. 1985; 37: 133–45.

52. Durnas C, Loi CM, Cusack BJ. Hepatic Drug Metabolism and Aging. Clin. Pharmacokinet. 1990; 19: 359–389; Woodhouse K, Wynne HA. Age-Related Changes in Hepatic Function: Implications for Drug Therapy. Drugs & Aging 1992; 2: 243.

53. Smit JW, Huisman MT, van Tellingen O, et al. Absence or pharmacological blocking of placental P-glycoprotein profoundly increases fetal drug exposure. J Clin Invest 1999; 104:1441–7.

54. Ingelmann-Sundberg M, Oscarson M, McLellan RA. Polymorphic Human Cytochrome P450 Enzymes: An Opportunity for Individualized Drug Treatment, Trends Pharmacol. Sci. 1999; 20:342–9.

55. Daly AK, Cholerton S, Gregory W, et al. Metabolic Polymorphisms. Pharmacol Ther 1993; 57: 129–160.

56. Gaedigk A. Interethic Differences of Drug Metabolizing Enzymes. Intern J Clin Pharmacol Therap 2000;38:61–68.

57. Myer UA, Skoda RC, Zanger UM. The Genetic Polymorphism of Debrisoquine/Sparteine Metabolism-Molecular Mechanisms et al. Pharmacol Ther 1990; 46: 297–308.

58. Kaminsky LS, Fasco MJ. Small Intestinal Cytochromes P450. Crit Rev Toxicol 1991; 21: 407–422.

59. Kane GC, Lipsky JJ. Drug-Grapefruit Juice Interactions. Mayo Clin Proc 2000; 75:933–942.

60. Yu Dk. The Contribution of P-glycoprotein to the Pharmacokinetics of Drug-Drug Interactions. J Clin Pharmacol 1999; 39: 1203–1211.

61. Silverman JA. Multi-drug Resistance Transporters. Pharm. Biotechnol. 1999; 12:353–386.

62. Oesch F. Metabolic transformation of clinically used drugs to epoxides: new perspectives in drug-drug interactions. Biochem Pharmacol 1976; 25: 1935–1937.

63. Ohnishi A, Matsuo H, Yamada S, et al. Effect of furanocoumarin derivatives in grapefruit juice on the uptake of vinblastine by Caco-2 cells and on the activity of cytochrome P450 3A4. Br J Pharmacol 2000; 130:1369–77.

64. Watkins PB. Role of Cytochrome P450 in Drug Metabolism and Hepatotoxicity. Semin Liver Dis 1990; 10: 235–250.

65. Roth RA, Vinegar A. Action by the Lungs on Circulating Xenobiotic Agents, with a Case Study of Physiologically Based Pharmacokinetic Modelling of Benzo[a]pyrene Disposition Pharmacol Ther 1990; 48: 143–155: Reed CJ. Action by the Lungs on Circulating Xenobiotic Agents, with a Case Study of Physiologically Based Pharmacokinetic Modelling of Benzo[a]pyrene Disposition. Drug Metab Rev 1993; 25: 173–205.

66. Sarkar MA. Drug Metabolism in the Nasal Mucosa Pharmacol Res 1992; 9: 1–8.

67. Testa B, Jenner P. eds. Drug Metabolism: Chemical and Biological Aspects. New York: M. Dekker 1976.

68. Gillette JR, et al. Role of chemically reactive metabolites of foreign compounds in toxicity. Ann Rev Pharmacol Toxicol 1974; 14: 271; Reed DJ. Cellular Defense Mechanisms Against Reactive Metabolites. In Anders M. ed. Bioactivation of Foreign Compounds Academic Press. New York: 1985 pp. 71–108.

69. Nelson SD et al. Role of Metabolic Activation in Chemical-Induced Tissue Injury. In. Jerina DM. ed. Drug Metabolism Concepts ACS Symposium Series 44 Washington D.C. American Chemical Society 1977 pp 155–185.

70. Dressor GK, Spence JD, Bailey DG. Pharmacokinetic-Pharmacodynamic Consequences and Clinical Relevance of Cytochrome P450 3A4 Inhibition. Clin. Pharmacokin. 2000; 38: 41–57.

71. Michalets EL. Update: Clinically Significant Cytochrome P450 Interactions. Pharmacotherapy 1998; 18:84–112.

72. Bailey DG, Dresser GK, Kreeft JH, et al. Grapefruit-felodipine interaction: effect of unprocessed fruit and probable active ingredients. Clin Pharmacol Ther 2000;68:468–77.

73. Evans AM. Influence of dietary components on the gastrointestinal metabolism and transport of drugs. Ther Drug Monit 2000;22:131–6.

SUGGESTED READINGS

Anders M ed. Bioactivation of Foreign Compounds. New York: Academic Press 1985.

Caldwell J, Jakoby W. eds. Biological Basis of Detoxication. New York: Academic Press 1983.

Jakoby W. ed. Enzymatic Basis of Detoxication Vols. I II. New York: Academic Press 1980.

Jakoby W, Bend JR, Caldwell J. eds. Metabolic Basis of Detoxication-Metabolism of Functional Groups. New York: Academic Press 1982.

Mulder GJ. ed. Conjugation Reactions in Drug Metabolism: An Integrated Approach. London: Taylor and Francis, 1990.

Ortiz de Montellano PR. ed. Cytochrome P450 Structure Mechanism and Biochemistry. 2nd Ed. New York: Plenum Press, 1995.

Testa B, Jenner P. eds. Drug Metabolism: Chemical and Biochemical Aspects. New York: Marcel Dekker, 1976.

Testa B, Jenner P. eds. Concepts in Drug Metabolism. New York: Marcel Dekker, 1981.

Wolf TF. ed. Handbook of Drug Metabolism. New York: Marcel Dekker 1999.

Williams RT. ed. Detoxication Mechanisms 2nd ed. New York: J Wiley and Sons, 1959.

9. U.S. Drug Regulation: An Overview

DOUGLAS J. PISANO

INTRODUCTION

Regulations and laws are central, social constructs that provide guidance for all societies around the globe. Governments create laws in a number of ways with various intents for a myriad of purposes. In the United States, laws are created by the Congress, a body of officials elected by the citizenry, who are charged with the governance of the country by representing the common, public good. The Congress proposes and passes laws that are relatively general in nature and intended to address some particular issue in a fashion that can be consistently applied by all who are affected by them. Once passed, laws are remanded to the appropriate government or administrative agency that then decides on how these laws are to be applied. These "applications of law" are called regulations. Regulations serve as the practical foundation from which citizens adhere to the law as it was originally intended.

In the United States, all food, drugs, cosmetics and medical devices, for both humans and animals, are regulated under the authority of the Food and Drug Administration (FDA). FDA and all of its regulations were created by the government in response to the pressing need to address the safety of the public with respect to its foods and medicinals. The purpose of this chapter is to describe and explain the nature and extent of these regulations as they apply to drugs in the U.S. A historical perspective is offered as a foundation for regulatory context. In addition, the chapter will discuss FDA's regulatory oversight and that of other agencies, the drug approval and development process, the mechanisms used to regulate manufacturing and marketing as well as various violation and enforcement schema.

BRIEF HISTORY OF DRUG LAWS AND REGULATIONS

Prior to 1902, the U.S. government took a hands off approach to the regulation of drugs. Many of the drugs available were so-called "patent medicines" which were so named because each had a more or less descriptive or patent name which was protected by a trademark whose contents were incompletely disclosed. No laws, regulations or standards existed to regulate drugs, their purity and strength any noticeable extend even though the United Stated Pharmacopia (USP) became a reality in 1820 as the first official compendia of the United States. The USP set standards for drug strength and purity which could be used by physicians and pharmacists who needed centralized guidelines to extract, compound and otherwise utilize drug components which existed at the time (1).

Biologics Control Act

However, in 1848, the first American drug law, the Drug Importation Act, was enacted when American troops serving in Mexico became seriously ill from the quinine that was administered to treat malaria. The quinine was subsequently discovered to be adulterated. This law required laboratory inspection, detention and even destruction of drugs that did not meet acceptable standards. Later, in 1902, the Virus, Serum and Toxins Act (Biologics Control Act) was passed in response to tetanus-infected diphtheria antitoxin serum which was manufactured by a small laboratory in St. Louis, Missouri. Ten school children died as a result of the infected serum. No national standards were as yet in place for establishing purity or potency of medicinal products.

Wiley Act

The Biologics Control Act authorized the Public Health Service to license and regulate the interstate sale of serum, vaccines and related biologic products used to prevent or treat disease.

This Act also spurred Dr. Harvey W. Wiley, Chief Chemist for the Bureau of Chemistry, a branch of the United States Department of Agriculture (USDA) and the forerunner for today's United States Food and Drug Administration (FDA), to investigate the country's foods and drugs. He established the Hygienic Table, a group of young men who volunteered to serve as human guinea pigs which would allow Dr. Wiley to feed them a controlled diet laced with a variety of preservatives and artificial colors. More popularly known as the "Poison Squad," they helped Dr. Wiley gather enough data to prove that many of America's foods and drugs were either "adulterated" and the products' strength or purity were suspect or, "misbranded" with inadequate or inaccurate labeling. Dr Wiley's efforts, along with publication of Upton Sinclair's *The Jungle* (a book revealing the putrid conditions in America's meat industry), were rewarded when Congress passed America's first food and drug law in 1906, the Pure Food and Drug Act (USPFDA) (also known as the Wiley Act). The Wiley Act prohibited interstate commerce of misbranded foods or drugs based on their labeling. This act did not affect unsafe drugs in that its legal authority would only come to bear when a product's ingredients were falsely labeled. Even intentionally false therapeutic claims were not prohibited.

SHERLEY AMENDMENT

Changes in the labeling of drugs began to change in 1911 with the enactment of the Sherley Amendment which

234

intended to prohibit the labeling of medications with false therapeutic claims that were intended to defraud the purchaser. These amendments however, required the government to find proof of intentional labeling fraud. Later, in 1937, a sentinel event occurred which changed the entire regulatory picture. Sulfa (e.g., sulfanilamide) became the miracle drug of the time and was used to treat many life threatening infections. It tasted bad and was hard to swallow which led entrepreneurs to seek a palatable solution. S.E. Massingill Co. of Bristol, TN developed what they thought was a palatable, raspberry flavored liquid product. However, they used diethylene glycol to solubilize the sulfa and six gallons of this dangerous mixture, "Elixir Of Sulfanilamide," killed approximately 107 people, mostly children.

Federal Food, Drug and Cosmetic Act of 1938

The result of these unnecessary deaths from ingestion of diethylene glycol was the passage of one of the most comprehensive statutes in the history of American health law, the Federal Food, Drug And Cosmetic Act Of 1938 (FDCA). The enactment of this act repealed the Sherley Amendments and required that all new drugs be tested by their manufacturers for human safety and then submit those results to the government for marketing approval via a New Drug Application. The FDCA also mandated that drugs be labeled with adequate directions if they were shown to have had harmful effects. In addition, the FDCA authorized the Food and Drug Administration (FDA) to conduct unannounced inspections of drug manufacturing facilities. Though amended many times since 1938, the FDCA is still the broad foundation for statutory authority for FDA as it exists today.

However, a new crisis loomed. Throughout the late 1950s, European and Canadian physicians began to encounter a number of infants born with a curious birth defect called, "phocomeglia," a defect which resulted in limbs which resembled "flippers" similar to those found on seals. These birth defects were traced back to mothers who had been prescribed the drug Thalidomide in an effort to relieve morning sickness while pregnant. The manufacturer of this drug applied for U.S. marketing approval as a sleep aid. However, due to the efforts of Dr. Frances O. Kelsey, FDA's chief medical officer at the time, the case was made that the drug was not safe for human consumption therefore not effective for release in the U.S. marketplace.

Kefauver-Harris Act

Dr. Kelsey's efforts and decisive work by the U.S. Congress resulted in yet another necessary amendment to the FDCA in 1962, the Kefauver-Harris Act. This Act essentially closed many of the loopholes regarding drug safety in American law. These "Drug Efficacy Amendments" now required drug manufacturers to prove safety and efficacy of their drug products registered with the FDA and be inspected at least every 2 years, have their prescription drug

advertising approved by the FDA (this authority being transferred from the Federal Trade Commission), provide and obtain documented "informed consent" from research subjects prior to human clinical trials, and increased controls over drug manufacturing and testing to determine drug effectiveness.

To address these new provisions of the Act, the FDA contracted the National Academy of Sciences along with the National Research Council to examine some 3,400 drug products approved between 1938 and 1962 based on safety alone. Called the Drug Efficacy Study Implementation Review of 1966 (DESI) it charged these organizations to make a determination as to whether post-1938 drug products were "Effective" for the indications claimed in their labeling or "Probably Effective," "Possibly Effective" or "Ineffective." Those products not deemed "Effective" were either removed from the marketplace, reformulated or sold with a clear warning to prescribers that the product was deemed not effective.

Over-The-Counter Product Review

Later in 1972, FDA began to examine Over-The-Counter (OTC) drug products. Phase II of the Drug Efficacy Amendments required FDA to determine the efficacy of OTC drug products. This project was much larger in scope than the analysis of prescription drugs. The 1970s American consumers could choose from more than 300,000 OTC drug products. FDA soon realized that it did not have the resources to evaluate each and every OTC drug product and hence, created advisory panels of scientists, medical professionals and consumers who were charged with evaluating the active ingredients used in OTC products within 80 defined therapeutic categories. After examining both the scientific and medical literature of the day, the advisory panels made decisions regarding active ingredients and their labeling. The result was a "monograph" which described, in detail, acceptable active ingredients and labeling for products within a therapeutic class. Products which complied with monograph guidelines were deemed "Category I: Safe and effective, not misbranded." However, products not in compliance with monograph guidelines were deemed "Category II: Not safe and effective" or "misbranded." Category II products were removed from the marketplace or reformulated. Products for which data was insufficient for classification were deemed Category III and were allowed to continue on the market until substantive data could be established or until they were reformulated and in compliance with the monograph. The OTC Drug Review took approximately 20 years to complete.

Federal Controlled Substances Act (CSA)

Though there were numerous other federal laws and regulations that were passed throughout the 1970s, many were based on regulating the professional practice of medical professionals or for the direct protection of consumers. For example, The Federal Controlled Substances Act (CSA), part of the Comprehensive Drug Abuse and Prevention Act of 1970, placed drugs with a relatively high potential for abuse into five federal schedules along with a "closed record keeping system" designed to track federally controlled substances via a definite paper trail as they were ordered, prescribed, dispensed and utilized throughout the healthcare system.

Orphan Drug Act of 1983

The 1980s also passed with significant regulatory change. Biotechnology had begun on a grand scale and the pharmaceutical industry was on its cutting edge. Many of the medicinal compounds being discovered were shown to very expensive and have limited use in the general U.S. population. However, these compounds could prove life saving to demographically small patient populations who suffered from diseases and conditions which were considered rare. In an effort to encourage these biotech pharmaceutical companies to continue to develop these and other products, congress passed the Orphan Drug Act in 1983. The Act continues to allow manufacturers to gain incentives for research, development and marketing of drug products used to treat rare diseases or conditions which would otherwise be unprofitable via a system of breaks and deductions in a manufacturers corporate taxes. Though the success of the Orphan Drug Act proved great medical benefit for a few, a scandal was looming in other parts of the pharmaceutical industry.

Price Competition and Patent Restoration Act of 1984 (Waxman-Hatch Act)

The generic pharmaceutical industry experienced steady growth as many of the exclusive patents enjoyed by major pharmaceutical companies for brand-named products were beginning to expire. Generic versions of these now freely copied products were appearing much more frequently in the marketplace. However, these generic copies were required to undergo the same rigorous testing that brand-name, pioneer or innovator products did. This led to a very public scandal in which a few unscrupulous generic pharmaceutical companies took short cuts in reporting data, submitted fraudulent samples and offered bribes to FDA officials to gain easy and rapid market approval of their products. As a result, Congress passed the Price Competition and Patent Restoration Act of 1984. This Act, also called the Waxman-Hatch Act after its sponsors, was designed to level the playing field in the prescription drug industry with regard to pioneer/innovator/brand name prescription drug products and their generic copies. The Act was composed of two distinct parts or "Titles." Title I was for the benefit of the generic pharmaceutical industry and it extended the scope of the Abbreviated New Drug Application (ANDA) to cover generic versions of post-1962 approved drug products. It required that generic versions of pioneer or innovator drugs have

the same relevant properties as those with regard to bioequivalence (rate and extent of absorption of the active drug in the human body) and pharmaceutical equivalence (same dosage form as the pioneer drug to which it is compared). Though somewhat simplified, the Waxman-Hatch Act permitted easier market access to generic copies of pioneer drugs provided they were not significantly different from the pioneer drug in its absorption, action and dosage form. In addition, Title II of the Act was designed to aid and encourage research based or innovator pharmaceutical companies in continuing their search for new and useful medicinal compounds by extending the patent life of pioneer drug products while in the FDA "review period."

Prescription Drug User Fee Act (PDUFA)

However, the patent extension benefit has become somewhat moot due to an overall reduction in FDA review time as a result of prescription drug user fees. In 1992, Congress passed the Prescription Drug User Fee Act (PDUFA). The Act was intended to help FDA generate additional funds to upgrade and modernize its operations and to accelerate drug approval. It authorized FDA to charge pharmaceutical manufacturers a "user fee" to accelerate drug review. As a result of the PDUFA legislation, FDA has been able to reduce approval time of new pharmaceutical products from more than 30 months to approximately 13 to 15 months. However, the Act had a "sunset" provision which limited FDA authority to charge user fees until the year 1997.

FDA Modernization Act (FDAMA) of 1997

After reviewing the successes of the PDUFA legislation, Congress extended the user fee provisions during passage of the FDA Modernization Act (FDAMA) of 1997. FDMA reauthorized the fees till the year 2002 in an effort to further reduce prescription drug approval time. The Act however, not only extended user fee provisions, it gave FDA the authority to conduct "fast track" product reviews to further speed lifesaving drug therapies to market, permitted an additional six month patent exclusivity for pediatric prescription drug products and required the National Institutes of Health to build a publicly accessible database on clinical studies of investigational drugs or life-threatening diseases. American drug law has come quite far since the early 1900s. Today, FDA continues to work with Congress and the pharmaceutical industry to regulate and evaluate new and existing drug, biologic and device products. The overriding regulatory challenge that FDA will face will be to keep current, through regulation and policy, with future technological advances by the science and the industry.

REGULATORY OVERSIGHT OF PHARMACEUTICALS

The primary responsibility for the regulation and oversight of pharmaceuticals and the pharmaceutical industry lies with U.S. Food and Drug Administration (FDA). FDA was created in 1931 and is one of several branches within the U.S. Department of Health and Human Services (HHS). FDA's counterparts within HHS include agencies such as the Centers for Disease Control and Prevention (CDC), the National Institutes of Health (NIH) and the Healthcare Financing Administration (HCFA).

U.S. Food and Drug Administration (FDA)

FDA is organized into a number of Offices and Centers headed by a Commissioner who is appointed by the President with consent of the Senate. It is a scientifically based law enforcement agency whose mission is to safeguard the public health and to ensure honesty and fairness between health regulated industries, i.e., pharmaceutical, device, biologic, and the consumer (2). It licenses and inspects manufacturing facilities, tests products, evaluates claims and prescription drug advertising, monitors research, creates regulations, guidelines, standards and policies. It does all of this through its Office of Operations which contains component Offices and Centers such as the Center for Drug Evaluation and Research (CDER), Center for Biologics Evaluation and Research (CBER), Center for Devices and Radiological Health (CDRH), Center for Food Safety and Applied Nutrition (CFSAN) and the Center for Veterinary Medicine (CVM), Office of Orphan Products Development, Office of Biotechnology, Office of Regulatory Affairs and the National Center for Toxicological Research. Each of these entities has a defined role, though sometimes their authorities overlap. For example, if a pharmaceutical company submits a drug that is contained and delivered to a patient during therapy by a device not comparable to any other, CDER and CDRH may need to coordinate that product's approval. Though most prescription drugs are evaluated by CDER, any other Center or Office may become involved with its review. One of the most significant resources to industry and consumers is the FDA's website www.fda.gov. Easily accessible and navigable, each Center and Office has its own HTML within the site.

Other Governmental Agencies

FDA isn't the only agency within the U.S. government with a stake in pharmaceutical issues. The Federal Trade Commission (FTC) has authority over general business practices in general such as deceptive and anti-competitive practices, i.e., false advertising. In addition, FTC regulates the advertising of OTC drugs, medical devices and cosmetics. To a lesser degree, the Consumer Product Safety Commission (CPSC) regulates hazardous substances and the containers of poisons and other harmful agents; the Environmental Protection Agency (EPA) regulates pesticides used in agriculture and FDA regulates food products; the Occupational Safety and Health Administration (OSHA) regulates the working environment of employees who may use FDA regulated commodities, i.e., syringes, chemotherapy, chemical reagents; the Healthcare Financing Administration (HCFA) regulates

the federal Medicaid and Medicare programs; the Drug Enforcement Administration (DEA) enforces the Federal Controlled Substances Act and is charged with controlling and monitoring the flow of licit and illicit controlled substances; and there are various state and local drug control agencies which establish their own regulations and procedures for manufacturing, research and development of pharmaceuticals.

NEW DRUG APPROVAL AND DEVELOPMENT

Prior to any discussion of how pharmaceuticals make their way through FDA for market approval, one needs to have an understanding of what constitutes a "drug." A "drug" is a substance which exerts an action on the structure or function of the body by chemical action or metabolism and is intended for use in the diagnosis, cure, mitigation, treatment or prevention of disease (3). The concept of "New Drug" stems from the Kefauver-Harris Amendments to the FDCA. A "New Drug" is defined as one that is not generally recognized as safe and effective for the indications proposed. However, this definition has much greater reach than simply a "new" chemical entity. The term "new drug" also refers to a drug product already in existence though never approved by FDA for marketing in the U.S.; new therapeutic indications; a new dosage form; a new route of administration; a new dosing schedule; or, any other significant clinical differences than those previously approved (4). Therefore, any chemical substance intended for use in humans or animals for medicinal purposes or any existing chemical substance which has some significant change associated with it, is considered not safe or effective and a "new drug" until proper testing and FDA approval is met.

FDA approval can be a fairly lengthy and expensive process. In order for a pharmaceutical manufacturer to place a product on the market for human use, a multiphasic procedure must be followed. It must be remembered that the mission of FDA is to protect the public and they take that charge very seriously. Hence, all drug products must at least follow the step-wise process.

PRECLINICAL INVESTIGATION

The testing of new drugs in humans cannot begin until there is solid evidence that the drug product can be used with reasonable safety in humans. This phase is called "preclinical investigation." The basic goal of preclinical investigation is to assess the potential therapeutic effects of the substance on living organisms and to gather sufficient data to determine reasonable safety of the substance in humans through laboratory experimentation and animal investigation (5). FDA requires no prior approval for investigators or pharmaceutical industry sponsors to begin a preclinical investigation on a potential drug substance. Investigators and sponsors are, however, required to follow Good Laboratory Practices (GLP) regulations (6). GLPs govern laboratory facilities, personnel, equipment and operations. Compliance with GLPs requires procedures and documentation of training, study schedules, processes and status reports which are submitted to facility management and included in the final study report to FDA. Preclinical investigation usually takes 1–3 years to complete. If at that time enough data is gathered to reach the goal of potential therapeutic effect and reasonable safety, the product sponsor must formally notify FDA of their wishes to test the potential new drug on humans.

INVESTIGATIONAL NEW DRUG APPLICATION (INDA)
Overview

Unlike the preclinical investigation stage, the INDA phase has much more direct FDA activity throughout. Since a preclinical investigation is designed to gather significant evidence of reasonable safety and efficacy of the compound in live organisms, the IND phase is the clinical phase where all activity is used to gather significant evidence of reasonable safety and efficacy data about the potential drug compound in humans. Clinical trials in humans are carefully scrutinized and regulated by FDA to protect the health and safety of human test subjects and to ensure the integrity and usefulness of the clinical study data (7). Numerous meetings between both the agency and sponsor will occur during this time. As a result, the clinical investigation phase may take as many as 12 years to complete. Only 1 in 5 compounds tested may actually demonstrate clinical effectiveness and safety and reach the U.S. marketplace.

The sponsor will submit to FDA the INDA. The INDA must contain information on the compound itself and information of the study. All INDAs must have the same basic components: a detailed cover sheet, a table of contents, an introductory statement and basic investigative plan, an investigators brochure, comprehensive investigation protocols, the compound's actual or proposed chemistry, manufacturing and controls, any pharmacology and toxicology information, any previous human experience with the compound and any other pertinent information FDA deems necessary. After submission, the sponsor company must wait 30 days to commence clinical trials. If FDA does not object within that period, the trials may begin.

Institutional Review Board (IRB)

Prior to the actual commencement of the clinical investigations however, a few ground rules must be established. For example, a clinical study protocol must be developed, proposed by the sponsor and reviewed by an Institutional Review Board (IRB). An IRB is required by regulation (8) and is a committee of medical and ethical experts designated by an institution such as a University Medical Center in which the clinical trial will take place. The charge of the IRB is to oversee the research to ensure that the rights of human test subjects are protected and that rigorous medical and scientific standards are main-

tained (9). IRBs must approve the proposed clinical study and monitor the research as it progresses. It must develop written procedures of its own regarding its study review process and its reporting of any changes to the ongoing study as they occur. In addition, an IRB must also review and approve documents for informed consent prior to commencement of the proposed clinical study. Regulations require that potential patients in a clinical study are informed adequately about the risks, benefits and treatment alternatives before participating in experimental research (10). An IRB's membership must be sufficiently diverse in order to review the study in terms of the specific research issue, community and legal standards, and professional and conduct and practice norms. All of its activities must be well documented and open to FDA inspection at any time.

Once the IRB is satisfied that the proposed trial is ethical and proper the clinical trial phase will begin. The clinical trial phase has three steps or phases. Each phase has a purpose requires numerous patients, and can take greater than one year to complete.

Phase I

A Phase I study is relatively small, less than 100 subjects, and brief (1 year or less). It's purpose is to determine toxicology, metabolism, pharmacologic actions and if possible any early evidence of effectiveness. The results of the Phase I study are used to develop the next step.

Phase II

Phase II studies are the first controlled clinical trial studies using several hundred subjects who are afflicted with the disease or condition being studied. The purpose of Phase II is to determine the compound's possible effectiveness against the targeted disease or condition and its safety in humans. Phase II may be divided into two subparts; Phase IIa, a pilot study which is used to determine initial efficacy and Phase IIb which uses controlled studies on several hundred patients. At the end of the Phase II studies, the sponsor and FDA will usually confer to discuss the data and plans for Phase III.

Phase III

Phase III studies are considered "pivotal" trials which are designed to collect all of the necessary data to meet the safety and efficacy standards the FDA requires to approve the compound for the U.S. marketplace. Phase III studies are usually very large consisting of several thousand patients in numerous clinical study centers with a large number of investigators who conduct long term trials over several months or years. Also, Phase III studies establish final formulation, marketing claims and product stability, packaging and storage conditions. On completion of Phase III, all clinical studies are complete, all safety and efficacy data has been analyzed, and, the sponsor is ready to submit the compound to FDA for market approval. This process begins with submission of a New Drug Application (NDA).

NEW DRUG APPLICATION (NDA)
Overview

A New Drug Application is a regulatory mechanism that is designed to give FDA sufficient information to make a meaningful evaluation of a new drug (11). All NDAs must contain the following information; preclinical laboratory and animal data, human pharmacokinetic and bioavailability data, clinical data, methods of manufacturing, processing and packaging, a description of the drug product and substance, a list of relevant patents for the drug, its manufacture or claims and any proposed labeling. In addition, an NDA must provide a summary of the application's contents and a presentation of the risks and benefits of the new drug (12). Traditionally, NDA's consisted of hundreds of volumes of information, in triplicate, all cross referenced. Since 1999, FDA has issued final guidance documents that allow sponsors to submit NDA's electronically in a standardized format. These electronic submissions facilitate ease of review and possible approval (13).

The NDA must be submitted complete, in the proper form and with all critical data. If "accepted," FDA will then determine the applications completeness. If "complete," the agency considers the application "filed" and will begin the review process within 60 days (14). The purpose of an NDA from FDA's perspective is to ensure that the new drug meets the criteria to be "safe and effective." Safety and effectiveness are determined through the Phase III pivotal studies based on "substantial evidence" gained from a well-controlled clinical study. Since FDA realizes there are no absolutely safe drugs, FDA looks to the new drug's efficacy as a measure of its safety. It weighs the risks vs. benefits of approving the drug for use in the U.S. market.

Also, the NDA must be very clear about the manufacture and marketing of the proposed drug product. The application must define and describe manufacturing processes, validate Current Good Manufacturing Practices (CGMPs), provide evidence of quality, purity, strength, identity and bioavailability (a pre-inspection of the manufacturing facility will be conducted by FDA). Finally, FDA will review all product packaging and labeling for content and clarity. Statements on a product's package label, package insert, media advertising or professional literature must be reviewed. Of note, "labeling" refers to all of the above and not just the label on the product container.

FDA is required to review an application within 180 days of filing. At the end of that time, the agency is required to respond with an "action letter." There are three kinds of action letters. An "Approval Letter" signifies that all substantive requirements for approval are met and that the sponsor company can begin marketing the drug as of the date on the letter.

An "Approvable Letter" signifies that the application substantially complies with the requirements but has some minor deficiencies which must be addressed before an approval letter is sent. Generally, these deficiencies are minor in nature and the product sponsor must respond within 10 days of receipt. At this point, the sponsor may amend the application and address the agency's concerns or request a hearing with the agency or withdraw the application entirely.

A "Non-Approvable Letter" signifies that FDA has major concerns with the application and will not approve the proposed drug product for marketing as submitted. The remedies that a sponsor can take for this type of action letter are similar to those as in the "Approvable Letter."

PDUFA/FDAMA Effects

The New Drug Application review has been significantly affected by both the PDUFA and FDAMA legislation. PDUFA allows FDA to collect fees from sponsor companies who submit applications for review. The fees are used to update facilities and hire and train reviewers. The fees only apply to NDA drug submissions, biologic drug submissions and any supplement thereto. The fees do not apply to generic drugs or medical devices. The results of the PDUFA legislation were significant, approval rates have increased from approximately 50% to near 80% and the review times have decreased to under 15 months for most applications (15).

Later, in 1997, the FDA Modernization Act (FDAMA) reauthorized PDUFA till the year 2002. It waives the user fee to small companies who have less than 500 employees and are submitting their first application and allows payment of the fee in stages and permits a some percentage of refund if the application is refused. Also, it exempts applications for drugs used in rare conditions (Orphan Drugs), supplemental applications for pediatric indications and applications for biologicals used as precursors for other biologics manufacture. In addition, FDMA permits a "fast track" approval of compounds who demonstrate significant benefit to critically ill patients such as those who suffer from AIDS (16).

BIOLOGICS

Biologics are defined as substances derived from or made with the aid of living organisms which include vaccines, antitoxins, serums, blood, blood products, therapeutic protein drugs derived from natural sources (i.e., anti-thrombin III), biotechnology (i.e., recombinantly-derived proteins), gene or somatic cell therapies (17). As with the more traditionally derived drug products, biologics follow virtually the same regulatory and clinical testing schema with regard to safety and efficacy. A Biologics License Application (BLA) is used rather than a New Drug Application (NDA) though the official FDA Form is designated 356h and is one and the same. The sponsor merely indicated in check box if the application is for a drug or a biologic. Compounds characterized as biologics are reviewed by CBER (18).

ORPHAN DRUGS

Orphan drugs are approved using many of the same processes as any other application. However, there are several significant differences. An Orphan Drug as defined under the Orphan Drug Act of 1993 is a drug used to treat a "rare disease" which would not normally be of interest to commercial manufactures in the ordinary course of business. A "rare disease" is defined in the law as any disease that affects fewer than 200,000 persons in the U.S. or one in which a manufacturer has no reasonable expectation of recovering the cost of its development and availability in the U.S. The Act creates a series of financial incentives that manufacturers can take advantage of. For example, the Act permits grant assistance for clinical research, tax credits for research and development and a seven year market exclusivity to the first applicant who obtains market approval for a drug designated as an orphan. This means that if a sponsor gains approval for an orphan drug, FDA will not approve any application by any other sponsor for the same drug for the same disease or condition for seven years from the date of the first applicant's approval, provided certain conditions are met such as an assurance of sufficient availability of drug to those in need or a revocation of the drugs' orphan status (19,20).

ABBREVIATED NEW DRUG APPLICATIONS (ANDA)

Abbreviated New Drug Applications (ANDAs) are used when a patent has expired for a product that has been on the U.S. market and another pharmaceutical company wishes to market a generic copy. In the U.S., a drug patent is good for 20 years. After that time, a manufacturer is able to submit an abbreviated application for the pioneer product provided that they certify that the product patent in question has already expired, is invalid, or will not be infringed.

The generic copy must meet with certain other criteria as well. The drug's active ingredient must already have been approved for the conditions of use proposed in the ANDA and nothing has changed to call into question the basis for approval of the original drug's NDA (21). Sponsors of ANDAs are required to prove that their version meets with standards of bio and pharmaceutical equivalence. FDA publishes a list of all approved drugs called, "Approved Drug Products with Therapeutic Equivalence Evaluations" also called the "Orange Book" because of its orange colored cover. It lists marketed drug products that are considered by FDA to be safe and effective and provides monthly information on therapeutic equivalence evaluations for approved multi source prescription drug products (22). The Orange Book rates drugs based on their therapeutic equivalence. For a product to be considered therapeutically equivalent, it must be both pharmaceutically equivalent (i.e., the same dose, dosage form, strength, etc.), and bioequivalent (i.e., rate and extent of its absorption is not significantly different than the rate and extent of absorption of the drug with which it is to be interchanged).

Realizing that there may be some degree of variability in patients, FDA allows pharmaceuticals to be considered bioequivalent in either of two methods. The first method studies the rate and extent of absorption of a test drug which may or may not be a generic variation and a reference or brand name drug under similar experimental conditions and in similar dosing schedules where the test results do not show significant differences. The second approach uses the same method and from which the results determine that there is a difference in the test drugs rate and extent of absorption, except, the difference is considered to be medically insignificant for the proper clinical outcome of that drug.

> "Bioequivalence of different formulations of the same drug substance involves equivalence with respect to the rate and extent of drug absorption. Two formulations whose rate and extent of absorption differ by 20% or less are generally considered bioequivalent. The use of the 20% rule is based on a medical decision that, for most drugs, a 20% difference in the concentration of the active ingredient in blood will not be clinically significant." (23).

FDA's Orange Book uses a two letter coding system which is helpful in determining which drug products are considered therapeutically equivalent. The first letter, either an "A" or a "B," indicates a drug product's therapeutic equivalence rating. The second letter describes dose forms and can be any one of a number of different letters.

The "A" codes are described in the "Orange Book" as follows:

> "Drug products that FDA considers to be therapeutically equivalent to other pharmaceutically equivalent products, i.e., drug products for which:
> 1. There are no known or suspected bioequivalence problems. These are designated **AA, AN, AO, AP** or **AT,** depending on the dose form; or
> 2. Actual or potential bioequivalence problems have been resolved with adequate in vivo and/or in vitro evidence supporting bioequivalence. These are designated **AB.**" (24)

The "B" codes are a much less desirable rating when compared to a rating of "A." Products which are rated "B" may still be commercially marketed, however, they may not be considered therapeutically equivalent. The Orange Book describes "B" codes as follows;

> "Drug products that FDA at this time does not consider to be therapeutically equivalent to other pharmaceutically equivalent products, i.e., drug products for which actual or potential bioequivalence problems have not been resolved by adequate evidence of bioequivalence. Often the problem is with specific dosage forms rather than with the active ingredients. These are designated **BC, BD, BE, BN, BP, BR, BS, BT,** or **BX.**" (25)

FDA has adopted an additional sub-category of "B" codes. The designation, "B*" is assigned to former "A" rated drugs "if FDA receives new information that raises a significant question regarding therapeutic equivalence." (26) Not all drugs are listed in the Orange Book. Drugs obtainable only from a single manufacturing source, DESI-drugs or drugs manufactured prior to 1938 are not included. Those that do appear, are listed by generic name.

PHASE IV AND POST-MARKETING SURVEILLANCE AND SUPPLEMENTAL NDA (SNDA)

Pharmaceutical companies who successfully gain marketing approval for their products are NOT exempt from further regulatory requirements. Many products are approved for market on the basis of a continued submission of clinical research data to FDA. This data may be required to further validate efficacy or safety, detect new uses or abuses for the product or to determine the effectiveness of labeled indications under conditions of widespread usage (27). FDA may also require a Phase IV study for drugs approved under FDAMA's "fast track" provisions.

Supplemental NDA (SNDA)

Any changes to the approved product's indications, active ingredients, manufacture, or labeling require the manufacturer to submit a supplemental NDA (SNDA) for agency approval. Also, "adverse drug reports" are required to be reported to the agency. All reports must be reviewed by the manufacturer promptly, and if found to be serious, life threatening or unexpected (not listed in the products labeling), the manufacturer is required to submit an "alert report" within 15 days working days of receipt of the information. All adverse reaction thought not to be serious or unexpected must be reported quarterly for three years after the application is approved, and annually thereafter (28).

OVER-THE-COUNTER (OTC) REGULATIONS (1951 DURHAM-HUMPHREY AMENDMENTS)

The 1951 Durham-Humphrey Amendments of the FDCA specified three criteria to justify prescription only status. If the compound is shown to be habit forming, require a prescribers supervision or has a NDA prescription only limitation, it will require a prescription. The principles used to establish OTC status (no prescription required) are a wide margin of safety, method of use, benefit-to-risk ratio and adequacy of labeling for self medication. For example, injectable drugs may not be used OTC with certain exceptions such as Insulin. OTC market entry is less restrictive than that for prescription drugs and does not require pre-market clearance. They pose many fewer safety hazards than prescription drugs because they are designed to alleviate symptoms rather than disease. Easier access to OTC drugs far outweighs the risks of side effects which can be adequately addressed through proper labeling.

As previously discussed, OTC products underwent an efficacy review in 1972. Though reviewing the therapeutic efficacy of more than 30,000 OTC drug products in existence at the time would be virtually impossible, FDA created OTC Advisory Panels to review data based on some 26 therapeutic categories. OTC drugs would only be examined by active ingredient within a therapeutic category. Inactive ingredients would only be examined provided they were shown to be safe and suitable for the product and not interfering with effectiveness and quality.

This review of active ingredients would result in the promulgation of a regulation or a "MONOGRAPH" which is a "recipe" or set of guidelines applicable to all OTC products within a therapeutic category. OTC Monographs are general and require that OTC products show "general recognition of the safety and effectiveness of the active ingredient." OTC products do not fall under prescription status if their active ingredients (or combinations) are deemed by FDA to be "Generally Recognized as Safe and Effective" (GRASE.). The monograph system is a public system with a public comment component included after each phase of the process. Any products for which a final monograph has not been established may remain on the market until one is determined.

There are four phases in the OTC monograph system. In Phase I, an expert panel is selected to review data for each active ingredient in each therapeutic category for safety, efficacy and labeling. Their recommendations are made in the federal register. A public comment period of 30–60 days is permitted and supporting or contesting data is accepted for review. Then the panel reevaluates the data and publishes a "Proposed Monograph" in the Federal Register which publicly announces the conditions for which the panel believed that OTC products in a particular therapeutic class are GRASE and not misbranded. A "Tentative Final Monograph" is then developed and published stating FDA's position on safety and efficacy of a particular ingredient within a therapeutic category and acceptable labeling for indications, warnings, and directions for use. Active ingredients are deemed: Category I—GRASE for claimed therapeutic indications and not misbranded; Category II—Not-GRASE and or misbranded; Category III—Insufficient data for determination.

After public comment, the final monograph was established and published with FDA's final criteria for which all drug products in a therapeutic class become GRASE and not misbranded. Following the effective date of the final monograph, all covered drug products that failed to conform to its requirements were considered misbranded and an unapproved new drug (29).

However, since the Monograph panels are no longer convened, many current products are switched from prescription to OTC status. A company who wishes to make this switch and offer an OTC product to the U.S. marketplace can submit an amendment to a monograph to FDA who will act as the sole reviewer. The company may also file an SNDA provided that they have three years of marketing experience as a prescription product, can demonstrate a relatively high use during that period and can validate that the product has a mild profile of adverse reactions. The last method involves a "Citizens Petition" which is rarely used (30).

REGULATING MARKETING

FDA has jurisdiction over prescription drug advertising and promotion. The basis for these regulations lies within the 1962 Kefauver-Harris Amendments. Essentially, any promotional information in any form must be truthful, fairly balanced and fully disclosed. FDA views this information as either "advertising" or "labeling." Advertising includes all traditional outlets in which a company places an ad. Labeling includes everything else including brochures, booklets, lectures, slide kits, letters to physicians, company sponsored magazine articles, etc. All information must be truthful and not misleading. All material facts must be disclosed in a manner that is fairly balanced and accurate. If any of these requirements are violated, the product is considered "misbranded" for the indications in which it was approved under its NDA. FDA is also sensitive to the promotion of a product for "off-label use." Off-label use occurs when a product is in some way presented in a manner that does not agree with or is not addressed in its approved labeling. Also, provisions of the Prescription Drug Marketing Act (PDMA) of 1987 apply. The Act prohibits company representatives from directly distributing or reselling prescription drug samples. Companies are required to establish a closed system of record keeping which will be able to track a sample from their control to that of a prescriber in order to prevent diversion. Prescribers are required to receive these samples and record and store them appropriately (31).

VIOLATIONS AND ENFORCEMENT

FDA has the power to enforce the regulations for any product as defined under the FDCA. It has the jurisdiction to inspect a manufacturers premises and their records. After a facilities inspection, an agency inspector will issue an FDA Form 483s which describes observable violations. Response to the finding as described on this form must be made promptly. A "Warning Letter" may be used when the agency determines that one or more of a company's practices, products, or procedures are in violation of the FDCA. The FDA district office has 15 days to issue a warning letter after an inspection. The company has 15 days in which to respond to this warning letter. If the company response is satisfactory to the FDA, no other action is warranted. If the response is not, the FDA may request a "recall" of the violated products. However, FDA has no authority to force a company to recall a product, but it may force removal of a product through the initiation of a seizure.

Recalls

Recalls can fall into one of three classes: A Class I recall exists when there is a reasonable possibility that the use of a product will cause either serious adverse effects on health or death; Class II recall exists when the use of a product may cause temporary or medically reversible adverse effects on health, or where the probability of serious adverse effects on health is remote; a Class III recall exists when the use of a product is not likely to cause adverse

health consequences. Recalls are also categorized as consumer level, where the product is requested to be recalled from the consumers homes or control; a retail level where the products are to be removed from retail shelves or control; and wholesale level, where the product is to be removed from wholesale distribution. Companies who conduct recall of their products are required to conduct "Effectiveness Checks" to determine the effectiveness of recalling the product from the marketplace.

An Injunction

If a company refuses to recall the product, FDA will seek an injunction against the company (32). An injunction is recommended to the Department of Justice (DOJ) by FDA who takes the request to federal court and issues the order that forbids a company from carrying out a particular illegal act, such as marketing a product that FDA considers a violation of the FDCA. Companies can either comply with the order and sign a "consent agreement," which will specify changes required by FDA in order for the company to continue operations, or litigate.

Seizure of Products

FDA may also initiate a seizure of violative products (33). A seizure is ordered by the federal court in the district that the products are located. The seizure order specifies products, their batch numbers and any records determined by FDA as violative. The U.S. Marshals carry out this action. FDA institutes a seizure to prevent a company from selling, distributing, moving or otherwise tampering with the product.

FDA may also debar individuals or firms from assisting or submitting an ANDA, or directly providing services to any firm with an existing or pending drug product application. Debarment may last for up to 10 years (34).

However, one of the more powerful deterrents that FDA uses is adverse publicity. The FDA has no authority to require a company to advertise adverse publicity, but it does publish administrative actions against a company in any number of federal publications such as the *Federal Register, the FDA Enforcement Report, the FDA Medical Bulletin and the FDA Consumer* (35).

SUMMARY

The laws and regulations that govern the U.S. pharmaceutical industry are both vast and complicated. Interpretation of the FDCA is in a constant state of flux. FDA is charged with this interpretation based on the rapid technologies changes that are everyday occurrences within the industry. Many may suggest that more rapid drug approval places the citizenry in greater danger of adverse events. Others may reply that technology offers newer and more effective therapies for deadly disease.

Historically, the U.S. congress has passed laws governing our medication based on a reaction to a crises. The Pure Food and Drug Act, The Food, Drug and Cosmetic

Act and the Price Competition and Patent Restoration Act are just a few. One hopes that this method of regulation will not continue as the norm. We can be proud of proactive legislation such as the Kefauver-Harris Amendments, the Orphan Drug Act, PDUFA and FDAMA. These Acts have paved the way for meaningful change within the drug investigation process as we continue in our battle against disease. The U.S. system of investigating new drugs is one which continues to have merit by allowing enough time to investigate benefit versus risk. The American public can look forward to great advances from the industry and should be comfortable that FDA is watching.

REFERENCES

1. Valentino, J, "Practical Uses for the USP: A Legal Perspective," in Strauss's Federal Drug Laws and Examination Review, 5th Ed., Technomic Publishing Co., Lancaster, PA, 1999, p.38.
2. Strauss, S, "Food and Drug Administration: An Overview," Strauss's Federal Drug Laws and Examination Review, 5th Ed., Technomic Publishing Co., Lancaster, PA, 1999, p.323.
3. FDCA, Sec.21(g)(1).
4. Strauss, S, ibid., p.176, 186.
5. Pinna, K, Pines, W, "The Drugs/Biologics Approval Process," A Practical Guide To Food and Drug Law and Regulation, FDLI, Washington, DC, 1998, p.96.
6. 21Code of the Federal Register Section 58.
7. Pinna, K,et al, ibid., p.98.
8. 21Code of the Federal Register Section 56.
9. Pinna, K, et al ibid., p.98.
10. 21Code of the Federal Register Section 50.
11. 21Code of the Federal Register Section 314.
12. Pinna, K, et al ibid., p.102–103.
13. Federal Register, V.64(18), January 28, 1999.
14. Pinna, K, et al ibid., p.103.
15. Strauss, S, ibid., p.280.
16. Food and Drug Administration Modernization Act of 1997, PL. 105, 1997.
17. 42U.S. Code, Sec. 262.
18. Form FDA 356h.
19. The Orphan Drug Act of 1982, PL 97–414.
20. The Orphan Drug Amendments of 1985, PL 99–91.
21. Pinna, K, at al ibid., p.119.
22. USP/DI, Volume III, 16th Edition, Preface, United States Pharmacopeia, Rockville, MD, 2000, p. v.
23. USP/DI, Volume III, 16th Edition, Preface, United States Pharmacopeia, Rockville, MD, 2000, p. I/7.
24. USP/DI, Volume III, 16th Edition, Preface, United States Pharmacopeia, Rockville, MD, 2000, p. I/9.
25. USP/DI, Volume III, 16th Edition, Preface, United States Pharmacopeia, Rockville, MD, 2000, p. I/10.
26. USP/DI, Volume III, 16th Edition, Preface, United States Pharmacopeia, Rockville, MD, 2000, p.I/12.
27. Pinna, K, et al ibid, p.111.
28. Pinna, K, et al, ibid., p.111.
29. Strauss, S, ibid., p.285.
30. Strauss, S, ibid., p.285.
31. 21U.S. Code301, et seq.
32. 21U.S. Code 302, et seq.
33. 21U.S. Code304, et seq.
34. Fundamentals of Regulatory Affairs, Regulatory Affairs Professions Society, 1999, p.199.
35. Fundamentals of Regulatory Affairs, p. 200.

PART II

Pharmacodynamic Agents

Overview: Drug Receptors: A Perspective

DAVID J. TRIGGLE

Pharmacodynamics is the study of drug action principally in terms of the structure of the drug, its site of action and the biological consequences of the drug-receptor interaction. Pharmacodynamics defines the selectivity, sites of action, concentration- and time-response relationships of a drug. These relationships are determined by several processes, including absorption, metabolism, distribution and excretion: these pharmacokinetic events are profoundly important in determining drug action, including the therapeutic and contraindication profile of a given agent and they can significantly modify the consequences of drug action at the specific site of action—the pharmacologic receptor. In this chapter a broad overview of the pharmacologic receptor is presented in terms of classification, recognition and transduction events, structures, and the relationship between structure and function and the alterations of receptor structure in discrete disease states. Separate chapters will provide more detailed application of these general concepts to specific receptors and classes of drugs.

HISTORICAL BACKGROUND

Two separate, but ultimately complementary, lines of evidence led in the late 19th century to the postulate of the existence of receptors serving as specific sites of interaction with which drugs interacted selectively to initiate or block a particular biological event—physiological or pathological. From his work on immunology and the chemotherapy of protozoan infections Paul Ehrlich speculated that the cell possessed specific protoplasmic side chains of defined and unique chemical and steric architecture and that these interacted specifically with complementary groups of a chemotherapeutic agent or antibody:

*"For the sake of brevity in what follows we shall in general always designate as **receptor** that binding group of the protoplasmic molecule to which a foreign, newly introduced group binds" (1).*

The concept of "lock-and-key" action, critical to the issue of specificity in the drug-receptor interaction, had previously been defined by Emil Fischer who observed:

"…I will say that enzyme and glucoside must fit together like lock and key in order to be able to exercise a chemical action on each other" (2).

Prior to these speculations John Newton Langley had written:

"We may, I think, without much rashness assume that there is some substance or substances in the nerve endings or gland cells with which both atropine and pilocarpine are capable of forming compounds. On this assumption, then, the atropine or pilocarpine compounds are formed according to some law of which their relative mass and chemical affinity for the substance are factors" (3).

Langley also recognized the receptor as a transducer that "… receives the stimulus and, by transmitting it causes contraction" (response) (4), thus serving to convert one form of information—the drug-receptor interaction—into another—the physiologic response. Later, and contemporaneously with the writings of Ehrlich, Langley used the term "receptive substance" for these compounds and speculated that separate receptors existed for atropine, pilocarpine, curare and other "autonomic agents" with which his physiologic research had been concerned.

Thus, by the beginning of the 20th Century the foundation had been laid for a definition of receptors that embodied the concepts of specificity, including stereoselectivity, dose-response relationships and transduction. These components of the definition are those that we use today, although they have been substantially refined and quantitated, notably with respect to definition of the location, structure and chemistry of the drug binding site, and the coupling of this site to response.

RECEPTOR CLASSIFICATION

In principle, receptors may be classified in a variety of ways: 1) by the physiological ligand which interacts with the receptor; 2) by the response that activation of the receptor induces; 3) by the biochemical changes that may link receptor activation to response; 4) by the structure of the receptor protein. Each of these schemes has, however, its own limitations. It is of little help to refer to the receptor that elevates blood pressure or increases heart rate since these are properties common to many receptors. Similarly, many receptors share a common biochemical cascade, for example activation of adenylyl cyclase, yet may produce similar or different physiologic responses. Furthermore, agonists at many receptors are pleiotropic, producing multiple biochemical consequences that may have different effects according to cell type. Additionally, since the coupling between receptor and effector depends upon intrinsic properties of the ligand the biochemical effect induced at the same receptor in the same cell can be agonist specific. Physiological ligands may interact with multiple receptors that are clearly unrelated, for example acetylcholine interacts with both the nicotinic and muscarinic classes of acetylcholine that are by all other criteria quite distinct receptor families and belonging to the transmitter-gated ion channel and guanine nucleotide binding protein-coupled [G protein-coupled receptors] classes respectively. Similar divisions occur with *gamma*-aminobutyric acid [GABA] where $GABA_A$ and $GABA_B$ receptors belong to the transmitter-gated channel and G protein-coupled classes respectively. Of particular interest, all receptors-$5-HT_{1-7}$- for serotonin belong to the G protein-coupled class, save for the $5-HT_3$ category, which is a ligand-gated ion channel. Finally, the same receptor may interact with ligands that are structurally and functionally totally unrelated. A prominent example is the chemokine family of receptors that recognize both the physiologic chemokine class of ligands, including interleukin-8, monocyte chemoattractant protein and other cytokines, and also is a co-receptor of the pathological human immunodeficiency virus [HIV].

The use of non-physiological ligands, notably selective agonists and antagonists, has permitted the sub-classification of receptor families and has allowed for the characterization of receptor subtypes. Thus, atropine and curare are classically known drugs and receptor antagonists that permitted the early subdivision of acetylcholine receptors into the "muscarinic" and "nicotinic" families. These families are now established, by structural information, to be quite distinct although they share a common physiological ligand—acetylcholine. Finally, it must be recognized that receptors exist that recognize signals other than chemical and that these receptors belong to the same classes as those for physiological ligands. Thus, rhodopsin, the visual light-recognizing pigment, is a member of the G protein-coupled class of receptors (Table II.1) and the visual cascade bears many similarities to the events initiated by, for example, catecholamine interaction at *beta*-adrenoceptors. Similarly, ion channels that are opened or closed by changes in membrane potential–voltage-gated channels—are similar in their fundamental construction to

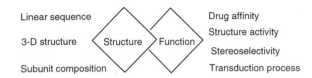

Fig. II.1. Defining structure-function factors that affect ligand binding sites and the transduction process.

ligand/transmitter-gated ion channels. Finally, receptors for odorant molecules, of which there may be many thousand, also belong to the G protein class.

Receptor structure, the linear amino acid sequence of the receptor protein inferred from the gene, provides a definitive identification and basis for classification of receptors. The degree of similarity between these sequences permits the establishment of "receptor families" and, through the techniques of molecular biology, has made possible the identification of receptors—so-called "orphan receptors"—for which physiological ligands may not yet have been identified. However, even linear and ultimately three-dimensional structure is not without its limitations. Post-translational modifications that are cell- or tissue-specific may contribute to the properties of the expressed receptor, including its coupling to effector systems. Additionally, receptors that are oligomeric assemblies of individual subunits may be heteromeric assemblies and thus the properties of the total receptor complex may depend upon the subunit composition. Because of the importance of receptor classification to the science and practice of pharmacology the International Union of Pharmacology (IUPHAR) has established a set of committees designed to report on receptor classification schemes and protocols and the total functional classification is dependent upon consideration of structural, recognition and transduction components (Fig. II.1). From these considerations four principal classes of pharmacologic receptors may be recognized (Table II.1).

1-Transmembrane Proteins

The first major class of pharmacologic receptors contains those that are intrinsically enzyme-associated, including those with guanylate cyclase activity or tyrosine kinase activity or which associate directly with a diffusible tyrosine kinase. These receptors include those for a number of growth factors, neurotrophins and cytokines (Table II.2). In these receptors there is but a single membrane-spanning domain and the receptor and the enzyme are components of the same peptide chain. In a variation on this structural theme the receptor and enzyme complexes are on separate chains that are closely associated. Activation of these receptors occurs through a process of dimerization. Several growth factors, including platelet-derived growth factor, can induce cross-linking of their corresponding receptors because they contain two binding sites. Other growth factors recruit accessory molecules to induce receptor oligomerization. This dimerization process has

Table II.1. Classification of Pharmacological Receptors*

Class	Receptor Type	Characteristics
1.	1-Transmembrane Proteins	Enzyme associated
2.	Transcriptional Regulators	Non-membrane, cytosolic protein with DNA-binding domains
3.	Ion Channels	Integral membrane; subunit composition; each subunit or domain has two or more membrane inserts as a pore region and four or more form the central pore of the channel.
4.	7-Transmembrane Proteins	G-protein coupled receptors

*For further explanations see text.

Table II.2. Receptors for Growth Factors and Related Ligands

Receptor Type	Ligand
Tyrosine kinase	Platelet derived growth factor (PDGF)
	Epidermal growth factor (EGF)
	Insulin-like growth factor (IGF)
	Fibroblast growth factor (FGF)
	Neurotrophins
Cytokines	Growth hormone
	Erythopoietin
	Interleukin 2, 3, 6
	Interferon
Tumor necrosis	Tumor necrosis factor
	Low affinity growth factor receptor
Serine/threonine kinase	Transforming growth factor beta (TGFB)
	Activin

A/B Variable transactivation	C Zn fingers DNA binding	D Hinge	E Ligand binding	F Variable

Fig. II.3. Structure of the nuclear hormone receptor made up of discrete regions or domains such as the C-terminal region for ligand binding and receptor dimeration (A/B), the central DNA binding region that contacts critical nucleotide sequences termed hormone response elements (C–E), and a variable region at the N-terminal domain (F).

been shown to be an integral component of the activation of many cell surface receptors associated with kinase activities. In contrast, the activity of tyrosine phosphatases is also controlled by dimerization, but dimerization decreases the enzyme activity.

Transcriptional Regulators

The intracellular hormone receptors constitute the second major class and include the receptors for steroid hormones, including estrogens and androgens, the glucocorticoids such as corticosterone, vitamin D, thyroxine and retinoic acid (Fig. II.2). There are in excess of 150 members of this receptor family which serve as transcription factors. This receptor super-family shares a number of common characteristics including the possession of multiple functional domains—ligand-binding, DNA-binding and transcriptional activation (Fig. II.3). Type I receptors for steroid hormones are localized in the cytoplasm and nucleus and form large macromolecular complexes with heat shock and other proteins: ligand binding induces dis-

sociation of the complex to form monomeric receptors which then homodimerize and bind to hormone response elements in the nuclear DNA. Type II receptors for vitamin D, thyroid hormone and retinoic acid, are exclusively localized in the nucleus and form heterodimers that can bind to DNA in the absence of ligand (Fig. II.4). These nuclear receptors may be associated with co-repressor proteins that inhibit basal transcription of the target genes. Several processes including the tissue-specific expression of receptors and the sequence and organization of the DNA target sequences presumably ensure selectivity of target gene activation.

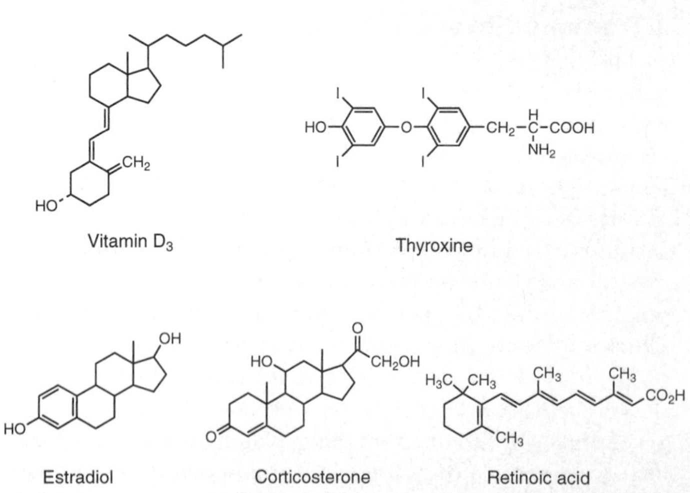

Ion Channel

The ion channel category of pharmacologic receptors includes voltage-gated channels and transmitter-gated channels (Table II.3): the latter include receptors for acetylcholine (nicotine), glycine and GABA, glutamate, serotonin, ATP, cyclic nucleotides and inositol *tris*-phosphate (IP_3).

7-Transmembrane Protein

The G protein-coupled receptors represent the largest single class of pharmacologic receptors; almost two hundred human receptors are known and there are an additional number for which no physiological function has yet been defined—"orphan receptors." G protein-coupled receptors are of major therapeutic significance since they are an established target of many therapeutic agents (Tables II.4 and II.5): it has been estimated that approximately 60% of existing therapeutically active drugs act on this class of receptor. Furthermore, an increasing number of structural and expression defects in these receptors are linked to defined disease states (see Receptors as Regulated Species).

These considerations permit the broad classification of receptors into several major classes. It is instructive to note that the detailed sub-classification of receptors, critical to

Vitamin D₃

Thyroxine

Estradiol   Corticosterone   Retinoic acid

Fig. II.2. Hormonal ligands that act as "nuclear receptors" of the transcriptional regulator receptors.

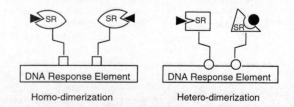

Homo-dimerization   Hetero-dimerization

Fig. II.4. Representation of nuclear hormone receptor dimers (SR = Steroid Receptor) and their interaction with DNA.

Table II.3. Classification of Ion Channels

Family	Ions	Functional Characteristics
Voltage-gated	Na^+, K^+ Ca^{2+}	Opened and closed by changes in membrane potential. Members of one structural super-family. Target of many toxins and therapeutic agents.
Transmitter-gated	Na^+, K^+, Ca^{2+} Cl^-	Opened by interaction with transmitter. Members of several structural classes.
ACh (nicotinc)	cation (Na^+, Ca^{2+}) channel	
Glycine	anion (Cl^-) channel	
$GABA_A$	anion (Cl^-) channel	
Glutamate	cation (Na^+, Ca^{2+}) channel	
Serotonin	cation channel	
ATP (purinergic)	cation (K^+) channel	
Cyclic-nucleotide	cation channel	
IP_3	cation (Ca^{2+}) channel	

Table II.4. G Protein-Coupled Receptors as Therapeutic Targets

Receptor	Drug	Indication
Acetylcholine (muscarinic)	Bethanchol Ipratropium	Gastrointestinal Pulmonary
Norepinephrine		
beta$_1$	Atenolol	Cardiovascular
beta$_1$/beta$_2$	Propranol	Cardiovascular
beta$_2$	Albuterol	Pulmonary
alpha$_1$	Terazosin	Cardiovascular
alpha$_2$	Clonidine	Cardiovascular
Angiotensin AT$_1$	Losartan	Cardiovascular
Dopamine, D$_2$	Haloperidol	Central Nervous System
Serotonin 5HT$_{ID}$	Sumatriptan	Central Nervous System
Histamine H$_2$	Cimetidine	Gastrointestinal
Opiod μ	Morphine	Central Nervous System

Table II.5. Drugs (Including Those Under Development) for Peptide G-Protein Coupled Receptors

Receptors	Clinical Status	Drugs	Indication
Opiod	In use	Morphine	Pain
Angiotensin II	In use	Losartan Valsartan	Hypertension
Endothelin [ETA,ETB]	In development	—	Heart failure
Tachykinin (NK1)	In development	—	Depression Asthma
Vasopressin (V$_2$)	In development	—	Heart failure
Cholecystokinin	In development	—	Anxiety Appetite
Neuropeptide Y, Y1, Y5	In development	—	Appetite
Neuropeptide Y, Y$_2$	In development	—	Depression
Chemokine CCR5 CXCR$_4$	In development	—	HIV

an understanding of the pharmacologic selectivity and the therapeutic efficacy of drugs, depends upon the simultaneous application of a number of considerations. This is seen with the receptors for the transmitter acetylcholine and for which two major structural classes exist—muscarinic and nicotinic receptors: these represent two major classes of receptors—the G protein-coupled receptors and the transmitter gated channels.

Muscarinic receptors are of five major classes—M$_1$ to M$_5$ —coded by separate genes, with differential expression, function, coupling and drug sensitivity (Table II.6). They are all members of the G protein-coupled receptor family that is characterized by a single protein with seven transmembrane spanning regions (see Receptor Structure). They are differentially recognized by synthetic drugs, although the greatest differential selectivity is demonstrated by antagonists rather than by agonists. Atropine is a nonselective antagonist, pirenzepine has selectivity for M$_1$ receptors, methoctramine and AF-DX 384 exhibit selectivity for M$_2$ receptors, and darifenacin for M$_3$ receptors; however, none of these antagonists (Fig. II.5) exhibits absolute

selectivity against a receptor subtype. In contrast, the nicotinic receptor is a transmitter-gated channel made up of a pentameric structure with *alpha, beta, gamma* and *delta* subunits. The classic curare-sensitive nicotinic acetylcholine receptor of skeletal muscle is made up of two *alpha,* one *beta,* one *gamma* and one *delta* subunit with the acetylcholine binding sites being carried on the alpha subunit. Nicotinic receptors found in the central and peripheral nervous system have a considerable diversity of subunit combination with *alpha$_{1-9}$* and *beta$_{2-4}$* expressed in combination (heteromeric) or, in a few cases, alone (homomeric). The major permutations found in the nervous system include *alpha$_4$beta$_2$* which is widespread in the CNS, and *alpha$_7$* which is also widespread in the CNS and is also found in ganglia and several other combinations (Table II.7).

Table II.6. Classification of Muscarinic Acetylcholine Receptors

| | Receptor Subtype | | | | |
	M_1	M_2	M_3	M_4	M_5
G protein coupling	√	√	√	√	√
	Simulation	Inhibition	Stimulation	Inhibition	Stimulation
Second Messenger	PLC/IP$_3$/DAG	c-AMP	PLC/IP3/DAG	c-AMP	PLC/IP3/DAG
Locations	CNS	CNS	CNS	CNS	CNS
	DNS	Heart	Glands		
	Glands	Smooth Muscle	Smooth Muscle		
Function	K$^+$ (M) current inhibition	Decrease heart rate and force	Glandular Secretion	—	—
Antagonist	Atropine	Atropine	Atropine	Atropine	Atropine
	Pirenzepine	—	—	—	—
	—	Methoctramine	—	Methoctramine	—
	—	—	Darifenacin	—	—
	—	AF-DX 384	—	AF-DX-384	—

PLC = Phospholipase C; IP$_3$ = 1,4,5-inositol triphosphate; DAG = Diacylglycerol; c-AMP = 3,5-cyclic adenosine monphosphate.

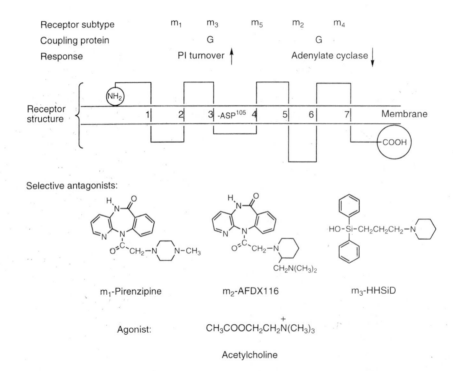

Fig. II.5. Schematic representation of the G protein-coupled muscarinic receptor family -m$_1$-m$_5$- and the selective antagonists that interact with the receptor.

Table II.7. Classification of Nicotinic Acetylcholine Receptors (5)

| | Receptor Subtype | | | | |
Subunit Composition	$\alpha_1 \beta_1 \delta_1$	$\alpha_4 \beta_2$	α_7	$\alpha_3 \beta_2 \beta_4$ (?)	$\alpha_3 \alpha_5 \beta_4$
Localization	Skeletal muscle	CNS	CNS	CNS	PNS
Function	Muscle contraction	Cognition NT Release	Cognition neuroprotection	NT release	Synaptic transmission
Selective drugs	α-Bungarotoxin	nicotine epibatidine cytosine	α-Bungarotoxin	Dihydro β-erythroidine	hexamethonium- n-bungarotoxin

Table II.8. Therapeutic Agents That Interact with Ion Channels

Drug	Channel	Therapeutic Use
Ligand-Gated Ion Channels		
Diazepam	GABA$_A$	Anti-anxiety
Phencyclidine	Glutamic acid	Tranquilizer
Minoxidil	K$^+_{ATP}$	Hair growth*
Glibenclamide	K$^+_{ATP}$	Diabetes
Pinacidil	K$^+_{ATP}$	Hypertension
Voltage-Gated Ion Channels		
Nifedipine	Ca^{2+}	Hypertension
Diltiazem	Ca^{2+}	Angina
Lidocaine	Na$^+$	Anti-anxiety Local anesthetic
Phenytoin	Na$^+$	Anti-convulsant
DDT	Na$^+$	Insecticide
Sotalol	K$^+$	Anti-arrhythmic
Quinidine	K$^+$	Anti-arrhythmic

*Not established to be related to any activity at the K$^+_{ATP}$ channel.

Considering the classification of voltage-gated ion channels can make a further useful comparison. These channels respond to an electrical signal rather than an endogenous chemical signal, but they can also be classified according to the specific toxins and synthetic chemicals with which they interact. A significant number of therapeutically useful drugs interact with both transmitter-gated and voltage-gated ion channels (Table II.8). Ion channels that permeate, with varying degrees of selectivity, Na$^+$, K$^+$, Ca^{2+} and Cl$^-$, may be sub-classified according to a number of criteria:

a. Structure and subunit composition
b. Voltage-gated or transmitter-gated
c. Ionic selectivity
d. Electrophysiological properties—conductance, kinetics of opening and closing, voltage-dependence and voltage-range of opening and closing
e. Sensitivity to drugs and toxins.

This classification scheme is shown in Table II.9 for voltage-gated Ca^{2+} channels. The L-type channel is the site of

action of a major group of cardiovascular drugs, the calcium channel blockers, that are antihypertensive, antianginal and selectively anti-arrhythmic, and interact at discrete receptors on the channel (Figure II.6).

RECEPTOR STRUCTURE

The majority of the pharmacologic receptors under discussion are integral membrane proteins and have not, until very recently, been amenable to high-resolution structural studies. However, considerable progress has been made in three areas—the structure of rhodopsin as a model for G protein-coupled receptors, the structure of the nicotinic acetylcholine receptor as an example of a ligand-gated ion channel, and a bacterial K$^+$ channel that serves to define the conductivity and ionic selectivity mechanisms of ion channels. In addition to such structural studies there are an increasing number of biochemical and mutational studies that serve to delineate particular protein regions and residues associated with ligand interaction. Regardless of receptor type under consideration structural studies have followed closely parallel pathways—biochemical studies that gave evidence of size and subunit composition, genomic and sequencing studies that described the primary structure of the proteins, modeling studies that provide descriptions of potential membrane organization and the final three-dimensional structural analyses.

Bacteriorhodopsin and G Protein-coupled Receptors

The G protein-coupled receptor superfamily is an extremely large family of integral membrane proteins receiving chemical information from odorants, neurotransmitters and polypeptide hormones and translating the information through the family of heterotrimeric G proteins into biologic response. This protein superfamily has a common 7 transmembrane helical (7-TM) structure that apparently evolved early in evolution since it is widely distributed from bacteria onwards.

Table II.9. Classification of Voltage-Gated Ca^{2+} Channels

Property	Channel Class			
	T	**L**	**N**	**P**
Conductance	Low	High	High	High
Voltage activating threshold	Low	High	High	High
Ion selectivity	Ba^{2+} = Ca^{2+}	Ba^{2+} > Ca^{2+}	Ba^{2+} > Ca^{2+}	Ba^{2+} > Ca^{2+}
Function	Pacemaking; cardiac and neuronal cells	Smooth muscle and cardiac contractability	←Neurotransmitter→ release	
Pharmacology	Mibefradil*	Verapamil Diltiazem Nifedipine and 1,4-Dihydropyridines	Conotoxins†	Agatoxins‡

*Cardiovascular drug now withdrawn.
†Polypeptide disulfide-bridged toxins from molluscs of Conus genus.
‡Polypeptide toxins from spiders including Agelenopsis aperta.

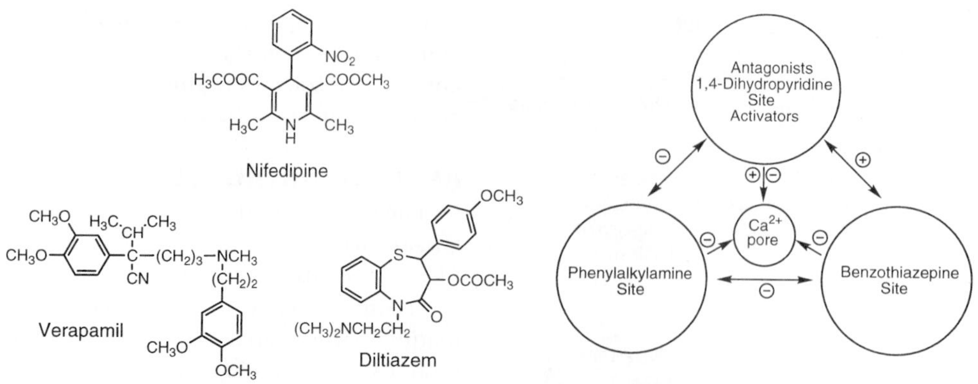

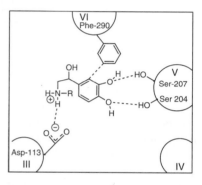

Fig. II.6. Interaction of calcium channel antagonists with the binding sites of the L-type voltage-gated calcium channel. Three distinct receptors interact with specific drug classes represented by the prototypical diltiazem, verapamil and nifedipine. The 1,4-dihydropyridine receptor is also the binding site for the 1,4-dihydropyridine activators and second-generation dihydropyridines.

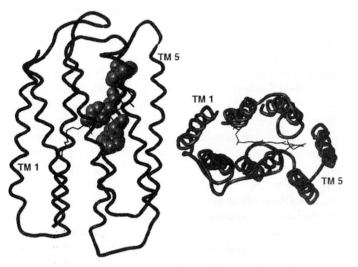

Fig. II.7. Representations of the structure of bacteriorhodospin, a template protein for G protein-coupled receptors. The left-hand representation depicts retinal covalently bound to transmembrane segment 7 [TM 7] and the right-hand representation depicts the helical arrangement of the protein. Reproduced with permission from: J.A. Bikker (6).

Fig. II.8. Representation of the binding site for catecholamines at the β-adrenergic receptor indicating the amino acid residues involved in agonist binding as determined from structure-activity and mutagenesis studies.

The basic model of the 7-TM receptor (over 700 sequences have been reported) is based on the established structures of bacteriorhodopsin and vertebrate rhodopsin. The structure of the template protein bacteriorhodopsin is shown in Figure II.7 and from this a number of models of G protein receptors have been constructed. The addition of mutagenesis studies to these model-building exercises has permitted the construction of several models of ligand interaction with their specific receptors. Such models do not permit, however, the full realization of the necessary dynamics of the receptor activation process. The availability of structures for G protein-coupled receptors will be a major advance for our understanding of receptor function.

The biogenic amine neurotransmitter receptors have been analyzed in some detail to generate models defining the critical interacting residues. Thus, for the *beta*-adrenoceptor critical interacting residues are defined as aspar-

tate-113 on helix III, serine-204 and 207 on helix V and phenylalanine-290 on helix VI (Fig. II.8). These and related studies have defined an homologous ligand "binding pocket" for cationic neurotransmitters and other small ligands which is shared by the catecholamines, histamine, serotonin, acetylcholine, as well as by other ligands. Similarly, these modeling and mutagenesis studies can produce models that accommodate the known stereoselectivity of interaction of the chiral species.

The interaction of peptides with G protein-coupled receptors presents, given the disparity in size, a scaling problem relative to the small neurotransmitter ligands. Small peptides, with as few as six residues, appear to define the minimally active fragment. The loop regions of the receptor may play a larger role in defining ligand interactions, although the binding site still shows similarity to the binding site for biogenic amines.

Nicotinic AChR (nAChR) and Ligand-gated Ion Channels

This channel was the first to have its amino acid sequence determined and it has been the subject of particularly intensive biochemical, electrophysiologic and pharmacologic analysis. Early work revealed the nicotinic

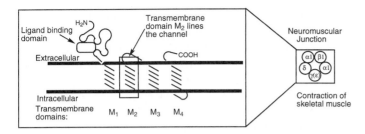

Fig. II.9. General organization of the nicotinic receptor depicting the four transmembrane domains, the M₂ domain that lines the ion channel and the extracellular ligand binding site.

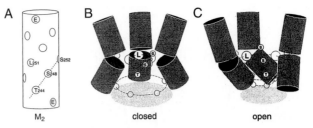

Fig. II.11. The structure of the nicotinic receptor. **A,** M₂ the pore-lining helix identifying the residues that face the pore; **B, C,** closed and open configurations of the receptor. Reproduced with permission from N. Unwin (8).

acetylcholine receptor to consist of a heteromeric association of five subunits—*alpha₂, beta, gamma* and *delta*. The *alpha* subunit bears the acetylcholine-binding site. The sequence analysis revealed the three types of subunits to be significantly homologous one to the other and to have likely originated from an ancestral subunit by gene duplication and independent mutation. Sequence analysis by consideration of the relative hydrophobic and hydrophilic balance of the residues indicates that each subunit comprises four membrane-spanning *alpha* helices (Fig. II.9). It is generally accepted that the M₂ helix of each subunit lines the channel pore and constitutes the pathway for ion translocation. A variety of biochemical studies have mapped out potential binding territories for cholinergic ligands and these are sketched in Figure II.10.

Ion channels are molecular machines and there is a great deal of interest in how they perform the conformational changes associated with opening, closing and the translocation of ions. In the case of the nAChR, high resolution electron micrographs of tubular arrays of receptors isolated from the electric organs of *Torpedo* have revealed major differences between the open and closed states (Fig. II.11). Although there is little change in the wide outer mouth of the channel there is a substantial change in the orientation of the M₂ helices that form the permeation pathway. At rest these helices are in a bent shape thus providing a narrow "stricture" in the path. In the open state the lower halves of the helices move to replace the hydrophobic leucine residues from the axis of the pore and replace them with smaller polar residues which results in an "opening" of the channel. Since there are clear homologies between the nAChR and other ligand-gated channels, including GABA, glycine and 5-HT₃, this activation mechanism may be quite general.

Bacterial K⁺ Channel and Ion Channel Permeation and Selectivity

A long series of electrophysiological studies, starting with the classic work of Hodgkin and Huxley, had established conceptually key features of ion channel function and organization. These are summarized in Figure II.12. There must be a pore through which ions permeate and this pore must have an ionic selectivity filter since channels can distinguish ions with remarkable fidelity: K⁺ channels select for K⁺ over Na⁺ by an approximately 10^3–10^4 factor. Channels open and close in response to specific signals, typically changes in membrane or chemical potential, and hence there are specific sensors that both recognize these signals and signal channel gates. Additional work has shown that these sensors may be integral to or remote from the channel structure proper and if the latter, are linked to the channel machinery by diffusible or membrane-associated signals.

The K⁺ channel from *Streptomyces lividans* is an integral membrane protein that shares sequence homology with other K⁺ channels. A solid state X-ray structure reveals an organization of four identical subunits, each with 2 trans-

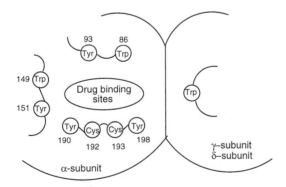

Fig. II.10. Representation of the drug binding sites of the nicotinic acetylcholine receptor. The acetylcholine binding sites are located at the interface between α- and γ- or δ- subunits. Depicted are a variety of residues that define drug binding sites as measured by covalent labeling studies (7).

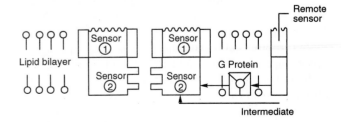

Fig. II.12. Schematic representation of an ion channel depicting the presence of gates that open and close in response to stimuli, sensors or receptors that respond to physical or chemical stimuli, and "remote" receptors linked to the channel via indirect pathways using cytosolic or membranal "second" messengers.

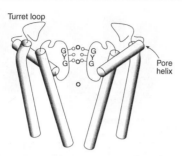

Fig. II.13. Representation of the structure of K⁺ channel. Two of the four subunits that comprise a function oligomeric assembly are shown. Each subunit contains an N-terminal *alpha*-helical region, an extracellular loop for toxin binding and a pore helix that contains the ionic selectivity filter Gly-Tyr-Gly. Reproduced with permission from D.A. Dougherty (9).

membrane units and a P or "pore region," that form an "inverted tepee" that contains within it the narrow ionic selectivity filter at the outer end (Fig. II.13). The selectivity filter is lined by polar amino acids from the so-called "signature sequence," a highly conserved set of amino acids that characterizes K⁺ channels—Thr-Xxx-Thr-Thr-Xxx-Gly-Tyr-Gly—and it is the carbonyl groups from the Gly-Tyr-Gly residues in the four subunits that bind K⁺ and are responsible for the ionic discrimination. Although this structure with two transmembrane helices represents only one class of existing K⁺ channels, it is highly probable that the conclusions drawn are applicable to other voltage gated channels.

GENOME STUDIES

Until very recently, the identification of receptors as targets for drug action, whether of physiologic or other origin, had followed the process depicted in Figure II.14 in which the initial characterization of a functional activity and identification of the responsible ligand, for example a neurotransmitter or hormone, led to the ultimate definition of the physiologic role of the receptor, its protein characterization and ultimately gene identification. This process then permits the characterized and expressed receptor to be used as a screen for the identification of novel structures. The genome project has now permitted the genomics-based process (Fig. II.14) whereby receptors can be identified and shown to have homology to existing receptors even though there may be no currently known physiological ligand with which these newly identified receptors interact. However, the cloned and expressed receptor can now be used to identify the putative physiological ligand and to identify novel structures—a process that is the reverse of that historically employed.

The G protein-coupled receptor class is of particular importance as a source of such "orphan receptors" since this class has a proven history of providing major therapeutic targets (Table II.5). At least 140 such receptors have been characterized from the human genome. Furthermore, there are an increasing number of diseases that

have been specifically associated with mutations in this class of receptors. The identification of a new human opiate receptor termed ORL1 [opiod receptor-like] which does not interact with known opiate ligands is an excellent example of this approach. This receptor has a specific endogenous agonist termed nociceptin, a 17-amino acid peptide with some similarity to the physiologic peptide dynorphin A (Fig. II.15). Nociceptin appears to have, consistent with the widespread distribution of the ORL1 receptor in the brain, corresponding widespread actions including nociception and stress reduction. Similarly, the orexins—orexin-A and orexin-B—are hypothalamic peptides that are involved in the complex process of regulation of feeding behavior and were discovered by screening brain extracts against the expressed orphan receptors, OX₁ and OX₂.

In a similar fashion, the steroid hormone receptor family has also generated a large number of orphan receptors—over 70 in all—and for the great majority of which no physiological ligand or function has yet been described. The retinoic acid receptor was first identified as an orphan species. These orphan receptors are widely expressed throughout animal species. Their widespread distribution indicates a fundamental importance to the processes of cellular activity. Thus, the RXR (Retinoid-X-Receptor) family of receptors does not bind the endogenous ligand, all-*trans*-retinoic acid, for the retinoic acid receptor (RAR), although these receptors share structural homology. Rather, the RXRs bind 9-*cis*-retinoic acid and from this discovery has come the development of new selective RXR ligands, including bexarotene.

RECEPTOR QUANTITATION

The receptor represents the locus of drug action and analysis of the kinetics of drug-receptor interaction is important from the perspective of defining the ability of a drug to interact with the receptor (affinity) and to activate the information encoded within the receptor (efficacy).

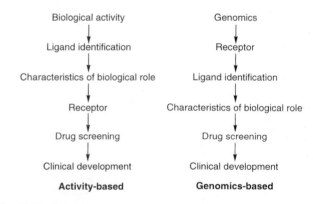

Fig. II.14. Comparison of "activity-based" and "genomics-based" drug discovery process. In "activity-based" a biologic, physiologic, pathologic activity is chosen which forms the "discovery target." "Genomics-based" discovery arises from a gene sequence discovery of a new putative receptor which is used to search for a physiological ligand from which is derived the physiologic function.

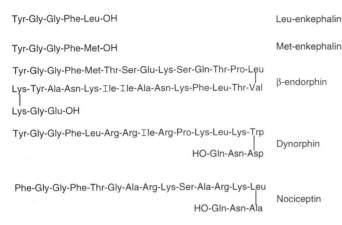

Tyr-Gly-Gly-Phe-Leu-OH   Leu-enkephalin

Tyr-Gly-Gly-Phe-Met-OH   Met-enkephalin

Tyr-Gly-Gly-Phe-Met-Thr-Ser-Glu-Lys-Ser-Gln-Thr-Pro-Leu
Lys-Tyr-Ala-Asn-Lys-Ile-Ile-Ala-Asn-Lys-Phe-Leu-Thr-Val   β-endorphin
Lys-Gly-Glu-OH

Tyr-Gly-Gly-Phe-Leu-Arg-Arg-Ile-Arg-Pro-Lys-Leu-Lys-Trp
HO-Gln-Asn-Asp   Dynorphin

Phe-Gly-Gly-Phe-Thr-Gly-Ala-Arg-Lys-Ser-Ala-Arg-Lys-Leu
HO-Gln-Asn-Ala   Nociceptin

Fig. II.15. The physiological ligands for the opiate-receptor—leu-enkephalin, met-enkephalin, β-endorphin and dynorphin. Nociceptin is the physiological agonist for the human opiod receptor termed ORL1 (opiod receptor-like-1).

The quantification of drug-receptor interaction is based upon the occupancy-response relationship which states that the more receptors occupied by a drug, the larger the drug response will be. However, the concentration of the drug at the receptor site in vivo is determined by the amount of drug administered and by the various pharmacokinetic processes, including metabolism, tissue binding and excretion as shown in Figure II.16. In this model, drugs are thought to interact with receptors via two mechanisms: drugs which stimulate the receptor and produce a biologic response (agonists); and drugs which bind to the receptor and do not produce an effect, but prevent agonists from binding (antagonists). Thus, agonists are drugs with affinity and efficacy while antagonists are drugs with affinity and zero efficacy.

A further complication exists in that some compounds behave as "partial" agonists. These are compounds which elicit a cellular response which is less than the response observed with other agonists. Partial agonists possess affinity and efficacy, but the efficacy is less than that of an agonist which produces a full response. The implications of this observation are that the total number of receptors becomes important for the overall generation of a biologic response and some drug-receptor couplings are very efficient whereby maximum response can be generated from occupancy of a small fraction of receptors. The fraction of receptors thus not occupied for response generation is termed the "receptor reserve" or "spare receptors." An agonist may, according to the density of receptors within a cell and the efficiency of receptor-effector coupling, be an agonist, partial agonist or antagonist according to the tissue and its physiologic or pathologic state.

In marked contrast the analysis of antagonists is more straightforward. Antagonists may be subdivided into competitive and non-competitive antagonists. Competitive antagonists can have their blocking effect overcome by addition of more agonist while this will not hold true for non-competitive antagonists. Almost all of the antagonists

in clinical use are competitive antagonists. Non-competitive antagonists can be further subdivided into irreversible and allosteric antagonists.

An extension of the simple division of receptor-active drugs into agonists/partial agonists and antagonists is provided by the recognition that receptors are considered as two-state devices [or more accurately as multi-state devices] that are conformationally mobile between activated and inactivated states. The function of ligands active at such receptors is then to influence the equilibrium between active and inactive receptor states. Accordingly, agonists shift the equilibrium to the activated state and antagonists do not exhibit selective affinity for either state and thus do not shift equilibria. There may thus exist a second class of antagonist species, termed "inverse agonists" whose function is to stabilize inactive conformations of receptors. In fact, the majority of competitive antagonists may actually be "inverse" agonists.

RECEPTORS AS RECOGNITION ENTITIES

The specificity of drug interaction, including stereoselectivity, at pharmacologic receptors has long been recognized as a distinguishing characteristic of both drug and receptor. The basic assumption in the analysis of structure-activity relationships is the existence of a definable mutual complementarity between the structure of a drug and its corresponding binding site. The specifics of such interactions are a central theme of the discipline of medicinal chemistry and are a major focus of this volume: structure-activity relationships are discussed individually for specific drug classes. The absence of such specificity, including stereoselectivity of recognition, is frequently employed as an argument against a biologic response being mediated through a receptor process. The definition of the action of general anesthetics has, for example, been intimately involved with questions of chemical specificity of the anesthetic interaction. Until the mid-1980s, the attempted correlation of chemical structure and biologic activity was the only available approach to the definition of receptor site structure. This has changed dramatically with the ability to determine protein sequences and the 3-dimensional structures of proteins both in the native state and liganded with substrates and antagonists.

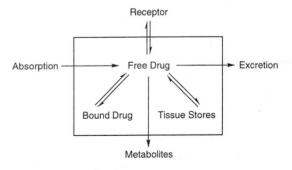

Fig. II.16. Concentration of drug at the receptor is greatly influenced by a number of pharmacokinetic processes depicted, including absorption, metabolism, distribution, storage and excretion.

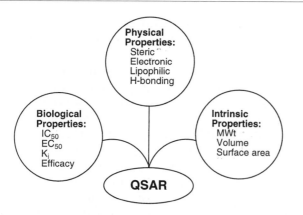

Fig. II.17. Definition of **Q**uantitative **S**tructure **A**ctivity **R**elationships—QSAR—is defined by Physical Properties, Intrinsic Properties and Biological Properties (10).

Quantitative Structure-Activity Relationships

Quantitative structure-activity relationships (QSARs) for drug-receptor interactions are a subset of structure-property correlations in which a variety of chemical and physical molecular properties is employed to define the association between structure and property. Such QSARs are widespread in medicinal chemistry since the advent of cheap and high-speed computing technologies in the past 20 years. They rely on the ability to examine multiple relationships between physical properties and biologic activities (Fig. II.17).

Classic quantitative structure-activity relationships, such as Hansch-type analyses, provide an equation defining biologic activity as a linear free energy relationship as, for example, in the description of cyclooxygenase inhibition by substituted phenylpropionic acids (Fig. II.18). A total of six variables is used to describe the biologic activity and an optimal compound occurs when R_1 = Cl, R_2 = Me and R_3 = H. This approach is clearly useful in probing, albeit indirectly, the nature of the interaction forces between drug and receptor as well as for predicting active compounds ahead of simple cumulative synthesis.

The QSAR approach can be extended with the recognition that the ligand occupies three-dimensional space. The ability to determine or predict a pharmacophore map by the use of molecular modeling techniques and the synthesis of rigid analogs then generates an hypothesis of bioactive conformation from which comparative molecular field analysis (CoMFA) can be used to calculate the intermolecular interaction fields that surround each molecule and subsequently the relationship between the biologic activity and the calculated fields is determined.

Structural Approaches

The increasing availability of protein and DNA structures determined by X-ray crystallographic and solution nmr approaches has greatly accelerated both the interpre-

tation of structure-activity relationships and structure-assisted drug design. The availability of these structures has not only permitted the analysis of key structural features that contribute to the activity of an enzyme or receptor, but has also identified binding areas for drug molecules that can be explored by *in silico* techniques to permit the more efficient synthesis of potentially active molecules. The majority of receptors are membrane proteins that have until recently been very resistant to 3-dimensional structure determination. However, this situation is rapidly changing and the recent elucidation of the structure of a potassium channel should greatly expedite our understanding of drug action at this important group of pharmacologic receptors.

Ion channels have become particularly important and exploited targets for drug action in recent years. Many agents from animal toxins, to natural and synthetic insecticides, cardiovascular drugs (Ca^{2+} channel antagonists and K^+ channel activators), anti-arrhythmic agents and local anesthetics are all active at one or more classes of ion channels. The properties of ion channels in terms of their ion selectivity, translocation properties, conductance, opening and closing kinetics and voltage-dependence of activation and inactivation have been well established from electrophysiological studies and have led to the construction of models of channel structure and function. However, as integral membrane proteins ion channels have, until recently, defied direct structural characterization. The recent elucidation of the structure of a K^+ channel has confirmed the essentials of the previous structural models and reveal this channel to have a flat outer mouth lined with negatively charged residues, a pore that progressively narrows and a "selectivity filter" consisting of a small series of five amino acids that coordinate the translocating ion through their carbonyl residues. Interestingly, the inward portion of the pore is lined by hydrophobic residues and the selectivity filter holds two K^+ ions. The selectivity filter provides the discriminating capacity of this channel for Na^+ over K^+ or Ca^{2+} and the multiple occupancy provides rapid transit, approximately diffusion-controlled, through mutual electrostatic repulsion (Fig. II.13).

Although the K^+ channel is the smallest of the cation channels, it is highly probable that the larger and more complex Na^+ and Ca^{2+} channels will mimic closely this fundamental structure. This will permit advances in structure-based drug discovery for these membrane effectors. Although the direct structures of these larger channels re-

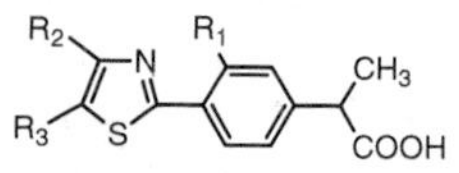

$$pIC_{50} = 1.03 \ \pi(R_1) - 4.48 \ \sigma_R(R_2) - 0.86 \ \Delta L(R_2)$$
$$+ 0.44 \ \pi(R_3) - 0.40 \ \Delta L(R_3) - 1.48 \ I_{180} + 6.11$$

Fig. II.18. QSAR for inhibition of cyclooxygenase by substituted propionic acid derivatives.

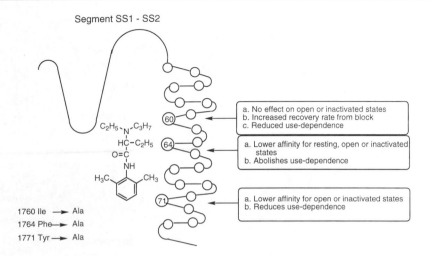

Segment SS1 - SS2

a. No effect on open or inactivated states
b. Increased recovery rate from block
c. Reduced use-dependence

a. Lower affinity for resting, open or inactivated states
b. Abolishes use-dependence

a. Lower affinity for open or inactivated states
b. Reduces use-dependence

1760 Ile → Ala
1764 Phe → Ala
1771 Tyr → Ala

Fig. II.19. Binding of a local anesthetic, etidocaine, to the voltage-gated Na^+ channel. Deduced from site-directed mutagenesis studies critical interactions of etidocaine depend upon residues 60, 64 and 71 and their replacement by alanine results in loss of specific site-dependent properties of etidocaine block. Reproduced with permission from D.S. Ragsdale (11).

main undetermined advances have been made, however, in the elucidation of the localization and function of drug binding sites. Local anesthetics serve as anti-arrhythmics by interacting in state-dependent manner with the voltage-gated Na^+ channel: the drug prefers to bind to the open or inactivated states of the ion channel. The binding site for etidocaine has been localized close to the pore-forming region and makes specific interactions with the aromatic residues phenylalanine and tyrosine (Fig. II.19). Presumably, conformational changes during channel opening (activation) position these residues such that they make tighter interactions than in the resting state.

The introduction of the "protease inhibitors" effective against HIV infection represents one of the recent triumphs of structure-based drug design. A critical component of the human immunodeficiency virus (HIV) genome codes for an aspartate protease. Inactivation of this enzyme resulted in the crippling of viral reproduction: hence, this protease was early recognized as a likely target for drug action. The structure reveals a dimer composed of two identical aspartate protease-like domains and it is thus essentially a symmetric structure (Fig. II.20).

This symmetry guided the development of the first inhibitors of the enzyme those shown in Figure II.21 and leading ultimately to the non-symmetric clinically available agents. A particularly interesting feature of the structural studies of enzyme-inhibitor complex is the presence of a water molecule that serves, through H-bonding interactions, to mediate contacts between enzyme and inhibitor. Potent protease inhibitors have been designed that include in the ligand groups that serve as a replacement for this water molecule, DMP-450 (Fig. II.21), an interesting, and possibly unique, example of structure-activity relationship around a water molecule.

Although these three-dimensional studies typically reveal that drug and receptor make intimate contact, a number of studies reveal that single residues can confer major

pharmacologic distinctions between receptor types or between species. Thus, the 5-HT$_{1B}$ receptor in rat and man shows major pharmacologic distinction that is conferred by residue 355; when the threonine of the human receptor is replaced by the asparagine of the rodent receptor the pharmacology becomes essentially indistinguishable (Table II.10). Similarly, the species specificity of the human growth hormone receptor is determined by a single arginine residue. Arg[43] in the human growth hormone receptor interacts with aspartate[171] of the hormone: in non-primates these residues are leucine and histidine respectively, and it is the non-comparability of arg[43] in the human receptor and his[171] in the non-primate hormone that determines the lack of interaction and hence the species specificity. There are important implications to these observations both for drug discovery where the use of human receptors becomes increasingly important: *"The proper study of mankind is man."* (Alexander Pope, 1688–1744), and in the determination of individual human variability to drugs where single nucleotide polymorphisms may control drug sensitivity. Thus, some 10% of the human population express an A118G nucleotide substitution at position 118 of the *mu*-opiod receptor gene and the expressed

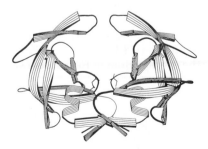

Fig. II.20. Structure of HIV protease-1 depicted as a ribbon backbone structure. The 2-fold axis of symmetry is vertical and the active site aspartate resides are depicted in the middle of the cleft. Reproduction with permission from J. Greer (12).

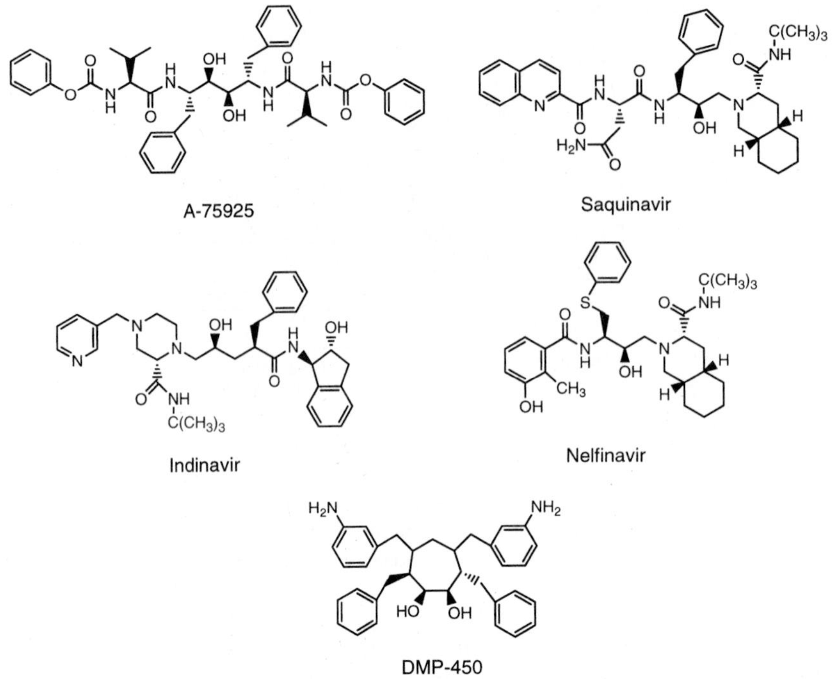

Fig. II.21. Inhibitors of HIV-1 protease. A-75925: Early symmetric inhibitor. Non-symmetric clinically available molecules: Saquinavir, Indinavir and Nelfinavir. DMP-450: Molecule that replaces bound water in protease active site.

variant receptor binds *beta*-endorphin with some three times higher affinity.

Stereochemistry of Drug-receptor Interactions

Chirality is a fundamental property of biologic systems, reflecting the fundamental asymmetry of matter. Drug-receptor interactions have long been recognized to be stereoselective: it is increasingly recognized that both pharmacokinetic and pharmacodynamic processes contribute to the clinically observed stereoselectivity. In fact, stereoselective drug-receptor interactions are so widely observed that they are frequently considered to be a defining component of the overall process of drug stereoselectivity.

In principle, stereoisomers may differ in several ways in their pharmacologic activities:

1. Both [all] enantiomers are equally active and there is no observed stereoselectivity of action. This situation is rare, but in some cases such as general anesthetics the stereoselectivity may be modest.
2. The enantiomers differ quantitatively in their pharmacologic activities: In the extreme situation one enantiomer is totally devoid of pharmacologic activity.
3. The enantiomers differ qualitatively in their pharmacologic activities and exhibit discrete activities at the same or different receptors.

In recognition of these differences drug regulatory agencies are issuing guidelines for drug evaluation and development that explicitly recognize racemic drugs as being composed of distinct chemical entities. Examples of all of these differences are known and are common (Fig. II.22). Thus, β-blockers exhibit stereoselectivity at β-adrenoceptors, whereby S-(−)-propranolol is some 40 times more potent than its R-(+)-enantiomer. However, in local anesthetic and anti-arrhythmic properties the enantiomers are essentially equipotent. The enantiomers of the Ca^{2+} channel antagonist verapamil, marketed as a racemate, exhibit stereoselectivity of interaction at its receptors in both vascular and cardiac tissue, but the stereoselectivity ratios are different in each tissue. Thus, S-verapamil has both vasodilating and cardiodepressant properties whereas R-verapamil is dominantly a vasodilating drug. The 1,4-dihydropyridine Bay K 8644 has both Ca^{2+} channel activator and antagonist properties associated with the S- and the R-isomers respectively.

Until recently, the issue of stereoselectivity of drug action was largely scientific: increasingly, it has become a regulatory issue. In particular, the use of single enantiomers may reduce undesired side effects that may be present in one enantiomer—the "inactive" enantiomer. The elimination or reduction of pharmacokinetic com-

Table II.10. Ligand Binding Properties of Human and Rodent 5-HT1B Receptors (wild-type) and the Mutant Human Receptor (13)

Ligand	Receptor K_i nM		
	Human	Rat	Mutant
5-HT	10	16	8
DHE	6	4	2
Metergoline	25	129	200
Sumatriptan	38	465	560
Methsergide	130	1,823	970
8-HO-DPAT	1,600	>10,000	25,000
RU 24 909	44	2	10

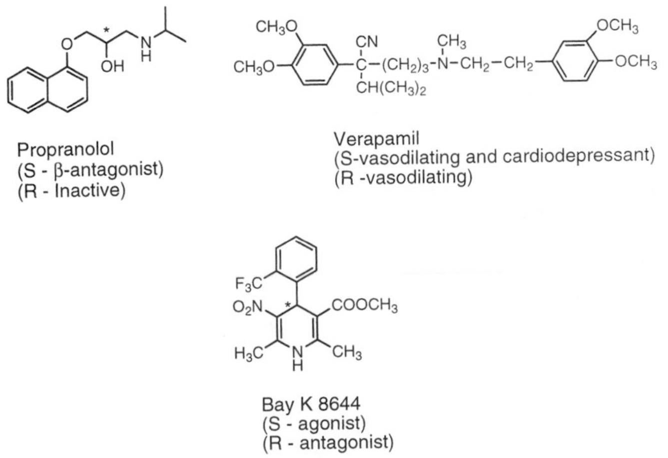

Propranolol
(S - β-antagonist)
(R - Inactive)

Verapamil
(S-vasodilating and cardiodepressant)
(R -vasodilating)

Bay K 8644
(S - agonist)
(R - antagonist)

Fig. II.22. Stereoselectivity of drug action at a variety of discrete receptor classes.

plexities that may arise from the differential metabolism, transport, protein binding, or elimination of the enantiomers may constitute a further, and significant, advantage. Furthermore, advances in synthetic chemistry, translatable to the process scale, have greatly simplified the production of enantiomerically pure chemicals. Although, and appropriately enough, there is no current regulatory prohibition on the development of racemic agents, it is increasingly likely that single enantiomer drugs will be the overwhelming future therapeutic choice.

Common Characteristics of Drug Structures

Until recently, the process of new drug discovery typically involved random screening of new compounds, synthetic or of natural origin, followed by the manual synthesis of modified structures typically "one molecule at a time" and with directed evaluation of pharmacologic activity.

There has been associated with this process a significant component of "chemical intuition," although this has been increasingly expanded with the advent of receptor structure availability and molecular modeling. With the advent of combinatorial chemistry and high throughput screening, opportunities exist for the rapid synthesis and evaluation of tens and hundreds of millions of molecules on a rapid time scale. In practice, such methodologies need to be focused to ensure that the "most profitable" chemical space is the most extensively exploited. The ability to delineate structural features that characterize "drug-like" molecules and distinguish these from "non-drug" molecules is therefore an important factor in the contemporary paradigm of drug discovery.

Several methodologies have been advanced that classify molecules in terms of sets of molecular descriptors, including molecular weight, functional groups, partition coefficients, hydrogen bonding groups, charge, atom type, etc. These methodologies have been reasonably successful in "predicting" "drug-like" molecules present in large chemical data-bases such as the Available Chemicals Directory, the World Drug Index and the Comprehensive Medicinal Chemistry Database. Prior to the development of these methodologies it had been realized that certain structures were indeed "pharmacophoric" and that when appropriately "decorated" with molecular features functioned as drugs active at a number of discrete receptors. One such early-recognized pharmacophore is the benzodiazepine nucleus active at receptors as diverse as GABA, opiate and cholecystokinin (Fig. II.23). A more recently recognized pharmacophore is the 1,4-dihydropyridine nucleus that is active also at a wide variety of receptors and ion channel types (Fig. II.24).

It is in fact likely that a number of basic "pharmacophoric structures" or "scaffolds" exist (Fig. II.25) and onto which are grafted the functional groups that define

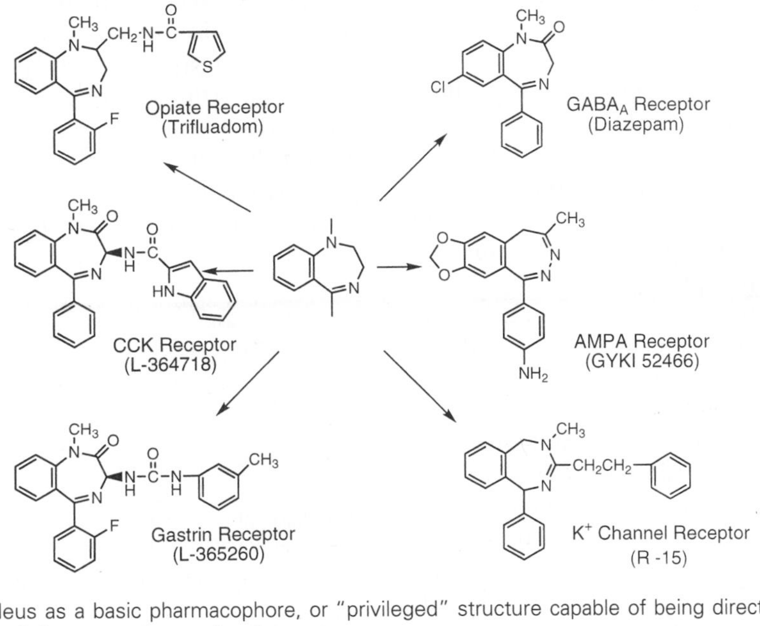

Opiate Receptor
(Trifluadom)

GABA_A Receptor
(Diazepam)

CCK Receptor
(L-364718)

AMPA Receptor
(GYKI 52466)

Gastrin Receptor
(L-365260)

K+ Channel Receptor
(R -15)

Fig. II.23. Benzodiazepine nucleus as a basic pharmacophore, or "privileged" structure capable of being directed, with appropriate molecular modification, against a number of discrete and non-related receptors.

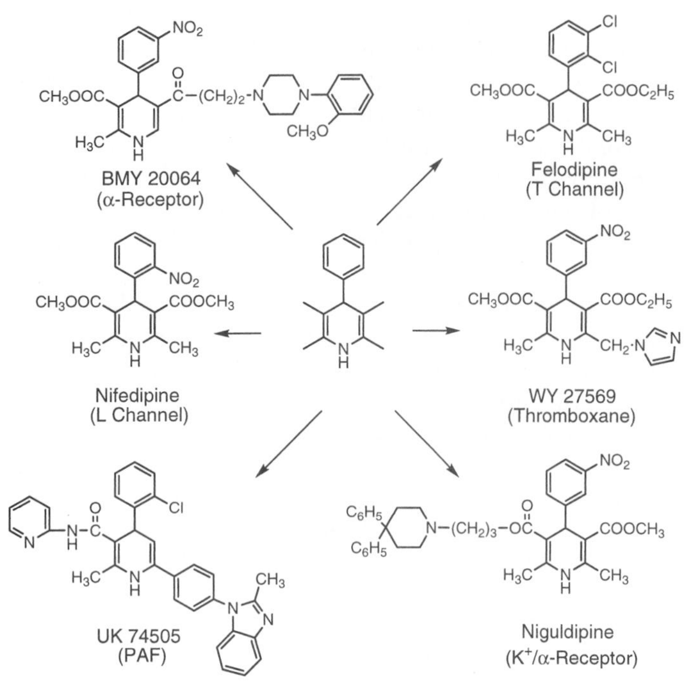

Fig. II.24. 1,4-dihydropyridine nucleus as a "privileged" structure.

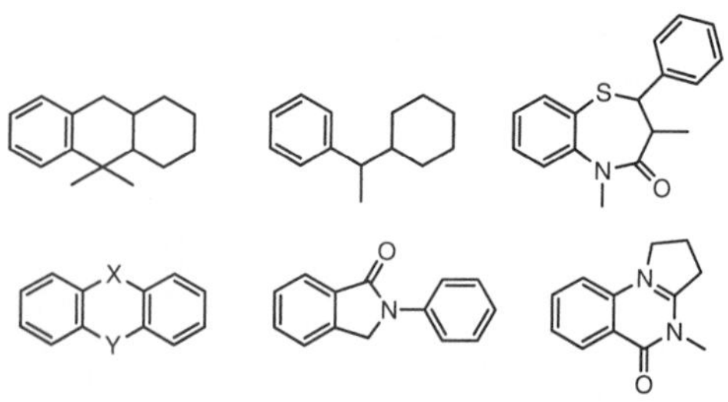

Fig. II.25. Number of basic "pharmacophoric structures" or "scaffolds" onto which may be grafted the functional groups that direct the ligand against a specific receptor type or subtype.

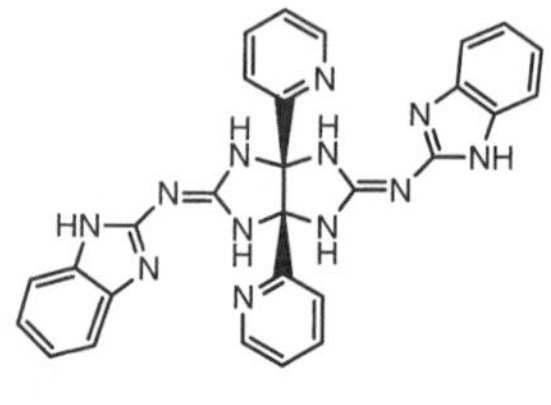

SB 247,464

specific individual drugs and drug families. It has been suggested that these scaffolds or templates are to be considered as structures that resist "hydrophobic collapse"—that is, they resist, through their conformational non-flexibility, the ability to self-associate to inactive species. This property is seen in the diphenylmethyl group, a popular molecular substructure of many active drugs of diverse classes.

From Proteins and Peptides to Small Molecule Drugs

One of the most challenging issues in drug-receptor recognition and in drug development is the translation of the receptor recognition properties of proteins and peptides to small molecules—"peptide mimetics" or "peptidomimetics"—without loss of the potency and specificity of action of the large parent molecule. Amongst the best known examples of this process is morphine and its various synthetic congeners that mimic the actions of the various opiate peptides (Fig. II.26). However, it is important to note that in this instance the small molecule mimetics were known long before the opiate peptides were discovered, and that the structural resemblance between the peptides and their non-peptide mimics is not immediately clear.

Peptide mimetics have been discovered by a variety of processes including routine screening and structure-based approaches designed to minimize the protein or polypeptide size or to reproduce in non-peptide molecules the essential conformation and functional characteristics of the binding epitopes (protein surface binding sites) of the polypeptide or protein. From the former process has been derived the benzodiazepine-based cholecystokinin (L 364,718) and gastrin (L 365,260) antagonists depicted in Figure II.23. Similarly, a small molecule mimetic agonist was discovered for the granulocyte-colony-stimulating factor receptor, SB 247464, activation of which stimulates the growth of white blood cells (14). This receptor, a member of the growth factor receptor family, is activated by oligomerization, and the symmetrical nature of this synthetic agonist suggests that it may be acting by mimicking the cross-linking capacity of the physiological ligand.

RECEPTORS AS TRANSDUCTION MACHINES

As recognized by John Newton Langley as early as 1906 a critical function of the receptor is to translate the information of the ligand-receptor interaction into a biologic response. With this translation comes very substantial amplification of the input information whereby a single ligand-receptor interaction is amplified in gain by several orders of magnitude. This is achieved by a variety of biochemical processes involving direct or indirect roles for second messengers—ions, cyclic nucleotides, lipid metabolites and the activation of protein kinases. The G protein-coupled receptors and ion chan-

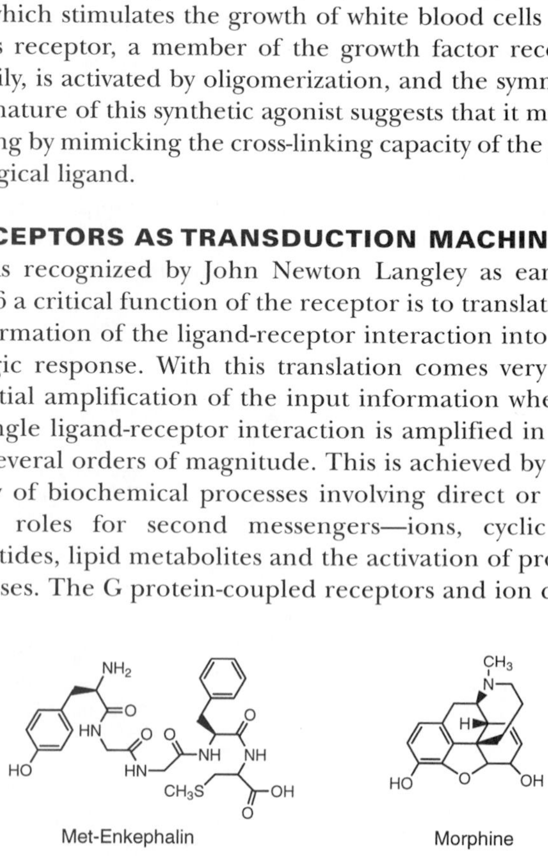

Fig. II.26. Structures of the physiologic peptide, met-enkephalin, and the non-peptide morphine, both of which are potently active at opiate receptors.

nels, representing the largest categories of membrane receptors, are increasingly well understood from a molecular standpoint and represent systems that frequently cross-communicate.

In the large family of G protein-coupled receptors heterotrimeric G proteins serve to translate the agonist-receptor interaction into a biologic response. The G proteins are a large "superfamily" of regulatory GTP hydrolase proteins and one that includes the receptor linked *alpha*-subunits, Ras and elongation factors. The interaction of an activated seven transmembrane helical receptor with the heterotrimeric G protein stimulates the G protein to release bound GDP and to associate with GTP leading to dissociation of the *beta*- and *gamma*-subunits and liberation of the activated GTP associated G protein *alpha*-subunit. This activated subunit and the dissociated *beta*- and *gamma*-subunits then interact with a number of effector systems, including adenylyl cyclase, phospholipases, phosphodiesterases and ion channels. Dissociation of the subunits from these effector systems and hydrolysis of the bound GTP by an intrinsic or extrinsic GTPase activity terminates the transduction process (Fig. II.27). This process can be further modulated by desensitization events (see following section).

RECEPTORS AS REGULATED SPECIES

Although the principal physiologic function of a receptor is to be activated by a physiological ligand to generate the corresponding biologic response, receptors are also

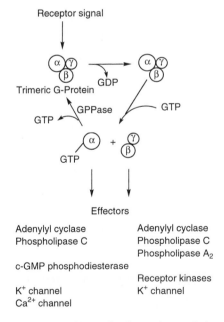

Fig. II.27. Transduction pathways for G protein-coupled receptors. The formation of the activated receptor (constitutively or through ligand interaction) interacts with the trimeric G protein in its GDP-ligated state. An exchange for GDP by GTP permits the formation of the GTP-bound α-subunit and the β, γ-subunits that are activators or inhibitors of a variety of biologic effectors. GTP hydrolysis and reassociation of the subunits terminates the process.

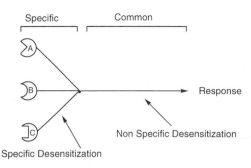

Fig. II.28. Process of specific- and non-specific desensitization. Depicted are three discrete receptors, **A**, **B** and **C**, linked to a common or shared transduction system and biologic response. The process of specific desensitization is assumed to be directed at the specific and discrete receptor components, whilst the process of non-specific desensitization is assumed to be directed through the common components of the receptor-response pathway.

controlled on a longer time frame through processes of desensitization and down-regulation. These processes may be viewed as elements of a homeostatic control system whereby the potentially deleterious effects of persistent receptor activation are reduced. In contrast, persistent occupancy of a receptor by an antagonist results in up-regulation of receptor number and function and this may also be viewed as a component of the same homeostatic control process designed to maintain balance between receptor number and receptor output or gain. Mutational defects in the structure of receptors or associated components are increasingly well characterized. These defects may cause persistent receptor activation in the absence of a ligand, "constitutively active receptors," may render the receptor unable to respond to a ligand, "constitutively silent receptors," or may simply shift the dose-response curve for the activated receptor in the directions of greater or lesser sensitivity to the ligand.

Desensitization and down-regulation appear to be common components to all receptor processes from bacterial chemotaxis, olfaction and neurotransmission to T-cell activation and may well be considered as a further characteristic property of receptors, together with specific ligand recognition and transduction mechanisms. Desensitization may be specific (homologous), or non-specific (heterologous), whereby the receptor is desensitized only to its receptor-specific ligand or to a series of unrelated ligands respectively (Fig. II.28). The processes of desensitization and down-regulation have, however, been particularly well described for G protein-coupled receptors where a series of biochemical events and cellular internalization processes operate to sequentially regulate receptor activity on the acute time scale of seconds and minutes. Longer-term control processes operate at the protein, translation and transcriptional levels to regulate the rates of degradation and synthesis of receptors.

Figure II.29 demonstrates a typical cycle of desensitization for a G protein-coupled receptor in which receptor phosphorylation mediated by a kinase activated by a second messenger product of receptor activation, c-AMP or

Ca^{2+}, renders the receptor uncoupled from the G protein. This process generates non-specific or heterologous regulation. In contrast, phosphorylation of the agonist-occupied receptor by a G protein-coupled receptor kinase (GRK_{1-6}) followed by association of the receptor with a member of the arrestin protein family yields agonist-specific or homologous desensitization. Subsequently, these receptors may be internalized and recycled to be reinserted into the plasma membrane, or they may be subject to lysosomal degradation processes. In the latter event, receptor restoration will be dependent upon *de novo* protein synthesis and export.

An increasing number of receptor diseases are known, many of which fall into the G protein receptor family. Mutations in the receptor protein or in associated signaling components may produce either loss-of-function or gain-of-function disorders. In loss-of-function mutations the receptor protein may not be delivered to the cell membrane, or may have impaired agonist binding or receptor coupling with G proteins. In contrast, gain-of-function mutations produce receptors that may be constitutively active, even in the absence of the physiological ligand. A number of these receptor diseases are listed in Table II.11. In addition, defects in the associated coupling components of these receptors may similarly alter the capacity of the receptor to achieve its signaling mission. Thus, a loss of function of the G protein $alpha_s$ subunit is associated with type 1a pseudohypoparathyroidism and a gain of function in this subunit is associated with acromegaly, hyperfunctional thyroid nodules and other disorders. Similarly, over- or under-expression of the GRKs can produce systems that show attenuated responses to agonists or that are not capable of showing homologous desensitization, respectively.

Similar diseases are now known to be associated with mutational defects in both ligand- and voltage-gated ion channels. Long QT syndrome, associated with ventricular arrhythmias and sudden death, is actually a group of dis-

Table II.11. G Protein-Coupled Receptor Diseases

Receptor	Disease	Mutation Type
Cone opsins	Color blindness	Loss
V_2 vasopressin	Nephrogenic diabetes insipidus	Loss
ACTH	Familial ACTH resistance	Loss
LH	Male precocious puberty	Gain
TSH	Pseudohermaphroditism	Loss
Ca^{2+}	Familial hypoparathyroidism	Gain
Thromboxane A_2	Congenital bleeding	Loss
Endothelin B	Hirschsprung disease	Gain

eases associated with defects in both K^+ and Na^+ channels, cystic fibrosis with defects in a chloride channel, hypokalemic periodic paralysis with defects in the L-type voltage-gated Ca^{2+} channel, and hyperinsulinemic hypoglycemia of infancy with defects in an ATP-sensitive K^+ channel. The form of long QT syndrome associated with defects in the HERG K^+ channel has assumed particular significance since this channel is blocked by a number of common drugs, including some antibiotics, antihistamines, and anti-fungal agents, that increase the chances of cardiac arrhythmias and sudden death.

REFERENCES

1. Ehrlich P. Chemotherapeutics: scientific principles, methods and results. Lancet 1913; Aug: 445–451.
2. Fischer E. Einfluss der konfiguration auf die wirkung der enzyme. Ber Dtsch Chem Ges 1894;27: 2985–2993.
3. Langley JN. On the physiology of salivary secretion. J. Physiol. 1878;1: 339–367.
4. Langley JN. Royal Society Croonian Lecture. On nerve endings and on special excitable substances in cells. Proc. Roy. Soc. London. Ser. B. 1906;78: 170–184.
5. Holladay MW, Dart MJ, Lynch JK. Neuronal nicotinic receptors as targets for drug discovery. J Med Chem 1997;40: 4169–4194.
6. Bikker JA, Trumpp-Kallmeyer S, Humblet C. G-Protein coupled receptors: models, mutagenesis and drug design. J Med Chem 1998;41: 2911–2927.
7. Galzi J.-L, Changeux J.-P. Neuronal nicotinic receptors: organization and regulation. Neuropharmacology 1995; 34: 563–572.
8. Unwin N. Acetylcholine receptor channel imaged in the open state. Nature 1995: 373: 37–43.
9. Dougherty DA, Lester HA. The crystal structure of a potassium channel-A new era in the chemistry of biological signaling. Angewandte Chemie [Inter Ed] 1998; 37: 2329–2331.
10. Van de Waterbeemd H. Quantitative approaches to structure-activity relationships, In: Wermuth CG, ed. The practice of Medicinal Chemistry. London and San Diego: Academic Press 1997; 367–389.
11. Ragsdale S, McPhee JC, Scheuer T, et al. Molecular determinants of state-dependent block of Na^+ channels by local anesthetics. Science 1994; 265: 1724–1728.
12. Greer J, Erickson JW, Baldwin JJ, et al. Application of the three-dimensional structures of protein target molecules in structure-based drug design. J Med Chem 1994; 37: 1035–1054.
13. Oksenberg D, Marrsters SA, O'Doud F, et al. A single amino-acid difference confers major pharmacologic variation between human and rodent 5-HT1$_B$ receptors. Nature 1992;360: 161–163.

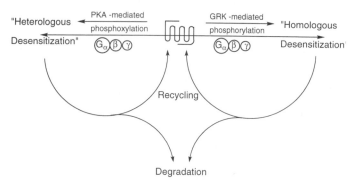

Fig. II.29. Biochemical events during desensitization and down-regulation of G protein-coupled receptors. In non-specific desensitization receptor phosphorylation uncouples the receptor from the G protein: in contrast, during specific desensitization the agonist-occupied receptor is phosphorylated by a G protein receptor kinase (GRK_{1-6}). Subsequent to phosphorylation receptors may be recycled to a patent form in the plasma membrane or may be subjected to degradation through the lysosomal machinery to generate receptor down-regulation.

14. Tian S-S, Lamb P, King AG, et al. A small nonpeptidyl mimic of granulocyte-colony-stimulating factor. Science 1998; 281: 257–259.

SUGGESTED READINGS

Ackerman MJ, Clapham, DE. Ion channels –basic science and clinical medicine. New Eng J Med 1997; 336:1575–1586.

Aidley DJ, Stanfield, PR. Ion channels: molecules in action. Cambridge: Cambridge University Press, 1996.

Banks MI, Pearce RA. Dual actions of volatile anesthetics on GABA$_A$ IPSCs. Dissociation of blocking and prolonging effects. Anesthesiology 1990; 90:120–134.

Bond C, LaForge KS, Tian M, et al. Single-nucleotide polymorphism in the human mu opiod receptor alters beta-endorphin binding and activity: possible implications for opiate addiction. Proc Nat Acad Sci 1998;95: 9608–9613.

Buscher R, Herrmann V, Insel PA. Human adrenoceptor polymorphism: evolving recognition of clinical importance. Trends Pharmacol Sci 1999;20: 94–100.

Colquhoun D. Binding, gating and efficacy: the interpretation of structure-activity relationships for agonists and the effects of mutating receptors. Brit J Pharmacol 1998; 125:924–947

Dietz III HC, Pyeritz RE. Molecular genetic approaches to the study of human cardiovascular disease. Ann Rev Physiol 1994;56: 763–796.

Doyle DA, Cabral JM, Pfuetzner RA, et al. The structure of the potassium channel: molecular basis of K$^+$ conduction and selectivity. Science 1998;280: 69–74.

Eckenhoff RG. Do specific or nonspecific interactions with proteins underlie inhalational anesthetic action? Mol Pharmacol 1998;54: 610–615.

Franks NP, Lieb WR. Molecular and cellular mechanisms of general anesthesia. Nature 1994;367: 607–614.

Greer J, Erickson JW, Baldwin JJ, et al. Application of the three-dimensional structures of protein target molecules—structure-based drug design. J Med Chem 1994;37: 1035–1054.

Guderman T, Kalkbrenner F, Shultz G. Diversity and selectivity of receptor-G-protein interaction. Ann Rev Pharmacol Toxicol 1996;36: 429–459.

Humphrey P, Spedding M, Vanhoutte P. Receptor classification and nomenclature: the revolution and the resolution. Trends Pharmacol Sci 1994;15: 203–204.

Jenkinson DH, Barnard EA, Hoyer D, et al. International Union of Pharmacology Committee on Receptor Nomenclature and Drug Classification. IX. Recommendations on terms and symbols in quantitative pharmacology. Pharmacol Revs 1995;47: 255–266.

Kenakin TP, Bond RA, Bonner TI. International Union of Pharmacology. II. Definition of pharmacological receptors. Pharmacol Revs 1992;44: 351–362.

Langley JN. On the reaction of cells and of nerve-endings to certain poisons, chiefly as regards the reaction of striated muscle to nicotine and to curari. J Physiol 1905; XXXIII: 374–413.

Laudet V. Evolution of the nuclear receptor superfamily: early diversification from an ancestral receptor. J Mol Endocrinol 1997;19: 207–226.

Meunier J.-C. Nociceptin/orphanin FQ and the opiod receptor-like ORL1 receptor. Eur J Pharmacol 1997;340: 1–15.

Meyer KH. Contributions to the theory of narcosis. Trans Farad Soc 1937;33: 1062–1068.

Oksenberg D, Marrsters SA, O'Doud F, et al. A single amino-acid difference confers major pharmacologic variation between human and rodent 5-HT1$_B$ receptors. Nature 1992;360: 161–163.

Overton E. Studien uber Die Narkose. 1907. Fischer, Jena Germany.

Pitcher JA, Freedman NJ, Lefkowitz RJ. G Protein-coupled receptor kinases. Ann Rev Biochem 1998;67: 633–692.

Souza SC, Frick GP, Wang X, et al. A single arginine residue determines species specificity of the human growth hormone receptor. Proc Nat Acad Sci USA 1995;92: 959–963.

Speigel AM. Defects in G protein-coupled signal transduction in human disease. Ann Rev Physiol 1995;58: 143–170.

Stadel JM, Wilson S, Bergsma DJ. Orphan G protein-coupled receptors: a neglected opportunity for pioneer drug discovery. Trends Pharmacol Sci. 1997;18: 430–437.

Trist DG, Humphrey PPA, Leff P, et al, eds. Receptor classification. The integration of operational, structural, and transductional information. Ann New York Acad Sci Vol 812, 1997.

Wiley RA, Rich DH. Peptidomimetics derived from natural products. Med Res Revs 1993;13: 327–384.

Wilson S, Bergsma DJ, Chambers JK, et al. Orphan G protein-coupled receptors: the next generation of drug targets. Brit J Pharmacol. 1998; 125: 1387–1392.

10. Drugs Affecting Cholinergic Neurotransmission

DANNY L. LATTIN AND E. KIM FIFER

INTRODUCTION AND HISTORY

The autonomic nervous system is divided into the parasympathetic and sympathetic divisions, which may be referred to by their anatomic origin of outflow as thoracolumbar and craniosacral, respectively. Neurons in these systems are classified according to the chemical neurotransmitters that they release to mediate a nerve impulse. Norepinephrine (noradrenaline) is the principle neurotransmitter of postganglionic neurons in the sympathetic nervous system. Hence, these neurons are sometimes classified as adrenergic. Acetylcholine is the neurotransmitter of all preganglionic fibers of the autonomic nervous system (both parasympathetic and sympathetic), postganglionic fibers of the parasympathetic division, and a few postganglionic fibers of the sympathetic division (e.g., sweat and salivary glands). It is also released by some neurons in the central nervous system as well as at the neuroeffector junction by neurons of the somatic nervous system. Neurons that release acetylcholine are collectively referred to as cholinergic. Figure 10.1 illustrates the sites of action of these neurotransmitters (1). As will be described later, receptors upon which cholinergic neurons synapse are referred to as cholinergic receptors and may be classified as either muscarinic or nicotinic.

Acetylcholine chloride

R(−) - Norepinephrine

Functioning as a chemical neurotransmitter, acetylcholine is released from the presynaptic nerve ending into the synapse. It traverses the synaptic space and interacts with a specific receptor at a postsynaptic site. This interaction leads to a receptor-mediated response. Synaptic acetylcholinesterase catalyzes the rapid hydrolysis of acetylcholine to afford acetate and choline. This hydrolytic inactivation of acetylcholine serves as the physiologic mechanism for terminating its effects.

The parasympathetic nervous system innervates both smooth and cardiac muscle as well as certain exocrine glands (e.g., salivary and sweat glands). Parasympathetic nerve impulses are responsible for stimulating contractions of smooth muscle in the gastrointestinal tract, urinary tract, and eye, as well as decreasing the heart rate and

relaxing smooth muscle of blood vessels. The parasympathetic nervous system causes relaxation of smooth muscle in the vasculature producing vasodilation.

Chemical compounds that stimulate the parasympathetic nervous system are called cholinomimetic or parasympathomimetic agents. Cholinergic agonists are cholinomimetic agents that act directly at receptors for acetylcholine. Compounds inhibiting acetylcholinesterase, the enzyme responsible for the hydrolysis of acetylcholine, are also cholinomimetic but are not receptor agonists. Those compounds that possess affinity for cholinergic receptors, but exhibit no intrinsic activity are termed cholinergic antagonists or parasympatholytic agents. This chapter is devoted to the discussion of both types of compounds as well as to the biochemistry of cholinergic neurotransmission.

Perhaps no other mammalian system or chemical neurotransmitter has been studied as exhaustively as the parasympathetic nervous system and acetylcholine. Scientists of all disciplines have been involved in this research, and their discoveries have found application to studies of all other systems in the human body. Studies of the parasympathetic nervous system and cholinergic agents led to the concept of neurochemical transmission, were instrumental in describing stereochemical influences on drug action, and pioneered the development of early drug receptor hypotheses and models. The history of research developments from the latter part of the 19th century to about 1940 makes interesting reading. An excellent summary of this history is presented in the first chapter of Waser (2).

In 1914, Dale defined the two fundamental subdivisions of the parasympathetic nervous system when he observed that ethers and esters (including acetylcholine) of choline produced effects similar to either muscarine (muscarinic effects) or nicotine (nicotinic effects) in different pharmacologic preparations (2). The initial experiments were performed using an ergot extract contaminated with acetylcholine, although Dale was unaware of this contamination. Ewins, a chemist who collaborated with Dale, isolated acetylcholine from the ergot extract and subsequently synthesized acetylcholine. This permitted Dale to prove that the unexpected muscarine-like effects he observed with the ergot preparation were due to acetylcholine. He proposed the term parasympathomimetic to describe the ability of acetylcholine to produce the same effects as electrical stimulation of parasympathetic nerves and suggested that acetylcholine was a chemical neurotransmitter in the parasympathetic nervous system. Dale also observed that the action of acetylcholine in his prepa-

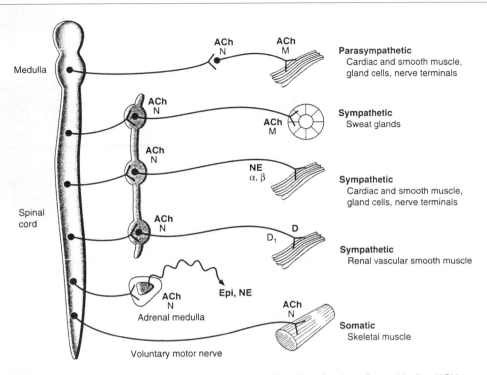

Fig. 10.1. Schematic representation of autonomic and somatic motor nerves. The sites of action of acetylcholine (ACh), norepinephrine (NE), epinephrine (Epi), and dopamine (D) are indicated. Cholinergic receptors are designated as nicotinic (N) or muscarinic (M). (Adapted from reference 1.)

rations was short-lived and proposed that the tissues contained an esterase that hydrolyzed acetylcholine to inactive products. Loewi's elegant experiments in 1921 were the first unequivocal demonstration that a chemical compound mediated impulses between nerves; he referred to the chemical substance in his preparation as *vagusstoff* (3). In 1926, Loewi and Navratil provided experimental evidence suggesting that vagusstoff was acetylcholine (4).

(+) Muscarine chloride

S(+) - Nicotine

These classic studies are the foundation for our current understanding of the role of acetylcholine in cholinergic nerve transmission and the recognition of muscarinic and nicotinic cholinergic receptors. These discoveries provided the stimulus for the subsequent studies of acetylcholine biochemistry, the synthesis of new organic compounds such as cholinergic and anticholinergic drugs, and the purification of cholinergic receptors.

The concept of muscarinic and nicotinic receptors to explain the different physiologic responses produced by acetylcholine was derived from the early research of Dale and Loewi. It is currently recognized that there may be many classes of muscarinic receptors, and perhaps of nico-

tinic receptors, but the general classification of two types of cholinergic receptors, muscarinic and nicotinic, continues to explain effectively the different physiologic responses produced by acetylcholine. Muscarinic receptors are those at which muscarine is the classic cholinergic agonist; nicotine is the classic cholinergic agonist at nicotinic receptors. Muscarinic receptors mediate cholinergic responses at all postganglionic parasympathetic nerve terminals and on autonomic presynaptic membranes. On the other hand, nicotinic receptors mediate responses on autonomic presynaptic nerve membranes, on autonomic ganglia, and at somatic neuromuscular junctions.

Because of the important role of acetylcholine as a chemical neurotransmitter in the autonomic nervous system, an imbalance in parasympathetic tone can lead to serious consequences and physiologic difficulties. Deficiencies of acetylcholine could conceptually be treated by administering the neurotransmitter itself, but acetylcholine is a poor therapeutic agent. It is nonselective in its actions, producing effects at all cholinergic receptor sites and leading to undesirable side effects, which could result in serious consequences for the patient. Acetylcholine is poorly absorbed across biologic membranes because it is a quaternary ammonium salt; this provides for poor bioavailability regardless of the route of administration. Furthermore, it is chemically labile owing to rapid hydrolysis of its ester functional group in aqueous solutions, in the gastrointestinal tract, and in blood, where hydrolysis is catalyzed by esterases. For these reasons, medicinal chemists have vigorously sought alternatives to acetylcholine as therapeutic agents from the time it was demonstrated to be a chemical neurotransmitter in the autonomic nervous system.

Most therapeutic cholinomimetic agents possess muscarinic effects. Muscarinic cholinergic agents are used postsurgically to reestablish smooth muscle tone of the gastrointestinal tract and the urinary tract in order to relieve abdominal distention and urinary retention. They are also used to treat some forms of glaucoma by enhancing the outflow of aqueous humor thereby reducing intraocular pressure. Cholinomimetic compounds possessing activity in the central nervous system are being evaluated for the treatment of cognitive disorders such as Alzheimer's disease. Cholinomimetic drugs having nicotinic effects are commonly used to treat myasthenia gravis.

The largest number of medicinal agents used to modify the effects of acetylcholine is the cholinergic antagonists or anticholinergic drugs. Cholinergic muscarinic antagonists

are sometimes referred to as antispasmodics because of their ability to reduce smooth muscle spasms resulting from over stimulation of the gastrointestinal smooth muscles.

One of the goals of medicinal chemistry research and drug discovery is to provide a rational basis for the design of new medicinal agents. As a result, many synthetic cholinergic agonists were designed using structure-activity relationships (SAR) based on the structure of acetylcholine. To design cholinergic agents selective for specific cholinergic receptors, it is necessary to have a more complete understanding of acetylcholine neurochemistry as well as of the chemical nature and role of cholinergic receptors.

ACETYLCHOLINE NEUROCHEMISTRY

The neurochemistry of acetylcholine includes its biosynthesis, storage, release, and metabolism, which are summarized in Figure 10.2.

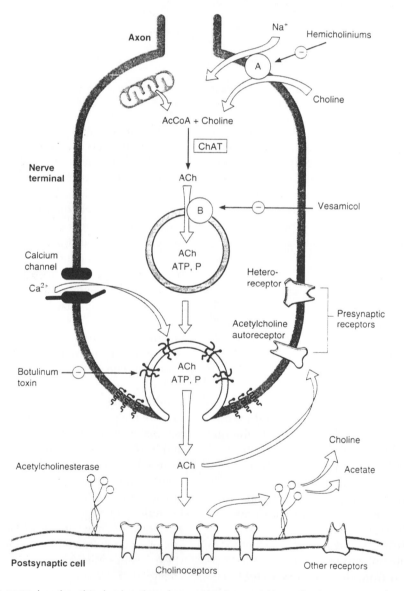

Fig. 10.2. General cholinergic nerve junction showing location of receptor sites and biosynthesis, storage, release, and hydrolysis of acetylcholine. (Adapted from reference 1.)

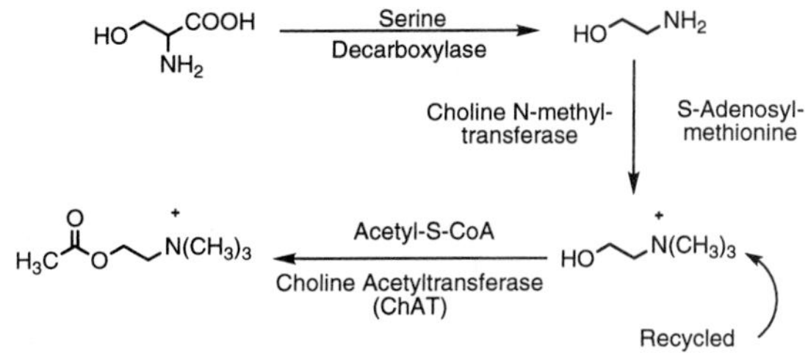

Fig. 10.3. Biosynthesis of acetylcholine.

Biosynthesis

Acetylcholine is biosynthesized in cholinergic neurons by the enzyme-catalyzed transfer of the acetyl group from acetyl coenzyme A (acetylCoA) to choline, a quaternary ammonium alcohol (5). The enzyme catalyzing this reaction, choline acetyltransferase (ChAT), is also biosynthesized in the cholinergic neuron. Some choline is biosynthesized from the amino acid serine (Fig. 10.3), but most of the choline used to form acetylcholine is recycled following the enzymatic hydrolysis of acetylcholine in the synaptic space. Extracellular choline is actively transported into the presynaptic nerve terminal by both high-affinity and low-affinity uptake sites. The high-affinity site, inhibited by hemicholinium, is probably responsible for most of the choline recycled from the synapse and used to biosynthesize acetylcholine. The active uptake of choline is considered to be the rate-determining step in the biosynthesis of acetylcholine.

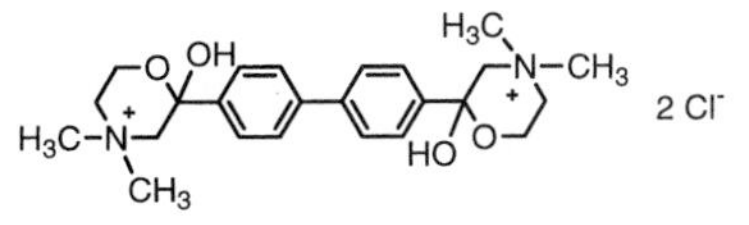

Hemicholinium chloride

Storage

Most newly biosynthesized acetylcholine is actively transported into cytosolic storage vesicles located in the presynaptic nerve endings, where it is maintained until it is released (6). Some acetylcholine remains in the cytosol and is eventually hydrolyzed to acetate and choline. Only the stored form of acetylcholine serves as the functional neurotransmitter.

Release

Acetylcholine release from the storage vesicles is initiated by an action potential that has been carried down the axon to the presynaptic nerve membrane. This action potential leads to the opening of voltage-dependent calcium channels affording an influx of Ca^{2+} and an exocytotic release of acetylcholine into the synapse. The increase in intracellular Ca^{2+} may induce fusion of the acetylcholine storage vesicles with the presynaptic membrane before release of the neurotransmitter. Each synaptic vesicle contains a quantum of acetylcholine; one quantum represents between 12,000 and 60,000 molecules of acetylcholine. A

Efforts to Modulate Acetycholine Biosynthesis

Efforts to develop therapeutic agents based on regulation of acetylcholine biosynthesis have not been successful. Dexpanthenol, the dextrorotatory enantiomer of the alcohol derived from pantothenic acid (a vitamin), was once used as a cholinomimetic agent to help reestablish normal smooth muscle tone in the gastrointestinal tract following surgery. Pantothenic acid is essential for the biosynthesis of coenzyme A. The apparent rationale for

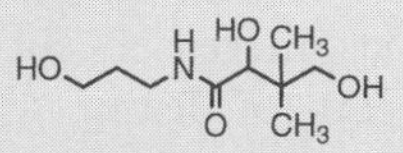

Dexpanthenol

the therapeutic use of dexpanthenol was that it would be biotransformed to pantothenic acid, which would be incorporated into coenzyme A. This would lead to increased intracellular levels of acetyl CoA, which would facilitate increased biosynthesis of acetylcholine. Limited therapeutic success of dexpanthenol, difficulty with administration, and the effectiveness of synthetic cholinergic agonists led to its discontinuation. The quaternary pyridinium salt, trans-N-methyl-4-(1-naphthylvinyl)pyridinium (MNPV) iodide, is an effective inhibitor of choline acetyltransferase in vitro, but it has proven to be a poor inhibitor in whole animal experiments.

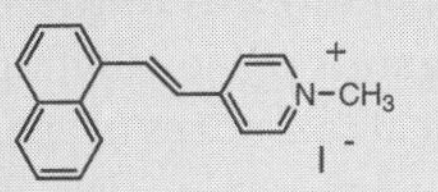

trans-N-Methyl-4-(1-naphthylvinyl)pyridinium iodide
(MNPV)

Although efforts have been made to design cholinergic agents based on the mechanism of biosynthesis of acetylcholine, such agents would be expected to have nonselective effects because it is currently thought that acetylcholine is biosynthesized by the same mechanism in all cholinergic neurons.

single action potential causes the release of several hundred quanta of acetylcholine into the synapse.

Metabolism

Acetylcholine in the synapse can bind with receptors on the postsynaptic or presynaptic membranes to produce a response. Free acetylcholine, that which is not bound to a receptor, is hydrolyzed by acetylcholinesterase. This hydrolysis is the physiologic mechanism for terminating the action of acetylcholine. There is enough acetylcholinesterase present in the synapse to hydrolyze approximately 3×10^8 molecules of acetylcholine in 1 msec; thus, there is adequate enzyme activity to hydrolyze all of the acetylcholine (approximately 3×10^6 molecules) released by one action potential. A number of useful therapeutic cholinomimetic agents have been developed based on the ability of the compounds to inhibit acetylcholinesterase. These agents are addressed later in this chapter.

ACETYLCHOLINE RECEPTORS
History

Medicinal chemists and other scientists have devoted a great deal of effort to understanding how cholinergic receptors carry out the two primary functions of all receptors—molecular recognition and signal transduction. A complete understanding of these phenomena is essential to achieve the desired goals of rational, efficient, and selective drug therapy.

Knowledge of the structure and function of acetylcholine receptors has increased substantially in the 80 years since the concept of distinct muscarinic and nicotinic receptors was first postulated. The earliest efforts to describe these receptors were hindered by the fact that receptors were only a concept. The location and fundamental chemical nature of the receptor was unknown because no one had isolated a receptor. Indeed, the existence of receptors was not established until 1973, when Snyder and Pert (7) provided demonstrable evidence for the existence of opiate receptors.

Early attempts by medicinal chemists to characterize cholinergic receptors were based on SAR and stereochemical studies of cholinergic agonists and antagonists. This research led to the synthesis of agonists and antagonists with exceptionally high affinity and selectivity for cholinergic receptors as well as to the synthesis of radiolabeled cholinergic ligands possessing high specific radioactivity. These chemical advances were paralleled by advances in biochemistry, molecular pharmacology, and molecular biology making possible the purification and sequencing of small quantities of protein, measurement of ligand binding to cell membranes and subcellular components of cells, and cloning and base sequencing of genes. These scientific and technologic advances culminated in the isolation, purification, and deduced amino acid sequencing of one of the nicotinic acetylcholine receptors—the first acetylcholine receptor, and the first neurotransmitter receptor, to be this completely characterized (8,9). Subsequently, muscarinic receptors have been isolated and purified, as well as sequenced, using these techniques.

Current evidence from pharmacologic and molecular biology research indicates that there are multiple muscarinic and nicotinic acetylcholine receptor subtypes (10,11). The traditional classification of muscarinic receptors and nicotinic receptors, however, is adequate to describe the actions of most cholinergic medicinal agents and is used throughout this chapter. Furthermore, most of the current therapeutic agents acting at muscarinic receptors exhibit little selectivity for the receptor subtypes.

Muscarinic Receptors

SAR were the basis for early models of the receptor structure that would account for the affinity and efficacy of cholinergic agonists. An early model of the muscarinic receptor, depicted in Figure 10.4, accounts for the importance of muscarinic agonists having an ester functional

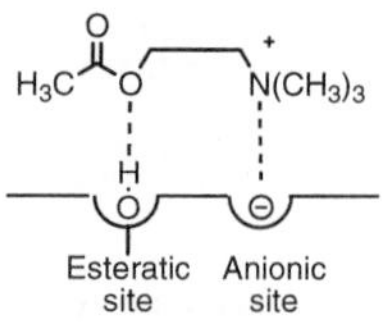

Fig. 10.4. Original representation of the muscarinic receptor.

group and a quaternary ammonium group separated by two carbons.

This model depicts ionic bonding of acetylcholine to the receptor by an electrostatic interaction between the positive charge of the quaternary nitrogen and a negative charge at the anionic site of the receptor. The negative charge was suggested to be due to a carboxylate ion from the free carboxyl group of a dicarboxylic amino acid (e.g., aspartate or glutamate) located at the binding site of the receptor protein. This model also involves a hydrogen bond between the ester oxygen of acetylcholine and a hydroxyl group contributed by the esteratic site of the receptor.

Although this early muscarinic receptor model accounted for two important SAR requirements for muscarinic agonists, it failed to explain the following: (1) at least two of the alkyl groups bonded to the quaternary nitrogen must be methyl groups; (2) the known stereochemical requirements for agonist binding to the receptor; and (3) the fact that all potent cholinergic agonists have only five atoms between the quaternary nitrogen and the terminal hydrogen atom. This latter point is known as Ing's rule of five (12).

Subsequent models of the cholinergic muscarinic receptor depicted the receptor as a binding site on a protein molecule and explained more completely the structural and stereochemical requirements for cholinergic agonist activity. Some scientists proposed that the muscarinic receptor and acetylcholinesterase were the same entity. This proposal was dispelled by experiments that demonstrated that interaction of cholinergic ligands with the muscarinic receptor did not lead to a chemical change (hydrolysis) of the ligand. None of these models, however, could explain completely the diverse pharmacologic effects produced by all the muscarinic agonists and antagonists.

Subsequent developments suggest that muscarinic receptor effects, like those of adrenergic receptors, are mediated by second messengers. Muscarinic receptors mediate at least two important biochemical events leading to second messengers: (1) inhibition of adenylyl cyclase and (2) activation of phospholipase C. Both of these biochemical events involve a guanosine triphosphate (GTP)-dependent mechanism. Two other important developments were the synthesis of radiolabeled muscarinic ligands and utilization of molecular biology techniques in the study of muscarinic receptors.

Heterogeneity in the muscarinic receptor population began to be realized in the late 1970s with studies of the pharmacology of the muscarinic antagonist pirenzepine.

At the time, pirenzepine was the only muscarinic antagonist to block gastric acid secretion at concentrations that did not block the effects of muscarinic agonists. This ob-

Pirenzepine

servation initiated research that ultimately led to discovery of five muscarinic receptor subtypes designated M_1, M_2, M_3, M_4, and M_5 based on their pharmacologic responses to various ligands. Rapid advances in molecular biology led to the cloning of cDNAs that encode for five muscarinic receptors. These, designated as m_1–m_5, corresponded to the respective M_1–M_5 receptors identified by their pharmacologic specificity. The International Union of Pharmacology Committee on Receptor Nomenclature and Drug Classification recently recommended that the upper case M_1–M_5 be used to designate both pharmacologic subtypes as well as the molecular subtypes (10).

All of the muscarinic receptor subtypes (M_1–M_5) are found in the CNS, and different tissues may contain more than one subtype. As the number of muscarinic receptor subtypes has increased it has become apparent that there is a lack of known antagonists exhibiting "very high subtype selectivity," and there "are no muscarinic agonists with high selectivity" (10). Thus, proof for involvement of any one receptor subtype in a given system requires the use of more than one antagonist. Additionally, if the selectivity of a novel muscarinic antagonist or putative agonist is to be assessed, it should be through use of recombinant muscarinic receptors expressed in cell lines rather than with native receptors.

Muscarinic M_1 receptors are located in neuronal tissue (the brain and presynaptic tissue of autonomic ganglia) and in various exocrine glands. They have been implicated in Alzheimer's disease and are thought to be involved with such functions as memory and learning. Early studies suggested that the agonist McN-A-343 was selective for the M_1 receptor, but more recent evidence indicates

McN-A-343

that is not the case; it may show moderate selectivity for M_4 receptors. M_2 receptors, located primarily on postganglionic membranes in the autonomic nervous system (smooth muscle, heart, and exocrine glands), decrease both the rate and force of contraction of the heart. Muscarinic M_3 receptors are found in brain, where they decrease neurotransmitter release. They are also found in

smooth muscle and secretory glands where stimulation leads to contraction and secretion, respectively. Stimulation of muscarinic M_4 receptors in smooth muscle and secretory glands leads to inhibition of calcium channels. Although there is evidence for the existence of the M_5 receptor in brain and peripheral tissue, a whole-tissue response at a location that matches that of the expressed gene product has not been observed (10).

Cloning and base sequencing of the genes encoding for muscarinic receptors have been major advances in the understanding of their chemical nature and function (10,13–15). These experiments demonstrated that muscarinic receptors belong to a group of receptors that are coupled to guanine nucleotide binding proteins and are referred to as G protein-coupled receptors (GPCR) (10,16,17). The β-adrenergic receptors are also members of the GPCR family. The guanine nucleotide regulatory protein to which these receptors are coupled is composed of three subunits (α, β, and γ) which link the receptor to effectors which produce second messenger molecules within the cell. Binding of muscarinic agonists to the GPCRs leads to a variety of effector responses, which include inhibition of adenylyl cyclase, stimulation of guanylyl cyclase, activation of phospholipase C, and regulation of potassium and calcium ion channel activity. The ultimate observable response is a function of the tissue where the receptor is located.

The amino acid sequences (primary structures) of the muscarinic receptor proteins expressed by the cloned genes for the GPCRs have been deduced from the base sequence of the respective genes. Application of molecular modeling programs to the deduced structures of the muscarinic GPCR suggests that they are components of the cell membrane and consist of seven transmembrane helical domains that are hydrophobic as well as four extracellular and four intracellular domains that are hydrophilic (18). The N-terminus of the GPCR protein is extracellular, and the C-terminus is intracellular. This proposed arrangement for the human type-1 muscarinic receptor, including its deduced amino acid sequence, is illustrated in Figure 10.5 (13). Computer-assisted molecular modeling has also made it possible to obtain three-dimensional models of the muscarinic receptor (18); a proposed top-view model of the M_1 muscarinic receptor is shown in Figure 10.6 (19). It is interesting to observe that this model suggests that the quaternary nitrogen of acetylcholine participates in an ionic bond with the free carboxylate group of an aspartate residue (D105)—one of the receptor functional groups that was hypothesized to be involved in receptor binding of acetylcholine almost 50 years ago using only SAR data and the powers of deduction.

The current model for muscarinic receptors is much more descriptive than earlier models of the relationship between ligand binding to the receptor molecule (molecular recognition) and the resulting effect (signal transduction). Figure 10.7 illustrates this relationship (15). In

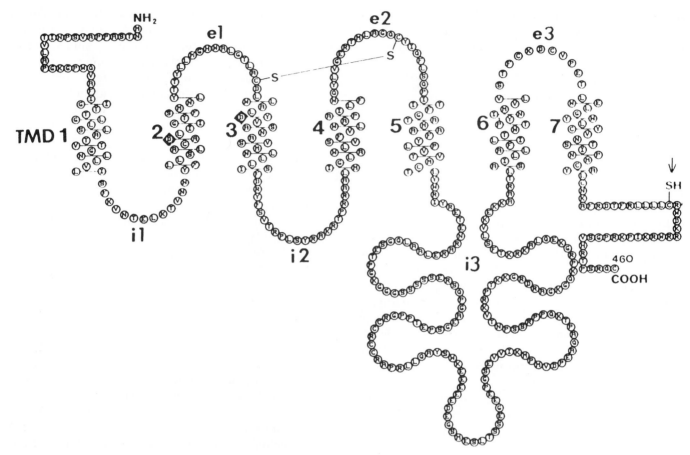

Fig. 10.5. Deduced amino acid sequence of human muscarininc acetylcholine receptor M_1 and putative arrangement of the seven transmembrane domains, three intracellular domains (i1–i3), three extracellular domains (e1–e3). (Adapted from reference 13.)

this model, acetylcholine (H) binds to the muscarinic receptor located in the cell membrane, and this ligand-receptor interaction is translated, presumably by a conformational perturbation, through the receptor protein to the receptor-coupled guanine nucleotide regulatory protein (G protein). A proposal for the relationship between the guanine nucleotide regulatory protein and the effector is shown in Figure 10.8 (20). In this proposal, the G protein is in the inactive state with GDP bound to its α subunit. Upon interaction of an agonist with the muscarinic receptor, the α subunit releases the GDP and binds to GTP. The α subunit-GTP complex then dissociates from the βγ subunits. Both the α subunit-GTP complex and the βγ subunits interact with membrane-bound effectors (phospholipase C and adenylate cyclase) or ion channels (K^+ and Ca^{2+}) either independently or in a parallel manner. The α subunit possesses GTPase activity, and quickly hydrolyzes the GTP to GDP to terminate signal transmission at which time the α, β, and γ subunits reassociate and migrate back to the receptor protein. Characteristics of the α subunit determine the classification of the particular G protein:

G_s increases adenylyl cyclase activity and increases Ca^{2+} currents

G_i decreases adenylyl cyclase activity and increases K^+ currents

G_o decreases Ca^{2+} currents

G_q increases phospholipase C activity

The βγ subunits are involved with receptor-operated K^+ currents with activity of adenylyl cyclase and phospholipase C.

Muscarinic agonist binding to "odd numbered" muscarinic receptor subtypes (M_1, M_3, and M_5) activates a G protein ($G_{q/11}$) whose α subunit is responsible for stimulation of phospholipase C. The "even numbered" subtypes

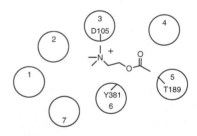

Fig. 10.6. Model of acetylcholine interaction with muscarinic M_1 receptor. Circles represent seven transmembrane domains; D105, T189, and Y381 are aspartate, threonine, and tyrosine residues. (Adapted from reference 19.)

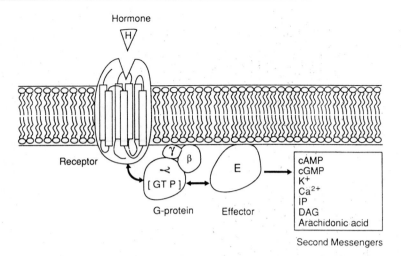

Fig. 10.7. Model of signal transduction by a G protein-coupled receptor. This illustrates a proposed relationship between receptor, G protein, the effector, and various second messengers. (Adapted from reference 15.)

(M_2 and M_4) are coupled to G proteins whose activation leads to inhibition of adenylyl cyclase (10).

Nicotinic Receptors

Nicotinic receptors have been the focus of intensive research interest even though the majority of clinically effective cholinergic medicinal agents have been designed as either agonist or antagonist ligands for muscarinic receptors (21). This interest is due both to the ready availability of nicotinic receptor protein from the electric organs of the electric eel *(Electrophorus electricus)* and the marine ray *(Torpedo californica)* and to the important role that nicotinic receptors play in myasthenia gravis, an autoimmune disease.

Pharmacologic and medicinal chemical evidence has long supported the concept of multiple nicotinic receptors based on the different anatomic sites (autonomic ganglia and skeletal neuromuscular junction) of these receptors and on the different structural requirements for nicotinic agonists and antagonists acting at these two receptor populations. Multiplicity of nicotinic receptors is also supported by more recent molecular biology research (21).

Acetylcholine nicotinic receptors belong to a group of receptors classified as ligand-gated ion channel receptors. The receptor creates a transmembrane ion channel (the gate), and acetylcholine (the ligand) serves as a gatekeeper by interacting with the receptor to modulate passage of ions, principally K^+ and Na^+, through the channel.

A nicotinic receptor was the first neurotransmitter receptor to be isolated and purified in an active form using the same molecular biologic techniques described for the isolation and characterization of the muscarinic receptors. The primary sequence of nicotinic receptors has been deduced from the cloning and sequencing of the genes that encode the nicotinic receptor proteins (22,23).

The nicotinic receptor of muscle tissue is a glycoprotein consisting of four distinct subunits—the α, β, γ, and δ. The

γ-subunit in mature muscle endplate may be replaced by an ϵ-subunit. In a single receptor molecule, there is a pentameric arrangement of two α-subunits in combination with one each of the β, γ (or ϵ), and δ-subunits, abbreviated $\alpha_2\beta\gamma\delta$ or $\alpha_2\beta\gamma\epsilon$, respectively. Neuronal nicotinic receptors in the CNS also exist as pentamers, but are composed of only heterogenic α- and β-subunits (24,25).

The five subunits of each receptor protein in muscle tissue are arranged around a central pore that serves as the ion channel. Based on molecular modeling of the deduced primary structure of the individual subunits, it is proposed that each subunit (α, β, γ, δ or ϵ) possesses a hydrophilic extracellular N-terminus, a hydrophilic intracellular C-terminus, and four alpha helical hydrophobic domains (M_1, M_2, M_3, M_4) that are in the cell membrane (Fig. 10.9) (24,26). It has been suggested that these five amphipathic domains make up the walls of the ion channel in the pentameric arrangement of the receptor subunits.

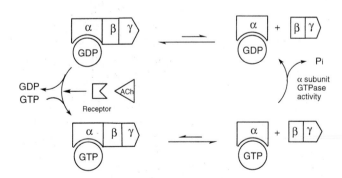

Fig. 10.8. Diagram of a GTPase cycle and subunit association/dissociation proposed to control signal transduction between muscarinic G protein-coupled receptors and the effector. ACh/receptor interaction facilitates GTP binding and activates the α-subunit. The α-subunit-GTP complex then dissociates from the $\beta\gamma$-subunit, and each is free to activate effector proteins. The duration of separation is determined by the rate of α subunit mediated GTP hydrolysis. (Adapted from reference 20.)

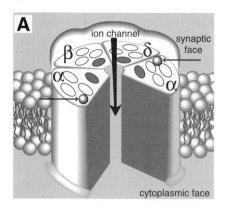
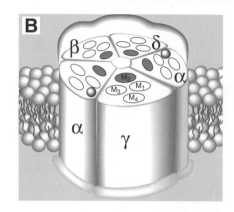
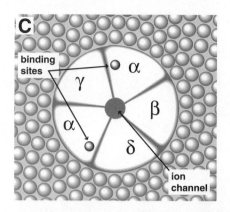

Fig. 10.9. Nicotinic cholinergic receptor: **A.** Longitudinal view (γ-subunit removed) showing the internal ion channel. Acetylcholine binding sites on the α-subunits are indicated by the arrows. These are located at the αγ and αδ interfaces. **B.** Each of the five transmembrane subunits (α, α, β, δ, γ) are composed of four hydrophobic membrane spanning segments (M₁–M₄). **C.** Top view of the nicotinic receptor showing the subunits surrounding the ion channel. (Adapted from references 24 and 26.)

There are two acetylcholine binding sites on the extracellular domain of each receptor molecule. One binding site is located on each α-subunit at the αγ and αδ interfaces (26); the binding sites possess a positive cooperativity even though the two binding sites are not adjacent to each other in the pentameric receptor.

Our knowledge and understanding of the muscarinic and nicotinic receptors has advanced tremendously from the time these receptors were only ethereal concepts, thanks to the dedicated efforts of many scientists. This understanding of cholinergic receptors provides the basis for the rational design of new selective therapeutic agents to treat diseases associated with cholinergic neurons.

Stereochemistry of Acetylcholine

One shortcoming of all the early models for cholinergic receptors was that they did not account for the observed stereoselectivity of the receptors for agonist and antagonist ligands. Even though acetylcholine does not exhibit optical isomerism, many of the synthetic and naturally occurring agonists and antagonists are optical isomers; usually one of the enantiomers is many times more active than the other. It was apparent to early receptor investigators that the stereochemistry of cholinergic ligands is important for receptor binding. In this regard, the stereochemical-activity relationships of cholinergic ligands has been studied extensively to provide a rational basis for the design of cholinergic drugs as well as to describe the properties and functions of cholinergic receptors.

The stereochemistry of acetylcholine resides in the different arrangements in space of its atoms by virtue of rotation about σ bonds, i.e., conformational isomerism. Because of the relatively unrestricted rotation about these single covalent bonds, acetylcholine can exist in a number of conformations. Most of the studies on the conformational isomerism of acetylcholine have focused on the torsion angles between the ester oxygen atom and the quaternary nitrogen resulting from rotation about the Cα-Cβ

bond. Four of these conformations are illustrated by Newman projections in Figure 10.10.

Techniques used to determine the thermodynamically preferred conformation of acetylcholine have included nuclear magnetic resonance spectrometry (NMR), X-ray crystallography (X-ray), and molecular orbital calculations. The NMR studies established the preferred conformation of acetylcholine in aqueous solution and indicated that the molecule assumes a synclinal (gauche or skew) conformational relationship between the ester oxygen and the quaternary nitrogen. This conformation is supported by the X-ray data, which established that the conformation of acetylcholine in the solid, crystalline state is also synclinal. Molecular orbital calculations of the preferred conformation of acetylcholine also resulted in the conclusion that the preferred conformation is synclinal, in keeping with the conformation derived from NMR and X-ray determinations. These experimental and theoretical determinations of the acetylcholine conformation differ from the antiperiplanar conformation that might be expected from molecular models by minimizing bond overlap. There is an intramolecular interaction, most probably an electrostatic

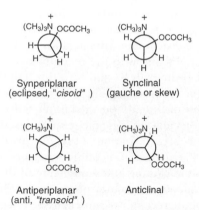

Fig. 10.10. Conformational isomers of acetycholine.

attraction, between the quaternary nitrogen and the carbonyl oxygen, which stabilizes the synclinal conformation.

It must be emphasized that the experimentally determined synclinal conformation of acetylcholine is only that measured in aqueous solution (NMR) or the crystalline state (X-ray). This may not be the conformation preferred by the receptors. Indeed, the conformation of receptor-bound acetylcholine could be much different and might not be a thermodynamically preferred conformation.

In recognition of this possibility, medicinal chemists have synthesized and tested conformationally restricted acetylcholine analogs. These compounds represent some of the possible conformations of acetylcholine. The most significant study in this regard is that of Armstrong and colleagues (27). They synthesized and evaluated the muscarinic and nicotinic activity of the *cis*- and *trans*-isomers of a conformationally rigid model of acetylcholine, *cis*- and *trans*-2-acetoxycyclopropyl-1-trimethylammonium iodide (ACTM). Because this model is based on the cyclopropane

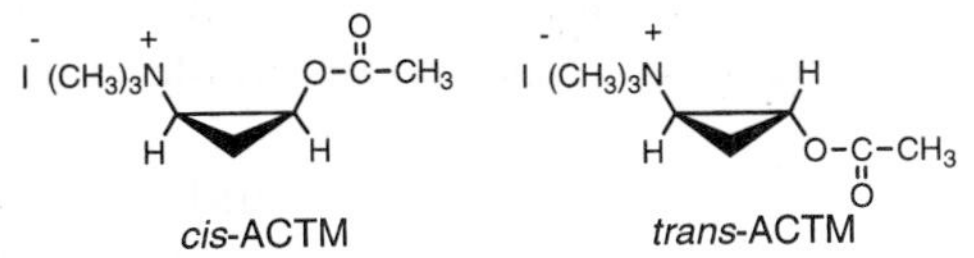

cis-ACTM   *trans*-ACTM

ring, the ester and quaternary ammonium functional groups cannot change their relative positions by bond rotation. The *cis*- and *trans*-isomers are rigidly constrained to the conformations shown. The *cis*-isomer is similar to the synperiplanar conformation of acetylcholine, and the *trans*-isomer approximates the anticlinal conformation. The (+)-*trans*-enantiomer was observed to be equally as potent or more potent, depending on the pharmacologic test used, than acetylcholine at muscarinic receptors; it was much more potent than the (−)-*trans*-enantiomer. The racemic cis-compound had almost no activity in the same muscarinic receptor test system, and all compounds were very weak nicotinic agonists.

The important conclusion drawn from this study was that acetylcholine would most probably interact with muscarinic receptors in its less favored anticlinal conformation. The most active isomer, the (+)-*trans*-enantiomer, of these cyclopropane analogs was found to have a torsion angle of 137° (anticlinal) between the ester oxygen and the quaternary nitrogen. This is significantly different from the 60° torsion angle in the synclinal conformation found by NMR and X-ray determinations to be the preferred conformation.

The stereochemistry of cholinergic ligands and stereoselectivity of the receptors has played an important role in the design of cholinergic ligands as therapeutic agents. This role becomes apparent in subsequent sections.

ACETYLCHOLINE MIMETICS— MUSCARINIC AGONISTS

The interaction of cholinergic agonists with muscarinic receptors leads to well-defined pharmacologic responses depending on the tissue or organ in which the receptor is located. These responses include contractions of smooth muscle, vasodilation of the vascular system, increased secretion from exocrine glands, miosis, and a decrease in both the cardiac rate and the force of contractions of the heart.

Acetylcholine

Acetylcholine is the prototypical muscarinic (and nicotinic) agonist because it is the physiologic chemical neurotransmitter. It is a poor therapeutic agent, however, because of the chemical and physicochemical properties associated with its ester and quaternary ammonium salt functional groups. Acetylcholine is quite stable in the solid crystalline form, but it undergoes rapid hydrolysis in aqueous solution. This hydrolysis is accelerated in the presence of catalytic amounts of either acid or base. For this reason, acetylcholine cannot be administered orally owing to rapid hydrolysis in the gastrointestinal tract. Even when administered by parenteral routes, its pharmacologic action is fleeting as a result of enzyme-catalyzed hydrolysis by serum and tissue esterases. The quaternary ammonium functional group imparts excellent water solubility to acetylcholine, but quaternary ammonium salts are poorly absorbed across lipid membranes because of the highly hydrophilic character imparted by the ionic quaternary ammonium functional group. Therefore, even if acetylcholine were chemically stable enough to be administered orally, it would be poorly absorbed. The pharmacologic effects of acetylcholine are not selective, inasmuch as it is the neurotransmitter at both muscarinic and nicotinic receptors. Acetylcholine is used during ocular surgery to produce complete miosis within seconds. It is not lipophilic enough to penetrate the cornea, so it cannot be administered topically. It must be instilled directly into the anterior chamber. Due to the aforementioned chemical lability, it requires aqueous reconstitution immediately prior to instillation.

Structure-activity Relationship

The necessity to design compounds that would serve as therapeutic alternatives to acetylcholine and as probes to study the role of acetylcholine in neurotransmission led to an exhaustive study of the structural features required for the action of acetylcholine. The SAR that developed from these studies have provided the basis for the design of all the muscarinic agonists currently used as therapeutic agents.

To review the SAR, it is logical to divide the structure of acetylcholine into the three components shown below to examine the effects of chemical modification of each group.

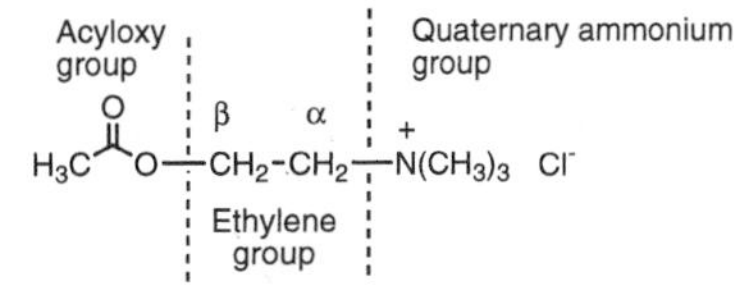

Modification of the Quaternary Ammonium Group

Analogs of acetylcholine in which the nitrogen atom was replaced by arsenic, phosphorus or sulfur have been synthesized (12,28). Although they exhibited some of the activity of acetylcholine, these compounds were less active and not used clinically. It was concluded that only compounds possessing a positive charge on the atom in the position of the nitrogen had appreciable muscarinic activity.

Compounds in which all three methyl groups on the nitrogen were replaced by larger alkyl groups were inactive as agonists. When the methyl groups are replaced by three ethyl groups, the resulting compound is a cholinergic antagonist. Replacement of only one methyl group by an ethyl or propyl group affords a compound that is active but much less so than acetylcholine (29). Furthermore, successive replacement of one, two or three of the methyl groups with hydrogen atoms to afford a tertiary, secondary, or primary amine, respectively, leads to successively diminishing muscarinic activity (31).

Modification of the Ethylene Bridge

Synthesis of acetic acid esters of quaternary ammonium alcohols of greater length than choline led to a series of compounds with activity that was rapidly reduced as the chain length increased. This observation led Ing to postulate his rule of five. This rule suggests that there should be no more than five atoms between the nitrogen and the terminal hydrogen atom for maximal muscarinic potency (12). Present concepts suggest that the muscarinic receptor cannot successfully accommodate molecules larger than acetylcholine and still produce its physiologic effect. Although larger molecules may bind to the receptor, they lack efficacy and demonstrate antagonist properties.

Replacement of the hydrogen atoms of the ethylene bridge by alkyl groups larger than methyl affords compounds that are much less active than acetylcholine. Introduction of a methyl group on the carbon beta to the quaternary nitrogen affords acetyl-β-methylcholine (methacholine), which has muscarinic potency almost equivalent to that of acetylcholine; it has selectivity for muscarinic receptors in that it possesses much greater muscarinic potency than nicotinic potency. Methacholine is used via inhalation as an effective diagnostic agent for the diagnosis of asthma. The resulting bronchospasm may be relieved with bronchodilators.

A methyl group on the carbon alpha to the quaternary nitrogen affords acetyl-α-methylcholine. Although activity relative to ACh is reduced at both muscarinic and nicotinic receptors, it exhibits greater nicotinic than muscarinic potency; this compound is not used currently as a therapeutic agent.

Acetyl-β-methylcholine chloride   Acetyl-α-methylcholine chloride

Addition of methyl groups to either one or both of the ethylene carbons results in asymmetric molecules exhibiting optical isomerism. Muscarinic receptors and acetyl-

cholinesterase (AChE) display stereoselectivity for the enantiomers of acetyl-β-methylcholine. The S(+)-enantiomer is equipotent with acetylcholine, and the R(−)-enantiomer is about 20-fold less potent. Acetylcholinesterase hydrolyzes the S(+)-isomer much slower (about half the rate) than acetylcholine. The R(−)-isomer is not hydrolyzed by AChE but is a weak competitive inhibitor of the enzyme. This stability to AChE hydrolysis as well as the AChE inhibitory effect of the R(−)-enantiomer may explain why methacholine (racemic acetyl-β-methylcholine) produces a longer duration of action than acetylcholine. The nicotinic receptor and AChE exhibit little stereoselectivity for the optical isomers of acetyl-α-methylcholine.

Modification of the Acyloxy Group

As would be predicted by Ing's rule of five (12), when the acetyl group is replaced by higher homologs (i.e., the propionyl or butyryl groups), the resulting esters are less potent than acetylcholine. Choline esters of aromatic or higher molecular-weight acids possess cholinergic antagonist activity.

The fleeting pharmacologic action and chemical instability of acetylcholine are due to its rapid hydrolysis. A logical approach to the development of better muscarinic therapeutic agents was to replace the acetyloxy functional group with a functional group resistant to hydrolysis. This led to the synthesis of the carbamic acid ester of choline (carbachol), which is a potent cholinergic agonist possessing both muscarinic and nicotinic activity. Esters derived from carbamic acid are referred to as carbamates and are more stable than carboxylate esters to hydrolysis, because the carbonyl carbon is less electrophilic. Carbachol is less readily hydrolyzed in the gastrointestinal tract or by acetylcholinesterase than acetylcholine and can be administered orally. Owing to its erratic absorption and pronounced nicotinic effects, however, its use has been limited to the treatment of glaucoma.

Carbachol   Bethanechol

This same chemical logic was extended to acetyl-β-methylcholine and led to the synthesis of its carbamate ester, bethanechol, an orally effective potent muscarinic agonist. Bethanechol must be administered orally or by subcutaneous injection since there is danger of a cholinergic crisis if it is given by intravenous or intramuscular injection. Therapeutically, it possesses almost no nicotinic activity and is used to treat postsurgical and postpartum urinary retention and abdominal distention. As would be expected, muscarinic receptors exhibit a stereoselectivity for the two optical isomers of bethanechol. The S(+)-enantiomer exhibits much greater binding to muscarinic receptors than the R(−)-enantiomer in isolated receptor preparations.

The profound muscarinic activity of the alkaloid muscarine provided substantial rationale for synthesizing ethers of choline. Muscarine, obtained from the red variety of mushroom, *Amanita muscaria* and other mushrooms, is one of the oldest known cholinergic agonists and is the compound for which muscarinic receptors were named. It was used in many pharmacologic experiments in the latter 19th century and early part of the 20th century, and its use preceded the discovery and chemical characterization of acetylcholine (2). The chemical structure of muscarine (see page 265), however, was not completely characterized until 1957. Muscarine possesses three chiral centers (C2, C3, and C5), or eight optical isomers (four enantiomeric pairs). Of these, only the naturally occurring alkaloid, (2S,3R,5S) (+)-muscarine (also called L (+)-muscarine), is correctly referred to as muscarine. The C5 carbon of (+)-muscarine has the same absolute configuration as the analogous chiral beta carbon in S(+)-methacholine.

Other choline ethers as well as alkylaminoketones have been synthesized and evaluated for muscarinic activity. Choline ethyl ether exhibits significant muscarinic activity and is chemically quite stable, but it has not been used clinically. The most potent ketone derivatives possess the carbonyl on the carbon delta to the quaternary nitrogen; this is the same relative position as the carbonyl in acetylcholine. This suggests that these carbonyl groups bind by either a hydrogen bond or other dipole-dipole interaction with an appropriate group on the muscarinic receptor. Furthermore, the activity of these ethers and ketones demonstrates that neither the ester functional group nor a carbonyl is required for muscarinic agonist activity.

Choline ethyl ether   Alkylaminoketones

The classic SAR for muscarinic agonist activity can be summarized as follows:

1. The molecule must possess a nitrogen atom capable of bearing a positive charge, preferably a quaternary ammonium salt.
2. For maximum potency, the size of the alkyl groups substituted on the nitrogen should not exceed the size of a methyl group.
3. The molecule should have an oxygen atom, preferably an ester-like oxygen, capable of participating in a hydrogen bond.
4. There should be a two-carbon unit between the oxygen atom and the nitrogen atom.

It is important to note that this SAR was based on pharmacologic evaluations using isolated tissues and whole animals and done over a 60 year period. Scientists conducting this research did not have the luxury of modern, highly refined biologic testing systems (i.e., protein binding assays, cell membrane binding assays, and single-cell models) that are considered state-of-the-art today for pharmacologic evaluation of new medicinal agents. This is why some classic muscarinic agonists and many of the more modern agents do not adhere to this SAR. Indeed, SAR rules are not meant to be static; they are expected to change as new experimental data refine the structural and stereostructural requirements for muscarinic agonist activity.

Pilocarpine hydrochloride, the salt of an alkaloid obtained from *Pilocarpus jaborandi*, is an example of a muscarinic agonist that does not adhere to the traditional SAR. Langley reported in 1876 that extracts containing the alkaloid stimulated the end organs of parasympathetic neurons and the structure of pilocarpine was reported in 1901.

Pilocarpine is marketed as an ophthalmic solution, gel, tablet, and Ocusert delivery system. It penetrates the eye well and is the miotic of choice for open-angle glaucoma and to terminate acute angle closure attacks. It is also used for the treatment of xerostomia resulting from radiation therapy of the head and neck, Sjogren's syndrome, or as a side effect of some psychotropic drugs.

Since pilocarpine is a lactone, its solutions are subject to chemical degradation by hydrolysis to afford the pharmacologically inactive pilocarpic acid, and by base-catalyzed epimerization at C3 in the lactone to isopilocarpine, and inactive stereoisomer of pilocarpine. This is not believed to be a serious problem if the drug is properly stored. Its solutions may be stored at room temperature, but the gel and Ocusert system should be stored in the refrigerator. In addition, the gel should be labeled with a two week expiration date when dispensed.

Future Muscarinic Agonists

Current research interest in the design and synthesis of new muscarinic agonists is focused on discovering agents that might be effective in the treatment of Alzheimer's disease and other cognitive disorders. In this regard, investigators are actively searching for muscarinic agonists that exhibit selectivity for muscarinic receptors in the brain. Among these compounds are analogs of arecoline, oxotremorine, and McN-A-343 as well as many other novel chemical structures possessing muscarinic agonist activity.

Arecoline   Oxotremorine

Arecoline is of historical interest because its structure, like those of many other early medicinal agents, was determined and confirmed by a 19th-century German pharmacist, E. Jahns (2). Xanomeline may be viewed as a non-classical bioisostere of arecoline. It is a muscarinic M_1/M_4 agonist that is showing promise in clinical trials for the treatment of Alzheimer's disease (32). Although not tolerated at orally effective doses, transdermal delivery systems are showing promise.

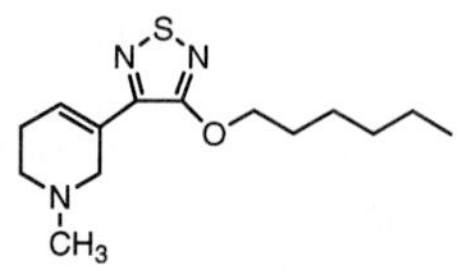

Xanomeline

ACETYLCHOLINESTERASE INHIBITORS (AChEIs)

Another means of producing an autonomic response is to interfere with the mechanism by which the action of the neurotransmitter is terminated. In the parasympathetic nervous system, the action of acetylcholine is terminated

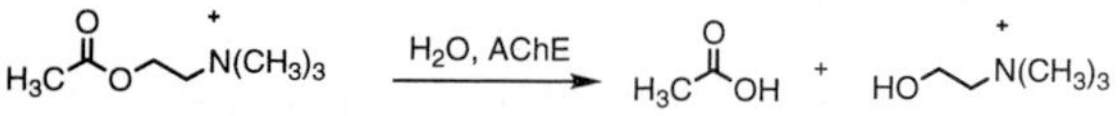

by its rapid, AChE-catalyzed hydrolysis to acetic acid and choline. Inhibition of AChE increases the concentration of acetylcholine in the synapse and results in production of both muscarinic and nicotinic responses.

Therapeutic Application

Acetylcholinesterase inhibitors (AChEIs), sometimes referred to as anticholinesterases, are classified as indirect cholinomimetics because their principle mechanism of action does not involve binding to cholinergic receptors. These agents are used therapeutically to improve muscle strength in myasthenia gravis. They are used clinically in open angle glaucoma to decrease intraocular pressure by stimulating contraction of the ciliary muscle and sphincter of the iris. This facilitates outflow of the aqueous humor into the canal of Schlemm. AChEIs have recently found use for the treatment of symptoms of Alzheimer's disease and similar cognitive disorders (33,34), conditions characterized by a cholinergic deficiency in the cortex and basal forebrain. They are used extensively as insecticides and have been used as chemical warfare agents.

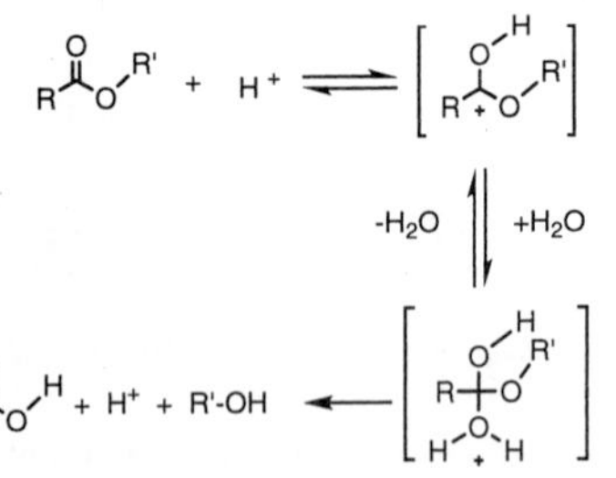

Fig. 10.11. Mechanism of acid-catalyzed hydrolysis of ACh by ACh esterase.

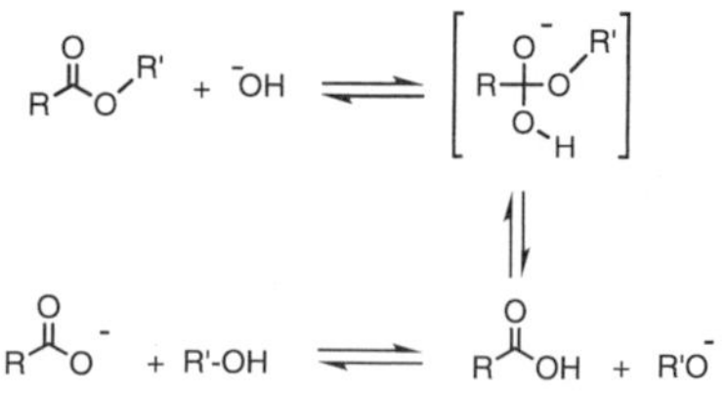

Fig. 10.12. Mechansim of base-catalyzed hydrolysis of ACh by ACh esterase.

Mechanism of Acetylcholinesterase Hydrolysis

Extensive studies of AChE have resulted in the purification and amino acid sequencing of the enzyme from several sources as well as the description of its quaternary structure from X-ray crystallographic and molecular modeling studies (35). To understand the mode of action of AChEIs, it is necessary to examine the mechanism by which AChE catalyzes hydrolysis of acetylcholine. This enzymatically controlled hydrolysis parallels the two chemical mechanisms for hydrolysis of esters. The first mechanism is acid-catalyzed hydrolysis, in which the initial step involves protonation of the carbonyl oxygen. The transition state is formed by the attack of a molecule of water at the electrophilic carbonyl carbon atom. Collapse of the transition state affords the carboxylic acid and the alcohol (Fig. 10.11).

The second mechanism, base-catalyzed hydrolysis, involves nucleophilic attack of hydroxide anion on the electrophilic carbonyl carbon (Fig. 10.12).

Both mechanisms for ester hydrolysis are proposed to be involved in the mechanism for AChE-catalyzed hydrolysis of acetylcholine. Figure 10.13 is a schematic illustration of the binding of acetylcholine to the catalytic (active) site of AChE, which consists of an esteratic binding site and an "anionic binding site." This figure reflects binding of the quaternary nitrogen of acetylcholine to an area that has been described as an "anionic site" on the enzyme. This

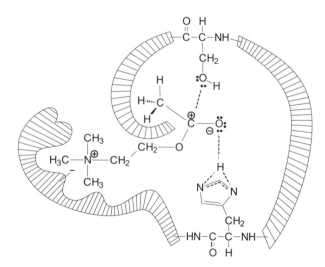

Fig. 10.13. Binding of acetylcholine to catalytic site of acetylcholinesterase; role of serine and histidine residues is illustrated.

"anionic site" was originally proposed to be contributed by the free carboxylate group of a glutamate residue. However, current evidence using selective mutagenesis suggests that rather than ionic bonding between the quaternary nitrogen and an anionic site, there is a cation-pi interaction between the quaternary nitrogen and a tryptophan moiety in the enzyme (36). In this illustration, there is a concerted protonation of the carbonyl oxygen by an imidazole proton from a histidine residue and nucleophilic attack on the partially positive carbon of the carbonyl group by the hydroxyl group of a serine residue. The remainder of the hydrolysis mechanism is described in Figure 10.14. Transition state B is unstable and collapses to form choline and acetylated AChE (C); this form of the enzyme is referred to as the acetylated enzyme. As long as the enzyme is acetylated, it cannot bind another molecule of acetylcholine; the enzyme is in an inactive state. The acetylated enzyme undergoes rapid hydrolysis to regenerate the original, active form of AChE (D) and a molecule of acetic acid.

The latter step in the mechanism, the regeneration of the active enzyme, is important in the development of AChEIs. If the enzyme becomes acylated by a functional group (i.e., carbamyl or phosphate) that is more stable to hydrolysis than a carboxylate ester, the enzyme remains inactive for a longer period of time. This chemical principle regarding the rates of hydrolysis led to the discovery and design of two classes of AChEIs, the reversible inhibitors and the irreversible inhibitors.

Reversible Inhibitors of Acetylcholinesterase
Mechanism of Action

Reversible AChEIs are those compounds that either (a) are substrates for and react with AChE to form an acylated enzyme which is more stable than the acetylated enzyme but still capable of undergoing hydrolytic regeneration or (b) bind to AChE with greater affinity than acetylcholine but do not react with the enzyme as substrates. Clinically useful inhibitors are those of the first type and include the aryl carbamates, e.g., esters of carbamic acid and phenols, such as physostigmine, the classic AChEI. Alkyl carbamates (esters of carbamic acid and alcohols), such as carbachol and bethanechol, both structurally related to acetylcholine, are also substrates for and competitively inhibit AChE because they are hydrolyzed very slowly by AChE. For reasons previously discussed, carbachol and bethanechol are more resistant to AChE-catalyzed hydrolysis than acetylcholine.

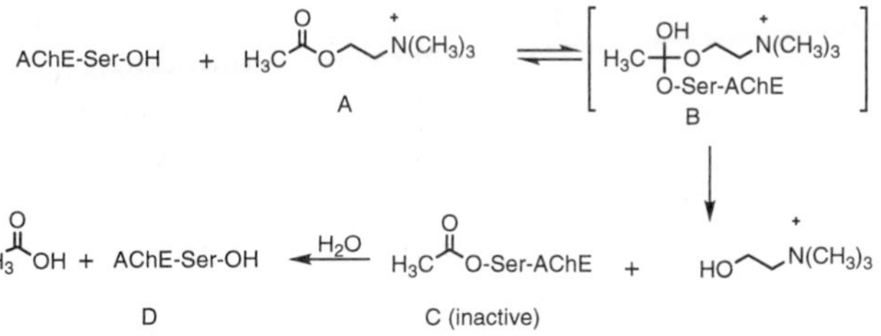

Fig. 10.14. Mechanistic steps in the hydrolysis of ACh.

When aryl carbamate AChEIs, such as physostigmine and its analogs, bind to the catalytic site of AChE, hydrolysis of the carbamate occurs, which transesterifies the serine residue with carbamic acid; this is referred to as the carbamylated enzyme. The rate of carbamylation follows the order of: carbamic acid esters > methylcarbamic acid esters > dimethylcarbamic acid esters (37).

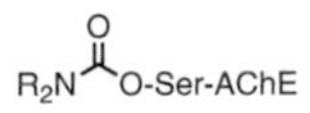

Carbamylated AChE

Regeneration of active AChE by hydrolysis of the carbamylated enzyme is much slower than hydrolysis of the acetylated enzyme. The rate for hydrolytic regeneration of the carbamylated AChE is measured in minutes (e.g., half-life for methyl carbamylated enzyme is about 15 minutes); the rate of hydrolytic regeneration of acetylated AChE is measured in milliseconds (half-life for acetylated enzyme is about 0.2 milliseconds). Despite the longer time required to regenerate the carbamylated enzyme, the fact remains that the active form of AChE is eventually regenerated. Therefore, these inhibitors are considered to be reversible.

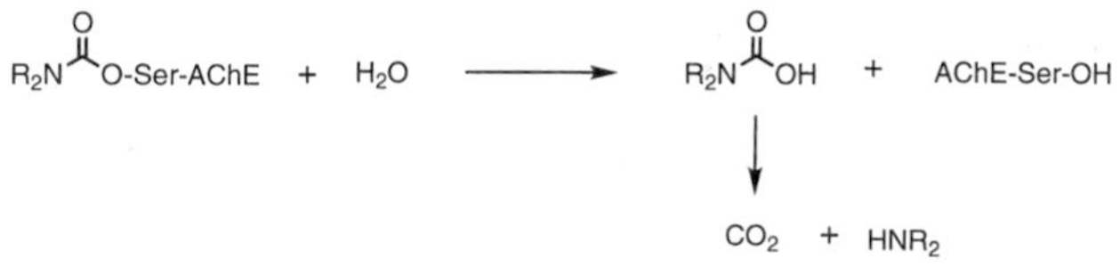

Aryl carbamates are superior to alkyl carbamates as AChEIs because they have better affinity for, and therefore carbamylate, AChE more efficiently. Physostigmine and other aryl carbamates exhibit inhibition constants (K_i) on the order of 10^{-9} to 10^{-8} M and are three to four orders of magnitude more effective than alkyl carbamates such as carbachol (approximate K_i of 10^{-5} M). This is to be expected owing to the fact that phenoxide anions are more stable and hence, are better leaving groups, than alkoxide anions. Phenoxide anions are stabilized through resonance with the aromatic ring. Thus, the therapeutically effective carbamate inhibitors of AChE are derived from phenols.

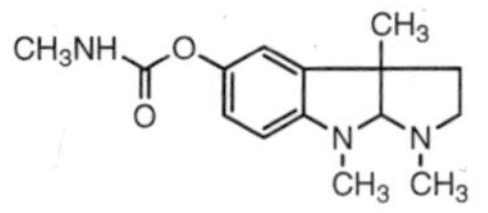

Physostigmine

Specific Agents

Physostigmine. The classic AChEI, physostigmine, is an alkaloid obtained from seeds of the Calabar bean, *Physostigma venenosum* (34). Its parasympathomimetic effects were recognized long before its structure was elucidated in 1923. In 1929, Stedman found that the mechanism of the parasympathomimetic effects of physostigmine was inhibition of AChE. It inhibits AChE by acting as its substrate and carbamylating the enzyme. AChE

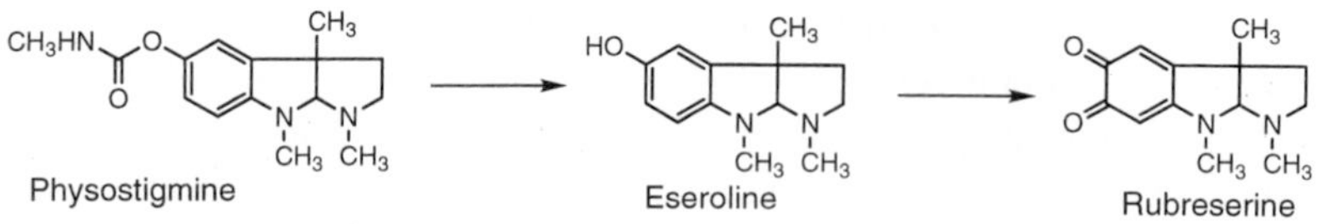

Fig. 10.15. In vitro degradation of physostigmine.

is carbamylated at a slow rate, but physostigmine has exceptionally high affinity (approximate K_i of 10^{-9} M) for the catalytic site of the enzyme; for comparison, the K_s for acetylcholine is on the order of 10^{-4} M. Thus, physostigmine is classified as a reversible AChEI that carbamylates the enzyme, but at a slow rate; the carbamylated AChE is also regenerated quite slowly.

Chemical Instability. Physostigmine undergoes hydrolytic decomposition in aqueous solutions to form eseroline, which is subject to light-catalyzed oxidation to form rubreserine, a red colored compound (Fig. 10.15). Both degradation products are inactive as AChEIs.

Therapeutic Application. Physostigmine has been used for many years in ophthalmology for the treatment of glaucoma. More recently, the salicylate salt has been used in hospital emergency rooms to treat overdoses of compounds possessing significant anticholinergic effects (depression) in the central nervous system, such as atropine and tricyclic antidepressants. Physostigmine, in contrast to many other AChEIs, is not a quaternary ammonium salt; therefore, it is more lipophilic and can readily diffuse across the blood-brain barrier into the central nervous system to inhibit AChE in the brain and reverse the effects of anticholinergic compounds. The ability of physostigmine to cross the blood-brain barrier has led to renewed interest in this molecule. It is used clinically to treat poisonings with anticholinergic agents. It is also one of a number of centrally active AChEIs being investigated as indirect cholinomimetics for use in the treatment of Alzheimer's disease and other cognitive disorders.

Neostigmine bromide   Pyridostigmine bromide

Neostigmine and Pyridostigmine. The discovery that physostigmine and other aryl carbamates inhibit AChE reversibly led to research to find other AChEIs possessing this activity. Most of this research involved the incorporation of the required structural features of both physostigmine and acetylcholine into the new molecules. This research led to the synthesis of neostigmine, a compound resembling physostigmine but having a much simpler structure. Neostigmine retains the substituted carbamate group, the benzene ring and the nitrogen atom

of the first heterocyclic ring of physostigmine. The distance between the ester and the quaternary ammonium group is approximately the same as that found in acetylcholine and physostigmine.

A closely related structure, pyridostigmine, incorporates the charged nitrogen into a pyridine ring. Both neostigmine and pyridostigmine are reversible AChEIs that act by the same mechanism as physostigmine but are chemically more stable with longer durations of action. Both are orally effective and are commonly used to treat myasthenia gravis because they lack central activity. Because pyridostigmine has a longer duration of action and a lower incidence of side effects than neostigmine, it is the better choice for oral therapy of myasthenia gravis. Both neostigmine and pyridostigmine are used by parenteral administration to reverse the effects of nondepolarizing neuromuscular blocking agents (see below).

Three AChEI compounds have been approved for the treatment of Alzheimer's disease. One, rivastigmine, is an arylcarbamate. The other two, tacrine and donepezil, lack the carbamate moiety and may be classified as nonclassic AChEIs.

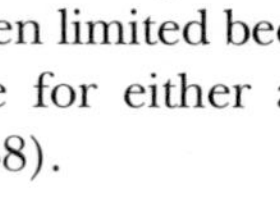

Tacrine

Tacrine (Cognex). Tacrine, an aminoacridine that was synthesized in the 1930s, is a nonclassic AChEI that was the first drug approved for the treatment of Alzheimer's disease. About 20% of tacrine-treated patients may show improvement, but its use has been limited because of hepatotoxicity. Tacrine is not selective for either acetylcholinesterase or butyrylcholinesterase (38).

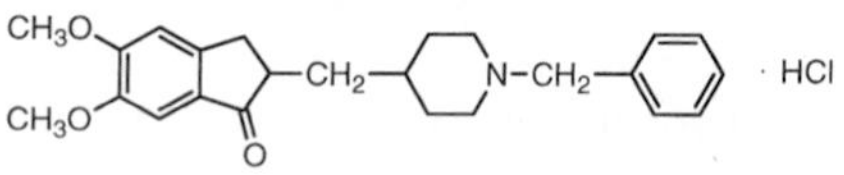

Donepezil hydrochloride

Donepezil (Aricept). Donepezil is another "nonclassic," centrally acting reversible, non-competitive AChEI that has recently been approved for treatment of Alzheimer's disease and dementia. Its selectivity for acetylcholinesterase is 570–1250 times that for butyrlcholinesterase, and it also exhibits greater affinity for AChE in the brain than in the periphery (39). When compared to tacrine, donepezil exhibits greater CNS

AChE selectivity, longer elimination half-life and little or no potential for hepatotoxicity.

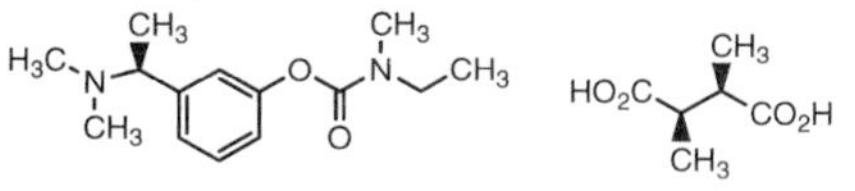

Rivastigminetartrate

Rivastigmine (Exelon). Rivastigmine is a centrally selective arylcarbamate AChEI that has recently been approved for the treatment of Alzheimer's disease. It has a half-life of 2 hours, but is able to inhibit AChE for up to 10 hours. Because of the slow dissociation of the carbamylated enzyme, it has been referred to as a pseudo-irreversible AChEI (39). Like donepezil, rivastigmine exhibits a low level of hepatotoxicity.

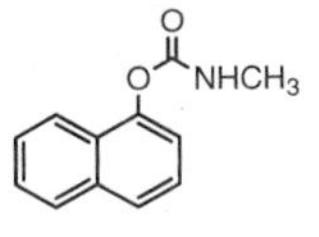

Carbaryl

Carbaryl. Carbaryl is a reversible carbamate-derived AChEI that has tremendous economic impact as an insecticide for use on house plants and vegetables, as well as for control of fleas and ticks on pets. Its structural relationship to physostigmine and neostigmine is readily apparent. A number of other carbamate AChEIs are also commercially available for this use.

Irreversible Inhibitors of Acetylcholinesterase
Mechanism of Action

The chemical logic involved in the development of effective AChEIs was to synthesize compounds that would be substrates for AChE and result in an acylated enzyme more stable to hydrolysis than a carboxylate ester. Phosphate esters are very stable to hydrolysis, being even more stable than many amides. Application of this chemical property to the design of AChEI compounds led to derivatives of phosphoric, pyrophosphoric, and phosphonic acids that are effective inhibitors of AChE. These act as inhibitors by the same mechanism as the carbamate inhibitors except that they leave the enzyme esterified as phosphate esters. The rate of hydrolytic regeneration of the phosphorylated enzyme is much slower than that of

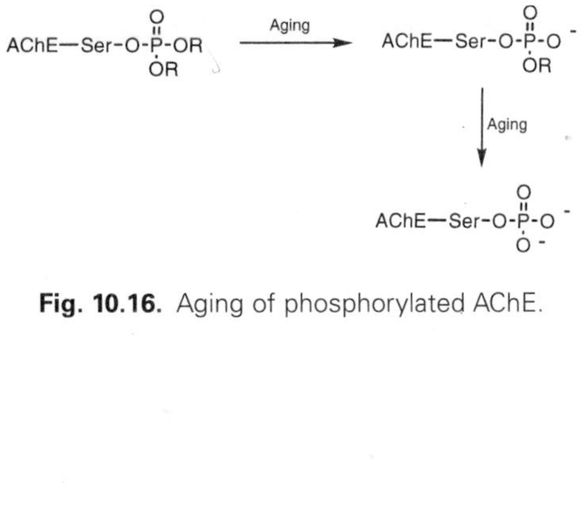

Fig. 10.16. Aging of phosphorylated AChE.

the carbamylated enzyme, and its rate is measured in hours (e.g., half-life for diethyl phosphates is about 8 hours). Because the duration of action of these compounds is much longer than that of the carbamate esters, they are referred to as irreversible inhibitors of AChE.

An important difference between irreversible phosphoester-derived AChEIs and reversible AChEIs is that the phosphorylated AChE can undergo a process known as aging (Fig. 10.16). This aging process, illustrated above, plays an important role in the toxicity of these irreversible AChEIs. Aging is the result of cleavage of one or more of the phosphoester bonds while the AChE is phosphorylated. This reaction affords an anionic phosphate that possesses a phosphorus atom which is much less electrophilic and therefore, much less likely to undergo hydrolytic regeneration than the original phosphoester. Thus, the aged phosphorylated enzyme does not undergo nucleophilic attack and regeneration by antidotes (see next section) for phosphate ester AChEIs. This aging process occurs over a period of time, which depends on the rate of the P-O bond cleavage reaction; during this time, the antidotes to phosphate ester poisoning may be effective.

Only those phosphorus-derived AChEIs that possess at least one phosphoester group undergo this aging process. Knowledge of the chemical mechanisms associated with irreversible inhibition of AChE and the aging process led to the development of deadly phosphorus-derived chemical warfare agents, one of which is sarin (GB). When this compound phosphorylates AChE, only one aging reaction takes

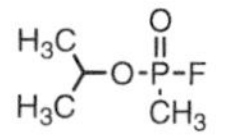

Sarin

place, and then the enzyme becomes completely refractory to regeneration by the currently available antidotal agents.

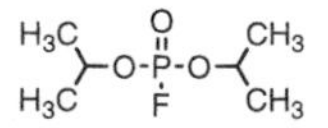

Diisopropylfluorophosphate (DFP) 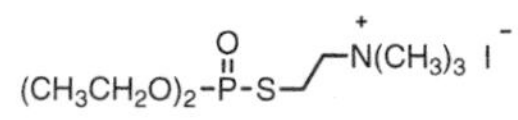   Echothiophate iodide

Specific Agents
Isoflurophate (Floropryl) and Echothiophate Iodide (Phospholine). Two phosphate ester AChEIs, diisopropylfluorophosphate or isoflurophate and echothiophate iodide have found therapeutic application for the treatment of open-angle glaucoma. Isoflurophate is applied topically to the eye as an ointment and is used primarily when other agents fail. Echothiophate iodide is applied topically as a solution and is the most widely used AChEI for the treatment of glaucoma. The decrease in intraocular pressure observed with both agents can last up to 4 weeks. AChEIs exhibit cataractogenic properties and have precipitated retinal detachment, thus their use should be reserved for patients

who are refractory to other forms of treatment, i.e., short-acting miotics, beta-blockers, epinephrine, and possibly carbonic anhydrase inhibitors. Because of their toxicity, these compounds are not used for their systemic action. Selectivity of echothiophate for the AChE catalytic site was enhanced by incorporation in the molecule of a quaternary ammonium salt functional group two carbons removed from the phosphoryl group.

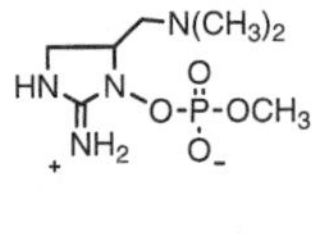

Anatoxin - a(s)

Anatoxin-a(s).   One novel phosphate ester AChEI, anatoxin-a(s), has been evaluated for its effects in animal models of cognitive disorders.

Insecticidal AChEIs.   A number of lipophilic derivatives of phosphoester AChEIs have been designed as insecticides; the structures of some of these are shown in Figure 10.17. This group of irreversible AChEI insecticides is beneficial to agricultural production throughout the world. In addition to being extremely lipophilic, another physicochemical property common to these compounds is a high vapor pressure. This combination of physicochemical properties makes it imperative that these compounds be used with extreme caution in the presence of humans and other mammals to prevent inhalation of the vapors and absorption of the compounds through the skin. Both routes of exposure cause a number of poisoning accidents every year, some of which are fatal.

Some of these irreversible AChEI insecticides possess a sulfur atom bonded to the phosphorus atom with a co-ordinate-covalent bond. These compounds exhibit little AChEI activity, but they are rapidly bioactivated (desulfurization) by microsomal oxidation in insects to afford the corresponding oxo derivatives (phosphate ester), which are quite potent. A good example of this bioactivation phenomenon is illustrated by commercially available parathion and its bioactivation to a toxic metabolite paraoxon. Malathion is a commercially available dithiophosphate ester insecticide and mitocide (treatment of lice) that was designed to take advantage of the selective toxicity between humans and insects. In humans

malathion is hydrolyzed by plasma esterases to less toxic hydrophilic carboxylic acid metabolites, but not in insects. Similar to parathion, malathion is bioactivated in insects to its toxic phosphate ester metabolite.

Antidotes for Irreversible AChEIs

Background.   The marked toxicity of the phosphate ester irreversible AChEIs, their widespread use as insecticides, and their proliferation as chemical warfare agents posed serious problems that stimulated research to develop antidotes for these agents. The solution of this problem required the rational use of reaction kinetics, organic reaction mechanisms, and synthetic organic chemistry. Water is a nucleophile capable of hydrolyzing acetylated AChE rapidly and regenerating the active enzyme. Phosphorylated AChE (irreversibly inhibited), however, was known to involve a phosphate ester of serine. It was well established from reaction kinetic studies that the rate of hydrolysis was much slower for organic phosphate esters than for carboxylate esters, and that a significantly stronger nucleophile than water would be required for efficient hydrolysis of phosphate esters. The problem required the design of reagents capable of efficiently catalyzing phosphate ester hydrolysis and regenerating active AChE, while being safe enough for use as therapeutic agents. The resolution of this problem is an elegant example of the application of chemical principles to the solution of a therapeutic problem (40–42).

Hydroxylamine (NH$_2$-OH) is a strong nucleophilic compound that efficiently cleaves phosphate esters. Hydroxylamine was demonstrated to increase significantly the rate of hydrolysis of phosphorylated AChE, but only at concentrations that were toxic (43). This prompted the development of a number of structurally related compounds in the hope of eliminating toxicity. The toxicity inherent in hydroxylamine would most probably be present in any structurally related compound, but might be minimized if sufficiently small doses could be used. It would be logical to design a compound that would (1) have a high degree of selectivity and strong binding affinity for AChE and (2) carry an hydroxylamine-like nucleophile into close proximity to the phosphorylated serine residue. This was achieved by synthesis of hydroxylamine derivatives of organic compounds, possessing a functional group bearing a positive charge.

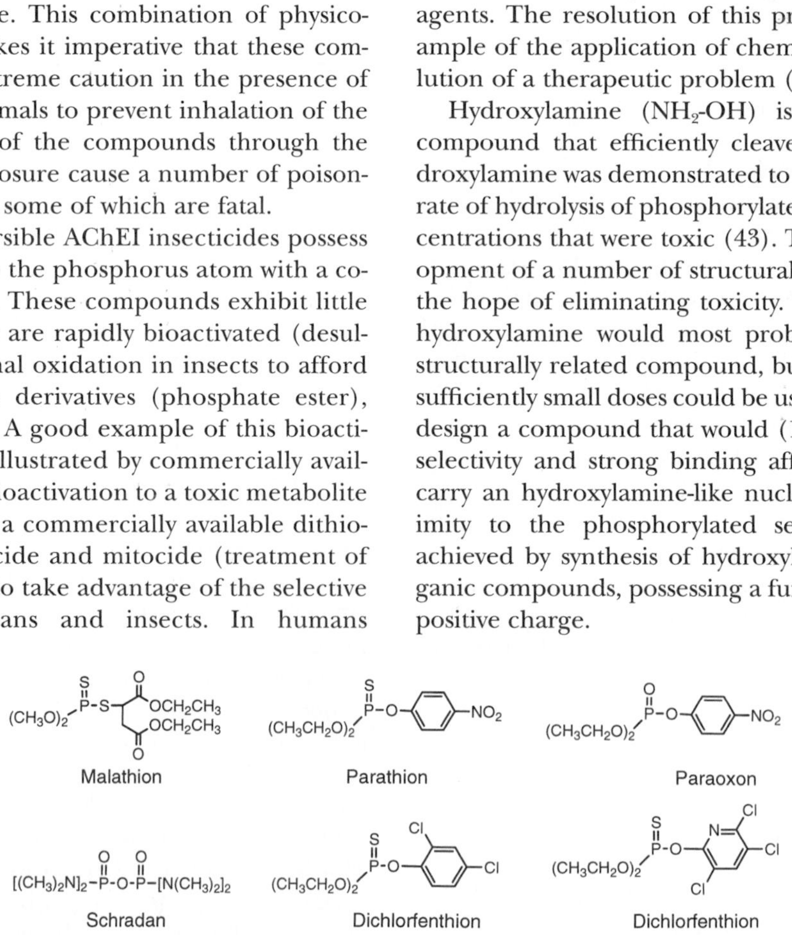

Fig. 10.17. Irreversible acetylcholinesterase inhibitors.

The reaction of hydroxylamine with aldehydes or ketones affords oximes, which possess the desired nucleophilic oxygen atom. A pyridine ring was considered an attractive carrier for the oxime function since such groups are common in a number of biochemical systems (e.g., NAD, NADP), indicating a possible low order of toxicity. Furthermore, there are three readily available positional isomers of pyridine aldehyde that can be converted easily to oximes. Finally, the nitrogen atom of the pyridine ring can be converted to a quaternary ammonium salt by treatment with methyl iodide. This cationic charge would be expected to increase affinity of the compound for the "anionic binding site" of the phosphorylated AChE.

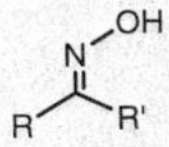

Oxime

The three isomeric pyridine aldoxime methiodides were synthesized and biologically evaluated. Of these, the most effective is the isomer derived from 2-pyridinylaldehyde. This compound, known as 2-PAM for 2-pyridine aldoxime methyl chloride (pralidoxime), is the only currently avail-

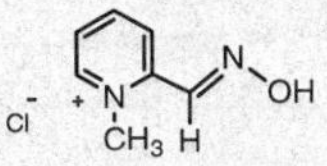

Pralidoxime chloride (2-PAM)

able agent proven to be clinically effective as an antidote for poisoning by phosphate ester AChEIs. The proposed mechanism for regeneration of AChE by 2-PAM is illustrated in Figure 10.18. The initial step involves binding of the quaternary ammonium nitrogen of 2-PAM to the "anionic binding site" of phosphorylated AChE. This places the nucleophilic oxygen of 2-PAM in close proximity to the electrophilic phosphorus atom. Nucleophilic attack of the oxime oxygen results in breaking of the ester bond between the serine oxygen atom and the phosphorus atom. The final products of the reaction are the regenerated active form of AChE and phosphorylated 2-PAM.

Pralidoxime must be given within a short period of time, after enzyme phosphorylation generally a few hours, for it to be effective because of the aging process of the phosphorylated enzyme. After aging has occurred, 2-PAM will not regenerate the enzyme. For this reason, as well as because new phosphate ester AChEIs capable of aging rapidly are being developed as insecticides and chemical warfare agents, there is a continuing research effort to discover new and better substitutes for 2-PAM. This research is focused on finding substitutes that are better nucleophiles than 2-PAM and, therefore, more effective generators of active AChE, as well as compounds that cross the blood-brain barrier to regenerate phosphorylated AChE in the brain.

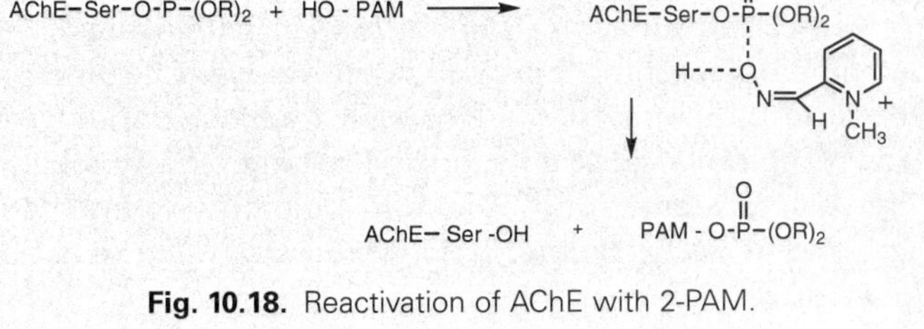

ACETYLCHOLINE ANTAGONISTS— MUSCARINIC ANTAGONISTS

Muscarinic antagonists are compounds that have high binding affinity for muscarinic receptors but have no intrinsic activity. When the antagonist binds to the receptor, it is proposed that the receptor protein undergoes a conformational perturbation that is different from that produced by an agonist. Therefore, antagonist binding to the receptor produces no response. Muscarinic antagonists are commonly referred to as anticholinergics, antimuscarinics, cholinergic blockers, antispasmodics, or parasympatholytics. The term anticholinergic refers in a pure sense to medicinal agents that are antagonists at both muscarinic and nicotinic receptors. Common usage of the term, however, has become synonymous with muscarinic antagonist, and it is used as such in this section.

Therapeutic Application

Muscarinic antagonists are frequently employed as both prescription drugs and over-the-counter medications. Because they act as competitive (reversible) antagonists of acetylcholine, these compounds have pharmacologic effects that are the opposite of the muscarinic agonists. The responses of muscarinic antagonists include decreased contractions of smooth muscle of the gastrointestinal and urinary tracts, dilation of the pupils, reduced gastric secretion, and decreased secretion of saliva. It follows that these compounds have therapeutic value in treating smooth muscle spasms, in ophthalmologic examinations, and in treatment of gastric ulcers. Compounds possessing muscarinic antagonist activity are common components of cold and flu remedies acting to reduce nasal and upper respiratory tract secretions.

Since agents of this type are mydriatics, they must be used with caution because of their effects on intraocular pressure. Drainage of the Canal of Schlemm is restricted by the iris when the pupil is dilated, and this can cause an increase in intraocular pressure. Hence, muscarinic antagonists are contraindicated in patients with glaucoma.

The earliest known anticholinergic agents are alkaloids found in the family Solanaceae, a large family of plants that includes potatoes. *Atropa belladonna* (Deadly Nightshade), *Hyoscyamus niger* (Black Henbane), and *Datura stramonium* (Jimsonweed, Thorn Apple) are plants that have significant historical importance to our understanding of the parasympathetic nervous system. Pharmacologic

Fig. 10.18. Reactivation of AChE with 2-PAM.

effects of extracts from these plants have been recognized since the Middle Ages, although these effects were not associated with the autonomic nervous system until the latter part of the 19th century.

Atropine   Scopolamine

Specific Agents—Atropine and Scopolamine

Atropine (pKa 9.8), an alkaloid isolated from *A. belladonna* and observed to block the effects of electrical stimulation and muscarine on the parasympathetic nervous system, became the first anticholinergic compound to be recognized as such. Scopolamine (pKa 7.6), another of the belladonna alkaloids, is chemically and pharmacologically similar to atropine but with different absorption and distribution properties.

Atropine is (±)-hyoscyamine, the tropic acid ester of tropine. The naturally occurring alkaloid is (−)-hyoscyamine. Atropine results from the base-catalyzed racemization of the chiral carbon of tropic acid, which occurs during the isolation process. Scopolamine is the generic name given to (−)-hyoscine, the naturally occurring alkaloid. The racemic compound isolated during extraction of the alkaloid from plants is atroscine.

Structural characterization of atropine and scopolamine and the discovery that these belladonna alkaloids are antagonists of acetylcholine were followed by introduction of a great many novel synthetic anticholinergic drugs. This research was stimulated by the need for additional chemical tools to probe the phenomenon of neurochemical transmission as well as the desire to develop the therapeutic potential of these agents. Efforts to discover new muscarinic antagonists remain unabated today, but the thrust is to design antagonists that are specific for the different muscarinic receptor subtypes.

Structure-activity Relationship

Atropine, the prototype anticholinergic agent, provided the structural model that guided the design of synthetic muscarinic antagonists for almost 70 years. The circled portion of the atropine molecule depicts the segment resembling acetylcholine.

Although the amine functional group is separated from the ester oxygen by more than two carbons, the conformation assumed by the tropanol ring orients these two atoms such that the intervening distance is similar to that in acetylcholine. One of the important structural differences between atropine and acetylcholine, both esters of amino alcohols, is the size of the acyl portion of the molecules. Based on the assumption that size was a major factor in blocking action, many substituted acetic acid esters of amino alcohols were prepared and evaluated for biologic activity.

It became apparent that the most potent compounds were those that possessed two lipophilic ring substituents on the carbon alpha to the carbonyl of the ester moiety. This is the first of the classic SAR for muscarinic antagonist activity, and this SAR became more precisely defined as research on these antagonists continued. The SAR for muscarinic antagonists can be summarized as follows:

$$R_2 - \overset{\displaystyle R_1}{\underset{\displaystyle R_3}{\text{C}}} - X-(CH_2)_n\text{-}N$$

1. Substituents R_1 and R_2 should be carbocyclic or heterocyclic rings for maximal antagonist potency. The rings may be identical, but the more potent compounds have different rings. Generally, one ring is aromatic and the other saturated or possessing only one olefinic bond. R_1 and R_2, however, may be combined into a fused aromatic tricyclic ring system such as that found in propantheline (Table 10.1). The size of these substituents is limited. For example, substitution of naphthalene rings for R_1 and R_2 affords compounds that are inactive apparently owing to steric hindrance of binding of these compounds to the muscarinic receptor.
2. The R_3 substituent may be a hydrogen atom, a hydroxyl group, a hydroxymethyl group, or a carboxamide, or it may be a component of one of the R_1 and R_2 ring systems. When this substituent is either a hydroxyl group or a hydroxymethyl group, the antagonist is usually more potent than the same compound without this group. The hydroxyl group presumably increases binding strength by participating in a hydrogen bond interaction at the receptor.
3. The X substituent in the most potent anticholinergic agents is an ester, but an ester functional group is not an absolute necessity for muscarinic antagonist activity. This substituent may be an ether oxygen, or it may be absent completely.
4. The N substituent is a quaternary ammonium salt in the most potent anticholinergic agents. This is not a requirement, however, because tertiary amines also possess antagonist activity presumably by binding to the receptor in the cationic (conjugate acid) form. The alkyl substituents are usually methyl, ethyl, propyl, or isopropyl.
5. The distance between the ring-substituted carbon and the amine nitrogen is apparently not critical, inasmuch as the length of the alkyl chain connecting these may be from two to four carbons. The most potent anticholinergic agents have two methylene units in this chain.

Muscarinic antagonists must compete with agonists for a common receptor. Their ability to do this effectively is because the large groups R_1 and R_2 enhance binding to the receptor. Because antagonists are larger than agonists, this suggests that groups R_1 and R_2 bind outside the binding site of acetylcholine. It has been suggested that the area surrounding the binding site of acetylcholine is hy-

Table 10.1. Anticholinergic Amino Alcohol Esters of General Structure, RCOOR

R	R′	Generic Name	Trade Name	Dose-Daily	Dosage Form (Strength in mg)
		Glycopyrrolate	Robinal Generic	3–6 mg 0.3–0.8 mg	Tab (1,2) Inj (0.2/ml)
		Propantheline	Pro-Banthine Generic	28.5–30 mg	Tab (7.5) Tab (15)
		Clidinium	Quarzan	7.5–20	Cap (2.5, 5)
		Ipratropium	Atrovent Generic	36 mcg q 4X 500 mcg q 3–4 X 168–252 mcg 505–672 mcg	Aer (18 mcg/actuation) Sol (0.2%–500 mcg/vial) Nasal (0.03%) Nasal (0.06%)
		Flavoxate	Urispas	300–800 mg	Tab (100)
		Oxyphencyclimine			

Tab = Tablet; Cap = Capsule; Aer = Aerosol; Inj = Injection; Sol = Solution.

drophobic in nature (44). This accounts for the fact that in potent cholinergic antagonists, the groups R_1 and R_2 must be hydrophobic (usually phenyl, cyclohexyl, or cyclopentyl). This concept is also supported by the current models for muscarinic receptors.

Pharmacokinetic Properties

Tables 10.1 and 10.2 include some of the anticholinergic agents that have found clinical application. These compounds reflect the SAR features that have been described. All of these compounds are effective when administered orally or by parenteral routes. Anticholinergic agents possessing a quaternary ammonium functional group are generally not well absorbed from the gastrointestinal tract because of their ionic character. These drugs are useful primarily in treatment of ulcers or other conditions in which a reduction in gastric secretions and reduced motility of the gastrointestinal tract are desired. Those antagonists having a tertiary nitrogen are much better absorbed and distributed following all routes of administration and are especially useful when systemic distribution is desired. The amino ether-derived and amino alcohol-derived anticholinergic agents readily cross the blood-brain barrier. These have proven particularly beneficial in the treatment of Parkinson's disease and other diseases requiring a central anticholinergic effect.

All these drugs display pronounced selectivity for muscarinic receptors; however, some of those possessing the quaternary ammonium functional group exhibit nicotinic antagonist activity at high doses. For the most part, these display no marked selectivity for muscarinic receptor subtypes.

Table 10.2. Anticholinergic Amino Alcohols and Amino Ethers

R	R'	Generic Name	Trade Name	Dose-Daily	Dosage Form (Strength in mg)
Amino alcohols of the general structure, R-CH₂-CH₂-R'					
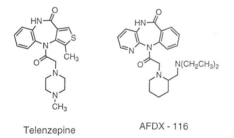		Procyclidine	Kemadrin	7.5–15 mg	Tab (5)
		Trihexyphenidyl	Artane	6–15 mg	Tab (2,5), Cap Sust (5) Elix (2/5 ml)
			Trihexy-5 Generic		Tab (5) Tab (2,5)
Amino ethers of the general structure, R-O-R'					
		Benztropine	Cogentin Generic	0.5–0.6 mg	Tab (0,5, 2), Inj (1 mg/ml) Tab (0.5, 1, 2)
		Orphenadrine	Norflex Generic Banflex, Flexojext, Flexon	200 mg Tab 60–120 mg Inj	Tab (100), Inj (30 mg/ml) Tab (100), Inj (30 mg/ml) Inj (30 mg/ml)

Tab = Tablet; Cap Sust = Capsule sustained release; Elix = Elixir; Inj = Injection.

Telenzepine

AFDX - 116

3-Quinuclidinylbenzilate (QNB)

d-Tubocurarine iodide

Recent Muscarinic Antagonists

More recently discovered muscarinic antagonists display higher affinity for the receptors than the older agents as exemplified by quinuclidinylbenzilate (QNB), which possesses structural features common to the classic anticholinergic agents. Radiolabeled QNB was instrumental in the development of muscarinic receptor labeling techniques as well as the discovery of subtypes of muscarinic receptors. This latter research also depended on the M_1-selective antagonist pirenzepine, a compound having a novel structure for muscarinic antagonist activity. A number of compounds structurally related to pirenzepine have demonstrated a similar M_1 selectivity; among these is telenzepine (45). Owing to their selectivity for muscarinic M_1 receptors, pirenzepine and telenzepine have been evaluated in clinical trials for the treatment of duodenal ulcers. It is of interest to note that AFDX-116, structurally similar to pirenzepine, is a muscarinic antagonist exhibiting selectivity for cardiac M_2 receptors.

NICOTINIC ANTAGONISTS— NEUROMUSCULAR BLOCKING AGENTS

Nicotinic antagonists are chemical compounds that bind to cholinergic nicotinic receptors but have no efficacy. All therapeutically useful nicotinic antagonists are competitive antagonists; i.e., the effects are reversible with acetylcholine.

There are two subclasses of nicotinic antagonists, skeletal neuromuscular blocking agents and ganglionic blocking agents, classified according to the two populations of nicotinic receptors. This section emphasizes nicotinic antagonists used clinically as neuromuscular blocking agents. These medicinal agents should not be confused with those skeletal muscle relaxant compounds that produce their effects through the central nervous system.

History

In terms of the historical perspective, tubocurarine, the first known neuromuscular blocking drug, was as important to the understanding of nicotinic antagonists as atropine was to muscarinic antagonists. The neuromuscular blocking effects of extracts of curare were first reported as early as 1510, when explorers of the Amazon River region of South America found natives using these plant extracts as arrow poisons. Early research with these crude plant extracts indicated that the active components caused muscle paralysis by effects on either the nerve or the muscle (the reader must remember that the concept of neurochemical transmission was not introduced until the late 19th century). In 1856, however, Bernard described the results of his experiments, which demonstrated unequivocally that curare extracts prevented skeletal muscle contractions by an effect at the neuromuscular junction and not on either the nerve innervating the muscle or the muscle itself (46).

Much of the early literature concerning the effects of curare is confusing and difficult to interpret. This is not at all surprising when it is realized that this research was performed using crude extracts, many of which came from different plants. It was not until the late 1800s that scientists recognized curare extracts contained quaternary ammonium salts. This knowledge prompted the use of other quaternary ammonium compounds to explore the neuromuscular junction. In the meantime, curare extracts continued to be used to block the effects of nicotine and acetylcholine at skeletal neuromuscular junctions and explore the nicotinic receptors.

In 1935, King (47) isolated a pure alkaloid which he named *d*-tubocurarine, from a tube curare of unknown botanical origin. The word tube refers to the container in which the South American natives transported their plant extract. It was almost 10 years later that the botanical source for *d*-tubocurarine was clearly identified as *Chondodendron tomentosum*. The structure that King assigned to tubocurarine possessed two nitrogen atoms, both of which were quaternary ammonium salts (e.g., a *bis*-quaternary ammonium compound). It was not until 1970 that the correct structure was reported by Everett and colleagues (48). The correct structure shown here has only one quaternary ammonium nitrogen; the other nitrogen is a tertiary amine salt. Nevertheless, the incorrect structure of tubocurarine served as the model for the synthesis of all the neuromuscular blocking agents in use today. These compounds have been of immense therapeutic value for surgical and orthopedic procedures and have been essential to research that led to the isolation and purification of nicotinic receptors. It is interesting to contemplate the consequences if no one had ever questioned the structure of tubocurarine as originally determined.

The potential therapeutic benefits of the neuromuscular blocking effects of tubocurarine as well as the difficulty in obtaining pure samples of the alkaloid encouraged medicinal chemists to design structurally related compounds possessing nicotinic antagonist activity. Using the *bis*-quaternary ammonium structure of tubocurarine (as reported by King) as a guide, a large number of compounds were synthesized and evaluated. It became apparent that a *bis*-quaternary ammonium compound, having two quaternary ammonium salts separated by 10 to 12 carbon atoms (similar to the distance between the nitrogen atoms in tubocurarine), was a requirement for neuromuscular blocking activity. The rationale for this structural requirement was that, in contrast to muscarinic receptors, nicotinic receptors possessed two anionic binding sites, both of which had to be occupied for a neuromuscular blocking effect. It is important to observe that the current transmembrane model for the nicotinic receptor protein has two anionic sites in the extracellular domain.

Some of the new *bis*-quaternary ammonium agents produced depolarization of the postjunctional membrane at the neuromuscular junction before causing blockade; other compounds, such as tubocurarine, did not produce this depolarization. Thus, the structural features of the remainder of the molecule determined whether the nicotinic antagonist was a depolarizing or a nondepolarizing neuromuscular blocker.

Therapeutic Application

Muscles producing rapid movements are the first to be affected by neuromuscular blocking agents. These include muscles of the face, eyes, and neck. Muscles of the limbs, chest and abdomen are affected next, with the diaphragm (respiration) being affected last. Recovery is generally in the reverse order.

As a result, the primary use of neuromuscular blocking agents is as an adjunct to general anesthesia. They produce skeletal muscle relaxation that facilitates operative procedures such as abdominal surgery. Furthermore, they reduce the depth requirement for general anesthetics; this decreases the overall risk of a surgical procedure and shortens post-anesthetic recovery time. Neuromuscular blocking agents have also found use in correction of dislocations and realignment of fractures. Short-acting neuromuscular blocking agents, such as succinylcholine, are routinely used to assist in tracheal intubation. When choosing a neuromuscular blocking agent four questions must be considered: 1) Will the compound produce the desired neuromuscular blockade? 2) What is its duration of action? 3) What are its adverse effects? and 4) What is its relative cost?

Side Effects

Adverse reactions to most, but not all, of the neuromuscular blocking agents may include hypotension, bronchospasm and cardiac disturbances. The depolarizing agents also cause an initial muscle fasciculation prior to relaxation. Many of these agents cause release of histamine and subsequent cutaneous (flushing, erythema, urticaria, pruritus), pulmonary (bronchospasm and wheezing), and cardiovascular (hypotension) effects.

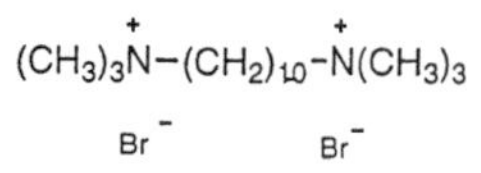

$$(CH_3)_3\overset{+}{N}-(CH_2)_{10}-\overset{+}{N}(CH_3)_3$$
$$Br^-\qquad Br^-$$

Decamethonium bromide

Specific Depolarizing Neuromuscular Blocking Agents
Decamethonium Bromide

One of the first neuromuscular blocking agents to be synthesized was decamethonium. A structure-activity study on a series of *bis*-quaternary ammonium compounds with varying numbers of methylene groups separating the nitrogen atoms demonstrated that maximal neuromuscular blockade occurred with 10 to 12 unsubstituted methylene groups. Activity diminished as the number of carbons was either decreased or increased. The compound with six methylene groups, hexamethonium, is a nicotinic antagonist at autonomic ganglia (ganglionic blocking agent). All the compounds in this series that possessed neuromuscular blocking activity also caused depolarization of the postjunctional membrane.

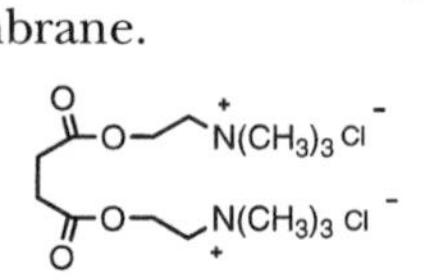

Succinylcholine chloride

Succinylcholine (Anectine)

Another depolarizing neuromuscular blocking agent is succinylcholine, which represents two molecules of acetylcholine connected at the carbons alpha to the carbonyl of the acetic acid moiety. The manner in which this compound is drawn gives the impression that the quaternary ammonium functional groups are not separated by the distance represented by decamethonium or tubocurarine. The molecule can exist, however, in an extended conformation (antiperiplanar) as shown in the Newman projection. This might account for the appropriate separation of

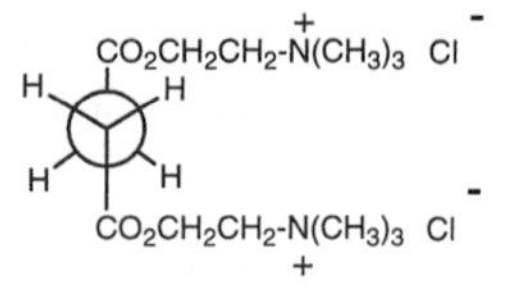

the quaternary nitrogens. Succinylcholine is rapidly hydrolyzed and rendered inactive, both in aqueous solution and by plasma esterases. This chemical instability must be considered when preparing solutions for parenteral administration. This same chemical property, however, gives the compound a brief duration of action. As a result, succinylcholine is used frequently for the rapid induction of neuromuscular blockade and when blockade of short duration is desired (Table 10.3). As such, it is used primarily to produce muscle relaxation during endotracheal intubation or endoscopic procedures. The depolarizing property is undesirable in neuromuscular blockers, so most research efforts have been directed toward the design of agents that are nondepolarizing.

Specific Nondepolarizing Neuromuscular Blocking Agents. Compounds in this class possess one or two quaternary ammonium groups. However, those with only one quaternary ammonium group exist as *bis*-cations in vivo due to having the second positive charge on a protonated

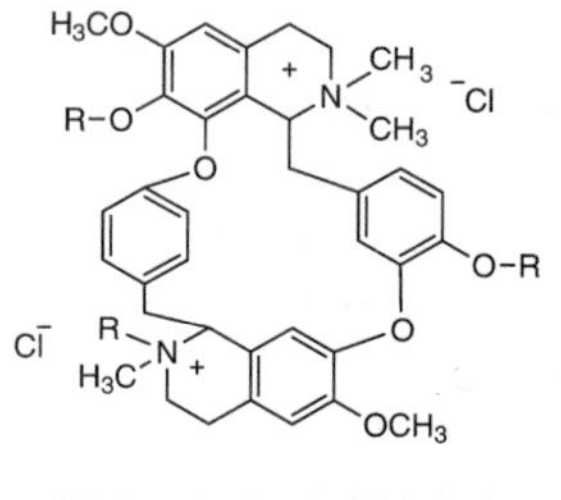

d-Tubocurarine iodide (R = H)
Metocurine iodide (R = CH₃)

Table 10.3. Properties of Clinically Useful Neuromuscular Blocking Agents

Agent	Time of Onset (min)	Duration of Action (min)	Mode of Elimination
Succinylcholine	1–1.5	6–8	Hydrolysis by plasma cholinesterases
d-Tubocurarine	4–6	80–120	Renal elimination, liver clearance
Vercuronium	2–4	30–40	Liver metabolism and clearance, renal elimination
Pancuronium	4–6	120–180	Renal elimination, liver metabolism and clearance
Pipecuronium	2–4	80–100	Renal elimination, liver metabolism and clearance
Rocuronium	1–2	30–40	Liver metabolism and clearance
Atracurium	2–4	30–40	Hofmann degradation, hydrolysis by plasma cholinesterases
Mivacurium	2–4	12–18	Hydrolysis by plasma cholinesterases
Doxacurium	4–6	90–120	Renal elimination, liver metabolism and clearance

Adapted from reference 24.

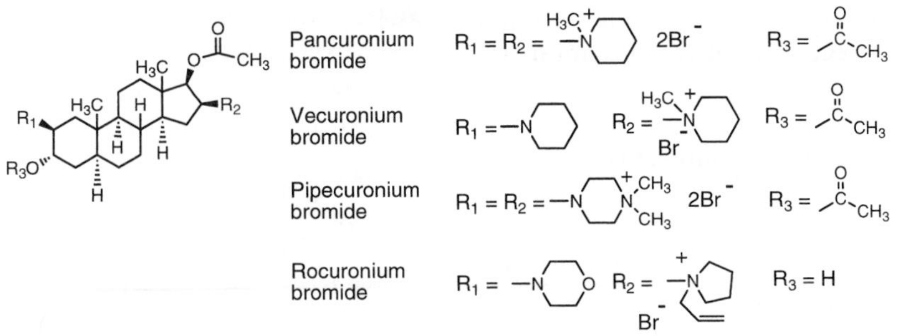

Fig. 10.19. Amino Steroid-based neuromuscular blocking agents.

tertiary amine. The various structures of these compounds serve primarily as a "scaffold" to position two positive charges in the correct three-dimensional orientation for interaction with the transmembrane nicotinic receptors.

d-Tubocurarine and Metocurine (Metubine iodide). The prototype of this class is d-tubocurarine. It is administered intravenously and has a relatively long duration of action. Only about 1% of a dose is demethylated in the liver and it is primarily excreted as unchanged drug in the urine and bile. Tubocurarine preparations contain bisulfites, and thus, may potentiate allergic reactions in patients with bisulfate allergy. It is the most potent inducer of histamine release of all the nondepolarizing neuromuscular blockers.

Reaction of d-tubocurarine with methyl iodide affords metocurine iodide (see structure on page 286), in which the two phenolic hydroxyl groups of tubocurarine are changed to the methyl ethers, and the tertiary amine becomes quaternary. This agent is about four times more potent than tubocurarine in neuromuscular blocking activity. Like tubocurarine it has a long duration of action and is eliminated (predominantly unchanged) via the kidney.

Steroid Based Neuromuscular Blocking Agents. An ideal neuromuscular blocking agent would be a nondepolarizing compound that is inactivated by metabolism and rapidly eliminated. Efforts to design the ideal neuromuscular blocker have resulted in development of several synthetic neuromuscular agents. Those that have found clinical use are either aminosteroids derived from (+) malouetine (an aminosteroid found in the rain forest of central Africa) (Fig. 10.19) or tetrahydroisoquinoline-based (Fig. 10.20).

Pancuronium (Pavulon). Pancuronium, a long acting agent, is more active than tubocurarine. It may cause increases in heart rate and blood pressure and should not be used in patients with coronary artery disease. Pancuronium undergoes hydrolysis in the liver to the active 3-hydroxy metabolite and the inactive 17-hydroxy and 3,17-dihydroxy metabolites and is primarily excreted in the urine with small amounts in the bile.

Vecuronium (Norcuron). Removal of the methyl group from the quaternary piperidine group at position number

three of pancuronium affords vecuronium, an intermediate-acting agent. Vecuronium has the advantage of not inducing histamine-release at normal doses and not exhibiting significant cardiovascular effects. One-third of an administered dose of vecuronium is hydrolyzed to the 3-hydroxy, 17-hydroxy, and 3,17-dihydroxy metabolites, all of which are active. Accumulation of the 3,17-dihydroxy metabolite is responsible for prolonged neuromuscular blockade in patients receiving long term therapy with vecuronium.

Pipecuronium bromide (Arduan). Pipecuronium bromide, a long-acting neuromuscular blocking agent, exhibits minimal cardiovascular effects. Like pancuronium and vecuronium, pipecuronium undergoes some hydrolysis but is primarily excreted unchanged in the urine with very small amounts in the bile. Pipecuronium may be used in patients with coronary artery disease, but neuromuscular blockade is prolonged in patients with renal failure.

Rocuronium Bromide (Zemuron). Rocuronium bromide is an intermediate-acting agent with a duration of action sim-

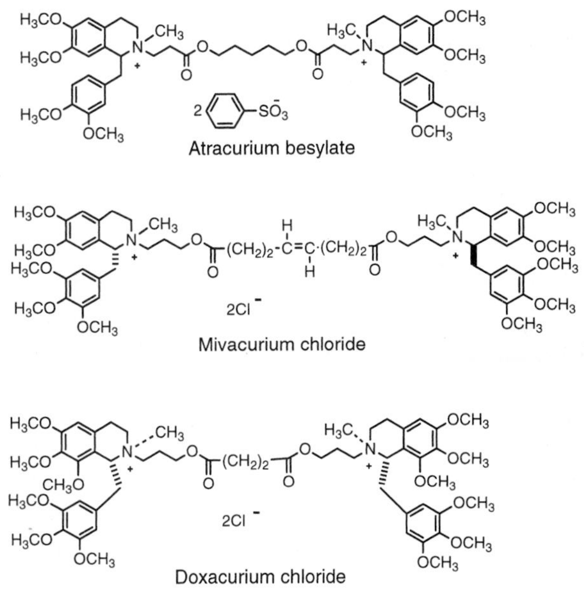

Fig. 10.20. Tetrahydroisoquinoline-based neuromuscular blocking agents.

ilar to vecuronium and atracurium, but with a more rapid onset. It does not appear to cause significant histamine release.

Tetrahydroisoquinoline Based Neuromuscular Blocking Agents

Atracurium Besylate (Tracrium [Glaxo Wellcome]). Atracurium besylate is a nondepolarizing neuromuscular blocker in which the quaternary ammonium groups are located in two substituted tetrahydroisoquinoline rings separated by an aliphatic diester. It has a duration of action slightly longer than that of succinylcholine. Atracurium is not metabolized in the liver, but undergoes hydrolysis of the ester functional groups that connect the two quaternary nitrogens. It also undergoes Hofmann elimination, a non-enzymatic base-catalyzed decomposition, to yield laudanosine which is inactive (Fig. 10.21) (49,50). Thus, termination of the effects of atracurium are independent of renal elimination. Because of this unusual metabolic profile, it is useful in patients with hepatic or renal disease.

Mivacurium Chloride (Mivacron) and Doxacurium (Nuromax). Mivacurium chloride, a short-acting neuromuscular blocking agent, and doxacurium, one of the longest acting agents, are structurally related to atracurium. However, unlike atracurium, they do not undergo Hofmann elimination. Mivacurium is rapidly hydrolyzed by plasma cholinesterases, while doxacurium appears to be only minimally metabolized and is primarily excreted unchanged by the kidneys.

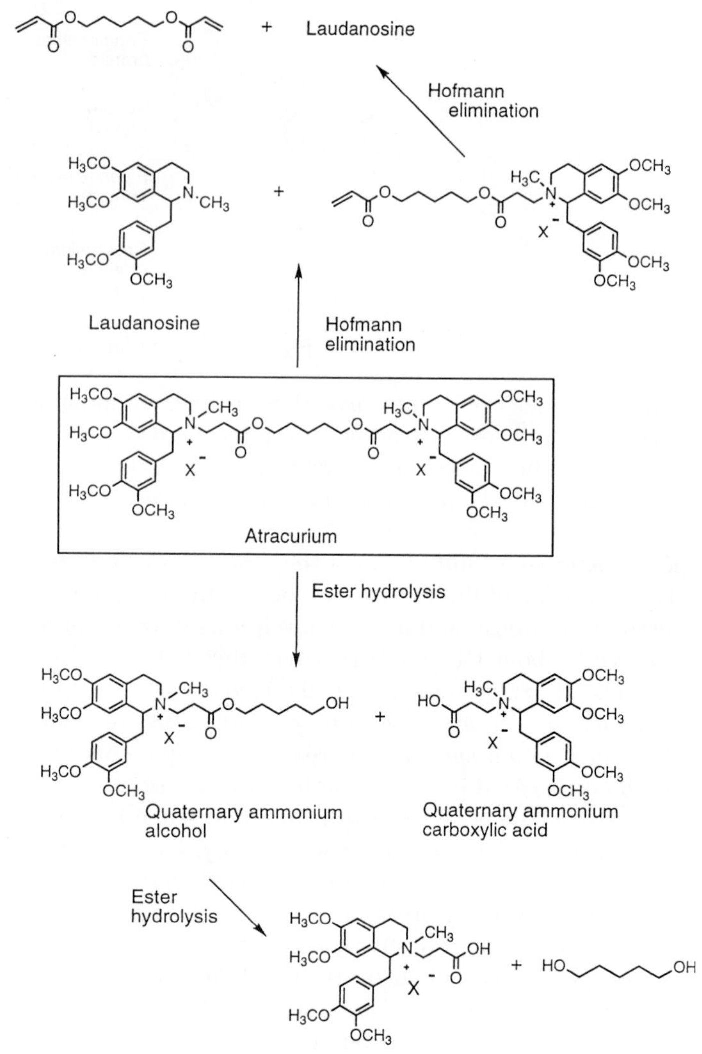

Fig. 10.21. Inactivation of atracurium by Hofmann elimination and hydrolysis.

CASE STUDY

Victoria F. Roche and S. William Zito

Dr. B. B. Orbius calls your pharmacy and requests your help in choosing a cholinesterase inhibitor. His patient, KR, is an 80-year-old, handicapped female residing in an assisted living facility. She is being treated for glaucoma with physostigmine sulfate (Eserine Sulfate, 1). The drug is being administered TID by her daughter, who, until recently, was working as an internet-based educator from her home one block away from the facility where KR resides. The daughter, in order to obtain healthcare insurance, has taken a job 25 miles from home at a community college as a full-time administrator. Because it will be difficult for KR's daughter to administer the noon dose of the medication and the assisted living facility staff will not take medication responsibility, a longer acting cholinesterase inhibitor is needed. Evaluate the structures given and make a suitable recommendation.

1. *Identify the therapeutic problem(s) where the pharmacist's intervention may benefit the patient.*

2. *Identify and prioritize the patient specific factors that must be considered to achieve the desired therapeutic outcomes.*

3. *Conduct a thorough and mechanistically oriented structure-activity analysis of all therapeutic alternatives provided in the case.*

4. *Evaluate the SAR findings against the patient specific factors and desired therapeutic outcomes and make a therapeutic decision.*

5. *Counsel your patient.*

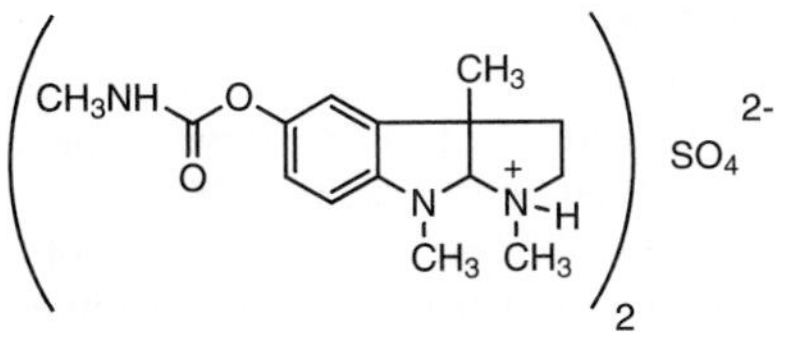

1 (Physostigmine)

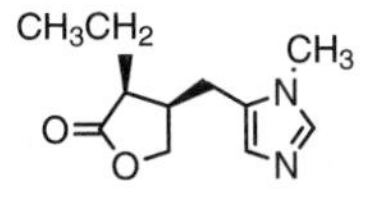

2

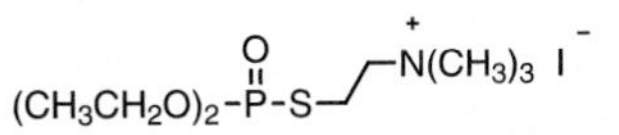

3

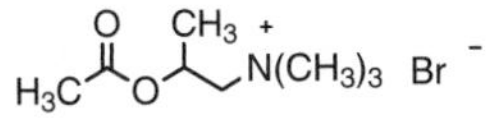

4

REFERENCES

1. Katzung BG. Introduction to autonomic pharmacology, In: Katzung BG, ed. Basic and Clinical Pharmacology, 7th ed. Norwalk, CT: Appleton & Lange, 1998.

2. Holmstedt G. Pages from the history of research on cholinergic mechanisms, In: Waser PG, ed. Cholinergic Mechanisms, New York: Raven Press, 1975, pp. 1–21.

3. Loewi O. Humoral transfer of heart action. Arch. Ges. Physiol., 1921;189:237–242.

4. Loewi O and Navratil E. Mechanism of the action of physostigmine and of ergotamine on vagus action. Arch. Ges. Physiol. 1926;214:689–696.

5. Tucek S. Choline acetyltransferase and synthesis of acetylcholine. In: Wittaker VP, ed. The Cholinergic Synapse, Handbook of Experimental Pharmacology, Berlin: Springer-Verlag, 1988.

6. Lefkowitz RJ, Hoffman BB, Taylor P. Neurotransmission: The autonomic and somatic motor nervous systems. In: Hardman JG, Limbird LE, Molinoff PB, et al, eds., Goodman and Gilman's The Pharmacological Basis of Therapeutics. 9th ed. New York: McGraw-Hill, 1996.

7. Pert CB, Snyder SH. Opiate receptor:demonstration in nervous tissue. Science 1973;179:1011–1114.

8. Changeaux JP, Devillers-Thiery A, Chemouilli P. Acetylcholine receptor: An allosteric protein. Science 1984;225:1335–1345.

9. Mishina M, et al. Expression of functional acetylcholine receptor from cloned cDNAs. Nature 1984;307:604–608.

10. Caulfield JP and Birdsall NJM. International Union of Pharmacology. XVII. Classification of Muscarinic Acetylcholine Receptors. Pharmacological Reviews 1998;50:279–290.

11. Lukas RJ, Bencherif M. Heterogeneity and regulation of nicotinic acetylcholine receptors. Int. Rev. Neurobiol. 1992;34:25–131.

12. Ing HR. The structure-action relationships of the choline group. Science 1949;109:264–266.

13. Lameh J, et al. Structure and function of G protein coupled receptors. Pharm. Res. 1990;7:1213–1221.

14. Drubbisch V, et al., Mapping the ligand binding pocket of the human muscarinic cholinergic receptor Hm1: contribution of tyrosine-82. Pharm. Res. 1992;9:1644–1647.

15. Dixon RAF, Strader CD, and Sigal IS. Structure and Function of G Protein-Coupled Receptors. Ann. Rep. Med. Chem. 1988;23:221–233.

16. Linder ME and Gilman AG. G Proteins Sci. Amer. 1992;267:56–65.

17. Ehlert FJ, Ostrom RS and Sawyer GW. Subtypes of the muscarinic receptor in smooth muscle. Life Sciences 1997;61:1729–1740.

18. Nordvall G and Hacksell U. Binding-site modeling of the muscarinic m1 receptor: A combination of Homology-based and indirect approaches. J. Med. Chem. 1993;36:967–976.

19. Humblet C and Mirzadegan T. Three-dimensional Models of G Protein-Coupled Receptors. Ann. Rep. Med. Chem. 1992;27:291–300.

20. Ross EM. Pharmacodynamics. Mechanisms of drug action and the relationship between drug concentation and effect. In: Hardman JG, Limbird LE, Molinoff PB, et al, eds., Goodman and Gilman's The Pharmacological Basis of Therapeutics. 9th ed. New York: McGraw-Hill, 1996.

21. Lindstrom J, et al. Neuronal nicotinic receptor subtypes. Ann. N. Y. Acad. Sci. 1995;757:100–116.

22. Changeux JP. The nicotinic acetylcholine receptor: an allosteric protein prototype if ligand-gated ion channels. Trends Pharmacol Sci., 1990;11:485–492.

23. Luyten WHML and Heinemann SG. Molecular cloning of the nicotinic acetylcholine receptor: New opportunities in drug design. Ann. Rep. Med. Chem. 1987;22:281–291.

24. Taylor P. Agents acting at the neuromuscular junction and autonomic ganglia. In: Hardman JG, Limbird LE, Molinoff PB, et al, eds., Goodman and Gilman's The Pharmacological Basis of Therapeutics. 9th ed. New York: McGraw-Hill, 1996.

25. Holladay MW, Dart MJ, Lynch JK. Neuronal nicotinic receptors as targets for drug discovery. J. Med. Chem. 1997;40:4170–4194.

26. Changeux JP. Chemical signaling in the brain. Scientific Amer. 1993;269:58–62.

27. Armstrong PD, Cannon JG, Long JP. Conformationally rigid analogues of acetylcholine. Nature 1968;220:65–66.

28. Ing HR, Kordik P, Williams DPHT. The structure-acton relationships of the choline group. Br. J. Pharmacol. 1952;7:103–116.

29. Welch AD, Roepke MH. A comparative study of choline and certain of its analogues I. The pharmacological activity of acetylphosphocholine and acetylarsenocholine relative to acetylcholine. J. Pharmacol. Exp. Ther. 1935;55:118–126.

30. Hotlon P, Ing HR. The specificity of the trimethylammonium group in acetylcholine. Br. J. Pharmacol. 1949;4:190–196.

31. Stehle RL, Melville KI, Oldham FK. Choline as a factor in the elaboration of adrenaline. J. Pharmacol. Exp. Ther. 1936;56:473–481.

32. Bodick NC, et al. Effects of xanomeline, a selective muscurinic receptor agonist, on cognitive function and behavioral symptoms in alzehimer disease. Arch. Neurology 1997;54:465–473.

33. John V, Lieberburg I, Thorsett ED. Alzheimer's disease: current therapeutic approaches. Ann Rep. Med Chem 1993;28:197–206.

34. Karczmar AG. Anticholinesterase agents: In: Raduoco-Thomas, C, ed. International Encyclopedia of Pharmacology and Therapeutics Section 13, Vol. 1, New York: Pergamon Press, 1970.

35. Sussman JL, et al. Atomic structure of acetylcholinesterase from Torpedo californca: a prototypic acetylcholine-binding protein. Science 1991;253:872–879.

36. Ordentlich A, et al. Dissection of the human acetylcholinesterase active center determinants of substrate specificity. Identification of residues constituting the anionic site, the hydrophobic site, and the acyl pocket. J. Biol. Chem. 1993;268:17083–17095.

37. Wilson IB, Harrison MA Ginsberg S. Carbamyl derivatives of acetylcholinesterase. J. Biol. Chem. 1961;236:1498–1500.

38. Shutske GM, et al. 9-Amino-1,2,3,4-tetrahydroacridin-1-ols: Synthesis and evaluation as potential alzheimer's disease therapeutics. J. Med. Chem. 1989;32:1805–1813.

39. Galatsis P. Market to Market–1997. Ann. Rep. Med Chem 1998;33:327–353.

40. Wilson IB, Ginsburg S. A powerful reactivator of alkylphosphate-inhibited acetylcholinesterase. Biochim. Biophys. Acta. 1955;18:168–170.

41. Wilson IB. Molecular complementarity and antidotes for alkyl phosphate poisoning. Fed. Proc. 1959;18:752–758.

42. Wilson IB. Acetylcholinesterase XI. Reversibility of tetraethylpyrophosphate inhibition. J. Biol. Chem.1951;190:111–117.

43. Hestrin S. Acetylation reactions mediated by purified acetylcholine esterase. J. Biol. Chem.1949;180:879–881.

44. Ariens EJ. Receptor theory and structure-activity relationships. Adv. Drug Res. 1966;3:235–285.

45. Mihm G, Wetzel B. Peripheral actons of selective muscarinic agonists and antagonists. Ann. Rep. Med. Chem. 1988;23:81–90.

46. McIntyre AR. History of curare, in Neuromuscular Blocking and Stimulating Agents. In: Cheymol J, ed. International Encyclopedia of Pharmacology and Therapeutics, Vol. 1, Sect. 14, Cheymol J, ed. Oxford: Pergamon Press 1972, pp. 187–203.

47. King H. Curarie alkaloids. I. Tubocurarine. J. Chem. Soc. 1935:1381–1389.

48. Everett AJ, Lowe AJ, Wilkinson S. Revision of the structures of (+)-tubocurarine chloride and (+)-chondrocurine. J. Chem. Soc. D 1970;16:1020–1021.

49. Stenlake JB, et al. Atracurium: condeption and inception. Br. J. Anaesth. 1983;55:3S-10S.

50. Basta SJ, et al. Clinical Pharmacology of atracurium besylate (BW33A): A new non-depolarizing muscle relaxnt. Anesth. Analg. 1983;61:723–729.

SUGGESTED READINGS

Belleau, B in Advances in Drug Research, Vol. 2, N. J. Harper and A. R. Simmons, Eds., New York, Academic Press, 1965, p. 143.
Cannon, JG. Cholinergics. In: Wolfe, ME, ed. Burger's Medicinal Chemistry, Vol. II, 5th ed. New York: John Wiley & Sons, 1996.
Rama Sastry, B.V. Anticholinergic Drugs. In: Wolfe, ME, ed. Burger's Medicinal Chemistry, Vol. II, 5th ed. New York: John Wiley & Sons, 1996.

11. Drugs Affecting Adrenergic Neurotransmission

ROBERT GRIFFITH

INTRODUCTION

Adrenergic drugs are a broad class of agents employed in the treatment of disorders of widely varying severity. Adrenergic drugs include popular prescription drugs such as albuterol for asthma and atenolol for hypertension (Table 11.1), as well as many common OTC cold remedies such as the nasal decongestant pseudoephedrine.

Adrenergic drugs act on effector cells through adrenoceptors that are normally activated by the neurotransmitter norepinephrine (noradrenaline), or they may act upon the neurons which release the neurotransmitter. The term adrenergic stems from the discovery early in the 20th century that administration of the hormone adrenaline (epinephrine) had specific effects on selected organs and tissues similar to the effects produced by stimulation of the sympathetic (adrenergic) nervous system (1). For a number of years adrenaline was thought to be the neurotransmitter in the sympathetic nervous system, but it was also recognized that the effects of administered epinephrine were not quite identical to sympathetic stimulation. Finally in the 1940s norepinephrine was identified as the true neurotransmitter at the terminus of the sympathetic nervous system (2). Today the terms adrenergic nervous system and sympathetic nervous system are generally used interchangeably.

Norepinephrins, R = H
Epinephrine, R = CH$_3$

Norepinephrine and epinephrine are members of a class of pharmacologically active substances known as catecholamines because they contain within their structures both an amine and *ortho*-dihydroxybenzene which is known by the common chemical name of catechol. Many adrenergic drugs are also catecholamines and their structure-activity-relationships (SAR) will be discussed.

From the spinal cord, neurons of the sympathetic nervous system do not connect directly to the affected tissues, but rather connect to a second set of neurons through a structure known as a ganglion. Thus the neurons leading from the spinal cord to the ganglia are known as preganglionic fibers and those leading from the ganglia to the innervated tissues are known as postganglionic fibers. The neurotransmitter between the preganglionic and postganglionic fibers is acetylcholine. The terminus of the postganglionic fiber releases norepinephrine to influence the

Table 11.1. Adrenergic Prescription Drugs in the Top 200

Drug	Application
albuterol (Ventolin)	bronchodilator
atenolol (Tenormin)	antihypertensive
metoprolol (Lopressor)	antihypertensive
propranolol (Inderal)	antihypertensive
clonidine (Catapress)	antihypertensive
terazosin (Hytrin)	antihypertensive, benign prostatic hyperplasia
nadolol (Corgard)	antihypertensive
labetolol (Normodyne)	antihypertensive
timolol (Timoptic)	glaucoma therapy
acebutolol (Sectral)	antihypertensive
methyldopa (Aldomet)	antihypertensive
levobunolol (Betagan)	glaucoma therapy
prazosin (Minipress)	antihypertensive

target tissue through binding to receptors on cells of the tissue or organ. The cells bearing the receptors are called effector cells since they produce the effect seen by sympathetic stimulation.

In general, stimulation of the sympathetic nervous system causes what is known as "fight or flight" responses. These effects include increased rate and force of heart contraction, a rise in blood pressure, a shift of blood flow to skeletal muscles, dilation of bronchioles and pupils, and an increase in blood glucose levels through gluconeogen-

History of the Sympathetic Nervous System

The term sympathetic nervous system is an anatomical description for a specific set of nerve fibers that dates from the time of the great physician Galen in the first century (3). Galen identified a set of nerve cords which were connected to, or "in sympathy with" certain internal organs. It was thought that these nerves were conduits for "humors" that flowed from the brain to the organs to which they were connected. Initially, the term sympathetic referred to the entire autonomic nervous system, but over time the nerves were divided into the sympathetic and parasympathetic nervous systems.

Early in the 20th Century investigators isolated from the adrenal cortex a substance that caused tissues to respond in the same manner as electrical stimulation of the Sympathetic Nervous System. The substance was initially called "sympathin," but later became known as adrenaline from its source in the adrenal cortex. Thus, adrenergic nervous system and sympathetic nervous system became synonymous terms.

292

esis and glycogenolysis. These responses are what one might predict in a mammal enraged and preparing to fight or in one frightened and preparing to flee. There are a variety of mechanisms of action through which drugs can influence adrenergic responses, and an understanding of these mechanisms requires knowledge of the details of norepinephrine biosynthesis, storage, release, and fate following release.

BIOSYNTHESIS, STORAGE, AND RELEASE OF NOREPINEPHRINE

Biosynthesis of norepinephrine takes place within adrenergic neurons near the terminus of the axon near the junction with the effector cell. The biosynthetic pathway (Fig. 11.1) begins with the active transport of the amino acid L-tyrosine into the adrenergic neuron cell (1). In the first step within the cytoplasm, the enzyme tyrosine hydroxylase (tyrosine-3-monooxygenase) oxidizes the 3' position of tyrosine to form the catechol-amino-acid L-dopa. This is the rate-limiting step in norepinephrine biosynthesis, and the activity of tyrosine hydroxylase is carefully controlled (4). The enzyme is under feedback inhibition control by product catecholamines and is controlled through a complex pattern of phosphorylation/dephosphorylation, in which phosphorylation by protein kinases activates the enzyme, and dephosphorylation by phosphatases decreases activity.

In the second step, L-dopa is decarboxylated to dopamine by aromatic-L-amino acid decarboxylase, another cytoplasmic enzyme. Aromatic-L-amino acid decarboxylase was discovered in the 1930s and originally named dopa decarboxylase. Researchers subsequently discovered that dopa decarboxylase is not specific for dopa and decarboxylates other aromatic amino acids having the L (or S) absolute configuration, such as 5-hydroxytryptophan, tryptophan, and tyrosine. Nevertheless the enzyme is still often referred to by the older name.

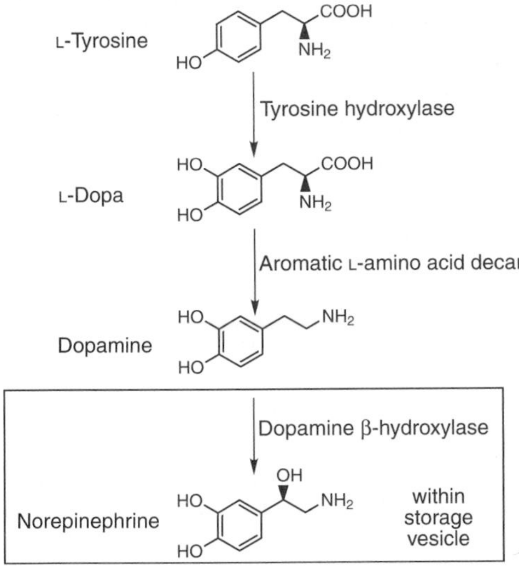

Fig. 11.1. Biosynthesis of norepinephrine.

The dopamine formed in the cytoplasm by decarboxylation of L-dopa is then taken up by active transport into storage vesicles or granules located near the terminus of the adrenergic neuron. Within these vesicles, the enzyme dopamine β-hydroxylase stereospecifically introduces a hydroxyl group in the R absolute configuration on the carbon atom beta to the amino group to generate the neurotransmitter norepinephrine. Norepinephrine is stored in the vesicles in a 4:1 complex with adenosine triphosphate (ATP) in such quantities that each vesicle in a peripheral adrenergic neuron contains between 6,000 and 15,000 molecules of norepinephrine (5). The norepinephrine remains in the vesicles until released into the synapse during signal transduction. When a wave of depolarization reaches the terminus of an adrenergic neuron, it triggers the transient opening of voltage-dependent calcium channels causing an influx of calcium ions. This influx of calcium ions triggers fusion of the storage vesicles with the neuronal cell membrane, spilling the norepinephrine and other contents of the vesicles into the synapse through exocytosis (Fig. 11.2). The pathway for epinephrine biosynthesis in the adrenal medulla is the same as for norepinephrine with the additional step of conversion of norepinephrine to epinephrine by the enzyme phenylethanolamine-N-methyltransferase.

REUPTAKE AND METABOLISM OF NOREPINEPHRINE FOLLOWING RELEASE

Following its release, norepinephrine diffuses through the intercellular space to bind reversibly to adrenoceptors (alpha or beta), on the effector cell, triggering a biochemical cascade that results in a physiologic response by the effector cell. In addition to the receptors on effector cells, there are also adrenoreceptors that respond to norepinephrine (α_2-receptors) on the presynaptic neuron, which, when stimulated by norepinephrine, act to inhibit the release of additional norepinephrine into the synapse. Once it has been released and is stimulating its various receptors, there must be mechanisms for removing the norepinephrine from the synapse and terminating the adrenergic impulse. By far the most important of these mechanisms for removing the norepinephrine is transmitter recycling through active transport uptake into the presynaptic neuron. This process, called uptake-1, is efficient, and in some tissues, up to 95% of released norepinephrine is likely removed from the synapse by this mechanism (6). Part of the norepinephrine taken into the presynaptic neuron by uptake-1 is metabolized to 3,4-dihydroxyphenylglycolaldehyde (DOPGAL) by mitochondrial monoamine oxidase (MAO) (see Fig. 11.3), and part of it is sequestered in the storage vesicles to be used again as neurotransmitter. A less efficient uptake process, uptake-2, operates in a variety of other cell types but only in the presence of high concentrations of norepinephrine. That portion of released norepinephrine which escapes uptake-1 diffuses out of the

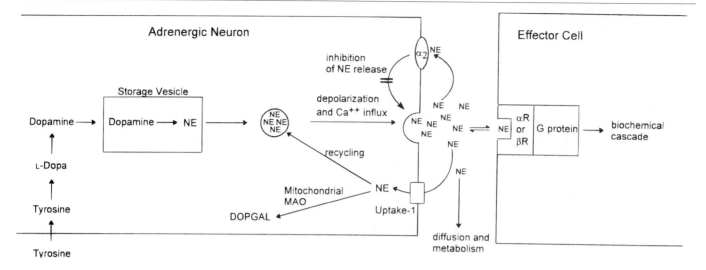

Fig. 11.2. Schematic of neurotransmission events in an adrenergic neuron and effector cell. NE, norepinephrine; αR, alpha adrenoceptor; βR, beta adrenoceptor; MAO, monoamine oxidase; DOPGAL, 3,4-dihydroxyphenylglycolaldehyde.

synapse and is metabolized in extraneuronal sites by catechol-O-methyltransferase, COMT, which methylates the meta hydroxyl group. Norepinephrine is also metabolized to DOPGAL by MAO present at extraneuronal sites, principally the liver and blood platelets. Both DOPGAL and normetanephrine are subject to further metabolism, as outlined in Figure 11.3 (7). These pathways are also important to drugs which are structural analogs of norepinephrine. In particular, drugs which are catechols are subject to metabolism by COMT and drugs with unsubstituted aliphatic amino groups are often substrates for MAO.

In summary (Fig. 11.3), following biosynthesis and storage in a vesicle, norepinephrine release into the synapse is triggered by depolarization-induced calcium influx. The norepinephrine in the synapse interacts with postsynaptic G protein-linked α- or β-receptors on the effector cell, triggering effector cell response, or with presynaptic α₂-receptors on the neuron, which inhibit release of more norepinephrine. Most of the synaptic neurotransmitter is taken back into the presynaptic neuron by uptake-1 active transport. Some of the norepinephrine is metabolized by monoamine oxidase and the remainder stored in a vesicle to be used again. That portion of norepinephrine not captured by uptake-1 diffuses out of the synapse and is metabolized by COMT and MAO.

CHARACTERIZATION OF ADRENERGIC RECEPTOR SUBTYPES

The discovery of subclasses of adrenergic receptors and the ability of relatively small molecule drugs to stimulate differentially or block these receptors represented a major advance in several areas of pharmacotherapeutics. Adrenergic receptors were subclassified by Ahlquist in 1948 into alpha and beta adrenoreceptor classes according to their responses to different adrenergic receptor agonists, principally norepinephrine, epinephrine, and isoproterenol (8).

These catecholamines are able to stimulate α-adrenoceptors in the descending order of potency epinephrine > norepinephrine > isoproterenol. In contrast, β-adrenoceptors are stimulated most potently by isoproterenol > epinephrine > norepinephrine.

Isoproterenol

In the years since Ahlquist's original classification, additional small molecule agonists and antagonists have been used to allow further subclassification of alpha and beta receptors into α_1 and α_2 subtypes of alpha receptors and β_1, β_2, and β_3 subtypes of beta adrenoceptors. The powerful tools of molecular biology have been used to clone and identify even more subtypes of alpha receptors for a total of six, three subtypes of α_1 and three subtypes of α_2 (9). This provides a wealth of information on the structures and biochemical properties of both alpha and beta receptors. Intensive research continues in this area, and the coming years may provide evidence of additional subtypes of both alpha and beta receptors. At this time, however, only the α_1, α_2, β_1, and β_2 receptor subtypes are sufficiently well differentiated by their small molecule binding characteristics to be considered clinically significant in pharmacotherapeutics.

The adrenoceptors, both alpha and beta, are members of a receptor superfamily of membrane-spanning proteins, including muscarinic, serotonin, and dopamine receptors, which are coupled to intracellular GTP-binding proteins (G proteins), which determine the cellular response to receptor activation (10). All of these receptors exhibit a common motif of a single polypeptide chain that is looped back and forth through the cell membrane seven times with an extracellular N-terminus and intracellular C-terminus. One of the most thoroughly studied of these receptors is the human β_2-adrenoreceptor (Fig. 11.4) (11). The seven transmembrane domains, TMD1–TMD7, are composed primarily of lipophilic amino acids arranged in α-helices connected by regions of hydrophilic amino acids. The hydrophilic regions form loops on the intracellular and extracellular faces of the membrane. In all of the adrenoceptors, the agonist/antagonist recognition site is located within the membrane-bound portion of the receptor. This binding site is within a pocket formed by the membrane spanning regions of the peptide, as illustrated in Figure 11.5 for epinephrine bound to the human β_2-receptor. All of the adrenoceptors are coupled to their effector systems through a G protein, which is linked through reversible binding interactions with the third intracellular loop of the receptor protein.

Salient features of the extensively studied β_2-adrenoreceptor are indicated in Figure 11.4. Binding studies with selectively mutated β_2-receptors have provided strong evidence for binding interactions between agonist functional groups and specific residues in the transmembrane domains of adrenoceptors. Such studies indicate that Asp_{113} in transmembrane domain 3, (TMD3), of the β_2-receptor is the acidic residue that forms a bond, presumably ionic or a salt bridge, with the positively charged amino group of catecholamine agonists. An aspartic acid residue is also found in a comparable position in all of the other adrenoceptors as well as other known G protein-coupled receptors that bind substrates having positively charged nitrogens in their structures. Elegant studies with mutated receptors and analogs of isoproterenol demonstrated that Ser_{204} and Ser_{207} of TMD5 are the residues that form hydrogen bonds with the catechol hydroxyls of β_2-agonists

(12). Furthermore, the evidence indicates that Ser_{204} interacts with the *meta* hydroxyl group of the ligand, whereas Ser_{207} interacts specifically with the *para* hydroxyl group. Serine residues are found in corresponding positions in the fifth transmembrane domain of the other known adrenoceptors. Evidence indicates that the phenylalanine residue of TMD6 is also involved in ligand-receptor bonding with the catechol ring. Studies such as these and others that indicated the presence of specific disulfide bridges between cysteine residues of the β_2-receptor led to the binding scheme shown in Figure 11.5.

Structural differences exist among the various adrenoceptors with regard to their primary structure, including the actual peptide sequence and length. Each of the adrenoceptors is encoded on a distinct gene, and this information was considered crucial to the proof that each adrenoreceptor is indeed distinct although related. The amino acids that make up the seven transmembrane regions are highly conserved among the various adrenoreceptors, but the hydrophilic portions are quite variable. The largest differences occur in the third intracellular loop connecting TMD5 and TMD6, which is the site of linkage between the receptor and its associated G protein. Compare the diagram of the β_2-receptor in Figure 11.4 with that of the α_2-receptor in Figure 11.6 (13).

Effector Mechanisms of Adrenergic Receptors

The receptors each are coupled through a G protein to effector mechanisms. Effector mechanisms are proteins that are able to translate the conformational change caused by activation of the receptor into a biochemical event within the cell. All of the beta adreno-

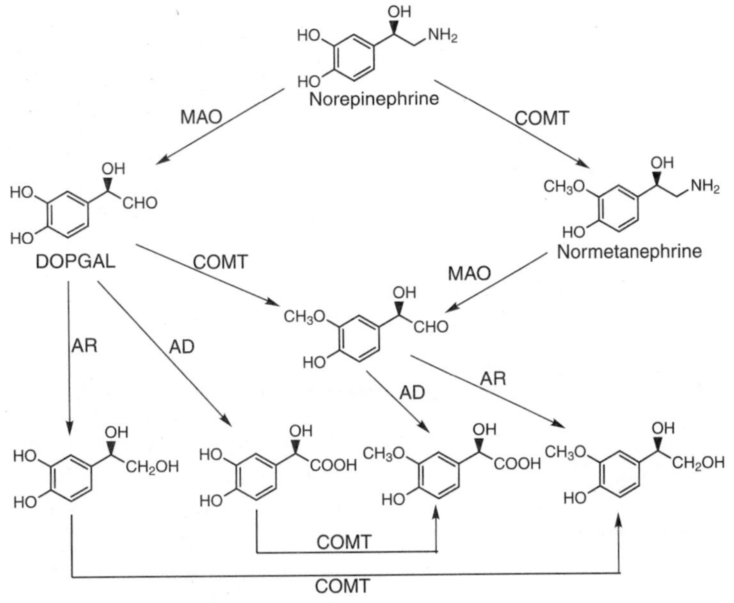

Fig. 11.3. Metabolism of norepinephrine. MAO, Monoamine oxidase; COMT, catechol-O-methyltransferase; AR, aldehyde reductase; AD, aldehyde dehydrogenase.

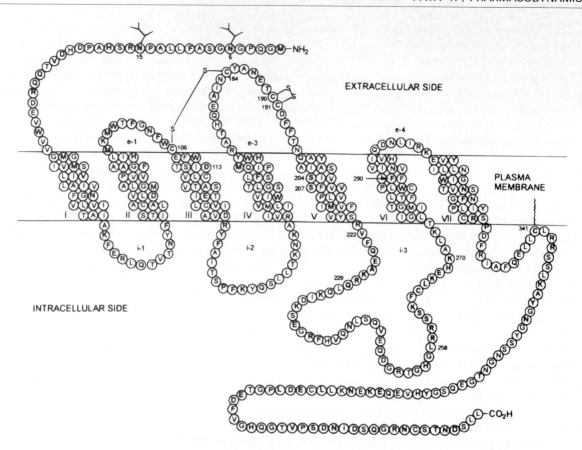

Fig. 11.4. Human β₂ adrenergic receptor. Amino acid sequence of the human β₂ receptor showing the seven transmembrane domains, I-VII, the connecting intracellular and extracellular loops, extracellular glycosylation sites at asparagines 6 and 15, and intrachain disulfide bonds between cysteines 106-184 and 190-191. Also indicated are the amino acids identified as participating in neurotransmitter binding—aspartate 113 in transmembrane domain III, which binds the positively charged amine of the neurotransmitter, and serines 204 and 207 of transmembrane domain V, which form H-bonds with the catechol hydroxyls. Phenylalanine 290 may also participate in agonist binding. Amino acids 222-229 and 258-270 of the third intracellular loop are critical for G protein-coupling, and palmitoylated cysteine 341 is critical for proper adenylyl cyclase activation. (Adapted from J. Ostrowski, et al., Annu. Rev. Pharmacol. Toxicol., 32, 167-183, [1992]).

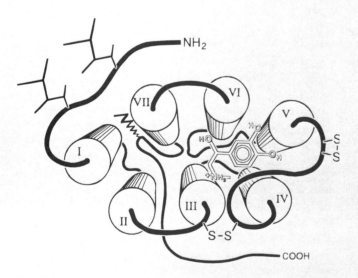

Fig. 11.5. Proposed arrangement for the transmembrane helices of the β₂-adrenergic receptor depicting the binding site for epinephrine as viewed from the extracellular side. (From J. Ostrowski, et al., Annu. Rev. Pharmacol. Toxicol., 32, 167-183 [1992]).

ceptors are coupled via specific G proteins (G_s) to the activation of adenylyl cyclase (14). Thus, when the receptor is stimulated by an agonist, adenylyl cyclase is activated to catalyze the formation of cyclic-adenosine monophosphate (cAMP) from ATP. cAMP, called a second messenger for the beta adrenoceptors, is known to function as a second messenger for a number of other receptor types. cAMP is considered a messenger because it can diffuse through the cell for at least short distances to modulate biochemical events remote from the synaptic cleft. Modulation of biochemical events by cAMP includes a phosphorylation cascade of other proteins. cAMP is rapidly deactivated by hydrolysis of the phosphodiester bond by the enzyme phosphodiesterase. The α_2-receptor may use more than one effector system depending on the location of the receptor. However, to date the best understood effector system of the α_2-receptor appears to be similar to that of the β-receptors except that linkage via a G protein (G_i) leads to inhibition of adenylyl cyclase instead of activation.

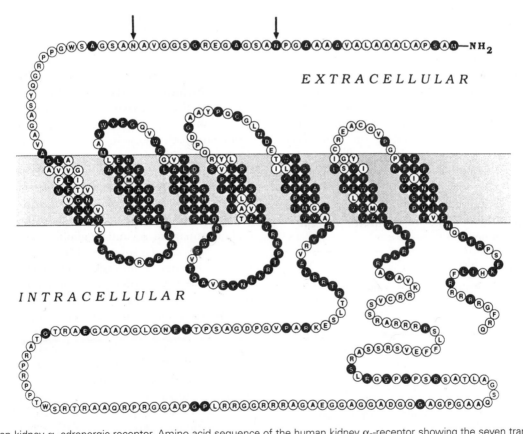

The α₁-adrenoreceptor is linked through yet another G protein to a complex series of events involving hydrolysis of polyphosphatidylinositol (15). The first event set in motion by activation of the α₁-receptor is activation of the enzyme phospholipase C. Phospholipase C catalyzes the hydrolysis of phosphatidylinositol-4,5-biphosphate (PIP₂). This hydrolysis yields two products, each of which has biologic activity as second messengers of the α₁-receptor. These are 1,2-diacylglycerol (DAG) and inositol-1,4,5-triphosphate (IP₃). IP₃ causes the release of calcium ions from intracellular storage sites in the endoplasmic reticulum resulting in an increase in free intracellular calcium levels. Increased free intracellular calcium is correlated with smooth muscle contraction. DAG is thought to activate cytosolic protein kinase C, which may induce slowly developing contractions of vascular smooth muscle. The end result of a complex series of protein interactions triggered by agonist binding to the α₁-receptor includes increased intracellular free calcium, which leads to smooth muscle contraction. When the smooth muscle innervated by α₁-receptors is in vascular walls, stimulation leads to vascular constriction.

Receptor Localization

The generalization made in the past about synaptic locations of adrenoreceptor subtypes was that all α₁, β₁, β₂, and β₃-receptors are postsynaptic receptors that are linked to stimulation of biochemical processes in the postsynaptic cell. However, presynaptic β-receptors are known to occur. The α₂-receptor has been traditionally viewed as a presynaptic receptor that resides on the outer membrane of the nerve terminus or presynaptic cell and reacts with released neurotransmitter. The α₂-receptor serves as a sensor and modulator of the quantity of neurotransmitter

Fig. 11.6. Human kidney α₂-adrenergic receptor. Amino acid sequence of the human kidney α₂-receptor showing the seven transmembrane domains and the connecting intracellular and extracellular loops. Note particularly the large third intracellular loop, which is the G protein binding site. The arrows point to the sites of glycosylation. Amino acids in black circles are those identical to the amino acids in the human platelet α₂-receptor. (From J. W. Regan, et al., Proc. Natl. Acad. Sci. USA, 85, 6301 [1988]).

present in the synapse at any given moment. Thus, during periods of rapid nerve firing and neurotransmitter release, the α_2-receptor is stimulated and causes an inhibition of further release of neurotransmitter. This is a well-characterized mechanism of modulation of neurotransmission, but not all α_2-receptors are presynaptic, and the physiologic significance of postsynaptic α_2-receptors is less well understood (16).

THERAPEUTIC RELEVANCE OF ADRENERGIC RECEPTOR SUBTYPES

The clinical utility of receptor-selective drugs becomes obvious when one considers the adrenoreceptor subtypes and effector responses of only a few organs and tissues innervated by the sympathetic nervous system. The major adrenoceptor subtypes are listed in Table 11.2. For example, the predominant response to adrenergic stimulation of smooth muscle of the peripheral vasculature is constriction causing a rise in blood pressure. Because this response is mediated through α_1-receptors, an α_1-antagonist would be expected to cause relaxation of the blood vessels and a drop in blood pressure with clear implications for treating hypertension. A smaller number of β-receptors on vascular smooth muscle mediate arterial dilation, particularly to skeletal muscle, and a few antihypertensives act through stimulation of these β_1-receptors. Adrenergic stimulation of the lungs causes smooth muscle relaxation and bronchodilation mediated through β_2-receptors. Drugs acting as β_2-agonists are useful for alleviating respiratory distress in persons with asthma or other obstructive pulmonary diseases. Activation of β_2-receptors in the uterus also causes muscle relaxation, and so some β_2-agonists are used to inhibit uterine contractions in premature labor. Adrenergic stimulation of the heart causes an increase in rate and force of contraction, which is mediated primarily by β_1-receptors. Drugs with β-blocking activity slow the heart rate and decrease the force of con-

traction. These drugs have utility in treating hypertension, angina, and certain cardiac arrhythmias.

From the preceding discussions of the biosynthesis, storage, release, and fate of norepinephrine, one can readily conceive of a number of possible sites of drug action for adrenergic drugs. As mentioned, there are drugs that act directly on the receptors as agonists and antagonists, drugs that affect storage and release from vesicles, drugs that affect neurotransmitter biosynthesis, and drugs that affect uptake and catabolism of norepinephrine and epinephrine. These categories are discussed in turn. Most adrenergic drugs fit into well-defined classes with readily defined structure-activity relationships (SAR), but a few adrenergic drugs do not permit such straightforward structural definition of their activity. We begin with a discussion of phenylethanolamine (or phenethanolamine) agonists, which do have reasonably clear SAR. Although many of these drugs directly stimulate adrenoceptors, others exhibit what is termed indirect activity. Indirect agonists do not directly bind to and activate adrenergic receptors, but rather, they are taken up into the presynaptic neuron, where they cause the release of norepinephrine, which can diffuse into the receptor causing the observed response. Mixed acting drugs have both a direct and an indirect component to their action, and the relative amount of direct versus indirect activity for a given drug varies considerably with its chemical structure, the tissue preparation examined and experimental animal species.

STRUCTURE-ACTIVITY RELATIONSHIPS OF ADRENERGIC AGONISTS
Phenylethanolamine Agonists

The structures of many clinically useful phenylethanolamine-type adrenergic agonists are summarized in Table 11.3. Agents of this type have been extensively studied over the years since the discovery of the naturally occurring prototypes, epinephrine and norepinephrine, and the structural requirements and tolerances for substitutions at each of the indicated positions have been established (2). In general, a primary or secondary aliphatic amine separated by two carbons from a substituted benzene ring is minimally required for high agonist activity in this class. Because of the basic amino groups, pKa range approximately 8.5 to 10, all of these agents are highly positively charged at physiologic pH. By definition agents in this class have a hydroxyl group on C1 of the side chain, β to the amine, as in epinephrine and norepinephrine. This hydroxyl-substituted carbon must be in the R absolute configuration for maximal direct activity as in the natural neurotransmitter, although most drugs are currently sold as mixtures of both (R) and (S) stereoisomers at this position (racemates). Given these features in common, the nature of the other substituents determines receptor selectivity and duration of action. In the following discussions, keep in mind that saying a drug is selective for a given receptor does not mean it has no activity

Table 11.2. Selected Tissue Responses to Stimulation of Adrenoceptor Subtypes

Organ Response	Major Receptor Type	Response
Arterioles, vascular smooth muscle	α_1, α_2	Constriction
	β_2	Dilation
Eye (radial muscle)	α_1	Contraction (pupillary dilation)
Fat cells	α_1, β_3	Lipolysis
Heart	β_1	Increased rate and force Increased conduction velocity
Intestine	α_1, β_2	Decreased motility
Liver	α_1, β_2	Increased gluconeogenesis and glycogenolysis
Lungs	β_2	Relaxation (bronchial dilation)
Uterus	α_1	Contraction (pregnant uterus)
	β_2	Relaxation

Table 11.3. Phenylethanolamine Adrenergic Agonists

Drug	R_1	R_2	R_3	Receptor Activity
Norepinephrine	H	H	3',4'-diOH	$\alpha_1, \alpha_2, \beta_1$
Epinephrine	CH_3	H	3',4'-diOH	$\beta_2 > \alpha, \alpha_2, \beta_1$
α-Methylnorepinephrine	H	CH_3	3',4'-diOH	$\alpha_2 > \alpha_1$
Ethylnorepinephrine	H	CH_2CH_3	3',4'-diOH	$\beta > \alpha$
Isoproterenol	$CH(CH_3)_2$	H	3',4'-diOH	$\beta_1 + \beta_2$
Isoetharine	$CH(CH_3)_2$	CH_2CH_3	3',4'-diOH	$\beta_2 > \beta_1$
Colterol	$C(CH_3)_3$	H	3',4'-diOH	$\beta_2 > \beta_1$
Metaproterenol	$CH(CH_3)_2$	H	3',5'-diOH	$\beta_2 > \beta_1$
Terbutaline	$C(CH_3)_3$	H	3',5'-diOH	$\beta_2 > \beta_1$
Albuterol	$C(CH_3)_3$	H	3'-CH_2OH, 4'-OH	$\beta_2 > \beta_1$
Phenylephrine	CH_3	H	3'-OH	α_1
Metaraminol	H	CH_3	3'-OH	α_1
Methoxamine	H	CH_3	2',5'-diOCH$_3$	α_1
Ephedrine,	CH_3	CH_3	H	$\alpha_1, \alpha_2, \beta_2$
Pseudoephedrine	CH_3	CH_3	H	0
Phenylpropanolamine	H	CH_3	H	0

at other receptors and that the clinically observed degree of selectivity is frequently dose-dependent.

R^1, Substitution on the Amino Nitrogen

We have already seen that as R^1 is increased in size from hydrogen in norepinephrine to methyl in epinephrine to isopropyl in isoproterenol, activity at α-receptors decreases, and activity at β-receptors increases. These compounds were used to define alpha and beta activity long before receptor proteins could be isolated and characterized. The activity at both α and β-receptors is maximal when R^1 is methyl as in epinephrine, but α-agonist activity is dramatically decreased when R^1 is larger than methyl and is negligible when R^1 is isopropyl as in isoproterenol, leaving only β-activity. In fact, the β-activity of isoproterenol is actually enhanced over norepinephrine and epinephrine. Presumably, the β-receptor has a large lipophilic binding pocket adjacent to the amine-binding aspartic acid residue, which is absent in the α-receptor. As R^1 becomes larger than butyl, affinity for α_1-receptors returns, but not intrinsic activity, which means large lipophilic groups can afford compounds with α_1-blocking activity, (e.g., see labetalol under mixed α/β-antagonists p. 309). In addition, the N-substituent can also provide selectivity for different β-receptors, with a t-butyl group affording selectivity for β_2-receptors. For example, with all other features of the molecules being constant, colterol is a selective β_2-agonist, whereas isoproterenol is a non-selective β-agonist. When considering use as a bronchodilator, a non-selective β-agonist such as isoproterenol has undesirable cardiac stimulatory properties owing to its β_1-activity that are greatly diminished in a selective β_2-agonist.

R^2, Substitution α to the Basic Nitrogen, Carbon-2

Small alkyl groups, methyl or ethyl, may be present on the carbon adjacent to the amino nitrogen, carbon-2 in Table 11.3. Such substitution slows metabolism by monoamine oxidase (MAO) but has little overall effect on duration of action in catecholamines because they remain substrates for catechol-O-methyltransferase (COMT). Resistance to MAO activity is more important in noncatechol indirect acting phenylethylamines. An ethyl group in this position diminishes α-activity far more than β-activity, affording compounds with β-selectivity such as ethylnorepinephrine. Substitution on this carbon also introduces another asymmetric center into these molecules producing pairs of diastereomers, which can have significantly different biologic and chemical properties. For example, maximal direct activity in the stereoisomers of α-methylnorepinephrine resides with the *erythro* stereoisomer with the

α–Methylnorepinephrine
direct acting stereoisomer

1R,2S absolute configuration (17). The configuration of C2 has a great influence on receptor binding because the 1R,2R diastereomer of α-methylnorepinephrine has primarily indirect activity even though the absolute configuration of the hydroxyl-bearing C1 is the same as in norepinephrine. In addition, with respect to α-activity, this additional methyl group makes the direct acting 1R,2S stereoisomer of α-methylnorepinephrine more selective for α_2-adrenoceptors than for α_1-adrenoceptors. This has important consequences in the anti-hypertensive activity of α-methyldopa, which is discussed later and in Chapter 24. The same stereochemical relationships hold for metaraminol and other phenylethanolamines, in which stereochemical properties have been investigated.

R³, Substitution on the Aromatic Ring

The natural 3,'4'-dihydroxy substituted benzene ring present in norepinephrine provides excellent receptor activity for both α and β-sites, but such catechol-containing compounds have poor oral activity because they are hydrophilic and rapidly metabolized by COMT. Alternative substitutions have been found that retain good activity but are more resistant to COMT metabolism. In particular, 3,'5'-dihydroxy compounds are not good substrates for COMT and, in addition, provide selectivity for β₂-receptors. Thus, because of its ring substitution pattern, metaproterenol is an orally active bronchodilator having little of the cardiac stimulatory properties possessed by isoproterenol.

Other substitutions are possible that enhance oral activity and provide selective β₂ activity, such as the 3'-hydroxymethyl, 4'-hydroxy substitution pattern of albuterol, which is also resistant to COMT. At least one of the groups must be capable of forming hydrogen bonds, and if there is only one, it should be at the 4' position to retain β-activity. For example, ritodrine has only a 4'-OH for R³, yet retains good β activity with the large substituent on the nitrogen making it β₂ selective.

Ritodrine

If R³ is only a 3'-OH, however, activity is reduced at α sites and almost eliminated at β sites, thus affording selective α agonists such as phenylephrine and metaraminol. Further indication that α sites have a wider range of substituent tolerance for agonist activity is shown by the 2,'5'-dimethoxy substitution of methoxamine, which is a selective α-agonist that also has β-blocking activity at high concentrations.

Phenylephrine   Metaraminol   Methoxamine

When the phenyl ring has no phenolic substituents, i.e., R³=H, these phenylethanolamines may have both direct and indirect activity. Direct activity (i.e., agonist) is the stimulation of an adrenoceptor by the drug itself while indirect activity is the result of displacement of norepinephrine from its storage granules or reuptake inhibition re-

sulting in non-selective stimulation of the adrenoceptors by the displaced norepinephrine. Since norepinephrine stimulates both α and β₁-adrenoceptors, indirect activity cannot be selective. Stereochemistry of the various substituents may also play a role.

For example ephedrine and pseudoephedrine have the same substitution pattern, but substitution of both carbons 1 and 2 means there are four possible stereoisomers. Racemic (±) ephedrine is a mixture of the *erythro* enantiomers 1R,2S and 1S,2R, whereas the *threo* pair of enantiomers, 1R,2R and 1S,2S, are known as racemic pseudoephedrine (ψ-ephedrine). As discussed for α-methylnorepinephrine, (−) ephedrine is the naturally occurring stereoisomer and has the 1R,2S absolute configuration with a mixed direct activity on both α and β receptors, and some indirect activity. Its 1S,2R (+) enantiomer exhibits primarily indirect activity. 1S,2S (+) Pseudoephedrine has virtually no direct receptor activity but is mostly indirectly acting.

(1R:2S)   Ephedrine   (1S:2R)

(1R:2R)   (1S:2S)

Pseudoephedrine

Norepinephrine and Epinephrine

Norepinephrine has limited clinical application because of the nonselective nature of its action, which causes both vasoconstriction and cardiac stimulation. In addition it must be given intravenously because it has no oral activity (poor oral bioavailability) as a result of its rapid metabolism by intestinal and liver COMT and MAO, and low lipophilicity. Rapid metabolism limits its duration of action to only 1 or 2 minutes even when given by infusion. The drug is used to counteract various hypotensive crises because its α activity raises blood pressure and as an adjunct treatment in cardiac arrest where its β activity stimulates the heart.

Epinephrine is far more widely used clinically than norepinephrine, although it also lacks oral activity for the same reasons as norepinephrine. Epinephrine, similar to norepinephrine, is used to treat hypotensive crises and, because of its greater β-activity, is used to stimulate the heart in cardiac arrest. Epinephrine's β₂ activity leads to its administration intravenously and in inhalers to relieve bronchoconstriction in asthma and to application in inhibiting uterine contractions. Because it has significant α activity, epinephrine had been used in nasal decongestants. Constriction of dilated blood vessels in mucous membranes shrinks the membranes and reduces nasal congestion although significant after-congestion may limit its utility.

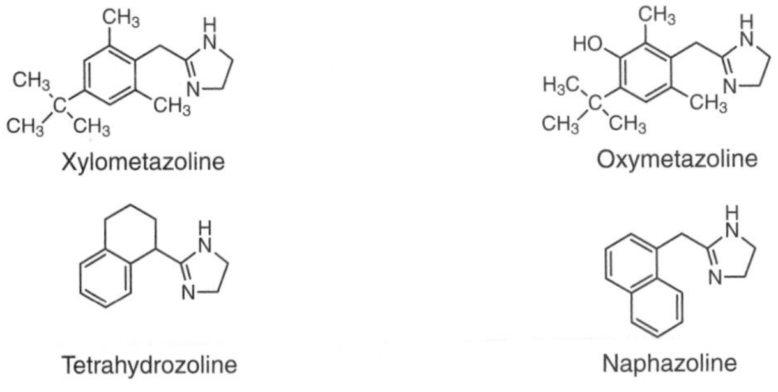

Fig. 11.7. Imidazoline α₁-adrenergic agonists.

Table 11.4. Imidazoline α₁-Agonists in OTC Vasoconstrictors

Drug	Nasal Decongestant	Eye Drops
xylometazoline	Otrivin, Inspire	na
oxymetazoline	Afrin, Duration, Neo-synephrine, Vicks Sinex	Visine L.R. Ocu Clear
tetrahydrozoline	na	Murine, Visine, Soothe
naphazoline	4-Way Fast Acting, Privine	Naphcon, Clear Eyes

α-Adrenergic Agonists

α₁-Agonist Phenylethanolamines—Metaraminol, Methoxamine and Phenylephrine

Metaraminol and methoxamine are selective for α₁-receptors and have little cardiac stimulatory properties. Because they are not substrates for COMT, their duration of action is significantly longer than norepinephrine, but their primary use is limited to treating hypotension during surgery or shock. Methoxamine is bioactivated by O-demethylation to an active m-phenolic metabolite. The β-blocking activity of methoxamine, which is seen at high concentrations, affords some use in treating tachycardia. Phenylephrine, is also a selective α₁-agonist, used similarly to metaraminol and methoxamine for hypotension. It also has widespread use as a nonprescription nasal decongestant in both oral and topical preparations. Its oral bioavailability is <10%. Phenylephrine preparations applied topically to the eye constricts the dilated blood vessels of bloodshot eyes and in higher concentrations are used to dilate the pupil during eye surgery.

2-Arylimidazoline α₁-Agonists

Although nearly all β-agonists are phenylethanolamine derivatives, α-receptors accommodate a more diverse assortment of structures. The imidazoline derivatives in Figure 11.7 are selective α₁-agonists and therefore vasoconstrictors/vasopressors. They all contain a one-carbon bridge between C-2 of the imidazoline ring (pKa 10-11) and a phenyl substituent, and therefore the general skeleton of a phenylethylamine is contained within the structures. Lipophilic substitution on the phenyl ring ortho to the methylene bridge appears to be required for agonist activity at α₁- and α₂-receptors (15). Presumably the bulky lipophilic groups attached to the phenyl ring at the meta or para positions provide selectivity for the α₁-receptor by diminishing affinity for α₂-receptors. These compounds are widely used only in topical preparations as nasal de-

congestants and eye drops some of which are listed in Table 11.4.

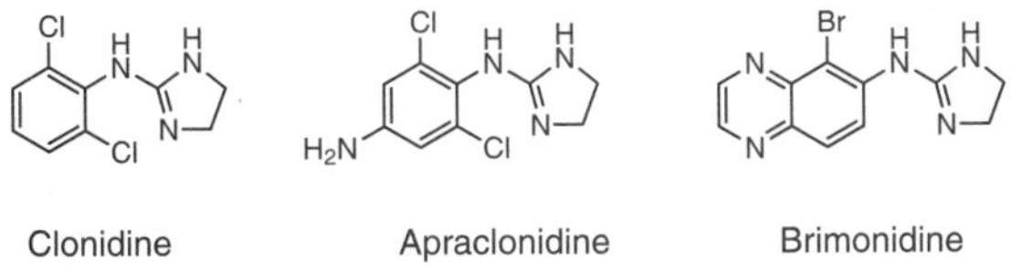

α₂-Adrenergic Agonists—2-Aminoimidazolines and Other α₂-Agonists

Clonidine. Closely related structurally to the imidazoline nasal decongestants is clonidine and other more recently developed analogs (Fig. 11.8). Clonidine was originally synthesized as a vasoconstricting nasal decongestant but in early clinical trials was found to have dramatic hypotensive effects in contrast to all expectations for a vasoconstrictor (22) (Chapter 24). Subsequent pharmacologic investigations showed not only that clonidine does have some α₁-agonist (vasoconstrictive) properties in the periphery, but also that clonidine is a powerful agonist at α₂-adrenoceptors and non-adrenergic imidazoline (I₁) receptors in the central nervous system. Through the use of imidazoline and α2-adrenoceptor antagonists, non-adrenergic imidazoline receptors have recently been discovered to be involved in central nervous system control of blood pressure (I₁-receptor) (Chapter 24). Because of its peripheral activity on extra-neuronal vascular postsynaptic α₁-receptors, initial doses of clonidine may produce a transient vasoconstriction and an increase in blood pressure that is soon overcome by vasodilation as clonidine penetrates the blood-brain barrier and interacts with central nervous system α₂-receptors.

Similar to the imidazoline α₁-agonists, clonidine has lipophilic ortho substituents on the phenyl ring. The o-chlorine groups afford better activity than o-methyl groups at α₂ sites. The most readily apparent difference between clonidine and the α₁-agonists in Figure 11.7, is the replacement of the CH₂ bridge on C-1 of the imidazoline by an amine NH. This makes the imidazoline ring part of a guanidino group, and the uncharged form of clonidine exists as a pair of tautomers as shown.

Clonidine has a pKa of 8.3 and is about 80% ionized at physiologic pH. The positive charge is shared through resonance by all three nitrogens of the guanidino group.

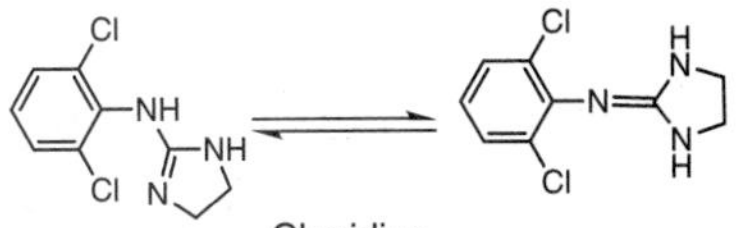

Clonidine   Apraclonidine   Brimonidine

Fig. 11.8. Imidazoline α₂-adrenergic agonists.

Clonidine

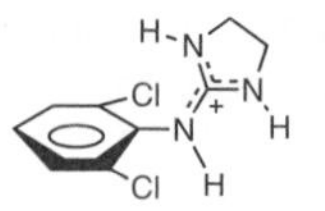

Fig. 11.9. Protonated clonidine.

Steric crowding by the bulky ortho chlorine groups does not permit a coplanar conformation of the two rings, as illustrated in Figure 11.9.

Apraclonidine, Brimonidine.   The other imidazoline α_2-agonists in Figure 11.8 are in clinical use, but not as antihypertensives. Apraclonidine (pKa 9.22) and brimonidine are selective α_2-agonists employed topically in the treatment of glaucoma. Stimulation of α_2-receptors in the eye reduces production of aqueous humor and enhances outflow of aqueous humor thus reducing intra-ocular pressure. Brimonidine is substantially more selective for α_2-receptors, than are clonidine or apraclonidine. Although both are applied topically to the eye, measurable quantities of these drugs are detectable in plasma so caution must be employed when cardiovascular agents are also being taken by the patient.

Guanfacine, Guanabenz.   Following the discovery of clonidine, extensive research into the SAR of central α_2-agonists showed that the imidazoline ring was not necessary for activity in this class, but the phenyl ring required at least one ortho chlorine or methyl group. Two clinically useful anti-hypertensive agents resulting from this effort are guanfacine and guanabenz (Chapter 24). These are ring-opened analogs of clonidine, and their mechanism of action is the same as that of clonidine.

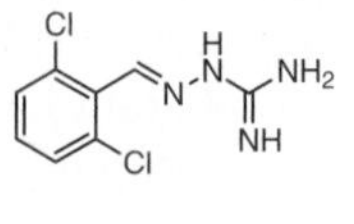

Guanabenz 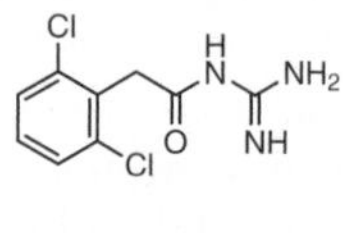   Guanfacine

Methyldopa.   Although it is structurally unrelated to clonidine, guanabenz or guanfacine, the pro-drug L-α-methyldopa (methyldopa) is another antihypertensive α_2-agonist acting in the central nervous system via its active metabolite, α-methylnorepinephrine (Fig. 11.10). Methyldopa is transported across the blood-brain barrier, where it is decarboxylated by aromatic L-amino acid decarboxylase to α-methyldopamine, which is stereospecifically hydroxylated to 1R,2S-α-methylnorepinephrine. As mentioned previously, this stereoisomer is an α_2-agonist and acts as an antihypertensive agent much like clonidine to inhibit sympathetic neural output from the central nervous system, thus lowering blood pressure. α-Methylnorepinephrine and α-methyldopamine do not cross the blood-brain barrier because of their hydrophilicity. Originally synthesized as a norepinephrine biosynthesis inhibitor (23), methyl-

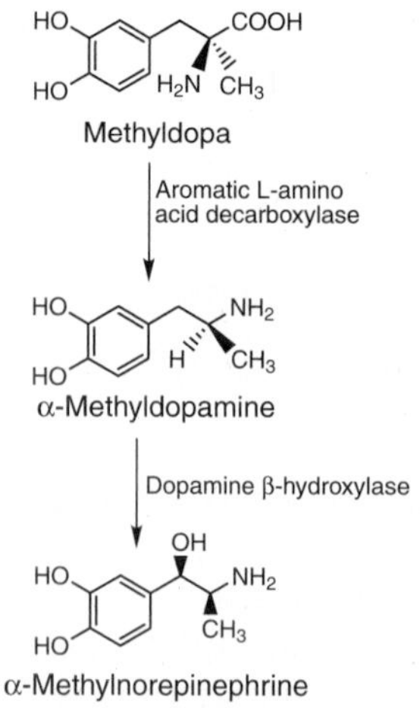

Fig. 11.10. Methyldopa bioactivation.

dopa was thought to act through a combination of inhibition of norepinephrine biosynthesis through dopa decarboxylase inhibition and metabolic decarboxylation to generate α-methylnorepinephrine. The latter was thought to replace norepinephrine in the nerve terminal and, when released, have less intrinsic activity than the natural neurotransmitter. This latter mechanism is an example of the concept of a false neurotransmitter. The antihypertensive mechanism for methyldopa, however, has since been shown to be due to α_2-agonist activity of its metabolite in the central nervous system (Chapter 24).

β-Adreneric Agonists
β_2-Agonist Phenylethanolamines

Most of the β-selective adrenergic agonists listed in Table 11.3 are used primarily as bronchodilators in asthma and other constrictive pulmonary conditions. Their pharmacologic and pharmacokinetic properties are described in Table 11.5. Isoproterenol is a non-selective β-agonist, and the cardiac stimulation caused by its β_1-activity and its lack of oral activity have led to its diminished use in favor of selective β_2-agonists.

Albuterol, Pirbuterol, Terbutaline.   Noncatechol selective β_2-agonists, such as albuterol, metaproterenol, and terbutaline, are available in oral dosage forms as well as in inhalers. All have similar activities and durations of action. Pirbuterol is an interesting analog of albuterol in which

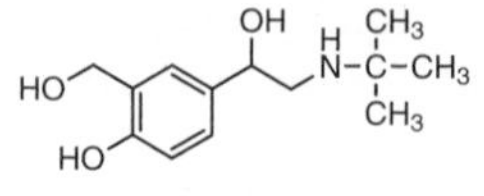

Albuterol

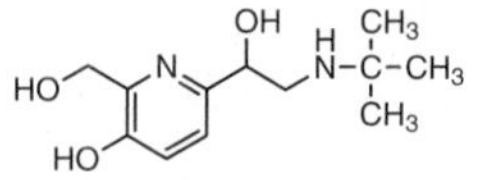

Pirbuterol

Table 11.5. Pharmacologic Effects and Pharmacokinetic Properties of Sympathomimetic Bronchodilators

Sympathomimetic	Adrenergic Receptor Activity	β_2 Potency[1]	Route	Onset (min)	Duration (hr)
Salmeterol[2] (Serevent)	$\beta_1 << \beta_2$	0.5	Inh	within 20	12
Albuterol[2] (Ventolin, Airet, Proventil)	$\beta_1 << \beta_2$	2	PO Inh[3]	within 30 within 5	4–8 3–6
Levalbuterol R-albuterol (Xopenex)	$\beta_1 <<< \beta_2$	3–4	Inh[3]	within 5	3–6
Bitolterol[2] (Tornalate)	$\beta_1 < \beta_2$	5	Inh	2–4	5–8
Isoetharine[2]	$\beta_1 < \beta_2$	6	Inh[3]	within 5	2–3
Metaproterenol[2] (Alupent)	$\beta_1 < \beta_2$	15	PO Inh[3]	≈30 5–30	4 1–6
Pirbuterol[2] (Maxair)	$\beta_1 < \beta_2$	5	Inh	within 5	5
Terbutaline[2] (Bricanyl, Brethine, Brethaire)	$\beta_1 < \beta_2$	4	PO SC	30 5–15	4–8 1.5–4
Isoproterenol (Isuprel, Medihaler-Iso)	$\beta_1 = \beta_2$	1	Inh IV Inh[3]	5–30 immediate 2–5	3–6 <1 1–3
Ephedrine	α β_1 β_2	—	PO SC IM IV	15–60 >20 10–20 immediate	3–5 ≤1 ≤1 —
Epinephrine (Adrenalin)	α β_1 β_2	—	SC IM Inh[3]	5–10 — 1–5	4–6 1–4 1–3

[1]Relative molar potency: 1 = most potent.
[2]These agents all have minor β_1 activity.
[3]May be administered via aerosol or bulb nebulizer or IPPB administration.
Table modified from Drug Facts and Comparisons 2000.

the benzene ring has been replaced by a pyridine ring. Similar to albuterol, pirbuterol is a selective β_2-agonist currently available only for administration by inhalation.

Bitolterol. Bitolterol is a prodrug form of colterol in which the catechol hydroxyl groups have been converted to 4-methylbenzoic (p-toloyl) acid esters, providing increased lipid solubility and prolonged duration of action. Bitolterol is administered by inhalation, and the ester groups are hydrolyzed by esterases to liberate the active drug, colterol. Colterol is then subject to metabolism by COMT, but the duration of action of a single dose of the produg bitolterol, up to 8 hours, is twice that of a single dose of colterol, permitting less frequent administration and greater convenience to the patient.

Salmeterol. A more recently developed selective β_2-agonist with an extended duration of action is salmeterol. Salmeterol has the same phenyl ring substitution R^3 as albuterol, but also an unusually long and lipophilic group

R^1 on the nitrogen. The octanol/water partition coefficient, logP for salmeterol is 3.88 vs. 0.66 for albuterol and the duration of action of salmeterol is 12 hours vs. 4 hours for albuterol (18). There is substantial evidence that the extended duration of action is due to a specific binding interaction ("anchoring") of the phenyl group at the end of the extended lipophilic side chain with a specific region of the β_2-receptor, affording salmeterol a unique binding mechanism (Fig. 11.11) (19).

Salmeterol

The long lipophilic nitrogen substituent of salmeterol has been shown through a series of site directed mutagenesis experiments to bind to a specific 10 amino-acid region of transmembrane domain 4 (TMD4) of the β_2-adrenoceptor. This region, amino-acids 149–158, is located at the interface of the cytoplasm and TMD4. Thus "anchored" by the lipophilic side chain, the remaining part of the molecule can pivot on and off the "normal" β_2 binding sites of aspartate 113 of TMD3 and serines 204/207 of TMD5 repetitively stimulating the receptor. This lipophilic anchoring keeps the drug localized at the site of action and produces the long duration of action of salmeterol.

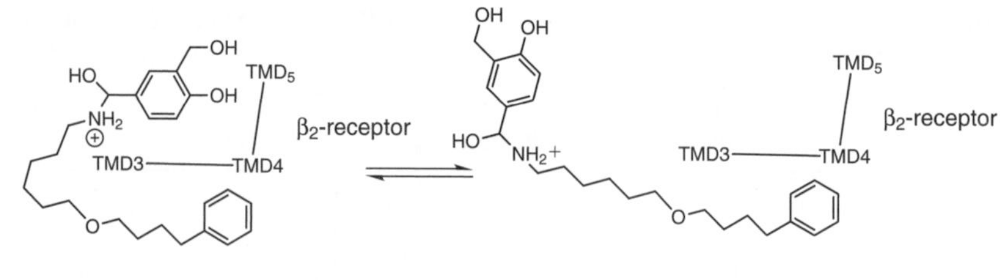

Fig. 11.11. Mechanism of action for salmeterol.

Ritodrine. The previously mentioned ritodrine is a selective β_2-agonist that is used exclusively for relaxing uterine muscle and inhibiting the contractions of premature labor. Terbutaline, in addition to its use as a bronchodilator has also been used for halting the contractions of premature labor.

β_1-Adrenergic Agonists
Dopamine. Dopamine, although not strictly an adrenergic drug, is a catecholamine with properties related to the cardiovascular activities of the other agents in this chapter. Dopamine acts on specific dopamine receptors to dilate renal vessels, increasing renal blood flow. Dopamine also stimulates cardiac β_1-receptors through both direct and indirect mechanisms. It is used to correct hemodynamic imbalances induced by conditions such as shock, myocardial infarction, trauma, or congestive heart failure. As a catechol and primary amine, dopamine is rapidly metabolized by COMT and MAO and, similar to dobutamine, has a short duration of action with no oral activity.

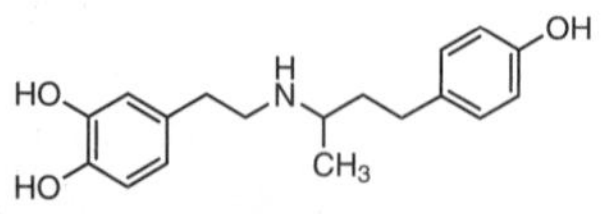

Dobutamine

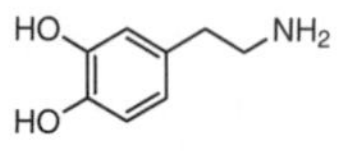

Dopamine

Dobutamine. Not all the adrenergic agonists with direct activity have an aliphatic β- hydroxyl group such as the agents discussed so far. One of these is the catechol dobutamine. Dobutamine is a dopamine analog with a bulky arylalkyl group on the nitrogen and one chiral (asymmetric) center. Racemic ($\pm$) dobutamine has direct activity on both α_1 and β_1-receptors, but because of some unusual properties of its two enantiomers, the overall pharmacologic response looks similar to that of a selective β_1-agonist (21). The S($-$)-isomer of dobutamine exhibits β_1-agonist activity and also is a powerful α_1-agonist and vasopressor. The R($+$)-isomer is an α_1-antagonist; thus, when the racemate is used clinically, the α-effects of the enantiomers cancel each other leaving primarily the β_1-effects. The stereochemistry of the methyl substituent does not affect the ability of the drug to bind to the α_1-receptor but does affect the ability of the molecule to activate the receptor. That is, the stereochemistry of the methyl group affects intrinsic activity but not affinity. Because both stereoisomers are β_1-agonists with the

($+$)-isomer about $\frac{1}{10}$ the potency of the ($-$)-isomer, the net effect is β_1 stimulation. Dobutamine is used as a cardiac stimulant after surgery or congestive heart failure. As a catechol, dobutamine is readily metabolized by COMT and has a short duration of action with no oral activity.

Mixed Acting Sympathomimetics
Ephedrine
($-$)Ephedrine is a natural product isolated from several species of ephedra plants, which were used for centuries in folk medicines in a variety of cultures worldwide (20). Its occurence in ephedra is about 80–90%. Other substances also found include ($+$)pseudo-ephedrine (10–15%) and N-methylephedrine (2–5%). Pure ephedrine was first isolated and crystallized in 1887 from a Chinese herbal medicine called Ma Huang. Its sympathomimetic activity was not recognized until 1917, and the pure drug was used clinically even before epinephrine and norepinephrine were isolated and characterized. Ephedrine does not have any phenolic substituents on the phenyl ring, giving it a mixed acting response and good oral activity because it is not a substrate for COMT. Lacking hydrogen-bonding phenolic substituents, ephedrine is less polar than the other compounds discussed thus far and crosses the blood-brain barrier far better than do catechols. Because of its ability to penetrate the central nervous system, ephedrine has been used as a stimulant and exhibits side effects related to its action in the brain. Ephedrine is widely used for many of the same indications as epinephrine, including use as a bronchodilator, vasopressor, cardiac stimulant, and nasal decongestant.

Herbal Remedies, Ma Huang and Ephedrine

In the United States the purified chemical ephedrine is considered a drug and regulated by the Food and Drug Administration (FDA). However the dried plant material, Ma Huang, is considered by law to be a dietary supplement, and not subject to FDA regulation. As a result there are a large number of Ma Huang containing herbal remedies and so-called "nutraceuticals" on the market whose active ingredient is the adrenergic agonist ephedrine. Some of these unregulated herbal remedies contain the same levels of the chemical ephedrine as FDA regulated drugs. Pharmacists must be aware that some patients may be taking such Ma Huang containing herbal remedies or dietary supplements in addition to regulated drugs which could lead to serious adverse reactions.

Pseudoephedrine

(+) Pseudoephedrine (Sudafed), the *threo* diastereomer of ephedrine, has virtually no direct activity and fewer central nervous system side effects than ephedrine. (+) Pseudoephedrine is widely used as a nasal decongestant.

Phenylpropanolamine

(±) Phenylpropanolamine (see Table 11.3) is the N-desmethyl analog of ephedrine that has many of the same properties. Lacking the N-methyl group, however, phenylpropanolamine has none of the β_2-agonist activity of ephedrine, is slightly less lipophilic, and therefore does not enter the central nervous system as well as ephedrine. Phenylpropanolamine, similar to ephedrine, is a mixture of erythro enantiomers with mixed direct and mostly indirect activity. The drug has been the active ingredient of a number of nasal decongestants and used as a nonprescription appetite suppressant (anorexian) until its U.S. FDA mandated recall in 2000 because of cerebral hemorrhages in women.

Amphetamine, Methamphetamine,

Other methyl substituted phenylethylamines (phenylisopropylamines), such as S(+) amphetamine and S(+)-methamphetamine, which lack both ring substituents and a side chain hydroxyl, are sufficiently lipophilic to cross the blood-brain barrier readily and cause dramatic central nervous system stimulation, which gives them serious abuse potential. The clinical utility of S(+)-amphetamine and its derivatives is entirely based on central nervous system stimulant and central appetite suppressant effects. These agents are discussed elsewhere in this textbook.

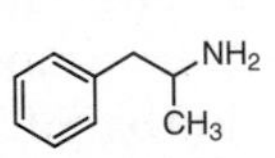

Amphetamine 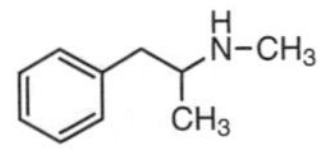   Methamphetamine

STRUCTURE-ACTIVITY RELATIONSHIPS OF ADRENERGIC ANTAGONISTS
General α-Antagonists
Phenoxybenzamine

Because α-agonists cause vasoconstriction and raise blood pressure, one would expect α-antagonists to be therapeutically used as antihypertensive agents. An old but powerful drug in this class is phenoxybenzamine (dibenzyline), a β-haloalkylamine that alkylates α-receptors. Beta-haloalkylamines are present in nitrogen mustard anticancer agents and are highly reactive alkylating agents. The acid salt of phenoxybenzamine is stable, but at physiologic pH there is equilibrium between protonated drug and free base. The unshared electrons of the unprotonated amino group is nucleophilic and displaces the β-chlorine atom in an intramolecular reaction to form a highly reactive aziridinium ion (Fig. 11.12). If this occurs in the vicinity of an α-receptor, a nucleophile group X on the receptor can open the aziridinium ion in a nucle-

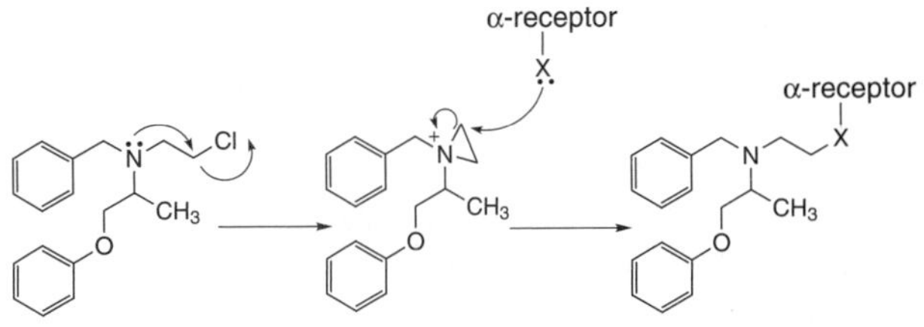

Fig. 11.12. Phenoxybenzamine alkylation of α-adrenoceptors. X is a nucleophile, such as S, N, or O.

ophilic reaction to form a covalent bond between the receptor and the drug. The substituents attached to the haloalkylamine provide selectivity for binding to α-adrenoceptors so that the nucleophile is generally part of the target receptor. The nucleophile X is presumably part of an amino acid side chain, such as a cysteine thiol, serine hydroxyl, or lysine amino group, but the specific site of covalent attachment to the α-receptor has not been determined. Because the reaction in which phenoxybenzamine forms covalent bonds with the receptors is irreversible, new receptors must be synthesized before the effects can be overcome. The α-blockade is therefore long lasting.

Unfortunately, other biomolecules besides the target α-receptor are also alkylated. Because of its receptor nonselectivity and toxicity, the use of phenoxybenzamine is largely limited to alleviating the sympathetic effects of pheochromocytoma. This tumor of chromaffin cells of the adrenal medulla produces large amounts of epinephrine and norepinephrine, which are released into the blood stream producing hypertension and generalized sympathetic stimulation.

Tolazoline and Phentolamine

Tolazoline and phentolamine are two imidazoline α-antagonists that also have antihypertensive activity, although they have been replaced in general clinical use by far better agents. Tolazoline has clear structural similarities to the imidazoline α_1-agonists, such as naphazoline and xylometazoline (see Fig. 11.7), but does not have the lipophilic substituents required for agonist activity. The resemblance of phentolamine is not as readily apparent, but extensive molecular modeling studies have provided a topologic scheme for α_1-antagonist SAR (22). This pattern, however, cannot be readily visualized without computer graphics and is beyond the scope of this chapter.

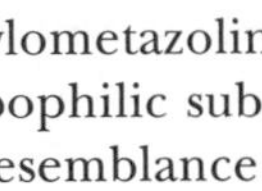

Tolazoline 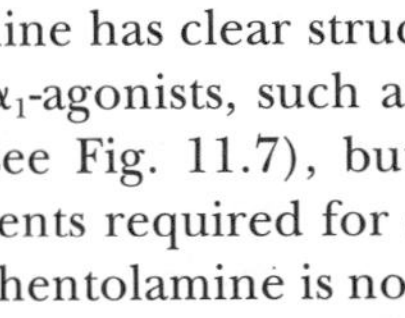   Phentolamine

Both phentolamine and tolazoline are potent but rather nonspecific α-antagonists. Both drugs stimulate gastrointestinal smooth muscle, an action blocked by atropine, which would indicate cholinergic activity, and they both stimulate gastric secretion, possibly through release of histamine. Because of these and other side effects, the clinical applications of tolazoline and phentolamine are also limited to treating the symptoms of pheochromocytoma.

Selective α₁-Antagonists
Prazosin, Doxazosin, Terazosin, Tamsulosin

Prazosin, the first known selective α₁-blocker, was discovered in the late 1960s (24) and is now one of a small group of selective α₁-antagonists which includes two other quinoxaline antihypertensives, terazosin, and doxazosin, and the structurally unrelated tamsulosin (Fig. 11.13). Prazosin is an antihypertensive agent, as are terazosin and doxazosin. The latter two were subsequently discovered to block α₁-receptors in the prostate gland and alleviate the symptoms of benign prostatic hyperplasia (BPH). The more recently developed tamsulosin is more selective for the subtype of α₁-adrenoceptor found in the prostate gland over those found in vascular tissue. Thus, tamsulosin has no utility in treating hypertension, but far fewer cardiovascular side effects than terazosin and doxazosin in treating BPH.

Structure-activity Relationship of the Quinazolines

Prazosin, doxazosin, and terazosin contain a 4-amino-6,7-dimethoxyquinazoline ring system attached to a piperazine nitrogen. The only structural differences are in the groups attached to the other nitrogen of the piperazine, and the differences in these groups afford dramatic differences in some of the pharmacokinetic properties of these agents. For example, when the furan ring of prazosin is reduced to form the tetrahydrofuran ring of terazosin, the compound becomes significantly more hydrophilic, (25) as would be expected because tetrahydrofuran is much more hydrophilic than furan.

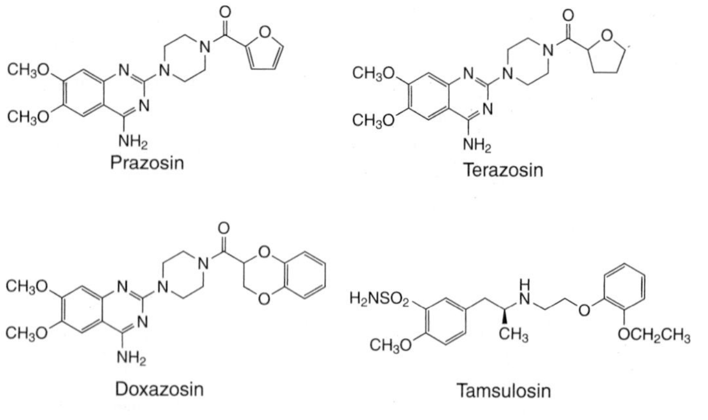

Some of the important clinical parameters of the quinazolines are shown in Table 11.6. Perhaps most significant are the long half-lives and durations of action for terazosin and doxazosin, which permit once-a-day dosing and generally lead to increased patient compliance.

Indoramin

An α₁-antagonist not available in the U.S. is indoramin, which is an indole derivative having a piperidine in the side chain instead of a piperazine. Although indoramin is more highly selective for α₁ than α₂-adrenoceptors, it also blocks histamine H₁ and serotonin receptors (25). In addition to its antihypertensive properties, it has other pharmacologic properties in the cardiovascular system that are not well understood. Indoramin's half-life and duration of action are also listed in Table 11.6.

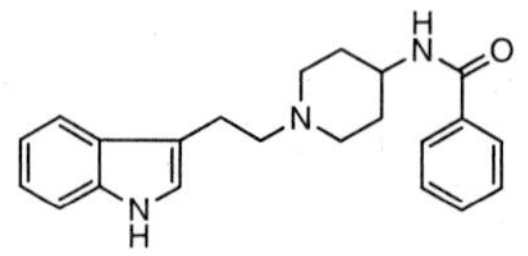

Indoramin

α₂-Adrenergic Antagonists
Yohimbine

Yohimbine, an indole alkaloid isolated from *Pausinystlia yohimbe* bark and *Rauwolfia* roots is an α₂-antagonist with greater selectivity for α₂ than for α₁-adrenoceptors; but it is also a serotonin antagonist. It has actions both in the central nervous system and in the periphery inducing hypertension and increases in heart rate. Yohimbine has no indications sanctioned by the United States Food and Drug Administration, but has been used to treat male impotence and postural hypotension. Yohimbine has also been used in research to induce anxiety. As was the case with ephedrine and the herbal Ma Huang, in the United States the purified chemical yohimbine is an FDA regulated drug, but herbal remedies and dietary supplements containing *yohimbe* bark are not regulated even though the active ingredient is the same chemical entity.

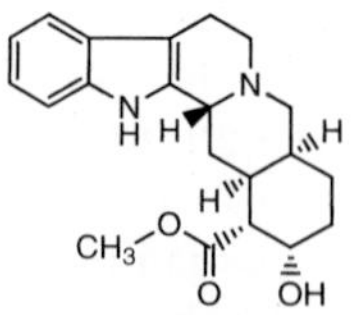

Yohimbine

β-Adrenergic Antagonists

In the 1950s, a derivative of isoproterenol in which the catechol hydroxyls had been replaced by chlorines, dichloroisoproterenol (DCI), was discovered to be a β-antagonist that blocked the effects of sympathomimetic amines on bronchodilation, uterine relaxation, and heart stimulation (26). Although DCI had no clinical utility, replacement of the 3,4-dichloro substituents with a carbon

Fig. 11.13. Selective α₁ adrenergic antagonists.

Table 11.6. Selected Clinical Parameters of α_1-adrenergic Antagonists

Drug	Trade Name	Therapeutic Dose (mg)	Half-life (hr)	Duration of Action (hr)	Frequency of Administration	Bioavailability (%)
Prazosin	Minipres	2–20	2–3	4–6	BID–TID	45–65
Terazosin	Hytrin	1–40	12	>18	QD–BID	90
Doxazosin	Cardura	1–16	22	18–36	QD–BID	65
Indoramin	Doralese	50–150	5	>6	BID–TID	30
Tamsulosin	Flomax	0.4–0.8	14–15	>24	QD	<50% with food 50–90% fasted

QD, Once daily; BID, twice daily; TID, three times daily.

bridge to form a naphthylethanolamine derivative did afford a clinical candidate, pronethalol, introduced in 1962 only to be withdrawn in 1963 because of tumor induction in animal tests.

Dichloroisoproterenol   Pronethalol

Structure-activity Relationships

Shortly thereafter, a major innovation in drug development for the β-adrenergic antagonists was introduced when it was discovered that an oxymethylene bridge, OCH_2, could be inserted into the arylethanolamine structure of pronethalol to afford propranolol, an aryloxypropanolamine and the first clinically successful β-blocker. Note that, along with the introduction of the oxymethylene bridge, the side chain has been moved from C2 of the naphthyl group to the C1 position. In general, the aryloxypropanolamines are more potent β-blockers than the corresponding arylethanolamines and most of the β-blockers currently used clinically are aryloxypropanolamines. β-blockers have found wide use in treating hypertension (Chapter 24) and certain types of glaucoma. Nine β-blockers are in the Top 200 prescription drugs in the United States (Table 11.1).

Propranolol

Initially, it might appear that lengthening the side chain would prevent appropriate binding of the required functional groups to the same receptor site. But molecular models show that the side chains of aryloxypropanolamines can adopt a conformation that places the hydroxyl and amine groups into approximately the same position in space (Fig. 11.14). The simple two-dimensional drawing in Figure 11.14 exaggerates the true degree of overlap; however, elaborate molecular modeling studies confirm that the aryloxypropanolamine side chain can adopt

a low-energy conformation that permits close overlap with the arylethanolamine side chain (27).

Propranolol

Propranolol was initially introduced for the treatment of angina pectoris, followed by trials as an antiarrhythmic. During clinical trials as an antianginal, propranolol was discovered to have antihypertensive properties and has been widely employed for that purpose for decades (28). Propranolol rapidly became widely used for a variety of cardiac arrhythmias as well. In addition, because of its high lipophilicity and ability to penetrate the CNS, propranolol has found use in treating disorders of the central nervous system such as anxiety.

At approximately this same time, a new series of 4-substituted phenyloxypropanololamines emerged, such as practolol, which selectively inhibited sympathetic cardiac stimulation. These observations led to the recognition that not all β-receptors were the same which led to the introduction of β_1 and β_2 nomenclature to differentiate cardiac β_1-receptors from others (29). Development of β-blockers proceeded rapidly, and there are now a large number of additional drugs available on the world market, both non-selective β-antagonists (Fig.

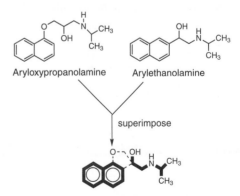

Aryloxypropanolamine   Arylethanolamine

superimpose

Fig. 11.14. Overlap of aryloxypropanolamines and arylethanolamines. The structures of prototype β-antagonists propranolol and pronethalol may be superimposed so the critical functional groups occupy the same approximate regions in space as indicated by the bold lines in the superimposed drawings. The dotted lines are those parts that do not overlap but are not necessary to receptor binding.

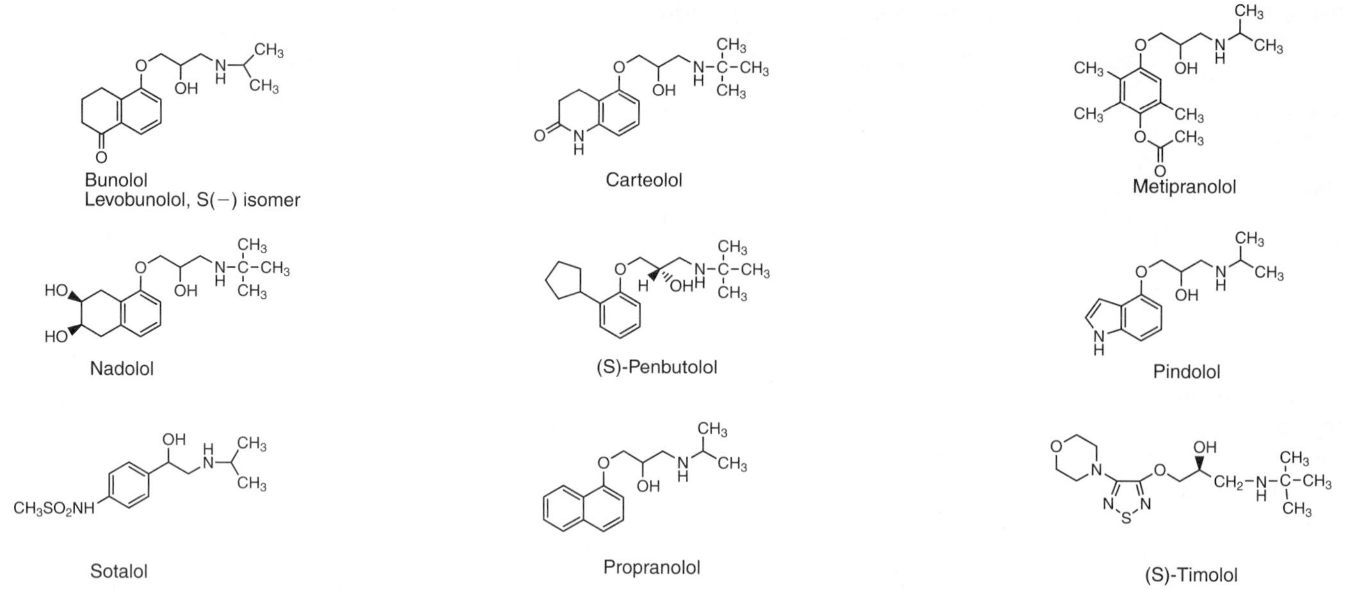

Fig. 11.15. Non-selective β-adrenergic antagonists.

11.15) and selective β₁-antagonists (Fig. 11.16). Although those antagonists are selective for the cardiac β₁-receptor, most also have some β₂-antagonist properties at the higher levels of therapeutic dosing (dose dependent). With the exception of sotalol, all of the drugs shown in Figures 11.15 and 11.16 are aryloxypropanolamines. Metipranolol (Fig. 11.15) is an exception to the general rule that 4-substituted aryloxypropanolamines are selective β₁-blockers.

Other than β₁-selectivity of 4-substituted aryloxypropanolamines, there is little obvious structural pattern to relate β-blockers to specific clinical applications with the exception of esmolol. Esmolol has a methyl ester at the end of the 4-substituent, which makes it susceptible to hydrolysis by serum esterases, and the acid metabolite generated by hydrolysis is essentially inactive and readily excreted as its zwitterion. For this reason, esmolol has a half-life of only about 8 minutes and is used to control supraventricular tachycardia during surgery when a short-acting β₁-adrenergic antagonist is desirable.

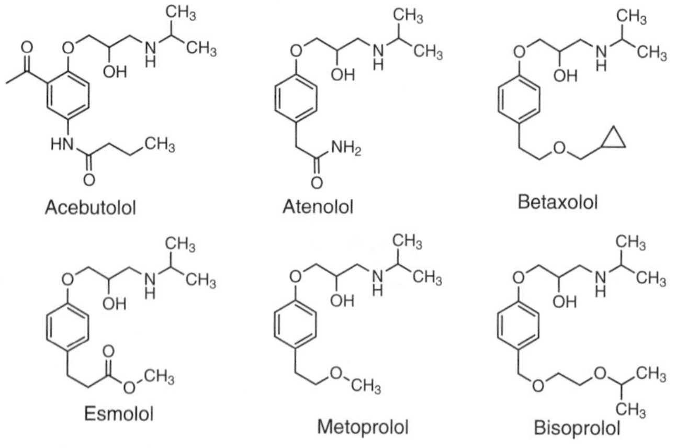

Another physicochemical parameter that has some clinical correlation is relative lipophilicity of different agents. Propranolol is by far the most lipophilic of the available β-blockers and enters the central nervous system far better than less lipophilic agents, such as atenolol or nadolol. Lipophilicity as measured by octanol/water partitioning also correlates with primary site of clearance as seen in Table 11.7 (31). The more lipophilic drugs are primarily cleared by the liver, whereas, the more hydrophilic agents are cleared by the kidney. This could have an influence on choice of agents in cases of renal failure or liver disease. Several of the β-blockers must be dose adjusted in patients with impaired renal function, as indicated in Table 11.7.

Mixed α/β-Adrenergic Antagonists— Labetalol and Carvedilol

Labetalol and carvedilol have an unusual activity in that they are antihypertensives with α₁-, β₁-, and β₂-blocking activity (Fig. 11.17) (Chapter 24). In terms of SAR, you will recall from the earlier discussion of phenylethanolamine agonists that although groups such as isopropyl and t-butyl eliminated α-receptor activity, still larger groups could bring back α₁-affinity but not intrinsic activity. Thus, these two drugs have structural features permitting binding to both the α₁ and non-selectively to both β-receptors. The β-blocking activity of labetalol is approximately 1.5 times that of its α-blocking activity. The more recently developed

Fig. 11.16. Selective β₁-adrenergic antagonists.

Table 11.7. Lipophilicity and Clearance Route of Representative β-Antagonists

Drug	Octanol/Buffer Partition Coefficient	Primary Clearance Route
Propranolol	20.4	Hepatic
Metoprolol	0.98	Hepatic
Pindolol	0.82	Hepatic plus Renal
Atenolol	0.008	Renal
Nadolol	0.006	Renal

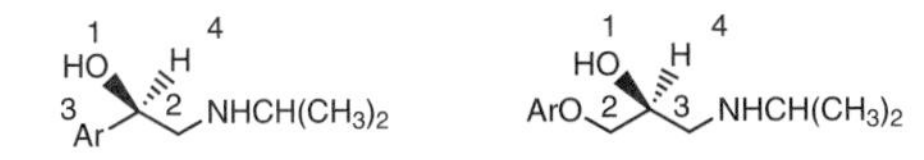

Fig. 11.18. Stereochemical nomenclature for arylethanolamines versus aryloxypropanolamines. The relative positions in space of the four functional groups are the same in the two structures; however, one is designated (R) and the other (S). This is because the introduction of an oxygen atom into the side chain of the aryloxypropanolamine changes the priority of two of the groups used in the nomenclature assignment.

carvedilol has an estimated β-blocking activity 10–100 times its α-blocking activity.

Stereochemistry of the β-Adrenergic Antagonists

A factor that sometimes causes confusion when comparing the structures of arylethanolamines with aryloxypropanolamines is the stereochemical nomenclature of the side chain carbon bearing the hydroxyl group. For maximum effectiveness in receptor binding, the hydroxy group must occupy the same region in space as it does for the phenylethanolamine agonists in the R absolute configuration. Because of the insertion of an oxygen atom in the side chain of the aryloxypropanolamines, the Cahn-Ingold-Prelog priority of the substituents around the asymmetric carbon changes, and the isomer with the required special arrangement now has the S absolute configuration. This is an effect of the nomenclature rules, and the groups still have the same spatial arrangements (Fig. 11.18).

Therapeutic Applications

β-blockers are widely used in the treatment of hypertension, angina, cardiac arrhythmias, and glaucoma (Table 11.8). Their application in the treatment of hypertension will be discussed in Chapter 24, Table 24.3. The ability of β-blockers to slow the heart rate and decrease force of contraction lowers the workload on the heart and relieves angina. Although the exact mechanism is less straightforward, these same effects may be the principal cause of the hypotensive effects of β-blockers. Lowered output from the heart is thought eventually to lead to relaxation of the peripheral vasculature, although an effect on renin output may be involved. The ability to decrease automaticity leads to their use in

treating arrhythmias. The action of β-blockers in treating glaucoma is more difficult to explain. The β-blockers lower intraocular pressure by decreasing the amount of aqueous humor fluid produced in the eye by the ciliary body, and β$_2$-receptors have been found in that tissue. However, observations have shown that the ciliary body has no adrenergic innervation; the effect is not stereoselective, and a correlation of activity exists with decreased ciliary blood flow and decreased dopamine levels indicate that the mechanism of action of β-blockers in treating glaucoma is unusual (30).

Even though β-blockers are widely used for a variety of ailments, certain precautions must be taken in the use of these agents in certain patient populations. Because the selectivity of β$_1$-antagonists is not absolute, at the higher range of recommended doses the compounds also block β$_2$-receptors. Therefore, extreme caution is advised in using these agents in persons with asthma or other pulmonary disease. Caution is also required with diabetics because the β-blockers inhibit catecholamine-induced glycogenolysis in response to insulin-induced hypoglycemia and may thus aggravate the condition.

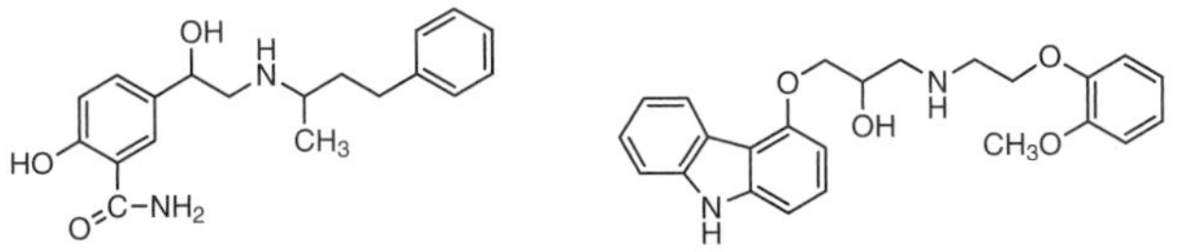

DRUGS AFFECTING NOREPINEPHRINE/EPINEPHRINE BIOSYNTHESIS

Hypothetically, inhibitors of any of the three enzymes involved in the conversion of L-tyrosine to norepinephrine could be used as drugs to moderate adrenergic transmission. Inhibitors of the rate-limiting enzyme tyrosine hydroxylase would be the most logical choice. One inhibitor of tyrosine hydroxylase, metyrosine or α-methyl-L-tyrosine, is in limited clinical use to help control hypertensive episodes and other symptoms of catecholamine overproduction in patients with the rare adrenal tumor pheochromocytoma (29). Metyrosine, a competitive inhibitor of tyrosine hydroxylase, inhibits the production of catecholamines by the tumor. Although metyrosine is useful in treating hypertension caused by excess catecholamine biosynthesis in pheochromocytoma tumors, it is not useful

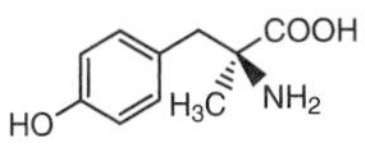

Labetalol   Carvedilol

Fig. 11.17. Mixed α/β-adrenergic antagonists.

Metyrosine

Table 11.8. Pharmacologic/Pharmacokinetic Properties of Beta-Adrenergic Blocking Agents

Drug	Adrenergic Receptor Blocking Activity	Membrane Stabilizing Activity	Intrinsic Sympathomimetic Activity	Lipid Solubility	Extent of Absorption (%)	Absolute Oral Bioavailability (%)	Half-life (hrs)	Protein Binding (%)	Metabolism/Excretion	Indications[1] (common)
Acebutolol (Sectral)	β_1[1]	+	+	Low	90	20–60	3–4	26	Hepatic; renal excretion 30 to 40%; nonrenal excretion 50 to 60% (bile)	H, Ar
Atenolol (Tenormin)	β_1[1]	0	0	Low	50	50–60	6–9	5–16	≈50 excreted unchanged in feces	H, An
Betaxolol (Kerlone, Betoptic)	β_1[1]	+	0	Low	≈100	80–90	14–22	≈50	Hepatic; >80% recovered as metabolites in urine, 15% unchanged in urine	H, G
Bisoprolol (Zebeta)	β_1[1]	0	0	Low	≥90	80–90	9–12	≈30	≈50% excreted unchanged in urine, remainder as inactive metabolites; <2% excreted in feces	H
Esmolol (Brevibloc)	β_1[1]	0	0	Low	na[5]	na[5]	0.15	55	Rapid metabolism by plasma and erythrocyte esterases	
Metoprolol (Lopressor)	β_1[1]	0[2]	0	Moderate	95	40–50	3–7	12	Hepatic; <5% excreted unchanged in urine	H, An, Ar
Metoprolol LA						77				
Carteolol (Cartrol, Ocupress)	β_1 β_2	0	++	Low	80	85	6	23–30	50 to 70% excreted unchanged in urine	H, G
Nadolol (Corgard)	β_1 β_2	0	0	Low	30	30–50	20–24	30	Mostly excreted unchanged in urine	H, An
Penbutolol (Levatol)	β_1 β_2	0	+	High	≈100	>90	5	80–98	Hepatic (conjugation, oxidation); renal excretion of metabolites (17% as conjugate)	H
Pindolol (Visken)	β_1 β_2	+	+++	Moderate	95	>90	3–4[3]	40	Urinary excretion of metabolites (60 to 65%) and unchanged drug (35 to 40%)	H
Propranolol (Inderal)	β_1 β_2	++	0	High	90	30	3–5	90	Hepatic; <1% excreted unchanged in urine	H, An, Ar
Propranolol LA						9–18	8–11			
Sotalol (Betapace)	β_1 β_2	0	0	Low	nd[6]	90–100	12	0	Not metabolized; excreted unchanged in urine	Ar
Timolol (Blocadren, Timoptic)	β_1 β_2	0	0	Low to moderate	90	75	4	10	Hepatic; urinary excretion of metabolites and unchanged drug	H, G
Labetalol[4] (Normodyne)	β_1 β_2 α_1	0	0	Moderate	100	30–40	5–8	50	55 to 60% excreted in urine as conjugates or unchanged drug	H
Carvedilol (Coreg)	β_1 β_2 α_1	0	0	Moderate to high	>90	25–35	7–10	98	Hepatic (oxidation, conjugation): <2% excreted unchanged in urine; conjugated metabolites excreted primarily into bile; exhibits stereoselective metabolism	H, An

[1]Inhibits β_2 receptors (bronchial and vascular) at higher doses.
[2]Detectable only at doses much greater than required for beta blockade.
[3]In elderly hypertensive patients with normal renal function, $t_{1/2}$ variable: 7 to 15 hours.
[4]Not labetalol monograph.
[5]Not applicable (available IV only).
[6]No data.
0 = none; + = low; ++ = moderate; +++ = high

Adapted from Drug Facts and Comparison 2000.

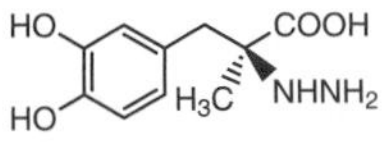

Carbidopa

for treating essential hypertension. The drug metyrosine is the L(S) stereoisomer of α-methyltyrosine. The enantiomer, D(R)-α-methyltyrosine, does not bind to the active site of tyrosine hydroxylase and thus has no useful pharmacologic activity.

Of far greater clinical significance in the treatment of hypertension is methyldopa, which is an inhibitor of aromatic L-amino acid decarboxylase action on dopa through its ability to serve as an alternative substrate for the enzyme. As previously discussed, the mechanism of antihypertensive activity of methyldopa is not due to norepinephrine biosynthesis inhibition but rather to metabolism to an $α_2$-agonist in the central nervous system. Other more powerful inhibitors of aromatic L-amino acid decarboxylase (e.g., carbidopa) have proven to be clinically useful, but not as modulators of peripheral adrenergic transmission. Rather these agents are used to inhibit the metabolism of exogenous L-dopa administered in the treatment of Parkinson's disease (Chapter 20).

The next enzyme in the biosynthetic pathway to norepinephrine and epinephrine, dopamine β-hydroxylase, has been the subject of extensive research into its chemical mechanism and the subject of many enzyme inhibition studies. The inhibitors known to date, however, are primarily of basic biochemical research interest and have no therapeutic relevance. The same is true of phenylethanolamine-N-methyltransferase, the last enzyme in the biosynthesis of epinephrine in the adrenal medulla.

ERGOT ALKALOIDS

The ergot alkaloids are a large group of indole alkaloids isolated from the ergot fungus, *Claviceps purpurea*, which is a plant parasite principally infecting rye. Eating grain contaminated with ergot caused a severely debilitating and painful disease during the Middle Ages called St. Anthony's Fire, but in small doses, ergot was known to midwives for centuries for its ability to stimulate uterine contraction. The pharmacology of the various ergot alkaloids is complex, involving actions on the adrenergic nervous system as well as a number of others. The structures of several ergot alkaloids are shown in Figure 11.19.

Ergotamine is a mixed agonist/antagonist of various peripheral and central adrenoceptors. It is a strong inducer of contractions in the pregnant uterus, which appears to be partially an α-effect because it is blocked by phentolamine, but other receptors may be involved. The drug is used to contract the postpartum uterus to prevent excessive bleeding. Ergotamine is also used to treat migraine headache. Ergonovine and methylergonovine are also strong inducers of uterine contractions and because of better oral absorption have largely replaced ergotamine for this purpose. Methysergide, structurally identical to methylergonovine except for the addition of a methyl group to the indole nitrogen, has far less of the uterine stimulatory properties of the other agents and is instead used exclusively for treatment of migraine headache. This is believed to be a serotonin antagonist effect.

All of these ergot alkaloids are amide derivatives of lysergic acid, but only the diethylamide LSD produces the profound hallucinatory effects for which it is so well-known.

XANTHINE BRONCHODILATORS

Although they are not truly adrenergic drugs, methylxanthines are extensively used as bronchodilators in asthma and so are included here (Fig. 11.20). The most widely used of the xanthines is theophylline and its salts. Aminophylline is the ethylemediamine salt of theophylline, and oxtriphylline is the choline salt. Enprofylline is widely used outside the United States.

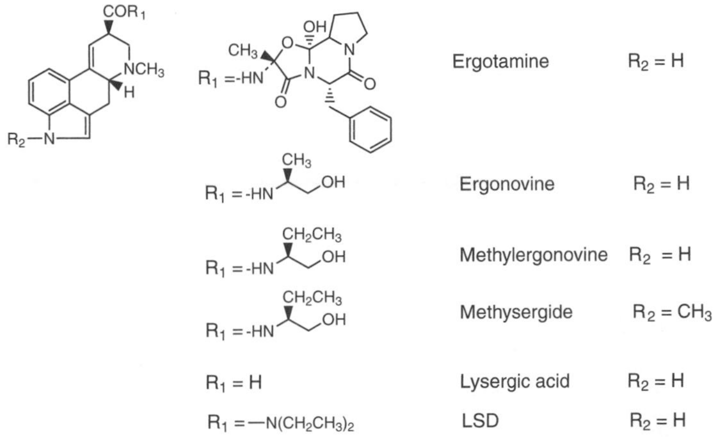

Fig. 11.19. Ergot alkaloids.

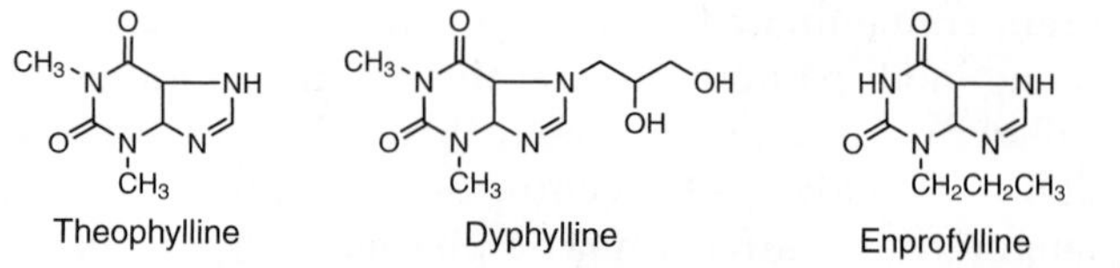

Fig. 11.20. Xanthine bronchodilators.

These xanthine derivatives are effective bronchodilators; however, their pharmacologic mechanism of action remains controversial despite many years of intensive study. Among the mechanisms of bronchodilation induction that have been suggested are inhibition of phosphodiesterase hydrolysis of cAMP, adenosine receptor antagonism, stimulation of increased secretion of endogenous catecholamines, inhibition of prostaglandins, and reduction of intracellular calcium ion concentrations. It is probable that the xanthines act by the sum of several actions or perhaps even by an as yet undiscovered mechanism.

CASE STUDY

Victoria F. Roche and S. William Zito

FC is a 28-year-old woman with a history of anorexia and bulimia. She was in therapy for a serious eating disorder until she finished high school. She was a member of a bulimia support group during college, but she has not seen a counselor for almost 6 years. During that time, her weight has fluctuated between 115 and 185 pounds (135 pounds has been recommended as her "ideal weight"). When heavy, she dedicates herself to "The Slim-Fast Plan," exercises like crazy and curbs her appetite with OTC Dexatrim, which contains phenylpropanolamine (PPA). She currently weighs 163 pounds, and came to the pharmacy yesterday in tears because of the FDA-mandated recall of all PPA-containing products. Her patient profile indicates no Rx medications, but she does take St. John's Wort when she's feeling depressed about her weight. FC wants you to recommend an OTC agent she can buy that will take the place of the PPA. She said she's also going to check with the "Herbs R Us" guy down the street to see what botanical product he might recommend

to help her. When doing a brief physical assessment, you note a moderately elevated blood pressure and a rapid heart rate. The adrenergic agents available on your OTC counter include drugs 1–3 drawn below.

1. *Identify the therapeutic problem(s) where the pharmacist's intervention may benefit the patient.*

2. *Identify and prioritize the patient specific factors that must be considered to achieve the desired therapeutic outcomes.*

3. *Conduct a thorough and mechanistically oriented structure-activity analysis of all therapeutic alternatives provided in the case.*

4. *Evaluate the SAR findings against the patient specific factors and desired therapeutic outcomes and make a therapeutic decision.*

5. *Counsel your patient*

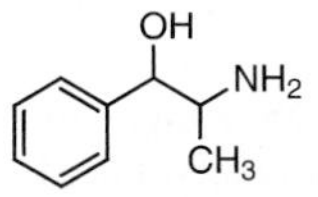

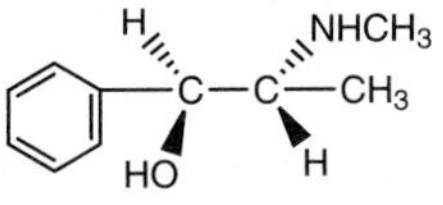

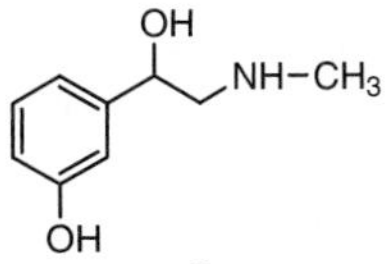

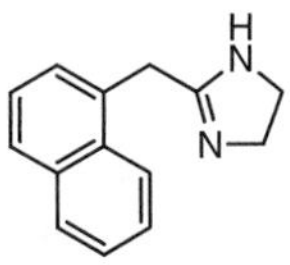

REFERENCES

1. von Euler, US, Synthesis, uptake and storage of catecholamines in adrenergic nerves, the effect of drugs, in Catecholamines, H. Blaschko and E. Marshall, Editors. 1972, Springer: New York. p. 186–230.
2. Triggle, DJ, Adrenergics: Catecholamines and related agents, in Burger's Medicinal Chemistry, M.E. Wolff, Editor. 1981, John Wiley & Sons: New York. p. 225–283.
3. Appezeller, O, The vegetative nervous system, in Handbook of Clinical Neurology, P.J. Vinken and G.W. Bruyn, Editors. 1969, North-Holland: Amsterdam. p. 427–8.
4. Kaufman, S and TJ Nelson, Studies on the regulation of tyrosine hydroxylase activity by phosphorylation and dephosphorylation, in Progress in Catecholamine Research, Part A: Basic Aspects and Peripheral Mechanisms, A. Dahlstrom, R.H. Belmaker, and M. Sandler, Editors. 1988, Alan R Liss: New York. p. 57–60.
5. Philippu, A and H Matthaei, Transport and storage of catecholamines in vessicles, in Catecholamines I, U. Trendelenburg and N. Weiner, Editors. 1988, Springer: New York. p. 1–42.
6. Trendelenburg, U, Factors influencing the concentration of catecholamines at the receptors, in Catecholamines, H. Blaschko and E. Marshall, Editors. 1972, Springer: New York. p. 726–761.
7. Kopin, IJ, Metabolic degradation of catecholamines, in Catecholamines, H. Blaschko and E. Marshall, Editors. 1972, Springer: New York. 270–282.
8. Ahlquist, RP, A study of the adrenotropic receptors. American J Physiol, 1948;153:586.
9. Harrison, JK, WR Pearson, and KR Lynch, Molecular characterization of alpha 1- and alpha 2-adrenoceptors. Trends Pharmacol Sci, 1991;12:62–7.
10. Trumpp-Kallmeyer, S, et al., Modeling of G protein-coupled receptors: application to dopamine, adrenaline, serotonin, acetylcholine, and mammalian opsin receptors. J Med Chem., 1992;35:3448–62.
11. Ostrowski, J, et al., Mutagenesis of the beta 2-adrenergic receptor: how structure elucidates function. Annu Rev Pharmacol Toxicol., 1992;32:167–83.
12. Strader, CD, et al., A single amino acid substitution in the beta-adrenergic receptor promotes partial agonist activity from antagonists. J Biol Chem., 1989;264:16470–7.
13. Regan, JW, et al., Cloning and expression of a human kidney cDNA for an alpha 2-adrenergic receptor subtype. Proc Natl Acad Sci U S A, 1988;85:6301–5.
14. Kobilka, B, Adrenergic receptors as models for G protein-coupled receptors. Ann Rev Neuroscience, 1992;15:87–114.
15. Nichols, AJ and RR Ruffolo, Jr, Structure-activity relationships for α-adrenoceptor agonists and antagonists, in α-Adrenoceptors: Molecular Biology, Biochemistry and Pharmacology, R.R. Ruffolo, Jr, Editor. 1991, Karger: New York. p. 75–114.
16. Timmermans, PB. and PA van Zwieten, Alpha 2 adrenoceptors: classification, localization, mechanisms, and targets for drugs. J Med Chem., 1982;25:1389–401.
17. Patil, PN and D. Jacobowitz, Steric aspects of adrenergic drugs. IX. Pharmacologic and histochemical studies on isomers of cobefrin (alpha-methylnorepinephrine). J Pharmacol Exp Ther., 1968;161:279–95.
18. Johnson, M. Salmeterol. Med Res Rev, 1995;15:225–57.
19. Green, SA, et al., Sustained activation of a G protein-coupled receptor via "anchored" agonist binding. J Biol Chem, 1996; 271:24029–24035.
20. Chen, KK and CF Schmidt, Ephedrine and related substances. Medicine, 1930;9:1–117.
21. Ruffolo, RRJ, et al., Alpha and beta adrenergic effects of the stereoisomers of dobutamine. J Pharmacol Exp Ther., 1981; 219:447–52.
22. Kobinger, W, Central α-adrenergic systems as targets for hypotensive drugs. Rev Physiol Biochem Pharmacol, 1978;81:39–100.
23. Henning, M and PA Van Zwieten, Central hypotensive effect of alpha-methyldopa. J Pharm Pharmacol., 1968;20:409–17.
24. Scriabine, A, et al., Pharmacological studies with some new antihypertensive aminoquinazolines. Experientia, 1968;24:1150–1151.
25. Cubeddu, LX, New alpha 1-adrenergic receptor antagonists for the treatment of hypertension: role of vascular alpha receptors in the control of peripheral resistance. Am Heart J., 1988; 116(1 Pt 1):133–62.
26. Moran, NC, New adrenergic blocking drugs: their pharmacological, biochemical and clinical actions. Ann N Y Acad Sci., 1967;139: 545–8.
27. Jen, T, et al., Adrenergic agents. 8.1 Synthesis and beta-adrenergic agonist activity of some 3-tert-butylamino-2-(substituted phenyl)-1-propanols. J Med Chem., 1977;20:1263–8.
28. Evans, DB, R Fox, and FP Hauck, β-Adrenergic receptor blockers as therapeutic agents. Ann Rep Med Chem, 1979;14:81–90.
29. Brogden, RN, et al., alpha-Methyl-p-tyrosine: a review of its pharmacology and clinical use. Drugs., 1981;21:81–9.
30. Lesar, T.S., Comparison of ophthalmic beta-blocking agents. Clin Pharm., 1987;6:451–63.
31. Kazierad, DJ, KD Schlanz, and MB Bottorff, Beta Blockers, in Applied Pharmacokinetics: Principles of Therapeutic Drug Monitoring, W.E. Evans, et al., Editors. 1992, Applied Therapeutics, Inc.: Vancouver, WA. p. 24/1–24/41.
32. Comer, WT, WL Matier, and MS Amer, Antihypertensive Agents, in Burger's Medicinal Chemistry, Part III, M.E. Wolff, Editor. 1981, John Wiley & Sons: New York. p. 285–337.

SUGGESTED READINGS

B. B. Hoffman and R. J. Lefkowitz, Catecholamines, Sympathomimetic Drugs, and Adrenergic Receptor Antagonists. In Goodman and Gilman's The Pharmacologic Basis of Therapeutics, 9th Ed., J.G. Hardman, L.E. Limbird, P. B. Molinoff, and R. W. Ruddon., Eds., New York, McGraw Hill, 1996, pp. 199–248.

D. J. Triggle, Adrenergics: Catecholamines and Related Agents, in Burger's Medicinal Chemistry, 4th Ed., Part III. Edited by M. E. Wolff. New York, John Wiley & Sons, 1981, pp. 225–283.

12. Serotonin Receptors and Drugs Affecting Serotonergic Neurotransmission

RICHARD A. GLENNON AND MALGORZATA DUKAT

SEROTONIN

Serotonin is the baby-boomer of neurotransmitters. Its adolescence was troubled and turbulent, it made the drug scene in the 1960s, and nearly died of an overdose in the early 1970s. At one point the remark was made that "serotonin doesn't do anything" (1). Upon reaching its middle years serotonin has matured and has become an important topic of study, a household name, and more complicated than ever. Serotonin has been associated with, among other things, anxiety, depression, schizophrenia, drug abuse, sleep, dreaming, hallucinogenic activity, headache, cardiovascular disorders, appetite control, and is now dabbling in acupuncture and transcendental meditation. This has prompted the comment: "… it almost appears that serotonin is involved in everything" (1). A review of the recent patent literature provides an indication of some of the newer claims being made for novel serotonergic agents (Table 12.1). Tens of thousands of papers have been published on serotonin; much is known—but an incredible amount remains to be learned.

Serotonin (5-HT)

Historical Perspectives

Serotonin was independently identified in the late 1940s by two groups of investigators: in the United States it was called serotonin whereas in Italy, enteramine (1). Its total synthesis in the early 1950s confirmed that both substances were 5-hydroxytryptamine (5-HT). Serotonin (5-HT) was

(+) Lysergic acid diethylamide (LSD)

detected in numerous plant and animal species and in the mid-1950s was identified in the central nervous system of animals. A neurotransmitter role was proposed for this substance (2). 5-HT was later implicated in a variety of central and peripheral physiologic actions. It seemed to be involved in vasoconstriction and vasodilation, regulation of body temperature, sleep, and hormonal regulation, and evidence suggested that it might be involved in depression. The structural similarity between 5-HT and the then recently discovered hallucinogenic agent (+)lysergic acid diethylamide (LSD) intrigued investigators. This observation led to speculation that 5-HT might be involved in the mechanism of action of psychoactive substances, and that it might play a seminal role in various mental disorders (2). LSD was shown to behave as a potent 5-HT agonist in some peripheral assays, and as a potent antagonist in others. However, the late 1960s and early 1970s witnessed a decline in 5-HT research as the result of three factors: 1) sophisticated techniques were still lacking for the investigation of the central actions of 5-HT, 2) apart from ergolines (LSD-related agents) only a few potent 5-HT agonists or antagonists had been developed, and 3) it was becoming increasingly difficult to understand how a single putative neurotransmitter substance could be involved in so many

Table 12.1. Some Indications and Treatment Claims for Novel Serotonergic Agents in Recent Patent Literature*

Aggression	Esophagitis	Obsessive-compulsive disorders
Alcoholism	Gastric motility	Pain
Alzheimer's disease	Head injury	Panic disorders
Amnesia	Headache	Parkinson's disease
Anorexia	Hypertension	Psychosis
Bulimia	Impotence	Raynaud's disease
Cardiac failure	Irritable bowel syndrome	Schizophrenia
Cardiovascular disorders	Ischemia	Sedation
Cerebrovascular disorders	Migraine	Sexual dysfunction
Cognition	Movement disorders	Sleep disorders
Depression	Nausea	Substance abuse
Drug abuse	Neurodegenerative disease	Substance dependence
Emesis	Obesity	Thromobembolism

*1997–1998 patent literature.

Radioligands

Radioligand binding techniques measure the affinity of agonists and antagonists for their respective receptors (i.e., Ki values). Radioligands are receptor agonists or antagonists to which a radioactive atom (label) is covalently attached.

different central and peripheral actions. The development of histochemical fluorescence techniques and radioligand binding methodology led to the mapping of serotonergic pathways and identifying binding sites in the brain, and to measuring the affinity (i.e., Ki values) of serotonergic agents for their respective serotonergic receptors.

Serotonin Biosynthesis, Catabolism, and Function as Targets for Drug Manipulation (3)

5-HT is biosynthesized from its dietary precursor L-tryptophan (Fig. 12.1). Serotonergic neurons contain tryptophan hydroxylase (L-tryptophan-5-monooxygenase) that converts tryptophan to 5-hydroxytryptophan (5-HTP) in what is the rate limiting step in 5-HT biosynthesis, and aromatic L-amino acid decarboxylase (previously called 5-HTP decarboxylase) that decarboxylates 5-HTP to 5-HT. This latter enzyme is also responsible for the conversion of L-DOPA to dopamine (Chapter 11). The major route of metabolism for 5-HT is oxidative deamination by monoamine oxidase (MAO-A) to the unstable 5-hydroxyindole-3-acetaldehyde which is either reduced to 5-hydroxytryptophol (~15%) or oxidized to 5-hydroxyindole-3-acetic acid (~85%). In the pineal gland, 5-HT is acetylated by 5-HT N-acetyltransferase

to N-acetylserotonin, which undergoes O-methylation by 5-hydroxyindole-O-methyltransferase to melatonin.

Each of the steps in 5-HT biosynthesis, metabolism, and function is a theoretical target for drug manipulation (Fig. 12.2). Tryptophan depletion, by reducing or eliminating dietary tryptophan, can result in decreased 5-HT biosynthesis. Conversely, tryptophan "loading," by increasing dietary tryptophan, can result in the overproduction of 5-HT. This latter effect can also occur in non-serotonergic

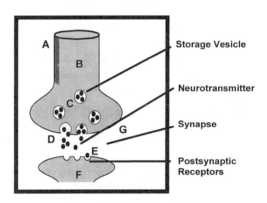

Fig. 12.2. Steps involved in serotonergic neurotransmission. The serotonin precursor tryptophan is taken up into the neuron **(A)** and converted to 5-HT **(B)**. Synthesized 5-HT is stored in synaptic vesicles **(C)**. Under the appropriate conditions, the synaptic vesicles migrate to and fuse with the cell membrane releasing their store of 5-HT **(D)**. Released neurotransmitter interacts with postsynaptic receptors **(E)** and, in the case of G protein-coupled receptors, activates second messenger systems **(F)**. The action of 5-HT is terminated **(G)** either by diffusion of 5-HT away from the synapse, with subsequent metabolism, or 5-HT is taken back up into the presynaptic neuron (i.e., reuptake) by a 5-HT transporter, where it can be stored or metabolized.

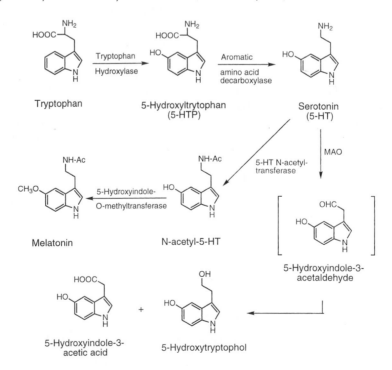

Fig. 12.1. Biosynthesis and catabolism of serotonin. In the pineal, serotonin is converted to melatonin. (Ac = acetyl.)

neurons, such as dopaminergic neurons, because of the non-selective nature of aromatic amino acid decarboxylase. Inhibitors of tryptophan hydroxylase such as *para*-chlorophenylalanine are used as pharmacologic tools and are not used therapeutically.

Therapeutically exploited serotonergic targets include the postsynaptic receptors, reuptake mechanisms, and metabolism. MAO inhibitors effectively interfere with the oxidative deamination of 5-HT to increase synaptic concentrations of 5-HT. The MAO inhibitor tranylcypromine, for example, has been used since the 1960s as an antidepressant. A problem associated with many MAO inhibitors is that they are notoriously nonselective and can interfere with the metabolism of other neurotransmitters, amines found in certain foods, and exogenously administered amine-containing therapeutic agents.

Tranylcypromine

SEROTONIN RECEPTORS

Seven families or populations of serotonergic receptors have been identified, 5-HT$_1$–5-HT$_7$, and several are divided into distinct subpopulations (see Table 12.2) (4–6, 13–15). The discovery of the individual populations and subpopulations of 5-HT receptors follows the approximate order of their numbering and, as a consequence, more is known about 5-HT$_1$ and 5-HT$_2$ receptors than about 5-HT$_6$ and 5-HT$_7$ receptors. Other factors contributing to our current lack of knowledge about certain receptor populations (i.e., 5-HT$_{1E}$ or 5-HT$_5$ receptors) is the absence of agonists/antagonists with selectivity for these receptors.

History

Tritiated LSD ([^{3}H]LSD) was the first radioligand used to identify a brain 5-HT binding site, suggesting it to be a "hallucinogen receptor." Tritiated 5-HT ([^{3}H]5-HT) labeled serotonergic sites displaying high affinity for LSD. Thus, not only did 5-HT and LSD share structural similarity, there now was evidence that these agents might be acting via a common receptor type. According to the *interconvertible receptor conformation hypothesis* popular at the time, 5-HT (known to be an agonist), interacted with the agonist conformation of the receptor whereas [^{3}H]LSD, LSD being known to be a partial agonist, labeled both the agonist and antagonist conformations (8). A search was initiated for 5-HT antagonists that could be used as radioligands for studying serotonergic receptors. Leysen and co-workers (7) made the serendipitous discovery that a tritiated version of the dopamine antagonist spiperone not only labeled dopaminergic receptors but also labeled nondopaminergic receptors in other brain regions. It was shown that 5-HT displayed modest affinity for these sites and that they might represent 5-HT receptors. Spiperone was also shown to antagonize some of the pharmacologic effects of 5-HT. These

data, coupled with the additional observation that 5-HT agonists tended to display higher affinity for [^{3}H]5-HT-labeled sites whereas 5-HT antagonists displayed higher affinity for [^{3}H]spiperone-labeled sites, led to the conclusion that [^{3}H]5-HT and [^{3}H]spiperone labeled two distinct populations of sites: termed 5-HT$_1$ and 5-HT$_2$ receptors, respectively (9). 5-HT$_1$ receptors were soon thereafter found to consist of 5-HT$_{1A}$ and 5-HT$_{1B}$ subpopulations. During the 1950s, Gaddum and Picarelli (11) had demonstrated the existence of two populations of serotonergic receptors in isolated guinea pig ileum and called these 5-HT-D (because the phenoxybenzamine, dibenzyline, blocked 5-HT at this receptor) and 5-HT-M receptors (because morphine and cocaine blocked the actions of 5-HT at the second population). 5-HT-D receptors were later found to be identical with 5-HT$_2$ receptors, and 5-HT-M receptors were later renamed 5-HT$_3$ receptors. By the early 1980s, 5-HT$_{1A}$, 5-HT$_{1B}$, (10) 5-HT$_2$ and 5-HT$_3$ (12) receptors had been identified, and interest in 5-HT research exploded. Molecular biology intervened in the late 1980s and early 1990s which allowed new populations of serotonergic receptors to be cloned and expressed. This led to attempts to develop selective agonists and antagonists for each subpopulation (13–17).

Table 12.2 lists the receptor classification and nomenclatures that have been employed for serotonergic receptors. Other 5-HT orphan receptors, that have not yet been cloned, include the 5-HT$_{1P}$ receptors which are found only in the gastrointestinal tract (15). Care should be used when reading the older primary literature because 5-HT receptor nomenclature has changed so dramatically and can often be confusing and very frustrating to comprehend.

Most of the seven serotonergic receptor populations have been cloned and, together with the cloning of other neurotransmitter receptors, has led to generalizations regarding amino acid sequence homology (18). Any two receptors whose amino acid sequences are about 70–80% identical in their transmembrane-spanning segments are called the *intermediate-homology group*. This group of receptors may be members of the same subfamily, and have highly similar, to nearly indistinguishable, pharmacologic profiles or second messenger systems. A *low-homology group* (~35–55% TM homology) consists of distantly related receptor subtypes from the same neurotransmitter family, and a *high-homology group* (~95–99% TM homology) consists of species homologs from the same gene in different species (18). Species homologs of the same gene reveal high sequence conservation in regions outside the transmembrane domains, whereas intraspecies receptor subtypes are usually quite different (18). Current 5-HT receptor classification and nomenclature require that several criteria be met before a receptor population can be adequately characterized. Receptor populations must be identified on the basis of drug-binding characteristics (*operational or recognitory criteria*), receptor-effector coupling (*transductional criteria*), and on gene and receptor structure sequences for the nucleotide and amino acid components, respectively (*structural criteria*) (15).

5-HT₁ Family

5-HT₁ receptors were one of the first two populations of 5-HT receptors to be identified (9), and 5-HT$_{1A}$, 5-HT$_{1B}$ (10), 5-HT$_{1C}$ (19) (later re-named 5-HT$_{2C}$), 5-HT$_{1D}$ (20), 5-HT$_{1E}$ (21) and 5-HT$_{1F}$ (22) receptor subfamilies have been subsequently defined and cloned. With the exception of 5-HT$_{1E}$ receptors, all 5-HT₁ receptors exhibit high affinity for 5-carboxamidotryptamine (5-CT).

5-CT

5-HT$_{1A}$ Receptors and Agents

5-HT$_{1A}$ receptors are G protein-coupled receptors that consist of seven transmembrane-spanning helices connected by intracellular and extracellular loops (see Fig. 12.3 for a schematic representation of a generalized G protein recep-

tor structure). The receptors are negatively coupled to an adenylate cyclase second messenger system, and the 5-HT$_{1A}$ receptors located in the raphe nuclei correspond to somatodendritic autoreceptors (see Fig. 12.4). 5-HT$_{1A}$ receptors differ significantly in structure from most other 5-HT receptors and exhibit a substantial similarity to adrenergic receptors which probably explains why a number of adrenergic agents bind at 5-HT$_{1A}$ receptors with high affinity. Cloned 5-HT$_{1A}$ receptors, and 5-HT$_{1A}$ ligands, have been extensively reviewed (5,13,23–26).

Structure-activity Relationship of 5-HT$_{1A}$ Agonists

Overview.   Numerous tryptamines bind with high affinity at 5-HT$_{1A}$ receptors but most are notoriously nonselective. The most selective 5-HT$_{1A}$ receptor agonist is the aminotetralin derivative 8-hydroxy-2-(di-n-propylamino)tetralin (8-OH DPAT), and its early discovery was significant in advancing an understanding of 5-HT$_{1A}$ receptors. Furthermore, because the structure of 8-OH DPAT is similar to that of 5-HT (8-OH DPAT/Serotonin), its activity indicated that an intact indole nucleus was not required for 5-HT$_{1A}$ actions. Although numerous 8-OH DPAT derivatives

Table 12.2. Classification and Nomenclature for the Various Populations of 5-HT Receptors

Populations and Subpopulations	Second Messenger System*	Currently Accepted Name†	Comments
5-HT₁			
5-HT$_{1A}$	AC(−)	5-HT$_{1A}$	Cloned and pharmacological 5-HT$_{1A}$ receptors.
5-HT$_{1B}$	AC(−)	5-HT$_{1B}$	Rodent homolog of 5-HT$_{1B}$ receptors.
5-HT$_{1Bβ}$			A mouse homolog of h5-HT$_{1B}$ receptors.
5-HT$_{1D}$			Sites identified in binding studies using human and calf brain homogenates.
5-HT$_{1Dα}$	AC(−)	h5-HT$_{1D}$	A cloned human 5-HT$_{1D}$ subpopulation.
5-HT$_{1Dβ}$	AC(−)	h5-HT$_{1B}$	A second cloned human 5-HT$_{1D}$ subpopulation; human counterpart of rat 5-HT$_{1B}$.
5-HT$_{1E}$	AC(−)	5-HT$_{1E}$	Sites identified in binding studies using brain homogenates and cloned receptors.
5-HT$_{1Eα}$			An alternate name that has been used for cloned human 5-HT$_{1E}$ receptors.
5-HT$_{1Eβ}$	AC(−)	5-ht$_{1F}$	A cloned mouse homolog of 5-HT$_{1F}$ receptors.
5-HT$_{1F}$			A cloned human 5-HT₁ receptor population.
5-HT₂			
5-HT₂	PI	5-HT$_{2A}$	Original "5-HT₂" (sometimes called 5-HT$_{2α}$) receptors.
5-HT$_{2F}$	PI	5-HT$_{2B}$	5-HT₂-like receptors originally found in rat fundus.
5-HT$_{1C}$	PI	5-HT$_{2C}$	Originally described as 5-HT$_{1C}$ (5-HT$_{2β}$) receptors.
5-HT₃			
5-HT₃	Ion Channel	5-HT₃	An ion channel receptor.
5-HT₄			
5-HT₄	AC(+)	5-HT₄	5-HT₄ population originally described in functional studies.
5-HT$_{4S}$			Short form of cloned 5-HT₄ receptors.
5-HT$_{4L}$			Long form of cloned 5-HT₄ receptors.
5HT$_{4(b)-4(d)}$			Recently identified human 5-HT₄ receptor isoforms.
5-HT₅			
5-HT$_{5A}$	?	5-ht$_{5A}$	Cloned mouse, rat and human 5-HT₅ receptors.
5-HT$_{5B}$	?	5-ht$_{5A}$	Cloned mouse and rat 5-HT$_{5A}$-like receptor.
5-HT₇			
5-HT$_{c}$	AC(+)	5-HT₆	Cloned rat and human 5-HT receptor.
5-HT₇			
5-HT₇	AC(+)	5-HT₇	Cloned rat, mouse, guinea pig and human 5-HT receptors.

*AC = adenylate cyclase, (−): negatively coupled and (+): positively coupled; PI = phospholipase coupled.
†From Hoyer et al (15).

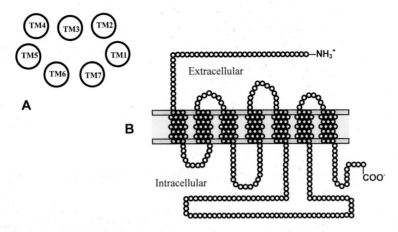

Fig. 12.3. Top view (**A**) and side view (**B**) of a schematic representation of a typical G protein-coupled receptor. In **B**, the transmembrane-spanning helical portions are numbered TM1-TM7 from left to right. The seven helices are connected by extracellular and intracellular loops. The large intracellular loop between TM5 and TM6 is believed to be associated with coupling to a second messenger system. The helices are arranged in such a manner that TM1 is adjacent to TM7 as shown in **A**. Molecular graphics studies suggest that agonists might bind in a manner that utilizes an aspartate residue in TM3 (common to all G protein-coupled 5-HT receptors) and residues in the TM4, TM5, and TM6 regions (Site 1), whereas antagonists likely utilize the aspartate moiety but residues in the TM2, TM1, and TM7 regions (Site 2).

have been reported, none is used therapeutically because of their low oral bioavailability. This has led to efforts to develop novel aminotetralins with greater oral availability.

8-OH DPAT

8-OH DPAT superimposed on Serotonin

Long-chain Arylpiperazines (LCAPs). Simple arylpiperazines (i.e., those bearing no N_4-substituent or only a small N_4-substituent), such as 1-(phenyl)piperazine (Fig. 12.5), bind with modest to reasonably high affinity at a multitude of receptor types and are nonselective agents. *Long-chain arylpiperazines* (LCAPs), those piperazines possessing an elaborated N_4 substituent, probably represent the largest class of 5-HT$_{1A}$ ligands (27). Buspirone (Fig. 12.5), the first arylpiperazine approved for clinical use as an anxiolytic agent, and the structurally related gepirone and ipsapirone, bind at 5-HT$_{1A}$ receptors and behave as agonists or partial agonists. Structure-activity and structure-affinity relationships (SAR and SAFIR, respectively) have been formulated and this has led to LCAPs with enhanced affinity and selectivity for 5-HT$_{1A}$ receptors (26–28). With the LCAPs there seems to be substantial structural latitude for 5-HT$_{1A}$ binding (28).

The **Aryl** portion of these agents (Fig. 12.6) is typically a phenyl, substituted phenyl, or a heteroaryl group such as 2-pyrimidinyl. The intact piperazine ring seems optimal for binding to 5-HT$_{1A}$ receptors. A **spacer** or linker separates the N_4-nitrogen atom of the piperazine and the **Terminus.** There has been controversy as to whether or not the spacer actively participates in binding to the receptor or whether it acts simply as a connector; in any event, a chain of two to five atoms is common. The **Terminus** is typically an amide or imide, but it has been shown that neither is required for

binding, or it may be a phenyl or some other aryl or heteroaryl substituent (28). With respect to spacer length, when the spacer is $-(CH_2)_n-$, two to four methylene groups appear optimal. Chain length (n) can influence affinity and selectivity. When the Terminus contains a heteroarylamide, $n = 4$ seems optimal, whereas when the Terminus is an alkylamide, optimal affinity is associated with $n = 2$ (27–29). A region of bulk tolerance is associated with the Terminus, or at least a portion thereof, and very bulky groups have been introduced into this part of the molecule (26,28). Some LCAPs are nonselective and may variously bind at other populations of 5-HT receptors, dopamine receptors, or adrenergic receptors.

Structure-activity Relationship of 5-HT$_{1A}$ Antagonists. Many 5-HT$_{1A}$ antagonists possess a 2-methoxy group with structural similarity to buspirone. BMY 7378 and NAN-190

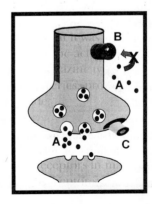

Fig. 12.4. Typical nerve ending showing the cell body (i.e., somatodendritic) autoreceptors (**B**) and the terminal autoreceptors (**C**). Neurotransmitter molecules are indicated by **A**. Neurotransmitters can interact with cell body autoreceptors **B** to regulate synthesis, and with terminal autoreceptors **C** to regulate release. Shown above is a drug molecule blocking the cell body autoreceptor and preventing an interaction with the neurotransmitter.

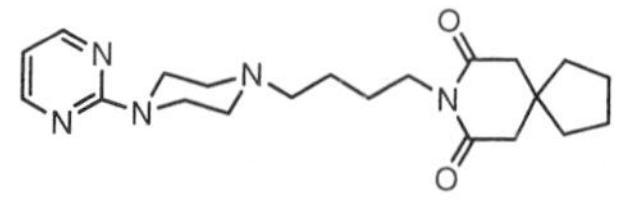

Buspirone

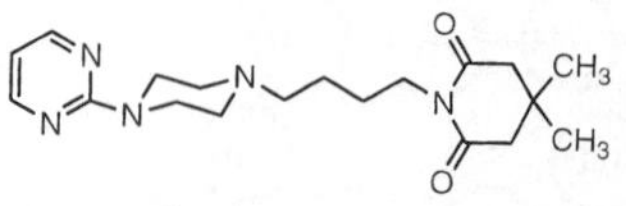

Gepirone

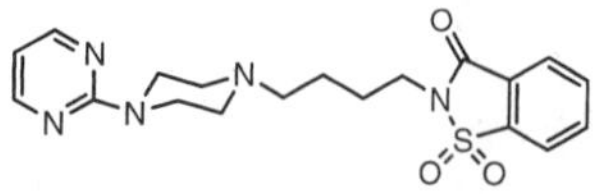

Ipsapirone

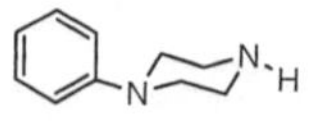

1-(Phenyl)piperazine

Fig. 12.5. 5-HT$_{1A}$ agonists-arylpiperaznies.

were among the first agents shown to be very weak partial agonists at 5-HT$_{1A}$ receptors and were used as antagonists (28) (Fig. 12.7). Certain aminotetralins (e.g., S(−)UH-301) and arylpiperazines (e.g., WAY 100135, WAY 100635) represent new classes of 5-HT$_{1A}$ antagonists that are termed "silent antagonists" because they are without any 5-HT$_{1A}$ agonist action. The alkylpiperidine spiperone is a 5-HT$_{1A}$ antagonist, but it displays even greater affinity for D$_2$ dopamine receptors and 5-HT$_{2A}$ receptors.

Molecular graphics studies suggest (30–33) that 5-HT and 5-HT$_{1A}$ agonists typically interact with amino acid residues associated with helices 4, 5 and 6 (*Site 1*) whereas 5-HT$_{1A}$ antagonists likely interact with amino acid residues in helices 1, 2, 7 and perhaps 6 (*Site 2*). The basic primary amine for both types of agents are thought to bind at a common aspartate residue found in TM helix 3 (see Fig. 12.3). The 5-hydroxy group of 5-HT forms a hydrogen bond with threonine residue in helix 5 (30,31).

5-HT$_{1A}$ Receptor Agonists: Clinical Significance. In preclinical studies, 5-HT$_{1A}$ agonists have demonstrated antianxiety, antidepressant, antiaggressive, and perhaps anticraving, anticataleptic, antiemetic, and neuroprotective properties (34). There is also evidence that 5-HT$_{1A}$ receptors might be involved in sleep, impulsivity, alcoholism, sexual behavior, appetite control, thermoregulation, and cardiovascular function (34–38). The main focus of drug development for 5-HT$_{1A}$ receptors is their therapeutic potential for the treatment of anxiety and depression (36). Buspirone (Buspar) was the first LCAP to become clinically available as an anxiolytic agent and a number of structurally-related agents hold promise as novel anxiolytics (25,26,39). 5-HT$_{1A}$ agents might also be useful in the treatment of depression and there may be a relationship between 5-HT metabolism, depression, and violent behavior. The antianxiety actions of 5-HT$_{1A}$ (partial) agonists may involve primarily presynaptic somatodendritic 5-HT$_{1A}$ receptors whereas the antidepressant actions of 5-HT$_{1A}$

agents may primarily involve postsynaptic 5-HT$_{1A}$ receptors (34). Gepirone was found to produce marked improvement in depressed patients, and buspirone has been found effective in the treatment of mixed anxious-depressive patients. 5-HT$_1$, possibly 5-HT$_{1A}$, receptors have been implicated in obsessive-compulsive disorders.

5-HT$_{1A}$ Receptor Antagonists: Clinical Significance. A new direction in 5-HT$_{1A}$ research targets the development of 5-HT$_{1A}$ antagonists (40). Agents such as the dopaminergic antagonist spiperone and the β-adrenergic antagonist propranolol were among the first to see application as 5-HT$_{1A}$ antagonists. However, these agents are obviously nonselective and bind at other populations of neurotransmitter receptors with higher affinities than they display at 5-HT$_{1A}$ receptors. The next generation of 5-HT$_{1A}$ antagonists, BMY 7378 and NAN-190, possessed postsynaptic antagonist character, but also some presynaptic agonist action (28,40) (Fig. 12.7). A third generation of agents—the "silent 5-HT$_{1A}$ antagonists"—has been developed and includes WAY 100635, WAY 100135 (a structural relative of BMY 7378 and NAN-190) and S(−)UH-301 (a derivative of the 5-HT$_{1A}$ agonist 8-OH DPAT); these are both presynaptic and postsynaptic 5-HT$_{1A}$ antagonists (40,41). The silent 5-HT$_{1A}$ antagonists, such as WAY 100135 and S(−)UH-301, are not intrinsically inactive and can indirectly produce non-5-HT$_{1A}$ serotonin-mediated actions (43,44). These antagonists presumably block 5-HT$_{1A}$ autoreceptors, increasing the postsynaptic concentration of 5-HT which results in the activation of other serotonergic receptor populations. Human evaluation of silent and selective 5-HT$_{1A}$ antagonists should prove interesting and could open new vistas in 5-HT$_{1A}$ research and therapeutics. For example, pretreatment of patients with 5-HT$_{1A}$ antagonists could accelerate the effects of selective 5-HT reuptake inhibitors (SSRIs) and enhance their clinical efficacy as antidepressants (45). The 5-HT$_{1A}$ antagonist WAY 100635 enhances the anorectic effect of citalopram in animals (46) and may thus be of benefit in weight reduction. Combination therapy using an SSRI plus a 5-HT$_{1A}$ antagonist, including the beta blocker pindolol which binds at 5-HT$_{1A}$ receptors, has been patented for the treatment of sleep disorders. However, recent studies suggest that pindolol may possess agonist, rather than antagonist, character at 5-HT$_{1A}$ autoreceptors (47). The therapeutic potential of 5-HT$_{1A}$ antagonists appears quite intriguing.

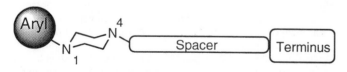

Fig. 12.6. General structure of long-chain arylpiperazines. (LCAPS)

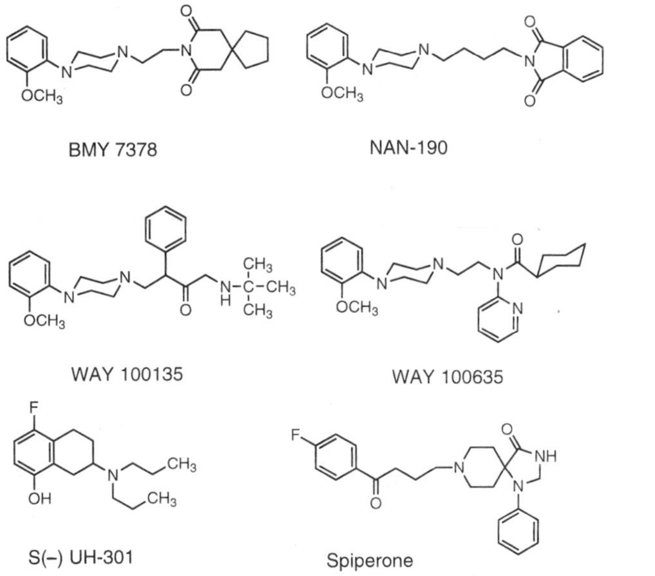

Fig. 12.7. 5-HT$_{1A}$ antagonists.

5-HT$_{1B}$ Receptors and Agents

Overview. Early studies identified 5-HT$_{1B}$ receptors in rodent brain using radioligand binding techniques, but failed to find them in human brain. 5-HT$_{1B}$ receptors are located both presynaptically, where they regulate the release of 5-HT (see Fig. 12.4), and postsynaptically (48). Like 5-HT$_{1A}$ receptors, they are negatively coupled to adenylate cyclase. See 5-HT$_{1D}$ receptors for further related discussion.

5-HT$_{1B}$ Receptors: Clinical Significance. Rodent 5-HT$_{1B}$ receptors have been implicated as playing roles in thermoregulation, respiration, appetite control, sexual behavior, aggression, locomotor activity, sleep regulation, sensorimotor inhibition, and anxiety (5,49).

5-HT$_{1D}$ Receptors

5-HT$_{1D}$ receptors were first identified by radioligand binding techniques and are widely distributed throughout the central nervous system (24,49,50). They are G protein-linked and are coupled to inhibition of adenylate cyclase. Two human subpopulations of 5-HT$_{1D}$ receptors, 5-HT$_{1D\alpha}$ and 5-HT$_{1D\beta}$ receptors, display about 77% sequence homology; their pharmacologic properties are nearly indistinguishable. Due to the high degree of species homology with rat and mouse 5-HT$_{1B}$ receptors, human 5-HT$_{1D\beta}$ receptors have been renamed h5-HT$_{1B}$ receptors. Human 5-HT$_{1D\alpha}$ receptors have been renamed h5-HT$_{1D}$ (15). Most agents that bind at 5-HT$_{1B}$ receptors typically bind at 5-HT$_{1D}$ receptors. Curious exceptions have been observed with certain aryloxyalkylamines such as the beta blockers, propranolol and pindolol, which exhibit very low affinity (Ki > 5,000 nM) for h5-HT$_{1D}$ receptors (51,52). The major functional difference between rat 5-HT$_{1B}$ receptors and human h5-HT$_{1B}$ receptors has been attributed to the presence of a threonine residue at position 355 (i.e., Thr 355)

in TM7 of the latter and the presence of an asparagine residue at the corresponding position in 5-HT$_{1B}$ receptors; site-directed mutagenesis studies have demonstrated that conversion of Thr 355 to an asparagine (i.e., a T355N mutant) accounts for the binding differences of certain ligands (e.g., aryloxyalkylamines such as propranolol). Combined ligand SAR, site-directed mutagenesis, and molecular modeling studies have led to the conclusion that although most typical serotonergic agonists bind in the central cavity formed by TM3, TM4, TM5 and TM6 (Site 1; see Fig. 12.3), propranolol most likely occupies the region defined by TM1, TM2, TM3, and TM7 (Site 2). The higher affinity of propranolol for the T355N mutant 5-HT$_{1B}$ receptors relative to the wild-type receptors was specifically attributed to the formation of two hydrogen bonds between the receptor asparagine and the ether and hydroxyl oxygen atoms of propranolol (52).

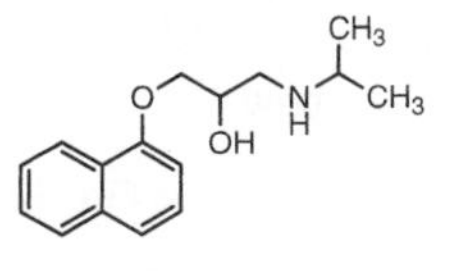

Propranolol 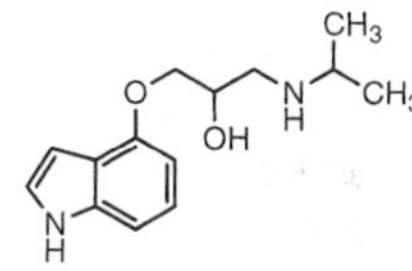   Pindolol

5-HT$_{1D}$ Agonists and Antagonists. There are few 5-HT$_{1D}$-selective agonists (55), but one agent commonly referred to as a prototypical 5-HT$_{1D}$ agonist is sumatriptan (Imitrex). However, sumatriptan exhibits 2- to 20-fold greater selectivity for the 5-HT$_{1D}$ receptors than for other populations of 5-HT$_1$ receptors, and binds at h5-HT$_{1D}$ and h5-HT$_{1B}$ receptors with nearly identical (ca 6–8 nM) affinity, and also binds at 5-HT$_{1F}$ receptors (55). Structure-activity relationships for 5-HT$_{1D}$ agonists have been reported for many indolealkylamines or tryptamine derivatives, which bind with high affinity but with little selectivity (49). New agents displaying high affinity and reasonable selectivity for h5-HT$_{1D}$/h5-HT$_{1B}$ receptors over other populations of 5-HT receptors (26,50,53) include, for example, zolmitriptan (Zomig), IS-159, naratriptan (Amerge), BMS-180048, rizatriptan (Maxalt), NOT(ALX-1323) and alniditan. Of these, all are tryptamine derivatives or sumatriptan-related structures except for the benzopyran alniditan. Many of these are commercially available or are currently undergoing clinical trials. Other investigational agonists are shown in Figure 12.8.

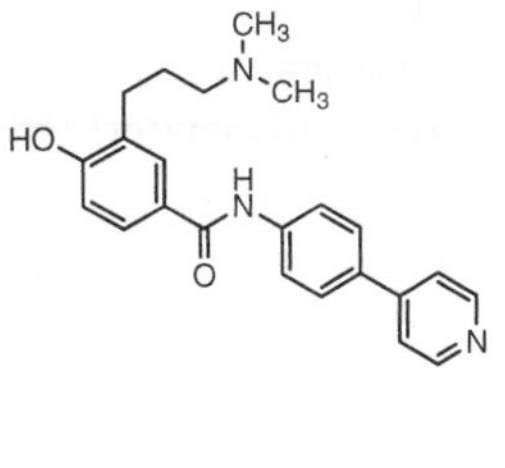

GR 55562 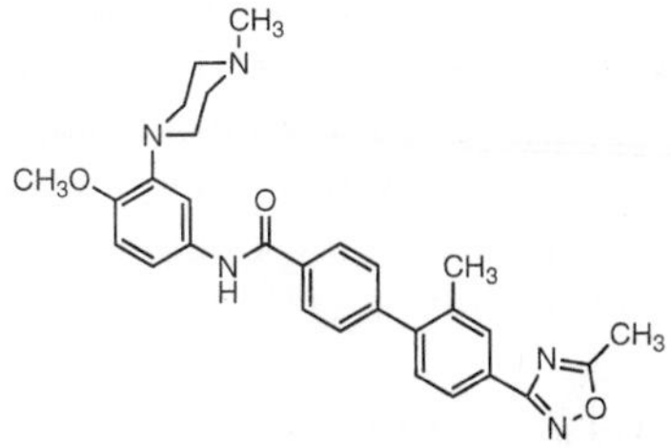   GR 127935

Several 5-HT$_{1D}$ receptor antagonists have been developed including GR127935 (high affinity for h5-HT$_{1D}$/h5-HT$_{1B}$ receptors but might be a low-efficacy partial agonist)

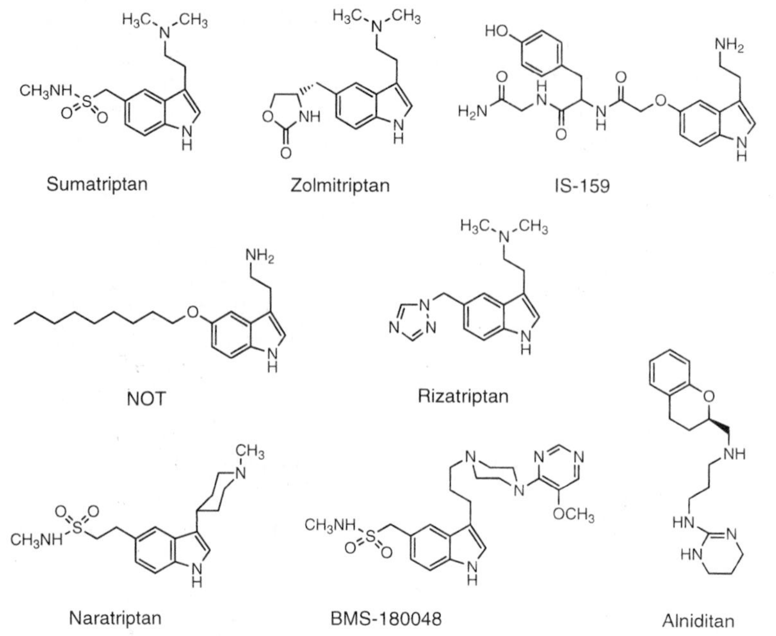

Fig. 12.8. 5-HT$_{1D}$ receptor agonists.

and GR55562 (54). Both of these agents antagonize many of the effects of sumatriptan (54).

5-HT$_{1D}$ Receptors: Clinical Significance. The clinical significance of 5-HT$_{1D}$ receptors remains largely unknown. There is speculation that these receptors might be involved in anxiety, depression, and other neuropsychiatric disorders, but this remains to be substantiated. Recent studies show that 5-HT$_{1D}$ receptors are the dominant species in human cerebral blood vessels. Sumatriptan, and several closely related agents, are clinically effective in the treatment of migraine and logical extrapolation implies a role for 5-HT$_{1D}$ receptors in this disorder. However, the finding that the sumatriptan-related agents bind nearly equally well at h5-HT$_{1D}$ and h5-HT$_{1B}$ receptors (53), and that sumatriptan also binds at 5-HT$_{1F}$ receptors, has further complicated this issue. It has been variously proposed that h5-HT$_{1D}$ (56) or h5-HT$_{1B}$ (55) receptors be targeted for the development of novel antimigraine agents, because h5-HT$_{1D}$ receptors might be primarily involved in neurogenic inflammation due to their preponderance in neuronal tissue whereas h5-HT$_{1B}$ receptors might be more involved in vasoconstriction. However, activation of h5-HT$_{1B}$-like receptors may account for some of the cardiovascular side effects associated with sumatriptan (57). Although this issue has yet to be resolved (58), there are now ongoing investigations to develop new agonists with h5-HT$_{1D}$ versus h5-HT$_{1B}$ selectivity.

5-HT$_{1E}$ Receptors and Agents

The masking of brain 5-HT$_{1A}$ and 5-HT$_{1B}$ receptors in radioligand binding studies using [^{3}H]5-HT as radioligand resulted in biphasic competition curves providing evidence of two additional 5-HT$_1$-like receptor populations. One of these was the 5-HT$_{1D}$ receptors and the other was termed 5-HT$_{1E}$. The low affinity of 5-CT and ergotamine for 5-HT$_{1E}$

receptors allowed their differentiation from 5-HT$_{1D}$ receptors. Simple O-methylation of 5-HT reduces the affinity of 5-HT for this receptor by about 100- to 300-fold (59,60). Typically, ergolines such as ergonovine and methylergonovine (60) bind to 5-HT$_{1E}$ receptors with Ki values of <100 nM. Studies indicate that these receptors are negatively coupled to adenylate cyclase. No 5-HT$_{1E}$-selective agonists or antagonists have been reported.

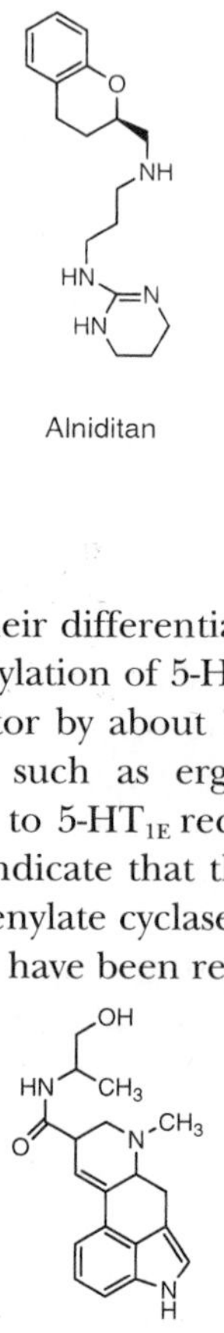

Ergonovine

5-HT$_{1F}$ Receptors

Overview. The newest 5-HT$_1$ receptor subpopulation to be cloned is the human 5-HT$_{1F}$ receptor (61) which exhibits intermediate (~50–70%) amino acid sequence homology with other 5-HT$_1$ receptor subpopulations. The receptors are coupled to inhibition of adenylate cyclase. Detection of these receptors in the uterus and mesentery suggest a possible role in vascular contraction. Although their distribution in the brain appears limited, there are distributional similarities with h5-HT$_{1B}$ receptors. A 4-(3-indolyl)piperidine, LY-334370, and an aminocarbazole, LY-344864, have been identified as the first 5-HT$_{1F}$-selective agonists (62). The nonselective 5-HT$_1$ antagonist methiothepin has been shown to also act as a 5-HT$_{1F}$ antagonist (22).

5-HT$_{1F}$ Receptors: Clinical Significance. The clinical significance of 5-HT$_{1F}$ receptors is unknown at this time. The binding of sumatriptan to this receptor population

LY-344864   LY-334370

suggests a relationship between 5-HT$_{1F}$ receptor binding and antimigraine activity (22,63). Other antimigraine agents currently undergoing clinical trials, including naratriptan, rizatriptan, and zolmitriptan, and LY-334370, bind at 5-HT$_{1F}$ receptors. Recent studies show that 5-HT$_{1D}$ receptors are the dominant species in human cerebral blood vessels and that 5-HT$_{1F}$ receptors are also expressed both in neural and vascular tissue (56).

5-HT$_2$ Family

Serotonin receptors were first divided into 5-HT$_1$ and 5-HT$_2$ receptor families in 1979 (9) and the latter were subsequently divided into subfamilies 5-HT$_{2A}$, 5-HT$_{2B}$, and 5-HT$_{2C}$ (formerly 5-HT$_{1C}$ receptors) receptors. The term "5-HT$_2$" now refers to a receptor family, not an individual population of receptors. Ketanserin was identified early as a 5-HT$_2$ antagonist with no affinity for 5-HT$_1$ receptors, and [^{3}H]ketanserin was introduced as a radioligand to label 5-HT$_2$ receptors. 1-(2,5-Dimethoxy-4X-phenyl)-2-aminopropane where X = -Br and -I (DOB and DOI, respectively) were introduced as 5-HT$_2$ agonists. A significant amount of pharmacology was published and structure-activity studies led to the development of many novel agents (64). Many of the original agents thought to be 5-HT$_2$-selective, including standard antagonists such as ketanserin and the agonists DOB and DOI, were later shown to bind nonselectively both to 5-HT$_{2A}$ and 5-HT$_{2C}$ receptors. Consequently, pharmacologic actions originally thought to be 5-HT$_2$-mediated might actually involve 5-HT$_{2A}$ receptors,

DOI   DOB

5-HT$_{2C}$ receptors, or a combination of 5-HT$_{2A}$ and 5-HT$_{2C}$ receptors. The structures of the three 5-HT$_2$ receptor subpopulations were found consistent with those of transmembrane-spanning G protein-coupled receptors, and the receptors all utilize a phospholipase C second messenger system. There is approximately 70–80% sequence homology among the three receptor subtypes. Only very recently have novel agents with subpopulation selectivity been reported.

5-HT$_{2A}$ Receptors

5-HT$_{2A}$ receptors, formerly 5-HT$_2$ receptors, have been extensively reviewed (6,24,64–66). 5-HT$_{2A}$ receptors have been cloned from various species, including

human, and exhibit a high degree (>90%) of species homology. There is significant (78%) amino acid sequence homology between the transmembrane portions of 5-HT$_{2A}$ receptors and cloned 5-HT$_{2C}$ receptors, which may explain the observed similarities in the binding of various ligands at the two receptor populations. Evidence was provided that 5-HT$_{2A}$ receptors exist in a high-affinity state and a low-affinity state (sometimes referred to as 5-HT$_{2H}$ and 5-HT$_{2L}$ states). Under normal conditions the low affinity state predominates. The tritiated antagonist, [^{3}H]ketanserin, has comparable affinity for both states whereas agonists display higher affinity for the high-affinity state (such as when a tritiated agonist is employed as radioligand).

5-HT$_{2A}$ Agonists. The structure-activity relationships for 5-HT$_{2A}$ binding have been reviewed (4,6,27,64). Most indolealkylamines are nonselective 5-HT$_{2A}$ ligands and typically bind with higher affinity at the tritiated agonist-labeled high-affinity state. Recent investigations suggest that all indolealkylamines may not bind in the same manner at 5-HT$_{2A}$ receptors (67). Phenylalkylamines, such as DOB and DOI, act as 5-HT$_{2A}$ agonists or high-efficacy partial agonists and are significantly more selective than the indolealkylamines due to their low affinity for non-5-HT$_{2A}$ sites, but do not differentiate between 5-HT$_2$ subpopulations.

5-HT$_{2A}$ Antagonists. One of the largest and more selective classes of 5-HT$_{2A}$ antagonists are the N-alkylpiperidines. The best known examples are ketanserin and ritanserin. Although numerous ketanserin-related derivatives have been reported, their structure-activity relationships still have not been well defined. Nevertheless, far less than the entire structure of ketanserin is required for high affinity (65). Even though spiperone (Fig. 12.7) has been employed as a 5-HT$_{2A}$ antagonist with 1,000-fold selectivity for 5-HT$_{2A}$ versus 5-HT$_{2C}$ receptors, it is also a dopamine antagonist, a 5-HT$_{1A}$ antagonist, and a 5-HT$_7$ antagonist. Other structurally-related agents, such as the piperazine derivative irindalone, also act as 5-HT$_{2A}$ antagonists. Many 5-HT$_{2A}$ antagonists, although fairly selective for 5-HT$_{2A/2C}$ receptors versus most other populations of 5-HT receptors, bind with modest to high affinity at dopaminergic, histaminergic or adrenergic neurotransmitter receptors. The tricyclic neuroleptics (risperidone, clozapine, olanzapine) (Fig. 12.8) and tricyclic antidepressants also bind at 5-HT$_{2A}$ receptors.

5-HT$_{2A}$ Receptors: Clinical Implications

Overview. The potential therapeutic roles of 5-HT$_{2A}$ ligands and the possible involvement of 5-HT$_{2A}$ receptors in modulating normal physiologic functions and various pathologic and psychopathologic conditions have been extensively reviewed (24,37,38). 5-HT$_{2A}$ receptors appear to play a role in thermoregulation and sleep, and might be involved in appetite control, learning (68), and, along with various other serotonergic receptor populations, in cardiovascular function and muscle contraction. Many of the clinical implications of 5-HT_{2A} receptors may actually involve 5-HT_{2C} receptors or a combination of 5-HT_{2A} and 5-HT_{2C} receptors because of the high homology between the two populations and because the investigations were conducted prior to the discovery of subpopulations of 5-HT_2 receptors. With the recent development of subpopulation-selective agents, this is currently an important area of research.

Antipsychotic Agents and Antidepressants. Various typical and atypical antipsychotic agents and antidepressants (Chapter 17) bind with relatively high affinity at 5-HT_{2A} receptors as antagonists. Although there is no direct correlation between their receptor affinities and clinically effective doses, there is strong evidence that these disorders involve, at least to some extent, 5-HT_{2A} receptors. For example, chronic administration of 5-HT_{2A} antagonists results in a paradoxical down regulation of 5-HT_{2A} receptors. Such a down regulation would be of benefit in the treatment of depression. Several 5-HT_{2A} antagonists, such as risperidone, seem to possess antipsychotic activity. Many 5-HT_{2A} antagonists also bind at dopamine receptors. Although this may obfuscate the role of 5-HT_{2A} antagonism versus dopamine antagonism as being the more important for antipsychotic activity, it has been suggested that certain types of schizophrenia might actually be more responsive to the combined effect. That is, D_2 dopaminergic antagonists seem more effective for treating the positive symptoms of schizophrenia whereas the 5-HT_{2A} antagonists might be more effective in treating the negative symptoms. Certain atypical antipsychotic agents bind to both dopamine and 5-HT_{2A} receptors, suggesting an *atypicality theory* of psychosis. This theory suggests that the 5-HT_{2A} component of binding may be related to the decrease in extrapyramidal side effects associated with these types of agents. Those drugs that display a $D_2/5\text{-HT}_{2A}$ ratio of >1 seem to produce fewer extrapyramidal effects than those with ratios of <1. The atypical antipsychotic agent clozapine, for example, has a $D_2/5\text{-HT}_{2A}$ ratio of 10–20 and (Ki values of 100–500 nM and 10–50 nM, respectively). Olanzapine and perosprione (SM-9018) (69) are other examples of an atypical antipsychotic agent that binds at 5-HT_{2A} receptors. From preclinical studies there are indications that 5-HT_{2A} antagonists possess anxiolytic properties, such as ritanserin (Fig. 12.9), which has been demonstrated to produce both antipsychotic and antianxiety effects in humans. The role of 5-HT receptors in anxiety has been reviewed (39).

5-HT_{2A} receptors may be involved in the actions of the classical hallucinogens (70; see also Chapter 18). Although indolealkylamine (e.g., 5-methoxy-N,N-dimethyltryptamine; 5-OMe DMT) and ergot-related (e.g. LSD) classical hallucinogens are fairly nonselective ligands that bind to multiple populations of serotonergic receptors, the phenylalkylamine hallucinogens (e.g., DOB, DOI) are much more 5-HT_2-selective agonists. Furthermore, there is a significant corre-

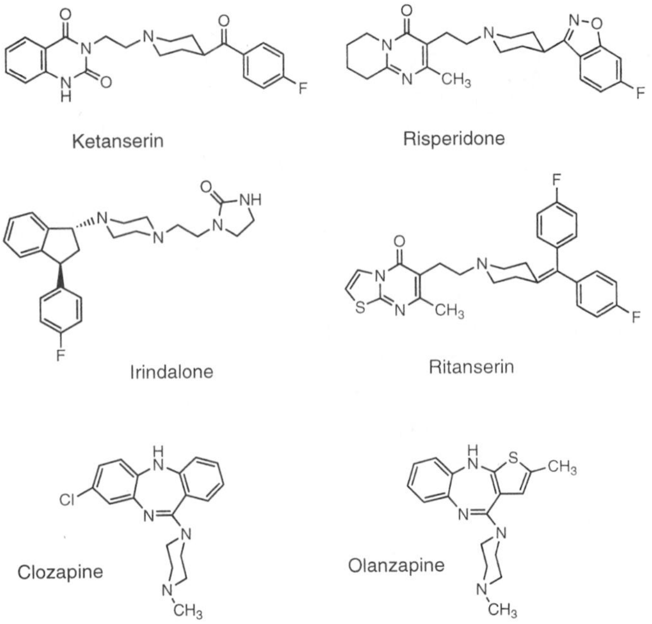

Fig. 12.9. 5-HT_{2A} antagonists.

lation between the human hallucinogenic potencies of classical hallucinogens and their 5-HT_{2A} receptor affinities (70). Interestingly, phenylalkylamine hallucinogens also bind at 5-HT_{2B} and 5-HT_{2C} receptors, and here, too, there is a significant correlation between human potency and receptor affinity for 17 different agents (71). Recent studies suggest that 5-HT_{2A} receptors may play a more prominent role than 5-HT_{2B} or 5-HT_{2C} receptors for the behavioral actions of hallucinogens (71), and differences may exist in the manner in which hallucinogens activate the different receptor populations (72,73). To date, there have been no attempts to block the effect of classical hallucinogens in humans with 5-HT_{2A} antagonists.

5-HT_{2B} Receptors

The rat fundus preparation is a peripheral tissue assay that has been used as a functional assay for serotonergic action for 40 years. Long-standing questions concerning the pharmacologic similarity of serotonergic fundus receptors (now termed 5-HT_{2B} receptors) to the 5-HT_2 family of receptors were answered once they were cloned (74–80). 5-HT_{2B} receptors exhibit about 70% homology to 5-HT_{2A} and 5-HT_{2C} receptors, and, like 5-HT_{2A} receptors, appear to couple functionally to phosphoinositol hydrolysis. Nevertheless, rat and human 5-HT_{2B} receptors display $>90\%$ transmembrane sequence homology. Therefore, most agents that bind at rat 5-HT_{2B} receptors also bind with similar affinity at human 5-HT_{2B} receptors. However, there are some exceptions (80). The standard 5-HT_{2A} antagonist ketanserin and the 5-HT_{2A} agonists DOI and DOB display higher affinity for 5-HT_{2A} and 5-HT_{2C} receptors than for 5-HT_{2B} receptors (71). Nevertheless, a number of DOI-related hallucinogens have been shown to bind at 5-HT_{2B} receptors with modest affinity (71). There is evidence that human 5-HT$_{2B}$ receptors, like human 5-HT$_{2A}$ receptors, also exist in high-affinity and low-affinity states (81).

5-HT$_{2C}$ Receptors

5-HT$_{2C}$ receptors, formerly 5-HT$_{1C}$ receptors, were originally identified in various regions of the brain using autoradiographic and radioligand binding techniques (6,24,64). Cloned human 5-HT$_{2C}$ receptors display a high amino acid sequence homology with 5-HT$_{2A}$ receptors, and like 5-HT$_{2A}$ receptors, they are coupled to phosphoinositol hydrolysis. A truncated version of 5-HT$_{2C}$ receptors, 5-HT$_{2C-tr}$, has been reported, but the truncated receptor failed to bind serotonergic ligands. As previously mentioned, some pharmacologic functions once attributed to 5-HT$_{2A}$ receptors might actually involve a 5-HT$_{2C}$ mechanism. For example the hyperthermic activity of a series of phenylisopropylamines is significantly correlated not only with 5-HT$_{2A}$ but also with their 5-HT$_{2C}$ receptor affinity (70). Numerous atypical antipsychotic agents bind at 5-HT$_{2C}$ receptors as well as at 5-HT$_{2A}$ receptors, however, there is no significant correlation between their atypical properties and binding affinity. 5-HT$_{2C}$ receptors may play a greater role than 5-HT$_{2A}$ receptors in migraine. Other preclinical studies also suggest that agents with 5-HT$_{2C}$ antagonist activity might possess anxiolytic activity (82). A role for 5-HT$_{2C}$ receptors in eating disorders and epilepsy has been identified using mutant mice lacking these receptors. The results with the mutant mice are consistent with earlier reports that the nonselective 5-HT$_{2C}$ agonist *m*CPP acts as an appetite suppressant.

Newer 5-HT$_2$ Subpopulation-selective Agents

Although numerous structure-activity studies for overall 5-HT$_2$ binding and pharmacology have been published, to date there are very few agents that can discriminate between subpopulations of 5-HT$_2$ receptors. In fact, relatively few agents have even been examined at all three 5-HT$_2$ subpopulations. Spiperone, MDL 100,907 and AMI-193 are among the most 5-HT$_{2A}$-selective antagonists available (65) (Fig. 12.10). Spiperone and AMI-193 bind at 5-HT$_{2A}$ receptors with 1,000- to 3,000-fold selectivity rela-

tive to 5-HT$_{2C}$ receptors, but display higher affinity for 5-HT$_{1A}$ and D$_2$ dopamine receptors (83,84). A newer member of this series, KML-010, is a spiperone-related derivative that lacks affinity for 5-HT$_{2C}$ and 5-HT$_{1A}$ receptors and binds at D$_2$ dopamine receptors with low affinity (85). MDL 11,939 displays >300-fold selectivity for 5-HT$_{2A}$ versus 5-HT$_{2C}$ receptors, and its affinity and selectivity are primarily associated with its R($-$)enantiomer: MDL 100,907 (86–88). The latter agent is one of the best investigated 5-HT$_{2A}$-selective antagonists and has been examined as a novel antipsychotic agent in humans. A series of 1-substituted β-carbolines (e.g., LY-23728, LY-287375, LY-266097) has been reported to be the first 5-HT$_{2B}$-selective antagonists. SB-221284 shows 100-fold selectivity for 5-HT$_{2C}$ versus 5-HT$_{2A/2B}$ receptors and is probably the most 5-HT$_{2C}$-selective antagonist to date.

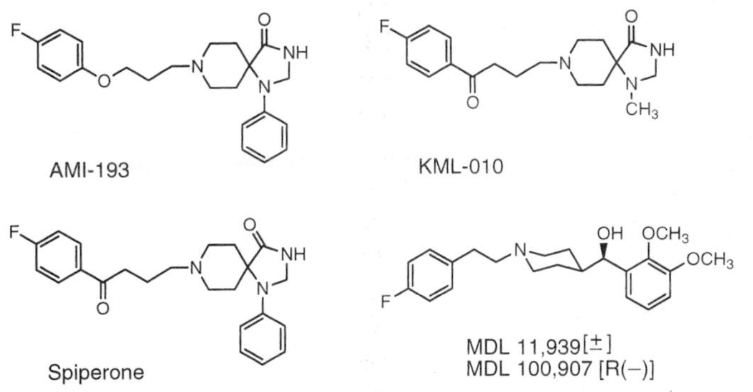

Much less work has been done with 5-HT$_2$ subpopulation-selective agonists. Mounting evidence suggests that many of the behavioral properties of DOB-like phenylisopropylamines are mediated by 5-HT$_{2A}$ receptors. A series of isotryptamine derivatives, including Ro 60-0175 (ORG-35030), has been shown to display up to 1000-fold selectivity for 5-HT$_{2C}$ versus 5-HT$_{2A}$ receptors and possesses 5-HT agonist activity; structurally related tricyclic analogs such as Ro 60-0332 (ORG-35035) have also been examined and display upwards of 100-fold selectivity (89). 10-Methoxy-9-methylpyrazino[1,2-a]indole, Ro 60-0175, and Ro 60-0332 all were active in animal models predictive of therapeutic utility for obsessive-compulsive disorders, panic disorders, and depression (89).

It is still not known with confidence specifically what pharmacologic effects are related to what 5-HT$_2$ subpopulation. Nevertheless, results with the newer agents indicate that 5-HT$_{2A}$ receptors might be involved in psychosis, depression, and hallucinogenic activity, and that 5-HT$_{2C}$ receptors may play a role in obsessive-compulsive disorders, panic, anxiety, and depression. In the periphery, 5-HT$_{2B}$ receptors seem to be involved in muscle contraction; however their function in the CNS is still a matter of speculation. On the basis of some preliminary studies, and on their central distribution in brain, 5-HT$_{2B}$ receptors might be involved in anxiety, cognition, food intake, neuroendocrine regulation, locomotor coordination, and balance (90). Several novel approaches may assist in further elucidating the roles of these subpopulations and in the development of site selective agents. For example, site directed mutagenesis and synthesis of chimeric receptors (66,92), coupled with the use of molecular graphics modeling studies (66,91), are beginning to identify what portions of the receptors are important for ligand binding.

5-HT$_3$ Receptors

Unlike most 5-HT receptor populations, early 5-HT$_3$ pharmacology relied almost exclusively on functional assays. It took a number of years before radioligands were available to identify 5-HT$_3$ receptors in brain. 5-HT$_3$ recep-

Fig. 12.10. Typical examples of newer 5-HT$_2$ subpopulation selective agents.

tors are unique among the families of serotonergic receptors in that they are nonselective Na⁺/K⁺ ion channel receptors (see Fig. 12.11). They are found in the periphery and in the central nervous system, and bear greater structural and functional similarity to nicotinic acetylcholinergic receptors than to other members of the 5-HT receptor family. Differences in the potencies and efficacies of various agonists and antagonists led to early speculation about 5-HT$_3$ receptor heterogeneity but, to date, subpopulations of 5-HT$_3$ receptors have not been identified. Postmortem studies indicate that the distribution of 5-HT$_3$ receptors in human brain is not identical to that in rodent brain, and further support for interspecies differences has come from molecular biological studies (93,94).

Structure-Activity Relationships of 5-HT$_3$ Agonists

Only a few 5-HT$_3$ agonists have been identified (95,96). Many indolealkylamine or tryptamine derivatives bind at 5-HT$_3$ receptors in a nonselective manner. However, simple O-methylation of 5-HT significantly decreases 5-HT affinity for 5-HT$_3$ receptors. Ergolines do not bind or bind only with very low affinity. 5-HT is a nonselective 5-HT$_3$ agonist that binds only with modest affinity (Ki = ca 500–1,000 nM). Its 2-methyl analog, 2-methyl-5-HT (Ki ~ 1,200 nM) is somewhat more selective, but binds with slightly lower affinity than 5-HT. Although 2-methyl 5-HT may be only a partial agonist, it has found widespread application in 5-HT$_3$ research due to its greater selectivity over 5-HT. But, recently, 2-methyl 5-HT was shown to bind at 5-HT$_6$ receptors. The N,N,N-trimethyl quaternary amine analog of 5-HT, 5-HTQ, binds with about 10 times greater affinity than 5-HT and is much more selective than 5-HT but, due to its quaternary nature, might not readily penetrate the blood-brain barrier when adminis-

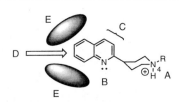

Fig. 12.12. Structure-activity composite for quipazine binding at 5-HT3 receptors (4,97,100,105): **(A)** the N4-piperazine nitrogen atom, but not the N1-piperazine nitrogen atom, is important for binding; an R5-CH3 is tolerated and results in somewhat greater 5-HT$_3$ selectivity, **(B)** the quinoline nitrogen atom is required for high affinity and its replacement by an sp2-hybridized carbon atom results in a > 100-fold decrease in affinity, **(C)** substituents in this region are tolerated and can influence intrinsic activity (105), **(D)** an aromatic moiety (e.g., benzene ring or isosteric structure), although not required for binding, results in optimal affinity, **(E)** regions of limited bulk tolerance.

tered systemically. Using cloned mouse 5-HT$_3$ receptors, 5-HT and 5-HTQ act as full agonists suggesting that the quaternary nature of 5-HTQ has little effect on efficacy, whereas 2-methyl 5-HT and tryptamine act as partial agonists. Another example of a low affinity (Ki *ca* 1,000 nM) 5-HT$_3$ agonist is phenylbiguanide. *m*CPBG or *meta*chlorophenylbiguanide, which binds in the low nanomolar range (Ki *ca* 20–50 nM) and retains agonist character, has largely replaced phenylbiguanide. *m*CPBG does not readily penetrate the blood-brain barrier because of its ionic properties. *m*CPG or *meta*chlorophenylguanidine is a newer more lipophilic analog of *m*CPBG (103). Adding multiple chloro groups to *m*CPBG or *m*CPG increases their lipophilicity and affinity.

Simple arylpiperazines were among the first serotonergic agents investigated at 5-HT$_3$ receptors. Many are nonselective 5-HT$_3$ ligands (see previous discussion of 5-HT$_{1A}$ receptors). Depending on the particular substitution pattern, they can behave as 5-HT$_3$ agonists, partial agonists, or antagonists (4,5,96,97,98). This nonselectivity probably accounts for the initial lack of interest in arylpiperazines as 5-HT$_3$ ligands, but today, however, there is renewed interest in these types of agents. Quipazine was the first arylpiperazine shown to bind at 5-HT$_3$ receptors (99) even though it is also a 5-HT$_{2A}$ agonist. It binds with much higher affinity than 5-HT at 5-HT$_3$ receptors (Ki ~ 1 nM), and was subsequently shown to act as an agonist in certain assays and as an antagonist in others. Interestingly, its structure was quite different from that of other 5-HT$_3$ antagonists known at that time. Early structure-affinity studies showed that its (pyridine-ring) centroid to N$_4$-piperazine nitrogen distance (~ 5.5 Å) was similar to that of 5-HT (4). Other findings indicated that (a) the N$_4$-piperazine nitrogen atom, but not the N$_1$-piperazine nitrogen atom, was important for binding, (b) the quinoline ring nitrogen atom was a major contributor to binding, (c) the benzene ring portion of the quinoline nucleus was not required for binding but that its presence was optimal for high affinity, and (d) N$_4$-methylation (N-methylquipazine or NMQ) enhances 5-

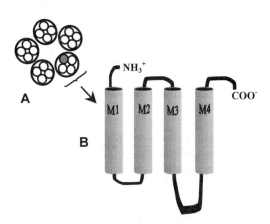

Fig. 12.11. Top view **(A)** and side view **(B)** of a schematic representation of an ion channel receptor. Ion channel receptors are pentameric units arranged to form a pore or ion channel. Each subunit consists of four transmembrane-spanning amino acid chains (M$_1$–M$_4$) constructed such that the M$_2$ chain faces the channel. The transmembrane portions are connected by extracellular and intracellular loops. In the serotonin family, only 5-HT$_3$ receptors have been identified as ion channel receptors.

HT$_3$ receptor selectivity (Fig. 12.12) (100). With the availability of newer arylpiperazines, it has been possible to conduct more comprehensive structure-activity studies (101,102). A summary of quipazine SAR is shown in Figure 12.12. Appropriate structural modification of arylpiperazines can result in rather selective 5-HT$_3$ agonists (Fig. 12.13) (96,98,104). For example, ring-fused quipazine-related analogs (MR 18445), such as the pyrrolo[1,2-a]quinoxalines, represent novel 5-HT$_3$ agonists. Some are full agonists whereas other (e.g., MR 18445) are partial agonists (105,106).

Structure-activity Relationship of 5-HT$_3$ Antagonists

Bemestron (MDL-72222) was the first selective 5-HT$_3$ antagonist (Fig. 12.14). Its development stems from the structural modification of cocaine, an agent that had been previously shown to be a weak 5-HT-M antagonist. Since then, a very large number, literally many hundreds, of 5-HT$_3$ antagonists have been identified. Many of these agents belong to the structural class of compounds broadly referred to as keto compounds and contain an amide, reverse amide, ester, reverse ester, carbamoyl, or ketone function. Typical of these 5-HT$_3$ antagonists is retention of the bulky tropane or tropane-like amine group. Some of the more widely used or newer agents include, in alphabetical order, dolasetron (Anzemet), granisetron (Kytril), itasetron, renzapride, ricasetron, tropisetron, WAY-100289, zacopride, and zatosetron. It should be noted that some of these keto compounds also bind at 5-HT$_{1P}$ and 5-HT$_4$ receptors.

A related group of antagonists that possess an imidazole or related heterocyclic terminal amine include ondansetron (Zofran), alosetron (Lotronex), fabesetron, and ramosetron (Fig. 12.15). Many others have been described (96,107). The structure-activity relationships of 5-HT$_3$ antagonists have been reviewed in detail (96,107,149).

Molecular modeling studies have identified a pharmacophore (Fig. 12.16) that is common to many 5-HT$_3$ antagonists (96,108). 5-HT$_3$ antagonists remain a very important area of research and refinements of the 5-HT$_3$ pharmacophore are very likely to lead to the development of novel therapeutic agents.

5-HT$_3$ Receptors: Clinical Implications

5-HT$_3$ antagonists have proven clinically effective for the treatment of chemotherapy-induced or radiation-induced nausea and vomiting (96,109) whereas they are ineffective against motion sickness and apomorphine-induced emesis (110). There are also indications that they may be effective in the treatment of migraine or the pain associated with migraine (96). Preclinical studies suggest that 5-HT$_3$ antagonists may enhance memory, and be of benefit in the treatment of anxiety, depression, pain, and dementia (110). There have been claims that 5-HT$_3$ antagonists may represent a novel class of atypical antipsychotics. However, additional clinical trials are required to substantiate these claims (110). 5-HT$_3$ receptors can control dopamine release and may also be involved with acetylcholine release and control of the GABA-ergic system (110,111). This intimate relationship could explain some of the unique pharmacologic properties of 5-HT$_3$ ligands. Finally, there is evidence that 5-HT$_3$ antagonists may suppress the behavioral consequences of withdrawing chronic treatment with drugs of abuse including alcohol, nicotine, cocaine, and amphetamine (96,110). It has been mentioned that one of the most attractive features of 5-HT$_3$ antagonists is their general lack of undesirable side effects characteristic of many psychotherapeutic agents. Very little is known about the possible therapeutic application of 5-HT$_3$ agonists, although some 5-HT$_3$ partial agonists possess an anxiolytic profile (98). One of the concerns associated

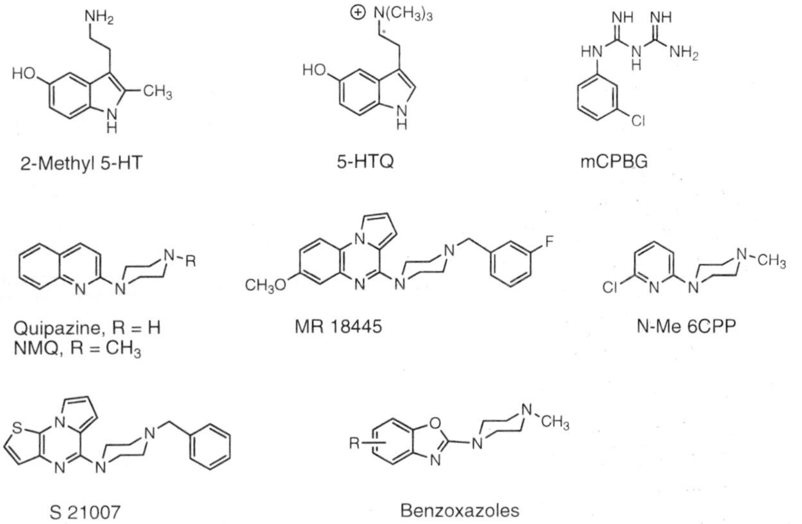

Fig. 12.13. 5-HT$_3$ agonists or partial agonists.

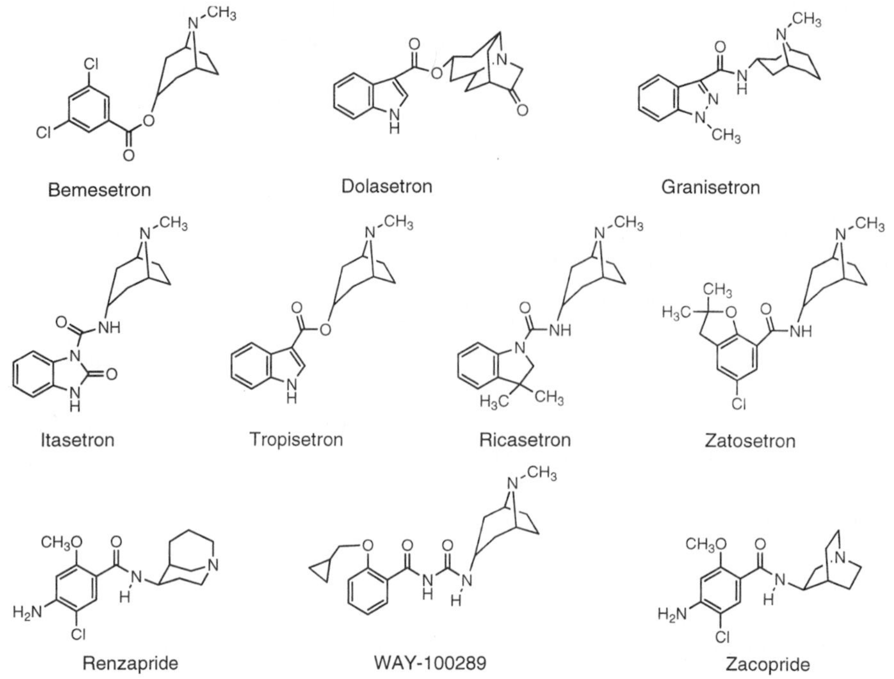

Fig. 12.14. 5-HT$_3$ antagonists.

with 5-HT$_3$ agonists is that they might produce emesis as an undesirable side effect.

5-HT$_4$ Receptors and Agents

A novel population of serotonergic receptors, originally identified in primary cell cultures of mouse embryo colliculi neurons, and later termed 5-HT$_4$ receptors, enjoys broad tissue distribution and are positively coupled to adenylate cyclase (112). In the brain, 5-HT$_4$ receptors appear to be localized on neurons and may mediate the slow excitatory responses to 5-HT. Peripherally, these receptors facilitate acetylcholine release in guinea pig ileum and may play a role in peristalsis. The uniqueness of this receptor type and its potential therapeutic utility spurred initial interests in drug development. Human 5-HT$_4$ receptors have been cloned and display low transmembrane sequence homology (<50%) with other 5-HT receptors (113). In fact, two 5-HT$_4$ isoforms have been isolated, a long form (5-HT$_{4L}$) and a short form (5-HT$_{4S}$). These isoforms are splice variants and differ only in their C-terminus ends with identical transmembrane regions (113). In general, the potency of agonists to stimulate cAMP was greater for the 5-HT$_{4S}$ receptor than for the 5-HT$_{4L}$ recep-

tor. It has been suggested that 5-HT$_4$ receptors might exist in high- and low-affinity states, as previously described for 5-HT$_2$ receptors (114). A mouse 5-HT$_{4L}$ receptor has been cloned and a human pseudogene has been identified that codes for a 5-HT$_4$-like receptor. Indeed, several new human 5-HT$_4$ receptor isoforms have been recently cloned and expressed (115). The new 5-HT$_4$ receptors have been termed 5-HT$_{4(b)}$, 5-HT$_{4(c)}$, and 5-HT$_{4(d)}$; the stimulatory pattern of cAMP formation in response to the 5-HT$_4$ agonist renzapride was found to be different for the various isoforms suggesting that the splice variants might differ in the manner in which they trigger signal transduction following receptor activation (115). In the rat gastrointestinal tract, both 5-HT$_{4L}$ and 5-HT$_{4S}$ receptors are expressed whereas only 5-HT$_{4S}$ receptors are found in the heart with localization almost exclusively in the atrium. 5-HT$_{4a}$ receptors have been cloned from human atrium and appear to correspond to the rodent 5-HT$_{4S}$ isoform. It has been proposed that the cardiac effects of 5-HT are mediated by this short splice variant whereas the 5-HT$_{4L}$ determine the neuronal effects of 5-HT (115).

Although 5-HT$_3$ receptors are ion channel receptors and 5-HT$_4$ receptors represent G protein-coupled recep-

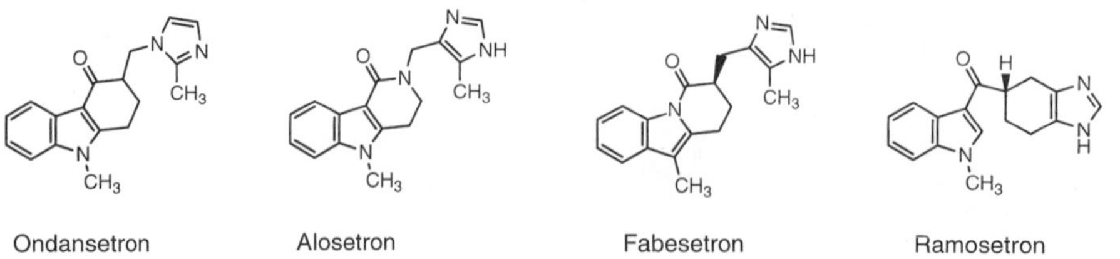

Fig. 12.15. Imadazole-containing 5-HT$_3$ antagonists.

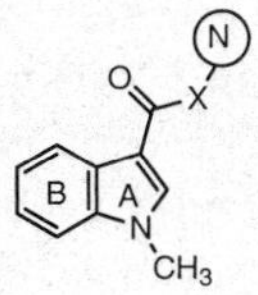

Fig. 12.16. A general pharmacophore model for 5-HT$_3$ antagonists (96). An aromatic centroid (A) to oxygen (O) distance of 3.3–3.5 Å is thought to be optimal. Distances calculated from the terminal amine (N) to the oxygen atom (O), and from the terminal amine N to centroid A, are 5.1–5.2 Å and 6.7–7.2 Å, respectively. It has been speculated that ring A is not required for binding and acts as a spacer; ring B may be more important for binding and associated hydrophobic binding regions has been proposed (Adapted from 106) (See also 149).

tors (Table 12.2). A number of 5-HT$_3$ ligands were demonstrated to be active at 5-HT$_4$ receptors. Even more interesting is that a number of 5-HT$_3$ antagonists, or what were considered at one time to be 5-HT$_3$–selective antagonists (including, for example, renzapride and zacopride), actually exhibited 5-HT$_4$ agonist activity. Even today, there is considerable structural similarity among the various 5-HT$_3$ and 5-HT$_4$ ligands. In addition to their lack of selectivity for 5-HT$_4$ versus other 5-HT receptors, many early 5-HT$_4$ ligands suffered from several other disadvantages such as their affinity for other receptor types, inability or difficulty in penetrating the blood brain barrier, and hydrolytic instability (116).

Structure-activity Relationships of 5-HT$_4$ Agonists

In general terms, 5-HT$_4$ agonists can be divided into several different categories (Fig. 12.17) (112): tryptamines (e.g., 5-HT, 5-CT; with 2-methyl 5-HT and 5-methoxy-N,N-dimethyltryptamine being nearly inactive), benzamides (in particular those bearing a 2-methoxy-4-amino-5-chloro substitution pattern such as SC 53116,

renzapride, zacopride and cisapride), benzimidazolones (e.g., BIMU 8), quinolines (e.g., SDZ 216,908), naphthalimides (e.g., S-RS 56532), benzoates (ML-10302), and ketones (e.g., RS 67333).

Structure-activity Relationships of 5-HT$_4$ Antagonists

The 5-HT$_3$ antagonist tropisetron was the first agent to see application as a 5-HT$_4$ antagonist and its low affinity for 5-HT$_4$ receptors prompted a search for higher affinity agents. Various agents now have been identified (112) and 5-HT$_4$ antagonists are derived from structural classes similar to those from which the 5-HT$_4$ agonists are derived. These include: indole esters and amides (e.g., GR 113,808), benzoates (e.g., SB 204070), benzimidazolones (e.g., DAU 6285), imidazoles (e.g., SC 53606) and ketones (e.g., RS 100235) (Fig. 12.18). These are just representative examples of the large number of agents that have been examined as 5-HT$_4$ antagonists. Structure-activity details for several different receptor preparations have been reviewed (112,117). It is worth noting that apart from 5-HT$_3$ receptors, 5-HT$_4$ receptors are the only other population of serotonergic sites that seem to accommodate quaternary amines.

5-HT$_4$ Receptors: Clinical Implications

Because it has been only relatively recently that selective 5-HT$_4$ agents have been developed, studies of the clinical potential of 5-HT$_4$ agents are still in their infancy. Peripheral actions currently being examined include: irritable bowel syndrome, gastrointestinal tract motility, bladder contraction, gastro-esophageal reflux, corticosteroid secretion, and atrial contractility (112,118). Cisapride was available as a prokinetic agent. With respect to

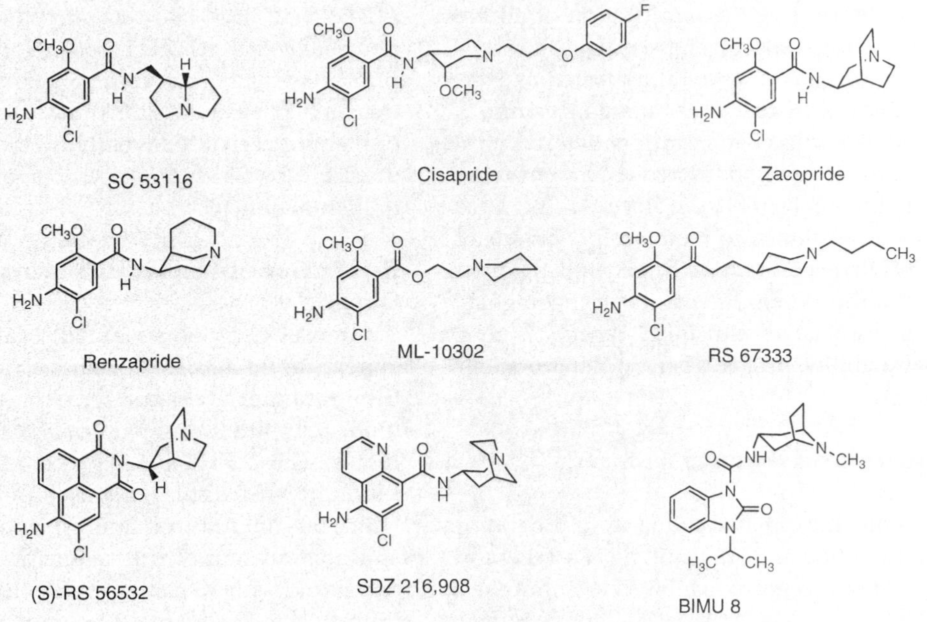

Fig. 12.17. 5-HT$_4$ agonists.

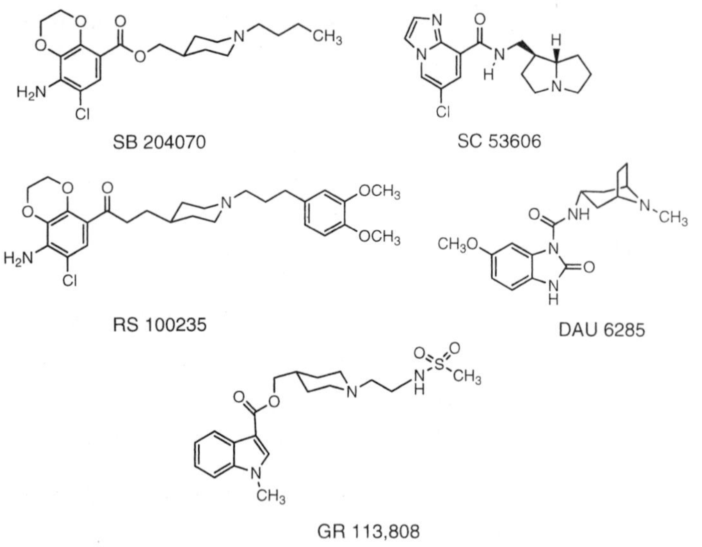

Fig. 12.18. 5-HT$_4$ antagonists.

their central effects, it has been suggested that 5-HT$_4$ agonists may restore deficits in cognitive function and that 5-HT$_4$ antagonists may be useful as anxiolytics or in the treatment of dopamine-related disorders. It is further speculated that 5-HT$_4$ receptors may be involved in memory and learning, and it has been noted that 5-HT$_4$ receptors are markedly decreased in patients with Alzheimer's disease (117). A high density of 5-HT$_4$ receptors in the nucleus accumbens has led some to speculate that these receptors may be involved in the reward system and that they might influence self-administration behavior, for example, GR 113,808 reduces alcohol intake in rats; and it has been suggested that ethanol-induced reinforcing properties may involve, at least in part, 5-HT$_4$ receptors (119). Other central roles are also beginning to emerge; for example, repeated administration of antidepressants decreases the responsiveness of central 5-HT$_4$ receptors to activation (120). It would appear that there are therapeutic roles both for 5-HT$_4$ antagonists and 5-HT$_4$ agonists. However, it has been cautioned that the use of highly potent and selective 5-HT$_4$ agonists might result in cardiovascular side effects (117). If different 5-HT$_4$ receptor isoforms can be shown to mediate the various effects for which 5-HT$_4$ receptors have been implicated, the potential exists for the development of selective agents. Another problem associated with 5-HT$_4$ agents is their lack of oral bioavailability; progress is now being made in this area (121,122).

5-HT$_5$ Receptors and Agents
Overview

Two 5-HT$_5$ receptors, expressed primarily in the mouse CNS, have been identified as 5-HT$_{5A}$ and 5-HT$_{5B}$ receptors (126). The two 5-HT$_5$ receptors exhibit 77% amino acid sequence homology, but less than 50% homology with other cloned serotonergic receptors. To some extent, the

5-HT$_5$ receptors appear to resemble 5-HT$_1$ receptors (e.g., high affinity for 5-HT and 5-CT), however their low homology with other 5-HT$_1$ receptors together with a failure to demonstrate G protein-coupling suggested that they represented a distinct family of receptors. Recent studies provide evidence that human 5-HT$_{5A}$ receptors might be G protein-coupled (123).

Radiolabeled LSD binds to both HT$_{5A}$ and 5-HT$_{5B}$ receptors with 5-CT having 10-fold greater affinity for human 5-HT$_{5A}$ receptors than 5-HT. 5-HT binds with modest affinity (Ki = 100–250 nM). Ergotamine and methiothepin bind with high affinity at human 5-HT$_{5A}$ receptors whereas agents such as spiperone, sumatriptan, yohimbine, ketanserin, propranolol, zacopride and clozapine bind with much lower affinity (Ki > 1,000 nM) (124). A structure-affinity study for the binding of tryptamine and related agents at 5-HT$_5$ receptors was recently published, and a comparative molecular field analysis was used to identify receptor features that might contribute to binding (125). 7-Hydroxy-1-naphthylpiperazine (7-OH 1-NP; Ki = 3 nM) was identified as binding with >50-fold greater affinity at 5-HT$_5$ receptors than 5-HT (125).

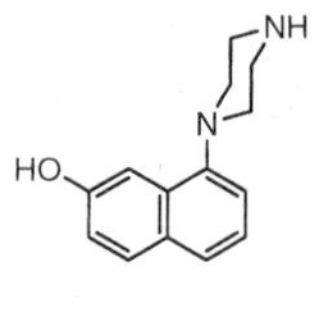

7-OH 1-NP

5-HT$_5$ Receptors: Clinical Implications

Pharmacologic functions of 5-HT$_5$ receptors are currently unknown. It has been speculated, on the basis of their localization, that they may be involved in motor control, feeding, anxiety, depression, learning, memory consolidation, adaptive behavior, and brain development (124,126,127). 5-HT$_{5A}$ receptors may also be involved in a neuronally-driven mechanism for regulating astrocyte physiology with relevance to gliosis; disruption of 5-HT neuronal-glial interactions may be involved in the development of certain CNS pathologies including Alzheimer's disease, Down's syndrome, and some drug-induced developmental deficits.

5-HT$_6$ Receptors and Agents
Overview

A novel G protein-coupled serotonergic receptor that appears to be localized exclusively in the CNS was cloned from rat brain (128) and termed 5-HT$_6$. This receptor exhibits only 40% transmembrane homology with 5-HT$_{1A}$, 5-HT$_{1B}$, 5-HT$_{1D}$, 5-HT$_{1E}$, 5-HT$_{2A}$, and 5-HT$_{2C}$ receptors. Both LSD and 5-HT display modest affinity for 5-HT$_6$ receptors (Ki ca 50–150 nM). Of interest is that a number of typical and atypical neuroleptic agents and tricyclic antidepressants bind with Ki values in the nM range. For example, lisuride acted as a partial agonist, and amoxapine, clozapine and methiothepin acted as antagonists (128).

More recently, the human 5-HT$_6$ receptor has been cloned and its gene structure, distribution, and pharmacology are similar to those of the rat receptor. Like the rat receptor, the human receptor is positively linked to adenylate cyclase. 5-HT binds at human 5-HT$_6$ receptors with moderate affinity (Ki = 65 nM), and one of the highest affinity, albeit nonselective, agents is methiothepin (Ki = 0.4 nM). Agents that bind at human 5-HT$_6$ receptors with Ki <50 nM include 5-methoxytryptamine, bromocriptine, octoclothepin, and the neuroleptics clozapine, olanzapine, chlorpromazine, loxapine, and fluphenazine (129). Agents with Ki >500 nM include 5-CT, sumatriptan, quipazine, ketanserin, 8-OH DPAT, haloperidol, risperidone, and mesulergine (129). A number of antipsychotic agents, typical and atypical, as well as antidepressants bind with low nanomolar affinity (129–131).

2-Ethyl-5-methoxy-N,N-dimethyltryptamine (EMDT) represents the first selective 5-HT$_6$ agonist. Ro 04-6790 and Ro 63-0563 represent the first 5-HT$_6$-selective antagonists and produced a behavioral syndrome in rodents that consists of yawning, stretching, and chewing (132).

Ro 63-0563, X = CH
Ro 04-6790, X = N

5-HT$_6$ Receptors: Clinical Implications

The exact clinical significance of 5-HT$_6$ receptors is unknown at this time. The high affinity of various antipsychotics, in particular atypical antipsychotics, and antidepressants, suggests a possible connection between 5-HT$_6$ receptors and certain psychiatric disorders (130). The different binding profiles of atypical antipsychotics may be responsible for their atypical nature (e.g., D$_2$/5-HT$_{2A}$ ratio); for example, certain agents such as clozapine may be classified as atypical on the basis of their binding with higher affinity at 5-HT$_{2A}$ than at D$_2$ receptors. However, antipsychotics that produce the fewest extrapyramidal side effects in humans (e.g., clozapine, olanzapine, fluperlapine) also possess high affinity for 5-HT$_6$ receptors (129). The atypical antipsychotic agent risperidone, which produces some extrapyramidal symptoms, binds with 1000-fold higher affinity at 5-HT$_{2A}$ than 5-HT$_6$ receptors; thus, the affinity of agents for 5-HT$_6$ receptors may contribute to the difference between typical and certain atypical antipsychotics (129). 5-HT$_6$ knock-out mice produce a behavioral syndrome that seems to involve an increase in cholinergic function. Blocking the receptors in rats with 5-HT$_6$ antagonists produced a similar effect. This has led to speculation that one of the roles of 5-HT$_6$ receptors may be to control cholinergic neurotransmission and that 5-HT$_6$-selective antagonists could be useful in the treatment of anxiety and memory deficits (132). Other studies suggest that 5-HT$_6$ receptors might be involved in motor func-

tion, mood-dependent behavior, anxiety disorders, and early growth processes involving 5-HT.

5-HT$_7$ Receptors and Agents
Overview

Two forms of the 5-HT$_7$ receptor, 5-HT$_{7(a)}$ and 5-HT$_{7(b)}$ have been identified and cloned from several species including rat, mouse, guinea pig and human. 5-HT$_7$ receptors are expressed mainly in the CNS. The two forms are probably splice variants in the rat and are positively coupled to adenylate cyclase. The long form of the 5-HT$_7$ receptor is referred to as 5-HT$_{7(a)}$ whereas the short form is called 5-HT$_{7(b)}$ (133). There is <50% transmembrane amino acid sequence homology between 5-HT$_7$ receptors and other 5-HT receptors.

Agents with Ki values of <10 nM include 5-HT, 5-methoxytryptamine, LSD, methiothepin and mesulergine; those with Ki values in the 10–100 nM range include 8-OH DPAT, spiperone, ritanserin, metergoline, mianserin, chlorpromazine; those in the 100–1,000 nM range include NAN-190, sumatriptan, haloperidol, and those with Ki >1,000 include 2-methyl 5-HT, tropisetron, pindolol, and ketanserin. 5-HT, 5-CT, 5-methoxytryptamine, and 8-OH DPAT reportedly act as agonists whereas methiothepin, mianserin, mesulergine, ritanserin, spiperone, NAN-190, and clozapine act as antagonists. Numerous antidepressants and antipsychotic agents bind at 5-HT$_7$ receptors with nanomolar or subnanomolar affinity (Ki values of <10 nM) include fluphenazine, acetophenazine, chlorprothixene, zotepine, clorotepine, clozapine, fluperlapine, pimozide, tiospirone, and risperidone (130). SB-258719 and the ergoline LY215840 have been identified as 5-HT$_7$ antagonists (134,135).

SB-258719   LY 215840

5-HT$_7$ Receptors: Clinical Implications

5-HT$_7$ receptors might be involved in mood and learning, as well as in neuroendocrine and vegetative behaviors. The 5-HT$_2$ ligand ritanserin, tricyclic antidepressants (e.g., amitriptyline), classical antipsychotic agents (e.g., chlorpromazine), and nonclassical antipsychotic agents (e.g., clozapine, loxapine) bind with Ki values of <100 nM (130,136). On this basis, it has been speculated that 5-HT$_7$ receptors may play a role in certain neuropsychiatric disorders. Consistent with these suggestions, 5-HT$_7$ receptors are sensitive to antidepressant treatment (137). 5-HT$_7$ receptors have been implicated in serotonergic-regulation of circadian rhythm leading to suggestions that 5-HT$_7$-selective agents might be effective in the treatment of jet lag or sleep disorders of a circadian nature (138). In the periphery, 5-HT produces both contraction and relaxation of coronary artery from various species (139). It has been proposed that relaxation of coronary artery may be mediated by 5-HT$_7$ receptors. Agents active at 5-HT$_7$ receptors might thus be effective in the treatment of coronary heart disease.

THE SEROTONIN TRANSPORTER

The actions of a neurotransmitter are terminated by diffusion away from the synapse, by enzymatic degradation, and by reuptake into the synaptic terminal. Following reuptake, once the neurotransmitter is inside the neuron, it can be re-stored in storage vesicles or it can be metabolized. The reuptake process involves a high-affinity transporter protein that is localized in the presynaptic terminal membrane. The transporter appears to regulate the duration and magnitude of postsynaptic response to the neurotransmitter. A different transporter is associated with different neurotransmitters. The 5-HT transporter (or SERT) has been cloned and expressed (140), and its putative structure is roughly similar to the general receptor structure shown in Figure 12.3 except that (a) it consists of 12 membrane-spanning helicies, (b) both the amino terminus and the carboxy terminus are located on the intracellular side, and (c) there is an exaggerated extracellular loop between TM3 and TM4 (Fig. 12.19). The 5-HT transporter possesses about 50% homology with the norepinephrine transporter (NET) and the dopamine transporter (DAT). For 5-HT transport, a ternary complex of protonated 5-HT, Na$^+$, and Cl$^-$ binds to the transporter protein to form a quaternary complex; the transporter undergoes a conformational change to release 5-HT into the cytoplasm of the neuron (140).

The 5-HT transporter has been implicated as playing a role in affective disorders. Agents that block the transporter, and thereby increase synaptic levels of 5-HT, are useful for the treatment of depression, obsessive-compulsive behavior, and panic disorders. Tricyclic antidepressants block the 5-HT transporter and the NET to varying degrees. Some display a preference for one transporter over the other, but most are nonselective (141). The selective 5-HT reuptake inhibitors (SSRIs) display greater selectivity for the 5-HT transporter over the NET. The first SSRI to be used clinically was fluoxetine. Several other agents have since become available. The structure-activity relationships of SSRIs have been reviewed (142); see also Chapter 17 for further discussion and examples. Certain drugs of abuse (e.g., cocaine) also block the 5-HT transporter.

Fluoxetine

Trazodone

Various tricyclic antidepressants and SSRIs, including fluoxetine, also bind at 5-HT$_{2A}$ and 5-HT$_{2C}$ receptors (143,144). The role, if any, derived from a direct interaction of these agents with 5-HT$_2$ receptors versus their interaction at the 5-HT transporter remains to be elucidated. In general, 5-HT$_2$ antagonists down-regulate 5-HT$_2$ receptors. The antidepressant trazodone, for example, is a weak reuptake blocker but binds at 5-HT$_2$ receptors and is a 5-HT$_2$ antagonist (144). The 5-HT$_{2C}$ agonist mCPP induces panic attacks in panic disorder patients and increases obsessive compulsions in obsessive-compulsive patients (145) implicating a role for this specific 5-HT$_{2C}$ subpopulation. 5-HT$_{2C}$ receptor antagonists might be useful targets for the development of novel agents to treat these disorders. However, this issue is complicated by findings that trazodone is metabolized to mCPP, and that in some instances trazodone possesses 5-HT$_{2C}$ agonist properties (146). In any event, long-term treatment with tricyclic antidepressants (and MAO inhibitors) leads to a down regulation in the number of 5-HT$_2$ receptors, the time course for which approximates the clinical response in depressed patients (141). Some SSRIs produce adaptive changes involving decreased responsiveness of 5-HT$_2$ receptors, whereas electroconvulsive therapy increases the number of 5-HT$_2$ receptors (141). Even though several 5-HT receptor populations have been implicated in the actions of antidepressants (e.g., 5-HT$_2$, 5-HT$_6$, 5-HT$_7$), the 5-HT transporter remains an attractive target for the development of novel psychotherapeutic agents.

SUMMARY

Serotonin is a major neurotransmitter in the brain and is also involved in a number of peripheral actions. Seven families or populations of 5-HT receptors have been identified, 5-HT$_1$ – 5-HT$_7$, and several are divided into distinct subpopulations (see Table 12.2). Excluding splice variants, 14 different populations and subpopulations of 5-HT receptors have been cloned. Over the past 20 years selective agonists and antagonists have been developed and identified for some of the subpopulations, but there still remain

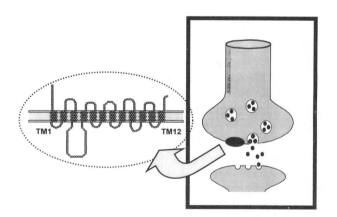

Fig. 12.19. Schematic of a neuron showing the general location and basic structure (enlarged in inset) of a serotonin transporter (SERT). Note that the transporter possesses 12 transmembrane-spanning helicies (TM1–TM12). Both the amine terminus (attached to TM1) and the carboxy terminus (attached to TM12) are on the intracellular side.

subpopulations for which selective agents have yet to be synthesized. The availability of such agents is important because it allows for functional investigations of the different 5-HT receptors. In addition to acting directly on 5-HT receptors, therapeutic agents with other mechanisms are available for influencing serotonergic transmission including SSRIs and inhibitors of MAO. Studies with 5-HT receptors have led to the introduction of agents useful for treating anxiety (e.g., buspirone), migraine (e.g., sumatriptan) and chemotherapy-induced emesis (e.g., ondansetron); numerous other agents are currently in clinical trials for the treatment of depression, schizophrenia, obsessive-compulsive and other disorders. Investigations have also led to a greater understanding of cardiovascular pharmacology, obesity, neurodegenerative disorders, aggression, sexual behavior, and drug abuse, just to mention a few examples. Serotonin may even play an indirect role in techniques as diverse as acupuncture (147) and transcendental meditation (148). To re-iterate a phrase from the introduction: "… it almost appears that serotonin is involved in everything" (1).

REFERENCES

1. Rapport MR. The discovery of serotonin. Perspect Biol Med 1997;40:260–273.
2. Woolley DW. Ed. The biochemical bases of psychoses; the serotonin hypothesis about mental diseases. New York: John Wiley and Sons, 1962.
3. Frazer A, Hensler JG. Serotonin. In: Siegel GJ, Agranoff BW, Albers RW, et al, eds. Basic neurochemistry. New York: Raven Press, 1993;283–308.
4. Glennon RA, Westkaemper RB, Bartyzel P. Medicinal chemistry of serotonergic agents. In: Peroutka SJ, ed. Serotonin receptor subtypes. New York: Wiley-Liss, 1991;19–64.
5. Glennon RA, Dukat M. Serotonin receptor subtypes. In: Bloom FE, Kupfer DJ, eds. Psychopharmacology: The fourth generation of progress. New York: Raven Press, 1995;415–429. CD ROM Version, 1998.
6. B. Olivier, van Wijngaarden I, Soudin W, eds. Serotonin receptors and their ligands. Amsterdam: Elsevier, 1997.
7. Leysen JE, Niemegeers CJE, Tollenaere JP, et al. Serotonergic component of neuroleptic receptors. Nature 1978;272:163–166.
8. Bennett JP, Snyder SH. Serotonin and lysergic acid diethylamide binding in rat brain membranes: relationship to postsynaptic serotonin receptors. Mol Pharmacol 1996;12:373–389.
9. Peroutka SJ, Snyder SH. Multiple serotonin receptors: differential binding of [³H]5-hydroxytryptamine, [³H]lysergic acid diethylamide and [³H]spiroperidol. Mol Pharmacol 1979;16:687–699.
10. Pedigo NW, Yamamura HI, Nelson DL. Discrimination of multiple [³H]5-hydroxytryptamine binding sites by the neuroleptic spiperone in rat brain. J Neurochem 1981;36:220–226.
11. Gaddum JH, Picarelli ZP. Two kinds of tryptamine receptors. Br J Pharmacol 1957;12:323–328.
12. Fozard JR. MDL 72222: A potent and highly selective antagonist at neuronal 5-hydroxytryptamine receptors. Naunyn-Schmiedeberg's Arch Pharmacol 1984;326:36–46.
13. Boess FG, Martin IL. Molecular biology of 5-HT receptors. Neuropharmacology 1994;33:275–317.

14. Hoyer D, Martin GR. Classification and nomenclature of 5-HT receptors: A comment on current issues. Behav Brain Res 1996;73:263–268.
15. Hoyer D, Clarke DE, Fozard JR, et al. International Union of Pharmacology Nomenclature and classification of receptors for 5-hydroxytryptamine (serotonin). Pharmacol Rev 1994;46:157–203.
16. Martin GR, Humphrey PPA. Receptors for 5-hydroxytryptamine: Current perspectives on classification and nomenclature. Neuropharmacology 1994;33:261–273.
17. Humphrey PPA, Barnard EA. International Union of Pharmacology. XIX. The IUPHAR receptor code: A proposal for an alphnumeric classification system. Pharmacol Rev 1998;50:271–277.
18. Hartig PR, Branchek TA, Weinshank RL. A subfamily of 5-HT$_{1D}$ receptor genes. Trends Pharmacol Sci 1992; 13:152–159.
19. Pazos A, Hoyer D, Palacios JM. The binding of serotonergic ligands to the porcine choroid plexus: characterization of a new type of serotonin recognition site. Eur J Pharmacol 1985;106:539–546.
20. Heuring RE, Peroutka SJ. Characterization of a novel [³H]5-hydroxytryptamine binding site subtype in bovine brain membranes. J Neurosci 1987;7:894–903.
21. Leonhardt S, Herrick-Davis K, Titeler M. Detection of a novel serotonin receptor subtype (5-HT$_{1E}$) in human brain: Interaction with a GTP-binding protein. J Neurochem 1989;53:465–471.
22. Adham N, Kao HT, Schechter LE, et al. Cloning of another human serotonin receptor (5-HT$_{1F}$): A fifth 5-HT$_1$ receptor subtype coupled to the inhibition of adenylate cyclase. Proc Nat Acad Sci (US) 1993;90:408–412.
23. Saudou F, Hen R. 5-HT receptor subtypes: Molecular and functional diversity. Med Chem Res 1994;4:16–84.
24. Zifa E, Fillion G. 5-hydroxytryptamine receptors. Pharmacol Rev 1992;44:401–458.
25. van Wijngaarden I, Soudijn W, Tulp MTM. 5-HT$_{1A}$ receptor ligands. In: Olivier B, van Wijngaarden I, Soudin W, eds. Serotonin receptors and their ligands. Amsterdam: Elsevier, 1997;17–43.
26. Glennon RA, Dukat M. 5-HT$_1$ Receptor Ligands: Update 1997. Investigaional Drugs Res Alerts 1997;2:351–372.
27. Glennon RA, Dukat M. 5-HT receptor ligands—Update 1992. Current Drugs: Serotonin 1993;1:1–45.
28. Glennon RA. Concepts for the design of 5-HT$_{1A}$ serotonin agonists and antagonists. Drug Dev Res 1992;6:251–274.
29. Orjales A, Alonso-Cires L, Labeaga L, et al. New (2-methoxyphenyl)piperazine derivatives as 5-HT$_{1A}$ receptor ligands with reduced α$_1$-adrenergic activity. Synthesis and structure-activity relationships. J Med Chem 1995;38:1273–1277.
30. Kuipers W, van Wijngaarden I, Ijzerman A P. A model of the serotonin 5-HT$_{1A}$ receptor: agonist and antagonist binding sites. Drug Design Discov 1994;11:231–249.
31. Kuipers W. Structural characteristics of 5-HT$_{1A}$ receptors and their ligands. In: Olivier B, van Wijngaarden I, Soudin W, eds. Serotonin receptors and their ligands. Amsterdam: Elsevier, 1997;45–64.
32. Glennon RA, Westkaemper RB. Serotonin receptors, 5-HT ligands, and receptor modeling. In: Angeli P, Gulini U, Quaglia W. eds. Trends in receptor research. Amsterdam: Elsevier, 1992;185–207.
33. Westkaemper RB, Glennon RA. Molecular modeling of the interaction of LSD and other hallucinogens with 5-HT$_2$ receptors. In: Lin G, Glennon RA, eds. Hallucinogens: An update. Rockville: National Institute on Drug Abuse, 1994:263–283

34. De Vry J. 5-HT$_{1A}$ receptor agonists: Recent developments and controversial issues. Psychopharmacology 1995; 121:1–26.

35. Neckelmann D, Bjorkum AA, Bjorvatn B, et al. Sleep and EEG power spectrum effects of the 5-HT$_{1A}$ antagonist NAN-190 alone and in combination with citalopram. Behav Brain Res 1996;75:159–168.

36. File SE. Recent developments in anxiety, stress, and depression. Pharmacol Biochem Behav 1996;54:3–12 and following papers.

37. Saxena P. Serotonin receptors: subtypes, functional responses and therapeutic relevance. Pharmac Ther 1995;66: 339–368.

38. Sleight AJ, Pierce PA, Schmidt AW, et al. The clinical utility of serotonin receptor active agents in neuropsychiatric disease. In: Peroutka SJ, ed. Serotonin receptor subtypes. New York: Wiley-Liss, 1991;211–227.

39. Perregaard J, Sanchez C, Arnt J. Recent developments in anxiolytics. Curr Opin Ther Pat 1993;3:101–126.

40. Fletcher A, Cliffe I, Dourish CT. Silent 5-HT$_{1A}$ receptor antagonists: utility as research tools and therapeutic agents. Trends Pharmacol Sci 1993; 14:441–448.

41. Assie M-B, Koek W. Effects of 5-HT$_{1A}$ receptor antagonists on hippocampal 5-hydtroxytryptamine levels: (S)-WAY100135, but not WAY100635, has partial agonist properties. Eur J Pharmacol 1996;304:15–21.

42. Newman-Tancredi A, Chaput C, Verriele L, et al. S 15535 and WAY 100,635 antagonize 5-HT-stimulated [^{35}S]GTPγS binding at cloned human 5-HT$_{1A}$ receptors. Eur J Pharmacol 1996;307:107–111.

43. Darmani NA, Reeves SL. The mechanism by which the selective 5-HT$_{1A}$ receptor antagonist S(−)UH-301 produces head-twitches in mice. Pharmacol Biochem Behav 1996; 55:1–10.

44. Mundey MK, Fletcher A, Marsden CA. Effects of 8-OH DPAT and 5-HT$_{1A}$ antagonists WAY 100135 and WAY 100635 on guinea pig behaviour and dorsal raphe 5-HT neurone firing. Br J Pharmacol 1996;117:750–756.

45. Arborelius L, Nomikos GG, Hertel P, et al. The 5-HT$_{1A}$ receptor antagonist (S)-UH-301 augments the increase in extracellular concentrations of 5-HT in the frontal cortex produced by both acute and chronic treatment with citalopram. Naunyn-Schmiedeberg's Arch Pharmacol 1996; 353:630–640.

46. Grignaschi G, Invernizzi RW, Fanelli E, et al. Citalopram-induced hypophagia is enhanced by blockade of 5-HT$_{1A}$ receptors: role of 5-HT$_{2C}$ receptors. Br J Pharmacol 1998;124: 1781–1787.

47. Clifford EM, Gartside SE, Umbers V, et al. Electrophysiological and neurochemical evi dence that pindolol has agonist properties at the 5-HT$_{1A}$ autoreceptor in vivo. Br J Pharmacol 1998;124:206–212.

48. Schoeffter P, Hoyer D. Interaction of arylpiperazines with 5-HT$_{1A}$, 5-HT$_{1B}$, 5-HT$_{1C}$, and 5-HT$_{1D}$ receptors. Do discriminatory 5-HT$_{1B}$ receptor ligands exist? Naunyn-Schmiedeberg's Arch Pharmacol 1989;339:675–683.

49. Glennon RA, Westkaemper RB. 5-HT$_{1D}$ receptors: A serotonin receptor population for the 1990's. Drug News Perspect 1993;6:390–405.

50. Middlemiss DN, Beer MS, Matassa VG. 5-HT$_{1D}$ receptors. In: Olivier B, van Wijngaarden I, Soudin W, eds. Serotonin receptors and their ligands. Amsterdam: Elsevier, 1997;101–138.

51. Adham N, Tamm JA, Salon JA, et al. A single point mutation increases the affinity of serotonin 5-HT$_{1D\alpha}$, 5-HT$_{1D\beta}$, 5-HT$_{1E}$ and 5-HT$_{1F}$ receptors for β-adrenergic antagonists. Neuropharmacology 1994;33:387–391.

52. Glennon RA, Dukat M, Westkaemper RB, et al. The binding of propranolol at 5-hydroxytryptamine$_{1D\beta}$ T355N mutant receptors may involve formation of two hydrogen bonds to asparagine. Mol Pharmacol 1996;49:198–206.

53. Weinshank RL, Zgombick JM, Macchi MJ, et al. Human serotonin$_{1D}$ receptor is encoded by a subfamily of two distinct genes: 5-HT$_{1D\alpha}$ and 5-HT$_{1D}$. Proc Nat Acad Sci (USA) 1992;89:3630–3634.

54. Skingle M, Beattie DT, Scopes DIC, et al. GR127935: A potent and selective 5-HT$_{1D}$ receptor antagonist. Behav Brain Res 1996; 73:157–161.

55. Hamel E. 5-HT$_{1D}$ receptors: Pharmacology and therapeutic potential. Serotonin 1996;1:19–29.

56. Bouchelet I, Cohen Z, Case B, et al. Differential expression of sumatriptan-sensitive 5-hydroxytryptamine receptors in human trigeminal ganglia and cerebral blood vessels. Mol Pharmacol 1996;50:219–223.

57. Kaumann AJ, Frenken M, Posival H, et al. Variable participation of 5-HT$_1$-like receptors in serotonin-induced contraction of human isolated coronary arteries. 5-HT$_1$-like receptors resemble cloned 5-HT$_{1D}$ receptors. Circulation 1994;90:1141–1153.

58. Wurch T, Pauwels PJ. Predominant expression of serotonin 5-HT$_{1B}$ receptor mRNA in pig coronary artery. Neurosci Res Commun 1998;23:45–53.

59. Gudermann T, Levy FO, Birnbaumer M, et al. Human S31 serotonin receptor clone encodes a 5-hydroxytryptamine$_{1E}$-like serotonin receptor. Mol Pharmacol 1993;43:412–418.

60. Zgombick JM, Schechter LE, Macchi M, et al. Human gene S31 encodes the pharmacologically defined serotonin 5-hydroxytryptamine-1E receptor. Mol Pharmacol 1992;42:180–185.

61. McAllister G, Castro JL. 5-HT$_{1E}$ and 5-HT$_{1F}$ receptors. In: Olivier B, van Wijngaarden I, Soudin W, eds. Serotonin receptors and their ligands. Amsterdam: Elsevier, 1997;141–157.

62. Phebus LA, Johnson KW, Zgombick JM, et al. Characterization of LY344864 as a pharmacological tool to study 5-HT$_{1F}$ receptors: Binding affinities, brain penetration and activity in the neurogenic dural inflammation model of migraine. Life Sci 1997;61:2117–2126.

63. Johnson KW, Schaus JM, Durkin MM, et al. 5-HT$_{1F}$ receptor agonists inhibit neurogenic dural inflammation in guinea pigs. Neuroreport 1997;8:2237–2240.

64. Herndon JL, Glennon RA. Serotonin receptors, agents, and actions. In: Kozikowsky A, ed. Drug design, molecular modeling, and the neurosciences, New York: Raven Press, 1993;167–212.

65. Glennon RA, Dukat M. Novel serotonergic agents: 5-HT$_2$—Update 1997. Investigational Drugs Res Alerts, 1997; 2:107–113.

66. Roth B, Willins DL, Kristiansen K, et al. 5-hydroxytryptamine$_2$-family receptors (5-hydroxytryptamine$_{2A}$, 5-hydroxytryptamine$_{2B}$, 5-hydroxytryptamine$_{2C}$): Where structure meets function. Pharmacol Ther 1998;79:231–257.

67. Johnson MP, Wainscott DB, Lucaites VL, et al. Mutations of transmembrane IV and V serines indicate that all tryptamines do not bind to rat 5-HT$_{2A}$ receptors in the same manner. Mol Brain Res 1997;49:1–6.

68. Meneses A, Terron JA, Hong E. Effects of the 5-HT receptor antagonists GR 127935 (5-HT$_{1B/1D}$) and MDL 100907 (5-HT$_{2A}$) in the consolidation of learning. Behav Brain Res 1997;89:217–223.

69. Takahashi Y, Kusumi I, Ishikane T, et al. In vivo occupation of D$_1$, D$_2$, and serotonin$_{2A}$ receptors by novel antipsychotic drug,

SM-9018 and its metabolite, in rat brain. J Neural Transm 1998;105:181–191.

70. Glennon RA. Do hallucinogens act as 5-HT$_2$ agonists or antagonists? Neuropsychopharmacology 1990;56:509–517.

71. Nelson DL, Lucaites VL, Wainscott DB, et al. Comparison of hallucinogenic phenylisopropylamine binding affinities at cloned human 5-HT$_{2A}$, 5-HT$_{2B}$ and 5-HT$_{2C}$ receptors. Naunyn-Schmiedeberg's Arch Pharmacol 1998, in press.

72. Smith RL, Canton H, Barrett RJ, et al. Agonist properties of N,N-dimethyltryptamine at serotonin 5-HT$_{2A}$ and 5-HT$_{2C}$ receptors. Pharmacol Biochem Behav 1998;61:323–330.

73. Newton RA, Phipps SL, Flanigan TP, et al. Characterisation of human 5-hydroxytryptamine$_{2A}$ and 5-hydroxytryptamine$_{2C}$ receptors expressed in the human neuroblastoma cell line SH-SY5Y: Comparative stimulation by hallucinogenic drugs. J Neurochem 1996;67: 2521–2531.

74. Wainscott DB, Cohen ML, Schenck KW, et al. Pharmacological characteristics of the newly cloned 5-hydroxytryptamine-2F receptor. Mol Pharmacol 1993;43: 419–426.

75. Kursar JD, Nelson DL, Wainscott DB, et al. Molecular cloning, functional expression, and pharmacological characterization of a novel serotonin receptor (5-hydroxytryptamine$_{2F}$) from rat stomach fundus. Mol Pharmacol 1992;42:549–557.

76. Foguet M, Hoyer D, Pardo LA, et al. Cloning and functional characterization of the rat stomach fundus serotonin receptor. EMBO J 1992;11:3481–3487.

77. Nelson DL. The serotonin2 (5-HT$_2$) subfamily of receptors: pharmacological challenges. Med Chem Res 1993; 3:306–316.

78. Schmuck K, Ullmer C, Engels P, et al. Cloning and functional characterization of the human 5-HT$_{2B}$ serotonin receptor. FEBS Lett 1994;342:85–90.

79. Bonhaus DW, Bach C, DeSouza A, et al. The pharmacology and distribution of human 5-hydroxytryptamine$_{2B}$ (5-HT$_{2B}$) receptor gene products: comparison with 5-HT$_{2A}$ and 5-HT$_{2C}$ receptors. Br J Pharmacol 1995;115:622–628.

80. Wainscott DB, Lucaites VL, Kursar JD, et al. Pharmacologic characterization of the human 5-hydroxytryptamine$_{2B}$ receptor: Evidence for species differences. J Pharmacol Exp Ther 1996;276:720–727.

81. Wainscott DB, Sasso DA, Kursar JD, et al. [^{3}H]Rauwolscine: an antagonist radioligand for the cloned human 5-hydroxytryptamine$_{2B}$ (5-HT$_{2B}$) receptor. Naunyn-Schmeideberg's Arch Pharmacol 1998;375:17–24.

82. Kennett GA, Bailey F, Piper DC, et al. Effect of SB 200646A, a 5-HT$_{2C}$/5-HT$_{2B}$ antagonist in two conflict models of anxiety. Psychopharmacology 1995;118:178–182.

83. Ismaiel AM, De Los Angeles J, Teitler M, et al. Antagonism of a 1-(2,5-dimethoxy-4-methylphenyl)-2-aminopropame stimulus with a newly identified 5-HT$_2$- versus 5-HT$_{1C}$-selective antagonist. J Med Chem 1993;36:2519–2525.

84. Ismaiel AM, Dukat M, Nelson DL,et al. Binding of N$_2$-substituted pyrido[4,3-b]indole analogs of spiperone at human 5-HT$_{2A}$, 5-HT$_{2B}$, and 5-HT$_{2C}$ serotonin receptors. Med Chem Res 1996;6:197–211.

85. Metwally KA, Dukat M, Egan CT, et al. Spiperone: Influence of spiro ring substituents on 5-HT$_{2A}$ serotonin receptor binding. J Med Chem 1998;41:5084–5093.

86. Kehne JH, Baron BM, Carr AA, et al. Preclinical characterization of the potential of the putative atypical antipsychotic MDL 100,907 as a potent 5-HT$_{2A}$ antagonist with a favorable CNS safety profile. J Pharmacol Exp Ther 1996;277: 968–981.

87. Baxter G, Kennett G, Blaney F, et al. 5-HT$_2$ receptor subtypes: A family reunited? Trends Pharmacol Sci 1995;18:105–110.

88. Sorensen SM, Kehne JH, Fadayel GM, et al. Characterization of the 5-HT$_2$ receptor antagonist MDL 100,907 as a putative atypical antipsychotic: Behavioral electrophysiological and neurochemical studies. J Pharmacol Exp Ther 1993;266: 684–691.

89. Martin JR, Bos M, Jenck F, et al. 5-HT$_{2C}$ receptor agonists: Pharmacological characteristics and therapeutic potential. J Pharmacol Exp Ther 1998;286:913–924.

90. Duxon MS, Flanigan TP, Reavley AC, et al. Evidence for expression of the 5-hydroxytryptamine-2B receptor system in the rat central nervous system. Neuroscience 1997;76:323–329.

91. Westkaemper RB. Guest Editor for Serotonin receptors: Molecular genetics and molecular modeling. Special issue of Med Chem Res 1993;3(5/6):269–418.

92. Branchek T. Site-directed mutagenesis of serotonin receptors. Med Chem Res 1993;3:287–296.

93. Belelli D, Balcarek JM, Hope AG, et al. Cloning and functional expression of a human 5-hydroxytryptamine type 3A receptor subunit. Mol Pharmacol 1995;48:1054–1062.

94. Miyake A, Mochizuki S, Takemoto Y, et al. Molecular cloning of human 5-hydroxytryptamine$_3$ receptor: Heterogeneity in distribution and function among species. Mol Pharmacol 1995;48:407–416.

95. Morain P, Abraham C, Portevin B, et al. Biguanide derivatives: Agonist pharmacology at 5-hydroxytryptamine type 3 receptors in vitro. Mol Pharmacol 1994;46:732–742.

96. Gozlan H. 5-HT$_3$ receptors. In: Olivier B, van Wijngaarden I, Soudin W, eds. Serotonin receptors and their ligands. Amsterdam: Elsevier, 1997;221–258.

97. Dukat M, Abdel-Rahman AA, Ismaiel AM, et al. Structure-activity relationships for the binding of arylpiperazines and arylbiguanides at 5-HT$_3$ serotonin receptors. J Med Chem 1996;39:4017–4035.

98. Rault S, Lancelot J-C, Prunier H, et al. Novel selective and partial agonists of 5-HT$_3$ receptors. Part 1. Synthesis and biological evaluation of piperazinopyrrolothienopyrazines. J Med Chem 1996;39:2068–2080.

99. Kilpatrick GJ, Butler A, Hagan RM, et al. [^{3}H]GR 67330, a very high affinity ligand for 5-HT$_3$ receptors. Naunyn-Schmeideberg's Arch Pharmacol 1990;342:22–30.

100. Glennon RA, Ismaiel AE-K, McCarthy BG, et al. Binding of arylpiperazines to 5-HT$_3$ serotonin receptors: Results of a structure-affinity study. Eur J Pharmacol 1989;168:387–392.

101. Cappelli A, Anzini M, Vemero S, et al. Novel potent and selective central 5-HT$_3$ receptor ligands provided with different intrinsic activity. 1. Mapping the central 5-HT$_3$ receptor binding site by arylpiperazine derivatives. J Med Chem 1998; 41:728–741.

102. Morreale A, Galvez-Ruano E, Iriepa-Canalda I, et al. Arylpiperazines with serotonin-3 antagonist activity: A comparative molecular field analysis. J Med Chem 1998;41: 2029–2039.

103. Dukat M, Young R, Glennon RA. MD-354: A new 5-HT3 agonist as training drug in drug discrimination studies. Behav Pharmacol 1998;9,S108.

104. Anzini M, Cappelli A, Vomero S, et al. Novel, potent, and selective 5-HT$_3$ receptor antagonists based on the arylpiperazine skeleton: Synthesis, structure, biological activity, and comparative molecular field analysis studies. J Med Chem 1995;38:2692–2704.

105. Campiani G, Cappelli A, Nacci V, et al. Novel and highly potent 5-HT₃ receptor agonists based on a pyrroloquinozaline structure. J Med Chem 1997;40:3670–3678.

106. Katounina T, Besret L, Dhilly M, et al. Synthesis and biological investigations of [¹⁸F]MR 18445, a 5-HT₃ receptor partial agonist. Bioorg Med Chem 1998;6:789–795.

107. King FD, Jones BJ, Sanger GJ, eds. 5-hydroxytryptamine-3 Receptor Antagonists. Boca Raton: CRC Press, 1994.

108. Evans SM, Huang B-S, Feng D, et al. Probing the 5-HT₃ receptor site using novel indole-3-glyoxylic acid derivatives. Med Chem Res 1993;3:386–406.

109. Gyermek L. 5-HT₃ receptors: Pharmacologic and therapeutic aspects. J Clin Pharmacol 1995;35:845–855.

110. Greenshaw AJ. Behavioural pharmacology of 5-HT₃ receptor antagonists: A critical update on therapeutic potential. Trends Pharmacol Sci 1993;14:265–270.

111. Bloom FE, Morales M. The central 5-HT₃ receptor in CNS disorders. Neurochem Res 1998;23:653–659.

112. Dumuis A, Ansanay H, Waeber C, et al. 5-HT₄ receptors. In: Olivier B, van Wijngaarden I, Soudin W, eds. Serotonin receptors and their ligands. Amsterdam: Elsevier, 1997;261–308.

113. Gerald C, Adham N, Kao H-T, et al. The 5-HT₄ receptor: molecular cloning and pharmacological classification of two splice variants. EMBO J 1995;14:2806–2815.

114. Adham N, Gerald C, Schechter L, et al. [³H]5-hydroxytryptamine labels the agonist high affinity state of the cloned rat 5-HT₄ receptor. Eur J Pharmacol 1996;304:231–235.

115. Blondel O, Gastineau M, Dahmoune Y, et al. Cloning, expression, and pharmacology of four human 5-hydroxytryptamine₄ receptor isoforms produced by alternative splicing in the carboxyl terminus. J Neurochem 1998;70:2252–2261.

116. Eglen RM, Bonhaus DW, Clark RD, et al. (R) and (S) RS 56532: Mixed 5-HT₃ and 5-HT₄ receptor ligands with opposing enantiomeric selectivity. Neuropharmacology 1994;33:515–526.

117. Eglen RM, Wong EHF, Dumuis A, et al. Central 5-HT₄ receptors. Trends Pharmacol Sci 1995;16:391–398.

118. Hedge S, Eglen R. Peripheral 5-HT₄ receptors. FASEB J 1996;10:1398–1407.

119. Panocka I, Ciccocioppo R, Polidori C, et al. The 5-HT₄ receptor antagonist GR113808 reduces ethanol intake in alcohol-preferring rats. Pharmacol Biochem Behav 1995;52:255–259.

120. Bijak M, Tokarski K, Maj J. Repeated treatment with antidepressant drugs induces subsensitivity to the excitatory effect of 5-HT₄ receptor activation in the rat hippocampus. Naunyn-Schmeideberg's Arch Pharmacol 1997;355:14–19.

121. Gaster LM, Joiner GF, King FD, et al. N-[(1-Butyl-4-piperidinyl)methyl]-3,4-dihydro-2H-1,3]oxazino[3,2-a]indole-10-carboxamide hydrochloride: The first potent and selective 5-HT₄ receptor antagonist with oral activity. J Med Chem 1995;38:4760–4763.

122. Schaus JM, Thompson DC, Bloomquist WE, et al. Synthesis and structure-activity relationships of potent and orally active 5-HT₄ receptor antagonists: Indazole and benzimidazolone derivatives. J Med Chem 1998;41:1943–1955.

123. Hurley PT, McMahon RA, Fanning P, et al. Functinal coupling of a recombinant human 5-HT₅ₐ receptor to G-proteins in HEK-293 cells. Br J Pharmacol 1998;124:1238–1244.

124. Rees S, den Daas I, Foord S, et al. Cloning and characterization of the human 5-HT₅ₐ serotonin receptor. FEBS Lett 1994;355:242–246.

125. Teitler M, Schieck C, Howard P, et al. 5-HT₅ₐ serotonin receptor binding: A preliminary structure-affinity investigation. Med Chem Res 1997;7:207–218.

126. Matthes H, Boschert V, Amlaiky N, et al. Mouse 5-hydroxytryptamine-5A and 5-hydroxytryptamine-5B receptors define a new family of serotonin receptors: Cloning, functional expression, and chromosomal localization. Mol Pharmacol 1993;43:313–319.

127. Wisden W, Parker EM, Mahle CD, et al. Cloning and characterization of the rat 5-HT₅ʙ receptor. FEBS Lett 1993;333:25–31.

128. Monsma FJ, Shey Y, Ward RP, et al. Cloning and expression of a novel serotonin receptor with high affinity for tricyclic psychotropic drugs. Mol Pharmacol 1993;43:320–327.

129. Kohen R, Metcalf MA, Khan N, et al. Cloning, characterization and chromosomal localization of a human 5-HT₆ serotonin receptor. J Neurochem 1996;66:47–56.

130. Roth BL, Craigo SC, Choudhary MS, et al. Binding of typical and atypical antipsychotic agents to 5-hydroxytryptamine-6 and 5-hydroxytryptamine-7 receptors. J Pharmacol Exp Ther 1994;268:1403–1410.

131. Glatt CE, Snowman A, Sibley DR, et al. Clozapine: selective labeling of sites resembling 5-HT₆ serotonin receptors may reflect psychoactive profile. Mol Med 1995;1:398–406.

132. Bourson A, Borroni E, Austin RH, et al. Determination of the role of 5-HT₆ receptors in the rat brain: A study using antisense oligonucleotides. J Pharmacol Exp Ther 1995;274:173–180.

133. Eglen RM, Jasper JR, Chang DJ, et al. The 5-HT₇ receptor: orphan found. Trends Pharmacol Sci 1997;18: 104–107.

134. Forbes IT, Dabbs S, Duckworth DM, et al. R-3,N-Dimethyl-N-[1-methyl-3-(4-methylpiperidin-1-yl)propyl]benzenesulfonamide: The first selective 5-HT₇ receptor antagonist. J Med Chem 1998;41:655–657.

135. Thomas DR, Gittins SA, Collin LL, et al. Functional characterisation of the human cloned 5-HT₇ receptor (long form); antagonist profile of SB-258719. Br J Pharmacol 1998;124:1300–1306.

136. Shen Y, Monsma Jr. FJ, Metcalf MA, et al. Molecular cloning and expression of a 5-hydroxytryptamine₇ serotonin receptor subtype. J Biol Chem 1993;268:18200–18204.

137. Sleight AJ, Carolo C, Petit N, et al. Identification of 5-hydroxytryptamine₇ receptor binding sites in rat hypothalamus: sensitivity to chronic antidepressant treatment. Mol Pharmacol 1995;47:99–103.

138. Lovenberg TW, Baron BM, de Lecea L, et al. A novel adenylyl cyclase-activating serotonin receptor (5-HT₇) implicated in the regulation of mammalian circadian rhythms. Neuron 1993;11:449–458.

139. Cushing DJ, Zgombick JM, Nelson DL, et al. LY215840, a high-affinity 5-HT₇ receptor ligand blocks serotonin-induced relaxation in canine coronary artery. J Pharmacol Exp Ther 1996;277:1560–1566.

140. Barker EL, Blakely RD. Norepinephrine and serotonin transporters. In: Bloom FE, Kupfer DJ, ed. Psychopharmacology: The Fourth Generation of Progress. New York: Raven Press, 1995;321–333.

141. Maes M, Meltzer HY. The serotonin hypothesis of major depression. In: Bloom FE, Kupfer DJ, ed. Psychopharmacology: The Fourth Generation of Progress. New York: Raven Press, 1995;933–944.

142. Soudjin W, van Wijngaarden I. 5-HT transporter. In: Olivier B, van Wijngaarden I, Soudin W, eds. Serotonin receptors and their ligands. Amsterdam: Elsevier, 1997;327–361.

143. Stanford SC. Prozac: Panacea or puzzle? Trends Pharmacol Sci 1996;17:150–154.
144. Jenck F, Moreau JL, Mutel V, et al. Brain 5-HT$_{1C}$ receptors and antidepressants. Prog Neuropsychopharmacol Biol Psychiat 1994;18:563–574.
145. Broekkamp CLE, Leysen D, Peeters BWMM, et al. Prospects for improved antidepressants. J Med Chem 1995;38:4615–4633.
146. Marcoli M, Maura G, Tortarolo M, et al. Trazodone is a potent agonist at 5-HT$_{2C}$ receptorπs mediating inhibition of the N-methyl-D-aspartate/nitric oxide/cyclic GMP pathway in rat cerebellum. J Pharmacol Exp Ther 1998;285:983–986.
147. Murray J. Evidence for acupuncture's analgesic effectiveness and proposals for the physiological mechanisms involved. J Psychol 1995;129:443–461.
148. Walton KG, PughND, Gelderloos P, et al. Stress reduction and preventing hypertension: preliminary support for a psychoneuroendocrine mechanism. J Altern Complement Med 1995;1:263–283.
149. Heidempergher F, Pillan A, Pinciroli V, et al. Phenylimidazolidin-2-one derivatives as selective 5-HT$_3$ receptor antagonists and refinement of the pharmacophore model for 5-HT$_3$ receptor binding. J Med Chem 1997;40:3369–3380.

13. Local Anesthetics

MATTHIAS C. LU

INTRODUCTION

A local anesthetic agent is a drug that, when given either topically or parenterally to a localized area, produces a state of local anesthesia by reversibly blocking the nerve conductances that transmit the feeling of pain from this locus to the brain. For this reason, local anesthetics play an important role clinically in dentistry and in other minor surgery for temporary relief of pain.

What Is Anesthesia?

The term anesthesia is defined as a loss of sensation with or without loss of consciousness. According to this definition, wide ranges of drugs with diverse chemical structures are anesthetics. The list includes not only the classic anesthetic agents, such as the general and local anesthetics, but also many central nervous system (CNS) depressants, such as analgesics, barbiturates, benzodiazepines, anticonvulsants, and muscle relaxants.

What Is the Difference Between a Local Anesthetic and Other Anesthetic Agents? How Does It Work at the Molecular Level?

Both general anesthetic and local anesthetic drugs produce anesthesia by blocking nerve conductance in both sensory and motor neurons. This blockade of nerve conduction leads to a loss of pain sensation as well as impairment of motor functions. The anesthesia produced by local anesthetics, however, is generally without loss of consciousness or impairment of vital central functions. It is generally accepted that a local anesthetic blocks nerve conductance by binding to selective site(s) on the sodium channels in the excitable membranes, thereby reducing sodium passage through the pores and thus interfering with the action potentials. Thus, a local anesthetic decreases the excitability of nerve membranes without affecting the resting potential. By contrast, a general anesthetic agent alters physical properties of nerve membranes through rather nonspecific interactions with the lipid bilayer or the receptor/ionic channel proteins. These, in turn, reduce membrane excitability through a number of possible mechanisms, including changes in membrane fluidity, permeability, and receptor/channel functions. Furthermore, local anesthetics, in contrast to analgesic compounds, do not interact with the pain receptors or inhibit the release or the biosynthesis of pain mediators.

How Modern Local Anesthetics Are Discovered

Similar to many modern drugs, the initial leads for the design of clinically useful local anesthetics were derived from natural sources. As early as 1532, the anesthetic properties of coca leaves (*Erythroxylon coca* Lam) became known to Europeans from the natives of Peru, who chewed the leaves for a general feeling of well-being and to prevent hunger. Saliva from chewing the leaves was often used by the natives to relieve painful wounds. The active principle of the coca leaf, however, was not discovered until 1860 by Niemann, who obtained a crystalline alkaloid from the leaves to which he gave the name cocaine and noted the anesthetic effect on the tongue. Although Moréno y Maiz in 1868 first asked the question whether cocaine could be used as a local anesthetic, it was Von Anrep, in 1880, who recommended that cocaine be used clinically as a local anesthetic after many animal experiments. The first report of successful surgical use of cocaine appeared in 1884 by Koller, an Austrian ophthalmologist. This discovery led to an explosive development of new anesthetic techniques and local anesthetic agents (1).

Although the structure of cocaine was not known until 1924, many attempts were made to prepare new analogs of cocaine without its addicting liability and other therapeutic shortcomings, such as allergic reactions, tissue irritations, and poor stability in aqueous solution. Also, cocaine is easily decomposed when the solution is sterilized (Fig. 13.1). Initially, analogs of ecgonine and benzoic acid, the hydrolysis products of cocaine, were prepared. When the chemical structure of ecgonine became known, the preparation of active compounds accelerated. It was soon realized that a variety of benzoyl esters of amino alcohols, including benzoyltropine, exhibited strong local anesthetic properties without any addicting liability. Thus, removal of the 2-carbomethoxy group of cocaine also abolished the addicting liability. This discovery eventually led to the synthesis of procaine (N, N-diethylaminoethyl ester of *p*-aminobenzoic acid) in 1905, which became the prototype for local anesthetics for nearly half a century largely because it did not have the severe local and systemic toxicities of cocaine.

Benzoyltropine   Procaine

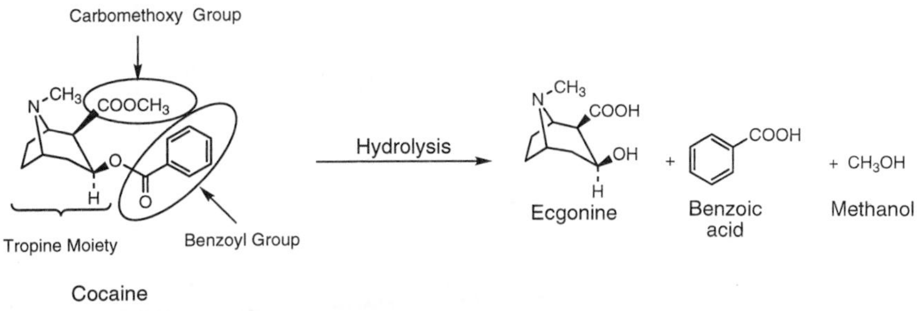

Fig. 13.1. Structures of cocaine and its hydrolysis products.

Study Question 1

Question: What is the biochemical and pharmacologic basis for the observation that co-administration of epinephrine with procaine leads to an increase in the duration of action as well as systemic toxicity of procaine?

Although the intrinsic potency of procaine was low and its duration of action was relatively short as compared with cocaine, it was found that these deficiencies could be remedied when it was combined with a vasoconstrictor such as epinephrine. Apparently, a vasoconstrictor agent reduces the local blood supply and thereby prolongs the residence time of the local anesthetic.

Following the introduction of procaine, hundreds of structurally related analogs were prepared and their local anesthetic properties examined. Most of these compounds were prepared for the purposes of enhancing the intrinsic potency and the duration of action of procaine. Among these compounds, tetracaine still is the most potent, long-acting ester-type local anesthetic agents used in spinal anesthesia.

Benzocaine, an effective topical anesthetic agent, was synthesized by Ritsert in 1890 and found to have good anesthetizing properties and low toxicity. Benzocaine, however, has limited water solubility except at low pH values owing to the lack of a basic aliphatic amino group, thereby disallowing the preparation of pharmaceutically acceptable parenteral solutions.

Study Question 2

Question: Explain, with your knowledge of acid–base chemistry, why benzocaine can only be used for topical applications.

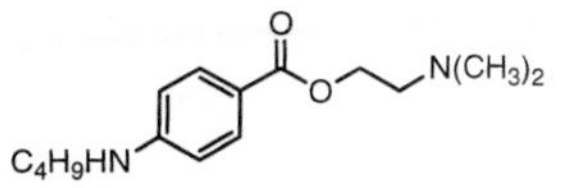

Tetracaine 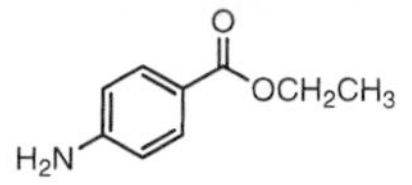   Benzocaine

The next major turning point in the development of clinically useful local anesthetic agents was the serendipitous discovery of the local anesthetic activity of another natural alkaloidal product, isogramine, in 1935 by von Euler and Erdtman. This observation led to the synthesis of lidocaine (Xylocaine) by Löfgren in 1946, the first non-irritating, amide-type local anesthetic agent with good local anesthetic properties and yet less prone to allergic reactions than procaine analogs. A further practical advantage of lidocaine is its stability in aqueous solution because of the more stable amide functionality. Structurally, lidocaine can be viewed as an open-chain analog of isogermine and thus is a bioisoteric analog of isogramine.

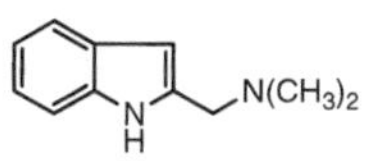

Isogramine 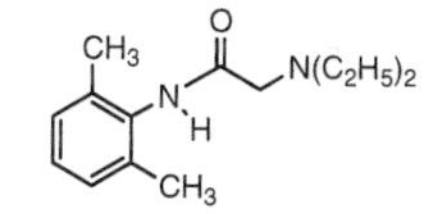   Lidocaine

In the years since 1948, extensive progress has been achieved primarily in the fields of neurophysiology and neuropharmacology rather than that of synthetic medicinal chemistry. Most of this research has significantly increased our understanding of how nerve conduction occurs and how compounds interact with the neuronal membranes to produce local anesthesia. It should be pointed out, however, that although a number of current clinically useful local anesthetic agents have been introduced into the market, unfortunately an ideal local anesthetic drug has not yet been realized.

Characteristics for an Ideal Local Anesthetic

An ideal local anesthetic should produce reversible blockade of sensory nerve fibers with a minimal effect on the motor fibers. It should also possess a rapid onset and have a sufficient duration of action for the completion of major surgical procedures without any systemic toxicity.

The realization of this goal, however, can only be attained through further structure-activity relationship studies, particularly with regard to their selective actions on the voltage-sensitive sodium channels. Additional leads for the design of ideal local anesthetics could also come from a more systematic metabolic and toxicity study of current available agents. To understand the chemical aspects of local anesthetics and thus provide a proper background for practical uses of these compounds, it is necessary to have a working knowledge of basic neuroanatomy and electrophysiology of the nervous system.

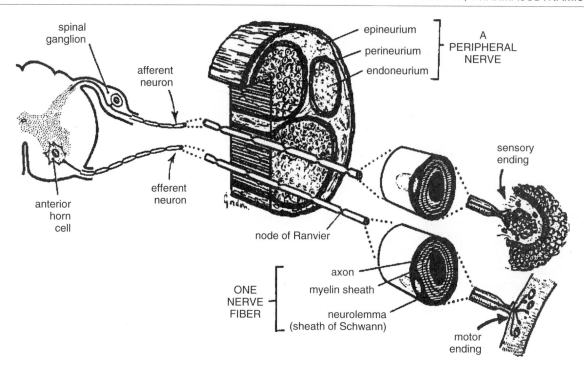

Fig. 13.2. Diagram showing the various parts of a peripheral nerve. (From A. W. Ham, Histology, 6th ed., Philadelphia, J. B. Lippincott.)

NEUROANATOMY AND ELECTROPHYSIOLOGY OF THE NERVOUS SYSTEM
Neuroanatomy

As can be seen in Figure 13.2, the sensory fibers (afferent neuron) course together in bundles with the motor fibers (efferent neuron) from the periphery to the spinal cord (2). The cell bodies of the sensory fibers are found at the point at which the nerve enters the vertebra and are seen as enlargements on the nerve bundles. The cell bodies of the motor fibers are found within the spinal cord. The bundles of sensory and motor fibers outside the spinal cord are wrapped in a connective tissue sheath, the epineurium. Groups of fibers are found within this "nerve" in small bundles, each of which is surrounded by connective tissue known as perineurium and in even smaller tubes of connective tissue called endoneurium.

Figures 13.2 and 13.3 also show that each nerve axon has its own membranous covering, often called the nerve membrane, tightly surrounded by a myelin sheath called a Schwann cell covering. The myelin is not continuous along the fiber. The interruptions are the nodes of Ranvier, which are of great importance for nerve functioning.

Electrophysiology of Nerve Membrane
Resting Potential

Most nerves have resting membrane potentials of about −70 to −90 mV as a result of a slight imbalance of electrolytes across the nerve membranes (i.e., between the cytoplasm and the extracellular fluid) (3). The origin of this membrane potential has been of great interest to neurophysiologists. The main electrolytes of nerve axons and cell bodies are sodium, potassium, calcium, magnesium, and chloride. At resting potential, the nerve membrane was believed to be impermeable to sodium because of the low sodium ion concentration in the excitable cell. Potassium ions may flow in and out of the cell with ease, indicating that the membrane is highly permeable to potassium ions. A high potassium ion concentration is retained intracellularly by the attractive forces provided by the negative charges on the protein molecules. Thus, the predominant intracellular cation is potassium (~110 to 170 mmol/L), and the predominant extracellular ions are sodium (~140 mmol/L) and chloride (~110 mmol/L). It would appear that changes in the intracellular or extracellular concentration of potassium ions markedly alter the resting membrane potential. For this reason, neurophysiologists treated an excitable cell as if it were an electrochemical, or Nernst, cell. The resting potential for one permeant species could therefore be explained by the familiar Nernst equation:

$$E = -RT/zF \ln [K^+]_i/[K^+]_o$$

in which E = membrane potential, inside minus outside; R = gas constant; T = temperature; z = valence of ion;

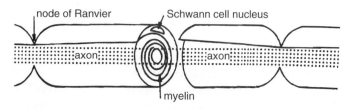

Fig. 13.3. Single myelinated nerve fiber.

F = Faraday's constant; $[K^+]_i$ = activity of potassium intracellularly, and $[K^+]_o$ = activity of potassium extracellularly.

Action Potential

Action potentials are transient membrane depolarizations that result from influx of sodium ions through a brief opening of the voltage-gated sodium channels on excitation of the cell (3). The transmembrane potential during an action potential goes from −70 to about +40 mV (a total net change of 110 mV) and promptly returns to the resting potential; the event lasts about 1 msec (Fig. 13.4).

The transmembrane potential at the peak of the action potential can be predicted from the Nernst equation by substituting appropriate sodium ion concentrations for those of potassium ions. It, therefore, appears that the excitable membrane can be transformed from a potassium electrode to a sodium electrode during the active process (4). As the cell approaches its peak action potential, the permeability to sodium again decreases (sodium inactivation or repolarization). If no other event occurred, this cell would slowly return to its resting potential, but the cell again becomes highly permeable to potassium ions, allowing potassium ions to flow out and quickly restore the membrane potential. After an action potential, the cell would therefore be left with a small increase in sodium ions and a decrease in potassium ions. To explain how the nerve is restored to its original electrolyte composition at the resting potential, it was necessary to postulate a mechanism by which sodium ions could be extruded and potassium ions could probably be accumulated. It has been suggested that by using the energy derived from splitting adenosine triphosphate (ATP), an ATPase system could serve this function and act as a sodium pump (5). Other investigators believe that, during excitation, the membrane goes from one stable state to another, functioning more like an ion exchanger (6). Koketsu suggests that during excitation the membrane goes from a calcium-associated to calcium-dissociated state, triggered by the depolarizing pulse, and that during recovery the membrane returns to the resting state by the reassociation as a result of outward movement of potassium ions (7).

Threshold

An electric stimulus of less than a certain voltage can result in only local electronegativity and cannot elicit a propagated action potential. The voltage necessary to change localized electronegativity into a propagated action potential is called the threshold voltage, which is closely related to the stimulus duration—the longer the stimulus, the lower the threshold voltage.

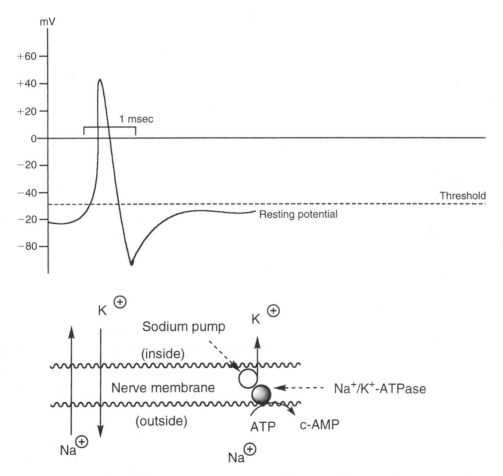

Fig. 13.4. Relationship between membrane action potential and ionic flux across the nerve membrane.

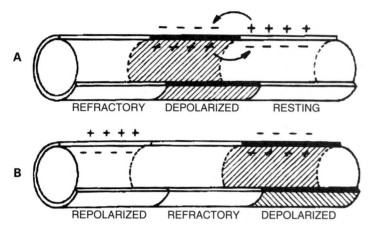

Fig. 13.5. Impulse propagation. **A,** The wave of depolarization passes down the nerve, followed by a wave of refractoriness. **B,** The wave of refractoriness is followed by a wave of repolarization. (After R. H. De Jong and F. G. Freund, Int. Anesthesiol. Clin., 8, 35[1970].)

Refractoriness

Immediately after an impulse has been propagated, the axon is *absolutely refractory,* or completely inexcitable, and no stimulus, no matter how strong or long, can excite it. Shortly thereafter, the axon becomes *relatively refractory;* it responds with a propagated impulse only to stimulation that is greater than the normal threshold. The length of the refractory period is affected by the frequency of stimulation and by many drugs (Fig. 13.5).

Conductance Velocity

This is the velocity at which an impulse is conducted along the nerve and is proportional to the diameter of the fiber.

Nodal Conduction

Because longitudinal resistance is inversely proportional to cross-sectional area, impulses are conducted faster in large-diameter fibers. The squid axon is unmyelinated and exceptionally large (approximately 800 μ); impulses are therefore conducted rapidly along it. Contraction of the mantle of a squid, however, is an uncomplicated procedure that does not require a complex sensorimotor system. Perhaps, during evolution, vertebrates developed a complicated input-output system of many fibers collected in bundles, as shown in Figure 13.2. Conduction in these fibers would be slow if they were not insulated with a myelin coat, interrupted at intervals by the nodes of Ranvier where current enters and exits. Ionic fluxes occur at these nodes. The impulse jumps along the fiber from node to node faster than in unmyelinated fiber (8).

Sodium Channel

The voltage-sensitive sodium channels are discrete membrane-bound glycoproteins that mediate sodium permeability (9–11). It consists of an aqueous pore spanning the axon membrane, which is narrow at one point (known as selective filter) to discriminate sodium ions from other ions

(i.e., sodium ions pass through this pore about 12 times faster than the potassium ions). Sodium channels open and close as they switch between several conformational states, i.e., the resting/closed form (nonconducting state), the open channel (conducting), and the inactivated form (nonconducting state). It is generally agreed that at resting potential, the sodium channels are in a rest/closed state and are impermeable to the passage of sodium ions. On activation, the channels undergo conformational changes to an open state, thus allowing rapid influx of sodium ions across the axonal membrane. Thus, when threshold potential is exceeded, most of the sodium channels are in an open or conducting state. At the peak of the action potential, the open channels spontaneously convert to an inactivated state (i.e., nonconducting, nonactivatable), leading to a decrease in sodium permeability. When a sodium channel is in the inactivated state, it cannot be opened without first transforming to the normal resting/closed form. The channel gating kinetics have been extensively studied with the use of the selective blockers of sodium channels such as tetrodotoxin (TTX) and saxitoxin (STX). These compounds bind stoichiometrically to the outer opening of the channels and are detected with patch-clamp electrophysiologic techniques on the cut-open squid giant axon (12). As a matter of fact, both Neher and Sakmann, two German scientists, were awarded the 1991 Nobel Prize in physiology and medicine for their work on ion channels.

(Lactone form)   (Hemiacetal form)

Tetrodotoxin (TTX)

Saxitoxin (STX)

What Are The Sources of These Neurotoxins?

Tetradotoxin is a potent neurotoxin isolated from the ovaries and liver of many species of *Tetraodontidae,* especially the Japanese fugu (or puffer-fish). Saxitoxin is a mussel or clam poison produced by certain marine dinoflagellates *Gonyaulax catenella* or *G. tamarensis,* the consumption of which cause the mussels or clams to become poisonous. These poisonous shellfish have been connected to a toxic "red-tides" environmental condition on the coastal region of California in early 1970.

MOLECULAR MECHANISM OF ACTION OF LOCAL ANESTHETICS

Local anesthetics decrease the excitability of nerve cells without affecting the resting potential. Because the action potential, or the ability of nerve cells to be excited, seems to be associated with the movement of sodium ions across the nerve membranes, anything that interferes with the movement of these ions interferes with cell excitability. For this reason, many hypotheses have been suggested to explain how local anesthetics regulate the sodium permeability changes that underlie the nerve impulse. These hypotheses include direct action on ionic channels that interferes with ionic fluxes, interaction with phospholipids and calcium that reduces membrane flexibility and responsiveness to changes in electrical fields, and competition with acetylcholine for the membrane-bound cholinergic receptor as well as rather nonspecific actions on the membrane structure (i.e., membrane expansion theory of anesthesia). The nonspecific membrane actions of local anesthetics can be easily ruled out because most clinically useful agents, in contrast to general anesthetics, possess a defined set of structure-activity relationships. As mentioned earlier, local anesthetic agents block nerve conductances and produce anesthesia as a result of their selective actions on membrane-bound sodium channels. It should be pointed out that at much higher drug concentrations local anesthetics also bind and block potassium channels. Before discussing where and how local anesthetics bind to the sodium channel to exert its action, the other hypotheses and the reason(s) why they may not be the molecular mechanism of action for the clinically useful local anesthetics are briefly reviewed.

Interaction with Phospholipids and Calcium

Calcium exists in the membrane in a bound state. Many investigators believe that the release of the bound calcium is the first step in membrane depolarization and that this release leads to the ionic permeability changes previously described. It has been suggested that local anesthetics displace the bound calcium from these sites and form more stable bonds, thereby inhibiting ionic fluxes. The following evidence has been offered in support of this theory. Both calcium and local anesthetics bind to phospholipids in vitro, reducing their flexibility and responsiveness to changes in electric fields (13,14). Also, membrane excitability and instability increase in calcium-deficient solutions. Local anesthetics counteract this abnormal increase in excitability, and more local anesthetic is necessary to block excitation in calcium-poor solutions (15). Direct proof of this hypothesis, however, is lacking because of the difficulty in measuring calcium movements in vivo. It is also possible that the aforementioned cause-and-effect relationship between intracellular free calcium and membrane excitability is the result of a sodium-calcium exchange reaction; i.e., the influx of sodium ions displaces the membrane-bound calcium, which leads to an increase of intracellular free calcium and thereby increases cellular excitability.

Interaction with Acetylcholine System

A quick comparison of the chemical structures of the clinically useful local anesthetics with the known cholinergic agents (Fig. 13.6) led various authors to suggest that perhaps a local anesthetic competes with acetylcholine for the cholinergic receptor as a mechanism of action of local anesthetics (16). Support for this hypothesis is derived from observations that local anesthetics antagonize the depolarizing action of acetylcholine on the nerve membrane. Lidocaine also modifies the kinetics of acetylcholine interactions at the myoneural junction. Again, there is no direct support for this hypothesis. The fact that most potent local anesthetic agents have only a weak anticholinergic activity weakens the argument for such a hypothesis. Perhaps the strongest evidence against such a mechanism can be obtained from the fact that attempts to increase anticholinergic activity by insertion of a substituted methylene group similar to that of propivacaine between the aromatic ring and the carbonyl function of the procaine molecule produces a compound with only weak local anesthetic activity.

Action on Voltage-Sensitive Sodium Channels

As mentioned before, the voltage-sensitive sodium channels are membrane-bound glycoproteins that mediate sodium permeability. On excitation, these channels undergo conformational changes from a closed state to an open state, thus allowing a rapid influx of sodium. The movement of sodium ions is blocked by neurotoxins TTX and STX and by local anesthetics (17). Most electrophysiologists and neuropharmacologists have now agreed that the mechanism of action of local anesthetics is due primarily to their binding to a site(s) within the sodium channels, thus blocking sodium conductance (18). The exact location of the binding site(s), however, and whether all local anesthetics interact with a common site remain a matter of dispute.

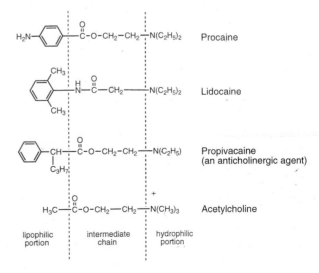

Fig. 13.6. Comparison of local anesthetics with cholinergic agents.

How Local Anesthetics Block Sodium Conductance

Local anesthetics block sodium conductance by two possible modes of action; the tonic and the phasic inhibition (19,20). Tonic inhibition results from the binding of local anesthetics to nonactivated closed channels and thus is independent of channel activation. Phasic inhibition may be accomplished when local anesthetics bind to either activated, open states (conducting) or inactivated (nonconducting) states of the channels. Thus, it is not surprising that a greater phasic inhibition is usually obtained with repetitive depolarization. Two reasons have been suggested to explain this observation: Channel inactivation during depolarization increases the number of binding sites normally inaccessible to local anesthetics at resting potential, or both the open and the inactivated channels possess binding sites with higher affinity and thereby bind local anesthetics more tightly and result in stronger nerve block. Furthermore, it is generally agreed that most of the clinically useful local anesthetics exert their actions by binding to the inactivated forms of the channels and thus prevent their transition to the original rest state (20). Because most of these drugs exhibit both tonic and phasic inhibitions, however, the question as to whether tonic and phasic block results from drug interaction at the same or different sites remains unclear.

Where Local Anesthetics Bind to Sodium Channels

Most of the clinically useful local anesthetics are tertiary amines with a pK_a value of 7.0–9.0. Thus, under physiologic conditions, both protonated forms (onium ions) and the unionized, molecular forms are available for binding to the channel proteins. In fact, the ratio between the onium ions [BH^+] and the unionized molecules [B] can be easily calculated based on the pH of the medium and the pK_a of the drug molecule by the Henderson-Hasselbalch equation:

$$pH = pK_a - \log [BH^+]/[B]$$

The effect of pH changes on the potency of local anesthetics has been extensively investigated (21). Based on these studies, it was concluded that local anesthetics block action potential by first penetrating the nerve membrane in their unionized forms and then binding to a site within the channels in their onium forms. Perhaps the most direct support for this hypothesis comes from the experimental results of Narahashi and co-workers (22,23), who studied the effects of internal and external perfusion of local anesthetics (both tertiary amines and quaternary ammonium compounds), at different pH values, on the sodium conductance of the squid axon. The observation that both tertiary amines and quaternary ammonium compounds produce greater nerve blockage when applied internally indicates an axoplasmic site for these compounds. Furthermore, only the tertiary amines exhibit a reduction in their local anes-

thetic activities when the internal pH is raised from 7.0–8.0. Because the increase of internal pH to 8.0 favors the existence of the unionized forms, this result again suggests that the onium ions are required for binding to the channel receptors. Narahashi and Frazier (24) further estimated that approximately 90% of the blocking actions of lidocaine may be attributed to onium forms of the drug molecule, whereas only about 10% may be due its unionized molecule and perhaps at a hydrophobic binding site other than the primary binding site. Benzocaine, owing to lack of a basic amine group ($pK_a = 2.78$) and other neutral anesthetics such as benzyl alcohol have been suggested to bind to this site.

In 1984, Hille proposed a unified theory involving a single receptor in the sodium channels for both onium ions (protonated tertiary amines and quaternary ammonium compounds) and unionized forms of local anesthetics (25). As depicted in Figure 13.7, a number of pathways are available, depending on the size, the pK_a and the lipid solubility of the drug molecules, and voltage and frequency-dependent modulation of the channel states, for a drug to reach its receptor binding sites. Protonated anesthetic molecules [BH^+] and quaternary ammonium compounds reach their target sites via the hydrophilic pathway externally (path b), which is available only during channel activation. The lipid-soluble anesthetic molecules, on the other hand, diffuse across the neuronal membrane in their unionized forms. They can interact with the same receptors from either the hydrophilic pathway (path b′) upon re-protonation to their onium ions [BH^+] (path b′) or via the hydrophobic pathway (path a) in their unionized forms. Benzocaine and other nonbasic local anesthetic molecules use this hydrophobic pathway and thus bind to the same receptor, though at the hydrophobic site of the receptor, to produce their actions. Again, this hypothesis is purely speculative, and its acceptance is still open for further debate. Recent studies by Ragsdale and co-workers (26) and Wang and his co-worker (27) have suggested that local anesthetics bind to the hydrophobic amino acid residues near the center and the intracellular end of the S6 segment in the domain IV, whereas the BTX receptor is within segment S6 in domain I, of the α subunit of the sodium channels.

Study Question 3

Question: In in vitro experiments with the frog sciatic nerve, the nerve blocking potency of tetrodotoxin (TTX) was potentiated 5-fold by benzyl alcohol and 10-fold by lidocaine. Furthermore, the concentrations of benzyl alcohol and lidocaine used in these experiments were just barely anesthetic by themselves. A small but consistent synergism was also observed between benzyl alcohol and lidocaine [Staiman AL, Seeman P. Can J. Physiol. Pharmacol. 1975; 53:513–524]. Explain these observations, with your knowledge of how local anesthetics bind to their receptor.

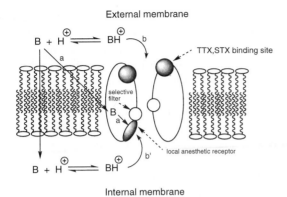

External membrane

TTX,STX binding site

selective filter

local anesthetic receptor

Internal membrane

Fig. 13.7. Model of a sodium channel, as suggested by Hille (25), depicting a hydrophilic pathway (denoted by "b" & "b'") and a hydrophobic pathway (denoted by "a") by which local anesthetics may reach their receptor site(s).

Toxicity and Side Effects

The side effects and toxicity of local anesthetics seem to be related to their actions on other excitable membrane proteins, such as in the sodium and potassium channels in the heart, the nicotinic acetylcholine receptors in the neuromuscular junctions, and the nerve cells in the CNS. In general, neuromuscular junctions and the CNS are more susceptible to the toxic effects of local anesthetics than the cardiovascular system. The actions on skeletal muscles are transient and reversible, whereas the CNS side effects can be deleterious. The primary effect of the toxicity seems to be convulsions, followed by severe CNS depression, particularly of the respiratory and cardiovascular centers. This may be related to an initial depression of inhibitory neurons such as GABAergic systems, causing convulsions, followed by depression of other neurons, leading to general depression of the CNS.

Amino amide-type local anesthetics (i.e., lidocaine derivatives) are, in general, more likely to produce CNS side effects than the amino ester-type compounds (procaine analogs). It should be pointed out, however, that the toxic effects observed depend heavily on the route and site of administration as well as the lipid solubility and metabolic stability of a given local anesthetic molecule. For example, most amide-type local anesthetics such as lidocaine are first degraded *via* N-dealkylations by the hepatic enzymes (see Fig. 13.9). However, unlike lidocaine, the initial metabolic degradation of prilocaine in humans is hydrolysis of the amide linkage to give *o*-toluidine and N-propylalanine. Formation of *o*-toluidine and its metabolites are said to cause methemoglobinemia in some patients (28). For this reason, prilocaine is more likely than other local anesthetics to cause methemoglobinemia.

In contrast, allergic reactions to local anesthetics, even though rare, are known to occur exclusively with *p*-aminobenzoic ester-type local anesthetics (29). Whether the formation of *p*-aminobenzoic acid (PABA) on ester hydrolysis is solely responsible for this hypersensitivity remains to be investigated. However, the preservative compounds

such as methyparaben used in the preparation of amide-type local anesthetics are metabolized to PABA-like substance, *p*-hydroxybenzoic acid. Thus, patients who are allergic to amino ester-type local anesthetics should be treated with a preservative-free amino amide-type local anesthetic.

Amide-type local anesthetics (e.g., procainamide and lidocaine) also possess antiarrhythmic activity when given parenterally and at a subanesthetic dosage. Although this action can also be attributed to their actions on sodium channels in cardiac tissues, current evidence suggests a distinctly different mechanism of action with respect to the modulation of channel receptors and the location of binding sites for these compounds (28,29).

CHEMICAL ASPECTS OF LOCAL ANESTHETIC AGENTS
Structure-activity Relationships

Since the discovery of cocaine in 1880 as a surgical local anesthetic, several thousand new compounds have been tested and found to produce anesthesia by blocking nerve conductance. Among these agents, only about 20 are clinically available in the United States as local anesthetic preparations (Table 13.1).

Table 13.2 contains chemical structures of the different types of agents in current or recent use. A quick perusal of Table 13.2 reveals that many diverse chemical structures possess local anesthetic properties, i.e., amino esters (procaine analogs), amino amides (lidocaine analogs), amino ethers (pramoxine), amino ketones (dyclonine), alcohols (benzyl alcohol and chlorobutanol), and phenols (eugenol and phenol). It would seem that there is no obvious structure-activity relationship among these agents. As mentioned earlier, however, most of the clinically useful local anesthetics are tertiary amines with pK_a values of 7.0–9.0. These compounds exhibit their local anesthetic properties by virtue of the binding of the onium ions to a selective site within the sodium channels. For this reason, any structural modifications that alter the lipid solubility, pK_a, and metabolic inactivation definitely have a pronounced effect on the ability of a drug molecule to reach or bind to the hypothetical receptor site(s), thus modifying its local anesthetic properties.

A brief discussion of known structure-activity relationships is presented according to the following structural characteristics according to Löfgren's classification (30) (see Fig. 13.6):

lipophilic portion—intermediate chain
—hydrophilic portion

Lipophilic Portion

The lipophilic portion of the molecule is essential for local anesthetic activity. For most of the clinically useful local anesthetics, this portion of the molecule consists of either an aromatic group directly attached to a carbonyl function (the amino ester series) or a 2,6-dimethylphenyl group attached to a carbonyl function through an —NH—

group (the amino amide series). Both of these groups are highly lipophilic and appear to play an important role in the binding of local anesthetics to the channel receptor proteins. Structural modification of this portion of the molecule is known to have a profound effect on its physical and chemical properties, which, in turn, alters its local anesthetic properties.

In the amino ester series, an electron-donating substituent in the *ortho* or *para* or both positions increases local anesthetic potency. Such groups as an amino (procaine, chloroprocaine, and propoxycaine), an alkylamino (tetracaine), or an alkoxy (proparacaine and propoxycaine) group can contribute electron density to the aromatic ring by both resonance and inductive effects, thereby enhancing local anesthetic potency over nonsubstituted analog (meprylcaine). As illustrated in Figure 13.8, using tetracaine as an example, through resonance we could expect that the structure of tetracaine is really between the two resonance forms; i.e., the electrons from the amino group can be resonance delocalized onto the carbonyl oxygen to create the resonance form as shown. Although neither structure may accurately represent the structure of tetracaine when it binds to the local anesthetic receptors, it is reasonable to assume that the greater the resemblance to the protonated onium resonance form, the greater the affinity for the receptor (i.e., binding from both the hydrophilic pathway b' and hydrophobic pathway a, Fig.

13.7). This is particularly true for the binding of benzocaine to its receptor. Thus, addition of any aromatic substitution that can enhance the formation of this resonance form through resonance or inductive effects will produce more potent local anesthetic agents. Electron-withdrawing groups such as nitro ($-NO_2$), carbonyl ($-CO-$), and nitrile ($-CN$) reduce the local anesthetic activity.

Insertion of a methylene group between the aromatic moiety and the carbonyl function in the procaine molecule, which prohibits the formation of the resonance form, has led to a procaine analog with greatly reduced anesthetic potency. This observation lends further support for the involvement of the resonance form when an ester-type local anesthetic binds to the receptor. It should be pointed out that a similar resonance form can also be envisioned in the amino amide series without the need for a direct attachment of the aromatic ring to the carbonyl function (see Fig. 13.8).

When an amino or an alkoxy group is attached to the *meta* position of the aromatic ring, however, no resonance delocalization of their electrons is possible. The addition of this function only increases (alkoxy group) or decreases (amino group) the lipophilicity of the molecule (such as benoxinate and proparacaine).

Furthermore, tetracaine, the most widely used analog of procaine, is approximately 50-fold more potent than procaine. This increase in potency cannot be correlated exper-

Table 13.1. Local Anesthetics in Current or Recent Use*

Generic Name	Proprietary Name	Recommended Application
Articaine†	Astracaine	Parenteral
Benoxinate§	Dorsacaine	Mainly in ophthalmology
Benzocaine†	Americaine	Topical
Bupivacaine†	Marcaine Sensorcaine	Parenteral
Butamben†	Butesin	Topical
Chloroprocaine†	Nesacaine	Parenteral
Cocaine†		Topical (mucosal only)
Dibucaine†	Nupercainal, Cinchocaine	Topical
Dyclonine	Dyclocaine, Dyclone, Sucrets	Topical (mucosal only)
Etidocaine†	Duranest	Parenteral
Lidocaine†	Xylocaine, Lignocaine, Anestacon, Dalacine, Dilocaine, Nervocaine, Nulicaine,	Parenteral, Topical
Mepivacaine†	Carbocaine, Polocaine, Isocaine	Parenteral, Topical
Meprylcaine*		
Pramoxine†	Anusol, Tronothane, Proxine, Tronolane, Pramocaine	Topical
Prilocaine†	Citanest	Parenteral
Procaine†	Novocain	Parenteral
Proparacaine†	Alcaine, Ophthaine, Ak-Taine	Mainly in ophthalmology
Propoxycaine‖	Blockaine	Parenteral
Ropivacaine†	Naropin	Parenteral
Tetracaine†	Pontocaine, Amethocaine, Prax	Parenteral, Topical
Benzyl alcohol‡		Topical, mainly in combination
Chlorobutanol‡		Topical, especially in dentistry
Eugenol‡		Topical, especially in dentistry
Phenol‡		Mainly topical (and for irreversible blocks)
Ethyl chloride‡		Extracutaneous, temperature decreasing

*United States Pharmacopoeia XXII (1990).
†USP DI 20th ed. (2000).
‡National Formulary 16 (2000).
§United States Pharmacopoeia 24 (2000).

Table 13.2. Structures of Local Anesthetics

Amino Esters

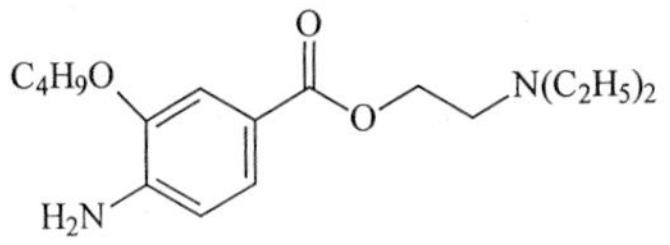

Benoxinate (pKa = 9.0)

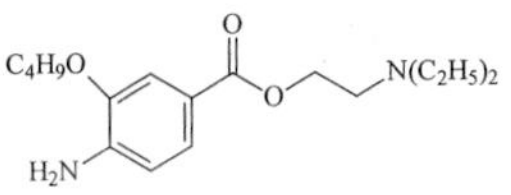

Benzocaine (pKa = 2.8)

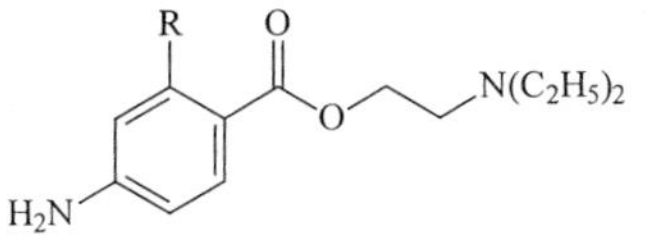

R = H, Procaine (pKa = 8.8)
R = Cl, Chloroprocaine (pKa = 9.0)
R = OC$_3$H$_7$, Propoxycaine (pKa = 9.1)

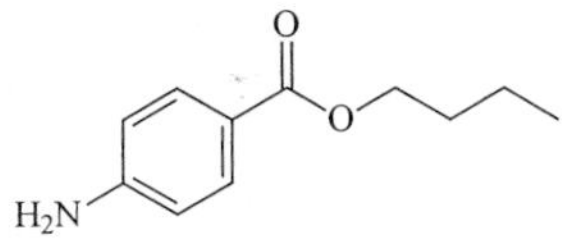

Butamben (pKa = 2.5)

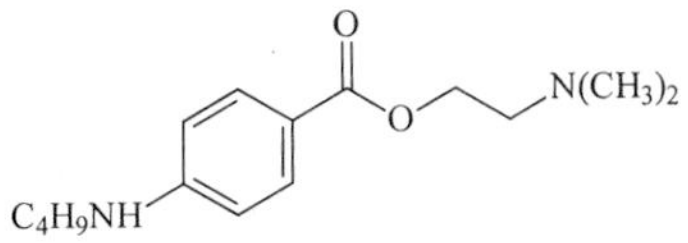

Tetracaine (pKa = 8.4)

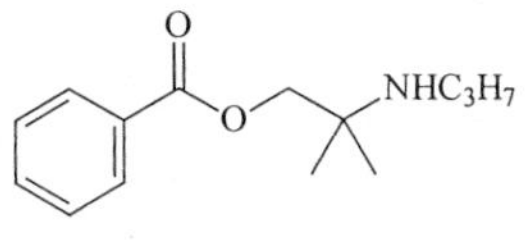

Meprylcaine (pKa = 7.8)

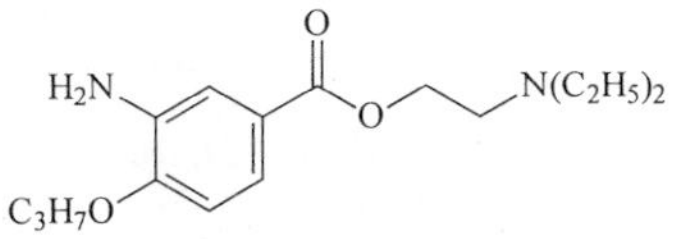

Proparacaine (pKa = 9.1)

Amino Amides

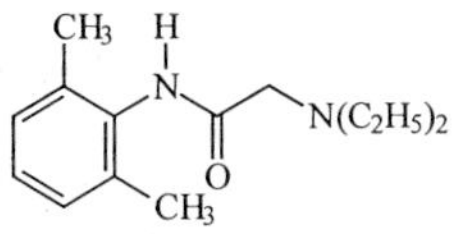

Lidocaine (pKa = 7.8)

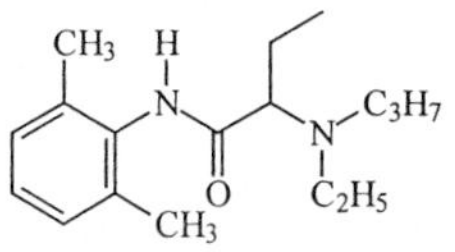

Etidocaine (pKa = 7.7)

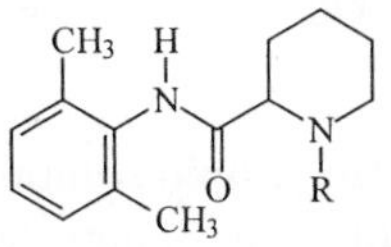

R = CH$_3$, Mepivacaine (pKa = 7.6)
R = C$_4$H$_9$, Bupivacaine (pKa = 8.1)

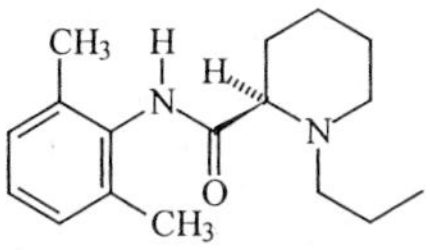

Ropivacaine [S (−) isomer]
(pKa = 8.2)

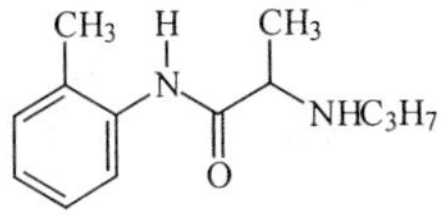

Prilocaine (pKa = 7.9)

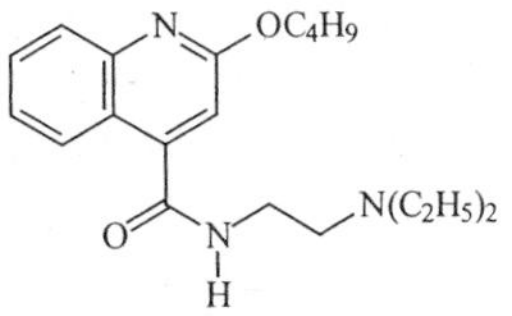

Dibucaine (pKa = 8.8)

Amino Ether

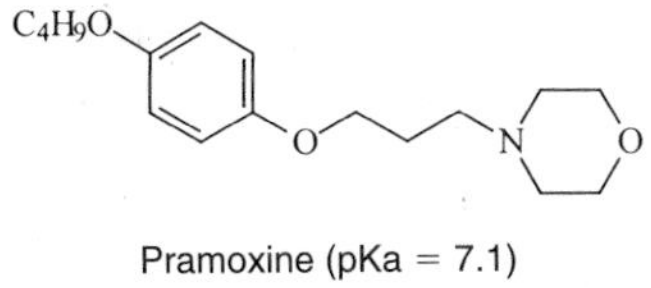

Pramoxine (pKa = 7.1)

Amino Ketone

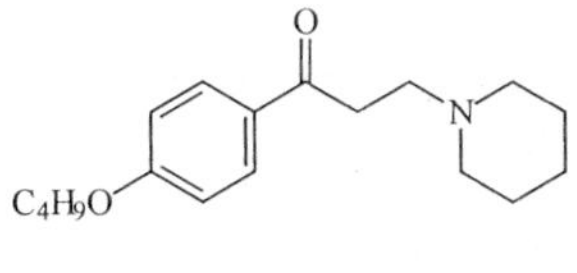

Dyclonine (pKa = 8.2)

Alcohols

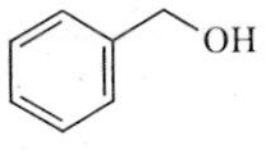

Benzyl alcohol

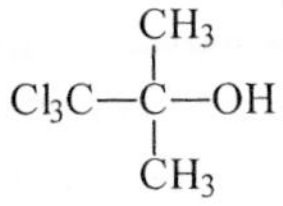

Chlorobutanol

Phenols

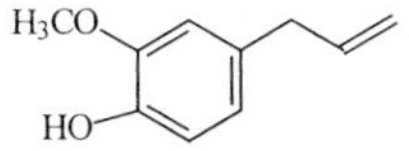

Eugenol

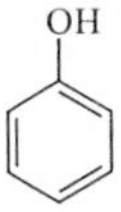

Phenol

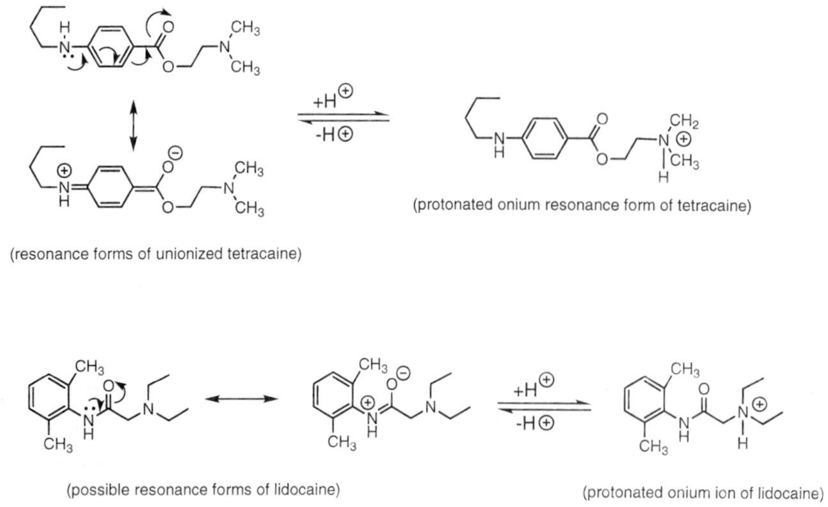

(resonance forms of unionized tetracaine)

(protonated onium resonance form of tetracaine)

(possible resonance forms of lidocaine)

(protonated onium ion of lidocaine)

Fig. 13.8. Possible resonance forms for procaine and lidocaine analogs.

imentally solely with the increase of lipid solubility of the n-butyl group. Perhaps part of this potentiation of local anesthetic activity can be attributed to the electron-releasing property of the n-butyl group via the inductive effect, which indirectly enhances the electron density of the *p*-amino group, which, in turn, increases the formation of resonance form available for binding to the receptor proteins.

Another important aspect of aromatic substitution has been observed from structure-activity relationship studies. In the amino amides (lidocaine analogs), the *o,o'*-dimethyl groups are required to provide suitable protection from amide hydrolysis to ensure a desirable duration of action. Similar conclusions can be made to rationalize the increase in the duration of action of propoxycaine by the *o*-propoxy group. The shorter duration of action, however, observed with chloroprocaine when it was compared with that procaine can only be explained by the inductive effect of the *o*-chloro group, which pulls the electron density away from the carbonyl function, thus making it more susceptible for nucleophilic attack by the plasma esterases.

Intermediate Chain

The intermediate chain almost always contains a short alkylene chain of one to three carbons in length linked to the aromatic ring via several possible organic functional groups. The nature of this intermediate chain determines the chemical stability of the drug. It also influences the duration of action and relative toxicity. In general, amino amides are more resistant to metabolic inactivation than the amino esters and thus are longer acting local anesthetics. The placement of small alkyl groups (i.e., branching), especially around the ester function (such as meprylcaine) or the amide function (such as etidocaine and prilocaine), also hinders esterase or amidase catalyzed hydrolysis prolonging the duration of action. It should be mentioned, however, that prolonging the duration of action of a compound usually also increases its systemic tox-

icities, and this is discussed in a later section under biochemical distribution.

In the lidocaine series, lengthening of the alkylene chain from one to two or three increases the pK_a of the terminal tertiary amino group from 7.7 to 9.0 or 9.5, respectively. Thus, lengthening of the intermediate chain effectively reduces local anesthetic potency as a result of a reduction of onium ions under physiologic conditions. As mentioned earlier, the onium ions are required for effective binding to the channel receptors.

Hydrophilic Portion

Most clinically useful local anesthetics have a tertiary alkylamine, which readily forms water-soluble salts with mineral acids, and this portion is commonly considered as the hydrophilic portion of the molecule. The necessity of this portion of the molecule for local anesthetic activity is still a matter of debate. The strongest opposition for requiring a basic amino group for local anesthetic action comes from the observation that benzocaine, which lacks the basic aliphatic amine function, has potent local anesthetic activity. For this reason, it is often suggested that the tertiary amine function in procaine analogs is needed only for the formation of water-soluble salts suitable for pharmaceutical preparations. With the understanding of the voltage-activated sodium channel and the possible mechanism of action of local anesthetics discussed previously, however, it is quite conceivable that the onium ions produced by protonation of the tertiary amine group are also required for binding to the receptors.

From Table 13.2, the hydrophilic group present in most of the clinically useful drugs can be in the form of a secondary or tertiary alkyl amine or as part of a nitrogen heterocycle (such as pyrrolidine, piperidine, morpholine). As mentioned earlier, most of the clinically useful local anesthetics have pK_a values of 7.5–9.0. As we learned in organic chemistry, the effects of an alkyl substituent on the pK_a depends on the size, length, and hydrophobicity of the

Study Question 4

Question: A pharmacist, in a biosphere space station with a limited supply of pharmaceutical products, is faced with making choices during a crisis.

a. Which of the following drugs after conversion to its salt, should NOT be administered as a local anesthetic for parenteral use? Explain.

A   B

b. Which of following drugs, hexylcaine or cyclomethycaine, should be selected to incorporate into an ointment for severe sunburn? Justify your choice.

Hexylcaine   Cyclomethycaine

N-Aminoalkyl spirotetralin succinimides

group; it is difficult to see a clear structure-activity relationship among these structures. It is generally accepted, however, that local anesthetics having higher lipid solubility and lower pK_a values appear to exhibit more rapid onset and lower toxicity.

Stereochemistry

Are there any stereochemical requirements of local anesthetic compounds when they bind to the sodium channel receptors? Although a number of clinically used local anesthetics do contain a chiral center (i.e., bupivacaine, etidocaine, mepivacaine, and prilocaine, Table 13.2), in contrast to cholinergic drugs, the effect of optical isomerism on isolated nerve preparations revealed a lack of stereospecificity. In a few cases (e.g., prilocaine, bupivacaine, and etidocaine), when they have been administered *in vivo*, however, small differences in total pharmacologic profile of optical isomers have been noted. Whether these differences are due to differences in uptake, distribution, and metabolism or due to direct binding to the receptor has not been determined. When structural rigidity has been imposed on the molecule, however, as in the case of some aminoalkyl spirotetraline succinimides (33), differences in local anesthetic potency of the enantiomers have been observed, ranging from 1:2–1:10. Although these differences in enantiomers are clearly not as pronounced as those in other pharmacologic agents, such as adrenergic blocking agents or anticholinergic drugs, steric requirements are necessary for effective interaction between a local anesthetic agent and its proposed channel receptors.

Stereochemistry of the local anesthetics, however, plays an important role in their observed toxicity and their pharmacokinetic properties. For example, ropivacaine, the only optically active local anesthetic marketed, has a considerable lower cardiac toxicity than its close structural analog, bupivacaine (34). Furthermore, the degree of separation between motor and sensory blockade is more apparent with ropivacaine relative to bupivacaine at a lower end of the dosage scale (35). Thus, the observed cardiac toxicity of bupivacaine has been attributed to the R(+)-bupivacaine enantiomer (36–38). The exact mechanism(s) for this enantiomeric difference remain unknown. Longobardo and co-workers observed a stereoselective blockade on the cardiac hKv1.5 channels by the R(+) isomers of bupivacaine, ropivacaine, and mepivacaine (39). It should be noted that the S(−)-bupivacaine is currently under FDA review and will be marketed under the name of Chirocaine. It has even less CNS toxicity than Ropivacaine.

Biochemical Distribution

A solution of a local anesthetic is commonly administered by injection to a site near the nerve trunk to allow maximum diffusion to the nerve ending to effect desirable local anesthesia. Thus, it is reasonable to assume that any diffusion of the drug from this site into the blood circulation only contributes to the toxicity and side effects of the administered drug. In the design of local anesthetic agents, many attempts have been made to maximize penetration of nerve membranes while minimizing the loss of drug to the systemic circulation by modifying the structure of a known drug. This has not been an easy task, however, even though the ability of a drug molecule to penetrate a membrane appears to correlate well with its lipid solubility, and this distribution coefficient can be measured experimentally. The difficulty arises from the fact that the in vivo system is normally more complex than the laboratory experiments used to assess the local anesthetic potency (i.e., isolated frog sciatic nerves or rabbit cornea). For example, increasing lipid solubility of a compound may well result in facilitated penetration of a nerve membrane, but it can also enhance the ability of the drug to pass through a blood vessel wall. This increased lipid solubility, therefore, reduces the anesthetic potency owing to the more rapid removal of the agent from the site, which thereby increases its systemic toxicity. Another complicating factor is the presence of adipose tissues in the area of drug deposition. Because of the lipoidal nature of the adipose tissue, any distribution of the drug into this lipid depot or site of loss also reduces local anesthetic activity.

Furthermore, the degree of vascularization or rate of blood flow at the site of application and the total dosage administered also play an important role in governing local anesthetic activity and the associated toxicities. Extraneuronal blood vessels near the site of drug application greatly affect the amount of drug that reaches the nerve trunk to establish anesthesia; thus, a larger dosage is required to elicit local anesthesia, which also affects the observed toxicity. After the establishment of anesthesia, however, a major contributing factor to the loss of the drug from the nerve may be the intraneuronal blood vessels. Thus, limitation of blood flow in the area of injection may substantially increase the amount of drug available to the nerve and thus improve the duration of successful anesthesia. A reduction in local blood flow also slows systemic uptake of the drug from the injection site and thus minimizes any potential toxicity.

Study Question 5

Question: Explain why alkalinization of local anesthetics to improve onset time is theoretically sound but clinically impractical?

Protein binding affinity of local anesthetic drugs seems to be correlated to the duration of local anesthetic activity. If the binding affinity is too great, however, the ability of the drug to reach its target site could be impeded, thereby leading to less active agents.

Metabolism

In discussing the metabolic fates of local anesthetics, most of the clinically available local anesthetics may be divided into two broad categories: the esters, of which procaine is an example, and the non-esters, exemplified by lidocaine.

The ester-type local anesthetics are hydrolyzed by esterases, which are widely distributed in body tissues. These compounds can therefore be metabolized in the blood, kidneys, and liver and, to a lesser extent, at the site of administration. For example, both procaine and benzocaine are easily hydrolyzed by esterases into p-aminobenzoic acid (PABA) and the corresponding alcohols. It is not surprising that potential drug interactions exist between the ester-type local anesthetics and other clinically important drugs, such as cholinesterase inhibitors or atropine-like anticholinergic drugs. These compounds either inhibit or compete with local anesthetics for esterases, therefore prolonging local anesthetic activity or toxicity. Another potential drug interaction with clinical significance may also be envisioned between benzocaine and sulfonamides; i.e., the hydrolysis of benzocaine to PABA may antagonize the antibacterial activity of sulfonamides.

The nonester-type local anesthetics, however, are primarily metabolized in the liver involving CYP450. A general metabolic scheme for lidocaine is shown in Figure

Study Question 6

Question: Patients who are dibucaine-resistant homozygotes or heterozygotes are more likely to experience toxic reactions to amino ester-type local anesthetics. Explain.

13.9. Marked species variations occur in the quantitative urinary excretion of these metabolites. For example, rats produce large quantities of the 3-hydroxy derivatives of both lidocaine and monoethylglycinexylidide, which are subsequently conjugated and recycled in the bile. Significant quantities of these two metabolites, however, are not produced by guinea pigs, dogs, or humans. It is therefore unlikely that biliary excretion is a major pathway of excretion of these species. Species variability is important primarily when the acute and chronic toxicity of nonester-type local anesthetic agents is being evaluated.

Although the exact mechanism of CNS toxicity of lidocaine is still unclear, the metabolic studies of lidocaine do provide some insight for future studies. Of all of the metabolites of lidocaine, only monoethylglycinexylidide but not glycinexylidide contributes to some of the CNS side effects of lidocaine. This observation suggests that, perhaps, the toxicities of lidocaine be related to the removal of the N-ethyl groups of lidocaine after crossing the

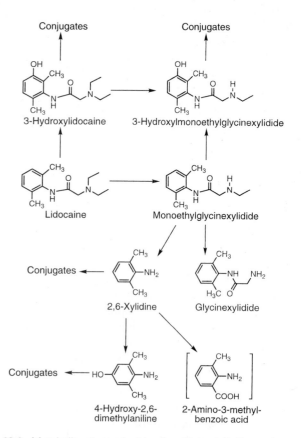

Fig. 13.9. Metabolic scheme for lidocaine. (From J. B. Keenaghan and R. N. Boyes: J. Pharmacol. Exp. Ther., 180, 454(1972).)

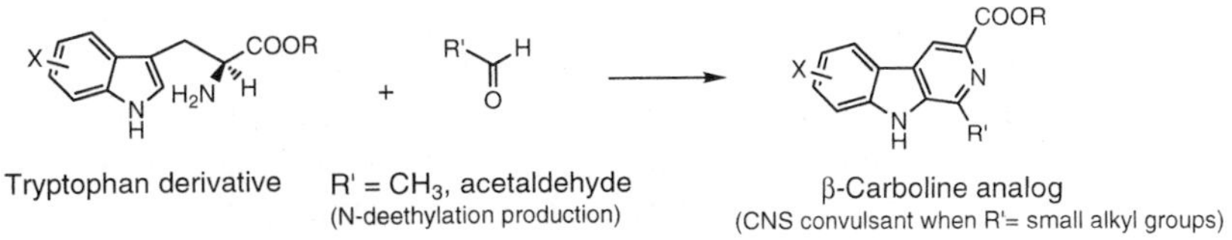

Fig. 13.10. Reaction of a tryptophan derivative with acetaldehyde under physiologic conditions.

blood-brain barrier. Support for this hypothesis can be obtained from the fact that reaction of a tryptophan derivative with formaldehyde under physiologic conditions will give a β-carboline derivative, which is a CNS convulsant (see Fig. 13.10). Recent advances in the GABA$_A$ receptor-benzodiazepine receptor-chloride ion channels and their role in the mechanism of action of benzodiazepine anticonvulsants further lends support to this hypothesis, i.e., β-carbolines are inverse agonists of benzodiazepines.

To minimize these unwanted side effects of lidocaine, tocainide and tolycaine have been prepared and found to possess good local anesthetic activity without any appreciable CNS side effects. Tocainide, which lacks the vulnerable N-ethyl group but has a α-methyl group to prevent degradation of the primary amine group from amine oxidase, has desirable local anesthetic properties. Tolycaine has an o-carbomethoxy substituted for one of the o-methyl group of lidocaine. The carbomethoxy group is fairly stable in tissues but is rapidly hydrolyzed in the blood to the polar carboxylic function and is thus unable to cross the blood-brain barrier. For this reason, tolycaine lacks any CNS side effects even though it still contains the N-ethyl groups. It should be pointed out, however, that both tocainide and tolycaine are primarily used clinically as antiarrhythmic agents.

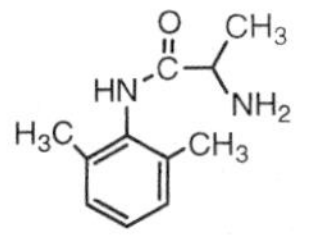

Tocainide 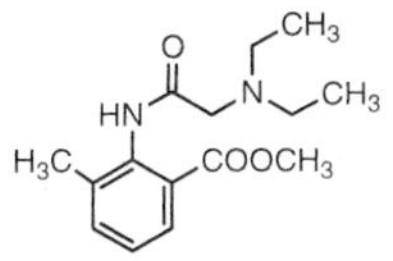   Tolycaine

Furthermore, nonester-type drugs, especially lidocaine derivatives, are also known to be more prone to enzyme induction or inhibition of other medications (e.g., cimetidine, barbiturates).

Pharmaceutical Considerations

Local anesthetic agents are generally prepared in various dosage forms: aqueous solutions for parenteral injection and creams and ointments for topical applications. Thus, chemical stability and aqueous solubility become primary factors in the preparations of suitable pharmaceutical dosage forms. As a rule, compounds containing an amide linkage have greater chemical stability than do the ester types. In this regard, an aqueous solution of an amino ester-type local anesthetic is more likely

Study Question 7

Question: Articaine (Ultracaine, Carticaine), a dental anesthetic available only in Europe and in Canada, is said to lack CNS and cardiovascular toxicity associated with lidocaine and other amide-type local anesthetics. Explain.

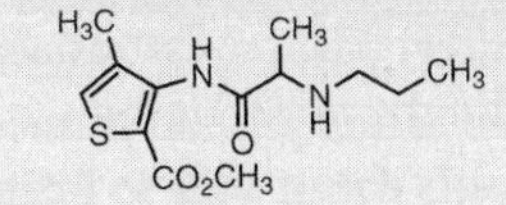

Study Question 8

Question: The metabolism of ropivacaine in human is mediated by CYP1A2 and to a minor extent by CYP3A4 [Arlander E, et al. Clin Pharmacol. Ther. 1998; 64:484–489]. The major metabolite is 3-hydroxyropivacaine and the minor metabolite is (S)-2',6'-pipecoloxylidide (a N-dealkylated product). Draw the chemical structures for these metabolites. Explain, based on your knowledge of drug metabolism, why severe drug-drug interactions between ropivacaine and fluvoxamine, a serotonin re-uptake inhibitor, were observed while ketoconazole, a known hepatic enzyme inhibitor, cause only minor decrease in ropivacaine renal clearance.

to decompose under normal conditions and cannot withstand heat sterilization because of base-catalyzed hydrolysis of the ester.

As stated before, local anesthetic activity usually increases with increasing lipid solubility. Unfortunately, this increase in lipid solubility is often inversely related to water solubility. For this reason, a suitable parenteral dosage form may not be available for these agents owing to poor water solubility under acceptable conditions. For example, benzocaine, which lacks an aliphatic amino group needed for salt formation, is practically insoluble in water at a neutral pH. Protonation of the aromatic amino group in benzocaine results in a salt with a pK$_a$ = 2.78, which is too acidic and therefore unsuitable for the preparation of a parenteral dosage form for injection. For this reason, benzocaine and its closely related analog, butamben, are used mostly in creams or ointments to provide topical anesthesia of accessible mucous membranes or skin for burns, cuts, or inflamed mucous surfaces.

Many attempts have been made to substitute oils, fats, or fluid polymers for the aqueous vehicle commonly used in injectable local anesthetics. Unfortunately, the pharmacologic results of these experiments have been quite disappointing, often as a result of the undesirable toxicity of the nonaqueous vehicle. Efforts have also been made to find additives that will potentiate the action of the classic local anesthetics. Substances such as quinine derivatives, caffeine, theobromine, antipyrine, aspirin, certain vitamins, and some quaternary ammonium compounds potentiate the action of local anesthetic drugs to various degrees. Unfortunately, these combinations are often associated with unacceptable levels of tissue irritation. The only commonly accepted organic additives to local anesthetics are vasoconstrictors, such as epinephrine. These compounds often increase the frequency of successful anesthesia and, to a limited degree, increase the duration of activity by reducing the rate of drug loss from the injection site. These agents are believed to function by constricting arterioles that supply blood to the area of the injection. The effect of these vasoconstrictors is less pronounced if the agents are added to a local anesthetic solution that is to be injected in an area that has profuse venous drainage but is remote from an arterial supply.

Because it is believed that local concentration of potassium in the vicinity of a nerve can affect the conduction of the nerve, mixtures of local anesthetic drugs enriched with potassium ions have been evaluated. The results of these experiments have also been disappointing. Ammonium sulfate, which is often used to denature proteins reversibly, has also been studied in combination with local anesthetics. Again, no substantial advantage has been established, and indications of possible irritation have been noted.

Administration of a local anesthetic in a carbonic acid-carbon dioxide solution rather than the usual solution of a hydrochloride salt appreciably improves the time of onset and duration of action. This change in solution form is apparently not associated with local or systemic toxicity. Current theories suggest that carbon dioxide potentiates the action of local anesthetics by initial indirect depression of the axon, followed by diffusion trapping of the active form of the local anesthetic within the nerve. Use of the carbonate salt appears to be one pharmaceutic modification of the classic local anesthetic agents that may result in significant clinical advantages.

Answer for Study Question 1

Answer: With the exception of cocaine (itself a vasoconstrictor), all local anesthetics are associated with arteriolar dilatation. Thus, in order to decrease the rate of removal of local anesthetics from site of administration and to maintain effective drug concentration to the site of action, a vasoconstrictor such as epinephrine is frequently used to reduce regional blood supply. Epinephrine is a potent adrenergic agonist at the α- and β-adrenergic receptors, however, its vasoconstricting action is due primarily to its action on the $α_1$-adrenergic receptors. A reduction of regional blood flow into and out of the site of action greatly reduces the systemic toxicity of procaine. Furthermore, as procaine and other ester-type local anesthetics are predominately inactivated by plasma esterase, a reduction of local blood flow also lowers the plasma esterases concentrations and thereby prolongs the duration of action of the local anesthetic.

Answer for Study Question 2

Answer: Benzocaine, which lacks an aliphatic amino group needed for salt formation, is practically insoluble in water. Protonation of the aromatic amino group in benzocaine results in a salt with a pKa = 2.78, which is too acidic and therefore unsuitable for the preparation of a parenteral dosage form for injection. Based on the acid–base chemistry principle, an aromatic amino group is a weak base because its nonbounded elections are delocalized into the aromatic ring. Thus, an aromatic amine salt such as benzocaine will not hold onto its proton as tightly as an aliphatic amine salt and therefore readily release the proton when dissolved in water.

Answer for Study Question 3

Answer: Tetrodotoxin (TTX) selectively blocks sodium channels from the external membrane while benzyl alcohol and lidocaine diffuse through the lipoidal membrane and bind via different membrane binding sites which are also part of the voltage-gated sodium channel. Thus, co-administration of TTX with benzyl alcohol or with lidocaine will have a synergistic effect on their nerve blocking action. A greater synergism occurred between TTX and lidocaine because lidocaine binds to its receptor via both hydrophobic (unionized form) as well as hydrophilic pathways (ionized form) while benzyl alcohol only binds to its receptor via hydrophobic pathway.

Answer for Study Question 4

Answer: a. Compound A is an ester-type local anesthetic with only an aromatic amine moiety for salt formation. The resulting dosage form will be too acidic for parenteral usage. On the other hand, compound B is an amide-type drug with an aliphatic amine function. The corresponding salt solution should have a pH approximately 6.0, which could easily be buffered to tissue pH. Thus, it is suitable for the preparation of a parenteral dosage form for injection.

b. Although both hexylcaine and cyclomethycaine have similar pKa values and lipid solubility, cyclomethycaine should be used for this preparation because it is more potent than hexylcaine. The electron-donating cyclohexyloxy group in cyclomethycaine enhances the formation of the resonance form of the drug molecule for binding to the local anesthetic receptors.

Answer for Study Question 5

Answer: Many in vitro studies have demonstrated that addition of sodium bicarbonate to solutions of local anesthetics decreases the ratio of ionized to unionized molecules, thereby allowing more rapid penetration of the local anesthetic through the lipid membrane (see Fig.13.7), thus shortening the onset time. However, addition of too much bicarbonate will cause precipitation of the drug molecules, and this may result in the injection of particulate unionized drug along with the solution. For this reason, routine alkalization of local anesthetics is not desirable.

Answer for Study Question 6

Answer: Patients with genetic anomalies of plasma cholinesterase in so called dibucaine-resistant homozygotes (lacks one such gene) or heterozygotes (lacks both genes) are unable to efficiently hydrolyze local anesthetics. Thus, an increased drug level in the blood circulation would lead to increased cardiac and CNS toxicity. For this reason, an individual with atypical plasma cholinesterase should wear a Medic-Alert bracelet so that complications can be avoided.

Answer for Study Question 7

Answer: Aricaine lacks the CNS and cardiovascular toxicity of lidocaine because it has a carbomethoxy group instead of a methyl group at the ortho position. It will protect amide hydrolysis in the site of local anesthetic action due to a lower tissue esterase concentration. However, when articaine is absorbed into the blood circulation, this carbomethoxy group is rapidly hydrolyzed to provide a carboxylic acid function. The presence of this carboxylic acid function with a basic amine group in the molecule will greatly decrease the concentration of neural unionized molecules needed to cross the lipoidal membranes in heart and in the blood-brain barrier. Furthermore, any unprotonated drug molecules present in blood circulation will probably exist in an internal salt similar to that of amino acid, thus greatly reducing their ability to cross lipid membranes.

Answer for Study Question 8

Answer: 3-Hydroxyropivacaine is produced via the microsomal aromatic hydroxylation catalyzed by CYP1A2 isozymes. This enzymatic reaction introduces a hydroxy group ortho to one of the methyl group of ropivacaine. Because CYP1A2 is the most important isozyme for the degradation of ropivacaine, a potent inhibitor of this isozyme such as fluvoxamine will greatly reduce the renal plasma clearance of ropivacaine. On the other hand, (S)-2'6'-pipecoloxylidide is formed by removal of N-propyl group of ropivacaine by isozymes CYP3A4. Because this is only a minor metabolite, an inhibitor of CYP3A4 like ketoconazole will have no relevance in total clearance of ropivacaine.

CASE STUDY

Victoria F. Roche and S. William Zito

AP, a pharmacist in a biosphere space station, is participating in a number of health-related experiments. Specifically, one experiment will test the effect of space travel on IOP and another will measure the rate of burn healing in a low gravity environment. She is asked to prepare a solution of a local anesthetic to decrease the pain associated with measurement of IOP and to prepare an ointment for topical application for the treatment of skin abrasions and burns. AP is limited to the following structures. Evaluate each for approriateness and make a recommendation.

1. Identify the therapeutic problem(s) where the pharmacist's intervention may benefit the patient.

2. Identify and prioritize the patient specific factors that must be considered to achieve the desired therapeutic outcomes.

3. Conduct a thorough and mechanistically oriented structure-activity analysis of all therapeutic alternatives provided in the case.

4. Evaluate the SAR findings against the patient-specific factors and desired therapeutic outcomes and make a therapeutic decision.

5. Counsel your patient.

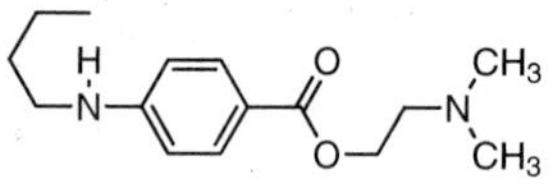

1

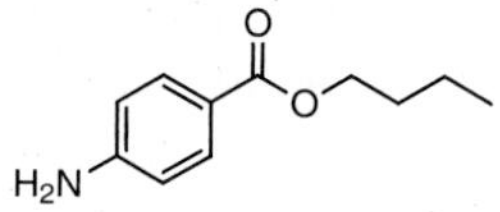

2

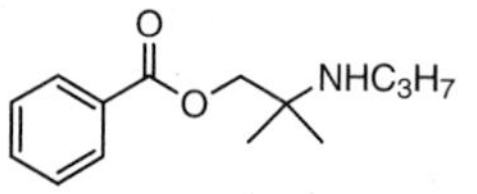

3

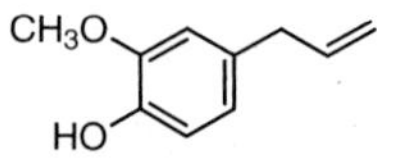

4

REFERENCES

1. Liljestrand G. The historical development of local anesthesia in local anesthetics. In: Lechat P, ed. International Encyclopedia of Pharmacology and Therapeutics. Oxford, Pergamon Press, 1971; 1:1–38.
2. Arey LB, Developmental Anatomy. 7th ed., Philadelphia, W. B. Saunders, 1965.
3. De Jong RH, Freund FG. Physiology of peripheral nerve and local anesthesia. Int Anesthesiol Clin 1979; 8: 35–53.
4. Hodgkin AL, Huxley AF. The dual effect of membrane potential on sodium conductance in the giant axon of *Loligo*. J Physiol (Lond) 1952; 116: 497–506.
5. Skou JC. Further investigations on a $Mg^{++} + Na^{+}$-activated adenosinetriphosphatase, possibly related to the active, linked transport of Na^{+} and K^{+} across the nerve membrane. Biochim Biophys Acta 1960: 42: 6–23.
6. Tasaki I, Singer I, Takenaka T. Effects of internal and external ionic environment on excitability of squid gaiant axon. A macromolecular approach. J Gen Physiol 1965; 48: 1095–1123.
7. Koketsu K. Calcium and the excitable cell membrane. Neurosci Res 1969; 2: 2–39.
8. Tasaki I. Nerve Transmission. Springfield, IL, Charles C Thomas, 1953.
9. Catterall WA. Structure and function of voltage-sensitive ion channels. Science 1988; 242: 50–61.
10. Timmer JS, Agnew WS. Molecular diversity of voltage-sensitive Na channels. Annu Rev Physiol 1989; 51: 401–418.
11. Catterall WA. Cellular and molecular biology of voltage-gated sodium channels. Physiol Rev 1992; 72 (suppl): 15–48.
12. Hamill OP, Marty A, Neher E, et al. Improved patch-clamp techniques for high-resolution current recording from cells and cell-free membrane patches. Pflügers Arch 1981; 391: 85–100.
13. Feinstein MB. Reaction of local anesthetics with phospholipids. A possible chemical basis for anesthesia. J Gen Physiol 1964; 48: 357–374.
14. Blaustein MP, Goldman DE. Competitive action of calcium and procaine on lobster axon. J Gen Physiol 1966; 49: 1043–1063.
15. Ritchie JM, Greengard P. On the mode of action of local anesthetics Annu Rev Pharmacol 1966: 6: 405–430.
16. Dettbarn WD. The acetylcholine system in peripheral nerve. Ann N Y Acad Sci 1967; 144: 483–503.
17. Tamkun MM, Talvenheimo JA, Catterall WA. The sodium channel from rat brain: Reconstitution of neurotoxin-activated ion flux and scorpion toxin binding from purified components. J Biol Chem 1984; 259: 1676–1688.
18. Butterworth IV JF, Strichartz GR. Molecular mechanisms of local anesthetics: A review. Anesthesiology 1990; 72: 711–734.
19. Strichartz GR. The inhibition of sodium currents in myelinated nerve by quaternary derivatives of lidocaine. J Gen Physiol 1973; 62: 37–57.
20. Courtney KR. Mechanism of frequency-dependent inhibition of sodium currents in frog myelinated nerve by the lidocaine derivative GEA 968. J Pharmacol Exp Ther 1975; 195: 225–236.
21. Narahashi T, Frazier DT, Site of action and active form of local anesthetics. In: Neurosciences Research, Ehrenpreis S, Solnitzky OC, eds., New York, Academic Press, 1971; 4: 65–99.
22. Narahashi T, Yamada M, Frazier DT. Cationic forms of local anesthetics block action potentials from inside the nerve membrane. Nature 1969; 223:748.
23. Narahashi T, Frazier DT, Yamada M. The site of activon and active form of local anesthetics. I. Theory and pH experiments with tertiary compounds. J Pharmacol Exp Ther 1970; 171: 32–44.
24. Narahashi T, Frazier DT. Site of action and active form of procaine in squid giant axons. J Pharmacol Exp Ther 1975; 194: 506–513.
25. Hille B. Ionic Channels of Excitable Membranes. Sunderland MA, ed. Sinauer Associates, Inc. 1984; pp. 272–302.
26. Ragsdale DR, McPhee JC, Scheuer T, et al. Molecular determinants of state-dependent block of Na^{+} channels by local anesthetics. Science 1994; 265: 1724–1728.
27. Wang GK, Quan C, Wang SY. Local anesthetic block of batrachotoxin-resistant muscle Na^{+} channels. Mol Pharmacol 1998; 54(2): 389–396.
28. Arthur GR. Pharmacokinetics. In: Local anesthetics. Strichartz GR. Ed. Handbook of Experimental Pharmacology 1987; 81: 165–186.
29. Eggleston ST, Lush LW. Understanding allergic reactions to local anesthetics. Ann Pharmacother 1996; 30 (7–8): 851–857.
30. Bean BP, Cohen CJ, Tsien RW. Lidocaine block of cardiac sodium channels. J Gen Physiol 1983; 81: 613–642.
31. Makielski JC, Alpert LA, Hanck DA, et al. An externally accessible receptor for lidocaine block of sodium current in canine cardiac Purkinje cells. Biophys J 1988; 53: 540.
32. Löfgren L. Studies on Local Anesthetics: Xylocaine, a New Synthetic Drug. Stockholm, Haegstroms, 1948.
33. Aåkerman SBA, Camougis G, Sandburg RV. Stereoisomerism and differential activitiy in excitation block by local anesthetics. Eur J Pharmacol 1969; 8: 337–347.
34. McClure JH. Ropivacaine. Br J Anesth 1996; 76:300–307.
35. Markham A, Faulds D. Ropivacaine. A review of its pharmacology and theraputic use in regional anesthesia. Drugs 1996; 52(3):429–449.
36. Rutten AJ, Mather LE, McLean CF. Cardiovascular effects and regional clearances of IV bupivacaie in sheep: enantiomeric analysis. Br J Anaesth 1991; 67:247–256.
37. Denson DD, Behbehani MM, Gregg RV. Enantiomer-specific effects of an intravenously administered arrhythmogenic dose of bupivacaine on neurons of the nucleus tractus solitarius and the cardiovascular system in the anesthetized rat. Reg Anesth 1992; 17:311–316.
38. Rutten AJ, Mather LE, McLean CF, et al. Tissue distribution of bupivacaine enantiomers in sheep. Chirality 1993; 5:485–491.
39. Longobardo M, Delpon E, Caballero R, et al. Structural determinants of potency and stereoselective block of hKv1.5 channels induced by local anesthetics. Mol Pharmacol 1998; 54(1):162–169.
40. Franqueza L, Longobardo M, Vicente J, et al. Molecular determinants of stereoselective bupivacaine block of hKv1.5 channels. Circulation Research, 1997; 81:1053–1064.

SUGGESTED READINGS

Akeson M, Deamer DW. Anesthetics and membranes: A critical review. In: Drug and Anesthetic Effects on Membrane Structure and Function, Aloia RC, Curtain CC, Gordon LM.eds., Wiley-Liss, New York, 1991, pp. 71–89.

Arthur GR. Pharmacokinetics of local anesthetics. In: Local Anesthetics. Handbook of Experimental Pharmacology, Strichartz GR. ed., Berlin, Springer, 1987; 81:165–186.

Courtney KR, Strichartz GR. Structural elements which determine local anesthetic activity. In: Local Anesthetics. Handbook of Experimental Pharmacology, Strichartz GR., ed., Berlin, Springer, 1987; 81:53–94.

Covino BG. Local anesthetics. In: Drugs in Anaesthesia: Mechanisms of Action. Feldman SA, Scurr CF, Paton W. eds., London, Edward Arnold, 1987, pp. 261–291.

Covino BG. Toxicity and systemic effects of local anesthetic agents. In: Local Anesthetics. Handbook of Experimental Pharmacology, Strichartz GR. ed., Berlin, Springer, 1987; 81:187–212.

Hille B. Ionic Channels of Excitable Membranes. Sunderland, MA, Sinauer Associates, 1984.

Strichartz R, Ritchie JM. The action of local anesthetics on ion channels of excitable tissues. In: Local Anesthetics. Handbook of Experimental Pharmacology, Strichartz GR. ed., Berlin, Springer, 1987; 81: 21–52.

Vandam LD. Some aspects of the history of local anesthesia. In: Local Anesthetics. Handbook of Experimental Pharmacology. Strichartz GR. ed., Berlin, Springer, 1987; 81:1–19.

14. Volatile Anesthetics

TIMOTHY J. MAHER

INTRODUCTION

Prior to the mid 1800s pain-producing surgical and dental procedures were typically undertaken without the aid of acceptable anesthetic agents. Chemical methods available at the time included intoxication with ethanol, hashish or opium, while physical methods included packing a limb in ice, creating ischemic conditions with tourniquets, inducing unconsciousness by a blow to the head, or the most common technique, employing strong-armed assistants to hold down the helpless patient during the entire surgical procedure. Additionally, at this time there were many physicians practicing who had been taught that pain was a requirement for effective healing, and therefore the observation of a patient in terrible pain was viewed as a part of the normal healing process. These factors, along with the lack of knowledge of sterile techniques or the availability of suitable infection fighting agents, made surgical procedures a method of last resort.

There have been many accounts of the first demonstration by the Hartford dentist Horace Wells of the use of nitrous oxide as a surgical anesthetic in 1844. Wells first observed the anesthetic actions of nitrous oxide at a public demonstration of "laughing gas." One of the volunteers, a pharmacy clerk named Samuel Cooley, injured his leg while under the influence of this gas and appeared to experience no pain. The next day Wells inhaled the gas himself and with the aid of a colleague had one of his own teeth extracted without any sensation of pain. Wells then began to routinely use nitrous oxide for dental procedures in his own practice. In 1845 he attempted to demonstrate the anesthetic effects of nitrous oxide at the Massachusetts General Hospital in Boston, however, the demonstration was considered a failure as the patient cried out during the procedure. Following this unfortunate incident, nitrous oxide use was minimal until it resurfaced in dental practice in the mid 1860s when it was combined with oxygen and made available in steel cylinders. This gas is still used today, especially in combination with other anesthetic and analgesic agents.

The anesthetic that gained greatest popularity shortly after the failed demonstration of Wells was diethyl ether. William Morton, a Boston dentist, was familiar at the time with the use of nitrous oxide by Wells. He also had heard of the interesting effects of diethyl ether and began to experiment on animals and himself with this volatile liquid. In 1846 he was allowed an opportunity to demonstrate the anesthetic actions of diethyl ether at the same Massachusetts General Hospital. In the famed "Ether Dome" (which still

stands today) Morton administered the ether with a specially designed delivery device to the nervous patient and the surgical procedure was performed without apparent pain. Following this demonstration the word of its success spread quickly and soon dental and medical practices throughout the United States and Europe were employing diethyl ether as an anesthetic agent. Today diethyl ether is no longer used in human procedures due to its toxicity and dangerous physical properties, e.g., flammable and explosive.

Another anesthetic agent that enjoyed some popularity early on was cyclopropane. However, like diethyl ether it is also explosive and is no longer used. As described below, the anesthetic agents used today are generally hydrocarbons and ethers with halogen (Cl, Br, F) substitutions. Nitrous oxide is the exception. Table 14.1 lists the characteristics of the "ideal" general anesthetic agent. Currently, the agent that fulfills all these characteristics is not known.

STAGES OF ANESTHESIA

The ideal anesthetic state is characterized by a loss of all sensations, and includes analgesia and muscle relaxation. Neuronal depression in specific central nervous system areas is believed to be largely responsible for such an anesthetic state. The areas involved include many cortical regions that are represented by excitatory pyramidal cells and inhibitory/excitatory stellate cells. Excitation of the pyramidal cells helps maintain consciousness, while the degree of inhibition or excitation of stellate cells determines the overall level of activity of the pyramidal cells they synapse with. As the concentration of anesthetic increases in the central nervous system, the degree of neuronal depression increases resulting in progressive stages of anesthesia. Based on observations using diethyether, Guedel in 1920 originally described this progression into four distinct stages, and subsequently Gillespie further subdivided these stages as described below:

Stage 1. Analgesia

Characterized by a mild depression of higher cortical neurons, this stage is suitable for surgical procedures that do not require significant neuromuscular relaxation. Depression of thalamic centers probably accounts for the observed analgesia as many of the neuronal systems that mediate pain sensation traverse through this anatomic area. While some general anesthetic agents do not possess significant analgesic activity, they all produce a loss of consciousness that may produce some insensitivity to painful stimuli.

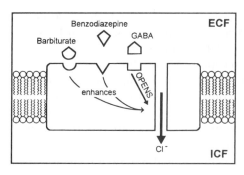

Fig. 14.4. GABA$_A$ receptor controls the chloride ion channel. GABA binds to its receptor, opening the chloride ion channel, resulting in hyperpolarization of the neuron. Benzodiazepines and barbiturates may produce anesthesia by allosterically enhancing GABA opening of chloride channels, which are located at inhibitory synapses on pyramidal cells. ECF = extracellular fluid; ICF = intracellular fluid. (Adapted from Wingard LB, Brody TM, Larner J, et al. *Human Pharmacology*: Molecular-To-Clinical. St Louis: Mosby-Year Book, 1991, 20–22.)

Chloride Channel

The ion channel that has received the most investigative attention is that for chloride (Fig. 14.4). Both the γ-amino butyric acid$_A$ (GABA$_A$) and the glycine$_A$ (strychnine-sensitive) receptors are linked to chloride channels and normally mediate inhibitory responses within the central nervous system. Halothane, isoflurane and other general anesthetics are capable of inhibiting the synaptic destruction of GABA, thereby increasing the GABA-ergic neurotransmission which is typically inhibitory in nature (16). Additionally, studies have demonstrated the ability of these anesthetics to enhance the binding of GABA or other allosteric modulators within the GABA receptor complex (17). In one such study (+)-isoflurane was significantly more potent than the (−)-enantiomer at enhancing GABA-ergic function (18). At therapeutic concentrations just about all of the general anesthetics are capable of enhancing GABA-ergic function, while at considerably higher concentrations many act directly as GABA-mimetics (19). Most of these agents also potentiate the actions of glycine, the other important inhibitory amino acid neurotransmitter (19). The combination of GABA-ergic and glycinergic potentiation by the general anesthetics probably accounts for much of their observed activity.

Halogenated Hydrocarbons and Ethers—Historical Aspects

Ether

The useful volatile anesthetics, with the exception of nitrous oxide, are halogenated hydrocarbons and ethers. Diethyl ether (Fig. 14.5), one of the first agents to be introduced as an anesthetic, has high potency with significant analgesic and neuromuscular relaxing effects. This agent is flammable, and when mixed with air, oxygen or nitrous oxide, it is explosive. Induction with diethyl ether is very slow such that significant time can be spent pro-

gressing through the delirium stage. Irritation of the respiratory tract by diethyl ether may lead to excessive bronchial secretions complicating adequate ventilation. In addition to the unpleasant induction and adverse effects, recovery is similarly prolonged and may be accompanied by vomiting. These pharmacologic and physical characteristics of diethyl ether limit the utility of this anesthetic in humans.

Short Chain Hydrocarbons

Many of the short-chain alkanes, alkenes and alkynes are capable of producing an anesthetic state when administered to patients. Potency generally increases as chain length increases. However, as a result of their flammability and increased propensity to cause cardiovascular toxicity, these non-substituted hydrocarbons are not useful as anesthetic agents.

Chloroform

Another of the earlier anesthetic agents to be employed was chloroform. This halogenated hydrocarbon was first officially used in the United States in 1847, however its toxicity seriously limited its utility. The addition of halogens to the hydrocarbon backbone increases potency and decreases flammability. Similar effects are observed with such substitutions on ethers also. As an anesthetic agent, chloroform is very potent and possesses significant analgesic and neuromuscular relaxing activity. Chloroform, a known carcinogen, has the disadvantage of being both hepatotoxic and nephrotoxic, in addition to producing adverse circulatory effects such as arrhythmias and severe hypotension. As a result of these toxicities chloroform has an unacceptable therapeutic index which prohibits its use in anesthesia. However, the knowledge of the influence of the halogen substitutions on the potency and flammability of hydrocarbons, and ethers, has significantly contributed to our understanding of the structure-activity relationship

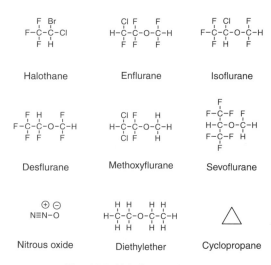

Fig. 14.5. Volatile anesthetics.

Table 14.4. Relative Flammability of "Nonflammable" Anesthetics (20,21)

	Halothane (%)	Enflurane (%)	Isoflurane (%)
Minimum flammable conc. (MFC) of agent in 30% O_2 with remaining atmosphere N_2O.	4.75	5.75	7.0
Minimum effective alveolar conc. (MAC) of agent given in above atmosphere.	0.28	0.65	0.46
MAC in man in absence of N_2O	0.75	1.68	1.15
MFC/MAC in N_2O	17	8.9	15.2

Table 14.5. Physical-Chemical Properties of Clinically Useful Volatile Anesthetics

Generic name (Trade name)	Structure	Boiling Point (°C)	Chemically Stable*
Desflurane (Suprane)	$F_2HC-O-CHF-CF_3$	23.5	Yes
Enflurane (Ethrane)	$F_2HC-O-CF_2-CHFCl$	56.5	Yes
Halothane (Fluothane)	$F_3C-CHBrCl$	50.2	No
Isoflurane (Forane)	$F_2HC-O-CHCl-CF_3$	48.5	Yes
Methoxyflurane (Penthrane)	$H_3C-O-CF_2-CHCl_2$	104.7	No
Nitrous oxide	N_2O	−88.0	Yes
Sevoflurane	$(CF_3)_2CH-O-CH_2F$	58.5	No

*Indicates stability to soda lime, UV light, and common metals.

of general anesthetics and the eventual design of substantially improved agents.

Flammability

The occurrence of fires in operating rooms is of great concern to all participants in the surgical procedure. Although the introduction of "nonflammable" agents such as halothane, enflurane, and isoflurane has substantially decreased the hazard, such fires still occur. Three essential ingredients are required for any combustion: 1) an ignition source such as a laser, 2) a combustible material (gauze, drapes, rubber tubes, etc.), and 3) an oxidizing agent (O_2, N_2O). Many substances are flammable in pure oxygen, N_2O, or mixtures, but not air. Certain substances are flammable in N_2O at concentrations that are too low to permit ignition in pure oxygen (20). The concentrations required for combustion as indicated in Table 14.4 are higher than those generally encountered, except possibly during induction.

CLINICALLY USEFUL AGENTS
Fluorinated Hydrocarbons

The structure and physical properties of the volatile anesthetics are given in Table 14.5.

Halothane

Halothane (Fig. 14.5) was introduced into medical practice in the United States in 1956 as a nonflammable, nonexplosive halogenated volatile anesthetic that is usually mixed with air or oxygen. The presence of the carbon-halogen bonds contributes to its nonflammability. This clear liquid with a sweet odor was developed based on predictions that its halogenated structure would provide

chemical stability, an intermediate blood solubility, and significant anesthetic potency. Halothane is the only useful volatile anesthetic possessing a bromine atom, which has been suggested to contribute to its potency. Similarly, the addition of fluorine atoms, of which halothane has three, is thought to contribute to the increased potency, volatility and increased chemical stability of the hydrocarbon skeleton (Table 14.5).

Halothane produces a rapid onset and recovery from anesthesia with high potency when used alone, or in combination with nitrous oxide. Most metals, with the exception of chromium, nickel and titanium, are easily tarnished by halothane. Although halothane is relatively stable, it is subject to spontaneous oxidative decomposition to hydrochloric acid, hydrobromic acid and phosgene. Because of this reason it is available in dark amber glass containers with thymol added as a preservative to minimize decomposition. Halothane may permeate into the rubber components of the anesthetic delivery devices, which might account for some slowing of the induction onset and recovery. Approximately 20% of an administered dose is metabolized which accounts partly for the increased hepatotoxicity observed with this agent (Fig. 14.6).

Enflurane

Enflurane (Fig. 14.5) was introduced into medical practice in the United States in 1973 and is a clear, colorless, nonflammable volatile liquid with a mild sweet odor. While enflurane is relatively stable chemically, it does not attack aluminum, copper, iron or brass, and is soluble in rubber (partition coefficient = 74), which can prolong induction/recovery times as seen with halothane (Table 14.5). Enflurane has an intermediate solubility in blood and has cle relaxant dantrolene, which blocks release of Ca^{2+} from the sarcoplasmic reticulum, reduces muscle rigidity and heat production, which significantly improves the prognosis of the patient. Besides the fluorinated general anesthetics, some depolarizing neuromuscular blocking agents (e.g., succinylcholine) and some neuroleptics (e.g., haloperidol) have also been reportedly associated with similar malignant hyperthermic syndromes, although the underlying mechanism mediating these may differ somewhat from those associated with the general anesthetics.

Nephrotoxicity

Fluorinated anesthetics that undergo metabolism to inorganic fluoride have the potential to produce damage to the renal tubular cells. Of the fluorinated anesthetics, methoxyflurane is the only agent commonly associated with nephrotoxicity. Methoxyflurane is subject to metabolism (Fig. 14.6) yielding plasma fluoride ion levels in excess of the threshold value for renal damage of 40 μM. Others, such as sevoflurane, have only very rarely been associated with nephrotoxicity and then usually in severely renally-compromised patients. Plasma levels of fluoride only reach 15–20 μM following 2.5 MAC hour exposure to enflurane (25). The rates of metabolic defluorination of the useful anesthetic agents are: methoxyflurane > enflurane = sevoflurane > isoflurane > desflurane = halothane.

Low Level Chronic Exposure

Typically patients are exposed to greater than MAC concentrations of the general anesthetics for limited periods of time, e.g., a number of hours during a surgical procedure and not for extended periods of time (days or weeks). However, as surgical and dental personnel may be exposed to low levels of the volatile anesthetics for prolonged periods over many years, or even decades, the ability of such agents to produce chronic toxicity is of paramount concern. Although the occupational exposure to these agents has been minimized with improved waste gas scavenging devices, some epidemiological studies have demonstrated increased levels of spontaneous abortions, congenital birth defects in offspring, and increased rates of certain cancers in chronically-exposed medical personnel (26).

Nitrous Oxide

Commonly called "laughing gas," nitrous oxide (dinitrogen monoxide, N_2O) is a gas at room temperature and is the least potent of the inhalation anesthetics utilized today (Table 14.5). With an MAC value in excess of 105%, this colorless, tasteless and odorless to slightly sweet-smelling gas is not normally capable of producing surgical anesthesia when administered alone. The MAC for nitrous oxide has been demonstrated to be between 105% and 140%, and thus cannot achieve surgical anesthesia under conditions at standard barometric pressure. To demonstrate that the MAC was greater than 100%, Bert in 1879 utilized a mixture of 85% nitrous oxide with oxygen at 1.2 atmospheres in a pressurized chamber. Only at this elevated pressure could an MAC adequate for surgical anesthesia be achieved. Decreasing the oxygen content of a nitrous oxide mixture to values less than 20% to allow for an increase in the concentration of nitrous oxide to greater than 80% can be dangerous as hypoxia would be expected to result. Thus, administered alone nitrous oxide finds utility as an anesthetic agent during certain procedures (e.g., dental) where full surgical anesthesia is not required. However, nitrous oxide is most commonly used in combination with other volatile anesthetics since it is capable of decreasing the concentration of the added anesthetic required to produce an adequate depth of anesthesia for surgical procedures.

While no firm underlying mechanisms have been demonstrated, some authors have suggested that irreversible oxidation of the cobalt atom in vitamin B_{12} by nitrous oxide can lead to inactivation of enzymes dependent upon this vitamin with resultant metabolic aberrations. Such examples have included methionine synthetase and thymidylate synthetase, which are essential in the synthetic pathways leading to the production of myelin and thymidine, respectively. Should these enzymes be impaired during the sensitive periods of *in utero* development, the potential for malformations may unfortunately be realized. While to date no studies have been able to demonstrate conclusively that low-level exposure to nitrous oxide is associated with a meaningful disruption of crucial metabolic functions to produce the above described toxicity, measures including improved waste gas scavenging systems should be taken to minimize personnel exposure.

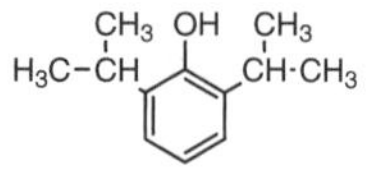

Propofol

Propofol

Used intravenously, propofol is not chemically related to the barbiturates or other intravenous anesthetics. Propofol appears to act via enhancing GABA-ergic neurotransmission within the central nervous system. This occurs most likely at the GABA-receptor complex, but at a site distinct from where the benzodiazepines bind. Because of its poor water solubility, propofol is formulated as a 1 or 2% emulsion with soybean oil, egg lecithin, and glycerol. Following intravenous administration of a dose of 2.0–2.5 mg/kg, a state of hypnosis is achieved within 1 minute, which lasts for approximately 5 minutes. A longer anesthetic state can be achieved by additional propofol dosing, or as typically is the case, maintenance with a volatile anesthetic agent. Blood pressure and heart rate are usually decreased following propofol administration. Metabolism of propofol proceeds rapidly via hepatic conversion to the glucuronide and sulfate conjugates with less than 0.3% excreted unchanged. As this agent produces a rapid induction and recovery, and is infrequently associated with episodes of vomiting, propofol has found utility as an anesthetic agent in outpatient surgical environments.

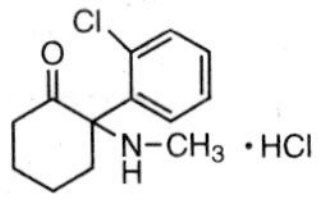

Ketamine

Ketamine

Ketamine hydrochloride is an injectable, very potent, rapidly-acting anesthetic agent. As with propofol above, its duration of anesthetic activity is also relatively short (10–25 minutes). Ketamine does not relax skeletal muscles and therefore can only be used alone in procedures of short duration that don't require muscle relaxation. Recovery from anesthesia may be accompanied by "emergence delirium" characterized by visual, auditory and confusional illusions. Disturbing dreams and hallucinations can occur for up to 24 hours after the administration of ketamine. Termination of the acute action of ketamine is largely due to its redistribution from the brain into other tissues, however the formation of the glucuronide conjugate and metabolism in the liver to a number of metabolites does occur. One of these metabolites of interest, norketamine, is formed via the action of cytochrome P450. This demethylated derivative retains significant activity at the NMDA receptor and may account for some of the longer lasting effects of this anesthetic agent. Eventual conversion of norketamine to hydroxylated metabolites and subsequent conjugation leads to metabolites that can be renally eliminated. Less than 4% of a dose is excreted unchanged in the urine.

Ketamine is capable of producing a "dissociative" anesthesia, which is characterized by EEG changes indicating a dissociation between the thalamocortical and limbic systems (27). These neuronal systems, which are normally associated with one another, help to maintain the neuronal connections required for consciousness. When disassociated the subject will appear cataleptic with the eyes open in a slow nystagmic gaze (1). A potent analgesic and amnesic effect is produced as is an increase in muscle tone in some areas. While the patient may appear to be awake, they are incapable of communicating and do not remember the event or the people around them. Blood pressure and heart rate are usually increased following ketamine administration.

Ketamine appears to act similarly to phencyclidine (PCP, Angel Dust) which acts as an antagonist within the cationic channel of the NMDA receptor complex (28). By preventing the flow of cations through this channel, ketamine prevents neuronal activation which is normally required for the conscious state. However, the analgesic activity of ketamine is more likely due to an interaction with an opioid receptor or the less-well understood sigma receptor. Other studies have suggested a possible involvement of serotonin receptors and muscarinic receptors (29). Ketamine, like PCP, has a significant potential for abuse.

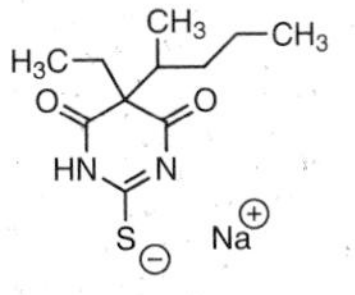

Thiopental

Ultrashort-acting Barbiturates

The ultrashort-acting barbiturates (e.g., thiopental) are used intravenously to produce a rapid unconsciousness for surgical and basal anesthesia. These agents may be used initially to induce anesthesia, which then can be maintained during the surgical procedure with a volatile anesthetic agent. The induction is typically very rapid and pleasant. (These ultrashort-acting barbiturates are discussed in Chapter 15.)

CASE STUDY

Victoria F. Roche and S. William Zito

MD is a 45-year-old, white female, who will be undergoing a lumpectomy to remove a malignancy in her right breast. MD has a history of reconstructive knee surgeries which have left her with one kidney as a result of the large doses of cephalosporins she was administered to control post-operative infections. The surgeon and the anesthesiologist want to use a rapid onset/recovery general anesthetic with a minimum risk for nephrotoxicity. Recommend one of the drawn structures 1–4.

1. Identify the therapeutic problem(s) where the pharmacist's intervention may benefit the patient.

2. Identify and prioritize the patient specific factors that must be considered to achieve the desired therapeutic outcomes.

3. Conduct a thorough and mechanistically oriented structure-activity analysis of all therapeutic alternatives provided in the case.

4. Evaluate the SAR findings against the patient specific factors and desired therapeutic outcomes and make a therapeutic decision.

5. Counsel your patient.

REFERENCES

1. Stoelting RK. Pharmacology and Physiology of Anesthetic Practice. 3rd Edition. Lippincott Williams and Wilkins, Philadelphia, 1999.
2. Stevens WC, Kingston HGG. Inhalation anesthesia, in Clinical Anesthesia, 2nd ed., PG Barash, BF Cullen, RK Stoelting, Eds. Lippincott, Philadelphia, 1992.
3. Harrison NL, Flood P. Molecular Mechanisms of General Anesthetic Action. Sci & Med 1998; (May:June): 18–27.
4. Meyer HH. The theory of narcosis. J Am Med Assoc 1906; 26: 1499–1502.
5. Overton E. Studien ueber die narkose, zugleich ein beitrag zur allgemeinem pharmakologie. Jena: Gustav Fischer, 1901.
6. Lysco GS, Robinson JL, Casto R, et al. The stereospecific effects of isoflurane isomers in vivo. Eur J Pharmacol 1994; 263: 25–29.
7. Graf BM, Boban M, Stowe DF, et al. Lack of stereospecific effects of isoflurane and desflurane isomers in isolated guinea pig hearts. Anesthesiology 1994; 81: 129–136.
8. Sidebotham DA, Schug SA. Stereochemistry in anaesthesia. Clin Exp Pharmacol Physiol 1997; 24: 126–130.
9. Flohr H, Glade U, Motzko D. The role of the NMDA synapse in general anesthesia. Toxicol Lett 1998; 100–101: 23–29.
10. Perouansky M, Kirson ED, Yaari Y. Mechanism of action of volatile anesthetics: effects of halothane on glutamate receptors in vitro. Toxicol Lett 1998; 100–101: 65–69.
11. Larsen M, Langmoen IA. The effect of volatile anaesthetics on synaptic release and uptake of glutamate. Toxicol Lett 1998; 100–101: 59–64.
12. Hudspith MJ. Glutamate: a role in normal brain function, anaesthesia, analgesia and CNS injury. Br J Anaesth 1997; 78: 731–747.
13. Narahashi T, Aistrup GL, Lindstrom JM, et al. Ion modulation as the basis for general anesthetics. Toxicol Lett 1998; 100–101: 185–191.
14. Franks NP, Lieb WR. Stereospecific effects of inhalational general anaesthetic optical isomers on nerve ion channels. Science 1991; 25: 427–430.
15. Doze VA, Chen BX, Ticklenberg JA, et al. Pertussis toxin and 4-aminopyridine differentially affect the hypnotic-anesthetic action of dexmedetomidine and pentobarbital. Anesthesiology 1990; 73: 304–307.
16. Cheng S-C, Brunner EA. Effects of anesthetic agents on synaptosomal GABA disposal. Anesthesiology 1981; 55: 34–40.
17. Olsen RW. The molecular mechanism of action of general anesthetics: structural aspects of interactions with GABAA receptors. Toxicol Lett 1998; 100–101: 193–201.
18. Moody EJ, Harris BD, Skolnick P. Stereospecific actions of the inhalation anaesthetic isoflurane at the GABAA receptor complex. Brain Res 1993; 615: 101–106.
19. Belelli D, Pistis M, Peters JA, et al. General anesthetic action at transmitter-gated inhibitory amino acid receptors. Trends Pharmacol Sci 1999; 20: 496–502.
20. Perry LB, et al. Case history number 82: "nonflammable" fires in the operating room. Anesth Analg 1975; 54: 152–154.
21. Eger EI II. Anesthetic Uptake and Action. Baltimore: Williams & Wilkins, 1974.
22. Christ DD, Kenna JG, Kammerer W, et al. Enflurane metabolism produces covalently bound liver adducts recognized by antibodies from patients with halothane hepatitis. Anesthesiology. 1988; 69:833–8.
23. Koblin DD. Characteristics and implications of desflurane metabolism and toxicity. Anesth Analg. 1992; 75:S10–S16.
24. Dodds C. General anesthesia: practical recommendations and recent advances. Drugs 1999; 58: 453–467.
25. Mazze RI, Calverely RK, Smith NT. Inorganic fluoride nephrotoxicity: prolonged enflurane and halothane anesthesia in volunteers. Anesthesiology 1977; 46: 265–271.
26. Lane GA Nahrwold ML, Tait AR. Anesthetics as teratogens: nitrous oxide is fetotoxic, xenon is not. Science 1980; 210: 899–901.
27. Reich DL, Silvay G. Ketamine: an update on the first twenty-five years of clinical experience. Can J Anaesth 1989; 36: 186–197.
28. Yamamura T, Harada K, Okamura A, et al. Is the site of action of ketamine anesthesia the N-methyl-D-aspartate receptor? Anesthesiology 1990; 72: 704–710.
29. Toro-Matos A, Redon-Platas AM, Avila-Valdez E, et al. Physostigmine antagonizes ketamine. Anesth Analg 1980; 59: 764–767.

SUGGESTED ADDITIONAL READINGS

Cooper JR, Bloom FE, Roth RH. The Biochemical Basis of Neuropharmacology, 7th ed., Oxford University Press, New York, 1996.
Hardman JG, Limbird LE, Molinoff PB, et al. The Pharmacological Basis of Therapeutics, 9th ed., McGraw Hill, New York, 1996.
Stoelting RK. Pharmacology and Physiology of Anesthetic Practice. 3rd Edition. Lippincott Williams and Wilkins, Philadelphia, 1999.

15. Hypnotics

WILLIAM SOINE

INTRODUCTION

Hypnotics are often referred to as sleeping pills, sedative medications and sedative-hypnotics. This class of drugs causes drowsiness and facilitates the initiation and maintenance of sleep. Classically, this chapter would be titled Sedative-Hypnotics, however, due to the extensive use of benzodiazepines as sedative-antianxiety (anxiolytic) drugs which are covered in Chapter 17, this chapter will be limited to drugs primarily used as hypnotics. The observed pharmacologic effects of the drugs in this class are dose related. Small doses cause sedation, larger doses cause hypnosis (sleep), and still larger doses may bring about surgical anesthesia. Drugs used as hypnotics are often sedative and anxiolytic (depending on dose), but not all anxiolytic drugs cause sedation. Refer to Chapter 17 for more information concerning sedative/anxiolytic use of the benzodiazepines. This chapter will emphasize the concepts important in sleep and wakefulness followed by presentation of current drugs used to initiate sleep.

Clinical situations are commonly encountered that require the use of hypnotics. The short-term "situational stress" variety of insomnia is appropriate for drug treatment to facilitate sleep. The drugs currently used as hypnotics are all very effective, however, there is ample need for newer and safer hypnotics. The introduction of supposedly a newer yet safer and more effective hypnotic drug has always been greeted with optimism, for example the piperidinedione, thalidomide (1). Thalidomide was proposed to be a substitute for the barbiturates in the 1950s. However, similar to most other drugs used as hypnotics or sedatives, it is only after its introduction and extensive clinical use that its limitations became better understood. The ideal hypnotic should cause a 1) transient decrease in the level of consciousness for the purpose of sleep without lingering effects, 2) have no potential for decreasing or arresting respirations (even at relatively high doses), and 3) produce no abuse, addiction, tolerance or dependence (2). A search for newer and better hypnotics is still needed.

PHYSIOLOGY OF SLEEP
Electrophysiology

At the start of the 20th century, sleep was considered a passive process. In the late 1920s and 1930s it was possible to monitor human electrical brain activity using the electroencephalogram (EEG). Using the EEG it was established that there occurred a passive nature of sleep that alternated with wakeful activity. This was followed by the discovery by Moruzzi and Magoun of the ascending reticular activating system and its relationship to the EEG (3). This discovery provided the basis for the modern theories of sleep and was validated by finding that sleeping animals could be awakened through stimulation of electrodes implanted in the midbrain reticular formation. Sleep is studied using related techniques that permit electronic monitoring of the head and neck muscles (electromyogram, EMG) and eye movements (electro-oculogram, EOG). From these and related studies three states have been defined: 1) wakefulness, 2) slow-wave sleep (SWS, nonrapid eye movement—NREM sleep), and 3) paradoxic sleep (PS, rapid eye movement—REM sleep). Wakefulness is characterized by low-voltage fast activity of the EEG, high muscle activity, and numerous rapid eye movements indicating intensive interaction with the environment.

The two states of sleep, NREM and REM, have been characterized, primarily using EEG. NREM sleep has been subdivided by Dement and Kleitman into four stages which are precisely defined (although somewhat arbitrarily) using the EEG (4). The EEG pattern is usually described as synchronous with characteristic waveforms as sleep spindles, K complexes, and high voltage slow waves. Stages 1 through 4 follow a sleep continuum with the ability to arouse an individual lowest in Stage 1 and highest in stage 4 sleep. When sleep overtakes wakefulness, the transition is gradual, indeed, there is not one single measure that is reliable all of the time. Stage 1 sleep is characterized by 8- to 12-cps α-rhythm in the EEG and by muscular tone relaxation and slow eyeball oscillation in the EOG. After a few minutes, stage 2 is reached, which involves definite sleep characterized by a 12- to 15-cps EEG pattern. From 45–50% of the total sleep period is spent in stage 2 sleep. As stage 3 sleep approaches, the EEG voltage continues to increase and the frequency continues to decrease. A gradual change into stage 4 sleep can then occur and is characterized by delta waves (high amplitude, slow waves). After the NREM sleep has been completed, a series of body movements signals an ascent through the sleep stages 4 through 1 into REM sleep. In humans REM sleep is associated with bursts of rapid eye movements that is associated with the mental activity of dreaming.

Sleep Cycle (4,5)

The simplest pattern of sleep is that associated with a normal young adult. The normal adult enters sleep through NREM sleep. After approximately 90 minutes of NREM sleep the first REM sleep occurs, with a mean duration of about 20 minutes. NREM and REM sleep alternate cyclically through the night with the average length of the NREM-REM sleep cycle being approximately 90–120 minutes. REM sleep tends to be greatest in the last third of the night. Therefore, a normal young adult displays a sleep pattern of 75–80% NREM and 20–25% REM sleep. The length of nocturnal sleep is dependant on a number of factors, of which voluntary control is the most significant. Other important factors are genetic determinants and processes associated with circadian rhythms. As sleep is extended the amount of REM sleep is increased.

There are a number of factors that modify sleep stage distribution: age, prior sleep history, drug ingestion, circadian rhythms, temperature, and pathology. Only the first four factors will be discussed in this chapter.

Age

Age related differences are seen in infants. The cyclic alteration of NREM-REM sleep at birth has a period of 50–60 minutes versus 90 minutes in adults. Infants gradually develop normal nocturnal slow wave sleep (stages 3 + 4 NREM) after 2–6 months of life. Slow wave sleep becomes maximal in young children and decreases markedly with age. Slow wave sleep may no longer be present by 60 years of age, more so in men than in women. The interindividual variability in the elderly is greatly increased and the generalizations made for young adults concerning "normal" sleep is no longer applicable.

Prior Sleep History and Drug Ingestion

Prior sleep history and the effects of drug ingestion on sleep history are important when comparing hypnotics. An individual experiencing sleep loss on one or more nights will show a sleep pattern of increased slow wave sleep during the first recovery night with REM sleep showing a rebound on the second or subsequent nights. When an individual becomes deprived of REM sleep by being awakened every time the EOG and EEG indicated that dreaming has begun, the individual becomes selectively deprived of REM sleep and a pressure for REM sleep builds up. A preferential rebound of REM sleep will occur. The cyclic patterns of sleep states and sleep stages can be affected by many common drugs, including the hypnotics. The ability of drugs to differentially affect one sleep stage over another can upon withdrawal produce rebound effects leading to exacerbation of the sleep disorder, comparable to deprivation of REM sleep.

Circadian Rhythms

The importance of the circadian phase at which sleep occurs and its affect on the distribution of sleep stages has become of interest due to the current popularity of melatonin. It has been shown that with individuals sleeping in situations free of all time cues, circadian phase can influence the timing of sleep onset and length of sleep. If sleep onset is delayed until the peak REM phase of circadian rhythm (early morning), REM sleep can predominate and may even occur at the onset of sleep. This abnormal sleep onset pattern or phase shift can occur due to a work shift change or a change resulting from jet travel across a number of time zones.

As a brief summary, the normal adult human enters sleep through NREM sleep. After approximately 80 minutes or longer the individual starts REM sleep after which NREM-REM sleep alternates through the remainder of the sleep period. Any situation that causes an alteration of this normal sleep cycle leads to compensation of REM or NREM sleep in subsequent nights.

Sleep Factors

The involvement of many autonomic, physiologic, and biochemical changes are associated with wakefulness, NREM and REM sleep. The relationship of cause and effect in relation to these systems is still somewhat controversial and a rapidly changing area of research. Several brain regions that regulate sleep have now been identified, however, the specific contribution on any one region to sleep is still controversial (6). The roles of the major systems are important to be familiar with in relation to sleep. This not only helps one understand the mechanism by which hypnotics work, but also provides some understanding of why unrelated drugs, such as neuroleptics, antihistamines, antidepressants, and antimanic drugs are occasionally used as hypnotics to facilitate sleep.

Neurotransmitter/Neuromodulator

Every neurotransmitter has at one time or another been implicated in sleep or wakefulness. The assumption is that if a neurotransmitter is involved in wakefulness it may be involved in initiation or maintenance of REM sleep. In contrast, an antagonist of the neurotransmitter would be anticipated to initiate or maintain NREM sleep. Studies of this type are rarely unambiguous due to the integration of the neural pathways. Some of the evidence for the involvement of these neurotransmitters in sleep or wakefulness is presented, however, the reader should consult reference 6 for details.

Catecholamines (7). It would be anticipated that catecholamines (originating from the locus ceruleus) would be involved in wakefulness and REM sleep. Initial experiments with reserpine suggested that a decrease in catecholamines involved in neurotransmission caused a decrease in REM sleep. However, contradictory and inconsistent findings with other compounds that modulate catecholamine synthesis gave ambiguous results on the relationship between monoamine levels and stages of sleep. The only consistent finding is that an intact catecholamine transmission system is needed for the REM component of sleep.

The catecholaminergic effects on sleep and wakefulness can be broken down in the following manner: a) drugs interfering with catecholaminergic transmission via the depletion or inhibition of the synthesis of the cate-cholamines; b) α_1- and α_2-agonists and antagonists and β-andrenergic agonists and antagonists; and c) dopamine 1 and 2 agonists and antagonists. Studies support the hy-pothesis that norepinephrine neurons aid in regulating wakefulness and REM sleep. For example, an α_1-agonist (e.g., methoxamine) decreased REM sleep while an α_1-an-tagonist increased REM sleep. Clonidine, primarily an α_2-agonist is associated with a sleep induction, but inhibits deep NREM (stage 3 and 4) sleep. Involvement of the β-adrenergic receptors for regulation of sleep is ambiguous. Propranolol in humans is often associated with the side ef-fect of insomnia that can be reversed by β-agonists and has been interpreted as suggesting these receptors are in-volved in regulation of REM sleep. It has been proposed that dopamine has a facilitative and active role in the sleep-wakefulness cycle. Waking appears to be a state maintained by D2 activation while decreased D2 activity appears to promote sleep. The D1 receptor may be im-portant in the regulation of REM sleep, but is not impor-tant in initiation or timing of REM sleep.

Serotonin (8). Initially serotonin was thought to be a sleep-promoting neurotransmitter or an "antiwaking" agent. The recognition of the numerous 5-HT receptor subtypes, often with unique anatomical distribution, has required that a more complex role for serotonin be devel-oped. Current studies indicate that conditions for sleep are now met when the serotoninergic system becomes in-active. The serotonin agonists for the 5-HT$_1$ (via the 5-HT$_{1A}$ and 5-HT$_{1B}$ types at the hypothalamic level), 5-HT$_2$, and 5-HT$_3$ receptors cause wakefulness and inhibit sleep. Blockade of the 5-HT$_2$ receptors (e.g., the 5-HT$_2$ antago-nist ritanserin) results in increased NREM and inhibition of REM sleep. It has been proposed that the 5-HT$_{1A}$ and 5-HT$_2$ may be involved in sleep by regulation of sleep pro-moting substances in the hypothalamus. With the devel-opment of newer and more selective ligands for use in studying the numerous serotonin receptor subtypes (see Chapter 12) a better understanding of the role of sero-tonin in sleep will evolve.

Histamine (9). It is proposed that histamine may have an involvement in wakefulness and REM sleep. Histamine related functions in the CNS are regulated at postsynaptic sites by both the H$_1$ and H$_2$ receptors while the H$_3$ recep-tors appear to be a presynaptic autoreceptor regulating the synthesis and release of histamine. These 3 receptors differ in molecular structure, distribution in the CNS and physiologic responses. The H$_1$ receptor agonists and the H$_3$ receptor antagonists increase wakefulness while the H$_1$ receptor antagonists (e.g., diphenhydramine) and H$_3$-re-ceptor agonists have the opposite effect. The H$_2$ receptor agonists and antagonists have not been shown to have any effect on wakefulness or sleep parameters. The H$_1$-recep-tor agonists do not modify sleep induction or mainte-nance, although it does increase Stage 4 NREM sleep and sleep latency. In controlled sleep laboratory studies, the H$_1$ receptor antagonists (e.g., diphenhydramine), when given before bedtime to normal subjects, have little effect on wakefulness. However, in equal doses given during the day they increase drowsiness, with an increased tendency to sleep and impair performance.

Acetylcholine (10). The cholinergic system was the first neurotransmitter system shown to have a role in wakeful-ness and initiation of REM sleep. Because of the poor pen-etration of the cholinergic drugs into the CNS, the role of this system in sleep have relied on animal studies using mi-croinjection into the brain, primarily in the area of the dorsal pontine tegmentum. Acetylcholine, cholinergic ag-onists (arecoline, bethanechol) and cholinesterase in-hibitors are effective in the initiation of REM sleep from NREM sleep after microinjection. Conversely, administra-tion of anticholinergic drugs (e.g., atropine or scopo-lamine) hinders the transition to REM sleep. Increase in the rate of discharge of these cholinergic cells (that acti-vate the thalamus, cerebral cortex and the hippocampus) during REM sleep parallel the same pattern seen with arousal and alertness.

Adenosine (11). Considerable evidence suggests that adenosine acts as neurotransmitter in the mammalian nervous system. Due to the highly polar nature of adeno-sine it also has to be injected into the brain (intracere-broventricular and preoptic). The stimulation of the adenosine A$_1$ receptors with adenosine causes a hypnotic effect. It has been proposed that the hypnotic effect oc-curs via suppression of calcium efflux into presynaptic nerve terminals and decreasing the amount of neuro-transmitters released into the synapse in brain regions crit-ical for sleep. This apparent induction and maintenance of sleep is associated with increases in both NREM and REM sleep. Consistent with the above proposal is that blocking of the central adenosine receptors with methyl-xanthines (e.g., caffeine, theophylline) is associated with wakefulness and a reduction in total sleep time. Studies also suggest that some of the actions of the benzodi-azepines may be related to their ability to inhibit adeno-sine uptake leading to down regulation of central adeno-sine receptors.

GABA (12). GABA probably represents the most impor-tant inhibitory transmitter of the mammalian CNS. Both types of GABAergic inhibition (pre- and postsynaptic) uti-lize the same GABA$_A$ receptor subtype, which acts by regu-lation of the chloride channel of the neuronal membrane. GABA$_B$, a second GABA receptor type that is a G protein-coupled receptor is not considered to be important in un-derstanding the mechanism of hypnotics. Activation of a GABA$_A$ receptor by an agonist increases the inhibitory synaptic response of central neurons to GABA through hyperpolarization. Since many if not all central neurons receive some GABAergic input, this leads to a mechanism by which CNS activity can be depressed. For example if the GABAergic interneurons are activated by an agonist that inhibits the monoaminergic structures of the brain stem, hypnotic activity will be observed. The specific neuronal structures in different brain regions affected by $GABA_A$ agonist is not well defined at this time due to the broad activity and lack of specificity of the current drugs (e.g., benzodiazepines, barbiturates) used as hypnotics.

Neurohumoral Modulators

Sleep and circadian rhythmicity, both controlled by the CNS can exhibit significant effects on hormonal release. Many of the hypophyseal hormones follow a circadian rhythm, however, both growth hormone (GH) and prolactin (PRL) appear to be most closely linked with sleep. This suggests that these hormones may affect sleep and contribute to the maintenance and quality of sleep.

Growth Hormone and Prolactin (13). In normal adult subjects the plasma level of GH remains very stable at a low level, however, a secretory pulse of GH occurs in association with the first phase of NREM sleep. Most of the GH pulse secretions occur during NREM sleep and a good correlation has been observed between the amount of GH secreted and the duration of NREM sleep. Studies in healthy elderly men (67–84 years) have observed that a decreased secretion of GH in the elderly parallels the decrease in NREM sleep and may be related to the decrease in sleep observed in the elderly.

Regardless of the time of day, sleep onset has a stimulatory effect on prolactin release. However, maximal effect is observed when sleep and circadian effects are superimposed. Due to pulse like secretions of prolactin there seems to be a relationship between the low prolactin levels and initiation of REM sleep or nocturnal awakenings, especially in the elderly.

Melatonin (13,14)

Melatonin, at times referred to as the hormone of darkness, is normally secreted during the night. It is synthesized in the pineal gland and its secretion is controlled by the suprachiasmatic nucleus (SCN) following an endogenous circadian rhythm. Recent studies indicate that melatonin may have effects on circadian rhythm and sleep processes. The presence of a pharmacologically specific receptor for melatonin is based on molecular cloning studies in which high affinity G protein-coupled receptors (mel_{1a}, mel_{1b} and mel_{1c}) have been characterized. Oral administration of melatonin has been associated with faster sleep onset and increased total sleep time, but the mecha-

nism by which this occurs and its role in sleep is not well understood. The secretion of melatonin can be decreased by bright light and physical activity in man. Melatonin is sold as a food supplement in the U.S., but has become increasingly popular for alleviating jet lag (a flight across five or more time zones) and helping to resynchronize individuals that have difficulty adapting to night shift work.

CNS Peptides (15). Endogenous peptide sleep substances (that are considered to be messengers of the humoral system) appear to modulate neuronal activity associated with sleep. Several CNS peptides have been associated with sleep modulation with delta-sleep-inducing peptide (DSIP) being the best known. A dialysate obtained from the cerebral blood of rabbits that were kept asleep by electrical stimulation of the thalamus could induce sleep in normal rabbits. The factor responsible was DSIP, a nonapeptide. The amino acid sequence is:

$$\text{Trp} - \text{Ala} - \text{Gly} - \text{Gly} - \text{Asp} - \text{Ala} - \text{Ser} \cdot \text{Gly} - \text{Glu}$$
$$\quad 1 \qquad 2 \qquad 3 \qquad 4 \qquad 5 \qquad 6 \qquad 7 \qquad 8 \qquad 9$$

A phosphorylated analog of DSIP (Ser in position 7), P-DSIP, also occurs and in rats is 5 times more active than DSIP. The ratio of DSIP/P-DSIP seems to be important in regulating the circadian time course of sleep and wakefulness in humans, i.e., high during daytime and low during the dark-night period. Both peptides enhance NREM and REM sleep. DSIP has been used clinically for insomnia and obstructive sleep apnea. Other physiologic effects observed for DSIP include thermoregulation, antinociception, relief of stress, and modulation of pituitary hormone secretion.

TESTING AND DEVELOPMENT OF NEW HYPNOTICS

As presented in the earlier section, a number of potential receptors can be identified that are associated with causing sleep with potential to be developed into a hypnotic. Initially, animal tests have been used for identifying new hypnotic drugs. In vitro receptor binding studies can then be used for screening of drugs that bind with improved specificity. The animal assays basically measure varying levels of CNS depression instead of sleep. The assumption is that CNS depression will relate to clinical hypnosis, although exceptions commonly occur. Common assays in mice or rats include an increase in sleeping time, a loss of righting reflex, rotorod impairment, decreased activity in an activity cage or potentiation of other CNS depressants (16). The observed pharmacologic effects of many drugs in this class are usually dose related such that small doses cause sedation, larger doses cause hypnosis, and still larger doses may bring about surgical anesthesia.

Larger animals, including rats, cats and monkeys, are studied in a sleep laboratory. In these studies electrophysiologic and electroencephalographic measurements are obtained and are often helpful in gaining information about the site of action of CNS depressants as well as about induced sleep patterns. Drug discrimination studies have also been useful in differentiating sites of action of CNS depressants (17).

Guidelines for the Clinical Evaluation of Hypnotic Drugs have been developed by the FDA for specific evaluation of this class of drugs. Human sleep laboratory studies have become increasingly valuable in determining a range of efficacy and defining an optimal dose. Because sleep laboratory studies are under closely controlled conditions, they are capable of continuous, electrophysiologic measurement throughout the night. This is then followed by objective measurement of pre- and post-sleep results to assess effectiveness and withdrawal effects of new hypnotics. The sleep laboratory studies coupled with clinical studies based on patients' subjective estimate of efficacy provide a thorough and clinically relevant approach to developing a new hypnotic (18).

CLASSIFICATION OF HYPNOTICS
Introduction to Classes of Hypnotics

The hypnotic drugs are not characterized by common structural features. Instead, a wide variety of chemical compounds have been used in clinical therapy. An arbitrary classification is as follows:

Benzodiazepines
Imidazopyridine and Cyclopyrrolone
Pyrazolopyrimidine
Barbiturates
Chloral
Tertiary Acetylenic Alcohols
Ureides
Piperidinediones

Benzodiazepines

Benzodiazepines are used as daytime anxiolytics, sleep inducers, anesthetics, anticonvulsants, and muscle relaxants. They will be discussed in depth in Chapter 17. Examination of the basic pharmacodynamic properties of the benzodiazepines (defined as receptor specific binding activity) show that the clinically useful benzodiazepines exhibit comparable sedative activity at therapeutically comparable doses, although clonazepam, desmethylclobazam, and desmethydiazepam are reported to be less sedative (Fig. 15.1) (12). Therefore, the use of a specific benzodiazepine as a hypnotic is based primarily on pharmacokinetic properties and marketing considerations. Hypnotics are unusual in that they are normally given as a single dose. The following variables will determine how well a benzodiazepine will work as a hypnotic: 1) is acute tolerance developed to the benzodiazepine that will diminish CNS effects before the drug is eliminated from the CNS, 2) is redistribution of the benzodiazepine from the CNS to other tissues very rapid, 3) is there a rapid drug elimination by biotransformation and is the metabolite also active. The benzodiazepines that are specifically promoted as sleep inducers

are listed in Table 15.1 (19); however, it is important to keep in mind that depending on dose any benzodiazepine may be used for its hypnotic effect.

Mechanism of Action

The initial studies suggesting a possible involvement of the benzodiazepines with GABA provided a basis for understanding the pharmacologic effects of this class of drugs. The identification of specific, high-affinity binding sites for the benzodiazepines (21,22) was then achieved by using radiolabeled benzodiazepines. The benzodiazepines were shown to bind at the $GABA_A$ receptors involved in the regulation of the chloride channel. Initial binding studies with the benzodiazepine derivatives were consistent with only one class or population of benzodiazepine receptors. Later studies suggested two subclasses of receptors, currently termed BZ_1 and BZ_2 receptors. Structurally distinct benzodiazepine receptor subclasses were confirmed using recombinant techniques in which $GABA_A$ receptor subclasses with different subunit composition identical to the BZ_1 and BZ_2 receptors were coexpressed (23,24). The $GABA_A$ receptor composed of $\alpha_1\beta_2\gamma_2$ comparable to BZ_1 subtype and accounted for 60–70% of the receptors and $\alpha_1\beta_3\gamma_2$ comparable to BZ_2 subtype accounted for 20–25% of the receptors. Although these biochemically distinct receptors are present, whether these subclasses are associated with a pharmacologic or therapeutic difference is still a matter of debate. It has been proposed, although certainly not proven, that compounds specific for the BZ_1 subclass would be "nonsedative" and the BZ_2 subclass is responsible for the sedative-hypnotic character of the benzodiazepines (12).

All of the benzodiazepines affect the normal sleep stages. They increase total sleep and EEG fast activity and decrease nocturnal wakefulness, body movements, number of awakenings, sleep latency (the time required to fall asleep), and stages 3 and 4 sleep (NREM). Upon withdrawal of the drug a gradual return to baseline values of

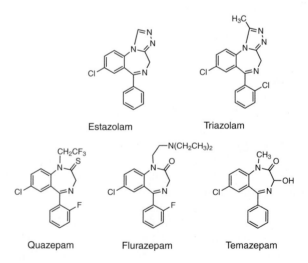

Fig. 15.1. Benzodiaepines commonly used as hypnotics.

Table 15.1. Comparison of Hypnotic Benzodiazepines (19)

Benzodiazepine	Trade Name	IC_{50} (nmol/l)(20)	Hypnotic Dose(mg)	$t_{1/2}$ (h)	Active Metabolite
Estazolam	Prosom	9	1–2	8–28	No
Flurazepam		15	15–30	2–3	Yes $t_{1/2}$ 47–100 h
Quazepam	Doral	30	7.5–15	41	Yes $t_{1/2}$ 47–100 h
Temazepam	Restoril	16	15–30	3.5–18.4	No
Triazolam	Halcion	4	0.125–0.5	1.5–5.5	No

NREM sleep returns. They also cause a mild suppression of REM sleep, especially during the first third of the night with rapid return to baseline upon withdrawal. Although these effects are documented from sleep studies, the physiologic or clinical significance of these drug induced alterations is not well understood.

Pharmacodynamic/Pharmacokinetic Balance

The onset of sedative or hypnotic activity of intravenously administered benzodiazepines is rapid, with a range of 15–30 seconds (a single circulation time) to a few minutes, depending on the patient's sensitivity, pharmacologic response, and size of the dose. The speed of onset of action of orally administered benzodiazepines can be very dependant on the drug dosage form. For example, temazepam when first introduced in the U.S. was formulated as a hard gelatin capsule. This formulation had a very slow rate of absorption following oral administration with peak plasma levels reached on average 1.8–4.7 hours after dosing (25) and exhibited little effect on sleep induction with most of its effect on sleep maintenance. Total wake time was slightly decreased with short-term drug administration and was similar to baseline with intermediate and long-term use. Temazepam has since been reformulated as a tablet or in a soft gelatin form. These formulations are now more effective in improving sleep by decreasing the time to sleep induction and improved sleep maintenance (25). Among the oral benzodiazepines formulations specifically indicated for the treatment of insomnia, flurazepam is absorbed most rapidly, triazolam has an intermediate rate of absorption, and temazepam is absorbed slowly and may be given 1 to 2 hours before bedtime.

Hypnotics can be used short term (1 week), intermediate term (2 weeks), and long term (4 weeks or greater) periods. The vast majority of the benzodiazepines are effective for inducing and maintaining sleep when used initially or for a short term. Differences are observed when they are used for longer terms and the proper balance between pharmacodynamics and pharmacokinetic effects become very important.

Benzodiazepines that have low specific activity (receptor binding affinity) and are slowly eliminated or are metabolized to slowly eliminated active metabolites can be used as hypnotics. For example, flurazepam is metabolized by N-dealkylation and hydroxylation α to the imine (26)

and quazepam is metabolized by oxidative loss of sulfur to oxygen (27) to form active metabolites that are slowly eliminated, and are associated with a slow development of tolerance to the hypnotic effects. These compounds exhibit good efficacy as hypnotics with long term use and are associated with little loss of initial effectiveness. Minimal rebound insomnia or rebound anxiety is observed when the drug is withdrawn due to the presence of the active metabolite. However, because of their slow elimination the presence of active agent or active metabolite in blood and brain tissue is responsible for the residual effects of hypnotics in the daytime. These effects may consist of "hangover" effects and oversedation, and may be so severe, especially in the elderly, as to cause tremors, ataxia, and confusion. A good example of this is flurazepam, which is metabolized to desalkylflurazepam (N-deethylation) (26). This metabolite has its own antianxiety and sedative activities and a long plasma half-life of 47–100 hours. Nitrazepam, a hypnotic drug used in Europe, has a moderately long elimination half-life of about 30 hours and may cause "hangover" effects as well as accumulation on repeated use. The presence of active agent or active metabolite in blood and brain tissue is responsible for the residual effects of hypnotics in the daytime.

Upon development of the newer benzodiazepines, such as triazolam, with high receptor-binding affinity and more rapid elimination, it was anticipated that the problem of daytime sedation would be eliminated. The duration of action for triazolam, which has an ultra-short half-life of less than 4 hours due to biotransformation to inactive metabolites, primarily hydroxylation of the triazole methyl group and phase 2 conjugation (28). Temazepam is rapidly metabolized via direct conjugation of the 3-hydroxyl with glucuronic acid (29). Both drugs have gained popularity as sleep inducers, especially in elderly individuals. However, sleep laboratory studies show that these compounds rapidly lose much of their initial effectiveness, often after only one week of continuous nightly administration. The effectiveness of some of the benzodiazepines have been shown to decrease when used long term. In addition these compounds are associated with hyperexcitability that is exhibited as daytime anxiety, tenseness or panic and early morning insomnia (25).

Although there exist some disadvantages to using the benzodiazepines as hypnotics, they have other advantages unique to this class of drug, the major advantage being their relative safety. Fatalities resulting from benzodiazepine overdosage alone are rare. When it is taken together with other drugs, intoxication probably depends largely on the type and quantity of nonbenzodiazepine (30). In addition, benzodiazepines do not cause significant hepatic enzyme induction in man, and therefore their tendency to interact with other drugs is less than that seen with other hypnotics.

Nonbenzodiazepine GABA$_A$ Agonists

Zolpidem   Zopiclone

Zolpidem (**Ambien**) and zopiclone possess nonbenzodiazepine structure and have been introduced as short-acting hypnotics in the U.S. and Europe. They act at the GABA$_A$ receptor high-affinity receptors comparable to the benzodiazepines. Zolpidem (classified as an imidazopyridine) binds with higher affinity at the BZR$_1$ receptor over the BZR$_2$ receptor, while zopiclone (classified as a cyclopyrrolone) binds with higher affinity at a slightly different recognition site on the GABA$_A$ receptor complex. The compounds show differences from the benzodiazepines in some pharmacologic tests, although the clinical differences are not readily apparent. They exhibit a reduced ability to cause physical dependence after treatment with high doses in animal models, but drug dependence has been reported for both compounds (12). Zolpidem has a rapid onset of action of 1.6 hours, a short elimination half-life of approximately 2.5 hours, and no rebound effects upon withdrawal of the drug. It has no ionizable groups at physiological pH and is extensively metabolized to inactive metabolites by CYP3A4 hydroxylation of the aryl methyl groups followed by further oxidation by aldehyde dehydrogenase to the carboxylic acid (31). These metabolites are eliminated in the urine. Its half-life in patients with liver disease is increased to about 10 hours. Zolpidem is available in the U.S. and is usually given in 5- to 10-mg dosages nightly.

Pyrazolopyrimidine

Zaleplon (**Sonata**), a pyrazolopyrimidine derivative, is a sedative and hypnotic agent structurally unrelated to the benzodiazepines and other sedative-hypnotic agents. Pharmacologically and pharmacokinetically, zaleplon is similar to zolpidem (32); both are hypnotic agents with short half-lives, and both have been shown to interact with the CNS gamma-aminobutyric acid (GABA$_A$)-receptor-chloride ionophore complex at benzodiazepine omega-1 (BZR$_1$, omega-1) receptors. Its partition coefficient in octanol/water is constant (log P = 1.23) over the pH range of 1–7.

Zaleplon is well absorbed following oral administration with an absolute bioavailability of approximately 30% because of significant first-pass metabolism (33). It exhibits a mean half-life of approximately 1 hour, with less than 1% of the dose excreted unchanged in urine. It is primarily metabolized by aldehyde oxidase to 5-oxo-zaleplon, and is also metabolized to a lesser extent by CYP3A4 N-deethylation to desethylzaleplon, which is quickly converted, presumably by aldehyde oxidase, to 5-oxo-desethylzaleplon. (34,35) These oxidative metabolites are then converted to glucuronides and eliminated in urine. All of zaleplon's metabolites are pharmacologically inactive. Zaleplon does not accumulate with once-daily administration and displays linear pharmacokinetics in the therapeutic range. Zaleplon is administered orally without regard to meals, although administration with a high-fat meal should be avoided because of a potential decreased rate of drug absorption. Such delay in GI absorption could result in decreased efficacy on sleep latency (32).

Zaleplon   5-Oxo zaleplon   Desethyl zaleplon

Barbiturates

The barbiturates have a different pharmacologic profile from that of the benzodiazepines. They exert a depressant effect on the cerebrospinal axis and depress neuronal activity, as well as skeletal muscle, smooth muscle, and cardiac muscle activity. Depending on the compound, dose, and route of administration, the barbiturates can produce different degrees of CNS depression and have found use as sedatives, hypnotics, anticonvulsants, or anesthetics.

Currently, the barbiturates get minimal use as sedatives and hypnotics (especially compared to the benzodiazepines) due to higher toxicity. This is associated with their ability to cause greater CNS depression and their ability to induce many of the liver drug metabolizing enzymes. In addition, the barbiturates cause tolerance and often dependence. Even with all these disadvantages, the barbiturates continue to find occasional clinical applications as sedatives and hypnotics. However, their primary use is as anesthetics (Chapter 14) and antiseizure drugs (Chapter 16). Due primarily to historical convention the general chemistry, structure-activity relationships, and metabolism of the barbiturates will be covered in this section.

Barbiturates exert their action on the central synaptic transmission process of the reticular activating system by reducing the excitability of the postsynaptic cell. In general, excitatory synaptic transmission is depressed by barbiturates, whereas inhibitory synaptic transmission is usually unaffected or enhanced. Barbiturates are antidepolarizing blocking agents that prevent the generation of excitatory postsynaptic potential by raising the threshold and extending the refractory period of the postsynaptic cell. A paradoxic effect of barbiturates also occurs in which small doses bring about hyperexcitation and agitation instead of sedation. This is because the barbiturate concentration is not sufficient to depress the reticular activating system, but is able to impede the inhibitory synapses normally present within the cortex. In addition to the effect on the reticular activating system, barbiturates act on the limbic, hypothalamic, and thalamic synaptic systems (36).

Mechanism of Action

The effects of the barbiturates is marked by a decrease in functional activities in the brain. At therapeutic doses the barbiturates enhance GABAergic inhibitory response, in a mechanism similar to that of the benzodiazepines, (i.e., by influencing conductance at the chloride channel). At higher concentrations, the barbiturates can potentiate the GABA$_A$-mediated chloride ion conductance and enhance both GABA and benzodiazepine binding. Therefore, the barbiturates and benzodiazepines display cross-tolerance and this can be seen with the barbiturates exhibiting weak anxiolytics and muscle relaxant properties. The barbiturate binding site is different from the benzodiazepines and is believed to occur at the picrotoxin binding site on the chloride channel (see Chapter 17). At higher concentrations the barbiturates also reduce glutaminergic transmission.

Other actions of the barbiturates at higher concentrations include uncoupling of oxidative phosphorylation, inhibition of the electron transport system, and inhibition of cerebral carbonic anhydrase activity. These drugs also affect the transport of sugars and are noted for their ability to induce liver microsomal enzymes that lead to an increased rate of biotransformation of many commonly used drugs, including the barbiturates. The biochemical effects of these drugs have been summarized (37,38).

Pharmacologic Effects

The effects of barbiturates on the sleep pattern are comparable to those of benzodiazepines. In short-term studies the barbiturates are equally effective as the benzodiazepines. Again the importance of the pharmacokinetic properties of the barbiturates determines their usefulness as hypnotics. The barbiturates that are slowly eliminated are capable of producing hangover and persistent psychomotor impairment. For example, amobarbital was once extensively used as a hypnotic but is no longer commercially available for oral dosing as a hypnotic (although still available in Tuinal, a combination of amobarbital and secobarbital) due to excessive daytime sedation. However, even amobarbital still finds clinical application as a parenteral formulation when used in the "intracarotid amobarbital procedure" to determine lateralization of language and memory prior to surgery (39).

The barbiturates also cause a physical dependence different from the opioid narcotics. In an individual addicted to barbiturates, the barbiturates should not be withdrawn abruptly, but tapered slowly. Sudden withdrawal of the barbiturates can precipitate extreme agitation and grand mal seizures. This can lead to a spasm of the respiratory musculature producing impaired respiration, cyanosis, and possibly death (40). As a rule, drug dependence is followed by tolerance, in which increasing doses are required to obtain the same pharmacologic effect. Because barbiturates cause tolerance and often dependence their use as a hypnotic is rarely justified.

Structure-Activity Relationships

Hundreds of barbiturates have been synthesized on a trial-and-error basis (41). Although many structural features required for hypnotic activity were recorded, no clear correlation between structure and activity emerged. In 1951, Sandberg (42) made his fundamental postulation that, to possess good hypnotic activity, a barbituric acid must be a weak acid and must have a lipid/water partition coefficient between certain limits. Therefore only the 5,5,-disubstituted barbituric acids, the 5,5,-disubstituted thiobarbituric acids, and the 1,5,5-trisubstituted barbituric acids possess acceptable hypnotic, anticonvulsant or anesthetic activity. All other substitution patterns such as 5-monosubstituted barbituric acids, 1,3-disubstituted barbituric acids, or 1,3,5,5-tetrasubstituted barbituric acids are inactive or produce convulsions.

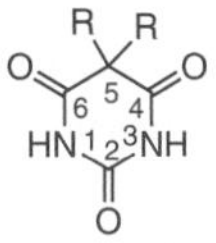

pKa and Structure of the Barbiturates. The 5,5-Disubstituted barbituric acid contains three lactam groups that can undergo pH dependent lactim—lactam tautomerization as shown in Figure 15.2.

Ultraviolet spectroscopic studies with 5,5-disubstituted barbituric acids (43) indicated that in aqueous solutions the dominant forms are either the dioxo tautomeric form (i.e., monolactam in alkaline medium) or the trioxo tautomeric form (barbituric acid structure in acid medium). The acidity of barbiturates in aqueous solution depends on the number of substituents attached to barbituric acid. The 5,5-disubstituted barbituric acids, 5,5-disubstituted thiobarbituric acids, and 1,5,5-trisubstituted barbituric acids are relatively weak acids and salts of these barbiturates are easily formed by treatment with bases. The pKa value of 5,5-disubstituted barbituric acids ranges from

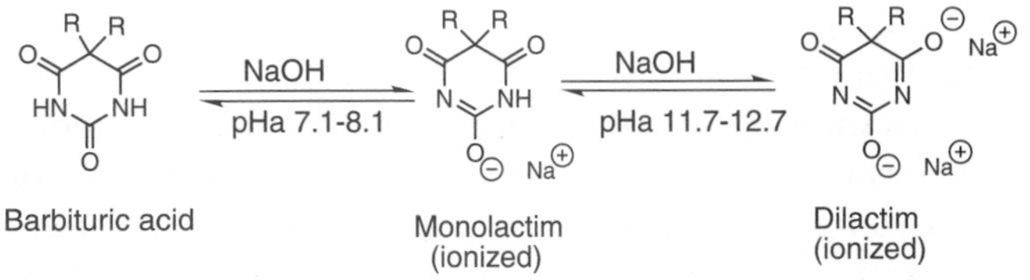

Fig. 15.2. pH dependent tautmerization of barbituates.

7.1–8.1 (44). The 5,5-disubstituted barbituric acids can undergo a second ionization (45), having pKa values in the range of 11.7–12.7. The alkali metal salts of the barbiturates coupled with their highly lipophilic character will cause chemical incompatibility reactions (precipitation) when these compounds are mixed with acid salts of weakly basic amines.

5,5-Disubstitution (43). As the number of carbon atoms at the fifth carbon position increases, the lipophilic character of the substituted barbituric acids also increases. Branching, unsaturation, replacement of alicyclic or aromatic substituents for alkyl substituents, and introduction of halogen into the alkyl substituents all increase the lipid solubility of the barbituric acid derivatives. A limit is reached, however, because as the lipophilic character increases, the hydrophilic character decreases. Although lipophilic character determines the ability of compounds to cross the blood-brain barrier, hydrophilic character is also important because it determines solubility in biologic fluids and ensures that the compound reaches the blood-brain barrier. Introduction of polar groups into the alkyl substituent decreases lipid solubility below desirable levels. Modifications at this position by variation of the alkyl substituents were of primary importance in the development of barbiturates with short (3–4 hour) to intermediate (6–8 hour) duration of action. These barbiturates were once extensively used as sedatives and hypnotics.

Substitution on Nitrogen (43). Substitution of one imide hydrogen by alkyl groups increases lipid solubility. The result is a quicker onset and a shorter duration of activity. As the size of the N-alkyl substituent increases (methyl -> ethyl -> propyl), the lipid solubility increases and the hydrophilic character decreases beyond limits. Furthermore, attachment of large alkyl groups (starting with the ethyl group) to the nitrogen imparts convulsant properties to barbiturates. Attachment of alkyl substituents to both N^1 an N^3 renders the drugs nonacidic, making them inactive. Modifications at this position are of primary importance in the barbiturates used as anticonvulsants and anesthetics.

Modification of Oxygen (43). Replacement of C^2 oxygen by sulfur increases lipid solubility. Because maximal thiobarbiturate brain levels are quickly reached, onset of activity is rapid. As a result, these drugs (i.e., thiopental) are used as intravenous anesthetics.

Metabolism (46)

Barbiturates lose their activities through metabolic transformations and redistribution. The metabolism of the barbiturates takes place primarily in the liver in the endoplasmic reticulum. After metabolism the lipophilic character of barbiturates decreases and this is associated with a loss in depressant activity. Although not used as a hypnotic, the metabolic pathway for mephobarbital (Fig. 15.3) is representative of the metabolic pathway for the barbiturates. The major pathways by which the activity of the barbiturates is terminated are the following:

1. Oxidation of substituents at carbon 5 by CYP450, often specifically by CYP2C19. The initial products are alcohols or phenols that form glucuronide and sulfate conjugates. The alcohols can undergo further oxidation to ketones or carboxylic acids, but these pathways are generally of minor importance in the biodisposition of the barbiturates. A pronounced product enantioselectivity is often observed for the chiral barbiturates. The barbiturates containing a propene at the 5-position (e.g., secobarbital) have been shown to inactivate the CYP450 by alkylation of the porphyrin ring of CYP450 (47).

2. Conjugation of the heterocyclic nitrogen with glucuronic acid. This unusual conjugation pathway can be as important as oxidative metabolism in the biotransformation of 5,5-disubstituted barbiturates (phenobarbital, amobarbital, pentobarbital). In humans a pronounced product enantioselectivity is observed for excretion of these metabolites (48).

3. Oxidative N-dealkylation at the nitrogen. CYP450 oxidation does not proceed rapidly. Introduction of an alkyl group on a barbiturate nitrogen introduces a site of asymmetry at the 5-position. The S-isomers of the these barbiturates primarily undergo N-dealkylation and the R-isomer primarily undergoes oxidation at the 5 position. The dealkylated products, however, may be excreted more slowly and therefore accumulate in the course of therapy with N-alkylated barbiturates. For example, a definite blood level of phenobarbital has been established in the course of mephobarbital therapy (49).

4. Oxidative desulfurization of 2-thiobarbiturates takes place readily to yield the more hydrophilic barbiturates. This occurs primarily following redistribution of the thiobarbiturate anesthetics.

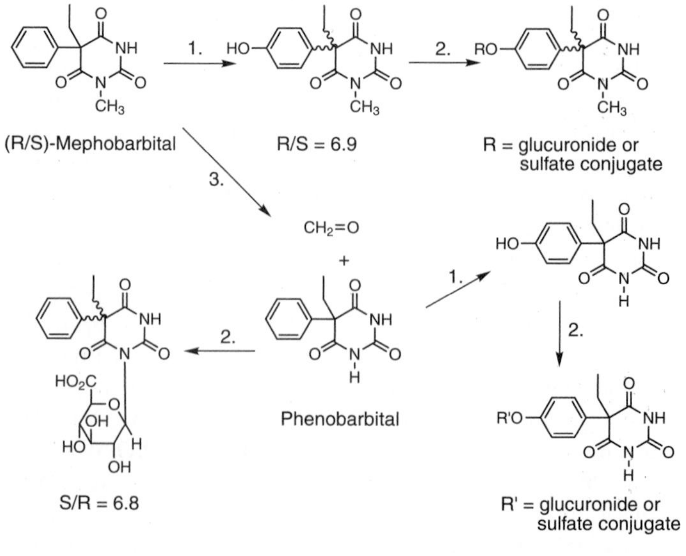

Fig. 15.3. Metabolism of mephobarbital and phenobarbital.

Table 15.2 Barbiturates Used Clinically as Hypnotics (19)

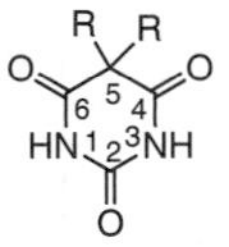

Barbiturate	R_5	R_5	Hypnotic Dose (mg)	Onset (min)	Duration (hr)
Amobarbital	C_2H_5	$(CH_3)_2CHCH_2CH_2$	100–200	45–60	6–8
Aprobarbital	$CH_2=CHCH_2$	$(CH_3)_2CH$	40–160	45–60	6–8
Butabarbital	C_2H_5	$CH_3CH_2CH(CH_3)$	50–100	45–60	6–8
Pentobarbital	C_2H_5	$CH_3(CH_2)_2CH(CH_3)$	100	10–15	3–4
Phenobarbital	C_2H_5	C_6H_5	100–320	30–$\geq$60	10–16
Secobarbital	$CH_2=CHCH_2$	$CH_3(CH_2)_2CH(CH_3)$	100	10–15	3–4

Clinical Applications

The currently available barbiturates are listed in Table 15.2. It must be concluded that a prescription for long-term use of the barbiturates as hypnotics is rarely indicated.

Chloral Derivative

During the 50s and 60s chloral hydrate was widely promoted as a hypnotic (doses of 500 mg) because it did not significantly suppress REM sleep (50). Today it still finds use as a sedative in nonoperating room procedures for the pediatric patient (51). Chloral hydrate does demonstrate initial and short term effectiveness for sleep induction and maintenance. Sleep occurs within 1 hour and lasts 4–8 hours. However, after 2 weeks of drug administration, a marked decrease in effectiveness is observed (52). The site of chloral hydrate action is the rostral reticular activating system. Chloral hydrate has no analgesic or tranquilizing effect and is devoid of adverse respiratory effects at therapeutic doses.

Chloral is a unique aldehyde due to the electron-withdrawing effect of the CCl_3 group. When chloral (an oily liquid) is treated with water or alcohol, a crystalline solid, chloral hydrate or chloral alcoholate is formed. Chloral hydrate is stable, but as indicated in Figure 15.3 when it is dissolved in water it is in equilibrium with the chloral form (equilibrium strongly favoring the chloral hydrate structure). The CCl_3 group is sufficiently electron withdrawing that chloral hydrate is a weak acid (pKa = 10.04) (44). This acidity makes it quite irritating to mucous membranes such as in the stomach. Therefore, it is not surprising that gastrointestinal upset commonly occurs for chloral if undiluted or taken on an empty stomach. This led to the development of adducts or complexes, or prodrugs that were widely used, but are now no longer available. Only chloral hydrate as a capsule, syrup or suppository is currently available.

Chloral hydrate is readily absorbed from the gastrointestinal tract following oral or rectal doses of 500 mg to 2 g. It is quickly reduced to trichloroethanol in the liver and other tissues. This metabolic transformation is so fast that it is difficult to detect appreciable chloral hydrate blood levels (53). It is believed that the initial hypnotic ef-

fect of chloral hydrate is exerted by the drug, but the more prolonged effect is caused by trichloroethanol. *In vitro* it has been shown that trichloroethanol can exert barbiturate like effects on the $GABA_A$ receptor channels (54). Trichloroethanol is metabolized by oxidation to chloral and then to the inactive metabolite, trichloroacetic acid (Fig. 15.4), which is also extensively metabolized to acyl glucuronides via conjugation with glucuronic acid (55).

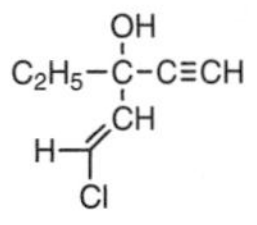

Ethchlorvynol

Tertiary Acetylenic Alcohol

Ethchlorvynol is a mild hypnotic with a quick onset and short duration of activity ($t_{1/2}$ = 5.6 hr) and a plasma half-life of 10–20 hours (56). It resembles the short-acting barbiturates (based on EEG), but it produces less initial arousal than barbiturates. The hypnotic dose of ethchlorvynol is 500–770 mg with chronic abuse leading to habituation and tolerance (57). The sedative dose is 100–200 mg, but its use as a sedative is not recommended due to its short duration of action. Ethchlorvynol also has anticonvulsant and muscle-relaxing properties. Due to its highly lipophilic character it is extensively metabolized to its secondary alcohol (app. 90%) prior to its excretion of free and unconjugated forms. It reportedly induces microsomal hepatic enzymes.

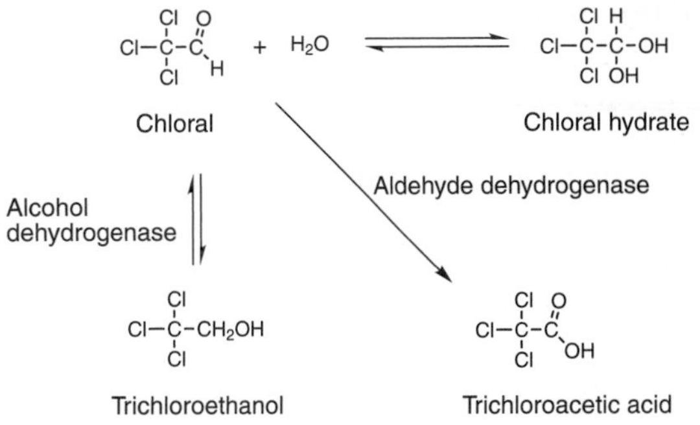

Fig. 15.4. Reactions and metabolism of chloral.

Ureide

Acecarbromal (acetylcarbromal)

The barbiturates are basically a cyclic urea in which malonic acid is condensed with urea. A similar reaction in which a mono carboxylic acid is used to acylate urea will yield the ureides. Although the ureides were once commonly used, only acetylcarbromal is still available. The usual oral dose of acetylcarbromal is 250–500 mg 2 or 3 times daily for sedation. Slightly higher doses are used for its hypnotic effect. It is metabolized to urea and is readily eliminated in the urine. Because bromide ion is released in vivo, prolonged use of these compounds is not recommended because of the possible development of bromidism in patients. This class of drugs is very rarely used due to their low therapeutic index (58).

Piperidinediones

Methyprylon   Glutethimide   Thalidomide

Encouraged by the success of barbiturates in sedative-hypnotic therapy, structurally related heterocyclic compounds containing the lactam functional group were prepared and tested for hypnotic activity. Of the piperidinediones, methyprylon and glutethimide, introduced in the middle 1950s, only glutethimide is still in use for its hypnotic activity: Both of these compounds are effective hypnotics that lack significant anesthetic, analgesic, tranquilizing, or muscle-relaxant properties. Their mechanism of action resemble that of barbiturates and they suppress REM sleep at hypnotic doses. At one time both compounds were considered to be safer than the barbiturates because they caused minimal respiratory depression at therapeutic doses. However, since their introduction both compounds have been shown to act as inducing agents of microsomal enzymes as well as leading to problems of habituation, tolerance, physical dependence and addiction. Basically, both compounds are general CNS depressant comparable to the barbiturates. It must be concluded that long-term use of this class of drugs as hypnotics is rarely indicated (57).

Methyprylon

Although no longer in therapeutic use, less is known about the pharmacology and toxicology of methyprylon. It

significantly reduces REM sleep at its hypnotic dose of 300 mg and is considered to be comparable to secobarbital (200 mg) or pentobarbital (100 mg). It is more water soluble than glutethimide, but it is unknown if this leads to better absorption. It is extensively metabolized (97%) to oxidized metabolites that are often further conjugated with glucuronic acid (57).

Glutethimide

Glutethimide is one of the most active nonbarbiturate hypnotics that is structurally similar to the barbiturates, especially phenobarbital. It was once considered to be safer than the barbiturates at the hypnotic dose of 500 mg because it did not affect respiration or blood pressure over a period of several hours. Due to glutethimide's low aqueous solubility (pKa = 11.8), its dissolution and absorption from the GI tract is highly variable. Consistent with its high lipid:water partition coefficient it undergoes extensive oxidative metabolism in the liver with a half-life of approximately 10 hours. Glutethimide is used as a racemic mixture with the (+) stereoisomer being primarily metabolized on the glutarimide ring and the (−) stereoisomer on the phenyl ring. The product of metabolic detoxification is excreted after conjugation with glucuronic acid at the hydroxyl group. Glutethimide poisoning is more dangerous than barbiturate poisoning (57).

Thalidomide (a member of this class of drugs) was also introduced in the middle 1950s, but was removed due to its teratogenic side effect (1).

Antihistamines and Anticholinergics

Diphenhydramine   Doxylamine

Some of the antihistamines (H1 receptor antagonists that can cross the blood-brain barrier) are used for their hypnotic activity. The primary antihistamines used for their sedative effect are diphenhydramine and doxylamine which belong to the ethanolamine class of antihistamines (see Chapter 33). Both drugs are sold without prescription. Sleep laboratory controlled studies indicate that the antihistamines (H1 receptor antagonists) have little effect on normal subjects when given before bedtime. However, the same doses during the day lead to drowsiness, increased tendency to sleep and impaired performance (9).

CASE STUDY

Victoria F. Roche and S. William Zito

WC is a 43-year-old, male recovering alcoholic who has been admitted into a residential halfway house following a 5 day stay in a detox unit. He is being treated with disulfiram to encourage him to stay off the "booze." Despite 5 years of alcohol abuse, WC is in relatively fine health. Liver function tests are normal. However, a physical exam revealed a slightly enlarged left atrium associated with mitral stenosis. Mitral stenosis is almost always caused by previous rheumatic fever, which WC confirms he had as a child. WC has not experienced any drowsiness with disulfiram, but instead complains of being unable to fall asleep. His physician wants to prescribe a hypnotic for a short period of time to help WC fall asleep at night. Evaluate the given hypnotics for use in this case.

1. *Identify the therapeutic problem(s) where the pharmacist's intervention may benefit the patient.*

2. *Identify and prioritize the patient specific factors that must be considered to achieve the desired therapeutic outcomes.*

3. *Conduct a thorough and mechanistically oriented structure-activity analysis of all therapeutic alternatives provided in the case.*

4. *Evaluate the SAR findings against the patient specific factors and desired therapeutic outcomes and make a therapeutic decision.*

5. *Counsel your patient.*

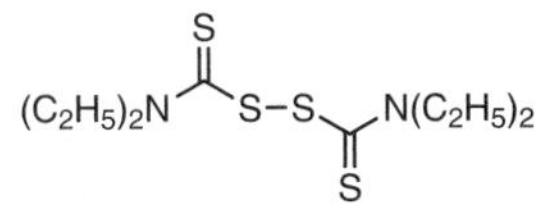

Disulfiram

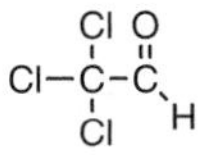

1

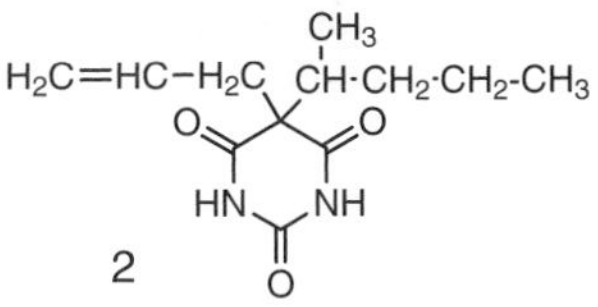

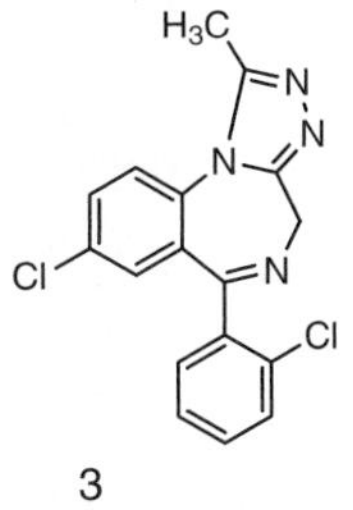

2

3

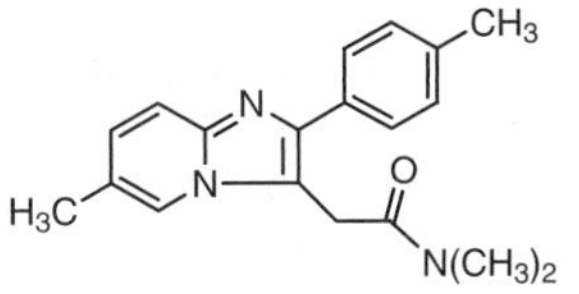

4

381

REFERENCES

1. Mellin GW, Katzenstein M. The Saga of Thalidomide. N Eng J Med 1962;267:1184–1192.
2. Miller NS, Gold MS. Sedative-hypnotics: pharmacology and use. J Fam Pract 1989;29:665–670.
3. Moruzzi G, Magoun H. Brain stem reticular formation and activation of the EEG. Electroencephalogr. Clin. Neurophysical 1949;1:455–473.
4. Carskadon MA, Dement WC. Normal Human Sleep: An Overview. In Kryger MH, Roth T, Dement WC, eds. Principles and practices of sleep medicine, 2nd edition. Philadelphia: WB Saunders Co, 1994;16–25.
5. Rosenthal MS. Physiology and neurochemistry of sleep. Am J Pharm Ed 1998;62:204–208.
6. Kales A, ed. The pharmacology of sleep, v. 116. Berlin: Springer-Verlag, 1995.
7. Wauquier A. Pharmacology of the catecholaminergic system. In: Kales A, ed. The pharmacology of sleep. Berlin: Springer-Verlag, 1995;116:65–90.
8. Adrien J. The serotoninergic system and sleep-wakefulness regulation. In: Kales A, ed. The pharmacology of sleep. Berlin: Springer-Verlag, 1995;116:91–116.
9. Monti JM. Pharmacology of the histaminergic system. In: Kales A, ed. The pharmacology of sleep. Berlin: Springer-Verlag, 1995;116:117–142.
10. Tononi G, Pompeiano O. Pharmacology of the cholinergic system. In: Kales A, ed. The pharmacology of sleep. Berlin: Springer-Verlag, 1995;116:143–210.
11. Radulovacki M. Pharmacology of the adenosine system. In: Kales A, ed. The pharmacology of sleep. Berlin: Springer-Verlag, 1995;116:307–322.
12. Muller WE. Pharmacology of the GABAergic/benzodiazepine system. In: Kales A, ed. The pharmacology of sleep. Berlin: Springer-Verlag, 1995;116:211–242.
13. Van Cauter E. Hormones and sleep. In: Kales A, ed. The pharmacology of sleep. Berlin: Springer-Verlag, 1995;116:279–306.
14. Mahle CD, Takaki KS, Watson AJ. Melatonin receptor ligands and their potential clinical applications. In: Bristol JA ed. Ann Rep Med Chem. 1997;32:31–40.
15. Inoue S. Pharmacology of the CNS peptides. In: Kales A, ed. The pharmacology of sleep. Berlin: Springer-Verlag, 1995;116:243–278.
16. Straw RN. Pharmacological Evaluation of Hypnotic Drugs in Infrahuman Species as Related to Clinical Utility. In: Hypnotics, Methods of Development and Evaluation, F. Kagan, et al., Eds. New York, Spectrum Publications, Inc. 1975; 65–85.
17. Young R, Glennon RA, Dewey WL. Stereoselective stimulus effects of 3-methylflunitrazepam and pentobarbital. Life Sci 1984;34:1977–1983.
18. Bixler EO, Vgontzas AN, Kales A. Methodological issues in pharmacological studies of sleep. In: Kales A, ed. The pharmacology of sleep. Berlin: Springer-Verlag, 1995;116:323–344.
19. Threlkeld, DS ed. Facts and Comparisons, St. Louis; Facts and Comparisons, 1998;269g–280a.
20. Haefely W. Tranquilizers. In: Grahame-Smith DG ed. Preclinical psychopharmacology. Amsterdam: Elsevier, 1985;92–182.
21. Squires RF, Braestrup C. Benzodiazepine receptors in rat brain. Nature 1977;266:732–734.
22. Mohler H, Okada T. Benzodiazepine receptor: Demonstration in the central nervous system. Science 1977;198:849–851.
23. Pritchett DB, Luddens H, Seeburg PH. Type I and type II GABA_A-benzodiazepine receptors produced in transfected cells. Science 1989;245:1389–1392.
24. Luddens H, Wisden W. Function and pharmacology of multiple GABAA receptor subunits. Trends Pharmacol Sci 1991;12:49–51.
25. Kales A, Vgontzas AN, Bixler EO. Hypnotic Drugs. In: Kagan F, Hatwood T, Rickels K, Rudzik AD, et al. eds., Hypnotics. New York: Spectrum Publication, Inc, 1975;345–385.
26. Clatworthy AJ, Jones LV, Whitehouse MJ. The gas chromatography mass spectrometry of the major metaboolites of flurazepam. Biomed Mass Spectrom 1977;4:248–254.
27. Zampaglione N, Hilbert JM, Ning J, et. al. Disposition and metabolic fate of 14C-quazepam in man. Drug Metab Dispos 1985;13:25–29.
28. Eberts FS Jr, Philopoulos Y, Reineke LM, et al. Triazolam Disposition. Clin Pharmacol Ther 1981;29:81–93.
29. Schwarz HJ. Pharmacokinetics and metabolism of temazepam in man and several animal species. Br J Clin Pharmacol 1979;8:23S-29S.
30. Greenblatt DJ, Allen MD, Noel BJ, et al. Acute overdosage with benzodiazepine derivatives. Clin Pharmacol Ther 1977;21;497–514.
31. Pichard L, Gillet G, Bonfils C, et. al. Oxidative metabolism of zolpidem by human liver cytochrome P450S. Drug Metab Dispos 1995;23:1253–62.
32. Greenblatt DJ, Harmatz JS, von Moltke LL, et. al. Comparative kinetics and dynamics of zaleplon, zolpidem, and placebo. Clin Pharmacol Ther 1998;64:553–61.
33. Rosen AS, Fournie P, Darwish M, et. al. Zaleplon pharmacokinetics and absolute bioavailability. Biopharm Drug Dispos 1999;20:171–5.
34. Renwick AB, Mistry H, Ball SE, et. al. Metabolism of Zaleplon by human hepatic microsomal cytochrome P450 isoforms. Xenobiotica 1998;28:337–48.
35. Kawashima K, Hosoi K, Naruke T, et. al. Aldehyde oxidase-dependent marked species difference in hepatic metabolism of the sedative-hypnotic, zaleplon, between monkeys and rats. Drug Metab Dispos 1999;27:422–8.
36. Richter JA, Holtman JR. Barbiturates: Their in vivo effects and potential biochemical mechanisms. Prog Neurobiol 1982;18:275–319.
37. Decsi, L. Biochemical effects of drugs acting on the central nervous system. Prog Drug Res 1965;8:53–194.
38. Knoll R. In: Lipton MA, et al., eds. Psychopharmacology, a generation of progress. New York, Raven Press, 1978;1337–1348.
39. Acharya JN, Dinner DS. Use of the intracarotid amobarbital procedure in the evaluation of memory. J Clin Neurophysiol 1997;14:311–25.
40. Wang RIH. Dependence liability of sedatives and hypnotics. In: Kagan F, Hatwood T, Rickels K, et al. eds., Hypnotics. New York: Spectrum Publication, Inc, 1975;297–310.
41. Mautner HG, Clemson HC. Hypnotics and Sedatives. In: Burger A, ed., Medicinal Chemistry, Part II. New York, Wiley-Interscience, 1970; 1365–1385.
42. Sandberg F. Anesthetic properties of some new N-substituted and N,N'-disubstituted derivatives of 5,5-diallylbarbituric acid. Acta Physiol Scand 1951;24:7–26.
43. Vida JA. Central nervous system depressants: sedative-hypnotics. In: Foye WO, Lemke TL, Williams DA, eds., Principles of medicinal chemistry, 4th Ed. Baltimore, MD, Williams & Wilkinson. 1995;154–180.
44. Drayton CJ, ed. Cumulative Subject Index & Drug Compendium, vol 6. In Hansch C, Sammes PG, Taylor JB, eds., Comprehensive Medicinal Chemistry, New York: Pergamon Press, 1990.
45. Butler TC, Ruth JM, Tucker, Jr. JF. The second ionization of 5,5-disubstituted derivatives of barbituric acids. J Am Chem Soc 1955;77;1488–1491.
46. Freudenthal RI, Carroll FI. Metabolism of certain commonly used barbiturates. Drug Metab Rev 1973;2:265–278.

47. He K, He YA, Szklarz GD, et al. Secobarbital-mediated inactivation of cytochrome P450 2B1 and its active site mutants. Partitioning between heme and protein alkylation and epoxidation. J Biol Chem 1996;271:25864–25872.

48. Soine WH, Soine PJ, England TM, et al. Identification of the diastereomers of pentobarbital N-glucosides excreted in human urine. Pharm Res 1994;11:1536–1540.

49. Lim WH, Hooper WD. Stereoselective metabolism and pharmacokinetics of racemic methylphenobarbital in humans. Drug Metab Disp 1989;17:212–217.

50. Kay DC, Blackburn AB, Buckingham JA, et al. Human pharmacology of sleep. In: Williams RL, Karacan I, eds. Pharmacology of sleep. New York: John Wiley & Sons, Inc, 1976; 83–210.

51. Warner TM. Clinical applications for pediatric sedation. CRNA 1997;8:144–151.

52. Kales A, Kales JD, Bixler EO, et al. Methodology of sleep laboratory drug evaluations: further considerations. In: Kagan F, Hatwood T, Rickels K, et al. eds., Hypnotics. New York: Spectrum Publication, Inc, 1975;109–126.

53. Marshall EK, Owens AH, Absorption, excretion and metabolic fate of chloral hydrate and trichloroethanol. Bull Hopkins Hosp, 1954;95:1–18.

54. Lovinger DM, Zimmerman SA, Levitin M, et al. J Pharmacol Exp Therap 1993;264:1097–1103.

55. Breimer DD. Clinical pharmacokinetics of hypnotics. Clin Pharmacokin 1977;2:93–109.

56. Cummins LM, Martin YC, Scherfling EE. Serum and urine levels of ethchlorvynol in man. J Pharm Sci 1971;60:261–263.

57. Harvey SC. Hypnotics and Sedatives. Goodman AG, Goodman LS, Gilman A. eds. Goodman and Gilman's The Pharmacological Basis of Therapeutics, 6th ed. New York: Macmillan Publishing Co., Inc., 1980;339–375.

16. Antiseizure Drugs

BARBARA LEDUC

INTRODUCTION

As early as 2000 B.C., it was recognized that some people suffered from convulsive seizures. The term epilepsy, based on the Greek word epilambanein (meaning "to seize"), is first mentioned by Hippocrates. In the world's first scientific monograph on epilepsy, entitled On the Sacred Disease (ca. 400 B.C.), Hippocrates disputed the myth that the cause of epilepsy is supernatural and the cure magic. He described epilepsy as a disease of the brain, which should be treated by diet. At the same time, Hippocrates provided the first classification of epilepsy, which is still used. He distinguished true (idiopathic) epilepsy (a disorder for which the cause is unknown) from symptomatic (organic) epilepsy (a disorder resulting from a physiologic abnormality, such as brain injury, tumor, infection, intoxication or metabolic disturbances).

Two opinions were put forward as to the causes of epilepsy. One was that epilepsy is a single disease entity, and all forms of it have a common cause. On the other hand, it was proposed that different types of epilepsy result from different chemical, anatomic, or functional disorders. At the Symposium on Evaluation of Drug Therapy in Neurologic and Sensory Disease, the general opinion was that "epilepsy is a symptom complex characterized by recurrent paroxysmal aberrations of brain functions, usually brief and self-limited" (1).

All forms of epilepsy originate in the brain and appear to be the result of changes in neuronal activity. These changes, such as an excessive neuronal discharge, may in turn be brought about by a disturbance of physicochemical function and electrical activity of the brain. The cause of this abnormality, however, is not clearly understood.

The most important property of the nerve cell is its excitability. It responds to excitation by generating an action potential, which may lead to repeated discharges. All normal neurons may become epileptic if subjected to excessive excitation. DeRobertis et al. list two possible mechanisms for convulsive disorders: a loss of the normal inhibitory control mechanism, and a chemical supersensitivity that increases excitability of neuronal elements (2).

The origin of the seizures was established as early as the 19th century by Jackson (3). According to him, an intense discharge of gray matter in various regions of the brain initiates the seizures. As a result, it is only a normal reaction of the brain to initiate convulsive seizures. The discharge of excessive electrical (nervous) energy has indeed been substantiated by brain-wave studies made possible by electroencephalography.

Attempts to classify epileptic seizures have been only partially successful, primarily because of limited knowledge of the pathologic processes of the brain. At the turn of the century, a classification of seizures had been published (4). Even more attempts appeared in the last two decades (5–9). In 1981, the Commission on Classification and Terminology of the International League Against Epilepsy put forward a new proposal (10). The classification outlined in Table 16.1 is a short version of this proposal, which is based on clinical seizure type, ictal (seizure induced) electroencephalographic (EEG) expression, and interictal (occurring between attacks or paroxysms) EEG expression.

SEIZURE CLASSIFICATION

Seizures result from the sudden, excessive firing of neurons. They are classified broadly as either partial seizures, in which the abnormal firing occurs initially in a small number of neurons but may spread to adjacent areas, or generalized seizures, in which virtually the entire brain is affected simultaneously (11). Seizures can be characterized by clinical symptoms and by electroencephalographic (EEG) patterns. In addition, computerized tomography (CT) and magnetic resonance imaging (MRI) of the head are used in virtually all patients with suspected epilepsy to aid in identifying the seizure type.

Partial (Local, Focal) Seizures

Partial seizures are divided into three categories: Simple Partial, Complex Partial, and Partial progressing to

Table 16.1. Classification of Epileptic Seizures

I. Partial (local, focal) seizures
  A. Simple (consciousness not impaired)
  B. Complex partial seizures (psychomotor seizures)
    1. Beginning as simple partial seizures, progressing to complex seizures
    2. With impairment of consciousness at onset
  C. Partial seizures evolving to secondarily generalized tonic-clonic convulsions
II. Generalized seizures (convulsive or nonconvulsive)
  A. Absence seizures
    Typical (petit mal)
    Atypical
  B. Myoclonic
  C. Clonic
  D. Tonic
  E. Tonic-clonic (grand mal)
  F. Atonic
III. Unclassified epileptic seizures (includes some neonatal seizures)

Generalized Seizures. The key distinction between simple and complex partial seizures is the level of consciousness of the person undergoing the seizure. In partial seizures, the initial neuronal discharge originates from a specific, limited cortical area, termed a "focus." Development of the focus is thought to be caused by scarring following head trauma, infection, or oxygen deprivation. The abnormal EEG seizure patterns are restricted to one region of the brain, at least at the onset. These types of seizures are possible at all ages but are most frequent in the elderly. Partial seizures respond fairly well to antiseizure drugs (most commonly referred to as AED).

Medications to combat partial seizures are effective against secondary or generalized tonic-clonic seizures as well. These seizures respond well to carbamazepine, hydantoins, and barbiturates, although this latter group unfortunately displays substantial sedative effects. The newer AED (gabapentin, lamotrigine, levetiracetam, oxcarbazepine, tiagabine, topiramate, and zonisamide) have been shown useful for either monotherapy or as adjunctive drugs. On the other hand, oxazolidinediones and succinimides are ineffective in the treatment of partial seizures. Valproate is appropriate when tonic-clonic seizures are combined with either myoclonic or absence seizures.

Simple Partial Seizures

The specific symptoms displayed during a simple partial seizure will depend on the area of the brain which is affected, and will occur on the opposite side of the body from the lesion. Combinations of symptoms are frequent, making accurate diagnosis a challenge. The temporal lobes are the most common origination site for partial seizures. Seizure foci located within the temporal lobe result in psychic symptoms such as fear, panic, or hallucinations, autonomic signs such as flushing and sweating, or unpleasant smells or tastes. Frontal lobe foci usually present with motor symptoms. Focal motor attacks most commonly start in one hand, one foot, or one side of the face. Often, however, the onset of focal seizures is not specific. Should the focal motor seizures spread to contiguous cortical areas, there may be an orderly sequence of repeated events (movement of hands, face, and legs) known as an epileptic march. This type of seizure is termed a "jacksonian seizure." If the unilateral movements characteristic of focal motor or jacksonian seizures steadily spread to the other half of the body, a generalized seizure may follow. In contrast, seizures beginning in the parietal lobes are termed sensory seizures, and present with altered sensations, tingling, numbness, or pain. Foci in the occipital lobes produce nystagmus, blinking, or visual disturbances such as flashing lights or the appearance of strange colors.

In simple partial seizures, the patient's consciousness is not impaired; thus the person remains able to respond to simple commands, perform simple deliberate movements, and recall events which occurred during the seizure.

Complex Partial Seizures

When consciousness is impaired, the seizure is classified as a complex partial seizure. Impaired consciousness will be manifested by the person's staring, inability to respond to simple commands, or by inaccurate recall or amnesia of events occurring during the seizure. Clouding of consciousness may be apparent initially, or appear subsequent to the start of a simple partial seizure. With the exception of the mental status, the other symptoms of complex partial seizures are similar to those outlined above. Many complex seizures have bilateral hemispheric involvement and are frequently accompanied by automatisms, i.e., repetitive involuntary movements such as chewing, swallowing, or wringing the hands.

Partial Seizures Evolving to Secondarily Generalized Seizures

The abnormal electrical activity responsible for any type of partial seizure can generalize throughout the brain, thus evolving into a secondary generalized tonic-clonic seizure. The diagnosis of partial seizures is therefore difficult. The generalization may occur rapidly, or slowly enough so that the symptoms of the partial seizure are experienced by the patient as an "aura" prior to the generalized tonic-clonic phase. Auras are comprised of symptoms such as seeing blinking lights, hearing unusual sounds, and serve as an important warning for the patient. The symptoms of tonic-clonic seizures are described below.

Generalized Seizures (Convulsive or Non-convulsive)

These disorders are generalized from the outset, show simultaneous involvement of both cerebral hemispheres, and loss of consciousness. It is not possible to single out one anatomic or functional system localized in one hemisphere of the brain that is responsible for the clinical symptoms. The initial neuronal discharge spreads quickly into the entire, or at least the greater part of, the gray matter. The EEG pattern consists of bilateral, essentially synchronous and symmetric discharges from the start and indicate the widespread nature of neuronal discharge. The cause is rarely known, but it is usually attributed to diffuse lesions, to toxic and metabolic disturbances, or to constitutional genetic factors. People of all ages are affected by generalized convulsions. There are several classes of generalized seizures, and useful drugs are selected according to the seizure type which transpires.

Absence (Petit Mal) Seizures

Both typical and atypical absence seizures bring about brief loss of consciousness. Typical absence seizures have a rapid onset and cessation which may cause them to be misinterpreted as daydreaming. However, the person cannot be alerted or awakened during the seizures. Absence seizures often begin with a change in facial expression, which is followed by a period of motionless, blank staring.

After the brief interruption in consciousness, typically about 10 seconds, the activity that was in progress before the seizure is resumed. The individuals have neither memory of events during the seizure nor postictal confusion. Typical absence seizures (petit mal) are more common in children than adults; they are particularly disabling since they tend to occur very many times daily. While most children will respond to drug treatment, a small percentage will go on to develop generalized tonic-clonic seizures as adults. Complex typical absence seizures may include additional phenomena, such as clonic or myoclonic motions, automatisms, or more elaborate behaviors. Between 25–40% of affected children have a family history of absence seizures.

Atypical absence seizures have a slower onset and cessation and last longer (up to several minutes) than typical absence seizures. They may include clonic motions, automatisms, or autonomic symptoms. Differential diagnosis between these types is made on the basis of the EEG. While typical absence seizures display a 3 Hz spike and wave EEG pattern, the pattern of atypical absence seizures is slower, usually in the 1.5–2.5 Hz range.

Both forms of absence seizure often occur as part of one of the recognized epilepsy syndromes. Typical absence seizures respond fairly well to AED; ethosuximide and valproate are first choice drugs. Clonazepam is effective but sedating, and tolerance to the anti-absence effects may develop; lamotrigine may be useful. AED treatment of atypical absence seizures is less successful.

Lennox-Gastaut syndrome is a mixed seizure disorder combining the atypical absence seizures with tonic, tonic-clonic or myoclonic motor patterns. The syndrome begins in childhood and usually includes mental retardation. Although adequate control of the seizures is rarely achieved, valproate, phenytoin, felbamate, lamotrigine, topiramate and clonazepam have been useful.

Myoclonic Seizures

Myoclonic seizures consist of sudden, very brief, jerking contractions which may involve the entire body, or be confined to limited areas such as the face and neck. The contractions may affect individual muscles or groups, with simultaneous contraction of both extensor and flexor muscles. These seizures occur in all age groups, the symptoms ranging from rapid tremors to falling down. No loss of consciousness is detectable due to the brief duration of the seizure. Myoclonic seizures often occur in combination with other seizure types. While valproate and clonazepam are used most often to treat myoclonic seizures, lamotrigine and topiramate have also shown some efficacy.

Tonic Seizures

Tonic seizures occur mostly in children and are characterized by increased tone in extensor muscles resulting in falling to the ground. Although brief, the duration of contractions is somewhat longer than in myoclonic seizures.

Vocalization may occur as a result of contraction of thoracic muscles forcing air past the larynx, and brief periods of apnea and postictal tiredness may be associated.

Atonic Seizures

In atonic seizures, a very sudden decrease in muscle tone occurs, leading to a head drop, drooping of a limb, or loss of all muscle tone resulting in falling. The risk of injury is high in these sudden "drop attacks." Atonic seizures are more common in children.

Attaining good control of tonic or atonic seizures is difficult. Valproate, felbamate, lamotrigine, benzodiazepines and topiramate have proven effective in some individuals.

Clonic Seizures

Clonic seizures nearly always occur in babies or young children. A loss or impairment of consciousness occurs simultaneously with a decrease in muscle tone, or with a generalized tonic contraction, and is followed by period of asymmetric jerking motions.

Tonic-Clonic (Grand Mal) Seizures

Generalized tonic-clonic seizures represent a maximal epileptic response of the brain. These seizures are characterized by the absence of an aura, tonic stiffening of all muscle groups causing the patient to fall. The initial contraction may be flexor and is rapidly followed by prolonged extension. Subsequently, there is a period of bilateral symmetric jerking of the extremities. The seizure may be associated with loss of bladder control and biting of the tongue or inside of the mouth. There is a pronounced postictal state following the seizure, and the person may pass directly into sleep before waking several hours later.

Status Epilepticus

Status epilepticus is a condition in which there is a single prolonged seizure lasting more than five minutes, or insufficient time between multiple seizures to permit recovery. Several types exist, depending on the type of seizure is involved, i.e., tonic-clonic, simple partial, complex partial or absence. Tonic-clonic status epilepticus is both the most common and most life-threatening. Pharmacologic treatment of most forms of status epilepticus may include intravenous administration of diazepam or lorazepam, fosphenytoin, and lastly phenobarbital. Although lorazepam is not approved by the FDA for this purpose, it is sometimes preferred due to its longer half-life.

Absence status epilepticus is a condition of impaired consciousness, perhaps including mild motor symptoms, which lasts from 30 minutes to 12 hours. It can be distinguished from ongoing seizures due to organic or toxic causes by the spike and wave EEG pattern characteristic of absence seizures. The usual pharmacologic treatment of absence status employs diazepam or lorazepam, followed by ethosuximide.

MECHANISMS OF ACTION FOR THE ANTISEIZURE DRUGS

Seizures are due to bursts of abnormal synchronous discharging by a network of neurons. Although the mechanisms of seizure generation are still poorly understood, the causes of abnormal firing appear to involve neuronal ion channels and an imbalance between excitatory and inhibitory synaptic function. Various AEDs exhibit different combinations of actions on neuronal function, causing them to show selective efficacy against different seizure types (12).

Ion Channels

Sodium and chloride ions are present at greater concentration outside the cell, while potassium, organic cations and charged proteins are more numerous within the cell. Since the membrane is permeable to only small ions but not large ions or proteins, the neuronal membranes maintain a charge separation, resulting in a "resting potential" in the range -50 to -80 mV vs the outside of the cell.

An increase in interior negativity, termed "hyperpolarization," decreases the resting potential (e.g., to -90 mV), thus making it more difficult for a neuron to reach threshold and subsequently fire.

A reduction in interior negativity, termed "depolarization," can result in generation of an action potential if the depolarization is sufficient to reach threshold (app. -40 mV). Neuronal firing is initiated by an influx of sodium ions.

After each depolarization, voltage-dependent sodium channels adopt an inactive state and remain refractory to re-opening for a period of time. While the channels are unable to open, rapid repetitive firing is diminished, and spread of electrical seizure activity to adjacent brain regions is suppressed (13). Stabilization and prolongation of this inactive state appears to be the primary mechanism of action of phenytoin, carbamazepine and lamotrigine, and may be instrumental in the antiseizure actions of phenobarbital, oxcarbazepine, valproate, topiramate and zonisamide (12).

Synaptic Inhibition and Excitation

For a neuron, whether or not an action potential is generated depends on the balance between excitatory and inhibitory stimulation. GABA is the predominant inhibitory neurotransmitter in the brain. It is synthesized from the amino acid, glutamic acid, by glutamic acid decarboxylase (GAD), and inactivated by GABA-transaminase (GABA-T). GABA binds to two receptor types, $GABA_A$ and $GABA_B$. $GABA_A$ receptors occur on chloride ion channels and the binding of GABA causes chloride influx and neuronal hyperpolarization. $GABA_B$ receptors are linked via G proteins and second messengers to potassium and calcium channel activity, also mediating inhibition in the CNS (14). $GABA_B$ receptors may also play a role in oscillatory rhythms in some forms of epilepsy (15).

A number of AEDs augment GABA-mediated inhibition or affect GABA concentration. Benzodiazepines, barbiturates, and perhaps topiramate enhance the action of GABA on the $GABA_A$ chloride channel. Tiagabine decreases the reuptake of GABA; vigabatrin (an investigational drug) and perhaps gabapentin decrease its metabolism.

Glutamate provides excitatory neurotransmission via the N-methyl-D-aspartate (NMDA), α-amino-3-hydroxy-5-methyl-4-isoxazole propionate (AMPA), and kainate receptors. Activation of these ligand-gated channels enables sodium and calcium influx, and potassium efflux, facilitating depolarization. Blockade of the NMDA receptor by felbamate and remacemide (an investigational drug) or of the AMPA receptor by phenobarbital and topiramate, inhibits depolarization (12,16).

Aberrant Calcium Signaling

Low threshold T-type calcium currents act as pacemakers for normal brain activity, particularly the thalamic oscillatory currents thought to be involved in the generation of absence seizures (15,17). Drugs such as ethosuximide, the oxazolidinediones, and zonisamide which inhibit T-type currents, are effective against absence seizures, but ineffective against partial or other seizure types.

ANTISEIZURE DRUGS
Introduction

The primary use of antiseizure drugs (most commonly referred to as AEDs) is in the prevention and control of epileptic seizures. According to Toman (18), the ideal AED among other things, should completely suppress seizures in doses that do not cause sedation or other undesired central nervous system toxicity. It should be well tolerated and highly effective against various types of seizures, and devoid of undesirable side effects on vital organs and functions. Its onset of action should be rapid after parenteral injection for control of status epilepticus, and it should have a long duration of effect after oral administration for prevention of recurrent seizures.

The first effective remedy, potassium bromide, was introduced by Locock (19) in 1857. This drug was largely replaced by phenobarbital in 1912 when Hauptmann (20) tried this sedative in epilepsy. Its great value was recognized at once, and it is still commonly prescribed.

The usefulness of both bromide and phenobarbital in convulsive disorders was discovered by chance, but phenytoin was developed in 1937 as the result of a study of potential AED in animals by Putnam and Merritt (21,22). Bromide is highly effective in man and is relatively nonsedating. Treatment of convulsive disorders by using bromide, phenobarbital, and phenytoin constitutes an important advance in clinical therapy.

Many of the standard AEDs that contain the ureide structure as shown in Figure 16.1 have been used clinically for more than 30 years without much change in their ureide structures. Small changes in the X substituent of the ureide

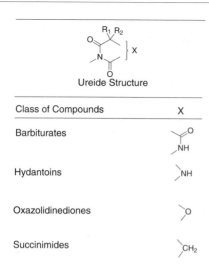

Fig. 16.1. Structure of anticonvulsant drugs containing the ureide structure.

structure can cause significant changes in the type of seizures controlled, which will be discussed for each of the respective drugs. As a result of rapid developments in molecular biologic techniques for the study of the neurophysiology of epilepsy and in the interactions of AEDs with neurotransmitters at ion channels or brain receptors (AMPA/kainate glutamate receptors), a new generation of clinically available AEDs have emerged (23). These AEDs include felbamate, gabapentin, lamotrigine, levetiracetam, oxcarbazepine, tiagabine, topiramate, and zonisamide; vigabatrin remains investigational. Their mechanisms of action are targeted towards ion channels and brain receptors by either enhancing brain GABA activity (e.g., tiagabine and vigabatrin) or inhibition of excitatory amino acids (GABA) (e.g., lamotrigine and felbamate). These new generation AEDs also exhibit limited drug interactions with fewer adverse effects (24). A rational approach to the drug discovery process is necessary in order to develop new leads to novel effective therapy, and to use structure-activity relationships to fine-tune the pharmacology of existing AEDs with the same or better efficacy and fewer adverse effects (25).

Approximately 60% of patients with epilepsy become seizure-free with monotherapy using frontline therapeutic drugs such as carbamazepine, phenytoin, valproate, ethosuximide, phenobarbital, and benzodiazepine; another 20% have their epilepsy controlled with more than one AED. Despite recent advances in neurobiology and significant insight into the molecular dysfunction of epilepsy, the remaining 20% do not completely respond to the current frontline therapeutic drugs, and are most often presribed more than two AEDs without any obvious benefit (11). Recently, much effort has been made to discover new AEDs effective in refractory seizures and partial complex seizures.

Seizure control requires continuous antiseizure action and is not achievable unless plasma concentrations remain relatively consistent at therapeutic levels throughout all 24 hours of the day. Therefore, a knowledge of the therapeutic

ranges of plasma concentrations, time to peak serum concentrations and elimination half-lives help guide AED administration to achieve consistent therapeutic serum concentrations that control seizures without causing intolerable toxicity (26). Enzymatic biotransformation is the principal determinant of the pharmacokinetic properties for most AEDs, although some drugs are excreted by the kidneys predominantly as unchanged drug. Most AEDs exhibit linear enzyme kinetics, in which changes in daily dose lead to proportional changes in serum concentration if clearance remains constant. However, the traditional concept of administering a drug at intervals equal to one elimination half-life does not apply to some drugs, where the half-life of biologic activity may exceed its elimination half-life. The standard AEDs have the greatest potential to be involved in pharmacokinetic drug interactions when they are co-administered with other AEDs or other drugs (27). These interactions usually involve changes in the rate of biotransformation or in the protein binding of one or both co-administered drugs (26). Drug-induced changes in the pharmacokinetics for many of the AEDs are particularly pronounced in children, requiring a higher oral dose/kg than in adults to obtain an effective plasma concentration (28).

This chapter surveys the SAR, mechanism of action, the metabolism and the pharmacokinetic parameters for the new generation of AEDs, felbamate, gabapentin, lamotrigine, oxcarbazepine, levetiracetam, tiagabine, topiramate, zonisamide and vigabatrin, and the standard AEDs, phenytoin, carbamazepine, phenobarbital, primidone, valproate, ethosuximide and the benzodiazepines, as well as several of the older AEDs that are less commonly used today. The application of AEDs in the treatment of various kinds of epilepsies is shown in Figure 16.2. This illustration is based on AEDs used in clinical therapy. Table 16.2 lists the AED, its mechanism of action and some of their pharmacokinetic properties. Table 16.3 lists the usual pediatric dosages and Table 16.4 the usual adult dosages for the antiseizure drugs.

Drugs Effective Against Partial and Generalized Tonic-Clonic Seizures
Hydantoins

The hydantoins have a 5-membered ring structure containing 2 nitrogens in an ureide configuration and were tested as antiepileptics by Merritt and Putnam (21,22). These drugs suppressed electrically induced convulsions in animals but were ineffective against convulsions induced by pentylenetetrazole, picrotoxin, or bicuculline. The structure for the clinically available hydantoins are listed in Figure 16.3.

Phenytoin (Diphenylhydantoin). Phenytoin is the prototype and most commonly prescribed member of the hydantoin family of drugs. Bioequivalency is a problem with the hydantoins because of their very poor water solubility and a low therapeutic ratio. In addition, phenytoin exhibits non-linear pharmacokinetics that exaggerate the

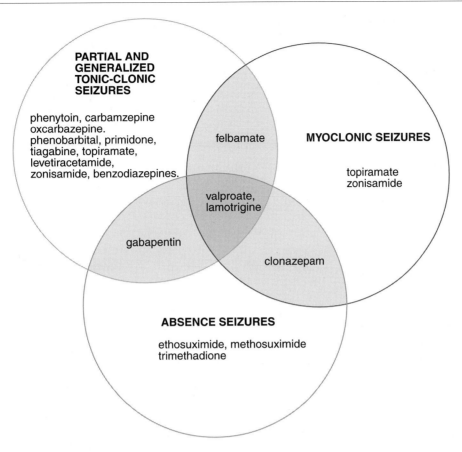

Fig. 16.2. The antiseizure drugs used in treatment of the various seizures.

Table 16.2. Mechanism(s) of Action and Pharmacokinetics for Antiseizure Drugs

Drug	Mechanism of Action*	Elimination Half-life in Children (hr)	Elimination Half-life in Adults (hr)	Time to Steady -state Plasma Concentration (hr)	Protein Binding (%)	Log P (pH 7.4)
Carbamazepine (Tegretol)	A	14–27 (children), 8–28 (neonates)	14–27	2–8	66–89	2.2
Clonazepam (Klonopin)	A,B	20–40	20–40	—	95–98	2.3
Diazepam (Diastat)	A,B	17	36	—	40	2.6
Ethosuximide (Zarontin)	C	20–60	20–60	7–10	0	0.38
Gabapentin (Neurontin)	E	—	5–7	—	0	
Lamotrigine (Lamictal)	A,D	—	See text	—	55	
Oxcarbazepine (Trileptal)	A	—	7–11†	2–3	40	
Phenobarbital	A,B	37–73	40–136	12–21	40–60	1.53
Phenytoin (Dilantin)	A	5–14 (children), 10–60 (neonates)	12–36	7–28	69–96	2.39 p OH metabolite 1.72
Primidone (Mysoline)	A,B	5–11	6–18	4–7	0	0.91
Tiagabine (Gabitril)	A	—	4–7	2	96	
Topiramate (Topamax)	A,B,D	10–15, 6–8‡	20–30 12–15‡	—	15	
Valproic acid (Depakene, Depakote, Depacon)	A,B	8–15	6–15	1–4 3–5 (sustained release)	80–95	0.13
Zonisamide (Zonegran)	A,C	—	27–46	10–12	40	

*See Mechanism of Action section of this chapter for discussion.
†Monohydroxy metabolite.
‡In the presence of enzyme-inducing drugs such as carbamazepine, phenobarbital, or primidone.
A, sodium currents; B, γ-aminobutiric acid-A receptor currents; C, T-calcium currents; D, glutamate receptor antagonist; E, unknown.

Table 16.3. Usual Pediatric Dosages for the Antiseizure Drugs

Drug	Starting Dose	Dosing Regimen	Daily Dose Increase/ Time Interval	Maintenance Dose	Therapeutic Range of Plasma conc. (μg/mL)
Carbamazepine Extended Release (Carbatrol, Tegretol-XR)	6–12: 200 mg/d >12 yr: 400 mg/d	b.i.d.	6–12: 100 mg/ 1 wk >12: up to 200 mg/ 1 wk	10–30 mg/kg/d	4–12
Carbamazepine (Tegretol)	<6yr: 10–15 mg/kg/d 6–12 yr: 100 mg b.i.d.	t.i.d.	<6 yr: 5 mg/kg/1 wk >6 yr: 100–200 mg/1 wk	10–30 mg/kg/d	4–12
Clonazepam (Klonopin)	<10 yr or <30 kg: 0.01–0.3 mg/kg/d>10 yr: 1–1.5 mg/d	t.i.d.–q.i.d.	<10 yr: 0.02 mg/kg/1 wk >10 yr: 0.5 mg/1 wk	0.1–0.3 mg/kg/d	0.02–0.08
Diazepam (Diastat)	See text				
Ethosuximide (Zarontin)	<6 yr: 10–15 mg/kg, not to exceed 250 mg/d >6 yr: 250 mg/d	t.i.d.–q.i.d.	125–250 mg/1 wk	15–40 mg/kg/d	40–100
Gabapentin (Neurontin)	10 mg/kg/d	t.i.d.	300 mg/1 d	30–100 mg/kg/d	Not established
Lamotrigine (Lamictal)	On enzyme inducers: 1 mg/kg/d On enzyme inducers and inhibitors (valproate): 0.3–0.5 mg/kg/d On enzyme inhibitor: 0.1–0.3 mg/kg/d Monotherapy: 0.5 mg/kg/	t.i.d.–b.i.d.	On enzyme inducers: 1 mg/kg/ 2 wk On enzyme inducers and inhibitors (valproate): 0.3–0.5 mg/kg/2 wk On enzyme inhibitor: 0.1–0.3 mg/kg/2 wk Monotherapy: 0.5 mg/kg/2 wk	On enzyme inducers: 15 mg/kg/d On enzyme inducers and inhibitors (valproate): 10 mg/kg/d On enzyme inhibitor: 5 mg/kg/d Monotherapy: 10 mg/kg/d	Not established
Phenobarbital	<1 yr: 3–5 mg/kg/d >1 yr: 2–4 mg/kg/d	b.i.d.–q.d.	1–2 mg/kg/2 wk	<1 yr: 3–5 mg/kg >1 yr: 2–4 mg/kg	10–40
Phenytoin (Dilantin)	5 mg/kg/d	b.i.d.	1–2 mg/kg/2 wk	5–8 mg/kg/d	10–25
Primidone (Mysoline)	<6 yr: 50 mg/d >12 yr: 100 mg/d	q.i.d.–t.i.d.	25–50 mg/2 wk	12–25 mg/kg/d	5–12
Tiagabine (Gabitril)	0.05–0.10 mg/kg/d (not to exceed 4 mg)	b.i.d.–q.i.d.	0.05–0.10 mg/kg/ 1wk	1–2 mg/kg/d	Not established
Topiramate (Topamax)	1–3 mg/kg/d	b.i.d.	1–3 mg/kg/wk or 2 wk	5–9 mg/kg/d	Not established
Valproic Acid (Depakene)	15–20 mg/kg/d	q.i.d.–t.i.d.	5–10 mg/kg/ 1 wk	30–80 mg/kg/d	50–150
Divalproex sodium (Depakote)	10–15 mg/kg/d	b.i.d.	5–10 mg/kg/ 1 wk	>60 mg/kg/d	50–100

Note: Only drugs marketed in September 1999 are included.

effects of changes in the fraction of dose absorbed (29). Its apparent pKa is in the range 8.06–8.33 and thus can form a water soluble sodium salt. Aqueous solutions of phenytoin sodium (pH 11–12) gradually absorb carbon dioxide neutralizing the alkalinity of the solution causing partial hydrolysis and crystallization of free phenytoin resulting in turbid solutions. When phenytoin sodium is administered I.M., its absorption may be erratic as a result of crystallization of insoluble phenytoin at the injection site because of the decrease in pH from 11.5. Phenytoin sodium injection is physically and chemically incompatible with parenteral solutions of many drugs, especially salts of basic drugs. The nature of the incompatibility depends on several factors, including the type of salt, concentrations of the drugs, diluents used, resulting pH, and temperature.

Mechanism of Action. Phenytoin is indicated for initial or adjunctive treatment of complex partial (psychomotor) or generalized tonic-clonic seizures, and status epilepticus. It is often selected for initial monotherapy due to its high efficacy and relatively low incidence of side effects (30).

Table 16.4. Usual Adult Dosages of Antiseizure Drugs (16 Years and Older)

Drug	Starting Dose (mg/d)	Dosing Regimen	Daily Dose Increase/ Time Interval	Maintenance Dose (mg/d)	Maximum Dose (mg/d)	Therapeutic Range of Plasma Concentration (μg/mL)
Carbamazepine (Tegretol)	200	Carbatrol or Tegretol-XR b.i.d.; other forms t.i.d.	200/1 wk	600–1,200	1,600	4–12
Clonazepam (Klonopin)	1.5	t.i.d.	0.5/4 d	2–6	20	0.02–0.08
Diazepam (Diastat)	See text					
Ethosuximide (Zarontin)	500	t.i.d.	250/1 wk	1,000–2,000	—	40–120
Gabapentin (Neurontin)	300	t.i.d.	300/daily	900–3,600	—	Not established
Lamotrigine (Lamictal)	See text	b.i.d.	See text	See text	700	Not established
Phenobarbital	90	q.d.[†]	30/4 wk	90–120	—	10–40
Phenytoin (Dilantin)	300	q.d.[†]	30–100/4 wk[‡]	300–500	—	10–40
Primidone (Mysoline)	100–125	t.i.d.	See text	750–1,000	2,000	5–12
Tiagabine (Gabitril)	4	b.i.d.–q.i.d.	4–8/1 wk	32–56	56	Not established
Topiramate (Topamax)	25–50	b.i.d.	See text	200–400	1,600	Not established
Valproic acid (Depakene) (Depakote)	1,000	Valproic acid t.i.d.; Divalproex sodium b.i.d.	250/1 wk	1,000–3,000	4,000 (60 mg/kg/d)	50–150

[†]Once-daily drugs are usually given at bedtime to avoid toxicity associated with peak plasma concentrations.
[‡]Increments of 100 mg/d if plasma concentration below 10 mg/mL; increments of 30 to 50 mg/d if plasma concentration is above 10 mg/mL.
Note: Only drugs marketed in September 1999 are included.

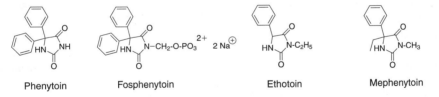

Fig. 16.3. Hydantoins.

Phenytoin is not used in the treatment of absence seizures as it may increase their frequency of occurrence (31). Phenytoin binds to and stabilizes the inactivated state of sodium channels, thus producing a use-dependent blockade of repetitive firing, and inhibition of the spread of seizure activity to adjacent cortical areas (32).

Pharmacokinetics. Phenytoin sodium from immediate release capsules is rapidly absorbed and generally attains peak serum concentration in 1.5–3 hours, while extended release phenytoin sodium is more slowly absorbed attaining peak serum concentration in 4–12 hours. The oral bioavailability for phenytoin may vary enough among formulations from different manufacturers to result in a subtherapeutic serum concentration and therefore ineffective in controlling seizures or a toxic blood concentration. Therapeutic plasma concentrations for phenytoin are usually 7.5–20 μg/mL, although in some patients, seizure control is not achieved at these plasma concentrations. Phenytoin is highly protein bound (Table 16.2).

Phenytoin is metabolized predominately by CYP2C9 to its primary metabolite, 5-(hydroxyphenyl)-5-phenylhydantoin (HPPH) (33). Approximately 60–75% of an oral dose is excreted as HPPH glucuronide or sulfate metabolites, about 1% is excreted unchanged in urine and some undergoes enterohepatic circulation. Other minor metabolites also appear in urine. Up to 10% of the oral phenytoin may be excreted unchanged by the kidneys at toxic doses. Phenytoin is notorious for displaying non-linear pharmacokinetics because the route of metabolism is a saturable process. Therefore, small increases in dosage may produce substantial increases in plasma phenytoin concentrations (refer to Fig. 7.7); the steady-state plasma concentration (C_p) may double or triple from a 10% or more increase in dosage, possibly resulting in toxicity. Phenytoin also induces CYP3A4 and UDP glucuronyltransferases (increased glu-

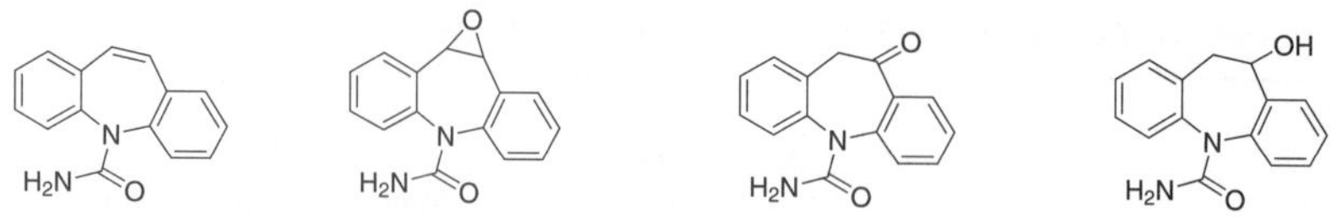

Carbamazepine   Carbamazepine   Oxcarbazepine   10-Hydroxy-
              10,11 epoxide   oxcarbazepine

Fig. 16.4. Iminostilbenes.

curonidation). Therefore, plasma concentrations for drugs metabolized by these isoforms will be affected (See Chapter 8). Thus, the addition of phenytoin to an AED regimen can reduce their plasma levels by inducing their CYP3A4 metabolism for carbamazepine, felbamate, lamotrigine, oxcarbazepine, tiagabine, valproate and zonisamide. Other drugs whose metabolism is induced by phenytoin include methadone, theophylline, warfarin, and oral contraceptives. On the other hand, plasma phenytoin levels are increased by carbamazepine, felbamate, cimetidine, warfarin, chloramphenicol, isoniazid and disulfiram. Plasma phenytoin levels are decreased by rifampin, antacids, valproate (free phenytoin levels remain the same).

The pharmacokinetics of phenytoin is significantly affected by age. Its rate of elimination is strongly dose-dependent (non-linear) at all ages. The elimination half-life for phenytoin in children increases with age due to an age-dependent decrease in its rate of metabolism (28). The combination of these factors makes it difficult to predict the phenytoin plasma concentrations following the administration of a dose (dose/kg) adjustments in neonates and children, particularly when phenytoin is co-administered with other liver enzyme-inducing AED, such as phenobarbital and carbamazepine.

Adverse Effects. Drug interactions, especially with other AED and CYP3A4 substrates, are extensive. Although toxic effects may begin in the upper normal plasma range (>20 µg/mL), serious toxicity is rare. Central nervous system effects are most frequent and include nystagmus, ataxia, dysarthria, and sedation. Gingival hyperplasia, usually reversible, is common. Idiosyncratic reactions such as rash, agranulocytosis, thrombocytopenia, lymphadenopathy, Stevens-Johnson syndrome, and hepatitis have occurred. Too rapid administration of I.V. phenytoin sodium can result in severe hypotension and fatal cardiotoxicity.

The incidence of phenytoin toxicity may be increased in the elderly, or in those patients with hepatic or renal impairment because of alterations in its pharmacokinetics. Plasma level determinations may be indicated in these cases. There is a 2–3% increase in the risk of fetal epilepsy syndrome if the mother is taking phenytoin. Phenytoin is contraindicated in cardiac patients with bradyarrhythmias.

Fosphenytoin (Cerebyx). Fosphenytoin sodium (Fig. 16.3) is a soluble prodrug phosphate ester of phenytoin which was developed as a replacement for parenteral phenytoin sodium to circumvent the pH and solubility problems associated with parenteral phenytoin sodium formulations (34). Unlike phenytoin, fosphenytoin is freely soluble in aqueous solutions and is rapidly absorbed by the IM route. It is rapidly metabolized (conversion half-life of 8–15 minutes) to phenytoin by in vivo phosphatases. Therapeutic free (unbound) and total plasma phenytoin concentrations are consistently attained following IM or I.V. administration of fosphenytoin (26). It is administered I.V. following benzodiazepines for control of status epilepticus, or whenever there is a need to rapidly achieve therapeutic plasma concentrations. Recently, severe cardiovascular adverse events to fosphenytoin, including some fatalities, have been reported. A dose reduction in the elderly or in renal or hepatic impairment has been suggested.

Ethotoin (Peganone). Ethotoin differs from phenytoin in that one phenyl substituent at position 5 has been replaced by hydrogen, and the N-H at position 3 is replaced by an ethyl group (Fig. 16.3). It may be indicated for treatment of tonic-clonic and complex partial (psychomotor) seizures. As it is considered less toxic but less effective and more sedating than phenytoin, ethotoin is usually reserved for use as an add-on drug (35). Ethotoin does not share phenytoin's profile of antiarrhythmic action. The metabolism of ethotoin, like phenytoin, is saturable and nonlinear. Its administration is contraindicated in patients with hepatic abnormalities and hematologic disorders.

Mephenytoin. Mephenytoin is N-methylated at position 3 with an ethyl group replacing one of the phenyl substituents at position 5 (Fig. 16.3). It is indicated for focal and Jacksonian seizures in patients refractory to less toxic AEDs. Mephenytoin produces more sedation than phenytoin, and should be used only when safer drugs have failed, as it is associated with an increased incidence of serious toxicities such as severe rash, agranulocytosis, and hepatitis (36). Its N-desmethyl metabolite, 5-phenyl-5-ethylhydantoin, contributes to both efficacy and toxicity for mephenytoin. The manufacturer has announced plans to discontinue production of this drug.

Iminostilbenes

Carbamazepine. Carbamazepine (CBZ) (Fig. 16.4) was approved by the U.S. FDA in 1974, and it is presently indicated as initial or adjunctive therapy for complex partial, tonic-clonic, and mixed-type seizures. It is one of the two safest and most effective of the older AEDs for these seizure types (phenytoin is the other) and is chosen for monotherapy due to its high effectiveness and relatively low incidence of side effects (36). Its tricyclic structure resembles that of the psychoactive drugs imipramine, chlorpromazine, and maprotiline and also shares some structural features with the AEDs phenytoin, clonazepam, and phenobarbital.

Mechanism of Action. In animals, the profile of antiseizure properties for CBZ is similar to that of phenytoin (12). CBZ is effective in the MES test (electrically induced seizure test) but ineffective against pentylenetetrazole-induced seizures. It is not effective for absence seizures, and may indeed exacerbate their onset (31). Like phenytoin, CBZ acts on voltage-dependent sodium channels to prevent the spread of seizures (37). CBZ depresses synaptic transmission in the reticular activating system, thalamus, and limbic structures. In a double-blind crossover study in patients whose seizures were not controlled completely by combinations of AED, CBZ was equal in efficacy to phenobarbital and phenytoin in controlling seizure frequency, and side effects were minimal.

Pharmacokinetics. Following the administration of an oral dose, CBZ is slowly absorbed with the attainment of peak concentration from immediate release tablets in 4–5 hours and from extended-release tablets in 3–12 hours. The normal half-life averages between 12–17 hours; however, because of autoinduction, the half-life may range from 8–29 hours. The half-life for carbamazepine-10,11-epoxide is 5–8 hours. Therapeutic plasma concentrations range from 4–12 μg/mL (in adults) and may require a month to achieve a stable therapeutic concentration for the desired antiseizure effect because of induction of hepatic metabolizing enzymes.

CBZ is principally metabolized by CYP3A4 its 10,11-epoxide, with CYP2C8 and CYP1A2 having minor roles. CBZ epoxide is hydrolyzed to inactive 10, 11-dihydroxyCBZ by epoxide hydrolase. CBZ epoxide is active and appears to be more toxic than CBZ(38). However, CBZ not only induces CYP3A4 activity but its own metabolism (an autoinducer), as well as inducing UDP-glucuronyltransferases (UGT) and the increased formation of glucuronide metabolites. Like phenytoin, CBZ is highly protein bound (Table 16.2), and extensively transformed. About 72% of an oral dose is excreted in the urine as metabolites and 3% as unchanged drug. The 28% found in the feces may be the result of incomplete absorption and enterohepatic cycling. As previously mentioned, interindividual variability in apparent plasma half-life and total body clearance is related to the phenomenon of autoinduction.

Adverse Effects. Gastric upset from CBZ may be diminished by taking the drug after meals. Common toxicities include blurred vision, dizziness, drowsiness ataxia and headache. Tremor, depression and cardiac disturbances are seen at high serum concentrations. Idiosyncratic rashes are common; rarer severe idiosyncratic effects include anemia, agranulocytosis, thrombocytopenia and jaundice. Therefore, patients receiving CBZ should have periodic blood count determinations and liver function tests. CBZ increases phenytoin levels, and decreases levels of felbamate, lamotrigine, oral contraceptives, theophylline, valproate, and zonisamide. CBZ levels are increased by propoxyphene, erythromycin, chloramphenicol, isoniazid, verapamil and cimetidine. CBZ levels are decreased by phenobarbital, phenytoin, felbamate, and primidone. Lamotrigine may elevate CBZ epoxide levels.

Macrolide antibiotics inhibit CBZ metabolism, thus increasing CBZ plasma levels and decreased clearance with the potential for toxicity effects. Drug-induced changes in CBZ pharmacokinetics are particularly pronounced in children (28).

CBZ should be used with caution in patients with a history of congestive heart failure or cardiac arrhythmias, as it may aggravate them, and with a history of hematologic reactions to other drugs or hypersensitivity to tricyclic antidepressants. Blood levels should be monitored in patients with renal or hepatic impairment.

Oxcarbazepine. Oxcarbazepine is the 10-keto analog of carbamazepine (Fig. 16.4) and is indicated as monotherapy or adjunctive therapy for partial seizures in adults with epilepsy, and adjunctive therapy for the treatment of partial seizures in children 4–16 years of age with epilepsy (40).

Mechanism of Action. Although oxcarbazepine is less potent that CBZ, its mechanism of action is similar (39). The majority of the pharmacologic activity for oxcarbazepine is attributed to its primary metabolite, 10-monohydroxycarbazepine (MHD) (Fig. 16.4), whose plasma levels may be nine times higher than that for CBZ. Both oxcarbazepine and MHD produce a blockade of voltage-dependent sodium channels, thus decreasing repetitive firing and spread of electrical activity. An additional action on calcium channels may contribute to the therapeutic effect (41).

Pharmacokinetics. Oxcarbazepine is completely absorbed and food has no effect on its absorption. Unlike CBZ, it does not cause autoinduction of its own metabolism. The metabolism of oxcarbazepine is different from that of CBZ. Oxcarbazepine is reduced by cytosolic enzymes to MHD prior to its O-glucuronidation. More than 95% of its oral dose is excreted as metabolites with approximately 4% of the drug converted to inactive 10,11-dihydroxyCBZ. Unlike CBZ, no epoxide metabolite is formed. The half-life for oxcarbazepine is 2 hours and for the active 10-monohydroxy metabolite, 9 hours. In patients with impaired renal function, the half-life for MHD is prolonged to 19 hours, with a doubling in its area under the plasma concentration curve (AUC). Peak plasma concentration following an oral dose occurs at about 4.5 hours.

Oxcarbazepine induces CYP3A4/5 and UDP-glucuronosyltransferase, and also inhibits CYP2C19 producing significant effects on plasma concentration of other drugs. Therefore, oxcarbazepine decreases felodipine bioavailability, and lowers plasma levels for lamotrigine, CBZ, CBZ epoxide, calcium channel blockers and oral contraceptives (42,43,44). Oxcarbazepine increases plasma levels of phenobarbital and phenytoin. The plasma levels for oxcarbazepine or MHD is decreased by CBZ, phenobarbital, phenytoin, valproate and verapamil. Oxcarbazepine clearance is decreased in renal impairment and the elderly. In children, a higher dose/kg for oxcarbazepine than for adults is required to obtain an effective plasma concentration.

Adverse Effects. Patients with hypersensitivity reactions to carbamazepine can be expected to show cross-sensitivity (e.g., rash) or related problems to oxcarbazepine. The improved toxicity profile for oxcarbazepine when compared to CBZ may be due to absence of the epoxide metabolite (39,45). The most common side effects are headache, dizziness, somnolence, nausea, ataxia, and fatigue. Adverse effects on cognitive status have been reported as well as hyponatremia. (46,47).

Barbiturates

The barbiturates are substituted pyrimidine derivatives with an ureide configuration (Fig. 16.1). They are lipophilic weak acids that are well distributed into brain (see Appendix I for the respective pKa). Although many barbiturates display sedative-hypnotic activity (Chapter 15), only a few have antiseizure properties. Paradoxically, many barbiturates cause convulsions at larger doses. The barbiturates clinically useful as AEDs are phenobarbital, mephobarbital, and primidone (Table 16.2 and Fig. 16.5). In laboratory animals, phenobarbital is effective by several tests in nontoxic doses. It is active against electrically induced seizures (MES), and it elevates the threshold for pentylenetetrazole stimulation. The mechanism of antiseizure action for the barbiturates is unknown, but thought to involve blockade of sodium channels and enhancement of GABA-mediated inhibitory transmission.

Phenobarbital. Phenobarbital is commonly used for convulsive disorders and is the drug of choice for seizures in infants up to 2 months old. Phenobarbital is indicated for the treatment of partial and generalized tonic-clonic seizures in all age groups, although it is less effective than phenytoin or CBZ in adults (36). Although occasionally used as monotherapy, it is usually combined with another AED (48). Phenobarbital may be administered parent-

erally as its sodium salt for emergency control of acute convulsive disorders associated with eclampsia (although magnesium sulfate is the standard treatment), meningitis, tetanus, and toxic reactions to strychnine or local anesthetics. Due to its slow onset of action, it is administered after benzodiazepines for the treatment of status epilepticus.

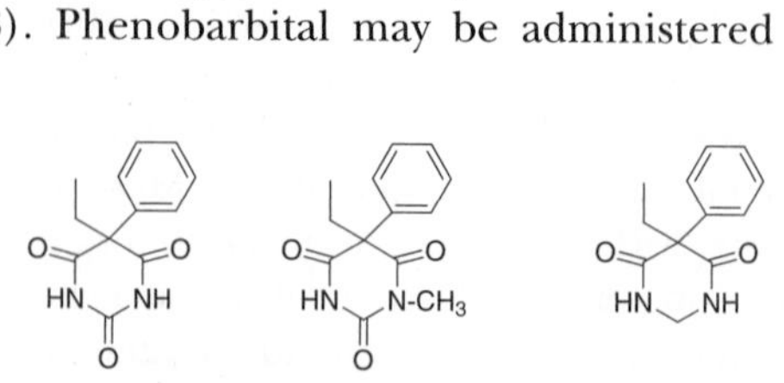

Pharmacokinetics. Phenobarbital is a weak acid (pKa 7.4) that is approximately 50% ionized at physiologic pH and is well distributed into the CNS. Its absorption is slow but nearly complete and shows linear kinetics. Phenobarbital is 40–60% protein bound and exhibits a long plasma half-life of 2–6 days, which yields an extremely stable plasma concentration. Approximately 25–50% of a phenobarbital dose is excreted unchanged in the urine. The remainder is metabolized primarily by hydroxylation to its inactive metabolite, 5-*p*-hydroxyphenyl-5-ethyl-barbituric acid, which is then conjugated as its glucuronide or sulfate and excreted in the urine. Some of the metabolites may appear in the feces from enterohepatic cycling. Alkalinization of the urine or increasing the urine flow substantially increases the rate of excretion of unchanged phenobarbital and its metabolites. Phenobarbital is a potent liver enzyme-inducing drug of CYP3A4 and increases the ability of the liver to metabolize many drugs when taken concurrently that are normally metabolized by CYP3A4. It also induces UDP-glucuronyltransferases and increased formation of glucuronidation. However, there is no conclusive evidence that phenobarbital induces its own metabolism (autoinducer) as does CBZ.

Because of its inducing effect on hepatic enzymes, phenobarbital has many drug interactions; decreasing plasma levels of CBZ, valproate, lamotrigine, tiagabine, zonisamide, warfarin, theophylline, cimetidine and those of other CYP3A4 substrates. Serum concentrations of phenobarbital are increased by valproate.

Adverse Effects. Serious toxicity is rare; however, drowsiness is the most common side effect reported for phenobarbital. Of the barbiturates, only phenobarbital, mephobarbital and primidone are antiseizure at subhypnotic doses. The sedative effect of phenobarbital limits its use in older children and adults, although tolerance to the sedative effects often develops. When compared to phenytoin or CBZ, phenobarbital shows more sedation, irritability, paradoxical hyperactivity and impaired intellectual function (49). This may prove particularly troublesome in children, especially those of school age, and in the elderly. Quite rare are idiosyncratic reactions to phenobarbital that include rash, agranulocytosis, aplastic anemia and hepatitis. Long term use of phenobarbital may precipitate folate, vitamin K or vitamin D deficiencies.

Phenobarbital should be used with caution in patients with hepatic impairment, and therefore a dose reduction may be needed. It should be avoided in patients with renal

Phenobarbital   Mephobarbital   Primidone

Fig. 16.5. Barbiturates.

impairment. Barbiturates are known to cause fetal abnormalities and a neonatal coagulation defect responsive to vitamin K.

Mephobarbital (Mebaral). Mephobarbital is a barbiturate-derivative AED with a pKa of 7.7 (log P 1.84 pH 7.4). Approximately 50% of an oral dose of mephobarbital is absorbed from the GI tract. The plasma concentrations required for its therapeutic effects are unknown. The principal route of mephobarbital metabolism is N-demethylation by the liver to form phenobarbital, which may be excreted in the urine unchanged and as its p-hydroxy metabolite and glucuronide or sulfate conjugates (see Chapter 15 Fig. 15.3 for more details). About 75% of a single oral dose of mephobarbital is converted to phenobarbital. It has not been determined whether mephobarbital contributes to the antiseizure effect or whether it is due to its active metabolite, phenobarbital. Similarly, it is unclear whether mephobarbital, like phenobarbital, is a potent inducer of the enzymes involved in the metabolism of other drugs, but because the drug is chemically and pharmacologically similar to phenobarbital as well as being metabolized to phenobarbital, this possibility is likely.

Mephobarbital is less commonly used in the treatment of generalized and partial seizures. Like phenobarbital, it is classified as a long-acting barbiturate. No evidence exists that it is more effective than phenobarbital in equivalent doses, however it may be less sedating in children.

Primidone (Mysoline). Primidone is the 2-deoxy derivative of phenobarbital (Fig. 16.5) and is approved for initial or adjunctive treatment of simple partial, complex partial and tonic-clonic seizures. It is less effective against these types of seizures than is phenytoin or CBZ and shares the antiseizure and sedative actions of phenobarbital.

Pharmacokinetics. Approximately 60–80% of an oral dose of primidone is absorbed and slowly metabolized by the liver to phenobarbital and phenylethylmalonamide (50,51). While all three molecules have antiseizure effects, PEMA appears to be weaker and to be the more toxic metabolite. During chronic therapy, approximately 15–25% of an oral dose of primidone is excreted in the urine unchanged, 15–25% metabolized to phenobarbital, and 50–70% excreted as PEMA (half-life of 24–48 hours). The phenobarbital metabolite may be excreted in the urine unchanged and as its p-hydroxy metabolite, and as glucuronide or sulfate conjugates. Following an oral dose, the peak plasma levels for primidone are reached in about 4 hours with a reported half-life of 10–12 hours. Plasma concentrations in the range of 8–12 µg/mL control seizures and minimize adverse effects. Primidone shows antiseizure activity before the phenobarbital levels reach therapeutic range. Only after chronic dosing of primidone are the levels of phenobarbital significant, suggesting autoinduction. Serum levels of chronically administered primidone exceed those of its metabolite,

phenobarbital, thus demonstrating that it has antiseizure activity independent of phenobarbital. When primidone is co-administered with enzyme inducing AEDs, the levels of its phenobarbital metabolite may be two to three times higher than in the noninduced state. Protein binding of primidone and PEMA is negligible and the phenobarbital metabolite is approximately 50% protein bound.

Primidone use is associated with decreases in CBZ, lamotrigine, valproate, tiagabine, and zonisamide serum levels. Primidone levels are increased by nicotinamide and isoniazid. Hydantoins increase the plasma concentrations of primidone, phenobarbital and PEMA. CBZ increases levels of phenobarbital derived from primidone. Primidone levels are decreased by succinimides, CBZ and acetazolamide.

Adverse Effects. As with phenobarbital, serious toxicity for primidone is rare, although it may cause disabling sedation, irritability and decreased mental functioning in a number of persons. Ataxia, dysphoria, idiosyncratic rash, leukopenia, agranulocytosis, lymphadenopathy, hepatitis, and a systemic lupus erythematosus-like syndrome have been reported adverse effects for primidone. Deficiencies of folic acid, and vitamins D and K are possible with long term therapy of primidone, as well as producing a folate-responsive megaloblastic anemia. Measurement of the complete blood cell count should be performed at 6 month intervals (36).

Benzodiazepines

This class of drugs has been widely used as sedative-hypnotics and antianxiety drugs (Chapters 15 and 19). In laboratory animals, benzodiazepines display outstanding antiseizure properties against seizures induced by maximal electroshock and pentylenetetrazole. The benzodiazepines diazepam, lorazepam, clonazepam, clorazepate dipotassium and midazolam are effective for seizure control (Table 16.2 and Fig. 16.6). All benzodiazepines enter cerebral tissue rapidly. Although the duration of action is short for diazepam (<2 hours), for midazolam (3–4 hours), longer for clonazepam (24 hours), and much longer for lorazepam (up to 72 hours), there is no correlation with the

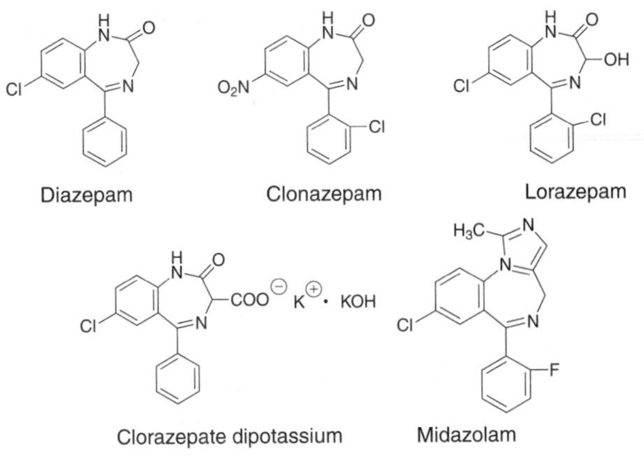

Fig. 16.6. Benzodiazepines.

plasma concentration-time profiles for these drugs (53). Diazepam and lorazepam can be administered either intravenously or intramuscularly for control of status epilepticus, however, absorption is slower from the intramuscular site (52). Midazolam is particularly useful for treating status epilepticus because its imidazole ring is open at low pH, allowing it to be dissolved in aqueous solution for intramuscular injection, but closed at physiologic pH, increasing lipophilicity with rapid intramuscular absorption, brain penetration, and fast onset of action. When administered intramuscularly, midazolam has a faster onset of action than diazepam and lorazepam because of its rapid absorption from the injection site with an efficacy at least equal to that of I.V. diazepam (53). Seizure arrest is usually attained within 5–10 minutes. Lorazepam, although not FDA approved for this purpose, is preferred by some clinicians for its longer duration of action (36).

Mechanism of Action. The benzodiazepines are thought to produce their antiseizure effects primarily by enhancing the effect of the inhibitory neurotransmitter GABA on the GABA$_A$ chloride channel. Additional evidence suggests that the benzodiazepines may diminish voltage-dependent sodium, potassium and calcium currents in a manner independent of the GABA$_A$/benzodiazepine receptor complex (54).

Diazepam. Diazepam is given orally for adjunctive control of convulsive disorders, as a rectal gel (Diastat) for refractory patients with epilepsy on a stable regimen of AEDs who require intermittent use of diazepam to control bouts of increased seizure activity, and parenterally as part of the regimen for treatment of status epilepticus or other severe recurrent seizures. Rectal diazepam gel is an effective and well-tolerated treatment for acute repetitive seizures (55,56).

Pharmacokinetics. Orally administered diazepam is less effective as an AED because tolerance to the antiseizure effects of diazepam develops within a short period. Diazepam gel (Diastat) is rapidly absorbed rectally, having greater than 90% bioavailability. In addition to cluster seizures, it has also been proven useful to control prolonged febrile seizures in children.

Intravenously administered diazepam is the route of choice for rapid control of status epilepticus (57.) Because of its high lipid solubility, intravenously administered diazepam enters the central nervous system rapidly, however the initial high brain concentration is reduced quickly because of its redistribution, thus status epilepticus may return (58). To prevent the return of status epilepticus, the initial diazepam dose is followed sequentially by parenteral phenytoin (fosphenytoin) and phenobarbital as needed for control of tonic-clonic status epilepticus. For absence status epilepticus, diazepam is usually followed by ethosuximide.

The half-life for diazepam is 46 hours and is metabolized by CYP2C19 and CYP3A4 to desmethyldiazepam, an active metabolite with a half-life of 71 hours. Diazepam is >95% protein bound. Cimetidine by inhibiting CYP3A4 decreases the metabolism and clearance of diazepam. Drugs which affect the activity of CYP2C19 or CYP3A4 may alter diazepam kinetics, and vice versa.

Adverse Effects. The most frequent side effect for diazepam is somnolence; dizziness, ataxia, headache, nervousness, euphoria and rash occur less frequently. Excessive use of rectal diazepam may produce rebound seizures (59). Intravenous administration may produce infrequent respiratory depression and hypotension. Other sedative drugs such as barbiturates, valproate, narcotics, phenothiazines, monoamine oxidase inhibitors and antidepressants can potentiate the effects of diazepam.

Because diazepam clearance is decreased in the elderly and in patients with hepatic insufficiency; a dosage reduction may be warranted. Intravenous diazepam should be used cautiously in patients who are elderly, very ill, or have limited pulmonary reserve, as respiratory depression has occurred. Rarely, I.V. diazepam is given to patients for absence status (typical and atypical) because it will precipitate tonic status epileptic.

Clonazepam. Clonazepam was approved in 1975 for monotherapy or adjunctive treatment of akinetic (atonic), myoclonic, and absence variant seizures (60). Clonazepam was also found to be effective in controlling absence seizures, but because of the high incidence of side effects, it is rated second to ethosuximide. It may be useful, however, in absence seizures when succinimide therapy has failed. It is considered a third-line drug after 1) ethosuximide or valproate and 2) lamotrigine or valproate for treatment of absence seizures.

Clonazepam is well-absorbed, 95–98% protein bound and extensively metabolized. Clonazepam displays a wide spectrum of antiseizure activities, and is one of the most potent AEDs. However, side effects are common, and the development of tolerance is more frequent than with ethosuximide or valproate. Sedation is prominent, especially early in treatment. Drowsiness, ataxia and behavioral changes may be disabling, but slowly increasing its dose over a two week period is recommended to minimize adverse effects. Diplopia, headaches, nystagmus and other neurologic effects have been reported with the use of clonazepam.

Serum levels of clonazepam are decreased by the enzyme inducing properties of phenobarbital, phenytoin and CBZ. Concurrent administration of amphetamines, methylphenidate, ethanol, antianxiety drugs or antipsychotics may cause CNS depression or altered respiration. The combined administration of clonazepam and valproate may cause absence status, and in patients displaying a mixed seizure pattern, clonazepam may precipitate grand mal seizures.

Clorazepate Dipotassium. Clorazepate dipotassium was approved for use as an AED by the U.S. Food and Drug Administration in 1981, and is less commonly used as adjunctive therapy for the management of partial seizures in adults and children over 9 years of age. Clorazepate is decarboxylated by the acidity of the stomach to desmethyldiazepam, which is also the major active metabolite of diazepam.

Therefore, clorazepate exhibits the profile and properties of diazepam.

Lorazepam (Ativan). Lorazepam is a benzodiazepine (Fig. 16.6) with a pKa value of 1.3 and 11.5. Its parenteral solutions are formulated with polyethylene glycol and dilution with diluents may cause its crystallization from solution. Lorazepam also is used intravenously or intramuscularly for the management of status epilepticus (61). Although intravenous diazepam has been used more extensively, some clinicians prefer intravenous lorazepam because of its more prolonged duration of effect. A long-acting AED such as intravenous phenytoin or fosphenytoin can be added to intravenous benzodiazepine therapy for the management of recurring seizures associated with status epilepticus.

Pharmacokinetics. Intramuscular lorazepam is slowly absorbed with peak plasma concentrations reached in approximately 60–90 minutes. The half-life for unconjugated lorazepam is about 16 hours when given intravenously or intramuscularly and is eliminated in the urine as its major metabolite, lorazepam 3-O-glucuronide. Lorazepam glucuronide has no demonstrable CNS activity in animals but has a half-life of about 18 hours. Lorazepam is 85% bound to plasma proteins. Drugs which inhibit or induce the oxidative metabolism of benzodiazepines (CYP3A4), are less likely to affect lorazepam because it undergoes only glucuronide conjugation.

Other Benzodiazepines. In addition to their anxiolytic and sedative-hypnotic properties, several other benzodiazepines also display antiseizure activity. They include clobazam and nitrazepam which are used outside the U.S.; they have not demonstrated any clinical advantage over clonazepam.

Felbamate (Felbatol)

Felbamate is a dicarbamate (Fig. 16.7) that is structurally similar to the antianxiety drug, meprobamate. It was FDA approved for antiseizure use in 1993. However, following the occurrence of rare cases of aplastic anemia and of severe hepatotoxicity associated with the use of felbamate during early 1994, a "black-box" warning was added to the drug's package insert (47,62). Despite this, felbamate continues to be used in many patients, although not as a first-line treatment. These toxicity effects may be attributed to the formation of toxic metabolites (63). Although felbamate use is now uncommon, it is reserved for severe refractory seizures, either partial, myoclonic or atonic, or in Lennox-Gastaut syndrome.

Mechanism of Action. Although its mechanism of action is unknown, felbamate antagonizes the NMDA receptor by binding to a glycine recognition site, and lowers voltage-gated calcium currents (41,64).

Metabolism and Pharmacokinetics. Although the metabolism of felbamate has not been fully characterized, felbamate is esterase hydrolyzed to its monocarbamate metabolite, 2-phenyl-1,3-propanediol monocarbamate, which is subsequently oxidized via aldehyde dehydrogenase to its major human metabolite 3-carbamoyl-2-phenylpropionic acid (Fig. 16.7). Other metabolites include the p-hydroxy and mercapturic acid metabolites of felbamate which have been identified in human urine (65). Felbamate is a substrate for CYP2C19 with minor activity for CYP3A4 and CYP2E1. Thompson (66) has provided evidence for the formation of the reactive metabolite, 3-carbamoyl-2-phenylpropionaldehyde, from the alcohol oxidation of 2-phenyl-1,3-propanediol monocarbamate. This aldehyde carbamate underwent spontaneous elimination to another reactive intermediate, 2-phenylpropenal (more commonly known as atropaldehyde), which is proposed to play a role in the development of toxicity during felbamate therapy. Evidence for in vivo atropaldehyde formation was confirmed with the identification of its mercap-

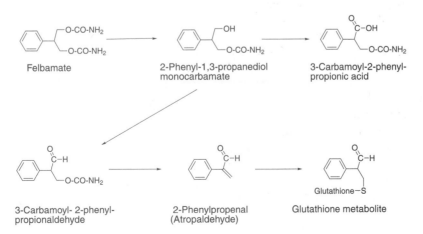

Fig. 16.7. Metabolism of felbamate.

turic acid conjugates in human urine after felbamate administration. This is consistent with the hypothesis that atropaldehyde reacts rapidly with thiol nucleophiles such as glutathione to form mercapturates (see subsection in Chapter 8). Felbamate administration exhibited linear kinetics with a half-life of 20–23 hours in the absence of enzyme-inducing AEDs. Approximately 50% of an oral dose of felbamate is excreted unchanged.

Adverse Effects. Felbamate has exhibited the rare occurrence of aplastic anemia and of severe hepatotoxicity which may be associated with the in vivo formation of reactive metabolites. Felbamate increases phenytoin and valproate serum levels, but decreases the level of CBZ. The increase in valproate plasma concentrations by felbamate is through the inhibition of beta-oxidation. No clinically relevant pharmacokinetic interactions were noted between felbamate and lamotrigine, clonazepam, vigabatrin, nor the active monohydroxy metabolite of oxcarbazepine (67). The enzyme inducers phenytoin, phenobarbital and CBZ decrease felbamate plasma levels by increasing its clearance.

Gabapentin

Mechanism of Action. Gabapentin is a water soluble amino acid originally designed to be a GABA-mimetic analog capable of penetrating the CNS (see Fig. 16.5). Surprisingly, it has no direct GABA-mimetic activity, nor is it active on sodium channels. The mechanism of action remains unknown, although it has been suggested that gabapentin may alter the metabolism or release of GABA. Gabapentin raises brain GABA levels in epilepsy patients (68). Recent studies have demonstrated gabapentin binding to calcium channels in a manner which can be allosterically modulated (69,70).

Gabapentin is indicated as an adjunct for use against partial seizures with or without secondary generalization, in patients more than 12 years of age.

Pharmacokinetics. The pharmacokinetic properties for gabapentin are generally favorable with a bioavailability of 60% when given in low doses, or somewhat less at higher doses due to saturable intestinal uptake by the L amino acid transporter (71). The L amino acid transporter is very susceptible to substrate saturation (low Km value). Its absorption and distribution into the CNS appears to be dependent on this amino acid transporter. Following the administration of an oral dose, gabapentin reaches peak plasma concentration in 2–3 hours. Additionally, it exhibits linear pharmacokinetics. Moreover, it is not extensively metabolized nor is it an inducer of he-

patic metabolizing enzymes. The elimination of unmetabolized gabapentin occurs by the renal route. Although its therapeutic range is not well characterized, gabapentin has a broad therapeutic index. This implies that a wide range of doses can be used, based on individual patient needs, without significant limitation due to dose-dependent side effects. Protein binding is negligible. Its elimination half-life of 5–7 hours is not affected by the dose or by other drugs, and its short half-life necessitates multiple daily administration.

Adverse Effects. Adverse effects of gabapentin are uncommon and not serious. CNS effects include mild to moderate sedation, fatigue, ataxia, headache, dizziness, and diplopia. Gabapentin may exacerbate myoclonus, but the effect is mild and does not require discontinuance of the drug. (47,72)

Drug interactions are infrequent with gabapentin. It does not induce hepatic metabolizing enzymes, nor do other AEDs affect its metabolism and elimination. Antacids may decrease absorption. Gabapentin dosage may need to be decreased in patients with renal disease or in the elderly.

Lamotrigine

Lamotrigine is a 5-phenyl-1,2,4-triazine derivative indicated as monotherapy or as an adjunct for partial seizures in adults, and for adjunctive use in patients with Lennox-Gastaut syndrome. Lamotrigine may have additional benefit in combating myoclonic and typical absence seizures.

Mechanism of Action. The most probable explanation for lamotrigine's efficacy is its ability to produce a blockade of sodium channel repetitive firing. In addition, lamotrigine appears to reduce glutaminergic excitatory transmission, although the mechanism for this action remains unclear. (73,74).

Pharmacokinetics. Following oral administration, lamotrigine is absorbed rapidly and completely, exhibiting linear pharmacokinetics, and modest protein binding (55%). Lamotrigine is metabolized predominantly by N-glucuronidation and subsequent urinary elimination of its major metabolite, the quaternary 2-N-glucuronide (80–90%), 8–10% of the minor 5-amino-N-glucuronide, and 8–10% of unchanged drug (75). Lamotrigine's usual elimination half-life of 24–35 hours is reduced to 13–15 hours in patients taking enzyme-inducing AEDs. The presence of valproate increases the lamotrigine half-life substantially by inhibiting N-glucuronidation, necessitating a reduction in dose to avoid toxicity. Hepatic disease patients may demonstrate a reduced capacity to for lamotrigine glucuronidation, thus reducing its rate of clearance.

Adverse Effects. The usefulness of lamotrigine is limited by the increased incidence of serious rashes, particularly in children or patients taking valproate (46,47). However, this increase may be attenuated by very slow dose escalation, as most rashes appear within the first 8 weeks of treatment. Also, lamotrigine may be associated with development of myoclonus after 2–3 years of drug treatment (76). Additional common side effects associated with lamotrigine therapy include dizziness, diplopia, headache, ataxia, blurred vision, somnolence, and nausea.

S(−) Levetiracetam

S(−) Levetiracetam is a pyrrolidone derivative unrelated to the structures of other AEDs. It is indicated as an adjunct in the treatment of partial onset seizures in adults.

Mechanism of Action. The mechanism of action for levetiracetam is unknown and does not appear to interact with any recognized excitatory or inhibitory neural mechanism. However, it has been found to have a stereospecific synaptic binding site in the central, but not peripheral, nervous system, (77) as well as antagonizing neuronal synchronization (72,78). In animal seizure models, levetiracetam protects against secondary generalization.

Pharmacokinetics. Levetiracetam displays rapid and complete absorption, although food slows the rate but not the extent of absorption. It exhibits linear pharmacokinetics and is minimally protein bound (79). Approximately 60% of an oral dose is excreted into the urine unchanged and 24–30% as its carboxylic acid metabolite, with an delimination half-life in adults of approximately 7 hours. Although levetiracetam is not metabolized by hepatic CYP450, UGT, or epoxide hydrolase, it is esterase hydrolyzed to its carboxylic acid metabolite (loss of amido group), which is not affected by the hepatic metabolizing enzymes.

Adverse Effects. The risk of clinically relevant drug interactions are minimal with levetiracetam because it does not alter the pharmacokinetics of co-administered drugs by inhibition or induction of hepatic enzymes (80). Toxic effects include mild to moderate somnolence, asthenia, ataxia, and dizziness; these effects seldom require discontinuance. A small increase in the incidence of psychosis was noted in clinical trials. Its use in the elderly or in patients with renal impairment will require an individualization of dose, and an additional dose is needed after renal dialysis. Levetiracetam was associated with developmental toxicity in the offspring of pregnant animals.

Tiagabine

Mechanism of Action. Tiagabine is a nipecotic acid derivative with an improved ability to cross the blood-brain barrier. It was rationally designed to be a GABA uptake inhibitor based on the fact that nipecotic acid (piperidine-3-carboxylic acid) inhibits GABA uptake by glial cells. Tiagabine binds to the GABA transporter GAT1, blocking the uptake of GABA into both neurons and glia, thus enhancing GABA-mediated inhibition (47,81,82). Tiagabine is presently approved for adjunctive use in epileptic patients more than 12 years of age with partial seizures which are not controlled by first line drugs.

Pharmacokinetics. Tiagabine is well absorbed with an oral bioavailability of 90–95% and displays linear pharmacokinetics with a plasma half-life of 5–8 hours necessitating a multiple daily dosing regimen (83). It is highly protein bound (96%). The major pathway of metabolism for tiagabine is oxidation by CYP3A4, followed by glucuronidation. Its pharmacokinetics are altered by the co-administration of enzyme inducing AED, even though tiagabine does not appear to induce or inhibit hepatic microsomal metabolizing enzymes (84).

Adverse Effects. Side effects are more common for tiagabine than with other adjunctive drugs, and most often involve the CNS. They include somnolence, headache, dizziness, tremor, abnormal thinking, depression, and psychosis. Furthermore, recent reports have implicated tiagabine in the development of absence status epilepticus (48,85,86).

Tiagabine does not affect the hepatic metabolism of other AEDs but its half-life is decreased by enzyme-inducing AEDs such as CBZ, phenytoin, and barbiturates. Other CYP3A4 inducing drugs may act similarly. Valproate decreases the protein binding of tiagabine increasing its plasma concentration in these patients.

Hepatic disease causes decreased clearance of tiagabine, and a dose reduction may be required. Renal disease does not affect elimination.

Topiramate

Topiramate is a sulfamate-substituted monosaccharide derived from fructose with a broad spectrum of AED activity. It is approved as an adjunctive drug for partial seizures and for primary generalized tonic-clonic seizures in adults, as adjunctive therapy in children aged 2–16 years with partial-onset seizures or primary generalized tonic-clonic seizures. Topiramate showed the highest responder rate in a controlled trial for refractory partial seizures, and may have utility in Lennox-Gastaut syndrome and typical absence seizures (36,47).

Mechanism of Action.   The mechanism of action for topiramate is unknown but several actions are thought to contribute to its AED activity (87). It blocks repetitive firing by acting on sodium channels, may enhance GABA$_A$-mediated chloride flux, and appears to be an antagonist at the AMPA and kainate receptors, thus blocking the effect of glutamate (88,89). In addition, there is recent evidence of inhibition of L-type calcium currents (90).

Pharmacokinetics.   Topiramate is rapidly absorbed with at least an 80–95% oral bioavailability which is unaffected by food. Following an oral dose of topiramate, peak plasma concentration is reached in 1–4 hours exhibiting linear pharmacokinetics (91,92). Protein binding is minimal (<20%) and the usual elimination half-life is 20–30 hours allowing for a twice daily dosing regimen. In the absence of enzyme-inducing drugs, approximately 70–80% of the drug is excreted unchanged in the urine and the remainder as metabolites resulting from oxidation and hydrolysis. Enzyme-inducing AEDs alter the pharmacokinetics of topiramate by reducing its plasma levels and increasing its rate of elimination (half-life 9–12 hours) (93).

In children 4–17 years of age, topiramate exhibits linear pharmacokinetics with a 50% increase in clearance rate compared with adults (92). Topiramate may require up to a 50% dose reduction in patients with renal insufficiency and a replacement dose may be needed after renal dialysis. Topiramate has demonstrated teratogenicity in animal studies.

Adverse Effects.   Common CNS side effects associated with topiramate therapy include drowsiness, dizziness, impaired concentration and memory, speech and language difficulties, and confusion (48,93). These effects develop during the first weeks of therapy and may decline over time. No hepatic or bone marrow effects have been noted thus far, however an increased incidence of renal stones is troublesome. A family history of nephrolithiasis may be a contraindication for using topiramate.

Topiramate is not devoid of potential interaction properties: it induces CYP3A4 and inhibits CYP2C19, thus significantly increasing plasma phenytoin levels (93). Topiramate may also decrease the effectiveness of oral contraceptives.

Valproic Acid and its Derivatives

| Valproic acid (dipropylacetic acid) | (E)-2-ene-valproic acid | 4-ene-valproic acid |

Valproate is available as valproic acid (Depakene), divalproex sodium (Depakote), and valproate sodium (Depacon) for I.V. use. Its AED properties were discovered serendipitously when it was used as a solvent for potential new AEDs undergoing testing. It is effective against both MES and pentylenetetrazole-induced seizures in animals and possesses a satisfactory margin of safety. Since the pKa of valproic acid is 4.7, the drug is completely ionized at physiologic pH, and thus the valproate ion is almost certainly the pharmacologically active species.

Mechanism of Action.   Although its mechanism of action is not clearly established, valproate is known to produce a blockade of high frequency repetitive firing in cultured neurons, a mechanism consistent with the actions of phenytoin and CBZ. In addition, valproate appears to increase the inhibitory effect of GABA, possibly by activation of GAD or inhibition of GABA-T, although the high drug concentrations required cast doubt on the clinical relevance of this effect (94). Furthermore, valproate has been recently shown to decrease uptake of GABA into cultured astrocytes; this action may contribute to the AED efficacy (95,96). The therapeutic utility of valproate is likely due to multiple effects.

Valproate is indicated for initial or adjunctive treatment for absence seizures, or as an adjunct when absence seizures occur in combination with either tonic-clonic seizures, myoclonic seizures, or both. It is also FDA approved for use in complex partial seizures, occurring with or without other seizure types. In new patients with typical absence seizures, ethosuximide is preferred to valproate due to the latter drug's risk of producing hepatotoxicity. In a comparative trial, sodium valproate and ethosuximide were equally effective when either drug was given alone or in combination with other AEDs in children with typical absence seizures. In atypical absence seizures (Lennox-Gastaut syndrome), sodium valproate is more effective, whereas in myoclonic seizures, it is less effective than clonazepam.

Pharmacokinetics.   Valproate undergoes rapid and complete absorption, which is only slightly slowed by food. It is 90% protein bound, and its clearance is dose-dependent due to an increase in the free fraction of the drug at higher doses. It is metabolized almost entirely by the liver, with 30–50% of an orally administered dose eliminated in the urine as its acyl glucuronide conjugate, 40% from mitochondrial β-oxidation, about 15–20% by omega-oxidation, and less than 3% is excreted unchanged in urine. Its major active metabolite is (E)-2-ene valproate (trans 2-ene valproate). Its 4-ene metabolite has been proposed to be a reactive metabolite responsible for the hepatotoxicity of valproate (see Chapter 8). Other metabolites found in the urine include 3-oxo- and 4-hydroxyvalproate. The elimination half-life for valproate ranged from 9–16 hours following oral dosing regimens of 250–1000 mg. Patients who are not taking enzyme-inducing AEDs (carbamazepine, phenytoin, and phenobarbital) will clear valproate more rapidly, and therefore, monitoring of AED plasma concentrations should be intensified whenever concurrent AEDs are introduced or withdrawn.

Adverse Effects. The most commonly observed side effects for valproate are gastrointestinal (anorexia, nausea and indigestion). These effects can be minimized by selecting divalproex sodium, which is enterically coated, and by initiating therapy at a low dose. More importantly, however, valproate is associated with the development of fatal hepatotoxicity, especially in children or when co-administered with other AEDs. Frequent monitoring of liver function tests is mandatory for onset of toxicity, particularly during the first six months of treatment. Tremors, hematologic dyscrasias, pancreatitis, stupor, depression, behavioral anomalies, and coma have been observed as well with valproate therapy.

Valproate has an extensive pattern of drug interactions. It increases the plasma concentrations of lamotrigine, CBZ and phenobarbital, and the free fraction of phenytoin by either displacing these drugs from plasma proteins or inhibiting their metabolism. Phenytoin, phenobarbital, and CBZ cause decreased plasma concentrations of valproate, while felbamate increases valproate levels.

Because of its propensity for causing liver damage, valproate therapy should be avoided in persons with liver disease. It should be used with caution before surgery, as it can produce thrombocytopenia and inhibition of platelet aggregation. In pregnancy, it has been associated with an increased risk of fetal epilepsy syndrome and spina bifida.

Zonisamide

Mechanism of Action. Zonisamide is a sulfonamide derivative which is indicated as an adjunct for partial seizures in patients over 12 years whose seizures are not controlled by first line drugs. In Japan, it is used for myoclonic seizures as well. The mechanism of action is unknown, but it produces blockade of both sodium and T-type calcium channels (97). As it also affects dopaminergic transmission, bipolar or schizoaffective disorder patients may improve.

Pharmacokinetics. The absorption for orally administered zonisamide is slow but nearly complete. Its pharma-cokinetics are linear with a half life of 50–70 hours when administered alone, or 27–46 hours when administered concurrently with enzyme inducing AEDs. Protein binding is moderate (<50%). An oral dose of zonisamide is completely absorbed with peak plasma concentration occurring in 2–6 hours. Although, the presence of food will delay the attainment of its peak plasma concentration, oral bioavailability does not appear to be altered. More than a third of each oral dose is excreted in the urine in an unchanged form. The routes of metabolism for zonisamide include acetylation to form its N-acetyl metabolite, reduction by CYP3A4/CYP2D6 and the formation of an open-ring metabolite, 2-sulfamoylacetyl phenol. These metabolites are subsequently eliminated unconjugated or glucuronidated in the urine with an elimination half-life of 63 hours. Its co-administration with enzyme-inducing AEDs such as phenytoin, CBZ, or phenobarbital, and with valproate will alter its pharmacokinetics by reducing its half-life and serum concentration. The half-life for zonisamide is decreased to 27 hours in the presence of phenytoin, to 38 hours in the presence of either CBZ or phenobarbital, and to 46 hours with valproate. Other drugs which inhibit or induce CYP3A4 could affect zonisamide's metabolism.

Zonisamide should be used with caution in patients with hepatic or renal disease. It has also shown to be teratogenic in animal studies.

Adverse Effects. Zonisamide is contraindicated in patients with a history of allergy to sulfonamides. The most frequent side effects include somnolence, anorexia, dizziness, agitation, confusion, headache, cognitive impairment, and memory loss. In addition, an incidence of drug-induced psychosis has been noted (98). Reports from both the U.S. and Europe have indicated that development of renal stones may occur with use of this drug. A family history of nephrolithiasis may be a contraindication, and urinary monitoring for hypercalcuria may be warranted in bedridden patients, or those receiving multiple AEDs (99). Although the incidence of severe rashes attributable to zonisamide is low, sulfonamides are associated with Stevens-Johnson syndrome. Thus, it is recommended to discontinue the drug immediately should a rash occur.

Drugs Effective Against Absence Seizures

Drugs effective against absence seizures include the 5-membered ureides, the oxazolidinediones and the succinimides (Fig. 16.1 and Fig. 16.8), and clonazepam and lamotrigine, which have been previously discussed. An examination of the SAR for the 5-membered heterocyclic ureides (Fig. 16.1) reveals that a small substructural difference between ring N (hydantoins), ring O (oxazolidinediones) and methylene (succinimides) results in switching from AEDs effective against partial and generalized tonic-clonic seizures to those effective against absence seizures.

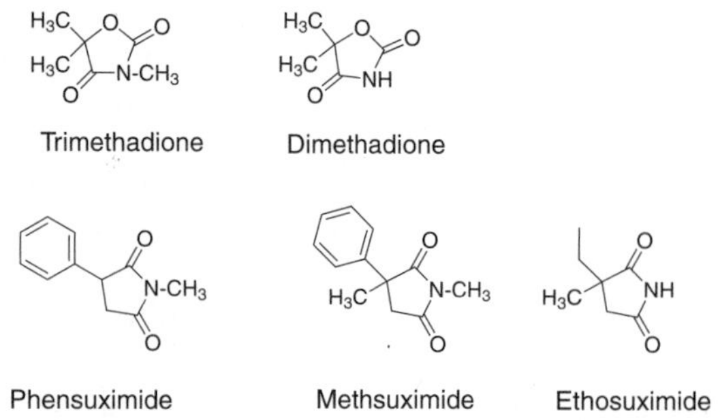

Fig. 16.8. Drugs effective against absence seizures.

Oxazolidinediones

These compounds are some of the oldest AEDs in use, having been introduced into antiseizure therapy between 1946 and 1948. At that time, no effective drugs were available to control absence seizures (petit mal disorders). Therefore the acceptance of trimethadione in 1946 and paramethadione in 1948 for the control of absence seizures was rapid. At present, trimethadione (Tridione) (Fig. 16.8) is indicated only for control of absence seizures refractory to treatment with other AEDs. It is ineffective against other seizure types. Trimethadione is a prodrug and is metabolized by N-demethylation to dimethadione, which is effective in the pentylenetetrazole test, which acts by decreasing T-type calcium currents. Trimethadione is rapidly absorbed, not protein bound, with a half-life of 16–24 hours. However, the half-life of dimethadione is substantially longer, i.e., 6–13 days, and accumulates to concentrations greater than the parent drug. Due to its potentially fatal side effects including aplastic anemia, nephrosis, idiosyncratic rashes and exfoliative dermatitis, trimethadione is rarely used today. It causes malformations or fetal death in up to 87% of pregnancies. Paramethadione is no longer clinically available in the U.S.

Succinimides

Because oxazolidinediones are toxic, an extensive search was undertaken to replace them with less toxic drugs. Substituting the ring O in the oxazolidinediones with a methylene group gave the AE succinimides. The clinically used succinimides include ethosuximide, methsuximide and phensuximide which were introduced between 1951 and 1958 (Fig. 16.8) and widely accepted for the treatment of absence seizures.

Mechanism of Action. Succinimides suppress the paroxysmal 3 Hz spike and wave activity associated with the lapses of consciousness associated with absence (petite mal) seizures, thus reducing the frequency of seizures and raising the threshold to seizures. The proposed mechanism of action involves a decrease in T-type calcium channel activity.

Succinimides are indicated for the monotherapy of absence seizures, or with concomitant therapy when additional forms of seizures occur in combination with absence seizures. These drugs are readily absorbed from the GI tract and display very low protein binding. The drug interactions for the succinimides are less extensive than with the oxazolidinediones. They may increase plasma phenytoin levels, decrease plasma primidone levels, and either increase or decrease valproate levels, although the changes may not be clinically significant.

Renal/hepatic disease does not appear to enhance their toxicity, although facts advise extreme caution as succinimides can cause morphological changes to kidneys and liver. Periodic monitoring of the blood count, hepatic function, and urinalysis are recommended with the use of succinimides.

Ethosuximide. Although ethosuximide is the drug of choice for treatment of simple absence seizures, it is not effective against partial complex or tonic-clonic seizures and may increase the frequency of grand mal attacks. Thus, it must be administered in combination with other AEDs when treating persons with mixed seizure types. Ethosuximide is a substrate for CYP3A4 and CYP2E1. The major metabolite for ethosuximide is the 3-(1-hydroxyethyl) metabolite and the minor metabolite is the ring hydroxylated metabolite, both of which are inactive products excreted unconjugated in the urine. Approximately 20% of an oral dose is excreted unchanged (100,101).

Although ethosuximide is thought to be the least toxic of the succinimides, it can cause gastrointestinal disturbances, dose-related CNS effects such as drowsiness, dizziness, ataxia, sleep disturbances and depression. Idiosyncratic reactions include severe rashes, leukopenia, agranulocytosis (some fatal), systemic lupus erythematosus, and parkinsonian-like symptoms. In addition to being less toxic than trimethadione, ethosuximide offers a wider range of protection against different kinds of absence seizures.

Methsuximide. Although methsuximide is less commonly used, it may be indicated for the control of absence seizures refractory to other drugs. Although it does not precipitate tonic-clonic convulsions, it is often combined with phenytoin or phenobarbital when absence seizures coexist with tonic-clonic symptoms. Much of the efficacy of methsuximide is attributed to its desmethyl metabolite. While the half-life of methsuximide is between 2.6–4 hours, the half-life for N-desmethylsuximide is 25 hours, causing it to accumulate substantially. Concentrations greater than 40 g/ml may be associated with toxicity. Methsuximide is considered to be more toxic than ethosuximide.

Phensuximide. Phensuximide is occasionally used for treatment of absence seizures refractory to other drugs, although it is considered less effective than ethosuximide. It is excreted in both urine and bile, and may cause harmless pink to red discoloration of the urine. It should be used with caution in patients with acute intermittent porphyria.

Drugs Effective Against Myoclonic Seizures

Clonazepam and valproate are commonly used to control myoclonic seizures. Studies suggest that lamotrigine and topiramate may be effective as well, although neither is FDA approved for this indication.

Drugs for Status Epilepticus

Intravenously or intramuscularly administered diazepam is a drug of choice for rapid control of status epilepticus (56). Lorazepam, although not FDA approved for the purpose, is preferred by some clinicians for its longer duration of action (36) and midazolam for its more rapid onset of action (64). Because of its high lipid solubility, intravenously administered diazepam enters the central nervous system rapidly. However, the initially high brain concentration is reduced quickly because of its redistribution, increasing the chance of recurring status epilepticus (57). Concomitant intravenous injection of diazepam and phenobarbital or fosphenytoin has been suggested to overcome this difficulty (102).

Investigational Antiseizure Drugs—Vigabatrin

Vigabatrin is a structural analog of the inhibitory neurotransmitter gamma-amino butyric acid (GABA). It is actively transported into the brain to produce its antiseizure effect by irreversibly inhibiting the degradative enzyme GABA-transaminase (GABA-T inhibitor) which produces an increase in central nervous system (CNS) GABA levels (103). This effect may exacerbate myoclonic seizures. Vigabatrin is among the few AEDs that was synthesized with a specific targeted mechanism in mind and was subsequently demonstrated to function by that mechanism. Tiagabine, a GABA reuptake blocker, is the only other "designer drug."

Following oral administration, vigabatrin is nearly completely absorbed, exhibits linear kinetics with approximately 70% of the dose eliminated unchanged in the urine. Its elimination half-life is 5–7 hours. Some studies have suggested that enzyme inducers increase its rate of clearance.

Among the adverse effects reported for vigabatrin is eye damage (47) which has limited its therapeutic use and availability. In most countries but not the U.S., psychosis and peripheral visual field constriction has been reported.

CASE STUDY

Victoria F. Roche and S. William Zito

IG is a 6-year-old, female child with a maternal family history of epilepsy. She has been diagnosed with absence seizures (formerly called petit mal) which have become quite frequent since she started school. Her symptoms consist of brief attacks of 10- to 30-second losses of consciousness with eyelid fluttering. IG doesn't convulse but abruptly stops activity and resumes it just as abruptly after her seizure. IG doesn't remember that an attack has occurred. Evaluate the following anti-seizure drugs for use in this case.

1. Identify the therapeutic problem(s) where the pharmacist's intervention may benefit the patient.

2. Identify and prioritize the patient specific factors that must be considered to achieve the desired therapeutic outcomes.

3. Conduct a thorough and mechanistically oriented structure-activity analysis of all therapeutic alternatives provided in the case.

4. Evaluate the SAR findings against the patient specific factors and desired therapeutic outcomes and make a therapeutic decision.

5. Counsel your patient.

1   2   3   4

REFERENCES

1. Forster FM. Ed., Report of the Panel on Epilepsy. Madison, WI, University of Wisconsin Press, 1961, p. 91.

2. DeRobertis E, DeLores-Arnaiz GR, and Alberici M. Ultrastructural neurochemistry, in Basic Mechanisms of the Epilepsies, H. H. Jasper, et al., Eds., Boston, Little, Brown and Co., 1969, pp. 137–158.

3. Jackson JH. in Selected Writings of John Hughlings Jackson, Vol. 1, J. Taylor, Ed., London, Hodder and Stoughton, 1931.

4. Gowers WR. Epilepsy and Other Chronic Convulsive Diseases: Their Causes, Symptoms and Treatment, 2nd ed., London, J. and A. Church, 1901.

5. Gastaut H. A Proposed International Classification of Epileptic Seizures. Epilepsia (Amst.), 5, 297–303(1964).

6. Lennox WG. Epilepsy and Related Disorders. Boston, Little, Brown and Co., 1960.

7. Penfield W, Jasper HH. Epilepsy and the Functional Anatomy of the Human Brain, Boston, Little, Brown and Co., 1954, p. 20.

8. Gastaut H. Classification of the epilepsies. Proposal for an international classification. Epilepsia. 1969;10:Suppl:14–21.

9. Masland RL. Comments on the classification of epilepsy. Epilepsia. 1969;10:Suppl:22–8.

10. Proposal for Revised Clinical and Electroencephalographic Classification of Epileptic Seizures, Epilepsia,, 22, 489(1981).

11. Browne TR, Holmes GL. Types of Seizures. In Handbook of Epilepsy, second edition, New York, Lippincott Williams & Wilkins, 1999: 19–41.

12. White HS. Comparative anticonvulsant and mechanistic profile of the established and newer antiepileptic drugs. Epilepsia 1999; 40Suppl 5:S2–10.

13. MacDonald RI, Meldrum B. Principles of Antiepileptic Drug Action. In Levy RH, Meldrum BS, eds., Antiepileptic drugs, 4th edition, New York, Raven Press, 1995, 61–78.

14. Jones KA, Tamm JA, Craig DA, et al. Signal transduction by GABA(B) receptor heterodimers. Neuropsychopharmacology 2000; 23 (4 Suppl):S41–9.

15. Bal T, Debay D, Destexhe A. Cortical feedback controls the frequency and synchrony of oscillations in the visual thalamus. J Neurosci. 2000; 20:7478–88.

16. Rho JM, Donevan SD, Rogawski MA. Mechanism of action of the anticonvulsant felbamate: opposing effects on N-methyl-D-aspartate and gamma-aminobutyric acid$_A$ receptors. Ann. Neurol. 1994; 35:229–34.

17. Browne TR, Holmes GL. Epilepsy: Definitions and Background. In Handbook of Epilepsy, second edition, New York, Lippincott Williams & Wilkins, 1999: 1–18.

18. Krall RL, Penry JK, White BG, et al. Antiepileptic drug development: II. Anticonvulsant drug screening. Epilepsia 1978; 19(4):409–28.

19. Swinyard EA, et al., General Principles, Experimental Selection, Quantification and Evaluation of Anticonvulsants. In Levy R. et al. eds. Antiepileptic Drugs, third edition New York, Raven Press, 1989, p. 88.

20. Vida JA. In: Foye WO ed. Central Nervous System Depressants: Sedative-Hypnotics. Principles of Medicinal Chemistry, second edition Philadelphia, Lea & Febiger, 1981.

21. Swinyard EA et al. Comparative assays of antiepileptic drugs in mice and rats. J Pharmacol Exp Ther 1952; 106: 319–330.

22. Woodbury LA, Davenport VD. Design and use of a new electroshock seizure apparatus, and analysis of factors altering seizure threshold and pattern. Arch Int Pharmacodyn 1952: 92:97–106.

23. Perucca E. The clinical pharmacokinetics of the new antiseizure drugs. Epilepsia 1999;40 Suppl 9:S7–13.

24. Gram L. Pharmacokinetics of new antiseizure drugs. Epilepsia 1996;37 Suppl 6:S12–6.

25. Emilien G, Maloteaux JM. Pharmacological management of epilepsy. Mechanism of action, pharmacokinetic drug interactions, and new drug discovery possibilities. Int J Clin Pharmacol Ther 1998;36:181–94.

26. Browne, TR. Pharmacokinetics of antiepileptic drugs. Neurology. 1998;51 Suppl 4:S2–7.

27. Benedetti MS. Enzyme induction and inhibition by new antiseizure drugs: a review of human studies. Fundam Clin Pharmacol 2000;14:301–19.

28. Battino D, Estienne M, Avanzini G. Clinical pharmacokinetics of antiseizure drugs in paediatric patients. Part II. Phenytoin, carbamazepine, sulthiame, lamotrigine, vigabatrin, oxcarbazepine and felbamate. Clin Pharmacokinet 1995;29:341–69.

29. Richens A. Impact of generic substitution of anticonvulsants on the treatment of epilepsy. CNS Drugs 1997; 8:124–133.

30. Mattson RH and the Department of Veterans Affairs Epilepsy Cooperative Study No. 118 Group. A comparison of carbamazepine, phenobarbital, phenytoin and primidone in partial and secondarily generalized tonic-clonic seizures. N Eng J Med. 1985; 313: 145–51.

31. Osorio I, Reed RC, Peltzer JN. Refractory idiopathic absence status epilepticus: a probable paradoxical effect of phenytoin and carbamazepine. Epilepsia 2000; 41:887–94.

32. Kuo CC. A common anticonvulsant binding site for phenytoin, carbamazepine, and lamotrigine in neuronal Na^1 channels. Mol. Pharmacol. 1998; 54: 712–21.

33. Cuttle L, Munns AJ, Hogg NA, et al. Phenytoin metabolism by human cytochrome P450: involvement of P450 3A and 2C forms in secondary metabolism and drug-protein adduct formation. Drug Metab Dispos. 2000; 28: 945–50.

34. DeToledo JC, Ramsay RE. Fosphenytoin and phenytoin in patients with status epilepticus: improved tolerability versus increased costs. Drug Saf. 2000, 22:459–66; Browne TR, Kugler AE, Eldon, MA. Pharmacology and pharmacokinetics of fosphenytoin. Neurology. 1996;46 Suppl 1:S3–7.

35. Biton, V, Gates JR, Ritter FJ, et al. Adjunctive therapy for intractable epilepsy with ethotoin. Epilepsia 1990, 31:433–7.

36. Browne TR, Holmes GL. Antiepileptic Drugs. In Handbook of Epilepsy, second edition, New York, Lippincott Williams & Wilkins, 1999: 163–96.

37. Mattson RH. Carbamazepine, In Engel J, Pedley TA, eds. Epilepsy: a comprehensive textbook. Philadelphia: Lippincott-Raven, 1997:1491–1502.

38. Potter JM, Donnelly A. Carbamazepine-10, 11-epoxide in therapeutic drug monitoring. Ther Drug Monit. 1998; 20:652–7.

39. Benes J, Parada A, Figueiredo AA, et al. Anticonvulsant and sodium channel-blocking properties of novel 10,11-dihydro-5H-dibenz[b,f]azepine-5-carboxamide derivatives. J Med Chem. 2000; 42:2582–7.

40. Beydoun A, Sachdeo RC, Rosenfeld WE, et al. Oxcarbazepine monotherapy for partial-onset seizures: a multicenter, double-blind, clinical trial. Neurology 2000; 54:2245–51.

41. Stefani A, Spadoni F, Bernardi G. Voltage-activated calcium channels: targets of antiepileptic drug therapy? Epilepsia 1997; 38:959–65.

42. Fattore C, Cipolla G, Gatti G, et al. Induction of ethinylestradiol and levonorgestrel metabolism by oxcarbazepine in healthy women. Epilepsia 1999; 40: 783–7.

43. May TW, Rambeck B, Jurgens U. Influence of oxcarbazepine and methsuximide on lamotrigine concentrations in epileptic patients with and without valproic acid comedication: re-

sults of a retrospective study. Ther Drug Monit. 1999; 21:175–81.

44. Wilbur K, Ensom MH. Pharmacokinetic drug interactions between oral contraceptives and second generation anticonvulsants. Clin Pharmacokinet 2000; 38:355–65.

45. Tecoma ES. Oxcarbazepine. Epilepsia 1999: 40 Suppl 5: S37–46.

46. Pellock JM. Treatment of epilepsy in the new millennium. Pharmacotherapy 2000; 20 (8 Pt 2):129S-138S.

47. Wong IC, Lhatoo SD. Adverse reactions to new anticonvulsant drugs. Drug Saf. 2000; 23; 35–56.

48. Lerman-Sagie T, Lerman P. Phenobarbital still has a role in epilepsy treatment. J Child Neurol 1999; 14:820–1.

49. Willis J, Nelson A, Black FW, et al. Barbiturate anticonvulsants: a neuropsychological and quantitative electroencephalographic study. J. Child Neurol. 1997; 12: 169–71.

50. Goodman LS, Swinyard EA, Brown WC, et al. Anticonvulsant properties of 5-Phenyl-5-Ethyl-Hexandropyrimidine-4,6-Dione (Mysoline), a new antiepileptic. J Pharmacol Exp Ther 1953; 108: 428–434.

51. Butler TC, Waddell WJ. Metabolic conversion of pyrimidone (Mysoline) to phenobarbital. Proc Soc Exp Biol Med 1956; 93: 544-546.

52. Belck TP. Management approaches to prolonged seizures and status epilepticus. Epilepsia 1999; 40 Suppl 1:S59–63.

53. Fountain NB, Adams RE . Midazolam treatment of acute and refractory status epilepticus. Clin Neuropharmacol 1999;22: 261–7; Towne AR, DeLorenzo RJ. Use of intramuscular midazolam for status epilepticus. J Emerg Med 1999;17:323–8.

54. Ishizawa Y, Furuya K, Yamagishi S, et al. Non-GABAergic effects of midazolam, diazepam and flumazenil on voltage-dependent ion currents in NG108–15 cells. Neuroreport 1997; 28: 2635–8.

55. Kriel RL, Cloyd JC, Pellock JM, et al. Rectal diazepam gel for treatment of acute repetitive seizures. The North American Diastat study group. Pediatr Neurol 1999; 20:282–8.

56. Shafer PO. New therapies in the management of acute or cluster seizures and seizure emergencies. J Neurosci Nurs 1999; 31:224–30.

57. Gastaut H, et al., Epilepsia (Amst.) 1956; 6: 167.

58. Mattson RH. In: Woodbury DM, et al. eds. Other antiepileptic drugs. The benzodiazepines. Antiepileptic Drugs. New York, Raven Press, 1972, 497–518.

59. Brodtkorb E, Aamo T, Henricksen O, Lossius R. Rectal diazepam: pitfalls of excessive use in refractory epilepsy. Epilepsy Res 1999; 35:123–33.

60. Schmidt D, Bourgeois B. A risk-benefit assessment of therapies for Lennox-Gastaut syndrome. Drug Saf 2000;22:467–77.

61. Di Lazzaro V, Oliviero A, Meglio M, et al. Direct demonstration of the effect of lorazepam on the excitability of the human motor cortex. Clin Neurophysiol 2000; 111:794–9.

62. Pellock JM. Felbamate. Epilepsia 1999; 40 Suppl5: S57–62.

63. Thompson CD, Barthen MT, Hopper DW, et al. Quantification in patient urine samples of felbamate and three metabolites: acid carbamate and two mercapturic acids. Epilepsia 1999;40:769–76.

64. Mazarati AM, Baldwin RA, Sofia RD, et al. Felbamate in experimental model of status epilepticus. Epilepsia 2000; 41:123–7.

65. Kapetanovic IM, Torchin CD, Thompson CD, et al. Potentially reactive cyclic carbamate metabolite of the antiseizure drug felbamate produced by human liver tissue in vitro. Drug Metab Dispos 1998; 26:1089–95.

66. Thompson CD, Gulden PH, Macdonald TL Identification of modified atropaldehyde mercapturic acids in rat and human urine after felbamate administration. Chem Res Toxicol 1997;10:457–62.

67. Glue P, Banfield CR, Perhach JL, et al. Pharmacokinetic interactions with felbamate. In vitro-in vivo correlation.Clin Pharmacokinet 1997;33:214–24.

68. Petroff OA, Hyder F, Rothman DL, et al. Effects of gabapentin on brain GABA, homocarnosine, and pyrrolidinone in epilepsy patients. Epilepsia 2000; 41:675–80.

69. Bryans JS, Davies N, Gee NS, et al. Identification of novel ligands for the gabapentin binding site on the alpha2delta subunit of a calcium channel and their evaluation as anticonvulsant agents. J Med Chem 1998; 41:1838–45.

70. Taylor MT, Bonhaus DW. Allosteric modulation of [(3)H] gabapentin binding by ruthenium red. Neuropharmacology 2000; 39:1267–73.

71. Luer MS, Hamani C, Dujovny M, et al. Saturable transport of gabapentin at the blood-brain barrier. Neurol Res 1999;21: 559–62.

72. Asconape J, Diedrich A, DellaBadia J. Myoclonus associated with the use of gabapentin. Epilepsia 2000; 41: 479–81.

73. Calabresi P, Centonze D, Marfia GA, et al. An in vitro electrophysiological study on the effects of phenytoin, lamotrigine and gabapentin on striatal neurons. Br J Pharmacol 1999; 126:689–96.

74. Lingamanemi R, Hemmings HC Jr. Effects of anticonvulsants on veratridine- and KCl-evoked glutamate release from rat cortical synaptosomes. Neurosci Lett 1999; 276:127–30.

75. Sinz MW, Remmel RP. Isolation and characterization of a novel quaternary ammonium-linked glucuronide of lamotrigine. Drug Metab Dispos 199;19:149–53; Magdalou J, Herber R, Bidault R, Siest G. In vitro N-glucuronidation of a novel antiepileptic drug, lamotrigine, by human liver microsomes. J Pharmacol Exp Ther 1992;260:1166–73.

76. Jansky J, Rasonyi G, Halasz P, et al. Disabling erratic myoclonus during lamotrigine therapy with high serum level—report of two cases. Clin Neuropharmacol 2000; 23:86–9.

77. Noyer M, Gillard M, Matagne A, et al. The novel antiepileptic drug levetiracetam (ucb LO59) appears to act via a specific binding site in CNS membranes. Eur J Pharmacol 1995; 286:137–46.

78. Georg Margineanu D, Klitgaard H. Inhibition of neuronal hypersynchrony in vitro differentiates levetiracetam from classical antiepileptic drugs. Pharmacol Res 2000; 42:281–5.

79. Patsalos PN. Pharmacokinetic profile of levetiracetam: toward ideal characteristics. Pharmacol Ther 2000;85:77–85.

80. Nicolas JM, Collart P, Gerin B, et al. In vitro evaluation of potential drug interactions with levetiracetam, a new antiseizure agent. Drug Metab Dispos 1999;27:250–4.

81. Eriksson IS, Allard P, Marcusson J. [3H] tiagabine binding to GABA uptake sites in human brain. Brain Res 1999; 85: 183–8.

82. Soudijn W, van Wijngaarden I. The GABA transporter and its inhibitors. Curr Med Chem 2000; 7:1063–79.

83. Gustavson LE, Mengel HB. Pharmacokinetics of tiagabine, a gamma-aminobutyric acid-uptake inhibitor, in healthy subjects after single and multiple doses. Epilepsia 1995;36: 605–11.

84. Adkins JC, Noble S. Tiagabine. A review of its pharmacodynamic and pharmacokinetic properties and therapeutic potential in the management of epilepsy. Drugs 1998;55: 437–60.

85. Knake S, Hamer HM, Schomburg U, et al. Tiagabine-induced absence status in idiopathic generalized epilepsy. Seizure 1999; 8:314–7.

86. Ettinger AB, Bernal OG, Andriola MR, et al. Two cases of non-convulsive status epilepticus in association with tiagabine therapy. Epilepsia 1999; 40:1159–62.

87. Shank RP, Gardocki JF, Streeter AJ, et al. An overview of the preclinical aspects of topiramate: pharmacology, pharmacokinetics, and mechanism of action. Epilepsia 2000;41 Suppl 1:S3–9.

88. Skradski S, White HS. Topiramate blocks kainate-evoked cobalt influx into cultured neurons. Epilepsia 2000; 41 Suppl 1:S45–7.

89. DeLorenzo RJ, Sombati S, Coulter DA. Effects of topiramate on sustained repetitive firing and spontaneous recurrent seizure discharges in cultured hippocampal neurons. Epilepsia 2000; 41 Suppl 1: S40–4.

90. Zhang X, Velumian AA, Jones OT, et al. Modulation of high-voltage-activated calcium channels in dentate granule cells by topiramate. Epilepsia 2000; 41 Suppl 1:S52–60.

91. Rosenfeld WE. Topiramate: a review of preclinical, pharmacokinetic, and clinical data. Clin Ther 1997; 19:1294–308.

92. Garnett WR. Clinical pharmacology of topiramate: a review. Epilepsia 2000;41 Suppl 1:S61–5.

93. Langtry HD, Gillis JC, Davis R. Topiramate. A review of its pharmacodynamic and pharmacokinetic properties and clinical efficacy in the management of epilepsy. Drugs 1997;54: 752–73.

94. Larsson OM, Gram L, Schousboe I, et al. Differential effects of gamma-vinyl GABA and valproate on GABA-transaminase from cultured neurons and astrocytes. Neuropharmacology 1986; 25:617–25.

95. Fraser CM, Sills GJ, Butler E, et al. Effects of valproate, vigabatrin and tiagabine on GABA uptake into human astrocytes cultured from foetal and adult brain tissue. Epileptic Disord 1999; 1:153–7.

96. Eckstein-Ludwig U, Fei J, Schwarz W. Inhibition of uptake, steady-state currents, and transient charge movements generated by the neuronal GABA transporter by various anticonvulsant drugs. Br J Pharmacol 1999; 128:92–102.

97. Oommen KJ, Mathews S. Zonisamide: a new antiepileptic drug. Clin Neuropharmacol 1999; 22:192–200.

98. Miyamoto T, Kohsaka M, Koyama T. Psychotic episodes during zonisamide treatment. Seizure 2000; 9:6570.

99. Kubota M, Nishi-Nagase M, Sakakihara Y, et al. Zonisamide-induced urinary lithiasis in patients with intractable epilepsy. Brain Dev 2000; 22:230–3.

100. Millership JS, Mifsud J, Collier PS. The metabolism of ethosuximide. Eur J Drug Metab Pharmacokinet 1993;18:349–53.

101. Bachmann K, Chu CA, Greear V. In vivo evidence that ethosuximide is a substrate for cytochrome P450IIIA. Pharmacology 1992;45:121–8.

102. Gallagher BB. In: Vida JA, et al. eds. Neuropharmacology and treatment of epilepsy. Anticonvulsants New York, Academic Press, 1977, 49.

103. French JA. Vigabatrin. Epilepsia 1999;40 Suppl 5:S11–6.

17. Psychotherapeutic Drugs: Antipsychotic and Anxiolytic Agents

RAYMOND G. BOOTH AND JOHN L. NEUMEYER

OVERVIEW OF MENTAL ILLNESSES

Mental illnesses that can be treated with psychotropic drugs are broadly categorized as psychoses, neuroses, and mood (depression, bipolar) disorders. Different classes of psychotropic agents differ in their ability to modify symptoms of these mental illnesses, thus, an appropriate diagnosis is critical to selecting an efficacious psychotropic drug. This chapter is focused on the medicinal chemistry of drugs used to treat psychosis and anxiety disorders. The definitive diagnostic criteria for psychiatric disorders in the United States are well described in the Diagnostic and Statistical Manual of Mental Disorders of the American Psychiatric Association (DSM IV-RT) (1). The psychoses (e.g., schizophrenia) are among the most severe mental illnesses and commonly include symptoms of delusions and sensory hallucinations. In anxiety disorders (neuroses), the ability to comprehend reality is retained, but mood changes (anxiety, panic, dysphoria) and thought (obsessions, irrational fears) and behavioral (rituals, compulsions, avoidance) dysfunction can be disabling. Mood and panic disorders usually include dysfunction of the autonomic nervous system (e.g., altered patterns of sleep and appetite) in addition to psychic abnormalities. Depression can lead to self-harm and suicide. In general, antipsychotic agents, which can have severe neurological side effects, should be used only to treat the most severe mental illnesses (i.e., psychoses such as schizophrenia).

SCHIZOPHRENIA
Definition

An historical definition of schizophrenia may begin about 100 years ago with the German psychiatrist Emil Kraepelin's description of a type of dementia that was characterized as a severe, chronic, mental disorder without known external causation wherein functional deterioration progresses with the symptoms of hallucinations, delusions, thought disorder, incoherence, blunted affect, negativism, stereotyped behavior and lack of insight (2). The deterioration progresses to catatonia and hebephrenia (illogical, incoherent, and senseless thought processes and actions, delusions, and hallucinations). Meanwhile, the Swiss psychiatrist Eugen Bleuler coined the term *schizophrenia* to take into account the perceived *schism* or splitting in mental functioning (3).

A modern definition of schizophrenia comes from DSM IV-RT(1). The diagnostic criteria for schizophrenia require two or more of the following characteristic symptoms to be present for a significant proportion of time during a one-month period: delusions, hallucinations, disorganized speech, or grossly disorganized or catatonic behavior. There is, however, flexibility in the diagnostic criteria that leaves room for professional psychiatric judgment. For example, it is enough if hallucinations consist of a voice maintaining a running commentary on the patient's behavior or there are two or more voices that converse with each other. Also, for a significant proportion of time, one or more areas of social functioning such as work, interpersonal relationships, or self-care are markedly below the level achieved prior to the onset of symptoms. Continuous symptoms must persist for six months. Finally, before a diagnosis of schizophrenia is made, affective disorders must be ruled out, as well as, drug/alcohol abuse or other medical conditions.

Etiology of Schizophrenia

A neurobiological basis for schizophrenia and related psychotic syndromes remains elusive. Compelling evidence linking genetic factors to the etiology of schizophrenia is not apparent despite enormous progress in the field of molecular genetics and numerous investigations of hereditary factors associated with psychotic illnesses. Investigations of environmental causative factors have focused on prenatal and perinatal risk factors for brain damage. For example, studies have examined the incidence of schizophrenics who were born under conditions of obstetrical complications, influenza epidemics, food shortages, and Rh factor incompatibility. Neuroanatomical hypotheses involve increased ventricular volume, however, neuropathological changes associated with schizophrenic brains are not obvious as in, for example, Alzheimer's disease. In contrast, neurochemical abnormalities are well documented. Alterations in brain dopaminergic neurotransmission in psychoses have been studied for more than 30 years and this field of psychobiological research generally revolves around the *dopamine hypothesis* of schizophrenia.

The connection between dopaminergic neurotransmission and schizophrenia is an example of a *pharmacocentric* approach to characterizing the etiology and neuropathology of mental illnesses (4–6). The dopamine hypothesis of schizophrenia arose from observations that the first relatively safe and effective antipsychotic drugs, the phenothiazines such as chlorpromazine, used in the early 1950s, affected brain dopamine metabolism (7). Simply put, the dopamine hypothesis of schizophrenia suggests that schizophrenia results from increased dopaminergic neurotransmission and that approaches which decrease dopaminergic neurotransmission will alleviate psychotic symptoms (8). Most antipsychotic agents have activity to limit dopaminergic neurotransmission, providing some indirect evidence to support the dopamine hypothesis of schizophrenia. In a seminal study by Seeman, the average daily dose of antipsychotic was found to correlate well with affinity for dopamine D_2-type receptors. Moreover, the extrapyramidal side effects of antipsychotic drugs certainly correlates with their D_2 antagonism effect (9).

While the dopamine hypothesis of schizophrenia and pharmacotherapy involving antagonism of dopamine receptors (especially D_2-type) has dominated the research directions, it should be noted, that the entire argument is somewhat circular. Consideration of potential new drugs as antipsychotic agents, both in academic and industrial research laboratories, is limited to compounds that have demonstrated behavioral or biochemical evidence of antidopaminergic actions. Of course, this somewhat conservative and exclusive approach is practical in view of the lack of proven alternative neuropharmacologic explanations of antipsychotic drug activity. Nevertheless, in light of the nearly 50 years of research focusing on brain dopaminergic systems, uncontested evidence linking the etiology of psychotic illnesses to the neurobiology of dopaminergic systems, has remained elusive. Alternative explanations, especially those involving adrenergic and serotonergic receptor systems, probably will gain popularity as more atypical antipsychotic drugs (e.g., clozapine) are introduced (by virtue of their antidopaminergic effects) and found also to have actions at these receptor systems, perpetuating and expanding the pharmacocentric approach to antipsychotic drug design and development.

Role of Dopamine Receptors in Schizophrenia

Until recently, compilation of histochemical, electrophysiological, biochemical, and behavioral evidence suggested that the physiologic effects of the neurotransmitter dopamine were mediated by only two subtypes of dopamine

receptors, D_1 and D_2 (10). Modern molecular biological methods involving recombinant DNA techniques, however, have resulted in the cloning of multiple receptor subtypes for several neurotransmitters, including dopamine. Currently, five different dopamine receptors have been cloned and characterized using molecular biologic and pharmacologic techniques (for a review see reference 11). The amino acid sequence of all these receptors, as deduced from their established nucleotide sequence, shows that they belong to the G protein-coupled superfamily of receptors that are structurally characterized by a seven transmembrane spanning region. Molecular biologic characterization of dopamine receptors has far outpaced pharmacologic characterization. There is a paucity of selective medicinal chemical probes of the various dopamine receptor subtypes, thus, it is still convenient to distinguish them as either D_1-type (D_1, D_5) or D_2-type ($D_{2\,short}$, $D_{2\,long}$, D_3, D_4), based on effects on adenylyl cyclase and affinity for known dopamine receptor ligands (Table 17.1).

Although compounds that can differentiate dopamine receptor subtypes (i.e., D_3, D_4, D_5) are scarce, there are available quite a few chemical probes that can distinguish between the general D_1-type and D_2-type receptor families. The $R(+)$-isomer of the benzazepine derivative, SKF 38393 (Fig. 17.1), is used for research as a selective D_1-type *partial* agonist. Meanwhile, the structurally related benzazepine derivative, $R(+)$-SCH 23390 (Fig. 17.1), is used as a selective D_1-type receptor antagonist. Although not very selective for D_1-type over D_2-type receptors, the rigid benzophenanthridine derivative $(+)$-dihydrexidine (Fig. 17.1) is a useful research tool because it is a D_1-type *full efficacy* agonist (produces stimulation of adenylyl cyclase equivalent to dopamine itself) (12, 13). Selective D_2-type full agonists, also shown in Figure 17.1, such as the pyrazole derivative $(-)$-quinpirole, and D_2-type antagonists such as $(-)$-sulpiride also are now available to researchers. The dopamine D_3 receptor subtype is of particular neuropharmacologic interest currently due to its preferential distribution in certain limbic regions of mammalian brain, notably in the nucleus accumbens of the basal forebrain. It is

Table 17.1. Cloned Dopamine Receptors

Criteria	D_1	D_2	D_3	D_4	D_5
No. of amino acids	446	414 ($D_{2\,short}$)	400	387	477
Effect of agonist on adenylyl cyclase	stimulate	443 ($D_{2\,long}$) inhibit	inhibit	inhibit	stimulate
Relative Affinity (K_i, nM) for: *Agonists*					
Dopamine	10	10^2	10^2	10^2	10
$(+)$-SKF 38393	10	10^2	10^2	10^3	10
$(-)$-Quinpirole	10^3	10	10	10	10^3
$(+)$-7-OH-DPAT	10^3	10	1.0	10^2	10^3
Antagonists					
$(+)$-SCH 23390	10^{-1}	10^3	10^3	10^3	10^{-1}
$(-)$Sulpiride	10^4	10	10	10^2	10^5
Clozapine	10^2	10^2	10^2	10	10^2

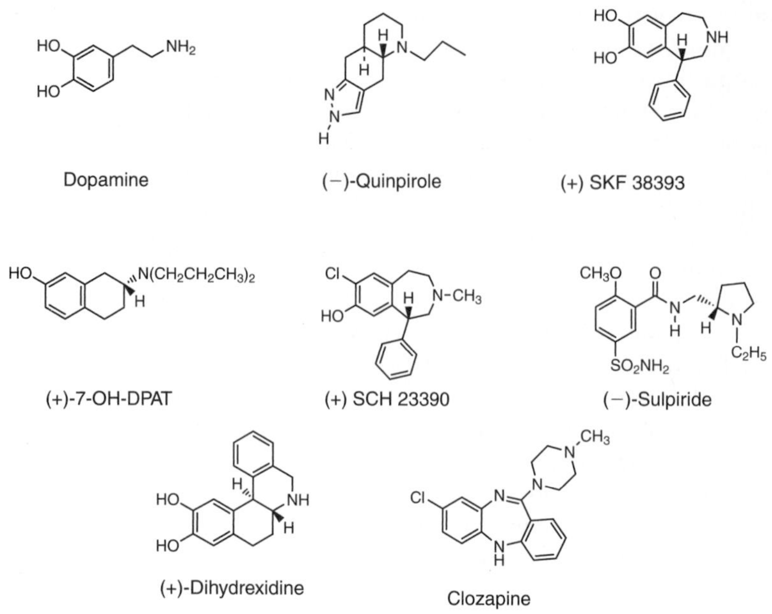

Dopamine   **(−)-Quinpirole**   **(+) SKF 38393**

(+)-7-OH-DPAT   **(+) SCH 23390**   **(−)-Sulpiride**

(+)-Dihydrexidine   **Clozapine**

Fig. 17.1. Structures of compounds useful for characterizing dopamine receptors.

proposed that highly D$_3$-selective drugs might be developed as antipsychotic agents with preferential limbic antidopaminergic actions, while sparing the extrapyramidal basal ganglia, presumably decreasing the neurological movement disorder side effects associated with antipsychotic drug therapy (*vide infra*). The tetrahydronaphthalene, (+)-7-hydroxy-*N,N*-di-*n*-propyl-2-aminotetralin (7-OH-DPAT) (Fig. 17.1), and some of its congeners are particularly promising D$_3$-selective lead agents. The dibenzodiazepine clozapine (Fig. 17.1), which is proposed to have a superior antipsychotic clinical profile with low incidence of extrapyramidal side effects, shows relatively greater affinity for the D$_4$ dopamine receptor subtype, in addition to its relatively high affinity for serotonin 5-HT$_2$, adrenergic α_1 and α_2, muscarinic M$_1$, and histamine H$_1$ receptors (14).

The dopamine D$_1$-type and D$_2$-type receptor families are differentially distributed in mammalian forebrain dopaminergic pathways. The extrapyramidal nigrostriatal pathway, which plays a key role in locomotor coordination, consists of neurons with cell bodies in the A9 pars compacta of the substantia nigra in the midbrain. These neurons project to the basal ganglia structures caudate nucleus and putamen (collectively referred to as striatum) in the forebrain (Fig. 17.2). Degeneration of neurons in the nigrostriatal pathway is the hallmark pathological feature of Parkinson's disease, clinically manifested as bradykinesia, muscular rigidity, resting tremor, and impairment of postural balance. Blockade of dopamine receptors on cholinergic neurons in striatum is associated with the sometimes severe extrapyramidal parkinsonian-like side effects (muscular rigidity, bradykinesia, akathisia) that frequently occur with antipsychotic drug treatment.

The mesolimbic and mesocortical pathway, involved in integration of emotions, behaviors, and higher thought processes, consists of neurons with cell bodies in the A10

ventral tegmentum. These neurons project to limbic forebrain structures, including the nucleus accumbens and amygdala, and to higher levels of cerebral function such as frontal cortex (Fig. 17.2). According to the dopamine hypothesis, increased dopaminergic neurotransmission in limbic pathways contributes to the "positive" symptoms (e.g., hallucinations and excited delusional behavior that can be reduced with typical antipsychotic drugs) but not necessarily the "negative" symptoms (e.g., catatonia) observed in the clinical manifestation of schizophrenia.

Typical antipsychotic drugs act in both extrapyramidal and limbic brain regions at D$_2$-type dopamine receptors that can be located postsynaptically (on cell bodies, dendrites, and nerve terminals of other neurons), as well as, presynaptically on dopamine neurons. Dopamine receptors located presynaptically on dopamine cell bodies and

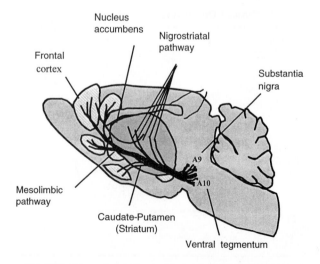

Fig. 17.2. Some dopamine pathways in mammalian brain.

nerve terminals are called *autoreceptors* that act to negatively modulate neuronal firing and dopamine synthesis and release (15) (Fig. 17.3). Low concentrations of certain dopamine agonists can *stereospecifically* activate dopamine D_2-type autoreceptors to decrease dopamine synthesis (16,17) and release (18), reducing dopaminergic neurotransmission. Consistent with the dopamine hypothesis of schizophrenia, selective dopamine autoreceptor agonists could be possible pharmacotherapeutic agents in the treatment of schizophrenia and related mental illnesses.

In addition to postsynaptic dopamine receptors and presynaptic dopamine D_2-type autoreceptors, heteroreceptors, such as adenosine (A_2) (19), histamine (H_1) (20,21), serotonin ($5-HT_{1A}$) (22), and putative sigma (σ_1) receptors (23), located on or near presynaptic dopaminergic nerve terminals in the striatum (extrapyramidal) or nucleus accumbens (limbic) regions of brain, can modulate dopamine synthesis (and release) by altering the activity of tyrosine hydroxylase, the rate-limiting step in catecholamine biosynthesis. Similarly, activation of adrenergic (α_2) autoreceptors in the limbic structure hippocampus negatively modulates the release of the neurotransmitter norepinephrine (24). It is proposed that atypical antipsychotic drugs, such as clozapine, may interact with these other neurotransmitter receptor systems (i.e., histamine, serotonin, adrenergic) instead of, or, in addition to dopamine receptor systems. Preceding the introduction of the first clinically successful phenothiazine-type neuroleptic, chlorpromazine, the first phenothiazine to be used to treat psychiatric patients in the 1940s (unsuccessfully) was promethazine, an "antihistamine" H_1 antagonist.

Treatment of Schizophrenia and Related Psychoses

The most widely used class of drugs in the treatment of psychotic disorders are the so-called *neuroleptics*. This term suggests that such medicines "take hold" (*lepsis*) of the central nervous system to suppress movement, as well as, behavior. Although the connotation has been stretched to include biochemical and clinical antagonism of dopamine D_2 receptors, debilitating extrapyramidal movement side effects are implicit in the clinical definition of neuroleptic antipsychotic drugs. Indeed, the term neuroleptic is so synonymous with neurologic side effects that newer antipsychotic drugs, without substantial risk of extrapyramidal effects, are referred to as *atypical neuroleptic* drugs. Also implied in the term *atypical* is a mechanism of antipsychotic action other than (or in addition to) postsynaptic D_2 receptor blockade.

In general, neuroleptic therapy benefits patients with schizophrenia or other psychiatric illnesses marked by agitation, aggressive and impulsive behavior, and impaired reasoning. Positive symptoms respond to treatment with typical neuroleptics, while negative symptoms are not appreciably affected. In general, neuroleptics provide calming, mood-stabilizing, and anti-hallucinatory effects and their beneficial impact on psychiatric medicine is unquestioned in spite of their sometimes severe extrapyramidal side effects. Chemical classes of neuroleptics include the phenothiazines, thioxanthenes, and the butyrophenones. The dibenzodiazepines and benzisoxazoles are examples of atypical neuroleptics that have less potential for ex-

Promethazine

Chlorpromazine

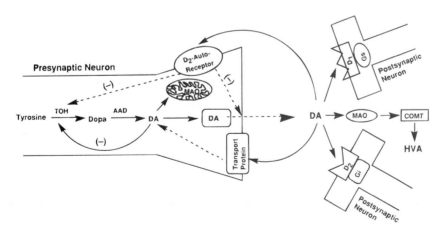

Fig. 17.3. Tyrosine is hydroxylated in a rate-limiting step by tyrosine hydroxylase (TOH) to form dihydroxylphenylalanine (DOPA), which is decarboxylated by L-aromatic amino acid decarboxylase (AAD) to form dopamine (DA). Newly synthesized DA is stored in vesicles, from which release occurs into the synaptic cleft by depolarization of the presynaptc neuron in the presence of Ca^{2+}. DA released into the synaptic cleft may go on to stimulate postsynaptic D_1- and D_2-type receptors or presynaptic D_2-type autoreceptors that negatively modulate DA synthesis (via inhibition of TOH) and release. The action of synaptic DA is inactivated largely via reaccumulation into the presynaptic neuron by high-affinity DA neurotransport proteins located on the nerve terminal membrane. Free cytoplasmic DA negatively modulates DA synthesis via end-product (feedback) inhibition of TOH by competition with biopterin cofactor. Cytoplasmic pools of DA may undergo metabolic deamination by monoamine oxidase (MAO), an enzyme bound to the outer membrane of mitochondria, to form dihydroxyphenylacetaldehyde, which oxides to dihydroxyphenylacetate (DOPAC). DA or DOPAC may undergo methylation by catechol-O-methyltransferase (COMT) ultimately to form homovanillic acid (HVA), a metabolite excreted in urine.

trapyramidal side effects and have activity at brain serotonin 5-HT$_2$, adrenergic α_1/α_2, or histamine H$_1$ receptors, in addition to dopamine receptors.

Mechanism of Action of Antipsychotic Drugs

Given that the pathogenesis of schizophrenia and related psychiatric disorders is unknown, it is perhaps naïve to suggest how drugs act at the molecular level to relieve the symptoms of these disorders. Nevertheless, it is generally agreed that the antipsychotic mechanism of action of neuroleptics involves antagonism of brain dopamine receptors (especially D$_2$-type) in the mesolimbic-mesocortical dopamine pathways. Antipsychotic drug interaction with dopamine D$_2$-type receptors, however, probably does not solely account for their antipsychotic activity and other CNS receptor systems (e.g., acetylcholine, histamine, norepinephrine, serotonin, and putative sigma) probably are involved, especially in light of the activity of newer atypical agents such as clozapine.

Side Effects of Neuroleptics

Many of the side effects associated with antipsychotic agents can be attributed to their antagonist activity of a variety of CNS receptors which include: histamine H$_1$, adrenergic α_1/α_2, cholinergic M$_1$ receptors, serotonin 5-HT$_2$ and dopamine D$_2$ receptors in the brain. For example, antipsychotic drug side effects such as sedation, hypotension, sexual dysfunction, and other autonomic effects, reflect blockade of adrenergic and histamine receptors. Meanwhile, the anticholinergic actions of neuroleptics on cardiac, ophthalmic, gastrointestinal, bladder, and genital tissue are due to antagonism of muscarinic acetylcholine receptors. Such anticholinergic actions also are characteristic of atypical antipsychotics such as clozapine and it has been proposed that anticholinergic activity may be beneficial in controlling negative symptoms in schizophrenics. The parkinsonian-like movement side effects of neuroleptics clearly are due to antagonism of dopamine receptors in the nigrostriatal pathway and the severity of these extrapyramidal side effects increases with the ratio of their antidopaminergic to anticholinergic potency. Extrapyramidal side effects occur in 30–50% of patients receiving standard doses of typical neuroleptics and tend to occur during the first to eighth week of therapy. Extrapyramidal side effects include acute dystonias (e.g., facial grimacing, torticollis, oculogyric crisis), akathisia (motor restlessness), and parkinsonian-type symptoms such as bradykinesia, cogwheel rigidity, tremor, masked face, and shuffling gait. The higher the potency of the neuroleptic, the worse the side effects, some of which can be reversed using anticholinergic drugs. Tardive dyskinesia occurs in 15–25% of patients after prolonged treatment with typical neuroleptics and is characterized by stereotyped, involuntary, repetitive, choreiform movements of the face, eyelids, mouth (grimaces), tongue, extremities, and trunk. There are also metabolic and endocrine side effects of neuroleptics such as weight gain, hyperprolactinemia, and gynecomastia.

Relatively common dermatologic reactions (e.g., urticaria, photosensitivity) are also observed especially with the phenothiazines. Interestingly, anticholinergic and dopaminergic agents worsen tardive dyskinesia while antidopaminergic agents tend to suppress the symptoms; the pathophysiology of tardive dyskinesia is not known and the disorder essentially is irreversible.

Meanwhile, antagonism of dopamine D$_2$-type receptors in the chemoreceptor trigger zone in the brainstem is responsible for beneficial antiemetic effects produced by neuroleptics; several phenothiazines (e.g., promethazine, prochlorperazine) are marketed to exploit this pharmacologic (side) effect.

Phenothiazine

Development of Phenothiazine and Related Neuroleptics

Although phenothiazine was synthesized in 1883 and had been used as an anthelmintic for many years, it has no antipsychotic activity. The basic structural type from which the phenothiazine antipsychotic drugs trace their origins is the antihistamines of the benzodioxane type I (Fig. 17.4). Bovet hypothesized in 1937 that specific substances antagonizing histamine ought to exist, tried various compounds known to act on the autonomic nervous system, and was the first to recognize antihistaminic activity (25). With the benzodioxanes as a starting point, many molecular modifications were carried out in various laboratories in a search for other types of antihistamines. The benzodioxanes led to ethers of ethanolamine of type II, which after further modifications led to the benzhydryl ethers (III) characterized by the clinically useful antihistamine, diphenhydramine, or to the ethylenediamine type IV, which led to antihistamine drugs such as tripelennamine (V). Further modification of the ethylenediamine type of antihistamine resulted in the incorporation of one of the nitrogen atoms into a phenothiazine ring system, which produced the phenothiazine (VI), a compound that was found to have antihistaminic properties and, similar to many other antihistaminic drugs, a strong sedative effect. Diethazine (VI) is more useful in the treatment of Parkinson's disease (owing to its potent antimuscarinic action) than in allergies, whereas promethazine (VII) is clinically used as an antihistaminic. The ability of promethazine to prolong barbiturate-induced sleep in rodents was discovered and the drug was introduced into clinical anesthesia as a potentiating agent.

To enhance the sedative effects of such phenothiazines, Charpentier and Courvoisier synthesized and evaluated many modifications of promethazine. This research effort eventually led to the synthesis of chlorpromazine (VIII) in 1950 at the Rhône-Poulenc Laboratories (26). Soon there-

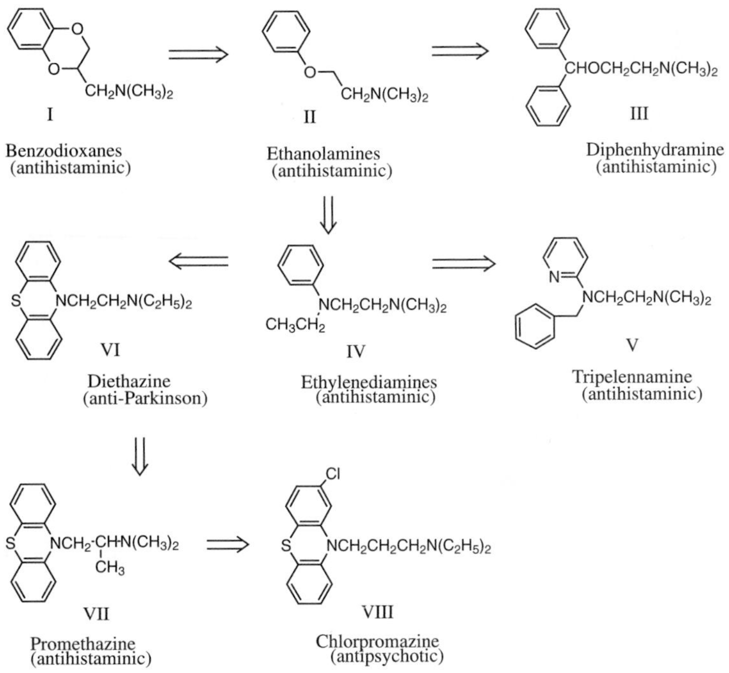

Fig. 17.4. Development of phenothiazine-type antipsychotic drugs.

after, the French surgeon Laborit and his co-workers described the ability of this compound to potentiate anesthetics and produce artificial hibernation (27). They noted that chlorpromazine by itself did not cause a loss of consciousness but produced only a tendency to sleep and a marked disinterest in the surroundings. The first attempts to treat mental illness with chlorpromazine alone were made in Paris in 1951 and early 1952 by Paraire and Sigwald. In 1952, Delay and Deniker began their important work with chlorpromazine (28). They were convinced that chlorpromazine achieved more than symptomatic relief of agitation or anxiety and that this drug had an ameliorative effect on psychosis. Thus, what initially involved minor molecular modifications of an antihistamine that produced sedative side effects resulted in the development of a major class of drugs that initiated a new era in the drug therapy of the mentally ill. More than anything else in the history of psychiatry, the phenothiazines and related drugs have positively influenced the lives of schizophrenic patients. They have enabled many patients, relegated in earlier days to a lifetime in mental institutions, to assume a greatly improved role in society.

More than 24 phenothiazine and the related thioxanthene derivatives are used in medicine, most of them for psychiatric conditions. The structures, generic and proprietary names, dose, and side effects of phenothiazines and thioxanthenes currently used as neuroleptics are listed in Table 17.2.

Structure-Activity Relationships of Phenothiazine and Thioxanthene Neuroleptics. It is presumed that phenothiazine and thioxanthene neuroleptics mediate their pharmacologic effects mainly through interactions at D_2-type dopamine receptors. Examination of the X-ray structures of dopamine (in the preferred *trans* α-rotamer conformation) and chlorpromazine shows that these two structures can be partly superimposed (Fig. 17.5) (29). In the preferred conformation of chlorpromazine, its side chain tilts away from the midline toward the chlorine-substituted ring.

The electronegative chlorine atom on ring *a* is responsible for imparting asymmetry to this molecule, and the attraction of the amine side chain (protonated at physiologic pH) toward the ring containing the chlorine atom indicates an important structural feature of such molecules. Phenothiazine and related compounds lacking a chlorine atom in this position are, in most cases, inactive as neuroleptic drugs. In addition to the ring *a* substituent, another major requirement for therapeutic efficacy of phenothiazines is that the side chain amine contain three carbons separating the two nitrogen atoms (Fig.17.5). Phenothiazines with two carbon atoms separating the two nitrogen atoms lack antipsychotic efficacy. Compounds such as promethazine (Fig.17.4, VII) are primarily antihistaminic and are less likely to assume the preferred conformation.

When thioxanthene derivatives that contain an olefinic double bond between the tricyclic ring and the side chain are examined, it can be seen that such structures can exist

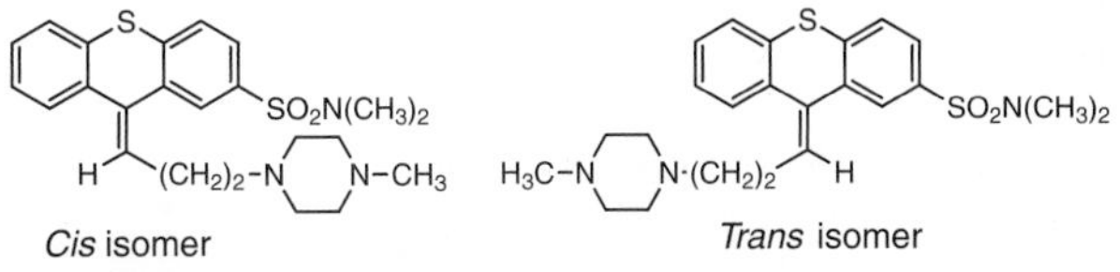

in either the *cis* or *trans* isomeric configuration. The *cis* isomer of the neuroleptic thiothixene is several times more

Table 17.2. Phenothiazine and the Thioxanthene Derivatives Used as Neuroleptics*

General phenothiazine nucleus: positions R_2 and R_{10}.

Phenothiazines Generic Name (Trade Name)	R_{10}	R_2	Adult Antipsychotic Oral Dose Range (mg/day)	Side Effects** Sedative Effects	Side Effects** Extra-pyramidal Effects	Side Effects** Hypertensive Effects	Other Effects
Chloropromazine hydrochloride (Thorazine)	$(CH_2)_3N(CH_3)_2 \cdot HCl$	Cl	300–800	+++	++	Oral ++ IM +++	Antiemetic dose 10–25 mg every 4–6 hrs
Triflupromazine hydrochloride (Vesprin)	$(CH_2)_3N(CH_3)_2 \cdot HCl$	CF_3	100–150	++	+++	++	Antiemetic dose 5–15 mg every 4–6 hrs
Thioridazine hydrochloride (Mellaril)	$(CH_2)_2$ [N-methylpiperidin-2-yl] $\cdot HCl$	SCH_3	200–600	+++	+	++	
Mesoridazine mesylate (Serentil)	$(CH_2)_2$ [N-methylpiperidin-2-yl] $\cdot C_6H_5SO_3H$	$O=SCH_3$	75–300	+++	+	++	
Perphenazine (Trilafon)	$(CH_2)_3N$ [piperazine] $N-CH_2CH_2OH$	Cl	8–32	++	+++	+	
Prochlorperazine edisylate maleate (Compazine)	$(CH_2)_3N$ [piperazine] NCH_3	Cl	75–100	++	+++	+	Antiemetic dose 5–10 mg every 4–6 hrs
Fluphenazine hydrochloride (Permitil, Prolixin)	$(CH_2)_3N$ [piperazine] $N-CH_2CH_2OH \cdot 2HCl$	CF_3	1–20	+	+++	+	
Trifluperazine hydrochloride (Stelazine)	$(CH_2)_3N$ [piperazine] $N-CH_3 \cdot 2HCl$	CF_3	6–20	+	+++	+	
Acetophenazine maleate (Tindal)	$(CH_2)_3N$ [piperazine] $N-CH_2CH_2OH$	$COCH_3$	60–120	++	++	+	
Thiethylperazine maleate (Torecan)	$(CH_2)_3N$ [piperazine] $N-CH_3$	SCH_2CH_3		+	+	+	Antiemetic dose 10–30 mg daily
Thioxanthene Thiothixene hydrochloride (Navane)	thioxanthene nucleus, $H-C-(CH_2)_2-N$ [piperazine] $N-CH_3 \cdot HCl$	$SO_2N(CH_3)_2$	6–30	++	++	++	

*The phenothiazine derivatives that are effective in the treatment of nausea and vomiting are included in this listing.

**+++, high; ++, medium; +, low.

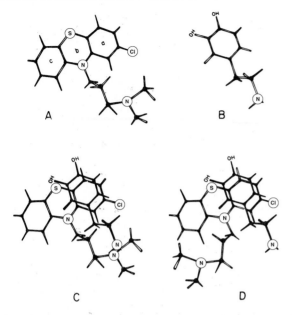

Fig. 17.5. Conformations of chlorpromazine **(A)**, dopamine **(B)**, and their superposition **(C)**, determined by X-ray crystallographic analysis. The a, b, and c in (A) designate rings. D shows another conformation in which the alkyl side chain of chlorpromazine is in the *trans* conformation (ring a and amino side chain), which is not superimposable on the dopamine. (Adapted from A.S. Horn and S.H. Snyder, *Proc. Natl. Acad. Sci. U.S.A., 68,* 2325[1971]).

active than both the *trans* isomer and the compound obtained from saturation of the double bond. Structure D in Figure 17.5 shows that the active structure of dopamine does not superimpose with a *trans*-like conformer of chlorpromazine that would be predicted to be inactive.

Long-acting Neuroleptics. The duration of action of many of the neuroleptics with a free hydroxyl (OH) moiety can be considerably prolonged by the preparation of long-chain fatty acid esters. Thus, fluphenazine decanoate and fluphenazine enanthate were the first of these esters to appear in clinical use and are longer acting with fewer side effects than the unesterified precursor. The ability to treat patients with a single intramuscular injection every 1–2 weeks with the enanthate or every 2–3 weeks with the decanoate ester means that problems associated with patient compliance to the drug regimens and with drug malabsorption can be reduced. Table 17.3 lists long-acting forms of phenothiazine and thioxanthene, derivatives available in the United States and other countries.

Metabolism of Phenothiazines and Thioxanthenes. There is increasing evidence that the metabolism of neuroleptic drugs is of major significance in the effects of these drugs. Although considerable information about the metabolism of the extensively studied chlorpromazine is available, information about many of the other drugs administered for prolonged periods is scant. Generally, however, the liver microsomal CYP450–catalyzed metabolic pathways for neuroleptics are similar to those for many other drugs. Some metabolic pathways for chlorpro-

mazine are shown in Figure 17.6. It should be kept in mind that, during metabolism, several processes can and do occur for the same molecule. For example, chlorpromazine can be demethylated, sulfoxidized, hydroxylated, and glucuronidated to yield 7-O-glu-nor-CPZ-SO. The combination of such processes leads to more than 100 identified metabolites. There is evidence that the 7-hydroxylated derivatives and possibly other hydroxylated derivatives, as well as, the mono- and di-desmethylated products (nor$_1$-CPZ, nor$_2$-CPZ), are active in vivo and at dopamine D$_2$ receptors, whereas the sulfoxide (CPZ-SO) is inactive. Although the thioxanthenes are closely related to the phenothiazines in their pharmacologic effects, there seems to be at least one major difference in metabolism; most of the thioxanthenes do not form ring-hydroxylated derivatives. Metabolic pathways for phenothiazines and thioxanthenes are significantly altered, both quantitatively and qualitatively, by a number of factors, including species, age, gender, interaction with other drugs, and route of administration.

Meperidine

Propiophenone analog

Butyrophenone analog

Development of Butyrophenone Neuroleptics

In the late 1950s, Janssen and co-workers synthesized the propiophenone and butyrophenone analogs of meperidine in an effort to increase its analgesic potency (30). The propiophenone analog had 200 times the analgesic potency of meperidine, but the butyrophenone analog also displayed activity resembling that of chlorpromazine. Janssen found that it was possible to eliminate the morphine type of analgesic activity and simultaneously to accentuate the chlorpromazine type of neuroleptic activity in the butyrophenone series, provided that certain structural changes are made.

Structure-activity Relationships. Haloperidol binds with equally high affinity to dopamine D$_2$, serotonin 5-HT$_2$, and putative σ$_2$ receptors in mammalian brain tissue and any or all of these receptor systems may be involved in mediating the antipsychotic activity of the butyrophenones. In most respects, the pharmacologic effects of haloperidol and other butyrophenones differ in degree but not in kind from those of the piperazine phenothiazines. Haloperidol produces a high incidence of extrapyramidal reactions, but its sedative effect in moderate doses is less than that observed with chlorpromazine. Haloperidol has less prominent autonomic effects than do

Table 17.3. Long-acting Neuroleptics for IM Depot Injection

Generic Name Phenothiazines	R	R$_2$	Dosage Range (mg)	Typical Duration of Action (weeks)
Fluphenazine enanthate	$(CH_2)_3N$ N-CH$_2$CH$_2$O·C(=O)-(CH$_2$)$_5$CH$_3$	CF$_3$	25–100	1–2
Fluphenazine decanoate	$(CH_2)_3N$ N-CH$_2$CH$_2$O-C(=O)-(CH$_2$)$_8$CH$_3$	CF$_3$	25–200	2–3
Perphenazine enanthate	$(CH_2)_3N$ N-CH$_2$CH$_2$O-C(=O)-(CH$_2$)$_5$CH$_3$	Cl	25–100	1–2
Thioxanthene Flupenthixol decanoate	H-C=(CH$_2$)$_2$-N N-(CH$_2$)$_2$-O-C(=O)-(CH$_2$)$_8$CH$_3$ (CF$_3$)		100–200	1–2

Adapted from Simpson and Lee (32) and Baldessarini (4).

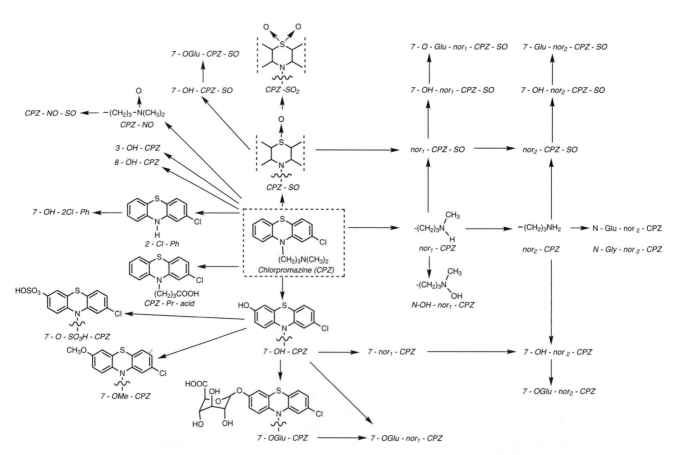

Fig. 17.6. Metabolism of chlorpromazine. Abbreviations: CPZ, chlorpromazine; NO, N-oxide; SO, sulfoxide; SO$_2$, sulfone; O-Glu, O-glucuronide; Ph, phenothiazine; Pr-acid, propionic acid; O-SO$_3$H, sulfate.

the other antipsychotic drugs and only mild hypotension occurs with the use of haloperidol even in high doses.

All butyrophenone derivatives displaying high neuroleptic potency have the following general structure:

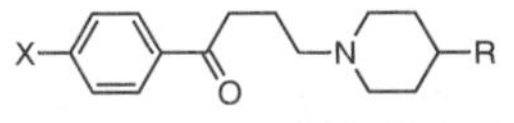

X = F or OCH_3

The attachment of a tertiary amino group to the fourth carbon of the butyrophenone skeleton is essential for neuroleptic activity; lengthening, shortening, or branching of the three-carbon propyl chain decreases neuroleptic potency. Replacement of the keto moiety (e.g., with the thioketone group as in the butyrothienones, with olefinic or phenoxy groups, or, reduction of the carbonyl group) decreases neuroleptic potency. In addition, most potent butyrophenone compounds have a fluorine substituent in the para position of the benzene ring. Variations are possible in the tertiary amino group without loss of neuroleptic potency; for example, the basic nitrogen usually is incorporated into a six-membered ring (piperidine, tetrahydropyridine, or piperazine) that is substituted in the *para* position.

Haloperidol was introduced for the treatment of psychoses in Europe in 1958 and the United States in 1967 (Fig. 17.7). It has proven to be an effective alternative to more familiar antipsychotic phenothiazine drugs, and also is used for the manic phase of bipolar (manic-depressive) disorder. Haloperidol decanoate has been introduced as depot maintenance therapy. When injected every 4–6 weeks, the drug appears to be as effective as daily orally administered haloperidol. Other currently available (mostly in Europe) butyrophenones include the very potent spiperone (spiroperidol), as well as, trifluperidol and droperidol. Droperidol, a short-acting, sedating butyrophenone, is used in anesthesia for its sedating and antiemetic effects and sometimes in psychiatric emergencies as a sedative-neuroleptic. Droperidol often is administered in combination with the potent narcotic analgesic fentanyl for preanesthetic sedation and anesthesia.

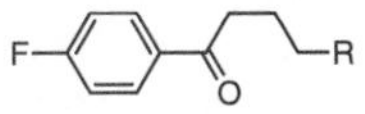

Generic names	Trade names	R
Haloperidol	Haldol	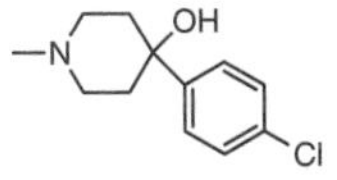
Haloperidol decanoate		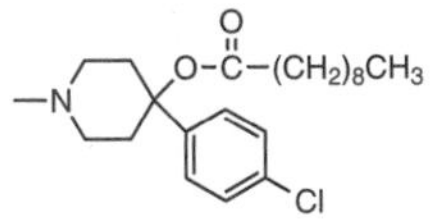
Spiperone		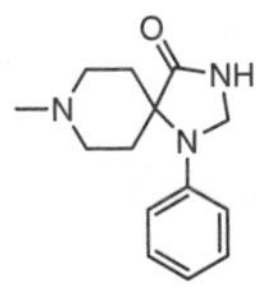
Trifluperidol		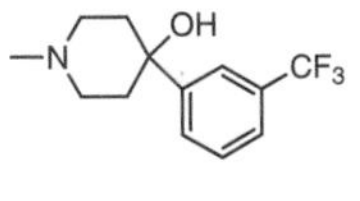
Droperidol	Inapsine	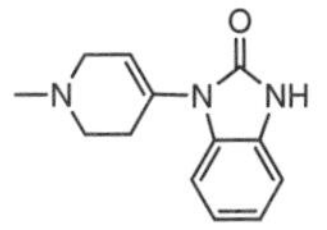

Fig. 17.7. Haloperidol and its analogs.

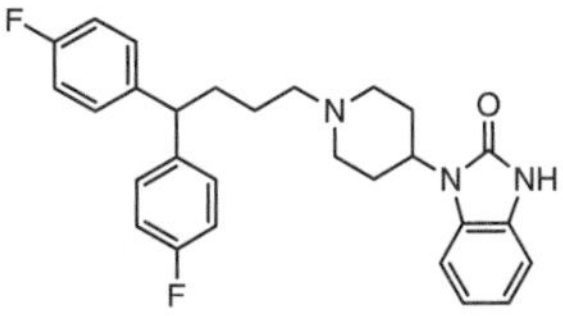

Pimozide

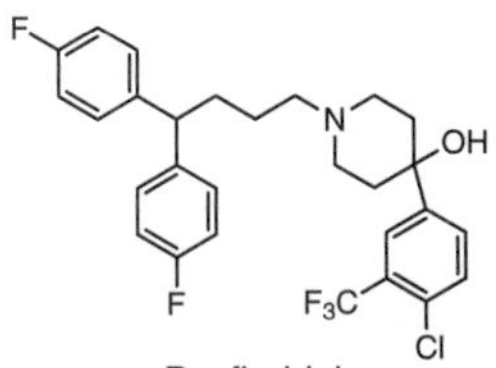

Penfluridol

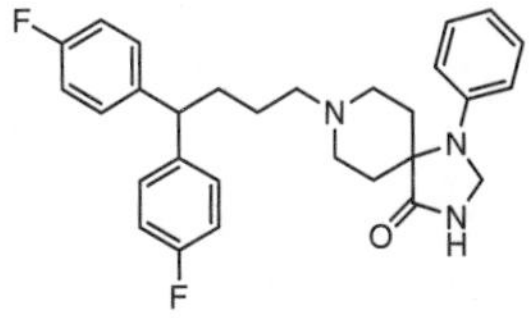

Fluspirilene

Modification of the haloperidol butyrophenone side chain by replacement of the keto function with a di-4-flurophenylmethane moiety results in diphenylbutyl piperidine neuroleptics, such as pimozide, penfluridol, and fluspirilene. The diphenylbutyl piperidines neuroleptics have a longer duration of action than the butyrophenone analogs. All are effective in the control of schizophrenia, and, in particular, pimozide has been shown to be useful in treating acute exacerbation of schizophrenia and in reducing the rate of relapse in chronic schizophrenic patients (32). Pimozide also is used for treatment of Tourette's syndrome, a movement disorder characterized by facial tics, grimaces, strange uncontrollable sounds, and sometimes the involuntary shouting of obscenities. This disorder may be misdiagnosed by clinicians as schizophrenia. Typically the onset of Tourette's syndrome occurs at age 10 and standard treatment for Tourette's syndrome in the past has been the neuroleptics such as haloperidol. Chronic treatment of Tourette's syndrome with haloperidol, as well as, pimozide, carries the risk of producing potentially irreversible tardive dyskinesia. Penfluridol and fluspiriline, although not currently available in the United States, are other examples of long-acting neuroleptics in this structure class.

Metabolism. Haloperidol is readily absorbed from the gastrointestinal tract. Peak plasma levels occur 2–6 hours after ingestion. The drug is concentrated in the liver and CNS, about 15% of a given dose is excreted in the bile, and about 40% is eliminated through the kidney. Figure 17.8 shows the typical oxidative metabolic pathway of butyrophenones as exemplified by haloperidol (31).

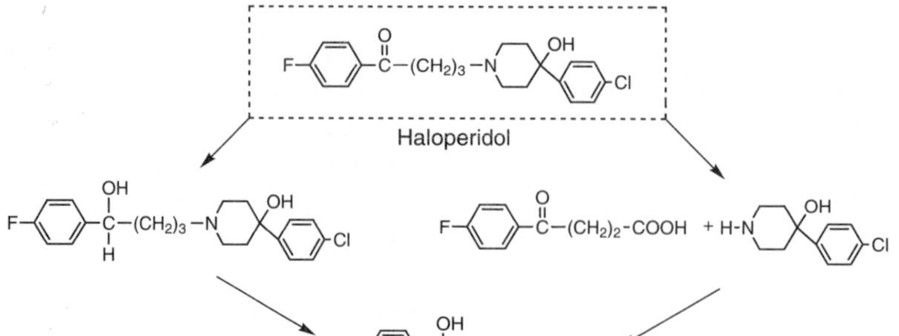

Fig. 17.8. Metabolism of haloperidol.

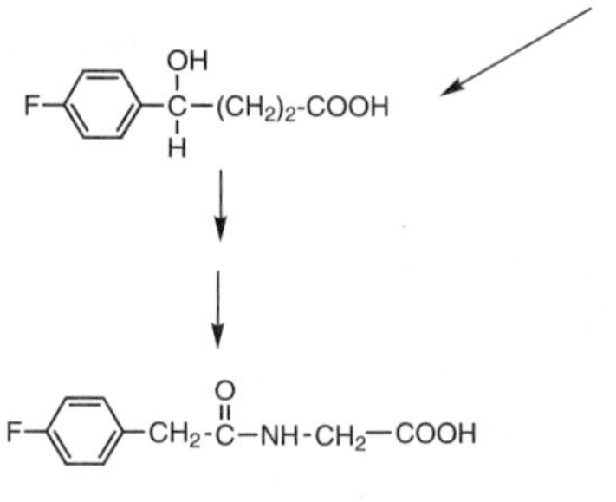

Toxicology

As described in the text (side effects of neuroleptics), extrapyramidal side effects occur in 30–50% of patients receiving standard doses of typical neuroleptics. Extrapyramidal side effects include acute dystonias, akathisia, and parkinsonian-type symptoms such as bradykinesia, cogwheel rigidity, tremor, masked face, and shuffling gait. Tardive dyskinesia is a severe extrapyramidal side effect that occurs in 15–25% of patients after prolonged treatment

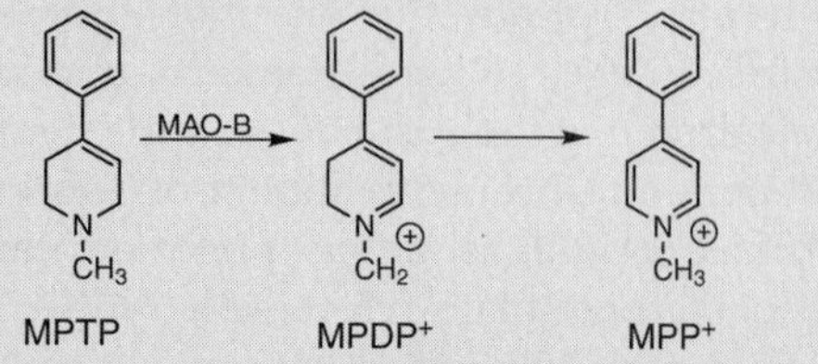

Haloperidol-induced dyskinesias may involve neurotoxicological mechanisms similar to the dopaminergic toxicant MPTP.

with typical neuroleptics. Tardive dyskinesia is characterized by stereotyped, involuntary, repetitive, choreiform movements of the face, eyelids, mouth, tongue, extremities, and trunk; the pathophysiology of tardive dyskinesia is not known and the disorder essentially is irreversible.

Haloperidol (HP, see Figure 17.8) is a potent neuroleptic associated with a high incidence of tardive dyskinesia. Microsomal catalyzed dehydration of haloperidol yields the

corresponding 1,2,3,6-tetrahydropyridine derivative, HPTP, a close analog of the parkinsonian-inducing neurotoxin 1-methyl-4-phenyl-1,2,3,6-tetrahydropyridine (MPTP). Long term (58 weeks) administration of HPTP to non-human primates alters both presynaptic and postsynaptic dopaminergic neuronal function, which may contribute to the neurotoxicologic effects of haloperidol (33). In humans, HPTP is oxidized in vivo to the corresponding pyridinium species HPP^+, similar to the oxidation of MPTP to its ultimate neurotoxic species MPP^+. The metabolite HPP^+ has been identified in the urine of humans treated with haloperidol (34).

Although there is no direct evidence of haloperidol induced brain lesions in humans, it is known that HPP^+ inhibits mitochondrial respiration and is toxic to dopaminergic neuronally-derived cells in vitro (35). Investigations currently are underway to determine if neuroleptic-induced pathology of the extrapyramidal motor system, such as that associated with tardive dyskinesia, may be related to production of MPP^+/HPP^+-type species in the brain.

See Chapter 20 for a related discussion of Parkinson's disease caused by MPTP.

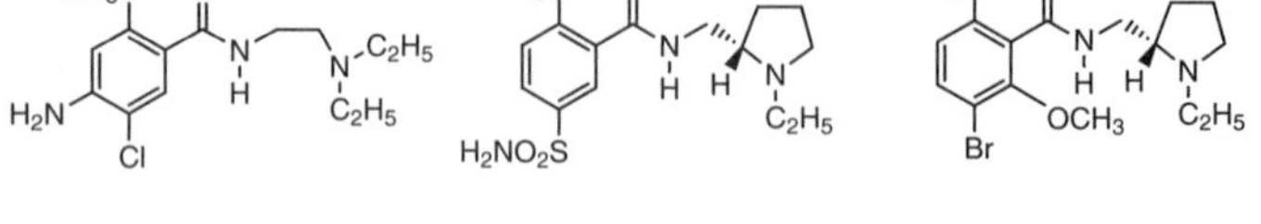

Metoclopramide (Reglan)   S-(−)-Sulpiride   S-(−)-Remoxipride

Miscellaneous Classes of Antipsychotic Agents

Benzamide Derivatives. Certain benzamide derivatives have both local anesthetic and antiemetic properties (36). The benzamide metoclopramide has limited local anesthetic activity but is an efficacious antiemetic drug that modifies gastric motility. Similar to the phenothiazine antiemetics (e.g., promethazine), metoclopramide was found to antagonize dopamine D_2-type receptors in the chemoreceptor trigger zone of the brainstem and subsequently was shown to be neuroleptic (37). Other pyrrolidinyl-containing benzamides such as S-(−)-sulpiride and S-$(-)$-remoxipride also are neuroleptic. Sulpiride produces a relatively low incidence of extrapyramidal side effects, putatively due to a preferential effect on limbic vs. extrapyramidal (striatum) tissue. The hydrophilic properties of sulpiride may account for its poor oral absorption, limited penetration into the central nervous system, and resulting low potency. Remoxipride, on the other hand, is orally well absorbed and is comparable to standard neuroleptics (e.g., haloperidol) in antipsychotic potency and efficacy, but with less incidence of extrapyramidal and autonomic side effects. Life-threatening aplastic anemia, however, has been reported with remoxipride use that may limit its popularity as an alternative antipsychotic drug.

Clozapine (Clozaril)

Olanzapine (Zyprexa)

Loxapine (Loxitane), (R = CH₃)
Amoxapine (Asendin), (R = H)

Quetiapine (Seraquel)

Benzazepine Derivatives. Clozapine, olanzapine, loxapine, and quetiapine are benzazepine-type derivatives with antipsychotic activity and atypically low risk of extrapyramidal side effects. The dibenzazepine clozapine is representative of the new generation of antipsychotic drugs that have greatly reduced or minimal extrapyramidal side effects and do not produce tardive dyskinesia with long term use. Clozapine also appears to effectively alleviate the negative symptoms of schizophrenia and has proven beneficial in treating patients who do not respond adequately to classical neuroleptic agents such as the phenothiazines or butyrophenones. A serious drawback to the use of clozapine, however, is the potentially fatal agranulocytosis that is reported to occur in 1–2% of unmonitored patients (38), necessitating weekly white blood cell counts for at least the first 6 months of pharmacotherapy. Clozapine has relatively low affinity for brain dopamine D_1 and D_2 receptors (moderate affinity for D_4) in comparison to its affinity at adrenergic α_1 and α_2, histamine H_1, muscarinic M_1 and serotonin $5\text{-}HT_{2A}$, receptors (14,39); thus, its special psychotherapeutic effects may be mediated through interactions with these other receptor systems. The thienobenzodiazepine olanzapine is an effective antipsychotic agent, however, its neuropharmacologic profile is somewhat different from clozapine in that it is a more potent antagonist at dopamine D_2 and especially serotonin $5\text{-}HT_{2A}$ receptors (14). The dibenzo-oxazepine loxapine is another antipsychotic in this structural class that has a more typical neuroleptic

biochemical profile with mainly antidopaminergic activity at D_2-type receptors. Loxapine undergoes phase-I aromatic hydroxylation to yield several phenolic metabolites that have higher affinity for D_2 receptors than the parent. Loxapine also undergoes N-demethylation to form amoxapine which is used clinically as an antidepressant. Amoxapine binds to D_2 receptors and inhibits the norepinephrine neurotransporter to block neuronal norepinephrine re-uptake, a correlate of antidepressant activity. Quetiapine is a dibenzothiazepine with a brain receptor binding profile similar to clozapine. Quetiapine binds most effectively to histaminergic H_1, adrenergic α_1 and α_2, and serotonergic $5\text{-}HT_{2a}$ receptors in the brain, and has even lower affinity than clozapine for dopaminergic D_2 receptors; unlike clozapine, quetiapine also has very low affinity for muscarinic receptors. Quetiapine is 100% bioavailable, but first pass metabolism yields at least 20 metabolites via CYP3A4, with a half-life of about 6 hours. Quetiapine is about as effective as haloperidol in treating the positive symptoms of schizophrenia, but also manages negative symptoms and induces a lower incidence of extrapyramidal side effects.

Risperidone (Risperdal)

BENZISOXAZOLES

Neuroanatomical and neurophysiologic interactions between dopaminergic and serotonergic systems, together with evidence that several atypical antipsychotic agents (e.g., clozapine, olanzapine) have high affinity for $5\text{-}HT_2$ receptors, led to the proposal that combination $D_2/5\text{-}HT_2$ antagonists may produce atypical antipsychotic effects (40, 41). Combining the chemical features present in the potent benzamide D_2 antagonists (e.g., remoxipride) with those of the benzothiazolyl piperazine $5\text{-}HT_2$ antagonists (e.g., tiospirone) led to the development of the 3-(4-piperidinyl)-1,2-benzisoxazole nucleus present in the $5\text{-}HT_2/D_2$ antagonist risperidone, which also has relatively high affinity at histamine H_1 and adrenergic α_1/α_2 receptors.

The anti-serotonergic effects of risperidone are proposed to un-inhibit dopaminergic neurotransmission in the striatum and cortex, reducing the severity of D_2 antagonist-induced extrapyramidal side effects and alleviating negative symptoms of schizophrenia, while maintaining a blockade of limbic system D_2 receptors (42). Risperidone is well absorbed orally and undergoes hepatic CYP2D6 catalyzed hydroxylation (active metabolite) and N-dealkylation.

Molindone. Molindone hydrochloride, a tetrahydroindolone derivative, is a neuroleptic agent that is structurally unrelated to any of the other marketed neuroleptics. Molindone is less potent than haloperidol at

Molindone (Moban)

blocking D_2 receptors, however, it nonetheless can produce extrapyramidal side effects. Metabolism studies in humans show molindone to be rapidly absorbed and metabolized when given orally. There are 36 recognized metabolites with less than 2–3% unmetabolized molindone being excreted in urine and feces. Clinical studies show that the antipsychotic effects of molindone last more than 24 hours, suggesting that one or more metabolites may contribute to its activity in vivo (43).

Sertindole (Serdolect)

Sertindole. Sertindole is an indole-containing compound that behaves as a high affinity serotonin 5-HT$_2$ receptor antagonist, with weak affinity for adrenergic α_1 receptors, and almost no affinity for dopaminergic D_2 receptors. It is about as effective as haloperidol in treatment of acute and chronic schizophrenia, but with much lower incidence of extrapyramidal side effects. Sertindole is relatively non-sedating and its effects are long lasting (several days) (44).

ANXIETY AND ANXIETY DISORDERS
Definitions

Anxiety can be defined as a sense of apprehensive expectation. In reasonable amounts and at appropriate times, anxiety is helpful (e.g., anxiety before an examination may cause a student to initiate an appropriate study plan). Too much anxiety, however, can be deleterious. Anxiety can be considered pathological when it is either completely inappropriate to the situation, or is in excess of what the situation normally should call for. An example of the former is nocturnal panic attacks—episodes of extreme anxiety that arise out of one of the most physiologically quiet times of the day, stage III/IV sleep (45). An example of the latter is specific phobias—an irrational fear to venture outside of one's home, for instance.

According to the DSM-IV-RT, abnormal anxiety is that level of anxiety that interferes with normal social or occupational functioning. This definition is helpful to distinguish between normal and pathologic levels of anxiety. To meet general DSM-IV-RT criteria, anxiety symptoms must not be caused by an exogenous factor (e.g., caffeine) or a medical condition (e.g., hyperthyroidism). Examples of anxiety disorders include specific phobias, generalized anxiety disorder (chronic abnormally high level of worry),

social phobia (e.g., fear of public speaking), obsessive-compulsive disorder (OCD), panic disorder with or without agoraphobia (avoidance of situations believed by the patient to precipitate panic attacks), and post-traumatic stress disorder.

Etiology of Anxiety Disorders

Studies of patients with anxiety disorders have not revealed a general gross neuroanatomic lesion. In vivo functional imaging studies, however, show altered blood flow or utilization of glucose in certain brain areas in patients with anxiety conditions, including OCD (46,47), panic disorder (48,49), specific phobia (50), generalized anxiety disorder (51), and post-traumatic stress disorder (52), mostly implicating the prefrontal cortex and hippocampus (and other limbic areas) as being involved in the anatomy of pathologic anxiety.

A variety of neurotransmitters, neuromodulators (e.g., adenosine), and neuropeptides (e.g., cholecystokinin, corticotropin-releasing factor, and neuropeptide Y) are suggested to be involved in the pathophysiology of anxiety. Currently, abundant evidence exists to document the involvement of the neurotransmitters γ-aminobutyric acid (GABA), norepinephrine, and serotonin in anxiety and research is increasingly revealing that these neurotransmitter systems have complex anatomical and functional interrelationships. For example, stimulation of the locus ceruleus, which contains the highest concentration of norepinephrine cell bodies in the central nervous system, generates a state of agitation and fear behaviors in laboratory animals (53). Meanwhile, data suggest that benzodiazepines influence norepinephrine release by stimulating inhibitory GABA receptors located on noradrenergic neurons (54).

GABA/Benzodiazepine Receptor Complex

GABA is the major inhibitory neurotransmitter in the mammalian central nervous system and is widespread, with approximately one-third of all synapses in the central nervous system utilizing this neurochemical for intercellular communication (55). There are two classes of receptors, GABA$_A$ and GABA$_B$. The neurobiologic role of GABA$_B$ receptors is not well understood. GABA$_A$ receptors have been extensively characterized. The GABA$_A$ receptor is a member of the gene superfamily of ligand-gated ion channels (56). The complex is a heteropentameric structure composed of several distinct subunits, or polypeptide types. The subunits have been labeled as α, β, γ, δ, and ρ and combine in varied proportions(57). These polypeptides are composed of an extra-cellular region, four membrane-spanning alpha-helical cylinders, and a large intracellular cytoplasmic loop. The extracellular region is thought to be the site to which ligands bind. The ion channel associated with GABA conducts chloride, and is defined by the second of the four membrane-spanning cylinders. So far, 16 distinct subunits of the $GABA_A$ receptor are identified: six α, four β, three γ, one δ, and two ρ (58). Available data, however, do not suggest that given receptors must have representative subunits from each class.

The $GABA_A$ receptor complex contains a number of distinct binding sites for neuroactive drugs. The benzodiazepines, among the most commonly prescribed antianxiety agents, interact with binding sites which are defined in large part by the α subunit of the $GABA_A$ receptor complex. The α subunit composition seems to govern not only affinity, but also the intrinsic potency of benzodiazepine receptor ligands (59). Previous to the discovery of the $GABA_A$ receptor, the site that benzodiazepines bind to was termed the benzodiazepine receptor (BZR). Early research on the BZR gave rise to the concept of agonists, inverse agonists, and antagonists. Agonist compounds bind to the $GABA_A$ receptor (BZR) and potentiate the action of GABA (e.g., sedation, anticonvulsant activity). Inverse agonists bind to the $GABA_A$ receptor and induce action opposite that of GABA (e.g., anxiogenesis, pro-convulsant action). Antagonists occupy the receptor, but have no intrinsic activity. A clinical example of the use of an antagonist is the compound flumazenil, which is used to reverse benzodiazepine-induced sedation in overdose. There also have been developed agents which are partial agonists and inverse partial agonists at the $GABA_A$ receptor. The existence of a $GABA_A$ receptor that recognizes benzodiazepines has implications for our understanding of both normal and pathologic anxiety states and suggests the existence of endogenous $GABA_A$ receptor ligands. Thus, anxiety could conceivably be either a lack of an endogenous $GABA_A$ receptor agonist, or a relative excess of a $GABA_A$ receptor antagonist or inverse agonist.

Drugs Used in the Treatment of Anxiety
Benzodiazepines

The benzodiazepines are the prototypic anti-anxiety agents. Chlordiazepoxide was the first benzodiazepine to be marketed for clinical use in 1960. Its effectiveness and wide margin of safety were major advances over compounds such as barbiturates used previously. A variety of new benzodiazepines followed, each with some minor differences from the competition. The major factors considered when selecting an agent include rate and extent of absorption, presence or absence of active metabolites, and degree of lipophilicity. These factors help determine how a benzodiazepine is marketed and used; e.g., an agent which is rapidly absorbed, highly lipid soluble, and without active metabolites would be useful as a hypnotic, but less useful for treatment of a chronic anxiety state. On the other hand, a compound with slower absorption, active metabolites, and low lipophilicity would be a more effective anti-anxiety agent, but less helpful as a soporific.

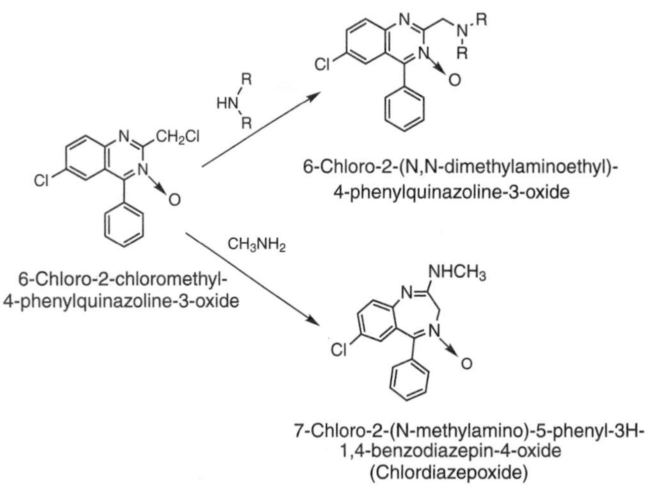

Fig. 17.9. Synthesis of chloradiazepoxide.

Despite their efficacy in a variety of pathologic anxiety syndromes, the benzodiazepines are not perfect anxiolytics. Such a hypothetical agent would selectively ameliorate anxiety without inducing other behavioral effects. Future efforts to enhance the efficacy of benzodiazepine anxiolytics may depend on a greater understanding of the heterogeneity of the $GABA_A$ receptor; for example, which specific clinical actions (anxiolytic, muscle relaxation, sleep facilitation) reside with which specific subunit composition.

Development of Benzodiazepine Anxiolytics. In the 1950s, the medicinal chemist Sternbach noted that "basic groups frequently impart biological activity" and in accordance with this observation, he synthesized a series of compounds by treating various chloromethylquinazoline N-oxides with amines to produce what he hoped would be products with "tranquilizer" activity at the New Jersey laboratories of Hoffman LaRoche (60,61). Sternbach's studies included the reaction of 6-chloro-2-chloromethyl-4-phenyl-quinazoline-3-oxide with methylamine, that yielded the unexpected rearrangement product, 7-chloro-2-(N-methylamino)-5-phenyl-3H-1,4,-benzodiazepin-4-oxide (Fig. 17.9). This product was given the code name RO 50690 and screened for pharmacologic activity in 1957. Subsequently, Randall (62,63) reported that RO 50690 was hypnotic and sedative, and, had antistrychnine properties similar to the propanediol meprobamate, a sedative with tranquilizer (anxiolytic) properties only at intoxicating doses. Renamed chlordiazepoxide, RO 50690 was marketed as Librium in 1960, a safe and effective anxiolytic agent.

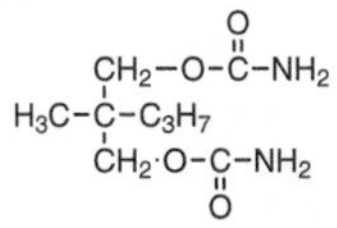

Meprobamate

Chlordiazepoxide turned out to have rather remarkable pharmacologic properties and tremendous potential as a

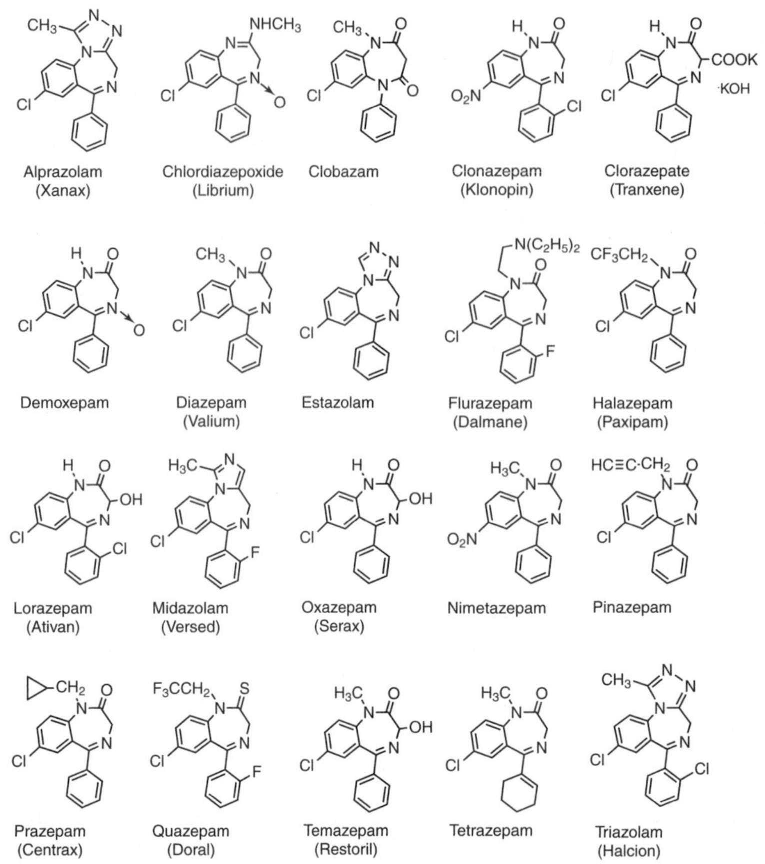

Fig. 17.10. Structures of some commercially available benzodiazepines.

pharmacotherapeutic product, but possessed a number of unacceptable physical chemical properties. In an effort to enhance its "pharmaceutical elegance," structural modifications of chlordiazepoxide were undertaken that eventually led to the synthesis of diazepam in 1959. In contrast to the maxim that basic groups impart biologic activity, diazepam contains no basic nitrogen moiety. Diazepam, however, was found to be 3–10 times more potent than chlordiazepoxide and was marketed in 1963 as the still enormously popular anxiolytic drug Valium. Subsequently, thousands of benzodiazepine derivatives were synthesized and more than two-dozen benzodiazepines are in clinical use in the United States, Figure 17.10.

Endogenous BZR Ligands

An endogenous ligand with affinity for the CNS benzodiazepine receptor (BZR) of the GABA$_A$ receptor complex has not been conclusively identified. Several compounds of endogenous origin, however, that inhibit the binding of radiolabeled benzodiazepines to the BZR, have been reported. In 1980, Braestrup (64) reported the presence in normal human urine of β-carboline-3-carboxylic acid ethyl ester (βCCE), that has very high affinity for the BZR complex. It was subsequently shown, however, that βCCE formed as an artifact from Braestrup's extraction procedure during which the urine extract was heated with ethanol at pH 1, a

condition favoring formation of the ethyl ester from β-carboline-3-carboxylic acid, a tryptophan metabolite.

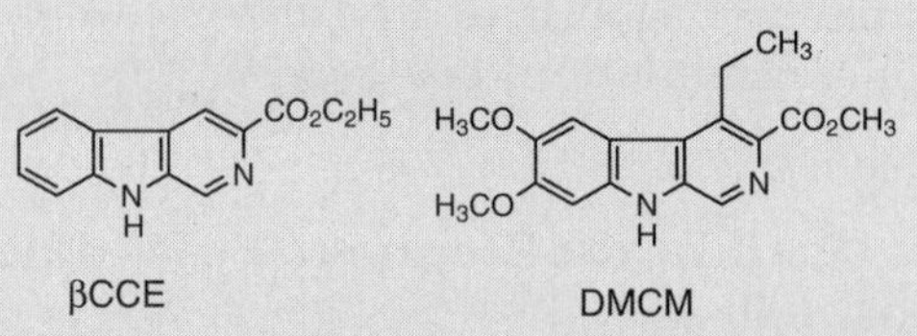

Although βCCE actually was shown not to be of endogenous origin, its discovery as a high affinity BZR ligand stimulated research that led to the synthesis of a series of β-carboline derivatives with a variety of intrinsic activities, presumably mediated through the BZR that is associated with the GABA$_A$ receptor complex. For example, while βCCE is considered to be a *partial* inverse agonist at this site, 6,7-dimethoxy-4-ethyl-β-carboline-3-carboxylic acid methyl ester (DMCM) appears to be a *full* inverse agonist (65). In fact, βCCE blocks the convulsions produced by the very potent convulsant DMCM (66). These effects are even more complex and interesting in light of the approximately 10-fold higher affinity that βCCE shows for the BZR labeled by [^{3}H]-diazepam when compared to DMCM (67). The β-carbolines currently are important research tools to probe the agonist, competitive antagonist, inverse agonist, and partial agonist/inverse agonist pharmacophores of the BZR/GABA receptor complex.

A major advance in the BZR field was made in 1981 with the first report that the imidazobenzodiazepinone derivative RO 15-1788 (flumazenil) (Fig. 17.11) binds with high affinity to the BZR and blocks the pharmacologic effects of the classi-

Flumazenil
(Romazicon)

cal benzodiazepines in vitro and in vivo (68). Unlike agonists, binding of [³H]-RO 15-1788 to the BZR is not affected by modulators such as GABA and several ions that induce changes in receptors (69). The insensitivity of RO 15-1788 to changes in BZR conformation suggests that the ligand does not induce a conformational change in the receptor to trigger a biologic response and is a pure antagonist (67). Such benzodiazepine antagonists are being used to characterize the pharmacologic nature of the BZR and several of these agents, including flumazenil, are used to treat benzodiazepine overdose. Other imidazobenzodiazepinone derivatives are not true BZR antagonists, but rather, have inverse agonist activity. For example, RO 15-4513 (Fig. 17.11), is reported to be a partial inverse agonist that produces anxiogenic-like effects in rats (65), pharmacologic activity quite different from a true BZR competitive antagonist such as flumazenil.

Mechanism of Action of Anxiolytic Benzodiazepines

Ligand Interaction with the Benzodiazepine Receptor (BZR). BZR ligands, regardless of intrinsic activity, do not directly alter transmembrane chloride conduction to produce

their observed characteristic physiologic anxiolytic or anxiogenic effects. BZR ligands act as modulators of GABA binding to its receptor, which then directly alters the gating of the GABA-dependent transmembrane chloride channel. A representation of the relationship between ligand interaction with the BZR and intrinsic activity to modulate GABA receptor function is shown in Figure 17.11. The BZR is indicated here as a single entity to simplify the presentation. It should be emphasized, however, that there is compelling evidence for the existence of subtypes of the BZR/GABA$_A$ receptor, based on relative binding affinity and intrinsic activity of BZR ligands. Accordingly, while the binding sites for functionally diverse BZR/GABA$_A$ receptor ligands may overlap, as previously described, the pharmacophores for agonist, inverse agonist, and antagonist functional activity must, by definition, differ (70). Although the functional significance of BZR subtypes is not well-established, subtype-selective ligands are functionally similar in that they interact with a BZR that is an integral part of the GABA$_A$ receptor-chloride channel complex to modulate the action of GABA (71). Of possible clinical importance, "uncoupling" of the BZR/GABA receptor complex has been observed in response to chronic benzodiazepine exposure both in vitro (72) and in vivo (73). In the absence of exogenous influences, however, coupling efficiency appears to be determined by the composition and stoichiometry of the α-subunits (74), while benzodiazepine affinity, intrinsic activity, and efficacy, is determined by the nature of both the α- and γ-subunits (75,76).

The BZR can be thought of as an allosteric modulatory "secondary" receptor that affects GABA binding to the GABA$_A$ receptor, which, in turn, modulates the transmembrane conductance of chloride. In the presence of BZR

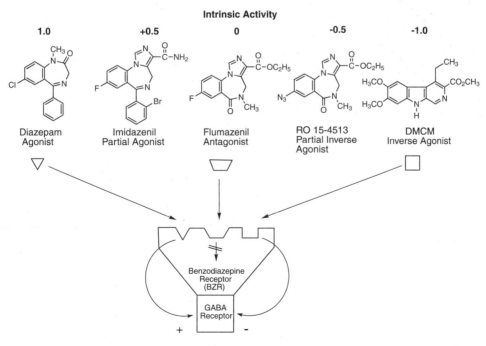

Intrinsic Activity

| 1.0 | +0.5 | 0 | -0.5 | -1.0 |

Diazepam
Agonist

Imidazenil
Partial Agonist

Flumazenil
Antagonist

RO 15-4513
Partial Inverse
Agonist

DMCM
Inverse Agonist

Fig. 17.11. Ligand interaction with the GABA$_A$/benzodiazepine receptor complex.

agonists or partial agonists, GABA potency at GABA$_A$ receptors is enhanced maximally or submaximally (respectively) and conductance of chloride by GABA is increased. Inverse agonists and partial inverse agonists reduce the effect of GABA and GABA$_A$ receptor-mediated conductance of chloride is accordingly decreased. GABA$_A$ receptor-chloride channels thus become either more or less sensitive to GABA in the presence of BZR agonists or inverse agonists, respectively. BZR competitive antagonists block access of agonists to the BZR, but presumably do not induce a conformational change in the BZR and have no intrinsic activity to affect GABA-modulated conductance of chloride.

The interaction of agonists, competitive antagonists, and inverse agonists with the BZR, as shown in Figure 17.11, is a simplistic rendering of the proposed three-state model of the BZR and GABA$_A$ receptor inter-relationship (77,78). This model is based on the hypothesis that the BZR and GABA$_A$ receptor exist in three spontaneously oscillating conformational states, functionally described as "active" or agonist; "neutral" or "resting"; and "inactive" or inverse agonist. BZR agonists and partial agonists bind to and stabilize the "active" state, inducing a conformational change in the GABA$_A$ receptor complex that results in chloride channel opening, that may lead to an anticonvulsant or anxiolytic effect. BZR inverse agonists and partial inverse agonists bind to and stabilize the "inactive" state, resulting in the chloride channel remaining closed, that may lead to a convulsant or anxiogenic effect. BZR competitive antagonists presumably bind equally well to both states (hence, they bind to a "neutral" state) and affect no change in GABA$_A$ receptor function or chloride conductance, but access of agonists to the BZR is blocked.

Structure-Activity Relationships. The structure-activity relationship (SAR) for classical 5-phenyl-1,4-benzodiazepine-2-one anxiolytic agents has been described by Sternbach and other investigators (60,67,77,79). Thousands of benzodiazepine derivatives with a variety of substituents have been synthesized that interact with the BZR, however, classical quantitative structure-activity relationship (QSAR) and molecular modeling techniques have been used to reduce this myriad of structures to the minimal common molecular features necessary for binding (70,80,81). It should be noted that this SAR for ligand binding is not meant to imply that the BZR is a separate or single entity. To reiterate, the BZR is an integral part of the GABA$_A$ receptor-chloride channel complex and subtypes of the BZR/GABA$_A$ receptor complex, with different subunit composition and stoichiometry, are known to exist. Accordingly, the functional pharmacophores for agonist, inverse agonist, and antagonist activity at different BZR subtypes can be expected to differ. In fact, this pharmacologic activity continuum (agonist, antagonist, inverse agonist) displayed by BZR ligands would seem to require that such diverse functional activity be mediated by ligand interaction with different receptors on the BZR/GABA$_A$

receptor-chloride channel complex. This continuum of activity, however, is displayed by ligands within the same chemical class and small modifications in the chemical structure of a ligand can shift the intrinsic activity from agonist to antagonist to inverse agonist. Moreover, each functional class of BZR ligands can competitively inhibit the binding of the other two classes and agonists and inverse agonists are functional antagonists of each other. These observations suggest that the binding sites of different BZR/GABA$_A$ receptor ligands, at least, overlap. Accordingly, most BZR pharmacophore models that describe ligand *functional* activity are based initially on the BZR pharmacophore for ligand *binding* activity at a single binding domain, and this approach is used here to summarize the SAR for benzodiazepine derivatives at the BZR/GABA$_A$ receptor.

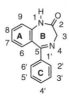

Ring A. In general, the minimum requirements for binding of 5-phenyl-1,4-benzodiazepin-2-one derivatives to the BZR includes an aromatic or heteroaromatic ring (ring A), believed to participate in π/π stacking with aromatic amino acid residues of the receptor. Substituents on ring A are known to have varied effects on binding of benzodiazepines to the BZR, however, such effects are not predictable on the basis of electronic or (within reasonable limits) steric properties. It is generally true, however, that an electronegative group (e.g., halogen, nitro) substituted at the 7-position markedly increases functional anxiolytic activity, albeit, effects on binding affinity *in vitro* are not as dramatic. On the other hand, substituents at positions 6, 8, or 9 generally decrease anxiolytic activity. Other 1,4-diazepine derivatives in which ring A is replaced by a heterocycle generally show weak binding affinity in vitro and even less pharmacologic activity in vivo when compared to phenyl-substituted analogs.

Ring B. A proton-accepting group (e.g., the carbonyl moiety) in the 2-position of ring B appears to be necessary, putatively to interact with a receptor histidine residue that serves as a proton source and is believed to be involved in ligand binding. It is thought that the electrons of the proton accepting group need to be in the same plane as the aromatic ring A, favoring a coplanar spatial orientation of the two moieties. Substitution of sulfur for oxygen at the 2-position (as in quazepam) may affect selectivity for binding to GABA BZR sub-populations, but, anxiolytic activity is maintained. Substitution of the methylene 3-position or the imine nitrogen is sterically unfavorable for antagonist activity, but has no effect on agonist (*i.e.*, anxiolytic) activity (*e.g.*, clobazam). Derivatives substituted with a 3-hydroxy moiety have comparable potency to nonhydroxylated analogs and are excreted faster. Esterification of a 3-hydroxy moiety also is possible without loss of potency. Neither the 1-position amide nitrogen, nor its substituent, is required for in vitro binding to the BZR and many clinically used analogs are not N-alkylated (Fig. 17.10). Although even relatively long N-alkyl side chains do not dramatically decrease BZR affinity, sterically bulky substituents like *tert*-butyl drastically reduce receptor affinity and in vivo activity. Neither the 4,5-double bond, nor the 4-position nitrogen (the 4,5-[methyleneimino] group) in ring B is required for in vivo anxiolytic activity, albeit, in vitro BZR affinity is decreased if the C = N bond is reduced to C – N. It is proposed that in vivo activity of such derivatives results from oxidation back to C = N (67). It follows that the 4-oxide moiety of chlordiazepoxide can be removed without loss of anxiolytic activity.

Ring C. The 5-phenyl ring C is not required for binding to the BZR in vitro , however, this accessory aromatic ring may contribute favorable hydrophobic or steric interactions to receptor binding and its relationship to ring A planarity may be important. Substitution at the 4'-(*para*)-position of an appended 5-phenyl ring is unfavorable for agonist activity, however, 2'-(*ortho*)-substituents are not detrimental to agonist activity, suggesting that limitations at the *para* position are steric, rather than electronic, in nature.

s-Triazolo[4,3a][1,4]benzodiazepine   Imidazo[1,5a][1,4]benzodiazepine

Annelating the 1,2 bond of ring B with an additional "electron-rich" (*i.e.*, proton acceptor) ring, such as s-triazole or imidazole, also results in pharmacologically active benzodiazepine derivatives with high affinity for the BZR (Fig. 17.11). For example, the s-triazolo-benzodiazepines, triazolam, alprazolam, and estazolam and the imidazo-benzodiazepine, midazolam, are popularly prescribed, clinically effective, anxiolytic agents (Fig. 17.10).

a   b

Stereochemistry

Most clinically useful benzodiazepines do not have a chiral center, however, the seven-membered ring B may adopt one of two possible boat conformations; a and b, that are "enantiomeric" (mirror images) to each other. Nuclear magnetic resonance studies indicate that the two confor-

mations can easily interconvert at room temperature, making it impossible to predict which conformation is active at the BZR, *a priori*. Evidence for stereospecificity for binding to the BZR was provided by introducing a 3-substituent into the benzodiazepine nucleus to provide a chiral center and enantiomeric pairs of derivatives (67). In vitro BZR binding affinity and in vivo anxiolytic activity of several 3-methylated enantiomers was found to reside in the S-isomer. Moreover, the S-enantiomer of 3-methyldiazepam was shown to stabilize conformation a for ring B, while the R-enantiomer stabilizes conformation b. Also, the 3-S configuration and a conformation for ring B is present in both the crystalline state (82) and in solution (83) for 3-methyldiazepam. In spite of the enantioselectivity demonstrated for benzodiazepines, the commonly used 3-hydroxylated derivatives (e.g., lorazepam, oxazepam) are commercially available only as racemic mixtures.

Physiochemical and Pharmacokinetics

The physiochemical and pharmacokinetic properties of the various benzodiazepines vary widely and these properties have clinical implications. For example, depending on the nature of substituents, particularly with regard to electronegative substituents, the lipophilicity of the benzodiazepines may vary by more than three orders of magnitude, affecting absorption, distribution, and metabolism of individual agents. In general, most benzodiazepines have relatively high lipid:water partition coefficients (log P values) and are completely absorbed after oral administration and rapidly distributed to the brain and other highly perfused organs. A notable exception is clorazepate, that first is rapidly decarboxylated at the 3-position to N-desmethyldiazepam and subsequently quickly absorbed. Also, most benzodiazepines and their metabolites bind to plasma proteins. The degree of protein binding is dependent on lipophilicity of the compound and varies from about 70% for more polar benzodiazepines, such as alprazolam, to 99% for very lipophilic derivatives, such as diazepam. Hepatic microsomal oxidation, including N-dealkylation and aliphatic hydroxylation, accounts for the major metabolic disposition of most benzodiazepines. Subsequent conjugation of microsomal metabolites by glucuronyl transferases yields polar glucuronides that are excreted in urine. In general, the rate and product of benzodiazepine metabolism varies, depending on route of administration and the individual drug.

Chlordiazepoxide is well absorbed after oral administration and peak blood concentration usually is reached in about 4 hours. Intramuscular absorption of chlordiazepoxide, however, is slower and erratic. The half-life of chlordiazepoxide is variable, but usually quite long, between 6 and 30 hours. The initial N-demethylation product, N-desmethylchloridiazepoxide, undergoes deamination to form the demoxepam (Fig. 17.12). Demoxepam is extensively metabolized and less than one-percent of a

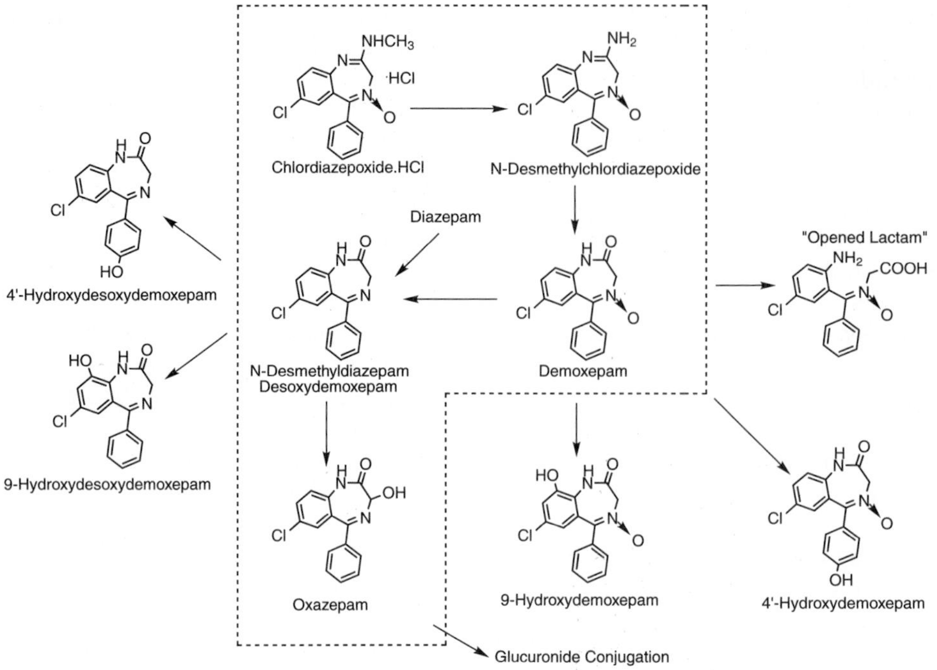

Fig. 17.12. Metabolism of chlordiazepoxide.

dose of chlordiazepoxide is excreted as demoxepam. Demoxepam can undergo four different metabolic fates. Removal of the *N*-oxide moiety yields the active metabolite, *N*-desmethyldiazepam (desoxydemoxepam). This product is a metabolite of both chlordiazepoxide and diazepam and can be hydroxylated to yield oxazepam, another active metabolite that is rapidly glucuronidated and excreted in the urine. Another possibility for metabolism of demoxepam is hydrolysis to the "opened lactam," that is inactive. The two other metabolites of demoxepam are the products of A ring hydroxylation (9-hydroxydemoxepam) or C ring hydroxylation (4'-hydroxydemoxepam), both inactive. The majority of a dose of chlordiazepoxide is excreted as glucuronide conjugates of oxazepam and other phenolic (9- or 4'-hydroxylated) metabolites. As with diazepam (*vide infra*), repeated administration of chlordiazepoxide can result in accumulation of parent drug and its active metabolites, that may have important clinical implications, including excessive sedation (4,5).

Diazepam is rapidly and completely absorbed after oral administration. Maximum peak blood concentration occurs in two hours and elimination is slow, with a half-life of about 20–50 hours. As with chlordiazepoxide, the major metabolic product of diazepam is *N*-desmethyldiazepam, that is pharmacologically active and undergoes even slower metabolism than its parent compound. Repeated administration of diazepam or chlordiazepoxide leads to accumulation of *N*-desmethyldiazepam, that can be detected in the blood for more than one week after discontinuation of the drug. Hydroxylation of *N*-desmethyldiazepam at the 3-position gives the active metabolite oxazepam (Fig. 17.12).

Oxazepam is an active metabolite of both chlordiazepoxide and diazepam and marketed separately as a short-acting anxiolytic agent. Oxazepam is rapidly inactivated to glucuronidated metabolites that are excreted in the urine. The half-life of oxazepam is about 4–8 hours and cumulative effects with chronic therapy are much less than with long-acting benzodiazepines such as chlordiazepoxide and diazepam. Lorazepam is the 2'-chloro derivative of oxazepam and has a similarly short half-life (2–6 hours) and pharmacologic activity.

Flurazepam is administered orally as the dihydrochloride salt. It is rapidly [1]*N*-dealkylated to give the 2'-fluoro derivative of *N*-desmethyldiazepam and subsequently follows the same metabolic pathways as chlordiazepoxide and diazepam (Fig. 17.12). The half-life of flurazepam is fairly long (about 7 hours) and consequently, it has the same potential as chlordiazepoxide and diazepam to produce cumulative clinical effects and side-effects (*e.g.*, excessive sedation) and residual pharmacologic activity, even after discontinuation. Chlorazepate is yet another benzodiazepine that is rapidly metabolized (3-decarboxylation) to *N*-desmethyldiazepam and so shares similar clinical and pharmacokinetic properties to chlordiazepoxide and diazepam.

Detailed pharmacokinetic analysis for most benzodiazepines is complex. Two-compartment models may be adequate to describe the disposition of most derivatives, but three-compartment models are necessary for highly lipophilic agents, such as diazepam. The distribution of such lipophilic drugs is further complicated by enterohepatic circulation. Thus, the usually stated elimination half-life of benzodiazepines may not adequately account for pharmacodynamics of the distributive phase of the drug, that can be clinically important. For example, the distributive (*alpha*) half-life of diazepam is about 1 hour, whereas the elimination (*beta*) half-life is about 1.5 days, acutely, and even longer after chronic dosing that results in accumulation of drug (4,5). Furthermore, plasma concentration and clinical effectiveness of benzodiazepines is difficult to correlate and only a 2-fold increase in clinically effective levels produces sedative side-effects. Consequently, in spite of the long half-life of many benzodiazepines, they are not safe or effective when given in one daily dose and are usually divided into two to four doses per day for treatment of daytime anxiety (4,5). Both therapeutic and toxic effects may persist several days after discontinuation of chronically administered long-acting benzodiazepines, such as chlordiazepoxide and diazepam. Thus, short-acting benzodiazepines, such as oxazepam, that are rapidly metabolized to inactive products, should be considered in elderly or hepato-compromised patients.

Nonbenzodiazepine Agonists at the Benzodiazepine Receptor (BZR)

There are relatively few structural classes of nonbenzodiazepine compounds that have reasonable affinity for the BZR and show pharmacologic activity in vivo. Examples of these classes include the β-carbolines, pyrazoquinolines, triazolopyridazines, and the imidazopyridines (Fig. 17.13). Of these structural classes, only the imidazopyridazines, zolpidem and alpidem, have been investigated in extensive clinical trials.

Several β-carbolines and pyrazoloquinolines have about 10-fold higher affinity for the BZR when compared to diazepam. As already mentioned, the ethyl ester of β-carboline-3-carboxylic acid (βCCE), identified in human urine extracts as an artifact of the extraction procedure, has very high affinity for the BZR. Although βCCE and other β-carbolines are not endogenous BZR ligands and have no clinical utility, β-carboline derivatives have been

useful to probe the agonist, competitive antagonist, inverse agonist, and partial agonist/inverse agonist pharmacophores of the BZR associated with the GABA receptor. Likewise, some derivatives of the pyrazoloquinoline class have been shown to be benzodiazepine antagonists, while others appear to be partial agonists with anxiogenic activity. No pyrazoloquinolines have yet been identified that show clinical promise, although the *para*-chloro derivative, CGS 9896 (Fig. 17.13), is a potent anticonvulsant (84). It should be noted that both the β-carbolines and the pyrazoloquinolines are planar ring systems that differ markedly in shape from the 1,4-benzodiazepines. Accordingly, it is expected that these compounds interact differently with the BZR and, in fact, the binding site for the β-carbolines and the pyrazoloquinolines may differ from that of the 1,4-benzodiazepines (67). Derivatives of the triazolopyridazine class include CL 218,872 (Fig. 17.13), that has only weak affinity for the BZR in vitro. In vivo, however, this agent is proposed to show selective affinity for a putative BZR subtype that mediates "anxioselective" activity, exclusive of sedative and muscle relaxant activity (85).

The imidazopyridine zolpidem (Fig. 17.13) initially was thought to be selective for the "BZ$_1$" receptor (86), which probably represents the GABA$_A$ receptor. After initial positive trials (87), it was placed on the market as a hypnotic. Another imidiazopyridine, alpidem (Fig. 17.13), has shown promise as an anxiolytic. Alpidem shows anxiolytic activity about one-eighth to one-tenth as potent as diazepam, but apparently induces no significant changes in sleep parameters (88) and has no effect on memory or muscle tone (89). Alpidem was found to be of at least equal efficacy to lorazepam in the treatment of patients with generalized anxiety disorder (90).

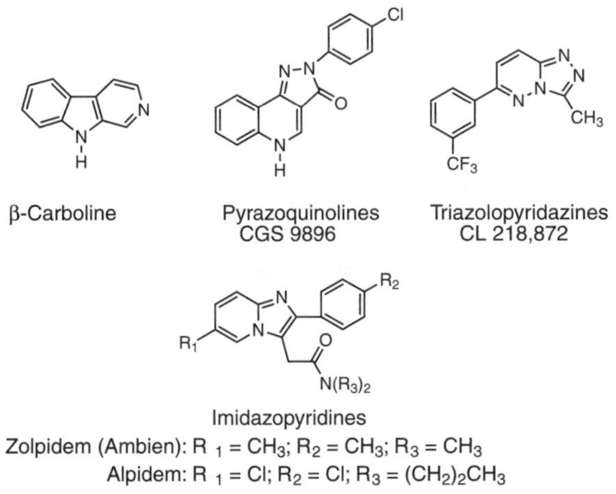

GABA$_A$ Partial Allosteric Modulators

Partial agonists of the GABA$_A$ receptor complex offer some theoretical and practical advantages over full agonists. For example, compared to the benzodiazepine-type full agonists, partial agonists seem to have lesser side effects such as sedation, ataxia, and potentiation of alcohol. Also, there may be less abuse potential associated with partial agonists. Three partial agonists of GABA$_A$ receptors currently are being investigated: imidazenil, bretazenil, and abecarnil (Fig. 17.14). Imidazenil is an imidazobenzodiazepine carboxamide that is more potent than diazepam, but only about one-half as efficacious at modulating GABA effects on chloride currents. When given concurrently with diazepam, imidazenil blocks the sedative, ataxic effects of diazepam (91), consistent with the general pharmacologic principle that partial agonists show antagonist effects in competition with a more potent agonist. Bretazenil has been shown to have similar binding and clinical characteristics to imidazenil (91), although it is less potent. Abecarnil is a β-carboline with anxiolytic properties. Typical of other partial allosteric

Fig. 17.13. Structures of nonbenzodiazepine agonists.

β-Carboline

Pyrazoquinolines
CGS 9896

Triazolopyridazines
CL 218,872

Imidazopyridines
Zolpidem (Ambien): R$_1$ = CH$_3$; R$_2$ = CH$_3$; R$_3$ = CH$_3$
Alpidem: R$_1$ = Cl; R$_2$ = Cl; R$_3$ = (CH$_2$)$_2$CH$_3$

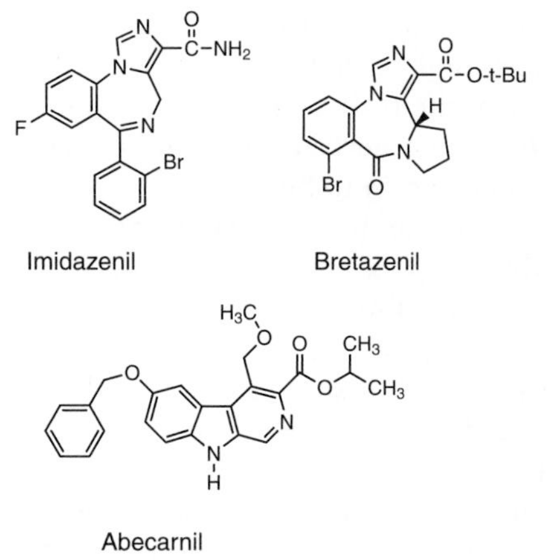

Fig. 17.14. Structures of GABA$_A$ receptor partial agonists.

modulators, abecarnil demonstrates potent antianxiety and anticonvulsant activities, with little or no development of tolerance to these effects (92).

Miscellaneous Anxiolytic Agents
Serotonin Receptor-Active Agents. In the development of anxiolytic agents that do not act via the GABA$_A$ receptor complex, serotonin receptors have been the focus of intensive research in recent years as preclinical and clinical evidence supports the involvement of serotonin in anxiety (93). For example, serotonin 5-HT$_{1A}$ receptors are found in relatively high density in the septohippocampal region of the brain, which is involved in the modulation of anxiety (94). In the structures of the limbic system, 5-HT$_{1A}$ receptors are predominantly postsynaptic, while presynaptic 5-HT$_{1A}$ are found in the dorsal and median raphe nuclei. Presynaptic 5-HT$_{1A}$ receptors function as autoreceptors to inhibit serotonergic neurotransmission; postsynaptic receptor activation also results in decreased neuronal activity. Thus, 5-HT$_{1A}$ receptors are an attractive target for design of anxiolytic drugs.

The best known ligands for brain 5-HT$_{1A}$ receptors are the pyrimidinylbutylpiperazine partial agonists buspirone, ipsaperone, and gepirone (Fig. 17.15). Buspirone is the only one of these agents currently marketed in the United States. It also has activity at central dopamine receptors, which, complicates an interpretation of its interaction with 5-HT$_{1A}$ receptors. All three of these compounds seem to have 5-HT$_{1A}$ partial agonist properties, and all three have anxiolytic activity in humans (95). Their anxiolytic effects appear only after several days of treatment and it is currently unclear whether their mechanism of action is to acutely increase serotonergic activity or chronically decrease serotonergic activity (96).

Ligands for other serotonin receptor subtypes also are being investigated for anxiolytic activity and their structures are shown in Figure 17.16. The 5-HT$_2$ antagonist ritanserin and the 5-HT$_3$ antagonist ondansetron show some anxiolytic activity (97). Pharmacotherapeutic exploitation of the myriad of serotonin receptor subtypes recently discovered by molecular biological techniques awaits functional characterization of the receptors and medicinal chemical approaches to provide selective agonist and antagonist ligands.

Serotonin Re-uptake Inhibitors. Several currently available selective serotonin re-uptake inhibitors (SSRIs), including fluoxetine, fluvoxamine, paroxetine, and sertraline (Fig. 17.17), are effective in some anxiety disorders. Specifically, the SSRIs have been shown to be effective in obsessive compulsive disorder (98), panic disorder (99), and social phobia (100). The mechanism of action of these agents in anxiety, however, may differ with their role in the treatment of depression and our understanding of the diverse psychobiologic effects of SSRIs will depend on a greater understanding of the function of serotonin receptor systems within different brain regions.

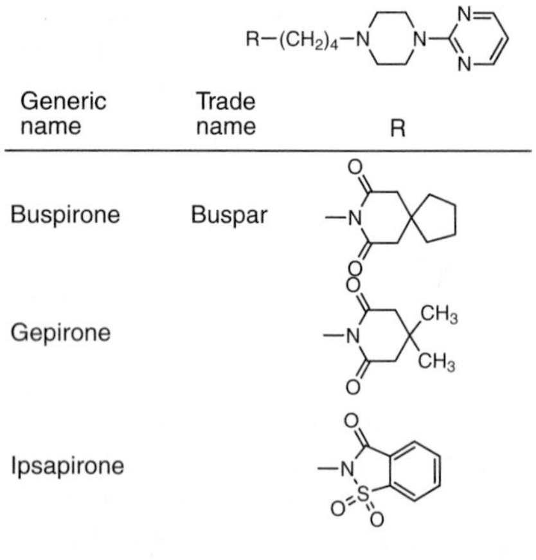

Generic name	Trade name	R
Buspirone	Buspar	
Gepirone		
Ipsapirone		

R—(CH$_2$)$_4$—N⟋⟍N—⟋pyrimidine

Fig. 17.15. Structures of 5-HT$_{1A}$ partial agonists.

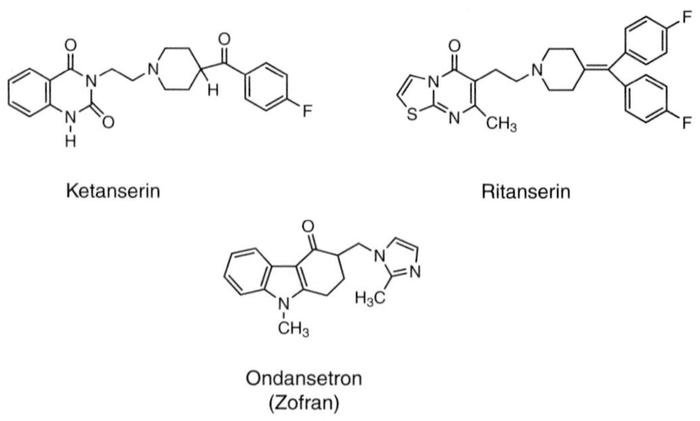

Ketanserin

Ritanserin

Ondansetron
(Zofran)

Fig. 17.16. Structures of 5-HT$_2$ antagonists ketansern and ritanserin, and the 5-HT$_3$ antagonist adansetron.

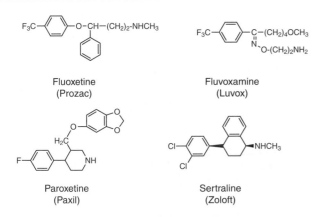

Fluoxetine
(Prozac)

Fluvoxamine
(Luvox)

Paroxetine
(Paxil)

Sertraline
(Zoloft)

Fig. 17.17. Structures of SSRIs fluoxetine, fluvoxamine, paroxetine, and sertraline.

Other Receptor-Active Agents. Tiagabine is a novel compound that functions as a GABA uptake blocker, with no typical benzodiazepine-like sedative effects (101). Less further along in development are agents such as *epalons* which are similar to endogenous steroids, and apparently interact with the GABA_A receptor. Also under development are receptor antagonists for the neuropeptides cholecystokinin-B and neurokinin, as well as, corticotropin releasing factor inhibitors. (101).

Tiagabine (Gabitril)

Acknowledgment. The authors wish to express their gratitude to Dr. Ross J. Baldessarini for reviewing this chapter manuscript.

CASE STUDY

Victoria F. Roche and S. William Zito

SN is a 23-year-old female who is in her dermatologist's office to have four rather deep plantar warts removed from the heel of her right foot. The procedure is painful and the area must be numbed by an injection of a local anesthetic before wart removal can begin. An injection in the bottom of the foot is, in itself, quite painful and SN, who is also afraid of needles, is extremely anxious about the procedure. Her behavior in the examining room is quite agitated, and she told the nurse she is so frightened that she's considering leaving without having the procedure done. The doctor suggests IV administration of a low dose of a benzodiazepine anxiolytic to calm her prior to the injection and surgery. Despite her dread of needles, she readily agrees when she learns that this injection would be painless. SN is in good health and is taking no medications. She drove herself to the clinic, and plans to return to her job as a bank teller after the short

(15–30 minute) procedure is finished. Therapeutic candidates 1–4 are being considered to assist her through this ordeal.

1. *Identify the therapeutic problem(s) where the pharmacist's intervention may benefit the patient.*

2. *Identify and prioritize the patient specific factors that must be considered to achieve the desired therapeutic outcomes.*

3. *Conduct a thorough and mechanistically oriented structure-activity analysis of all therapeutic alternatives provided in the case.*

4. *Evaluate the SAR findings against the patient specific factors and desired therapeutic outcomes and make a therapeutic decision.*

5. *Counsel your patient*

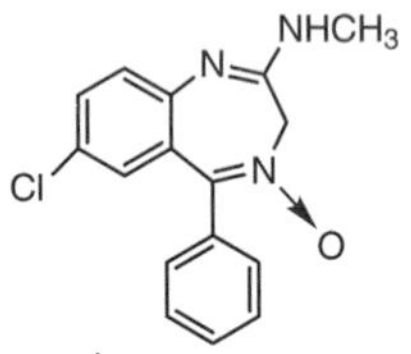

430

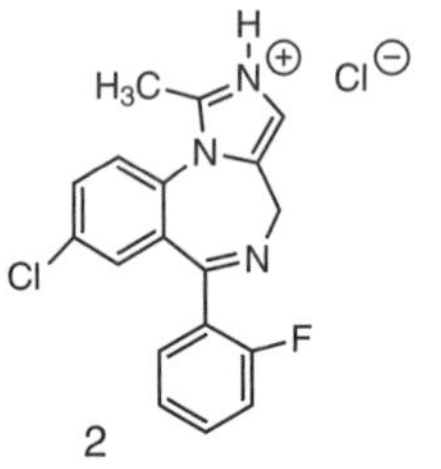

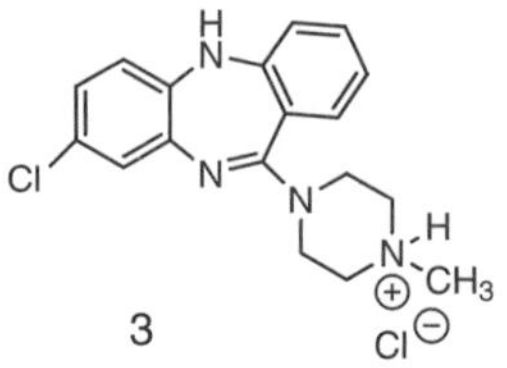

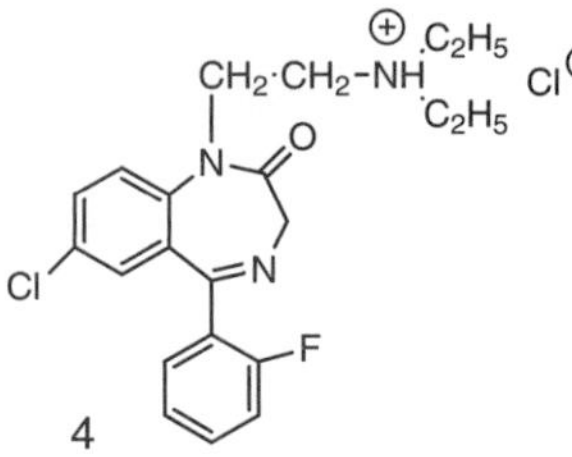

REFERENCES

1. American Psychiatric Association. Diagnostic and Statistical Manual of Mental Disorders. 4th ed. Washington, DC: APA Press, 1994. Revised text, 2000.
2. Kraepelin E. Dementia Praecox and Paraphrenia (Barclay RM, Roberston GM, trans.). Edinburgh: Livingstone, 1919.
3. Bleuler E. Dimentia Praecox oder Gruppe der Schizophrenien. In Aschaffenberg G, ed. Handbuch der Geisleskrankheiten. Leipzig: Denticke, 1911.
4. Baldessarini RJ, Tarazi FI. Chemotherapy in Psychiatry: Principles and Practice. 3nd ed. Cambridge, MA: Harvard University Press, 1996.
5. Baldessarini RJ, Tarazi FI. Drugs and the treatment of psychiatric disorders: Psychosis and mania. In: Hardman JG, Limbird LE, Gilman AG, eds. The Pharmacological Basis of Therapeutics. 9th ed. New York: McGraw-Hill, 2001:485–520.
6. Baldessarini RJ, Tarazi FI. Brain dopamine receptors: A primer on their current status, basic and clinical. Harvard Rev Psychiatry 1996; 3:301–325.
7. Carlsson A, Lindquist M. Effect of chlorpromazine and haloperidol on formation of 3-methoxytyramine and normetanephrine in mouse brain. Acta Pharmacol Toxicol 1963;20:140–144.
8. Seeman P. Dopamine receptors and the dopamine hypothesis of schizophrenia. Synapse 1987; 1:133–52.
9. Seeman P, Lee T, Chau-Wong M, et al. Antipsychotic drug doses and neuroleptic/dopamine receptors. Nature 1976; 261:717–719.
10. Kebabian J, Calne D. Multiple receptors for dopamine. Nature 1979; 277:93–96.
11. Hartman DS, Civelli O. Dopamine receptor diversity: molecular and pharmacological perspectives. Progress in Drug Research 1997; 48:173–94.
12. Lovenberg TW, Brewster WK, Motolla DM, et al. Dihydrexidine, a novel selective high potency full dopamine D1 receptor agonist. Eur J Pharmacol 1989; 166:111–113.
13. Knoerzer TA, Nichols DE, Brewster WK, et al. Dopaminergic Benzo[a]phenanthridines: Resolution and pharmacological evaluation of the enantiomers of dihyrexidine, the full efficacy D1 dopamine receptor agonist. J Med Chem 1994;37:2453–2460.
14. Richelson, E. Preclinical pharmacology of neuroleptics: focus on new generation compounds. J Clin Psychiatry 1996; 57(Suppl 11):4–11.
15. Wolf, ME, Roth RH. Autoreceptor regulation of dopamine synthesis. Annal NY Acad Sci 1990; 604:323–342.
16. Tissari AH, Atzori L, Galdieri MT. Inhibition of dopamine synthesis in striatal synaptosomes by lisuride: Stereospecific reversal by (−)-sulpiride. Naunyn-Schmiedeberg Arch Pharmacol 1983; 322:89–91.
17. Booth RG, Baldessarini R J, Kula NS, et al. Presynaptic inhibition of dopamine synthesis in rat striatal tissue by enantiomeric mono- and dihydroxyaporphines. Mol Pharmacol 1990; 38:92–101.
18. Arbilla S, Langer SZ. Stereoselectivity of presynaptic autoreceptors modulating dopamine release. Eur J Pharmacol 1981; 76:345–351.
19. Booth RG, Baldessarini RJ. Adenosine A2 stimulation of tyrosine hydroxylase activity in rat striatal minces is reversed by dopamine D2 autoreceptor activation. Eur J Pharmacol 1990; 185:217–221.
20. Booth RG, Owens CE, Brown RL, et al. Putative σ_3 sites in mammalian brain have histamine H_1 receptor properties: Evidence from ligand binding and distribution studies with the novel H_1 radioligand [^{3}H]-(−)-trans-1-phenyl-3-aminotetralin (PAT). Br Res 1999; 837:95–105.
21. Choksi NY, Nix William B, Wyrick SD, et al. A novel phenylaminotetralin recognizes histamine H_1 receptors and stimulates dopamine synthesis in vivo in rat brain. Br Res 2000; 852:151–160.
22. Johnson EA, Tsai CE, Shahan YH, et al. Serotonin 5HT1A receptors mediate inhibition of tyrosine hydroxylase in rat striatum. J Pharmacol Exp Ther 1993; 266:133–141.
23. Booth RG, Baldessarini RJ (+)-Benzomorphan sigma ligands stimulate dopamine synthesis in rat corpus striatum tissue. Br Res 1991; 557:349–352.
24. El Tamer A, Prokopenko I, Wulfert E, et al. Mivazerol, a novel alpha2-agonist and potential anti-ischemic drug, inhibits KC1-stimulated neurotransmitter release in rat nervous tissue preparations. J Neurochemistry 1996; 67:636–644.
25. Bovet D, Staup AM. C R Soc Biol (Paris) 1937; 124:547.
26. Charpentier P, Gailliot P, Jacob R, et al. Rescherches sur les di methylaminopropyl-N-phenothiazines substituees. C R Acad Sci (Paris) 1952; 235:59–60.
27. Laborit H, Huguenard P, Alluaume R. A new vegetative stabilizer. Presse Med 1952; 60:206–208.
28. Delay J, Deniker P, Harl J. Utilization therapeutique psychiatrique d'une phenothiazine d'action centrale elective. Ann Med Psychol (Paris) 1952; 110:112–117.
29. Horn AS, Snyder SH. Chlorpromazine and dopamine: Conformational similarities that correlate with the antischizophrenic activity of phenothiazine drugs. Proc Natl Acad Sci USA 1971; 68:2325–2328.
30. Janssen PA. In Ayd FI, Blackwell B, eds. Discoveries in Biological Psychiatry. Philadelphia: Lippincott, 1970.
31. Janssen PAJ, Van Bever, FM. Applications. In Usdin E, Forrest IS, eds. Psychotherapeutic Drugs. Part II. New York: Marcel Decker, 1977:839–921.
32. Simpson GM, Lee JH. In Lipton MA, ed. Psychopharmacology: A Generation of Progress. New York: Raven Press, 1978:1131–1137.
33. Subramanyam B, Pond S, Eyles D, et al. N. Identification of a potentially neurotoxic pyridinium metabolite in the urine of schizophrenic patients treated with haloperidol. Biochem Biophys Res Commun 1990; 181:573–578.
34. Rollema H, Skolnick M, D'Engelbronner J, Igarashi K, Usuki E, Castagnoli Jr. N. MPP$^+$-like neurotoxicity of a pyridinium metabolite derived from haloperidol: In vivo microdialysis and in vitro mitochondrial studies. J Pharmacol Exp Ther 1994 268:380–387.
35. Fang J, Zuo D, Yu PH. Comparison of the cytotoxicity of a quaternary pyridinium metabolite of haloperidol (HP$^+$) with the neurotoxin N-methyl-4-phenylpyridinium (MPP$^+$) toward cultured dopaminergic neuroblastoma cells. Psychopharmacology 1995; 121:373–378.
36. Augrist BM. In: Rotrosen J, Stanley M, eds. The Benzamides: Pharmacology, Neurobiology and Clinical Effects. New York: Raven Press, 1982:1.
37. Jenner P, Marsden CD. In. Horwell DC, ed. Drugs in Central Nervous System Disorders. New York: Marcel Dekker, 1985:149–262.
38. Alvir JMJ, Jeffrey PH, Lieberman J A, et al. Clozapine-induced agranulocytosis. Incidence and risk factors in the United States. N Engl J Med 1993; 329:162–167.
39. Kinon BJ, Lieberman JA. Mechanisms of action of atypical antipsychotic drugs: a critical analysis. Psychopharmacology 1996; 124:2–34.
40. Meltzer HY, Matsubara S, Lee JC. The ratios of serotonin2 and dopamine2 affinities differentiate atypical and typical an-

tipsychotic drugs. Psychopharmacology Bulletin 1989; 25:390–2.

41. Busatto GF, Kerwin RW. Perspectives on the role of serotonergic mechanisms in the pharmacology of schizophrenia. J Psychopharmacol 1997; 11:3–12.

42. Kapur S, Remingotn G. Serotonin-dopamine interaction and its relevance to schizophrenia. Am J Psychiatry 1996; 153:466–476.

43. Owen RR Jr. Cole JO. Molindone hydrochloride: A review of laboratory and clinical findings. J Clin Psychopharmacology 1989 9:268–276.

44. Galatsis P. Market to market. In Bristol JA, ed. Annual Reports in Medicinal Chemistry. Vol. 32. San Diego: Academic Press, 1997; 318.

45. Mellman TA, Uhde TW. Electroencephalographic sleep in panic disorder. Arch Gen Psych 1989; 46:178–184.

46. Rapoport JL. The neurobiology of obsessive-compulsive disorder. JAMA 1988; 260:2888–2890.

47. Baxter L. Positron emission tomography studies of cerebral glucose metabolism in obsessive compulsive disorder. J Clin Psychiatry 1994; 55:54–59.

48. Nordahl TE, Semple WE, Gross M, et al. Cerebral glucose metabolic differences in patients with panic disorder. Neuropsychopharmacology 1990; 3:261–272.

49. Nickell PV, Uhde TW. Dose-response effects of intravenous caffeine in normal volunteers. Anxiety 1995; 4:161–168.

50. Rauch S, Savage C, Alpert N, et al. A positron emission tomographic study of simple phobic symptom provocation. Arch Gen Psych 1995; 52:20–28.

51. Wu JC, Buchsbaum MS., Hershey TG, et al. PET in generalized anxiety disorder. Biol Psychiatry 1991; 29:1181–1199.

52. Semple WE, Goyer P, McCormick R. Preliminary report: brain blood flow using PET in patients with posttraumatic stress disorder and substance abuse histories. Biol Psychiatry 1993; 34:115–118.

53. Redmond DEJ, Huang YH. New evidence for a locus ceruleus-norepinephrine connection with anxiety. Life Sci 1979; 25:2149–2162.

54. Harary N, Kellogg C. The relationship of benzodiazepine binding sites to the norepinephrine projection of the adult rat. Brain Res 1989; 492:293–299.

55. Haefely W. Actions and interactions of benzodiazepine agonists and antagonists at GABAergic synapses. In Bower NG, ed. Actions and Interactions of GABA and Benzodiazepines. New York: Raven Press, 1984; 263–285.

56. Olsen RW Tobin AJ. Molecular biology of GABA A receptors. FASEB J 1990; 4:1469–1480.

57. DeLorey TM, Olsen RW. Gamma-aminobutyric acid A receptor structure and function. J Biol Chem 1992; 267:16747–16750.

58. Macdonald R, Olsen R. GABAa Receptor Channels. Annual Review of Neuroscience 1994; 17:569–602.

59. Sanger DJ, Benavides J, Perrault G, et al. Recent developments in the behavioral pharmacology of benzodiazepine (omega) receptors: evidence for the functional significance of receptor subtypes. Neurosci Biobeh Rev 1994; 18:355–372.

60. Sternbach LH. In Garattini S, Mussini E, Randall LD, eds. The Benzodiazepines. New York: Raven Press, 1973:1–25.

61. Sternbach LH. The benzodiazepine story. J Med Chem 1979; 22:1–7.

62. Randall LO, Schallek W, Heise GA, et al. J. Pharmacol Exp Ther 1960; 129:163.

63. Randall LO, Scheckel CL, Banziger RF. Pharmacology of the metabolites of chlordiazepoxide and diazepam. Current Therapeutic Research, Clinical & Experimental 1965; 7:590–606.

64. Braestrup C, Nielsen M, Olsen CE. Urinary and brain beta-carboline-3-carboxylates as potent inhibitors of brain benzodiazepine receptors. Proc Natl Acad Sci USA 1980; 77: 2288–2292.

65. Cole BJ, Hillman M, Seidelmann D, et al. Effects of benzodiazepine receptor partial inverse agonists in the elevated plus maze test of anxiety in the rat. Psychopharmacology 1995; 121:118–126.

66. Braestrup C, Schmiechen R, Neef G, et al. Interaction of convulsive ligands with benzodiazepine receptors. Science 1982; 216:1241–1243.

67. Haefely W, Kyburz E, Gerecke M, et al. Advances in Drug Research, Vol. 14. London: Academic Press, 1985; 166–322.

68. Hunkeler W, Möhler H, Pieri L, et al. Selective antagonists of benzodiazepines. Nature 1981; 290:514–6.

69. Möhler H, Richards JG. Agonist and antagonist benzodiazepine receptor interaction in vitro. Nature 1981; 294:763–765.

70. Zhang W, Koehler KF, Zhang P, et al. Development of a comprehensive pharmacophore model for the benzodiazepine receptor. Drug Des Discovery 1995; 12:193–248.

71. Schoch P, Richards JG, Häring P, et al. Co-localization of GABA receptors and benzodiazepine receptors in the brain shown by monoclonal antibodies. Nature 1985; 314: 168–171.

72. Wong G, Lyon T, Skolnick P. Chronic exposure to benzodiazepine receptor ligands uncouples the gamma-aminobutyric acid type A receptor in WSS-1 cells. Mol Pharmacol 1994; 46:1056–1062.

73. Tietz EI, Chiu TH, Rosenberg HC. Regional GABA/benzodiazepine receptor/chloride channel coupling after acute and chronic benzodiazepine treatment. Eur J Pharmacol 1989; 167:57–65.

74. Huh KH, Delorey TM, Endo S, et al. Pharmacological subtypes of the gamma-aminobutyric acid$_A$ receptors defined by a gamma-aminobutyric acid analogue 4,5,6,7-tetrahydroisoxazolo[5,4-c] pyridin-3-ol and allosteric coupling: characterization using subunit-specific antibodies. Mol Pharmacol 1995; 48:666–675.

75. Pritchett DB, Sontheimer H, Shivers BD, et al. Importance of a novel GABAA receptor subunit for benzodiazepine pharmacology. Nature 1989; 338:582–585.

76. Pritchett DB Seeburg PH. Gamma-aminobutyric acid A receptor alpha 5-subunit creates novel type II benzodiazepine receptor pharmacology. J Neurochem 1990; 54:1802–1804.

77. Fryer RI. Ligand interaction at the benzodiazepine receptor. In Hansch C, ed. Comprehensive Medicinal Chemistry. Vol. 3. New York: Pergamon Press, 1990; 539–566.

78. Haefely W. The GABA-benzodiazepine interaction fifteen years later. Neurochemical Res 1990; 15:169–174.

79. Crippen GM. Distance geometry analysis of the benzodiazepine binding site. Mol Pharmacol 1982; 22:11–19.

80. Diaz-Arauzo H, Koehler KF, Hagen TJ, et al. Synthetic and computer assisted analysis of the pharmacophore for agonists at benzodiazepine receptors. Life Sci 1991; 49: 207–216.

81. Villar, HO, Davies MF, Loew, GH, et al. Molecular models for recognition and activation at the benzodiazepine receptor: a review. Life Sci 1991; 48:593–602.

82. Blount JF, Fryer RI, Gilman NW, et al. Quinazolines and 1,4-benzodiazepines. 92. Conformational recognition of the receptor by 1,4-benzodiazepines. Mol Pharmacol 1983; 24:425–428.

83. Sunjic V, Lisin A, Sega A, et al. Heterocyc Chem 1979; 16:757.

84. Yokoyama N, Ritter B, Neubert AD. 2-Arylpyrazolo[4,3-c]-quinolin-3-ones: novel agonist, partial agonist, and antagonist of benzodiazepines. J Med Chem 1982; 25:337–339.

85. Lippa AS, Coupet J, Greenblatt EN, et al. A Synthetic non-benzodiazepine ligand for benzodiazepine receptors: a probe for investigating neuronal substrates of anxiety. Pharmacol Biochem Behav 1979; 11:99–106.

86. Arbilla S, Allen J, Wick A, et al. High affinity [^{3}H]zolpidem binding in the ratbrain: an imidazopyridine with agonist properties at central benzodiazepine receptors. Eur J Pharmacol 1986; 130 :257–263.

87. Nicholson AN, Pascoe PA. Hypnotic activity of an imidazopyridine (zolpidem). Br J Clin Pharmacol 1986; 21:205–211.

88. Saletu B, Schultes M, Grunberger J. Sleep laboratory study of a new antianxiety drug, alpidem: short-term trial. Curr Ther Res 1986; 40:769–779.

89. Bartholini G. Nonbenzodiazepine anxiolytics and hypnotics, concluding remarks. Pharmacol Biochem Behav 1988; 29:833–834.

90. Diamond BI, Nguyen H, et al. A comparative study of alpidem, a nonbenzodiazepine, and lorazepam in patients with nonpsychotic anxiety. Psychopharm Bull 1991; 27:67–71.

91. Puia G, Ducic I, Vicini S, Costa E. Molecular mechanisms of the partial allosteric modulatory effects of bretazenil at gamma-aminobutyric acid type A receptor. Proc Natl Acad Sci USA 1992; 89:3620–3624.

92. Ozawa M, Sugimachi K, Nakada-Kometani Y, et al. Chronic pharmacological activities of the novel anxiolytic beta-carboline abecarnil in rats. J Pharmacol Exp Ther 1994; 269:457–462.

93. Lucki I. Serotonin receptor specificity in anxiety disorders. J Clin Psychiatry 1996; 57 (Suppl 6):5–10.

94. Gray JAG: The Neuropsychology of Anxiety: An Enquiry Into the Functions of the Septo-Hippocampal System. New York: Oxford University Press, 1982.

95. Traber J, Glaser T. 5-HT$_{1A}$ receptor-related anxiolytics. Trends Pharmacol Sci 1987; 8:432–437.

96. Peroutka SJ. 5-hydroxytryptamine receptors. J Neurochem 1993; 60:408–416.

97. Eison AS, Eison MS. Serotonergic mechanisms in anxiety. Prog Neuro-Psychopharmacol Biol Psychiat 1994; 18:47–62.

98. Pigott TA, Pato BT, Bernstein SE, et al. Controlled Comparisons of Clomipramine and Fluoxetine in the Treatment of Obsessive-Compulsive Disorder. Arch Gen Psych 1990; 47:926–932.

99. Schneirer FR, Liebowitz MR, Davies SO, et al. Fluoxetine in panic disorder. J Clin Psychopharm 1990;10:119–121.

100. Black B, Uhde TW, Tancer ME. Fluoxetine for the treatment of social phobia. J Clin Psychopharm 1992; 12:293–295.

101. Mosconi M, Chiamulera C, Recchia G. New anxiolytics in development. Int J Clin Pharm Res 1993; 13:331–344.

18. Hallucinogens, Stimulants, and Related Drugs of Abuse

RICHARD A. GLENNON

PSYCHOTOMIMETIC/ HALLUCINOGENIC AGENTS
Introduction

Why study psychotomimetic agents? In the past it was argued that investigations of such agents might shed light on mental illness and its treatment. Although studies with psychotomimetic agents have certainly contributed to our current understanding of these disorders, it is now recognized that there are many kinds of mental illnesses and that the actions, and putative mechanisms of action, of psychotomimetic agents are only tangentially related to their etiology or treatment. It also has been argued that investigations of psychotomimetic agents might contribute to a greater general understanding of basic neurochemical mechanisms and neurotransmitter function. This research approach has been more rewarding. Studies with psychotomimetic agents have contributed significantly to what is currently known about G protein receptors (e.g., cannabinoid receptors, serotonin receptors) and ion channel receptors (e.g., PCP receptors, excitatory amino acid receptors). Subsequent work with these receptors has identified new receptor subtypes that are being targeted for the development of novel therapeutic agents. Indeed, the past 10 years have witnessed an explosion of interest in the investigation of psychoactive substances because of their relevance to neurochemical mechanisms. But, perhaps the most important reason to study psychotomimetic agents is because these agents represent a large group of abused substances, and because pharmacists generally serve as one of the first lines of defense for the dissemination of drug abuse prevention and treatment information. In addition, the past one or two decades have seen the popularization of controlled substance analogs (i.e., designer drugs), and the future will likely witness the introduction of yet more designer drugs. So, a second reason to study these agents is to prepare for the future; an understanding of the presently available agents, and their structure-activity relationships, will be instructive because many designer drugs are the result of the clandestine application of these same structure-activity principles at the street level.

Definitions and Classification

Psychotomimetic and *hallucinogenic* are commonly used terms, and they are frequently used interchangeably; and yet there is little agreement as to what constitutes such agents or exactly what they do. Because the actions of these agents are largely subjective, the best information should come from those experiencing the agents; yet, by experiencing their effect, one may not be in a position to accurately describe the effects they produce (1). In contrast, an outside observer can never fully and accurately describe the effects of the agents. This has led to problems of definition. Perhaps the best and most widely accepted definition of a psychotomimetic substance is that provided by Hollister (2): psychotomimetic/hallucinogenic agents are those which upon administration of a single effective dose (a) consistently produce changes in thought, mood, and perception with little memory impairment, (b) produce little stupor, narcosis or excessive stimulation, (c) produce minimal autonomic side effects, and (d) are nonaddicting. Although certain opiate analgesics occasionally produce psychotomimetic effects, they are effectively eliminated from this category of agents because they do not meet the necessary criteria (e.g., they can be addicting). Likewise, chronic administration of high doses of stimulants such as amphetamine and cocaine sometimes produce hallucinogenic episodes (i.e., "amphetamine psychosis," "cocaine psychosis"); these agents are not considered hallucinogens, however, because multiple doses are typically required to produce this effect. Thus, the Hollister criteria have served a very useful function in narrowing the list of agents that belong to this category of drugs. Nevertheless, Hollister was still able to identify several classes of psychotomimetic agents: lysergic acid derivatives (such as lysergic acid diethylamide; LSD), phenylethylamines (such as mescaline), indolealkylamines (such as N,N-dimethyltryptamine; DMT), other indolic derivatives (such as ibogaine and the harmala derivatives), piperidyl benzilate esters (such as JB-329), phenylcyclohexyl compounds (such as phencyclidine; PCP), and miscellaneous agents (such as kawain, dimethylacetamide, and cannabinoids) (2).

Over time it has been demonstrated that psychotomimetic agents represent a behaviorally heterogeneous class of psychoactive agents. For example, human subjects can differentiate between the actions produced by certain compounds in this category, and cross-tolerance develops among some of these agents, but not between others. Likewise, it is possible to differentiate between certain of these agents using various animal procedures. Subcategorization was necessary. Today, it is recognized that some hallucinogens act primarily via a serotonergic mechanism, that the cannabinoids probably produce their behavioral effects via cannabinoid receptors, and that phencyclidine likely produces its effects via PCP receptors. This is not to imply that there now is a full understanding of how these agents work, but it does support the concept that the agents do not belong to a homogeneous mechanistic class.

Human Versus Animal Studies: Applicability of Animal Models

As mentioned above, human subjects should be best suited to provide the most reliable assessment of the actions and potency of psychotomimetic agents, and considerable human data are available on some agents. However, much less information is available on most. Often, what information is available comes from studies that might not have been well controlled, studies that included limited subject populations, or studies that investigated few drug doses. Some of what is known even comes from anecdotal reports. Very few clinical studies with psychotomimetic agents were sanctioned following the early 1960s. Although some limited human evaluation has been allowed beginning in the early 1990s, for a period of about 30 years information on psychotomimetic substances relied (and continues to rely) heavily on the use of animal studies. This raises several questions. Do animal models exist that can accurately reflect human hallucinogenic activity? Indeed, do animals hallucinate? Many attempts have been made to develop animal models of psychotomimetic or hallucinogenic activity, but to date, no single animal model accounts for the actions of these agents as a class (3).

Drug Discrimination Paradigm. One animal technique that has seen widespread application for the investigation of psychoactive agents is the *drug discrimination paradigm* (4). It must be emphasized at the outset that this method does not represent a model of psychotomimetic activity. Indeed, the technique has general applicability and has been employed to study a wide variety of centrally acting agents including stimulants, barbiturates, anxiolytics, opiates, and many other drug classes. The technique may be viewed as a "drug detection" procedure. Specifically, animals (typically rats, pigeons, or monkeys) are trained to recognize or discriminate the stimulus effects of a *training drug* from vehicle; humans also have been used as subjects in some drug discrimination studies. Many centrally-acting agents seemingly produce an interoceptive cue or stimulus that subjects recognize. When animals are used, they are taught to make a particular response (e.g., to respond on one lever of a two-lever operant apparatus or Skinner box) when administered training drug and to make a different response (e.g., to respond on the second of the two levers) when administered saline vehicle. After a period of time the animals learn the stimulus cue and associate it with one of the two levers; that is, the animals make > 80% of their responses on the training-drug lever (i.e., > 80% drug-appropriate responding) when administered the training dose of the training drug, and make < 20% of their responses on the same lever when administered vehicle. Training drug doses less than those of the training dose result in a decrease in percent drug-appropriate responding. The effect is dose related and a dose-response curve can be constructed; an ED50 dose can be calculated as a measure of potency. Once trained, these animals can be used in what are referred to as tests of substitution or stimulus transfer, or more commonly, as tests of *stimulus generalization*. In such tests, other agents (i.e., challenge drugs) are administered to the animals to determine if they produce stimulus effects similar to those of the training drug. Stimulus generalization is said to have occurred when animals make >80% of their responses on the training-drug-appropriate lever following administration of some dose of challenge drug. Stimulus generalization or substitution implies that the challenge drug and the training drug are producing similar stimulus effects in the animals. It should be noted that no claim has ever been made that the agents—the training drug and a challenge drug—are producing identical effects; rather, there is an implication that the agents are capable of producing a common stimulus effect or that they are capable of producing a behavioral cue common to the two agents (for example, a drug that produces effects A and B may be recognized by animals trained to a drug that produces effects B and C; although this may not be a common occurrence, it should be recognized that it is possible). Thus, not only is it possible to determine if two agents are producing similar stimulus effects, it is also possible to compare their relative potencies by calculating an ED50 value for the challenge drug. Other studies that can be conducted are tests of *stimulus antagonism*. That is, a specific training drug can be administered together with another agent; if the combination results in <20% training-drug-appropriate responding, stimulus antagonism is said to have occurred. Although this technique can be employed in the development of novel antagonists for a series of agents for which an antagonist is unknown, it is more common to use a receptor-selective antagonist to investigate mechanisms of action. Drug discrimination, then, is a very powerful tool to investigate the actions and mechanisms of action of many different kinds of centrally acting agents. Specific examples of stimulus generalization and stimulus antagonists will be described later.

The drug discrimination procedure has seen broad application in the investigation of centrally acting agents and a wide variety of different training drugs has been employed. When a psychotomimetic agent is used as the training drug, it should be possible to identify other agents that produce similar stimulus effects (5). In this manner, it has been demonstrated that the psychotomimetics represent a behaviorally heterogeneous group of agents, much in the same way that humans have been able to differentiate the effects of these agents. Animals trained to discriminate LSD, for example, do not recognize PCP, and animals trained to discriminate PCP do not recognize LSD. Neither LSD- nor PCP-trained animals recognize THC. LSD-trained animals, however, recognize mescaline, 1-(2,5-dimethoxy-4-methylphenyl)-2-aminopropane (DOM), and certain other hallucinogens. Using this technique, then, it has been possible to identify what are termed the *classical hallucinogens* (6). The classical hallucinogens are LSD-like agents that share common stimulus properties and may act via a common mechanism of action. The remaining psychotomimetic agents will be referred to here as nonclassical agents; these groups of agents act by different mechanisms and produce distinct effects common to members within each group.

Psychoactive Drugs of Abuse: Nonclassical Hallucinogens

The term nonclassical hallucinogen is used here to differentiate these psychoactive agents from the classical hallucinogens that will be discussed later in this chapter. There are several categories of agents described here, but there is no implication that these classes produce similar effects or act via similar mechanisms.

Cannabinoids

The marihuana or cannabis plant represents one of the oldest and most widely used psychoactive substances in the world. Botanically, there are three major species of the plant: *Cannabis sativa, Cannabis indica,* and *Cannabis ruderalis,* and cannabis has been cultivated since about 6,000 B.C. Reference is made to three preparations, listed here in order of increasing potency: bhang, ganja, and hashish. Bhang typically refers to the leaves and stems of the plant, ganja is prepared from the flowering tops of the plant, and hashish is the pure resin. Although marihuana is active orally, inhalation by smoking is a more frequently used route of administration. One of the major active constituents of the plant is Δ^9-tetrahydrocannabinol (Δ^9-THC; often referred to simply as THC). THC is rapidly and efficiently absorbed by inhalation; it is absorbed into body tissue and slowly released back into circulation. Deuterium-labeled THC has been detected in human plasma up to nearly two weeks post administration. A major metabolite of THC is 11-hydroxy-Δ^9-THC. There is evidence that tolerance develops to THC, and that THC does not generally lead to physical dependence. Marihuana can produce impairment of per-

formance, memory, and learning; there is controversy over whether it produces an amotivational syndrome. There are many claims for the medicinal use of marihuana and THC but these will not be addressed here.

Over the years many cannabinoids and related structures, such as CP-55,940, were synthesized and evaluated. Noncannabinoids such as WIN-55,212-2 were also shown to possess THC-like actions. Few compounds displayed cannabinoid antagonist properties and there was an extensive search for possible candidates that would be useful for better defining the actions of THC. A number of compounds were explored, and the pyrazole analog SR141716A has been found to be one of the most effective. SR141716A attenuates the effects of WIN-55,212-2 (7) and THC (8), as well as the stimulus effects of THC (9). Thus, in addition to cannabinoids and cannabinoid-related structures such as CP-55,940, there are three other structural classes of cannabinoid ligands: indolic derivatives such as WIN-55,212–2, pyrazoles such as SR141716A, and fatty acid derivatives such as anandamide (discussed below).

CP-55,940   WIN-55,212-2   SR141716A

Mechanism of Action. For many years it was thought that cannabinoids were acting in a nonspecific manner, but in the early 1990s two populations of cannabinoid receptors were identified: CB-1 and CB-2 (10,11). Human forms of these receptors have been cloned. Both types are G protein-coupled, seven helix transmembrane-spanning receptors. These receptors are differentially expressed; CB-1 receptors, which may mediate the psychoactive effects of THC-related agents, are found primarily in the brain whereas CB-2 receptors, possibly involved in immunomodulatory actions, are found almost exclusively in the periphery. The identification of such receptors suggested the possible existence of endogenous ligands and claims for several have been published. The best investigated of these is the eicosanoid derivative arachidonylethanolamide or anandamide which was initially isolated from porcine brain. Anandamide (Ki = 52 nM) binds at CB-1 receptors with an affinity similar to that of THC (46 nM) (12). Related structures have also been detected in brain including docosatetraenylethanolamide (Ki = 34.4 nM) and homo-γ-linolenyllathanolamide (Ki = 53.4 nM) (12). A related compound, palmitoylethanolamide, may show selectivity for CB-2 receptors. Anandamide seems to be a THC-like agent. Although the actions of anandamide may not be identical to those of THC, particularly in *in vivo* studies, it is possible that differences may be related to the metabolic instability

Δ^9-Tetrahydrocannabinol (Δ^9-THC)

Δ^8-Tetrahydrocannabinol

Cannabidiol

11–Hydroxy-Δ^9-Tetrahydrocannabinol (11-OH-Δ^9-THC)

of anandamide. For example, in drug discrimination studies a THC stimulus failed to consistently or reliably generalize to anandamide (9); however, the more metabolically stable methanandamide, a chain-methylated analog of anandamide, produced THC-like effects; furthermore, methanandamide has been used as a training drug and the methanandamide stimulus generalizes to THC (13).

Anandamide

Docosatetraenylethanolamide

Homo-γ-linolenylethanolamide

Structure-activity Relationships. Structure-activity relationships both for THC-like actions and CB-1 binding are being formulated. Structure-activity studies can be discussed on the basis of several different types of behavioral assays in rodents, and it has been shown, for 60 cannabinoids, that behavioral potencies are highly correlated with receptor binding affinities (14). THC-like discriminative effects probably offer a more specific method of detecting and measuring cannabimimetic effects and are particularly useful for formulating structure-activity relationships (15). Using this approach, it has been demonstrated that structure-activity relationships for THC-like stimulus effects are not necessarily identical to those for the analgesic, antiemetic, or anticonvulsant actions of cannabinoids. An early study showed that animals trained to discriminate intraperitoneal (ip) dosing of THC recognized hashish smoke, and animals trained to discriminate hashish smoke recognized THC, supporting the concept that THC likely accounts for the stimulus actions of hashish. A number of cannabinoids now have been evaluated. Cannabidiol, for example, does not produce THC-like stimulus effects. Relative to Δ^9-THC (ED50 = 0.43 mg/kg, ip), some 11-hydroxy metabolites are quite potent: 11-OH Δ^9-THC (ED50 = 0.10 mg/kg), 11-OH Δ^8-THC (ED50 = 0.38 mg/kg). One of the more potent cannabinoids is Δ^8-THC-DMH (ED50 = 0.05 mg/kg) where the 4-pentyl moiety of THC has been replaced with a 1,1-dimethylheptyl (i.e., DMH) group; its 11-hydroxyl analog 11-OH Δ^8-THC-DMH (ED50 = 0.002 mg/kg) is even more potent (15). One of the most extensively studied cannabinoid ligands is WIN-55,212-2 (16). Molecular modeling and site-directed mutagenesis studies suggest that cannabinoids, CP-55,940 and anandamide bind in a similar fashion but in a manner that differs from the binding of WIN-55,212-2. Two distinct pharmacophores have been proposed (16–18). Attempts are also being made to identify CB-1 versus CB-2 pharmacophoric features (17).

The discovery of CB receptors, and novel chemical tools with which to investigate these receptors, has generated renewed interest in the cannabinoids. In particular, the discovery of cannabinoid antagonists, endogenous cannabinoids, and subpopulations of CB receptors, finally promise that the mechanism of action of THC will be unraveled and that novel therapeutic agents lacking THC's psychoactive effects eventually may be developed.

PCP-related Agents

Phencyclidine or 1-(1-phenylcyclohexyl)piperidine (PCP) was introduced as a dissociative anesthetic in the late 1950s. Shortly after its introduction, clinical studies were terminated due to the occurrence of schizophrenic-like psychotomimetic effects, particularly during emergence from anesthesia (19). This might have been the end of the story except that (a) additional attempts were made to exploit the anesthetic effects of PCP, leading to the development of novel agents such as ketamine, (b) it was theorized that PCP-like states might provide a good model to investigate schizophrenia, leading to studies of PCP's mechanism of action, and (c) PCP (e.g., "Angel Dust"), administered by inhalation, injection, or smoking (as with PCP-laced parsley, tobacco, or marihuana) and ketamine (e.g., "Special K") emerged as drugs of abuse, leading to investigations of their abuse liability. Shortly thereafter it was discovered that PCP behaves as an N-methyl-D-aspartate (NMDA) antagonist. Because NMDA receptors had been implicated in seizures and trauma, phencyclidine and related arylcycloalkylamines were explored as potential antiepileptics and neuroprotective agents.

Phencyclidine   Ketamine
(PCP)

Actions. In humans, PCP can produce disorientation, confusion, incoordination, delirium, impaired memory, and euphoria (20). PCP also has a history of producing aggression and violent behavior. However, because PCP is often consumed together with other substances it sometimes has been difficult to establish exactly which effects are produced by PCP, and which may be related to possible drug interactions. PCP has seen extensive investigation in animals and it appears to produce effects similar both to those of amphetamine-like stimulants and central depressants. PCP is self-administered by animals, and tolerance develops to the behavioral effects of PCP upon repeated exposure to the drug (20). PCP has both direct and indirect effects on dopaminergic systems; this may account, at least in part, for some of the amphetamine-like effects of PCP and may contribute to the production of its schizophrenic-like actions. The PCP model of schizophrenia was particularly attractive because PCP seemed to produce both the positive and negative symptoms associated with this disorder. PCP has also been widely investigated as a training drug in animals in drug discrimination studies.

Mechanism of Action. N-Allylnormetazocine (NANM, SKF-10047) produces some effects reminiscent of PCP. At one time NANM was considered a prototypic sigma (σ) opiate receptor ligand (21,22). It is now recognized that the σ receptors are likely not a class of opiate receptors, and that the low-affinity NANM is only one of very few opiates that binds at these receptors. Subsequent structure-activity studies showed that NANM simply possesses certain minimal pharmacophoric features that are required for σ receptor binding (23). Nevertheless, the behavioral similarities between NANM and PCP led to early investigations of the binding of PCP at σ receptors and because of its affinity, albeit low, for these receptors, the σ receptors were renamed NANM-PCP receptors or σ/PCP receptors. This confusion continued for several years until it was demonstrated that agents with much higher affinity and selectivity than PCP for σ receptors failed to produce PCP-like actions in animals (20). Later, it was shown that PCP antagonizes the effects of the excitatory amino acid NMDA. [³H]PCP has been used to label putative PCP binding sites, and PCP binding and NMDA binding displayed similar regional distribution in brain. It now has been established that PCP is a noncompetitive NMDA receptor antagonist.

The NMDA receptor (Fig. 18.1) is a ligand-gated ion channel receptor that regulates the flow of cations (Na$^+$, Ca^{++}) into certain neurons. The receptor complex possesses multiple binding sites, similar to the benzodiazepine/GABA receptor complex, that allows the binding of glutamate, glycine, polyamines, and other ligands that can modulate the actions of NMDA. PCP, like the NMDA antagonist dizocilpine (MK-801), binds at a site (i.e., the PCP site) that is believed to be located within the ion channel. Drug discrimination studies have shown that PCP-trained animals recognize NMDA antagonists that bind at PCP receptors; for example, MK-801 is nearly 10 times more potent than PCP. Furthermore, animals trained to discriminate MK-801 recognize PCP and other PCP-related agents.

Structure-activity Relationships. Structure-activity relationships for PCP-like actions have not been particularly well worked out and what little is known stems primarily from drug discrimination studies. The PCP stimulus does not generalize to opioids, sympathomimetic stimulants, anticholinergic agents, classical hallucinogens, and only partially generalizes to depressants such as barbiturates; in general, the stimulus properties of PCP are not shared by members of other drug classes (24). The PCP stimulus generalizes to ketamine and other structurally-related derivatives of PCP such as TCP, an analog of PCP where the phenyl ring has been replaced by the isosteric 2-thienyl group.

PCP does not possess a chiral center. Several 1,3-dioxolanes possessing an asymmetric center produce PCP-like effects and have proven useful for investigating PCP-like actions. Dioxadrol, or 2-(2,2-diphenyl-1,3-dioxolan-4-yl) piperidine, and etxadrol (i.e., dioxadrol where one of the phenyl groups has been replaced by an ethyl group) are examples of such dioxolanes. The (+)-isomer of dioxadrol, dexoxodrol, but not the (−)-isomer levoxadrol, binds at PCP receptors and is recognized by PCP-trained animals (24).

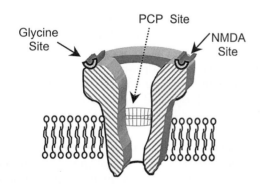

N-Allylnormetazocine   Dizocilpine   Dioxadrol
(NANM)   (MK-801)

Psychoactive Drugs of Abuse: Classical Hallucinogens

Classical hallucinogens are agents that meet the Hollister definition (2) and, in addition, (a) bind at 5-HT$_2$ serotonin receptors, and (b) are recognized by DOM-trained animals in tests of stimulus generalization (5). The classical hallucinogens all possess the general structure **Ar-C-C-N** where **Ar** is a substituted phenyl, 3-indolyl, or substituted 3-indolyl moiety, **C-C** is an ethyl or branched ethyl chain, and **N** is a primary, secondary or tertiary amine. This will be further discussed. (See also Chapter 12 for additional information on serotonin receptors.)

Classification

There are two major structural categories of classical or arylalkylamine hallucinogens: the indolealkylamines (IAAs) and the phenylalkylamines (PAAs). The indolealkylamines are further divided into the simple N-substituted tryptamines, the α-alkyltryptamines, the ergolines (or lysergamides), and, tentatively, the β-carbolines. The phenylalkylamines consist of the phenylethylamines (PEAs) and the phenylisopropylamines (PIAs). In humans, examples from the different categories seem to produce similar effects. It should be noted, however, that relatively few agents have been examined in comprehensive and carefully controlled clinical situations. Furthermore,

Figure 18.1. NMDA ion channel receptor showing binding sites for glycine, NMDA, and PCP.

Table 18.1. Results of Stimulus Generalization Studies with Examples from the Various Categories of Classical Hallucinogens Using Animals Trained to Discriminate DOM from Vehicle

Category	Example*	ED50 Value for DOM-Stimulus Generalization (mg/kg)[†]
N-Alkyltryptamines	DMT	5.8
α-Alkyltryptamines	α-MeT	3.1
Lysergamides	(+)LSD	0.05
β-Carbolines	Harmaline	6.2
Phenylethylamines	Mescaline	14.6
Phenylisopropylamines	DOB	0.2

*See text for explanation of abbreviations.
[†]Data from Glennon (5,27).

no claim is made that these agents produce identical effects in humans. Each category and, indeed, even certain examples from within a given category, may produce effects that make them somewhat different from the others. However, as if to underscore that there is behavioral similarity among these agents, examples from each of the above categories produce common DOM-like stimulus effects in animals (see Table 18.1).

Indolealkylamines

N-Alkyltryptamines. One of the best investigated hallucinogens is N,N-dimethyltryptamine (DMT; see Table 18.2), and DMT is considered the prototype of this subclass of agents. DMT is a naturally occurring substance and is also readily synthesized in the laboratory. Its actions are characterized by a rapid onset (typically < 5 minutes) and short duration of action (about 30 minutes). DMT, like some other members of this family, are not active via oral administration; DMT is generally administered by inhalation or by smoking. Although less common, DMT can also be injected. Some indolealkylamines are sensitive to the acidic conditions of the stomach. The corresponding secondary amine, N-monomethyltryptamine, and primary amine, tryptamine, are inactive as psychoactive substances because they are not sufficiently lipophilic to readily penetrate the blood-brain barrier, and because what little does get into the brain is rapidly metabolized by monoamine oxidase. Other tertiary amine derivatives, such as the N-ethyl-N-methyltryptamine, N,N-diethyltryptamine (DET), N,N-di-*n*-propyltryptamine (DPT), and some secondary amines, are also hallucinogenic in humans. If the N-alkyl or N,N-dialkyl substituents are bulky and lipophilic enough, these tryptamines can be orally active (see Table 18.2).

The effect of substitution in the pyrrole portion of DMT has not been extensively investigated in humans. In contrast, substitution in the benzenoid ring can enhance or diminish potency depending on the specific nature and location of the substituents. Table 18.2 shows some of the more frequently encountered derivatives of DMT, their common names, and their approximate human potency. Serotonin is not hallucinogenic and does not readily penetrate the blood-brain barrier when administered

Table 18.2. Psychoactive Phenylisopropylamines and Related Agents

Agent	Common Name	R₁/R₂	R	X	Approximate Hallucinogenic Dose (mg)*	DOM Stimulus Generalization Potency (mg/kg)[†]
Tryptamine		H/H	H	H	Likely Inactive	Inactive
N-Methyltryptamine	NMT	CH₃/H	H	H	Likely Inactive	Inactive
(±)α-Methyltryptamine	α-MeT	H/H	CH₃	H	5–20 (smoke) 15–30 (po)	3.13
N,N-Dimethyltryptamine	DMT	CH₃/CH₃	H	H	60–100 (smoke) 4–30 (iv)	5.80
N,N-Diethyltryptamine	DET	C₂H₅/C₂H₅	H	H	50–100 (po)	2.45
N-Ethyl-N-methyltryptamine	MET	CH₃/C₂H₅	H	H	Unknown	—
N,N-Di-n-propyltryptamine	DPT	nC₃H₇/nC₃H₇	H	H	100–250 (po)	2.20
N,N-Di-isopropyltryptamine	DIPT	iC₃H₇/iC₃H₇	H	H	25–100 (po)	2.60
(±)α-Ethyltryptamine	α-EtT	H/H	CH₂CH₃	H	100–150 (po)	6.62
4-Hydroxy DMT	Psilocin	CH₃/CH₃	H	4-OH	10–20 (po)	—
4-Methoxy DMT	4–OMe DMT	CH₃/CH₃	H	4-OCH₃	Unknown	3.53
5-Hydroxytryptamine	5–HT	H/H	H	5-OH	Inactive	Inactive
5-OH DMT	Bufotenine	CH₃/CH₃	H	5-OH	Likely Inactive	Inactive
5-Methoxy DMT	5-OMe DMT	CH₃/CH₃	H	5-OCH₃	6–20 (smoke) 2–3 (iv)	1.22
(±)5-Methoxy-α-MeT	5-OMe α-MeT	H/-H	CH₃	5-OCH₃	2.5–4.5 (po)	0.50
6-Methoxy DMT	6-OMe DMT	CH₃/CH₃	H	6-OCH₃	Likely Inactive	Inactive
7-Methoxy DMT	7-OMe DMT	CH₃/CH₃	H	7-OCH₃	Likely Inactive	Inactive

* Data primarily from 25,26. Key: po = oral, iv = intravenous.
[†] Drugs were administered via the ip route. (reference 5,27.)

systemically. N,N-Dimethylserotonin (bufotenine, 5-OH DMT) has been reported to be a weak hallucinogen but the results of human studies are controversial. It, too, likely does not readily penetrate the blood-brain barrier and produces considerable peripheral effects (e.g., facial flushing, cardiovascular actions) that prevented evaluation of an extended dose range. O-Methylation of bufotenine results in 5-OMe DMT, one of the more potent N-alkyltryptamines. 5-OMe DMT is a naturally-occurring substance and is a constituent of a number of plants used in various concoctions prepared by South American Indians for ceremonial and visionary purposes. Bufotenine and 5-OMe DMT are also found in the skin of certain frogs and may have given rise to the phenomenon of "toad licking." Psilocin is 4-hydroxy DMT; like bufotenine with a polar hydroxyl group, psilocin might not have been expected to enter the brain. Yet, it is hallucinogenic. Although this phenomenon has never been adequately explained, it has been speculated that the 4-hydroxyl group forms a hydrogen bond with the terminal amine and that this reduces polarity just enough that psilocin penetrates the blood-brain barrier. Psilocin and its phosphate ester, psilocybin, are widely found in certain species of mushrooms and have given rise to the terms "shrooms" and "shrooming." There are no reports that 6-methoxy DMT or 7-methoxy DMT are hallucinogenic. It is quite difficult to make strict potency comparisons within this series due to the different routes of administration that have been used (see Table 18.2).

In tests of stimulus generalization, the DOM-stimulus has been shown to generalize to DMT, DET, DPT, 4-OMe DMT, 5-OMe DMT, and a number of other DMT analogs, but not to 5-OH DMT, 6-OMe DMT or 7-OMe DMT.

The metabolism of these agents has not been well investigated. The indolealkylamine 5-HT is a substrate for oxidative deamination by monoamine oxidase (MAO) and what evidence exists suggests that other indolealkylamines are also substrates for this enzyme system.

α-Alkyltryptamines. Tryptamine, as mentioned above, is not psychoactive. Introduction of an α-methyl group seemingly enhances lipophilicity, and sufficiently protects against metabolism, such that α-methyltryptamine (α-MeT; see Table 18.2) is about twice as potent as DMT. As a general rule of thumb, α-methyltryptamines, where such agents have been investigated, are typically twice as potent as their corresponding DMT counterpart. Otherwise, their SAR is essentially the same as that of the DMT analogs. For example, 5-methoxy-α-methyltryptamine (5-OMe α-MeT) is about twice as potent as 5-OMe DMT. Introduction of the α-methyl group results in the creation of an asymmetric center and the $S(+)$-isomers of α-methyltryptamines are more potent than their $R(-)$-enantiomers. Homologation of the α-methyl group to an α-ethyl group affords α-ethyltryptamines. α-Ethyltryptamine (α-EtT) has been reported to be hallucinogenic with effects somewhat distinguishable

by human subjects from those of LSD and mescaline (28). Interestingly, α-EtT was clinically available in the early 1960s as an antidepressant because of its actions as a monoamine oxidase (MAO) inhibitor; however, it was removed from the market about a year after its introduction. It may be the MAO inhibitory effect that allowed the actions of α-EtT to be distinguished from those of LSD and mescaline (but see also the section below on Designer Drugs). α-ET made an appearance on the clandestine market in the mid-1990s as a designer drug (i.e., "ET"). (±)α-Methyltryptamine, (±)5-methoxy-α-methyltryptamine and both of its optical isomers, and (±)α-ethyltryptamine are recognized by DOM-trained animals in tests of stimulus generalization.

Ergolines or Lysergamides. (+)Lysergic acid diethylamide (LSD) is perhaps the best known, and certainly one of the most potent, of the classical hallucinogens. Although LSD itself is not naturally occurring, many related ergolines are found in nature. Potencywise, LSD is at least 3000 times more potent than mescaline with doses of <100 micrograms showing activity. Certain structurally modified analogs of LSD retain hallucinogenic activity; although many derivatives are possible, relatievly few have been investigated in humans. Structural changes can often reduce the activity of a pharmacologically-active substance. Here is an instance where a structural change resulting in even a 1000-fold decrease in potency can afford a very active agent. Some work has been reported on the structure-activity relationships of LSD (29,30).

(+)Lysergic acid diethylamide
(LSD)

LSD has been thoroughly investigated in humans (29) and no hallucinogen has been as extensively studied as this agent. Its actions in humans can be divided into three major categories: perceptual (altered shapes and colors, heightened sense of hearing), psychic (alterations in mood, depersonalization, visual hallucinations, altered sense of time), and somatic (nausea, blurred vision, dizziness). In terms of principal effects, there seems to be little difference between LSD, psilocybin, and mescaline.

Although LSD has been sold on the clandestine market in tablet form, it is not uncommon to find this material available on "blotter paper" due to its high potency. A sheet of porous paper is impregnated with a solution of LSD and the sheet can later be cut to afford the appropriate dose.

β-Carbolines. The β-carbolines represent a very interesting and controversial class of agents generally referred to as the harmala alkaloids. Several are naturally occurring. In South America, β-carbolines are found in certain vines and lianas (e.g., *Banisteriopsis caapi*), and in the Old World β-carbolines are constituents of Syrian Rue (*Pegnum harmala*). South American Indians prepare a variety of concoctions and snuffs, the most notable of which is Ayahuasca, that are used for their hallucinogenic and visionary healing properties. In fact, the first written account of the use of these substances was made by a member of the Columbus expedition in 1493. There is little question that the concoctions are psychoactive; however, these plant preparations usually consist of admixtures in which certain tryptamines, such as DMT or 5-OMe DMT, sometimes have been identified. Some β-carbolines possess activity as MAO inhibitors; thus, the MAO inhibitory effect of the β-carbolines might be simply potentiating the effect of any tryptaminergic hallucinogens possibly present in an admixture by interfering with their metabolism. Studies with individual β-carbolines, especially under carefully controlled clinical settings, have been very limited. The three most commonly occurring β-carbolines are harmine, harmaline, and tetrahydroharmine, and evidence suggests that harmine and harmaline are hallucinogenic in humans (with potencies not greater than that of DMT) (32,33). Harmaline has seen some limited experimental application as an adjunct to psychotherapy (34). Like other classical hallucinogens, certain β-carbolines bind at 5-HT$_{2A}$ receptors and, in animal studies, DOM-stimulus generalization occurs to harmaline (33). Using harmaline-trained animals, harmaline-stimulus generalization occurs to DOM. However, very few β-carbolines have been investigated to date, so they are only tentatively categorized as classical hallucinogens.

Harmine   Harmaline   Tetrahydroharmine

Although the scientific community has been aware of the psychoactive effects of the β-carbolines or β-carboline-containing natural substances for over 100 years, it is only in the past decade or so that they are becoming popular "on the street." The use of β-carboline-containing plants has moved out of the jungle and has given rise to a variety of religious movements in some South American cities. Recent books and movies are also helping popularize the use of these preparations and they are now being encountered in North America.

Phenylalkylamines. Phenylalkylamines, the phenylethylamines and the phenylisopropylamines, represent the largest group of classical hallucinogens (35). The phenylethylamines are the α-*des*methyl counterparts of the phenylisopropylamines; as with the indolealkylamines, the presence of the α-methyl group increases the agent's

lipophilicity and reduces its susceptibility to metabolism by monoamine oxidase. As a consequence, the phenylethylamines typically produce effects that are qualitatively similar to those of their corresponding phenylisopropylamines but are typically less potent. Phenylethylamine counterparts of weak phenylisopropylamines might be inactive. Literally hundreds of analogs have been examined in human and in animal studies (e.g., see ref. 31).

Phenylethylamines. As mentioned above, the phenylethylamines are usually less-potent analogs of the phenylisopropylamines. Some hallucinogenic phenylisopropylamines are claimed to possess some stimulant character that may be minimized or altogether absent in the corresponding phenylethylamines. The phenylisopropylamines also possess a chiral center that is absent in the phenylethylamines. Otherwise, the SAR of the two groups of agents are relatively similar and, consequently, the phenylethylamines will not be discussed in detail here. The most common, and indeed one of the oldest known, phenylethylamine hallucinogens is mescaline. Mescaline, a constituent of peyote (and other) cactus, is a relatively weak hallucinogenic agent (total human dose approximately 350 mg). Like many of the hallucinogens, mescaline is listed as a Schedule I substance; however, the use of peyote in certain native American Indian religious practices is sanctioned.

Mescaline

Phenylisopropylamines. Structural modification of mescaline and related substances by introduction of an α-methyl group and by deletion or rearrangement of the position of its methoxy groups resulted in a series of agents known as the phenylisopropylamines. As might have been expected, introduction of an α-methyl group, to afford 3,4,5-TMA or α-methylmescaline, doubled the potency of mescaline. Although there exist different nomenclatures for the dimethoxy- and trimethoxyphenylisopropylamines, that used herein is a commonly used nomenclature; the position of methoxy groups is given by indicating its position, and the number of methoxy groups is indicated by a prefix. For example, α-methylmescaline is 3,4,5-TMA indicating that it is a **tri**methoxy **a**nalog and that the methoxy groups are situated at the 3-, 4-, and 5-positions. Dimethoxy analogs are referred to as DMAs.

There are three possible monomethoxyphenylisopropylamines: the *ortho*-methoxy analog OMA, the *meta*-methoxy analog MMA, and the *para*-methoxy analog PMA (Table 18.3). Although PMA is specifically listed as a Schedule I substance, none of these three analogs is hallucinogenic. PMA possesses weak central stimulant actions and is an abused sub-

Table 18.3. Psychoactive Phenylisopropylamines and Related Agents

Agent	R$_2$	R$_3$	R$_4$	R$_5$	R$_6$	Human Hallucinogenic Dose (mg)*	DOM-stimulus Generalization Potency (μmol/kg)†
Amphetamine	H	H	H	H	H	NH	NSG
OMA	OCH$_3$	H	H	H	H	NH	NSG
MMA	H	OCH$_3$	H	H	H	NH	NSG
PMA	H	H	OCH$_3$	H	H	NH	NSG
2,3-DMA	OCH$_3$	OCH$_3$	H	H	H	(?)	NSG
2,4-DMA	OCH$_3$	H	OCH$_3$	H	H	> 60 (?)	21.0
2,5-DMA	OCH$_3$	H	H	OCH$_3$	H	120 (80–160)	23.8
2,5-DMA, R(−)-	OCH$_3$	H	H	OCH$_3$	H	(?)	14.0
2,6-DMA	OCH$_3$	H	H	H	OCH$_3$	(?)	NSG
3,4-DMA	H	OCH$_3$	OCH$_3$	H	H	> 500 (?)	NSG
3,5-DMA	H	OCH$_3$	H	OCH$_3$	H	(?)	NSG
2,3,4-TMA	OCH$_3$	OCH$_3$	OCH$_3$	H	H	> 100 (?)	29.8
2,3,5-TMA	OCH$_3$	OCH$_3$	H	OCH$_3$	H	> 80 (?)	63.0
2,3,6-TMA	OCH$_3$	OCH$_3$	H	H	OCH$_3$	> 30 (?)	—
2,4,5-TMA	OCH$_3$	H	OCH$_3$	OCH$_3$	H	30 (20–40)	13.7
2,4,6-TMA	OCH$_3$	H	OCH$_3$	H	OCH$_3$	38 (25–50)	13.9
3,4,5-TMA	H	OCH$_3$	OCH$_3$	OCH$_3$	H	175 (100–250)	24.2
MEM	OCH$_3$	H	OC$_2$H$_5$	OCH$_3$	H	35 (20–50)	22.9
DOM	OCH$_3$	H	CH$_3$	OCH$_3$	H	7 (3–10)	1.8
DOM, R(−)-	OCH$_3$	H	CH$_3$	OCH$_3$	H	(?)	0.9
DOM, S(+)-	OCH$_3$	H	CH$_3$	OCH$_3$	H	(?)	6.9
DOET	OCH$_3$	H	C$_2$H$_5$	OCH$_3$	H	4 (2–6)	0.9
DOPR	OCH$_3$	H	nC$_3$H$_7$	OCH$_3$	H	4 (2.5–5)	0.6
DOIP	OCH$_3$	H	iC$_3$H$_7$	OCH$_3$	H	(?)	2.9
DOBU	OCH$_3$	H	nC$_4$H$_9$	OCH$_3$	H	(?)	3.2
DOAM	OCH$_3$	H	nC$_5$H$_{11}$	OCH$_3$	H	(?)	NSG
DOT	OCH$_3$	H	SCH$_3$	OCH$_3$	H	8 (5–10)	—
DON	OCH$_3$	H	NO$_2$	OCH$_3$	H	4 (3–4.5)	2.7
DOF	OCH$_3$	H	F	OCH$_3$	H	(?)	5.8
DOC	OCH$_3$	H	Cl	OCH$_3$	H	2.5 (1.5–3)	1.2
DOB	OCH$_3$	H	Br	OCH$_3$	H	2 (1–3)	0.6
DOB, R(−)-	OCH$_3$	H	Br	OCH$_3$	H	1.0–1.5 (?)	0.3
DOI	OCH$_3$	H	I	OCH$_3$	H	2.5 (1.5–3)	1.2
DOOC	OCH$_3$	H	COOH	OCH$_3$	H	(?)	NSG
DOOH	OCH$_3$	H	OH	OCH$_3$	H	(?)	NSG

*Data are primarily from Shulgin and co-workers (26,31). Where a dose range was reported in the original literature, the arithmetic mean is also provided here to facilitate comparison and the original range is given in parenthesis; the values should not be taken as a measure of precision. In fact, doses are approximate and no implication is made that the different agents produce an identical effect. Key: NH indicates that the material is not a hallucinogen, (?) indicates that the material has not been well investigated or that its actions or potency are essentially unknown.

†Drug discrimination data represent ED50 values and are from Glennon (5,27,35). NSG: No stimulus generalization.

stance; several deaths have been attributed to PMA overdose within the past few years.

There are six isomeric DMA analogs. These have not been thoroughly investigated in humans, and few produce DOM-like stimulus effects in animals (Table 18.3); none is more potent than DOM. The most potent agent, and one that has been evaluated in humans, is 1-(2,5-dimethoxyphenyl)-2-aminopropane or 2,5-DMA. There are also six different TMA analogs (Table 18.3). Here, most show some activity but the 2,4,5-timethoxy analog 2,4,5-TMA (sometimes referred to simply as TMA) is the most potent of the series. Most of the trimethoxy analogs are recognized by DOM-trained animals but none is more potent than DOM itself (5). The presence of the 2,5-methoxy substitution pattern in 2,5-DMA and 2,4,5-TMA might be noted.

The DMAs and TMAs are methoxy-substituted derivatives of the parent phenylisopropylamine known as amphetamine (Fig. 18.2). Amphetamine undergoes several different routes of metabolism; one of these is *para*-hydroxylation (a route that seems more important in rodents than in humans). Initially, it was thought that the greater potency of 2,4,5-TMA over that of 2,5-DMA might be related to the 4-position of the former being blocked to metabolism by *para*-hydroxylation. Keeping the 2,5-dimethoxy substitution intact, different 4-position substituents were examined. This led to a series of agents such as DOM and DOB (see Table 18.3). These 4-substituted 2,5-dimethoxy analogs represent some of the most potent members of the series.

1-(2,5-Dimethoxy-4-methylphenyl)-2-aminopropane (DOM) represents the prototype member of this family of agents. Increasing the length of this 4-methyl group to an ethyl or n-propyl group (i.e., DOET and DOPR, respectively) results in enhanced potency on a molar basis. Further extension of the alkyl chain results in a decrease in potency or loss of action. Substitution at the 4-position by electron-withdrawing groups, particularly those with hydrophobic character, also results in active agents such as DOB (see Table 18.3). DOB is quite a potent agent and has been misrepresented on the clandestine market as LSD both in tablet and "blotter" form.

Where optical isomers have been examined, activity resides primarily with the R(−)isomer; the S(+)isomers are typically less active, inactive, or have received little study. For example, although not well investigated, it appears that R(−)DOM and R(−)DOB show activity at total human doses of < 4 mg and < 1 mg, respectively. N-Monomethylation reduces potency or abolishes activity; for example the N-monomethyl analogs of DOM and DOB are about 1/10th as potent as their primary amine counterparts. Structure-activity relationships for the DOM-like actions of phenylisopropylamines are summarized in Table 18.3 and Figure 18.2.

Table 18.3 provides a comparison of the approximate human doses of various phenylisopropylamines when administered via the oral route. These agents represent a mere sampling of the agents that have been examined; it can be imagined, using only those functional groups shown in the table, how many different analogs are possible on the basis of structural rearrangement. There is no reason to suspect that each of these agents produces identical effects. In fact, the actions of some of these agents have been reported to be quite unique, and range from hallucinations and closed-eye imagery to intellectual and sensory enhancement to erotic arousal (31).

Classical Hallucinogens: Mechanism of Action

Given that the arylalkylamines may not be producing identical effects, a common mechanism of action may not be expected. LSD was one of the first hallucinogens to be investigated mechanistically; another agent to see extensive investigation is mescaline. Interestingly, from a potency perspective, these two agents seem to represent opposite extremes. LSD has been proposed to produce its effects via numerous mechanisms including those involving serotonergic, dopaminergic, histaminergic, adrenergic, and other receptors. LSD binds with high affinity at many different receptor populations and acts as an agonist at some, an antagonist at others, and as a partial agonist at yet others. For many years it was supposed that mescaline might be acting via a dopaminergic or adrenergic mechanism because of its structural similarity to dopamine and norepinephrine. As early as the late 1950s it was speculated, because of its structural similarity to 5-HT, that LSD might be working through a serotonergic mechanism. Significant experimental evidence supported this claim. However, there was controversy as to whether LSD was a serotonergic agonist or antagonist. Furthermore, later studies revealed the existence of at least 14 populations of 5-HT receptors (see Chapter 12). With the subsequent availability of 5-HT$_2$-selective antagonists, it was demonstrated that several of these antagonists (e.g., ketanserin, pirenperone) were particularly effective in blocking the stimulus effects of DOM, and of DOM-stimulus generalization to other hallucinogens such as LSD, in tests of stimulus antagonism. It was later shown that the classical hallucinogens bind at 5-HT$_2$ serotonin receptors and that their receptor affinities were significantly correlated with both their DOM-stimulus generalization potencies and their human hallucinogenic potencies (35). The classical hallucinogens are now thought to produce their effect by acting as agonists at 5-HT$_2$ receptors in the brain—the *5-HT$_2$ hypothesis of hallucinogen action*. Radiolabeled analogs of DOB and DOI (e.g., [^{3}H]DOB, [^{125}I]DOI) now are available for the investigation of 5-HT$_2$ pharmacology.

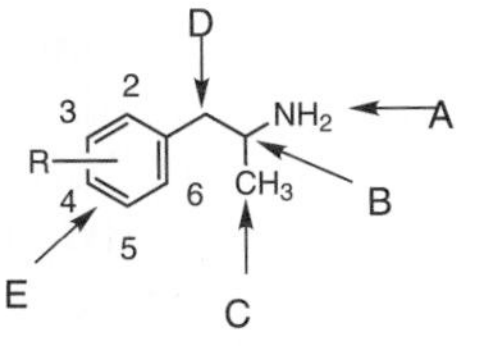

Position	Amphetamine-like action	DOM-like actions
A: Terminal amine	N-Methyl > NH$_2$ > NHR > NR$_2$	NH$_2$ > NHR > NR$_2$
B: Chiral center	S(+) > (±) > R(−)	R(−) > (±) > S(+)
C: α-Methyl group	Homologation decreases potency Replacement by H decreases potency	Homologation decreases potency Replacement by H decreases potency
D: β-Position	β-OH: reduces potency β =O: retains activity and potency	β-OH: not well investigated β =O: not well investigated
E: Aromatic substitution	Unsubstituted aromatic ring prefered	2,5-Dimethyl-substitution preferred 4-Substitution further modulates activity

Figure 18.2. Comparative SAR for the amphetamine-like stimulant actions and the DOM-like action of the phenylisopropylamines (27,40).

It has been more recently demonstrated that 5-HT$_2$ receptors actually represent a family of 5-HT receptors that consist of 5-HT$_{2A}$, 5-HT$_{2B}$ and 5-HT$_{2C}$ receptor subpopulations. Fewer that three dozen arylalkylamines have been compared but it appears that they show little selectivity for one subpopulation versus the others. Various pharmacologic studies with selective antagonists or by employing antagonist correlation analysis studies, however, suggest that it may be the 5-HT$_{2A}$ subtype that plays a predominant role in the behavioral actions of these agents (36). Although the 5-HT$_{2A}$ receptors might be responsible for those actions that the classical hallucinogens have in common, it may be other neurochemical mechanisms that account for their differences. For example, LSD is a very promiscuous agent that binds with high affinity at many receptor populations for which most other classical hallucinogens show little to no affinity. Many of the indolealkylamines bind with high affinity at multiple populations of 5-HT receptors and some display comparable or higher affinity at these receptors (e.g., 5-HT$_{1A}$, h5-HT$_{1D}$, 5-HT$_6$) than they do at 5-HT$_{2A}$ receptors. The phenylalkylamines are quite selective for 5-HT$_2$ receptors but, as mentioned above, display little selectivity for the three 5-HT$_2$ subpopulations. Some β-carbolines, although they bind at 5-HT$_2$ receptors, also possess activity as MAO inhibitors. Thus, these differences might account for their somewhat different actions. The one feature that all the classical hallucinogens have in common (i.e., the *common component hypothesis*) is that they bind at 5-HT$_{2A}$ receptors.

CENTRAL STIMULANTS
Introduction, Classification, and Definitions

Stimulants can be divided into several categories. The term *stimulant* or *behavioral stimulant* typically refers to agents with a central stimulatory effect whose actions are manifested mostly in motor activity, whereas *analeptics* are agents that have a stimulant effect primarily on autonomic centers such as those involved in the regulation of respiration and circulation (37). Nicotine and related nicotinic agents also possess stimulant properties but are best discussed with other cholinergic agents. Analeptics include agents such as pentylenetetrazol, nikethamide, and strychnine. The boundary between analeptics and behavioral stimulants is not sharply defined; caffeine, for example, has been classified as an analeptic but high doses produce a stimulant effects (37). Caffeine is probably the best known of a series of xanthines; in fact, caffeine, which is found in coffee, tea, chocolate, and other naturally-occurring substances, is probably the most widely used psychoactive substance in the world. Although most analeptics do not represent significant abuse problems, there is evidence for caffeine abuse (38). However, because caffeine, particularly in the form of its naturally-occurring products, is not subject to legal constraints it will not be discussed here.

The term stimulant typically conjures up substances such as the phenylisopropylamine amphetamine and the tropane analog cocaine. The following discussion will focus primarily on such substances.

Phenylisopropylamine Stimulants—Amphetamine-related Agents

The simplest unsubstituted phenylisopropylamine is 1-phenyl-2-aminopropane or amphetamine. Amphetamine possesses central stimulant, anorectic, and sympathomimetic actions, and is the prototype member of this class (39). It is common to refer to *amphetaminergic* structures and *amphetaminergic* activity, but amphetamine may be more of an exception than a rule. Most substituted derivatives of amphetamine (i.e., phenylisopropylamine) lack central stimulant activity; in fact, pharmacologically there are a greater number of "non-amphetamine-like" derivatives of amphetamine than there are "amphetamine-like" derivatives of amphetamine. Relatively few derivatives of amphetamine retain the activity of amphetamine; still fewer retain the potency of amphetamine. The present section will focus almost exclusively on the central stimulant actions of amphetamine and it should be recognized that these structure-activity relationships are not necessarily identical to those for anorectic or sympathomimetic actions.

Structure-activity Relationships for Amphetamine-like Stimulant Action

In general, the structure-activity relationships for amphetamine-like actions of the phenylisopropylamines are quite distinct from those for the DOM-like actions of the phenylisopropylamines. The structure-activity relationships for the two actions are summarized in Figure 18.2. The stimulus effects of amphetamine analogs have been reviewed (40).

Aryl-substituted Derivatives. In general, incorporation of substituents into the aromatic ring of amphetamine reduces or abolishes amphetamine-like stimulant activity. The sympathomimetic agent 4-hydroxyamphetamine lacks central stimulant action and is unlikely to penetrate the blood-brain barrier due to the presence of the polar aromatic hydroxyl group. Masking of the hydroxyl group in the form of its methyl ether affords the Schedule I substance PMA (*para*-methoxyamphetamine, also known as 4-methoxyamphetamine). PMA is a weak central stimulant with approximately one-tenth the potency of amphetamine. 4-Methylamphetamine (1-(*para*-tolyl)-2-aminopropane or *p*TAP) has also been found on the clandestine market and is, at best, a weak central stimulant. Incorporation of electron-withdrawing substituents results in agents that generally lack central stimulant properties. For example, PCA or *para*-chloroamphetamine is a 5-HT releasing agent that saw evaluation as a potential antidepressant. Another related analog is the 5-HT releasing agent fenfluramine that was used for some time as an appetite suppressant. Both of these latter agents are still widely employed as pharmacologic tools in basic neuroscience research.

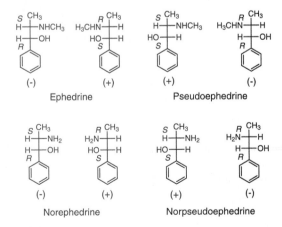

S(+)Amphetamine   p-Chloroamphetamine   Fenfluramine
(PCA)

Amine Substitution. In general, the primary amines are more potent than secondary amines, and secondary amines are more potent than tertiary amines as central stimulants. With regard to secondary amines, as the length of the amine substituent increases, activity decreases; the N-monoethyl and N-mono-*n*-propyl amines retain stimulant character but are somewhat less potent than amphetamine itself. Larger substituents typically result in agents with little to no stimulant character. The one exception is the N-monomethyl derivative methamphetamine. Methamphetamine ("crystal," "ice," "meth") is at least as potent as amphetamine as a central stimulant; in most studies it may be two to three times more potent than amphetamine. N-Hydroxylation of amphetamine has little effect on stimulant action. N,N-Dimethylamphetamine has been seized from clandestine laboratories but it has never been certain whether this agent was being prepared for its possible stimulant actions or whether it was a by-product of methamphetamine synthesis.

α-Substituents. Amphetamine possesses an α-methyl group. As already mentioned at the beginning of this chapter, α-demethylation (to afford phenylethylamine or 2-phenyl-1-aminoethane in the case of amphetamine) results in agents with decreased lipophilicity and increased susceptibility to metabolism. Phenylethylamine lacks central stimulant activity. Homologation of the α-methyl group, to for example an α-ethyl or α-*n*-propyl group, results in a decrease or loss of central stimulant activity. The presence of the α-methyl group in amphetamine creates a chiral center; hence, amphetamine exists as a pair of optical isomers. With respect to central stimulant actions, the S(+)isomer (i.e., dextroamphetamine) is several times more potent than its R(−)enantiomer (i.e., levamphetamine); this is not necessarily the case with other actions produced by amphetamine, particularly those produced in the periphery such as its cardiovascular actions.

β-Substituents. The β-position has not been all that well investigated. Perhaps the best studied derivatives are ephedrine and norephedrine (and even these agents have not been especially well investigated). Ephedrine and norephedrine are phenylpropanolamines that may be viewed as the β-hydroxy analogs of methamphetamine and amphetamine, respectively. Actually, β-hydroxylation of

amphetamine or methamphetamine results in the creation of a new chiral center; hence, there are a total of four optical isomers resulting from hydroxylation in each case. These eight structures are shown in Figure 18.3. Relatively little comparative information is available on the central stimulant actions of these phenylpropanolamine isomers.

In the 1970s there was a problem with what were termed "look-alike drugs." Look-alikes available on the clandestine market were made to resemble amphetamine and methamphetamine, both in action and physical appearance, to circumvent the control of amphetamine. The major constituents of these agents were various combinations of ephedrine, norephedrine, and caffeine. Although the look-alikes are no longer a major problem, the 1990s have witnessed the introduction of "herbal dietary supplements." These supplements are legally available in some health food and herbal shops; approximately two dozen such preparations have appeared on the market. The major ingredients of many of these preparations are various combinations of ephedrine and caffeine (or of ephedrine-containing natural products such as ma huang or ephedra, or caffeine-containing natural products such as guarana or kola nut). Interestingly, although ephedrine and caffeine possess stimulant character of their own, there is evidence that these agents may potentiate one another's actions (41). The exact mechanism by which they do so is unknown.

Although β-hydroxylation of amphetamine results in decreased central stimulant actions, this may be the result of the decreased ability of norephedrine to penetrate the blood-brain barrier, or it may be a clue that the presence of a β-oxygen substituent is inherently detrimental to activity. Support for the former possibility is derived from the shrub *Catha edulis. Catha edulis,* commonly known as khat or kat, is a plant indigenous to certain regions of the Middle East and eastern portion of Africa. The fresh shrub is sold openly in local markets, and is used for its central

Figure 18.3. Structures of β-oxidized analogs of methamphetamine (i.e., ephedrine and pseudoephedrine) and amphetamine (norephedrine and norpseudoephedrine). Note: norpseudoephedrine is also known as cathine.

stimulant character, much in the same way as the West uses coffee. Khat is used to prepare an infusion, or the fresh leaves are simply chewed. For more than 50 years it was thought that the active constituent was the phenyl-propanolamine cathine or (+)norpseuroephedrine (Fig. 18.3). However, in the late 1970s a more potent compound was isolated from fresh leaves and shown to be what is now termed cathinone. Cathinone, which is simply β-ketoamphetamine or an oxidized analog of norephedrine, is at least as potent as amphetamine as a central stimulant. Certain anorectic agents, such as diethypropion, also possess a benzylic keto group. The anorectic agent phenmetrazine or 3-methyl-2-phenylmorpholine and aminorex possess a benzylic oxygen atom in the form of an ether. All three of these agents possess stimulant character. A related stimulant is pemoline (available as a magnesium salt). Hence, it is specifically the hydroxyl analogs that seem to possess weak stimulant actions and this is likely due to their reduced lipophilicity and not because they simply possess an oxygen atom at the β- or benzylic position.

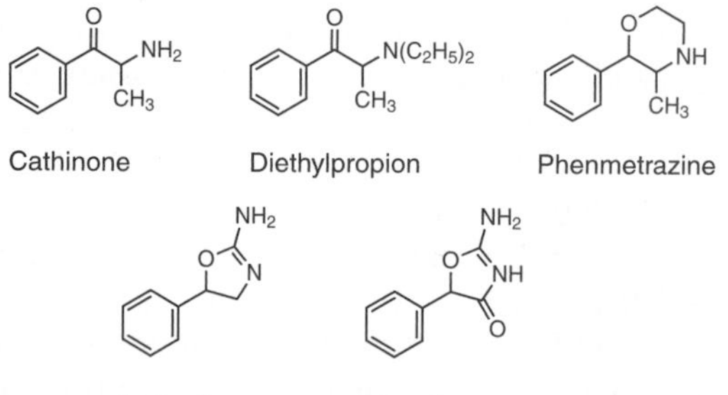

Metabolism of Amphetamine

In humans, (+)amphetamine has a half-life of about 7 hours. Some of the metabolic products of amphetamine metabolism are shown in Figure 18.4. Although a significant portion of amphetamine is excreted unchanged, it also undergoes both Phase I (functionalization to more polar derivatives) and Phase II (conjugation) metabolism (42). The Phase I metabolism of amphetamine analogs is catalyzed by two enzyme systems: cytochrome P450 and flavin monooxy-genase. The latter system oxidizes secondary and tertiary amine analogs of amphetamine. Amphetamine undergoes hydroxylation on the α-carbon, the β-carbon, the terminal amine, and on the aromatic ring. These metabolites are subsequently oxidized, where possible, or conjugated.

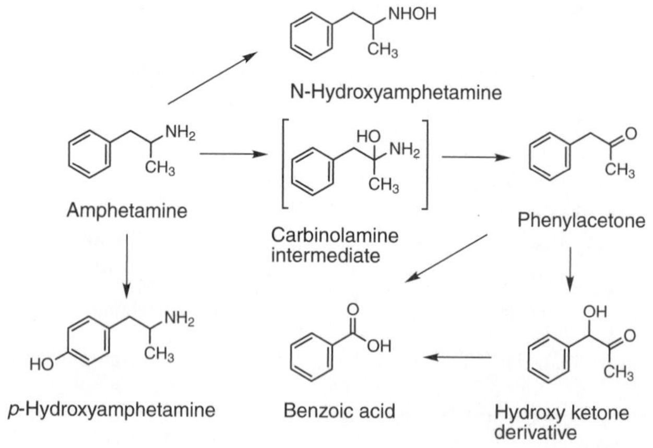

Amphetamine is oxidized to phenylacetone via a presumed carbinolamine intermediate. The phenylacetone is further oxidized directly to benzoic acid, or first to a hydroxy keto analog which is subsequently converted to benzoic acid. Amphetamine can also undergo aromatic hydroxylation to parahydroxyamphetamine. Initial work with rats indicated that para-hydroxylation was a major route of metabolism; subsequent studies showed, however, that benzoic acid is the major metabolite in humans. Subsequent oxidation at the benzylic position by dopamine β-hydroxylase affords parahydroxynorephedrine. Alternatively, direct oxidation of amphetamine by dopamine β-hydroxylase can afford norephedrine. Amphetamine and related derivatives also undergo N-hydroxyalation, and the N-hydroxy derivatives can be further oxidized to nitroso, nitro, and oximino compounds. There is some evidence that the oximino derivative is hydrolyzed to phenylacetone. Additional metabolites are possible. In Phase II reactions, ring hydroxylated metabolites are conjugated to their corresponding glucuronides. Sulfation of the enol form of phenylacetone has been reported. About 23% of methamphetamine is excreted unchanged; 18% is excreted as parahydroxymethamphetamine and 14% is excreted as the demethylated product (42).

Mechanism of Action of Amphetamine

Amphetamine is an indirect-acting dopaminergic and noradrenergic agonist; that is, amphetamine causes an increase in the synaptic concentrations of these neurotransmitters. The central stimulant actions of amphetamine primarily involve the dopamine system; amphetamine enhances the release of dopamine and, to a lesser extent, prevents the re-uptake of dopamine into presynaptic terminals (Fig. 18.5). The stimulant actions of amphetamine can be attenuated by the administration of dopamine antagonists such as the antipsychotic phenothiazine chlorpromazine and the butyrophenone haloperidol. Chronic administration of high doses of amphetamine may result in "amphetamine psychosis" which exhibits symptoms similar to acute paranoid psychosis. This is consistent with a role for dopamine in the central actions of amphetamine and, further, with the dopamine antagonist mechanisms proposed for certain antipsychotic agents. Similar psychotic episodes have been associated with khat ("khat psychosis" or "cathinone psychosis") and cocaine ("cocaine psychosis").

Cocaine-related Agents

There are eight possible stereoisomeric forms of methyl 3-(benzoyloxy)-8-methyl-azabicyclo[3.2.1]octan-2-carboxylate of which one, R-cocaine, is simply referred to as "cocaine." Chemically, cocaine is known as 2R-carbomethoxy-3S-benzyl-

Figure 18.4. Some products of amphetamine metabolism.

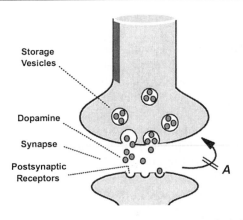

Figure 18.5. Schematic of a dopaminergic nerve terminal. Amphetamine increases synaptic concentration of dopamine primarily by causing its release from presynaptic terminals whereas cocaine increases synaptic concentration by preventing its re-uptake ("A").

oxy-1*R*-tropane. Cocaine is naturally occurring in a variety of plants belonging to the *Erythroxylon coca* species indigenous to some countries in South America. In addition to its stimulant actions, cocaine possesses vasoconstrictor actions and is a local anaesthetic; it has served as a template for the development of other therapeutically useful agents including local anesthetics and 5-HT$_3$ serotonin antagonists.

Cocaine has a very interesting history. The coca plant was used by South American Indians for religious and mystical purposes and as a stimulant to increase endurance and alleviate hunger. It was introduced into Europe in the 1800s and at the end of the 19th century cocaine use was popular and socially acceptable. Various cocaine-containing preparations were available and it was also used to "fortify" wines (e.g., Vin Coca). For a period of about 20 years, until just after the turn of the century, it was a constituent of the soft drink Coca-Cola. Cocaine was also used for therapeutic reasons but was later supplanted by amphetamine.

Cocaine is active via nearly every possible route of administration; however, insufflation of "snow" or "coke" represents one of the most popular routes. Administered in this manner, peak effects and plasma levels are achieved within 30 minutes (43). Smoking the free base form of cocaine ("crack") results in an even more rapid effect. The free base form rather than the hydrochloride salt is used for smoking because temperatures required for vaporization of the salt result in considerable decomposition (43). Intravenously administered cocaine can achieve peak blood levels within a few minutes. Cocaine is metabolized to benzoylecgonine and the methyl ester of ecgonine, and to a lesser extent to ecgonine, norcocaine, and hydroxylated derivatives.

Cocaine: Mechanism of Action

Cocaine has been shown to block the re-uptake of norepinephrine, serotonin, and dopamine; however, the reinforcing and stimulant nature of cocaine seem primarily related to blockade of dopamine re-uptake leading to the "dopamine hypothesis" of cocaine's actions (44). [³H]Co-

caine was used in an attempt to identify the "cocaine receptor" and this was later shown to be similar to the dopamine transporter. It is currently thought that cocaine produces it reinforcing effects by interfering with dopamine re-uptake (see Fig. 18.5) by blocking the dopamine transporter (45). Although the human dopamine transporter has been cloned, it is unknown if the dopamine and cocaine binding domains are identical or how much they overlap (44).

Cocaine-like Structure-activity Relationships and Cocaine-like Agents. Because cocaine binds at the dopamine transporter, this provides a convenient method for the investigation and formulation of structure-activity relationships; these have been recently reviewed (44,45). Important features for the binding of cocaine analogs include a) configuration, b) substituent at C$_2$, c) stereochemistry at C$_2$, d) substituent at N$_8$, and e) substituents at C$_3$. With respect to cocaine analogs, inversion of configuration can decrease activity. The C$_2$-position is quite important; epimerization from β to α reduces activity by 30- to 200-fold, and hydrolysis of the ester to the acid (i.e., benzoylecgonine) reduces activity by >1,500-fold. Although an ester function seems to be important, the methyl group can be replaced by other substituents (e.g., phenyl, benzyl) with relatively little effect. A basic nitrogen atom appears to be optimal; replacement of the N$_8$-methyl group by other substituents, such as small alkyl or benzyl, has only a small negative influence on activity whereas quaternization or acylation (of norcocaine) reduces activity by 33- and 111-fold, respectively (44).

Other dopamine transport blockers are known and their structure-activity relationships have been investigated (45). One of the oldest and most widely investigated is WIN 35,428 (44–49) and [³H]WIN 35,428 is available as a radioligand. Others include benztropine (45), GBR 12909 (50), mazindol (51), and methylphenidate (52). These latter compounds produce varying degrees of cocaine-like actions and are thus being examined as structural leads for the development of therapies for the treatment of cocaine abuse (45).

DESIGNER DRUGS
Introduction

Designer drugs, or controlled substance analogs, are the end result of the application of structure-activity relationships at the clandestine level. That is, knowledge of

WIN 35,428

Benztropine

GBR 12909

Mazindol

Methylphenidate

the established structure-activity relationships of a particular class of abused substances can be applied at the clandestine level for the development of novel agents of abuse. What is particularly frightening about this concept is that the novel agents are not necessarily, or even commonly, examined for action or toxicity before they are put on the illicit market. The term "designer drug" was first introduced in reference to novel opiate-related analogs that appeared on the clandestine market about two decades ago; today, the term is applied more generically to any class of abusable substance. Furthermore, the term is now commonly applied to nearly any substance, novel or not, that is new to the street scene. Designer drugs have appeared that are structurally related to the hallucinogens and stimulants discussed above; the present discussion will focus on some of these agents.

Specific Examples

Because some designer drugs result from the clandestine application of structure-activity relationships, it should be possible to legitimately forecast the actions, and perhaps even the approximate potencies, of novel street drugs on the basis of the same structure-activity data. This is sometimes the case. For example, "Nexus" made an appearance on the East coast of the United States in the early 1990s. Nexus is α-desmethyl DOB or 2-(4-bromo-2,5-dimethoxyphenyl)-1-aminoethane. Knowing that DOB is a potent phenylisopropylamine hallucinogen and that α-demethylation typically reduces the potency of phenylisopropylamines, it might be suspected that Nexus would be a DOB-like agent with reduced potency. This has been supported by the results of drug discrimination studies in animals. Furthermore, this material, also known as 2C-B, has been shown to be active in humans at 12–24 mg relative to about 2 mg for DOB (31).

Stimulant designer drugs have also appeared. For example, "CAT" or methcathinone has been found on the illicit American market. Interestingly, it seems that methcathinone was a popular drug of abuse in the former Soviet Union (where it was known under a variety of names including ephedrone) but reports of this agent were never published in either the scientific or lay literature of that time. Methcathinone is the N-monomethyl

analog of cathinone. Indeed, structurally, methcathinone is to cathinone what methamphetamine is to amphetamine. Methcathinone, which may be viewed as an oxidation product of ephedrine (hence the name ephedrone) is a potent central stimulant that is at least as potent as methamphetamine. Another example of a stimulant designer drug is 4-methylaminorex (4-MAX; "U4Euh") which has been misrepresented on the illicit market as cocaine or methamphetamine. 4-Methylaminorex, an alkylated version of the anorectic/stimulant aminorex, contains two chiral centers and, hence, exists as four optical isomers. Typically, it is a mixture of the two cis isomers that has been confiscated by law enforcement officials, and cis 4-methylaminorex is now classified as a Schedule I substance. On the basis of known structure-activity data, it might have been suspected that 4-methylaminorex would possess amphetamine-like actions. In tests of stimulus generalization employing (+)amphetamine-trained animals, all four isomers behaved as amphetamine-like agents with the trans(4S,5S) isomer being the most active (ED50 = 0.25 mg/kg) with a potency slightly greater than that of (+)amphetamine itself (ED50 = 0.42 mg/kg) (53).

cis(4S,5R)   cis(4R,5S)   trans(4S,5S)   trans(4R,5R)

4-Methylaminorex

Not all designer drugs result in actions that are entirely predictable. One of the most popular of such agents is MDMA or N-methyl-1-(3,4-methylenedioxyphenyl)-2-aminopropane ("Ecstasy," "XTC," "Adam"). MDMA is the N-monomethyl analog of MDA. MDA or 1-(3,4-methylenedioxyphenyl)-2-aminopropane was popular during the 1960s where it was known on the street as the "Love Drug." It was reported to produce effects in humans akin to a combination of cocaine and LSD. It has since been shown that MDA produces both amphetamine-like and DOM-like stimulus effects in animals and, further, that animals trained to discriminate MDA recognize central stimulants such as amphetamine and cocaine as well as classical hallucinogens such as LSD, mescaline, and DOM. Interestingly, the stimulant actions of MDA appear associated with the S(+)-isomer whereas the DOM-like actions are associated with the R(−)-isomer. Knowing that N-monomethylation of phenylisopropylamine stimulants enhances their potency whereas the corresponding change is detrimental to DOM-like actions it would have been predicted that MDMA would probably behave as an amphetamine-like stimulant. Consistent with this prediction, amphetamine-trained, but not DOM-trained, animals recognized MDMA in tests of stimulus generalization. Furthermore, animals trained to discriminate MDMA recognized amphetamine but not DOM. However, MDMA was claimed to produce empathogenic effects in humans (i.e., increased empathy and sociability, enhanced feelings of well being) and was used for several years as an adjunct to psychotherapy prior to emergency scheduling under the Controlled Substances Act as a Schedule I substance. It was argued that MDMA produced a unique non-amphetamine-like effect (54). Although both optical isomers are active, the $S(+)$-isomer is the more active of the two. A closely related agent is its N-ethyl homolog MDE ("Eve"). The general consensus today is that MDMA is probably an empathogen with amphetamine-like stimulant side effects. Homologation of the α-methyl group of phenylisopropylamine stimulants and hallucinogens typically diminishes their potency or abolishes their activity; however, the α-ethyl analog of MDMA, MBDB or N-methyl-1-(3,4-methylenedioxyphenyl)-2-aminobutane, retains MDMA-like actions (55).

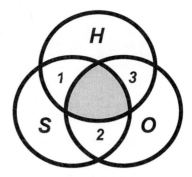

Figure 18.6. The behavioral effects of arylalkylamines may be described as falling into one or more of three different stimulus categories: classical hallucinogen (**H**), central stimulant (**S**) or "other" (**O**). See text for further discussion.

A closely related agent is PMMA or N-methyl-1-(4-methoxyphenyl)-2-aminopropane. PMMA is a hybrid structure of two phenylisopropylamine stimulants: PMA and methamphetamine. Surprisingly, PMMA lacks significant central stimulant actions and, unlike PMA and methamphetamine, PMMA is not recognized by (+)amphetamine-trained animals. Because PMMA is structurally related to metabolites of MDMA it was examined in MDMA-trained animals and found to be several-fold more potent than MDMA. Animals have been trained to discriminate PMMA from vehicle and PMMA stimulus generalization occurred to (±)MDMA and $S(+)$MDMA, but not to DOM, (+)amphetamine, R(−)MDMA, or R(−)PMMA. Another psychoactive agent that has not been well investigated is 3,4-DMA (Table 18.3). 3,4-DMA may be viewed as an O-methyl ring-opened analog of MDA. Although 3,4-DMA was not recognized by either DOM- or (+)amphetamine-trained animals, it was recognized by MDA- and PMMA-trained animals. These results, coupled with the above discussion of MDMA, suggest that phenylisopropylamines may not be best described as merely central stimulants or hallucinogens, but that there is yet a third action that needs to be accounted for. Although MDMA is widely abused, a contributing factor may be related to its amphetaminergic actions. It is not yet known if agents that fall into this third

pharmacologic category possess abuse potential; consequently they have been referred to simply as "other" agents. It has been proposed that the behavioral actions of the phenylisopropylamines can be described by the Venn diagram shown as Figure 18.6. The three types of actions are classical hallucinogen (**H**), stimulant (**S**), and "other" (**O**) (56); DOM is a prototypical phenylisopropylamine hallucinogen, (+)amphetamine is a prototypical phenylisopropylamine stimulant, and the "other" activity is, at least for the time being, associated with PMMA. Because MDMA possesses both PMMA-like and (+)amphetamine-like activity, it is perhaps best represented by *Intersect 2*. As mentioned above, R(−)MDA is hallucinogenic and $S(+)$MDA is a stimulant; both isomers possess "other" activity. Thus, R(−)MDA is best represented by *Intersect 3* whereas $S(+)$MDA is best represented by *Intersect 2;* the common intersect (shaded area) describes the actions of (±)MDA. Using this classification system, it should be possible to classify the various phenylisopropylamines as falling into one or more categories. Furthermore, there is no reason to suspect that this classification system will be limited to the phenylisopropylamines; that is, there is evidence that the indolealkylamines might be classified in a similar manner. For example, $S(+)$α-EtT produces both DOM- and PMMA-like effects but not (+)amphetamine-like effects, whereas R(−)α-EtT produces (+)amphetamine- and PMMA-like effects but not DOM-like effects (57). The classification scheme suggests that there will be three different structure-activity relationships and three different mechanisms of action. Certain agents, because they fall into more than one category, may represent mechanistic and structure-activity composites. The same may be said of arylalkylamine designer drugs; indeed, it may be the particular "mix" of actions that makes certain designer drugs so attractive as drugs of abuse.

Acknowledgement. Work from the author's laboratory was supported by PHS grant DA 01642.

CASE STUDY

Victoria F. Roche and S. William Zito

You are working the late shift on Saturday night at your local supermarket pharmacy. JG, the pharmacology lab technician from your school, asks you about the relative merits of OTC eye drops for his congested and red eyes. You notice that his shopping basket contains several bottles of water and 26 packages of Oreo cookies, and that the bright store lights seem to bother his eyes. JG, always laid-back, seems more so than usual, and everything you say makes him laugh. Chuckling to himself, JG takes the package of eye drops and deliberately weaves his way to the checkout register. Back at school on Monday you remember that JG is the research technician of Dr. R, who is studying cannabinoid binding to the CB-1 receptor. Based on his recent and past behaviors, you become concerned that JG may have helped himself to some of the lab's cannabinoids and approach Dr. R with your concerns. Dr. R checks the lab inventory of test chemicals and indeed finds one of them to be missing. Which of the following structures is most likely the missing one?

1. Identify the therapeutic problem(s) where the pharmacist's intervention may benefit the patient.

2. Identify and prioritize the patient specific factors that must be considered to achieve the desired therapeutic outcomes.

3. Conduct a thorough and mechanistically oriented structure-activity analysis of all therapeutic alternatives provided in the case.

4. Evaluate the SAR findings against the patient specific factors and desired therapeutic outcomes and make a therapeutic decision.

5. Counsel your patient.

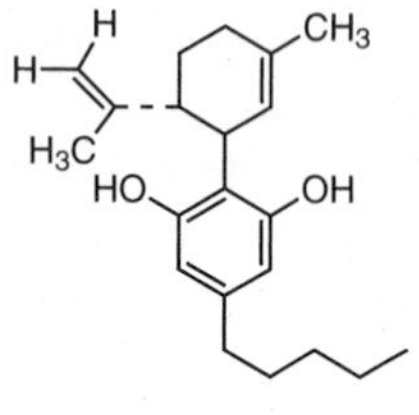

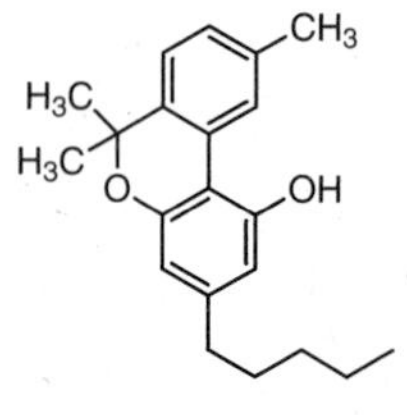

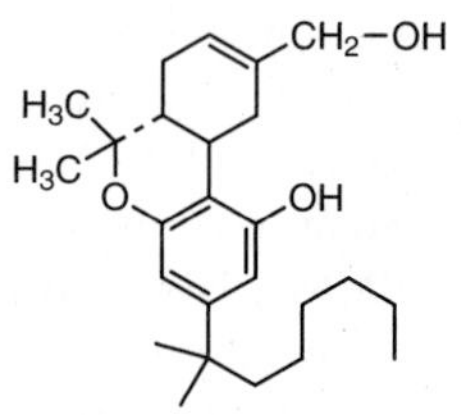

REFERENCES

1. Brimblecombe RW, Pinder RM. Hallucinogenic agents. Bristol: Wright-Scientechnica, 1975.
2. Hollister LE. Chemical psychoses. Springfield, (IL): Charles C. Thomas, 1968.
3. Glennon RA. Animal models for assessing hallucinogenic agents. In: Boulton AA, Baker GB, Wu PH, eds. Animal models of drug addiction. Totowa (NJ): Humana Press, 1992; 345–381.
4. Glennon RA, Jarbe TUC, Frankenheim J, eds. Drug discrimination: Applications to drug abuse research. Rockville (MD): National Institute on Drug Abuse, 1991.
5. Glennon RA. Discriminative stimulus properties of hallucinogens and related designer drugs. In: Glennon RA, Jarbe TUC, Frankenheim J, eds. Drug discrimination: Applications to drug abuse research. Rockville (MD): National Institute on Drug Abuse, 1991; 25–44.
6. Lin JC, Glennon RA. eds. Hallucinogens: An update. Rockville (MD): National Institute on Drug Abuse, 1994.
7. Rinaldi-Carmna M, Barth F, Heaulme M, et al. SR141716A, a potent and selective antagonist of the brain cannabinoid receptor. FEBS Lett 1994;350: 240–244.
8. Dutta AK, Sard H, Ryan W, et al. The synthesis and pharmacological evaluation of the cannabinoid antagonist SR 141716A. Med Chem Res 1994;5: 54–62.
9. Wiley JL. Cannabis: Discrimination of 'Internal Bliss'? Behavioural Pharmacology (1998);9: S125.
10. Matsuda L, Lolait SJ, Brownstein MJ, et al. Structure of a cannabinoid receptor and functional expression of the cloned cDNA. Nature 1990;246: 561–564.
11. Munro S, Thomas KL, Abu-Shaar M. Molecular characterization of a peripheral receptor for cannabinoids. Nature 1993;365: 61–64.
12. Hanus L, Gopher A, Almog S, et al. Two new unsaturated fatty acid ethanolamides in brain that bind to the cannabinoid receptor. J Med Chem 1993;36: 3032–3034.
13. Jarbe TUC, Lamb RL, Makriyannis A, et al. (R-)-Methanandamide as a discriminative stimulus in rats: Tests with anandamide and Δ⁹-THC. Behavioural Pharmacology 1998;9: S47.
14. Martin BR. Marijuana. In: Bloom FE, Kupfer DJ, eds. Psychopharmacology: The fourth generation of progress. New York: Raven Press, 1995; 1757–1765.
15. Jarbe TUC, Mathis DA. Discriminative stimulus functions of cannabinoids/cannabimimetics. In: Glennon RA, Jarbe TUC, Frankenheim J, eds. Drug discrimination: Applications to drug abuse research. Rockville (MD): National Institute on Drug Abuse, 1991; 75–99.
16. Reggio PH, Panu AM, Miles S. Characterization of a region of steric interference at the cannabinoid receptor using the active analog approach. J Med Chem 1993;36: 1761–1771.
17. Reggio PH, Wang T, Brown AE, et al. Importance of the C-1 substituent in classical cannabinoids to CB2 receptor selectivity: synthesis and characterization of a series of O,2-propano-Δ⁸-tetrahydrocannabinol analogs. J Med Chem 1997;40: 3312–3318.
18. Lagu SG, Varona A, Chambers JD, et al. Construction of a steric map of the binding pocket for cannabinoids at the cannabinoid receptor. Drug Design Discovery 1995;12: 179–192.
19. Gorelick DA, Balster RL. Phencyclidine (PCP). In: Bloom FE, Kupfer DJ, eds. Psychopharmacology: The fourth generation of progress. New York: Raven Press, 1995; 1767–1776.
20. Balster RL, Willetts J. Phencyclidine: A drug of abuse and a tool for neuroscience research. In: Schuster CR, Kuhar MJ, eds. Pharmacological Aspects of Drug Dependence. Handbook of Experimental Pharmacology Series, Volume 118. Berlin: Springer, 1996; 233–262.
21. Abou-Gharbia M, Ablordeppey SY, Glennon RA. Sigma receptors and their ligands: The sigma enigma. Ann Rep Med Chem 1993;28: 1–10.
22. Itzhak Y., ed. Sigma Receptors. London: Academic Press, 1994.
23. Glennon RA, Ablordeppey SY, Ismaiel AM, et al. Structural features important for σ₁ receptor binding. J Med Chem 1994;37: 1214–1219.
24. Balster RL. Discriminative stimulus properties of phencyclidine and other NMDA antagonists. In: Glennon RA, Jarbe TUC, Frankenheim J, eds. Drug discrimination: Applications to drug abuse research. Rockville (MD): National Institute on Drug Abuse, 1991; 163–180.
25. Shulgin AT, Shulgin A. Tihkal. Berkeley (CA): Transform Press, 1997.
26. Jacob P, III, Shulgin AT. Structure-activity relationships of classical hallucinogens and their analogs. In: Lin JC, Glennon RA. eds. Hallucinogens: An update. Rockville (MD): National Institute on Drug Abuse, 1994, 74–91.
27. Glennon RA. Classical hallucinogens: An introductory overview. In: Lin JC, Glennon RA. eds. Hallucinogens: An update. Rockville (MD): National Institute on Drug Abuse, 1994.
28. Murphree HB, Dippy RH, Jenney EH, et al. Effects in normal man of α-methyltryptamine and α-ethyltryptamine. Clin Pharmacol Ther, 1961;2: 722–726.
29. Siva Sankar DV. ed. LSD: A total study. Westbury (NY): PJD Publications, 1975.
30. Pfaff RC, Huang X, Marona-Lewicka D, et al. Lysergamides revisited. In: Lin JC, Glennon RA. eds. Hallucinogens: An update. Rockville (MD): National Institute on Drug Abuse, 1994, 52–73.
31. Shulgin AT, Shulgin A. Pihkal. Berkeley (CA): Transform Press, 1991.
32. Naranjo C. Psychotropic properties of harmala alkaloids. In: Efron DK, Holmstedt B, Kline NS, eds. Ethnopharmacologic search for psychoactive drugs. Washington DC: U S Government Printing Office, 1967; 385–391.
33. Grella B, Dukat M, Young R, et al. Investigation of hallucinogenic and related β-carbolines. Drug Alcohol Dependence, 1998;50: 99–107 and references therein.
34. Naranjo C. The healing journey. New York: Pantheon Books, 1973.
35. Glennon RA, Classical hallucinogens. In: Schuster CR, Kuhar MJ, eds. Pharmacological Aspects of Drug Dependence. Handbook of Experimental Pharmacology Series, Volume 118. Berlin: Springer, 1996; 343–371.
36. Nelson DL, Lucaites VL, Wainscot DB, et al. Comparisons of hallucinogenic phenylisopropylamine binding affinities at cloned human 5-HT$_{2A}$, 5-HT$_{2B}$, and 5-HT$_{2C}$ receptors. Naunyn-Schmeideberg's Arch Pharmacol, 1998; 359:1–6.
37. Van Praag HM. Psychotropic drugs. New York: Brunner/Mazel Publishers, 1978.
38. Griffiths RR, Mumford GK. Caffeine reinforcement, discrimination, tolerance, and physical dependence in laboratory animals and humans. In: Schuster CR, Kuhar MJ, eds. Pharmacological Aspects of Drug Dependence. Handbook of Experimental Pharmacology Series, Volume 118. Berlin: Springer, 1996; 315–341.
39. Cho AK, Segal DS, eds. Amphetamine and its analogs. San Diego: Academic Press, 1994; 43–77.
40. Young R, Glennon RA. Discriminative stimulus properties of amphetamine and structurally-related phenalkylamines. Med Res Rev, 1986;6: 99–130.
41. Young R, Gabryszuk M, Glennon RA. (−)Ephedrine and caffeine mutually potentiate one another's amphetamine-like stimulus effects. Pharmacol Biochem Behav 1998;61: 169–173.

42. Cho AK, Kumagai Y. Metabolism of amphetamine and other arylisopropylamines. In: Cho AK, Segal DS, eds. Amphetamine and its analogs. San Diego: Academic Press, 1994; 43–77.

43. Fischman MW, Johanson CE. Cocaine. In: Schuster CR, Kuhar MJ, eds. Pharmacological Aspects of Drug Dependence. Handbook of Experimental Pharmacology Series, Volume 118. Berlin: Springer, 1996; 159–195.

44. Carroll FI, Lewin AH, Boja JW, et al. Cocaine receptor: Biochemical characterization and structure-activity relationships of cocaine analogues at the dopamine transporter. J Med Chem;35: 969–981.

45. Newman AH. Novel dopamine transporter ligands: The state of the art. Med Chem Res 1998;8: 1–11, and following articles.

46. Meltzer PC, Blundell, Madras BK. Structure-activity relationships of inhibition of the dopamine transporter by 3-arylbicyclo[3.2.1]octanes. Med Chem Res 1998;8: 12–34.

47. Lomenzo SA, Izenwasser S, Katz J, et al. The effects of alkyl substituents at the 6-position of cocaine analogues on dopamine transporter binding affinity and dopamine uptake inhibition. Med Chem Res 1998;8: 35–42.

48. Prakash KRC, Araldi GL, Smith MP, et al. Synthesis and biological activity of new 6- and 7-substituted 2β-butyl-3-phenyltropanes as ligands for the dopamine transporter. Med Chem Res 1998;8: 43–58.

49. Carroll FI, Lewin AH, Kuhar MJ. 3β-Phenyl-2β-substituted tropanes—An SAR analysis. Med Chem Res 1998;8: 59–65.

50. Zhang Y. The identification of GBR 12909 as a potential therapeutic agent for cocaine abuse. Med Chem Res 1998;8: 66–76.

51. Houlihan WJ, Boja JW, Kopajtic TA, Kuhar MJ, et al. Positional isomers and analogs of mazindol as potential inhibitors of the cocaine binding site on the dopamine transporter site. Med Chem Res 1998;8: 77–90.

52. Deutsch HM, Shi Q, Gruszecka-Kowalik E, et al. Synthesis and pharmacology of potential cocaine antagonists. 2. Structure-activity relationship studies of aromatic ring-substituted methylphenidate analogs. J Med Chem 1996;39:1201–1209.

53. Glennon RA, Misenheimer B. Stimulus properties of a new designer drug: 4-methylaminorex ("U4Euh"). Pharmacol, Biochem, Behav 1990;35: 517–521.

54. Nichols DE, Oberlender R. Structure-activity relationships of MDMA-like substances. In: Ashgar K, De Souza E. eds. Pharmacology and toxicology of amphetamine and related designer drugs. Washington DC: U S Government Printing Office, 1989, 1–29.

55. Oberlender R, Nichols DE. (+)N-Methyl-1-(1,3-benzodioxol-5-yl)-2-butanamine as a discriminative stimulus in studies of 3,4-methylenedioxyamphetamine-like behavioral activity. J Pharmacol Exp Ther, 1990;255: 1098–1106.

56. Glennon RA, Young R, Dukat M, et al. Initial characterization of PMMA as a discriminative stimulus. Pharmacol Biochem Behav, 1997;57: 151–158.

57. Glennon RA. Arylalkylamine drugs of abuse: An overview of drug discrimination studies. Pharmacol Biochem Behav 1999; 64:251–256.

19. Opioid Analgesics

DAVID S. FRIES

INTRODUCTION

Agents that decrease pain are referred to as analgesics or as analgetics. Although analgetic is grammatically correct, common use has made the term analgesic preferable to analgetic for the description of the pain killing drugs. Pain relieving agents are also called antinociceptives.

There are a number of classes of drugs that are used to relieve pain. The nonsteroidal anti-inflammatory agents have primarily a peripheral site of action, are useful for mild to moderate pain, and often have an anti-inflammatory effect associated with their pain killing action. Anesthetics (general or local) inhibit pain transmission by inhibition of voltage-regulated sodium and calcium channels. These agents are often highly sedating or toxic when used in concentrations sufficient to relieve chronic or acute pain in ambulatory patients. Dissociative anesthetics (ketamine), and other compounds that act as inhibitors of N-methyl-D-aspartate (NMDA) activated glutamate receptors in the brain, are effective antinociceptive agents when used alone or in combination with opioids. Compounds, such as the antiseizure drug gabapentin, which inhibit voltage regulated Ca²⁺ ion channels, are useful in treating some types of pain. Most CNS depressants (e.g., ethanol, barbiturates, and antipsychotics) will cause a decrease in pain perception. Inhibitors of serotonin and norepinephrine re-uptake (i.e., antidepressant drugs) are useful alone and in combination with opiates in treating certain cases of chronic pain. Current research into the antinociceptive effects of centrally acting α-adrenergic-, cannabinoid- and nicotinic-receptor agonists may yield clinically useful analgesics working by new mechanisms. Preliminary research with inhibitors to neurokinin (tachykinin) receptors shows promise of yielding new analgesic agents. While research in one or more of the above areas may lead to new drugs, at the present time, severe acute or chronic pain generally is treated most effectively with opioid agents.

Opioid analgesics historically have been called narcotic analgesics. Narcotic analgesic literally means that the agents cause sleep or loss of consciousness (narcosis) in conjunction with their analgesic effect. The term narcotic has become associated with the addictive properties of opioids and other CNS depressants. Since the great therapeutic value of the opioids is their ability to induce analgesia without causing narcosis, and not all opioids are addicting, the term narcotic analgesic is misleading and will not be used further in this chapter.

History

The use of the juice (opium in Greek) or latex from the unripe seed pods of the poppy *Papaver Somniferum* is among the oldest recorded medications. The writings of Theophrastus around 200 B.C. describe the use of opium in medicine; however, there is evidence that opium was used in the Sumerian culture as early as 3500 B.C. The initial use of opium was as a tonic or it was smoked. The pharmacist Surtürner first isolated an alkaloid from opium in 1803. He named the alkaloid morphine, after Morpheus, the Greek god of dreams. Codeine, thebaine and papaverine are other medically important alkaloids that were later isolated from the latex of opium poppies.

Morphine was among the first compounds to undergo structure modification. Ethylmorphine (the 3-ethyl ether of morphine) was introduced as a medicine in 1898. Diacetylmorphine, which may be considered to be the first synthetic prodrug, was synthesized in 1874 and marketed as a nonaddicting analgesic, antidiarrheal and antitussive agent in 1898.

Opiate/Opioid

The use of the terms opiate and opioid requires some clarification. The term opiate was used extensively until the 1980s to describe any natural or synthetic agent that was derived from morphine. One could say an opiate was any compound that was structurally related to morphine. The discovery, in the mid-1970s, of peptides in the brain that had pharmacologic actions similar to morphine prompted a change in nomenclature. The peptides were not easily related to morphine structurally; yet, their actions were like those produced by morphine. At this time the term opioid, meaning opium- or morphine-like in terms of pharmacologic action, was introduced. The broad group of opium alkaloids, synthetic derivatives related to the opium alkaloids, and the many naturally occurring and synthetic peptides with morphine-like pharmacologic effects are called opioids. In addition to having pharmacologic effects similar to morphine, a compound must be antagonized by an opioid antagonist such as naloxone to be classed as an opioid. The neuronal-located proteins to which opioid-agents bind and initiate biologic responses are called opioid receptors.

ENDOGENOUS OPIOID PEPTIDES AND THEIR PHYSIOLOGIC FUNCTIONS

Scientists had postulated for some time, based on structure-activity relationships, that opioids bound to specific receptor sites to cause their actions. It also was reasoned that morphine and the synthetic opioid derivatives were not the natural ligands for the opioid receptors and that some analgesic substance must exist within the brain. Techniques to prove these two points were not developed until the mid-1970s. Hughes, Kosterlitz and coworkers (1) used the electrically stimulated contractions of guinea pig ileum (GPI) and the mouse *vas deferens* (MVD), that are very sensitive to inhibition by opioids, as bioassays to follow the purification of compounds with morphine-like activity from mammalian brain tissue. These researchers were able to isolate and determine the structures of two pentapeptides, Tyr-Gly-Gly-Phe-Met (Met-enkephalin) and Tyr-Gly-Phe-Leu (Leu-enkephalin), that caused the opioid activity. The compounds were named enkephalins after the Greek word "Kaphale" that translates "from the head."

At about the same time as Hughes and Kosterlitz were making their discoveries, three other laboratories, using a different assay technique, were able to identify endogenous opioids and opioid receptors in the brain (2–4). These laboratories used radiolabeled opioid compounds (radioligands), with high specific activity, to bind to opioid receptors in brain homogenates (5). One can demonstrate saturable binding (i.e., the tissue contains a finite number of binding sites that can all be occupied) of the radioligands and the bound radioligands can be displaced stereoselectively by nonradiolabeled opioids. Discovery of the enkephalins was soon followed by the identification of other endogenous opioid peptides, including β-endorphin (6) the dynorphins (7) and the endomorphins (8).

The opioid peptides isolated from mammalian tissue are known collectively as endorphins, a word derived from a combination of endogenous and morphine. The opioid alkaloids and all of the synthetic opioid derivatives are called exogenous opioids. Interestingly, the isolation of morphine and codeine in small amounts has been reported from mammalian brain (9). The functional significance of endogenous morphine remains unknown.

Opioid Peptides

The endogenous opioid peptides are synthesized as part of the structures of large precursor proteins (10). There is a different precursor protein for each of the major types of opioid peptides (Fig. 19.1). Proopiomelanocortin (PMOC) is the precursor for β-endorphin. Proenkephalin A is the precursor for Met- and Leu-enkephalin. Proenkephalin B (prodynorphin) is the precursor for dynorphin and α-neoendorphin. The pronociceptin protein has been identified and contains only one copy of the active peptide, while the precursor protein for morphaceptin remains to be identified. All of the pro-opioid proteins are synthesized in the cell nucleus and transported to the terminals of the nerve cells from which they are released. The active peptides are hydrolyzed from the large proteins by processing proteases that recognize double basic amino acid sequences positioned just before and after the opioid peptide sequences.

Peptides with opioid activity have been isolated from sources other than mammalian brain. The hexapeptide β-casomorphin (Tyr-Pro-Phe-Pro-Gly-Pro-Ile), found in cow's milk, is a mu opioid agonist (11). Dermorphin (Tyr-D-Ala-Phe-Gly-Tyr-Pro-Ser-NH2), a mu selective peptide isolated from the skin of South American frogs, is about 100 times more potent than morphine in *in vitro* tests (12).

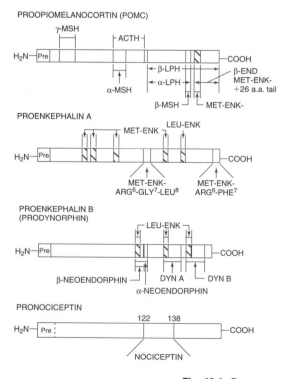

Met-enkephalin = Tyr-Gly-Gly-Phe-Met

Leu-Enkephalin = Tyr-Gly-Gly-Phe-Leu

β-Endorphin = Tyr-Gly-Gly-Phe-Met-Thr-Ser-Glu-Lys-Ser^{10}-Gln-Thr-Pro-Leu-Val-Thr-Leu-Phe-Lys-Asn^{20}-Ala-Ile-Ile-Lys-Asn-Ala-Tyr-Lys-Lys-Gly-GluOH^{31}

Dynorphin(dyn$^{1-17}$) = Tyr-Gly-Gly-Phe-Leu-Arg-Arg-Ile-Arg-Pro-Lys-Leu-Lys-Trp-Asp-Asn-Gln

Dynorphin(dyn$^{1-8}$) = Tyr-Gly-Gly-Phe-Leu-Arg-Arg-Ile

Dynorphin(dyn$^{1-13}$) = Tyr-Gly-Gly-Phe-Leu-Arg-Arg-Ile-Arg-Pro-Lys-Leu-Lys

α-Neoenodorphin = Tyr-Gly-Gly-Phe-Leu-Arg-Lys-Tyr-Pro-Lys

β-Neoendorphin = Tyr-Gly-Gly-Phe-Leu-Arg-Lys-Tyr-Pro

Nociceptin = Phe-Gly-Gly-Phe-Thr-Gly-Ala-Arg-Lys-Ser-Ala-Arg-Lys-Leu-Ala-Asn-Gln

Fig. 19.1. Precursor proteins to the endogenous opioid peptides.

The endogenous opioids exert their analgesic action at spinal and supraspinal sites (Fig. 19.2). They also produce analgesia by a peripheral mechanism of action associated with the inflammatory process. In the central nervous system, the opioids exert an inhibitory neurotransmitter or neuromodulator action on afferent pain signaling neurons in the dorsal horn of the spinal cord and on interconnecting neuronal pathways for pain signals within the brain. In the brain, the arcuate nucleus, periaqueductal gray and the thalamic areas are especially rich in opioid receptors and are sites where opioids exert an analgesic action. In the spinal cord, concentrations of endogenous opioids are high in laminae 1, laminae 2 and trigeminal nucleus areas. All of the endogenous opioid peptides and the three major classes of opioid receptors appear to be at least partially involved in the modulation of pain. The actions of opioids at the synaptic level are described in Figure 19.3.

Analgesia that results from acupuncture or is self-induced by a placebo or biofeedback mechanisms is caused by release of endogenous endorphins. Analgesia produced by these procedures can be prevented by the prior dosage of a patient with an opioid antagonist. Electrical stimulation from electrodes properly placed in the brain causes endorphin release and analgesia. This procedure is used for the "self-stimulated" release of endorphins in chronic pain patients who do not respond to any other medical treatment. As with exogenously administered opioid drugs, tolerance develops to all procedures that work by release of endogenous opioids.

OPIOID RECEPTORS

There are the three major types of opioid receptors: mu (μ), kappa (κ) (13) and delta (δ) (14). All three of the receptor types have been well characterized and cloned (15). A recently adopted nomenclature classifies the three opioid receptors in the order which they were cloned (16). By this classification, delta opioid receptors are OP$_1$ receptors,

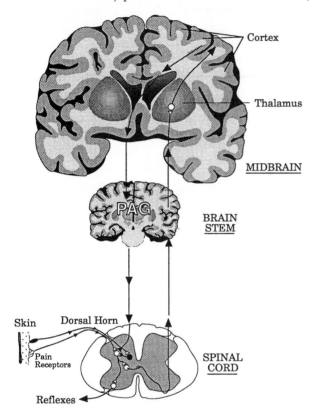

Fig. 19.2. Location of endogenous opioid nerve tracts in the CNS. Endorphins and opioid receptors in the dorsal horn of the spinal cord, thalamus, and periaqueductal gray (PAG) areas are associated with the transmission of pain signals.

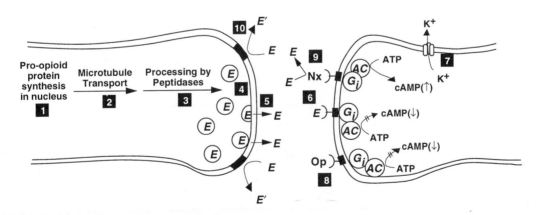

Fig. 19.3. Schematic representation of a delta enkephalinergic nerve terminal. 1. Pro-opioid proteins (proenkephalin A) are synthesized in the cell nucleus. 2. Pro-opioid proteins undergo microtubular transport to the nerve terminal. 3. Active endogenous opioids (E) are cleaved from the pro-opioid proteins by the action of "processing" proteases. 4. The active peptides (E) are taken up and stored in presynaptic vesicles. 5. The peptides are released when the presynaptic neuron fires. 6. The endogenous opioid peptides bind to postsynaptic receptors and activate second message systems. 7. For mu opioid receptors, the second messenger effect is mediated by a G-inhibitory (Gi/o) protein complex which promotes the inactivation of adenylate cyclase, a decrease in intracellular cyclic-adenosine-3,' 5'-monophosphate (cAMP), and finally an efflux of potassium ions (K$^+$) from the cell. The net effect is the hyperpolarization of the postsynaptic neuron and inhibition of cell firing. 8. Exogenous opioids (Op) such as morphine combine with opioid receptors and mimic the actions of E. 9. Opioid antagonists such as naloxone (Nx) combine with opioid receptors and competitively inhibit the actions of E or Op. 10. The action of E is terminated by a membrane-bound endopeptidase [EC3.4.24.11] (enkephalinase) which hydrolyze the Gly3-Phe4 peptide bond of enkephalin. Other endopeptidases may be employed in the metabolism of different endogenous opioid peptides.

Table 19.1. Opioid Receptor Types and Subtypes

Receptor Type (Natural Ligand)	Selective Agonists	Agonist Properties	Selective Antagonists
μ, mu, OP$_3$ (endormorphin 1) (endomorphin 2) (β-endorphin)*	Morphine Sufentanil DAMGO (Tyr-D-Ala-MePhe-NH-(CH$_2$)$_2$OH PLO17 (Tyr-Pro-MePhe-D-Pro-NH$_2$ BIT (affinity label)	Analgesia (morphine-like) Euphoria Increased gastrointestinal transit time Immune suppression Respiratory depression (volume)	Naloxone Naltrexone CTOP Cyprodime β-FNA (affinity label)
μ_1 (high affinity)	Meptazinol Etonitazene	Emetic effects Tolerance Physical dependence	Naloxonazine
μ_2 (low affinity)	TRIMU-5 (Tyr-D-Ala-Gly-NH-(CH$_2$)$_2$-CH-(CH$_3$)$_2$		
κ, kappa, OP$_2$ (dynorphins) (β-endorphin)*	Ethylketocyclazocine (EKC) Bremazocine Mr2034 dyn (1–17) Trifluadom	Analgesia Sedation Miosis Diuresis Dysphoria	TENA nor-BNI
κ_1 (high affinity)	U-50,488 Spiradoline (U-62,066) U-69,593 PD 117302		UPHIT
κ_2	dyn 1–17		
κ_3	NalBzOH		
δ, delta, OP$_1$ (enkephalins) (β-endorphin)*	DADLE (D-Ala^2-D-Leu^5-enkephalin) DSLET (Tyr-D-Ser-Gly-Phe-Leu-Thr) DPDPE (D-Pen^2-D-Pen^5-Enkephalin)	Analgesia Immune stimulation Respiratory depression (rate)	ICI 174864 FIT (affinity label) SUPERFIT (affinity label)
δ_2	DADLE		Naltrindole (NTI) BNTX
δ_2	D-Ala^2-deltorphin II		Naltriben (NTB) Naltrindol isothiocynate (NTII)

kappa opioid receptors are OP$_2$ receptors, and mu opioid receptors are OP$_3$ receptors. There is evidence for subtypes of each of these receptors; however, the failure of researchers to find genetic evidence for additional receptors indicates that the receptor subtypes are post-translational modifications of known receptor types. Receptor subtypes also may be known receptor types that are coupled to different signal transduction systems. Table 19.1 lists the opioid receptor types and subtypes, their known physiologic functions and selective agonists and antagonists for each of the receptors. All three of the opioid receptor types are located in human brain or spinal cord tissues and each has a role in the mediation of pain. At this time, mu and kappa agonists are in clinical use and several delta receptor selective compounds are in clinical trials.

Orphan Opioid Receptor

A fourth receptor has been identified and cloned based on homology with cDNA sequence of the known (mu, delta and kappa) opioid receptors (17). Despite the homology in cDNA sequence with known opioid receptors, this new receptor did not bind the classical opioid peptide or nonpeptide agonists or antagonists with high affinity. Thus the receptor was called the orphan opioid receptor. In subsequent studies, two research groups found a hep-

tadecapeptide (Phe-Gly-Gly-Thr-Gly-Ala-Arg-Lys-Ser-Ala-Lys-Ala-Asn-Gln) to be the endogenous peptide for the orphan opioid receptor. One of the research groups (18) named the heptadecapeptide nociceptin, because they determined it caused hyperalgesia (nociception) after i.c.v. injection into mice. The other research group (19) named the heptapeptide orphanin FQ after its affinity for the orphan opioid receptor and the first and last amino acids in the peptides sequence (i.e., F = Phe and Q = Gln.) Nociceptin/orphanin FQ resembles dynorphin-A in structure with the most notable difference being the replacement of Tyr at the N-terminus with Phe. Conflicting results have now been published on the ability of nociceptin/orphanin FQ to produce hyperalgesia vs. analgesia in rodent pain assay models. One study has established this compound to be a potent initiator of pain signals in periphery where it acts by releasing substance P from nerve terminals (20). Years of research will be required to establish the importance of this system in pain transmission and its relationship to the classical opioid systems.

Identification and Activation of Opioid Receptors

Identification of multiple opioid receptors has depended upon the discovery of selective agonists and antagonists, the identification of sensitive assay techniques (21) and ultimately the cloning of the receptor proteins (15). The techniques that have been especially useful are the radioligand binding assays on brain tissues and the electrically stimulated peripheral muscle preparations. Rodent brain tissue contains all three opioid receptor types and special evaluation procedures (computer assisted line fitting) or selective blocking (with reversible or irreversible binding agents) of some of the receptor types must be used to sort out the receptor selectivity of test compounds. The myenteric plexus-containing longitudinal strips of guinea pig ileum (GPI) contain mu and kappa opioid receptors. The contraction of these muscle strips is initiated by electrical stimulation and is inhibited by opioids. The *vas deferens* from mouse contains mu, delta, and kappa receptors and reacts similarly to the GPI to electrical stimulation and to opioids. Homogenous populations of opioid receptors are found in rat (μ), hamster (δ) and rabbit (κ) *vas deferentia*.

The signal transduction mechanism for mu, delta and kappa receptors is through $G_{i/o}$ proteins. Activation of opioid receptors is linked through the G protein to an inhibition of adenylate cyclase activity. The resultant decrease in cAMP production causes an efflux of potassium ions, and results in hyperpolarization of the nerve cell (22,23). Cells also show an increase in Ca^{2+} activity.

Mu Opioid Receptors

Endomorphin-1 (Tyr-Pro-Trp-Phe-NH$_2$) and endomorphin-2 (Try-Pro-Phe-Phe-NH$_2$) are endogenous opioid peptides with a high degree of selectivity for mu (OP$_3$) receptors (8). A number of therapeutically useful compounds have been found that are selective for mu opioid receptors (Fig. 19.4). All of the opioid alkaloids and most of their synthetic derivatives are mu selective agonists. Morphine, normorphine, and dihydromorphinone have 10–20-fold mu receptor selectivity and were particularly important in early studies to differentiate the opioid receptors. Sufentanil and the peptides DAMGO (24) and dermorphin (25), all with 100-fold selectivity for mu over other opioid receptors, are frequently used in the laboratory studies to demonstrate mu receptor-selectivity in cross-tolerance, receptor

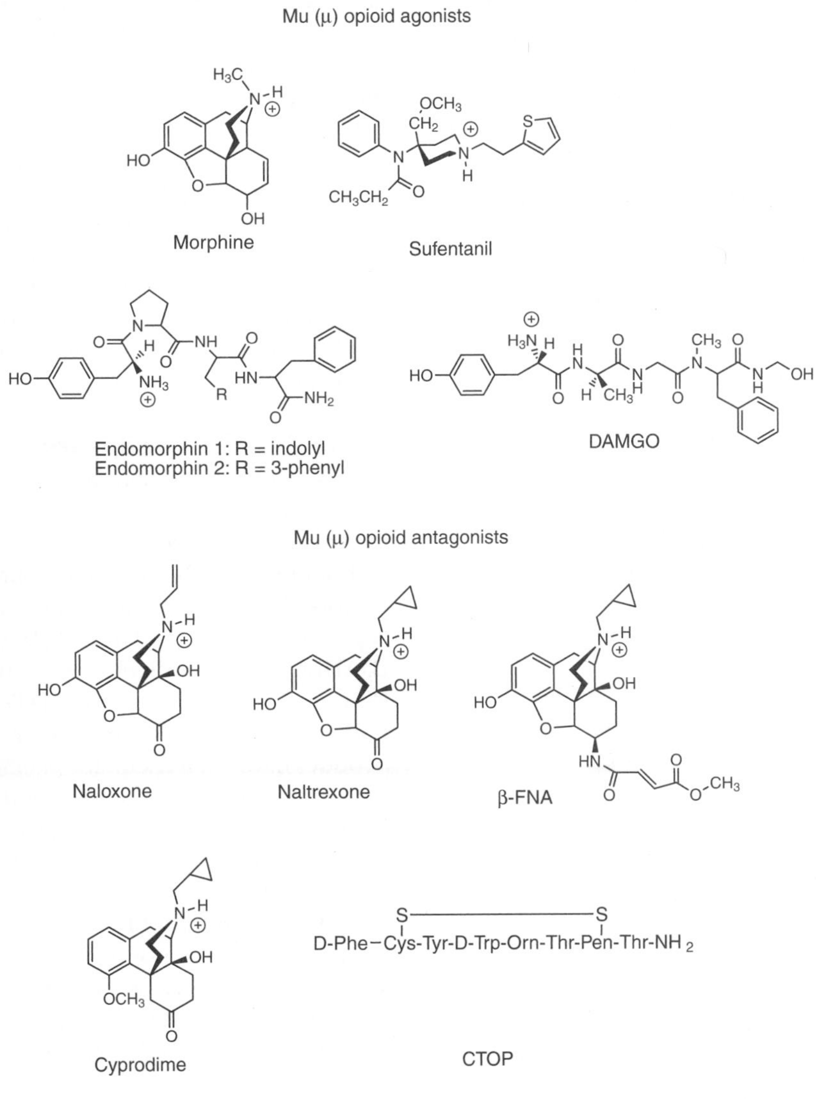

Fig. 19.4. Structures of compounds selective for mu (OP$_3$) opioid receptors.

binding, and isolated smooth muscle assays. Studies with mu receptor knockout mice have confirmed that all the major pharmacologic actions observed on injection of morphine (analgesia, respiratory depression, tolerance, withdrawal symptoms, decreased gastric motility, emesis, etc.) occur by interactions with mu receptors (26).

Naloxone and naltrexone are antagonists that have slight (5–10-fold) selectivity for mu receptors. Cyprodime is the most selective nonpeptide mu antagonist (about 30-fold selective for mu over kappa and 100-fold selective for mu over delta) available for laboratory use (27). CTOP, a cyclic peptide analog of somatostatin, is a selective mu antagonist (28). There is evidence that mu_1 receptors are high affinity binding sites that mediate pain neurotransmission, while mu_2 receptors control respiratory depression. Naloxoneazine is a selective inhibitor of mu_1 opioid receptors (29).

Kappa Opioid Receptors

Ethylketazocine and bremazocine are 6,7-benzomorphan derivatives with kappa opioid receptor selectivity (Fig. 19.5). These two compounds were used in early studies to investigate kappa receptors; however, they are not highly selectivity and their use in research has diminished. More recently, a number of arylacetamides derivatives, having a high selectivity for kappa over mu or delta receptors, have been discovered. The first of these compounds, (±) U50488, has a 50-fold selectivity for kappa over mu receptors and has been extremely important in the characterization of kappa opioid activity (30). Other important agents in this class are (±) PD-117302 (31) and (−) CI-977 (32). Each of these agents has 1000-fold selectivity for kappa over mu or delta receptors. There is evidence that the arylacetamides bind to a subtype of kappa receptors. Kappa agonists, in general, produce analgesia in animals including humans. Other prominent effects are diuresis, sedation and dysphoria. Compared to mu agonists, kappa agonists lack respiratory depressant, constipating and strong addictive (euphoria and physical dependence) properties. It was hoped that kappa agonists would become useful strong analgesics that lacked addictive properties; however, clinical trials with several highly selective and potent kappa agonists have been aborted due to the occurrence of unacceptable sedative and dysphoric side effects. Kappa selective opioids with only a peripheral action have been shown to be effective in relieving inflammation and the pain associated with it (33). The scientific evidence suggesting κ_1, κ_2 and κ_3 subtypes of kappa receptors leaves some researchers still hopeful of finding nonaddicting analgesics related to this class of opioid agents (34). The physiologic effects initiated by the kappa receptor subtypes are not well defined.

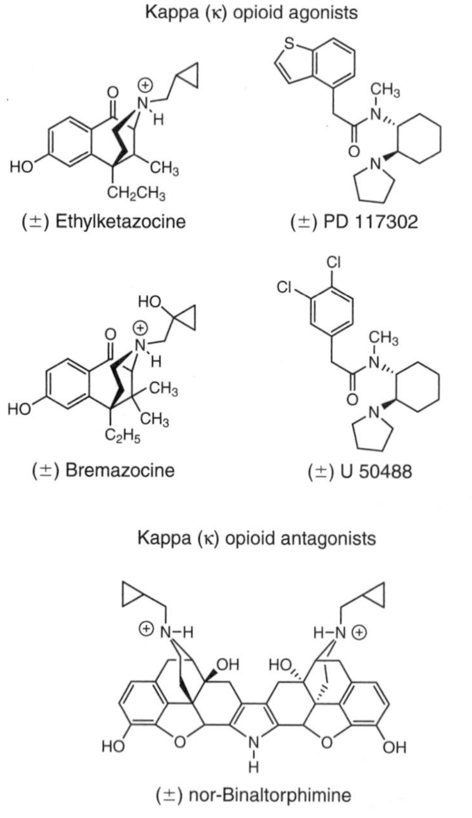

The peptides related to dynorphin are the natural agonists for kappa receptors. Their selectivity for kappa over mu receptors is not very high. Synthetic peptide analogues have been reported that are more potent and more selective than dynorphin for kappa receptors (35, 36)

The only antagonist with good selectivity for kappa receptors is nor-binaltorphimine (35). This compound has about a 100-fold selectivity for kappa over delta receptors and an even greater selectivity for kappa vs. mu receptors when tested in competitive binding studies in monkey brain homogenate. No medical use for a kappa antagonist has been found.

Delta Opioid Receptors

Enkephalins, the natural ligands at delta receptors, are only slightly selective for delta over mu receptors. Changes in the amino acid composition of the enkephalins can give compounds with high potency and selectivity for delta receptors. The peptides most often used as selective delta receptor ligands (Fig. 19.6) are [D-Ala^2, D-Leu^5] enkephalin (DADLE) (38), [D-Ser^2, Leu^5] enkephalin-Thr (DSLET) (39), and the cyclic peptide [D-Pen^2, D-Pen^5] enkephalin (DPDPE) (40). These and other delta receptor selective peptides have been useful for in vitro studies, but their metabolic instability and poor distribution properties (i.e., penetration of the blood-brain barrier is limited by their hydrophilicity) has limited their usefulness for in vivo studies. Nonpeptide agonists that are selective for delta receptors have been reported. Derivatives of morphindoles (nor-OMI) were the first nonpeptide molecules to show delta selectivity in in vitro assays (41). SNC-80 is a newer and more selective delta opioid receptor agonist (42). This compound produces analgesia after oral dose in several rodent

Kappa (κ) opioid agonists

(±) Ethylketazocine

(±) PD 117302

(±) Bremazocine

(±) U 50488

Kappa (κ) opioid antagonists

(±) nor-Binaltorphimine

Fig. 19.5. Structures of compounds selective for kappa (OP$_2$) opioid receptors. (−) Stereoisomers are the most active compounds.

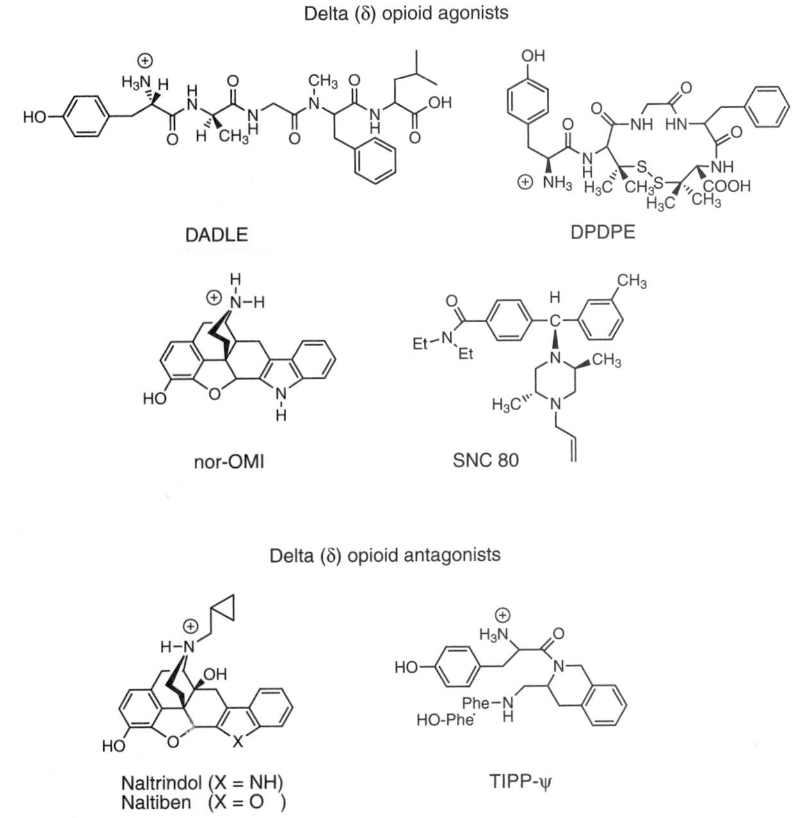

Delta (δ) opioid agonists

DADLE

DPDPE

nor-OMI

SNC 80

Delta (δ) opioid antagonists

Naltrindol (X = NH)
Naltiben (X = O)

TIPP-ψ

Fig. 19.6. Structures of compounds selective for delta (OP$_1$) opioid receptors.

models and side effects appear minimal. Clinical trials with SCN-80 and other nonpeptide delta receptor agonists are in progress. Radioligand binding studies in rodent brain tissue and in electrically stimulated *vas deferentia* have provided evidence of δ$_1$ and δ$_2$ receptors (43). The functional significance of this differentiation has not been determined.

Naltrindol and naltriben are highly selective nonpeptide antagonist for delta receptors (44,45). Naltrindol penetrates the CNS and displays antagonist activity that is selective for delta receptors in *in vitro* and *in vivo* systems. Peptidyl antagonists TIPP and TIPP-ψ are selective for delta receptors (46,47); however; their usefulness for *in vivo* studies and as clinical agents is limited by their poor pharmacokinetic properties. Delta opioid receptor antagonists have shown clinical potential as immunosuppressants and in treatment of cocaine abuse.

Receptor Affinity Labeling Agents

A number of opioid receptor selective affinity labeling agents (i.e., compounds that form an irreversible covalent bond with the receptor protein) have been developed (Fig. 19.7). These compounds have been important in the characterization and isolation of the opioid receptor types. Each of the affinity-labeling agents contains a pharmacophore that allows initial reversible binding to the receptor. Once reversibly bound to the receptor an affinity labeling agent must have an electrophilic group positioned so that it can react with a nucleophilic group on the receptor protein.

The receptor selectivity of these agents is dependent upon 1) the receptor type selectivity of the pharmacophore, 2) the location of the electrophile within the pharmacophore structure so that, when bound to the receptor it is positioned near a nucleophile, and 3) the relative reactivities of the electrophilic and nucleophilic groups.

Examples of important affinity labeling agents are β-CAN which, due to its highly reactive 2-chloroethylamine electrophilic group, irreversibility binds to all three opioid receptor types (48). The structurally related compound β-FNA has a less reactive fumaramide electrophilic group and reacts irreversibly with only mu receptors (49). Derivatives of the fentanyl series, FIT and SUPERFIT bind mu and delta receptors but only the delta receptor is bound irreversibly (50–51). Apparently, when these agents are bound to mu receptors the electrophilic isothiocyanate group is not oriented in proper juxtaposition to a receptor nucleophile for covalent bond formation to occur. Incorporation of the electrophilic isothiocyanate into the structure of the highly kappa receptor selective benzacetamides has provided affinity labeling agents (UPHIT and DIPPA) for kappa receptors (52,53).

NEUROBIOLOGY OF DRUG ABUSE AND ADDICTION

The factors that drive some individuals to abuse drugs, with resultant tolerance and psychological and physical dependence, remains unknown. It has been proposed that

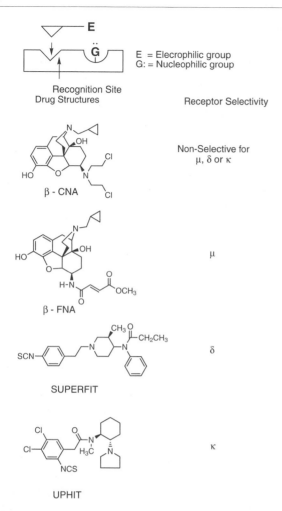

E = Elecrophilic group
G: = Nucleophilic group

Recognition Site
Drug Structures

Receptor Selectivity

β - CNA

Non-Selective for
μ, δ or κ

β - FNA

μ

SUPERFIT

δ

UPHIT

κ

Fig. 19.7. A representation of the concept of affinity labeling of receptors and affinity labeling agents for opioid receptors.

a deficiency exists in the opioid mediated self-reward system of individuals who have a predisposition to abuse addictive drugs (54). In the United States, the use of highly addictive drugs such as heroin and cocaine is treated as a crime, rather than as a medical problem. New insights into the neurobiology of drug addiction is now providing an understanding of why individuals abuse drugs and how drug abuse and addiction can be avoided and treated.

Self-Reward Response

It is now evident that all forms of drug addiction are driven by the stimulation of the brain's self-reward system (55), which originates in the ventral tegmental nucleus (VTN) and extends to the nucleus accumbens (NAC) area of the midbrain (Fig. 19.8). Self-reward is initiated by the release of dopamine (DA) from the mesocorticolimbic DA neurons originating in the VTN and stimulating D_1 and D_2 receptors in the NAC. Cocaine acts by inhibiting the re-uptake of DA at nerve terminals, thus increasing the intensity and duration of the reward response. Amphetamine, methamphetamine, and similar indirect acting adrenergic stimulants cause inhibition of DA re-uptake,

DA release, and an inhibition of MAO-mediated mediated of DA at this site. Mu opioid agonists work upstream in the reward neuronal system by exerting an inhibitory action on GABAergic neurons, thus removing the inhibitory GABAergic tonus on DA neurons and initiating the self-reward response. Kappa opioid agonists work at a site more downstream in the system and cause the opposite effect of mu agonists. The kappa neurons synapse directly onto the DA nerve terminal in the NAC and exert an inhibitory effect (negative tonus) on DA release. Thus, a mu agonist will cause a self-reward and euphoric stimulus and a kappa agonist will cause an aversive and dysphoric stimulus. Alcohol (ethanol) also causes a stimulation of the self-reward system, partially by acting on the mu opioid neurons to facilitate the release of endogenous opioids (56). Nicotine, acting through nicotinic cholinergic receptors, also has been shown to stimulate the DA self-reward system. (57).

Thus, the common driving pathway in drug addiction is the euphoria experienced when a drug is taken and the self-reward system is activated by DA release. The self-reward response tends to be self-limiting, because feedback (adaptive) mechanisms in the nerve cells attenuate the reward delivered after prolonged or repeated activation of the system. Agents that slowly distribute to the brain have minor abuse potential because the adaptive mechanisms in the self-reward neuronal system are able to respond quickly enough to attenuate the euphoric response. Highly abused substances tend to have high potency, full efficacy and a fast onset of action so that the reward signal is initiated and fully activated before the adaptive process can take effect. Factors that contribute to fast onset of action are high lipophilicity of the drug and a dosing method that allows rapid distribution to the brain. Most abused drugs are highly lipophilic so that they rapidly cross the blood-brain barrier. The dosage routes preferred by drug addicts (smoking and intravenous injection) meet the criteria for fast distribution to the brain. Of course, agents that are rapidly distributed to, and absorbed by, the brain are also rapidly redistributed from the brain to other body tissues. Because of the redistribution phenomenon, the intense euphoric rush experienced by the addict is short-lived and must be frequently reinduced. Repeated exposure of the reward system to the drugs activates the adaptive mechanisms, which results in desensitization (tolerance) of the system to the abused substance. The addict must take a larger dose of the drug to get the euphoric high she/he seeks, which results in increased tolerance, and propagation of the addiction cycle.

Opioid Tolerance and Withdrawal

Tolerance to and withdrawal from the opioids is explained by the cellular adaptation that occurs upon repeated activation of mu opioid receptors (58). When an agonist binds to the mu receptor, $G_{i/o}$ second messenger proteins are activated and inhibition of adenylate cyclase occurs. Continual activation of the receptors results in an up-regulation of adenylate cyclase to compensate for the decrease in cellular concentrations of cAMP. In addition, cellular mechanisms are activated that result in a decrease in the synthesis of $G_{i/o}$ protein subunits and an internalization of the mu receptor protein. Together, these adaptations cause a decrease in the magnitude of the opioid response to a given dose of agonist and explain the development of tolerance in the system and the need for ever higher doses to get the same degree of euphoric response.

When the nerve cells are pushed into a highly tolerant state, they have a great capacity to make cAMP due to the up-regulation in adenylate cyclase; however, the capacity is held in check by inhibitory effect of the opioids on adenylate cyclase. Upon cessation of dosing the opioid (about 4–6 hours with heroin), the inhibitory effect on the up-regulated adenylate cyclase system is removed and the cells over produce cAMP. The increase in cellular cAMP induces a number of abnormal and unpleasant effects that are recognized collective as opioid withdrawal symptoms. The acute phase of withdrawal lasts for days; the time required for cAMP levels and receptor mechanisms to return to a normal state. The long-term effect of drug addiction is a learned drug-craving behavior, which can last for a lifetime and is thought to be responsible for the high incidence of stress induced relapses into drug abuse.

Rehabilitation of Opioid Addiction

Therapeutic programs that employ drugs in the rehabilitation of drug addicts have been in use for some time. The best known treatment is the use of methadone maintenance in the rehabilitation of the opioid addict. In a well run program, daily treatment with oral methadone maintains the addicted (tolerant) state while allowing minimal euphoric/aversive mood swings, attenuates drug craving,

decreases the spread of HIV, and minimizes the social destructive behavior (prostitution, theft, etc.) of the addicted patient (59). Other agents such as the mu agonist L-α-acetylmethadol and the partial mu agonist buprenorphine can be substituted for methadone and offer the advantage of dosing every third day (60). The biggest problem with addiction treatment programs is their failure to alleviate the drug-craving behavior of the recovering addict and she/he resumes the habit of drug abuse. There is evidence that treatment of a detoxified opioid addict (i.e., an individual who has been weaned from opioid dependence through a methadone or other treatment program) with a long-acting opioid antagonist such as naltrexone cannot only pharmacologically block readdiction but also curb the addict's drug craving urge (61). Interestingly, naltrexone treatment has been shown to inhibit alcohol craving in the recovering alcoholic (62). Naltrexone and buprenorphine have shown promise in treatment of cocaine abuse (63,64).

A number of possible neurobiological mechanisms have been identified by which drug intervention might prevent drug abuse or aid in the recovery of the addict (Fig. 19.8). The use of mu opioid agonists, partial agonists and antagonists has been described in the preceding paragraph. Additional opioid-related mechanisms may be effective in the prevention of drug abuse and addiction. When a delta opioid agonist is given in combination with a mu opioid agonist, analgesia is enhanced while there is minimal induction of tolerance and physical dependence (65). It has also been shown that administration of a mu agonist along with a delta antagonist to rodents resulted in analgesia without inducing tolerance and physical dependence (66). Alpha-adrenergic agonists are known to interact with many of the same neuronal systems as the opioids. The centrally acting α-agonist clonidine works through the same $G_{i/o}$ second messenger system as the opioids and it is used clinically to

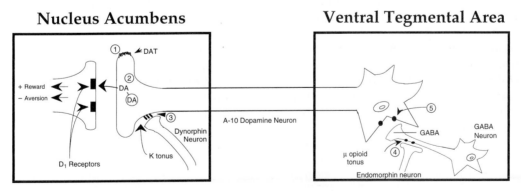

Fig. 19.8. The neurochemical basis of drug abuse and addiction. The diagram is a representation of the brain's self-reward system. According to this theory, any agent that promotes stimulation of type-1 dopamine (D_1) receptors in the nucleus accumbens (NCA) potentiates self-reward and has the potential to be abused. Major drugs of abuse exert their actions at various sites within the self-reward system to increase dopamine (DA) in the NCA and stimulate D_1 receptors. Site 1. Cocaine inhibits DA re-uptake by the DA transporter (DAT) and greatly enhances DA action at D_1. Site 2. Amphetamine, methamphetamine and related drugs cause DA release with the resultant stimulation of D_1. Site 3. Opioid kappa agonists exert an inhibitory effect on DA neuronal firing, resulting in a decrease in DA release and aversion in animals. Site 4. Opioid mu agonists, such as morphine and heroin, exert an inhibitory action on GABA interneurons in the VAT; thus, removing the GABAergic inhibition on DA neuronal firing. Site 5. GABA agonists, such as gabapentin, enhance DA neuronal firing and DA release, and these agents may be useful in treating or preventing drug abuse and addiction. Other abused agents, such as nicotine and cannabis, also cause an increase in DA release in the NAC, but their exact neuronal connections to the self-reward system is not yet understood.

inhibit withdrawal symptoms in patients addicted to opioids. Testing of the long acting indirect GABAergic agent vigabatrin (a suicide inhibitor of GABA aminotransferase) has been proposed for the treatment of drug addiction (67). One additional area of promise is the proposal that a high-affinity, slow-onset inhibitor of the DA transporter will be effective for the treatment of cocaine abuse (68).

STRUCTURE-ACTIVITY RELATIONSHIPS (SAR) OF MU RECEPTOR AGONISTS
SAR—Morphine

Morphine is the prototype opioid (see Table 19.2). It is selective for mu opioid receptors. The structure of morphine is composed of five fused rings and the molecule has five chiral centers with absolute stereochemistry 5(R), 6(S), 9(R), 13(S) and 14(R). The naturally occurring isomer of morphine is levo- [(−)] rotatory. (+)-Morphine has been synthesized and it is devoid of analgesic and other opioid activities (67).

It is important to remember that a minor change in the structure of morphine (or any other opioid) will likely cause a different change in the affinity and intrinsic activity of the new compound at each of the opioid receptor types. Thus, the opioid receptor selectivity profile of the new compound may be different than the structure from which it was made or modeled (i.e., a selective mu agonist may shift to become a selective kappa agonist, etc.) In addition, the new compound will have different physicochemical properties than its parent. The different physicochemical properties (solubility, partition coefficient, pK$_a$, etc.) will result in different pharmacokinetic characteristics for the new drug and can affect its *in vivo* activity profile. For example, a new drug (Drug A) that is more lipophilic than its parent (Drug B) may distribute better to the brain and appear to be more active, while in actuality it may have lower affinity or intrinsic activity for the receptor. The greater concentration of Drug A reaching the brain is able to overcome its decreased agonist effect at the receptor. The SARs discussed in the following paragraphs describe the relative therapeutic potencies of the compounds and are a combination of pharmacokinetic and receptor binding properties of the drugs.

The A-ring and the basic nitrogen, which exists predominantly in the protonated (ionized) form at physiologic pH, are the two most common structural features found in compounds displaying opioid analgesic activity. The aromatic A ring and the cationic nitrogen may be connected either by an ethyl linkage (9,10–positions of the B ring) or a propyl linkage (either edge of the piperidine ring that forms the D ring). The A ring and the basic nitrogen are necessary components in every potent mu agonist known; however, these two structural features alone are not sufficient for mu opioid activity and additional pharmacophoric groups are required. In compounds having rigid structures (i.e., fused A, B and D rings), the 3-hydroxy group and a tertiary nitrogen either greatly enhance or are essential for activity. A summary of other important SAR features for morphine is given in Table 19.2.

SAR—Nitrogen Atom

The substituent on the nitrogen of morphine and morphine-like structures is critical to the degree and type of activity displayed by an agent. A tertiary amine is usually necessary for good opioid activity. The size of the N-substituent can dictate the compound's potency and its agonist verses antagonist properties. N-Methyl substitution generally results in a compound with good agonist properties. Increasing the size of the N-substituent to three to five carbons (especially where unsaturation or small carbocyclic rings are included) results in compounds that are antagonists at some or all opioid receptor types. Larger substituents on nitrogen return agonist properties to the opioid. An N-phenylethyl substituted opioid is usually on the order of 10 times more potent as a mu agonist than the corresponding N-methyl analog.

Ideal Opioid

Thousands of derivatives of morphine and other mu agonists have been prepared and tested (70–71). The objective of most of the synthetic efforts has been to find an analgesic with improved pharmacologic properties over known mu agonists. Specifically, one would like to have an orally active drug that retains the strong analgesic properties of morphine, yet lacks its ability to cause tolerance, physical dependence, respiratory depression, emesis and constipation. The success of this search has been limited. Many compounds that are more potent than morphine

Table 19.2. Structure, Numbering and Selected SAR for (−)-Morphine

(−)-Morphine

Substituent Change	Analgesic Activity
3-H for -OH	10x Decrease
6-OH to 6-keto	Decrease activity or increase w/7,8-dihydro
6-OH to 6-H	Increase activity
7,8-dihydro	Increase activity
14 β-OH	Increase activity
3-OCH$_3$ for OH	Decrease activity
CH$_3$CO- ester at 3	Decrease activity
CH$_3$CO- ester at 6	Increase activity
NCH$_2$CH$_2$Ph for NCH$_3$	Increase activity (10x)
NCH$_2$CH=CH$_2$ for NCH$_3$	Becomes a μ antagonist

have been discovered. Also, compounds with pharmacodynamic properties different from morphine have been discovered and some of these compounds are preferred to morphine for selected medical uses. However, the ideal analgesic drug is yet to be discovered. Research to find new centrally acting analgesics has turned away from classic mu agonists and now is focused on agents that act through other types or subtypes of opioid receptors or through nonopioid neurotransmitter systems.

SAR—3-Hydroxy Group

The SARs of compounds structurally related to morphine are outlined in Table 19.2. A number of the structural variations on morphine have yielded compounds that are available as drugs in the United States. The most important of these agents, in terms of prescription volume, is the alkaloid codeine. Codeine, the 3-methoxy derivative of morphine, is a relatively weak mu agonist, but it undergoes slow metabolic O-demethylation to morphine which accounts for much of its action. Codeine is also a potent antitussive agent and it is used extensively for this purpose.

Heroin

The 3,6-diacetyl derivative of morphine is known commonly as heroin. Heroin was synthesized from morphine in 1874 and was introduced to the market in 1898 by the Friedrich Bayer Co. in Germany. The 1906 Squibb's Materia Medica lists 10 mg tablets of heroin at $1.20/1000. At the time of its introduction, heroin was described as "preferable to morphine because it does not disturb digestion or produce habit readily." Heroin itself has relatively low affinity for mu opioid receptors; however, its high lipophilicity compared to morphine results in enhanced penetration of the blood-brain barrier. Once in the body (including the brain), serum and tissue esterases hydrolyze the 3-acetyl group to produce 6-acetylmorphine. This latter compound has mu agonist activity in excess of morphine. The combination of rapid penetration by heroin into the brain after intravenous dose and rapid conversion to a potent mu agonist provide an "euphoric rush" that makes this compound a popular drug of abuse. Repeated use of heroin results in the development of tolerance, physical dependence, and the acquisition of a drug habit that is often destructive to the user and to society. In addition, the use of unclean or shared hypodermic needles for self-administering heroin often results in the transmission of the human immunodeficiency virus (HIV), hepatitis and other infectious diseasess.

SAR—Ring C

Changes in the C-ring chemistry of morphine or codeine can lead to compounds with increased activity. Hydromorphone is the 7,8-dihydro-6-keto derivative of morphine and it is 8–10 times more potent than morphine on a weight basis. Hydrocodone, the 3-methoxy derivative of hydromorphone, is considerably more active than codeine.

SAR—14β-Hydroxy-6-Keto Derivatives

The opium alkaloid thebaine can be synthetically converted to 14β-hydroxy-6-keto derivatives of morphine. The 14β-hydroxy group generally enhances mu agonist properties and decreases antitussive activity, but activity varies with the overall substitution on the structure. Oxycodone, the 3-methoxy-N-methyl derivative, is about as potent as morphine when given parenterally but its oral to parenteral dose ratio is better than for morphine. Oxymorphone is the 3-hydroxy-N-methyl derivative and it is 10 times as potent as morphine on a weight basis. Substitution of an N-cyclobutylmethyl for N-methyl and reduction of the 6-keto group to 6β-OH of oxymorphone gives nalbuphine. Nalbuphine acts through kappa receptors to produce about one-half the analgesic potency as morphine. Nalbuphine is an antagonist at mu receptors. Interestingly, N-allyl- (naloxone) and N-cyclopropylmethyl-(naltrexone) noroxymorphone are "pure" opioid antagonists. Naloxone and naltrexone are slightly mu receptor selective and are antagonists at all opioid receptor types.

Figure 19.9 contains some of the diverse chemical structures that produce mu agonist activity. The structures shown in the figure illustrate that the morphine structure may be built up or broken down to yield compounds that produce potent agonist activity. Reaction of thebaine with dienophiles (i.e., Diels-Alder reactions) results in 6, 14-endo-ethenotetrahydrothebaine derivatives, which are commonly called oripavines (72). Some of the oripavine derivatives are extremely potent mu agonists. Etorphine and buprenorphine are the best known of these derivatives. Etorphine is about 1000 times more potent than morphine as a mu agonist. Etorphine has a low therapeutic index in humans and its respiratory depressant action is difficult to reverse with naloxone or naltrexone; thus, the compound is not useful in medical practice. Etorphine (M-99) is available for use in veterinary medicine for the immobilization of large animals. The oripavine structure based antagonist diprenorphine is used to reverse the tranquilizing effect of etorphine. Buprenorphine, a marketed oripavine derivative, is a partial agonist at mu receptors with a potency of 20–30 times that of morphine. The compound's uses and properties are described in the section on clinically available agents.

SAR—3,4-epoxide Bridge and the Morphinans

Removal of 3,4-epoxide bridge in the morphine structure results in compounds that are referred to as morphinans. One cannot remove the epoxide ring from the morphine structure by simple synthetic means. Rather, the morphinans are prepared by total synthesis using a procedure described by Grewe (73). The synthetic procedure yields compounds as racemic mixtures and only the levo (−) isomers possess opioid activity. The dextro isomers have useful antitussive activity. The two morphinan derivatives that are marketed in the United States are levorphanol and butorphanol. Levorphanol is about eight times more potent as an analgesic in humans than morphine. Levorphanol's increased activity is due to an increase in affinity for mu opioid receptors and its greater lipophilicity that allows higher peak concentrations to reach the brain. Butorphanol is a mu antagonist and a kappa agonist. These mixed agonist/antagonists are described in more detail later in this chapter.

SAR—Benzomorphans

Synthetic compounds that lack both the epoxide ring and the C ring of morphine retain opioid activity. Compounds having only the A, B and D rings are named chemically as derivatives of 6,7-benzomorphan (Fig. 19.9) or, using a different nomenclature system, as 2,6-methano-3-benzazocine. They are commonly referred to simply as benzomorphans. The only agent from this structural class that is marketed in the United States is pentazocine. Pentazocine has an agonist action on kappa opioid receptors—an effect that produces analgesia. Pentazocine is a weak antagonist at mu receptors. The dysphoric side effects that are produced by higher doses of pentazocine are due to actions at kappa opioid receptors and also at sigma (PCP) receptors. The benzomorphan derivative phenazocine (*N*-phenylethyl) is about 10 times as potent as morphine as a mu agonist and is marketed in Europe.

Aminotetralins represent A, B ring analogs of morphine. A number of active compounds in this class have been described, but only dezocine, a mixed agonist/antagonist, has been marketed.

SAR—4-Phenylpiperidines

Analgesic compounds in the 4-phenylpiperidine class may be viewed as A, D ring analogs of morphine (Fig. 19.9). The opioid activity of these agents was discovered serendipitously. The first of these agents, meperidine, was synthesized in 1937 by Eislab who was attempting to prepare antispasmodic agents (74). The compound produced an S-shaped tail (Straub tail) in cats, an effect that had been recognized as a response caused by morphine and its derivatives. Meperidine proved to be a typical mu agonist with about one-fourth the potency of morphine on a weight bases. It is particularly useful in certain medical procedures because of its short duration of action. Reversed esters of meperidine have greater potency and several of these derivatives have been marketed. The 3-methyl reversed ester derivatives of meperidine, α- and β-prodine, were available in the United States but have been removed from the market because of their low prescription volume and their potential to undergo elimination reactions to compounds that resemble the neurotoxic agent MPTP (see Chapter 20). Trimeperidine or γ-promedol, the 1,2,5-trimethyl reserved ester of meperidine, is used in Russia as an analgesic.

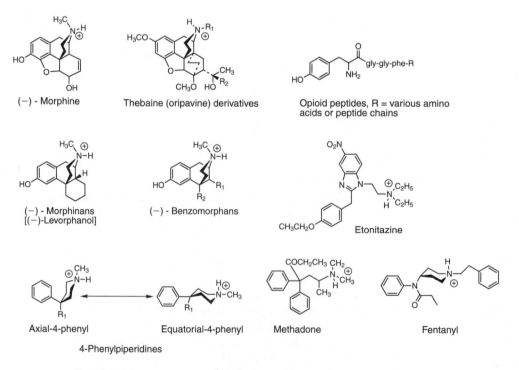

Fig. 19.9. Diverse structural families that yield potent opioid agonists.

SAR—Anilidopiperidines

Structural modification of the 4-phenylpiperidines has led to discovery of the 4-anilidopiperidine or the fentanyl group of analgesics (Fig. 19.9). Fentanyl and its derivatives are mu agonists and they produce typical morphine-like analgesia and side effects. Structural variations of fentanyl that have yielded active compounds are substitution of an isosteric ring for the phenyl group, addition of a small oxygen containing group at the 4-position of the piperidine ring, and introduction of a methyl group onto the 3-position of the piperidine ring. Newer drugs that illustrate some of these structural changes are alfentanil and sufentanil. Both of these drugs have higher safety margins than other mu agonists. For unknown reasons, the compounds produce analgesia at much lower doses than is necessary to cause respiratory depression.

SAR—Diphenylheptanone

In the period just before or during the Second World War, German scientists synthesized another series of open chain compounds as potential antispasmodics. In an analogous manner to meperidine, animal testing showed some of the compounds to possess analgesic activity. Methadone was the major drug to come from this series of compounds (Fig. 19.9). Methadone is especially useful for its oral activity and its long duration of action. These properties make methadone useful for maintenance therapy of opioid addicts and for pain suppression in the terminally ill (i.e., Hospice programs). Methadone is marketed in the United States as a racemic mixture but the (−)-isomer possesses almost all of the analgesic activity. Many variations on the methadone structure have been made, but little success in finding more useful drugs in class has been achieved. Reduction of the keto and acetylation of the resulting hydroxyl group gives the acetylmethadols (see below). Variations of the methadone structure have led to the discovery of the useful antidiarrheal opioids diphenoxylate and loperamide.

Propoxyphene is an open chain compound that was discovered by structural variation of methadone. Propoxyphene is a weak mu opioid agonist having only one-fifteenth the activity of morphine. The (+)-isomer produces all of the activity.

SAR—Mu Antagonists

The SAR for mu antagonists is relatively simple if one focuses just on marketed compounds. All of the marketed rigid-structured opioid analogs that have the 3-phenolic group and a N-allyl, N-cyclopropylmethyl (CPM), or N-cyclobutylmethyl (CBM) substituent replacing the N-methyl are mu antagonists (Fig. 19.5). Compounds behaving as mu antagonists may retain agonist activity at other opioid receptor types. The only exception to this rule is buprenorphine which has an N-CPM substituent and is a potent partial agonist (or partial antagonist) at mu receptors. Only two compounds are pure antagonists (i.e., act as antagonists at all opioid receptors). These compounds are the N-allyl (naloxone) and N-

CPM (naltrexone) derivatives of noroxymorphone. The 14β-hydroxyl group is believed to be important for the pure antagonistic properties of these compounds. It is not understood how the simple change of an N-methyl to an N-allyl group can change an opioid from a potent agonist into a potent antagonist. The answer may lie in the ability of opioid receptor protein to effectively couple with signal transduction proteins (G proteins) when bound by an agonist but not to couple with the G proteins when bound by an antagonist. This explanation infers that an opioid having an N-substituent of three to four carbon size, induces a conformational change in the receptor or blocks essential receptor areas that prevent the interaction of the receptor and the signal transduction proteins.

Those interested in an in-depth understanding of the SAR for mu receptor antagonists should be aware that properly substituted N-methyl-4-phenylpiperidines, N-methyl-6, 7 benzomorphans and even nonphenolic opioid derivatives that have good antagonist activity are known.

SAR—KAPPA RECEPTOR AGONISTS

The SAR for marketed kappa agonists is somewhat related to that of mu antagonists (Fig. 19.5). All of the marketed kappa agonists have structures related to the rigid opioids and N-allyl, N-CPM or N-CBM substitutions. The compounds are all mu receptor antagonists and kappa receptor agonists. The kappa agonist activity is enhanced if there is an oxygen group placed at the 8-position (e.g., ethylketazocine) or into the N-substituent (e.g., bremazocine). The oxygen group in a N-furanylmethyl substituent also enhances kappa activity.

Potent and selective kappa agonists that lack antagonistic properties at any of the opioid receptors are found in a number of trans-1-arylacetamido-2-aminocyclohexane derivatives. There are not enough compounds reported in this class to develop strong trends in structure-activity relationships. The relative mode of receptor binding for the morphine-related verses the arylacetamide kappa agonists is not known. Evidence exists for the selective binding of the arylacetamides to κ_1 and the benzomorphan compounds (e.g., bremazocine) to κ_2 and κ_3 opioid receptor subtypes.

SAR—DELTA RECEPTOR AGONISTS

Structure-activity relationships for delta receptor agonists are the least developed among the opioid compounds. Nonpeptide delta selective agonists are just beginning to be discovered (Fig. 19.6). Peptides with high selectivity for delta receptors are known. The SARs for some of these peptides are discussed in the following paragraphs. Several selective delta agonists are in clinical trials, but none appears to be headed for quick entry into medical practice.

SAR—OPIOID PEPTIDES

Thousands of derivatives related to the endogenous opioid peptides have been prepared since the discovery of the enkephalins in 1975 (75) (Fig. 19.1). A thorough discussion of the SAR of these peptides would be a major task; however, there are some major trends that have emerged and easily can be discussed. Some selected general SAR points for peptide opioids are:

1. All of the endogenous opioid peptides, except for the morphaceptins, have Leu- or Met-enkephalin as their first five amino acid residues.
2. The tyrosine at the first amino acid residue position of all the endogenous opioid peptides is essential for activity. Removal of the phenolic hydroxyl group or the basic nitrogen (amino terminus group) will abolish activity. The Tyr^1 free amino group may be alkylated (methyl or allyl groups to give agonists and antagonists) but it must retain its basic character. The structural resemblance between morphine and the Tyr^1 group of opioid peptides is especially obvious.
3. In additional to the phenol and amine groups of Tyr^1, the next most important moiety in the enkephalin structure is the phenyl group of Phe^4. Removal of this group or changing its distance from Tyr^1 results in full or substantial loss in activity.
4. The enkephalins have several low energy conformations and it is likely that different conformations are bound at different opioid receptor types and subtypes.
5. The replacement of the natural L-amino acids with unnatural D-amino acids can make the peptides resistant to the actions of several peptidases that generally rapidly degrade the natural endorphins. The use of a D-Ala in place of Gly^2 has been especially useful for protecting the peptides from the action of nonselective aminopeptidases. The placement of bulky groups into the structure (e.g., the addition of N-Me to Phe^4) will also slow the action of peptidases. When evaluating new peptides for opioid activity, it is often difficult to tell if changes are due to metabolic stability or receptor affinity.
6. Conversion of the terminal carboxyl group into an alcohol or an amide will protect the compound from carboxy peptidases.

7. Any introduction of unnatural D- or L-amino acids or bulky groups into the enkephalin structure will affect its conformational stability. The resultant peptides will have an increase or decrease in affinity for each of the opioid receptor types. The right combination of receptor affinity increases and/or decreases will result in selectivity for a receptor type.
8. Structural changes that highly restrict the conformational mobility of the peptides (e.g., substitution of proline for Gly^2 or cyclization of the peptide) have been especially useful for the discovery of receptor selective opioid peptides.

For examples of the above structure-activity relationships, see the structures of the peptides given in Figures 19.4, 19.5 and 19.6.

Enkephalin Peptides

The effect of lengthening the amino acid chain of the enkephalin peptides deserves special consideration. As previously noted, all of the endogenous opioids found in mammals have Leu- or Met-enkephalin at their amino terminus end. Lengthening the carboxyl terminus can give the peptide greater affinity or selectivity for an opioid receptor type. This effect can be illustrated by the dynorphins, where incorporation of the basic amino acids (especially Arg^7) into the C-terminus chain results in a marked increase in affinity for kappa receptors. The message-address analogy has been used to describe this effect. The first four amino acids [Tyr-Gly-Gly-Phe] are essential for peptide ligands to bind to and to activate all opioid receptor types. The N-terminus amino acids can then be referred to as carrying the "message" to the receptors. Adding additional amino acids to the C-terminus can "address" the message to a specific receptor type. The additional peptide chain may be affecting the address (selectivity) by providing new and favorable binding interactions to one of the receptor types. Alternatively, the additional peptide could be inducing a conformational change in the

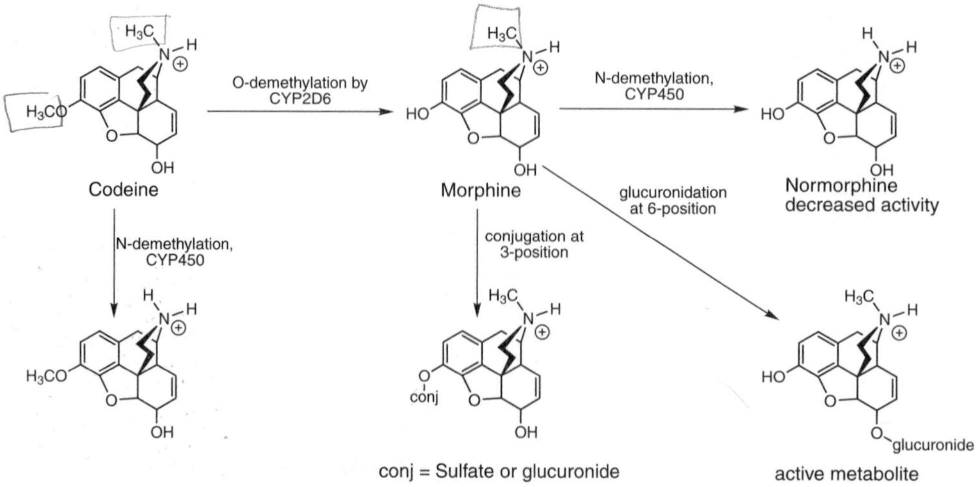

Fig. 19.10. Metabolism of morphine and codeine.

message portion of the peptide that favors interaction with one of the receptor types.

METABOLISM OF THE OPIOIDS

Knowledge of the metabolism of the opioid drugs is essential to the understanding of the uses of these agents. The poor oral versus parenteral dose ratio (about 6:1) of morphine is caused by extensive first pass metabolic conjugation of morphine at the phenolic (3-OH) position (Fig. 19.10). The metabolism occurs predominantly in the liver and requires the action of sulfotransferase or glcuronyltransferase enzymes. The conjugates have low activity and poor distribution properties. The 3-glucuronide does undergo enterohepatic cycling, which explains the need for high initial oral doses of morphine followed by lower maintenance doses. Glucuronidation of morphine at the 6-OH position results in the formation of an active metabolite. Morphine is also N-demethylated to give normorphine, a compound that has decreased opioid activity and decreased bioavailability to the CNS. Normorphine undergoes N- and O-conjugations and excretion. Geriatric patients metabolize morphine at a slower rate than normal adult patients, thus they are likely to show greater sensitivity to the drug and require lower doses.

In human subjects, about 10% of an oral dose of codeine is O-demethylated by CYP2D6 to produce morphine. The morphine produced as a metabolite of codeine is essential for the analgesic effect. A significant portion of the American population (8–10%) lack CYP2D6 and these individuals do not experience analgesia when dosed with codeine. The antitussive activity of codeine is produced by the unmetabolized drug at non-opioid receptors and is not affected by the lack of CYP2D6. The bioactivation of codeine (versus the bioinactivation of morphine) results in an oral/parenteral dose ratio for codeine of 1.5 to 1; however, codeine is seldom given parenterally because of its strong effect to release histamine from mast cells.

Other rigid-structured opioid analogs undergo similar routes of metabolism as morphine. The amount of first pass 3-O-conjugation varies from compound to compound, thus the relative oral/parenteral usefulness of the agents will vary. In general compounds that are more potent and lipophilic than morphine (e.g., levorphanol) tend to have better oral activity. Compounds with N-alkyl groups larger than methyl get N-dealkylated as a major route of inactivation.

The short duration of action of meperidine is the result of rapid metabolism. Esterases cleave the ester bond to leave the inactive 4-carboxylate derivative. Meperidine also undergoes N-demethylation to give normeperidine. Normeperidine has little analgesic activity but it contributes significantly to the toxicity of meperidine.

The metabolism of methadone, as outlined in Figure 19.11, is important to its action. The major route of inactivation results from N-demethylation and cyclization of the secondary amine into an inactive pyrrole derivative. If

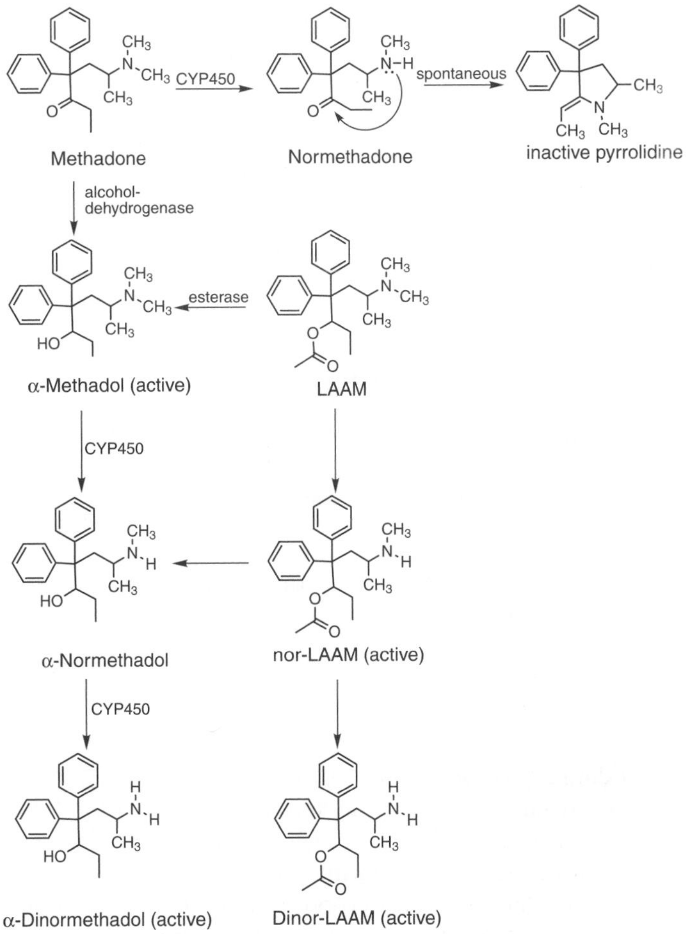

Figure 19.11. Metabolism of methadone and L-α-acetylmethadol (LAAM).

the keto group is reduced by alcohol dehydrogenase to give methadol, the demethylation product can no longer cyclize to the pyrrole derivatives. Methadol is less active than methadone as an analgesic, but the N-demethylation products of methadol, normethadol and dinormethadol, are active analgesics with increased half-lives compared to methadone. The build up of these metabolites is responsible for the long duration of action and mild prolonged withdrawal symptoms produced by methadone.

Levo-alpha-acetylmethadol (LAAM) is longer acting than methadone. Its slow onset of action after oral dose, and the isolation of at least three active metabolites, suggests that LAAM itself is a prodrug. The relative contributions of LAAM and its active metabolites to the analgesic and addition maintenance properties in humans has not been determined. It is clear that a 75–100 mg oral dose of this agent will suppress withdrawal symptoms in opioid addicts for 3 to 4 days.

MU OPIOID RECEPTOR MODELS

A number of models have been proposed to represent the bonding interactions of agonists at mu opioid receptors. These models are "reflections" of complementary

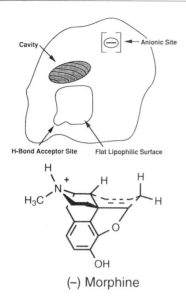

Fig. 19.12. A representation of the original model for the opioid receptor as proposed by Beckett and Casy (see reference 76). The morphine structure would have to rotate 180° about a vertical axis before it could bind to the receptor site. The model is only good for mu selective agents.

bonding interactions of mu agonists to the receptor as revealed from SAR studies. Beckett and Casy published the first such receptor drawing in 1954 (76). They studied the configurations and conformations of the mu agonists known at that time, and proposed that all opioids could bind to the template (receptor model) shown in Figure 19.12. The model presumed that nonrigid opioids (e.g., meperidine and methadone) took a shape like morphine's when binding to the receptor. It soon became apparent that the most stable conformations of meperidine and methadone were not superimposible on the structure of morphine. New compounds that could not assume the shape of morphine were also being discovered and it became apparent that the Beckett and Casy model could not explain the activity of all mu agonists.

In the mid-1960s, Portoghese attempted to correlate the structures and analgesic activities of rigid and nonrigid opioids that contained the same series of N-substituents (7). He argued that if all opioids bound the receptor in the same conformation, then a substituent at a like position on any of the compounds should fall on the same surface area of the receptor. One would expect the same structure modification on any opioid structure to give the same type and degree of bonding interaction, and thus, the same contribution to analgesic activity. Portoghese found that parallel changes of the N-substituent on rigid (morphine, morphinan or benzomorphan) analgesic parent structures gave parallel changes in activity. This finding supported the notion that rigid-structural opioid compounds bound to the receptor for analgesia in the same manner. However, when the same test was applied to nonrigid (meperidine-like) opioid structures, varying the N-substituent did not produce an activity change that paralleled that seen for the rigid-structured series. Apparently the N-substituents in the rigid and nonrigid opioid series were falling on different surfaces of a receptor and thus making different contributions to analgesic activity. Portoghese concluded that the rigid and nonrigid series of compounds were either binding to different receptors, or they were interacting with the same receptor by different binding modes. He introduced the bimodal receptor binding model (Fig. 19.13) as one possible explanation of the results. Later it was discovered that the activity of the rigid opioid compounds (Series 1) was enhanced by a 3-OH substituent on the aromatic ring, while a like substituent in some nonrigid opioids (Series 2) caused a loss of activity. Again, like substituents produced nonparallel changes in activity, indicating that the aromatic rings in the two series were not binding to the same receptor site. To provide an explanation for these results, the bimodal binding model was modified to incorporate the structure of the enkephalin (Fig. 19.14) (78). The rigid-structured opioids that benefit from the inclusion of a phenolic hydroxyl group, were proposed to bind the mu receptor in a manner equivalent to the tyrosine (Tyr[1] or T-subsite) of enkephalin. The nonrigid-structure opioids, that lose activity on introduction of a phenolic hydroxyl group into their structure, were proposed to interact with the receptor in a manner equivalent to the phenylalanine (Phe[4] or P-subsite) of enkephalin. The free amino group of Tyr[1] occupies the anionic binding site of the receptor that is the common binding point of both opioid series. This model closely resembles original bimodal binding proposal.

Models that attempt to explain the ability of Na[+] to decrease the binding affinity of agonists but not antagonists

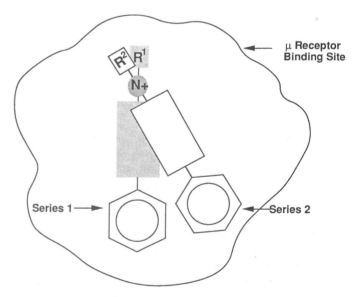

Fig. 19.13. A representation of the bimodal binding model of the mu opioid receptor as proposed by Portoghese (see reference 77). Different opioid series bind to different surface areas of the same receptor protein.

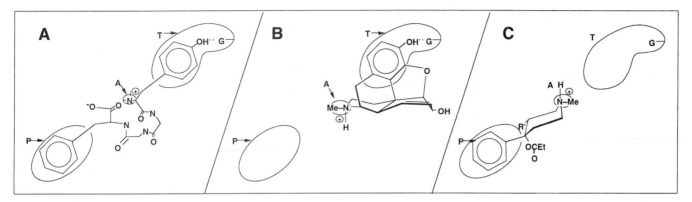

Fig. 19.14. A representation of the enkephalin binding site of mu opioid receptors (see reference 78). Panel A shows an enkephalin bound to the receptor. Panel B shows morphine binding the receptor by utilizing the T-subsite (i.e., the tyrosine binding site). Panel C shows a meperidine-type opioid binding the receptor by utilizing the P-subsite (i.e., the phenylalanine binding site).

for the opioid receptor have been made (79). Sodium ions also protect the receptor from alkylation by nonselective alkylating agents.

The Beckett and Casy model was extended to explain the increased potency of the oripavine analogs such as etorphine (Fig. 19.15) (72). The affinity of the oripavines for the mu opioid receptor can be much greater than that seen for morphine. It is likely that the increased receptor affinity comes from auxiliary drug-receptor bonding interactions similar to those depicted in the receptor model.

Martin has proposed a receptor model for kappa opioid receptors (80). Martin's model considers just the binding of rigid morphine-related opioid structures. The relationship of how rigid morphine-related agents interact with the kappa receptor compared to the arylacetamide kappa agonist derivatives has not been well studied.

Models for the delta opioid receptors have not been proposed.

CLINICALLY AVAILABLE AGENTS
Mu Agonists

Structures of morphine, codeine and related opioid compounds are given in Table 19.3.

(−)-Morphine Sulfate

Morphine sulfate is the most often used analgesic for severe, acute and chronic pain. Morphine is a mu agonist and is a Schedule II drug. It is available in intramuscular, subcutaneous, oral, rectal, epidural and intrathecal dosage forms. The epidural and intrathecal preparations are formulated without a preservative. Morphine is three to six times more potent when given intramuscularly than when it is given orally. The difference in activity is due to extensive first pass 3-0-glucuronidation of morphine—an inactive metabolite. The half-life of intramuscularly dosed (10 mg) morphine is about 3 hours. The dose of morphine, by any dosage route, must be reduced in patients with renal failure and in geriatric and pediatric patients. The enhanced effects of morphine in renal failure is believed due to a build up of the active 6-glucuronide metabolite, which depends on renal function for elimination.

The analgesic effect of orally dosed morphine can equal that obtained by parenteral administration, if proper doses are given. When given orally, the initial dose of morphine is usually 60 mg, followed by maintenance doses of 20–30 mg every 4 hours. Addiction to clinically used morphine by the oral route is generally not a problem.

Overdoses of morphine, as well as all mu agonists in this section, can be effectively reversed with naloxone.

(−)-Codeine Phosphate

Codeine is used extensively to treat moderate to mild pain. Codeine is a weak mu agonist but about 10% of an oral dose (30–60 mg) is metabolized to morphine (see Metabolism Section), which contributes significantly to its analgesic effect. The plasma half-life of codeine after oral dose is 3.5 hours. The dose of codeine needed to produce analgesia after parenteral dose causes releases of histamine sufficient to produce hypotension, pruritus and other allergic responses. Thus, administration of codeine by parenteral route is not recommended.

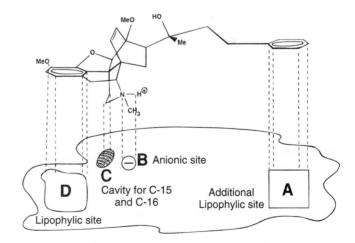

Fig. 19.15. A representation of the binding of an oripavine-type analgesic to the mu opioid receptor (see reference 72). The hydroxyl and phenyl groups in the side chain are believed to form additional bonding interactions with the receptor compared to the Beckett and Casy receptor model.

Table 19.3. Marketed Drugs That Are Derivatives of Morphine

Generic Drug Name	R_1	R_2	R_3	X	Other
(−)-Morphine	H	OH	CH_3	H	None
(−)-Codeine	CH_3	OH	CH_3	H	None
(−)-Hydromorphone	H	Keto	CH_3	H	No 7,8–double bond
(−)-Oxymorphone	H	Keto	CH_3	OH	No 7,8–double bond
(−)-Hydrocodone	CH_3	Keto	CH_3	H	No 7,8–double bond
(−)-Oxycodone	CH_3	Keto	CH_3	OH	No 7,8–double bond
(−)-Nalbuphine	H	OH	CH_2–cBu	H	No 7,8–double bond
(−)-Naloxone	H	Keto	CH_2–CH=CH_2	OH	No 7,8–double bond
(−)-Naltrexone	H	Keto	CH_2–cPr	OH	No 7,8–double bond

(−)-Hydromorphone Hydrochloride (Dilaudid)

Hydromorphone is a potent mu agonist (eight times morphine) used to treat severe pain. It is available in intramuscular, intravenous, subcutaneous, oral and rectal dosage forms. Like all strong mu agonists, hydromorphone is addicting and is a Schedule II drug. Hydromorphone has an oral to parenteral potency ratio of 5:1. The plasma half-lives, after parenteral and oral dosage are 2.5 and 4 hours, respectively.

(−)-Oxymorphone Hydrochloride (Numorphan)

Oxymorphone is a potent mu agonist (10 times morphine) that is used to treat severe pain. It is used by intramuscular, subcutaneous, intravenous and rectal routes of administration. The intramuscular dose of oxymorphone (1 mg) has a half-life of 3–4 hours. It is a Schedule II drug. Oxymorphone, because of its 14-hydroxy group, has low antitussive activity.

(−)-Levorphanol Bitartrate (Levo-Dromoran)

Levorphanol is a potent mu agonist (about six times morphine) and its uses, side effects and physical dependence liability are like oxymorphone or hydromorphone. Levorphanol is available in oral, subcutaneous and intravenous dosage forms. The oral dose of levorphanol is about twice the parenteral dose. This drug is unique among the mu agonists in that its analgesic duration of action is 4–6 hours while its clearance half-life is 11.4 hours. Thus, effective analgesic doses of this agent can lead to a build up of the drug in the body and result in excessive sedation.

(−)-Hydrocodone Bitartrate (Lortab, Vicodin in Mixtures With Acetaminophen)

Hydrocodone is a Schedule III drug that is used to treat moderate pain. It is used mostly by the oral route (5 mg tablets & solutions) in combination with acetaminophen. The compound has good oral bioavailability and is metabolized in a manner similar to codeine.

(−)-Oxycodone Hydrochloride (Roxicodone, Oxycontin sustained release; and Percocet, Percodan, Tylox; in Mixtures)

Oxycodone is about equipotent with morphine, but because of the 3-OCH group it has a much lower oral to parenteral dose ratio. Thus, oxycodone is used orally to treat severe to moderate pain. It is a Schedule II drug as a single agent and when it is combined in strong analgesic mixtures. Oxycodone has a plasma half-life of about 4 hours and requires dosing every 4–6 hours. Metabolism of this agent is comparable to that of codeine.

Meperidine Hydrochloride (Demerol)

Meperidine is a mu agonist with about one-tenth the potency of morphine after intramuscular dose. Meperidine produces the analgesia, respiratory depression and euphoria caused by other mu opioid agonists, but it causes less constipation and it does not inhibit cough. When given orally, meperidine has 40–60% bioavailability due to significant first pass metabolism. Because of the limited bioavailability, it is one-third as potent after an oral dose compared to a parenteral dose.

Meperidine has received extensive use in obstetrics because of its rapid onset and short duration of action. When it is given intravenously in small (25 mg) doses during delivery, the respiratory depression in the newborn child is minimized. Meperidine is used as an analgesic in a variety of non-obstetric anesthetic procedures. Meperidine is extensively metabolized in the liver with only 5% of the drug being excreted unchanged. Prolonged dosage of meperidine may cause an accumulation of the metabolite normeperidine (see Metabolism section). Normeperidine has only weak analgesic activity but it causes CNS excitation and can initiate grand mal seizures. It is recommended that meperidine be discontinued in any patient who exhibits signs of CNS excitation.

Meperidine has a strong adverse reaction when given to patients receiving a monoamine oxidase (MAO) inhibitor. This drug interaction has been seen recently in Parkinson's Disease patients taking the MAO-selective inhibitor selegiline (Eldepryl).

The elimination half-life of meperidine is 3–4 hours and it can double in patients with liver disease. Acidification of the urine will cause an enhancement of the clearance of meperidine but there is a lesser effect on the clearance of the toxic metabolite normeperidine.

Tramadol HCl (Ultram)

The analgesic activity of tramadol is attributed to a synergistic effect caused by the opioid activity of the (+)-isomer and the neurotransmitter re-uptake blocking effect of the (−)-isomer. The (+)-isomer possesses weak mu opioid agonist activity equivalent to about 1/3800 that of morphine. The O-desmethyl metabolite of (±)-tramadol has improved mu opioid activity equivalent to 1/35 that of morphine. Affinity for both delta and kappa receptors is improved. Despite its higher opioid potency, the contribution of O-desmethyltramedol to the overall analgesic effect has been questioned, but not well studied. The fact that naloxone causes a decrease in the analgesic potency of tramadol argues strongly for an opioid component to the analgesic activity. (−)-Tramadol possesses only 1/20 the opioid activity of its (+)-isomer, but it has good activities for inhibition of norepinephrine ($K_I = 0.78\ \mu M$) and serotonin ($K_I = 0.99\ \mu M$) re-uptake. Tramadol's neurotransmitter re-uptake activity is only about 1/20 that of imipramine, a tricyclic antidepressant agent that is used widely in pain management. Though none of the individual activities of tramadol is impressive, they interact to give a synergistic analgesic effect that is clinically useful.

Tramadol is a drug that has been used for about 20 years in Europe, but was just introduced to the U.S. market in 1995. The drug is nonaddicting and thus is not a scheduled agent. In addition, tramadol does not cause respiratory depression or constipation.

(±) Methadone Hydrochloride (Dolophine Hydrochloride)

Methadone is a synthetic agent with about the same mu opioid potency as morphine. The drug is used as a racemic mixture in the USA, but nearly all of the activity is due to the (−)-isomer. Methadone's usefulness is a result of its greater oral potency and longer duration compared to most other mu agonists. When given orally, a 20 mg dose

every 8–12 hours can give effective analgesia. Methadone is an excellent analgesic for use in the cancer patient and it is often used in the Hospice program. Oral doses of 40 mg are commonly used for 24 hour suppression of withdrawal symptoms (addiction maintenance) in opioid addicts. When given parenterally in doses of 2.5–10 mg, methadone (Schedule II drug) has all of the effects of morphine and other mu agonists.

The metabolism of methadone is extremely important in determining its long duration of action (see the section on metabolism in this chapter). The elimination of methadone is dependent upon liver function and urinary pH. The typical half-life is 19 hours. When urinary pH is raised from normal values of 5.2 to 7.8, the half-life becomes 42 hours. At the higher pH, a lower percentage of methadone exists in the ionized form and there is more renal reabsorption of the drug. The metabolism of methadone by liver enzymes is extensive and there are at least two active metabolites. CYP3A4 is the major enzyme catalyzing methadone metabolism. Enzyme inducers (e.g., phenytoin, rifampin) can lead to withdrawal in patients using methadone for maintenance of addiction. Toxic concentrations of methadone can accumulate in patients with liver disease, in geriatric patients who have a decreased oxidative metabolism capacity, or in patients taking an inhibitor of CYP2A4 (nifedipine, diazepam, fluvoxamine).

Though methadone is a good drug for maintenance of addiction, it is not ideal. Methadone requires once a day dosing, usually at a clinic, to suppress withdrawal symptoms. Once a day dosing is expensive and sometimes logistically difficult to achieve. Levo-alpha-acetylmethadol (LAAM) is available and is used in some treatment programs to overcome the problems of methadone. LAAM is more potent than methadone and it has a longer duration of action. A single oral dose of this agent can suppress abstinence withdrawal for up to three days.

Propoxyphene Hydrochloride or Napsylate (Darvon, Dolene, Darvon-N & Generics).

Propoxyphene is a weak mu agonist that is used as a single agent and in mixtures with nonsteroidal anti-inflammatory agents to treat mild or moderate pain. The active (+)-isomer has 2S, 3R absolute configuration. Propoxyphene is only available in oral dosage forms. Propoxyphene has about one-twelfth the potency of morphine and most studies show it to be equal or less effective than aspirin as an analgesic. Doses of propoxyphene that approach the analgesic efficacy of morphine are toxic. Propoxyphene's popularity is due to the fact that physicians prescribe it for its lower abuse potential (Schedule IV) compared to codeine.

Fentanyl Citrate (Sublimaze; Also in Combination With Droperidol)

The structure of fentanyl and related compounds are given in Table 19.4. Fentanyl is a mu agonist with about 80 times the potency of morphine. Fentanyl has been used in combination with nitrous oxide for "balanced" anesthesia and in combination with droperidol for "neurolepalgesia." The advantages of fentanyl over morphine for anesthetic procedures are its shorter duration of action (1–2 hours) and the fact that it does not cause histamine release upon intravenous injection.

A fentanyl patch has recently been released for the treatment of severe chronic pain. This dosage form delivers fentanyl transdermally and provides effective analgesia for periods up to 72 hours. In 1999, fentanyl also became available in a lollipop dose form for absorption from the oral cavity.

Fentanyl's short duration of action after parenteral dose is due to redistribution, rather than to metabolism or excretion. Repeated doses of fentanyl can result in accumulation and toxicities. Elderly patients are usually more sensitive to fentanyl and require lower doses.

Sufentanil Citrate (Sufenta)

Addition of the 4-methoxymethyl group and bioisosteric replacement of the phenyl with a 2-thiophenyl on the fentanyl structure results in a 10-fold increase in mu opioid activity (Table 19.4). The resultant compound, sufentanil is 600–800 times more potent than morphine. Despite its greater sedative and analgesic potency, sufentanil produces less respiratory depression at effective anesthetic doses. Sufentanil is available in an intravenous dosage form and it is used for anesthetic procedures. It has a faster onset and shorter duration of action than fentanyl. The short duration is due to redistribution from brain tissues.

Alftentanil Hydrochloride (Alfenta)

Substitution of tetrazol-5-one for the thiophene ring in sufentanil results in a decrease in potency (~25 × morphine) and a decrease in the pKa of the resultant compound, alfentanil (Table 19.4). The lower pKa of alfentanil results in a lower percentage of the drug existing in the ionized form at physiologic pH. Being more unionized, alfentanil penetrates the blood-brain barrier even faster than other fentanyl derivatives and has a faster onset and shorter duration of action. In addition, alfentanil is metabolized 99% in the liver and has a half-life of only 1.3 hours. Alfentanil is available as an intravenous dosage form for use in ultrashort anesthetic procedures.

Remifentanil HCl (Ultiva)

Remifentanil is much like alfentanil in its pharmacodynamic effects. It is a selective mu opioid agonist with 15- to 20-fold greater potency than alfentanil (Table 19.4). Remifentanil has an onset of action of 1–3 minutes when given intravenously. Its unique property is its rapid offset of effects which is independent of the duration of administration of the compound. Thus, it is very useful for titration of antinociceptive effect, followed by a rapid and predictable recovery time of 3–5 minutes. The short duration of action is a result of the ester group which has been rationally designed into the substituent on the piperidine nitrogen. This ester group is rapidly hydrolyzed to the inactive carboxylic acid by serum and tissue esterases, making the drug's duration of action essentially independent of the liver or renal function of the patient. Remifentanil is used extensively for analgesia associated with general anesthesia procedures. It

Table 19.4. Analogues Related to Fentanyl [4-(phenylpropionamido)piperidines]

Generic Name	Trade Name	R₁	R₂
Fentanyl	Sublimaze Duragesic	H	—CH₂·CH₂— (phenyl)
Sufentanil	Sufenta	—CH₂—OCH₃	—CH₂·CH₂— (thiophene)
Alfentanil	Alfenta	—CH₂—OCH₃	—CH₂·CH₂—N (tetrazolone) N–Et
Remifentanil	Ultiva	—C(O)—OCH₃	—CH₂·CH₂—C(O)—OCH₃

is often used in combination with injectable general anesthetic agents such as midazolam or propofol.

Mixed Agonist-Antagonists
(−)-Buprenorphine Hydrochloride (Buprenex)

Buprenorphine is 20–50 times more potent than morphine in producing an ED50 analgesic effect in animal studies; however, it cannot produce an ED100 in these tests. Thus, buprenorphine is a potent partial agonist at mu opioid receptors. It is also a partial agonist at kappa receptors but more of an antagonist at delta receptors. Buprenorphine, at 0.4 mg im. dose, will produce the same degree of analgesia as 10 mg of morphine. Due to its partial agonist properties, it has a lower ceiling on its analgesic action but also produces less severe respiratory depression. It is incapable of producing tolerance and addiction comparable to full mu agonists. In fact, buprenorphine's partial agonist action, very high affinity for opioid receptors, and high lipophilicity combine to give buprenorphine a tolerance, addiction and withdrawal profile that is unique among the opioids. When given by itself to opioid naive patients, little tolerance or addictive potential (Schedule 5) is observed. A mild withdrawal can occur some two weeks after the last dose of buprenorphine. Buprenorphine will precipitate withdrawal symptoms in highly addicted individuals, but it will suppress symptoms in individuals who are undergoing withdrawal from opioids. It effectively blocks the effect of high doses of heroin. Because of these properties, buprenorphine has been used in opioid addict treatment programs. It has also been reported to suppress cocaine use and addiction.

Buprenorphine undergoes extensive first pass 3-0-glucuronidation which negates its usefulness after oral dose. It is available in parenteral dosage forms in the USA and as a sublingual preparation in Europe. Its typical dose is 0.3 to 0.6 mg three times per day by intramuscular injection. The duration of analgesic effect is 4–6 hours. After parenteral dose, about 70% of the drug is excreted in the feces and the remainder appears as N-dealkylated and conjugated metabolites in the urine.

Naloxone is not an effective antagonist to buprenorphine because of the latter's high binding affinity to opioid receptors.

(−)-Butorphanol Tartrate (Stadol)

Butorphanol is a strong agonist at kappa opioid receptors and through this interaction it is five times more potent than morphine as an analgesic. Kappa agonists have a lower ceiling analgesic effect than full mu agonists, thus they are not as effective in treating severe pain. Butorphanol is an antagonist at mu opioid receptors with about one-sixth the potency of naloxone. If given to a person addicted to a mu agonist, butorphanol will induce an immediate onset of abstinence syndrome.

Butorphanol has a different spectrum of side effects than mu opioid analgesics. Respiratory depression occurs but there is a lower ceiling on this effect and it is not generally lethal as is the case with high doses of mu agonists. Major side effects after normal analgesic doses are sedation, nausea, sweating and dysphoric (hallucinogenic) effects at higher doses. Butorphanol causes an increase in pulmonary arterial pressure and pulmonary vascular resistance. There is an overall increased workload on the heart and it should not be used in patients with congestive heart failure or to treat pain from acute myocardial infarction. Butorphanol has low abuse potential and is not a scheduled drug.

Because of first pass metabolism, butorphanol is not used in an oral dose form. Given parenterally, it has a plasma half-life and a duration of analgesic effectiveness of 3–4 hours. The outpatient use of butorphanol has been greatly increased by the introduction of a metered inhalant dosage form of the drug. The major metabolite of butorphanol is the inactive trans-3-hydroxycyclobutyl product, which is excreted primarily in the urine.

Nalbuphine Hydrochloride (Nubain)

Nalbuphine (see Table 19.3 for structure) is an antagonist at mu receptors and an agonist at kappa receptors. As an antagonist it has about one-fourth the potency of naloxone and it does produce withdrawal when given to addicts. On a weight basis, the analgesic potency of nalbuphine approaches that of morphine. An intramuscular injection of 10 mg will give about the same degree and duration of analgesia as an equivalent dose of morphine.

Side effects of nalbuphine are like other kappa agonists. Dysphoria is not as common as with pentazocine. Sedation is the most common side effect. Nalbuphine does not have the adverse cardiovascular properties found with pentazocine and butorphanol. Nalbuphine has low abuse potential and is not listed under the Controlled Substances Act.

Nalbuphine is only available for parenteral dosage. Its elimination half-life is 2–3 hours. Metabolism of nalbuphine is by conjugation of the 3-OH group and greater than 90% of drug is excreted as conjugates in the feces.

(−)-Pentazocine Hydrochloride and Lactate (Talwin Nx and Talwin)

Pentazocine is a weak antagonist (one-thirtieth naloxone) at mu receptors and an agonist at kappa receptors.

Pentazocine is one-sixth as potent as an analgesic compared to morphine after parenteral doses. Pentazocine also is dosed orally and has an oral to parenteral dose ratio of about 2 to 1. It is used to treat moderate pain. The mu antagonist properties of pentazocine are sufficient to produce abstinence signs in opioid addicts.

The side effects of pentazocine are like other kappa agonists. It has a greater tendency to produce dysphoric episodes and it causes an increase in blood pressure and heart rate similar to butorphanol. Pentazocine is a Schedule IV drug. The major abuse of pentazocine has been its injection along with the antihistaminic drug tripelennamine (the "T's and blues"). Inclusion of the antihistaminic drug reportedly causes an increase in the euphoric, while decreasing the dysphoric effects, of the pentazocine. The manufacturers of pentazocine have attempted to thwart this use by including naloxone in the oral dose formulation of pentazocine. When taken orally, as intended, the naloxone has no bioavailability and the pentazocine is able to act as normal. When the tablet is dissolved and injected, the naloxone will effectively block the opioid actions of the pentazocine.

The elimination half-life of pentazocine is about 4 hours after parenteral dosage and 3 hours after oral dosage. Bioavailability after oral dose is only 20–50% due to first pass metabolism. Pentazocine is metabolized extensively in the liver and excreted via the urinary tract. The major metabolites are 3-0-conjugates and hydroxylation of the terminal methyl groups of the N-substituent. All metabolites are inactive.

Dezocine (Dulgan)

Dezocine is classified as a mixed agonist/antagonist. The SAR of dezocine is unique among the opioids. It is a primary amine while all other nonpeptide opioids are tertiary amines. Its exact receptor selectivity profile has not been reported; however, its pharmacology is most similar to that of buprenorphine. It seems to be a partial agonist at mu receptors, to have little effect at kappa receptors, and to exert some agonist effect at delta receptors. On a weight basis, it is about equipotent with morphine, and like morphine it is useful for the treatment of moderate to severe pain. It is available for intramuscular and intravenous dose. The drug is indicated for postoperative and cancer induced pain.

Dezocine has a half-life of 2.6–2.8 hours in healthy patients and 4.2 hours in patients with liver cirrhosis. The onset of action of dezocine is faster (30 minutes) than equivalent analgesic doses of morphine and its duration of action is longer (4–6 hours). Dezocine is extensively metabolized by glucuronidation of the phenolic hydroxyl group and by N-oxidation. Metabolites are inactive and excreted mostly via the renal tract.

Dezocine causes respiratory depression, but like buprenorphine there is a ceiling to this effect. Presumably, there is also a ceiling to the analgesic effect of dezocine, but this point is not well documented. Dezocine does not have the very high affinity for mu receptors that buprenorphine has and its respiratory depressant effect can be reversed readily by naloxone.

The major side effects of dezocine are dizziness, vomiting, euphoria, dysphoria, nervousness, headache, pruritus and sweating. Normal volunteers and recovered addicts report the subjective effects of single doses of dezocine to be like morphine. Because of the partial agonist mechanism of dezocine, one would not expect it to have a high abuse potential.

Opioids Used as Antidiarrheal Agents

Structure modification of 4-phenylpiperidines has led to the discovery of opioid analogs that are used extensively as antidiarrheal agents. Opioid agonists that act on mu and delta receptors have a strong inhibitory action on the peristaltic reflex on the intestine. This action occurs because endogenous opioid tracts innervate the intestinal wall where they synapse onto cholinergic neurons. When opioids are released onto cholinergic neurons, they inhibit the release of acetylcholine and thus inhibit peristalsis. Any mu agonist used in medicine causes constipation as a side effect. Most mu agonists are not used as antidiarrheal agents because of their potential for abuse and addiction.

Opium tincture and camphorated opium tincture (paregoric) have long been used as effective antidiarrheal agents. The bad taste of these liquid preparations and their abuse potential (Schedule II and III, respectively) serve to limit their use and to favor newer agents. Codeine sulfate or phosphate salt, as a single agent, is sometimes used for the short term treatment of mild diarrhea.

Synthetic agents that are structural combinations of meperidine and methadone are used extensively as antidiarrheal agents. Structures and uses of these agents are given below.

Diphenoxylate HCl with Atropine Sulfate: (Lomotil)

Diphenoxylate HCl (2.5 mg) and atropine (0.025 mg) are combined in tablets or 5 mL liquid and used effectively as symptomatic treatment for diarrhea. The typical dose is 2 tablets or 10 mL every 3–4 hours. The combination with atropine enhances the block of acetylcholine stimulated peristalsis and the adverse effects of atropine helps to limit the abuse of the opioid. The combination is Schedule V under the Controlled Substance Act. Diphenoxylate itself has low mu opioid agonist activity. It is metabolized rapidly by ester hydrolysis to the free carboxylate (difenoxin) which is 5-fold more potent after oral dosing. The high polarity of difenoxin probably limits its penetration of the CNS and explains the low abuse potential of this agent. High doses of diphenoxylate (40–60 mg) will cause euphoria and addiction.

Difenoxin HCl with Atropine Sulfate: (Motofen)

Difenoxin, the active metabolite of diphenoxylate (as described above), is also used as an antidiarrheal agent. Tablets contain 1 mg of difenoxin and 0.025 mg of atropine sulfate. Dosage, uses, and effectiveness are similar to that of diphenoxylate.

Loperamide HCL (Imodium)

Loperamide is a safe and effective opioid-derived antidiarrheal agent and it is not listed under the Controlled Substance Act. This medication is now available as a nonprescription item in the United States. It is used extensively for traveler's diarrhea. Loperamide is marketed as capsules (2 mg) and liquid (1 mg/5 mL) preparations. The recommended dose is 4 mg initially and an additional 2 mg following each diarrheal stool. The dose should not exceed 16 mg/day. The reason for the low abuse potential of loperamide has not been determined. The compound is highly lipophilic and undergoes slow dissolution, thus limiting the bioavailability of the agent to about 40% of the dose. The combination of a slow absorption rate, poor overall bioavailability and first pass metabolism could explain the low abuse potential after an oral dose. The compound is too lipophilic to dissolve in water for an intravenous dosage form, a property that limits its abuse potential.

Enkephalinase Inhibitors as Antidiarrheal Agents

Though not available in the United States, inhibitors of enkephalinase, the major enzyme for the inactivation of endogenous opioid peptides, are available in Europe and are under investigation in Japan for the treatment of diarrhea. Acetorphan, a prodrug of thiorphan, is a good example of a clinically useful enkephalinase inhibitor used to treat diarrhea. The free thio-group of thiorphan binds tightly to the zinc ion in the active site of the enzyme and inhibits its proteolytic action. Orally dosed acetorphan causes its antidiarrheal effect by inhibition of intestinal secretions and has a complementary effect when used in combination with loperamide which exerts its effects by decreasing gastrointestinal transit time.

Opioid Agents Used as Cough Suppressants (Antitussives)

Many of the rigid-structured opioids have cough suppressant activity. This action is not a true opioid effect in that it is not antagonized by opioid antagonists, and the (+)-isomers are equally effective with the analgesic (−)-isomers as cough suppressants. The 3-methoxy derivatives of morphine (codeine and hydrocodone) are nearly as effective antitussive agents as free phenolic agents. The better oral activity and decreased abuse potential of the methoxy derivatives make them preferred as antitussive agents. Incorporation of the 14β-hydroxyl into the structure (oxycodone) greatly decreases antitussive activity. If no cough suppression is desired in a patient being treated for pain, meperidine is the preferred agent.

Codeine is used extensively as a cough suppressant. It is available as a single agent or as mixtures in a variety of tablet and liquid cough suppressant formulations. As a simple agent, codeine is Schedule II and in mixtures it is Schedule V under the Controlled Substance Act. When used properly as a cough suppressant, codeine has little abuse potential; however, cough formulas of codeine are often abused.

Hydrocodeine bitartrate is about three times more effective on a weight basis compared to codeine as an oral antitussive medication. Hydrocodone also has greater analgesic activity and abuse potential than codeine. Hydrocodone is only available as a Schedule III prescription agent in combination formulations for cough suppression.

Dextromethorphan HBr is the (+)-isomer of the 3-methoxy form of the synthetic opioid levorphanol. It lacks the analgesic, respiratory depressant and abuse potential of mu opioid agonists but retains the centrally acting antitussive action. Dextromethorphan is not an opioid and is not listed in the Controlled Substance Act. Its effectiveness as an antitussive is less than that of codeine. Dextromethorphan is available in a number of nonprescription cough formulations.

CASE STUDY

Victoria F. Roche and S. William Zito

You are moonlighting at a local hospital inpatient pharmacy when JB, a 37-year-old nightclub owner, is rushed in to the emergency room, unconscious, unresponsive and breathing shallowly. JB is a locally well-known wheeler-dealer who lives in the fast lane of life, drinks heavily, and has even been arrested once for distributing cocaine and heroin to his cronies in the back room of his club. The "friend" who drove JB to the hospital dumped him off on the ER sidewalk, honked the horn and sped off, so the care staff has no information on what happened to this "party czar." The paramedic who reached him first lifted his eyelids and noted pinpoint pupils. As he is being wheeled into the ER, JB experiences a mild convulsion.

1. *Identify the therapeutic problem(s) where the pharmacist's intervention may benefit the patient.*

2. *Identify and prioritize the patient specific factors that must be considered to achieve the desired therapeutic outcomes.*

3. *Conduct a thorough and mechanistically oriented structure-activity analysis of all therapeutic alternatives provided in the case.*

4. *Evaluate the SAR findings against the patient specific factors and desired therapeutic outcomes and make a therapeutic decision.*

5. *Counsel your patient*

REFERENCES

1. Hughes J, Smith TW, Kosterlitz HW, et al. Identification of two related pentapeptides from the brain with potent opiate agonist activity. Nature (Lond.) 1975;258: 577–579.

2. Terenius L. Stereospecific interaction between narcotica nalgesics and synaptic plasma membrane fraction of rat cerebral cortex. Acta Pharmacol Toxicol 1973;32:317–320.

3. Pert CB, Snyder SH. Opiate receptor: demonstration in nervous tissue. Science 1973;70:2243–2247.

4. Simon EJ, Hiller JM, Edelman I. Stereospecific binding of the potent narcotic analgesic [³H] etorphine to rat brain homogenate. Proc Natl Acad Sci USA 1973;70: 1947–1949.

5. Goldstein A, Lowney LI, Pal BK. Stereospecific and nonspecific interactions of the morphine cogener levorphanol in subcellular fractions of mouse brain. Proc Natl Acad Sci USA 1971;68:1742–1747.

6. Li CH, Lemaire S, Yamashiro D, et al. The synthesis and opiate activity of beta-endorphin. Biochem Biophys Res Commun 1976;71:19–25.

7. Goldstein A, Tachibana S, Lowney LI, et al. Procaine pituitary dynorphin: complete amino acid sequence of the biologically active heptadecapeptide. Proc Natl Acad Sci USA 1979;76: 6666–6670.

8. Zadina JE, Hackler L, Ge LJ, et al. A potnet and selective endogenous agonist for the mu-opiate receptor. Nature 1997;386: 499–502.

9. Goldstein A, Barrett RW, James IF, et al. Morphine and other opiates from beef brain and adrenal. Proc Natl Acad Sci USA 1985;82:5203–5207.

10. Akil H, Watson SJ, Young E, et al. Endogenous opioids: biology and function. Annu Rev Neurosci 1984;7:233–255.

11. Brantl V, Teshemacher H. A material with opioid activity in bovine milk and milk products. Naunyn Schmiedebergs Arch Pharmacol 1979;306:301–4.

12. Montecucchi PC, de Castiglioni R, Piani S, et al. Amino acid composition and sequence of dermorphin, a novel opiate-like peptide from the skin of Phyllomedusa sauvagei. Int J Pept Protein Res 1981;17:275–83.

13. Gilbert PE, Martin WR. The effects of morphine and nalorphine-like drugs in the nondependent, morphine-dependent and cyclazocine-dependent chronic spinal dog. J Pharmacol Exp Ther 1976;198:66–82.

14. Lord JAH, Waterfield AA, Hughes J, et al. Endogenous opioid peptides: multiple agonists and receptors. Nature (Lond.) 1977:267:495–499.

15. Satoh M, Minami M. Molecular pharmacology of the opioid receptors. Pharmacol Ther 1995;68:343–64.

16. Dhawan BN, Cesselin R, Raghbir R, et al. International Union of Pharmacology. XII. Classification of opioid receptors. Pharmacol Rev 1996;48:567–592.

17. Henderson G, McKnight AT. The orphan opioid receptor and its endogenous ligand—nociceptin/orphanin FQ. Trends Pharmacol Sci. 1997;18:293–300.

18. Meunier JC, Mollereau C, Toll L, et al. Isolation and structure of the endogenous agonist of opioid receptor-like ORL1 receptor. Nature 1995;377:532–5.

19. Reinscheid RK, Nothacker HP, Bourson A, et al. Orphanin FQ: a neuropeptide that activates an opioidlike G protein-coupled receptor. Science 1995;270:792–794.

20. Inoue M, Kobayashi M, Kozaki S, et al. Nociceptin/orphanin FQ-induced nociceptive responses through substance P release from peripheral nerve endings in mice. Proc Natl Acad Sci USA 1998;95:10949–10953.

21. Leslie FM. Methods used for the study of opioid receptors. Pharmacol Rev 1987;39:197–249.

22. Childers SR. Opioid receptor-coupled second messengers systems. Life Sci 1991;48:1991–2003.

23. Georgoussi Z, Milligan G, Zioudrou C. Immunoprecipitation of opioid receptor-Go-protein complexes using specific GTP-binding-protein antisera. Biochem J 1995;306 (Pt 1):71–5.

24. Handa BK, Land AC, Lord JA, et al. Analogues of beta-LPH61–64 possessing selective agonist activity at mu-opiate receptors. Eur J Pharmacol 1981;70:531–40.

25. Negri L, Erspamer GF, Severini C, et al. Dermorphin-related peptides from the skin of Phyllomedusa bicolor and their amidated analogs activate two mu opioid receptor subtypes that modulate antinociception and catalepsy in the rat. Proc Natl Acad Sci USA 1992;89:7203–7

26. Kieffer BL. Opioids: first lessons from knockout mice. Trends Pharmacol Sci 1999;20:19–25.

27. Schmidhammer H, Burkhard WP, Eggstein-Aeppi L, et al. Synthesis and biological evaluation of 14–alkoxymorphinans. 2. (−)-N-(cyclopropylmethyl)-4,14-dimethoxymorphinan-6-one, a selective mu opioid receptor antagonist. J Med Chem 1989;32: 418–421.

28. Pelton JT, Kazmierski W, Gulya K, et al. Design and synthesis of conformationally constrained somatostatin analogues with high potency and specificity for mu opioid receptors. J Med Chem 1986;29:2370–2375.

29. Paul D, Pasternak GW. Differential blockade by naloxonazine of two mu opiate actions: analgesia and inhibition of gastrointestinal transit. Eur J Pharmacol 1988;149:403–404.

30. Szmuszkovicz J, Von Voigtlander PF. Benzeneacetamide amines: structurally novel non-m mu opioids. J Med Chem 1982;25:1125–1126.

31. Clark CR, Halfpenny PR, Hill RG, et al. Highly selective kappa opioid analgesics. Synthesis and structure-activity relationships of novel N-[(2-aminocyclohexyl)aryl]acetamide and N-[(2-aminocyclohexyl)aryloxy]acetamide derivatives. J Med Chem 1988;31:831–836.

32. Hunter JC, Leighton GE, Meecham KG, et al. CI-977, a novel and selective agonist for the kappa-opioid receptor. Br J Pharmacol 1990;101:183–189.

33. Barber A, Bartoszyk GD, Bender HM, et al. A pharmacological profile of the novel, peripherally-selective κ-opioid receptor agonist, EMD 61753. Br J Pharmacol 1994;113:843–851.

34. Rothman RB, Bykov V, de Costa BR, et al. Evidence for four opioid kappa binding sites in guinea pig brain. Prog Clin Biol Res 1990;328:9–12.

35. Choi H, Murray TF, DeLander GE, et al. N-terminal alkylated derivatives of [D-Pro¹⁰]dynorphin A-(1–11) are highly selective for κ-opioid receptors. J Med Chem 1992;35:4638–4639.

36. Lung FDT, Meyer JP, Li G, et al. Highly κ receptor-selective dynorphin A analogues with modifications in position 3 of dynorphin A(1–11)-NH₂. J Med Chem 1995;38:585–586.

37. Portoghese PS, Lipkowski AW, Takemori AE. Bimorphinans as highly selective, potent kappa opioid receptor antagonists. J Med Chem 1987;30:238–9

38. James IF, Goldstein A. Site-directed alkylation of multiple opioid receptors. I. Binding selectivity. Mol Pharmacol. 1984;25: 337–342.

39. Gacel G, Fournie-Zaluski M-C, Roques BP. D-Tyr–Ser–Gly–Phe–Leu–Thr, a highly preferential ligand for delta-opiate receptors. FEBS Lett 1980;118:245–7.

40. Mosberg HI, Hurst R, Hruby VJ, et al. Bis-penicillamine enkephalins possess highly improved specificity toward delta opioid receptors. Proc Natl Acad Sci U S A 1983;80:5871–4.

41. Portoghese PS, Larson DL, Sultana M, et al. Opioid agonist and antagonist activities of morphindoles related to naltrindole. J Med Chem 1992;35:4325–9.

42. Bilsky EJ, Calderon SN, Wang T, et al. SNC 80, a selective, nonpeptidic and systemically active opioid delta agonist. J Pharmacol Exp Ther 1995;273:359–66.

43. Jiang Q, Takemori AE, Sultana M, et al. Differential antagonism of opioid delta antinociception by [D-ala2,Leu5,Cys6]-enkephalin and naltrindole 5′-isothiocyanate: evidence for delta receptor subtypes. J Pharmacol Exp Ther 1991;257:1069–75.

44. Portoghese PS, Sultana M, Takemori AE. Naltrindole, a highly selective and potent non-peptide delta opioid receptor antagonist. Eur J Pharmacol 1988;146:185–6.

45. Takemori AE, Sultana M, Nagase H, et al. Agonist and antagonist activities of ligands derived from naltrexone and oxymorphone. Life Sci 1992;149:1–5.

46. Schiller PW, Nguyen TM, Weltrowska G, et al. Differential stereochemical requirements of mu vs. delta opioid receptors for ligand binding and signal transduction: development of a class of potent and highly delta-selective peptide antagonists. Proc Natl Acad Sci USA 1992;89:11871–5.

47. Schiller PW, Weltrowska G, Nguyen TM, et al. TIPP[4]: a highly potent and stable pseudopeptide delta opioid receptor antagonist with extraordinary delta selectivity. J Med Chem 1993;36:3182–7.

48. Portoghese PS, Larson DL, Jiang JB, et al. Synthesis and pharmacologic characterization of an alkylating analogue (chlornaltrexamine) of naltrexone with ultralong-lasting narcotic antagonist properties. J Med Chem 1979;22:168–73.

49. Portoghese PS, Larson DL, Sayre LM, et al. A novel opioid receptor site directed alkylating agent with irreversible narcotic antagonistic and reversible agonistic activities. J Med Chem. 1980;23:233–4.

50. Burke TR Jr, Bajwa BS, Jacobson AE, et al. Probes for narcotic receptor mediated phenomena. 7. Synthesis and pharmacological properties of irreversible ligands specific for mu or delta opiate receptors. J Med Chem 1984;27:1570–1574.

51. Burke TR Jr, Jacobson AE, Rice KC, et al. Probes for narcotic receptor mediated phenomena. 12. cis-(+)-3-Methylfentanyl isothiocyanate, a potent site-directed acylating agent for delta opioid receptors. Synthesis, absolute configuration, and receptor enantioselectivity. J Med Chem 1986;29:1087–93.

52. de Costa BR, Band L, Rothman RB, et al. Synthesis of an affinity ligand ('UPHIT') for in vivo acylation of the kappa-opioid receptor. FEBS Lett 1989;249:178–82.

53. Chang AC, Takemori AE, Ojala WH, et al. Kappa opioid receptor selective affinity labels: electrophilic benzeneacetamides as kappa-selective opioid antagonists. J Med Chem 1994;37:4490–8.

54. Goldstein A. Some thouthts about endogenous opioids and addiction. Drug Alcohol Depend 1983;11:11–14.

55. Nestler EJ, Aghajanian GK. Molecular and Cellular Basis of Addiction. Science 1997;278:58–63.

56. Hyytia P. Involvement of μ-opioid receptors in alcohol drinking by alcohol-preferring AA rats. Pharmacol Biochem Behav 1993;45:697–701.

57. Epping-Jordan MP, Watkins SS, Koob GF, et al. Dramatic decreases in brain reward function during nicotine withdrawal. Nature 1998;393:76–9.

58. Sharma SK, Klee WA, Nirenberg M. Dual regulation of adenylate cyclase accounts for narcotic dependence and tolerance. Proc Natl Acad Sci USA 1975;72:3092–6.

59. Marsch LA. The efficacy of methadone maintenance interventions in reducing illicit opiate use, HIV risk behavior and criminality: a meta-analysis. Addiction 1998;93:515–32.

60. Rawson RA, Hasson AL, Huber AM, et al. A 3-year progress report on the implementation of LAAM in the United States. Addiction 1998;93:533–40.

61. Gonzalez JP, Brogden RN. Naltrexone. A review of its pharmacodynamic and pharmacokinetic properties and therapeutic efficacy in the management of opioid dependence. Drugs 1988;35:192–213.

62. Volpicelli JR, Alterman AI, Hayashida M, et al. Naltrexone in the treatment of alcohol dependence. Arch Gen Psychiatry 1992;49:876–80.

63. Walsh SL, Sullivan JT, Preston KL, et al. Effects of naltrexone on response to intravenous cocaine, hydromorphone and their combination in humans. J Pharmacol Exp Ther 1996;279:524–38.

64. Compton PA, Ling W, Charuvastra VC, et al. Buprenorphine as a pharmacotherapy for cocaine abuse: a review of the evidence. J Addict Dis 1995;14:97–114.

65. Horan PJ, Mattia A, Bilsky EJ, et al. Antinociceptive profile of biphalin, a dimeric enkephalin analog. J Pharmacol Exp Ther 1993;265:1446–54.

66. Miyamoto Y, Portoghese PS, Takemori AE. Involvement of delta 2 opioid receptors in acute dependence on morphine in mice. J Pharmacol Exp Ther 1993;265:1325–7.

67. Dewey SL, Morgan AE, Ashby CR Jr, et al. A novel strategy for the treatment of cocaine addiction. Synapse 1998;30:119–29.

68. Kreek MJ. Opiate and cocaine addictions: Challenge for pharmacotherapies. Pharmacol Biochem Behav 1997;57:551–569.

69. Iigima I, Minamikawa J, Jacobson AE, et al. Studies in the (+)-morphine series. 4. A markedly improved synthesis of (+)-morphine. J Org Chem 1978;43;1462–1463.

70. Casy AF, Parfitt RT. Opioid Analgesics: Chemistry and Receptors. Plenum Press, New York, 1986.

71. Rees DC, Hunter JC. Opioid receptors. In Emment JC, ed. Comprehensive medicinal chemistry: The rational design, mechanistic study and therapeutic application of chemical compounds. Vol. 3, Membranes and receptors. Pergamon Press, Oxford, England, 1990:805–846.

72. Lewis JW, Bently KW, Cowan A. Narcotic analgesics and antagonists. Annu Rev Pharmacol 1971;11:241–270.

73. Grewe R. Synthetic drugs with morphine action. Angew Chem 1947;A59:194–99.

74. Eisleb O, Schaumann O. Dolantin, a new antispasmodic and analgesic. Dtsch Med Wschr 1939;65: 967–968.

75. Schiller PW. Development of receptor-specific opioid peptide analogues. In Ellis GP, West GB. Progress in mecicinal chemistry. Amsterdam: Elsevier, 1988;28:301–340.

76. Beckett AH, Casy AF. Synthetic analgesics: stereochemical considerations. J Pharm Pharmacol 1954;6:986–1001.

77. Portoghese PS. A new concept on the mode of interaction of narcotic analgesics with receptors. J Med Chem 1965;8:609–616.

78. Portoghese PS, Alreja BD, Larson DL, Allylprodine analogues as receptor probes. Evidence that phenolic and nonphenolic ligands interact with different subsites on identical opioid receptors. J Med Chem 1981;24:782–787.

79. Feinberg AP, Creese I, Snyder SH. The opiate receptor: a model explaining structure-activity relationships of opiate agonists and antagonists. Proc Natl Acad Sci USA 1976;73:4215–4219.

80. Martin WR, Pharmacology of opioids. Pharmacol Rev 1984;35:283–318.

SUGGESTED READINGS

Aldrich JV. Analgesics. In: Wolff ME, ed. Burger's medicinal chemistry and drug discovery, 5th edition. New York: John Wiley, 1996;321–441.

Bloom FE. The endorphins: a growing family of pharmacologically pertinent peptides. Annu Rev Pharmacol Toxicol 1983;23:151–70.

Carr DJ, Rogers TJ, Weber RJ. The relevance of opioids and opioid receptors on immunocompetence and immune homeostasis. Proc Soc Exp Biol Med 1996 Dec;213(3):248–57.

Childers SR. Opioid receptors: pinning down the opiate targets. Curr Biol 1997;7:R695–697.

Collier HOJ, Hughes J, Rance MJ, et al, eds. Opioids: past, present and future. London: Tayler and Frances, 1984.

Darland T, Grandy DK. The orphanin FQ system: an emerging target for the management of pain? Br J Anaesth 1998;81:29–37.

Dhawan BN, Raghaubir R, Harman M. Opioid receptors. In IUPHAR receptor compendium. London: IUPHAR Media 1998;218–226.

Eisenstein TK, Hilburger ME. Opioid modulation of immune responses: effects on phagocyte and lymphoid cell populations. J Neuroimmunol 1998;83:36–44.

Fowler CJ, Fraser GL. μ-, δ-, κ-opioid receptors and their subtypes. A critical review with emphasis on radioligand binding experiments. Neurochem Intl 1994;24:836–846.

Fries DS, In: Cannon JG, ed. CNS drug-receptor interactions. Greenwich, CT: JAI Press, 1991:1,1–21.

Harrison C, Smart D, Lambert DG. Stimulatory effects of opioids. Br J Anaesth 1998;81:20–8.

Höllt VR. Opioid peptide processing and receptor selectivity. Annu Rev Pharmacol Toxicol 1986:26:59–77.

Hruby VJ, Gehrig CA. Recent developments in the design of receptor specific opioid peptides. Med Res Rev 1989;9:343–401.

Jordan B, Devi LA. Molecular mechanisms of opioid receptor signal transduction. Br J Anaesth 1998;81:12–9.

Koob GF, Nestler EJ. The neurobiology of drug addiction. J Neuropsychiatry Clin Neurosci 1997;9:482–97.

Kowaluk EA, Arneric SP. Novel molecular approaches to analgesia. In: Bristol JA, ed. Annual reports in medicinal chemistry. New York: Academic Press, 1998;33:11–20.

Lentz R, Evans SM, Walters DE, et al. Opiates. Orlando: Academic Press, 1986.

May EL. Alfred Burger Award address. A half century in medicinal chemistry with major emphasis on pain-relieving drugs and their antagonists. J Med Chem 1992;35:3587–3594.

Olson GA, Olson RD, Kastin AJ. Endogenous opiates: 1996. Peptides 1997;18:1651–88.

Portoghese PS. Edward E. Smissman-Bristol-Myers Squibb Award Address. The role of concepts in structure-activity relationship studies of opioid ligands. J Med Chem 1992;35:1927–1937.

Reisine T, Bell GI. Molcular biology of opioid receptors. Trends Neurosci 1993;16:506–510.

Reisine T, Pasternak G. Opioid analgesics and antagonists. In: Hardman JG, Limbird, eds-in chief. Goodman and Gilman's; The pharmacological basis of therapeutics; 9th edition. New York: McGraw-Hill 1996;521–555.

Reitz AB, Jetter MC, Wild KD, et al. In: Bristol AJ, ed. Annual reports in medicinal chemistry. New York: Academic Press, 1995; 30:11–20.

Schnitzer TJ. Non-NSAID pharmacologic treatment options for the management of chronic pain. Am J Med 1998;105:45S-52S.

Ulett GA, Han S, Han JS. Electroacupuncture: mechanisms and clinical application. Biol Psychiatry 1998;44:129–38.

Williams M, Kowaluk EA, Arneric SP. Emerging molecular approaches to pain therapy. J Med Chem 1999:42:1481–1500.

Zimmerman DM and Leander JD. Selective opioid receptor agonists and antagonists: research tools and potential therapeutic agents. J Med Chem 1990;33:895–902.

20. Drugs Used to Treat Neuromuscular Disorders: Antiparkinsonian and Spasmolytic Agents

RAYMOND G. BOOTH AND JOHN L. NEUMEYER

OVERVIEW OF NEUROMUSCULAR DISORDERS

Pharmacotherapy of neuromuscular disorders covered in this chapter include the neurodegenerative movement disorder Parkinson's disease and various spasticity disorders. Parkinson's disease affects about 1% of the general population, primarily senior citizens, and clinically presents as debilitating tremor, rigidity, and bradykinesia. The neuropathology (but not the etiology) of Parkinson's disease with resulting neurotransmitter (dopamine) deficit has been well defined for decades, however, pharmacotherapy of the disorder remains far from satisfactory. The development of prophylactic and perhaps curative pharmacotherapy of Parkinson's disease requires advances in our understanding of the causes and pathogenesis of the disease and this chapter reviews some current research in these areas in addition to available drugs.

Spasticity disorders are generally characterized by an increase in tonic stretch reflexes and flexor muscle spasms together with muscle weakness. Muscle spasticity may accompany a number of different disorders but mostly is associated with cerebral palsy, multiple sclerosis, spinal cord injury, and stroke. These disorders do not share a similar pathophysiology with neurodegenerative diseases such as parkinsonism. Accordingly, drugs used to treat spastic neuromuscular disorders have mechanisms of action that differ from those used to treat Parkinson's disease. Nevertheless, most drugs described in this chapter to treat neurodegenerative or spastic neuromuscular disorders have in common the ability to reduce muscle tone by virtue of their action on the central nervous system.

PARKINSON'S DISEASE
Clinical Features and Neuropathology

Parkinson's disease, first described by James Parkinson in 1817, affects over one million people in North America. In 90% of cases, the disease becomes manifest after age 55 and presents clinically as a classic triad of signs: resting tremor, rigidity, and bradykinesia. Dementia also is a common feature of Parkinson's disease and occurs 6.6 times more frequently in elderly patients with the disease than without. Along with this morbidity, mortality is two to five times higher among Parkinson's disease patients than in age-matched controls, greatly reducing life expectancy among affected individuals (1).

Neuropathologically, Parkinson's disease is a slowly progressive neurodegenerative disorder of the extrapyramidal dopaminergic nigrostriatal pathway (Fig. 20.1). The disease is characterized by the destruction of dopaminergic cells in the pars compacta region of the substantia nigra, leading to a deficiency of dopamine in the nerve terminals of the striatum (2). Degenerative changes in the pigmented nuclei of the noradrenergic locus ceruleus region also are typical, as well as, the appearance of intraneuronal inclusions called Lewy bodies.

Neurochemically, the striatal dopamine deficiency accounts for the major motor symptoms of the disease and the mainstay of pharmacologic treatment (3) continues to be replacement therapy with the α-amino acid L-dihydroxyphenylalanine (L-dopa) (the immediate biochemical precursor to dopamine (Fig. 20.2), developed in the mid-1960s.

Pathophysiology

In the normal striatum, dopamine, released from nerve terminals of dopaminergic cells originating in the substantia nigra, modulates activity of inhibitory GABA*ergic* neurons. In turn, striatal GABAergic neurons, through a series of complex neuronal connections, modulate neuronal outflow to the motor cortex via so-called "direct" and "indirect" pathways (1). In the normal striatum, dopamine, released from nerve terminals of dopaminergic cells originating in the substantia nigra, modulates activity of inhibitory GABAergic neurons. In turn, striatal GABAergic neurons, through a series of complex neuronal connections, modulate neuronal outflow via so-called "direct" and "indirect" pathways to the thalamus,

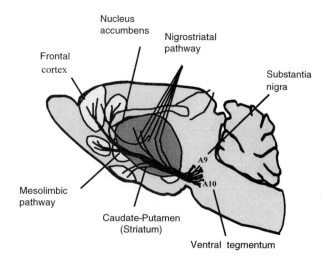

Fig. 20.1. Some dopaminergic pathways in the brain. The nigrostriated pathway (A9 cell bodies in substantia nigra; nerve terminals in striatum) is degenerated in Parkinson's disease.

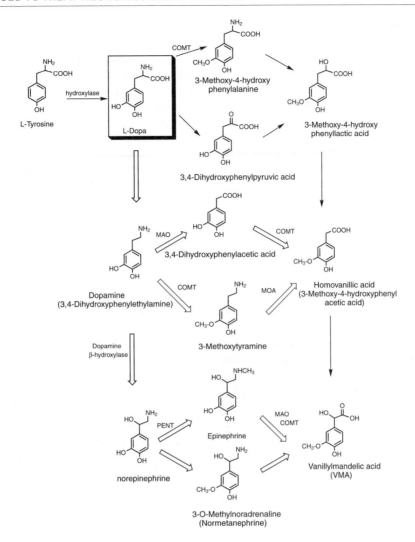

Fig. 20.2. Important pathways in the biosynthesis and metabolism of levodopa. Major pathways are shown by heavy arrows: COMT, catechol-O-methyltransferase; monoamine oxidase, PENT, phenylethanolamine N-methyltransferase.

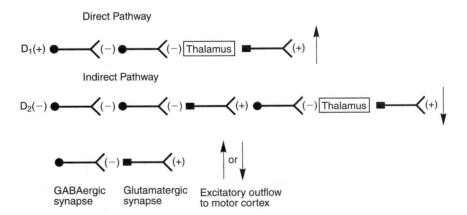

Fig. 20.3. Striatal dopaminergic stimulation of the direct and indirect pathways modulates the thalamus excitatory outflow to the motor cortex.

which provides excitatory (glutamatergic) input to the motor cortex. In the direct pathway, striatal GABAergic neurons activate a second set of inhibitory GABAergic neurons. The first set of striatal GABAergic neurons in this direct pathway contain a predominance of excitatory

dopamine D_1-type receptors; thus, the net effect of D_1-mediated stimulation of striatal GABAergic neurons in the direct pathway is to increase excitatory outflow from the thalamus to the motor cortex (Fig. 20.3). In the indirect pathway, striatal GABAergic neurons activate a second set of inhibitory GABAergic neurons, which in turn modulate excitatory glutamatergic neurons. The first set of striatal GABAergic neurons in this indirect pathway contain a predominance of inhibitory D_2-type receptors; thus, the net effect of dopamine D_2-mediated modulation of striatal GABAergic neurons in the indirect pathway is to reduce excitatory outflow from the thalamus to the motor cortex (Fig. 20.3). In the normal condition, dopamine released in the striatum tends to increase activity of the direct pathway and decrease activity of the indirect pathway. In Parkinson's disease, the striatal dopamine deficiency results in diminished activity of the direct pathway and increased activity of the indirect pathway; the net effect is decreased excitatory input to the motor cortex (Fig. 20.3).

Etiology

Although the neuropathology is well defined, the cause of Parkinson's disease is unknown. The development of effective pharmacotherapeutic and prophylactic therapy will require advances in our understanding of the etiology of the disease. Currently, there are several, sometimes convergent, theories regarding the cause of Parkinson's disease; environmental and/or endogenous neurotoxicants, mitochondrial dysfunction, and oxidative metabolism—any and all of which may lead to "oxidative stress." This section describes these and some alternative proposals regarding the etiology of Parkinson's disease.

Since several neurodegenerative disorders (including the movement disorder Huntington's disease) are genetically determined, researchers have investigated a possible genetic influence in Parkinson's disease. Epidemiological studies have found that, apart from age, a family history of Parkinson's disease is the strongest predictor of an increased risk of the disorder (4), however, the role of shared environmental exposure in families must be considered. Recently, the identification of distinct mutations in the α-synuclein gene located on chromosome 4q was reported in a single large Italian family, three smaller Greek families, and a German family (5,6). The α-synuclein protein is a highly conserved, abundant 140-amino acid protein of unknown function that is expressed mainly in presynaptic nerve terminals in the brain (7). Several other studies, however, have failed to detect mutations in the α-synuclein gene in a larger number of other families (8, 9) or in sporadic cases (6), suggesting that Parkinson's disease is only

rarely caused by such mutations. Studies using both identical and heterozygous twins provide a rigorous genetic analysis, however, these studies too have failed to reveal a genetic component of Parkinson's disease (10). There also is little evidence to suggest the disease is autoimmune related (11) and studies on a form of Parkinson's disease in villages in New Guinea (12) indicate that neither a genetic nor a communicable infectious etiology is involved.

There is, however, direct evidence to suggest that environmental toxicants may cause some types of Parkinson's disease. For instance, manganese miners in South America are at a high risk of developing a form of Parkinson's disease characterized by tremor, bradykinesia, postural difficulties, dystonia, and psychiatric disturbances (13). In another case, in the major agricultural region of the Quebec province of Canada, investigators showed there was a remarkably high correlation between the incidence of Parkinson's disease and the sale of pesticides (14).

One of the best characterized epidemiologic findings in Parkinson's disease is its lower incidence in cigarette smokers than in nonsmokers (15). Something in cigarette smoke may protect against a toxicant (environmental or endogenous) relevant to parkinsonian neuropathology. For example, the carbon monoxide in cigarette smoke may detoxify free radicals from environmental or endogenous sources. It also has been suggested that compounds present in cigarette smoke or metabolites of these compounds may inhibit monoamine oxidase (MAO)-B activity (16), the main enzyme responsible for metabolism of monoamine neurotransmitters such as dopamine.

In fact, dopamine itself has been implicated in the disease process through production of chemically reactive oxidation products, suggesting that endogenously formed substances may be etiologic factors in Parkinson's disease (17). For example, the MAO catalyzed oxidation of the monoamine neurotransmitters (dopamine, norepinephrine, serotonin) generates hydrogen peroxide (Equation 1, Fig. 20.4) which can undergo a redox reaction with superoxide in the Haber-Weiss reaction (18) to form the extremely cytotoxic hydroxy radical (Equation 2, Fig. 20.4). Moreover, the auto-oxidation of dopamine to the corresponding electrophilic semiquinone and quinone (Fig. 20.4) species has received attention since these oxidation products also are cytotoxic (19). Manganese ion can catalyze oxidation of dopamine, and the resulting semi-

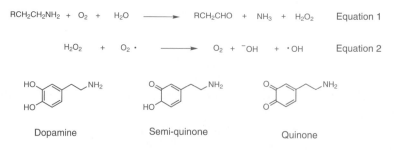

$$RCH_2CH_2NH_2 \; + \; O_2 \; + \; H_2O \longrightarrow RCH_2CHO \; + \; NH_3 \; + \; H_2O_2 \qquad \text{Equation 1}$$

$$H_2O_2 \; + \; O_2 \cdot \longrightarrow O_2 \; + \; {}^-OH \; + \; \cdot OH \qquad \text{Equation 2}$$

Dopamine   Semi-quinone   Quinone

Fig. 20.4. Formation of cytotoxic chemical species.

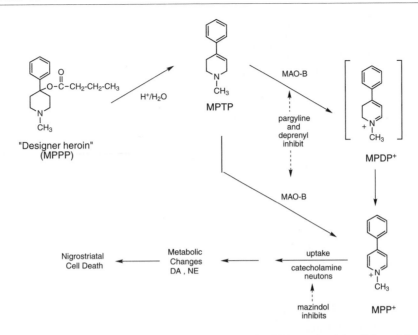

Fig. 20.5. Chemical conversion of MPPP and probable mechanism of MPTP neurotoxicity. (Adapted from reference 37)

quinone and quinone species have been implicated in manganese neurotoxicity (20). The auto-oxidation of dopamine also leads to the formation of the polymeric black pigment neuromelanin (19). The physiologic role of neuromelanin is poorly understood but the pigment is increasingly deposited in catecholaminergic neurons with advancing age and it has been suggested that its accumulation in nigral neuronal cells eventually causes cell death (2).

It has been postulated that Parkinson's disease might be the consequence of normal aging superimposed on a lesion in the substantia nigra that took place earlier in life (21). For example, it is known that dopamine neurons degenerate with advancing age and in normal adults dopamine levels in striatum decline about 13% per decade (22). Parkinsonian symptoms usually become apparent when striatal dopamine levels decline by about 80% (23). Conceivably, the symptoms of parkinsonism could be produced by two processes, a specific disease-related insult combined with pathological changes due to normal aging. This two-pronged pathophysiology may explain why Parkinson's disease is a progressive disorder of late onset. The discovery of the potent and selective dopaminergic neurotoxicant N-methyl-4-phenyl-1,2,3,6-tetrahydropyridine (MPTP) has greatly aided scientists conducting studies to determine the etiology of Parkinson's disease.

Parkinsonism Caused by MPTP

The cyclic tertiary amine MPTP (Fig. 20.5), induces a form of parkinsonism in humans and monkeys similar in neuropathology and motor abnormalities to idiopathic Parkinson's disease (24-26). The role of MPTP in parkinsonian disorders was revealed by a serendipitous series of events. In 1977, a 23-year-old college student suddenly developed parkinsonian symptoms with severe rigidity, bradyki-

nesia, and mutism. The abrupt and early onset of symptoms was so atypical that the patient initially was thought to have catatonic schizophrenia. The subsequent diagnosis of parkinsonism was substantiated by a therapeutic response to L-dopa, whereupon the patient was referred to the National Institute of Mental Health in Bethesda, Maryland. He admitted having synthesized and used several illicit drugs. The psychiatrist who had elicited the patient's history visited his home and collected glassware that had been used for chemical syntheses. Chemical analysis revealed several pyridines, including MPTP, formed as by-products in synthesizing the reverse ester of the narcotic analgesic meperidine known as MPPP (N-methyl-4-propionoxy-4-phenylpiperidine), "designer heroin," or "synthetic heroin." This substance is also an analog of another narcotic analgesic, α-prodine (Fig. 20.6). It was initially unclear, however, whether MPTP or other constituents of the injected mixture accounted for the neurotoxicity.

After the patient returned home, he continued to abuse drugs and died of an overdose; autopsy revealed degeneration of the substantia nigra—the hallmark neuropathological feature of Parkinson's disease. Subsequently, other patients were identified with virtually identical parkinsonian symptoms who had also been receiving intravenous injec-

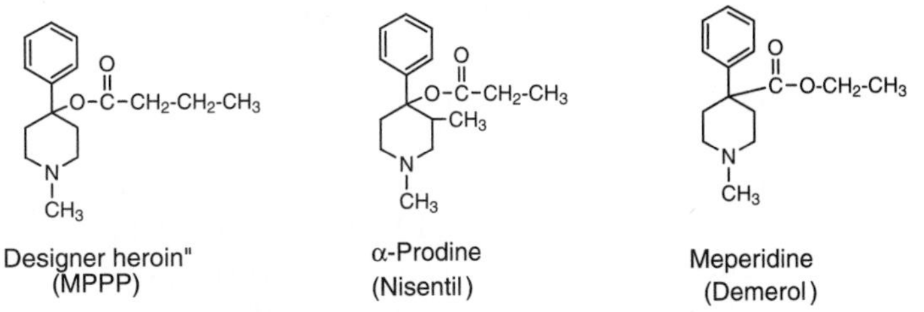

Fig. 20.6. Phenylpiperidine synthetic analgesics.

tions of preparations of MPPP containing varying amounts of MPTP. In several patients, MPTP was the principal or sole constituent injected, providing the first definitive evidence that MPTP is a parkinsonism-producing neurotoxicant. More than 400 people now are known to have self-administered MPTP, but only a few have developed parkinsonian symptoms. Many of these individuals who are presently asymptomatic, however, may be at risk for developing parkinsonism as they age.

Both the clinical and neuropathological features of MPTP-induced parkinsonism resemble idiopathic Parkinson's disease more closely than any previous animal or human disorder elicited by toxins, metals, viruses, or other means. Accordingly, understanding the molecular pathophysiology of MPTP neurotoxicity has shed light on the neurodegenerative mechanisms present in idiopathic parkinsonism.

Mechanisms of Neuronal Cell Death in MPTP-induced Parkisonism

Consideration of the chemical structure of MPTP would suggest the compound to be relatively chemically inert since no highly reactive functional group is present. Almost immediately, it was recognized that MPTP might undergo some type of metabolic activation to a more reactive metabolite. Researchers soon discovered that brain MAO-B catalyzes the two-electron oxidation of MPTP at the allylic α-carbon to give the unstable intermediate product, 1-methyl-4-phenyl-2,3-dihydropyridinium (MPDP$^+$), which subsequently undergoes a further two-electron oxidation to the stable 1-methyl-4-phenylpyridinium species (MPP$^+$) via auto-oxidation, disproportionation, and enzyme-catalyzed mechanisms (27–29) (Fig. 20.5). Inhibitors of MAO-B subsequently were shown to prevent MPTP-induced parkinsonism in primates (30) and it is currently accepted that MPP$^+$ is the major metabolite of MPTP responsible for the destruction of dopamine neurons (although a role for the unstable dihydropyridinium species MPDP$^+$ has not been ruled out).

The relationship of MAO and MPTP has neurobiological relevance beyond MPTP neurotoxicity. MAO catalyzes the α-carbon oxidation of the monoamine neurotransmitters (e.g., dopamine, norepinephrine, serotonin) (see Fig. 20.2). Oxidation of a heterocyclic tertiary amine (i.e., MPTP) by MAO is unprecedented and suggests a novel physiologic role for this enzyme. For example, MAO could be important in regulating the oxidation state of pyridine systems, such as those involving nucleic acids and NADH (31), which may be involved in the neurotoxicity of MPTP (vide infra). Interestingly, too, is biochemical and epidemiologic evidence that cigarette smokers have depressed MAO-B activity (32) and a lower incidence of Parkinson's disease (33). Nicotine is not a particularly potent inhibitor of MAO, and, in fact, nicotine increases neurotoxicity of MPTP (34). Other components of cigarette smoke, however, do inhibit MAO and cigarette smoke protects against MPTP-induced depletion of striatal dopamine in mice (35).

Although extensive metabolic, biochemical, and toxicologic investigations have established that the nigrostriatal neurodegenerative properties of MPTP are mediated by the MAO-B derived metabolite, MPP$^+$, this bioactivation reaction must proceed outside of the target nigrostriatal dopamine neurons since they apparently do not contain MAO-B (36). It is thought that MPTP is oxidized to MPDP$^+$ in MAO-B rich glial cells near striatal nerve terminals and nigral cell bodies; the conjugate base MPDP presumably diffuses out of glial cells and is subsequently oxidized to the MPP$^+$ metabolite. MPP$^+$ is sequestered into striatal dopaminergic nerve terminals via the dopamine neurotransporter, which accepts MPP$^+$ as a substrate (Fig. 20.5) (37). Intraneuronally, MPP$^+$ is concentrated into mitochondria where it selectively inhibits complex I of the electron transport chain, inhibiting NADH oxidation and eventually depleting the nigrostriatal neuronal cell of ATP (38,39). The depletion of ATP following inhibition of complex I currently is the accepted mechanism of nigrostriatal cell death induced by MPTP (via MPP$^+$) (40). In this regard, there is increasing evidence for a defect of mitochondrial respiratory chain function in idiopathic Parkinson's disease and specific NADH CoQ1 reductase (complex I) deficiency, which has been documented in the substantia nigra of parkinsonian brains (41).

Several sequential factors may account for the selective damage of nigrostriatal dopamine neurons by MPTP (37) (Fig. 20.5). First, MPTP binds selectively to MAO-B, which is highly concentrated in glial cells in human substantia nigra and corpus striatum. Then, the MPP$^+$ produced from MPTP is selectively accumulated by dopamine neurotransporters into nigral dopamine cells and striatal dopamine nerve terminals. Finally, within nigral cell bodies, MPP$^+$ binds to neuromelanin, and may be gradually released in a depot-like fashion, maintaining a toxic intracellular concentration of MPP$^+$ that inhibits mitochondrial respiration.

The serendipitous discovery and subsequent scientific investigation of the mechanism of parkinsonism produced by MPTP has refocused study of the etiology and pathogenesis of idiopathic Parkinson's disease. For example, it has been documented that there is a 30–40% reduction in mitochondrial complex I activity in the substantia nigra of patients with Parkinson's disease (42). In general, mitochondrial dysfunction and oxidative metabolism (e.g., oxidation of dopamine to electrophilic quinone-type species) now are considered critical components of most theories of nigral cell degeneration in Parkinson's disease (3). Moreover, discovery of the selective ability of MPTP to induce nigral cell death has stimulated broad interest in identifying potential environmental or endogenous compounds that may be causative agents in Parkinson's disease.

Pharmacotherapy of Parkinson's Disease

No currently available treatment slows the progression of the neurodegeneration in Parkinson's disease. Based in part on the discovery of parkinsonism produced by MPTP, selective MAO-B inhibitors were hypothesized to slow the progression of idiopathic Parkinson's disease. Clinical evidence, however, has not been encouraging regarding the effectiveness of the MAO-B inhibitor selegiline (Eldepryl), the antioxidant vitamin E to slow progression of the disease (43,44).

(−)R-Selegiline (Eldepryl)

Thus, available pharmacotherapy continues to be symptomatic, involving replacement of the dopamine deficiency in striatum by one or more of the following means: (1) augmentation of the synthesis of brain dopamine, (2) stimulation of dopamine release from presynaptic sites, (3) direct stimulation of dopamine receptors, (4) decreasing re-uptake of dopamine at presynaptic sites, or (5) decreasing dopamine catabolism.

Levodopa Therapy

More than 30 years after its introduction, levodopa remains the most effective pharmacotherapy in Parkinson's disease (3). Despite controversy regarding long term efficacy, side effects, and even potential neurotoxicity, most patients derive a substantial benefit from levodopa over the entire course of their illness. Moreover, levodopa increases life expectancy among patients with Parkinson's disease and survival is significantly reduced if there is a delay in initiation of levodopa therapy (45).

The seminal report by Cotzias and co-workers in 1967 (46), describing dramatic symptomatic improvement of parkinsonian patients given high oral doses of racemic dopa, was followed by more clinical trials that confirmed the efficacy and safety of the *levo* isomer. The effectiveness of levodopa requires penetration of the drug into the central nervous system and its subsequent enzymatic decarboxylation to dopamine. Dopamine does not cross the blood-brain barrier because it exists primarily in its protonated form under physiologic conditions (pKa 10.6 [NH₂]) (47). The precursor amino acid levodopa, however, is less basic (pKa 8.72 [NH₂]) (47) and thus can penetrate the central nervous system.

Biosynthesis and Metabolism of Levodopa. Levodopa is an intermediary metabolite in the biosynthesis of catecholamines, formed from L-tyrosine in a rate-limiting hydroxylation step by tyrosine hydroxylase (Fig. 20.2). Levodopa subsequently is decarboxylated by the cytoplasmic enzyme L-aromatic amino acid decarboxylase (dopa decarboxylase) to form dopamine. The effects observed following systemic administration of levodopa have been attributed to its catabolites, dopamine, norepinephrine, and epinephrine, acting at various sites in the periphery and in the brain. The principal metabolic pathways for levodopa are shown in Figure 20.2. A small amount is methylated to 3-O-methyldopa, which accumulates in the central nervous system due to its long half-life. Most levodopa, though, is decarboxylated to dopamine, small amounts of which are metabolized to norepinephrine and epinephrine. The activity of dopa decarboxylase, however, is greater in the liver, heart, lungs, and kidneys than in the brain (48). Therefore, ingested levodopa is converted to dopamine in the periphery in preference to the brain. It is thought that, in humans, levodopa thus enters the brain only when administered in doses high enough to overcome losses caused by peripheral metabolism (3–6 g daily). Inhibition of peripheral decarboxylase activity, by co-administration of a peripheral decarboxylase inhibitor such as carbidopa, can markedly increase the proportion of levodopa that crosses the blood-brain barrier (Fig. 20.7).

S(−)-Carbidopa

The greater amount of dopamine that is formed in the brain after orally administered levodopa/carbidopa presumably provides symptomatic relief of parkinsonian symptoms such as rigidity and bradykinesia. Parkinsonian patients not previously treated with levodopa usually are started on a combination therapy with Sinemet, which is available in a fixed ratio of 1 part carbidopa and 10 parts levodopa, either 10/100 mg or 25/250 mg. Once formed from levodopa, metabolism of dopamine then proceeds relatively rapidly to the principal excretion products 3,4-dihydroxyphenylacetic acid (DOPAC) and 3-methoxy-4-hydroxyphenylacetic acid (homovanillic acid, HVA) (Fig. 20.2).

Pyridoxine (a coenzyme for dopa decarboxylase) can reverse the therapeutic effects of levodopa by increasing decarboxylase activity, which results in more levodopa being converted to dopamine in the periphery and consequently less being available for penetration into the central nervous system. When peripheral dopa decarboxylation is blocked with carbidopa, however, the pyridoxine effect on peripheral levodopa metabolism is negligible.

Side Effects of Levodopa. One of the most common side effects of levodopa therapy is gastric upset with nausea and vomiting. This appears to be the result of direct gastrointestinal irritation, as well as stimulation by dopamine of the chemoreceptor trigger zone (CTZ) in the area postrema of the brain stem that activates the emetic center of the medulla. The blood-brain barrier is poorly developed in the area postrema and the CTZ is accessible to emetic substances in the circulation. One of the advantages of combining levodopa with a peripheral decarboxylase inhibitor such as carbidopa is that a 75–80% reduction of the dosage of levodopa is permitted, thus, some side effects may be avoided or lessened in severity. Administration of carbidopa with levodopa results in a significant decrease in the incidence and severity of nausea and vomiting associated with levodopa alone. Other side effects of levodopa involve activation of peripheral adrenergic and dopaminergic receptors by dopamine (Fig. 20.7). For example, dopamine stimulation of peripheral α-adrenergic receptors causes vasoconstriction and stimulation of β-adrenergic receptors enhances heart rate; either may lead to increased blood pressure. Stimulation of peripheral dopamine receptors causes renal and mesenteric vasodilation. These cardiovascular side effects of levodopa (via dopamine) also can be diminished by co-administration of carbidopa to allow a lower dose of levodopa.

After about 5 years of levodopa therapy, 50 percent of patients develop motor fluctuations; the proportion of patients affected increases to 70 percent after 15 years of therapy (49). Motor complications include "off" periods of immobility or greater severity of other parkinsonian symptoms and various abnormal involuntary movements. This phenomenon may be due to progression of the disease with resulting striatal nerve terminal degeneration and decreased synthesis and storage of dopamine generated from endogenous or exogenous levodopa. In addition to these presynaptic changes, changes in postsynpatic D_1-type and D_2-type receptor systems in the striatum also may occur.

Psychiatric disturbances such as visual hallucinations, mania, hypersexuality, and paranoid psychosis also are complications of levodopa therapy. It is generally believed that these psychiatric disturbances are due to dopamine (produced from levodopa) stimulation of dopamine receptors outside the motor striatum, i.e., in the mesolimbic dopaminergic system.

MAO-B and COMT Inhibitors

Selegiline (commonly referred to as L-deprenyl in the clinical literature), the levo isomer of N-α-dimethyl-N-2-propynylbenzenethanamine, is a selective inhibitor of MAO-B, which inactivates dopamine. Selegiline can extend the duration of response to levodopa by reducing the metabolism of dopamine, thus, the dose of levodopa can be reduced without loss of therapeutic benefit (3). In contrast to nonspecific MAO-A and MAO-B inhibitors (e.g., pargyline, phenelzine, and isocarboxazid), selegiline does not cause profound and potentially lethal potentiation of the effects of catecholamines when administered concurrently with a centrally active amine. In addition to inhibition of MAO-B, selegiline also inhibits re-uptake of dopamine and norepinephrine into presynaptic nerve terminals and increases the turnover of dopamine, thus adding to its potentiation of the pharmacologic effects of levodopa (50). It is hypothesized that use of MAO-B inhibitors may prevent formation of neurotoxic oxidation products of dopamine and slow neurodegeneration in Parkinson's disease, however, data from recent clinical studies does not supported this "neuroprotective" hypothesis (43,44).

Tolcapone and entacapone are catechol-O-methyltransferase (COMT) inhibitors that prolong the action of levodopa by inhibiting the methylation and subsequent inactivation of dopamine (Fig. 20.2). COMT inhibitors may produce increased dyskinesias or induction of hallucinations that may require a reduction in the dose of levodopa (51). Severe diarrhea also is a side effect of the COMT inhibitors and liver dysfunction may occur, requiring moni-

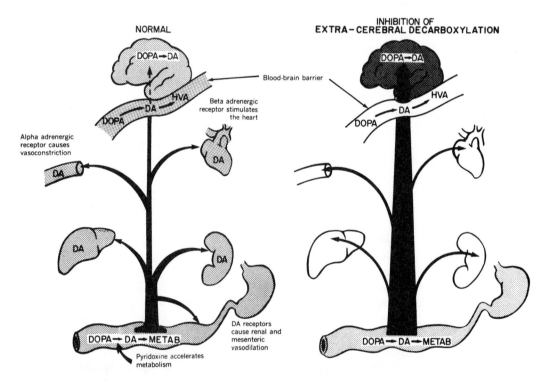

Fig. 20.7. Diagrammatic representation of the peripheral decarboxylation of levodopa to form dopamine (DA) and the mode of action of extra-cerebral decarboxylase on levodopa metabolism and distribution in vivo. The concurrent administration of levodopa and a decarboxylase inhibitor decreases the amount of levodopa required to elicit a therapeutic response in parkinsonism. HVA, homovanillic acid.

toring through liver function tests at baseline and every 6 weeks for the first 6 months of therapy (3).

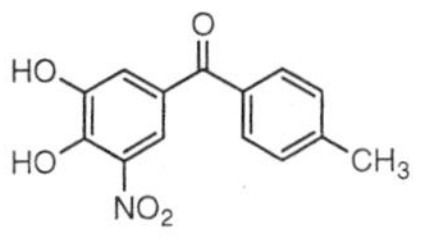

Tolcapone (Tasmir)

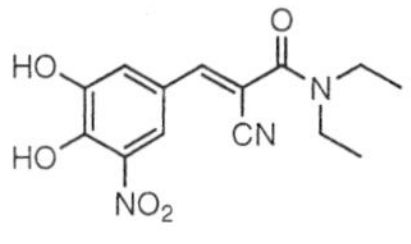

Entacapone (Comtun)

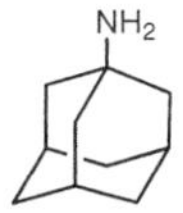

Amantadine
(Symmetrel)

Amantadine

Amantadine can release dopamine from intraneuronal storage sites and has clinically significant antiparkinsonian effects, which are enhanced in the presence of levodopa. Amantadine has been shown to delay the re-uptake of dopamine by nerve terminals and has glutamic acid (NMDA receptor) antagonist effects (3), as well.

Amantadine is a primary amine with a pK_a of 10.8 and most of the drug is in the protonated form at physiologic pH. Nevertheless, the drug may enter the brain due to its cage-like structure that not only increases its lipophilicity, but also precludes its catabolism by oxidative enzymes; metabolism studies have shown that amantadine is excreted in the urine unchanged.

Dopamine Receptor Agonists

Therapy and Side Effects.   The nigrostriatal neurodegeneration that proceeds over the course of Parkinson's disease limits the number of striatal nerve terminals that are available to decarboxylate levodopa to dopamine. Drugs that act directly to stimulate dopamine receptors, however, do not require functioning dopaminergic nerve terminals and can be useful in management of late-stage disease problems during levodopa therapy.

Bromocriptine is an ergot peptide derivative that is a partial agonist at D_1-type and a full agonist at D_2-type postsynaptic dopamine receptors, usually given in combination with levodopa therapy (Fig. 20.8). Pergolide is a nonpeptide ergot derivative that also is a partial D_1 agonist and full D_2 agonist, and acts similar to bromocriptine. Side effects of both bromocriptine and pergolide include hallucinations and other psychiatric disturbances that are more common and more severe than with levodopa alone. Nausea and vomiting also are common side effects associated with these agents, presumably due to D_2 agonist activation of the CTZ. Both drugs also are used to inhibit lactation via D_2-mediated suppression of prolactin secretion.

Ropinirole and pramipexole are non-ergot agents that are selective full agonists at dopamine D_2 and D_3 receptors, in contrast to ergot alkaloids which also have activity at other non-dopaminergic neurotransmitter receptors.

Peripheral and central dopaminergic side effects similar to the ergot derived dopamine agonists can be expected for these drugs.

Use of dopamine agonist monotherapy (i.e., without levodopa) has been suggested as initial therapy for Parkinson's disease based on the hypothesis that oxidative metabolites of dopamine (formed from exogenous and endogenous levodopa) may be neurotoxic. At present, however, there is no substantial evidence to support an indirect neuroprotective effect of dopamine receptor agonists and these drugs generally are given in combination with a reduced dose of levodopa/carbidopa (3).

Structure-activity Relationships of Dopamine Receptor Agonists.   As described in Chapter 17, molecular cloning technology has been used to identify five genes that code for dopamine receptor proteins: two D_1-type receptors (D_1, D_5) and three D_2-type receptors (D_2, D_3, D_4). While antipsychotic drug design (see Chapter 17) is directed toward discovery of molecules that act as *antagonists* at especially dopamine D_2-type receptors (albeit, an important role for the D_1 family has not been ruled out), the dopamine deficiency that characterizes Parkinson's disease naturally directs research toward discovery of ligands that act as *agonists* at dopamine D_1-type and especially at D_2-type receptors. Currently, however, no validated three-dimensional orientation of the amino acid residues at the dopamine binding site has been reported for D_1-type or D_2-type receptors. Thus, development of selective agonists and antagonists for dopamine receptors still is guided by quantitative structure-activity relationships (QSAR) based on a lead molecule.

The side chain of dopamine possesses unlimited flexibility and unrestricted rotation about the β-carbonphenyl bond, thus, little information can be obtained concerning the conformational requirements for activation of dopamine receptors using the endogenous ligand. Accordingly, various compounds in which the catechol ring and the amino-ethyl moiety of dopamine are held in rigid conformation have been synthesized. For example,

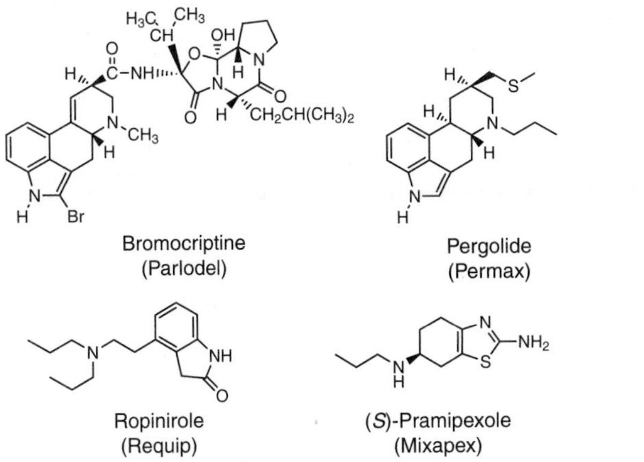

Bromocriptine
(Parlodel)

Pergolide
(Permax)

Ropinirole
(Requip)

(S)-Pramipexole
(Mixapex)

Fig. 20.8. Structures of the dopamine agonists bromocriptine, pergolide, ropinirole, and pramipexole.

the aporphine alkaloid apomorphine, obtained by the acid-catalyzed rearrangement of morphine and recognized for years as a powerful centrally acting emetic by its action on the medullary CTZ, was found to produce effects similar to those of dopamine by direct stimulation of central dopamine receptors.

Although the pKa of apomorphine is about 9 (thus, mostly protonated at physiologic pH), the molecule apparently is lipophilic enough to pass across the blood-brain barrier, whereas dopamine (pKa = 10.6) cannot. In the brain, (R)-$(-)$-apomorphine is a potent D_1 and D_2 agonist and produces an antiparkinsonian effect equivalent to that of levodopa. Interestingly, $S(+)$-apomorphine is a postsynaptic D_2-type antagonist and a presynaptic D_2-type autoreceptor agonist that decreases dopamine synthesis (theoretically, such neurobiochemical activity would be desirable in an antipsychotic drug) (52). Unfortunately, apomorphine is difficult to administer because of first-pass enterohepatic metabolism and potent emetic effects. Nevertheless, apomorphine can be administered by subcutaneous injection and is approved to treat late-stage Parkinson's disease (53).

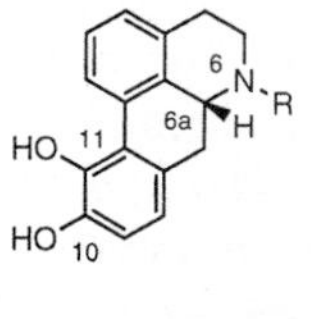

R = CH_3: $R(-)$-Apomorphine
R = (CH_2)_2CH_3: $R(-)$-N-n-propylnorapomorphine (NPA)

Of other apomorphine analogs examined, N-n-propylnorapomorphine was found to be nearly 100-times more active than apomorphine as a dopamine agonist. Such aporphines have enabled medicinal chemists to examine the structural requirements of dopamine receptors using a rigid molecular

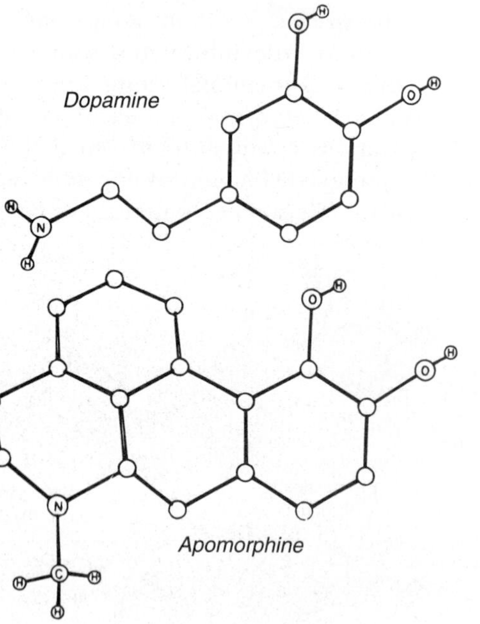

Fig. 20.9. Model of apomorphine molecule as determined by the X-ray crystal data of Giesecke (54) showing the structural relationship to dopamine in the *trans* α-rotameric conformation.

system. Examination of a structural model of apomorphine, based on the X-ray crystal structure (54), shows that it contains molecular features in common with the structure of dopamine in the *trans* α-rotamer conformation (Fig. 20.9).

Meanwhile, isoapomorphine, which contains the structure of dopamine in the *trans* β-rotameric conformation (Fig. 20.10), is less active as a dopamine agonist. The 1,2-dihydroxyaporphine analog, which mimics the *cis* α-rotamer conformation of dopamine, also is inactive (55). In other studies, the semi-rigid aminotetralin 2-amino-6,7-dihydroxy-1,2,3,4-tetrahydronaphthalene (A-6,7-DTN), which has a *trans* β-rotamer conformation between the benzene ring and the amino side chain (Fig. 20.10), was found to be a more potent dopamine agonist than 2-amino-5,6-dihydroxy-1,2,3,4-tetrahydronaphthalene (A-5,6-DTN), which has a *trans* α-rotamer conformation (Fig. 20.10) (56). Thus, results of experiments using these rigid dopamine-mimetic compounds suggest that the preferred conformation of dopamine is the extended *trans* conformation (α- or β-rotamer). While it is unclear if side chain rotameric conformation makes a significant contribution to *binding* at D_1-type receptors, it has been suggested that the *trans* β-rotamer conformation of dopamine is an important determinant of agonist *activation* of D_1-type receptors (57). Meanwhile, at D_2-type receptors, rigid benzoquinoline derivatives containing the *trans* β-rotamer conformation of dopamine were determined to bind more potently than benzoquinolines containing the *trans* α-rotamer conformation (58). Recent research suggests that the nitrogen moiety, rather than the catechol group, is a more important determinant of activity at dopamine receptors (*vide infra*).

Recently, a computational method (comparative molecular field analysis; CoMFA) was used to establish a three-dimensional quantitative structure-activity relationship (3D-QSAR) for activation of D_1-type and D_2-type dopamine receptors using 16 structurally diverse dopamine agonists (59). A molecular database was established for proposed receptor-bound conformations of the agonists using prototypical template D_1 and D_2 agonists. It was determined that the interaction of a D_1 or D_2 agonist with its receptor could best be described by a three-point pharmacophore consisting of one protonated nitrogen (at physiologic pH) and at least one electronegative center (e.g., catechol or equivalent electronegative moieties) able to participate in hydrogen bonding. The pharmacophore maps for the D_1 vs. D_2 receptor differed primarily in the height (higher for D_1) of the nitrogen atom above the plane of the electronegative hydrogen bonding group. Thus, it appears that the cationic nitrogen moiety is more important than rotameric conformation of the catechol (hydrogen bonding) group in determining pharmacophore differences between dopamine D_1 and D_2 receptors.

Adjunct Therapy—Anticholinergic and Antihistamine Drugs

Cholinergic interneurons in the striatum exert mainly excitatory effects on GABAergic output from the striatum.

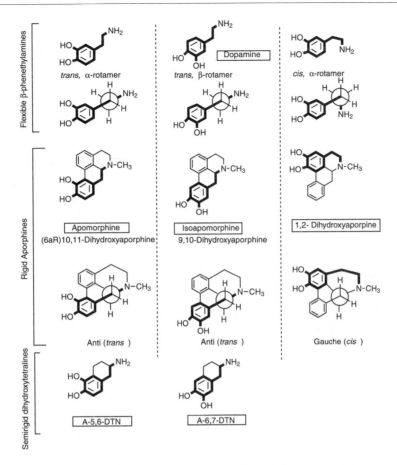

Fig. 20.10. Conformations of dopamine in the trans α-rotameric, trans β-rotameric, and cis α-rotameric forms and structural relationships to the rigid dopamine analogs apomorphine, isoapomorphine, and 1,2-dihydroxyaporphine. Also shown are the corresponding semirigid analogs of dopamine, the dihydroxytetralins, A-5,6-DTN and A-6,7-DTN.

Historically, it had been observed that drugs which increase cholinergic neurotransmission (e.g., the cholinesterase inhibitor physostigmine and the cholinergic agonist carbachol) aggravate parkinsonism in humans. Accordingly, before the discovery of levodopa, drug therapy for parkinsonism depended primarily on the limited efficacy of the natural belladonna alkaloids (e.g., atropine), which are cholinergic muscarinic receptor antagonists. With newer synthetic alkaloids (Table 20.1), attempts were made to increase central anticholinergic effects, as well as, to reduce undesirable peripheral effects, such as dry mouth, blurred vision, constipation, urinary retention, and tachycardia. Unfortunately the central nervous system side effects of these agents also are very troublesome and include delusions, hallucinations, somnolence, ataxia, and dysarthria. In general, anticholinergic drugs rarely produce more than 20% improvement, and, despite continued use, the symptoms of the disease continue to progress. The most important present usage of the anticholinergic agents is as adjunct therapy with L-dopa. The antihistamines, particularly those with central anticholinergic effects, are generally better tolerated in the elderly and may produce slightly greater relief from tremor, but this therapy is rarely used today.

SPASTICITY DISORDERS
Clinical Evaluation

Spasticity is characterized by skeletal muscle spasms and increase in tonic stretch reflexes, sometimes with accompanying muscle weakness. Spasticity often is associated with cerebral palsy, multiple sclerosis, spinal cord injury, or stroke. The mechanisms that underlie clinical spasticity appear to involve damage to descending pathways in the spinal cord that results in hyperexcitability of alpha motor neurons. A limiting factor in identifying the pathophysiology of spasticity is a lack of quantitative methodology to demonstrate neurophysiologic improvement in the drug treatment of spastic states in humans, as well as, accurate experimental models. Simple tests of muscle tone or reflex latency have not been fruitful, however, global clinical assessments, such as the number of painful spasms per day, have been more useful. Even the combined subjective impressions of improvement by patient, family, and physician, however, cannot establish that the drug is working. A straightforward strategy to establish whether a spasmolytic drug produces any benefit is gradual withdrawal of the drug (66). Nevertheless, the diversity of neurological disorders that culminate in spasticity and the subjectivity of many of the measurements make it difficult to establish the superiority of any one of the spasmolytic drugs

Table 20.1. Drugs Used for Parkinsonism

Class and Nonproprietary Name	Chemical Structure	Trade Name	Initial Single Oral Dose
Synthetic anticholinergic agents			
Benztropine mesylate		Cogentin	0.5–1.0 mg
Trihexyphenidyl hydrochloride		Artane Pipanol Tremin	1.0–2.0 mg
Procyclidine hydrochloride		Kemadrin	2.0–5.0 mg
Biperiden hydrochloride		Akineton	1.0–2.0 mg
Antihistamine			
Diphenhydramine hydrochloride		Benadryl	25.0 mg
Phenothiazine (Antihistamine)			
Ethopropazine hydrochloride		Parsidol	50.0 mg
Dopamine agonist Levodopa		Bendopa Dopar Larodopa	0.1–1.0 g

Table 20.1—continued

Class and Nonproprietary Name	Chemical Structure	Trade Name	Initial Single Oral Dose
Decarboxylase inhibitors Carbidopa (MK 486)		Sinemet (contains Levodopa)	
Benserazide hydrochloride			
Dopamine-releasing agent Amantadine hydrochloride		Symmetrel	100 mg

Clinical Applications: Radiopharmaceuticals in Diagnosis of Parkinson's Disease

Even for an experienced neurologist, a diagnosis of Parkinson's disease can be difficult to confirm, especially in the early stages of this disease. Disease progression is highly variable; the degree of disability can fluctuate dramatically, and no two people have exactly the same symptoms. In addition, there are a number of conditions that mimic Parkinson's disease, but cannot be treated effectively with antiparkinsonism drugs.

Imaging techniques are increasingly applied to neuropharmacologic studies of brain function. Positron emission tomography (PET) and single photon emission computed tomography (SPECT) are sensitive methods which can be used in such studies. Though spatial resolution remains somewhat greater with PET, several advantages are offered by SPECT technology. Positron emitting nuclides have such short half-lives (^{11}C, 20 min; ^{18}F, 109 min) that they usually require an on-site cyclotron for their production, whereas, SPECT nuclides have longer half-lives (^{123}I, 13 hr) so that they can be supplied commercially. Quantitative assessment of nigrostriatal presynaptic dopaminergic nerve terminal function also has been a useful diagnostic tool for the early diagnosis of Parkinson's disease (60). Previously, 6-[^{18}F]fluoro-L-dopa ([^{18}F]-DOPA) has been used in PET to assess dopamine nerve terminal function in human brain. Meanwhile, it has been known for some time that cocaine and its radiolabeled derivatives bind to the dopamine neurotransporter located on presynaptic dopaminergic nerve terminals. Researchers have investigated whether it might be possible to image these dopamine neurotransporter proteins using radiolabeled analogs of cocaine (61). Although radiolabeled cocaine analogs have been shown to bind to the neurotransporter, rapid hydrolysis of its benzoyl ester function limits its use in SPECT imaging. By removal of the ester group and directly linking the phenyl ring to the heterocyclic ring system, more stable tropane molecules are obtained which can be radiolabeled for imaging purposes.

Phenyltropanes used for imaging the dopamine neurotransporter and their relationship to cocaine.

The first radiopharmaceutical to emerge from this research, [^{123}I]2-β-carbomethoxy-3β-(4-iodophenyl)tropane, is known as [^{123}I]β-CIT or RTI-55 (62,63); [^{123}I]β-CIT contains a radioactive iodine atom in the *para* position of the phenyl ring. [^{123}I]-β-CIT, however, requires 8 hours for peak uptake prior to imaging. Thus, Neumeyer and coworkers (64) developed the N-3-fluoropropyl analog of β-CIT, known as [^{123}I]FP-CIT, which has the advantage of more favorable kinetics for clinical use since the patient can be imaged 1–2 hours after injection of the isotope. Moreover, a radioligand suitable for PET imaging is obtained by replacing the fluorine atom of the fluoropropyl group with [^{18}F] and replacing the [^{123}I] atom with iodine in FP-CIT (65). Both [^{123}I]-β-CIT and [^{123}I]-FP-CIT are being studied in patients with Parkinson's disease and DAT Scan has been approved for clinical use in Europe.

(67). Furthermore, spasm frequently coexists with pain and spasmolytic drug efficacy may be related to both skeletal muscle relaxation and analgesia (68).

Spasmolytic Drugs
Skeletal Muscle Relaxants

The spasmolytic drugs are diverse in their chemical structures and their sites and mechanisms of action. The first drug recognized to exhibit spasmolytic activity was antodyne or 3-phenoxy-1,2-propanediol. In guinea pigs and rabbits, antodyne produced prolonged paralysis without impairing consciousness. Antodyne was introduced into clinical medicine in 1910 as an analgesic and antipyretic. The duration of its skeletal muscle relaxant effect, however, was too short-lived to be clinically useful. In 1943, SAR studies of a series of simple glyceryl ethers related to antodyne, led to the development and introduction of mephenesin (3-[o-toloxy]-1,2-propanediol; Table 20.2) in 1946 (69). Pharmacologic studies revealed that mephenesin selectivity depressed polysynaptic while sparing monosynaptic spinal cord reflexes. Because of its safety and selective action on the spinal cord, mephenesin became the first widely prescribed centrally acting skeletal muscle relaxant. Accordingly, mephenesin is the prototype of the interneuronal blocking type of muscle relaxant.

The efficacy of propanediol carbamates in treatment of spasticity is difficult to assess because of the lack of well-controlled clinical studies. These agents largely have been replaced by diazepam, sedatives, or analgesics. The pharmacology of the mephenesin-like muscle relaxants is remarkably similar to that of the sedative-hypnotics. Indeed, the only apparent difference is that the spasmolytics have greater selectivity for modulating effects mediated by the spinal cord, thus, producing less sedation than general sedative-hypnotics. Nevertheless, both classes produce a reversible nonspecific depression of the central nervous system.

Several other compounds with mephenesin-like pharmacologic profiles, some longer-lasting, were developed and marketed as muscle relaxants. These include chlorphenesin carbamate, methocarbamol, meprobamate, carisoprodol, metaxalone, chlorzoxazone, orphenadrine, and cyclobenzaprine (Table 20.2). Most of these drugs are promoted for relief of acute muscle spasm caused by local trauma or strain and are not effective in treating spasms associated with cerebral palsy or spinal cord injuries (67). Most are centrally acting sedatives, some with mainly antihistamine (i.e., orphenadrine) or antimuscarinic (i.e., cyclobenzaprine) activity.

Diazepam (Valium)

The second group of antispastic drugs to be developed are the benzodiazepines, diazepam in particular. Diazepam exerts its skeletal muscle relaxant effect by binding as an agonist at the benzodiazepine receptor (BZR) of the $GABA_A$ receptor complex which enhances GABA potency to increase chloride conductance (see Chapter 17). Diazepam probably has both supraspinal and spinal sites

of spasmolytic action; its actions are sufficient to relieve spasticity in patients with lesions affecting the spinal cord and occasionally in patients with cerebral palsy (70). Diazepam is effective in the treatment of spasticity as well as nonspastic disorders (e.g., tetanus), however, diazepam produces sedation in most patients at doses required to significantly reduce muscle tone.

Baclofen

Baclofen (Lioresal, generic)

In an attempt to elevate GABA activity in the brain more directly, the GABA structural analog baclofen (β-[4-chlorophenyl]GABA) was developed. In contrast to GABA, baclofen is lipophilic, completely absorbed after oral administration, and penetrates the blood-brain barrier. Baclofen appears to act as an agonist at $GABA_B$ receptors, causing neuronal hyperpolarization in the brain and spinal cord to reduce the release of excitatory neurotransmitters (67). It may also reduce pain in patients with spasticity by inhibiting release of substance-P in the spinal cord (70). Baclofen is at least as effective as diazepam in reducing spasticity and produces less sedation; intrathecal administration via an implanted infusion pump is used to control severe spasticity and pain that is not responsive to medication given by oral or other parenteral routes. Baclofen is effective in the treatment of spasticity in paraplegia and quadriplegia, patients with multiple sclerosis, and traumatic lesion to the spinal cord (70).

Dantrolene sodium

Dantrolene (Dantrium)

Dantrolene is a hydantoin derivative that acts peripherally to reduce spasticity. The site of action of dantrolene is believed to be at the sarcoplasmic reticulum in skeletal muscle cells (66). Dantrolene binds to a calcium channel protein (called the ryanodine receptor) on the sarcoplasmic reticulum to close the channel and inhibit release of calcium; the alkaloid ryanodine activates the same receptor to open the channel. Cardiac muscle and smooth muscle are minimally affected by dantrolene, perhaps because calcium release from sarcoplamic reticulum of these muscle cell types occurs via a mechanism that differs from skeletal muscle. The muscle relaxant effect of dantrolene on skeletal muscle, however, is not specific and generalized muscle weakness occurs as a major adverse side effect. Like other hydantoins, dantrolene is a weak base (pKa = 7.5) that can cross the blood-brain barrier, thus, central nervous system depressant side effects (e.g., sedation) are common. Dantrolene sodium salt is slowly absorbed from the gastrointestinal tract. The mean half-life of the drug in adults is about 9 hours after a 100-mg dose. It is slowly metabolized by the liver to give the 5-hydroxy and ac-

Table 20.2. Skeletal Muscle Relaxants

Class and Nonproprietary Name	Chemical Structure	Trade Name	Single Dose
Glycerol monoethers and derivatives Mephenesin			1–2 g (oral)
Chlorphenesin carbamate		Maolate	800 mg (oral)
Methocarbamol		Robaxin	1–2 g (oral) 500 mg IM 1–3 g daily (IV)
Substituted alkanediols and derivatives Meprobamate		Equanil Miltown	400 mg
Carisoprodol		Rela Soma	250–350 mg
Metaxalone		Skelaxin	800 mg
Benzazole Chlorzoxazone		Paraflex	250–750 mg
Miscellaneous Orphenadrine citrate		Norflex	100 mg (oral) 60 mg IM or IV
Cyclobenzaprine		Flexaril	10 mg

etamido (nitro reduction and acetylation) metabolites, as well as, unchanged drug excreted in the urine. Interestingly, dantrolene is also valuable in alleviating the signs of malignant hyperthermia. This rare genetically determined condition, which can be triggered by a variety of stimuli including inhalation anesthetics and neuromuscular blocking drugs, involves an impaired ability of the sarcoplasmic reticulum to sequester calcium. For treating malignant hyperthermia, dantrolene is administered intravenously.

Acknowledgement. The authors wish to express their gratitude to Dr. Ross J. Baldessarini for reviewing this chapter manuscript.

CASE STUDY

Victoria F. Roche and S. William Zito

You are a 25-year-old, second-year pharmacy student working two jobs trying to put yourself through school. Last weekend you strained a muscle in your lower back unloading a truck of stock for the pharmacy at which you work as an intern. You have considerable pain, but can't take aspirin because you have a hypersensitivity to it. The acetaminophen you've been taking isn't helping you feel any better, and you are hesitant to take other OTC NSAIDs due to the aspirin sensitivity. In addition, you experience difficulty sitting for long periods of time. This obviously is cramping your study habits. Your physician, knowing that you are taking medicinal chemistry, challenges you to evaluate the following choices and recommend your own treatment!

1. Identify the therapeutic problem(s) where the pharmacist's intervention may benefit the patient.

2. Identify and prioritize the patient specific factors that must be considered to achieve the desired therapeutic outcomes.

3. Conduct a thorough and mechanistically oriented structure-activity analysis of all therapeutic alternatives provided in the case.

4. Evaluate the SAR findings against the patient specific factors and desired therapeutic outcomes and make a therapeutic decision.

5. Counsel your patient.

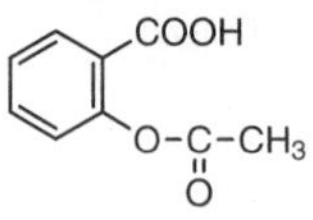

Aspirin

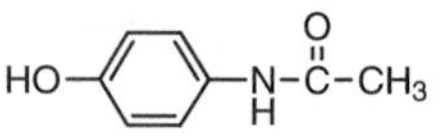

Acetaminophen

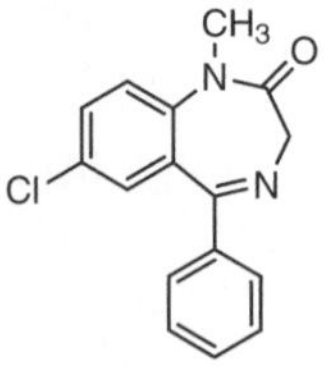

1 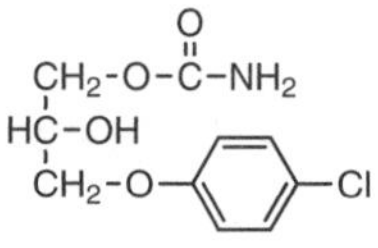   2 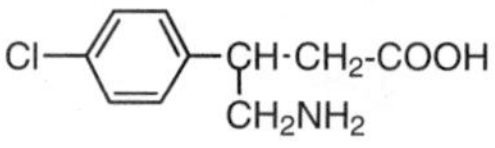   3 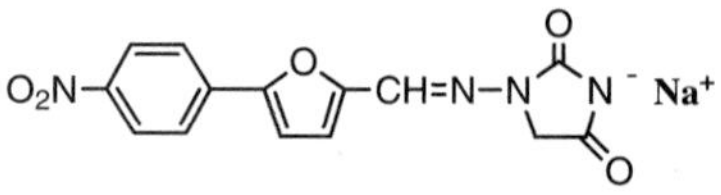   4

REFERENCES

1. Lang AE, Lozano AM. Parkinson's disease, part 1. New Eng J Med 1998; 339:1044–1053.
2. Forno LS. The neuropathology of Parkinson's disease. In Marsden CD, Fahn S, eds. Movement Disorders. London: Butterworth Scientific, 1982:25–40.
3. Lang AE, Lozano AM. Parkinson's disease, part 2. New Eng J Med 1998; 339:1130–1143.
4. Semchuk KM, Love EJ, Lee RG. Parkinson's disease: a test of the multifactorial etiologic hypothesis. Neurology 1993; 43:1173–1180.
5. Polymeropoulos MH, Lavedan C, Leroy E, et al. Mutation in the alpha-synuclein gene identified in families with Parkinson's disease. Science 1997; 276:2045–2047.
6. Kruger R, Kuhn W, Muller T, et al. Ala30Pro mutation in the gene encoding alpha-synuclein in Parkinson's disease. Nature Genetics 1998; 18:106–108.
7. Goedert M. Familial Parkinson's disease. The awakening of alpha-synuclein. Nature 388:232–233 (1997).
8. Gasser T, Muller-Myhsok B, Wszolek ZK, et al. Genetic complexity and Parkinson's disease. Science 1997; 277:388–389.
9. Scott WK, Staijich JM, Yamaoka LH, et al. Genetic complexity and Parkinson's disease. Deane Laboratory Parkinson Disease Research Group. Science 1997; 277:387–388.
10. Ward CD, Duvoisin RC, Ince SE, et al. Parkinson's disease in 65 pairs of twins and in a set of quadruplets. Neurology 1983; 33:815–824.
11. Duvoisin RC. The cause of Parkinson's disease. In Marsden CD, Fahn S, eds. Movement Disorders. London: Butterworth Scientific, 1982:8–24.
12. Gajdusek DC, Salazar AM. Amyotrophic lateral sclerosis and parkinsonian syndromes in high incidence among the Auyu and Jakai people of West New Guinea. Neurology 1982; 32:107–126.
13. Cotzias GC. Manganese in health and disease. Physiol Rev 1958; 38:503–532.
14. Barbeau A, Roy M, Cloutier T, et al. Environmental risk and gentic factors in the etiology of Parkinson's disease. In Yahr M, Bergmann K, eds. Advances in neurology. Vol 45. New York: Raven Press, 1986.
15. Kessler II, Diamond EL. Epidemiologic studies of Parkinson's disease. I. Smoking and Parkinson's disease: a survey and explanatory hypothesis. Am J Epidemiol 1971; 94:16–25.
16. Yu PH, Boulton AA. Irreversible inhibition of monoamine oxidase by some components of cigarette smoke. Life Sci 1987; 41:675–682.
17. Langston JW, Irwin I, Ricaurte GA. Neurotoxins, parkinsonism and Parkinson's disease. Pharmacology and Therapeutics 1987; 32:19–49.
18. Haber F, Weiss J. Naturwissenschaften 1932; 5:45–92.
19. Graham DG, Tiffany SM, Bell WR Jr, et al. Autoxidation versus covalent binding of quinones as the mechanism of toxicity of dopamine, 6-hydroxydopamine, and related compounds toward C1300 neuroblastoma cells in vitro. Mol Pharmacol 1978; 14:644–653.
20. Graham DG. Catecholamine toxicity: a proposal for the molecular pathogenesis of manganese neurotoxicity and Parkinson's disease. Neurotoxicology 1984; 5:83–95.
21. Calne DB, Langston JW, Martin WR, et al. Positron emission tomography after MPTP: observations relating to the cause of Parkinson's disease. Nature 1985; 317:246–248.
22. Carlsson A, Winblad B. Influence of age and time interval between death and autopsy on dopamine and 3-methoxytyramine levels in human basal ganglia. J Neural Transmission 1976; 38:271–276.
23. Riederer P, Woketich S. Time course of nigrostriatal degeneration in parkinson's disease. A detailed study of influential factors in human brain amine analysis. J Neural Transmission 1976; 38:277–301.
24. Davis GC, Williams AC, Markey SP, et al. Chronic Parkinsonism secondary to intravenous injection of meperidine analogues. Psychiatric Res 1979; 1:249–254.
25. Langston JW, Ballard P, Tetrud JW, et al. Chronic Parkinsonism in humans due to a product of meperidine-analog synthesis. Science 1983; 219:979–980.
26. Burns RS, Chiueh CC, Markey SP, et al. A primate model of parkinsonism: selective destruction of dopaminergic neurons in the pars compacta of the substantia nigra by N-methyl-4-phenyl-1,2,3,6-tetrahydropyridine. Proc Natl Acad Sci USA 1983; 80:4546–4550.
27. Chiba K, Trevor A, Castagnoli N Jr. Metabolism of the neurotoxic tertiary amine, MPTP, by brain monoamine oxidase. Biochem Biophys Res Comm 1984; 120:574–578.
28. Salach JI, Singer TP, Castagnoli N Jr, et al. Oxidation of the neurotoxic amine 1-methyl-4-phenyl-1,2,3,6-tetrahydropyridine (MPTP) by monoamine oxidases A and B and suicide inactivation of the enzymes by MPTP. Biochem Biophys Res Comm 1984; 125:831–835.
29. Peterson LA, Caldera PS, Trevor A, et al. Studies on the 1-methyl-4-phenyl-2,3-dihydropyridinium species 2,3-MPDP+, the monoamine oxidase catalyzed oxidation product of the nigrostriatal toxin 1-methyl-4-phenyl-1,2,3,6-tetrahydropyridine (MPTP). J Med Chem 1985; 28:1432–1436.
30. Langston JW, Irwin I, Langston EB, et al. Pargyline prevents MPTP-induced parkinsonism in primates. Science 1984; 225:1480–1482.
31. Snyder SH, D'Amato RJ. MPTP: a neurotoxin relevant to the pathophysiology of Parkinson's disease. The 1985 George C. Cotzias lecture. Neurology 1986; 36:250–258.
32. Yong VW, Perry TL. Monamine oxidase B, smoking, and Parkinson's disease. J Neurol Sci 1986; 72:265–272.
33. Nefzger MD, Quadfasel FA, Karl VC. A retrospective study of smoking in Parkinson's disease. Am J Epidemiol 1968; 88:149-158.
34. Behmand RA, Harik SI. Nicotine enhances 1-methyl-4-phenyl-1,2,36-tetrahydropyridine neurotoxicity. J Neurochem 1992; 58:776–779.
35. Shahi GS, Das PN, Moochhala SM. 1-Methyl-4-phenyl-1,2,36-tetrahydropyridine-induced neurotoxicity: partial protection against striato-nigral dopamine depletion in C57BL/6J mice by cigarette smoke exposure and by β-naphthoflavone-pretreatment. Neuroscience Letters 1991; 127:247–250.
36. Berry MD, Juorio AV, Paterson IA. The functional role of monoamine oxidases A and B in the mammalian central nervous system. Progress in Neurobiology 1994; 42:375–391.
37. Javitch JA, D'Amato RJ, Strittmatter SM, et al. Parkinsonism-inducing neurotoxin, N-methyl-4-phenyl-1,2,3,6-tetrahydropyridine: uptake of the metaboliteN-methyl-4-phenylpyridine by dopamine neurons explains selective toxicity. Proc Natl Acad Sci USA 1985; 82:2173–2177.
38. Vyas I, Heikkila RE, Nicklas WJ. Studies on the neurotoxicity of 1-methyl-4-phenyl-1,2,3,6-tetrahydropyridine: inhibition of NAD-linked substrate oxidation by its metabolite, 1-methyl-4-phenylpyridinium. J Neurochem 1986; 46:1501–1507.
39. Ramsay RR, McKeown KA, Johnson EA, et al. Inhibition of NADH oxidation by pyridine derivatives. Biochem Biophys Res Comm 1987; 146: 53–60.
40. Castagnoli N Jr, Rimoldi JM, Bloomquist J, et al. Potential metabolic bioactivation pathways involving cyclic tertiary amines and azaarenes. Chem. Res. Toxicol. 10:924-940 (1997).

41. Schapira AH, Mann VM, Cooper JM, et al. Mitochondrial function in Parkinson's disease. The Royal Kings and Queens Parkinson's Disease Research Group. Annals of Neuroloy 1992; 32:S116–124.

42. Mann VM, Cooper JM, Krige D, et al. Brain, skeletal muscle and platelet homogenate mitochondrial function in Parkinson's disease. Br Res 1992; 115:33–42.

43. The Parkinson's disease study group. Impact of tocopherol and deprenyl in DATATOP subjects not requiring levodopa. Annals of Neurology 1996; 39:29–36.

44. The Parkinson's disease study group. Impact of tocopherol and deprenyl in DATATOP subjects requiring levodopa. Annals of Neurology 1996; 39:37–45.

45. Rajput AH, Uitti RJ, Offord KO. Timely levodopa administration prolongs survival in Parkinson's disease. Parkinsonism and Related Disorders 1997; 3:159–165.

46. Cotzias GC, Van Woert MH, Schiffer LM. Aromatic amino acids and modification of parkinsonism. N Eng J Med 1967; 276: 374–379.

47. Nagatssu, T. In Biochemistry of Catecholamines, Baltimore: University Park Press, 1973:289.

48. Vogel WH. Determination and physiological disposition of p-methoxyphenylethylamine in the rat. Biochem Pharmacolo 1970; 19:2663–2665.

49. Miyawaki E, Lyons K, Pahwa R. Motor complications of chronic levodopa therapy in Parkinson's disease. Clin Neuropharmacol 1997; 20:523–530.

50. Heinonen EH, Lammintausta R. A review of the pharmacology of selegiline. Acta Neurologica Scandinavica Supplementum 1991; 136:44–59.

51. Kurth MC, Adler CH, St. Hilaire MS, et al. Tolcapone improves motor function and reduces levodopa requirement in patients with Parkinson's disease experiencing motor fluctuations: a multicenter, double-blind, randomized, placebo-controlled trial. Neurology 1997; 48:81–87.

52. Booth RG, Baldessarini RJ, Kula NS, et al. Presynaptic inhibition of dopamine synthesis in rat striatal tissue by enantiomeric mono- and dihydroxyaporphines. Mol Pharmacol 1990; 38: 92–101.

53. Neumeyer JL, Baldessarini RJ. Apomorphine: new uses for and old drug. Pharmaceutical News 1997; 4:12–16.

54. Giesecke J. The absolute configuration of apomorphine. Acta Cryst 1977; B33:302–303.

55. Neumeyer JL, McCarthy M, Battista S, et al. Aporphines 9. The synthesis and pharmacological evaluations of (±)-9,10-dihyroxyaporphine, ([±]-isoapomorphine), (±)-, (−)-, and (+)-1,2-dihydroxyaporphine, and (+)-1,2,9,10-tetrahydroxyaprophine. J Med Chem 1973; 16:1228.

56. Westerink, BHC, Dijkstra D, Feenstra MGP, et al. Dopaminergic prodrugs: brain concentrations and neurochemical effects of 5,6- and 6,7-ADTN after administration as dibenzoyl esters. Eur J Pharmacol 1980; 61:7–15.

57. Snyder SE, Aviles-Garay FA, Chakraborti R, et al. Synthesis and evaluation of 6,7-dihydroxy-2,3,4,8,9,13b-hexahydro-1H-benzo[6,7]cyclohepta[1,2,3-ef][3] benzazepine, 6,7-dihydroxy-1,2,3,4,8,12b-hexahydroanthr [10,4a,4-cd]azepine, and 10-(aminomethyl)-9,10-dihydro-1,2-dihydroxyanthracene as conformationally restricted analogs of beta-phenyldopamine. J Med Chem 1995; 38:2395–2409.

58. Craig JC, Torkelson SM, Findell PR, et al. Synthesis and dopaminergic activity of 2-substituted octahydrobenzo[f]quinolines. J Med Chem 1989; 32:961–968.

59. Wilcox RE, Tseng T, Brusniak MY, et al. CoMFA-based prediction of agonist affinities at recombinant D1 vs D2 dopamine receptors. J Med Chem 1998; 41:4385–4399.

60. Garnett ES, Firnau G, Chan PKH, et al. [18F]-Fluoro-dopa, and analogue of dopa, and its use in direct external measurements of storage, degradation, and turnover of intracerebral dopamine. Proc Natl Acad Sci USA 1978; 75:464–467.

61. Volkow N, Fowler J, Wang G, et al. Decreased dopamine transporters with age in healthy human subjects. Ann Neurol 1994; 36:237–239.

62. Neumeyer JL, Wang S, Milius R, et al. [123I]-2β-carbomethoxy-3β-(4-iodophenyl)tropane: High-affinity SPECT radiotracer of monoamine reuptake sites in brain. J Med Chem 1991; 34: 3144–3146.

63. Innis R, Seibyl J, Scanley B, et al. Single photon emission computed tomographic imaging demonstrates loss of striatal dopamine transporters in Parkinson disease. Proc Natl Acad Sci USA 1993; 90:11965–11969.

64. Neumeyer JL, Wang S, Gao Y, et al. N-(ω-Fluoroalkyl Analogs of (1R)-2βCarbomethoxy-3β-(4-Iodophenyl) tropane (β-CIT): Radiotracers for PET and SPECT Imaging of Dopamine Transporters. J Med Chem 1994; 37:1558–1561.

65. Ishikawa T, Dhawan V, Kazumata K, et al. Comparative Nigrotriatal Dopaminergic Imaging with [123I] β-CIT-FP/SPECT and [18F]F-DOPA/PET. J Nucl Med 1996; 37:1760–1765.

66. Young RR, Delwaide PJ. Drug therapy: spasticity (first of two parts). N Eng J Med 1981; 304:28–33.

67. Gracies JM, Nance P, Elovic E, et al. Traditional pharmacological treatments for spasticity. Part II: General and regional treatments. Muscle and Nerve Supplement 1997; 6:S92–120.

68. Elenbaas JK. Centrally acting oral skeletal muscle relaxants. Am J Hosp Pharm 1980; 37:1313–1323.

69. Berger FM, Bradley W. Br J Pharmacol Chemother 1946; 1:265.

70. Young RR, Delwaide PJ. Drug therapy: spasticity (second of two parts). N Eng J Med 1981; 304:96.

21. Cardiac Agents: Cardiac Glycosides, Antianginal, and Antiarrhythmic Drugs

AHMED S. MEHANNA

Heart diseases are grouped into three major disorders: cardiac failure, ischemia (with angina as its primary symptom) and cardiac arrhythmia.

CARDIAC GLYCOSIDES IN THE TREATMENT OF HEART FAILURE
Congestive Heart Failure

Cardiac failure can be described as inability of the heart to pump blood effectively at a rate that meets the needs of metabolizing tissues. This is the direct result of a reduced contractility of the cardiac muscles, especially those of the ventricles which causes a decrease in cardiac output, increasing the blood volume of the heart (hence the name congested). As a result, the systemic blood pressure and the renal blood flow are both reduced, which often lead to the development of edema in the lower extremities and the lung (pulmonary edema) as well as renal failure. A group of drugs known as the cardiac glycosides were found to reverse most of these symptoms and complications.

Cardiac Glycosides

The cardiac glycosides are an important class of naturally occurring drugs whose actions include both beneficial and toxic effects on the heart. Their desirable cardiotonic action is of particular benefit in the treatment of congestive heart failure and associated edema and their preparations have been used as medicinal agents as well as poisons since 1500 B.C. This dual application serves to highlight the toxic potential for this class of life-saving drugs. Despite the extended use and obvious therapeutic benefits of the cardiac glycosides, it was not until the famous monograph by William Withering in 1785, entitled "An Account of the Foxglove and Some of its Medical Uses," that cardiac glycoside therapy started to become

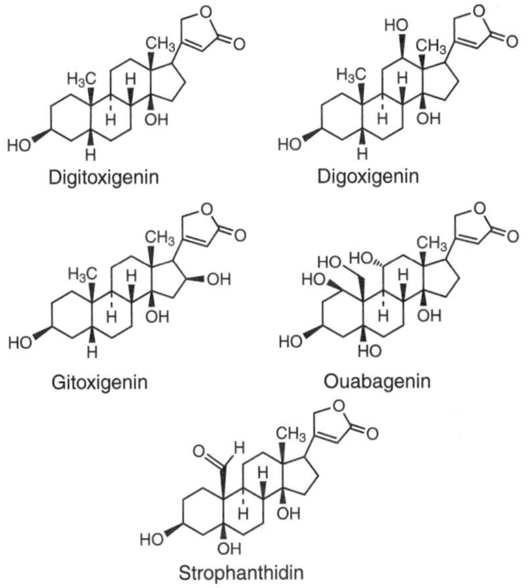

Fig. 21.2. Major cardenolide aglycones.

more standardized and rational (1,2). The therapeutic use of purified cardiac glycoside preparations has occurred only over the last century. Today the cardiac glycosides represent one of the most important drug classes available to the physician to treat congestive heart failure.

Chemistry of the Cardiac Glycosides

Cardiac glycosides and similar other glycosides are composed of two portions: the sugar and the non-sugar (the aglycone) moiety.

Aglycones. The aglycone portion of the cardiac glycosides is a steroid nucleus with a unique set of fused rings, which makes these agents easily distinguished from the other steroids. Rings A-B and C-D are cis fused, while rings B-C have a trans configuration. Such ring fusion gives the aglycone nucleus of cardiac glycosides the characteristic "U-shape" as shown in Figure 21.1. The steroid nucleus also carries, in most cases, two angular methyl groups at C-10 and C-13. Hydroxyl groups are located at C-3, the site of the sugar attachment, and at C-14. The C-14 hydroxyl is normally unsubstituted. However, additional hydroxyl groups may be found at C-12 and C-16, the presence or absence of which distinguishes the important genins: digitoxigenin, digoxigenin, and gitoxigenin (Fig. 21.2). These additional hydroxyl groups have significant impact on the partitioning and pharmacokinetics for each glycoside as

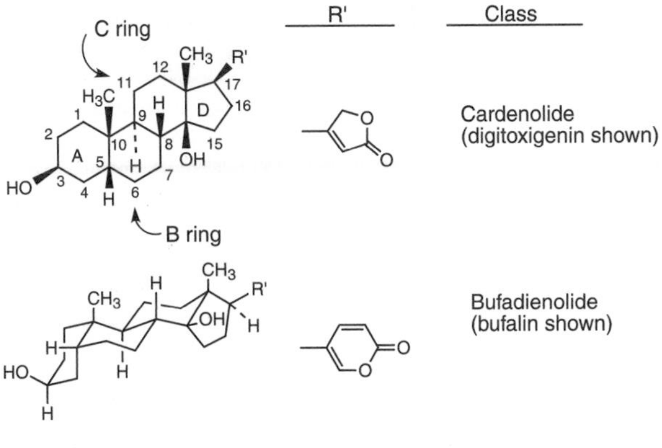

Fig. 21.1. Cardenolide and bufadienolide aglycones.

497

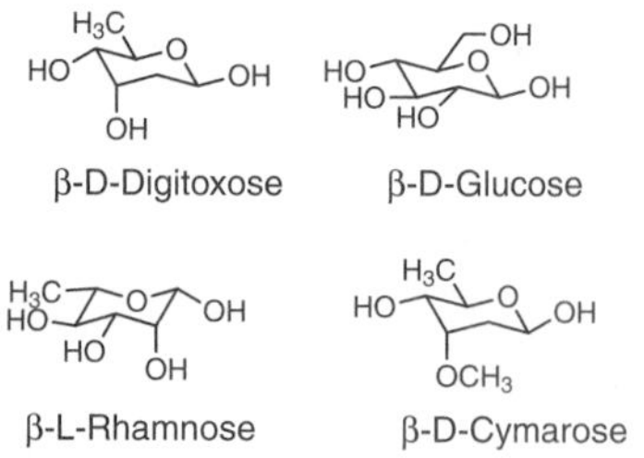

Fig. 21.3. Selected sugars found in naturally occurring cardiac glycosides.

discussed later. The lactone ring at C-17 is another major structural feature of the cardiac aglycones. The size and degree of unsaturation of the lactone ring varies with the source of the glycoside. In most cases, the cardiac glycosides of plant origin, the cardenolides, possess a five-membered α,β-unsaturated lactone ring, whereas those derived from animal origin, the bufadienolides, possess a six-membered lactone ring with two conjugated double bonds (generally referred to as α-pyrone) (see Fig. 21.1).

Sugars. The hydroxyl group at C-3 of the aglycone portion is usually conjugated to a monosaccharide or a polysaccharide with β-1,4-glucosidic linkages. The number and identity of sugars vary from one glycoside to another as detailed subsequently. The most commonly found sugars in the cardiac glycosides are D-glucose, D-digitoxose, L-rhamnose, and D-cymarose (Fig. 21.3). These sugars predominately exist in the cardiac glycosides in the β-conformation. In some cases, the sugars exist in the acetylated form. The presence of an O-acetyl group on a sugar greatly affects the lipophilic character and pharmacokinetics of the entire glycoside as discussed subsequently.

Sources and Common Names of Cardiac Glycosides

The cardiac glycosides occur mainly in plants and in rare cases in animals, such as poisonous toads. *Digitalis Purpurea* or the foxglove plant, *Digitalis Lanata, Strophan-*

thus Gratus, and *Strophanthus Kombe'* are the major plant sources of the cardiac glycosides. Based on the nature and number of sugar molecules and the number of hydroxyl groups on the aglycone moiety, each combination of sugars and aglycones assumes different generic names. The site of the glycosides concentration in the plant, types of glycosides, and the names of the structural components of these glycosides are summarized in Table 21.1.

Digitalis Lanata. Lanatoside A is composed of the aglycone digitoxigenin (genin indicates no sugar) connected to three digitoxose sugar molecules, the third of which carries a 3-acetyl group, and a terminal glucose molecule; i.e., the structure sequence is glucose$_4$-3-acetyldigitoxose$_3$-digitoxose$_2$-digitoxose$_1$-digitoxigenin.

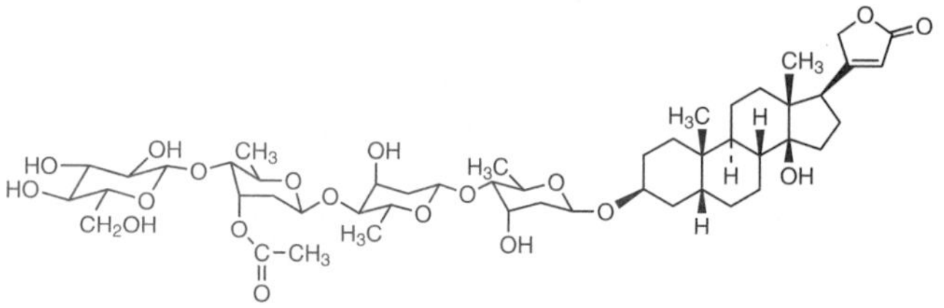

Lanatoside A

Lanatoside B has the identical sugar portion to Lanatoside A, except that the aglycone has extra hydroxyl group at C-16 and is given the name gitoxigenin. The structural sequence is glucose$_4$-3-acetyldigitoxose$_3$-digitoxose$_2$-digitoxose$_1$-gitoxigenin.

Lanatoside C also has the same sugars found in both lanatosides A and B; however, the aglycone has the nucleus of lanatoside A plus an additional hydroxyl group at C-12. This cardenolide is named digoxigenin. The structural sequence is glucose$_4$-3-acetyldigitoxose$_3$-digitoxose$_2$-digitoxose$_1$-digoxigenin.

Partial hydrolysis of the glucose molecule and the acetate group from the lanatosides A and C produces respectively two new and most important cardiac glycosides, digitoxin and digoxin with the following sequences: Digitoxin: (digitoxose)$_3$-digitoxigenin and digoxin: (digitoxose)$_3$-digoxigenin.

Table 21.1. Selected Natural Cardiac Glycosides and Their Sources

Source	Glycoside	Aglycone	Sugar*
Digitalis lanata (leaf)	Lanatoside A (digilanide A)	Digitoxigenin	Glucose-3-acetyldigitoxose-digitoxose-digitoxose
	Lanatoside B (digilanide B)	Gitoxigenin	
	Lanatoside C (digilanide C)	Digoxigenin	
Digitalis purpurea (leaf)	Purpurea glycoside A (desacetyl digilanide A)	Digitoxigenin	Glucose-digitoxose-digitoxose-digitoxose
	Purpurea glycoside B (desacetyl digilanide B)	Gitoxigenin	
Strophanthus gratus (seed)	G-Strophanthin	Oubagenin	Rhamnose
Strophanthus Kombe' (seed)	k-Strophanthoside	Strophanthidin	Glucose-Glucose-Cymarose

*Conjugated with the C-3 hydroxyl of the aglycone via the sugar to the far right. All sugars are conjugated via β-1,4–glucosidic bond.

Digitoxin

Digoxin

Digitalis Purpurea. Purpurea glycosides A and B have identical structures to the lanatosides A and B but with no acetyl group on the third digitoxose. Therefore, the purpurea glycosides A and B are sometimes called desacetyl digilanides A and B. Their sequences are as follows: Purpurea glycoside A: glucose-(digitoxose)₃-digitoxigenin and purpurea glycoside B: glucose-(digitoxose)₃-gitoxigenin. There is no purpurea glycoside C.

Strophanthus Gratus and Strophanthus Kombe'. The glycosides extracted from the plants *Strophanthus gratus* and *Strophanthus Kombe'* are called g-strophanthin (or ouabain) and k-strophanthoside, respectively. The corresponding aglycone for ouabain is ouabagenin and for k-strophanthoside is strophanthidin. Ouabagenin has a polyhydroxylated steroidal nucleus and strophanthidin has an additional hydroxyl group at C-5 with an angular aldehyde group at C-10, replacing the traditional methyl group at that position (see Fig. 21.2). Ouabagenin is conjugated only to a single molecule of L-rhamnose, whereas strophanthidin is conjugated to a molecule of cymarose, which is further linked to two molecules of glucose.

Ouabain

The medicinally used preparations are mainly obtained from *Digitalis purpurea* and *Digitalis lanata* plants. These glycosides are generally referred to as digitalis glycosides, cardiac glycosides or simply as cardenolides. Strophanthus glycosides (e.g., Ouabain) are no longer used therapeutically but had been previously administered only intravenously because of poor oral absorption. Cardiac glycosides from animal sources (generally referred to as

bufadienolides) are rare and of far less medicinal importance due to their high toxicity. Pharmaceutical preparations of whole plants and partially hydrolyzed glycosides of *Digitalis lanata* and *Digitalis purpurea* have been widely used clinically. The advancement in isolation and purification techniques, however, has made it possible to obtain highly purified digoxin preparations.

Pharmacology

Cardiac glycosides affect the heart in a dual fashion, both directly (on the cardiac muscle and the specialized conduction system of sinoatrial (S-A) node, atrioventricular (A-V) node and His-Purkinje system), and indirectly (on the cardiovascular system mediated by the autonomic nervous reflexes). The combined direct and indirect effects of the cardiac glycosides lead to changes in the electrophysiological properties of the heart, including alteration of the contractility; heart rate; excitability; conductivity; refractory period; and automaticity of the atrium, ventricle, Purkinje fibers, A-V node, and S-A node. The heart response to the cardiac glycosides is a dose dependent process and varies considerably between normal and the congestive heart failure (CHF) diseased heart. The effects observed after the administration of low doses (therapeutic doses) differ considerably from those observed at high doses (cardio-toxic doses). The pharmacologic effects discussed consequently relate mainly to therapeutic doses administered to CHF patients. The effects of cardiac glycosides on the properties of the heart muscle and different sites of the conduction system are summarized in Table 21.2. The increased force and rate of myocardial contraction (positive inotropic effect) and the prolongation of the refractory period of the A-V node are the most relevant effects to the CHF problem. Both of these effects are due to the direct action of the cardiac glycosides on the heart. The indirect effects are manifested as increased vagal nerve activity, which probably results from the glycoside-induced sensitization of the baroreceptors of the carotid sinus to changes in the arterial pressure; i.e., any given increase in the arterial blood pressure results in an increase in the vagal activity (parasympathetic) coupled with a greater decrease in the sympathetic activity. The vagal effect with uncompensated sympathetic response results in decreased heart rate, and decreased peripheral vascular resistance (afterload). Therefore, cardiac glyco-

Table 21.2. Effects of Cardiac Glycosides on the Heart*

	Atrium	Ventricle	Purkinje Fiber	A-V Node	A-S Node
Contractility	↑	↑	—	—	—
Excitability	0	Variable	↑	—	—
Conductivity	↑	↑	↓	↓	—
Refrac.period	↓	↓	↑	↑	—
Automaticity	—	—	↑	—	↓

*Modified from facts and comparisons.
↑ = increased action; ↓ = decreased action; 0 = no action; — = no data available.

sides reverse most of the symptoms associated with CHF as a result of increased sympathetic system activity, including increased heart rate, vascular resistance, and afterload. The administration of cardiac glycosides to a patient with CHF increases cardiac muscle contraction, reduces heart rate, and decreases both edema and the heart size.

Biochemical Mechanism of Action

The mechanism whereby cardiac glycosides cause a positive inotropic effect and electrophysiological changes is still not completely known despite years of active investigation. Several mechanisms have been proposed, but the most widely accepted mechanism involves the ability of cardiac glycosides to inhibit the membrane-bound Na^+, K^+ adenosine triphosphatase (Na^+, K^+ -ATPase) pump responsible for sodium/potassium exchange. To understand better the correlation between the pump and the mechanism of action of cardiac glycosides on the heart muscle contraction, one has to consider the sequence of events associated with cardiac action potential that ultimately leads to muscular contraction. The process of membrane depolarization/repolarization is controlled mainly by the movement of the three ions, Na^+, K^+, and Ca^{++}, in and out of the cell.

At the resting state (no contraction), the concentration of sodium is high outside the cell. On membrane depolarization, Na^+ fluxes-in, leading to an immediate elevation of the action potential. Elevated intracellular sodium triggers the influx of Ca^{++} which occurs slowly and is represented by the plateau region of the cardiac action potential. The influx of calcium results in efflux of potassium out of the myocardium. The Na^+/K^+ exchange occurs at later stage of the action potential to restore the membrane potential to its normal level (for further detail see antiarrhythmic agents and their classification at the end of this chapter). The Na^+/K^+ exchange requires energy and is catalyzed by the enzyme K^+, Na^+ATPase. Cardiac glycosides are proposed to inhibit this enzyme with a net result of reduced sodium exchange with potassium, i.e., increased intracellular sodium, which, in turn, results in increased intracellular calcium. Elevated intracellular calcium concentration triggers a series of intracellular biochemical events that ultimately result in an increase in the force of the myocardial contraction, or a positive inotropic effect. The events that lead to muscle contraction are discussed in further detail elsewhere in this chapter under the mechanism of action of the calcium channel blockers.

This mechanism of the cardiac glycosides via inhibiting the Na^+, K^+- ATPase pump is in agreement with the fact that the action of the cardiac glycosides is enhanced by low extracellular potassium and inhibited by high extracellular potassium. The cardiac glycosides- induced changes in the electrophysiology of the heart can also be explained based on the inhibition of Na^+, K^+ -ATPase. It has been suggested that the intracellular loss of potassium owing to inhibition of the pump causes a decrease in the cellular transmembrane potential approaching zero. This decrease in the membrane potential is sufficient to explain the increased excitability and other electrophysiological effects observed following cardiac glycosides administration.

Structural Requirements for Intrinsic Activity

Many hypotheses have been put forth to explain the cardiac glycoside structure-activity relationships (SAR). Some of the difficulty in arriving at a universally acceptable SAR model has been attributed to the early method of testing cardiac glycoside preparations and the lack of a well-characterized cardiac glycoside "receptors." Until the early 1970s, nearly, all the cardiac glycosides were evaluated based on their cardiac toxicity rather than on the more therapeutically relevant criteria. This was partly because of the belief that the cardiac toxicity was, in fact, an extension of the desired cardiotonic action. Thus, comparisons of cardiac glycoside preparations were based on the amount of drug required to cause cardiac arrest in test animals, usually anesthetized cats. More recently, most SAR studies rely, at least initially, on results obtained with isolated cardiac tissue or whole-heart preparations. In these models, inotropic activity, contractility, and so forth can be directly assessed. In addition, the recognition of cardiac Na^+, K^+ ATPase as the probable receptor for the cardiac glycosides has made the inhibition of this enzyme system an important criterion for the cardiac glycosides activity.

Much of the interest in the effects of structural modification on cardiotonic activity is due to the desire to develop agents with less toxic potential. Early studies based primarily on cardiac toxicity testing data suggested the importance of the steroid "backbone" shape, the 14-β-hydroxyl and the 17-unsaturated lactone for activity. More recent studies have been directed toward characterizing the interaction of the cardiac glycosides with Na^+, K^+ ATPase, the putative cardiac glycoside receptor. Using this enzyme model with enzyme inhibition as the biological end point, a number of hypotheses for cardiac glycoside receptor binding interactions have been put forth. Many of these suggested that the 17-lactone plays an important role in receptor binding. Using synthetic analogs, it was found that unsaturation in the lactone ring was important, with the saturated lactone analog showing diminished activity (3,4). Further investigations of synthetic compounds in which the lactone was replaced with open chain structures of varying electronic and steric resemblance to the lactone showed that, in fact, the α, β-unsaturated lactone ring at C-17 was not an absolute requirement and that several α, β-unsaturated open chain groups could be replaced with little or no loss in activity (3,4). For example, analogs possessing an α, β-unsaturated nitrile at the 17-β position had high activity. In light of this, most current theories point to a key interaction of the carbonyl oxygen (or nitrile nitrogen) with the cardiac glycoside binding site on Na^+, K^+ ATPase (5,6). Some controversy, however, exists over this point. The importance of the "rest" of the cardiac glycoside molecule must not be ignored. Despite the apparently dominant role of the 17-lactone, it is the steroid (A-B-C-D) ring system that provides the lead structure for cardiac glycoside activity. Lactones alone, when not attached to the steroid ring system, show no Na^+, K^+ ATPase inhibitory activity. Some important steroid structural features have become apparent. The C-D cis ring juncture appears critical for activity in compounds possessing the unsaturated butyrolactone in the normal 17-β position. This apparent requirement may be a reflection of changes in the spatial orientation of the 17-substituent (6). Moreover, the 14-β-OH is now believed to be dispensable. The contribution to activity previously attributed to this group is now thought to be related to the need to retain the sp^3 and cis character of the C-D ring juncture. The earlier interpretation arose from the fact that 14-deoxy analogues often had unsaturation in the D ring in place of the 14-OH. This double bond markedly influenced the position of the C-17 substituent, thereby complicating interpretation of 14-OH group importance. Finally, the A-B cis ring juncture also appears not to be mandatory for cardiac glycosides activity. This feature, however, is characteristic of all clinically useful cardiac glycosides, and conversion to an A-B trans ring system generally leads to a marked drop in activity, unless compensating modifications are made elsewhere in the molecule.

Pharmaceutical Preparations

The cardiac glycoside preparations that have been used range from powdered digitalis leaf to purified individual glycosides, including gitalin, lanatoside C, its partially hydrolyzed product deslanatoside C (desacetyl lanatoside C), digoxin, and ouabain. Currently, digoxin is the only cardiac glycoside commercially available for therapeutic use in the U.S. Dosage forms and adult doses for digoxin are summarized in Table 21.3.

To arrive at an effective plasma concentration, often a large initial dose (i.e., digitalizing or loading dose) is given (Table 21.3). The purpose of this large initial dose is to achieve a therapeutic blood and tissue level in the shortest possible time. Depending on the condition of the patient and the desired therapeutic goal, the loading dose may be much less than the dose likely to cause toxicity, or almost equal to it. Once the desired effect is obtained, the amount of drug lost from the body per day is replaced with a maintenance dose. For digoxin, this is approximately 35% of the total body store (Table 21.3).

Absorption, Metabolism, and Excretion of Digoxin

The therapeutic effects of all cardiac glycosides on the heart are qualitatively similar; however, the glycosides largely differ in their pharmacokinetic properties. The latter are greatly influenced by the lipophilic character of each glycoside. In general, cardiac glycosides with more lipophilic character are absorbed faster and exhibit longer duration of action as a result of a slower urinary excretion rate. The lipophilicity of a cardiac glycoside is measured by its partitioning between chloroform and water mixed with methanol. The higher is the concentration of the cardiac glycoside in the chloroform phase the higher will be its partition coefficient, and the more lipophilic it is. The partition coefficients for five cardiac glycosides are listed in Table 21.4. It is evident from a comparison of the coefficients that their lipophilicity is markedly influenced by the number of sugar molecules and the number of hydroxyl groups on the aglycone part of a given glycoside. Lanatoside C with a partition coefficient of 16.2 is far less lipophilic than that of acetyldigoxin (98), which structurally differs only in lacking the terminal glucose molecule. Likewise, a comparison of digitoxin and digoxin structures reveals that they differ only by an extra hydroxyl in digoxin at C-12. This seemingly minor difference in their partition coefficients from 96.5 to 81.5 for digitoxin and digoxin, respectively,

Table 21.3. Cardiac Glycosides and Their Dosage Forms

Name	Dosage Forms	Typical Dosages*
Digoxin USP and BP	Tablets: 0.125, 0.25, 0.5 mg; elixir, pediatric: 0.05 mg/mL; injection: 2 mL ampules, 0.25 mg/mL; injection, pediatric: 1 mL ampules, 0.1 mg/mL	Loading Dose: IV, 0.5–1.0 mg total in increments of 0.25 mg at 6 hour intervals; or loading: oral, 0.75–1.5 mg total in increments of 0.25–0.5 mg cautiously every 8 hours; maintenance, IV, 0.125–0.5 mg/day; or maintenance, oral, 0.125–0.5 mg/day
Digitalis Powder (Leaf) BP	Tablets: 32.5, 48, 75, 65, 100 mg; capsules: 100 mg	Loading Dose: 1.2 g total in divided doses at 6 hour intervals; maintenance: 100–200 mg/day
Digitoxin BP	Tablets: 0.05, 0.1, 0.1, 0.2 mg; injection: 1mL ampules, 0.2 mg/mL	Loading dose: 0.8–1.2 mg total oral or IV (starting with 0.6 mg, then 0.4 mg at six hours and 0.2 mg every six hours thereafter as needed); maintenance: 0.05–0.2 mg orally per day
Lanatoside C BP	Tablets: 0.5 mg	Loading Dose: 3.5 mg on 1st day, 2.5 mg on second day, 2 mg on third day, then 1.5 mg/day until digitalized; maintenance: 0.5–1.5 mg/day
Ouabain BP (G-Strophanthin)	Injection: 2 mL ampules, 0.25 mg/mL	Loading Dose: IV, 0.25 mg followed by 0.1 mg hourly until desired effect. Ouabain is not suitable for maintenance therapy
Deslanatoside C BP (desacetyl lanatoside C)	Injection: 2 mL ampules, 0.2 mg/mL	Loading Dose: 1.6 mg IV or 1.6 mg IM at two different sites; not appropriate for maintenance therapy

Those cardiac glycosides with only BP (British Pharmacopeia) designation are available only in Canada and other countries except the United States.
*All dosages are subject to modification according to patient condition and response.

Table 21.4. Effect of Glycoside Structure on Partition Coefficient

Glycoside	Partition Coefficient (CHCl$_3$/16% aq.MeOH)
Lanatoside C (glucose-3-acetyldigitoxose–digitoxose$_2$–digoxigenin)	16.2
Digoxin (digitoxose$_3$-digoxigenin)	81.5
Digitoxin (digitoxose$_3$-digitoxigenin)	96.5
Acetyldigoxin (3-acetyldigitoxose-digitoxose$_2$-digoxigenin)	98.0
G-Strophanthin (rhamnose-ouabagenin)	very low

results in significant differences in their pharmacokinetic behavior (Table 21.5). Table 21.4 also illustrates that the presence of the 3-O-acetyl group on acetyldigoxin enhances its lipophilic character more than that of desacetyl analog, digoxin (partition coefficients of 98 and 81.5, respectively). The glycoside G-strophanthin (ouabain), possesses a very low lipophilic character owing to the presence of five free hydroxyl groups on the steroid nucleus of the aglycone ouabagenin.

Digoxin is the most frequently used cardiac glycoside. The absorption of digoxin from the gastrointestinal tract is a passive process that depends on its lipid solubility, dissolution and membrane permeability of the drug. The oral bioavailability of digoxin following oral administration exhibits interindividual variability, ranging from 70–85% of an administered dose. Although digoxin is not extensively metabolized, it is known to be transported from intestinal enterocytes along its epithelium into the intestinal lumen (effluxed) by P-glycoprotein (P-gp), which is also expressed in the kidney and liver. This interindividual variability has been attributed to intestinal P-gp efflux and P-gp dependent renal elimination. Alterations in P-gp transport may be the basis for several digoxin-drug interactions. For this reason, it is important to establish carefully the effective dose of digoxin for each patient to avoid digitalis toxicity.

Once the cardiac glycosides are absorbed, they bind to plasma proteins; digoxin has only 30% binding. The half-life of digoxin in patients with normal renal function is 1.5–2 days. Biliary excretion of digoxin is minimal. Digoxin is primarily eliminated unchanged by renal tubule excretion.

Contributing to the discontinuance of digitoxin as a therapeutic agent was a half-life range between 5 and 7 days because of its enterohepatic circulation. Approximately 25% of an absorbed dose of digitoxin is excreted in the bile unchanged to be reabsorbed via enterohepatic circulation. Digitoxin, however, is extensively metabolized by the liver to a variety of metabolites, (digitoxose)$_2$-digitoxigenin, (digitoxose)$_1$-digitoxigenin and (digitoxose)$_1$-digitoxigenin. Trace amounts of digoxin have been discovered in the urine. The pharmacokinetic data for digoxin and digitoxin is summarized in Table 21.5.

Drug Interactions

Digoxin-drug interactions are common causes of digitalis toxicity. Recently, the clinical significance of the renal tubular secretion of digoxin associated with the well documented digoxin-quinidine has been reported (29). The discovery that digoxin is actively secreted into the urine by the renal tubular cell via the P-gp efflux pump has led to the conclusion that the digoxin-quinidine interaction can be attributed to inhibition of renal tubular secretion of digoxin by quinidine (a P-gp substrate). Quinidine competitively binds to P-gp in the renal tubule reducing the renal secretion of digoxin by as much as 60%, raising digoxin's plasma concentration to toxic levels. Other drugs that are substrates for renal P-gp are also likely to be associated with digoxin-drug interactions. Another documented digoxin-drug interaction associated with increased digoxin blood levels and toxicity is with verapamil. Verapamil, unlike quinidine, inhibits intestinal P-gp efflux of digoxin, thereby blocking the intestinal secretion of digoxin into the lumen of the intestine, and raising digoxin blood levels to toxic levels. On the other hand, the rifampin-digoxin drug interaction involves the rifampin induction of intestinal P-gp expression, thereby increasing the P-gp mediated secretion of digoxin. This results in the lowering of digoxin blood levels to subtherapeutic concentrations. P-gp transporters and their substrates, inhibitors or inducers (see Table 8.16 for list) appear to play an important role in controlling the digoxin AUC values through the renal tubular and intestinal secretion of digoxin, and subsequently to digoxin-drug interactions and digitalis toxicity. Concurrent use of the cardiac glycosides with antiarrhythmics, sympathomimetics, β-adrenergic blockers, and calcium channel blockers that are substrates for P-gp may alter control of arrhythmias.

The absorption of digoxin after oral administration can also be significantly altered by other drugs concurrently present in the gastrointestinal tract. For example, laxatives may interfere with the absorption of digoxin because of increased intestinal motility. The presence of the drug cholestyramine, an agent used to treat hyperlipoproteinemia, decreases the absorption of digoxin by binding to

Table 21.5. Comparison of the Pharmacokinetic Properties for Digoxin and Digitoxin

	Digoxin	Digitoxin
Gastrointestinal absorption	70–85%	95–100%
Average half life	1–2 days	5–7 days
Protein binding	25–30%	90–95%
Entero-hepatic cycling	5%	25%
Excretion	Kidneys; largely unchanged	Liver metabolism
Therapeutic plasma level	0.5–2.5 ng/ml	20–35 ng/ml
Digitalizing dose (mg)	Oral: 0.75–1.5 IV: 0.5–1.0	Oral: 0.8–1.2 IV: 0.8–1.2
Maintenance dose (oral mg)	0.125–0.5	0.05–0.2

and retaining digoxin in the gastrointestinal tract. Antacids, especially magnesium trisilicate, and antidiarrheal adsorbent suspensions may also inhibit the absorption of the digoxin. Potassium depleting diuretics, such as thiazides, may increase the possibility of digitalis toxicity owing to the additive hypokalemia. Several other drugs which are known to bind to plasma proteins, such as thyroid hormones, have the potential to displace digoxin from its plasma-binding sites, thereby increasing its free drug concentration to a toxic level.

Therapeutic Uses

Although the primary clinical use for digoxin is for the treatment of congestive heart failure, this agent is also used in cases of atrial flutter or fibrillation, and paroxysmal atrial tachycardia.

Toxicity

All cardiac glycosides preparations have the potential to cause toxicity. Because the minimal toxic dose of the glycosides is only two to three times the therapeutic dose, intoxication is quite common. In mild-to-moderate toxicity, the common symptoms are: anorexia, nausea and vomiting, muscular weakness, bradycardia, and ventricular premature contractions. The nausea is a result of excitation of the chemoreceptor trigger zone (CTZ) in the medulla. In severe toxicity, the common symptoms are: blurred vision, disorientation, diarrhea, ventricular tachycardia, and AV block, which may progress into ventricular fibrillation. It is generally accepted that the toxicity of the cardiac glycosides is due to inhibition of the Na^+/K^+-ATPase pump, which results in increased intracellular levels of Ca^{++}. Hypokalemia (decreased potassium), which can be induced by co-administration of thiazide diuretics, glucocorticoids, or by other means can be an important factor in initiating a toxic response. It has been shown that low levels of extracellular K^+ partially inhibit the Na^+, K^+-ATPase pump. In a patient stabilized on a cardiac glycoside, the Na^+, K^+-ATPase pump is already partially inhibited, and the hypokalemia only further inhibits the pump, causing an intracellular buildup of sodium, which leads to an increase in intracellular calcium levels. The high levels of calcium are responsible for the observed cardiac arrhythmias characteristic of the cardiac glycosides toxicity.

A common procedure used in treating cardiac glycosides toxicity is to administer potassium salts to increase extracellular potassium level, which stimulates the Na^+, K^+-ATPase pump, resulting in decreased intracellular sodium levels and thus decreased intracellular calcium. In treating any cardiac glycoside-induced toxicity, it is important to discontinue administration of the drug, in addition to administering a potassium salt. Other drugs that may be useful in treating the tachyarrhythmias present during toxicity are lidocaine, phenytoin, and propranolol. Specific antibodies directed toward digoxin (Dig-Bind) have been used experimentally and proven very effective.

Additional Positive Inotropic Agents

Inamrinone and Milrinone. Although the digitalis glycosides may be the principal therapeutic agents for the treatment of congestive heart failure, they are not the only positive inotropic agents available. Among several types of "non glycoside" inotropic agents, a few have emerged as potentially useful drugs (7). The first of these agents was inamrinone (formerly known as amrinone; name changed in 2000) (Fig. 21.4), introduced in 1978. Inamrinone produces both positive inotropic and concentration-dependent vasodilatory effects. Despite similar positive inotropic action of the cardiac glycosides, inamrinone appears to act through a distinctly different mechanism. This agent and related compounds are thought to elicit their effects by the inhibition of a specific phosphodiesterase (phosphodiesterase fraction III) in the myocardium. This inhibition leads to elevated levels of cAMP, which through a complex chain of biochemical events leads to an increase in the intracellular Ca^{++} and ultimately an increase in muscle contractility. Inamrinone was approved in 1984 by the FDA for short-term intravenous administration in patients with severe heart failure refractory to other measures. The compound undergoes some conjugative metabolism in the liver and is excreted in the urine. Although inamrinone is orally active, several adverse side effects have dampened enthusiasm for long-term oral inamrinone therapy. These effects include gastrointestinal disturbances, thrombocytopenia, and impairment of the liver function.

The promising, although limited, success of inamrinone led to the development of structurally related newer agents such as milrinone (Fig. 21.4). Milrinone produces similar pharmacologic effects and probably acts through the same mechanism as inamrinone. Milrinone, however, is an order of magnitude more potent than inamrinone. Furthermore, preliminary reports show it to be better tolerated, with no apparent thrombocytopenia or gastrointestinal disturbances. Milrinone is excreted largely unchanged in the urine, and accordingly, patients with impaired renal function require reduced dosages.

β-adrenergic Receptor Agonists. Another promising area for the development of new positive inotropic agents is that of β-adrenergic receptor agonists. Adrenergic nervous system activity is mediated by two distinct receptor types, designated α and β. In addition, these receptors are further

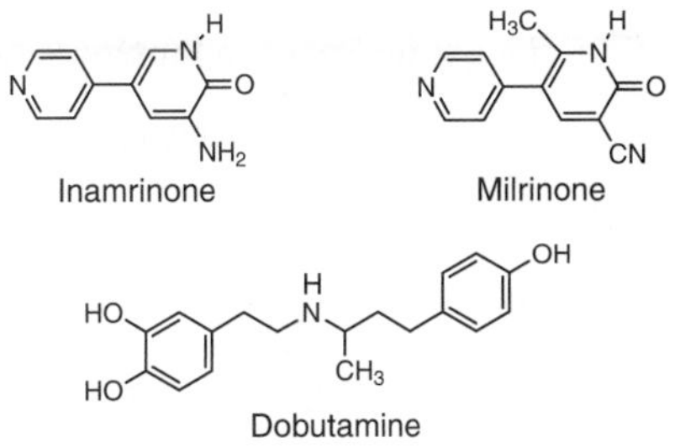

Fig. 21.4. Miscellaneous inotropic agents.

differentiated into α_1, α_2, β_1, β_2 subtypes (8). The distribution of these receptor subtypes depends greatly on the tissue in question. The myocardium has mostly β-adrenergic receptors of the β_1 subtype and stimulation of these receptors by a variety of β-adrenergic agonists produces a potent positive inotropic response. The mechanism underlying this effect is believed to involve elevation of cAMP levels, this time through the indirect stimulation of the enzyme adenylate cyclase. Elevated cAMP levels lead to a cascade of events ultimately producing an increase in intracellular Ca^{++} and thereby increased myocardial contractility. Although many agents possess β-adrenergic agonist activity, most have side effects that make them inappropriate for the treatment of CHF. For example, the well-known catecholamines, norepinephrine and epinephrine, are potent β-receptor agonists. Because the actions of these agents are not limited to the myocardial β_1 receptors, however, they produce undesirable positive chronotropic effects, exacerbate arrhythmias, and produce vasoconstriction. These effects limit their utility in the treatment of CHF.

Among the most promising β_1 adrenergic agonists are those derived from dopamine, the endogenous precursor to norepinephrine. Dopamine itself is a potent stimulator of the β_1-receptors, but it results in many of the undesirable side effects described previously. The new analogs of dopamine that have been developed retain the potent inotropic effect, but possess fewer effects on heart rate, vascular tone, and arrhythmias. Dobutamine (Fig. 21.4) is a prime representative of this group of agents. Dobutamine is a potent β_1-adrenergic agonist and beneficial effects, although largely attributed to its β_1 agonistic activity on the myocardium, are likely the composite of a variety of actions on the heart and the peripheral vasculature (Chapter 11). Dobutamine is active only by the intravenous route because of its rapid first-pass metabolism via COMT. Therefore, its use is limited to critical care situations. Nonetheless, its parenteral success has led to the search and development of orally active drugs. One of the major limitations associated with β_1 agonists is the phenomenon of myocardial β-receptor desensitization. This lowered responsiveness (desensitization) of the receptors appears to be due to a decrease in the number of β_1 receptors and partial uncoupling of the receptors from adenylate cyclase. Table 21.6 lists dosage forms and typical adult doses for the nonglycosidic inotropic agents.

DRUGS FOR THE TREATMENT OF ANGINA
Angina Pectoris

Angina pectoris is the disease affecting the coronary arteries, which supply oxygenated blood from the left ventricle to all heart tissues including the ventricles themselves. When the lumen of the coronary artery becomes restricted it becomes less efficient in supplying blood and oxygen to the heart; the heart is said to be ischemic (short in oxygen). Angina is the primary symptom of ischemic heart disease, characterized by a sudden, severe pain originating in the chest, often radiating to the left shoulder and down the left arm. Angina is further subclassified into typical or variant angina based on the precipitating factors and the electrophysiological changes observed during the attack. Typical angina usually is the result of an advanced state of atherosclerosis and is provoked by food, exercise, and emotional factors. It is characterized by low S-T segment of the electrocardiogram. Variant or acute angina results from sudden spasm in the coronary artery, unrelated to atherosclerotic narrowing of the coronary circulation and can occur at rest. It is characterized by an increase in the S-T segment of the electrocardiogram.

Antianginal Drugs

Therapy of angina is directed mainly to alleviating and preventing anginal attacks by dilating the coronary artery. Three classes of drugs are found to be very efficient in this regard, although via different mechanisms. These include: organic nitrates, calcium channel blockers, and β-adrenergic blockers.

Organic Nitrates

Organic nitrates have dominated the treatment of acute angina over the last hundred years. Although the recent introduction of the calcium channel blockers, and the β-blockers as antianginal agents has expanded the physician therapeutic arsenal, organic nitrates are still the class of choice to treat acute anginal episodes.

Chemistry

Overview. Organic nitrates are esters of simple organic alcohols or polyols with nitric acid. This class was developed after the antianginal effect of amyl nitrite (ester of isoamyl alcohol with nitrous acid) was first observed in 1857. Five members of this class are in clinical use today: amyl nitrite

Table 21.6. Non-glycosidic Positive Inotropic Agents

Name	Dosage Forms	Typical Adult Dosages*
Inamrinone Lactate (Inocor)	Injection: 20 mL ampules, 5 mg/mL	Intially 0.5 mg/kg IV over 2–3 minutes, then 5–10 μg/kg/min IV infusion (not to exceed 10 mg/kg per day)
Dobutamine (Dobutrex) hydrochloride	Injection: 20 mL vials, 12.5 mg/mL (250 mg total)	IV infusion: 2.5–10 μg/kg/minute
Milrinone Lactate (Primacor)	Injection: 5 mL, 1 mg/mL	Intially 0.05 mg/kg every 10 minutes Maintenance 0.59–1.13mg/kg over 24 hrs

*All dosages are subject to modification according to patient condition and response.

Table 21.7. Antianginal Nitrates and Nitrites

Name	Dosage Forms	Typical Adult Dose*
Amyl nitrite (isoamyl nitrite)	Inhalant: 0.18, 0.3 ml	0.18 or 0.3 ml inhaled as needed
Nitroglycerin (glyceryl trinitrate) (Nitro-Bid, Deponit, Nitro-Dur, Nitrogard)	Sublingual tablets: 0.15, 0.3, 0.4, 0.6mg extended release capsules / tablets: 1.3, 2.5, 2.6, 6.5, 9.0 mg; ointment: 2%; transdermal systems: many (eg. 26,51,77,104,154 mg disks which release 2.5,5.0,7.5,10,15mg/ 24h, respectively) IV infusion 5mg/mL	0.15–0.6 mg sublingually; 2.5–9mg orally, extended release every 8–12 hours; 1.25–5 cm topical ointment every 4–8; one transdermal disk/day (2.5–15mg/ day)
Isosorbide dinitrate (Iso-Bid, Sorate, Sorbigtrate,Isordil, Novosorbide, Dilatrate)	Sublingual tablets: 2.5, 5, 10 mg; sustained release tablets/capsules: 40mg; chewable tablets: 5,10 mg; oral tablets: 5,10, 20,30 mg	2.5–10 mg sublingually every 4–6 hours; 40 mg sustained release every 6–12 hours; 5–10 mg chewable every 2–3 hours; 5–30 mg orally every 6 hours
Erythrityl tetranitrate (Cardilate)	Oral/sublingual tablets:5,10,15 mg; chewable tablets;10mg	5–10 mg oral/sublingual 3 times a day; 10 mg chewable 3 times a day
Pentaerythritol tetranitrate (Duotrate, Pentol, pentritol, Pentylan, Peritrate)	Oral tablets: 10, 20, 40 mg; sustained release tablets/capsules: 30, 45, 60, 80 mg	10–40 mg orally 4 times a day; 30–80mg sustained release every 12 hours

*All dosages are subject to modification according to patient condition and response.

(amyl nitrite inhalant USP), nitroglycerin, isosorbide dinitrate, erythrityl tetranitrate, and pentaerythritol tetranitrate (Table 21.7). The chemical structures of these agents are shown in Figure 21.5. This class is usually referred to as organic nitrates because all of these agents, except amyl nitrite, are nitrate esters. It should be noted that the generic names do not always precisely describe the chemical nature of the drug though used for simplicity. For example, the drug nitroglycerin is not really a nitro compound because nitro compound means nitro group attached to a carbon atom i.e., NO_2-C; the correct chemical name of nitroglycerin is glyceryltrinitrate. Another example is amyl nitrite, whose structure indicates that it is an ester of isoamyl alcohol with nitrous acid; the correct chemical name of this drug is isoamyl nitrite.

The chemical nature of these molecules as esters constitutes some problems in formulating these agents for clinical use. The small non-polar ester character make them volatile. Volatility is an important concern in drug formulation owing to the potential loss of the active principle from the dosage form. In addition, moisture should be avoided during storage to minimize the hydrolysis of the ester bond which can lead to a decrease in the therapeutic effectiveness. Lastly, since these agents are nitrate esters, they possess explosive properties, especially in the pure concentrated form. Dilution in a variety of vehicles and excipients eliminates this potential hazard. The nonpolar nature of these esters, however, make these agents very efficient in emergency treatment of anginal episodes as a result of rapid absorption through bio-membranes.

Pharmacologic Actions. The oxygen requirements of the myocardial tissues are related to the workload of the heart, which is, in part, a function of the heart rate, the systolic pressure, and the peripheral resistance of the blood flow. Myocardial ischemia occurs when the oxygen is insufficient to meet the myocardial workload. This can occur, as explained previously, because of atherosclerotic narrowing of the coronary circulation (typical) or vasospasm of the coronary artery (variant). The nitrates have been shown to be effective in treating angina resulting from either cause. The vasodilating effect of organic nitrates on the veins leads to pooling of the blood in the veins and decreased venous return to the heart (decreased preload), whereas vasodilation of the arteries decreases the resistance of the peripheral tissues (decreased afterload). The decrease in both preload and afterload results in a generalized decrease in the myocardial workload, which translates into a reduced oxygen demand by the myocardium. Organic nitrates restore the balance between oxygen supply (by vasodilating the coronary artery) and oxygen demand (by decreasing the myocardial workload).

Biochemical Mechanism of Action

Although the physiologic effects of the organic nitrates are clearly due to its vasodilating effect on the vascular smooth muscles, the underlying molecular mechanism remains elusive. The presence of nitrate receptors on vascular smooth muscle has been postulated by Needleman and Johnson (9). These investigators suggested that the nitrate-receptor interaction is accompanied by the oxidation of a critical receptor sulfhydryl groups, which initiate vascular relaxation. The involve-

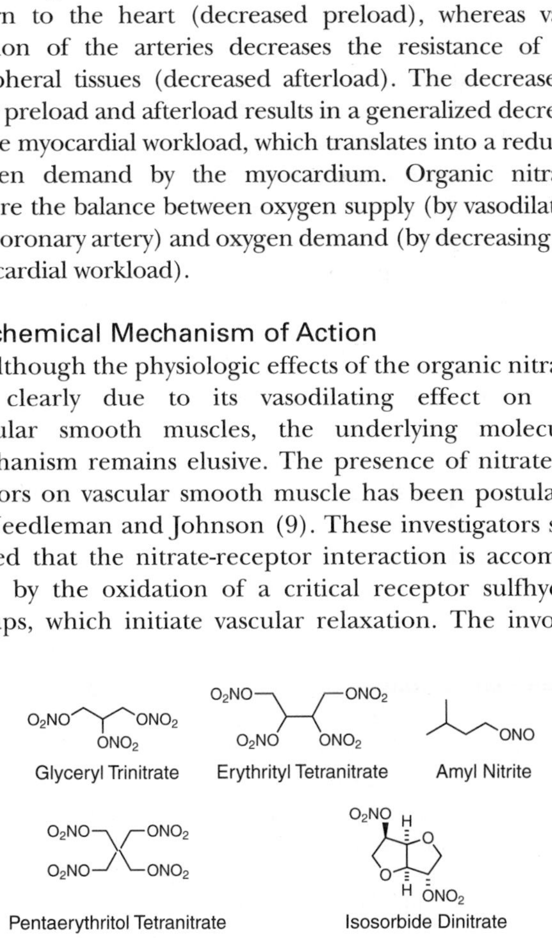

Fig. 21.5. Organic nitrates and nitrites.

ment of free tissue sulfhydryl groups was supported by experimental evidence showing that prior administration of N-acetylcysteine, which should increase the availability of free sulfhydryl groups, resulted in an increase in the vasodilating effect of organic nitrates. Similarly, pretreatment with reagents that react with free sulfhydryl groups such as ethacrynic acid blocked glyceryl trinitrate vasodilation in vitro (10). A more complex mechanism for nitrate vasodilation, however, was proposed by Ignarro and co-workers (11). They suggested that the nitrates act indirectly by stimulating the enzyme guanylate cyclase, thereby producing elevated levels of cyclic guanosine monophosphate (cGMP), which, in turn, leads to vasodilation. The initial stimulation of guanylate cyclase is believed to be mediated by a nitrate-derived nitrosothiol metabolite produced intracellularly. In support of this mechanism is the observation that a variety of synthetic nitrosothiols were found to increase markedly guanylate cyclase activity and produce vasodilation in vitro (12–16). Such a mechanism is consistent with the requirement for free sulfhydryl groups described previously. A unifying mechanism suggests that the organic nitrates through the release of nitrous oxide activate guanylate cyclase, causing an increase in cGMP, which, in turn, reduces the Ca^{++} catalyzed vascular contractions (17–20). It is clear that much research is required to clarify this complex process.

Pharmaceutical Preparations and Dosage Forms

Organic nitrates are administered by inhalation; by infusion; as sublingual, chewable, and sustained release tablets; as capsules; as transdermal disks; and as ointments. Table 21.7 summarizes different dosage forms and typical adult doses of organic nitrates as antianginal drugs.

Absorption, Metabolism, and Therapeutic Effects

Organic nitrates are used for both treatment and prevention of painful anginal attacks. The therapeutic approaches to achieve these two goals, however, are distinctly different. For the treatment of acute anginal attacks, that is, attacks which have already begun, a rapid-acting preparation is required. In contrast, preventative therapy requires a long-acting preparation with more emphasis on duration and less emphasis on onset. The onset of organic nitrate action is influenced not only by the specific agent chosen, but also by the route of administration. Sublingual administration is used predominantly for a rapid onset of action. The duration of nitrate action is strongly influenced by metabolism. All of the organic nitrates are subject to fairly rapid first-pass metabolism, not only in the liver by the action of glutathione-nitrate reductase, but also in extrahepatic tissues such as the blood vessels themselves (21,22). In addition, avid uptake into the vessel walls plays a significant role in the rapid disappearance of organic nitrates from the bloodstream. Sublingual, transdermal, and buccal administration routes have been used in an attempt to avoid at least some of the hepatic metabolism.

Acute angina is most frequently treated with sublingual glyceryl trinitrate. This sublingual preparation is rapidly absorbed from the sublingual, lingual, and buccal mucosa and provides relief usually within 2 minutes. The duration of action is also short, lasting about 30 minutes. Other treatments include amyl nitrite by inhalation and sublingual isosorbide dinitrate. Amyl nitrite is by far the fastest-acting preparation, with an onset of about 15–30 seconds, but lasts only about one minute. Isosorbide dinitrate, although usually used as a long-acting agent, may be used to treat acute angina. Sublingually administered isosorbide dinitrate has a somewhat slower onset than glyceryl trinitrate (about 3 minutes), but its action may last for 4–6 hours. Although the onset appears to be almost as rapid as that of glyceryl trinitrate, to wait an additional minute for relief may be deemed unacceptable by some patients.

To prevent recurring angina, long-acting organic nitrate preparations are used. Several agents fall into this category, such as orally administered isosorbide dinitrate, pentaerythritol tetranitrate, and erythrityl tetranitrate. In addition, a number of long-acting glyceryl trinitrate preparations are available. These include oral sustained release forms, glyceryl trinitrate ointment, transdermal patches, and buccal tablets. Of these therapeutic options, isosorbide dinitrate and glyceryl trinitrate preparations are by far the most frequently used. The whole concept of prophylactic nitrate use was at first met with skepticism by many physicians because early studies indicated that oral nitrates were nearly completely broken down by first-pass metabolism (21,22), and blood levels of the parent drug appeared to be virtually nil. These findings, in conjunction with several clinical studies showing equivocal efficacy, led Needleman and co-workers (22) to conclude that "There is no rational basis for the use of 'long-acting' nitrates (administered orally) in the prophylactic therapy of angina pectoris." More recent studies, however, suggest that oral prophylactic nitrates may be effective if appropriate doses are used (23). Moreover, some metabolites of long-acting nitrates are active as vasodilators, albeit less potent than the parent drug. Isosorbide dinitrate is an example of this. Isosorbide dinitrate is metabolized primarily in the liver by glutathione-nitrate reductase, which also participates in the metabolism of other organic nitrates, catalyzing the denitration of the parent drug to yield two metabolites, 2- and 5-isosorbide mononitrate (24). Of these, the 5-isomer is still a potent vasodilator, and its plasma half-life of about 4.5 hours is much longer than that of isosorbide dinitrate itself. The extended half-life, owing to the metabolite's resistance to further metabolism, has suggested that it may be contributing to the prolonged duration of action associated with isosorbide dinitrate use (24).

Adverse Effects

Most patients tolerate the nitrates fairly well. Headache and postural hypotension are the most common side effects of organic nitrates. Dizziness, nausea, vomiting, rapid pulse, and restlessness are among the additional side effects reported. These symptoms may be controlled by administering low doses initially and gradually increasing the dose. Fortunately, tolerance to nitrate-induced headache develops after a few days of therapy. Because postural hypotension may occur in some individuals, it is wise to advise the patient to sit down when taking a rapid-acting nitrate preparation for the first time. An effective dose of nitrate usually produces a fall in upright systolic pressure of 10 mm Hg and a reflex rise in heart rate of 10 beats per minute.

Another concern associated with prophylactic nitrate use is the development of tolerance (23,25). Tolerance, usually in the form of shortened duration of action, is commonly observed with chronic nitrate use. The clinical importance of this tolerance is, however, a matter of controversy. Because tolerance to nitrates has not been reported to lead to a total loss of activity, some physicians feel it is not clinically relevant. In addition, an adjustment in dosage can compensate for the reduced response (23). It has also been reported that intermittent use of long-acting and sustained release preparations may limit the extent of tolerance development.

Drug Interactions

The most significant interactions of organic nitrates are with those agents which cause hypotension such as other vasodilators, alcohol, and tricyclic antidepressants, where a potential of orthostatic hypotension may arise. On the other hand, concurrent administration with sympathomimetic amines, such as ephedrine and norepinephrine, may lead to a decrease in the antianginal efficacy of the organic nitrates.

Calcium Channel Blockers

The second major therapeutic approach to the treatment of angina is the use of calcium channel blockers (26,27) (also see corresponding subsection in Chapter 23 for more discussion). The recognition that inhibition of calcium ion (Ca^{++}) influx into myocardial cells may be advantageous in preventing angina occurred in the 1960s. Three classes of calcium channel blockers are currently approved for use in the prophylactic treatment of angina, the dihydropyridines nifedipine, nicardipine, and amlodipine; the benzothiazepine derivative diltiazem; and the aralkyl amine derivatives verapamil, and the diaminopropanol ether bepridil (Fig. 21.6). The last-mentioned are reserved for treatment failures in that serious arrhythmias may occur.

Chemistry

The structural dissimilarity of these agents is apparent and serves to emphasize the fact that each is distinctly different from the others in its profile of effects. Although nifedipine and similar drugs belong to the so-called dihydropyridine family, diltiazem belongs to the benzo[b-1,5]thiazepine family. Verapamil is structurally characterized by a central basic nitrogen to which alkyl and aralkyl groups are attached. It is noteworthy that diltiazem and verapamil are both chiral, possessing asymmetric centers. In each case, the dextro-rotatory, i.e., the (+) enantiomer is about an order of magnitude more potent as a calcium channel blocker than the levo-rotatory, (−) enantiomer.

Pharmacologic Effects

Calcium ions are known to play a critical role in many physiologic functions. Physiologic calcium is found in a variety of locations, both intracellular and extracellular. Because calcium plays such a ubiquitous role in normal physiology, the overall therapeutic effect of the calcium channel blockers is often the composite of numerous pharmacologic actions in a variety of tissues. The most important of these tissues associated with angina are the myocardium and the arterial vascular bed. Because of the dependency of the myocardium contraction on calcium, these drugs have a negative inotropic effect on the heart. Vascular smooth muscle also depends on calcium influx for contraction. Although the underlying mechanism is somewhat different, inhibition of calcium channel influx into the vascular muscles by the calcium channel blockers leads to vasodilation, particularly in the arterial smooth muscles. The venous beds appear to be less affected by the calcium channel blockers. The negative

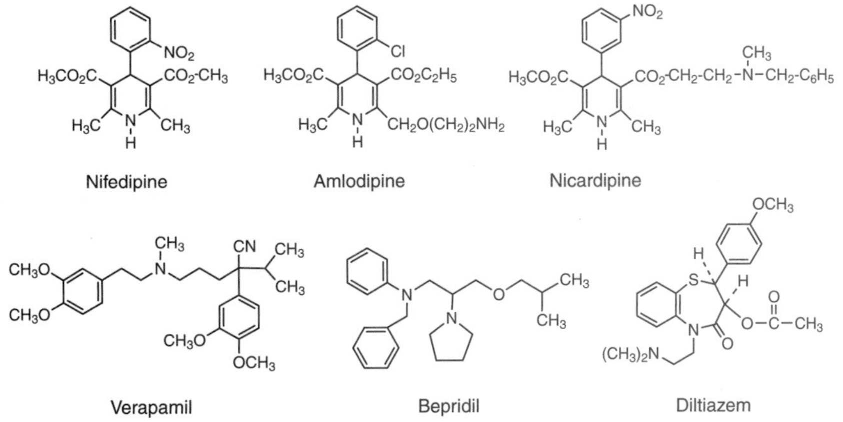

Fig. 21.6. Calcium channel blockers.

inotropic effect and arterial vasodilation result in decreased heart workload and afterload respectively. The preload is not affected due to lesser sensitivity of the venous bed to the calcium channel blockers.

Mechanism of Action

The depolarization and contraction of the myocardial cells are mediated in part by calcium influx. As previously explained, the overall process consists of two distinct inward ion currents. The first of these is the rapid flow of sodium ions into the cell through the "fast channels" and subsequently, calcium enters more slowly through the "slow channels." The calcium ions trigger contraction indirectly by binding and inhibiting troponin, a natural suppressor of the contractile process. Once the inhibitory effect of troponin is removed, actin and myosin can interact to produce the contractile response. The calcium channel blockers produce negative inotropic effect by interrupting the contractile response. In vascular smooth muscles, calcium causes constriction by binding to a specific intracellular protein calmodulin to form a complex which initiates the process of vascular constriction. The calcium channel blockers inhibit vascular smooth muscle contraction by depriving the cell from the calcium ions.

The effects of the three classes of calcium channel blockers on the myocardium and the arteries varies from one class to the other. Although verapamil and diltiazem affect both the heart and the arterial bed, the dihydropyridines have much less effect on the cardiac tissues and higher specificity for the vascular bed. Therefore, both verapamil and diltiazem are clinically used in the management of angina, hypertension, and cardiac arrhythmia, whereas the dihydropyridines are more frequently used as antianginal and antihypertensive agents. Because nicardipine has a less negative inotropic effect than nifedipine, it may be preferred over nifedipine for patients with angina pectoris or hypertension who also have CHF dysfunction.

The recognition of the pivotal role of calcium flux on biologic functions led to the reexamination of several therapeutic agents already in clinical use to see if their effects were also mediated through calcium-dependent mechanisms. Interestingly, many drugs were found to influence calcium movement and availability. In many cases, however, this effect was not found to significantly contribute to the desirable pharmacologic activity, with other mechanisms playing more dominant roles.

Pharmaceutical Preparations

Calcium channel blockers are administered as oral tablets and capsules as regular or sustained-release forms. Verapamil and diltiazem are also administered by injection. The pharmaceutical dosage forms and the corresponding adult doses are summarized in Table 21.8.

Absorption, Metabolism, and Excretion

The calcium channel blockers are rapidly and completely absorbed after oral administration (see Table 23.11 for summary of pharmacokinetic parameters). Pre-hepatic first-pass metabolism by CYP3A4 enzymes occurs, with some orally administered calcium channel blockers, especially for verapamil, with its low bioavailability of 20–35%. For diltiazem, its bioavailability is 40–67%; for nicardipine 35%; for nifedipine 45–70%; and for amlodipine 64–90%. Verapamil is metabolized by N-demethylation to norverapamil (CYP3A4), which retains approximately 20% of verapamil activity and by O-demethylation (CYP2C9) into inactive metabolites. Diltiazem is metabolized to the desacetyl derivative which retains approximately 25–50% of the diltiazem activity.

Norverapamil

Desacetyldiltiazem

Table 21.8. Calcium Channel Blockers and Their Dosage Forms

Name	Dosage Forms	Typical Adult Dosage*
Verapamil (Calan, Isoptin, Verelan)	Tablets: 80, 120 mg; Injection: 5 mg/2 ml	IV: 5–10 mg over 2 minutes; Orally: 80 mg three or four times a day (usually 320–480 mg/day)
Diltiazem (Cardizem)	Tablets: 30, 60 mg	30 mg orally 4 times a day, then if necessary, increased to 60 mg, 3 or 4 times a day
Nifedipine (Adalat, Procardia)	Capsules: 10 mg	10 mg orally 3 times a day, may be increased to 20 mg 3 times daily, not to exceed 180 mg/day
Nicardipine (Cardene)	Capsules: 20 mg	20 mg 3 times a day, allow 3 days before increasing the dose to 40 mg 3 times a day
Amlodipine (Norvasc)	Tablets: 2.5, 5, 10mg	5 to 10 mg/day
Bepridil (Vascor)	Tablets: 200, 300, 400 mg	Intially 200 or 300 mg qd, maximum 400 mg/day

*All dosages are subject to modification according to patient condition and response.

The dihydropyridines are metabolized largely to a variety of inactive metabolites. Their binding to plasma proteins is high ranging from 70–98% depending on the individual agent: for verapamil protein binding is 90%; for diltiazem, 70–80%; for nifedipine, 92–98%; for nicardipine, it is greater than 90%; and for amlodipine, greater than 90%. Less than 4% of the dihydropyridine dose is excreted unchanged into the urine. The duration of action of the calcium channel blockers ranges from 4–8 hours (verapamil 4 hours, diltiazem 6–8 hours, nifedipine 4–8 hours, nicardipine 6–8 hours). Amlodipine has a 24-hour duration of action. Thus, it is the only calcium channel blocker that can be given once daily as non-sustained-release product.

Adverse Effects

The most common side effects of the calcium channel blockers include: dizziness, hypotension, headache, peripheral and pulmonary edema. These symptoms are mainly related to the excessive vasodilation, especially with the dihydropyridines. Verapamil was reported to cause constipation to some patients.

Drug Interactions

Clinically significant drug interactions between calcium channel blockers and co-administration of CYP3A4 inhibitors such as 6–8 oz. grapefruit juice, HIV protease inhibitors and erythromycin have resulted in 100–200-fold increase in the AUC for some calcium channel blockers (30). On the other hand, the co-administration of CYP3A4 inducers such as rifampin or phenobarbital, result in approximately a 50% decrease in the AUC of calcium channel blockers. With other vasodilators, antihypertensive drugs, and alcohol excessive hypotension may arise due to an additive effect. The high protein-binding nature of these drugs precipitates a potential of mutual plasma displacement with other drugs known to possess the same property, such as oral anticoagulants, digitalis glycosides, oral hypoglycemic agents, sulfa drugs, and salicylates. Dose adjustment may be necessary in some cases.

Therapeutic Uses

Calcium channel blockers are clinically used as antianginal, antiarrhythmic, and antihypertensive agents (see corresponding subsection in Chapter 23).

β-Adrenergic Blocking Agents

The use of β-adrenergic blockers as antianginal agents is limited to the treatment of exertion-induced angina. Propranolol is the prototype drug in this class, but several newer agents have been approved for clinical use in the United States (see Chapter 11). Although these agents may be used alone, they are often used in combination therapy with nitrates, calcium channel blockers, or both. In several instances, combination therapy was found to provide more improvement than did either agent alone. This, however, is not always the case.

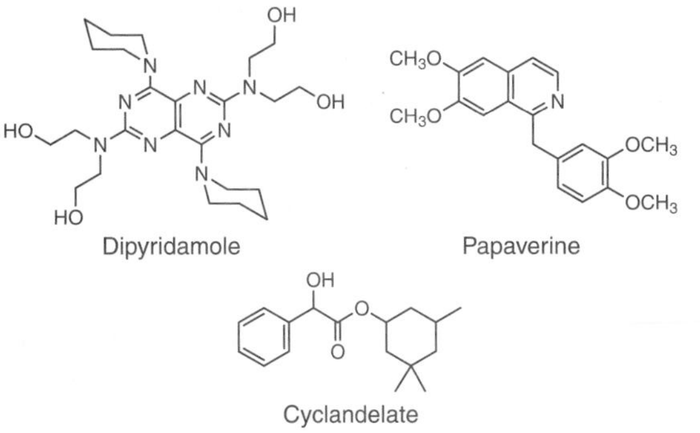

Fig. 21.7. Miscellaneous coronary vasodilators.

Miscellaneous Coronary Vasodilators

Another approach to the treatment of myocardial insufficiency is the use of the coronary vasodilators dipyridamole, papaverine, and cyclandelate. Dipyridamole (Fig. 21.7) causes a long-acting and selective coronary vasodilation, presumably through inhibition of adenosine uptake by the red blood cells and vasculature. Adenosine is a natural vasodilatory substance released by the myocardium during hypoxic episodes. Inhibition of its uptake is therefore believed to prolong its vasodilatory effects. Some structural similarity of adenosine to dipyridamole is apparent and substantiates this mechanism. Dipyridamole is generally used prophylactically, but its efficacy in reducing the incidence and severity of anginal attacks is not universally accepted. Cyclandelate and papaverine (Fig. 21.7), although structurally unrelated to one another, appear to act similarly by the relaxation of vascular smooth muscle. The exact mechanism of action of these agents is unclear. Despite few studies supporting their efficacy, they still remain in clinical use.

DRUGS FOR THE TREATMENT OF CARDIAC ARRHYTHMIA
Arrhythmia

Arrhythmia is an alteration in the normal sequence of electrical impulse activation that leads to the contraction of the myocardium. It is manifested as an abnormality in the rate, the site from which the impulses originate, or in the conduction through the myocardium. This process is controlled by the so-called pacemaker cells in the A-V and S-A nodes; however, both the atria and the ventricles are also involved.

Causes of Arrhythmias

Many factors influence the normal rhythm of electrical activity in the heart. Arrhythmias may occur because pacemaker cells fail to function properly or because of a blockage in transmission through the AV-node. Underlying diseases such as atherosclerosis, hyperthyroidism, or lung disease may also be initiating factors. Some of the more common arrhythmias are those termed ectopic, which occur when electrical signals spontaneously arise in regions other than the pacemaker and then compete with the normal impulses. Myocardial ischemia, excessive myocardial catecholamine release, stretching of the myocardium, and cardiac glycoside toxicity have all been shown to stimulate ectopic foci. A second mechanism for the generation of arrhythmias is from a phenomenon called re-entry. This occurs when the electrical impulse does not die out after firing, but continues to circulate and re-excite resting heart cells into depolarizing. The result of this reexcitation may be a single, premature beat or runs of ventricular tachycardia. Re-entrant rhythms are common in the presence of coronary atherosclerosis.

Antiarrhythmic Agents and Their Classification

It is widely accepted that most currently available antiarrhythmic drugs may be classified into four categories, grouped on the basis of their effects on the cardiac action potential (Table 21.9), and consequently on the electrophysiological properties of the heart. To understand the basis of classification and the pharmacology of these agents, an understanding of normal cardiac electrophysiology is necessary.

Normal Physiologic Action

Normal cardiac contractions are largely a function of: the action of a single atrial pacemaker, a fast and generally uniform conduction in predictable pathways, and a normal duration of the action potential and refractory period. Figure 21.8 depicts a normal cardiac action potential from a Purkinje fiber. The resting cell has a membrane potential of approximately -90 mV, with the inside of the cell being electronegative relative to the outside of the cell. This is called the transmembrane resting potential. On excitation, the transmembrane potential reverses, and the inside of the membrane rapidly becomes positive with respect to the outside. On recovery from excitation, the resting potential is restored. These changes have been divided into five phases: phase 0 represents depolarization and reversal of the transmembrane potential, phases 1–3 represent different stages of repolarization, and phase 4 represents the resting potential. During phase 0, also referred to as rapid depolarization, the permeability of the membrane for sodium ions increases, and sodium rapidly enters the cell, causing it to become depolarized. Phase 1 results from the ionic shift, which creates an electrochemical and concentration gradient which reduces the rate of sodium influx but favors the influx of chloride and efflux of potassium. Phase 2, the plateau phase, results from the slow inward movement of calcium, which is triggered by the rapid inward movement of sodium in phase 0. During this time, there is also an efflux of potassium which balances the influx of calcium, thus resulting in little or no change in membrane potential. Phase 3 is initiated by a slowing of the calcium influx coupled with a continued efflux of potassium. This continued efflux of potassium from the cell restores the membrane potential to normal resting potential levels. During phase 4 the Na^+, K^+-ATPase pump restores

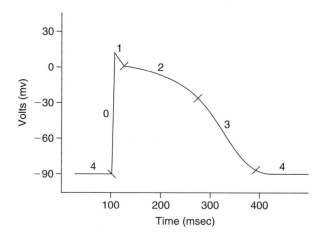

Fig. 21.8. Cardiac action potential recorded from a Purkinje fiber.

Table 21.9. Classification of Antiarrhythmic Agents

Class	Agent	Primary Pharmacologic Effect
IA	Quinidine Procainamide Disopyramide	Decrease maximal rate of depolarization; increases duration of action potential
IB	Lidocaine Phenytoin Tocainide Mexiletine	Decrease maximal rate of depolarization; decrease duration of action potential
IC	Flecainide Encainide Propafenone Moricizine	Decrease maximal rate of depolarization; no change in duration of action potential
II	Propranolol	Inhibition of sympathetic activity
III	Sotalol Ibutilide Bretylium Amiodarone	Prolongation of duration of action potential
IV	Verapamil Diltiazem Bepridil	Inhibition of inward slow calcium current

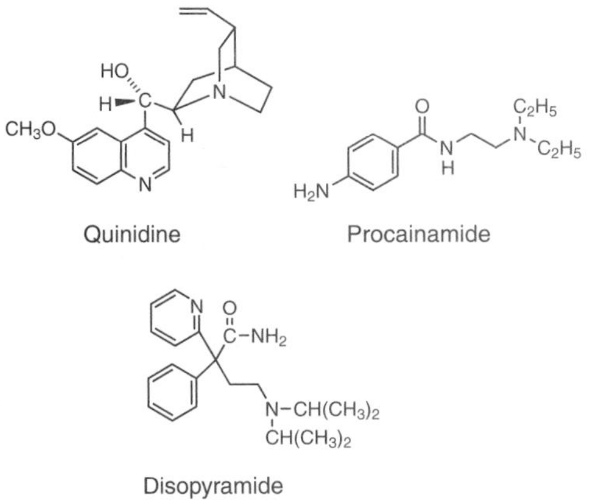

Fig. 21.9. Class IA Antiarrhythmics.

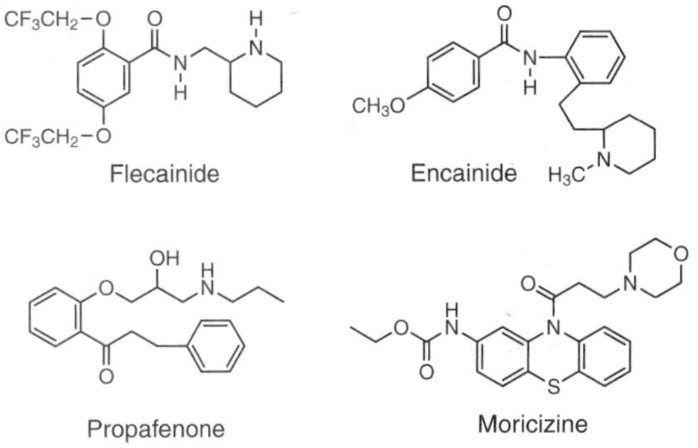

Fig. 21.11. Class IC Antiarrhythmics.

the ions to their proper local concentrations. The action potential is a coordinated sequence of ion movements where sodium initially enters the cell, followed by a calcium influx, and finally a potassium efflux that returns the cell to its resting state. Several antiarrhythmic agents exert their effects by altering these ion fluxes.

Classification of Antiarrhythmic Agents

Class I drugs are generally local anesthetics acting on nerve and myocardial membranes to slow conduction by inhibiting phase 0 of the action potential (Fig. 21.8). Myocardial membranes show the greatest sensitivity. Class I drugs decrease the maximal rate of depolarization without changing the resting potential. They also increase the threshold of excitability, increase the effective refractory period, decrease conduction velocity, and decrease spontaneous diastolic depolarization in pacemaker cells. The decrease in diastolic depolarization tends to suppress ectopic foci activity. Prolongation of the refractory period tends to abolish re-entry arrhythmias. This class is further subclassified into class IA, IB, and IC based on the primary pharmacologic effect. Table 21.9 summarizes those effects, and Figures 21.9 to 21.11 illustrate the chemical structures of members of each subclass. Quinidine is considered the prototype drug for class I.

Class II antiarrhythmic drugs are, β-adrenergic receptor blocking agents, which block the role of the sympathetic nervous system in the genesis of certain cardiac arrhythmias. Their dominant electrophysiological effect is to depress adrenergically enhanced calcium influx through β-receptor blockade. Drugs in this class decrease neurologically induced automaticity at normal therapeutic doses. At higher doses, these drugs may also exhibit anesthetic properties, which cause decreased excitability, decreased conduction velocity, and a prolonged effective refractory period. In normal therapeutic situations, the β-blocking effects are more important than any local anesthetic effects these drugs may have. Propranolol is the prototype β-adrenergic blocker drug for class II (Chapter 11).

Class III drugs cause a homogeneous prolongation of the duration of the action potential. This results in a prolongation of the effective refractory period. It is believed that most of Class III antiarrhythmic agents act through phase 3 of the action potential by blocking potassium channels. Figure 21.12 illustrates the chemical structures of members of class III. Bretylium is the prototype drug for this class.

Class IV antiarrhythmic drugs comprise a group of agents which selectively block the slow inward current carried by calcium, i.e., calcium channel blockers. The slow inward current in cardiac cells has been shown to be of importance for the normal action potential in pacemaker cells. It has also been suggested that this inward current is involved in the genesis of certain types of cardiac arrhythmias. Administration of a Class IV drug causes a prolongation of the refractory period in the A-V node and the atria, a decrease in atrioventricular conduction, and a decrease in spontaneous diastolic depolarization. These effects block conduction of premature impulses at the AV node and thus are very effective in treating

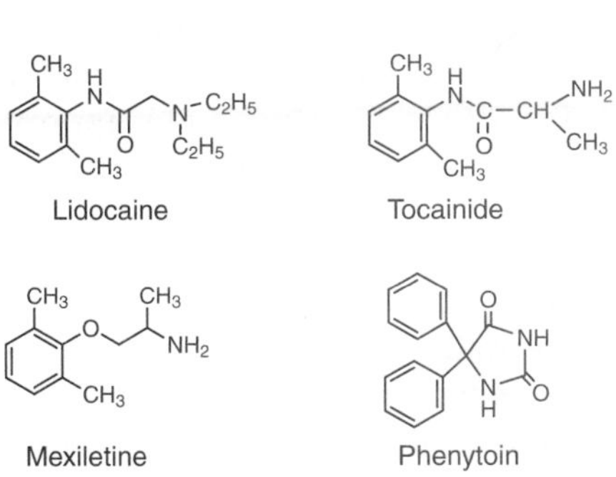

Fig. 21.10. Class IB Antiarrhythmics.

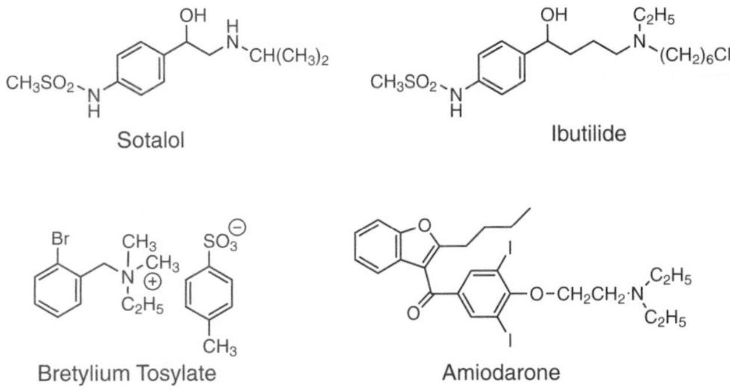

Fig. 21.12. Class III Antiarrhythmics.

Table 21.10. Class I Antiarrhythmic Drugs and Their Dosage Forms

Name	Dosage Forms	Typical Adult Dosage*
Quinidine sulfate, (Cardioquin, Cin-Quin, Dura-Quin, Quinora)	Tablets: 100, 200, 300 mg; tablets, extended release 300 mg; capsules: 200, 300 mg; solution for injection, 200 mg/mL	200–300 mg orally 3 or 4 times daily; a loading dose of 600–1000 mg may be used
Quinidine gluconate	10 mL ampules, 80 mg/mL	IV: slow infusion, 0.3–0.4 mg/kg/min
Procainamide hydrochloride, (Procan, Promine, Pronestyl, Rhythmin)	Capsules: 250, 375, 500 mg; tablets: 250, 375, 500 mg; 10 mL ampules: 100, 500 mg/mL	Initially, 1.25 g orally then 0.5–1.0 g every 4 hours; 0.5–1.0 g IM; 0.2–0.5 g IV, not exceeding 50 mg/min, then maintenance of 2–6 mg/min
Disopyramide phosphate, (Norpace)	Capsules: 100, 500 mg	100–200 mg 4 times a day
Lidocaine hydrochloride, (Baylocaine, Lido Pen, Xylocaine)	Ampules: 5 and 50 ml, 10, 20, 40, 100, 200 mg/mL	50–100 mg IV, then 1–4 mg/min infusion
Phenytoin (diphenylhydantoin sodium) (Dilantin, Diphenylhydantoin)	Capsules: 30,100 mg; vials (to be reconstituted): 100, 200 mg; oral suspension: 125 mg/5 mL	50–100 mg IV over 5 min, not to exceed 50 mg/min; 5–6 mg/kg/day orally in 1 or 2 divided doses
Tocainide hydrochloride (Tonocard)	Tablets: 400, 600 mg	400–600 mg orally 3 times a day
Mexiletine hydrochloride (Mexitil)	Capsules: 100, 200, 250 mg	200 mg orally every 8 hours with incremental increase of 50 mg each if needed
Flecainide (Tambocor)	Tablets: 100 mg	100 mg orally every 12 hours with incremental increases of 50 mg each as needed to a maximum of 400 mg/day

*All doses required individual adjustment according to patient condition and response.

Table 21.11. Class II-IV Antiarrhythmic Drugs and Their Dosage Forms

Name	Dosage Forms	Typical Adult Dosage*
Propranolol (Inderal, Betachrom)	Tablets: 10, 40, 80 mg; ampules: 2 ml, 2.5 mg/mL	20–80 mg orally per day; 0.5–3 mg IV
Bretylium tosylate (Bretylol)	Ampules: 10 ml, 50 mg/mL	5–10 mg/kg IV infusion over 10–30 min, repeated every 6 hours
Amiodarone (Cordarone)	Tablets: 200 mg; Concentrate for injection, for IV infusion: 50 mg/mL	800–1600 mg orally per day, gradually decreased over 1–3 weeks to 600–800 mg/day, then further decreased to 400 mg/day
Verapamil (Calan, Isoptin)	Tablets: 80,120 mg; ampules: 2 mL, 2.5 mg/mL	5–10 mg IV over 2 minutes, then 80–120 mg orally 4 times a day

*All doses required individual adjustment according to patient condition and response.

supraventricular arrhythmias. Verapamil is the prototype drug for this class (see Fig. 21.6). Dosage forms and typical adult dosages of class-I drugs are summarized in Table 21.10, and those of classes II-IV, are summarized in Table 21.11.

Quinidine

Quinidine is widely used for acute and chronic treatment of ventricular and supraventricular arrhythmias, especially supraventricular tachycardia. It is a member of a family of alkaloids found in Cinchona bark (*Cinchona Offici-nalis L.*) and is the diastereomer of quinine. Despite their structural similarity, quinidine and quinine differ markedly in their effects on the cardiac muscles, with quinidine's effects being much more pronounced. Structurally, quinidine is composed of a quinoline ring and the bicyclic quinuclidine ring system with a hydroxymethylene bridge connecting these two components. Examination of quinidine reveals two basic nitrogens, with the quinuclidine nitrogen (pKa 11) being the stronger of the two. Because of quinidine's basic character, it is always used in a water-soluble salt forms. These salts include quinidine sulfate, gluconate, and

polygalacturonate. Good absorption (approximately 95%) is observed with each of these forms after oral administration. In special situations, quinidine may be administered intravenously as the gluconate salt. The use of intravenous quinidine, however, is rare. The gluconate salt is particularly suited for parenteral use because of its high water solubility and lower irritant potential.

Quinidine's bioavailability appears to depend on a combination of metabolism and P-gp efflux. The bioavailabilities of quinidine sulfate and gluconate are 80–85% and 70–75%, respectively. Once absorbed, quinidine is subject to hepatic first pass metabolism and is approximately 85% plasma protein bound, with an elimination half-life of about 6 hours. Quinidine is metabolized mainly in the liver, and renal excretion of unchanged drug is also significant (approximately 10–50%). The metabolites are hydroxylated derivatives at either the quinoline ring through first pass O-demethylation, or at the quinuclidine ring through oxidation of the vinyl group. These metabolites possess only about one-third the activity of quinidine. Their contribution to quinidine's overall therapeutic effect is unclear. Recently, the clinical significance of the well documented digoxin-quinidine was previously described under digoxin drug interactions. Apparently quinidine (a P-gp substrate) inhibits the renal tubular secretion of digoxin via the P-gp efflux pump, resulting in increased plasma concentration for digoxin.

O-Demethylquinidine

Oxydihydroquinidine

In addition, a common contaminant in quinidine preparations, dihydroquinidine (derived from reduction of the quinuclidine vinyl group at C-3 to an ethyl group), may also contribute to its activity (28). Although similar to quinidine in pharmacodynamic and pharmacokinetic behavior, this contaminant is both more potent as an antiarrhythmic and more toxic. Thus, levels of this contaminant may contribute to variability between commercial preparations. The most frequent adverse effects associated with quinidine therapy are gastrointestinal disturbances, such as nausea, diarrhea, and vomiting.

Procainamide

Procainamide is effective in the treatment of several types of cardiac arrhythmias. Its actions are similar to those of quinidine, and yet procainamide may be effective in patients who are unresponsive to quinidine. The initial development of procainamide was stimulated by the observation that the local anesthetic procaine (the ester bioisostere of procainamide), when administered intravenously, produced significant though short-lived antiarrhythmic effects. Unfortunately, considerable central nervous system toxicity, in addition to the short duration, limited the usefulness of this agent. Moreover, procaine is not active orally because of its short duration of action caused by both chemical and enzymatic (catalyzed by plasma esterases) hydrolysis. A logical modification of this molecule was the isosteric replacement of the ester with an amide group. This produced orally active procainamide, which is more resistant to both enzymatic and chemical hydrolysis. Peak plasma levels of procainamide are observed within 45–90 minutes after oral administration, and about 70–80% of the dose is bioavailable. About half of this dose is excreted unchanged, and the remaining half undergoes acetylation metabolism in the liver. Metabolites of procainamide include p-aminobenzoic acid and N-acetylprocainamide. Interestingly, the acetylated metabolite is also active as an antiarrhythmic. Its formation accounts for up to one-third of the administered dose and is catalyzed by the liver enzyme, N-acetyl transferase. Because acetylation is strongly influenced by an individual's genetic background, marked variability in the amounts of this active metabolite may be observed from patient to patient. Renal excretion dominates, with about 90% of a dose excreted as unchanged drug and metabolites. The elimination half-life is about 3.5 hours. A substantial percentage (60–70%) of patients on procainamide show elevated levels of antinuclear antibodies after a few months. Of these patients, between 20 and 30% develop a drug-induced lupus syndrome if therapy is continued. These adverse effects which are attributed to the aromatic amino group, are observed more frequently and more rapidly in "slow acetylators." Usually, the symptoms associated with procainamide-induced lupus syndrome subside fairly rapidly after the drug is discontinued. These problems, however, have discouraged long-term procainamide therapy.

Disopyramide

Disopyramide phosphate is used orally for the treatment of certain ventricular and atrial arrhythmias. Despite its structural dissimilarity to quinidine and procainamide (Fig. 21.9), its cardiac effects are very similar. Disopyramide is rapidly and completely absorbed from the gastrointestinal tract. Peak plasma level is usually reached within 1–3 hours, and a plasma half-life of 5–7 hours is common. About half of an oral dose is excreted unchanged in the urine. The remaining drug undergoes hepatic metabolism, principally to the corresponding N-dealkylated form. This metabolite retains about half of disopyramide's antiarrhythmic activity and is also subject to renal excretion. Adverse effects of disopyramide are frequently observed. These effects are primarily anticholinergic in nature, and include dry mouth, blurred vision, constipation, and urinary retention.

Lidocaine

Lidocaine, similar to procaine, is an effective, clinically used local anesthetic (see Fig. 21.10) (Chapter 13). Its cardiac effects, however, are distinctly different from those of procainamide or quinidine. Lidocaine is normally reserved for the treatment of ventricular arrhythmias and is, in fact, usually the drug of choice for emergency treatment of ventricular arrhythmias. Its utility in these situations is due to the rapid onset of antiarrhythmic effects on intravenous infusion. In addition, these effects cease soon after the infusion is terminated. Thus, lidocaine therapy may be rapidly modified in response to changes in the patient's status. Lidocaine is effective as an antiarrhythmic only when given parenterally, and the intravenous route is the most common. Antiarrhythmic activity is not observed after oral administration because of the rapid and efficient first-pass metabolism by the liver. Parenterally administered lido-

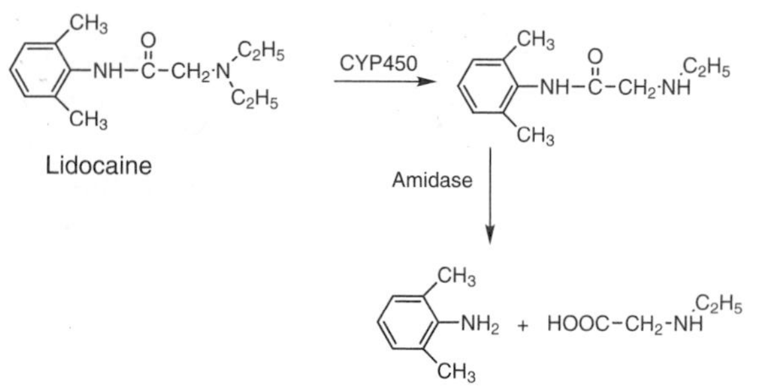

Fig. 21.13. Metabolism of lidocaine.

caine is about 60–70% plasma protein-bound. Hepatic metabolism is rapid (plasma half-life is about 15–30 minutes) and primarily involves deethylation to yield monoethylglycinexylide, followed by amidase-catalyzed hydrolysis into N-ethylglycine and 2,6-dimethylaniline (2,6-xylidine) (see Fig. 21.13).

Monoethylglycinexylide has good antiarrhythmic activity, but is not clinically useful, because it undergoes rapid enzymatic hydrolysis. Lidocaine's adverse effects include emetic and convulsant properties that predominantly involve the central nervous system and heart. The central nervous system effects may begin with dizziness and paresthesia and, in severe cases, ultimately lead to epileptic seizures.

Tocainide

Tocainide (see Fig. 21.10) is an α-methyl analog structurally related to monoethylglycinexylide, the active metabolite of xylocaine which possesses very similar electrophysiologic effects to lidocaine. In contrast to lidocaine, tocainide is orally active and its oral absorption is excellent. Like lidocaine, it is usually reserved for the treatment of ventricular arrhythmias. The α-methyl group is believed to slow the rate of metabolism and thereby contributes to oral activity. The plasma half-life of tocainide is about 12 hours, and nearly 50% of the drug may be excreted unchanged in the urine. Adverse effects associated with tocainide are like those observed with lidocaine, specifically, gastrointestinal disturbances and central nervous system effects.

Mexiletine

Mexiletine (Fig. 21.10) is similar to both lidocaine and tocainide in its effects and therapeutic application. It is used principally to treat and prevent ventricular arrhythmias. Like tocainide, mexilitine has very good oral activity and absorption properties. Clearance depends on metabolism and renal excretion. A relatively long plasma half-life of about 12–16 hours is common. Adverse effects are similar to those experienced with tocainide and lidocaine.

Phenytoin

For 50 years, phenytoin (Fig. 21.10) has seen clinical use in the treatment of epileptic seizures (Chapter 16). During this time, it was noticed that phenytoin also pro-

duced supposedly adverse cardiac effects. On closer examination, these adverse effects were actually found to be beneficial in the treatment of certain arrhythmias. Currently, phenytoin is used in the treatment of atrial and ventricular arrhythmias resulting from digitalis toxicity. It is, however, not officially approved for this use.

Phenytoin may be administered either orally or intravenously and is absorbed slowly after oral administration, with peak plasma levels achieved after 3–12 hours. It is extensively plasma protein bound (approximately 90%) and the elimination half-life is between 15 and 30 hours. These large ranges reflect the considerable variability observed from patient to patient. Parenteral administration of phenytoin is usually limited to the intravenous route. Phenytoin for injection is dissolved in a highly alkaline vehicle (pH 12). This alkaline vehicle is required because phenytoin is weakly acidic and has very poor solubility in its un-ionized form. However, its phosphate ester fosphenytoin reportedly has some advantages over phenytoin for injection. Intramuscular phenytoin is generally avoided because it results in tissue necrosis at the site of injection and erratic absorption. In addition, intermittent intravenous infusion is required to reduce the incidence of severe phlebitis.

Phenytoin metabolism is relatively slow and predominantly involves aromatic hydroxylation to p-hydroxylated inactive metabolites (see subsection Chapter 16 for metabolism details). Phenytoin also induces its own metabolism and is also subject to large interindividual variability. The major metabolite, 5-p-hydroxyphenyl-5-phenylhydantoin, accounts for about 75% of a dose. This metabolite is excreted through the kidney as the β-glucuronide conjugate. Phenytoin clearance is strongly influenced by its metabolism, and therefore agents that affect phenytoin metabolism may cause intoxication. In addition, since phenytoin is highly plasma protein-bound, agents that displace phenytoin may also cause toxicity.

Flecainide

Flecainide is a relatively new drug that exhibits properties distinctly different from those of Class IA (e.g., quinidine) or Class IB (e.g., lidocaine) antiarrhythmic agents. Flecainide is a fluorinated benzamide derivative (Fig. 21.11), available as the acetate salt. Flecainide has been approved by the FDA for the treatment of ventricular arrhythmias. Clinical studies suggest that this agent may be more effective than either quinidine or disopyramide in suppressing premature ventricular contractions. Oral flecainide is well absorbed and the plasma half-life is about 14 hours. About half of an oral dose is metabolized in the liver, and a third is excreted unchanged in the urine. As with other antiarrhythmics, flecainide may produce adverse effects. The most severe is flecainide's tendency to occasionally aggravate existing arrhythmias or induce new ones. Although fewer than 10% of patients experience this effect, it may be life-threatening. Accordingly, it may be desirable to start therapy in the hospital. Other less serious side effects include: blurred vision, headache, nausea, and abdominal pain.

Encainide

Encainide (Enkaid) (Fig. 21.11) represents another benzamide derivative, with similar pharmacologic properties to encainide, however, with less negative inotropic effect.

Propafenone

Propafenone (Rythmol) (Fig. 21.11) is a class I, local anesthetic-type antiarrhythmic agent. Propafenone is structurally related to other class IC antiarrhythmic drugs and also to adrenergic β-receptor blockers. It is used primarily for ventricular and supraventricular arrhythmias. The drug is administered orally and IV, however, the parenteral dosage forms are not commercially available in the United States. After oral administration, the drug is rapidly and almost completely absorbed from the gastrointestinal tract. Propafenone metabolism involves hepatic CYP2D6 enzymes. Its rate of metabolism is genetically determined by an individual's ability to metabolize the so called phenotype compounds (fast or slow metabolizers) (Chapter 8).

Moricizine

Moricizine (Ethmozine) (Fig. 21.11) is a phenothiazine analog which processes the same electrophysiological effects on the heart as those of class IC antiarrhythmics. Despite its short half-life after oral administration, its antiarrhythmic effects can persist for many hours, suggesting that some of its metabolites may be active.

Propranolol

Propranolol, a β-adrenergic blocker, is the prototype for Class II antiarrhythmics. Its pharmacology is discussed in detail in Chapters 11 and 24. Its use as an antiarrhythmic is usually for the treatment of supraventricular arrhythmias, including atrial flutter, paroxysmal supraventricular tachycardia, and atrial fibrillation. Propranolol is also reported to be effective in the treatment of digitalis-induced ventricular arrhythmias. Moreover, beneficial results may be obtained when propranolol is used in combination with other agents. For example, in certain cases quinidine and propranolol together have proved more successful in alleviating atrial fibrillation than either agent alone. Few serious adverse effects are associated with propranolol therapy.

Sotalol

Sotalol (Betapace, Sotacor), a β-adrenergic blocker, is methansulfonanilide antiarrhythmic agent (Fig. 21.12). As an antiarrhythmic, it is dually classified as class II and III due to the similarity of its cardiac effects to both classes. Sotalol is used orally to suppress and prevent the recurrence of life-threatening ventricular arrhythmia.

Ibutilide

Ibutilide (Corvert) is another methanesulfonanilide derivative (Fig. 21.12), but unlike sotalol it lacks any β-adrenergic blocking activity. Like sotalol, it exhibits electrophysiologic effects characteristic of class III. Ibutilide is used only by IV infusion as its fumarate salt.

Bretylium Tosylate

Bretylium tosylate is a quaternary ammonium salt derivative (Fig. 21.12), originally developed for use as an antihypertensive. Its antiarrhythmic use is limited to emergency life-threatening situations where other agents, such as lidocaine and procainamide, have failed. Generally, bretylium is used only in intensive care units and may be administered either intravenously or intramuscularly. The plasma elimination half-life is usually about 10 hours, and is eliminated largely unchanged in the urine. The major adverse effect associated with bretylium tosylate is hypotension, including orthostatic hypotension, which may be very severe.

Amiodarone

Amiodarone (Fig. 21.12), initially developed as an antianginal (coronary vasodilator), has antiarrhythmic effects which are somewhat similar to those of bretylium. It is approved by the FDA for the treatment of life-threatening ventricular arrhythmias that are refractory to other drugs. Its cardiac effects are not well characterized, but clinical studies indicate that it is a promising new class III agent. Its severe toxicity, however, makes it the drug of last choice. As with bretylium tosylate, use of this agent should be initiated in a hospital setting.

Verapamil

Verapamil (Fig. 21.6), like amiodarone, was originally conceived as a coronary vasodilator for angina. It is, however, also effective and widely used for the treatment of supraventricular arrhythmias. Therapeutic effects after oral administration are observed within 2 hours. Considerable variability may be observed in the elimination half-life of 1.5–7 hours. In addition, the plasma half-life may not always accurately predict the duration of action due to the presence of active metabolites. Verapamil is subject to extensive pre-hepatic first-pass oxidative metabolism mediated by intestinal CYP3A4 enzymes (N-demethylation) and CYP2C9 (O-demethylation). Less than 5% of an orally administered dose is excreted unchanged into the urine.

A well documented drug interaction between digoxin and verapamil that increases the AUCs for digoxin has been attributed to verapamil blocking the intestinal P-gp secretion of digoxin (previously described under digoxin drug interactions). The fact that verapamil is a substrate for P-gp transport of drugs may be a potential source of other drug interactions. The oral co-administration of verapamil with CYP3A4 inhibitors (see Table 8.10 for a list of inhibitors) has resulted in at least a 100–200-fold increase in the blood AUCs for verapamil and thereby, a toxic dose.

CASE STUDY

Victoria F. Roche and S. William Zito

LM is an 80-year-old, black female resident in the Sweet Azalea's assisted living facility where you are the consulting pharmacist. LM is a bright, intelligent widow, who visits with her children through cyberspace on her laptop. Her stage 1 (mild) hypertension is controlled with an ACE inhibitor, enalapril. However, LM has just been diagnosed with congestive heart failure (CHF) characterized by loss of appetite, constipation, ankle edema and slight hepatomegaly, indicative of right ventricular dysfunction. Her physician wants to begin treatment with a cardiac glycoside or other positive inotropic agent and a diuretic, furosemide (1). Evaluate the following structures (1–5) for appropriate use in this case.

1. *Identify the therapeutic problem(s) where the pharmacist's intervention may benefit the patient.*

2. *Identify and prioritize the patient specific factors that must be considered to achieve the desired therapeutic outcomes.*

3. *Conduct a thorough and mechanistically oriented structure-activity analysis of all therapeutic alternatives provided in the case.*

4. *Evaluate the SAR findings against the patient specific factors and desired therapeutic outcomes and make a therapeutic decision.*

5. *Counsel your patient.*

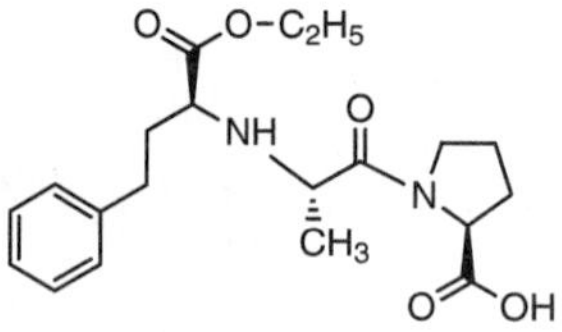

Enalapril

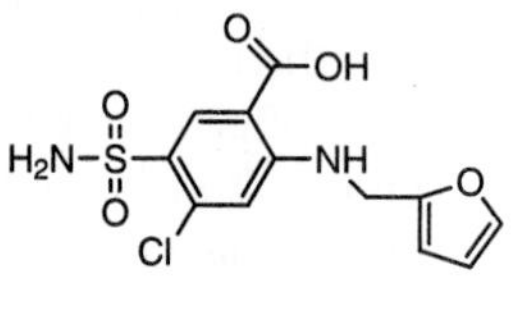

1

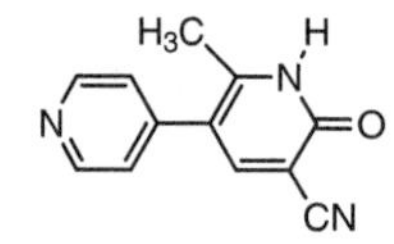

2

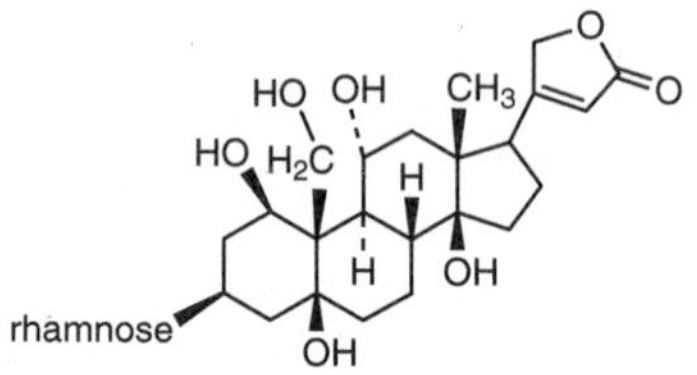

3

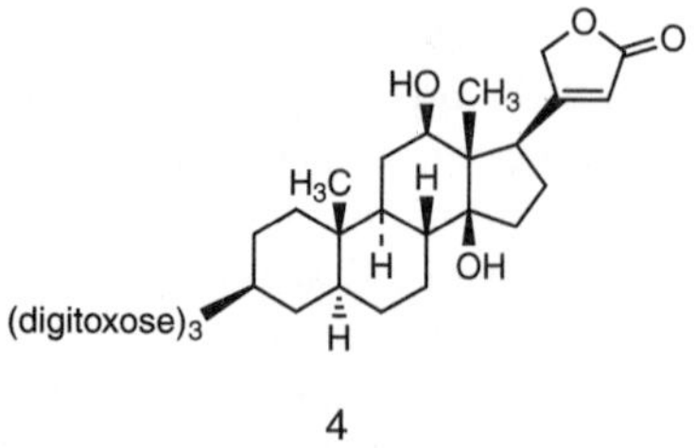

4

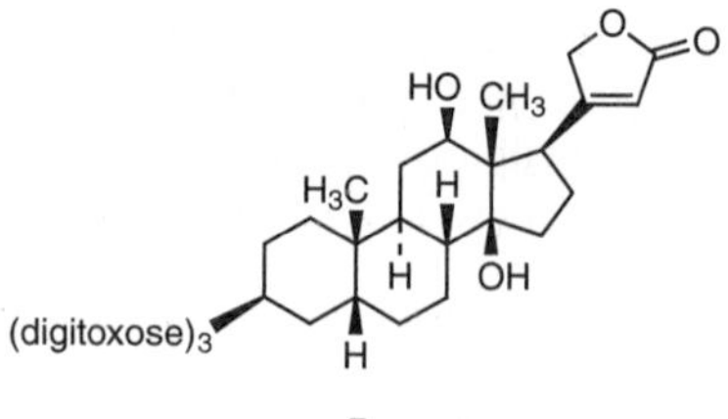

5

REFERENCES

1. TW Smith. EM Antman, PL Friedman, et al. Digitalis glycosides: mechanisms and manifestations of toxicity. Part II. Prog Cardiovasc Dis. 1984;26:495–540. Digitalis glycosides: mechanisms and manifestations of toxicity. Part III. Prog Cardiovasc Dis. 1984;27:21–56.

2. N Rietbrock, BG Woodcock. Two Hundred Years of Foxglove Therapy: *Digitalis Purpurea* 1785–1985. Trends Pharmacol Sci, 1985;6:267–269.

3. R Thomas, J Bontagy, A Gelbart. Synthesis and biological activity of semisynthetic digitalis analogs. J. Pharm. Sci., 1974;63:1649–1683.

4. R Thomas, in Burger's Medicinal Chemistry, 4th ed., M. E. Wolff, Ed., Part III, New York, John Wiley and Sons, 1981.

5. K Repke, New Developments in Cardiac Glycoside Structure-Activity Relationships. Trends Pharmacol. Sci., 1985;6:275–278.

6. DS Fullerton, JF Griffin, DC Rohrer, et al. Using Computer Graphics to Study Cardiac glycoside-receptor Interactions. Trends Pharmacol Sci, 1985;6:279–282.

7. WS Colucci, RF Wright, E Braunwald. New positive inotropic agents in the treatment of congestive heart failure. 1. Mechanisms of action and recent clinical developments. N Engl J Med, 1986;314:290–299; New positive inotropic agents in the treatment of congestive heart failure. 2. Mechanisms of action and recent clinical developments. N Engl J Med, 1986;314:349–358.

8. BF Hoffman and RJ Lefkowitz, in Coodman and Gilman's The Pharmacological Basis of Therapeutics, 8th ed., AG Gilman, TW Rall, AS Nies, et al, Eds. Pergamon Press Inc., New York, 1990.

9. P Needleman, EM Johnson, Jr., Mechanism of tolerance development to organic nitrates. J Pharmacol Exp Ther, 1973;184:709–715.

10. P Needleman, B Jakschik, and EM Johnson, Jr., Sulfhydryl requirement for relaxation of vascular smooth muscle. J Pharmacol Exp Ther, 1973;187:324–331.

11. LJ Ignarro, H Lippton, JC Edwards, et al. Mechanism of vascular smooth muscle relaxation by organic nitrates, nitrites, nitroprusside and nitric oxide: evidence for the involvement of S-nitrosothiols as active intermediates. J Pharmacol Exp Ther, 1981;218:739–749.

12. LJ Ignarro, BK Barry, DY Grueter, et al. Guanylate cyclase activation of nitroprusside and nitroguanidine is related to formation of S-nitrosothol intermediates. Biochem Biophys Res Commun, 1980;94:93–100.

13. LJ Ignarro, BK Barry, DY Grueter, et al. Selective alterations in responsiveness of guanylate cyclase to activation by nitroso compounds during enzyme purification. Biochim Biophys Acta, 1981;673:394–407.

14. LJ Ignarro, JC Edwards, DY Gruetter, et al. Possible involvement of S-nitosothiols in the activation of guanylate cyclase by nitroso compounds. FEBS Lett, 1980; 110:275–278.

15. LJ Ignarro, CA Gruetter. Requirement of thiols for activation of coronary arterial guanylate cyclase by glyceral trinitrate and sodium nitrite: possible involvement of S-nitrosothiols. Biochim Biophys Acta, 1980; 631:221–231.

16. LJ Ignarro, PJ Kadowitz, WH Baricos. Evidence that regulation of hepatic guanylate cyclase activity involves interactions between catalytic site -SH groups and both substrate and activator. Arch Biochem Biophys, 1981;208:75–86.

17. Moncada S, Plamer RM, Higgs EA. Nitric oxide: physiology, pathophysiology, and pharmacology. Pharmacol Rev, 1991;43, 109–142.

18. SH Synder, DS Bredt. Nitric oxide as a neuronal messenger. Trends Pharmacol Sci, 1991;12, 125.

19. T McCall, P Vallance. Nitric oxide takes centre-stage with newly defined roles. Trend Pharmacol Sci, 1992;13, 1.

20. PL Feldman, et al., Chem Eng News, 1993;26.

21. HL Fung, SC Sutton, A Kamiya. Blood vessel uptake and metabolism of organic nitrates in the rat. J Pharmacol Exp Ther, 1984;228:334–341.

22. P Needleman, S Lang and EM Johnson Jr. Organic nitrates: relationship between biotransformation and rational angina pectoris therapy. J Pharmacol Exp Ther, 1972;181:489–497.

23. J Abrams. Pharmacology of nitroglycerin and long-acting nitrates. Am J Cardiol, 1985;56:12A-18A, and refs. therein.

24. HL Fung. Pharmacokinetics of nitroglycerin and long-acting nitrate esters. Am J Med, 1983;72(Suppl.):13–19.

25. S Corwin, JA Reiffel. Nitrate therapy for angina pectoris. Current concepts about mechanism of action and evaluation of currently available preparations. Arch Intern Med, 1985;145:538–543.

26. RG Rahwan, DT Witiak, W W Muir. Newer Antiarrhythymics. Ann Rep Med Chem, 1981;16:257–268.

27. KC Yedinak. Use of calcium channel antagonists for cardiovascular disease. Am Pharm, 1993;33:49–65.

28. HL Conn, Jr., RJ Luchi. Some Cellular and Metabolic Considerations Relating to the Action of Quinidine as a Prototype Antiarrhythymic Agent. Am J Med, 1964;37:685.

29. G Koren, C Woodland, S Ito. Toxic digoxin-drug interactions: the major role of renal P-glycoprotein. Vet Human Toxicol 1998;40: 45–6.

30. EL Michalets. Update: clinically significant cytochrome P-450 drug interactions. Pharmacotherapy, 1998;18: 84–112.

SUGGESTED READINGS

Fozzard HA and Sheets MF, "Cellular Mechanism of Action of Cardiac Glycosides," J. Am. Coll. Cardiol., 5:10A-15A (1985).

Hansten PD, Ed., "Drug Interactions: Clinical Significance of Drug-drug Interactions," 5th ed., Philadelphia, Lea and Febiger, 1985.

Kaplan HR, "Advances in Antiarrhythmic Drug Therapy Changing Concepts," Federation Proc. 45:2184–2213(1986).

Katz AM, "Effects of Digitalis on Cell Biochemistry: Sodium Pump Inhibition," J. Am. Coll. Cordiol., 5:16A-21A(1985).

Kowey PR, Pharmacological Effects of Antiarrhythmic Drugs, Archives of Internal Medicine, 158 n4-325 (1998).

Mangini RJ, Ed., "Drug Interaction Facts," St. Louis, J. B. Lippincott, 1983.

Robertson RM and Robertson D, "Drugs Used for the Treatment of Myocardial Ischemia" (Chapter 32); RA Kelly and TW Smith, "Pharmacological Treatment of Heart Failure" (Chapter 34); DM Roden, "Antiarrhythmic Drugs" (Chapter 35); in Goodman and Gilman's The Pharmacological Basis of Therapeutics, 9th ed., JG Hardman, LE Limbrid, Eds-in-Chief, PB Molinoff, RW Ruddon, Eds., and AG Gilman, consulting Ed., McGraw-Hill, New York, 1996.

Thomas RE, "Cardiac Drugs" (Chapter 28), in Burger's Medicinal Chemistry and Drug Discovery, 5th ed., Part IIA, Volume 2, M. E. Wolff, Ed., New York, John Wiley and Sons, Inc., 1996.

22. Diuretics

GARY O. RANKIN

INTRODUCTION

Diuretics are chemicals that increase the rate of urine formation (1). By increasing the urine flow rate, diuretic usage leads to the increased excretion of electrolytes (especially sodium and chloride ions) and water from the body without affecting protein, vitamin, glucose or amino acid reabsorption. These pharmacologic properties have led to the use of diuretics in the treatment of edematous conditions resulting from a variety of causes (e.g., congestive heart failure, nephrotic syndrome, chronic liver disease) and in the management of hypertension. Diuretic drugs also are useful as the sole agent or as adjunctive therapy in the treatment of a wide range of clinical conditions, including hypercalcemia, diabetes insipidus, acute mountain sickness, primary hyperaldosteronism, and glaucoma.

The primary target organ for diuretics is the kidney, where these drugs interfere with the reabsorption of sodium and other ions from the lumina of the nephrons, the functional units of the kidney. The amount of ions and accompanying water that are excreted as urine following administration of a diuretic, however, is determined by many factors, including the chemical structure of the diuretic, the site or sites of action of the agent, the salt intake of the patient and the amount of extracellular fluid present. In addition to the direct effect of diuretics to impair solute and water reabsorption from the nephron, diuretics can also trigger compensatory physiological events that have an impact on either the magnitude or the duration of the diuretic response. Thus, it is important to be aware of the normal mechanisms of urine formation and renal control mechanisms to understand clearly the ability of chemicals to induce a diuresis.

NORMAL PHYSIOLOGY OF URINE FORMATION

Two important functions of the kidney are (1) to maintain a homeostatic balance of electrolytes and water and (2) to excrete water-soluble end products of metabolism. The kidney accomplishes these functions through the formation of urine by the nephrons (Fig. 22.1). Each kidney contains approximately 1 million nephrons and is capable of forming urine independently. The nephrons are composed of a specialized capillary bed called the glomerulus and a long tubule divided anatomically and functionally into the proximal tubule, loop of Henle, and distal tubule. Each component of the nephron contributes to the normal functions of the kidney in a unique manner, and thus all are targets for different classes of diuretic agents.

Urine formation begins with the filtration of blood at the glomerulus. Approximately 1200 mL of blood per minute flows through both kidneys and reaches the nephron by way of afferent arterioles. About 20% of the blood entering the glomerulus is filtered into Bowman's capsule to form the glomerular filtrate. The glomerular filtrate is composed of blood components with a molecular weight less than albumin (approximately 69,000) and not bound to plasma proteins. The glomerular filtration rate (GFR) averages 125 mL/minute in humans but can vary widely even in normal functional states.

The glomerular filtrate leaves Bowman's capsule (BC) and enters the proximal convoluted tubule (PCT; S1, S2), where the majority (50–60%) of filtered sodium is reabsorbed osmotically. Sodium reabsorption is coupled electrogenetically with the reabsorption of glucose, phosphate, and amino acids and nonelectrogenetically with bicarbonate reabsorption. Glucose and amino acids are completely reabsorbed in this portion of the nephron, whereas phosphate reabsorption is between 80 and 90% complete. The early proximal convoluted tubule is also the primary site of bicarbonate reabsorption (80–90%), a process that is mainly sodium dependent and coupled to hydrogen ion secretion. The reabsorption of sodium and bicarbonate is facilitated by the enzyme carbonic anhydrase which is present in proximal tubular cells and catalyzes the formation of carbonic acid from water and carbon dioxide. The carbonic acid provides the hydrogen ion, which drives the reabsorption of sodium bicarbonate. Chloride ions are reabsorbed passively in the proximal tubule, where they follow actively transported sodium ions into tubular cells.

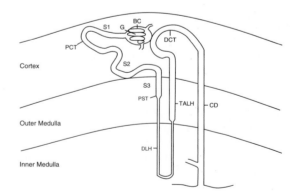

Fig. 22.1. The nephron. BC, Bowman's capsule; G, glomerulus; PCT, proximal convoluted tubule; PST, proximal straight tubule; DLH, descending limb of the Loop of Henle; TALH, thick ascending limb of the Loop of Henle; DCT, distal convoluted tubule; CD, collecting duct.

518

Reabsorption of electrolytes and water also occurs isosmotically in the straight proximal tubule or pars recta (PST; S3). By the end of the straight segment, between 65 and 70% of water and sodium, chloride, and calcium ions; 80–90% of bicarbonate and phosphate; and essentially 100% of glucose, amino acids, vitamins, and protein have been reabsorbed from the glomerular filtrate. The proximal tubule is also the site of active secretion of weakly acidic and weakly basic organic compounds. Thus, many of the diuretics can enter luminal fluid not only by filtration at the glomerulus, but also by active secretion.

The descending limb of the loop of Henle (DLH) is impermeable to ions, but water can freely move from the luminal fluid into the surrounding medullary interstitium, where the higher osmolality draws water into the interstitial space and concentrates luminal fluid. Luminal fluid continues to concentrate as it descends to the deepest portion of the loop of Henle, where the fluid becomes the most concentrated. The hypertonic luminal fluid next enters the water-impermeable thick ascending limb of the loop of Henle. In this segment of the nephron, approximately 20–25% of the filtered sodium and chloride ions are reabsorbed via a cotransport system ($Na^+/K^+/2 Cl^-$) on the luminal membrane. Reabsorption of sodium and chloride in the medullary portion of the thick ascending limb is important for maintaining the medullary interstitial concentration gradient. Reabsorption of sodium chloride in the cortical component of the thick ascending limb (TALH) and the early distal tubule (DCT) contributes to urinary dilution, and as a result these two nephron sections are sometimes called the cortical diluting segment of the nephron.

Luminal fluid leaving the early distal tubule next passes through the late distal tubule and cortical collecting tubule (CD), where sodium is reabsorbed in exchange for hydrogen and potassium ions. This process is partially controlled by mineralocorticoids (e.g., aldosterone) and accounts for the reabsorption of between 2 and 3% of filtered sodium ions. Although the reabsorption of sodium ions from these segments of the nephron is not large, this sodium-potassium/hydrogen ion exchange system determines the final acidity and potassium content of urine. Several factors, however, can influence the activity of this exchange system, including the amount of sodium ions delivered to these segments, the status of the acid-base balance in the body, and the levels of circulating aldosterone.

The urine formed during this process represents only about 1–2% of the original glomerular filtrate, with more than 98% of electrolytes and water filtered at the glomerulus being reabsorbed during passage through the nephron. Thus, a change in urine output of only 1–2% could double urine volume. Urine leaves the kidney through the ureters and travels to the bladder, where the urine is stored until urination removes the urine from the body.

NORMAL REGULATION OF URINE FORMATION

The body contains several control mechanisms that regulate the volume and contents of urine. These systems are activated by changes in solute or water content of the body, by changes in systemic or renal blood pressure, and by a variety of other stimuli. Activation of one or more of these systems by diuretic drugs can modify the effectiveness of these drugs to produce their therapeutic response and may require additional therapeutic measures to ensure a maximal response.

The kidney has the ability to respond to changes in the GFR through the action of specialized distal tubular epithelial cells called the macula densa. These cells are in close contact with the glomerular apparatus of the same nephron and detect changes in the rate of urine flow and luminal sodium chloride concentration. An increase in the urine flow rate at this site (as can occur with the use of some diuretics) activates the macula densa cells to communicate with the granular cells and vascular segments of the juxtaglomerular (JG) apparatus. Stimulation of the JG apparatus causes renin to be released, which leads to the formation of angiotensin II and subsequent renal vasoconstriction. Renal vasoconstriction leads to a decrease in GFR and possibly a decrease in the effectiveness of the diuretic. Renin release also can be stimulated by factors other than diuretics, including decreased renal perfusion pressure, increased sympathetic tone, and decreased blood volume.

Another important regulatory mechanism for urine formation is antidiuretic hormone (ADH), also known as vasopressin. ADH is released from the posterior pituitary in response to reduced blood pressure and elevated plasma osmolality. In the kidney, ADH acts on the collecting tubule to increase water permeability and reabsorption. As a result, the urine becomes more concentrated, and water is conserved in the presence of ADH.

DIURETIC DRUG CLASSES
History

Compounds that increase the urine flow rate have been known for centuries. One of the earliest substances known to induce diuresis is water, an inhibitor of ADH release. Calomel (mercurous chloride) was used as early as the 16th century as a diuretic, but because of poor absorption from the gastrointestinal tract and toxicity, calomel was replaced clinically by the organomercurials (e.g., chlormerodrin). The organomercurials represented the first group of highly efficacious diuretics available for clinical use. The need to administer these drugs parenterally, the possibility of tolerance, and their potential toxicity, however, soon led to the search for newer, less toxic diuretics. Today the organomercurials are no longer used as diuretics, but their discovery began the search for many of the diuretics used today. Other compounds previously used as diuretics include the acid-forming salts (ammonium chloride) and methylxanthines (theophylline).

Structure Classification

The diuretics currently in use today (Table 22.1) are classified by their chemical class (thiazides), mechanism of action (carbonic anhydrase inhibitors, osmotics), site of action (loop diuretics), or effects on urine contents (potassium-sparing diuretics). These drugs vary widely in their efficacy (ability to increase the rate of urine formation) and their site of action within the nephron. Efficacy is often measured as the ability of the diuretic to increase the excretion of sodium ions filtered at the glomerulus (i.e., the filtered load of sodium) and should not be confused with potency, which is the amount of the diuretic required to produce a specific diuretic response.

Efficacy is determined in part by the site of action of the diuretic. Drugs (e.g., carbonic anhydrase inhibitors) that act primarily on the proximal tubule (PCT) to induce diuresis are weak diuretics because of the ability of the nephron to reabsorb a significant portion of the luminal contents in latter portions of the nephron. Likewise, drugs (potassium-sparing diuretics) that act at the more distal segments of the nephron are weak diuretics because most of the glomerular filtrate has already been reabsorbed in the proximal tubule and ascending limb of the loop of Henle before reaching the distal tubule. Thus, the most efficacious diuretics discovered so far, the high-ceiling or loop diuretics, interfere with sodium chloride reabsorption at the ascending limb of the loop of Henle, which is situated after the proximal tubule but before the distal portions of the nephron and collecting tubule.

Osmotic Diuretics

Mechanism of Action

Osmotic diuretics are low-molecular-weight compounds that are freely filtered through Bowman's capsule into the renal tubules, are non-reabsorbable solutes, and are not extensively metabolized except for glycerin and urea (see Table 22.2 for their pharmacokinetic proper-

ties). Once in the renal tubule, osmotic diuretics have a limited reabsorption because of their high water solubility. When administered as a hypertonic (hyperosmolar) solution, these agents cause water to pass from the body into the tubule, producing a diuretic effect.

Polyols such as mannitol, sorbitol, and isosorbide provide this effect. Sugars such as glucose and sucrose can also have a diuretic effect by this mechanism. Although not a polyol, urea has a similar osmotic effect and has been used in the past as an osmotic diuretic.

Osmotic diuretics are not frequently used in medicine today except in the prophylaxis of acute renal failure where these drugs inhibit water reabsorption and maintain urine flow. They may also be helpful in cases where urinary output is diminished because of severe bleeding or traumatic surgical experiences. They are not considered primary diuretic agents in treating ordinary edemas since osmotic diuretics can expand extracellular fluid volume.

Mannitol   Sorbitol

Isosorbide

Mannitol

Mannitol is the agent most commonly used as an osmotic diuretic. Sorbitol can also be used for similar reasons. These compounds can be prepared by the electrolytic reduction of glucose or sucrose.

Mannitol is administered intravenously in solutions of 5–50% at a rate of administration that is adjusted to main-

Table 22.1. Diuretics: Sites and Mechanisms of Action

Class of Diuretic	Site of Action	Mechanism of Action
Osmotics	Proximal tubule	Osmotic effects decrease sodium and water reabsorption
	Loop of Henle	Increases medullary blood flow to decrease medullary hypertonicity and reduce sodium and water reabsorption
	Collecting tubule	Sodium and water reabsorption decreases because of reduced medullary hypertonicity and elevated urinary flow rate
Carbonic anhydrase inhibitors	Proximal convoluted tubule	Inhibition of renal carbonic anhydrase decreases sodium bicarbonate reabsorption
Thiazides and thiazide-like	Cortical portion of the thick ascending limb of loop of Henle and distal tubule	Inhibition of Na$^+$-Cl$^-$ symporter
Loop or high-ceiling	Thick ascending limb of the loop of Henle	Inhibition of the luminal Na$^+$/K$^+$/2 Cl$^-$ transport system
Potassium-sparing	Distal tubule and collecting duct	Inhibition of sodium and water reabsorption by: Competitive inhibition of aldosterone (spironolactone) Blockade of sodium channel at the luminal membrane (triamterene and amiloride)

Table 22.2. Pharmacokinetic Properties of the Non-Thiazide Diuretics

Drug	Trade Name	Relative Potency	Oral Absorption (%)	Peak Plasma	Duration of Effect	$t_{1/2}$	Route of Elimination
Osmotic diuretics							
Glycerin			>80	1–1.5 h	4–6 h	0.5–0.75 h	>90% metabolism
Isosorbide			>80	NA	NA	5–9.5 h	urine unchanged
Mannitol			<20	1–3 h iv	3–8 h	1.5 h	urine unchanged
Urea			<10	1–2 h iv	3–10 h	NA	metabolized
Loop diuretics: High-ceiling diuretics							
Furosemide	Lasix	1	11–90*	4–5 h	6–8 h	0.5–4 h (>3 h)‡	80% urine unchanged (20% metabolized)
Bumetanide	Bumex	40	80–100	<2 h	5–6 h	0.3–1.5 h (>3 h)‡	50% urine unchanged 45% metabolized
Ethacrynic acid	Edecrin	0.7	>90	2 h	6–8 h	0.5–1 h	30–50% urine unchanged 30% mercapturate
Torsemide	Demadex	3	80–100%	NA	NA	0.8–4 h	30% urine 70% metabolized
Inhibitor of carbonic anydrase							
Acetazolamide	Diamox		>90	1–3 h	NA	<6 h	urine unchanged
Potassium-sparing diuretics (Inhibitors of renal epithelial Na⁺ channels)							
Amiloride	Midamor	1	~50*	3–4 h	10–24 h	6–9 h normal (21 h)‡	50% urine unchanged
Triameterene	Dyrenium	0.1	>70	2–4 h	>24 h	2–3 h	metabolized to active metabolites
Aldosterone antagonists; Potassium-sparing diuretics (Mineralocorticoid receptor antagonists)							
Spironolactone	Aldactone		>90†	1–2 h	2–3 d	1–3 h	active metabolite
Canrenone (7α-thiospironolactone) active metabolite			NA		13–24 h	3–4 h	urine

NA: no data available.
*Food affects bioavailability.
†Formulation affects bioavailability.
‡In patients with renal insufficiency.
Data from McEvoy GK, ed. AHFS 2000 Drug Information. Bethesda, MD: American Society of Health-System Pharmacists, 2000.

tain the urinary output at 30–50 ml per hour. Mannitol is filtered at the glomerulus and is poorly reabsorbed by the kidney tubule. The osmotic effect of mannitol in the tubule inhibits the reabsorption of water, and the rate of urine flow can be maintained.

Isosorbide

Isosorbide is basically a bicyclic form of sorbitol, used orally to cause a reduction in intraocular pressure in glaucoma cases. Although a diuretic effect is noted, its ophthalmologic properties are its primary value.

Carbonic Anhydrase Inhibitors
Mechanism of Action

It was proposed in 1937 that the normal acidification of urine was caused by secretion of hydrogen ions by the tubular cells of the kidney. These ions were provided by the action of the enzyme carbonic anhydrase, which catalyzes the formation of carbonic acid (H_2CO_3) from carbon dioxide and water.

$$CO_2 + H_2O \longrightarrow H_2CO_3 \longrightarrow H^+ + HCO_3^-$$

It was also observed that sulfanilamide rendered the urine of dogs alkaline because of the inhibition of carbonic anhydrase. This inhibition of carbonic anhydrase re-

sulted in a lesser exchange of hydrogen ions for sodium ions in the kidney tubule. The sodium ions, along with bicarbonate ions, and associated water molecules were then excreted, and a diuretic effect was noted. The large doses required and the side effects of sulfanilamide prompted a search for more effective carbonic anhydrase inhibitors as diuretic drugs.

It was soon learned that the sulfonamide portion of an active diuretic molecule could not be monosubstituted or disubstituted. It was reasoned that a more acidic sulfonamide would bind more tightly to the carbonic anhydrase enzyme. Synthesis of more acidic sulfonamides produced compounds more than 2500 times more active than sulfanilamide. Acetazolamide was introduced in 1953 as an orally effective diuretic drug. Previous to that time, the organic mercurials, which commonly required intramuscular injection, were the principal diuretics available.

Carbonic anhydrase inhibitors induce diuresis by inhibiting the formation of carbonic acid within proximal (PCT, S2) and distal tubular cells to limit the number of hydrogen ions available to promote sodium reabsorption. For a diuretic response to be observed, more than 99% of the carbonic anhydrase must be inhibited. Although carbonic anhydrase activity in the proximal tubule regulates the reabsorption of about 20–25% of the filtered load of sodium, the carbonic anhydrase inhibitors are not highly efficacious diuretics. An increased excretion of only 2–5% of the filtered load of sodium is seen with carbonic anhydrase inhibitors due to increased reabsorption of sodium ions by the ascending limb of the loop of Henle and more distal nephron segments.

With prolonged use of the carbonic anhydrase inhibitor diuretics, the urine becomes more alkaline, and the system becomes more acidic. When acidosis occurs, the carbonic anhydrase inhibitors lose their effectiveness as diuretics. They remain ineffective until normal acid-base balance in the body has been regained. For this reason, this class of compounds is limited in its diuretic use. Today they are most commonly used in the treatment of glaucoma where they reduce the rate of aqueous humor formation, and subsequently reducing the intraocular pressure. These compounds have also found some limited use in the treatment of absence seizures, to alkalinize the urine and prophylactically to reduce acute mountain sickness.

Acetazolamide

Methazolamide

Ethoxzolamide

Dichlorphenamide

Acetazolamide

Acetazolamide was the first of the carbonic anhydrase inhibitors to be introduced as an orally effective diuretic with a diuretic effect that lasts about 8–12 hours (see Table 22.2 for its pharmacokinetic properties). As mentioned earlier, its diuretic action is limited because of the systemic acidosis it produces. Acetazolamide reduces the rate of aqueous humor formation, and is used primarily in reducing intraocular pressure in the treatment of glaucoma and absence seizures. The dose is 250 mg to 1 g per day.

Glaucoma

The following carbonic anhydrase inhibitors are used orally in the treatment of glaucoma.

Methazolamide. Methazolamide is a derivative of acetazolamide in which one of the active hydrogens has been replaced by a methyl group. This decreases the polarity and permits a greater penetration into the ocular fluid, where it acts as a carbonic anhydrase inhibitor, reducing intraocular pressure. Its dose for glaucoma is 50–100 mg two to three times a day.

Ethoxzolamide and Dichlorphenamide. Ethoxzolamide is another carbonic anhydrase inhibitor whose properties and uses resemble those of acetazolamide. Dichlorphenamide is a disulfonamide derivative that shares the same pharmacologic properties and clinical uses as the

previously discussed compounds. The dose of dichlorphenamide is 25–100 mg one to three times a day.

Benzothiadiazine or Thiazide Diuretics

Further study of these benzene disulfonamide derivatives provided some compounds with a high degree of diuretic activity. Chloro and amino substitution gave compounds with increased activity, but these compounds were weak carbonic anhydrase inhibitors. When the amino group was acylated, an unexpected ring closure took place. These compounds possessed a diuretic activity independent of the carbonic anhydrase inhibitory activity, and a new series of diuretics called the benzothiadiazines was discovered.

Structure-activity Relationship

The thiazide diuretics are weakly acidic (see Appendix I for their pKa values) with a benzothiadiazine 1,1-dioxide nucleus.

The structure for the thiazide diuretics, relative activities and the pharmacokinetic properties for the thiazides are shown in Table 22.3. Chlorothiazide is the simplest member of this series having a pKa of 6.7 and 9.5. The hydrogen atom at the 2-N is the most acidic because of the electron-withdrawing effects of the neighboring sulfone group. The sulfonamide group that is substituted at C-7 provides an additional point of acidity in the molecule but is less acidic than the 2-N proton. These acidic protons make possible the formation of a water-soluble sodium salt that can be used for intravenous administration of the diuretics.

An electron-withdrawing group is necessary at position 6 for diuretic activity. Little diuretic activity is seen with a hydrogen atom at position 6, whereas compounds with a chloro or trifluoromethyl substitution are highly active. The trifluoromethyl-substituted diuretics are more lipid-soluble and have a longer duration of action than their chloro-substituted analogs. When electron-releasing groups, such as methyl or methoxyl, are placed at position 6, the diuretic activity is markedly reduced.

Replacement or removal of the sulfonamide group at position 7 yields compounds with little or no diuretic activity. Saturation of the double bond to give a 3,4-dihydro derivative produces a diuretic that is 10 times more active than the unsaturated derivative. Substitution with a lipophilic group at position 3 gives a marked increase in the diuretic potency. Haloalkyl, aralkyl, or thioether substitution increases the lipid solubility of the molecule and yields compounds with a longer duration of action. Alkyl

Table 22.3. Pharmacologic and Pharmacokinetic Properties for the Thiazide Diuretics

Generic Name	Trade Name	Structure	Relative Potency*	Carbonic Anhydrase Inhibition†	Bioavailability	Peak Plasma (hr)	$t_{1/2}$ (hr)	Duration (hr)	Route of Elimination
Chlorothiazide	Diuril	Structure I: R_1 = H	0.8	2×10^{-6}	<25%	4	1–2	6–12	U
Benzthiazide	Exna	Structure I: R_1 = $-S-CH_2-$phenyl	1.3	$\sim 10^{-7}$	NA	NA	e: 13 / NA	12–18	NA
Hydrochlorothiazide	HydroDiuril Esidrix Oretic	Structure II: R_1 = H; R_2 = Cl; R_3 = H	1.4	2×10^{-5}	>80%	4	6–15	6–12	U
Trichloromethiazide	Diurese Metahydrin Naqua	Structure II: R_1 = $CHCl_2$; R_2 = Cl; R_3 = H	1.7	6×10^{-5}	var.	6	NA	24	U
Methyclothiazide	Enduron Aquatensen	Structure II: R_1 = CH_2Cl; R_2 = Cl; R_3 = CH_3	1.8	—	var.	6	NA	>24	U
Polythiazide	Renese	Structure II: R_1 = $-CH_2-S-CH_2-CF_3$; R_2 = Cl; R_3 = CH_3	2.0	5×10^{-7}	var	6	NA	24–48	U 30% M
Hydroflumethiazide	Saluron Diucardin	Structure II: R_1 = H; R_2 = CF_3; R_3 = H	1.3	2×10^{-4}	inc	3–4	17 active metab.	18–24	U active metab.
Bendroflumethiazide	Naturetin	Structure II: R_1 = benzyl; R_2 = CF_3; R_3 = H	1.8	3×10^{-4}	>90%	4	8.5	6–12	U

*The numerical values refer to potency ratios (in humans) with the natriuretic response to that of a standard dose of meralluride, given a value of 1. Data from AHFS 2000 Drug Information. Bethesda, MD: American Society of Health-System Pharmacists; 2000 and USPDI Vol. I Drug Info. for the Hlth Care Prof. 20th ed. Rockville, MD; United States Pharmacopeial Convention. 2000.

†50% inhibition of carbonic anydrase in vitro.

U = urine unchanged; M = metabolized. NA = data not available. var. = variables absorption. inc. = incomplete absorption.

substitution on the 2-N position also decreases the polarity and increases the duration of diuretic action. Although these compounds do have carbonic anhydrase activity, there is no correlation of this activity with their saluretic activity (excretion of sodium and chloride ions).

Mechanism of Action

The mechanism of action of the benzothiadiazine diuretics is primarily related to their ability to inhibit the Na^+-Cl^- symporter located in the distal convoluted tubule (DCT). These diuretics are actively secreted in the proximal tubule and are carried to the loop of Henle and to the distal tubule. The major site of action of these compounds is in the distal tubule, where these drugs compete for the chloride binding site of the Na^+-Cl^- symporter and inhibit the reabsorption of sodium and chloride ions. For this reason, they are referred to as saluretics. They also inhibit the reabsorption of potassium and bicarbonate ions but to a lesser degree.

Therapeutic Applications

The thiazide diuretics are administered once a day or in divided daily doses. Some have a duration of action that permits administration of a dose every other day. Some of these compounds are rapidly absorbed orally and can show their diuretic effect in an hour (Table 22.3). These compounds are not extensively metabolized and are primarily excreted unchanged in the urine. Thiazide diuretics are used to treat edemas caused by cardiac decompensation as well as in hepatic or renal disease. They are also commonly used in the treatment of hypertension. Their effect may be attributed to a reduction in blood volume and a direct relaxation of vascular smooth muscle.

When the thiazide diuretics are administered for long periods, they can cause an increase in the elimination of potassium ions as well as sodium, chloride and magnesium ions. Hypokalemia and hypomagnesemia may result. Potassium and magnesium supplements may be administered in such cases, but their use is controversial. These supplements are usually administered as potassium chloride, potassium gluconate, potassium citrate, magnesium oxide, or magnesium lactate. The salts are administered as solutions, tablets or timed-release tablets. Generally, about 20 mEq of potassium is given daily. In cases of hypokalemia, 40–100 mEq per day may be administered. Potassium-sparing diuretics (e.g., triamterene, amiloride) may also be used to prevent hypokalemia. Combination preparation of hydrochlorothiazide and a potassium-sparing diuretic are available (e.g., Diazide, Moduretic).

Thiazide diuretics may induce side effects, including hypersensitivity reactions, gastric irritation, nausea, and electrolyte imbalances such as hypokalemia and hypochloremic alkalosis. Individuals who exhibit hypersensitivity reactions to one thiazide are likely to have a hypersensitivity reaction to other thiazides and sulfamoyl-containing diuretics (e.g., thiazide-like and some high-ceiling diuretics).

Quinazolinone Derivatives—Quinethazone and Metolazone
Overview

The quinazolin-4-one molecule has been structurally modified in a manner similar to the modification of the thiazide diuretics. Quinethazone and metolazone (pKa 9.7) are examples of this class (Table 22.4). The structural difference between the quinazolinone diuretics is the replacement of the 4-sulfone group (—SO_2—) with a 4-keto group (—CO—).

quinazolin-4-one

Because of their similar structures, it is not surprising that the quinazolinones have a diuretic effect similar to that of the thiazides. The side effects are also the same.

Mechanism of Action and Therapeutic Applications

The pharmacokinetic properties for the quinazolinone diuretics are listed in Table 22.4. They have a long duration of action usually as a result of protein binding. Although chlorothiazide has a duration of action of 6–12 hours, quinethazone has a duration of 18–24 hours, and metolazone has a duration of 12–24 hours. Metolazone has a bioavailability <65% (Zaroxolyn) and a prolonged onset to reach peak plasma concentrations of action ranging from 8–12 hours. However, when reformulated as for Mykrox, metolazone is almost completely absorbed with peak plasma concentrations reached in 2–4 hours. Thus, other versions of metolazone cannot be interchanged with Mykrox. Approximately 50–70% of metolazone is bound to carbonic anhydrase in the erythrocytes. Metolazone also has an increased potency and its mode of action of both compounds is similar to that of the thiazide derivatives. The dose of quinethazone is 50–100 mg daily, and that of metolazone is 2.5–20 mg given as a single oral dose.

Phthalimidine Derivatives—Chlorthalidone
Overview

Chlorthalidone (pKa 9.4) is an example of a diuretic in this class of compounds that bears a structural analogy to the quinazolinones (see Table 22.4) This compound may be named as a1-oxo-isoindoline or a phthalimidine. Although the molecule exists primarily in the phthalimidine form, the ring may be opened to form a benzophenone derivative.

The benzophenone form illustrates the relationship to the quinazolinone series of diuretics. It may be regarded as an open ring variation.

Table 22.4. Pharmacokinetic Properties for the Thiazide-like Diuretics

Generic Name	Trade Name	Structure	Bioavailability	Peak Plasma	$t_{1/2}$	Duration	Route of Elimination
Metolazone	Zaroxylon Mykrox#		<65% >90%	8–12 h 2–4 h	14	12–24 h	U: 70—95% EHC: 10–30%
Quinethazone	Hydromox		NA	6 h	6–15 h	18–24 h	U
Chlorthalidone	Hygroton Thalitone#		inc/var. >90%	4 h	35–50* e: 54	48–72 h	U: 30–60%
Indapamide	Lozol		>90%	2–3 h	14–18 h	8 wks	M: 60–70% EHC: 20–30%

Data from AHFS 2000 Drug Information. Bethesda, MD: American Society of Health-System Pharmacists; 2000 and USPDI Vol. I Drug Info. for the Hlth Care Prof. 20th ed. Rockville, MD; United States Pharmacopeial Convention. 2000.
* Strongly bound to red blood cells. # = not interchangeable with similar drug. U = urine unchanged; M = metabolized. NA = data not available. var. = variable absorption. inc. = incomplete absorption.

Therapeutic Application

Chlorthalidone has a long duration of action, 48–72 hours (see Table 22.3 for its other pharmacokinetic properties). Although quinethazone and metolazone are administered daily, chlorthalidone may be administered in doses of 25–100 mg three times a week. When chlorthalidone is formulated with the excipient povidone, the product, Thalitone, has greater bioavailability (>90%) and reaches peak plasma concentrations in a shorter time when compared to its other products. Similar to the quinazolinones, it is also extensively bound to carbonic anhydrase in the erythrocytes.

Indolines—Indapamide
Mechanism of Action

The prototypic indoline diuretic is indapamide, reported as a diuretic in 1984. Indapamide contains a polar chlorobenzamide moiety and a nonpolar lipophilic methylindoline group. In contrast to the thiazides, indapamide does not contain a thiazide ring, and only one sulfonamide group is present within the molecular structure (pKa 8.8). It is rapidly and completely absorbed from the GI tract and reaches its peak plasma level in 2–3 hours with a duration of action up to 8 weeks. This prolonged duration of action is associated with its extensive binding to carbonic anhydrase in the erythrocytes. It exhibits biphasic kinetics with a half-life of 14–18 hours and an elimination half-life of 24 hours. Indapamide is extensively metabolized with 60–70% of the oral dose being eliminated in the urine as glucuronide and sulfate metabolites and <10% excreted unchanged. The remaining 20–30% is eliminated via extrahepatic cycling.

Therapeutic Application

Uses of indapamide include the treatment of essential hypertension and edema due to congestive heart failure. The duration of action is approximately 24 hours with the normal oral adult dosage starting at 2.5 mg given each morning. The dose may be increased to 5.0 mg per day, but doses beyond this level do not appear to provide additional results.

High-ceiling or Loop Diuretics
Mechanism of Action

This class of drugs is characterized more by its pharmacologic similarities than its chemical similarities. These diuretics produce a peak diuresis much greater than that observed with the other commonly used diuretics, hence the name high-ceiling diuretics. Their main site of action is believed to be on the thick ascending limb of the loop of Henle (TALH), where they inhibit the luminal $Na^+/K^+/2Cl^-$ symporter. These diuretics are commonly referred to as loop diuretics. Additional effects on the proximal and distal tubules are also possible. High-ceiling diuretics are characterized by a quick onset and short duration of activity. Their diuretic effect appears in about 30 minutes and lasts for about 6 hours. The pharmacokinetic properties for the loop diuretics are listed in Table 22.2.

Furosemide

Structure-activity Relationships. Furosemide is an example of a high-ceiling diuretic and may be regarded as a derivative of anthranilic acid or o-aminobenzoic acid.

Research on 5-sulfamoylanthranilic acids at the Hoechst Laboratories in Germany showed them to be effective diuretics. The most active of a series of variously substituted derivatives was furosemide.

Furosemide

5-Sulfamoyl-
anthranilic acid

The chlorine and sulfonamide substitutions are features seen also in previously discussed diuretics. Because the molecule possesses a free carboxyl group, furosemide is a stronger acid than the thiazide diuretics (pKa 3.9). This drug is excreted primarily unchanged. A small amount of metabolism, however, can take place on the furan ring, which is substituted on the aromatic amino group (see Table 22.2 for its other pharmacokinetic properties).

Therapeutic Applications. Furosemide has a saluretic effect 8–10 times that of the thiazide diuretics, however, it has a shorter duration of action, about 6–8 hours. Furosemide causes an excretion of sodium, chloride, potassium, calcium, magnesium, and bicarbonate ions. It is effective for the treatment of edemas connected with cardiac, hepatic, and renal sites. Because it lowers the blood pressure similar to the thiazide derivatives, one of its uses is in the treatment of hypertension.

Furosemide is orally effective but may be used parenterally when a more prompt diuretic effect is desired. The dosage of furosemide, 20–80 mg per day, may be given in divided doses because of the short duration of action of the drug and carefully increased up to a maximum of 600 mg per day. Clinical toxicity of furosemide involves abnormalities of fluid and electrolyte balance. Hyperuricemia, ototoxicity and gastrointestinal side effects are also observed.

Bumetanide

Therapeutic Application. A diuretic structurally related to furosemide is bumetanide.

Bumetanide

This compound also functions as a high-ceiling diuretic in the ascending limb of the loop of Henle. It has a duration of action of about 4 hours. The uses of this compound are similar to those described for furosemide. The dose of bumetanide is 0.5–2 mg per day, given as a single dose.

Structure-activity Relationships. For bumetanide, a phenoxy group has replaced the customary chloro or trifluoromethyl substitutions seen in other diuretic molecules. The phenoxy group is an electron-withdrawing group similar to the chloro or trifluoromethyl substitutions. The amine group that had been customarily seen at position 6 has been moved to position 5. These minor variations from furosemide produced a compound with a mode of action similar to that of furosemide, but with a marked increase in diuretic potency. The short duration of activity is similar, but the compound is about 50 times more potent. Replacement of the phenoxy group at position 4 with a C_6H_5NH- or C_6H_5S- group also gives compounds with a favorable activity. When the butyl group on the C_5 amine is replaced with a furanylmethyl group, such as in furosemide, however, the results are not favorable.

Torsemide

Torsemide—Mechanism of Action and Therapeutic Applications

Further modification of furosemide-like structures has led to the development of torsemide. Instead of the sulfonamide group found in furosemide and bumetanide, torsemide contains a sulfonylurea moiety. Similar to other high-ceiling diuretics, torsemide inhibits the luminal $Na^+/K^+/2\ Cl^-$ symporter in the ascending limb of the loop of Henle to promote the excretion of sodium, potassium, chloride, calcium, and magnesium ions and water. An additional effect on the peritubular side at chloride channels may enhance the luminal effects of torsemide. Torsemide, however, does not act at the proximal tubule, in contrast to furosemide and bumetanide, and therefore does not increase phosphate or bicarbonate excretion. Peak diuresis is observed in 1–2 hours following oral or intravenous administration with a duration of action of about 6 hours. Torsemide was recommended for approval by the Food and Drug Administration's Cardiovascular and Renal Drug's Advisory Committee for the treatment of hypertension and edema associated with congestive heart failure and cirrhosis.

Ethacrynic acid

Ethacrynic Acid

Structure-activity Relationship. Another major class of high-ceiling diuretics is the phenoxyacetic acid derivatives. These compounds were developed at about the same time as furosemide but were designed to act mechanistically similar to the organomercurials (i.e., via inhibition of sulfhydryl-containing enzymes involved in solute reabsorption). Optimal diuretic activity was obtained when an oxyacetic acid group was positioned para to an α,β-unsaturated carbonyl (or other sulfhydryl-reactive group) and chloro or methyl groups were placed at the 2- or 3-position of the phenyl ring. In addition, hydrogen atoms on the terminal alkene carbon also provided maximum reactivity. Thus, a molecule with a weakly acidic group to direct the drug to the kidney and an alkylating moiety to react with sulfhydryl groups and lipophilic groups seemed to provide the best combination for a diuretic in this class. These features led to the development of ethacrynic acid as the prototypic agent in this class.

Mechanism of Action. The mode of action of ethacrynic acid appears to be more complex than the simple addition of sulfhydryl groups of the enzyme to the drug molecule. When the double bond of ethacrynic acid is reduced, the resultant compound is still active, although the diuretic activity is diminished. The sulfhydryl groups of the enzyme would not be expected to add to the drug molecule in the absence of the α,β,-unsaturated ketone. The pharmacokinetic properties for ethacrynic acid are listed in Table 22.2.

In 1984, a new series of diuretics was reported (2,3). The following substance is representative of this series.

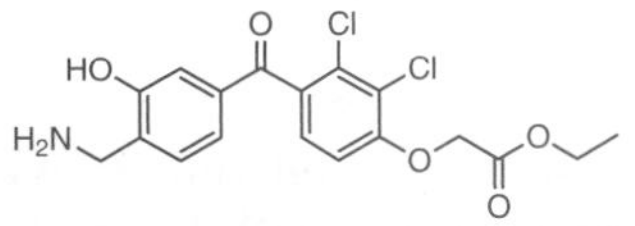

These compounds are potent high-ceiling diuretics that resemble ethacrynic acid in their mechanism of action. The ethyl ester group represents a prodrug that can be easily hydrolyzed to the free carboxyl group. As in ethacrynic acid, a 2,3-dichloro substitution is necessary. In addition, a para-hydroxyl group and an unsubstituted aminomethyl group on the benzene ring are highly beneficial. The carbonyl group can be replaced with an ether or sulfide group. These compounds have no ability to add the sulfhydryl groups of the kidney enzymes. The complete mechanism of action of these compounds remains in doubt.

Similar to the other high-ceiling diuretics, ethacrynic acid inhibits the $Na^+/K^+/2Cl^-$ symporter in the ascending limb of the loop of Henle (TALH) to promote a marked diuresis. Sodium, chloride, potassium, and calcium excretion are increased following oral or intravenous administration of ethacrynic acid. Oral administration of ethacrynic acid results in diuresis within 1 hour and a duration of action of 6–8 hours. Toxicity induced by ethacrynic acid is similar to that induced by furosemide and bumetanide. Ethacrynic acid, however, is not widely used because it induces a greater incidence of ototoxicity and more serious gastrointestinal effects than furosemide or bumetanide.

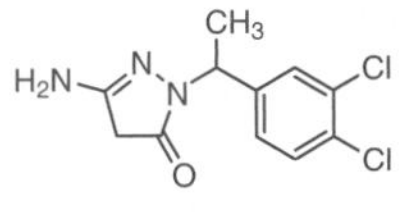

Muzolimine

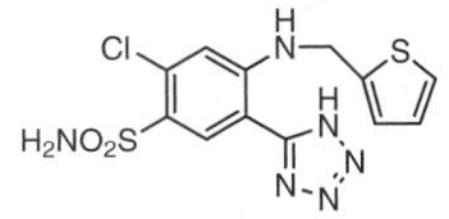

Azosemide

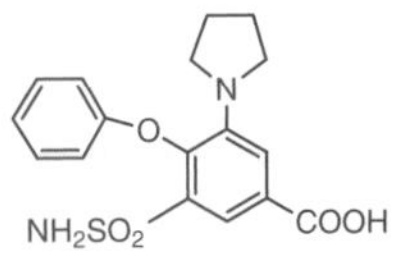

Piretanide

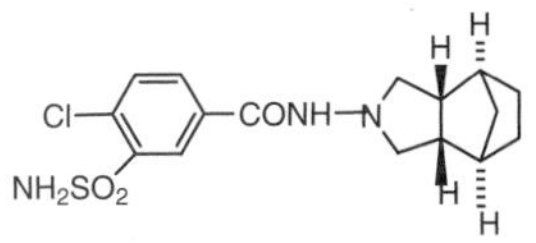

Tripamide

New Drugs

Four additional high-ceiling diuretics reported are azosemide, muzolimine, piretanide and tripamide.

As can be seen by these varied structures, the high-ceiling diuretics are characterized more by their pharmacologic similarities than by their chemical similarities.

Potassium-sparing Diuretics (Mineralocorticoid Receptor Antagonists)— Antihormone Diuretics

Mechanism of Action

The adrenal cortex secretes a potent mineralocorticoid called aldosterone which promotes salt and water retention and potassium and hydrogen ion excretion.

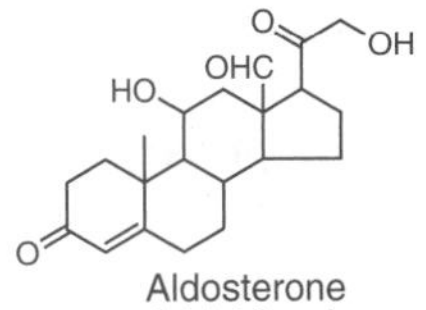

Aldosterone
(aldol form)

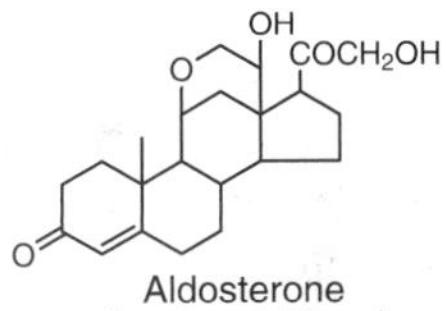

Aldosterone
(hemiacetal form)

Other mineralocorticoids have an effect on the electrolytic balance of the body, but aldosterone is the most potent. Its ability to cause increased reabsorption of sodium and chloride ion and increased potassium ion excretion is about 3000 times that of hydrocortisone. A substance that antagonizes the effects of aldosterone could conceivably be a good diuretic drug. Spironolactone is such an antagonist.

Spironolactone

Spironolactone is a competitive antagonist to the mineralocorticoids such as aldosterone. The mineralocorticoid receptor is an intracellular protein that can bind

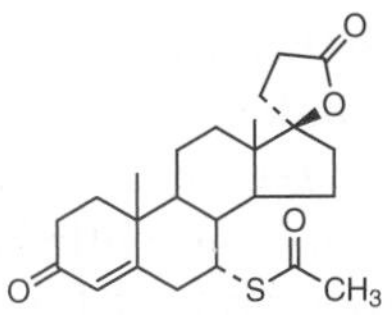

Spironolactone

aldosterone. Spironolactone binds to the receptor and competitively inhibits aldosterone binding to the receptor. The inability of aldosterone to bind to its receptor prevents reabsorption of sodium and chloride ions and the associated water. The most important site of these receptors is in the late distal tubule and collecting system (DCT, CD).

Metabolism. On oral administration, about 90% of the dose of spironolactone is absorbed and is significantly metabolized during its first passage through the liver to its major active metabolite, canrenone (see Table 22.2 for their pharmacokinetic properties), which is interconvertible with its canrenoate anion. Canrenone is an antagonist to aldosterone.

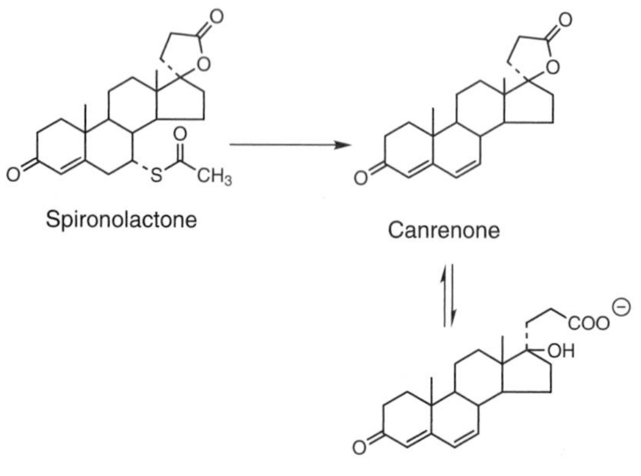

Spironolactone   Canrenone

Canrenoic acid anion

The canrenoate anion is not active per se but acts as aldosterone antagonist because of its conversion to canrenone, which exists in the lactone form. Canrenone has been suggested as the active form of spironolactone as an aldosterone antagonist. The formation of canrenone, however, cannot account fully for the total activity of spironolactone. Both canrenone and potassium canrenoate are used as diuretics in other countries, but they are not yet available in the United States.

Therapeutic Applications. The most serious side effect of spironolactone is hyperkalemia because it has a potassium-sparing effect. Potassium levels should be monitored during the use of this drug. The dose of spironolactone is 100 mg per day given in single or divided doses. Spironolactone can also be administered in a fixed-dose combination with hydrochlorothiazide. Spironolactone has been implicated in tumor production in chronic toxicity studies in rats.

Pteridines—Triamterene

Pteridines have a marked potential for influencing biologic processes. Early screening of pteridine derivatives revealed that 2,4-diamino-6,7-dimethylpteridine was a fairly potent diuretic. Further structural modification led to the development of triamterene.

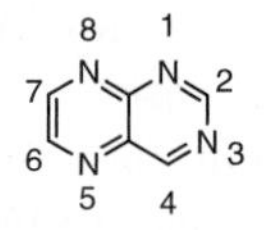

Pteridine

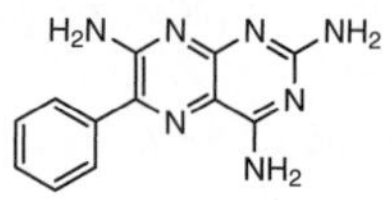

Triamterene

Mechanism of Action

Triamterene interferes with the process of cationic exchange by blocking luminal sodium channels in the distal tubule (DCT). Sodium channel inhibitors block the reabsorption of sodium ion and block the secretion of potassium ion. Aldosterone is not antagonized by triamterene. The net result is increased sodium and chloride ion excretion in the urine and almost no potassium excretion. In fact, hyperkalemia may result from the use of triamterene. Triamterene is more than 70% absorbed on oral administration (see Table 22.2 for its other pharmacokinetic properties). The diuretic effect occurs rapidly, in about 30 minutes, and reaches a peak plasma concentration in 2–4 hours, with a duration of action of more than 24 hours. Triamterene is extensively metabolized, and some of the metabolites are active as diuretics. Both the drug and its metabolites are excreted in the urine.

Therapeutic Applications

Triamterene is administered initially in doses of 100 mg twice a day. A maintenance dose for each patient should be individually determined. This dose may vary from 100 mg a day to as low as 100 mg every other day.

The most serious side effect associated with the use of triamterene is hyperkalemia. For this reason, potassium supplements are contraindicated, and serum potassium levels should be checked regularly. Triamterene is also used in combination with hydrochlorothiazide. Here the hypokalemic effect of the hydrochlorothiazide counters the hyperkalemic effect of the triamterene. Other side effects seen with the use of triamterene are nausea, vomiting, and headache.

Modifications of the triamterene structure are not usually beneficial in terms of diuretic activity. Activity is retained if an amine group is replaced with a lower alkylamine group. Introduction of a para-methyl group on the phenyl ring decreases the activity about one-half. Introduction of a para-hydroxyl group on the phenyl ring yields a compound that is essentially inactive as a diuretic.

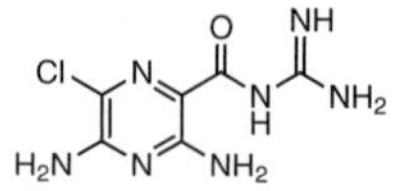

Amiloride

Aminopyrazines—Amiloride

Amiloride, another potassium-sparing diuretic, is an aminopyrazine structurally related to triamterene as an open-chain analog. Similar to triamterene, it interferes with the process of cationic exchange in the distal tubule (DCT) by blocking luminal sodium channels. It blocks the reabsorption of sodium ion and the secretion of potassium ion. It has no effect on the action of aldosterone. Oral amiloride is about 50% absorbed (see Table 22.2 for its other pharmacokinetic properties) with a duration of action of 10–12 hours, slightly longer than that for triamterene. Although triamterene is extensively metabolized, about 50% of amiloride is excreted unchanged. Renal impairment can increase its elimination half-life. As with triamterene, the most serious side effect associated with amiloride is hyperkalemia, and it also has the other side effects associated with triamterene. The dose of amiloride is 5–10 mg per day. Amiloride is also combined with hydrochlorothiazide in a fixed dose combination.

Therapeutic application of diuretics

B.D. is a 67-year-old man who was admitted with a complaint of shortness of breath which has increased over the last few months. He also indicated that he has recently gained over 12 pounds without changing eating or exercise habits, and that he often has trouble breathing when climbing stairs at home. Physical examination reveals signs and symptoms consistent with both right-sided (systemic edema, hepatomegaly, neck vein distension) and left-sided (weakness, fatigue, rales, cyanosis) heart failure. A diagnosis of congestive heart failure (CHF) is made, and a decision is made to limit sodium intake (low sodium diet) and initiate oral therapy with digitalis to improve heart function. A diuretic will also be added to help remove edema fluid and decrease the workload on the heart. What diuretics would be appropriate to use in this patient?

ANSWER:
Selection of a diuretic would be based on the drug's ability to mobilize edema fluid and to help reduce the workload on the heart. Thiazide and loop (high-ceiling) diuretics are effective in mobilizing edema fluid and could be used in this patient. Osmotic diuretics are not effective at mobilizing edema fluid and will expand extracellular fluid which would worsen the workload on the heart. Carbonic anhydrase inhibitors are weak diuretics and would not provide adequate diuresis to effectively reduce the workload on the heart. Potassium-sparing diuretics are also less effective than thiazides or loop diuretics in mobilizing edema fluid, and would not be a diuretic of first choice in this patient.

Choosing between a thiazide or a loop diuretic depends on many factors including the amount of edema present, severity of symptoms, and the patient's renal function. Loop diuretics (e.g. furosemide, torsemide) are more efficacious than thiazides and can remove edema fluid faster than thiazides to provide quicker relief. Loop diuretics also have direct effects on the pulmonary venous system to help improve pulmonary symptoms related to the failing heart. However, loop diuretics also can cause more dramatic imbalances in extracellular volume and electrolyte levels than thiazides, and loop diuretics can alter these levels sooner than with thiazide use. Thus, loop diuretic use should be employed when moderate to severe CHF is present, while thiazides may be preferred when mild CHF is present. Since this patient has moderate to severe symptoms, furosemide is chosen as the diuretic to use in this patient.

If B.D. had been seen when his CHF was mild, but his renal function was already impaired (GFR 25 ml/min), how would these circumstances affect your selection of a diuretic?

ANSWER:
Although a thiazide diuretic would normally be the diuretic of choice in treating mild CHF, a thiazide generally is less effective in patients with renal insufficiency. Thiazides can reach their site of action (the luminal sodium ion-chloride ion symporter of the distal convoluted tubule) following filtration at the glomerulus. The amount of drug filtered at the glomerulus depends on the extent of plasma protein binding for that drug. In addition, since thiazides are weakly acidic drugs (pKas around 7.0 to 9.0), they are substrates for active secretion by the organic anion transport system of the proximal tubular cells. However, with the exception of metolazone and indapamide, most thiazides are ineffective as diuretics when the glomerular filtration rate (GFR) is <30 to 40 ml/min (normal - 125 ml/min).

Loop diuretics reach their site of action (luminal sodium ion-potassium ion-2 chloride ion transporter of the ascending limb of the loop of Henle) primarily via active secretion by the organic anion transport system of proximal tubular cells. As stronger organic acids than thiazide diuretics (e.g. pKa of furosemide = 4.7), loop diuretics are good substrates for secretion. Extensive plasma protein binding by these drugs limits their access to the lumina of nephrons via filtration. Thus, a marked reduction in GFR does not limit access of loop diuretics to tubular lumina or markedly alter the therapeutic efficacy of these drugs. As a result, a loop diuretic would still be a preferred choice for treating B.D. if his CHF had been mild, but his renal function had been reduced.

Following six weeks on his low salt diet and drug therapy, B.D.'s condition seems greatly improved. However, his serum potassium levels have decreased from 4.2 mEq/liter to 3.1 mEq/liter (normal - 3.8 to 5.6 mEq/liter). What caused his serum potassium levels to decrease over time? Why is this change a concern? What can be done to remedy this problem?

ANSWER:
One of the major side effects of using a loop diuretic is excessive excretion of electrolytes, including potassium ions. Loss of potassium can eventually lead to hypokalemia (low blood potassium), and hypokalemia alone can lead to the development of cardiac arrhythmias. However, potassium loss also potentiates the actions of digitalis (cardiac sodium-potassium ATPase inhibition) and can lead to digitalis-induced cardiac arrhythmias as well. Hypokalemia can be treated/prevented by the use of potassium supplements _or_ the use of a potassium-sparing diuretic (e.g. triamterene, amiloride). Since potassium-sparing diuretics are weakly basic drugs, they do not alter the active secretion of loop diuretics.

CASE STUDY

Victoria F. Roche and S. William Zito

ON, a 67-year-old male with moderate to severe CHF has been doing extremely well on his low salt diet and drug therapy (furosemide (1) and digoxin (2)). He visits his physician complaining that over the past few weeks he has experienced difficulty breathing, muscle weakness and cramps. Clinical tests show a plasma potassium of 3.2 mEq/l, indicative of borderline hypokalemia. Reccomend a remedy for ON from the structures drawn for you given below (3–5).

1. *Identify the therapeutic problem(s) where the pharmacist's intervention may benefit the patient.*

2. *Identify and prioritize the patient specific factors that must be considered to achieve the desired therapeutic outcomes.*

3. *Conduct a thorough and mechanistically oriented structure-activity analysis of all therapeutic alternatives provided in the case.*

4. *Evaluate the SAR findings against the patient specific factors and desired therapeutic outcomes and make a therapeutic decision.*

5. *Counsel your patient.*

REFERENCES

1. Jackson EK. Diuretics. In: Goodman and Gilman's The Pharmacological Basis of Therapeutics, 10th ed., JG Hardman et al., Eds., New York, McGraw-Hill, 2001.

2. Lee CM, Plattner JJ, Ours CW, et. al. [(Aminomethyl)aryloxy]acetic acid esters. A new class of high-ceiling diuretics. 1. Effects of nitrogen and aromatic nuclear substitution. J Med Chem 1984; 27:1579–1587.

3. Plattner JJ, Fung AK, Smital JR, et al. [(Aminomethyl)aryloxy]acetic acid esters. A new class of high-ceiling diuretics. 2. Modifications of the oxyacetic side chain. J Med Chem 1984; 27:1587–1596.

SUGGESTED READINGS

Acara MA. Renal pharmacology–Diuretics. In: Smith CM, Reynard AM, eds. Textbook of Pharmacology. Philadelphia, W. B. Saunders, 1992.

Berndt WO, Friedman PA. Diuretic drugs. In: Craig CR, Stitzel RE, eds. Modern Pharmacology, 5th ed. Boston, Little, Brown & Co., 1997.

Brenner BM, Rector FC Jr. eds. The Kidney, 4th ed., Philadelphia, W. B. Saunders, 1991.

Breyer J, Jacobson HR. Molecular mechanisms of diuretic agents. Annu. Rev. Med., 41, 265(1990).

Diuretics. In: Bennett DR, ed. Drug Evaluations, Annual 1994, Chicago, American Medical Association, 1994.

Jackson EK. Diuretics. In: Hardman JG et al. eds. Goodman and Gilman's The Pharmacological Basis of Therapeutics, 10th ed. New York, McGraw-Hill, 2001.

23. Angiotensin Converting Enzyme Inhibitors, Antagonists and Calcium Blockers

MARC HARROLD

THE RENIN-ANGIOTENSIN PATHWAY

The renin-angiotensin system is a complex, highly regulated pathway that is integral in the regulation of blood volume, electrolyte balance, and arterial blood pressure. It consists of two main enzymes, renin and angiotensin converting enzyme (ACE), whose primary purpose is to release angiotensin II from its endogenous precursor, angiotensinogen (Fig. 23.1). Angiotensin II is a potent vasoconstrictor which affects peripheral resistance, renal function, and cardiovascular structure (1).

> ### Compounds Listed in the Top 200 Drugs Which Effect The Renin-Angiotensin Pathway (2)
>
> Benazepril (Lotensin), enalapril (Vasotec), fosinopril (Monopril), lisinopril (Zestril, Prinivi), lisinopril/ hydrochlorothiazide (Zestaretic), losartan (Cozaar), quinapril (Accupril), ramipril (Altace).

History and Overview of Pathway

Historically, the renin-angiotensin system dates back to 1898 when Tiegerstedt and Bergman demonstrated the existence of a pressor substance present in crude kidney extracts. A little over 40 years later, two independent research groups discovered that this pressor substance, which had previously been named renin, was actually an enzyme and that the true pressor substance was a peptide formed by the catalytic action of renin. This peptide pressor substance was initially assigned two different names, angiotonin and hypertensin; however, these names were eventually combined to produce the current designation, angiotensin. In the 1950s, it was discovered that angiotensin exists as both an inactive decapeptide, angiotensin I, and an active octapeptide, angiotensin II and that the conversion of angiotensin I to angiotensin II was catalyzed by an enzyme distinct from renin (3).

Angiotensinogen is an α_2-globulin with a molecular weight of 58,000–61,000. It contains 452 amino acids, is abundant in the plasma, and is continually synthesized and secreted by the liver. A number of hormones including glucocorticoids, thyroid hormone and angiotensin II stimulate its synthesis. The most important portion of this compound is the N-terminus, specifically the Leu_{10}-Val_{11} bond. This bond is cleaved by renin and produces the decapeptide angiotensin I. The Phe_8-His_9 peptide bond of angiotensin I is then cleaved by ACE to produce the octapeptide angiotensin II. Aminopeptidase can further convert angiotensin II to the active heptapeptide angiotensin III by removing the N-terminal arginine residue. Further actions of carboxypeptidases, aminopeptidases, and endopeptidases result in the formation of inactive peptide fragments. An additional compound can be formed by the action of a prolyl-endopeptidase on angiotensin I. Cleavage of the Pro_7-Phe_8 bond of angiotensin I produces a heptapeptide known as angiotensin 1-7. The actions of all of these compounds are discussed below.

Actions and Properties of Renin-Angiotensin Pathway Components

Renin is an aspartyl protease that determines the rate of angiotensin II production. It is a much more specific enzyme than ACE. Its primary function is to cleave the leucine-valine bond located at residues 10 and 11 of angiotensinogen. The stimulation of renin release is controlled very closely by hemodynamic, neurogenic and humoral signals (Fig. 23.2). Hemodynamic signals involve the renal juxtaglomerular cells. These cells are sensitive to the hemodynamic stretch of the afferent glomerular arteriole. An increase in the stretch implies a raised blood pressure and results in a reduced release of renin, while a decrease in the stretch increases renin secretion. Additionally, these cells are also sensitive to NaCl flux across the adjacent macula densa. Increases in NaCl flux across the macula densa inhibit renin release, while decreases in the flux stimulate release. Further, neurogenic enhancement of renin release occurs via activation of β_1-receptors. Finally, a variety of hormonal signals influence the release of renin. Somatostatin, atrial natriuretic factor, and angiotensin II inhibit renin release, while vasoactive intestinal peptide, parathyroid hormone, and glucagon stimulate renin release (4).

In contrast, ACE, also known as kininase II, is a zinc protease which is under minimal physiologic control. It is not a rate-limiting step in the generation of angiotensin II. It is a relatively nonspecific dipeptidyl carboxypeptidase that requires only a tripeptide sequence as a substrate. The only structural feature required by ACE is that the penultimate amino acid in the peptide substrate cannot be proline. It is for this reason that angiotensin II, which contains a proline in the penultimate position, is not further metabolized by ACE. The lack of specificity and control exhibited by ACE results in its involvement in the bradykinin pathway (Fig. 23.3). Bradykinin is a nonapeptide which acts locally to produce pain, cause vasodilation, increase vascular permeability, and stimulate prostaglandin synthesis. Similar to angiotensin II, bradykinin is produced by proteolytic cleavage of a precursor peptide. Cleavage of kininogen by the protease kallikrein produces a decapeptide known as either kallidin or lysyl-bradykinin. Subsequent cleavage of the N-terminal lysine by aminopeptidase produces bradykinin. The degradation of bradykinin to inactive peptides occurs through the actions of ACE. Thus ACE not only produces a potent vasoconstrictor but also inactivates a potent vasodilator (1,4,5).

Angiotensin II is the dominant peptide produced by the renin-angiotensin pathway (Fig. 23.2). It is a potent vasoconstrictor that increases total peripheral resistance through a variety of mechanisms: direct vasoconstriction, enhancement of both catecholamine release and neurotransmission within the peripheral nervous system, and increased sympathetic discharge. The result of all these actions is a rapid pressor response. Additionally, angiotensin II causes a slow pressor response resulting in a long term stabilization of arterial blood pressure. This long term effect is accomplished by the regulation of renal function. Angiotensin II directly increases sodium reabsorption in the proximal tubule. It also alters renal hemodynamics and causes the release of aldosterone from the adrenal cortex. Finally, angiotensin II causes the hypertrophy and remodeling of both vascular and cardiac cells through a variety of hemodynamic and nonhemodynamic effects (1).

Although secondary peptides, angiotensin III and angiotensin 1-7 are also thought to contribute to the overall effects of the renin-angiotensin pathway. Angiotensin III is equipotent with angiotensin II in stimulating aldosterone secretion; however, it is only 10–25% as potent in increasing blood pressure. In contrast, angiotensin 1-7 does not cause either aldosterone secretion or vasoconstriction, but has potent effects which are distinct from angiotensin II.

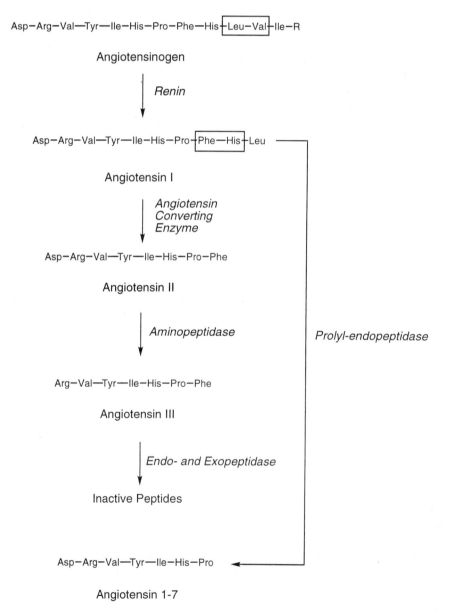

Fig. 23.1. Schematic representation of the renin-angiotensin pathway. The labile peptide bonds of angiotensinogen and angiotensin I are highlighted.

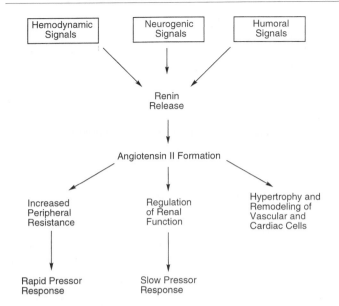

Fig. 23.2. Summary of the factors involved in renin release and the effects medicated by angiotensin II.

Similar to angiotensin II, angiotensin 1-7 causes neuronal excitation and vasopressin release. Additionally, it enhances the production of prostaglandins via a receptor-mediated process that does not involve an increase in intracellular calcium levels. It has been proposed to be important in the modulation of cell-to-cell interactions in cardiovascular and neural tissues (6).

ROLE OF THE RENIN-ANGIOTENSIN PATHWAY IN CARDIOVASCULAR DISORDERS

Due to the fact that the renin-angiotensin pathway is central to the maintenance of blood volume, arterial blood pressure, and electrolyte balance, abnormalities in this pathway (*e.g.,* excessive release of renin, overproduction of angiotensin II) can contribute to a variety of cardiovascular disorders. Specifically, overactivity of this pathway can result in hypertension or congestive heart failure (CHF) via the mechanisms previously described. Abnormally high levels of angiotensin II can contribute to hypertension through both rapid and slow pressor responses. Additionally, high levels of angiotensin II can cause cellular hypertrophy and increase both afterload and wall tension. All of these events can cause or exacerbate CHF.

High blood pressure is a relatively common disorder, affecting more than 50 million Americans. It is more prevalent in males than in females and in blacks than in Caucasians. Onset usually begins during the third, fourth, and fifth decades of life, and the incidence of the disorder increases with age. Hypertension is classified as either primary or secondary. Primary hypertension, also known as essential hypertension, is the most prevalent form of the disorder and is defined as high blood pressure of an unknown etiology. Most cases of primary hypertension are thought to be due to a variety of underlying pathophysiologic mechanisms and not to a single, specific cause. Ad-

ditionally, genetic factors appear to be important in the development of primary hypertension. Secondary hypertension is associated with a specific disorder (e.g., chronic renal disease, pheochromocytoma, and Cushing's syndrome), is present in approximately 5% of individuals with high blood pressure, and in some instances is potentially curable. Secondary hypertension is much more common in children than in adults (7).

Congestive heart failure affects approximately 4 million Americans and is the most common hospital discharge diagnosis in patients over 65 years of age. Average survival from the time of diagnosis is 1.7 and 3.2 years in men and women, respectively. The disease results from conditions in which the heart is unable to supply blood at a rate sufficient to meet the demands of the body. Similar to hypertension, this pathophysiologic state can occur via a variety of mechanisms. Any pathophysiologic event which causes either systolic or diastolic dysfunction will result in CHF. Systolic dysfunction, or decreased contractility, can be caused by dilated cardiomyopathies, ventricular hypertrophy, or a reduction in muscle mass. Diastolic dysfunction, or restriction in ventricular filling, can be caused by increased ventricular stiffness, mitral or tricuspid valve stenosis, or pericardial disease. Both ventricular hypertrophy and myocardial ischemia can contribute to increased ventricular stiffness (8).

OVERVIEW OF DRUG THERAPY AFFECTING THE RENIN-ANGIOTENSIN PATHWAY

Since angiotensin II produces the majority of the effects attributed to the renin-angiotensin pathway, compounds which can block either the synthesis of angiotensin II or the binding of angiotensin II to its receptor should attenuate the actions of this pathway. Indeed, enzyme inhibitors of both renin and ACE, as well as receptor antagonists of angiotensin II have all been shown to produce beneficial effects in decreasing the actions of angiotensin II. Inhibitors of ACE were the first class of compounds to be marketed. This occurred in 1981 with the FDA approval of captopril. Fourteen years later, losartan was approved as the first angiotensin II receptor antagonist. The development, SAR, physicochemical properties,

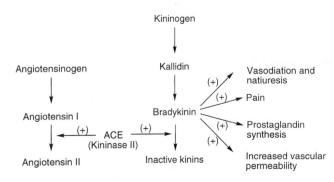

Fig. 23.3. Schematic representation of the bradykinin pathway and its relationship to ACE and the renin-angiotensin pathway.

interactions and indications of these classes of drugs are discussed below.

Attempts to develop orally active, bioavailable renin inhibitors actually predate the development of ACE inhibitors. Research in this area continues today; however one of the main attractions of renin inhibitors, specificity, has proven to be a significant hurdle to the clinical development (9) of these agents.

ANGIOTENSIN-CONVERTING ENZYME INHIBITORS

There are currently 11 ACE inhibitors approved for therapeutic use in the United States. These compounds can be subclassified into three groups based on their chemical composition: sulfhydryl-containing inhibitors exemplified by captopril, dicarboxylate-containing inhibitors exemplified by enalapril, and phosphonate-containing inhibitors exemplified by fosinopril. Captopril and fosinopril are the lone representatives of their respective chemical subclassifications, while the majority of the inhibitors contain the dicarboxylate functionality. All of these compounds effectively block the conversion of angiotensin I to angiotensin II and have similar therapeutic and physiologic effects. The compounds differ primarily in their potency and pharmacokinetic profile (1). Additionally, the sulfhydryl group in captopril is responsible for certain effects not seen with the other agents. Detailed descriptions of the rationale for the development of captopril, enalapril, and fosinopril are provided below.

Sulfhydryl-containing Inhibitors: Development of Captopril

In 1965, Ferreira reported that the venom of the South American pit viper, *Bothrops jararaca*, contained factors which potentiated the action of bradykinin. These factors, originally designated as bradykinin potentiating factors (BPFs), were isolated and found to be a family of peptides containing 5–13 amino acid residues (13). Their actions in potenti-

---

Development of Orally Active Renin Inhibitors

Renin is a very specific enzyme. The octapeptide, His-Pro-Phe-His-*Leu-Leu*-Val-Tyr, is the smallest substrate recognized by the enzyme and is similar to the eight amino acid sequence, His_6-Pro_7-Phe_8-His_9-Leu_{10}-Val_{11}-Ile_{12}-His_{13}, which is found in angiotensinogen. Using this octapeptide, Boger and coworkers (9) replaced the labile Leu-Leu bond with the stable dipeptide mimic statine and replaced the two C-terminal residues (Val–Tyr) with similar hydrophobic amino acids (Leu-Phe).

The resulting compound, *N*-isovaleryl-His-Pro-Phe-His-*Sta*-Leu-Phe-NH$_2$ (aka SCRIP), showed effective, though short-lived, inhibition of renin when given intravenously. Infusion experiments with SCRIP were the first to demonstrate that a small molecule renin inhibitor could maintain a lowered blood pressure for an extended period of time. However, susceptibility to proteolytic cleavage limited the therapeutic utility of SCRIP and other analogous peptides.

Structure-activity studies with SCRIP revealed that the N-terminal His-Pro-Phe sequence could be replaced with an acylated phenylalanine or tyrosine without any significant loss in inhibitor activity. Additional changes to SCRIP resulted in the clinical drug candidate enalkiren, also known as A-64662 (Fig. 23.4). The histidine residue (His$_6$), present in angiotensinogen and all previous inhibitors, was thought to be essential for enzyme recognition and was left unchanged. The acylated tyrosine protects the compound from aminopeptidase enzymes and also contributes to enzyme active site recognition. The remainder of the molecule is a stable dipeptide isostere. The cyclohexylmethylene and *iso*-butyl side chains are lipophilic and approximate the lipophilic side chains present in Leu$_{10}$ and Val$_{11}$ of angiotensinogen. Additionally, the use of a C-terminal alcohol instead of a C-terminal carboxylate protects enalkiren from carboxypeptidase enzymes (10,11).

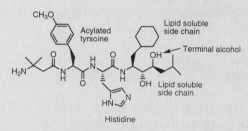

Fig. 23.4. Structures of enalkiren and zankiren.

Enalkiren has been extensively studied in preclinical and clinical trials and has been shown to be efficacious if given intravenously. However, it lacks significant bioavailability due mainly to a lack of lipid solubility. A more lipophilic analog, zankiren (A-72517, Fig. 23.4), has demonstrated increased oral bioavailability and efficacy. Preclinical and clinical trials with orally administered zankiren showed good bioavailability and significant reduction in blood pressure (11,12). Zankiren has since been withdrawn from clinical trials for undisclosed reasons; however, other orally active renin inhibitors are still under development.

ating bradykinin were subsequently linked to their ability to inhibit the enzymatic degradation of bradykinin. Soon thereafter, Bakhle and co-workers (14) reported that these same peptides also inhibited the enzymatic conversion of angiotensin I to angiotensin II. This latter enzyme, angiotensin converting enzyme (ACE), is now known to be identical with the former bradykininase enzyme (kininase II); however, even at the time of these initial discoveries, BPFs were seen as lead compounds for the development of new antihypertensive agents since they possessed dual activities—inhibition of the degradation of bradykinin, a potent vasodilator, and inhibition of the biosynthesis of angiotensin II, a potent vasoconstrictor (15).

A nonapeptide, SQ 20,881 (teprotide), isolated from the original BPFs had the greatest *in vivo* potency in inhibiting ACE and was shown to consistently lower blood pressure in patients with essential hypertension. It also exerted beneficial effects in patients with heart failure; however, due to its peptide nature and lack of oral activity, teprotide had limited activity in the therapeutic treatment of these diseases (15,16).

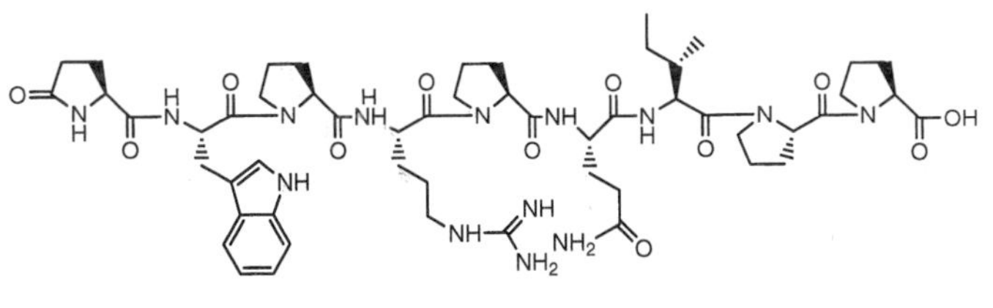

SQ 20,881

Cushman, Ondetti and coworkers (17–19) used SQ 20,881 and other peptide analogs to provide an enhanced understanding of the enzymatic properties of ACE. Using a knowledge of substrate binding specificities and the fact that ACE has properties similar to those of pancreatic carboxypeptidases, these researchers developed a hypothetical model of the enzyme active site. Carboxypeptidase A, like ACE, is a zinc-containing exopeptidase. The binding of a substrate to carboxypeptidase A involves three major interactions (Fig. 23.5, part A). First, the negatively charged carboxylate terminus of the amino acid substrate binds to the positively charged Arg-145 present on the enzyme. Second, a hydrophobic pocket present in the enzyme provides specificity for a C-terminal aromatic or nonpolar residue. Third, the zinc atom is located close to the labile peptide bond and serves to stabilize the negatively charged tetrahedral intermediate which results when a molecule of water attacks the carbonyl bond between the C-terminal and penultimate amino acid residues (20). Similarly, the binding of substrates to ACE was proposed to involve three or four major interactions (Fig. 23.5, part B). First, the negatively charged carboxylate terminus of angiotensin I, and other substrates, was assumed to occur via an ionic bond with a positively charged amine present on ACE. Second, the role of the zinc atom in the mechanism of ACE hydrolysis was assumed to be similar to that of carboxypeptidase A. Since ACE cleaves dipeptides instead of single amino acids, the position of the zinc atom was assumed to be located two amino acids away from the cationic center in order for it to be adjacent to the labile peptide bond. Third, the side chains R_1 and R_2 could contribute to the overall binding affinity; however ACE, unlike carboxypeptidase A, does not show specificity for C-terminal hydrophobic amino acids and was not expected to have a hydrophobic binding pocket. Finally, the terminal peptide bond is nonlabile and was assumed to provide hydrogen bonding between the substrate and ACE.

The development of captopril and other orally active ACE inhibitors began with the observation that D-2-benzylsuccinic acid was an extremely potent inhibitor of carboxypeptidase A (17–19). The binding of this compound to carboxypeptidase A (Fig. 23.6, part A) is very similar to that seen for substrates with the exception that the zinc ion binds to a carboxylate group instead of the labile peptide bond. Byers and Wolfenden proposed that this compound is a byproduct analog that contains structural features of both products of peptide hydrolysis. Most of the structural features of the compound are identical to the terminal amino acid of the substrate (Fig. 23.5, part A), while the additional carboxylate group is able to mimic the carboxylate group which would be produced during peptide hydrolysis (21). Applying this concept to the hypothetical model of ACE described above resulted in the synthesis and evaluation of a series of succinic acid derivatives (Fig. 23.6, part B). Since proline was present

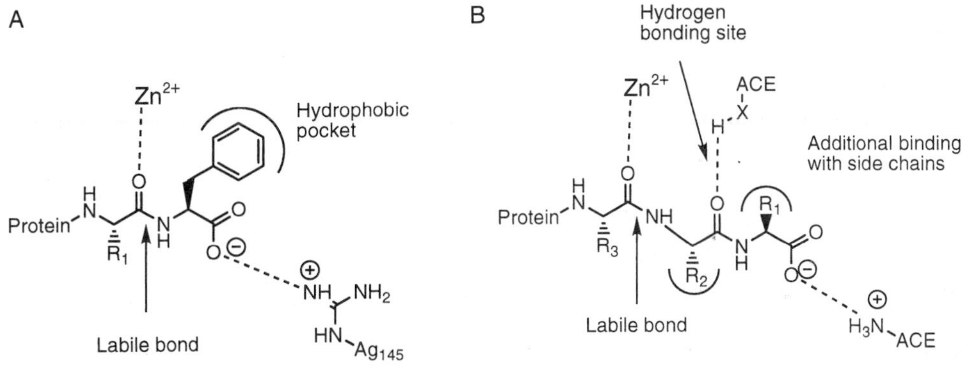

Fig. 23.5. A model of substrate binding to carboxypeptidase A (**A**) and ACE (**B**).

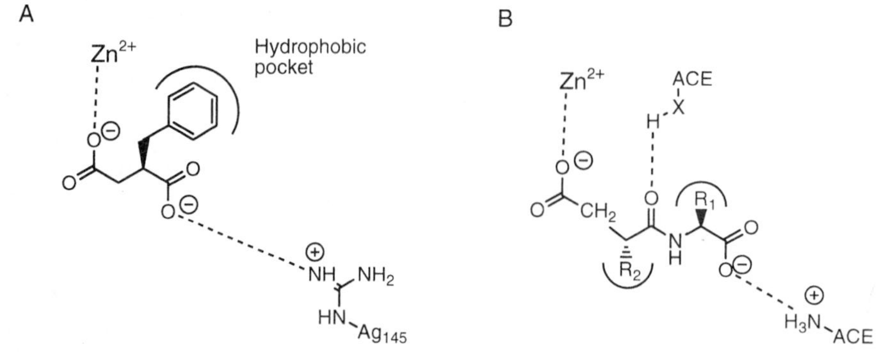

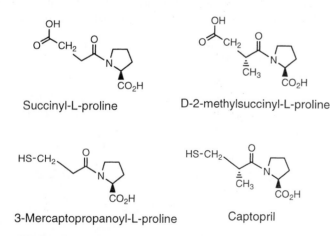

Fig. 23.6. Inhibitor binding models of (**A**) D-2-benzylsuccinic acid to carboxypeptidase A and (**B**) succinic acid derivatives to ACE.

as the C-terminal amino acid in SQ 20,881 as well as in other potent, inhibitory snake venom peptides, it was included in the structure of newly designed inhibitors. The first inhibitor to be synthesized and tested was succinyl-L-proline (Fig. 23.7). This compound proved to be somewhat disappointing. Although it provided reasonable specificity for ACE, it was only about 1/500 as potent as SQ 20,881.

Substitution of other amino acids in place of proline produced compounds which were even less potent; hence all subsequent SAR studies were conducted using analogs of L-proline (Fig. 23.7). The addition of a methyl group to the 2 position of succinyl-L-proline in order to mimic the amino acid side chain, R_2, of the substrate enhanced activity but only marginally. D-2-Methylsuccinyl-L-proline had effects similar to SQ 20,881 but was still only 1/300 as potent. The D-isomer, rather than the L-isomer normally seen for amino acids, was necessary because of the isosteric replacement of an NH_2 with a CH_2 present in succinyl-L-proline. A comparison of the R_2 group of the substrate (Fig. 23.5, part B) with the methyl group of D-2-methylsuccinyl-L-proline, illustrates that this methyl group occupies the same binding site as the side chain of an L-amino.

One of the most important alterations to succinyl-L-proline was the replacement of the succinyl carboxylate with other groups having enhanced affinity for the zinc atom bound to ACE. Replacement of this carboxylate with

a sulfhydryl group produced 3-mercaptopropanoyl-L-proline. This compound has an IC_{50} value of 200 nM and is more than 1000 times as potent than succinyl-L-proline (Fig. 23.7). Additionally, it is 10–20 times more potent than SQ 20,881 in inhibiting contractile and vasopressor responses to angiotensin I. Addition of a 2-D-methyl group further enhanced activity. The resulting compound, captopril (Fig. 23.7), is a competitive inhibitor of ACE with a K_i value of 1.7 nM and was the first ACE inhibitor to be marketed.

The sulfhydryl group of captopril proved to be responsible not only for the excellent inhibitory activity of the compound but also for the two most common side effects, skin rashes and taste disturbances (e.g., metallic taste, loss of taste). These side effects usually subsided upon dosage reduction or discontinuation of captopril. They were attributed to the presence of the sulfhydryl group since similar effects had been observed with penicillamine, a sulfhydryl containing agent used to treat Wilson's disease and rheumatoid arthritis (22,23).

Dicarboxylate-containing Inhibitors
Development of Enalapril

Researchers at Merck (24) sought to develop compounds which lacked the sulfhydryl group of captopril yet maintained some ability to chelate zinc. Compounds having the general structure shown below were designed to meet this objective.

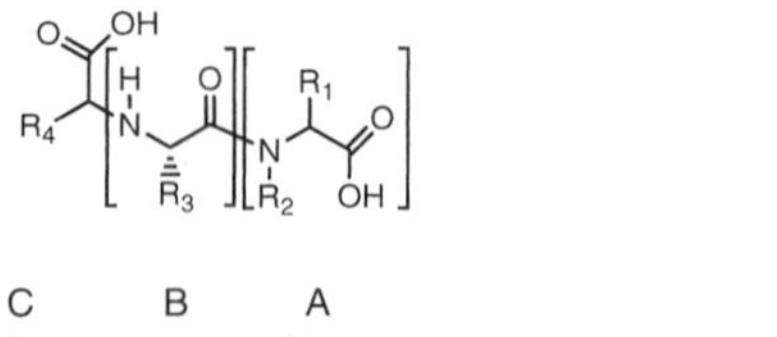

These compounds are tripeptide substrate analogs in which the C-terminal (A) and penultimate (B) amino acids are retained but the third amino acid is isosterically replaced by a substituted N-carboxymethyl group (C). Similar to the results seen in the development of captopril, C-terminal proline analogs provided optimum activity. The use of a methyl group at R_3 (i.e., B = Ala) and a phenylethyl group at R_4 re-

Succinyl-L-proline

D-2-methylsuccinyl-L-proline

3-Mercaptopropanoyl-L-proline

Captopril

Fig. 23.7. Compounds prepared in the development of captopril.

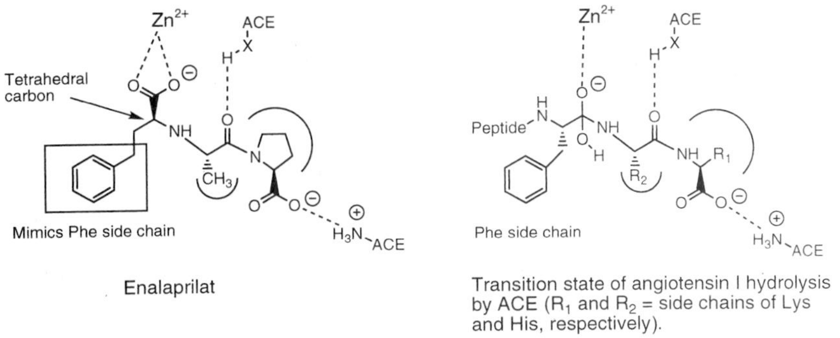

Fig. 23.8. A comparison of enalaprilat and the transition state of angiotensin I hydrolysis by ACE.

sulted in enalaprilat (Fig. 23.8). In comparing the activity of captopril and enalaprilat, it was found that enalaprilat, with a K_i of 0.2 nM, was approximately 10-fold more potent than captopril. Studies investigating the binding of enalaprilat revealed that its ability to chelate the enzyme-bound zinc atom was significantly less than that of captopril. The enhanced binding was proposed to be due to a mimicking of the transition state of angiotensin I hydrolysis. As shown in Figure 23.8, enalaprilat possess a tetrahedral carbon in place of the labile peptide bond. The secondary amine, the carboxylic acid and phenylethyl groups all contribute to the overall binding of the compound to ACE. The secondary amine is located at the same position as the labile amide nitrogen, the ionized carboxylic acid can form an ionic bond with the zinc atom, and the phenylethyl group mimics the hydrophobic side chain of the Phe amino acid which is present in angiotensin I.

Despite excellent intravenous activity, enalaprilat has very poor oral bioavailability. Esterification of enalaprilat produced enalapril (Fig. 23.9), a compound with superior oral bioavailability. The combination of structural features present in enalaprilat, especially the two carboxylate groups and the secondary amine, are responsible for its overall low lipophilicity and poor oral bioavailability. Zwitterion formation has also been suggested to contribute to the low oral activity (25), and a comparison of the pKa values for the secondary amine of enalaprilat and enalapril supports this explanation. Ionization of the adjacent carboxylate in enalaprilat greatly enhances the basicity of the secondary amine such that the pKa of the amine in this compound is 8.02, while in enalapril, it is only 5.49. Thus in the small intestine, the amine in enalaprilat will be primarily ionized and form a zwitterion with the adjacent carboxylate, but the amine in enalapril will be primarily un-ionized (26).

Intravenous administration of either enalapril or enalaprilat produced similar effects on angiotensin II production despite the fact that enalapril showed a 1000-fold decrease in *in vitro* activity. Subsequent studies showed that enalapril undergoes bioactivation and is thus a prodrug of enalaprilat. Since human plasma was reported to lack enalapril esterolytic activity, bioactivation by hepatic esterases (Fig. 23.9) has been suggested as the most probable mechanism for enalaprilat formation (27,28).

Additional Dicarboxylate Inhibitors

Eight other dicarboxylate inhibitors (Table 23.1) have been approved for various therapeutic indications; however, spirapril has never been marketed. Lisinopril is chemically unique in two respects. First, it contains the basic amino acid lysine ($R_1 = CH_2CH_2CH_2CH_2NH_2$) instead of the standard nonpolar alanine ($R = CH_3$) residue. Second it does not require bioactivation since neither of the carboxylic acid groups are esterified (i.e., $R_2 = H$). Lisinopril was developed at the same time as enalapril. Despite the addition of another ionizable group, the oral absorption of lisinopril was found to be superior to that of enalaprilat, but less than that of enalapril. *In vitro* studies of enalaprilat and lisinopril showed lisinopril to be slightly more potent than enalaprilat (27,28). Lisinopril, along with captopril, are currently the only two ACE inhibitors which are not prodrugs.

The major structural difference among the remaining ACE inhibitors is in the ring of the C-terminal amino acid. Lisinopril, like enalapril and captopril, contains the pyrrolidine ring of proline while all of the other compounds contain larger bicyclic or spiro ring systems. Studies of indoline analogs of captopril indicated that a hydrophobic pocket similar to that seen in carboxypeptidase A was also present in ACE. This led to a modification (Fig. 23.10) of Ondetti and Cushman's original model and the development of inhibitors which contained larger hydrophobic ring systems (29). Even though this modified model was proposed for captopril analogs, it is readily adaptable to include enalaprilat analogs. In general, the varied ring systems seen in benazepril, moexipril, perindopril, quinapril, ramipril, spirapril, and trandolapril provide enhanced binding and potency. They also lead to differences in absorption, plasma protein binding, elimination, onset of action, duration of action and dosing among the drugs. These differences are discussed in more detail in the Pharmacokinetic Properties section below.

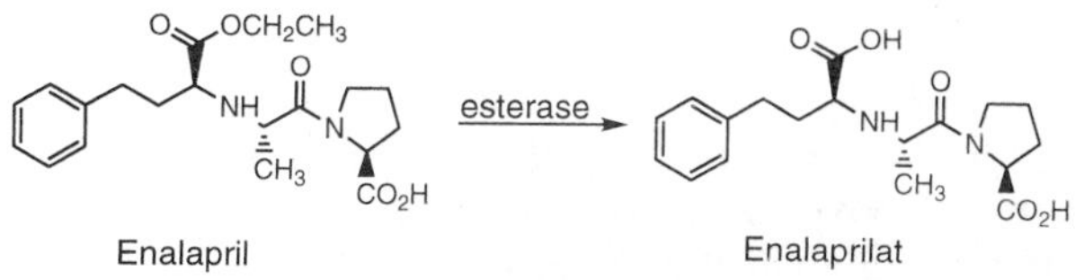

Fig. 23.9. Bioactivation of enalapril.

Table 23.1. Additional Dicarboxylate-containing Angiotensin Converting Enzyme Inhibitors

General Structure:

Benazepril

Compounds	Ring	R_1	R_2	R_3
Lisinopril		$(CH_2)_4NH_2$	H	
Moexipril		CH_3	CH_2CH_3	
Perindopril		CH_3	CH_2CH_3	CH_3
Quinapril		CH_3	CH_2CH_3	
Ramipril		CH_3	CH_2CH_3	
Spirapril		CH_3	CH_2CH_3	
Trandolapril		CH_3	CH_2CH_3	

Phosphonate-containing Inhibitors: the Development of Fosinopril

The search for ACE inhibitors which lacked the sulfhydryl group also lead to the investigation of phosphorous containing compounds (30). The phosphinic acid shown in Figure 23.11 is capable of binding to ACE in a manner similar to enalapril. The interaction of the zinc atom with the phosphinic acid is similar to that seen with sulfhydryl and carboxylate groups. Additionally, this compound is capable of forming the ionic, hydrogen, and hydrophobic bonds similar to those seen with enalapril and other dicarboxylate analogs. A feature unique to this compound is the ability of the phosphinic acid to more truly mimic the ionized, tetrahedral intermediate of peptide hydrolysis. However, unlike enalapril and other dicarboxylate analogs, the spacing of this tetrahedral species is shorter, being only two atoms removed from the proline nitrogen. Additionally, the spacing between the proline nitrogen and the hydrophobic phenyl ring is one atom longer than that seen in the dicarboxylates.

Structural modification to investigate more hydrophobic, C-terminal ring systems, similar to that described above for the dicarboxylate compounds, lead to a 4-cyclohexyl-proline analog of the original phosphinic acid. This compound, fosinoprilat (Fig. 23.12), was more potent than captopril but less potent than enalaprilat. The above mentioned differences in the spacing of the phosphinic acid and phenyl groups may be responsible for this latter

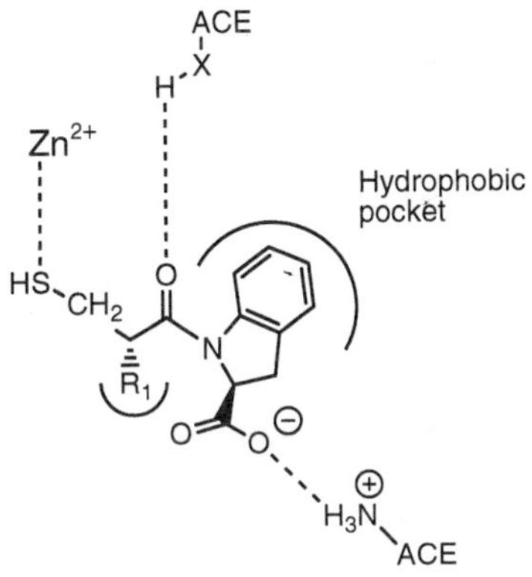

Fig. 23.10. A modified model of ACE inhibitor binding.

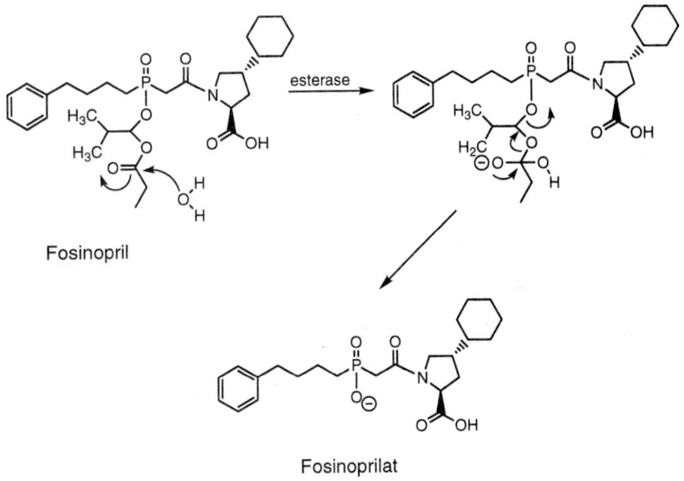

Fig. 23.12. Bioactivation of fosinopril.

difference in potency. Similar to the dicarboxylates, fosinoprilat was too hydrophilic and exhibited poor oral activity. The prodrug fosinopril contains an (acyloxy)alkyl group which allows for better lipid solubility and improved bioavailability (30). Bioactivation via esterase activity in the intestinal wall and liver produces fosinopril (Fig. 23.12).

Mechanism of Action

Angiotensin converting enzyme inhibitors attenuate the effects of the renin-angiotensin system by inhibiting the conversion of angiotensin I to angiotensin II (Fig. 23.1). They also inhibit the conversion of [des-Asp[1]]angiotensin I to angiotensin III; however, this action has only a minor role in the overall cardiovascular effects of these drugs. They are selective in that they do not directly interfere with any other components of the renin-angiotensin system; however, they do cause other effects which are unrelated to the decrease in angiotensin II concentration. Inhibitors of ACE increase bradykinin levels which in turn stimulate prostaglandin biosynthesis (Fig. 23.3). Both of these compounds have been proposed to contribute to the overall action of ACE inhibitors. Additionally, decreased angiotensin II levels increase the release of renin and the production of angiotensin I. Since ACE is inhibited, angiotensin I is shunted towards the production of angiotensin 1-7 and other peptides. The contribution of these peptides to the overall effect of ACE inhibitors is unknown (1).

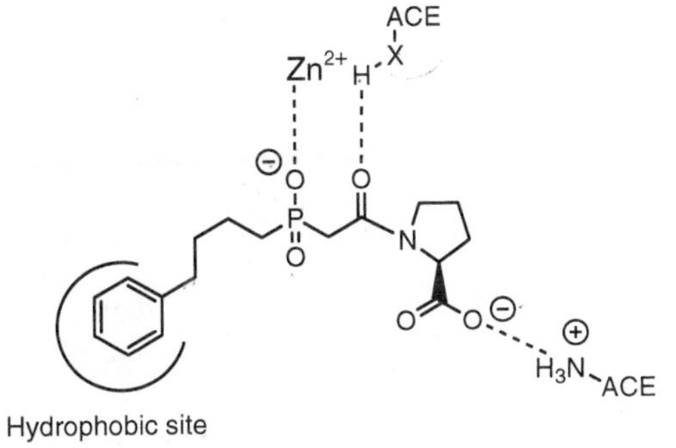

Structure-activity Relationships

The structural characteristics for ACE inhibitory activity are given in Table 23.2. Angiotensin converting enzyme is a stereoselective drug target. Since currently approved ACE inhibitors act as either di- or tripeptide substrate analogs, they must contain a stereochemistry that is consistent with the L-amino acids present in the natural substrates. This was established very early in the development of ACE inhibitors when compounds with carboxyl-terminal D-amino acids were discovered to be very poor inhibitors (31). Later work by Patchett et al. (24) reinforced this idea. They reported a 100- to 1000-fold loss in inhibitor activity whenever the configuration of either the carboxylate or the R_1 substituent (Table 23.1) was altered. The S,S,S configuration seen in enalapril and other dicarboxylate inhibitors meets the above stated criteria and provides for optimum enzyme inhibition.

Physicochemical Properties

Captopril and fosinopril are acidic drugs, while all other ACE inhibitors are amphoteric. The carboxylic acid attached to the N-ring is a common structural feature in all ACE inhibitors. It has a pKa in the range of 2.5–3.5 and will be primarily ionized at physiologic pH. As discussed above with enalapril, the pKa and ionization of the secondary amine present in the dicarboxylate series depends upon whether the adjacent functional group is in the prodrug or active form. In the prodrug form, the amine is adjacent to an ester, is less basic, and is primarily un-ionized at physiologic pH. Following bioactivation, the amine is adjacent to an ionized carboxylic acid which enhances both the basicity and ionization of the amine. Similarly, the basic nitrogen enhances the acidity of the adjacent carboxylic acid such that it usually has a lower pKa than the carboxylic acid attached to the N-ring. As an example, the pKa values of enalapril are 3.39 and 2.30. These values correspond to the carboxylic acid on the N-ring and the carboxylic acid adjacent to the amine, respectively. The

Fig. 23.11. The binding of phosphinate analogs to ACE.

Table 23.2. Structure-activity Relationship of ACE Inhibitors

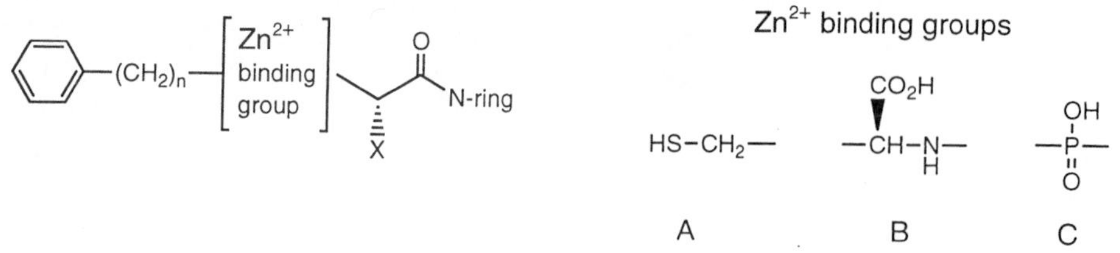

a. The N-ring must contain a carboxylic acid to mimic the C-terminal carboxylate of ACE substrates.
b. Large hydrophobic hetercyclic rings in the N-ring increase potency and alter pharmacokinetic parameters.
c. Groups A, B, or C can serve as zinc binding groups.
d. The sulfhydryl group shows superior binding to zinc (Phe in carboxylate and phosphinic acid side chain compensates for sulfhydryl group).
e. Sulfhydryl-containing compounds produce high incidence of skin rash and taste disturbances.
f. Sulfhydryl-containing compounds can form disulfides which may shorten duration of action.
g. Binding to zinc through either a carboxylate or phosphinate mimics the peptide hydrolysis transition state.
h. Esterification of the carboxylate or phosphinate produces an orally bioavailable prodrug.
i. X is usually methyl to mimic the side chain of alanine. Within the dicarboxylate series, when X equals n-butylamine (lysine side chain) this produces a compound which is orally active without being a prodrug.
j. Optimum activity occurs when stereochemistry of inhibitor is consistent with L-amino acid stereochemistry.

analogous values for these functional groups in lisinopril are 3.3 and 1.7 (26).

The calculated log P values along with other pharmacokinetic parameters for the ACE inhibitors are shown in Table 23.3 (see pharmacokinetic parameters below) (26). With two notable exceptions, enalaprilat and lisinopril, all of the compounds possess good lipid solubility. Compounds which contain hydrophobic bicyclic ring systems are more lipid soluble than those which contain proline. A comparison of the log P values of benazepril, perindopril, quinapril, ramipril, and trandolapril to those for captopril and enalapril illustrates this fact. As previously discussed, enalaprilat is much more hydrophilic than its ester prodrug and is currently the only ACE inhibitor marked for intravenous administration. In terms of solubility, lisinopril is probably the most interesting compound in that it is the most hydrophilic inhibitor, yet unlike enalaprilat, it is orally active. One possible explanation for this phenomenon is that in the duodenum, lisinopril will exist as a di-zwitterion in which the ionized groups can internally bind to one another. In this manner, lisinopril may be able to pass through the lipid bilayer with an overall net neutral charge.

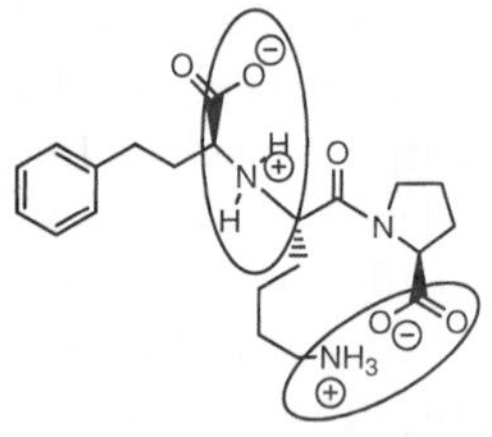

Metabolism

Lisinopril and enalaprilat are excreted unchanged while all other ACE inhibitors undergo some degree of metabolic transformation (1,32–34). As previously discussed and illustrated (Figs 23.9, 23.12), all dicarboxylate and phosphonate

prodrugs must undergo bioactivation via hepatic esterases. Additionally, based on their structural features, specific compounds can undergo metabolic inactivation via various pathways (Fig. 23.13). Due to its sulfhydryl group, captopril is subject to oxidative dimerization or conjugation. Approximately 40–50% of a dose of captopril is excreted unchanged, while the remainder is excreted as either a disulfide dimer or a captopril-cysteine disulfide. Glucuronide

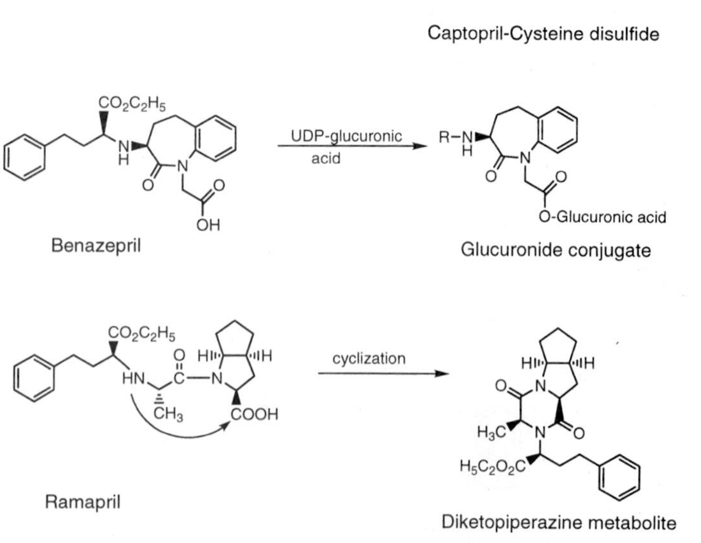

Fig. 23.13. Metabolic routes of ACE inhibitors.

conjugation has been reported for benazepril, fosinopril, quinapril, and ramipril. This conjugation can occur with either the parent prodrug or with the activated drug. Benazepril, with the N-substituted glycine, is especially susceptible to this reaction. This is due to a difference in steric hindrance. For all ACE inhibitors, except benazepril, the carbon atom directly adjacent to the carboxylic acid is part of a ring system and provides some steric hindrance to conjugation. The unsubstituted methylene group (*i.e.*, $-CH_2-$) of benazepril provides less steric hindrance and thus facilitates conjugation. Moexipril, perindopril and ramipril can undergo cyclization to produce diketopiperazines. This cyclization can occur with either the parent or active forms of the drugs.

A comparative study of the metabolism and biliary excretion of lisinopril, enalapril, perindopril, and ramipril revealed that while neither lisinopril nor enalapril underwent any appreciable metabolism beyond bioactivation of enalapril to enalaprilat, both perindopril and ramipril were extensively metabolized beyond the initial bioactivation. It was proposed that these differences in hepatic metabolism could in part be explained by the larger, more hydrophobic rings present on perindopril and ramipril (35).

Pharmacokinetic Parameters

The pharmacokinetic parameters and dosing information for ACE inhibitors are summarized in Tables 23.3 and 23.4, respectively (1,32–34,36–39). The oral bioavailability of this class of drugs ranges from 13%–95%. Differences in both lipid solubility and first pass metabolism are most likely responsible for this wide variation. Both parameters should be considered when comparing any two or more compounds. With the exceptions of enalapril, lisinopril and fosinopril, the concurrent administration of food adversely effects the oral absorption of ACE inhibitors. Product literature specifically instructs that captopril should be taken one hour before meals and that moexipril should be taken in the fasting state. Although not specifically stated, similar instructions should also benefit patients taking an ACE inhibitor whose absorption is affected by food.

The extent of protein binding also exhibits wide variability among the different compounds. Currently available data suggests that this variation has some correlation with the calculated log P values for the compounds. The three most lipophilic compounds—trandolapril, quinapril, and benazepril—exhibit protein binding greater than 90%, while three of the least hydrophilic compounds—lisinopril, enalapril, and captopril—exhibit much lower protein binding. The lack of a log P value for fosinopril and a protein binding value for spirapril prevents a more definitive statement on this correlation.

Renal elimination is the primary route of elimination for most ACE inhibitors. With the exceptions of fosinopril and spirapril, altered renal function significantly diminishes the plasma clearance of ACE inhibitors. Therefore, the dosage of most ACE inhibitors should be reduced in patients with renal impairment (1). Studies of fosinopril in patients with CHF demonstrated that it is eliminated by both renal and hepatic pathways and does not require a dosage reduction in patients with renal dysfunction (40). Spirapril also exhibits similar properties; however, it is not currently available for use. It should be noted that the literature data for the elimination of moexipril, quinapril, ramipril, and trandolapril is both confusing and inconclusive. While it is clear that renal elimination is of primary importance for these drugs, it is difficult to correlate what some sources call renal/hepatic elimination with what others call renal/fecal elimination. Additionally, it is uncertain whether or not the designation of fecal elimination also includes unabsorbed drug. Since the designation renal/fecal

Table 23.3. Pharmacokinetic Parameters of ACE Inhibitors

Drug	Calculated Log P	Oral Bioavailability	Effect of Food on Absorption	Active Metabolite	Protein Binding	Onset of Action (hr)	Duration of Action (hr)	Major Route(s) of Elimination
Benazepril	1.74	37%	reduced rate, same extent	Benazeprilat	>95%	1	24	Renal (primary) Biliary (secondary)
Captopril	1.02	60–75%	reduced	na*	25–30%	0.25–0.50	6–12	Renal
Enalapril	0.71	60%	none	Enalaprilat	50–60%	1	24	Renal
Enalaprilat	0.01	na*	na*	na*	—†	0.25	6	Renal
Fosinopril	—†	36%	none	Fosinoprilat	95%	1	24	Renal (50%) Hepatic (50%)
Lisinopril	−1.77	25–30%	none	na*	25%	1	24	Renal
Moexipril	—†	13%	reduced	Moexiprilat	50–90%	1	24	Renal/Fecal
Perindopril	1.26	65–95%	reduced	Perindoprilat	60–80%	1	24	Renal
Quinapril	1.84	60%	reduced	Quinaprilat	97%	1	24	Renal/Fecal
Ramipril	1.59	50–60%	reduced	Ramiprilat	73%	1	24	Renal/Fecal
Spirapril	0.61	50%	—†	Spiraprilat	—†	1	24	Renal (50%) Hepatic (50%)
Trandolapril	2.14	80%	reduced rate, same extent	Trandolaprilat	65–94%	0.5–1.0	24	Renal/Fecal

*Not applicable
†Data not available

was the most prevalent in the literature, it is also used in Table 23.3.

With one exception, all ACE inhibitors have a similar onset of action, duration of action and dosing interval. Captopril has a more rapid onset of action; however, it also has a shorter duration and requires a more frequent dosing interval than any of the other compounds. When oral dosing is inappropriate, enalaprilat can be used intravenously. The normal dose administered to hypertensive patients is 0.625–1.25 mg every six hours. The dose is usually administered over 5 minutes.

Therapeutic Applications

Angiotensin converting enzyme inhibitors have been approved for the treatment of hypertension, CHF, left ventricular dysfunction or hypertrophy (LVD or LVH), acute myocardial infarction, and diabetic nephropathy. Although all ACE inhibitors possess the same physiologic actions and should thus produce similar therapeutic effects, the approved indications differ among the currently available agents (Table 23.4). Inhibitors of ACE are one of many chemical/pharmacologic agents used to treat hypertension and are effective for a variety of situations. They can be used either individually or with other classes of compounds. They are especially useful in treating hypertensive patients who also suffer from CHF, LVD, or diabetes. Arterial and venous dilation seen with ACE inhibitors not only lowers blood pressure but also has favorable effects on both preload and afterload in patients with CHF. Additionally, the ability of ACE inhibitors to cause regression of LVH has been demonstrated to reduce the incidence of further heart disease in hypertensive patients. The use of ACE inhibitors in patients with myocardial infarction is similarly based on the ability of ACE inhibitors to decrease mortality by preventing postinfarction LVH and CHF. Current recommendations to give ACE inhibitors to all patients with impaired left ventricular systolic impairment regardless of the presence of observable symptoms are also based on the ability of these inhibitors to block the vascular and cardiac hypertrophy and remodeling caused by angiotensin II. Inhibitors of ACE have also been reported to slow the progression of diabetic nephropathy and thus are preferred agents in the treatment of hypertension in a diabetic patient. It has also been suggested that ACE inhibitors be used in patients with diabetic nephropathy regardless of the presence or absence or hypertension (1,7,8).

Chemical/Pharmacologic Classes Used to Treat Hypertension

Diuretics (Chapter 22), ACE Inhibitors, Angiotensin II Antagonists, Calcium Channel Blockers (Chapter 23), Central α_2 Agonists, Peripheral α_1 Antagonists, β-Blockers, Ganglionic Blockers, Vasodilators (Chapter 24)

Combination Products Which Include an ACE Inhibitor:

ACE Inhibitor/Diuretic: benazepril/hydrochlorothiazide, captopril/hydrochlorothiazide, enalapril/hydrochlorothiazide, lisinopril/hydrochlorothiazide, moexipril/hydrochlorothiazide

ACE Inhibitor/Calcium Channel Blocker: benazepril/amlodipine, enalapril/diltiazem, enalapril/felodipine, trandolapril/verapamil

---

Table 23.4. Dosing Information for Orally Available ACE Inhibitors.

Generic Name	Brand Name(s)	Approved Indications	Dosing Range (Treatment of Hypertension)	Maximum Daily Dose	Dose Reduction with Renal Dysfunction	Available Tablet Strengths (mg)
Benazepril	Lotensin	Hypertension	20–40 mg qd or bid	80 mg	yes	5, 10, 20, 40
Captopril	Capoten	Hypertension, CHF, Left ventricular dysfunction, Diabetic nephropathy	25–150 mg bid or tid	450 mg	yes	12.5, 25, 50, 100
Enalapril	Vasotec	Hypertension, CHF, Left ventricular dysfunction	5–40 mg qd or bid	40 mg	yes	2.5, 5, 10, 20
Fosinopril	Monopril	Hypertension, CHF	10–40 mg qd	80 mg	no	10, 20
Lisinopril	Prinivil, Zestril	Hypertension, CHF, Acute MI	10–40 mg qd	40 mg	yes	2.5, 5, 10, 20, 40
Moexipril	Univasc	Hypertension	7.5–30 mg qd or bid	30 mg	yes	7.5, 15
Quinapril	Accupril	Hypertension, CHF	10–80 mg qd or bid	80 mg	yes	5, 10, 20, 40
Ramipril	Altace	Hypertension, CHF	2.5–20 mg qd or bid	20 mg	yes	1.25, 2.5, 5, 10
Trandolapril	Mavik	Hypertension	1–4 mg qd	4 mg	yes	1, 2, 4
Perindopril	Aceon	Hypertension	4–8 mg qd	16 mg	yes	2, 4, 8

Unlabeled Uses

Hypertensive crises, neonatal and childhood hypertension, rheumatoid arthritis, diagnosis of anatomic renal artery stenosis, scleroderma renal crisis, diagnosis of primary aldosteronism, idiopathic edema, Bartter's syndrome, Raynaud's syndrome, hypertension of Takayasu's disease (36).

Adverse Effects

The most prevalent or significant side effects of ACE inhibitors are listed here (1,36). Some can be attributed to specific functional groups within individual agents, while others can be directly related to the mechanism of action of this class of compounds. The higher incidence of maculopapular rashes and taste disturbances observed for captopril have been linked to the presence of the sulfhydryl group in this compound. All ACE inhibitors can cause hypotension, hyperkalemia, and a dry cough. Hypotension results from an extension of the desired physiologic effect, while hyperkalemia results from a decrease in aldosterone secretion secondary to a decrease in angiotensin II production. Cough is by far the most prevalent and bothersome side effect seen with the use of ACE inhibitors. It is seen in 5%–20% of patients, is usually not dose related, and is apparently due to the lack of selectivity of this class of drugs. As previously discussed, ACE inhibitors also prevent the breakdown of bradykinin (Fig. 23.3), and since bradykinin stimulates prostaglandin synthesis, prostaglandin levels also increase. The increased levels of both bradykinin and prostaglandin have been proposed to be responsible for the cough (41).

Adverse Effects of ACE Inhibitors

Hypotension, hyperkalemia, cough, rash, taste disturbances, headache, dizziness, fatigue, nausea, vomiting, diarrhea, acute renal failure, neutropenia, proteinuria, and angioedema.

The use of ACE inhibitors during pregnancy is contraindicated. While this class of compounds is not teratogenic during the first trimester, administration during the second and third trimester is associated with an increased incidence of fetal morbidity and mortality. Inhibitors of ACE can be used in women of child bearing age; however, they should be discontinued as soon as pregnancy is confirmed.

ANGIOTENSIN II RECEPTOR ANTAGONISTS

From a historical perspective, the angiotensin II receptor was the initial target for developing compounds which could inhibit the renin-angiotensin pathway. Efforts to develop angiotensin II receptor antagonists began in the early 1970s and focused on peptide based analogs of the natural agonist. The prototypical compound which resulted from these studies was saralasin, an octapeptide in which the Asp_1 and Phe_8 residues of angiotensin II were replaced with Sar (sarcosine, *N*-methylglycine) and Ile, respectively. Saralasin as well as other peptide analogs demonstrated the ability to reduce blood pressure; however, these compounds lacked oral bioavailability and expressed unwanted partial agonist activity. More recent efforts have utilized peptide mimetics to circumvent these inherent problems with peptide based antagonists. The culmination of these efforts was the 1995 approval of losartan, a non-peptide angiotensin II receptor antagonist (1,42).

Development of Losartan

The development of losartan can be traced back to two 1982 patent publications (45) which described the antihypertensive effects of a series of imidazole-5-acetic acid analogs. These compounds are exemplified by S-8308 (Fig. 23.15) and were later found to specifically block the angiotensin II receptor. Although these compounds were relatively weak antagonists, they did not possess the unwanted agonist activity previously seen in peptide analogs. A computerized molecular modeling overlap of angiotensin II with the structure of S-8308 revealed three common structural features. The ionized carboxylate of S-8308 correlated

Table 23.5. Drug Interactions for ACE Inhibitors

Drug	ACE Inhibitor	Result of Interaction
Allopurinol	All	Increased risk of hypersensitivity
Antacids	All	Decreased bioavailability of ACE inhibitor
Capsaicin	All	Exacerbation of cough
Digoxin	All	Increased plasma digoxin levels
Indomethacin	All	Decreased hypotensive effects
K^+ Preparations or K^+ Sparring Diuretics	All	Elevated serum potassium levels
Lithium	All	Increased serum lithium levels
Phenothiazides	All	Increased pharmacological effects of ACE inhibitor
Probenecid	Captopril	Decreased clearance and increased blood levels of captopril
Rifampin	Enalapril	Decreased pharmacological effects of enalapril
Tetracycline	Quinapril	Decreased absorption of tetracycline (may be due to high magnesium content of quinapril tablets)

Peptide Mimetics: Design of Agonists/Antagonists

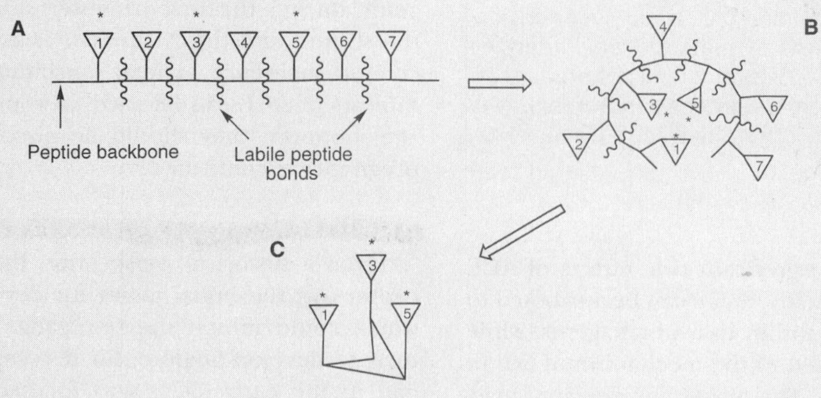

Fig. 23.14. A general process for the rational design of peptide mimetics: (**A**) identification of crucial pharmacophoric groups, (**B**) determination of the spatial arrangement of these groups, and (**C**) use of a template to mount the key functional groups in their proper conformation. Groups highlighted with an asterisk comprise the pharmacophore of the heptapeptide. Reprinted by permission (44).

Peptide mimetics have been defined as molecules which mimic the action of peptides, have no peptide bonds (*i.e.,* no amide bonds between amino acids), and a molecular weight less than 700 Daltons. In comparison with peptide drugs, peptide mimetics have numerous pharmaceutical advantages. Foremost among these are increased bioavailability and increased duration of action. The majority of known peptide mimetics have been discovered by random screening techniques; however, this process is costly, labor intensive, and unpredictable. A more logical and rational approach is *de novo* peptide mimetic design (43). An example of this approach is illustrated in Figure 23.14. In this example, the overall process is divided into three steps (A–C). Initially, the amino acids which comprise the pharmacophore of the peptide must be identified. Thus, a knowledge of the structure-activity relationships for the peptide under consideration is essential. In Figure 23.14A, the side chains present on amino acid residues 1,3, and 5 of a hypothetical heptapeptide are assumed to comprise the pharmacophore while the remainder of the peptide is assumed to provide the proper structural support for these key groups. In the second step of this *de novo* design process, the proper spatial arrange-

ment of the pharmacophoric groups must be elucidated. Nuclear magnetic resonance spectroscopy, X-ray diffraction studies and molecular modeling programs which allow for energy minimization procedures and molecular dynamics simulation can be used to construct a model of the biologically active conformation. Returning to the example, the side chains representing the pharmacophore are assumed to be located on the inside of the peptide, while the remaining residues are assumed to be located on the outside of the peptide (Fig. 23.14B). In the final step of the process, the pharmacophoric groups must be mounted on a nonpeptide template in such a manner that they retain the proper spatial arrangement found in the original peptide. This is shown in Figure 23.14C where side chains 1, 3, and 5 of the original peptide are connected to a rigid template (represented by the polygon). A variety of aromatic ring systems (*e.g.,* benzene, biphenyl, phenanthrene, and benzodiazepine) can be used to provide the rigid template, while appropriately placed alkyl groups can be used to enhance spacing and increase flexibility. Additionally, isosteres of the original pharmacophoric groups may be used to circumvent specific synthetic problems.

with the C-terminal carboxylate of angiotensin II, the imidazole ring of S-8308 correlated with the imidazole side chain of the His$_6$ residue, and the *n*-butyl group of S-8308 correlated with the hydrocarbon side chain of the Ile$_5$ residue (Fig. 23.15). The benzyl group of S-8308 was proposed to lie in the direction of the N-terminus of angiotensin II; however, it was not believed to have any significant receptor interactions.

From S-8308, a number of molecular modifications were carried out in an attempt to improve receptor binding and lipid solubility. The latter being important to assure adequate oral absorption. These changes resulted in preparation of losartan, a compound with high receptor affinity (IC$_{50}$ = 0.019 M) and oral activity (Fig. 23.16).

Additional Angiotensin II Receptor Antagonists

Valsartan, irbesartan, candesartan, and telmisartan are biphenyl analogs of losartan (Fig. 23.17). Each of these compounds has a structural feature unique from those seen in losartan. Valsartan, named for the valine portion of the compound, is the first nonimidazole containing angiotensin II antagonist, and is slightly more potent (IC$_{50}$ = 0.0089 μM) than losartan. The amide carbonyl of valsartan is isosteric with the imidazole nitrogen of losartan and can serve as a hydrogen bond acceptor similar to the imidazole nitrogen. Irbesartan is a spiro-compound which lacks the primary alcohol of losartan but which has a 10-fold greater binding affinity (IC$_{50}$ = 0.0013 μM) for the angiotensin II receptor. Hydrogen bonding, or ion-dipole binding, of the carbonyl group can mimic the interaction of the primary alcohol of losartan, while the spirocyclopentane can provide enhanced hydrophobic binding. Candesartan cilexitil and telmisartan are the newest agents to be approved. Both contain benzimidazole rings which allow for enhanced hydrophobic binding and an increase in potency, as compared to losartan. Candesartan cilexitil is a prodrug which is rapidly and completely metabolized to the active metabolite, candesartan.

Eprosartan was developed using a different hypothesis than that for losartan (Fig. 23.18). Similar to the rationale for losartan, the carboxylic acid of S-8308 was thought to mimic the Phe$_8$ (i.e., C-terminal) carboxylate of angiotensin II. The benzyl group of S-8308 was proposed to

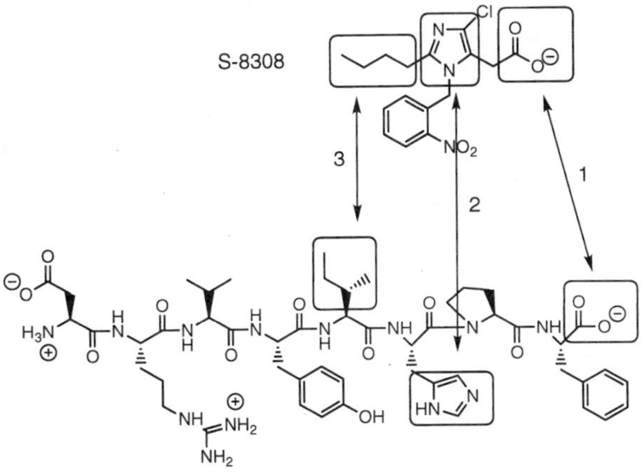

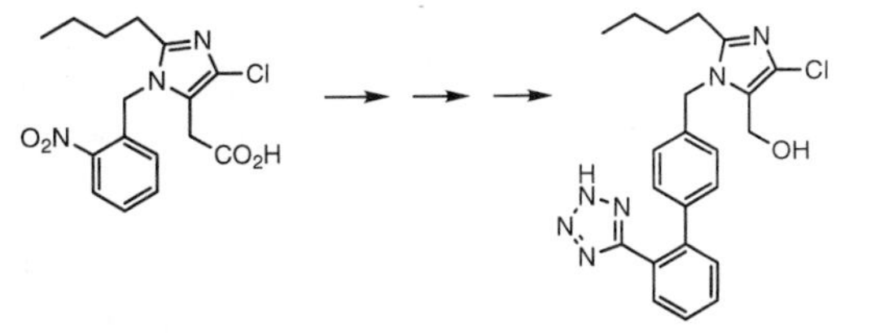

S-8308 (IC$_{50}$ = 15 μM)   Losartan (IC$_{50}$ = 0.019μM)

Fig. 23.16. The development of losartan from S-8308.

be an important structural feature which mimicked the aromatic side chain of Tyr$_4$ present in the agonist. Thus the major structural change was not extension of the N-benzyl group but enhancement of the compound's ability to mimic the C-terminal end of angiotensin II. This was accomplished by substituting the 5-acetic acid group with an α-thienylacrylic acid. In addition, a *para*-carboxylate, a functional group investigated during the development of losartan, was also added. The thienyl ring isosterically mimics the Phe$_8$ phenyl ring of angiotensin II and along with the *para*-carboxylate is responsible for the excellent potency (IC$_{50}$ = 0.0015 μM) of this compound (42).

Mechanism of Action

The angiotensin II receptor exists in at least two subtypes, type 1 (AT$_1$) and type 2 (AT$_2$). The AT$_1$ receptors are located in brain, neuronal, vascular, renal, hepatic, adrenal, and myocardial tissues and mediate the cardiovascular, renal, and CNS effects of angiotensin II. Losartan, valsartan, irbesartan, and eprosartan all show selectivity for this receptor subtype. They prevent and reverse all of the known effects of angiotensin II, including rapid and slow pressor responses, stimulatory effects on the peripheral

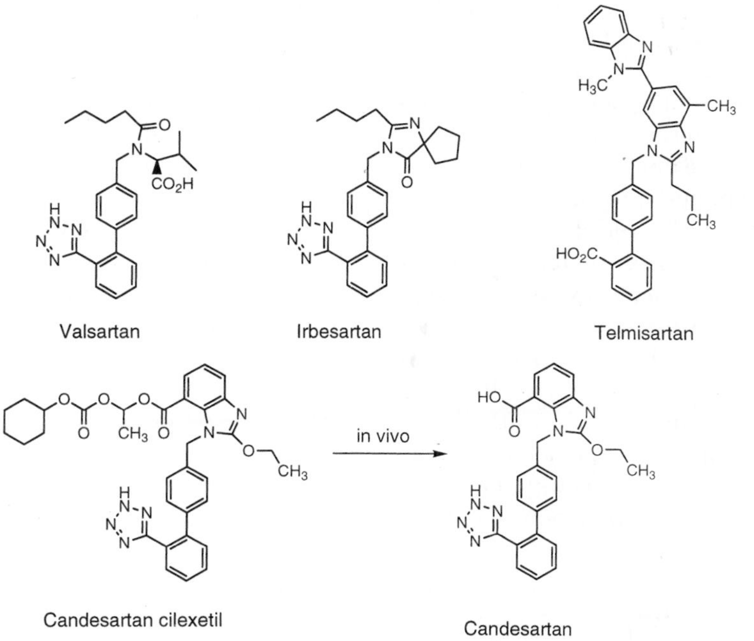

Fig. 23.15. Structural comparison of S-8308, an imidazole-5-acetic acid analog, with angiotensin II. Modified with permission from Timmermans et. al. (42).

Valsartan   Irbesartan   Telmisartan

Candesartan cilexetil   in vivo   Candesartan

Fig. 23.17. Structures of losartan analogs.

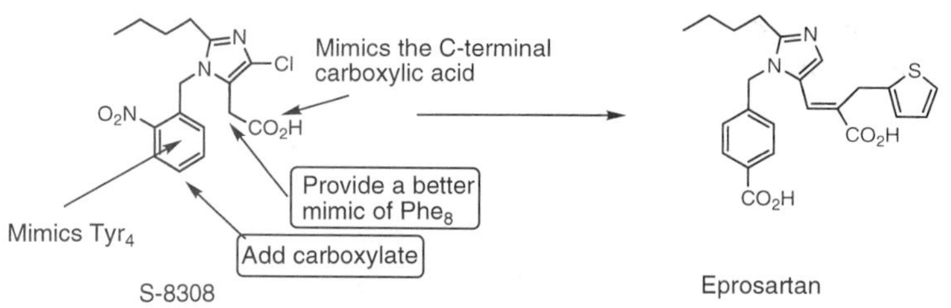

Fig. 23.18. The development of eprosartan from S-8308. The Phe₈ residue of angiotensin II contains the C-terminal carboxylic acid.

sympathetic nervous system, CNS effects, release of catecholamines, secretion of aldosterone, direct and indirect renal effects, and all growth-promoting effects. The function of the AT_2 receptors is not as well characterized; however, they have been proposed to mediate a variety of growth, development and differentiation processes. Some concern has arisen that unopposed stimulation of the AT_2 receptor in conjunction with AT_1 receptor antagonism may cause long-term adverse effects. As a result, compounds which exhibit balanced antagonism at both receptor subtypes are currently being sought (2,46).

Structure-activity Relationships

All commercially available angiotensin II antagonists are analogs of the following general structure:

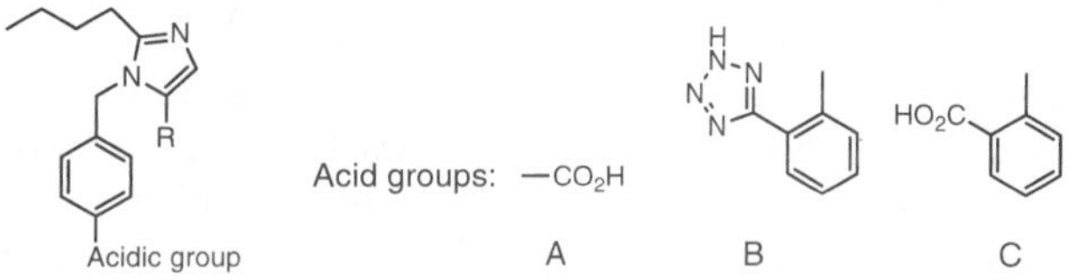

1) The "acidic group" is thought to mimic either the Tyr_4 phenol or the Asp_1 carboxylate of angiotensin II. Groups capable of such a role include the carboxylic acid (A), a phenyl tetrazole (B), or a phenyl carboxylate (C). 2) In the biphenyl series, the tetrazole and carboxylate groups must be in the ortho position for optimal activity (the tetrazole group is superior in terms of metabolic stability, lipophilicity, and oral bioavailability). 3) The *n*-butyl group of the model compound provides hydrophobic binding and most likely mimics the side chain of Ile_5 of angiotensin II. As seen with candesartan and telmisartan, this *n*-butyl group can be replaced with a substituted benzimidazole ring. 4) The imidazole ring, or an isosteric equivalent, is required to mimic the His_6 side chain of angiotensin II. 5) Substitution with a variety of R groups including a carboxylic acid, methyl alcohol, an ether, or an alkyl chain is required to mimic the Phe_8 of angiotensin II. All of these groups are thought to interact with the AT_1 receptor, some through ionic or ion-dipole bonds and others through hydrophobic interactions.

Physicochemical Properties

All angiotensin II receptor antagonists are acidic drugs. The tetrazole ring found in losartan, valsartan, irbesartan,

and candesartan has a pKa of approximately 6 and will be at least 90% ionized at physiologic pH. The carboxylic acids found on valsartan, candesartan, telmisartan, and eprosartan have pKa values in the range of 3–4 and will also be primarily ionized. Currently, available agents have adequate, but not excellent, lipid solubility. As previously mentioned, the tetrazole group is more lipophilic than a carboxylic. Additionally, the four nitrogen atoms present in the tetrazole ring can create a greater charge distribution than that available for a carboxylic acid. These properties have been proposed to be responsible for the enhanced binding and bioavailability of the tetrazole containing compounds (47). Similar to ACE inhibitors, the stereochemistry of valsartan is consistent with the L-amino acids present in the natural agonist.

Metabolism

Approximately 14% of a dose of losartan is oxidized by the isozymes CYP2C9 and CYP3A4 to produce EXP-3174, a noncompetitive AT_1 receptor antagonist that is 10–40 times more potent than losartan (Figure 23.19). The overall cardiovascular effects seen with losartan are due to the combined actions of the parent drug and the active metabolite, thus losartan should not be considered a prodrug (1). As previously mentioned, candesartan cilexetil is rapidly and completely metabolized to candesartan in the intestinal wall.

None of the other compounds are converted to active metabolites. All of these compounds are primarily (80%) excreted unchanged. About 20% of valsartan is metabolized to inactive compounds via mechanisms that do not appear to involve the CYP450 system. The primary circulating metabolites for irbesartan, telmisartan and eprosartan are inactive glucuronide conjugates. A small amount of irbesartan is oxidized by CYP2CP; however, irbesartan does

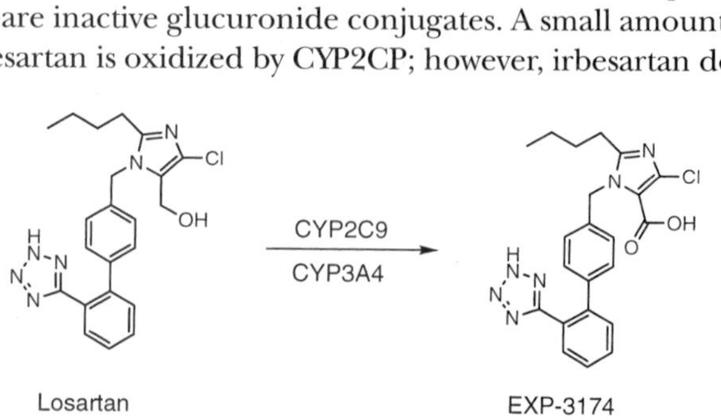

Fig. 23.19. The metabolic conversion of losartan to EXP-3174 by cytochrome P450 isozymes.

not substantially induce or inhibit CYP450 enzymes normally involved in drug metabolism (48–52).

Pharmacokinetic Parameters

The pharmacokinetic parameters and dosing information for angiotensin receptor antagonists are summarized in Tables 23.6 and 23.7, respectively (33, 36, 48–52). With the exception of irbesartan (60–80%), and possibly telmisartan (42%), all of the compounds have low, but adequate, oral bioavailability (15–33%). Given the fact that most of the compounds are excreted unchanged, the most probable reasons for the low bioavailability are poor lipid solubility and incomplete absorption. Effects of food on the absorption of losartan, valsartan, and eprosartan have been noted. These effects have however been deemed clinically insignificant, and thus the compounds can be taken either with or without food. All of the compounds have similar onsets, are highly protein bound, have elimination half-lives which allow once or twice daily dosing, and are primarily eliminated via the fecal route. The two newest agents appear to require a slightly longer time in order to reach peak plasma concentrations. As with ACE inhibitors, literature designation of fecal elimination is unclear as to whether or not it includes unabsorbed drug.

Losartan and candesartan cilexetil are different from the other compounds in several respects. They are the only compounds with active metabolites, and they have the highest renal elimination of all of the agents. While product labeling indicates that renal impairment does not require a dosage reduction for losartan, area under the curve (AUC) values are increased by 50% in patients with creatinine clearance less than 30 mL/min and doubled in hemodialysis patients. These increases are not seen for the other agents. Losartan and telmisartan are the only two agents which require initial dose reductions in patients with hepatic impairment. Due to significantly increased plasma concentration, patients with impaired hepatic function or biliary obstructive disorders, should avoid the use of telmisartan.

Therapeutic Applications

Angiotensin II receptor antagonists are currently approved for the treatment of hypertension, either alone or in combin-

Combination Products Which Include an Angiotensin II Receptor Antagonist

Angiotensin II Antagonist/Diuretic:
  losartan/hydrochlorothiazide
  irbesartan/hydrochlorothiazide

Table 23.6. Pharmacokinetic Parameters of Angiotensin II Antagonists

Drug	Oral Bioavailability (%)	Effect of Food on Absorption	Active Metabolite	Protein Binding (%)	Time to Peak Plasma Conc. (hrs)	Elimination Half-life (hrs)	Major Route(s) of Elimination (%)
Losartan	33	Reduced	EXP-3174	98.7 (losartan) 99.8% (EXP-3174)	1 (losartan) 3–4 (EXP-3174)	1.5–2 (losartan) 6–9 (EXP-3174)	Fecal (60) Renal (35)
Valsartan	25	Reduced	None	95	2–4	6	Fecal (83) Renal (13)
Irbesartan	60–80	None	None	90	1.5–2	11–15	Fecal (80) Renal (20)
Candesartan Cilexetil	15	None	Candesartan	99	3–4	9	Fecal (67) Renal (33)
Telmisartan	42	None	None	100	5	24	Fecal (97)
Eprosartan	15	Variable	None	98	1–2	5–7	Fecal (90) Renal (10)

Table 23.7. Dosing Information for Angiotensin II Antagonists*

Generic Name	Brand Name(s)	Dosing Range (Treatment of Hypertension) (mg)	Maximum Daily Dose (mg)	Initial Dose Reduction with Hepatic Dysfunction	Dose Reduction with Renal Dysfunction	Available Tablet Strengths (mg)
Losartan	Cozaar	25–100 qd or bid	100	yes	no	25, 50
Valsartan	Diovan	80–320 qd	320	no	no	80, 160
Irbesartan	Avapro	150–300 qd	300	no	no	75, 150, 300
Candesartan Cilexetil	Atacand	8–32 qd	32	no	no	4, 8, 16, 32
Telmisartan	Micardis	40–80 qd	80	yes (avoid)	no	40, 80
Eprosartan	Teveten	300–800 qd or bid	1200	—[†]	—[†]	—[†]

[†] = not available.
*All compounds approved for treatment of hypertension.

ation with other antihypertensive agents. Based on their ability to attenuate the renin-angiotensin system, one should expect a gradual increase in the number of uses and approved indications for this class of agents. As an example, the marketing of eprosartan has been voluntarily delayed by the manufacturer while the FDA completes a review on recently completed studies. It is anticipated that a favorable review will have a significant impact on the product's labeling (51).

Unlabeled Uses

Heart failure, diabetic nephropathy

Adverse Effects

Adverse Effects of Angiotensin II Receptor Antagonists

Headache, dizziness, fatigue, hypotension, hyperkalemia, GI upset, diarrhea, upper respiratory tract infection, myalgia, back pain, pharyngitis

The most prevalent side effects of angiotensin II antagonists are listed here (1,48–50,52). Overall, this class of agents is well tolerated, with CNS effects being the most commonly reported complaint. Similar to ACE inhibitors, some of the adverse effects seen here are directly related to attenuation of the renin-angiotensin pathway. Notably absent are the dry cough and angioedema seen with ACE inhibitors. Since angiotensin II antagonists are specific in their actions, this class of drugs does not affect the levels of bradykinin or prostaglandins and thus does not cause these bothersome side effects. Like ACE inhibitors, the use of angiotensin II antagonists during pregnancy is contraindicated, especially during the second and third trimesters. The use of angiotensin II antagonists should be discontinued as soon as pregnancy is confirmed unless the benefits outweigh the potential risks.

Drug Interactions

Despite the oxidative metabolism of some angiotensin II receptor antagonists, no clinically significant drug interactions involving CYP450 enzymes have been reported. Telmisartan has been reported to increase digoxin levels and slightly decrease warfarin levels; however, the reduced warfarin levels were not sufficient to alter the international normalized ratio (INR).

ROLE OF CALCIUM AND CALCIUM CHANNELS IN VASCULAR SMOOTH MUSCLE CONTRACTION

Calcium is a key component of the excitation-contraction coupling process which occurs within the cardiovascular system. It acts as a cellular messenger to link internal or external excitation with cellular response. Increased cytosolic concentrations of Ca^{2+} result in the binding of Ca^{2+} to a regulatory protein, either troponin C in cardiac and skeletal muscle or calmodulin in vascular smooth muscle.

This initial binding of Ca^{2+} uncovers myosin binding sites on the actin molecule, and subsequent interactions between actin and myosin result in muscle contraction. All of these events are reversed once the cytosolic concentration of Ca^{2+} decreases. In this situation, Ca^{2+} binding to troponin C or calmodulin is diminished or removed, myosin binding sites are concealed, actin and myosin can no longer interact and muscle contraction ceases (53,54).

Mechanisms of Calcium Movement and Storage

The regulation of cytosolic calcium levels occurs via specific influx, efflux, and sequestering mechanisms (Fig. 23.20). The influx of calcium can occur through receptor-operated (ROC) channels (site 1), the Na^+/Ca^{2+} exchange process (site 2), "leak" pathways (site 3), and potential-dependent (PDC) channels (site 4). Influx via either receptor-operated or voltage-dependent channels has been proposed to be the major entry pathway for Ca^{2+}. Receptor-operated channels have been defined as those associated with cellular membrane receptors and activated by specific agonist-receptor interactions. In contrast, potential-dependent channels, also known as voltage dependent or voltage gated calcium channels, have been defined as those activated by membrane depolarization. The Na^+/Ca^{2+} exchange process can promote either influx or efflux since the direction of Ca^{2+} movement depends upon the relative intracellular and extracellular ratios of Na^+ and Ca^{2+}. The "leak" pathways, which include unstimulated Ca^{2+} entry as well as entry during the fast inward Na^+ phase of an action potential, play only a minor role in calcium influx.

Efflux can occur through either an ATP-driven membrane pump (site 5) or via the Na^+/Ca^{2+} exchange process previously mentioned. In addition to these influx and efflux mechanisms, the sarcoplasmic reticulum (site 6) and the mitochondria (site 7) function as internal storage/release sites. These storage sites work in concert with the influx and efflux processes to assure that cytosolic calcium

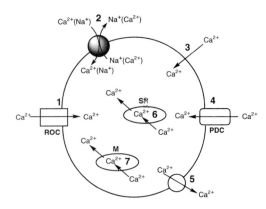

Fig. 23.20. Cellular mechanisms for the influx, efflux, and sequestering of Ca^{2+}. Key: ROC = receptor-operated Ca^{2+} channels; PDC = potential-dependent Ca^{2+} channels; SR = sarcoplasmic reticulum; M = mitochondria.

levels are appropriate for cellular needs. While influx and release processes are essential for excitation-contraction coupling, efflux and sequestering processes are equally important for terminating the contractile process and for protecting the cell from the deleterious effects of Ca^{2+} overload (55,56).

Potential-dependent Calcium Channels

Compounds listed in the Top 200 Drugs which block potential-dependent calcium channels (2)

Amlodipine (Norvasc), diltiazem (Cardizem CD), nifedipine (Adalat CC, Procardia XL), verapamil (Calan SR, Verapamil SR).

The pharmacologic class of agents known as calcium channel blockers produce their effects through interaction with potential-dependent channels. To date, six functional subclasses, or types, of potential-dependent Ca^{2+} channels have been identified: T, L, N, P, Q, and R. These types differ in location and function and can be divided into two major groups: low-voltage activated (LVA) channels and high-voltage activated (HVA) channels. Of the six types, only the T (transient, tiny) channel can be rapidly activated and inactivated with small changes in the cell membrane potential. It is thus designated as an LVA channel. All of the other types of channels require a larger depolarization and are thus designated as HVA channels. The L (long-lasting, large) channel is the site of action of currently available calcium channel blockers and has therefore been extensively studied. It is located in skeletal, cardiac, and smooth muscle and is thus highly involved in organ and vessel contraction within the cardiovascular system. The N channel is found in neuronal tissue and exhibits kinetics and inhibitory sensitivity distinct from both L and T channels. The functions, sensitivities, and properties of the other three types of channels are not as well known. The P channel has been named for its presence in the Purkinje cells, while the Q and R channels have been characterized by their abilities to bind to certain polypeptide toxins (57,58).

The L channel is a pentameric complex consisting of α_1, α_2, β, γ, and δ polypeptides. The α_1 subunit is a transmembrane spanning protein which consists of four domains and which functions as the pore-forming subunit. The α_1 subunit also contains binding sites for all of the currently available calcium channel blockers. The other four subunits surround the α_1 portion of the channel and contribute to the overall hydrophobicity of the pentamer. This hydrophobicity is important in that it allows the channel to be embedded in the cell membrane. Other types of potential-dependent channels are similar to the L channel. They all have a central α_1 subunit; however, molecular cloning studies have revealed that there are at least six α_1 genes: α_{1S}, α_{1A}, α_{1B}, α_{1C}, α_{1D}, and α_{1E}. Three of these genes, α_{1S}, α_{1C} and α_{1D}, have been associated with L channels. The L channels found in skeletal muscle result from the α_{1S} gene, those in the heart, aorta, lung, and fibroblast result from the α_{1C} gene, while those in endocrine tissue result from the α_{1D} gene. Both α_{1C} and α_{1D} are used for L channels in the brain. Thus, there are some differences among the L channels located in different organs and tissues. Additionally, differences in α_1 genes as well as differences among the other subunits are responsible for the variations seen among the other five types of potential-dependent channels. As an example, the N channel lacks the γ subunit and contains an α_1 subunit derived from the α_{1B} gene (57).

CARDIOVASCULAR DISORDERS ASSOCIATED WITH POTENTIAL-DEPENDENT CALCIUM CHANNELS

As described above, the movement of calcium underlies the basic excitation-contraction coupling process. Thus, vascular tone and contraction are primarily determined by the availability of calcium from extracellular or intracellular sources. Potential-dependent Ca^{2+} channels are important in regulating the influx of Ca^{2+}; therefore, inhibition of Ca^{2+} flow through these channels results in both vasodilation and decreased cellular response to contractile stimuli. Arterial smooth muscle is more sensitive to this action than venous smooth muscle. Additionally, coronary and cerebral arterial vessels are more sensitive than other arterial beds (56,59). As a result of these actions, calcium channel blockers are useful in the treatment of hypertension, CHF (unapproved), and ischemic heart disease (IHD). Brief overviews of both hypertension and CHF are provided in the renin-angiotensin section of this chapter.

The term IHD encompasses a variety of syndromes. These include angina pectoris, silent myocardial ischemia, acute coronary insufficiency, and myocardial infarction (MI). In a 1992 study, IHD was shown to be responsible for over 20% of total mortality in the United States. More specifically, MIs accounted for over 10% of all deaths. The overall incidence of IHD is higher in men than in women and increases with age. The average annual incidence rate (i.e., number of new cases/population) of angina pectoris is 1.5%, while the average mortality from this disease is 4% (60).

Angina pectoris is a clinical manifestation that results from coronary atherosclerotic heart disease. It is characterized by a severe constricting pain in the chest that often radiates to the left shoulder, the left arm, or the back. Clinically, angina pectoris can be classified as either exertional, variant, or unstable. Exertional angina, otherwise known as stable angina or exercise-induced angina, is the most common form and is due to an imbalance between myocardial oxygen supply and demand. Variant angina, otherwise known as Prinzmetal's angina, results from the vasospasm of large, surface coronary vessels or branches. Unstable angina is the most difficult to treat and may occur as a result of advanced atherosclerosis and coronary vasospasm (61).

Excitation-contraction coupling in the heart is different from that in vascular smooth muscle in that a portion of

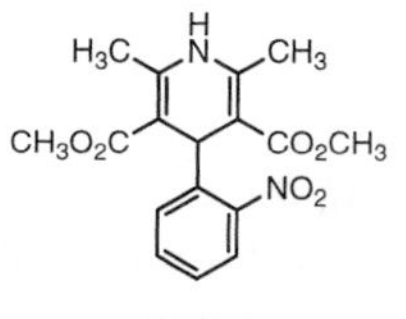

Nifedipine
(a 1,4-dihydropyridine)

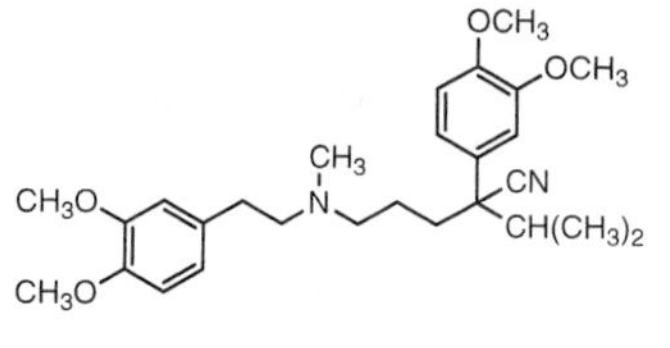

Verapamil
(a phenylalkylamine)

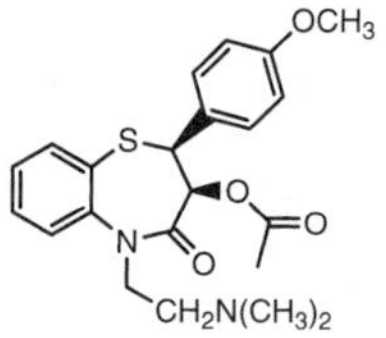

Diltiazem
(a benzothiazepine)

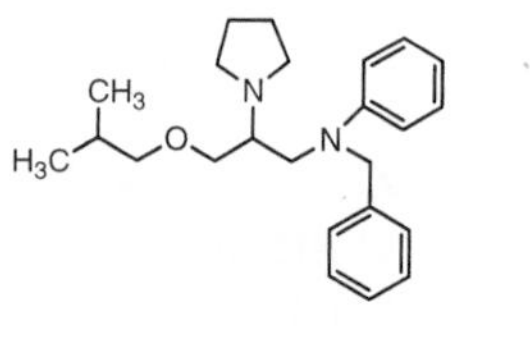

Bepridil
(a diaminopropanol ether)

Fig. 23.21. Chemical classes of calcium channel blockers.

the inward current is carried by Na^+ through the fast channel. In the SA and AV nodes, however, depolarization depends primarily on the movement of Ca^{2+} through the slow channel. Attenuation of this Ca^{2+} movement produces a negative inotropic effect and decreased conduction through the AV node. This latter effect is especially useful in treating paroxysmal supraventricular tachycardia (PSVT), an arrhythmia primarily caused by AV nodal reentry and AV reentry (59).

CALCIUM CHANNEL BLOCKERS

Historical Overview

Identification of compounds that could block the inward movement of Ca^{2+} through slow cardiac channels occurred in the early 1960s. Verapamil and other phenylalkylamines were shown to possess negative inotropic and chronotropic effects which were distinct from other coronary vasodilators. Further investigations revealed that these agents mimicked the cardiac effects of Ca^{2+} withdrawal: they reduced contractile force without affecting the action potential. The effects of these compounds could be reversed by the addition of Ca^{2+}, thus suggesting that the negative inotropic effect was linked to an inhibition of excitation-contraction coupling. Subsequently, derivatives of verapamil, as well as other chemical classes of compounds, were shown to competitively block Ca^{2+} movement through the slow channel and thus alter the cardiac action potential. Thus, calcium channel blockers are also known as slow channel blockers, calcium entry blockers, and calcium antagonists (55,59).

Chemical Classifications

Overview

There are currently 10 calcium channel blockers available for therapeutic use. These compounds have diverse chemical structures and can be grouped into one of four chemical classifications (Fig. 23.21), each of which produces a distinct pharmacologic profile: 1,4-dihydropyridines (e.g., nifedipine), phenylalkylamines (e.g., verapamil), benzothiazepines (e.g., diltiazem), and diaminopropanol ethers (e.g., bepridil). The majority of calcium channel blockers are 1,4-dihydropyridines (1,4-DHPs), and a detailed description of the SAR for this chemical class is provided below. In contrast, verapamil, diltiazem, and bepridil are the lone representatives of their respective chemical classes, and are thus discussed as individual agents. Verapamil and diltiazem are discussed along with the 1,4-DHPs. Bepridil is unique in that it is a nonselective agent, and it is discussed separately at the end of this chapter.

1,4-Dihydropyridines

History and Development. The chemistry of dihydropyridines can be traced back to an 1882 paper in which Hantzsch described their utility as intermediates in the synthesis of substituted pyridines. Fifty years later, interest in this chemical class of compounds increased when it was discovered that a 1,4-dihydropyridine ring was responsible for the "hydrogen-transfer" properties of the coenzyme NADH. Numerous biochemical studies followed this discovery; however, it was not until the early 1970s that the pharmacologic properties of 1,4-DHPs were fully investigated. Loev and coworkers at Smith, Klein & French laboratories investigated the activities of "Hantzsch-type" compounds. As shown in Figure 23.22, the Hantzsch reaction produced a symmetrical compound in which both the esters (i.e., CO_2R_2) and the C_2 and C_6 substituents (i.e., CH_3) are identical with each other. Structural requirements necessary for activity were identified by sequentially modifying the C_4 substituent (i.e., the R_1 group), the C_3- and C_5-esters (i.e., the R_2 groups), the C_2- and C_6-alkyl groups, and the N_1-H substituent (62–65).

Structure-activity Relationships. The structure-activity relationships for 1,4-DHP derivatives (see General Structure in Table 23.8) indicates that the following structural features are important for activity: 1) A substituted phenyl ring at the C_4 position optimizes activity (heteroaromatic rings, such as pyridine, produce similar therapeutic ef-

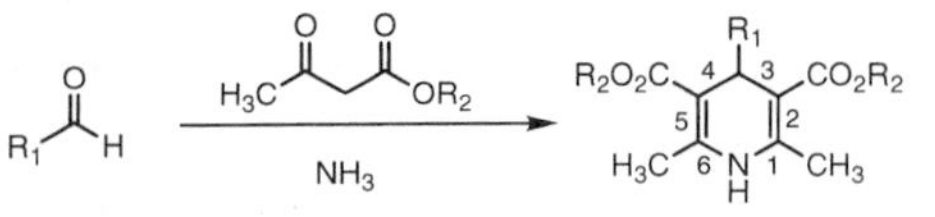

General structure for
1,4-dihydropyridines

Fig. 23.22. Synthesis of 1,4-DHPs using the Hantzsch reaction.

Table 23.8. Structure of the Dihydropyridine Calcium Channel Blockers

General structure:

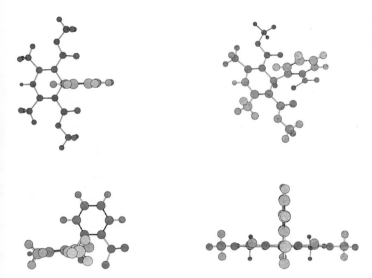

Isradipine:

Compounds	R_1	R_2	R_3	X
Amlodipine	CH₂OCH₂CH₂NH₂	CO₂CH₂CH₃	CO₂CH₃	2-Cl
Felodipine	CH₃	CO₂CH₂CH₃	CO₂CH₃	2,3-Cl₂
Nicardipine	CH₃	CO₂CH₂CH₂–NH–CH₂·C₆H₅	CO₂CH₃	3-NO₂
	CH₃	CH₃		
Nifedipine	CH₃	CO₂CH₃	CO₂CH₃	2-NO₂
Nimodipine	CH₃	CO₂CH₂CH₂OCH₃	CO₂CH(CH₃)₂	3-NO₂
Nisoldipine	CH₃	CO₂CH₂CH(CH₃)₂	CO₂CH₃	2-NO₂

Fig. 23.23. Molecular models of nifedipine. The ortho-nitro group of nifedipine provides steric bulk and ensures that the required perpendicular nature of the phenyl and dihyropyridine rings is maintained.

fects; but are not used due to observed animal toxicity). C_4 substitution with a small nonplanar alkyl or cycloalkyl group decreases activity. 2) Phenyl ring substitution (X) is important for size and position rather than for electronic nature. Compounds with *ortho-* or *meta-*substitutions possess optimal activity, while those which are unsubstituted or contain a *para-*substitution show a significant decrease in activity. Electron withdrawing *ortho-* or *meta-*substituents or electron donating demonstrated good activity. The importance of the *ortho-* and *meta-*substituents is to provide sufficient bulk to "lock" the conformation of the 1,4-DHP such that the C_4 aromatic ring is perpendicular to the 1,4-dihydropyridine ring (Fig. 23.23). This perpendicular conformation has been proposed to be essential for the activity of the 1,4-DHPs. 3) The 1,4-dihydropyridine ring is essential for activity. Substitution at the N_1 position or the use of oxi-

dized (piperidine) or reduced (pyridine) ring systems greatly decreases or abolishes activity. 4) Ester groups at the C_3 and C_5 positions optimize activity. Other electron-withdrawing groups show decreased antagonist activity and may even show agonist activity. For example, the replacement of the C_3 ester of isradipine with a NO_2 group produces a calcium channel activator, or agonist (Fig. 23.24). Thus the term, calcium channel modulators, is a more appropriate classification for the 1,4-DHPs. 5) When the esters at C_3 and C_5 are nonidentical, the C_4 carbon becomes chiral and stereoselectivity between the enantiomers is observed. Additionally, there is evidence that the C_3 and C_5 positions of the dihydropyridine ring are not equivalent positions. Crystal structures of nifedipine, a symmetrical 1,4-DHP, have shown that the C_3 carbonyl is *synplanar* to the C_2-C_3 bond, but that the C_5 carbonyl is *antiperiplanar* to the C_5-C_6 bond (Fig. 23.25). Asymmetrical compounds have shown enhanced selectivity for specific blood vessels and are preferentially being developed. Nifedipine, the first 1,4-DHP to be marketed, is the only symmetrical compound in this chemical class. 6). With the exception of amlodipine, all 1,4-DHPs have C_2 and C_6 methyl groups. The enhanced potency of amlodipine (vs. nifedipine) suggests that the 1,4-DHP receptor can tolerate larger substituents at this position and that enhanced activity can be obtained by altering these groups.

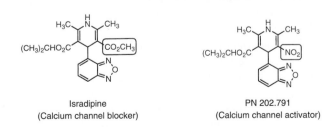

Isradipine
(Calcium channel blocker)

PN 202.791
(Calcium channel activator)

Fig. 23.24. Structures of isradipine and its analogous 3-nitro derivative.

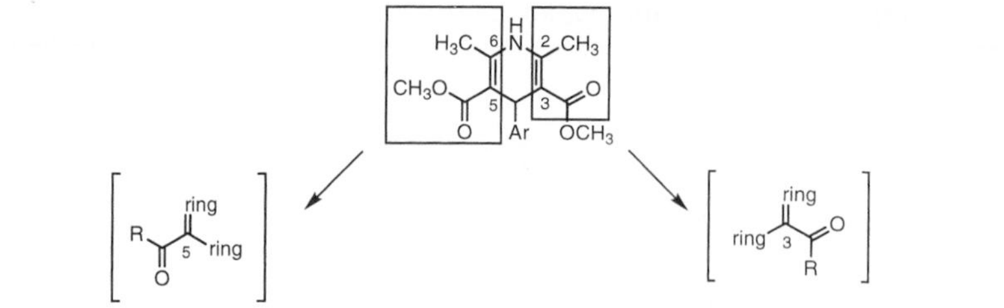

Antiperiplanar relationship
between carbonyl and double bond

Synplanar relationship
between carbonyl and double bond

Fig. 23.25. Conformation of the C_3 and C_5 esters of nifedipine (Ar = 2-nitrophenyl). The C_3 carbonyl is synplanar to the C_2–C_3 bond, and the C_5 carbonyl antiperiplanar to the C_5–C_6 bond.

Table 23.9. Actions of Calcium Channel Blockers and Interactions Among Their Receptor Sites

Calcium Channel Blocker	Effect on Ca^{2+} Channel	Allosteric Effect on the Binding of:		
		Verapamil	Diltiazem	1,4-DHPs
Verapamil	Antagonist; blocks channel	na	Inhibits	Inhibits
Diltiazem	Antagonist; blocks channel	Inhibits	na	Enhances
1,4-Dihydropyridines	Antagonist/agonist; can either block or open channel	Inhibits	Enhances	na

Table 23.10. Comparison of the Cardiovascular Effects of Verapamil, Diltiazem, and Nifedipine

Cardiovascular Effect	Verapamil	Diltiazem	Nifedipine (a 1,4-DHP)
Peripheral vasodilation	○○	○	○○○
Blood pressure	●	●	●
Heart rate	Variable	●	○○
Coronary vascular resistance	●	●	●
Coronary blood flow	○○	○○	○○○
Atrioventricular (AV) node conduction	●●	●	NE
Contractility	●	NE/●	NE/○

○ = increase; ● = decrease, NE = no effect.
The number of circles represents the magnitude of response.
Adapted from references 56,62.

Mechanism of Action

Despite the name, calcium channel blockers do not simply "plug the hole" and physically block the Ca^{2+} channel. Instead, they exert their effects by binding to specific receptor sites located within the central α_1 subunit of L type, potential-dependent channels. Three distinct but allosterically interacting receptors have been identified for verapamil, diltiazem, and the 1,4-DHPs. As shown in Table 23.9, the binding of verapamil to its receptor inhibits the binding of both diltiazem and the 1,4-DHPs to their respective receptors. Likewise, the binding of either diltiazem or the 1,4-DHPs inhibits the binding of verapamil. In contrast, diltiazem and the 1,4-DHPs mutually enhance the binding of each other (62).

Potential-dependent channels can exist in one of three conformations: a resting state which can be stimulated by membrane depolarization, an open state which allows the Ca^{2+} to enter, and an inactive state which is refractory to further depolarization. Calcium channel blockers have been shown to be more effective when membrane depolarization is either longer, more intense, or more frequent. This use-dependency suggests that these compounds preferentially interact with their receptors when the Ca^{2+} channel is in either the open or inactive state. This state dependence is not identical for all classes of Ca^{2+} blockers, and in combination with the different binding sites, allosteric interactions, acidity and solubility, may be responsible for the pharmacologic differences among verapamil, diltiazem, and the 1,4-DHPs. A summary of these differences are listed in Table 23.10. The 1,4-DHPs, exemplified by nifedipine, are primarily vasodilators, while verapamil and diltiazem have both vasodilator and cardiodepressant actions. The increased heart rate seen with nifedipine is due to a reflex mechanism which tries to overcome the vasodilation and subsequent drop in blood pressure caused by this 1,4-DHP. In contrast, the compensatory mechanism does not occur to the same extent with either verapamil and diltiazem. This is in part due to the ability of verapamil and diltiazem to block AV nodal conductance, and in part due to the increased ability of 1,4-DHP's to activate the baroreceptor reflex. These pharmacologic differences are ultimately reflected in the clinical use of these agents (56,61,62).

Physicochemical Properties

A comparison of the acid/base properties of verapamil, diltiazem, and the 1,4-DHPs reveals that while all of the compounds are basic, the 1,4-DHPs are considerably less basic than verapamil and diltiazem. Verapamil and diltiazem both contain tertiary amines with pKa values of 8.9 and 7.7, respectively (26). In contrast, the nitrogen of the 1,4-DHPs is part of a conjugated carbamate. Its electrons are involved in resonance delocalization and are much less available for protonation. Thus, at physiologic pH, verapamil and diltiazem are primarily ionized, while 1,4-DHPs are primarily un-ionized. There are two exceptions to this. Amlodipine and nicardipine contain basic amine groups as part of the side chains connected to the 1,4-DHP ring. While the 1,4-DHP ring of these compounds is un-ionized, the side chain amines will be primarily ionized at physiologic pH. Since ionic attraction is often the initial interaction between a drug and its receptor, the differences in basicity between the 1,4-DHP ring and the tertiary amines of verapamil and diltiazem are consistent with the previously noted fact that the binding site for the 1,4-DHPs is distinct from those for verapamil and diltiazem.

The calculated log P values for the calcium channel blockers are listed in Table 23.11 (26). As evidenced by the data, all of these compounds possess good lipid solubility and hence excellent oral absorption (not shown in table). Within the 1,4-DHP class, enhanced lipid solubility occurs in compounds which contain either larger ester groups or disubstituted phenyl rings. A comparison of the log P values of nifedipine and nisoldipine illustrates this fact. It should be noted that the calculated log P values listed in Table 23.11 are for the un-ionized compounds. These values significantly decrease for the ionized forms of amlodipine, nicardipine, verapamil and diltiazem, such that the latter three agents possess sufficient water solubility to be used both orally and parenterally.

All calcium channel blockers, with the exception of nifedipine, contain at least one chiral center; however, they are all marketed as their racemic mixtures. As previously noted, 1,4-DHPs with asymmetrically substituted esters exhibit stereoselectivity between the enantiomers. Additionally, the S (−) enantiomers of verapamil and other phenylalkylamines are more potent than the R (+) enantiomers. Very few SAR studies are available for diltiazem; however, the *cis* arrangement of the acetyl ester and the substituted phenyl ring is required for activity (62).

Metabolism

All calcium channel blockers undergo extensive first-pass metabolism in the liver (33,52). With the exception of nisoldipine, 1,4-DHPs are oxidatively metabolized by the hepatic cytochrome P450 system to a variety of inactive compounds. Nifedipine is metabolized by the CYP3A4 isozyme; however, reports for other 1,4-DHPs are less specific. In many cases, the dihydropyridine ring is initially oxidized to an inactive pyridine analog (Fig. 23.26). These

Table 23.11. Pharmacokinetic Parameters of Calcium Channel Blockers

Drug	Calculated Log P	Oral Bioavailability (%)	Effect of Food on Absorption	Active Metabolite	Protein Binding (%)	Onset of Action (min)	Elimination Half-life (hr)	Major Route(s) of Elimination (%)
1,4-Dihydropyridines								
Amlodipine	2.76	64–90	None	None	93–97	360	35–50	Renal (60%) Fecal (20–25%)
Felodipine	4.69	10–25	None	None	>99	120–300	10–16	Renal (70%) Fecal (10%)
Isradipine	3.19	15–34	Reduced rate, same extent	None	95–97	120	8	Renal (90%) Fecal (10%)
Nicardipine	4.27	35	Reduced	None	>95	20	2–4	Renal (60%) Fecal (35%)
Nifedipine	2.40	45–70 86 (SR)	None	None	92–98	20	2–5	Renal (60–80%) Biliary/Fecal (Minor)
Nimodipine	3.14	13	Reduced	None	>95	nd	1–2	Renal
Nisoldipine	3.86	5	Reduced rate, same extent	Hydroxylated analog	>99	60–180	7–12	Renal (70–75%) Fecal (6–12%)
Phenylalkylamines								
Verapamil	3.53	20–35	Reduced (SR form only)	Norverapamil	83–92	30 3–5 (IV)	3–7	Renal (70%) Fecal (16%)
Benzothiazepines								
Diltiazem	3.55	40–67	Enhanced	Deacetyl-diltiazem	70–80	30–60	3.5–6 5–7 (SR)	Renal
Diaminopropanol Ethers								
Bepridil	5.8	59	None	4-OH-phenyl bepridil	>99	60	24	Renal (70%) Fecal (22%)

SR = sustained released product.
IV = intravenous administration.
nd = not determined.

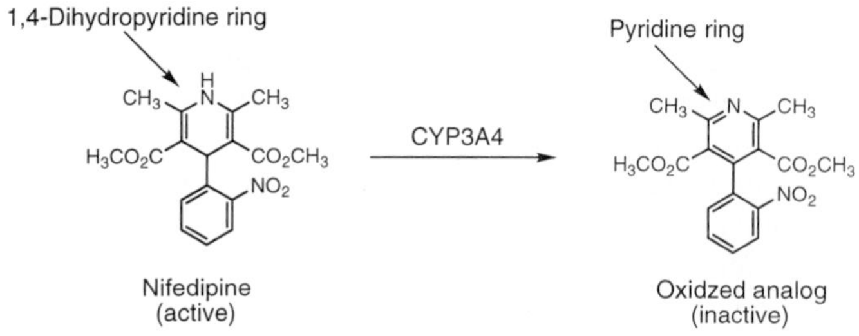

1,4-Dihydropyridine ring

Pyridine ring

Nifedipine
(active)

Oxidzed analog
(inactive)

Fig. 23.26. Oxidation of the 1,4-dihydropyridine ring of nifedipine.

initial metabolites are then further transformed by hydrolysis, conjugation, and additional oxidation pathways. Nisoldipine is also subject to these processes; however, hydroxylation of its isobutyl ester produces a metabolite which retains 10% of the activity of the parent compound. In addition to the drug-drug interactions listed below (see Table 23.13), an interesting drug-food interaction occurs with the 1,4-DHPs and grapefruit juice (66). Co-administration of 1,4-DHPs with grapefruit juice produces an increase systemic concentration of the 1,4-DHPs. The mechanism of this interaction appears to be due to inhibition of intestinal CYP450 by flavanoids and furanocoumarins specifically found in grapefruit juice (see Chapter 8).

Verapamil is primarily metabolized to the N-demethylated compound, norverapamil. Norverapamil retains approximately 20% of the pharmacologic activity of verapamil and can reach or exceed the steady state plasma levels of verapamil. Interestingly, the more active $S(-)$ isomer undergoes more extensive first-pass hepatic metabolism than does the less active $R(+)$ isomer. This is important to note because when given IV, verapamil prolongs the PR interval to a greater extent than when it is given orally (67). This is because the preferential metabolism of the more active enantiomer does not occur with parenteral administration. Diltiazem is primarily hydrolyzed to deacetyldiltiazem. This metabolite retains 25–50% of the coronary vasodilatory effects of diltiazem and is present in the plasma at levels of 10–45% of the parent compound.

Pharmacokinetic Parameters

The pharmacokinetic parameters and oral dosing information for calcium channel blockers are summarized in Tables 23.11 and 23.12, respectively (32,33,36,52). Some doses, specifically those for diltiazem and verapamil, may vary for either specific indications (*i.e.*, hypertension versus angina) or different brand names, and the reader should consult the product literature for additional information. The primary differences among the compounds are onset of action, half-life, and oral bioavailability. All calcium channel blockers have excellent oral absorption; however, since they are also subject to rapid first pass metabolism in the liver, the actual oral bioavailability of these compounds varies considerably depending upon the extent of metabolism. All compounds are highly plasma protein bound and primarily eliminated as inactive metabolites in the urine. Due to extensive hepatic transformation, calcium channel blockers

Table 23.12. Oral Dosing Information for Calcium Channel Blockers

Generic Name	Trade Name(s)	Approved Indications	Normal Dosing Range	Maximum Daily Dose	Precautions with Hepatic Dysfunction	Available Tablet or Capsule Strengths (mg)
1,4–Dihydropyridines						
Amlodipine	Norvasc	Angina (V,CS), Hypertension	5–10 mg qd	10 mg	Reduce dosage	2.5, 5, 10
Felodipine	Plendil	Hypertension	2.5–10 mg qd	20 mg	Reduce dosage	2.5, 5, 10
Isradipine	DynaCirc	Hypertension	2.5–5 mg bid	20 mg	Titrate dosage	2.5, 5
Nicardipine	Cardene	Angina (CS), Hypertension	20–40 mg tid (SR: 30–60 mg bid)	120 mg	Titrate dosage	20, 30 (SR: 30, 45, 60)
Nifedipine	Procardia, Adalat	Angina (V), Hypertension	10–20 mg tid (SR: 30–60 mg qd)	180 mg (SR: 90–120 mg)	Reduce dosage	10, 20 (SR: 30, 60, 90)
Nimodipine	Nimotop	Subarachnoid hemorrhage	60 mg q 4 hours for 21 days	—	Titrate dosage	30
Nisoldipine	Sular	Hypertension	20–40 mg qd	60 mg	Closely monitor blood pressure	10, 20, 30, 40
Phenylakylamines						
Verapamil	Calan, Isoptin	Angina (V,CS, U), Hypertension, Arrhythmias (IV)	240–480 mg tid or qid (SR: 240–480 mg qd or bid)	480 mg	Reduce dosage	40, 80, 120 (SR: 120, 180, 240, 360)
Benzothiazepines						
Diltiazem	Cardizem, Tiamate, Dilacor	Angina (V, CS), Hypertension, Arrhythmias (IV)	30–120 mg tid or qid (SR: 120–480 mg qd)	540 mg	Titrate dosage	30, 60, 90, 120 (SR: 60, 90, 120, 180, 240, 300, 360)
Diaminopropanol Ethers						
Bepridil	Vascor	Angina (CS)	200–300 mg qd	400 mg	Titrate dosage	200, 300, 400

Types of angina: V = vasospastic, CS = chronic stable, U = unstable.
SR = sustained release formulation.
IV = Intravenous Administration.

should be used cautiously in patients with hepatic disease. Recommendations for these patients include dosage reductions, careful titrations, and close therapeutic monitoring. Diltiazem and verapamil also require dosage adjustments in patients with renal dysfunction because renal impairment can significantly increase the concentrations of the active metabolites of these compounds. Dosage adjustments are usually not required for the other eight compounds since six of them produce inactive metabolites and the other two, nisoldipine and bepridil, produce active metabolites with significantly lower activity.

Nifedipine, nicardipine, verapamil, and diltiazem are the only four compounds which are available as both immediate release and sustained release formulations. The latter three compounds are also available as parenteral preparations. Unlike regular tablets and capsules, sustained release formulations cannot be chewed or crushed since this may lead to an immediate, rather than a sustained, release of the compound. This effect will not only decrease the duration of the dose, but could produce an overdose and subsequent toxicities in the patient. Parenteral preparations of nicardipine and verapamil are incompatible with IV solutions containing sodium bicarbonate. In each case, sodium bicarbonate increases the pH of the solution resulting in the precipitation of the calcium channel blocker. While this interaction is not listed for diltiazem, it is reasonable to assume that a similar interaction may occur. Additionally, nicardipine is incompatible with lactated Ringer's solution, and verapamil will precipitate in solutions having a pH greater than or equal to six (32,36).

Chemical/pharmacologic classes used to treat angina pectoris

Organic Nitrates, β-Blockers (Chapter 24), Calcium Channel Blockers

Therapeutic Applications

As illustrated in Table 23.12, calcium channel blockers have been approved for the treatment of hypertension, angina pectoris, subarachnoid hemorrhage, and specific types of arrhythmias (32,36). All calcium channel blockers cause vasodilation and decrease peripheral resistance. With the exceptions of nimodipine and bepridil, all are approved to treat hypertension. Recent studies have indicated that immediate release formulations of short acting calcium channel blockers, especially nifedipine, can cause an abrupt vasodilation which can result in myocardial infarction. As a result, only the sustained release formulations of nifedipine and diltiazem should be used in the treatment of essential hypertension (68). Six of the ten agents are approved for the treatment of angina pectoris. Verapamil is the most versatile agent in that it is indicated for all three types of angina—vasospastic, chronic stable and unstable. All of the other agents are indicated for either vasospastic or chronic stable angina. Nimodipine is

unique in that it has a greater effect on cerebral arteries than on other arteries. As a result, nimodipine is indicated for the improvement of neurological deficits due to spasm following subarachnoid hemorrhage from ruptured congenital intracranial aneurysms in patients who are otherwise in good neurological condition following the episode. Verapamil and diltiazem are pharmacologically different from the 1,4-DHPs in that they block sinus and AV nodal conduction. As a result, IV formulations of verapamil and diltiazem are indicated for the treatment of atrial fibrillation, atrial flutter, and paroxysmal supraventricular tachycardia (PSVT). Verapamil can also be used orally, either alone, for prophylaxis of repetitive PSVT, or in combination with digoxin, for atrial flutter or atrial fibrillation.

Unlabeled Uses

Migraine headache, Raynaud's syndrome, CHF, cardiomyopathy.

Adverse Effects

Adverse Effects of Calcium Channel Blockers

Edema, flushing, hypotension, nasal congestion, palpitations, chest pain, tachycardia, headache, fatigue, dizziness, rash, nausea, abdominal pain, constipation, diarrhea, vomiting, shortness of breath, weakness, bradycardia, AV block.

The most prevalent or significant side effects of calcium channel blockers are listed here (32,56,59,61). In most instances, these side effects do not cause long term complications, and they often resolve with time or dosage adjustments. Many of these effects are simply extensions of the pharmacologic effects of this class of compounds. Excessive vasodilation results in edema, flushing, hypotension, nasal congestion, headache, and dizziness. Additionally, the palpitations, chest pain, and tachycardia seen with 1,4-DHPs are a result of sympathetic responses to the vasodilatory effects of this chemical class. The use of a β-blocker in combination with a 1,4-DHP can minimize these compensatory effects and can be very useful in treating hypertension. Verapamil and diltiazem can cause bradycardia and AV block due to their ability to depress AV nodal conduction. Due to risks associated with additive cardiodepressive effects, they should not be used in combination with β-blockers.

Bepridil

Bepridil (Fig. 23.21) is unique from all of the above agents in that its actions are not solely based on its ability to block potential-dependent L-type (i.e., slow) Ca^{2+} channels (32,33,69). Unlike other calcium channel blockers, bepridil also blocks fast Na^+ channels as well as receptor-operated calcium channels. These additional actions are

Table 23.13. Drug Interactions for Calcium Channel Blockers

Drug	Calcium Blocker(s)	Result of Interaction
Amiodarone	Diltiazem, Verapamil	Increased bradycardia and cardiotoxicity; decreased cardiac output
Aspirin	Verapamil	Increased incidence of bruising
β-Blockers	All	Increased cardiodepressant effects (more extensive with verapamil and diltiazem)
Carbamazepine	Felodipine, Diltiazem, Verapamil	Carbamazepine decreases felodipine and diltiazem levels; verapamil increases carbamazepine levels
Cyclosporine	Amlodipine, Isradipine, Nicardipine, Diltiazem, Verapamil	Increased cyclosporine levels
Diclofenac	Isradipine	Decreased antihypertensive response
Digoxin	Felodipine, Nifedipine, Nisoldipine, Diltiazem, Verapamil	Increased digoxin levels
Doxorubicin	Verapamil	Increased doxorubicin levels
Encainide	Diltiazem	Increased effects of encainide, severe hypotension
Erythromycin	Felodipine (possibly other 1,4-DHPs)	Increased felodipine levels and increased toxicity
Fentanyl	All	Severe hypotension and increased fluid volume requirements
Histamine H₂ Antagonists	All	Increased bioavailability of calcium channel blocker
Imipramine	Diltiazem	Increased imipramine levels
Lovastatin	Isradipine	Decreased effects of lovastatin
Nitroprusside	Diltiazem	Increased nitroprusside levels
Omeprazole	Nimodipine, Nisoldipine	Increased bioavailability of calcium channel blocker
Phenobarbital	Felodipine, Nifedipine, Verapamil	Decreased bioavailability of calcium channel blocker
Phenytoin	Nifedipine	Increased phenytoin levels
Quinidine	Nifedipine, Verapamil	Increased levels of calcium channel blocker; nifedipine may decrease quinidine levels
Rifampin	Nifedipine, Verapami	Decreased levels of calcium channel blocker
Theophylline	Felodipine, Nifedipine, Diltiazem, Verapamil	Felodipine decreases the effects of theophylline; all others increase theophylline levels
Valproic acid	Nimodipine	Increased nimodipine levels
Vecuronium	Verapamil, Diltiazem	Increased vecuronium levels
Vincristine	Nifedipine	Increased vincristine levels

responsible for bepridil's ability to inhibit cardiac conduction, slow AV nodal conduction, increase the refractory period, slow the heart rate, and prolong the QT interval.

Bepridil possesses physicochemical and pharmacokinetic properties (Table 23.11) similar to those of previously discussed calcium channel blockers. Bepridil is a basic compound. Its pyrrolidine ring has a pKa of approximately 10 and is primarily ionized at physiologic pH (70). Bepridil is also highly lipid soluble. The calculated Log P for the un-ionized form of the drug is 5.8, while the measured Log P of the drug at physiologic pH is 2.0 (26). Bepridil contains one chiral center; however, information pertaining to enantiomeric differences is currently lacking. The oral absorption of bepridil is greater the 90%; however, the drug is subject to first-pass metabolism and shows an oral bioavailability of 59%. The drug is extensively metabolized with less than 1% excreted unchanged. At least one of the metabolites, the 4-hydroxyphenyl analog, is active. Compared to other calcium channel blockers, bepridil has an intermediate onset of action and a longer elimination half-life. It also demonstrates high plasma protein binding similar to other agents.

Bepridil is indicated for the oral treatment of chronic stable angina pectoris. Due to potential adverse effects, it is recommended for use only in patients who are intolerant of or fail to optimally respond to other treatment. It can be used alone or in combination with nitrates or β-blockers. While caution should be taken for patients with either renal or hepatic impairment, specific recommendations are not currently available. Dosing information is provided in Table 23.12.

Bepridil is contraindicated in patients with ventricular or atrial arrhythmias, sick-sinus syndrome, A-V block, cardiogenic shock, hypotension, uncompensated cardiac insufficiency, congenital Q-T interval prolongation, or patients taking other drugs that prolong the Q-T interval. Bepridil has also been shown to increase cyclosporin and digitalis levels.

Adverse Effects of Bepridil

Dizziness, headache, nausea, dyspepsia, diarrhea, tremor, weakness, nervousness, dry mouth, bradycardia, and palpitations.

Victoria F. Roche and S. William Zito

Two days ago HW, a 64-year-old, white, male postal worker, was brought unconscious to the emergency room of the hospital where you work. His wife told the ER physician that they were spending their usual Wednesday night at home watching "Law & Order" on television when HW, who had been complaining of a bad headache and stiff neck ever since he got home, suddenly "passed out." A brief medical history provided by Mrs. HW indicated mild hypertension that HW treated rather poorly with diet and occasional exercise. A call to HW's family physician uncovered a brief history of arrhythmia that was treated successfully with flecainide, and recent complaints of erectile dysfunction. Physical examination showed marked rigidity of the neck, and there were traces of blood in his CSF. His liver and kidney function are normal. A diagnosis of intracranial hemorrhage secondary to cerebral hypertension was made. Although the prognosis for most patients with this diagnosis is poor, fortune smiled on HW as he survived and is now on the road to recovery. HW's physician has put him on atenolol (a polar β_1-selective antagonist) for his hypertension. Because atenolol has an unlabeled use in treating supraventricular arrhythmia and tachycardia and can interact with flecanide to augment the pharmacologic action of both agents, the flecanide was discontinued. The doctor is now looking for your input on an appropriate calcium channel blocker to decrease the risk of neurological deficit from cerebral vasospasm which is a common, posthemorrhagic event. Consider the three calcium channel blocker structures provided.

1. Identify the therapeutic problem(s) where the pharmacist's intervention may benefit the patient.

2. Identify and prioritize the patient specific factors that must be considered to achieve the desired therapeutic outcomes.

3. Conduct a thorough and mechanistically oriented structure-activity analysis of all therapeutic alternatives provided in the case.

4. Evaluate the SAR findings against the patient specific factors and desired therapeutic outcomes and make a therapeutic decision.

5. Counsel your patient.

REFERENCES

1. Jackson EK and Garrison JC. Renin and angiotensin. In: Hardman JG, Limbird LE, Molinoff PB, et al, eds. The pharmacological basis of therapeutics. 9th ed. New York: McGraw-Hill, 1996; 733–758.
2. Zoeller, J. The Top 200 Drugs. American Druggist 1998; 215(2): 46–53.
3. Skeggs L. Historical overview of the renin-angiotensin system. In: Doyle AE, Bearn AG, eds. Hypertension and the antiotensin system: therapeutic approaches. New York: Raven Press, 1984; 31–45.
4. Vallotton MB. The renin-angiotensin system. Trends Pharmacol Sci 1987;8, 69–74.
5. Babe KS, Serafin WE. Histamine, bradykinin, and their antagonists. In: Hardman JG, Limbird LE, Molinoff PB, et al, eds. The pharmacological basis of therapeutics. 9th ed. New York: McGraw-Hill, 1996; 593–598.
6. Ferrario CM, Brosnihan KB, Diz DI, et al. Angiotensin-(1–7): a new hormone of the angiotensin system. Hyperten 1991; 18: III126–III133.
7. Hawkin DW, Bussey HI, Prisant LM. Hypertension. In: Dipiro JT, Talbert RL, Yee, GC, et al, eds. Pharmacotherapy, a pathophysiologic approach, 3rd ed. Stamford, CT: Appleton & Lange, 1997; 195–218.
8. Johnson JA, Lalonde RL. Congestive Heart Failure. In: Dipiro JT, Talbert RL, Yee, GC, et al. eds. Pharmacotherapy, a pathophysiologic approach, 3rd ed. Stamford, CT: Appleton & Lange, 1997; 219–256.
9. Boger J. Clinical goal in sight for small molecule renin inhibitors. Trends Pharmacol Sci 1987;8, 370–372.
10. Petrillo EW, Jr., Trippodo NC, DeForrest JM. Antihypertensive Agents. Ann Rep Med Chem 1990;25: 51–60.
11. Kleinert HD, Rosenberg SH, Baker WR, et al. Discovery of a peptide-based renin inhibitor with oral bioavailability and efficacy. Science 1992;257: 1940–1943.
12. Buchholz RA, Lefker BA, Ravi Kiron MA. Hypertension therapy: what next? Ann Rep Med Chem 1993;28: 69–78.
13. Ferreira SH, Bartelt DC, Lewis LJ. Isolation of bradykinin-potentiating peptides from Bothrops jararaca venom. Biochemistry 1970;9: 2583–2593.
14. Bakhle YS. Conversion of angiotensin I to angiotensin II by cell-free extracts of dog lung. Nature 1968;220: 919–21.
15. Garrison JC and Peach MJ. Renin and angiotensin. In: Gilman AG, Rall TW, Nies AS, et al, eds. The pharmacological basis of therapeutics. 8th ed. New York: Pergamon Press, 1990; 749–763.
16. Silverman RB. The organic chemistry of drug design and drug action. San Diego: Academic Press, 1992; 162–170.
17. Ondetti MA, Rubin B, Cushman DW. Design of specific inhibitors of angiotensin-converting enzyme: new class of orally active antihypertensive agents. Science 1977;196: 441–444.
18. Cushman DW, Cheung HS, Sabo EF, et al. Design of potent competitive inhibitors of angiotensin-converting enzyme. Carboxyalkanoyl and mercaptoalkanoyl amino acids. Biochemistry 1977;16: 5484–5491.
19. Ondetti MA, Cushman DW. Enzymes of the renin-angiotensin system and their inhibitors. Ann Rev Biochem 1982;51: 283–308.
20. Stryer L. Biochemistry. 4th ed. New York: Freeman and Company, 1995; 218–222.
21. Byers LD, Wolfenden R. Binding of the by-product analog benzylsuccinic acid by carboxypeptidase A. Biochemistry 1973;12: 2070–2078.
22. Klaassen CD. Heavy metals and heavy-metal antagonists. In: Hardman JG, Limbird LE, Molinoff PB, et al, eds. The pharmacological basis of therapeutics. 9th ed. New York: McGraw-Hill, 1996; 1667–1668.
23. Atkinson AB and Robertson JIS. Captopril in the treatment of clinical hypertension and cardiac failure. Lancet 1979;2: 836–839.
24. Patchett AA, Harris E, Tristram EW, et al. A new class of angiotensin-converting enzyme inhibitors. Nature 1980;288: 280–283.
25. Gringauz A. Introduction to medicinal chemistry. New York: Wiley, 1997; 450–461.
26. Craig PN. Drug Compendium. In: Hansch C, Sammes PG, Taylor JB, eds. Comprehensive Medicinal Chemistry. Volume 6. Oxford: Permagon Press, 1990; 237–991.
27. Gross DM, Sweet, CS, Ulm EH, et al. Effect of N-[(S)-1-carboxy-3-phenylpropyl]-L-Ala-L-Pro and its ethyl ester (MK-421) on angiotensin converting enzyme in vitro and angiotensin I pressor responses in vivo. J Pharmacol Exp Ther 1981;216: 552–557.
28. Ulm EH, Hichens M, Gomez HJ, et al. Enalapril maleate and a lysine analogue (MK-521): disposition in man. Br J clin Pharmac 1982;14: 357–362.
29. Kim DH, Guinosso CJ, Buzby GC, Jr., et al. (Mercaptopropanoyl)indoline-2–carboxylic acids and related compounds as potent angiotensin converting enzyme inhibitors and antihypertensive agents. J Med Chem 1983;26: 394–403.
30. Krapcho J, Turk C, Cushman DW, et al. Angiotensin-converting enzyme inhibitors. Mercaptan, carboxyalkyl dipeptide, and phosphinic acid inhibitors incorporating 4-substituted prolines. J Med Chem 1988;31: 1148–1160.
31. Oparil S, Koerner T, Tregear GW, et al. Substrate requirements for angiotensin I conversion in vivo and in vitro. Circ Res 1973;32: 415–423.
32. Clinical Reference Library [CD-ROM]. Version 98.1. Hudson, OH: Lexi-Comp, 1998.
33. Clinical Pharmacology [CD-ROM]. Reents S, ed. Tampa, FL: Gold Standard Multimedia, 1998.
34. Borne RF, Vinson MC. New drugs of 1992, Part 2. Drug Topics 1994;138(5): 71–73.
35. Drummer OH, Nicolaci J, Iakovidis D. Biliary excretion and conjugation of diacid angiotensin-converting enzyme inhibitors. J Pharmacol Exp Ther 1990;252: 1202–1206.
36. Drug Facts and Comparisons. St. Louis, MO: Facts and Comparisons, 1998; 999–1026.
37. Riley TN, DeRuiter J. New drugs. U.S. Pharmacist 1992;17(3): 42–46.
38. Riley TN, DeRuiter J. New drugs. U.S. Pharmacist 1997;22(3): 175–176.
39. Annon. Trandolapril: an ACE inhibitor for treatment of hypertension. The Medical Letter 1996;38: 104–105.
40. Kostis JB, Garland WT, Delaney C, et al. Fosinopril: pharmacokinetic and pharmacodynamics in congestive heart failure. Clin Pharmacol Ther 1995;58: 660–665.
41. Lacourciere Y, Brunner H, Irwin R, et al. Effects of modulators of the renin-angiotensin-aldosterone system on cough. Losartan Cough Study Group. J Hypertens. 1994;12: 1387–1393.
42. Timmermans PB, Wong PC, Chiu AT, et al. Angiotensin II receptors and angiotensin II receptor antagonists. Pharmacol Rev 1993;45: 205–213.
43. Moore GJ. Designing peptide mimetics. Trends Pharmacol Sci 1994;15: 124–129.
44. Harrold MW. Preparing students for future therapies: the development of novel agents to control the renin-angiotensin system. Am J Pharm Educ 1997;61: 173–178.
45. Furakawa Y, Kishimoto, S, Nishikawa, K. Hypotensive imidazole derivatives and hypotensive imidazole-5-acetic acid derivatives. U.S. Patents 4,340,598 and 4,355,040. Osaka, Japan, 1982.

46. Bauer JH, Reams GP. The angiotensin II type 1 receptor antagonists: a new class of antihypertensive drugs. Arch Intern Med 1995;155: 1361–1368.

47. Carini DJ, Duncia JV, Aldrich PE, et al. Nonpeptide angiotensin II receptor antagonists: the discovery of a series of N-(biphenylylmethyl)imidazoles as potent, orally active antihypertensives. J Med Chem 1991;35: 2525–2547.

48. Hussar DA. New drugs of 1997. J Am Pharm Assoc 1998;38: 166–167.

49. Annon. New product bulletin: Avapro (irbesartan). Washington DC: American Pharmaceutical Association, 1998.

50. McClellan KJ, Balfour JA. ADIS new drug profile: eprosartan. Drugs 1998; 55: 713–718.

51. Personal communication, SmithKline Beecham Pharmaceuticals, 1998.

52. Gelman CR, Rumack BH, Klasco R, eds. Drugdex system [CD-ROM] Englewood, CO: Micromedex, 1999.

53. Cocolas GH. Cardiovascular agents. In: Delgado, JN, Remers, WA, eds. Textbook of organic medicinal and pharmaceutical chemistry. 10th ed. Philadelphia: Lippincott-Raven, 1998, 589–593.

54. Silverthorn DU. Human physiology: an integrated approach. Upper Saddle River, NJ: Prentice Hall, 1998, 325–361.

55. Janis RA, Triggle DJ. New developments in Ca^{+2} channel antagonists. J Med Chem 1983;26: 775–785.

56. Swamy VC, Triggle DJ. Calcium channel blockers. In: Craig CR, Stitzel RE, eds. Modern pharmacology with clinical applications. 5th ed. Boston: Little, Brown, 1997, 229–234.

57. Varadi G, Mori Y, Mikala G, et al. Molecular determinants of Ca^{2+} channel function and drug action. Trends Pharmacol Sci 1995;16, 43–49.

58. Gilmore J, Dell C, Bowman D, et al. Neuronal calcium channels. Ann Rep Med Chem 1995;30, 51–60.

59. Robertson RM, Roberson D. Drugs used for the treatment of myocardial ischemia. In: Hardman JG, Limbird LE, Molinoff PB, et al, eds. The pharmacological basis of therapeutics. 9th ed. New York: McGraw-Hill, 1996; 759–779.

60. Talbert RL. Ischemic heart disease. In: Dipiro JT, Talbert RL, Yee GC, et al. eds. Pharmacotherapy, a pathophysiologic approach. 3rd ed. Stamford, CT: Appleton & Lange, 1997; 257–294.

61. Vaghy PL. Calcium antagonists. In: Brody TM, Larner J, Minneman KP, et al, eds. Human pharmacology: molecular to clinical. 2nd ed. St. Louis: Mosby, 1994; 203–213.

62. Triggle DJ. Drugs acting on ion channels and membranes. In: Hansch C, Sammes PG, Taylor JB, eds. Comprehensive Medicinal Chemistry. Volume 3. Oxford: Permagon Press, 1990; 1047–1099.

63. Loev B, Ehrreich SJ, Tedeschi RE. Dihydropyridines with potent hypotensive activity prepared by the Hantzsch reaction. J Pharm Pharmac 1972;24, 917–918.

64. Loev B, Goodman MM, Snader KM, et al. "Hantzsch-type" dihydropyridine hypotensive agents. J Med Chem 1974;17, 956–965.

65. Triggle AM, Shefter E, Triggle DJ. Crystal structures of calcium channel antagonists: 2,6-dimethyl-3,5-dicarbomethoxy-4-[2-nitro, 3-cyano-, 4-(dimethylamino)-, and 2,3,4,5,6-pentafluorophenyl]-1,4-dihydropyridine. J Med Chem 1980; 23, 1442–1445.

66. Bailey DG, Arnold JMO, Spence JD. Grapefruit juice and drugs: how significant is the interaction? Clin Pharmacokinet 1994; 26, 91–98.

67. Roden DM. Antiarrhythmic drugs. In: Hardman JG, Limbird LE, Molinoff PB, et al, eds. The pharmacological basis of therapeutics. 9th ed. New York: McGraw-Hill, 1996; 854–855.

68. Annon. Safety of calcium-channel blockers. The Medical Letter 1997;39: 13–14.

69. Annon. Bepridil for angina pectoris. The Medical Letter 1991;33: 54–55.

70. Lemke TL. Review of organic functional groups. 3rd ed. Philadelphia: Lea & Febiger, 1988; 45–56.

24. Central and Peripheral Sympatholytics and Vasodilators

DAVID A. WILLIAMS

INTRODUCTION
Overview of Hypertension

Hypertension is the most common cardiovascular disease and is the major risk factor for coronary artery disease, heart failure, stroke, and renal failure. Approximately 50 million Americans have a systolic or diastolic blood pressure above 140/90. The onset of hypertension is defined as having a blood pressure ≥ 140/90 and most commonly appears during the fourth, fifth, and sixth decades of life (1).

The importance of controlling blood pressure is well documented (1), although the rates of awareness, treatment and control of hypertension have not risen as had been expected (National Health and Nutrition Examination Survey) (2). This survey showed that 68% of Americans are aware that they have high blood pressure but only 53% are receiving treatment, and only 27% have their blood pressure under control. Since 1976 there had been a significant improvement in the rates of awareness, treatment and control of hypertension, but since 1990, whatever progress had been achieved has now reached a plateau (2). Although the age-adjusted death rates from stroke and coronary heart disease during this period have fallen by 59% and 53% respectively, these rates of decline also appear to have reached a plateau (2). These troubling trends should awaken clinicians to be more aggressive in the treatment of patients with hypertension.

When the decision to initiate hypertensive therapy is made, physicians are often presented with the dilemma of which of more than 80 antihypertensive products representing more than 8 different drug classes to use for their patients (1,3) (Table 24.2). Those factors which can affect the outcomes from the treatment of hypertension include potential adverse effects, clinically significant drug-drug interactions(especially when so many different drug classes are involved), patient compliance, affordability (especially for the elderly and those on fixed incomes), risk/benefit ratios, dosing frequency, etc. must be considered (3). Having considered these factors the healthcare provider (clinician, pharmacist) arrives at an appropriate choice of antihypertensive drug (3). Once the patient is stabilized on a antihypertensive medication, some of these issues need to be re-evaluated. Patients should be continually asked about side effects because many of the antihypertensive drugs possess side effects that the patient may not tolerate (1). This problem and the cost of drug therapy can affect compliance to drug therapy especially for the elderly and those on fixed incomes (4).

Drug therapy in the management of hypertension must be individualized and adjusted based on coexisting risk factors including the degree of blood pressure elevation, severity of the disease (e.g., presence of target organ damage), presence of underlying cardiovascular or other risk factors, response to therapy (single or multiple drugs), and tolerance to drug-induced adverse effects (1,3). Antihypertensive therapy is generally reserved for patients who fail to respond to nondrug therapies along with lifestyle modifications such as diet including sodium restriction and adequate potassium intake, regular aerobic physical activity, moderation of alcohol consumption and weight reduction (3).

It is not surprising that compliance with antihypertensive therapy may be as low as 40% when one considers that the patient, if they have other chronic diseases, may be taking as many as 10 different drugs and up to 40 tablets/capsules per day (4). To achieve better compliance requires educating the patient and simplification of the drug regimen by reducing the number of drugs being taken.

Hypertension in pregnancy presents a formidable therapeutic challenge and requires comprehensive management with close monitoring for both maternal and fetal welfare (5). Mechanisms involved with pregnancy-related hypertension include a hyperadrenergic state, plasma volume reduction, a reduction in uteroplacental perfusion, hormonal control of vascular reactivity and prostacyclin deficiency may result from or may activate the mechanisms that elevate blood pressure. Effective blood pressure control for pregnancy-related hypertension can often be achieved with β-blockers, mixed α/β-blockers, combinations of β-blockers with α-blockers, methyldopa or vasodilating agents such as hydralazine (1,8). The presence or development of proteinuria (preeclampsia) in a hypertensive pregnant woman implies a major increase in risk to the fetus and warrants immediate admission to a hospital for specialist management (5).

Combination Therapy

It is well-documented that monotherapy adequately controls hypertension in only about 50% of patients (6,7). Therefore, a large percentage of patients will require at least two drugs to control their blood pressure and the symptoms of hypertension. By combining different antihypertensive drug classes in low doses, their different mechanisms of action result in synergistic blood pressure lowering as well as minimizing the adverse effects and improving compliance issues (1,7). For example, the addition of a low-dose thiazide diuretic dramatically increases the response rates to methyldopa, ACE inhibitors and a β-blockers without producing the undesirable side effects. In the latest guidelines for treatment of hypertension, the Joint National Committee for Prevention, Detection, Evaluation, and Treatment of High Blood Pressure (JNC VI), clinicians are encouraged to use either diuretics or β-blockers for initial monotherapy for patients with uncomplicated hypertension since both of these drug classes have been shown to decrease morbidity and mortality in long-term clinical trials (2). However, in the presence of other cardiovascular diseases, the other antihypertensive classes that could be used as first-line agents include angiotensin-converting-enzyme (ACE) inhibitors, calcium-channel blockers, α_1 blockers or mixed α/β-blockers. In patients with risk factors for heart disease or with clinical manifestations of cardiovascular disease (Table 24.1), treatment should be more aggressive with the goal to reduce blood pressure to less than 140/90 mm Hg (1). These recommendations reflect the current awareness of the importance of addressing other cardiovascular conditions aside from just lowering the blood pressure.

Arterial pressure is the product of cardiac output and peripheral vascular resistance, and therefore can be lowered by decreasing or inhibiting either or both of these physiologic responses with the drug classes represented in Table 24.2. This chapter will discuss those antihypertensives that are classified as sympatholytics having a central or peripheral mechanism of action and vasodilators. Although these classes of drugs are less commonly used because of higher incidence of side effects associated with inhibition of the sympathetic nervous system or vasodilation, they have been replaced by availability of newer and more effective antihypertensive drugs with fewer side effects, such as ACE inhibitors.

DRUG THERAPY OF HYPERTENSION
Peripheral Acting Sympatholytics
β-Adrenergic Receptor Blockers

The structures for the β-blockers available for the treatment of uncomplicated hypertension are included in Figure 24.1 (non-selective β-blockers) and Figure 24.2 (β_1 selective blockers) and their SAR, pharmacokinetics and metabolism are discussed in Chapter 11 and also presented in Table 24.3. However, they may also be used as

Table 24.1. Risk Factors for Cardiovascular Disease

Correctable	Noncorrectable
Cigarette Smoking	Age >60 years
Hypertension	Sex (men and postmenopausal women)
Elevated cholesterol	Family history of cardiovascular disease or stroke (women <65 years, men <55 years)
Reduced HDL cholesterol	
Diabetes mellitus	Target organ damage
Obesity	

Table 24.2. Classification of Antihypertensive Activity According to Mechanism of Action

I. Diuretics (Chapter 22)
II. Sympatholytic Drugs
  1. Centrally acting drugs (methyldopa, clonmidine, guanabenz, guanfacine) (Chapter 24)
  2. Ganglionic Blocker Drugs
  3. Adrenergic neuron blocking drugs (Chapter 24)
  4. Beta adrenergic blocking drugs (Chapters 11 and 24)
  5. α-Adrenergic blocking drugs (Chapters 11 and 24)
  6. Mixed α/β-adrenergic blocking drugs (Chapters 11 and 24)
III. Vasodilator (Chapter 24)
  Arterial (hydralazine, minoxidil, diazoxide)
  Arterial and venous (sodium nitroprusside)
IV. Calcium Channel Blockers (Chapter 23)
V. Angiotensin Converting Enzyme Inhibitors (Chapter 23)
VI. Angiotensin Receptor Antagonists (Chapter 23)

monotherapy in the treatment of angina, arrhythmias, mitral valve prolapse, myocardial infarction, migraine headaches, performance anxiety, excessive sympathetic tone or "thyroid storm" in hyperthyroidism (8).

Mechanism of Action. The mechanism of action for the β-blockers in lowering blood pressure is attributed to their competitive inhibition of cardiac and vascular β_1 and β_2 receptors thereby reducing the contractility of the myocardium (negative inotropic), decreasing heart rate (negative chronotropic), blocking sympathetic outflow from the CNS, and suppression of renin release (9). The antianginal and antiarrhythmic effects of the β-blockers are discussed in Chapter 21.

Therapeutic Applications (1,8,10). The selection of oral β-blockers as monotherapy for uncomplicated hypertension is based upon several factors, including their cardioselectivity and pre-existing conditions, intrinsic sympathomimetic activity (ISA), lipophilicity, metabolism, and adverse effects (exception is esmolol) (Table 24.3). Esmolol is a very short-acting cardioselective β_1 blocker administered by infusion because of its rapid hydrolysis by plasma esterases to a rapidly excreted zwitterionic metabolite (plasma half-life 9 minutes). Following the discontinuation of esmolol infusion, blood pressure returns to pre-existing conditions in about 30 minutes. Oral beta blockers are recommended as initial therapy for uncomplicated hypertension or in the stepped-care approach to antihypertensive drug therapy, as step 1. The elderly hypertensive patient (>65 years old) may not tolerate or respond to these drugs due to their mechanism of lowering cardiac output and increasing systemic vascular resistance (11).

Adverse Effects. Common adverse effects for the β-blockers include decreased exercise tolerance, cold extremities, depression, sleep disturbance, and impotence, although these side effects may be less severe with the β_1 selective blockers such as metoprolol, atenolol or biso-

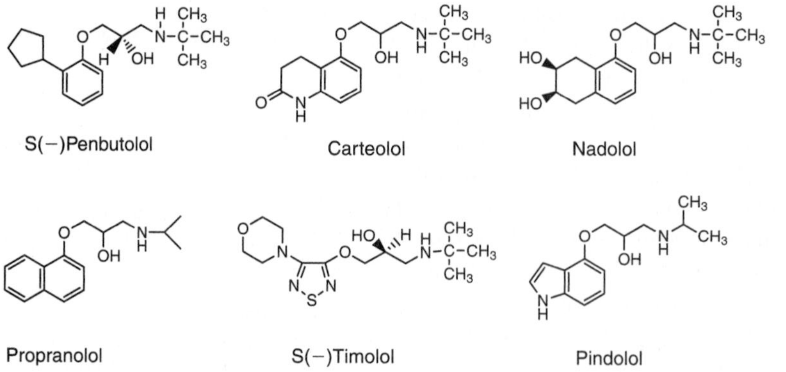

Fig. 24.1. Nonselective β-adrenergic blockers.

prolol (12). The use of lipid soluble β-blockers such as propranolol (Table 24.3) has been associated with more central nervous system side effects such as dizziness, confusion, or depression (1,8). However, these side effects can be avoided with the use of hydrophilic drugs such as nadolol or atenolol. The use of β₁ selective drugs also helps to minimize adverse effects associated with β₂ blockade including suppression of insulin release and increasing the chances for bronchospasms(asthma) (1,8). It is important to emphasize that none of the β-blockers, including the cardioselective ones, are cardiospecific. At high doses, these cardio-selective agents can still adversely affect asthma, peripheral vascular disease, and diabetes (1,8). Nonselective β-blockers are contraindicated in patients with bronchospastic disease (asthma) and β₁ selective blockers should be used with caution in these patients. Beta blockers with intrinsic sympathomimetic activity (ISA) such as acebutolol, pindolol, carteolol, or penbutolol (Table 24.3) partially stimulate the β-receptor while also blocking it (13). The proposed advantages of β-blockers with ISA over those without ISA include less cardiodepression and resting bradycardia as well as neutral effects on lipid and glucose metabolism. However, neither cardioselectivity nor ISA influence the efficacy of β-blockers in lowering blood pressure (8).

α₁ Adrenergic Blockers

The structures for α₁ receptor blockers available are shown in Figure 24.3 and include prazosin, doxazosin, and temazosin, whose SAR was previously discussed in Chapter 11, along with their pharmacokinetics and metabolism.

Mechanism of Action. The primary mechanism of action for the α₁ blockers is peripheral vasodilation by inhibiting post-synaptic α₁ receptors in vascular smooth muscle (9). These receptors are also abundant in the smooth muscle of the bladder neck and prostate, which when inhibited, cause relaxation of the bladder muscle increasing urinary flow rates and the relief of symptoms of benign prostatic hyperplasia (BPH) (8).

Therapeutic Applications (8,14). α₁ blockers are effective agents for the initial management of hypertension, and are especially advantageous for older men who also suffer from symptomatic BPH. In the stepped-care approach to antihypertensive drug therapy, α₁ blockers are suggested as a step 1 drug. They have been shown to be as effective as other major classes of antihypertensives in lowering blood pressure in equivalent doses. α₁ blockers possess a characteristic "first-dose" effect, which means that orthostatic hypotension frequently occurs with the first few doses of the drug. This side effect can be minimized by slowly increasing the dose, and by administering the first few doses at bedtime.

Mixed α/β-Blockers

The two available mixed α/β-receptor blockers are carvedilol (15) and labetalol (17) (pKa 9.3) (Fig 24.4) and their SAR was previously discussed in Chapter 11, along with their pharmacokinetics and metabolism (Table 24.3). The α-methyl substituent attached to the N-arylalkyl group appears to be responsible for the α-adrenergic blocking effect. Carvedilol is administered as its racemate. Its S(−) enantiomer is both an α and nonselective β-blocker, whereas its R(+) enantiomer is an α₁ blocker. Labetalol possesses two chiral centers and therefore is administered as a mixture of four stereoisomers, of which R(CH₃),R(OH) is the active β-

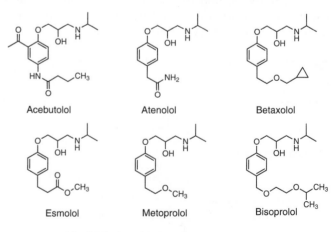

Fig. 24.2. β₁ selective adrenergic blockers.

Table 24.3. Pharmacologic/Pharmacokinetic Properties of Antihypertensive β-Adrenergic Blocking Agents

Drug	Adrenergic Receptor Blocking Activity	Membrane Stabilizing Activity	Intrinsic Sympathomimetic Activity	Lipid Solubility	Extent of Absorption (%)	Absolute Oral Bioavailability (%)	Half-life (hr)	Protein Binding (%)	Metabolism/Excretion
Acebutolol (Sectral)	β$_1$[1]	+	+	Low	90	20–60	3–4	26	Hepatic; renal excretion 30 to 40%; nonrenal excretion 50 to 60% (bile)
Atenolol (Tenormin)	β$_1$[1]	0	0	Low	50	50–60	6–9	5–16	≈50% excreted unchanged in feces
Betaxolol (Kerlone)	β$_1$[1]	+	0	Low	≈100	80–90	14–22	50	Hepatic; >80% recovered as metabolites in urine, 15% unchanged in urine
Bisoprolol (Zebeta)	β$_1$[1]	0	0	Low	≥0	80–90	9–12	30	≈50% excreted unchanged in urine, remainder as inactive metabolites; <2% excreted feces
Esmolol (Brevibloc)	β$_1$[1]	0	0	Low	na[5]	na[5]	0.15	55	Rapid metabolism by plasma and erythrocyte esterases
Metoprolol (Lopressor)	β$_1$[1]	0[2]	0	Moderate	95	40–50	3–7	12	Hepatic; <5% excreted unchanged in urine
Metoprolol, LA						77			
Carteolol (Cartrol)	β$_1$,β$_2$	0	++	Low	80	85	6	23–30	50 to 70% excreted unchanged in urine
Nadolol (Corgard)	β$_1$,β$_2$	0	0	Low	30	30–50	20–24	30	Mostly excreted unchanged in urine
Penbutolol (Levatol)	β$_1$,β$_2$	0	+	High	≈100	>90	5	80–98	Hepatic (conjugation, oxidation); renal excretion of metabolites (17% as conjugate)
Pindolol (Visken)	β$_1$,β$_2$	+	+++	Moderate	95	>90	3–4[3]	40	Urinary excretion of metabolites (60 to 65%) and unchanged drug (35 to 40%)
Propranolol (Inderal)	β$_1$,β$_2$	++	0	High	90	30	3–5	90	Hepatic; 1% excreted unchanged in urine
Propranolol, LA						9–18	8–11		
Timolol (Blocadren)	β$_1$,β$_2$	0	0	Low to moderate	90	75	4	10	Hepatic; urinary excretion of metabolites and unchanged drug
Labetalol[4] (Normodyne)	β$_1$,β$_2$ α$_1$	0	0	Moderate	100	30–40	5–8	50	55 to 60% excreted in urine as conjugates or unchanged drug
Carvedilol (Coreg)	β$_1$,β$_2$ α$_1$	0	0	Moderate to high	>90	25–35	7–10	98	Hepatic (oxidation, conjugation): <2% excreted unchanged in urine; conjugated metabolites excreted primarily into bile; exhibits stereoselective metabolism

[1] inhibits β$_2$ receptors (bronchial and vascular) at higher doses., [2] Detectable only at doses much greater than required for beta blockade., [3] In elderly hypertensive patients with normal renal function, t1/2 variable: 7 to 15 hours, [4] Not labetalol monograph, [5] Not applicable (available IV only), [6] No data.
Adapted from Drug Facts and Comparison 2000
0 = none; + = low; ++ = moderate; +++ = high.

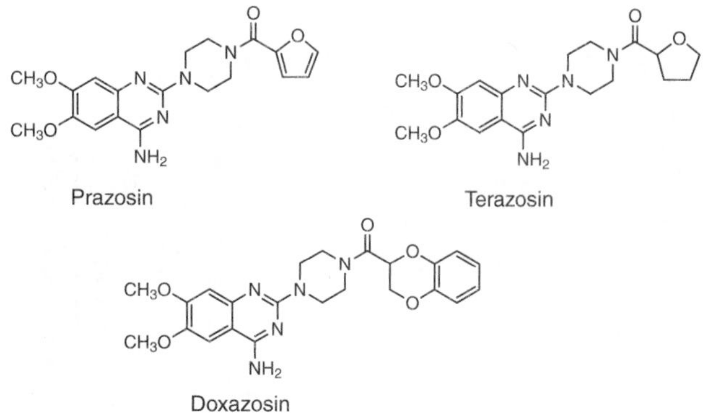

Fig. 24.3. α_1 selective adrenergic blockers.

blocker diastereomer with minimal α_1-blocking activity and the S(CH$_3$),R(OH) diastereomer is predominantly an α_1 blocker. The R,R diastereomer is also known as dilevalol. The S(CH$_3$),S(OH) and R (CH$_3$),S(OH) diastereomers are both inactive. The comparative potency for labetalol reflects the fact that 25% of the diastereomeric mixture is the active R,R-diastereomer.

Mechanism of Action. The mixed α/β-receptor blocking properties in the same molecule confer some advantages in the lowering of blood pressure. Vasodilation via α_1 blockade lowers peripheral vascular resistance to maintain cardiac output, thus preventing bradycardia more effectively when compared to β-blockers (16). Beta blockade helps to avoid the reflex tachycardia sometimes observed with the other vasodilators listed below.

Therapeutic Applications. Monotherapy with these mixed acting antihypertensive drugs reduces blood pressure as effectively as other major antihypertensives and their combinations (15,16,17). In the stepped care approach to antihypertensive drug therapy, mixed α/β-blockers are recommended for initial management of mild to moderate hypertension (step 1). Both drugs effectively lower blood pressure in essential and renal hypertension. Carvedilol is also effective in ischemic heart disease.

Adverse Effects. Any adverse effects are usually related to β_1 or α_1 blockade, and the β-effects are usually less bothersome because the α_1 blockade reduces the effects of β-blockade.

Centrally Acting Sympatholytics
Methyldopa
Methyldopate Ester Hydrochloride

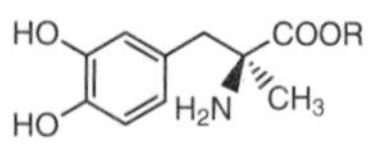

L-Methyldopa R = H
Methyldopate ethyl ester hydrochloride R = C$_2$H$_5$

Methyldopa is structurally and chemically related to L-dopa and the catecholamines. To increase its water solubility for

parenteral administration, the zwitterion methyldopa is esterified and converted to its hydrochloride salt, methyldopate ethyl ester hydrochloride (referred to as methyldopate). Methyldopate ester hydrochloride is used to prepare parenteral solutions of methyldopa having a pH in the range of 3.5–6. Methyldopa is unstable in the presence of oxidizing agents (i.e., air), alkaline pH and light. Being related to the catecholamines which are subject to air oxidation, metabisulfite/sulfite may be added to dosage formulations to prevent oxidation. Some patients especially asthmatic patients, may exhibit sulfite-related hypersensitivity reactions. Methyldopate hydrochloride injection has been reported to be physically incompatible with drugs that are poorly soluble in an acidic medium (e.g., sodium salts of barbiturates and sulfonamides) and with drugs that are acid labile. Incompatibility depends on several factors (e.g., concentrations of the drugs, specific diluents used, resulting pH, temperature).

Mechanism of Action. As previously discussed in Chapter 11, the central mechanism for the antihypertensive activity of the pro-drug methyldopa is not due to its inhibition of norepinephrine biosynthesis but rather to its metabolism in the CNS to α-methylnorepinephrine, an α_2 adrenergic agonist (9). Other more powerful inhibitors of aromatic L-amino acid decarboxylase (e.g., carbidopa) have proven to be clinically useful, but not as antihypertensives. Rather, these agents are used to inhibit the metabolism of exogenous L-dopa administered in the treatment of Parkinson's disease (Chapter 20).

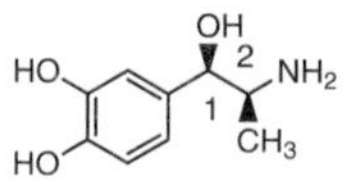

α–Methylnorepinephrine
direct acting stereoisomer

The mechanism of the central hypotensive action for methyldopa is attributed to its transport into the CNS via an aromatic amino acid transport mechanism where it is decarboxylated and hydroxylated into α-methylnorepinephrine (9). This active metabolite of methyldopa decreases total peripheral resistance with little change in cardiac output and heart rate, through its stimulation of central inhibitory α_2 adrenoceptors. A reduction of plasma renin activity may also contribute to the hypotensive action of methyldopa. Postural hypotension and sodium and water retention are also effects related to a reduction in blood pressure. If a diuretic is not administered concurrently with methyldopa, tolerance to the

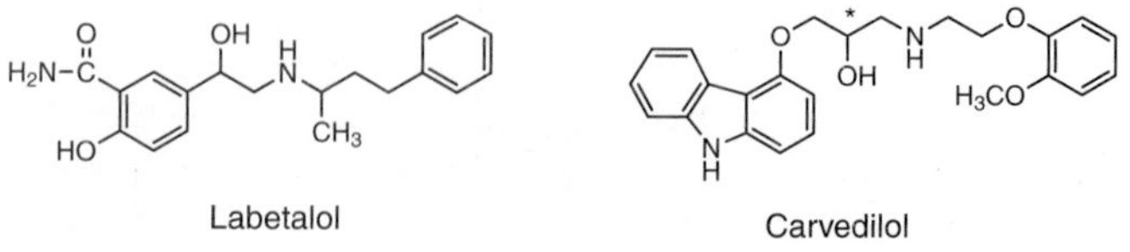

Fig. 24.4. Mixed α/β selective adrenergic blockers.

antihypertensive effect of the methyldopa during prolonged therapy can result.

Pharmacokinetics (18). The oral bioavailability of methyldopa ranges from 20–50% and varies among individuals. Optimum blood pressure response occurs in 12–24 hours in most patients. After withdrawal of the drug, blood pressure returns to pretreatment levels within 24–48 hours. Methyldopa and its metabolites are weakly bound to plasma proteins. Although 95% of a dose of methyldopa is eliminated in hypertensive patients with normal renal function with a plasma half-life of about 2 hours, in patients with impaired renal function, the half-life is doubled to approximately 3–4 hours with about 50% of it excreted. Orally administered methyldopa undergoes presystemic first pass metabolism in the GI tract to its 3-O-monosulfate metabolite. Sulfate conjugation occurs to a greater extent when the drug is given orally than when it is given intravenously. Its rate of sulfate conjugation is decreased in patients with renal insufficiency. Methyldopa is excreted in urine as its mono-O-sulfate conjugate. Any peripherally decarboxylated α-methylnorepinephrine is metabolized by COMT and MAO.

Methyldopate is slowly hydrolyzed in the body to form methyldopa. The hypotensive effect of intravenous methyldopate begins in 4–6 hours and lasts 10–16 hours.

Therapeutic Applications (1,8). Methyldopa is used in the management of moderate to severe hypertension, and is considered to be a step 2 drug reserved for patients who fail to respond to therapy with step 1 drugs. Methyldopa is also co-administered with diuretics and other classes of antihypertensive drugs, permitting a reduction in the dosage of each drug and minimizing adverse effects while maintaining blood pressure control. Methyldopa has been used in the management of hypertension during pregnancy without apparent substantial adverse effects on the fetus, and also for the management of pregnancy-induced hypertension (i.e., pre-eclampsia) (5).

Intravenous methyldopate may be used for the management of hypertension when parenteral hypotensive therapy is necessary. However, because of its slow onset of action, other agents such as sodium nitroprusside are preferred when a parenteral hypotensive agent is employed for hypertensive emergencies.

Adverse Effects (8). The most common adverse effect for methyldopa is drowsiness which occurs within the first 48–72 hours of therapy and may disappear with continued administration of the drug. Sedation commonly recurs when its dosage is increased. A decrease in mental acuity, including impaired ability to concentrate, lapses of memory, and difficulty in performing simple calculations, may occur and usually necessitates withdrawal of the drug. Patients should be warned that methyldopa may impair their ability to perform activities requiring mental alertness or physical coordination (e.g., operat-

ing machinery, driving a motor vehicle). Nightmares, mental depression, orthostatic hypotension, and symptoms of cerebrovascular insufficiency may occur during methyldopa therapy and is an indication for dosage reduction. Orthostatic hypotension may be less pronounced with methyldopa than with guanethidine but may be more severe than with reserpine, clonidine, hydralazine, propranolol, or thiazide diuretics. Nasal congestion occurs commonly in patients receiving methyldopa. Positive direct antiglobulin (Coombs') test results have been reported in about 10–20% of patients receiving methyldopa, usually after 6–12 months of therapy. This phenomenon is dose related. Methyldopa should be used with caution in patients with a history of previous liver disease or dysfunction, and should be stopped if unexplained drug-induced fever and jaundice occurs. These effects commonly occur within 3 weeks after initiation of treatment.

Dosage forms of methyldopa and methyldopate may contain sulfites, which can cause allergic-type reactions, including anaphylaxis and life-threatening or less severe asthmatic episodes. These allergic reactions are more frequently observed in asthmatic than in nonasthmatic individuals. Methyldopa is contraindicated in patients receiving monoamine oxidase (MAO) inhibitors.

α₂ Adrenergic Agonists

The mechanism of action, therapeutic applications and adverse effects common to the α₂ adrenergic agonists clonidine, guanabenz, and guanfacine (Fig. 24.5) and will be discussed together, but any significant differences between these specific agents will be included under the individual drugs.

Mechanism of Action. The overall mechanism of action for the centrally active sympatholytics, clonidine, guanabenz and guanfacine appears to be stimulation of α₂ adrenoceptors and nonadrenergic imidazoline (I₁) receptors in the CNS (mainly in the medulla oblongata) causing inhibition of sympathetic output (19,20). This effect results in reduced peripheral and renovascular resistance and leads to a decrease in systolic and diastolic blood pressure. Through the use of imidazoline and α₂ adrenergic antagonists, nonadrenergic imidazoline receptors have recently been discovered to be involved in

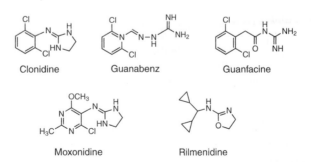

Fig. 24.5. Centrally acting sympatholytics.

central nervous system control of blood pressure (I_1 receptor) (21). Thus, the central hypotensive action for clonidine, other 2-aminoimidazolines and structurally related compounds need both the I_1 and α_1 adrenoceptors to produce their central sympatholytic response (20). As a result of this discovery, a new generation of central-acting antihypertensive agents selective for the I_1 receptor has been developed; moxonidine (a pyrimidinyl amino-imidazoline) and rilmenidine (an alkylaminooxazoline) (Fig. 24.5). Rilmenidine and moxonidine are both highly selective for the I_1 receptor, while having low affinity for α_2 adrenoceptors, and control blood pressure effectively without the adverse effects of sedation, bradycardia and mental depression that are usually associated with central-acting antihypertensives (20). Clonidine appears to be more selective for α_2-adrenoceptors than for I_1 receptors.

The effective oral dose range for rilmenidine is 1–3 mg with a dose dependent duration of action of 10–20 hours. Moxonidine is administered once a day at a dose range of 0.2–0.4 mg. The oral bioavailability of moxonidine in humans is greater than 90% with approximately 40–50% of the oral dose excreted in the urine unmetabolized (24). The principal route of metabolism for moxonidine is oxidation of the 2-methyl group in the pyrimidine ring to 2-hydroxymethyl and 2-carboxylic acid derivative, as well as the formation of corresponding glucuronides. Following an oral dose of monoxidine, peak hypotensive effects occur within 2 hours with an elimination half-life of greater than 8 hours (22,24). Rilmenidine is readily absorbed from the GI tract with an oral bioavailability greater than 95%. It is poorly metabolized and is excreted unchanged in the urine with an elimination half-life of 8 hours (25,26).

Following intravenous or oral administration of these drugs in normotensive patients, an initial hypertensive response to the drug occurs which is caused by activation of the peripheral α_2 adrenoceptors and the resulting vasoconstriction. However, this response is not observed in hypertensive patients.

Therapeutic Applications (1,8).   The selection of these drugs for monotherapy or in the stepped care approach is based upon several factors, including their similar mechanism of action, pre-existing conditions, pharmacokinetics, distribution and metabolism. The α_2 adrenergic antagonists show a similarity in adverse effects.

Clonidine, guanabenz and guanfacine are used in the management of mild to moderate hypertension (1,8). They have been used as monotherapy or to achieve lower dosages when used in combination with other classes of antihypertensive agents. In the stepped-care approach to antihypertensive drug therapy, central-acting sympatholytics are generally step 2 drugs and reserved for patients who fail to respond to therapy with a step 1 drug (e.g., diuretics, β-adrenergic blocking agents, angiotensin-converting enzyme (ACE) inhibitors, α_1 blockers). Clonidine, guanabenz,

and guanfacine have been used in conjunction with diuretics and other hypotensive agents permitting a reduction in the dosage of each drug, minimizing adverse effects while maintaining blood pressure control. However, geriatric patients may not tolerate the adverse cognitive effects of these sympatholytics. All three drugs reduce blood pressure to essentially the same extent in both supine and standing patients, thus orthostatic effects are mild and infrequently encountered. Exercise does not appear to affect the blood pressure response to guanabenz and guanfacine in hypertensive patients. Plasma renin activity may be unchanged or reduced during long-term therapy with these drugs.

Adverse Effects (8).   Overall, the frequency of adverse effects produced by clonidine, guanabenz and guanfacine are similar and appear to be dose related. Drowsiness, tiredness, dizziness, weakness, bradycardia, headache and dry mouth are common adverse effects for patients receiving clonidine, guanabenz, and guanfacine. The sedative effect for these centrally acting sympatholytics may result from their central α_2 agonist activity. The dry mouth induced by these drugs may result from a combination of central and peripheral α_2 adrenoceptor mechanisms, and the decreased salivation may involve inhibition of cholinergic transmission via stimulation of peripheral α_2 adrenoceptors. Orthostatic hypotension does not appear to be a significant problem with these drugs since there appears to be little difference between supine and standing systolic and diastolic blood pressures in most patients. Other adverse effects include urinary frequency and sexual dysfunction (e.g., decreased libido, impotence), nasal congestion, tinnitus, blurred vision, and dry eyes. These symptoms most often occur within the first few weeks of therapy and tend to diminish with continued therapy or may be relieved by a reduction in dosage. Although adverse effects of the drug generally are not severe, discontinuance of therapy has been necessary in some patients because of intolerable sedation or dry mouth. Sodium and fluid retention may be avoided or relieved by administration of a diuretic.

Drug Interactions (8).   The hypotensive actions for clonidine, guanabenz and guanfacine may be additive with, or may potentiate the action of, other CNS depressants such as opiates or other analgesics, barbiturates or other sedatives, anesthetics, or alcohol. Co-administration of opiate analgesics with clonidine also may potentiate the hypotensive effects of clonidine. Tricyclic antidepressants (i.e., imipramine, desipramine) have reportedly inhibited the hypotensive effect of clonidine, guanabenz and guanfacine and the increase in blood pressure usually occurs during the second week of tricyclic antidepressant therapy; dosage should be increased to adequately control hypertension if necessary. Sudden withdrawal of clonidine, guanabenz and guanfacine may result in an excess of circulating catecholamines; therefore, caution should be exercised in concomitant use of drugs which affect the metabolism or tissue uptake of these amines (monoamine oxidase inhibitors or tricyclic antidepressants, respectively). Because clonidine, guanabenz and guanfacine may produce bradycardia, the possibility of additive effects should be considered if these drugs are given concomitantly with other drugs, hypotensive drugs or cardiac glycosides.

Specific Drugs—Clonidine. Clonidine is an aryl-2-aminoimidazoline that is more selective for α_2 adrenoceptors than for I_1 receptors (Fig. 24.5) in producing its hypotensive effect. It is available as oral tablets, injection, or as a transdermal system.

Mechanism of Action. In addition to its central stimulation of noradrenergic I_1 and α_2 adrenoceptors (20,21), when administered epidurally clonidine (as well as other α_2 adrenergic agonists) produce analgesia by stimulation of spinal α_2 adrenoceptors inhibiting sympathetically mediated pain pathways that are activated by nociceptive stimuli, thus preventing transmission of pain signals to the brain (9). Activation of α_2 adrenoceptors apparently also stimulates acetylcholine release and inhibits the release of substance P, an inflammatory neuropeptide. Analgesia resulting from clonidine therapy is not antagonized by opiate antagonists.

Pharmacokinetics. Clonidine has an oral bioavailability of more than 90% with a pKa of 8.3 (8). It is also absorbed when applied topically to the eye. Clonidine is well absorbed percutaneously following topical application of a transdermal system to the arm or chest (27,28,29). Following application of a clonidine transdermal patch, therapeutic plasma concentrations are attained within 2–3 days. Studies indicated that release of clonidine from the patch averaged 50–70% after 7 days of wear. Plasma clonidine concentrations attained with the transdermal systems are generally similar to twice-daily oral dosing regimens of the drug. Percutaneous absorption of the drug from the upper arm or chest is similar, but less drug is absorbed from the thigh (29). Replacement of the transdermal system at a different site at weekly intervals continuously maintains therapeutic plasma clonidine concentrations. Following discontinuance of transdermal therapy, therapeutic plasma drug concentrations persist for about 8 hours and then decline slowly over several days; over this time period, blood pressure returns gradually to pretreatment levels.

Blood pressure begins to decrease within 30–60 minutes after an oral dose of clonidine with the maximum decrease in approximately 2–4 hours (8). The hypotensive effect lasts up to 8 hours. Following epidural administration of a single bolus dose of clonidine, it is rapidly absorbed into the systemic circulation and into CSF with maximal analgesia within 30–60 minutes. Although the CSF is not the presumed site of action of clonidine-mediated analgesia, the drug appears to diffuse rapidly from

the CSF to the dorsal horn. After oral administration, clonidine appears to be well distributed throughout the body with the lowest concentration in the brain. Clonidine is approximately 20–40% bound to plasma proteins, and crosses the placenta. The plasma half-life of clonidine is 6–20 hours in patients with normal renal function and for patients with impaired renal function the range is 18–41 hours. Clonidine is metabolized in the liver to its inactive major metabolite, 4-hydroxyclonidine and its glucuronide and sulfate conjugates (10–20%) (Fig. 24.6). In humans, 40–60% of an orally or intravenously administered dose of clonidine is excreted in urine as unchanged drug within 24 hours. Approximately 85% of a single dose is excreted within 72 hours, with 20% of the dose excreted in feces, probably via enterohepatic circulation.

Therapeutic Applications (8). Clonidine is administered twice a day for the management of mild to moderate hypertension (8). Transdermal clonidine has also been successfully substituted for oral clonidine in some patients with mild to moderate hypertension whose compliance with a daily dosing regimen may be a problem (28).

Clonidine when administered by epidural infusion is used as adjunctive therapy in combination with opiates in the management of severe cancer pain that is not relieved by opiate analgesics alone. Other nonhypertensive uses for clonidine include the prophylaxis of migraine headaches, the treatment of severe dysmenorrhea, menopausal flushing, rapid detoxification in the management of opiate withdrawal in opiate-dependent individuals, in conjunction with benzodiazepines for the management of alcohol withdrawal, and for the treatment of tremors associated with the adverse effects of methylphenidate in ADD patients. Clonidine has been used to reduce intraocular pressure in the treatment of open-angle and secondary glaucoma.

Adverse Effects (8). Adverse effects occurring with transdermal clonidine generally appear to be similar to those occurring with oral therapy (28,29). They have been mild

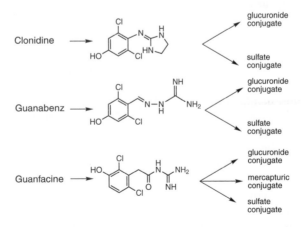

Fig. 24.6. Metabolic products formed from clonidine, guanabenz, and guanfacine.

and have tended to diminish with continued treatment. Hypotension occurred in patients receiving clonidine by epidural infusion as adjunctive therapy with epidural morphine for the treatment of cancer pain. With the transdermal system, localized skin reactions have occurred in some patients, such as erythema and pruritus.

Within 2–3 hours following the abrupt withdrawal of oral clonidine therapy, a rapid increase in systolic and diastolic blood pressures occurred and blood pressures may exceed pretreatment levels. Associated with the clonidine withdrawal syndrome, the symptoms observed include nervousness, agitation, restlessness, anxiety, insomnia, headache, sweating, palpitation, increased heart rate, tremor, and increased salivation. The exact mechanism of the withdrawal syndrome following discontinuance of α_2 adrenergic agonists has not been determined but may involve increased concentrations of circulating catecholamines, increased sensitivity of adrenoceptors, enhanced renin-angiotensin system activity, decreased vagal function, failure of autoregulation of cerebral blood flow, and failure of central α_2 adrenoceptor mechanisms to regulate sympathetic outflow from the CNS (8). The clonidine withdrawal syndrome is more pronounced after abrupt cessation of long-term therapy and with administration of high oral dosages (greater than 1.2 mg daily). Withdrawal symptoms have been reported following discontinuance of transdermal therapy or when absorption of the drug was impaired because of dermatologic changes (e.g., contact dermatitis) under the transdermal system. Epidural clonidine may prolong the duration of the pharmacologic effects, including both sensory and motor blockade, of epidural local anesthetics.

Guanabenz Acetate. Guanabenz is a centrally active hypotensive agent that is pharmacologically related to clonidine, but differs structurally from clonidine by the presence of an aminoguanidine side chain rather than an aminoimidazoline ring (Fig. 24.5). At pH 7.4, guanabenz (pKa 8.1) is predominately (80%) in the nonionized lipid soluble base form. Guanabenz can be given as a single daily dose administered at bedtime to minimize adverse effects.

Pharmacokinetics (30). The oral bioavailability of guanabenz is 70–80%. Following an oral dose, the hypotensive effect of guanabenz begins within 1 hour, peaks within 2–7 hours, and is diminished within 6–8 hours. It has an elimination half-life averaging 4–14 hours. The blood pressure response can persist for at least 12 hours. Following intravenous dosing, guanabenz is distributed into the CNS with brain concentrations 3–70 times higher than concurrent plasma concentrations. Guanabenz is approximately 90% bound to plasma proteins. In patients with hepatic or renal impairment, its elimination half-life may be prolonged.

Guanabenz is metabolized principally by hydroxylation to its inactive metabolite, 4-hydroxyguanabenz, which is eliminated in the urine as its glucuronide (major) and sul-

fate conjugates (Fig. 24.6). Guanabenz and its inactive metabolites are excreted principally in urine, with approximately 70–80% of its oral dose excreted in urine within 24 hours and about 10–30% of the dose excreted in feces via enterohepatic cycling. About 40% of an oral dose of guanabenz is excreted in urine as 4-hydroxyguanabenz and its glucuronide and less than 5% is excreted unchanged. The remainder is excreted as unidentified metabolites and their conjugates.

Therapeutic Applications (8,30). Overall, the therapeutic applications for guanabenz are similar to those of clonidine and other α_2 adrenergic agonists. One advantage for guanabenz is its once a day dosing schedule. Guanabenz has been used in diabetic hypertensive patients with no adverse effect on control or therapy of diabetes, and has been effective in hypertensive patients with chronic obstructive pulmonary disease (COPD), including asthma, chronic bronchitis, or emphysema. Guanabenz has been used alone or in combination with naltrexone in the management of opiate withdrawal in patients physically dependent on opiates and undergoing detoxification. Guanabenz has also been used as an analgesic in a limited number of patients with chronic pain

Adverse Effects (8,30). Overall, the frequency of adverse effects produced by guanabenz is similar to that produced by clonidine and the other α_2 adrenergic agonists, but the incidence is less. As with the other centrally active sympatholytics (e.g., clonidine), abrupt withdrawal of guanabenz may result in rebound hypertension, but the withdrawal syndrome symptoms appear to be less severe.

Drug Interactions (8). Overall, the frequency of adverse effects produced by guanabenz is similar to that produced by the other α_2 adrenergic agonists.

Guanfacine Hydrochloride. Guanfacine, a phenylacetyl guanidine derivative (pKa 7.7) (Fig. 24.5), is a centrally acting sympatholytic that is more selective for α_2 adrenoceptors than is clonidine. Its mechanism of action is similar to clonidine and is an effective alternative to the other centrally acting antihypertensive drugs. Although guanfacine is 5–20 times less potent than clonidine on a weight basis, comparable blood pressure lowering effects have been achieved when the two drugs were given in equipotent dosages. Its relatively long elimination half-life time permits a once-a-day dosing schedule. Guanfacine activates peripheral α_2 adrenoceptors because a transient increase in blood pressure is observed in normotensive patients, but not in hypertensive patients.

Pharmacokinetics (31,32,33). The pharmacokinetic properties for guanfacine differ from those of clonidine, guanabenz and α-methyldopa. At pH 7.4, guanfacine is predominately (67%) in the nonionized lipid soluble base form, which accounts for its high oral bioavailability greater than 80%. Following an oral dose, peak plasma concentrations occur in 1–4 hours with a relatively long elimination half-life of 14–23 hours. The maximum blood pressure response occurs in 8–12 hours after oral administration and is maintained up to 36 hours following its discontinuation. Following intravenous dosing, guanfacine achieves highest concentrations in liver and kidney, with low concentrations in the brain. Guanfacine is 64% bound to plasma proteins. In patients with hepatic or renal impairment, its elimination half-life may be prolonged.

Guanfacine is metabolized principally by hepatic hydroxylation to its inactive metabolite, 3-hydroxyguanfacine, which is eliminated in the urine as its glucuronide, sulfate or mercapturic acid conjugate (Fig. 24.6). Its nearly complete bioavailability suggests no evidence of any first pass effect. Guanfacine and its inactive metabolites are excreted principally in urine, with approximately 80% of its oral dose excreted in urine within 48 hours. An oral dose of guanfacine is excreted in urine as 3-hydroxyguanabenz (20%) and its glucuronide (30%), sulfate (8%) and mercapturic acid (10%) conjugates, and 24–37% as unchanged guanfacine. The remainder are unidentified metabolites and their conjugates.

Therapeutic Applications (8,32).   Overall, the therapeutic applications for guanfacine are similar to those of the other centrally acting α_2 adrenergic agonists and methyldopa. It has been effective as monotherapy in the treatment of patients with mild to moderate hypertension. One advantage for guanfacine is its once-a-day dosing schedule. The use of diuretics to prevent accumulation of fluid may allow for a reduction in the dosage for guanfacine.

Adverse Effects (8,32).   Overall, although the frequency of troublesome adverse effects produced by guanfacine is similar to that produced by clonidine and the other centrally acting sympatholytics, their incidence and severity is lower with guanfacine. Unlike clonidine, abrupt discontinuation of guanfacine rarely results in rebound hypertension. When a withdrawal syndrome has occurred, its onset was slower and symptoms less severe than the syndrome observed with clonidine.

Metyrosine

Metyrosine

Hypothetically, inhibitors of any of the three enzymes involved in the conversion of L-tyrosine to norepinephrine (Chapter 11, Fig. 11.1) could be used as drugs to moderate adrenergic transmission. Inhibitors of the rate-limiting enzyme tyrosine hydroxylase would be the most logical choice. One inhibitor of tyrosine hydroxylase, metyrosine or α-methyl-L-tyrosine, a competitive inhibitor of tyrosine hydroxylase, is in limited clinical use to help control hypertensive episodes caused by excess catecholamine biosynthesis and other symptoms of catecholamine overproduction in patients with the rare adrenal tumor pheochromocytoma. Although metyrosine is useful in treating hypertension associated with pheochromocytoma it is not useful for treating essential hypertension. The drug metyrosine is the S-enantiomer of α-methyltyrosine. The R-enantiomer, R-α-methyltyrosine, does not bind to the active site of tyrosine hydroxylase and thus has no useful pharmacologic activity.

ADRENERGIC NEURON BLOCKING AGENTS

Bretylium, guanethidine, and guanadrel are three drugs whose similar mechanisms involve norepinephrine storage granules. These drugs are transported into the adrenergic neurons by uptake-1, where they bind to the storage vesicles and prevent release of neurotransmitter in response to a neuronal impulse. Reserpine, guanethidine and guanadrel are orally active antihypertensives that actually replace norepinephrine in the storage vesicles resulting in a slow release in the amount of norepinephrine present. At usual doses guanethidine and guanadrel act as "false neurotransmitters" in that they are released into the synapse but do not effectively stimulate the receptors. At higher acute doses their principal mechanism is a poorly understood inhibition of neurotransmitter release. Bretylium is a quaternary ammonium salt and must be given intravenously because it has poor oral absorption. Initially, it can cause a release of norepinephrine and a transient rise in blood pressure, but its clinical utility is limited to cardiac arrhythmias and will not be discussed in this chapter (see Chapter 21).

Reserpine

Reserpine

An old and historically important drug that affects the storage and release of norepinephrine is reserpine. Reserpine is one of several indole alkaloids isolated from the roots of *Rauwolfia serpentina*, a plant whose roots were used in India for centuries as a remedy for snake bites and as a sedative. The antihypertensive effects of the root extracts were first reported in India in 1918 and in the West in 1949. Shortly thereafter, reserpine was isolated and identified as the principal active agent. Reserpine was the first effective antihypertensive drug introduced into Western medicine, although it has largely been replaced in clinical use by agents with fewer side effects.

Mechanism of Action (9)

Reserpine acts to replace and deplete the adrenergic neurons of their stores of norepinephrine by inhibiting the active transport Mg-ATPase responsible for sequestering norepinephrine and dopamine within the storage vesicles. The norepinephrine and dopamine that are not sequestered in vesicles are destroyed by MAO. As a result the storage vesicles contain little neurotransmitter, adrenergic transmission is dramatically inhibited, and sympathetic tone is decreased leading to vasodilation. Reserpine has the same effect on epinephrine storage in the adrenal medulla. Reserpine readily enters the central nervous system, where it also depletes the stores of norepinephrine and serotonin. The central nervous system neurotransmitter depletion led to the use of reserpine in treating certain mental illnesses.

Pharmacokinetics (8,9)

Limited information is available on the pharmacokinetics of reserpine. Peak blood concentrations for reserpine occur within 2 hours following oral administration and the full effects for reserpine are usually delayed for at least 2–3 weeks. CNS and cardiovascular effects may persist several days to several weeks after chronic oral therapy is discontinued. Reserpine appears to be widely distributed in body tissues, especially adipose tissue, crosses the blood-brain barrier and the placenta, and is distributed into milk. The elimination of reserpine appears to be biphasic, with a plasma half-life averaging 4.5 hours during the first phase and about 11.3 days during the second phase. Reserpine is metabolized to unidentified inactive compounds. Unchanged reserpine and its metabolites are excreted slowly in urine and feces, with an average of 60% reserpine recovered in feces within 96 hours after oral administration of 0.25 mg of radiolabeled reserpine. An average of about 10% of the total radioactivity was recovered from urine during this study.

Therapeutic Application (8)

Reserpine has been used in the management of mild to moderate hypertension, but because of very significant CNS adverse effects and its cumulative action in the adrenergic neurons, reserpine is rarely used. Reserpine and related Rauwolfia alkaloids have been used in the symptomatic treatment of agitated psychotic states such as schizophrenic disorders, although other antipsychotic agents have generally replaced reserpine and the alkaloids.

Adverse Effects (8)

The common adverse CNS effects for reserpine include drowsiness, fatigue, or lethargy. Mental depression is one of the most serious potential adverse effects for reserpine, which may be severe enough to require hospitalization or result in suicide attempts. Reserpine-induced depression may persist for several months after the drug is discontinued.

Guanethidine Monosulfate

Guanethidine contains 2 basic nitrogen atoms with pKa values of 9.0 and 12.0, and can therefore form guanethi-

Guanethidine

dine monosulfate ($C_{10}H_{22}N_4 \cdot H_2SO_4$) or guanethidine sulfate [$(C_{10}H_{22}N_4)_2 \cdot H_2SO_4$]. Caution should be exercised when interchanging between these sulfate forms because the potency of guanethidine may be expressed in terms of guanethidine sulfate or guanethidine monosulfate, a significant difference in molecular weight.

Mechanism of Action

Guanethidine is a adrenergic neuronal blocking agent that produces a selective block of peripheral sympathetic pathways by replacing and depleting norepinephrine stores from adrenergic nerve endings (but not from the adrenal medulla) (8,9). It prevents the release of norepinephrine from adrenergic nerve endings in response to sympathetic nerve stimulation. The chronic administration of guanethidine results in an increased sensitivity of these effector cells to catecholamines. Following the oral administration of usual doses of guanethidine, depletion of the catecholamine stores from adrenergic nerve endings occurs at a very slow rate, producing a more gradual and prolonged fall in systolic blood pressure than diastolic pressure. Associated with the decrease in blood pressure is an increase in sodium and water retention and expansion of plasma volume (edema). If a diuretic is not administered concurrently with guanethidine, tolerance to the antihypertensive effect of the guanethidine during prolonged therapy can result.

Pharmacokinetics (8)

Guanethidine is incompletely absorbed from the GI tract and is metabolized in the liver to several metabolites including guanethidine N-oxide (from FMN monooxygenase). These metabolites of guanethidine are excreted in the urine and have less than 10% of its hypotensive activity. The amount of drug which reaches the systemic circulation after oral administration is highly variable from patient to patient and may range from 3–50% of a dose. Guanethidine accumulates in the neurons with an elimination half-life of 5 days.

Therapeutic Applications (8)

Guanethidine is used in the management of moderate to severe hypertension and in the management of renal hypertension. In the stepped-care approach to antihypertensive drug therapy, guanethidine has been suggested as a step 2 or 3 drug and is generally reserved for patients who fail to respond adequately to an antihypertensive regimen that includes a diuretic and other step 1 drugs such as β-blocker, angiotensin-converting enzyme (ACE) inhibitor or calcium-channel blocking agent. Its co-administration with other hypotensive agents permits a reduction in the dosage of each drug and minimizing adverse effects while maintaining blood pressure control. It has been administered as ophthalmic drops in the treatment of chronic open-angle glaucoma and for endocrine ophthalmopathy, ophthalmoplegia, lid lag, and lid retraction.

Adverse Effects (8)

Adverse effects of guanethidine are frequently dose related including dizziness, weakness, lassitude, and syncope resulting from postural or postexercise hypotension. A hot environment (i.e., hot bath) may aggravate postural hypotension. Patients should be warned about possible orthostatic hypotension and about the effect of rapid postural changes on blood pressure (such as arising in the morning) which may cause fainting, especially during the initial period of dosage adjustment. Sodium retention (edema) is usually controlled by the co-administration of a diuretic.

Drug Interactions (8)

Diuretics and other hypotensive drugs can potentiate the hypotensive effects of guanethidine. Monoamine oxidase inhibitors reportedly antagonize the hypotensive effect of guanethidine. Oral sympathomimetic, nasal decongestants and other vasopressor agents should be used cautiously in patients receiving guanethidine because guanethidine may potentiate their pressor effects. The mydriatic response to ophthalmic administration of phenylephrine is markedly increased in patients receiving guanethidine ophthalmically or orally. Tricyclic antidepressants and some phenothiazines block the uptake of guanethidine into adrenergic neurons and thus prevent the hypotensive activity of guanethidine. Orthostatic hypotension may be increased by concomitant administration of alcohol with guanethidine, and patients receiving guanethidine should be cautioned to limit alcohol intake.

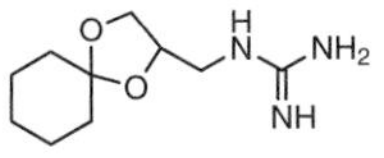

Guanadrel

Guanadrel Sulfate

Guanadrel sulfate is a adrenergic neuronal blocking agent that is structurally and pharmacologically related to guanethidine: both are guanidine derivatives. Guanadrel differs structurally from guanethidine by the presence of a dioxaspirodecyl ring system linked to guanidine by a methyl group rather than a hexahydroazocinyl ring linked by an ethyl group.

Mechanism of Action

Guanadrel, like guanethidine, produces a selective block of efferent, peripheral sympathetic pathways by replacing and depleting norepinephrine stores from adrenergic nerve endings, thus preventing the release of norepinephrine from adrenergic nerve endings in response to sympathetic nerve stimulation (9,34). Unlike guanethidine, it doesn't release norepinephrine from the adrenal medulla and reportedly depletes norepinephrine stores in the GI tract to a lesser extent than does guanethidine. Guanadrel decreases systolic blood pressure more than diastolic blood pressure.

Pharmacokinetics (34)

Guanadrel, unlike guanethidine, is rapidly and almost completely absorbed following oral administration. Following oral administration, its peak plasma concentrations are usually achieved in about 2 hours and its hypotensive effect usually has an onset of 0.5–2 hours with peak activity at 4–6 hours and a duration of action of 4–14 hours. Approximately 20% of guanadrel is bound to plasma proteins and little, if any, of the drug crosses the blood-brain barrier or distributes into the eye. Guanadrel has a plasma half-life of approximately 2 hours and an elimination half-life of about 10–12 hours in patients with normal renal function. Approximately 40–50% of guanadrel is metabolized in the liver to 2,3-dihydroxypropylguanidine and several unidentified metabolites which are excreted principally in the urine (Fig. 24.7). Unlike guanethidine, approximately 85% of an oral dose of the drug is excreted in the urine within 24 hours with 40–50% of the dose excreted in the urine unchanged. In patients with impaired renal function, the half-life of guanadrel is prolonged, and apparent total body clearance and renal clearances are decreased.

Therapeutic Application (8,34)

Guanadrel is used in the management of hypertension and its efficacy is similar to that of guanethidine. Guanadrel is generally considered as a step 2 drug and is reserved for patients who fail to respond to therapy with a step 1 drug or in cases requiring more prompt or aggressive therapy. Postural and postexercise hypotension is common in patients receiving guanadrel and it is also likely that heat-induced vasodilation will augment its hypotensive effect. There is a possibility that geriatric patients may not tolerate the postural hypotensive effects of guanadrel. Being a peripheral adrenergic neuron blocking drug, guanadrel shares the toxic potentials of guanethidine and the usual precautions of this drug should be observed.

Adverse Effects (8)

Overall, the frequency of adverse effects produced by guanadrel is similar or less than those produced by guanethidine and by methyldopa. In patients with impaired renal function, the elimination half-life of unmetabolized guanadrel is prolonged and its clearance is decreased, thus increasing the incidence of adverse effects if usual dosage is maintained in these patients.

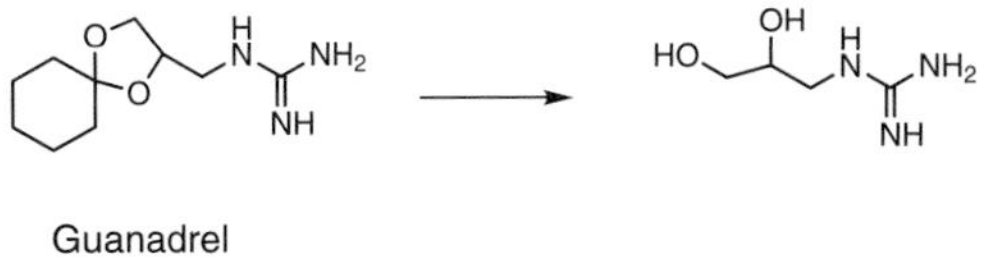

Guanadrel

Fig. 24.7. Metabolism of guanadrel.

Drug Interactions

Being a peripheral adrenergic neuron blocking drug, guanadrel shares the same potential for drug interactions as guanethidine and the usual precautions of this drug should be observed.

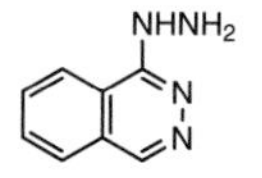

NHNH$_2$

Hydralazine

Arterial Vasodilators

Hydralazine Hydrochloride

Mechanism of Action. Hydralazine is a phthalazine substituted hydrazine antihypertensive drug with a pKa of 7.3. It has been suggested that hydralazine (similar to minoxidil O-sulfate and diazoxide) reduces peripheral resistance and blood pressure by a direct vasodilating effect on vascular smooth muscle by activating (opening) the ATP-modulated potassium channel (9,35). Activation, therefore increases the efflux of potassium ions from the cells causing hyperpolarization of vascular smooth muscle cells, thus prolonging the opening of the potassium channel and sustaining a greater vasodilation on arterioles than on veins (9). Diastolic blood pressure is usually decreased more than is systolic pressure. The hydralazine-induced decrease in blood pressure and peripheral resistance causes a reflex response which is accompanied by increased heart rate, cardiac output, stroke volume and an increase in plasma renin activity. It has no direct effect on the heart (8). This reflex response could offset the hypotensive effect of arteriolar dilation limiting its antihypertensive effectiveness. Hydralazine also causes sodium and water retention and expansion of plasma volume which could develop tolerance to its antihypertensive effect during prolonged therapy. Thus, the co-administration of a diuretic improves the therapeutic outcome.

Pharmacokinetics (8,9). Hydralazine is well absorbed from the GI tract and is metabolized in the GI mucosa (prehepatic systemic metabolism) and in the liver by acetylation, hydroxylation, and conjugation with glucuronic acid (Fig. 24.8, Table 8.17). Little of the hydralazine dose is excreted unchanged in urine but mainly as metabolites, which are without significant therapeutic activity. A small amount of hydralazine is reportedly converted to a hydrazone most likely with Vitamin B$_6$ (pyridoxine) which may be responsible for some its neurotoxic effects. Following the oral administration of hydralazine, its antihypertensive effect begins in 20–30 minutes and lasts 2–4 hours. The plasma half-life of hydralazine is generally 2–4 hours, but may be up to 8 hours in some patients (i.e., slow acetylators). In slow acetylator patients or those with impaired renal function, the plasma concentrations for hydralazine are increased and possibly prolonged. Approximately 85% of hydralazine in the blood is bound to plasma proteins following administration of usual doses.

First-pass acetylation in the GI mucosa and liver is related to genetic acetylator phenotype (8). Acetylation phenotype is an important determinant of the plasma concentrations of hydralazine when the same dose of hydralazine is administered orally. Slow acetylators have an autosomal recessive trait which results in a relative deficiency of the hepatic enzyme N-acetyl transferase, thus, prolonging the elimination half-life of hydralazine (Chapter 8). This population of hypertensive patients will require an adjustment in dose to reduce its increased overactive response. About 50% of African-Americans, Caucasians and the majority of American Indians, Eskimos, and Orientals are rapid acetylators of hydralazine. This population of patients will have subtherapeutic plasma concentrations of hydralazine because of its rapid metabolism to inactive metabolites and shorter elimination times. Patients with hydralazine-induced SLE are frequently slow acetylators.

Therapeutic Applications (8). Hydralazine is used in the management of moderate to severe hypertension. In the stepped-care approach to antihypertensive drug therapy, hydralazine has been suggested as a step 2 or 3 drug and is generally reserved for patients who fail to respond adequately to an antihypertensive regimen that includes a diuretic and other hypotensive drugs such as β-blockers, angiotensin-converting enzyme (ACE) inhibitors or calcium-channel blockers. Hydralazine is recommended to be used in conjunction with a diuretic and another hypotensive drugs such as β-adrenergic blocker and has been effectively used in conjunction with cardiac glycosides, diuretics, and other vasodilators for the short-term treatment of severe congestive heart failure. Patients who engage in potentially hazardous activities such as operating machinery or driving motor vehicles should be warned about possible faintness, dizziness, or weakness. Hydralazine should be used with caution in patients with cerebrovascular accidents or with severe renal damage.

Parenteral hydralazine may be used for the management of severe hypertension when the drug cannot be given orally or when blood pressure must be lowered immediately. Other agents (e.g., sodium nitroprusside) are preferred for the management of severe hypertension or hypersensitive emergencies when a parenteral hypotensive agent is employed.

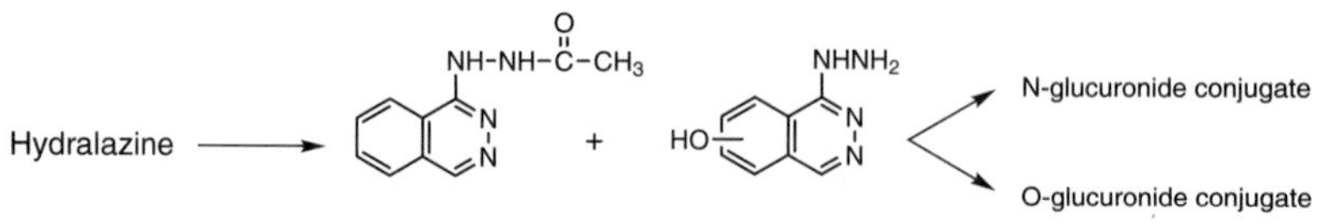

Hydralazine ⟶

Fig. 24.8. Metabolism of hydralazine.

Drug Interactions. The co-administration of diuretics and other hypotensive drugs may have a synergistic effect resulting in a marked decrease in blood pressure.

Minoxidil

Minoxidil is the N-oxide of a piperidinopyrimidine hypotensive agent with a pKa of 4.6 and is not an active hypotensive drug until it is metabolized by hepatic sulfotransferase to minoxidil N-O-sulfate (9).

Minoxidil   Minoxidil N-O-sulfate   Minoxidil N-O-glucuronide

Mechanism of Action. Minoxidil as its active metabolite minoxidil O-sulfate, causes a direct vasodilating effect on vascular smooth muscle by activating (opening) the ATP-modulated potassium channel, thereby increasing the efflux of potassium ions from the cells causing hyperpolarization of vascular smooth muscle cells (35,36). Thus, minoxidil O-sulfate prolongs the opening of the potassium channel, sustaining greater vasodilation on arterioles than on veins. The drug decreases blood pressure in both the supine and standing positions, and there is no orthostatic hypotension. Associated with the decrease in peripheral resistance and blood pressure, there is a reflex response which is accompanied by increased heart rate, cardiac output, and stroke volume, which can be attenuated by the co-administration of a β-blocker (8). Along with this decrease in peripheral resistance, is increased plasma renin activity and sodium and water retention which can result in expansion of fluid volume, edema, and congestive heart failure. The sodium and water retaining effects of minoxidil can be reversed by the co-administration of a diuretic. When used in conjunction with a β-adrenergic blocker, pulmonary artery pressure remains essentially unchanged.

Pharmacokinetics (36). Minoxidil is absorbed from the GI tract and metabolized to its active sulfate metabolite. Peak plasma concentrations for minoxidil sulfate peak within 1 hour and then decline rapidly. Following an oral dose of minoxidil, its hypotensive effect begins in 30 minutes, is maximal in 2–8 hours, and persists for about 2–5 days. The delayed onset of the hypotensive effect for minoxidil is attributed to its metabolism to its active metabolite. The drug is not bound to plasma proteins. The major metabolite for minoxidil is its N-O-glucuronide, which unlike the sulfate metabolite, is inactive as a hypotensive agent. Approximately 10–20% of an oral dose of minoxidil is metabolized to its active metabolite, minoxidil O-sulfate, and about 20% minoxidil is excreted unchanged.

Therapeutic Applications

Hypertension (8,36). Minoxidil is used in the management of severe hypertension and is considered a step 3 drug. It is generally reserved for resistant cases of hypertension that have not been managed with maximal therapeutic dosages of a diuretic and two other hypotensive drugs or who fail to respond adequately to step 3 therapy that includes hydralazine. To minimize sodium retention and increased plasma volume, minoxidil must be used in conjunction with a diuretic. A β-adrenergic blocker (e.g., propranolol) must be given before minoxidil therapy is begun and should be continued during minoxidil therapy to minimize minoxidil-induced tachycardia and increased myocardial workload.

Androgenetic Alopecia (8,37). Minoxidil is used topically to stimulate regrowth of hair in patients with androgenic alopecia (male pattern alopecia, hereditary alopecia, common male baldness) or alopecia areata. Commercially available topical minoxidil preparations should be used rather than the extemporaneous topical formulations from tablets to reduce the potential of minoxidil being absorbed systemically.

Drug Interactions. When minoxidil is administered with diuretics or other hypotensive drugs, the hypotensive effect of minoxidil increases and their concurrent use may cause profound orthostatic hypotensive effects.

Diazoxide

Diazoxide

Diazoxide is a nondiuretic hypotensive and hyperglycemic agent that is structurally related to the thiazide diuretics. Being a sulfonamide with a pKa of 8.5, it can be solubilized in alkaline solutions (pH of injection is 11.6). Solutions or oral suspension of diazoxide are unstable to light and will darken when exposed to light. Such dosage forms should be protected from light, heat, and freezing. Darkened solutions may be subpotent and should not be used.

Mechanism of Action. Diazoxide reduces peripheral vascular resistance and blood pressure by a direct vasodilating effect on vascular smooth muscle by activating (opening) the ATP-modulated potassium channel, thereby increasing the efflux of potassium ions from the cells causing hyperpolarization of vascular smooth muscle cells (35). Thus, diazoxide prolongs the opening of the potassium channel, sustaining greater vasodilation on arterioles than on veins (9). The greatest hypotensive effect is observed in patients with malignant hypertension. Although oral or slow intravenous administration of diazoxide can produce a sustained fall in blood pressure, rapid intravenous administration is required for maximum hypotensive effects, especially in patients with malignant hypertension (8). Diazoxide-induced decreases in blood pressure and peripheral vascular resistance are accompanied by a reflex response resulting in an increased heart rate, cardiac output, and left ventricular ejection rate. In contrast to the thiazide diuretics, diazoxide causes sodium and water retention and decreased urinary output which can result in expansion of plasma and extracellular fluid volume, edema, and congestive heart failure, especially during prolonged administration.

Diazoxide increases blood glucose concentration (diazoxide-induced hyperglycemia) by several different mechanisms, inhibiting pancreatic insulin secretion, by stimulating release of catecholamines, or by increasing hepatic release of glucose (8,9). The precise mechanism of inhibition of insulin release has not been elucidated, but may possibly result from an effect of diazoxide on cell-membrane potassium channels and calcium flux.

Pharmacokinetics (8). Following rapid intravenous administration, diazoxide produces a prompt reduction in blood pressure with maximum hypotensive effects occurring within 5 minutes. The duration of its hypotensive effect varies from 3–12 hours, but ranges from 30 minutes–72 hours have been observed. The elimination half-life of diazoxide following a single oral or intravenous dose has been reported to range from 21–45 hours in adults with normal renal function. Patients with renal impairment, the half-life is prolonged. Approximately 90% of the diazoxide in the blood is bound to plasma proteins. About 20–50% of diazoxide is eliminated unchanged in the urine, along with its major metabolites resulting from the oxidation of the 3-methyl group to its 3-hydroxymethyl- and 3-carboxyl-metabolites.

Therapeutic Applications

Severe Hypertension (8). Intravenous diazoxide has been used in hypertensive crises for emergency lowering of blood pressure when prompt and urgent decrease in diastolic pressure is required in adults with severe, nonmalignant and malignant hypertension and in children with acute severe hypertension. However, other intravenous hypotensive agents generally are preferred for the management of hypertensive crises. Diazoxide is intended for short-term use in hospitalized patients only. Although diazoxide has also been administered orally for the management of hypertension, its hyperglycemic and sodium-retaining effects make it unsuitable for chronic therapy.

Hypoglycemia (8). Diazoxide is administered orally in the management of hypoglycemia caused by hyperinsulinism associated with inoperable islet cell adenoma or carci-

noma, or extrapancreatic malignancy in adults.

ARTERIAL AND VENOUS VASODILATORS
Sodium Nitroprusside (Sodium Nitroferricyanide; Nitropress; Nipride)

Sodium nitroprusside has been known as a rapid-acting hypotensive agent since 1929 when administered as an infusion. It is chemically and structurally unrelated to other available hypotensive agents. As a reminder in preparing extemporaneous infusions, the potency of sodium nitroprusside is expressed in terms of the dihydrated drug. When reconstituted with 5% dextrose injection, sodium nitroprusside solutions are reddish-brown in color with a pH of 3.5–6. Its crystals and solutions are sensitive and unstable to light and should be protected from extremes of light and heat. The exposure of sodium nitroprusside solutions to light causes deterioration which may be evidenced by a change from a reddish-brown to a green to a blue color indicating a reduction of the ferric complex to the inactive ferrous complex. Sodium nitroprusside solutions in glass bottles undergo approximately 20% degradation within 4 hours when exposed to fluorescent light, and even more rapid degradation in plastic bags. Sodium nitroprusside solutions should be protected from light by wrapping the container with aluminum foil or other opaque material. When adequately protected from light, reconstituted solutions are stable for 24 hours. Trace metals such as iron and copper can catalyze the degradation of nitroprusside solutions. Any change in color for the nitroprusside solutions is an indication of degradation and the solution should be discarded. No other drug or preservative should be added to stabilize sodium nitroprusside infusions.

Mechanism of Action

Sodium nitroprusside, a nitric oxide generator or nitrovasodilator, is not an active hypotensive drug until metabolized to its active metabolite, nitric oxide (9). Nitric oxide activates guanylate cyclase leading to increased cGMP formation which triggers vasodilation of both arterioles and veins (9). The hypotensive effect of sodium nitroprusside is augmented by concomitant use of other hypotensive agents and is not blocked by adrenergic blocking agents. It has no direct effect on the myocardium, but it may exert a direct coronary vasodilator effect. When sodium nitroprusside is administered to hypertensive patients, a slight increase in heart rate commonly occurs and cardiac output is usually decreased slightly. Moderate doses of sodium nitroprusside in hypertensive patients produce renal vasodilation without appreciable increase in renal blood flow or a decrease in glomerular filtration (8).

Intravenous infusion of sodium nitroprusside produces an almost immediate reduction in blood pressure. Blood pressure begins to rise immediately when the infusion is

$$\left(\begin{array}{c} CN \\ | \quad {\cdot}^{CN} \\ NC\!\!-\!\!Fe{\cdot}\!\!-\!\!CN \\ O\!\!=\!\!N\;| \\ CN \end{array} \right)^{2-} Na_2 \;\cdot\; 2H_2O$$

Sodium nitroprusside

slowed or stopped and returns to pretreatment levels within 1–10 minutes.

Pharmacokinetics

Sodium nitroprusside is rapidly metabolized to its active metabolite, nitric oxide probably by glutathione and/or interaction with sulfhydryl groups in the erythrocytes and tissues, and to cyanide (8,9). The cyanide that is produced is rapidly converted into thiocyanate in the liver by the enzyme thiosulfate sulfurtransferase (rhodanese) and excreted in the urine (8,9). The rate-limiting step in the conversion of cyanide to thiocyanate is the availability of sulfur donors especially thiosulfate. Toxic symptoms of thiocyanate begin to appear at plasma thiocyanate concentrations of 50–100 mg/mL. The elimination half-life of thiocyanate is 2.7–7 days when renal function is normal but is longer in patients with impaired renal function.

Therapeutic Applications (8)

Intravenous sodium nitroprusside is used as an infusion for hypertensive crises and emergencies. The drug is consistently effective in the management of hypertensive emergencies, irrespective of etiology, and may be useful even when other drugs have failed. It may be used in the management of acute congestive heart failure.

Adverse Effects (8)

The most clinically important adverse effects of sodium nitroprusside are profound hypotension and the accumulation of cyanide and thiocyanate. Thiocyanate may accumulate in the blood of patients receiving sodium nitroprusside therapy, especially in those with impaired renal function. Thiocyanate is mildly neurotoxic at serum concentrations of 60 µg/mL and may be life-threatening at concentrations of 200 µg/mL. Other adverse effects of thiocyanate includes inhibition of both the uptake and binding of iodine producing symptoms of hypothyroidism.

Sodium nitroprusside can bind to vitamin B_{12} interfering with its distribution and metabolism, and should be used with caution in patients with low plasma vitamin B_{12} concentrations. Excess cyanide can also bind to hemoglobin producing methemoglobinemia.

CASE STUDY

Victoria F. Roche and S. William Zito

VD is an 81-year-old, white, female housewife with rheumatoid arthritis. Her RA is treated with low-dose methotrexate (10mg/week) and celecoxib (100mg bid). She manages to cook but her cantankerous 77-year-old husband does the housework and shopping. VD also suffers from type 2 diabetes and her plasma glucose is well maintained with glipizide. VD visits her physician every three months and during her last visit her cholesterol was elevated (250mg/dl) so therapy with simvastatin (20mg/day at bedtime) was initiated. VD has always had normal blood pressure but during her most recent examination her pressure was 150/95 mm Hg which persisted over the next three days. VD already maintains a healthy diet in controlling her type 2 diabetes but her RA and age precludes strenuous exercise. Her physician wants to initiate antihypertensive therapy and contemplates the following 4 possible therapeutic agents. Evaluate each in relation to this case and make a recommendation.

1. *Identify the therapeutic problem(s) where the pharmacist's intervention may benefit the patient.*

2. *Identify and prioritize the patient specific factors that must be considered to achieve the desired therapeutic outcomes.*

3. *Conduct a thorough and mechanistically oriented structure-activity analysis of all therapeutic alternatives provided in the case.*

4. *Evaluate the SAR findings against the patient specific factors and desired therapeutic outcomes and make a therapeutic decision.*

5. *Counsel your patient.*

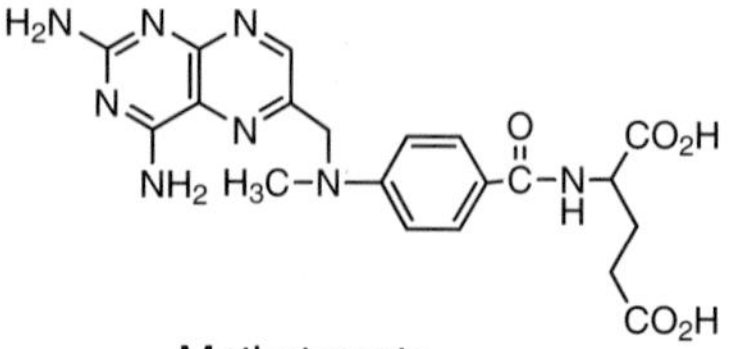

Methotrexate

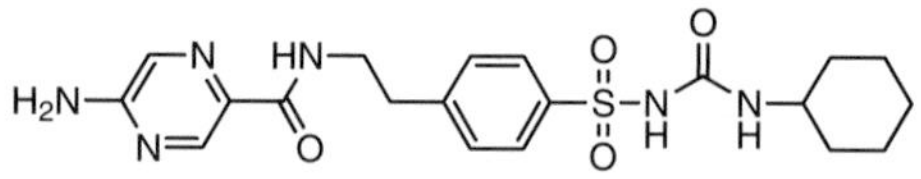

Glipizide

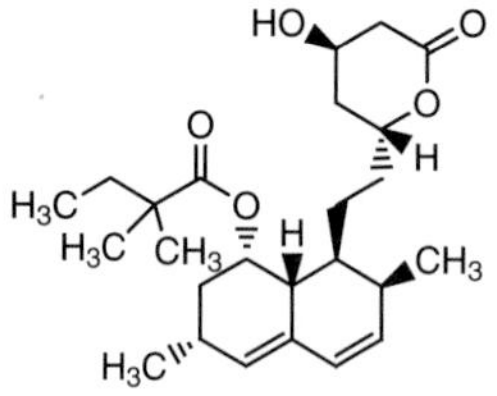

Simvastatin

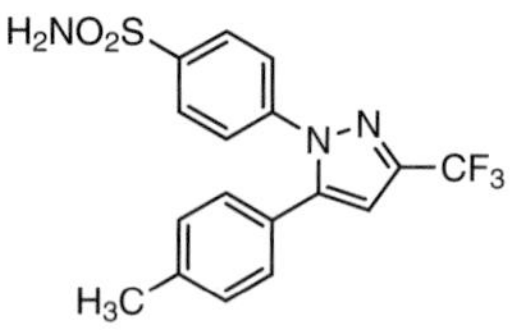

Celecoxib

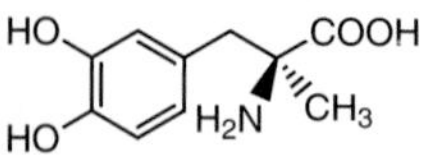

1

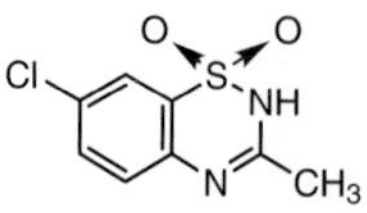

2

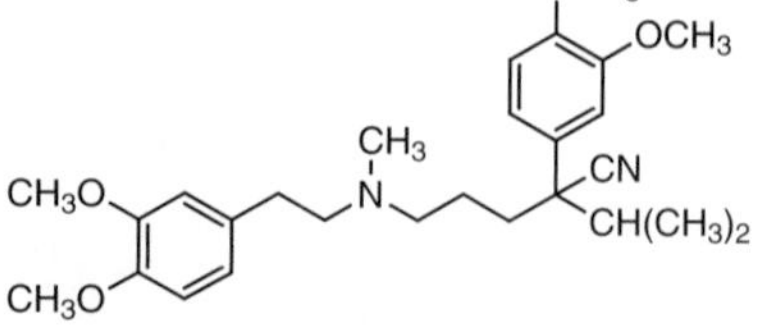

3

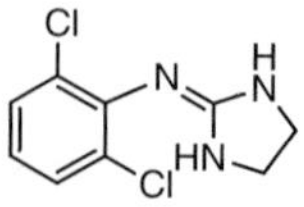

4

REFERENCES

1. Weibert RT, Hypertension. In: Herfindal ET, Gourley DR, eds. Textbook of Therapeutics: Drug and Disease Management, 7th Ed. Baltimore, MD: Lippincott Williams & Wilkins, 2000, 795–824.

2. The Sixth Report of the Joint National Committee on Prevention, Detection, Evaluation, and Treatment of High Blood Pressure (JNC VI). Arch Intern Med. 1997;157,2413–2446.

3. Brown MJ. Haydock S. Pathoaetiology, epidemiology and diagnosis of hypertension. Drugs, 2000; 59(SUPPL. 2), 1–12.

4. Morgan TO, Nowson C, Murphy J, et al. Compliance and the elderly hypertensive. Drugs. 1986. 31, 174–183.

5. Lubbe WF. Hypertension in pregnancy. Pathophysiology and management. Drugs, 1984, 28, 170–188.

6. Kaplan NM. Combination therapy for systemic hypertension. Am J Cardiol. 1995;76:595–597.

7. Abernethy DR. Pharmacological properties of combination therapies for hypertension. Am J Hypertens. 1997; 10,13–16S.

8. McEvoy GK, ed. AHFS 2000 Drug Information. Bethesda, MD: American Society of Health-System Pharmacists; 2000, 1658–1726.

9. Oates JA. Antihypertensive Agents and the Drug Therapy of Hypertension. In: Hardman JG, Limbird LE, Molinoff PB, et al, eds. Goodman and Gilman's The Pharmacologic Basis of Therapeutics, 9th Ed. New York: McGraw Hill, 1996, 780–808.

10. Robertson JIS. State-of-the-art review: beta-blockade and the treatment of hypertension. Drugs. 1983; 25(Suppl. 2), 5–11).

11. Freis ED, Papademetriou V. Current drug treatment and treatment patterns with antihypertensive drugs. Drugs. 1996;52, 1–16.

12. Husserl FE, Messerli FH. Adverse effects of antihypertensive drugs. Drugs, 1981; 22, 188–210.

13. Goldberg M, Fenster PE. Clinical significance of intrinsic sympathomimetic activity of beta blockers. Drug Therapy. June 1991:35–43.

14. Cauffield JS, Gums JG, Curry RW. Alpha blockers: A reassessment of their role in therapy. Am Fam Phys. 1996;54, 263–270.

15. Dunn CJ. Lea AP. Wagstaff AJ. Carvedilol. A reappraisal of its pharmacological properties and therapeutic use in cardiovascular disorders. Drugs.1997; 54, 161–185.

16. Van Zwieten PA. An overview of the pharmacodynamic properties and therapeutic potential of combined alpha and beta-adrenoreceptor antagonists. Drugs. 1993;45:509–517.

17. Goa KL, Benfield P, Sorkin EM. Labetalol: A reappraisal of its pharmacology, pharmacokinetics and therapeutic use in hypertension and ischemic heart disease. Drugs, 1989; 37, 583–627.

18. Skerjanec A, Campbell NRC, Robertson S, et al. Pharmacokinetics and presystemic gut metabolism of methyldopa in healthy human subjects. J Clin Pharmacol. 1995; 35, 275–280.

19. Yu A. Frishman WH. Imidazoline receptor agonist drugs: A new approach to the treatment of systemic hypertension. J Clin Pharmacol. 1996, 36, 98–111.

20. Bousquet P. Feldman J. Drugs acting on imidazoline receptors. A review of their pharmacology, their use in blood pressure control and their potential interest in cardioprotection. Drugs. 1999; 58, 799–812.

21. Molderings GJ. Imidazoline Receptors: Basic Knowledge, Recent Advances and Future Prospects for therapy. Drugs Future, 1997; 22, 757–72.

22. Chrisp P, Faulds D. Moxonidine: A review of its pharmacology, and therapeutic use in essential hypertension. Drugs. 1992; 44, 993–1012.

23. Ziegler D, Haxhiu MA, Kaan EC, et al. Pharmacology of moxonidine, an I1–imidazoline receptor agonist. J Cardiovascular Pharmacol. 1996; 27(SUPPL. 3), S26–S37).

24. Theodor R, Weimann HJ, Weber W, et al. Absolute bioavailability of moxonidine. Eur J Drug Metab Pharmacokin. 1991; 16, 153–159).

25. Genissel P, Bromet N, Fourtillan JB, et al. Pharmacokinetics of rilmenidine in healthy subjects. Amer J Cardiol. 1988; 61, 47D-53D.

26. Genissel P, Bromet N. Pharmacokinetics of rilmenidine. Amer J Med. 1989; 87, 8S-23S.

27. Langley MS, Heel RC. Transdermal clonidine. A preliminary review of its pharmacodynamic properties and therapeutic efficacy. Drugs, 1988; 35, 123–142.

28. Fujimura A, Ebihara A, Ohashi K-I, et.al. Comparison of the pharmacokinetics, pharmacodynamics, and safety of oral (Catapres) and transdermal (M-5041T) clonidine in healthy subjects. J Clin Pharmacol. 1994; 34, 260–265.

29. Ebihara A, Fujimura A, Ohashi K-I, et.al. Influence of application site of a new transdermal clonidine, M-5041T, on its pharmacokinetics and pharmacodynamics in healthy subjects. J Clin Pharmacol. 1993; 33, 1188–1191.

30. Holmes B, Brogden RN, Heel RC, et.al. Guanabenz. A review of its pharmacodynamic properties and therapeutic efficacy in hypertension. Drugs. 1983; 26, 212–229.

31. Sorkin EM, Heel RC. Guanfacine: A review of its pharmacodynamic and pharmacokinetic properties, and therapeutic efficacy in the treatment of hypertension. Drugs. 1986; 31, 301–336.

32. Cornish LA. Guanfacine hydrochloride. A centrally acting antihypertensive agent. Clinical Pharmacy. 1988; 7, 187–197.

33. Carchman SH, Crowe JT Jr, Wright GJ. The bioavailability and pharmacokinetics of guanfacine after oral and intravenous administration to healthy volunteers. J Clin Pharmacol 1987, 27, 762–767.

34. Finnerty FA Jr, Brogden RN. Guanadrel. A review of its pharmacodynamic and pharmacokinetic properties and therapeutic use in hypertension. Drugs. 1985; 30, 22–31.

35. Duty S, Weston AH. Potassium channel openers. Pharmacological effects and future uses. Drugs.1990; 40, 785–791.

36. Campese VM. Minoxidil: A review of its pharmacological properties and therapeutic use. Drugs. 1981; 22, 257–278.

36. Clissold SP, Heel RC. Topical minoxidil: A preliminary review of its pharmacodynamic properties and therapeutic efficacy in alopecia areata and alopecia androgenetica. Drugs. 1987, 33, 107–122.

25. Antihyperlipoproteinemics and Inhibitors of Cholesterol Biosynthesis

MARC HARROLD

THE CHEMISTRY AND BIOCHEMISTRY OF PLASMA LIPIDS

The major lipids found in the bloodstream are cholesterol, cholesterol esters, triglycerides, and phospholipids. Excess plasma concentrations of one or more of these compounds is known as hyperlipidemia. Since all lipids require the presence of soluble lipoproteins in order to be transported in the blood, hyperlipidemia ultimately results in an increased concentration of these transport molecules, a condition known as hyperlipoproteinemia. Hyperlipoproteinemia has been strongly associated with atherosclerotic lesions and coronary heart disease (1,2). Prior to discussing lipoproteins, their role in cardiovascular disease, and agents to decrease their concentrations, it is essential to examine the biochemistry of cholesterol, triglycerides, and phospholipids.

Compounds Listed in the Top 200 Drugs that Affect Plasma Lipids (3)

Atorvastatin (Lipitor), fluvastatin (Lescol), lovastatin (Mevacor), pravastatin (Pravachol), simvastatin (Zocor).

Synthesis and Degradation of Cholesterol

Cholesterol is a C_{27} steroid which serves as an important component of all cell membranes and as the precursor for androgens, estrogens, progesterone, and adrenocorticoids (Fig. 25.1). It is synthesized from acetyl CoA as shown in Figure 25.2 (4,5). The first stage of the biosynthesis is the formation of isopentenyl pyrophosphate from three acetyl CoA molecules. The conversion of 3-hydroxy-3-methylglutaryl CoA (HMG CoA) to mevalonic acid is especially important because it is a primary control site for cholesterol biosynthesis. This reaction is catalyzed by HMG CoA reductase and reduces the thioester of HMG CoA to a primary hydroxyl group. The second stage involves the coupling of six isopentenyl pyrophosphate molecules to form squalene. Initially, three isopentenyl pyrophosphate molecules are condensed to form farnesyl pyrophosphate, a C_{15} intermediate. Two farnesyl pyrophosphate molecules are then combined using a similar type of reaction. The next stage involves the cyclization of squalene to lanosterol. This process involves an initial epoxidation of squalene followed by a subsequent cyclization requiring a concerted flow of four pairs of electrons and the migration of two methyl groups. The final stage involves the conversion of lanosterol to cholesterol. This process removes three methyl groups from lanosterol, reduces the side chain double bond, moves the other double bond within the ring structure, and requires approximately 20 steps.

Squalene Synthase: A Potential Drug Target

Inhibitors of squalene synthase, the enzyme responsible for catalyzing the two-step conversion of two molecules of farnesyl pyrophosphate to squalene, are currently being investigated as antihyperlipidemic agents. Squalene synthase catalyzes the first committed step in sterol biosynthesis and offers some potential advantages over HMG CoA reductase as a drug target. The latter group of compounds inhibit cholesterol synthesis at an early stage of the pathway and thus lack specificity. Mevalonic acid, the immediate product of HMG CoA reductase, is a common intermediate in the biosynthesis of other isoprenoids such as ubiquinone (an electron carrier in oxidative phosphorylation), dolichol (a compound involved in oligosaccharide synthesis), and farnesylated proteins (the farnesyl portion targets the protein to cell membranes as opposed to the cytosol). Inhibitors of squalene synthase target an enzyme involved in a later stage of cholesterol biosynthesis and could potentially accomplish the same desired outcomes as currently available agents without interfering with the biosynthesis of other essential, nonsteroidal compounds. One class of compounds currently under investigation are the squalestatins. These compounds were originally isolated as fermentation products produced by a species of *Phoma*. Squalestatin 1 is a potent inhibitor of squalene synthetase and has been shown to produce a marked decrease in serum cholesterol. Additional analogs as well as other structural classes continue to be investigated and may ultimately produce alternatives to currently available therapy (6,7).

Squalestatin 1

Cholesterol is enzymatically transformed by two different pathways. As illustrated in Figure 25.1, cholesterol can be oxidatively cleaved by the enzyme desmolase (side chain cleaving enzyme). The resulting compound, pregnenolone, serves as the common intermediate in the biosynthesis of all other endogenous steroids. As illustrated in Figure 25.3, cholesterol can also be converted to bile acids and bile salts. This pathway represents the most important mechanism for

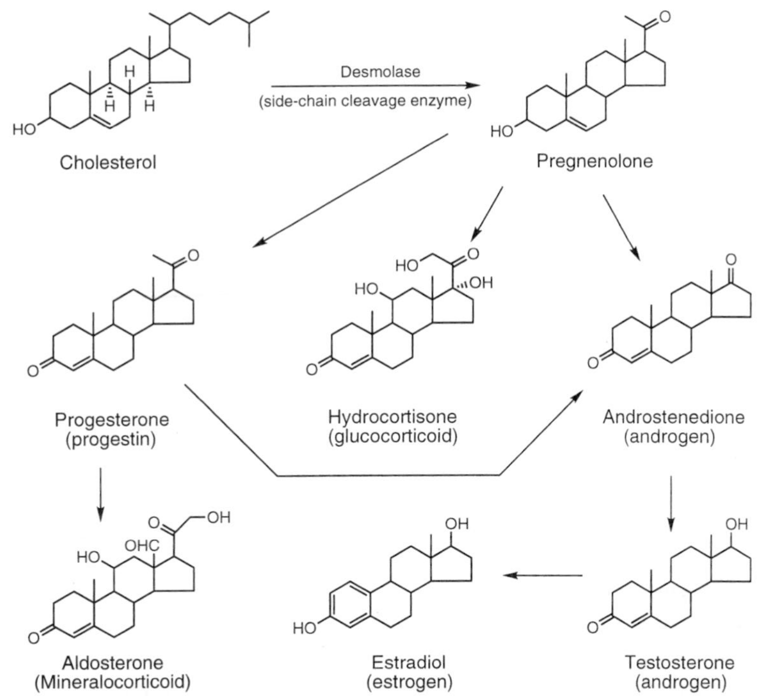

Fig. 25.1. Cholesterol's role as a key intermediate in the biosynthesis of endogenous steroids.

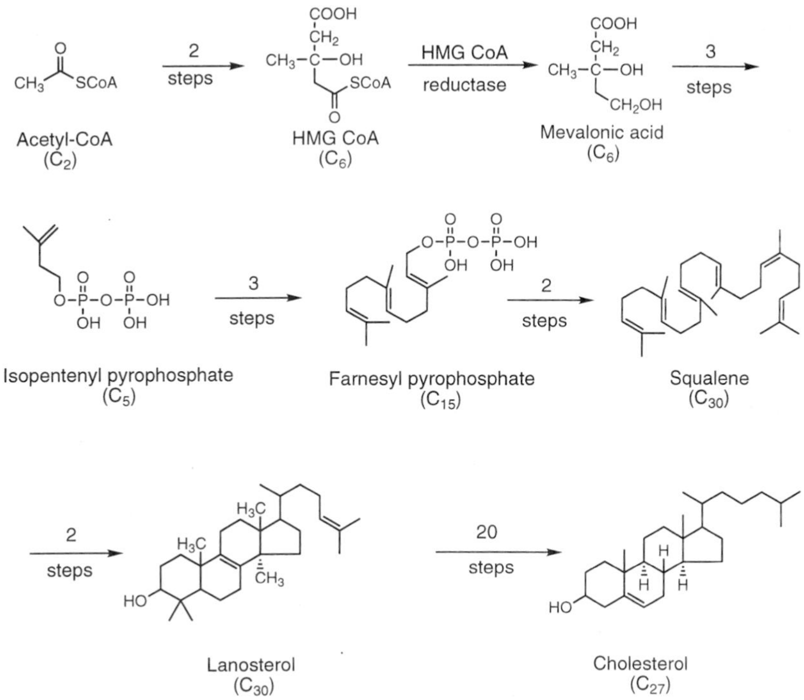

Fig. 25.2. The biosynthesis of cholesterol.

cholesterol catabolism. It is controlled by the enzyme 7α-hydroxylase which catalyzes the initial, rate-limiting step in this metabolic pathway. Cholic acid and its derivatives are primarily (99%) conjugated with either glycine (75%) or taurine (24%). Bile salts, such as glycocholate, are surface-active agents that act as anionic detergents.

They are synthesized in the liver, stored in the gallbladder, and released into the small intestine where they emulsify dietary lipids and fat-soluble vitamins. This solubilization promotes the absorption of these dietary compounds through the intestinal mucosa. Bile salts are predominantly reabsorbed through the enterohepatic circulation

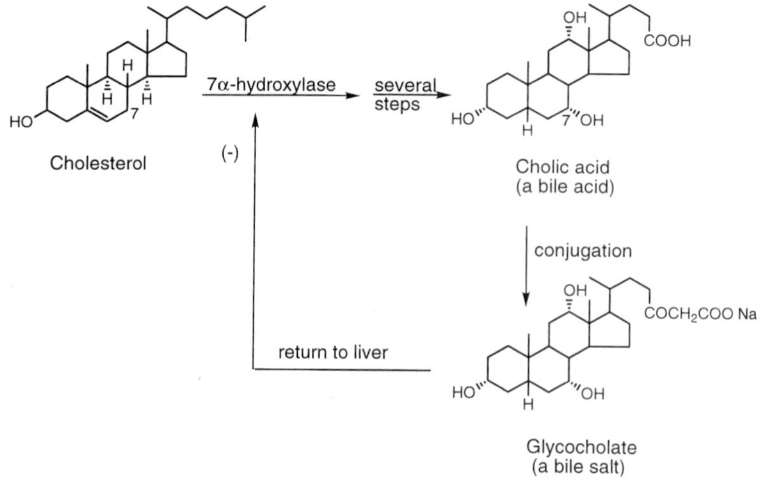

Fig. 25.3. The conversion of cholesterol to bile acids and bile salts.

and returned to the liver where they exert a negative feedback control on 7α-hydroxylase and thus regulate any subsequent conversion of cholesterol (4,5,8).

The terms bile acid and bile salt refer to the un-ionized and ionized forms of these compounds, respectively. For illustrative purposes only, Figure 25.3 shows cholic acid as a un-ionized bile acid and glycocholate as an ionized bile salt (as the sodium salt). At physiologic and intestinal pHs, both of these compounds would exist almost exclusively in their ionized forms.

Overview of Triglycerides and Phospholipids

Triglycerides, or more appropriately triacylglycerols, are highly concentrated stores of metabolic energy. They are formed from glycerol 3-phosphate and acylated coenzyme A (Fig. 25.4) and accumulate primarily in the cytosol of adi-

pose cells. When required for energy production, triglycerides are hydrolyzed by lipase enzymes to liberate free fatty acids which are then subjected to β-oxidation, the citric acid cycle, and oxidative phosphorylation.

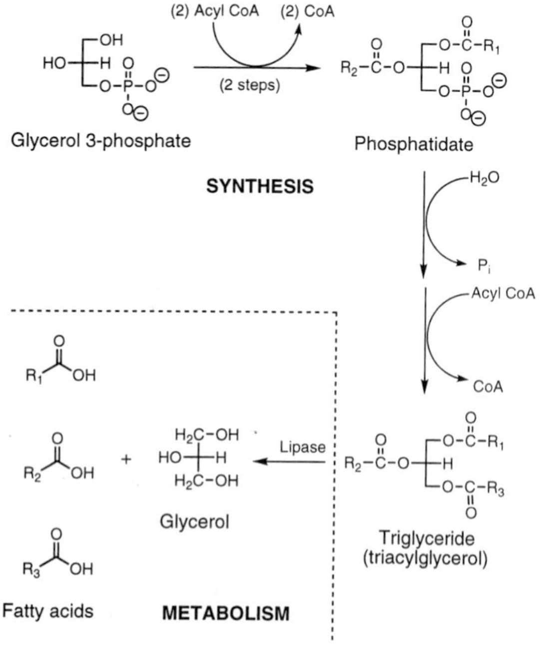

Phospholipids, or phosphoglycerides, are amphipathic compounds which are used to make cell membranes, generate second messengers, and store fatty acids for use in the generation of prostaglandins. They can be synthesized from phosphatidate, an intermediate in triglyceride synthesis. Two common phospholipids, phosphatidyl choline and phosphatidyl inositol, are shown below (4,5).

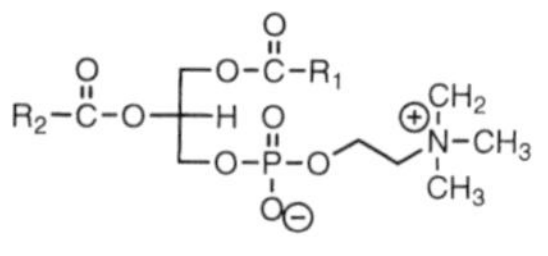

Phosphatidyl choline 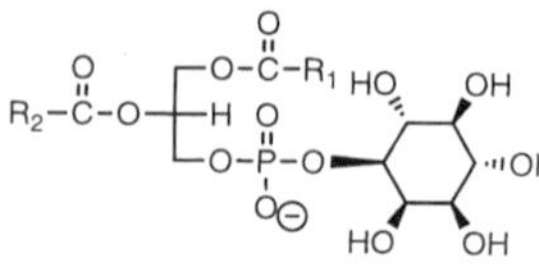   Phosphatidyl inositol

Lipoproteins and Transport of Cholesterol and Triglycerides

Cholesterol, triglycerides, and phospholipids are freely soluble in organic solvents such as isopropanol, chloroform, and diethyl ether but are relatively insoluble in aqueous, physiologic fluids. In order to be transported within the blood, these lipids are solubilized through association with macromolecular aggregates known as lipoproteins. Each lipoprotein is associated with additional proteins, known as apolipoproteins, located on their outer surface. These apolipoproteins provide structural support and stability, bind to cellular receptors, and act as cofactors for enzymes involved in lipoprotein metabolism. The compositions and primary functions of the six major lipoproteins are listed in Table 25.1 (8–11).

Lipoprotein nomenclature is based on mode of separation. When preparative ultracentrifugation is used, lipoproteins are separated according to their density and identified as very low density lipoproteins (VLDL), intermediate density lipoproteins (IDL), low density lipopro-

Fig. 25.4. The biosynthesis and metabolism of triglycerides.

teins (LDL), and high density lipoproteins (HDL). When electrophoresis is employed in the separation, lipoproteins are designated as pre-β, β, and α. IDL is mainly found in the pre-β fraction as a second electrophoretic band and is currently believed to be an intermediate lipoprotein in the catabolism of VLDL to LDL. Chylomicron remnants and IDL may show similar electrophoretic and ultracentrifugation separation characteristics. In general, VLDL, LDL and HDL correspond to pre-β, β, and α-lipoproteins, respectively.

The interrelationship among the lipoproteins is shown in Figure 25.5 (8–11). As illustrated, the pathway can be divided into both exogenous (dietary intake) and endogenous (synthetic) components. The exogenous pathway begins following the ingestion of a fat-containing meal or snack. Dietary lipids are absorbed in the form of cholesterol and fatty acids. The fatty acids are then re-esterified within the intestinal mucosal cells, and along with the cholesterol, are incorporated into chylomicrons, the largest lipoprotein. During circulation, chylomicrons are degraded into remnants by the action of lipoprotein lipase, a plasma membrane enzyme located on capillary endothelial cells in adipose and muscle tissue. The liberated free acids are then available for either storage or energy generation by these tissues. The remnants are predominantly cleared from the plasma by liver parenchymal cells via recognition of the apoE portion of the carrier.

The endogenous pathway begins in the liver with the formation of VLDL. Similar to chylomicrons, triglycerides are present in a higher concentration than either cholesterol or cholesterol esters; however, the concentration difference between these lipids is much less than that seen in chylomicrons. The metabolism of VLDL is also similar to chylomicrons in that lipoprotein lipase reduces the triglyceride content of VLDL and increases the availability of free fatty acids to the muscle and adipose tissue. The resulting lipoprotein, IDL, can either be further metabolized to LDL or be transported to the liver for receptor-mediated endo-

cytosis. This latter effect involves an interaction of the LDL receptor with the apolipoproteins, apoB-100 and apoE, present on IDL. The amount of IDL delivered to the liver is approximately the same as that converted to LDL. The half-life of IDL is relatively short as compared to LDL and thus accounts for only a small portion of total plasma cholesterol. In contrast, LDL accounts for approximately two-thirds of total plasma cholesterol and serves as the primary source of cholesterol for both hepatic and extrahepatic cells. As with IDL, the uptake of LDL by these cells is mediated by a receptor interaction with the apoB-100 apolipoprotein present on LDL. Regulation of cellular

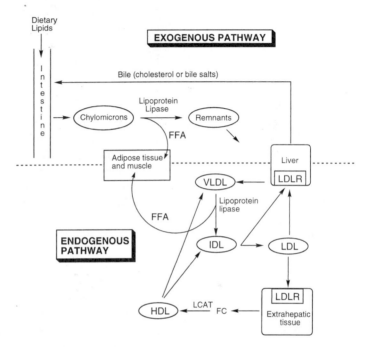

Fig. 25.5. Endogenous and exogenous pathways for lipid transport and metabolism. Abbreviations: FFA = free fatty acids; LDLR = LDL receptor; FC = free unesterified cholesterol; LCAT = lecithin-cholesterol acyltransferase.

Table 25.1. Classification and Characteristics of Major Plasma Lipoproteins

Classification	Composition	Major Apolipoproteins	Primary Function(s)
Chylomicrons	Triglycerides 85–95%, Free Cholesterol 1–3%, Cholesterol Esters 2–4%, Phospholipids 3–6%, Apoproteins 1–2%	apoA-I, apoA-II, apoA-IV, apoB-48, apoC-II/C-III	Transport dietary triglycerides to adipose tissue and muscle for hydrolysis by lipoprotein lipase
Chylomicron Remnants	Primarily composed of dietary cholesterol esters	apoB-48, apoE	Transport dietary cholesterol to liver for receptor-mediated endocytosis
VLDL	Triglycerides 50–65%, Free Cholesterol 4–8%, Cholesterol Esters 16–22%, Phospholipids 15–20%, Apoproteins 6–10%	apoB-100, apoE, apoC-II/C-III	Transport endogenous triglycerides to adipose tissue and muscle for hydrolysis by lipoprotein lipase
IDL	Intermediate between VLDL and LDL	apoB-100, apoE, apoC-II/C-III	Transport endogenous cholesterol for either conversion to LDL or receptor-mediated endocytosis by the liver
LDL	Triglycerides 4–8%, Free Cholesterol 6–8%, Cholesterol Esters 45–50%, Phospholipids 18–24%, Apoproteins 18–22%	apoB-100	Transport endogenous cholesterol for receptor-mediated endocytosis by either the liver or extrahepatic tissues
HDL	Triglycerides 2–7%, Free Cholesterol 3–5%, Cholesterol Esters 15–20%, Phospholipids 26–32%, Apoproteins 45–55%	apoA-I, apoA-II, apoC-II/C-III-	Removal of cholesterol from extrahepatic tissues via transfer of cholesterol esters to IDL and VLDL

LDL uptake is mediated by the number of LDL receptors present on the cell surface. Cells requiring increased amounts of cholesterol will increase the biosynthesis of LDL receptors. Conversely, it has been demonstrated that increased hepatic concentrations of cholesterol will inhibit both HMG CoA reductase as well as the production of LDL receptors. This latter effect is mediated through a metabolite, 25-hydroxycholesterol (12). As previously discussed, hepatic cholesterol can be converted to bile acids and bile salts and re-enter the endogenous pathway through the bile and enterohepatic circulation.

Synthesized in the liver and intestine, HDL initially exists as a phospholipid disc containing apolipoproteins apoA-I and apoA-II. The primary function of HDL is to act as a scavenger to remove cholesterol from extrahepatic cells and to facilitate its transport back to the liver. Nascent HDL accepts free, unesterified cholesterol. A plasma enzyme, lecithin-cholesterol acyltransferase (LCAT) then esterifies the cholesterol. This process is important because it increases the lipid solubility of cholesterol, allows it to move from the surface to the core, and thus exposes more of the HDL surface for the uptake of subsequent cholesterol molecules. The ultimate return of cholesterol from HDL to the liver is known as reverse cholesterol transport and is accomplished via an intermediate transfer of cholesterol esters to either VLDL or IDL. Thus HDL serves to prevent the accumulation of cholesterol in arterial cell walls and other tissue and may serve as the basis for its cardioprotective properties (8).

Classification of Hyperlipoproteinemias

Hyperlipoproteinemia can be divided into primary and secondary disorders. Primary disorders are the result of genetic deficiencies or mutations, while secondary disorders are the result of other conditions or diseases. Secondary hyperlipoproteinemia has been associated with diabetes mellitus, hypothyroidism, renal disease, liver disease, alcoholism, and certain drugs (1,8).

In 1967, Fredrickson and co-workers classified primary hyperlipoproteinemias into six phenotypes (I, IIa, IIb, III, IV, V) based upon which lipoprotein(s) and lipids were elevated (13). Current literature and practice, however, appear to favor the more descriptive classifications and subclassifications listed in Table 25.2. Primary disorders are currently classified as those that primarily cause hypercholesterolemia, those that primarily cause hypertriglyceridemia, and those that cause a mixed elevation of both cholesterol and triglycerides. Subclassifications are based upon the specific biochemical defect responsible for the disorder. Classifications developed by Fredrickson have been included in Table 25.2 under the heading "Previous Classification" for comparative and reference purposes.

As shown in Table 25.2, some disorders are well characterized while others are not (1,8). Familial hypercholesterolemia is caused by a deficiency of LDL receptors. This results in a decreased uptake of IDL and LDL by hepatic and extrahepatic tissues and an elevation in plasma LDL levels. The homozygous form of this disorder is rare but results in extremely high LDL levels and early morbidity and mortality due to the total lack of LDL receptors. A related disorder, familial defective apoB-100, also results in elevated LDL levels but is caused by a genetic mutation rather than a deficiency. Alteration of apoB-100 decreases the affinity of LDL for the LDL receptor and thus hinders normal uptake and metabolism. Elevations in chylomicron levels can result from a deficiency of either lipoprotein lipase or apoC-II. These deficiencies cause decreased or impaired triglyceride hydrolysis and result in a massive accumulation of chylomicrons in the plasma. Dysbetalipoproteinemia results from the presence of an altered form of apolipoprotein E and is the only mixed hyperlipoproteinemia with a known cause. Proper catabolism of chylomicron and VLDL remnants requires apoE. The presence of a binding-defective form of apoE, known as apoE$_2$, results in elevated levels of VLDL and IDL triglyceride and cholesterol levels.

DISEASES AND DISORDERS CAUSED BY HYPERLIPIDEMIAS

Coronary heart disease (CHD), which includes acute myocardial infarction (MI), ischemic heart disease, and angina pectoris, is the leading cause of mortality in the

Table 25.2. Characteristics of the Major Primary Hyperlipoproteinemias

Current Classification	Biochemical Defect	Elevated Lipoproteins	Previous Classification
Hypercholesterolemias			
Familial hypercholesterolemia	Deficiency of LDL receptors	LDL	IIa
Familial defective apoB-100	Mutant apoB-100	LDL	IIa
Polygenic hypercholesterolemia	Unknown	LDL	IIa
Hypertriglyceridemias			
Familial hypertriglyceridemia	Unknown	VLDL	IV
Familial lipoprotein lipase deficiency	Deficiency of lipoprotein lipase	Chylomicrons	I (chylomicron elevation only), V
Familial apoC-II deficiency	Deficiency of apoC-II	Chylomicrons	I (chylomicron elevation only), V
Mixed Hypercholesterolemia and Hypertriglyceridemia			
Familial combined hyperlipidemia	Unknown	VLDL, LDL	IIb
Dysbetalipoproteinemia	Presence of apoE$_2$ isoforms	VLDL, IDL	III

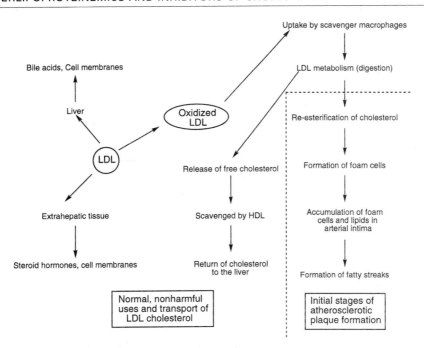

Fig. 25.6. The role of LDL cholesterol in the development of atherosclerotic plaques. The mechanism by which HDL provides a cardioprotective action is also shown.

United States. In 1996, more than 470,000 deaths were caused by CHD. Additionally, mortality from CHD often occurs rapidly. Annually, over 250,000 deaths occur within one hour after the onset of symptoms. The highest mortality is seen in patients over the age of 65; however, the vast majority of deaths in patients under the age of 65 occur during an initial attack. Risk factors associated with CHD include cigarette smoking, elevated plasma cholesterol levels, physical inactivity and obesity (14).

Atherosclerosis, which is named from the Greek terms for "gruel" (*athere*) and "hardening" (*sclerosis*), is the underlying cause of CHD. It is a gradual process in which an initial accumulation of lipids in the arterial intima leads to thickening of the arterial wall, plaque formation, thrombosis, and occlusion (15–17). The involvement of LDL cholesterol in this process is shown in Figure 25.6. Within the extracellular space of the intima, LDL is more susceptible to oxidative metabolism because it is no longer protected by plasma antioxidants. This metabolism alters the properties of LDL such that it is readily scavenged by macrophages. Unlike normal LDL, the uptake of oxidized LDL is not regulated; thus macrophage cells can readily become engorged with oxidized LDL. Subsequent metabolism produces free cholesterol which can either be released into the plasma or re-esterified by the enzyme acyl CoA:cholesterol acyltransferase (ACAT). Cholesterol released into plasma can be scavenged by HDL and returned to the liver, thus preventing any accumulation or damage. In this manner, HDL acts as a cardioprotective agent, because high concentrations of re-esterified cholesterol can morphologically change macrophages into foam cells. Accumulation of lipid-engorged foam cells in the arterial intima results in the formation of fatty streaks, the initial lesion of atherosclerosis. Later, the deposition of lipoproteins, cholesterol, and phospholipids causes the formation of softer, larger plaques. Associated with this lipid deposition is the proliferation of arterial smooth muscle cells into the intima and the laying down of collagen, elastin, and glycosaminoglycans leading to fibrous plaques. Ultimately, the surface of the plaque deteriorates and an atheromatous ulcer is formed with a fibrous matrix, accumulation of necrotic tissue, and appearance of cholesterol and cholesterol ester crystals. A complicated lesion also shows calcification and hemorrhage with the formation of organized mural thrombi. Thrombosis results from changes in the arterial walls and in the blood-clotting mechanism.

Obviously, individuals with higher cholesterol and LDL levels are more susceptible to these detrimental effects than those with normal cholesterol and LDL levels. Total plasma cholesterol levels less than 200 mg/dL are considered desirable. Levels above 240mg/dL are considered high, and levels between 200 and 239 mg/dL are considered border-line. For LDL, plasma levels less than 100 mg/dL are considered optimal, plasma levels equal to or greater than 160 are considered high, plasma levels between 130 and 159 mg/dL are considered border-line (8,14), and plasma levels between 100–129 are considered above optimal (new guidelines summer 2001).

Elevated plasma triglyceride levels can contribute to atherosclerosis and CHD in mixed hyperlipoproteinemias while pure hypertriglyceridemias are primarily associated with pancreatitis and show little to no relationship to CHD (18).

ACAT: A Potential Drug Target

Inhibitors of acyl CoA:cholesterol acyltransferase (ACAT) are currently being investigated as cholesterol lowering or antiatherosclerotic agents. In addition to its role in foam cell formation, ACAT is also required for esterification of cholesterol in intestinal mucosal cells and for synthesis of cholesterol esters in hepatic VLDL formation. Thus, ACAT inhibitors have the potential of providing three beneficial effects in patients with hypercholesterolemia: decreased cholesterol absorption, decreased hepatic VLDL synthesis, and decreased foam cell formation. Initial successes at inhibiting ACAT were dampened by the discovery of accompanying adrenal toxicity. Subsequent structural modifications have lead to the development of potent, orally active ACAT inhibitors (e.g., CI1011) which lack this toxicity and have given new hope that inhibitors of this enzyme may provide an alternative treatment of atherosclerotic disorders (16,19).

CI1011

OVERVIEW OF DRUG THERAPY AFFECTING LIPOPROTEIN METABOLISM

Bile acid sequestrants, HMG CoA reductase inhibitors, fibrates, and niacin are all used in the treatment of hyperlipoproteinemia. In general, successful use of these compounds depends upon proper identification and classification of the hyperlipoproteinemia affecting the patient. With the possible exceptions of niacin and atorvastatin, currently available compounds do not have equal efficacy in reducing both hypercholesterolemia and hypertriglyceridemia, and are thus used primarily for their ability to decrease either cholesterol or triglyceride levels. Bile acid sequestrants and inhibitors of HMG CoA reductase are effective in decreasing plasma cholesterol and LDL levels. The fibrates also have some actions on plasma cholesterol; however, their main effect is to stimulate lipoprotein lipase and increase the clearance of triglycerides. Niacin, through its ability to decrease VLDL formation, has been shown to decrease the plasma levels of both triglycerides and cholesterol. All of these compounds are discussed below. References for these sections have been limited to current reviews and texts, selected papers, and product literature, both traditional and electronic. Readers requiring additional references for any of these compounds should consult either the previous edition of this text or the references contained within the cited reviews and texts.

BILE ACID SEQUESTRANTS
Historical Overview

Cholestyramine was originally developed in the 1960s to treat pruritus secondary to elevated plasma concentra-

tions of bile acids in patients with cholestasis. Its ability to bind (i.e., hold, sequester) bile acids and increase their fecal elimination was subsequently shown to produce beneficial effects in lowering serum cholesterol levels. In 1973, cholestyramine was approved for the treatment of hypercholesterolemia in patients who did not respond to dietary modifications. Colestipol, which retains the key structural features required to bind bile acids, was approved in 1977 (8,20).

Cholestyramine and colestipol are chemically classified as anion-exchange resins. This term arises from their ability to selectively bind and exchange negatively charged atoms or molecules with one another. The selectivity comes from the fact that these positively charged resins do not bind equally to all anions. For example, the chloride ion of cholestyramine can be displaced by, or exchanged with, other anions (e.g., bile acids) which have a greater affinity for the positively charged functional groups on the resin.

Mechanism of Action

Cholestyramine and colestipol lower plasma LDL levels by indirectly increasing the rate at which LDL is cleared from the bloodstream. Under normal circumstances, approximately 97% of bile acids are reabsorbed into the enterohepatic circulation. As previously discussed, these compounds are returned to the liver where they regulate their own production. Bile acid sequestrants are not orally absorbed but act locally within the gastrointestinal tract to interrupt this process. They bind the two major bile acids, glycocholic acid and taurocholic acid, and greatly increase their fecal excretion. As a result, decreased concentrations of these compounds are returned to the liver. This removes the feedback inhibition of 7α-hydroxylase and increases the hepatic conversion of cholesterol to bile acids (see Fig. 23.3). The decrease in hepatic cholesterol concentrations leads to several compensatory effects: increased expression of LDL receptors, increased hepatic uptake of plasma LDL, induction of HMG CoA reductase, and increased biosynthesis of cholesterol. The latter two effects are insufficient to counteract the increases in cholesterol clearance and catabolism; however, the concurrent use of an HMG CoA reductase inhibitor can provide an additive effect in lowering LDL cholesterol. Bile acid sequestrants do not alter the removal of plasma LDL by nonreceptor-mediated mechanisms and are thus ineffective in treating homozygous familial hypercholesterolemia (8,20–22).

The decreased return of bile acids to the liver will also produce an increase in triglyceride synthesis and a transient rise in VLDL levels. Subsequent compensatory mechanisms will increase VLDL removal, most likely through the increased LDL receptors, and return VLDL levels to pre-drug levels. For those patients with preexisting hypertriglyceridemia, the compensatory mechanisms are inadequate and a persistent rise in VLDL levels occurs (8).

Structure-activity Relationships

Cholestyramine (Fig. 25.7) is a copolymer consisting primarily of polystyrene with a small amount of divinylbenzene as the cross-linking agent. In addition, it contains approximately 4 meq of fixed quaternary ammonium groups per gram of dry resin. These positively charged groups function as binding sites for anions. Virtually all of these sites are accessible by bile acids. Increasing the amount of divinylbenzene from 2% to 4% to 8% increases the cross linkage and reduces the porosity of the resin. This prevents binding of bile acids to interior sites and decreases the efficacy of the compound.

Colestipol (Fig. 25.7) is a copolymer of tetraethylenepentamine and epichlorhydrin and is commercially marked as its hydrochloride salt. The key functional groups on colestipol are the basic secondary and tertiary amines. Although the total nitrogen content of colestipol is greater than that of cholestyramine, the functional anion exchange capacity of the resin depends upon intestinal pH and may be less than cholestyramine. Recent in vitro studies indicate that cholestyramine has a higher adsorption capacity than colestipol for bile salts (24). Quaternization of colestipol with methyl iodide increases the capacity in vitro for glycocholate (25).

Physicochemical Properties

Both cholestyramine and colestipol are large, hygroscopic, water-insoluble resins. The molecular weight of cholestyramine is reported to be greater than 1,000,000; however, no specific molecular weight has been assigned to colestipol. Cholestyramine contains a large number of quaternary ammonium groups and thus has multiple permanent positive charges. Colestipol contains a large number of secondary and tertiary amines. Normal pKa values for these functional groups range from 9–10.5; thus, all of these groups should be primarily ionized at intestinal pH.

Pharmacokinetic Parameters, Metabolism and Dosing

Cholestyramine and colestipol are not orally absorbed and are not metabolized by gastrointestinal enzymes. They are excreted in the feces as an insoluble complex with bile acids. Their onset of action occurs within 24–48 hours; however, it may take up to one month to achieve peak response (8,20,26).

Cholestyramine is available as a powder which is mixed with water, juice or other noncarbonated beverages to create a slurry to drink. Patients should experiment with various liquids in order to find the most palatable combination; however, patient acceptance and compliance with this dosage formulation can limit its use. Each packet or scoop of cholestyramine is equivalent to 4 grams of cholestyramine. The recommended daily dose for the treatment of hypercholesterolemia is 16–24 grams (4–6 packets or scoops) per day divided into 2 or 3 doses and taken with meals. Colestipol is available as either granules or 1 gram tablets. The granules should be taken in a manner similar to that described for the cholestyramine powder. The starting dose for the granules is 5 grams once or twice daily. This dose can be increased in 5 gram increments every 1 to 2 months until therapeutic goals are reached or a maximum of 30 grams per day has been reached. The starting dose for the tablets is 2 grams once or twice daily. This dose can then be increased in 2 gram segments up to a maximum daily dose of 16 grams. Patients must be advised that colestipol tablets should not to be chewed, crushed, or cut and should be taken with plenty of water (20,27).

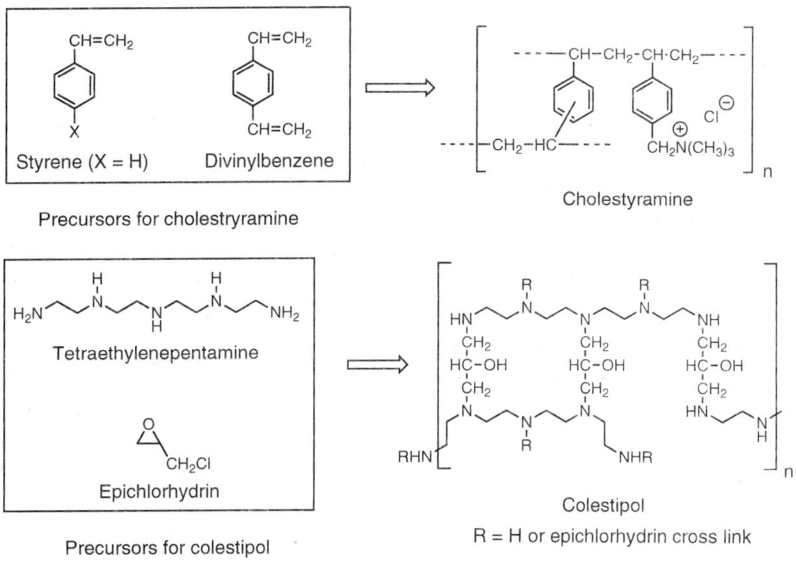

Fig. 25.7. Structures of cholestyramine, colestipol, and the precursors for these polymeric resins. Note that cholestyramine will contain a fraction of unsubsituted aromatic rings (i.e., those that are neither cross-linked nor contain a quaternary ammonium group).

Therapeutic Applications

Bile acid sequestrants are indicated for the treatment of hypercholesterolemia in patients who do not adequately respond to dietary modifications. They may be used either alone or in combination with HMG CoA reductase inhibitors or niacin. These combinations can often achieve a 50% reduction in plasma LDL levels. Cholestyramine, but not colestipol, is also approved for the relief of pruritus associated with partial biliary obstruction. Bile acid sequestrants should not be used to treat hypertriglyceridemias or mixed hyperlipoproteinemias where hypertriglyceridemia is the primary concern. These compounds are also contraindicated in patients with cholelithiasis or complete biliary obstruction due to the impaired secretion of bile acids caused by these conditions (8,20,27).

Unlabeled Uses

Diarrhea, digitalis toxicity, pseudomembranous colitis

Adverse Effects

Since bile acid sequestrants are not orally absorbed, they produce minimal systemic side effects and are thus one of the safest drugs to use for hypercholesterolemia. Constipation is by far the most frequent patient complaint. This can often be minimized by increasing dietary fiber or using bulk-producing laxatives such as psyllium. Other gastrointestinal symptoms, such as bloating and abdominal discomfort, usually disappear with continued use; however, the possibility of fecal impaction requires that extreme caution be used in patients with preexisting constipation. Both cholestyramine and colestipol release chloride ions as part of their exchange mechanism and can cause hyperchloremic acidosis. While this is not a common occurrence, it may limit the use of bile acid sequestrants in patients with renal disease. Hypoprothrombinemia and bleeding are caused by the ability of bile acid sequestrants to bind with and impair the absorption of dietary vitamin K. These effects are also rare, but may limit the use of these agents in patients with preexisting clotting disorder and those concurrently treated with anticoagulants (8,20,27).

Adverse Effects of Bile Acid Sequestrants

Bloating, abdominal discomfort, constipation, bowel obstruction, steatorrhea, anorexia, cholelithiasis, pancreatitis, hyperchloremic acidosis, hypoprothrombinemia, and bleeding

Drug Interactions

Due to their mechanism of action, cholestyramine and colestipol can potentially bind with and decrease the oral absorption of almost any other drug. Since these anion-exchange resins contain numerous positive charges, they are much more likely to bind to acidic compounds than to basic compounds or nonelectrolytes. This is not an absolute since cholestyramine and colestipol have been reported to decrease the oral absorption of propranolol (a base) and the lipid soluble vitamins, A, D, E, and K (nonelectrolytes). As a result, the current recommendation is that all other oral medication should be administered at least 1 hour before or 4–6 hours after cholestyramine and colestipol. Interestingly, this drug interaction has been used in a beneficial manner to treat digitalis overdose and toxicity (8,20).

HMG CoA REDUCTASE INHIBITORS

There are currently six HMG CoA reductase inhibitors (HMGRIs) approved for therapeutic use in the United States. Chemically, they can be divided into two groups, natural products and synthetic agents. All of these com-

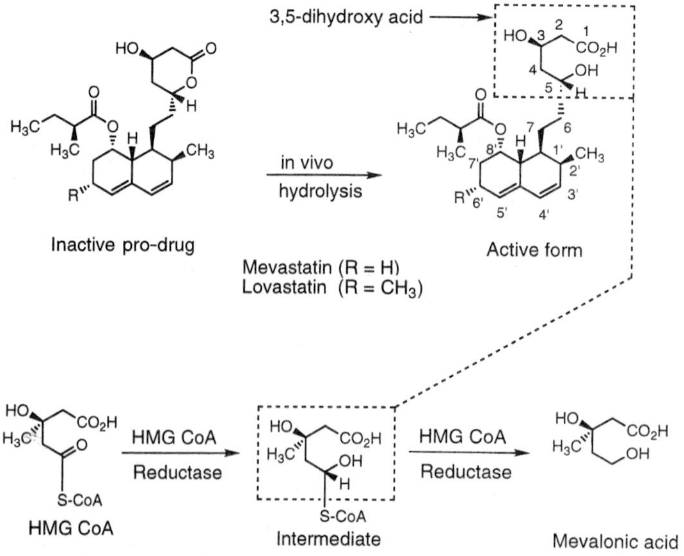

Fig. 25.8. Mechanism of action of mevastatin and lovastatin. Hydrolysis of these pro-drugs produces a 3,5-dihydroxy acid which mimics the tetrahedral intermediate produced by HMG CoA reductase.

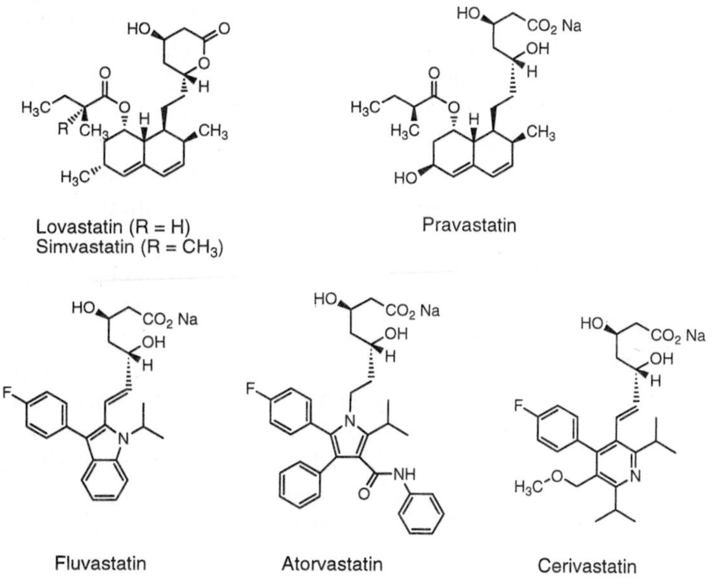

Fig. 25.9. Commercially available HMG CoA reductase inhibitors (Note: Cerivastatin was voluntarily withdrawn in 2001).

pounds effectively block the conversion of HMG CoA to mevalonic acid and have similar effects on plasma cholesterol levels. The compounds differ somewhat in their indications, potencies and pharmacokinetic profiles. They are often referred to as "statins" or, more recently, "vastatins." Due to the potential confusion of the terms "statin" and "statine," (a stable dipeptide mimic, see Chapter 23), it is suggested here that classifying an HMGRI as a vastatin is preferable to classifying it as a statin.

Historical Overview and Development

The development and use of HMGRIs began in 1976 with the discovery of mevastatin. Originally named compactin, this fungal metabolite was isolated from two different species of *Penicillium* and demonstrated potent, competitive inhibition of HMG CoA reductase. Its affinity for the enzyme was shown to be 10,000 times greater than that of the substrate HMG CoA (28). Several years later, a structurally similar compound was isolated from *Monascus ruber* and *Aspergillus terreus*. This compound was originally known as mevinolin, was later renamed lovastatin, and was over 2-fold more potent than mevastatin (Fig. 25.8). Structurally, it differed from mevastatin only by the presence of a methyl group at the 6′ position of the bicyclic ring. As illustrated in Figure 25.8, mevastatin and lovastatin can bind very tightly with HMG CoA reductase because their hydrolyzed lactones mimic the tetrahedral intermediate produced by the reductase enzyme (8). Studies published in 1985 confirmed this theory and also established that the bicyclic portions of these compounds bind to the coenzyme A site of the enzyme (29). Clinical trials of mevastatin were halted due to reports of altered intestinal morphology in dogs (30); however, lovastatin received FDA approval in 1987 as the first HMGRI to be available for therapeutic use.

Structure-activity Relationship

Mevastatin and lovastatin served as lead compounds in the development of additional HMGRIs. Initial research published by Merck Pharmaceuticals examined alterations of the lactone and bicyclic rings as well as the ethylene bridge between them. Their results demonstrated that the activity of HMGRIs is sensitive to the stereochemistry of the lactone ring, the ability of the lactone ring to be hydrolyzed, and the length of bridge connecting the two ring systems. Additionally, it was found that the bicyclic ring could be replaced with other lipophilic rings and that the size and shape of these other ring systems were important to the overall activity of the compounds (31).

Minor modifications of the bicyclic ring and side chain ester of lovastatin produced simvastatin and pravastatin (Fig. 25.9). Pravastatin, a ring-opened dihydroxyacid with a 6′-hydroxyl group, is much more hydrophilic than either lovastatin or simvastatin. Proposed advantages of this enhanced hydrophilicity are minimal penetration into the lipophilic membranes of peripheral cells, better selectivity for hepatic tissues, and a reduction in the incidence of side effects seen with lovastatin and simvastatin. (32,33).

The replacement of the bicyclic ring with various substituted, aromatic ring systems led to the development of fluvastatin, atorvastatin, and cerivastatin (Fig. 25.9). The initial rationale centered on a desire to simplify the structures of mevastatin and lovastatin. The 2,4-dichlorophenyl analog (compound A) shown below was one of the first compounds to demonstrate that this type of substitution was possible; however, compound A was considerably less potent than mevastatin (30). Subsequent research investigated a variety of aromatic substitutions and heterocyclic ring systems in order to optimize HMGRI activity. The substituted pyrrole (compound B) shown below retained 30% of the activity of mevastatin (34) and was a key intermediate in the development of atorvastatin. The 4-fluorophenyl and iso-propyl substitutions found in compound B are also seen in the indole and pyridine ring systems of fluvastatin and cerivastatin, respectively, and thus most likely represent the optimum substitutions at their respective positions. The design of all three of these compounds included the ring-opened dihydroxyacid functionality first seen in pravastatin.

Compound A   Compound B

All HMGRIs can be chemically classified as 7-substituted-3,5-dihydroxyheptanoic acids, the general structure of which is shown in Table 25.3. Additionally, these compounds can be subclassified based upon their lower ring. Compounds structurally related to the natural products mevastatin and lovastatin have structural features common to ring A, while those which are completely synthetic have structural features common to ring B (31,33,34,35–41).

Mechanism of Action

Inhibitors of HMG CoA reductase lower plasma cholesterol levels by three related mechanisms: inhibition of cholesterol biosynthesis, enhancement of receptor-mediated LDL uptake, and reduction of VLDL precursors (8,42). As previously discussed, HMG CoA reductase is the rate-limiting step in cholesterol biosynthesis. Inhibition of this enzyme causes an initial decrease in hepatic cholesterol. Compensatory mechanisms result in an enhanced expression of both HMG CoA reductase and LDL receptors. The net result of all of these effects is a slight to modest decrease in cholesterol synthesis, a significant increase in receptor-mediated LDL uptake, and an overall lowering of plasma LDL levels. Evidence to support the theory that enhanced LDL receptor expression is the primary mechanism for lowering LDL levels comes from the fact that most statins do not lower LDL levels in patients unable to produce LDL receptors (i.e., homozygous familial hypercholesterolemia). The increased number of LDL receptors may also increase the direct removal of VLDL and IDL. Since these lipoproteins are precursors to LDL, this action may contribute to the overall lowering of plasma LDL cholesterol.

Atorvastatin appears to have some effects beyond those seen by the other HMGRIs. It has been shown to decrease plasma LDL levels in patients with homozygous familial hypercholesterolemia, an effect which is proposed to be due to its ability to produce a more significant decrease in the hepatic production of LDL cholesterol. Additionally, atorvastatin produces a marked lowering in plasma triglycerides. This effect has been attributed to its ability to produce an enhanced removal of triglyceride-rich VLDL (42).

Physicochemical Properties

In their active forms, all HMGRIs contain a carboxylic acid. This functional group is required for inhibitory activity, has a pKa in the range of 2.5–3.5, and will be prima-

Table 25.3. Structure-activity Relationship of HMG CoA Reductase Inhibitors

7-substituted-3,5-dihydroxyheptanoic acid   Ring A   Ring B

Common for all HMGRIs
1. The 3,5-dihydroxycarboxylate is essential for inhibitory activity. Compounds containing a lactone are pro-drugs requiring in vivo hydrolysis.
2. The absolute stereochemistry of the 3- and 5-hydroxyl groups must be the same as that found in mevastatin and lovastatin.
3. Altering the two carbon distance between C5 and the ring system diminishes or fails to improve activity.
4. A double bond between C6 and C7 can either increase or decrease activity. The ethyl group provides optimal activity for compounds containing ring A and some heterocyclic rings (e.g., pyrrole ring of atorvastatin). The ethenyl group is optimal for compounds with other ring systems, including the indole and pyrimidine rings seen in fluvastatin and cerivastatin, respectively.

Ring A subclass
- The decalin ring is essential for anchoring the compound to the enzyme active site. Replacement with a cyclohexane ring resulted in a 10,000-fold decrease in activity
- Stereochemistry of the ester side chain is not important for activity; however, conversion of this ester to an ether results in a decrease in activity.
- Methyl substitution at the R2 position increases activity (i.e., simvastatin is more potent than lovastatin).
- β-Hydroxl group substitution at the R1 position enhances hydrophilicity and may provide some cellular specificity.

Ring B subclass
- Substituents W, X, and Y can be either carbon or nitrogen, n is equal to either zero or one (i.e., five or six member heterocyclic).
- The para-fluorophenyl cannot be coplanar with the central aromatic ring. (Structural restraints to cause coplanarity have resulted in a loss of activity.)
- R substitution with aryl groups of hydrocarbon chains enhances lipophilicity and inhibitory activity.

rily ionized at physiologic pH. Lovastatin and simvastatin are neutral, lactone pro-drugs and should be classified as nonelectrolytes. Pravastatin, fluvastatin, and atorvastatin can be classified as acidic drugs. The nitrogen atoms in the indole and pyrrole rings of fluvastatin and atorvastatin, respectively, are aromatic nitrogens that are not ionizable. This is because the lone pair electrons of these atoms are involved in maintaining the aromaticity of their respective rings and are not available to bind protons. Cerivastatin is an amphoteric compound; however, its pyridine nitrogen is a weak base and most likely will not be ionized at physiologic pH.

The calculated log P values for the HMGRIs are shown in Table 25.4. Those values shown in parentheses were calculated using the CLOGP program and were previously reported in the literature (43). Since literature references were incomplete, the LOGKOW program was used to calculate values for all compounds (44). While there is some variation among the values for lovastatin, pravastatin, and simvastatin, general trends are the same regardless of what program was used to calculate the values. The pro-drugs lovastatin and simvastatin have the highest lipid solubility. Hydrolysis of the lactone ring to produce the 3,5-dihydroxycarboxylate significantly improves water solubility. The most hydrophilic compound is pravastatin which contains a 6′-hydroxyl group along with a ring-opened dihydroxy acid.

HMG CoA reductase is a stereoselective enzyme. The 3R, 5R stereochemistry seen in the active forms of mevastatin and lovastatin (Fig. 25.8) is required for inhibitory activity and is present in all other HMGRIs. Stereochemistry of the substituents on the bicyclic rings of lovastatin, simvastatin, and pravastatin is less crucial to activity as indicated in the SAR summary.

Metabolism

As previously mentioned, lovastatin and simvastatin are inactive pro-drugs which must undergo in vivo hydrolysis in order to produce their effects (Fig. 25.8). The active forms of these two compounds as well as all other HMGRIs undergo extensive first-pass metabolism (20,26,42,45). The CYP3A4 isozyme is responsible for the oxidative metabolism of atorvastatin, cerivastatin, lovastatin, and simvastatin. In the case of atorvastatin, the ortho- and para-hydroxylated metabolites are equiactive with the parent compound and contribute significantly to the overall activity of the drug (Table 25.4). Similarly, demethylation of the ether and hydroxylation of an isopropyl group provide metabolites of cerivastatin which retain 50% and 100% activity, respectively. These compounds have been given the abbreviations M1 and M23 by the manufacturer. In contrast, the activity of lovastatin and simvastatin resides primarily in the initial hydrolysis product (i.e., further oxidation decreases activity). Fluvastatin is metabolized by the CYP2C9 isozyme to active hydroxylated metabolites; however, these metabo-

lites do not circulate systemically and do not contribute to the overall activity. Pravastatin also undergoes oxidative metabolism; however, the resulting compounds retain only minimal activity and are not significant. Pravastatin is not metabolized by CYP3A4; however, further information regarding specific isozymes is currently lacking.

Pharmacokinetic Parameters

The pharmacokinetic parameters and dosing information for HMGRIs are summarized in Tables 25.4 and 25.5, respectively (8,20,26,27,42,45,46). With a few exceptions, all of these compounds have similar onsets of action, durations of action, dosing intervals, and plasma protein binding. Despite the ability to attain a peak plasma concentration in 1–4 hours, HMGRIs require approximately 2 weeks to demonstrate an initial lowering of plasma cholesterol. Peak reductions of plasma cholesterol occur after 4–6 weeks of therapy for most compounds. Studies with atorvastatin indicate that it may only need 2 weeks to produce its peak reduction. Atorvastatin is also unique in that it has a much longer duration of action than the other compounds. Its normal half-life is 14 hours; however, this may increase to 19 hours in older patients. Most HMGRIs bind extensively to plasma proteins. The lone exception is pravastatin which is much more hydrophilic than the other compounds in this class.

Due to first-pass metabolism, the oral bioavailability of this class of drugs is generally low and does not reflect the actual absorption of the individual drugs. For example, 60–80% of a dose of simvastatin is orally absorbed but only 5% is actually available to produce an effect. The same is true with fluvastatin, pravastatin, and lovastatin which have oral absorptions of 90%, 34%, and 35%, respectively, but much lower bioavailabilities (Table 25.4). With the exception of lovastatin, the concurrent administration of food does not affect the overall therapeutic effects of HMGRIs. Lovastatin should always be administered with food to maximize oral bioavailability. Failure to do this results in a 33% decrease in plasma concentrations. In general, HMGRIs should be administered in the evening or at bedtime to counteract the peak cholesterol synthesis which occurs in the early morning hours. An exception to this is atorvastatin which, due to its long half-life, is equally effective regardless of when it is administered.

The primary route of elimination of these compounds is through the feces. Due to extensive hepatic transformation and the ability to elevate hepatic enzymes, HMGRIs are contraindicated in patients with active hepatic disease or unexplained persistent elevations in serum aminotransferase concentrations. Dosage reductions in patients with renal dysfunction depends upon the individual agent. Atorvastatin, which has minimal renal excretion, requires no dosage reduction and may be the best agent for patients with renal disorders. Fluvastatin and simvastatin re-

Table 25.4. Pharmacokinetic Parameters of HMG CoA Reductase Inhibitors

Drug	Calculated Log P	Oral Bioavailability (%)	Effect of Food on Absorption	Active Metabolite(s)	Protein Binding (%)	Time to Peak Concentration (hr)	Elimination Half-Life (hr)	Major Route(s) of Elimination
Atorvastatin	2.84	12–14	clinically insignificant	ortho- and para-hydroxylated metabolites	98	1–2	14–19	Biliary/Fecal (> 90%) Renal (<2%)
†Cerivastatin	1.02	60	none	demethylated (M1) and hydroxylated (M23) metabolites	>99	2.5	2–3	Fecal (70%) Renal (24%)
Fluvastatin	1.04	20–30	clinically insignificant	none	98	0.5–1	1	Biliary/Fecal (95%) Renal (5%)
Lovastatin	4.74 (4.04)	5	increased	3,5-dihydroxy acid	>95	2	3–4	Fecal (83%) Renal (10%)
Pravastatin	−0.71 (0.5)	17	clinically insignificant	none	43–55	1–1.5	2–3	Fecal (70%) Renal (20%)
Simvastatin	5.19 (4.2)	5	none	3,5-dihydroxy acid	95	4	3	Fecal (60%) Renal (13%)

†Removal from the market in 2001.

Table 25.5. Dosing Information for HMG CoA Reductase Inhibitors

Generic Name	Brand Name(s)	Approved Indications	Dosing Range	Dose Reduction Maximum Daily Dose	Available with Renal Dysfunction	Tablet Strengths (mg)
Atorvastatin	Lipitor	Hypercholesterolemia, Mixed dyslipidemia	10–80 mg qd	80 mg	No	10, 20, 40
Cerivastatin[†]	Baycol	Hypercholesterolemia, Mixed dyslipidemia	0.2–0.4 mg qd	0.8 mg	Yes	0.2, 0.3, 0.4
Fluvastatin	Lescol	Hypercholesterolemia, Mixed dyslipidemia, Atherosclerosis	20–80 mg qd or BID	80 mg	Caution in severe impairment	20, 40
Lovastatin	Mevacor	Hypercholesterolemia, Atherosclerosis	20–80 mg qd or BID	80 mg	Yes	10, 20, 40
Pravastatin	Pravachol	Hypercholesterolemia, Mixed dyslipidemia, Atherosclerosis, MI and stroke prophylaxis	10–40 mg qd	40 mg	Yes	10, 20, 40
Simvastatin	Zocor	Hypercholesterolemia, Mixed dyslipidemia, Atherosclerosis, MI and stroke prophylaxis	5–40 mg qd	80 mg	Only with severe impairment	5, 10, 20, 40

[†]Removal from the market in 2001.

quire dosage reductions only in cases of severe renal impairment and are better choices than which require dosage reductions in mild or moderate impairment.

Therapeutic Applications

HMG CoA reductase inhibitors are approved for the treatment of hypercholesterolemia and familial combined hyperlipidemia (Fredrickson's type IIa and IIb, see Table 25.2) in patients who have not responded to diet, exercise, and other nonpharmacologic methods (20,27). They may be used alone or in combination with bile acid sequestrants or niacin. As previously mentioned, they should be administered at least 1 hour before or 4–6 hours after bile acid sequestrants when this combination is desired. Fluvastatin, lovastatin, pravastatin, and simvastatin have been specifically indicated to reduce the mortality of coronary heart disease and stroke. By reducing plasma LDL levels, these compounds slow the progression of atherosclerosis and reduce the risk of MI and other ramifications of vascular occlusion. Since Atorvastatin, the newest agent, acts via the same mechanism as the above four compounds, it is reasonable to predict that its uses and approved indications will gradually increase as more information becomes available. Inhibitors of HMG CoA reductase are contraindicated in pregnancy. Fetal development requires cholesterol as a precursor for the synthesis of steroids and cell membranes; thus, inhibition of its synthesis may cause fetal harm. Additionally, HMGRIs are excreted in breast milk and should not be used by nursing mothers.

Unlabeled Uses

Hypertriglyceridemia, stroke paralysis

Potential Nonlipid-lowering Uses of HMGRIs

Cellular metabolites derived from mevalonic acid are required for cell proliferation. Cholesterol is an essential component of cell membranes, farnesyl pyrophosphate is required to covalently bind to intracellular proteins and modify their function, ubiquinone is required for mitochondrial electron transport, and dolichol phosphates are required for glycoprotein synthesis.

Ubiquinone

Dolichol phosphate
(n = 15-19)

Farnesyl pyrophosphate (Fig. 25.2) is an intermediate in the biosynthesis of cholesterol, ubiquinone, and dolichol phosphates. Based on their site of action, HMGRIs will decrease the availability of all four of these compounds and thus decrease cell proliferation. Potential applications of this antiproliferative effect include the prevention of restenosis following angioplasty, prevention of glomerular injury in renal disease, treatment of malignant disease, and prevention of organ transplantation rejection (47).

Adverse Effects

The most prevalent or significant side effects of HMGRIs are listed here (8,20,27). In general, this class of drugs is well tolerated. Gastrointestinal disturbances are the most common complaint; however, these and other adverse reactions tend to be mild and transient. Elevations in hepatic transaminase levels can occur with all HMGRIs. These in-

Adverse Effects of HMGRIs

Constipation, flatulence, dyspepsia, abdominal pain, diarrhea, nausea, vomiting, headache, rhinitis, sinusitis, elevated hepatic enzymes, arthralgia, myalgia, myopathy, muscle cramps, rhabdomyolysis

creases usually occur shortly after the initiation of therapy and resolve after the discontinuation of medication. In a small percentage of patients, these levels can increase to more than three times the upper limit of normal. Therefore, liver function tests should be done at the initiation of therapy, 6 and 12 weeks after the initiation of therapy, and at periodic intervals (e.g., 6 months) thereafter. Similar testing should be done with dosage increases. Approximately 5–10% of patients will experience mild increases in creatine phosphokinase (CPK) levels; however, less than 1% will develop symptoms of myalgia and myopathy (e.g., fever, muscle aches or cramps, unusual tiredness or weakness). Tests for CPK levels should be performed in patients reporting muscle complaints. Rhabdomyolysis, massive muscle necrosis with secondary acute renal failure, has occurred, but is rare. The risk of this very serious adverse effect increases when an HMGRI

Drug Interactions

Drug interactions for HMGRIs are listed in Table 25.6

is taken with certain other medications, such as cyclosporin, erythromycin, niacin, or the fibrates (Table 25.6). In August 2001, Bayer Pharmaceuticals voluntarily withdrew cerivastatin from the U.S. market due to 31 deaths associated with rhabdomyolysis. Of these deaths, 12 involved the concomitant use of the fibrate, gemfibrozil (48).

FIBRATES
Historical Overview and Development

The use of this class of drugs to treat hyperlipoproteinemias can be traced back to 1962 and thus predates the use of bile acid sequestrants and HMGRIs. A random screening test on a series of aryloxyisobutyric acids demonstrated that these compounds could lower both plasma cholesterol and total lipid levels (49). The compound which produced the best balance between activity and toxicity was ethyl *p*-chlorophenoxyisobutyrate (Fig. 25.10). Later renamed clofibrate, this compound was subsequently shown to be a pro-drug for *p*-chlorophenoxyisobutyric acid (clofibric acid). It was approved for therapeutic use in 1967, and for a time, it was a very popular and widely prescribed drug. Results from a 1978 World Health Organization trial changed the acceptance of clofibrate and dramatically decreased its use. These trials indicated that despite a 9% lowering of cholesterol, patients taking clofibrate showed no reduction of cardiovascular events and actually had an increase in overall mortality (8). Despite this, clofibrate has served as the prototype for the design of safer and more effective fibrates. Structural modifications, focused primarily on ring

Table 25.6. Drug Interactions for HMG CoA Reductase Inhibitors

Drug	HMGRI(s)	Result of Interaction
Antacids	Atorvastatin	Decreased levels of atorvastatin; no change in plasma LDL reduction
Azole antifungal agents	All	Increased risk of severe myopathy or rhabdomyolysis; increased plasma levels of atorvastatin, cerivastatin, lovastatin, and simvastatin due to inhibition of CYP3A4; Additive decreases in concentrations or activity of endogenous steroid hormones
Bile acid sequestrants	All	Decreased bioavailability of HMGRI if administration is not adequately spaced
Cimetidine	All	Additive decreases in concentrations or activity of endogenous steroid hormones; increase in plasma fluvastatin levels
Cyclosporine	All	Increased risk of severe myopathy or rhabdomyolysis
Danazol	Lovastatin	Increased risk of severe myopathy or rhabdomyolysis
Digoxin	All	Slight elevation in plasma concentrations of digoxin
Erythromycin	All	Increased risk of severe myopathy or rhabdomyolysis; increased plasma levels of atorvastatin, cerivastatin, lovastatin, and simvastatin due to inhibition of CYP3A4
Ethanol	Fluvastatin, Lovastatin	Increased risk of hepatotoxicity
Fibrates	All	Increased risk of severe myopathy or rhabdomyolysis
Isradipine	Lovastatin	Increased clearance of lovastatin and its metabolites
Niacin	All	Increased risk of severe myopathy or rhabdomyolysis
Omeprazole	Fluvastatin	Increase in plasma fluvastatin levels
Oral contraceptives	Atorvastatin	Increased plasma concentrations of norethindrone and ethinyl estradiol
Propranolol	All	Decreased antihyperlipidemic effect
Ranitidine	Fluvastatin	Increase in plasma fluvastatin levels
Rifampin	Fluvastatin	Increased plasma clearance of fluvastatin
Spironolactone	All	Additive decreases in concentrations or activity of endogenous steroid hormones
Warfarin	All	Anticoagulant effect of warfarin may be increased

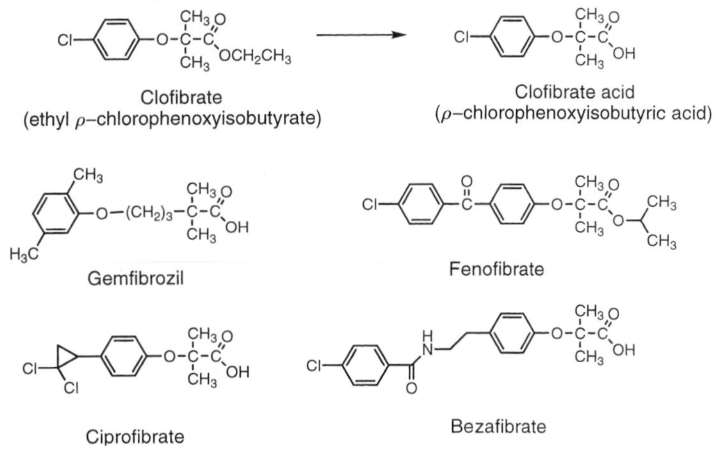

Fig. 25.10. Bioactivation of clofibrate and chemical structures of other fibrates.

substitutions and the addition of spacer groups, have produced a number of active compounds (Fig. 25.10). Gemfibrozil and fenofibrate became available for therapy in 1981 and 1998, respectively. Fenofibrate was actually approved in 1993; however, its marketing was voluntarily delayed until a more bioavailable, micronized formulation of the drug was available (50). Both of these compounds are more effective than clofibrate in lowering plasma triglyceride levels and increasing plasma HDL levels. Additional compounds, such as ciprofibrate and bezafibrate, are not currently available in the U.S. but have been used in other countries.

Mechanism of Action

Overall, fibrates decrease plasma triglyceride levels much more dramatically than plasma cholesterol levels. They significantly decrease VLDL levels, cause a moderate increase in HDL levels, and have variable effects on LDL concentrations. As an example of this latter point, gemfibrozil will raise LDL levels in patients with hypertriglyceridemia, but lower LDL levels in patients with normal triglyceride levels. The exact mechanisms for these actions have not been fully elucidated; however, studies have shown that this class of compounds can produce a variety of beneficial effects on lipoprotein metabolism (8,20,21,50). Many of these effects have been proposed to be mediated through the activation of peroxisome proliferator activated receptors (PPARs) and an alteration of gene expression (8,20).

Decreases in plasma VLDL are primarily due to the ability of these compounds to stimulate the activity of lipoprotein lipase, the enzyme responsible for removing triglycerides from plasma VLDL (Fig. 25.5). Additionally, fibrates can lower VLDL levels through inhibition of triglyceride synthesis, inhibition of hepatic VLDL production, and inhibition of VLDL release. They can also alter the composition of VLDL by decreasing the production of apolipoproteins B and C-III. Decreasing the amounts of apoC-III aids in the stimulation of lipoprotein lipase since this apolipoprotein inhibits the enzyme.

Favorable effects on HDL levels may be related to the induction of lipoprotein lipase and VLDL catabolism. High levels of VLDL lead to the exchange of VLDL triglycerides with HDL cholesterol esters and cause an overall reduction in HDL cholesterol. A reduction in VLDL levels through the mechanisms described above leads to a decreased exchange and a rise in HDL cholesterol. Additionally, fenofibrate has been shown to increase HDL production through a PPAR-induced increase in gene transcription.

Clofibrate decreases serum cholesterol by inhibiting cholesterol biosynthesis prior to mevalonate formation. All fibrates accelerate the turnover and removal of cholesterol from the liver. This increases the biliary secretion of cholesterol, enhances its fecal excretion, and may cause cholelithiasis (i.e., gallstone formation).

Structure-activity Relationships

Fibrates can be chemically classified as analogs of phenoxyisobutyric acid. Literature references to SAR for this class of drugs is sparse; however, all compounds are analogs of the following general structure.

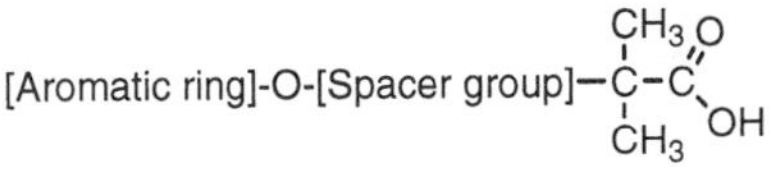

$$[Aromatic\ ring]-O-[Spacer\ group]-\underset{CH_3}{\overset{CH_3}{C}}-\overset{O}{C}\diagdown OH$$

The isobutyric acid group is essential for activity. Compounds containing an ester, such as clofibrate and fenofibrate, are pro-drugs and require in vivo hydrolysis. Substitution at the *para* position of the aromatic ring with a chloro group or a chlorine containing isopropyl ring produces compounds with significantly longer half-lives. While most compounds contain a phenoxyisobutyric acid, the addition of an m-propyl spacer, as seen in gemfibrozil, results in an active drug.

Physicochemical Properties

Similar to HMGRIs, the active forms of all fibrates contain a carboxylic acid. The pKa of this functional

Table 25.7. Pharmacokinetic Parameters of Fibrates

Drug	Calculated Log P	Oral Bioavailability (%)	Effect of Food on Absorption	Active Metabolite(s)	Protein Binding (%)	Time to Peak Concentration (hr)	Elimination Half-Life (hr)	Major Route(s) of Elimination
Clofibrate	3.65	95–99	Increased	Clofibric acid	95–97	3–6	18–22	Renal (95–99)
Fenofibrate	5.24	60–90	Increased	Fenofibric acid	99	4–6	20–22	Renal (60–90) Fecal (5–25)
Gemfibrozil	3.9	>90	Increased	None	99	1–2	1.5	Renal (70) Fecal (6)

Table 25.8. Dosing Information for Fibrates

Generic Name	Brand Name(s)	Approved Indications	Dosing Range	Maximum Daily Dose	Dose Reduction with Renal Dysfunction	Available Tablet/Capsule Strengths (mg)
Clofibrate	Atromid-S	Dysbetalipoproteinemia, Hypertriglyceridemia	1–2 g/daily divided into 2–4 doses	2g	yes	500
Fenofibrate	TriCor	Hypertriglyceridemia	67–201 mg qd	201 mg	only with severe impairment	67
Gemfibrozil	Lopid	Familial combined hyperlipidemia, hypertriglyceridemia	900 mg qd or 600 mg BID	1500 mg	yes	300, 600

group on clofibric acid is reported to be 3.5 (43), and will thus be primarily ionized at physiologic pH. Although not reported, the pKa and ionization values of gemfibrozil and fenofibric acid can reasonably be assumed to be similar. Both clofibrate and fenofibrate are neutral, ester pro-drugs and should be classified as non-electrolytes. Gemfibrozil can be classified as an acidic drug. The calculated log P values for the fibrates are shown in Table 25.7 (43). All three compounds are highly lipid soluble, despite the fact that gemfibrozil contains a water soluble carboxylic acid. This can be partially explained by examining the π values for the substituents present on clofibrate and gemfibrozil (51). The 2,5-dimethyl ring in gemfibrozil is predicted to be much more hydrophobic than the 4-chloro ring of clofibrate. Additionally, the propyl bridge seen in gemfibrozil, but not clofibrate, significantly adds to its hydrophobicity. All currently available fibrates are achiral molecules and not subject to stereochemical concerns.

Metabolism

The pro-drugs, clofibrate and fenofibrate, undergo rapid hydrolysis to produce clofibric acid and fenofibric acid, respectively. These active compounds can then be further metabolized by oxidative or conjugative pathways. Gemfibrozil is slightly different in that it does not require initial bioactivation; however similar to the other agents, it can be oxidized or conjugated. Oxidation of the aromatic methyl groups produces inactive, hydroxymethyl and carboxylic acid analogs. As a drug class, fibrates and their oxidized analogs are primarily excreted as glucuronide conjugates in the urine. Oxidization requires the CYP3A4 isozyme; however, due to the ability of these compounds to be conjugated and eliminated either with or without oxidation, drug interactions with other compounds affecting the CYP3A4 system are less important here than with other drug classes.

Pharmacokinetic Parameters

The pharmacokinetic parameters and dosing information for the fibrates are summarized in Tables 25.7 and 25.8, respectively (8,20,26,27,43,52). The pro-drugs, clofibrate and fenofibrate, require a longer time to reach peak concentrations than does gemfibrozil. Due to differences in aromatic substitution, they also have a much longer half-life than gemfibrozil. As previously mentioned, the 2,5-dimethyl substitution present in gemfibrozil is much more susceptible to oxidative metabolism than the para-chloro groups present in clofibrate and gemfibrozil. Similar to HMGRIs, initiation of fibrate therapy does not produce an immediate effect. Clofibrate therapy requires 2–5 days to cause an initial decrease in plasma triglyceride levels and 3 weeks to produce maximum clinical effects. Fenofibrate may require up to 6–8 weeks to determine efficacy.

Fibrates have excellent bioavailability and are extensively bound to plasma proteins. Because food can significantly enhance their oral absorption, these compounds should be taken either with or just prior to meals. Fenofibrate was available in Europe and other countries as standard tablet and capsule formulations for many years prior to U.S. approval and marketing. It was introduced in the U.S. only after the development of a micronized formulation which allowed for better oral absorption, a lower daily dose, and a once daily administration. A 67 mg dose of micronized fenofibrate is bioequivalent to a 100 mg dose of nonmicronized drug.

Renal elimination is the primary route through which these compounds are excreted from the body. Patients with mild renal dysfunction can often be managed with minor dosage adjustments while those with severe impairment or renal failure may have to discontinue use.

Therapeutic Applications

Fibrates are approved to treat hypertriglyceridemia, familial combined hyperlipidemia, and dysbetalipoproteinemia (Fredrickson's type IIb, III, IV, and V, see Table 25.2) in patients who are at risk of pancreatitis and have not responded to dietary adjustments or in patients who are at risk of coronary heart disease and have not responded to weight loss, dietary adjustments, and other pharmacologic treatment. They can be used either alone or in combination with niacin, bile acid sequestrants, or HMGRIs. If used with bile acid sequestrants, fibrates must be taken either 1 hour before or 4–6 hours after the sequestrant. As discussed previously and re-emphasized below, caution should be used if fibrates are combined with HMGRIs. Fibrates are not effective in the treatment of hypertriglyceridemia associated solely to elevated chylomicron levels (Fredrickson's type I).

Unlabeled Uses

Diabetes insipidus

Adverse Effects

The most prevalent or significant side effects caused by the fibrates are listed here (8,20,21). Despite the potential to cause serious side effects, fibrates are usually well tolerated. Gastrointestinal complaints are the most common, but do not usually cause discontinuation of therapy. In general, gemfibrozil and fenofibrate appear to be safer agents than clofibrate. In fact, many of the concerns regarding fibrate therapy are based upon the effects of clofibrate and the results of a 1978 clinical trial in which patients taking clofibrate had a significantly higher morbidity and mortality from causes other than coronary heart disease. These included malignancy, gall bladder disease, pancreatitis, and post-cholecystectomy complications. Studies with gemfibrozil and fenofibrate have not shown similar increases; however, since all fibrates have similar pharmacologic actions, cautions and

Adverse Effects

Abdominal pain, dyspepsia, nausea, vomiting, diarrhea, cholestasis, jaundice, cholelithiasis, pancreatitis, headache, dizziness, drowsiness, blurred vision, mental depression, impotence, decreased libido, myopathy, myositis, rhabdomyolysis, anemia, leukopenia, eosinophilia, pruritus, rash

contraindications are generally applied to the entire drug class. As an example, even though gemfibrozil and fenofibrate have not demonstrated a significant increase in gallbladder disease seen with clofibrate, all three of these compounds are contraindicated in patients with preexisting gall bladder disease or cholelithiasis. Similar to HMGRIs, fibrates can cause myopathy, myositis, and rhabdomyolysis. Although rare, the risk of these serious effects increases when these two classes of agents are used together.

NICOTINIC ACID
Historical Overview

The history of nicotinic acid (niacin) began in 1867 when it was first synthesized by oxidation of nicotine. The name niacin was derived later from the words *ni*cotinic *ac*id and vitam*in* in an effort to avoid confusing nicotinic acid and nicotinamide with nicotine. Although the terms niacin and nicotinic acid are today used interchangeably, only the more chemically descriptive term, nicotinic acid, will be used in the following discussions.

Nicotine   Nicotinic acid   Nicotinamide

The biochemical and pharmacologic actions of nicotinic acid began in the early 1900s when brewer's yeast was demonstrated to prevent pellagra in humans. The subsequent isolation of nicotinic acid from brewer's yeast established its role as an essential dietary requirement. In the 1930s, its amide metabolite, nicotinamide, was isolated from liver extracts and found to be a required structural feature of nicotinamide adenine dinucleotide phosphate (NADP$^+$), a cofactor involved in electron transport and intermediary metabolism (53). In 1955, Altschul and coworkers (54) observed that high doses of nicotinic acid lowered cholesterol levels in humans, an activity unrelated to its properties as a vitamin. Subsequent studies have

Table 25.9. Drug Interactions for Fibrates

Drug	HMGRI(s)	Result of Interaction
Bile acid sequestrants	All	Decreased bioavailability of fibrate if administration is not adequately spaced
Cyclosporine	Fenofibrate	Increased potential for nephrotoxicity
Dantrolene	Clofibrate	Reduction of dantrolene plasma protein binding
Furosemide	Clofibrate	Possible exaggeration of diuretic response in patients with hypoalbuminemia
HMG CoA reductase inhibitors	All	Increased risk of severe myopathy or rhabdomyolysis
Insulin	Clofibrate	Increased effects of insulin resulting in hypoglycemia
Oral Anticoagulants	All	Increased hypoprothrombinemic effect
Oral contraceptives	Clofibrate	Increased elimination of clofibric acid
Probenecid	Clofibrate	Increased plasma levels of clofibrate
Rifampin	Clofibrate	Decreased clofibrate concentrations due to enhanced metabolism
Sulfonylurea	All	Increased effects of the sulfonylurea resulting in hypoglycemia
Ursodiol	Clofibrate	Increased hepatic cholesterol secretion which may increase the possibility of gallstone formation and counteract the effectiveness of ursodiol

shown that nicotinic acid also lowers serum triglyceride levels and is effective against a variety of hyperlipoproteinemias. None of these antihyperlipidemic effects are seen with nicotinamide.

Mechanism of Action

Nicotinic acid exerts a variety of effects on lipoprotein metabolism (8,21,55). One of its most important actions is the inhibition of lipolysis in adipose tissue. This initial inhibition, like those of previously discussed antihyperlipidemic agents, produces a sequence of events which ultimately result in the lowering of plasma triglycerides and cholesterol. Impaired lipolysis decreases the mobilization of free fatty acids thus reducing their plasma levels and their delivery to the liver. This in turn decreases hepatic triglyceride synthesis and results in a decreased production of VLDL. Enhanced clearance of VLDL through stimulation of lipoprotein lipase has also been proposed to contribute to the reduction of plasma VLDL levels. Since LDL is derived from VLDL (Fig. 25.5), the decreased production of VLDL ultimately leads to a decrease in LDL levels. The sequential nature of this process has been clinically demonstrated. The reduction in triglyceride levels occurs within several hours after initiation of nicotinic acid therapy, while the reduction in cholesterol does not occur until after several days of therapy. Unlike bile acid sequestrants and HMG CoA reductase inhibitors, nicotinic acid does not have any effects on cholesterol catabolism or biosynthesis.

Physicochemical Properties

Nicotinic acid (niacin) is a stable, nonhygroscopic, white, crystalline powder. Its carboxylic acid has a pKa of 4.76 and is thus predominantly ionized at physiologic pH. The pyrimidine nitrogen is a very weak base (pKa 2.0) and thus primarily exists in the un-ionized form. Nicotinic acid is freely soluble in alkaline solutions and has a measured Log P of -0.20 at pH 6.0 (43).

Metabolism

Nicotinic acid is a B-complex vitamin which is converted to nicotinamide, NAD^+, and $NADP^+$. The latter two compounds are coenzymes and are required for oxidation/reduction reactions in a variety of biochemical pathways. Additionally, nicotinic acid is metabolized to a number of inactive compounds, including nicotinuric acid and N-methylated derivatives. Normal biochemical regulation and feedback prevent large doses of nicotinic acid from producing excess quantities of NAD^+ and $NADP^+$. Thus, small doses of nicotinic acid, such as those used for dietary supplementation, will be primarily excreted as metabolites, while large doses, such as those used for the treatment of hyperlipoproteinemia, will be primarily excreted unchanged by the kidney (20).

Pharmacokinetic Parameters

Nicotinic acid is readily absorbed. Peripheral vasodilation is seen within 20 minutes and peak plasma concentrations occur within 45 minutes. The half-life of the compound is approximately one hour, thus necessitating frequent dosing or an extended release formulation. Extended release tablets produce peripheral vasodilation within one hour, reach peak plasma concentrations within four to five hours, and have a duration of 8–10 hours.

Dosing of nicotinic acid should be titrated to minimize adverse effects. An initial dose of 50–100 mg TID is often used with immediate release tablets. The dose is then gradually increased by 50–100 mg every 3–14 days, up to a maximum of 6 grams/day, as tolerated. Therapeutic monitoring to assess efficacy and prevent toxicity is essential until a stable and effective dose is reached. Similar dosing escalations are available for extended release products (8,20,26).

Therapeutic Applications

Nicotinic acid is approved for the treatment of hypercholesterolemia, hypertriglyceridemia, and familial combined hyperlipidemia (Fredrickson's type IIa, IIb, IV and V, see Table 25.2) in patients who have not responded to diet, exercise, and other nonpharmacologic methods. It is also approved for nutritional supplementation, the prevention of pellagra, and as adjunctive therapy for peripheral vascular disease and circulatory disorders. It is contraindicated in patients with hepatic disease and peptic ulcer disease. Additionally, due to its ability to elevate glucose and uric acid levels, especially when taken in large doses, nicotinic acid should be used with caution in patients with or predisposed to diabetes mellitus and gout (26).

Adverse Effects of Niacin

Flushing, pruritus, headache, nausea, vomiting, diarrhea, flatulence, hepatic dysfunction, jaundice, hyperglycemia, hyperuricemia, blurred vision, and tachycardia

Adverse Effects

The most common, and often dose-limiting, side effects of nicotinic acid treatment are cutaneous vasodilation (flushing and pruritus) and gastrointestinal intolerance, which may occur in 20–50% of treated patients. Flushing and pruritus are prostaglandin-mediated effects and may be prevented by taking aspirin or indomethacin prior to nicotinic acid. Gastrointestinal side effects such as flatulence, nausea, vomiting, and diarrhea, can be minimized if nicotinic acid is taken either with or immediately after meals. As previously mentioned, all of these effects can be minimized by slowly titrating the dose of nicotinic acid. Hepatic dysfunction is one of the more serious complications of high dose nicotinic acid. Plasma aspartate transaminase (AST), alanine transaminase (ALT), lactate dehydrogenase (LDH), and alkaline phosphatase levels are often elevated, but usually return to normal when therapy is either adjusted or discontinued (8,20).

Drug Interactions

Drug Interactions for niacin are listed in Table 25.10

Table 25.10. Drug Interactions for Nicotinic Acid

Drug	Result of Interaction
Adrenergic blocking agents	Enhance vasodilation and postural hypotension
Ethanol	Potential enhanced hepatoxicity and excessive peripheral or cutaneous vasodilation
Lovastatin	Increased risk of myopathy and rhabdomyolysis. Caution should be used with all HMG CoA reductase inhibitors

CASE STUDY

Victoria F. Roche and S. William Zito

TLH is a 35-year-old, full-blooded, female member of the Navajo tribe. An artisan, she lives and works outside of Taos, New Mexico and spends her days making and selling jewelry in a silver and turquoise shop. Like many women of Native American heritage, TLH has cholelithiasis (gallstones). Fortunately, her condition has been, for the most part, asymptomatic, and she has declined to have her gall bladder surgically removed. Her medical history also includes adult onset diabetes mellitus, for which she is taking the sulfonylurea hypoglycemic agent chlorpropamide (250 mg qd). She has a family history of cardiovascular disease, and her father died after suffering a severe MI secondary to atherosclerosis at the age of 63. Her liver and kidney function is normal. TLH tries to keep her blood sugar and the symptoms of her cholelithiasis under control by monitoring her diet but finds it difficult to exercise regularly. In fact, she is getting no exercise at all these days, as she has been recuperating from surgery to repair a torn ligament in her left knee. Oral warfarin therapy has also been started to treat deep vein thrombosis that commonly occurs after mobility-limiting surgery of this type. Her physician is recommending a longer course of therapy than usual (e.g., 4–6 months) due to her sedentary life style.

TLH's pre-surgery blood work-up showed normal triglyceride levels, but a significant elevation of her total serum cholesterol (280 mg/dL) and LDL (190 mg/dL). Her HDL level is borderline-low (52 mg/dL). Blood lipid-lowering therapy is indicated. Consider the relative merit of the following drug candidates for the treatment of this patient.

1. *Identify the therapeutic problem(s) where the pharmacist's intervention may benefit the patient.*

2. *Identify and prioritize the patient specific factors that must be considered to achieve the desired therapeutic outcomes.*

3. *Conduct a thorough and mechanistically oriented structure-activity analysis of all therapeutic alternatives provided in the case.*

4. *Evaluate the SAR findings against the patient specific factors and desired therapeutic outcomes and make a therapeutic decision.*

5. *Counsel your patient.*

REFERENCES

1. Ginsberg HN, Goldberg IJ. Disorders of lipoprotein metabolism. In: Fauci AS, Braunwald E, Isselbacher KJ, et al, eds. Harrison's principles of internal medicine. 14th ed. New York: McGraw Hill, 1998; 2138–2149.
2. Annon. Choice of lipid-lowering drugs. The Medical Letter 1998;40:117–122.
3. Zoeller J. The top 200 drugs. American Druggist 1999;216:41–48.
4. Stryer L. Biochemistry. 4th ed. New York: Freeman and Company, 1995; 685–712.
5. Zubay GL. Biochemistry. 4th ed. Dubuque, IA: Wm. C. Brown, 1998; 532–560.
6. Bamford MJ, Chan C, Craven AP, et al. The squalestatins: synthesis and biological activity of some C3–modified analogues; replacement of a carboxylic acid or methyl ester with an isoelectronic heterocyclic functionality. J Med Chem 1995;38: 3502–3513.
7. Chan C, Andreotti D, Cox B, et al. The squalestatins: decarboxy and 4-deoxy analogues as potent squalene synthase inhibitors. J Med Chem 1996;39:207–216.
8. Witztum JL. Drugs used in the treatment of hyperlipoproteinemias. In: Hardman JG, Limbird LE, Molinoff PB, et al, eds. The pharmacological basis of therapeutics. 9th ed. New York: McGraw-Hill, 1996; 875–897.
9. Brown MS, Goldstein JL. Drugs used in the treatment of hyperlipoproteinemias. In: Gilman AG, Rall TW, Nies AS, et al, eds. The pharmacological basis of therapeutics. 8th ed. New York: Pergamon Press, 1990; 874–896.
10. Talbert RL. Hyperlipidemia. In: Dipiro JT, Talbert RL, Yee GC, et al, eds. Pharmacotherapy, a pathophysiologic approach, 3rd ed. Stamford, CT: Appleton & Lange, 1997; 459–489.
11. McKenney JM. Dyslipidemias. In: Young LY, Koda-Kimble MA, eds. Applied therapeutics: the clinical use of drugs. 6th ed. Vancouver, WA: Applied Therapeutics, Inc., 1995.
12. Orci L, Brown MS, Goldstein JL, et al. Increase in membrane cholesterol: a possible trigger for degradation of HMG CoA reductase and crystalloid endoplasmic reticulum in UT-1 cells. Cell 1984;36:835–45.
13. Fredrickson DS, Levy RI, Lees RS. Fat transport in lipoproteins–an integrated approach to mechanisms and disorders. N Engl J Med 1967;276:34–42.
14. (a)American Heart Association. 1999 Heart and stroke statistical update. In: http://www.americanheart.org/statistics. Accessed June 1999; (b) McKenney JM. New guidelines for managing hypercholesterolemia. J Am Pharm Assoc 2001;41:596–607.
15. Libby P. Atherosclerosis. In: Fauci AS, Braunwald E, Isselbacher KJ, et al, eds. Harrison's principles of internal medicine. 14th ed. New York: McGraw Hill, 1998; 1345–1352.
16. Sliskovic DR, White AD. Therapeutic potential of ACAT inhibitors as lipid lowering and anti-atherosclerotic agents. Trends Pharmacol Sci 1991;12:194–199.
17. Annon. APhA special report: Primary and secondary prevention of atherosclerotic vascular disease; a continuing education program for pharmacists. Washington DC: American Pharmaceutical Association, 1998.
18. Berkow R, Fletcher AJ, eds. Merck Manual. 16th ed. Rahway, NJ: Merck Research Laboratories, 1992; 1038–1048.
19. Roth B. ACAT inhibitors: evolution from cholesterol-absorption inhibitors to antiatherosclerotic agents. Drug Discov Today 1998;3:19–25.
20. Clinical Pharmacology [CD-ROM]. Reents S, Seymour J, eds. Tampa, FL: Gold Standard Multimedia, 1999.
21. Cendella RJ. Cholesterol and hypocholesterolemic drugs. In: Craig CR, Stitzel RE, eds. Modern pharmacology with clinical applications. 5th ed. Boston: Little, Brown, 1997, 279–289.
22. Brown MS, Goldstein JL. A receptor-mediated pathway for cholesterol homeostasis. Science 1986;232:34–47.
23. Blanchard J, Nairn JG. The binding of cholate and glycocholate anions by anion-exchange resins. J Phys Chem 1968;72:1204–1208.
24. Zhu XX, Brown GR, St-Pierre LE. Polymeric sorbents for bile acids. I: Comparison between cholestyramine and colestipol. J Pharm Sci 1992;81:65–69.
25. Clas SD. Quaternized colestipol, an improved bile salt adsorbent: in vitro studies. J Pharm Sci 1991;80:128–131.
26. Gelman CR, Rumack BH, Klasco R, eds. Drugdex system [CD-ROM] Englewood, CO: Micromedex, 1999.
27. Drug Facts and Comparisons. St. Louis, MO: Facts and Comparisons, 1998; 1065–1092.
28. Heathcock CH, Hadley CR, Rosen T, et al. Total synthesis and biological evaluation of structural analogues of compactin and dihydromevinolin. J Med Chem 1987;30:1858–1873.
29. Adams JL, Metcalf BW. Therapeutic consequences of the inhibition of sterol metabolism. In: Hansch C, Sammes PG, Taylor JB, eds. Comprehensive Medicinal Chemistry. Volume 2. Oxford: Permagon Press, 1990;333–363.
30. Cocolas GH. Cardiovascular agents. In: Delgado JN, Remers WA, eds. Textbook of organic medicinal and pharmaceutical chemistry. 10th ed. Philadelphia: Lippincott-Raven, 1998; 616–620.
31. Stokker GE, Hoffman WF, Alberts AW, et al. 3-Hydroxy-3-methylglutaryl-coenzyme A reductase inhibitors. 1. Structural modification of 5-substituted 3,5-dihydroxypentanoic acids and their lactone derivatives. J Med Chem 1985;28:347–358.
32. Sliskovic DR, Blankley CJ, Krause BR, et al. Inhibitors of cholesterol biosynthesis. 6. trans-5-[2-(N-Heteroaryl-3,5-disubstituted-pyrazol-4-yl)ethyl/ethenyl]tetrahydro-4-hydroxy-2H-pyran-2-ones. J Med Chem 1992;35:2095–2103.
33. Bone EA, Davidson AH, Lewis CN, et al. Synthesis and biological evaluation of dihydroeptastatin, a novel inhibitor of 3-hydroxy-3-methylglutaryl coenzyme A reductase. J Med Chem 1992;35:3388–3393.
34. Roth BD, Ortwine DF, Hoefle ML, et al. Inhibitors of cholesterol biosynthesis. 1. trans-6-(2-Pyrrol-1-ylethyl)-4-hydroxypyran-2-ones, a novel series of HMG-CoA reductase inhibitors. 1. Effects of structural modifications at the 2-and 5-positions of the pyrrole nucleus. J Med Chem 1990;33:21–31.
35. Hoffman WF, Alberts AW, Cragoe Jr EJ, et al. 3-Hydroxy-3-methylglutaryl-coenzyme A reductase inhibitors. 2. Structural modification of 7-(substituted aryl)-3,5-dihydroxy-6-heptenoic acids and their lactone derivatives. J Med Chem 1986;29: 159–169.
36. Stokker GE, Alberts AW, Anderson PS, et al. 3-Hydroxy-3-methylglutaryl-coenzyme A reductase inhibitors. 3. 7-(3,5-Disubstituted [1,1′-biphenyl]-2-yl)-3,5-dihydroxy-6-heptenoic acids and their lactone derivatives. J Med Chem 1986;29:170–181.
37. Heathcock CH, Davis BR, Hadley CR. Synthesis and biological evaluation of a monocyclic, fully functional analogue of compactin. J Med Chem 1989;32:197–202.
38. Lee TJ, Holtz WJ, Smith RL, et al. 3-Hydroxy-3-methylglutaryl-coenzyme A reductase inhibitors. 8. Side chain ether analogues of lovastatin. J Med Chem 1991;34:2474–2477.
39. Hoffman WF, Alberts AW, Anderson PS, et al. 3-Hydroxy-3-methylglutaryl-coenzyme A reductase inhibitors. 4. Side chain ester derivatives of mevinolin. J Med Chem 1986;29:849–852.
40. Stokker GE, Alberts AW, Gilfillan JL, et al. 3-Hydroxy-3-methylglutaryl-coenzyme A reductase inhibitors. 5. 6-(Fluoren-9-yl)- and 6-(fluoren-9-ylidenyl)-3,5-dihydroxyhexanoic acids and their lactone derivatives. J Med Chem 1986;29:852–855.

41. Procopiou PA, Draper CD, Hutson JL, et al. Inhibitors of cholesterol biosynthesis. 2. 3,5-Dihydroxy-7-(N-pyrrolyl)-6-heptenoates, a novel series of HMG-CoA reductase inhibitors. J Med Chem 1993;36:3658–3662.

42. Annon. Atorvastatin–a new lipid-lowering drug. The Medical Letter 1997;39:29–31.

43. Craig PN. Drug Compendium. In: Hansch C, Sammes PG, Taylor JB, eds. Comprehensive Medicinal Chemistry. Volume 6. Oxford: Permagon Press, 1990; 237–991.

44. Values calculated by author using LOGKOW program, Version 1.03 (Meylan W and Howard PH. Syracuse Research Corporation: Syracuse NY, 1993) and SMILES notation obtained from http://clogp.pomona.edu/medchem/chem/master/search.html.

45. Annon. Baycol (cerivastatin sodium tablets) product literature. Bayer Corporation, 1999.

46. Annon. Zocor (simvastatin) product literature. Merck, 1999.

47. Wheeler DC. Are there potential non-lipid-lowering uses of statins? Drugs 1998;56:517–522.

48. FDA Talk Paper. Bayer voluntarily withdraws Baycol. http://www.fda.gov/bbs/topics/ANSWERS/2001/ANS1095.html. Accessed August, 2001.

49. Thorp JM, Waring WS. Modification and distribution of lipids by ethyl chlorophenoxyisobutyrate. Nature 1962;194:948–949.

50. Hussar DA. New drugs of 1998. J Am Pharm Assoc 1999;39:170–172.

51. Hansch C, Leo A. Substituent constants for correlation analysis in chemistry and biology. New York: Wiley, 1979; 49–54.

52. Clinical Reference Library [CD-ROM]. Version 98.1. Hudson, OH: Lexi-Comp, 1998.

53. Garrett RH, Grisham CM. Biochemistry. Fort Worth, TX: Saunders College Publishing, 1995; 468–473.

54. Altschul R, Hoffer A, Stephen JD. Influence of nicotinic acid on serum cholesterol in man. Arch Biochem 1955;54:558–559.

55. Drood JM, Zimetbaum PJ, Frishman WH. Nicotinic acid for the treatment of hyperlipoproteinemia. J Clin Pharmacol 1991; 31:641–650.

26. Antithrombotics, Thrombolytics, Coagulants, and Plasma Extenders

ROBERT B. PALMER, Ph.D.

INTRODUCTION

Question: What do heart attack therapy, porcine intestinal mucosa and rat poison have in common with sweet clover? Answer: Anticoagulation. The discovery, development and eventual therapeutic use of drugs that affect the clotting capabilities of blood is diverse. In 1916, a young coal-miner turned medical student, Jay McLean, was paying his tuition bill for the John's Hopkins medical school by working in the research laboratory of Professor W. H. Howell when he inadvertently isolated heparin (1). In 1933, Dr. K. P. Link discovered that hydroxycoumarins are contained in sweet clover after finding cattle hemorrhaging to death (1). This lead to the development of therapeutic agents such as warfarin and dicoumarol for oral inhibition of blood coagulation.

But, through what mechanism(s) do these and other compounds alter the ability of blood to clot? In order to understand the answer to this question, it is necessary to first understand the normal process of blood coagulation. The formation of a blood clot is not a solitary event. In fact, it is the result of an intricate and elegant cascade of biochemical events (Fig. 26.1).

Two sources of coagulation initiation exist. They are referred to as the intrinsic and extrinsic pathways. These two pathways eventually coalesce into a common pathway in the final stages of clot formation. Initiation of the intrinsic pathway involves the sequential activation of factors XII, XI and IX. (The activated form of a coagulation factor is indicated by a lower case "a.") Factor IXa initiates the activation of factor X to Xa. In addition, initiation of the extrinsic pathway involves activation of factor VII which, like factor IXa, also catalyzes the conversion of factor X to Xa. The underlying purpose of the intrinsic pathway is maintenance of homeostasis while the extrinsic pathway is activated by trauma. The intrinsic and extrinsic pathways come together with the conversion of factor X to its activated form, Xa. The coagulation cascade is unique in that the product of a given reaction (i.e., activated form of a specific factor) catalyzes the activation of the next factor in the cascade. The final steps in the coagulation cascade involve the conversion of prothrombin (factor II) to thrombin (factor IIa) by factor Xa (Fig. 26.2). Thrombin in turn catalyzes the conversion of fibrinogen to soluble fibrin, which then becomes insoluble fibrin through the action of factor XIIIa. In its activated state, factor XIIIa is actually a transamidase enzyme. This enzyme catalyzes the formation of isopeptide bonds between lysine and glutamine side chains of distinct fibrin molecules resulting in crosslinked (insoluble) fibrin aggregates (Fig. 26.3)(2).

Once a clot has formed, its location becomes important. Two terms commonly used to describe specific thrombotic conditions are thrombus (plural, thrombi) and embolus (plural, emboli). A thrombus is a clot adhered to the vascular wall while an embolus is a free-floating clot within the vasculature. Therefore, if a thrombus detaches from the vascular wall, it becomes an embolus. Both thrombi and emboli can occlude vessels resulting in decreased oxygen and nutrient availability to tissues distal to the clot. Arterial thrombi usually form in medium sized vessels as a result of surface lesions on endothelial cells roughened by atherosclerosis. In most cases, circulating platelets adhere to the areas of abnormal vascular endothelium. More platelets then aggregate with those stuck to the vascular wall forming a clot known as a white thrombus (3). This growing white thrombus reduces arterial blood flow through the vessel distal to the clot. Venous thrombi typically result either from inappropriate activation of the coagulation cascade or due to some disease process or venous pooling (stasis) of the blood. These thrombi, called red thrombi, are initiated in much the same fashion as white thrombi (i.e., platelet aggregation) except the bulk of the clot is formed of long fibrin tails that enmesh red blood cells (3). It is also possible for a red thrombus to form around a nidal white thrombus as the blood flow distant to a white thrombus tends to be significantly more static. This stasis allows the formation of the fibrin tails. Regardless of specific origin (arterial or venous) of the red thrombus, the tails easily fragment and embolize, typically into the pulmonary arteries if venous or distal extremity if arterial. As a general rule, arterial thrombi cause serious conditions through localized occlusive ischemia while venous thrombi fragment giving rise to pleural embolic complications.

MEDICAL CONDITIONS REQUIRING ANTICOAGULANT THERAPY

A number of serious medical conditions are thrombotic in nature. In fact, in Western society, thrombotic conditions are the single largest medical cause of morbidity and mortality and it is speculated that these disorders will be the leading cause of death worldwide within 20 years (4). As would be expected from the gravity of thrombotic disorders, many of the conditions involve the major vasculature, heart, brain and lungs.

604

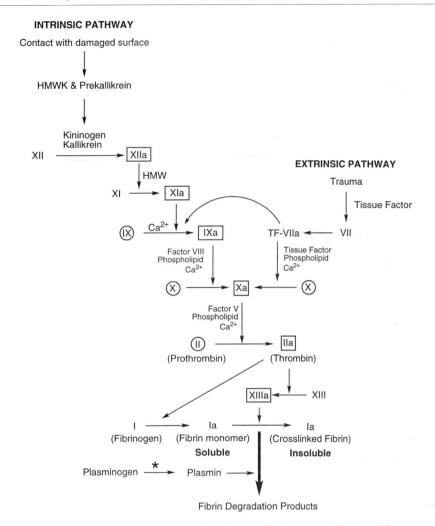

Fig. 26.1. The coagulation cascade. Circled factors are those inhibited by warafin-like drugs while boxed factors are affected by heparin. The star indicates the site of action of thrombolytic drugs such as streptokinase and urokinase.

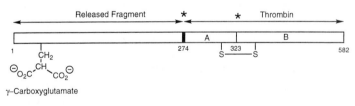

Fig. 26.2. Structure of prothrombin. Thrombin is liberated through the cleavage of the Arg 274-Thr 275 and Arg 323-Ile 324 peptide bonds (indicated with stars). The γ-carboxyglutamate residues are in the released N-terminal portion of prothrombin and are not part of thrombin. The A and B chains of thrombin are joined by a disulfide bond.

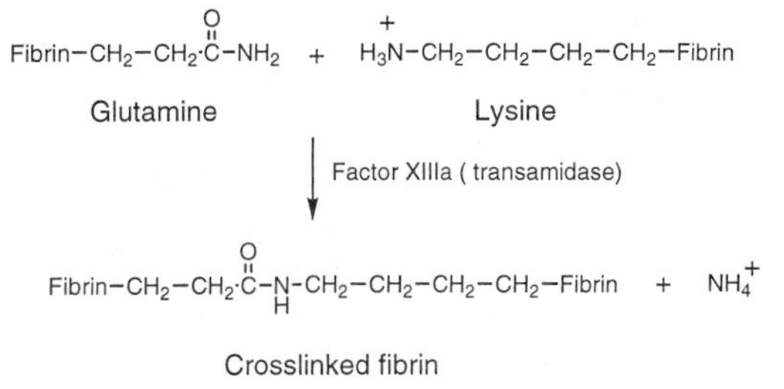

$$Fibrin-CH_2-CH_2\overset{\overset{\displaystyle O}{\|}}{C}-NH_2 \quad + \quad \overset{+}{H_3N}-CH_2-CH_2-CH_2-CH_2-Fibrin$$

Glutamine   Lysine

↓ Factor XIIIa (transamidase)

$$Fibrin-CH_2-CH_2\overset{\overset{\displaystyle O}{\|}}{C}-\underset{H}{N}-CH_2-CH_2-CH_2-CH_2-Fibrin \quad + \quad NH_4^+$$

Crosslinked fibrin

Fig. 26.3. Crosslinking of soluble fibrin monomers (factor Ia) through the activity of factor XIIIa, a transamidase enzyme.

Cardiac conditions involving thrombotic disorders include acute myocardial infarction, valvular heart disease, unstable angina and atrial fibrillation as well as surgical procedures such as percutaneous transluminal coronary angioplasty (PTCA) and prosthetic heart valve replacement. In these cases, therapy is designed to prevent reocclusion after circulation has been restored or to prevent thrombus formation or dislodging (embolization). Thrombotic conditions involving the vasculature include venous thromboembolism, primary and secondary prevention of arterial thromboembolism and peripheral vascular disease. The most significant such condition involving the lungs is pulmonary embolism and in the brain, cerebrovascular accidents (CVAs). Anticoagulation therapy is indicated for all of these conditions. Other miscellaneous indications for anticoagulation therapy include preventing occlusion of intravenous catheters and vascular access shunts and therapy for small cell lung carcinoma and disseminated intravascular coagulation (DIC).

GENERAL APPROACHES TO ANTICOAGULANT THERAPY
Overview

Several factors are used to determine the most appropriate therapeutic regimen for a given patient with a coagulation-based complaint. Considerations such as the patient's medical and drug history, age and location of the clot and underlying diagnosis, to name a few, must be thoroughly investigated. One important point to consider with respect to anticoagulants (also referred to as antithrombotics) such as the orally active vitamin K antagonists and heparin, is that these drugs do not dissolve thrombi that have already formed. Rather, the goal of anticoagulation is prevention of the formation of new thrombi or reocclusion/extension at an existing thrombus. In cases where dissolving an existing clot is necessary, thrombolytic drugs may be of benefit.

There are a few specific areas within the coagulation cascade that are therapeutic targets. The selection of the appropriate portion of the coagulation cascade for attack is based primarily on the ultimate goal of the therapeutic intervention. For example, if lysis of an existing clot is needed, activation of plasminogen, which will degrade insoluble fibrin, is the typical approach. However, if the therapeutic goal is prevention of thrombus formation or extension, inhibition of factor activation higher in the cascade is most appropriate.

Laboratory Assessment and Monitoring

Anticoagulant drug dosing represents a fine balance between reducing the morbidity and mortality associated with the thrombotic condition and minimizing the risk of serious hemorrhage from excessive therapeutic anticoagulation. Due to the potentially life-threatening consequences of either inadequate or excessive anticoagulation, patients receiving antithrombotic medications are often closely monitored with specific clinical laboratory assays. A baseline assessment of the patient's coagulation features is performed prior to the initiation of anticoagulant therapy. This allows detection of congenital coagulation factor deficiencies, thrombocytopenia, hepatorenal insufficiency and vascular abnormalities which could prove catastrophic if anticoagulant therapy was instituted empirically.

For monitoring oral anticoagulant therapy (i.e., vitamin K antagonists), the prothrombin time (PT) is measured(5). This test is used to assess the activity of the vitamin K dependent clotting factors (II, VII, IX and X). The PT is particularly sensitive to factor VII which, though not of great clinical significance in itself, serves as a rough estimate of the ability of the liver to synthesize proteins or the extent of vitamin K depletion from warfarin therapy. The PT assay measures the time it takes for a clot to form in citrated plasma after the addition of tissue thromboplastin and calcium. In normal (i.e., warfarin free) plasma, this clot formation takes 10–13 seconds (5). Due to variances in commercially available thromboplastins, most clinical laboratories now report PT results in terms of International Normalized Ratios (INR's). The INR is calculated using the formula:

$$INR = (PT_{pt}/PT_{ctrl})^{ISI}$$

Where PT_{pt} is the measured PT value for the patient, PT_{ctrl} is the measured PT value for control plasma and ISI is the index of sensitivity for the thromboplastin reagent compared to an international standard and provided for each reagent lot by the manufacturer. Patients on warfarin therapy are optimally maintained with an INR value of 2.0–3.0. In cases of patients that have had mechanical prosthetic heart valves placed, an INR of 2.5–3.5 is often recommended. At the initiation of warfarin therapy, daily PT's are performed. As the drug dosage is adjusted appropriately based on these results, the length of time between PT assessments can be extended to weekly. Finally, after warfarin therapy has been optimized and the patient's PT results have stabilized within an acceptable range, monthly or bimonthly PT checks are reasonable.

Heparin directly deactivates clotting factors II and X. Therapy with this drug is monitored based on the activated partial thromboplastin time (aPTT) assay (5). This assay monitors factors II and X as well as several others. Deficiencies of clotting factors that affect the aPTT result can be of little clinical significance (e.g., prekallikrein and factor XII), potential clinical significance (e.g., factor XI), or great clinical significance (e.g., factors VIII, IX and the hemophilic factors). In the aPTT assay, a surface activator such as elegiac acid, kaolin or silica, is used to activate the intrinsic pathway. When this activator comes in contact with citrated plasma in the presence of calcium and phospholipid, clot formation begins. As with the PT, the time taken for this clot to form is measured. In normal (nonheparinized) plasma, the average aPTT result is 25–45 seconds. A therapeutic aPTT in a patient receiving heparin is typically 70–140 seconds. In vivo, the platelet membrane rather than the phospholipid is the source of several clotting factors and site of many of the coagulation reactions in the intrinsic pathway. The phospholipid used in the aPTT assay does not completely substitute for the in vivo actions of the platelets. While this phospholipid does potentiate the intrinsic pathway, it does so without activating factor VII. This "partial activation" of the intrinsic pathway is the genesis of the name of the assay (activated partial thromboplastin time).

Several other laboratory assays are used to assess function at various points within the clotting cascade. Quantitative levels of fibrinogen and fibrin degradation products are used to assess the extent of the effects of conditions such as acute inflammation DIC and severe liver disease. The specific clotting factor(s) in which a given patient may be deficient can also be determined using various mixing studies(5). These assessments are far more specialized and performed much less frequently than the PT and aPTT.

ORAL ANTICOAGULANTS
Mechanism of Action

The coagulation of blood is dependent upon the cyclic interconversion of vitamin K and vitamin K 2,3-epoxide (Fig. 26.4)(6). Vitamin K is a cofactor necessary for the postribosomal synthesis of several clotting factors including II, VII, IX and X. The vitamin K sensitive step in this process involves the carboxylation of 10 or more glutamate residues on the N-terminal portions of important precursor proteins. This carboxylation results in a new amino acid, γ-carboxyglutamate, which through chelation of calcium ions, causes the proteins to undergo a conformational change. This change in tertiary structure allows the four vitamin K dependent clotting factors to bind to phospholipid membranes during clotting cascade activation.

The specific enzyme that carboxylates vitamin-K dependent coagulation factors requires reduced vitamin K (vitamin K hydroquinone, KH₂), molecular oxygen and carbon dioxide as cofactors. In the process of this reaction, KH₂ is oxidized to vitamin-K 2,3-epoxide. The return of the epoxide to the active KH₂ form is the result of a two step reduction. First, the epoxide is reduced to vitamin-K quinone by vitamin-K 2,3-epoxide reductase in the presence of NADH. This quinone intermediate is then further reduced back to KH₂ by vitamin K quinone reductase. The

warfarin-like anticoagulants (i.e., vitamin K antagonists) exert their anticoagulant activity through the inhibition of vitamin-K 2,3-epoxide reductase and possibly through inhibition of vitamin-K quinone reductase which results in inhibition of the activation of the four affected coagulation factors. In other words, the clotting factors affected are structurally incomplete and incapable of promoting the coagulation cascade. Unlike heparin, and as a direct result of their mechanism of action, the vitamin K antagonists only inhibit blood coagulation in vivo.

Structure-activity Relationship

All of the coumarin derivatives (Fig. 26.5) are water insoluble lactones (7). Though coumarin is a neutral compound, the clinically utilized derivatives are weakly acidic due to a 4-hydroxy substitution. Therefore, reaction of the 4-hydroxycoumarin derivatives with an appropriate base yields water-soluble salts. Because of the acidity of the proton on the 4-hydroxy group of warfarin and the proximity of the side chain carbonyl six atoms away, the possibility of another ring closure exists. If the acidic 4-hydroxy proton is removed, the resulting oxyanion can act as a nucleophile and attack the electrophilic carbonyl carbon forming a hemiketal called cyclocumarol which is neutral.

Structure-activity relationship (SAR) requirements are typically based on substitution of the lactone ring, specifically, in positions 3 and 4. Initial investigation into the anticoagulant activity requirements of coumarin derivatives

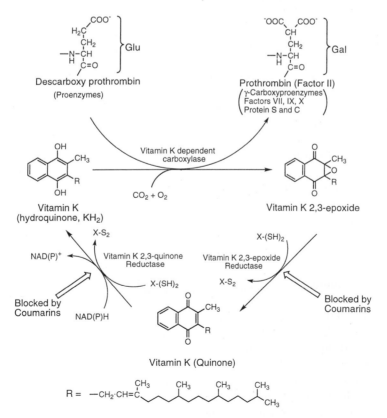

Fig. 26.4. Redox cycling of vitamin K in the activation of blood clotting which involves conversion of glutamate residues to γ-carboxyglutamates.

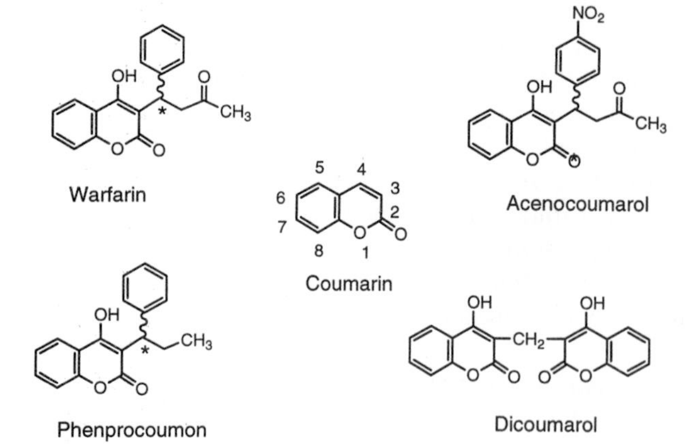

Fig. 26.5. Chemical structures of coumarin and coumarin-derived drugs.

led Link to suggest that a 3-substituent, a 4-hydroxy group and a bis molecule were all necessary (7). Though a bis compound (bishydroxycoumarin, dicoumarol) fits these requirements, it is no longer used clinically. Additional studies have concluded that the methoxy group addition to position 8 increases anticoagulant activity (8).

The conformation of warfarin has been studied by nuclear magnetic resonance spectroscopy. These studies suggest that there are three conformations of the drug in solution—two diastereomeric cyclic hemiketals and one open form. Since it has been suggested that vitamin K forms an active hemiketal in vivo, vitamin K antimetabolite compounds such as warfarin may well be active as the cyclic hemiketals (Fig. 26.6) (9).

Warfarin is a chiral compound. Though the clinically utilized preparation is racemic, the enantiomers are not equipotent. In fact, (S)-warfarin is at least 4-fold more potent as an anticoagulant than the (R)-warfarin. The difference in the activities and metabolism of the enantiomers is key to understanding several stereoselective drug interactions including those with zileuton, miconazole, sulfinpyrazone and cimetidine (10,11,12).

Derivatives of 1,3-indandione are also known to cause anticoagulation through mechanisms similar to warfarin in that they inhibit the synthesis of active clotting factors VII, IX, X and plasma prothrombin.

Specific Agents

Warfarin (Coumadin)

Pharmacokinetics.   Warfarin sodium is rapidly and completely absorbed following oral administration and is 100% bioavailable. This compound is highly protein bound (95–99%) and, as a result, has numerous interactions with other drugs. The free drug (i.e., that not bound to plasma proteins) is the active constituent. Therefore, any other substance that displaces bound drug from protein binding sites increases the levels of free drug and, as a result, can cause warfarin toxicity which is usually manifested by hemorrhage. The volume of distribution is quite

small (V_d = 0.1–0.2 L/kg) and the plasma half-life quite long ($t_{1/2}$ = 15–70 hrs) both presumably due to the high degree of plasma protein binding (13).

The kinetics of the onset of warfarin's therapeutic action deserve comment. Diminished coagulation is not immediately present following initiation of therapy. Instead, a delay in onset of anticoagulation occurs while the clotting factors with normal activity are cleared and those that have not been carboxylated due to the actions of warfarin reach physiologically significant levels. On average, this delay is approximately 5 hours for factor V turnover and 2–3 days for factor II (thrombin). Consequently, because of the rapid decline in protein C levels, the anticoagulated state is frequently preceded by a period of hypercoagulability.

Metabolism.   Hepatic formation of metabolites that are excreted in the bile and then the intestine terminates the action of warfarin. The metabolites are 6- and 7-hydroxy-warfarins which are inactive as anticoagulants, and pharmacologically active diastereomeric alcohols formed through reductive metabolism (Fig. 26.7)(13). Almost no unchanged drug is excreted in the urine. As expected, those individuals with compromised hepatic function are at greater risk for warfarin toxicity secondary to diminished clearance. Many additional drugs and conditions have profound effects on warfarin therapy. A partial list of these factors is shown in Table 26.1(14).

Coumarin Derivatives

Significant differences between warfarin and its derivatives are their relative half lives and toxicities. Dicoumarol has an onset time of 1–5 days, duration of action of 2–10 days and a $t_{1/2}$ = 1–4 days (14). Dicoumarol is not completely absorbed from the GI tract and is often associated with gastrointestinal discomfort and is now very rarely used clinically. Phenprocoumon has a slower onset and longer duration of action (7–14 days) than warfarin and a half-life of 5–6 days(14). In contrast, acenocoumarol has a half-life of only 10–24 hours, a rapid effect on prothrombin time and a duration of action of only 2 days. Ethylbiscoumacetate has a very short half-life of only 2–3 hours (14).

Indandiones

Indan-1,3-dione derivatives such as phenindione and diphenadione are also lipophilic orally active anticoagulants (Fig. 26.8). These compounds have significant pharmaco-

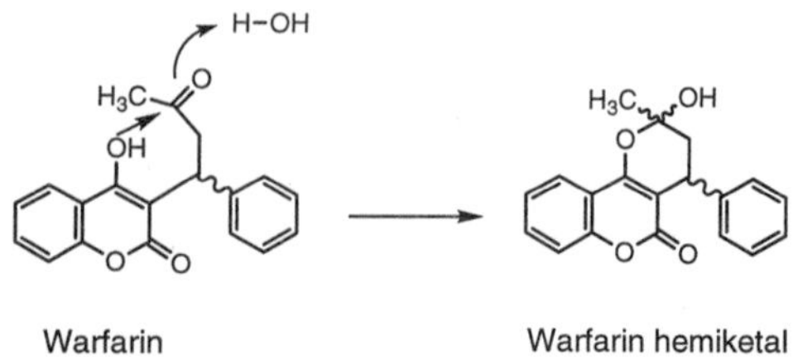

Fig. 26.6. Formation of cyclic hemiketal of warfarin.

logic actions in addition to anticoagulation including hypermetabolic, analgesic, uricosuric and anti-inflammatory properties. Depending upon the substitution of the phenyl moiety, the acidity of the proton on C2 can be altered. For example, in anisindione, the electron withdrawing character of the *p*-methoxy group combined with that of the carbonyls on C1 and C3 makes the C2 proton more ionizable relative to the unsubstituted phenindione (7). Numerous other derivatives with a variety of substituents in the 4 or 5 position on the indandione nucleus have been screened for activity. However, no cohesive structural motif correlated well with any observed pharmacologic response (15). Therefore,

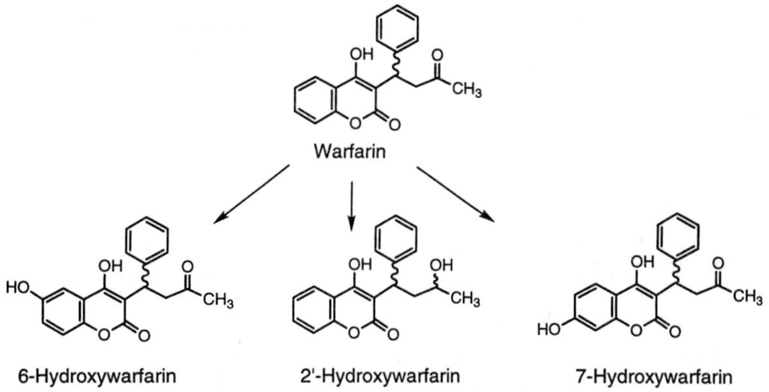

Fig. 26.7. Metabolism of warfarin.

Table 26.1. Factors Affecting Warfarin Therapy

Potentiate Anticoagulation		Antagonize Anticoagulation	Drugs Enhanced by Oral Anticoagulants
Drugs:		Drugs:	Phenytoin
Acetaminophen	Ketoconazole	Alcohol (chronic abuse)	Sulfonylureas
Alcohol (acute intoxication)	Lovastatin	Aminoglutethimide	
Allopurinol	Mefenamic acid	Antacid	
Amiodarone	Metronidazole	Antihistamines	
Anabolic & androgenic steroids	Miconazole	Barbiturates	
Aspirin	Nalidixic acid	Carbamazepine	
Bromelains	Naproxen	Chlordiazepoxide	
Cephalosporins	Omeprazole	Cholestyramine	
Chenodiol	Oral hypoglycemics	Colestipol	
Chloral hydrate	Pentoxiphylline	Corticosteroids	
Cimetidine	Phenylbutazone	Dextrothryroxine	
Clofibrate	Phenytoin	Griseofluvin	
Clorpropamide	Piroxicam	Haloperidol	
Cotrimoxazole	Propafenone	Meprobamate	
Dextran	Propranolol	Nafcillin	
Diazoxide	Quinidine, quinine	Oral contraceptives	
Diflunisal	Ranitidine	Penicillins (large doses)	
Disulfiram	Sulfamethoxazole/	Phenytoin	
Erythromycin	trimethoprim	Primadone	
Ethacrynic acid	Sulfonylureas	Rifampin	
Ethanol	Sulfinpyrazone	Sucralfate	
Fenoprofen	Sulindac	Trazodone	
Fluconazole	Tamoxifen	Vitamin K (large doses)	
Glucagon	Thyroxine		
Heparin	Ticlopidine	Other Factors:	
Ibuprofen	Tolmetin	High Vitamin K Diet	
Indomethacin	Tricyclic anti-	Spinach	
Inhalation anesthetics	depressants	Cheddar cheese	
Isoniazid		Cabbage	
		Edema	
Other Factors:		Hypothyroidism	
Fever	Diarrhea	Nephrotic syndrome	
Stress	Cancer		
Congestive heart failure	X-rays		
Radioactive compounds	Hyperthyroidism		
Hepatic dysfunction			

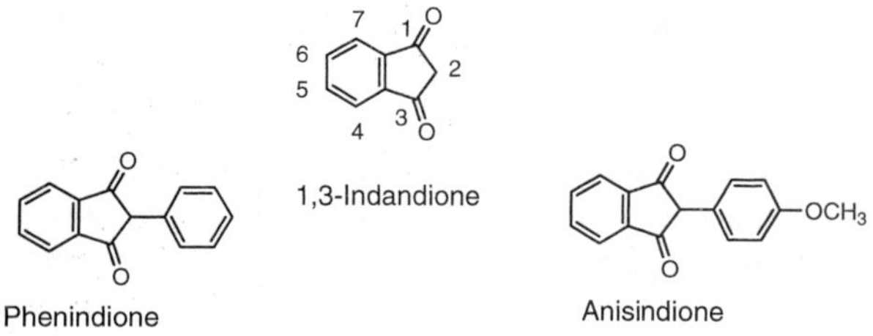

Fig. 26.8. Chemical structures of 1,3-indandione and 3,4-indandione-derived drugs.

structural modification of a single lead compound was determined to be impractical and was largely abandoned. Attempts at developing a clear SAR for the indandiones in order to improve the anticoagulant therapeutic index have been made (15). However, the toxicities of these compounds limit their clinical utility.

The kinetics and metabolism of the indandione drugs have not been extensively studied. The urine of patients taking phenindione and its congeners will frequently take on an orange-red tint. This discoloration of the urine is due to the metabolites of the drugs. Though it may initially cause alarm, the unusual color of the urine is easily removed by acidification thereby allowing a distinction from true hematuria.

The indandiones are associated with significant renal and hepatic toxicities. Though anisindione reportedly has the fewest significant side effects, it is rarely used clinically. Due to these toxicities, most clinicians prefer warfarin over the indandiones for oral anticoagulation.

HEPARIN
Mechanism of Action

Heparin inhibits blood coagulation at a different site within the coagulation cascade than the vitamin K antagonists. Specifically, heparin accelerates binding of antithrombin III (a protease inhibitor) to thrombin as well as other serine proteases necessary for normal blood coagulation. Antithrombin inhibits proteases necessary for clotting by forming a stable 1:1 complex with them. While the rate of this reaction is slow in the absence of heparin, binding is accelerated 1000-fold when heparin is added (3). When heparin binds the antithrombin, it induces a conformational change resulting in increased accessibility of its active site and more rapid interaction with its protease substrates (the activated clotting factors). Interestingly, heparin is catalytic in this action (i.e., it is not consumed, inactivated or degraded by the reaction). In fact, once the complex of antithrombin and protease is formed, the heparin is released with no loss of activity, to catalyze formation of more antithrombin:protease complexes. Only 30–35% of the polysaccharides present in clinically utilized heparin actually possess the accelerating and catalytic effects (3). The remaining polysaccharides lack the specific sugar sequence necessary for high-affinity binding to antithrombin. The end result of heparin's actions are the inhibition of clotting

"Superwarfarin" Rodenticides

Brodifacoum is a member of the second-generation anticoagulant rodenticides known as "superwarfarins"(16). This compound and others like it (e.g., bromadiolone, difenacoum, chlorophacinone [see figure]) were developed to combat rodent resistance to warfarin (16).

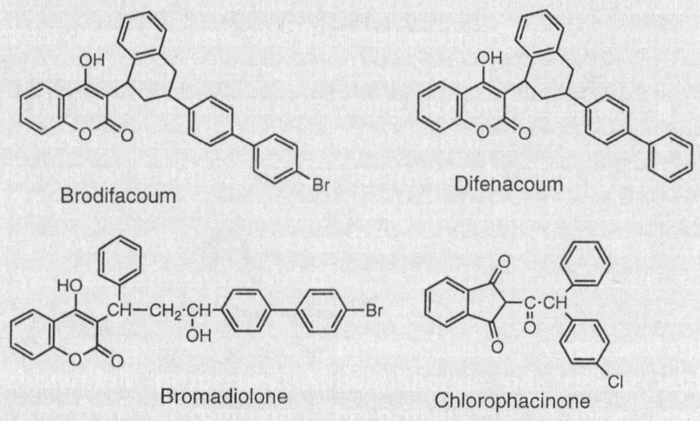

Chemical structures of long-acting "superwarfarin" rodenticides.

Human ingestion of brodifacoum is typically accidental in children and suicidal in adults (17). In large ingestions, severe and potentially fatal hemorrhage can result. Brodifacoum is readily available over-the-counter in hardware stores and supermarkets and is marketed under numerous trade names in North America, Europe, Australia and New Zealand. Brodifacoum, like warfarin, is thought to exhibit its anticoagulant effects through inhibition of vitamin K epoxide reductase. Despite the similarity in mechanism of action between brodifacoum and warfarin, brodifacoum is at least five times more potent as an anticoagulant rodenticide (16,18). The half-life of brodifacoum in humans is approximately 24.2 days which is roughly nine times longer than that of warfarin (16,19,20). Brodifacoum also has a volume of distribution roughly six times that of warfarin (19). For these reasons, vitamin K therapy may be needed for weeks to months after ingestion of a superwarfarin rodenticide (21).

Coumarin

Derivatives of 4-hydroxycoumarin such as warfarin are effective anticoagulants for therapeutic use or pest control. However, the coumarin moiety itself is not effective as an anticoagulant. In fact, its use is quite different. Coumarin is present in woodruff, sweet clover and lavender oil as well as many other plants. It has a pleasant odor similar to that of vanilla beans and is often used in cosmetics and lotions as a fragrance additive (22).

factors IX, X, XI and XII, kallikrein and thrombin. Additional effects of heparin on the coagulation of blood are a result of heparin's effects on plasminogen activator inhibitor, protein C inhibitor and others.

Chemistry

Heparin is composed of a heterogenous mixture of sulfated mucopolysaccharides of molecular weight range

5–30 kD typically isolated from bovine lung or porcine intestinal mucosa. Heparin (also known as heparinic acid) is an acidic molecule similar to chondroitin and hyaluronic acid. The polysaccharide polymer chains are composed of two alternating sugar units, N-acetyl-D-glucosamine and D-glucuronic acid, linked by $\alpha,1{\rightarrow}4$ bonds (Fig. 26.9).

These chains are called glycosaminoglycans and are typically composed of 200–300 monosaccharide units. In mast cells, approximately 10–15 of these chains are bound to a core protein to yield a proteoglycan (i.e., a protein-sugar conglomerate molecule) with a molecular weight of 750–1000 kD. Before the molecule is capable of binding to antithrombin, the proteoglycan must undergo a series of structural modifications. These modifications include: O-sulfation and N-sulfation of the D-glucosamine residues at carbons 6 and 2, respectively; O-sulfation of the D-glucuronic acid at carbon 2; epimerization of the D-glucuronic acid at carbon 5 to form L-iduronic acid; O-sulfation at carbon 2 of the L-iduronic acid; N-deacetylation of the glucosamine and O-sulfation of the glucosamine at position 3. However, none of these reactions goes to completion so the resulting polysaccharide chains are structurally quite diverse (23). The heparin proteoglycan then undergoes degradation by an endo-β-glucuronidase in mast cell granules to release the active 5–30 kD polysaccharide chains.

At physiologic pH, heparin exists primarily as the polysulfate anions and is therefore usually administered as a salt. Clinically utilized standard heparin is most often the sodium salt though calcium heparin is also effective. Lithium heparin is used in blood sample collection tubes to prevent clotting of the blood samples in vitro but not in vivo. The use of heparin salts is also important to maintain aqueous solubility which is necessary for injection. Heparin can be administered intravenously or subcutaneously but not orally as the polysaccharide chains are broken down by gastric acid. Intramuscular injection of heparin is associated with a high risk of hematoma formation and is not recommended.

Forms of Heparin
High Molecular Weight Heparin (HMWH)

Standard heparin is unfractionated and contains mucopolysaccharides ranging in molecular weight from 5–30 kD, and is referred to as high molecular weight heparin. This group of compounds has a very high affinity for antithrombin III and causes significant in vivo anticoagulant effects. Since HMWH is a heterogenous mixture of poly-

saccharides with different affinities for the target receptor, dosing based on mg weight of drug is inappropriate (i.e., there is frequently a limited correlation between the concentration of heparin given and anticoagulant effect produced). Therefore, heparin is dosed in terms of standardized activity units that must be established by bioassay. One USP unit for heparin is the quantity of heparin required to prevent 1.0 mL of citrated sheep blood from clotting for 1 hour after the addition of 0.2 mL of 1% calcium chloride (5). Commercially available heparin sodium USP must contain at least 120 USP units per milligram. Heparin therapy is typically monitored by the activated partial thromboplastin time (aPTT). A therapeutic aPTT is represented by a clotting time in the assay that is 1.5–2.5 times the normal mean aPTT value (5). Monitoring therapy with laboratory testing is critical.

Low Molecular Weight Heparins (LMWH)

In the past two decades, an increased interest has surfaced in a group of compounds known as low molecular weight heparins (LMWH) (24). The LMWH are typically in the 4–6 kD molecular weight range and are isolated as fractions from HMWH using gel filtration chromatography or differential precipitation with ethanol (3). The LMWH have more favorable pharmacokinetic and pharmacodynamic profiles relative to standard heparins. The mechanism of action of LMWH is somewhat similar to conventional heparin but LMWH binding is more specific. LMWH has a targeted activity against activated factor X and less against activated factor II (thrombin). Though all LMWH's inactivate Xa, only 25–50% also inactivate IIa (24). This factor selectivity is typically defined as a higher factor Xa:thrombin (anti-Xa:anti-IIa) activity ratio. In fact, while standard (unfractionated) heparin has an anti-Xa:anti-IIa ratio of 1:1, the same ratio in the LMWH's varies from 2:1–4:1 (24).

Three LWMH's are commercially available in the U.S. These are enoxaparin (MW = 2–6 kD) (Lovenox), dalteparin (MW = 2–9 kD) (Fragmin) and tinzaparin (average MW = 5.5–7.5 kD) (Innohep). The three drugs differ slightly in their medical indications for use as well as their molecular weight ranges. All three compounds are indicated for perioperative thromboembolism prevention for specific abdominal and orthopedic surgeries. Enoxaparin and dalteparin are approved for use in unstable angina and non-Q-wave myocardial infarction. Enoxaparin is also used in therapy for deep venous thrombosis (DVT) with or without concomitant pulmonary embolism. Because of

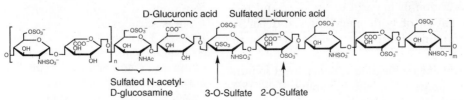

Fig. 26.9. Chemical structure of heparin polymer.

the increased homogeneity of enoxaparin compared to HMWH, dosing of this drug is based on drug weight rather than U.S.P. unitage. A typical dosing scheme for enoxaparin is the administration of 1 mg/kg once or twice daily. In the cases of dalteparin and ardeparin, dosage is based on anti-factor Xa units (a-Xa U). Dalteparin is given as a once daily subcutaneous injection at a dose of 2500–5000 a-Xa U. Typical dosing for tinzaparin is 175a–Xa U/kg once daily. The LMWH compounds have a limited anticoagulant effect on in vitro clotting assays such as the aPTT. In contrast to the HMWH's, coagulation parameters such as aPTT are not usually monitored in patients receiving LMWH nor is monitoring these assays really necessary as the LMWH compounds have a highly predictable dose response relationship (24).

The pharmacokinetic profiles of HMWH and LMWH are quite different. While HMWH is only 30% absorbed following subcutaneous injection, >90% of LMWH is systemically absorbed (17). The binding affinity of HMWH to various protein receptors such as those on plasma proteins, endothelial cells, platelets, platelet factor 4 and macrophages is very high. However, these same affinities are quite low in the case of LMWH's. These parameters explain several of the LMWH benefits. The favorable absorption kinetics and low protein binding affinity of the LMWH's results in a greater bioavailability over HMWH. The lowered affinity of LMWH's for platelet factor 4 seems to correlate with a reduced incidence of heparin-induced thrombocytopenia. HMWH is subject to fast zero-order metabolism in the liver followed by slower first-order clearance from the kidneys (24,25). LMWH is renally cleared and follows first order kinetics. This makes the clearance of LMWH more predictable as well as resulting in a prolonged half-life. Finally, the incidence of heparin mediated osteoporosis is significantly diminished with use of LMWH's as opposed to HMWH's.

Metabolism

Independent of molecular weight, the metabolic fate of heparin is essentially the same. The distribution of the compounds is limited primarily to the circulation but heparins are also taken up by the reticuloendothelial system (13). Once this uptake occurs, rapid depolymerization of the polysaccharide chains ensues resulting in products that are inactive as anticoagulants. Desulfation also occurs in mononuclear phagocytes also providing inactive metabolites. These metabolites, as well as some parent compound, are then excreted in the urine (13). Because of the depolymerization of heparin in the liver and ultimate renal elimination of both metabolites and parent drug, half-life is prolonged in patients with hepatic or renal dysfunction.

Another heparin-like medication is danaparoid sodium (26). The drug is composed of 84% heparan sulfate, 12% dermatan sulfate and 4% chondroitin sulfate. The average molecular weight is 5.5 kD and, like the LMWH's, dana-

paroid is dosed in terms of anti-factor Xa activity. Danaparoid is completely bioavailable intravenously or subcutaneously and attains maximal anti-factor Xa activity 2–5 hours after administration. The elimination half-life is approximately 24 hrs and clearance is through the kidneys. Coagulation assays (e.g., PT, aPTT) are not routinely monitored in patients receiving danaparoid therapy as the drug has a very limited effect on factor II (thrombin) activity.

Newer Heparin Developments

Many recent studies involving heparin have been directed toward either increasing oral bioavailability or decreasing unwanted side effects (27). The poor bioavailability of heparin is due to its high molecular weight and high anionic charge density. These properties combined with the instability of the polysaccharides to gastric acid, make penetration of biological membranes such as the gut wall extremely difficult for heparin. Various approaches to modify heparin absorption following oral administration have been investigated (28). Formulations of heparin including the use of amine salts in enteric-coated tablets (29), salts from organic bases such as lipophilic amines (30), oil-water emulsions (31,32), liposomes (33), and microsphere encapsulation (34,35) have been examined. Combinations of heparin with assorted calcium binding substances and nonalpha amino acids (N-acylatedaminoalkanoic acids) for simultaneous oral administration have also been studied (28). None of these formulations has yet been approved for clinical use.

Attempts to use structural modifications to heparin in order to attenuate undesirable side effects have also been investigated (27). Heparin induced thrombocytopenia is caused by the interaction of heparin with platelet factor 4 (PF4). The PF4 binding domain appears to be distinct from the thrombin binding domain. Therefore, it should be possible to use shorter oligosaccharides that bind specifically to the thrombin inhibitory sites without binding to

Hirudin

Hirudin is a small protein (65 amino acids) that was originally isolated from the salivary glands of the medicinal leech, *Hirudo medicinalis* (36). This protein has potent and specific inhibitory effects on thrombin through the formation of a 1:1 complex with the clotting factor. The anticoagulant activity of hirudin seems to be contained within its highly anionic C-terminus. Several clinical studies have compared hirudin and a small peptidomimetic analog, hirulog, with heparin in the treatment of several thrombotic disorders. In many cases, hirudin seems to be more efficacious and the responses to it more predictable. Furthermore, some of the studies also indicated a lower incidence of bleeding complications with hirudin compared with heparin. Hirudin is now produced by recombinant technology and many hirulogs continue to be screened (37,38). Development of hirudin and its analogs into therapeutically useful agents is quite promising.

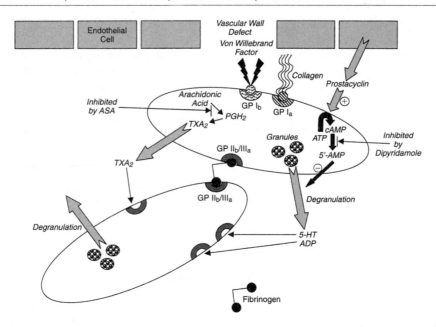

Fig. 26.10. Scheme describing platelet activation as it relates to blood clot formation. The thrombus is formed at the site of a damaged wall in the vasculature. Normal endothelial cells in the vascular wall provide prostacyclin which stimulates the conversion of ATP to cAMP preventing platelet aggregation. In injury, glycoprotein (GP) receptors bind substances such as von Willebrand factor and collagen activating the platelet. The GP IIb/IIIa receptors crosslink platelets via fibrinogen binding. As the platelet degranulates, additional aggregating substances including thromboxane A2 (TXA2), serotonin (5-HT) and adenine diphosphate (ADP) are released. These substances bind to other platelets activating them and resulting in a cascade effect. Sites of inhibition of platelet aggregation.

PF4 (27). These observations were utilized to develop and synthetically produce a series of oligosaccharides with good thrombin binding profiles that have limited interaction with PF4. Though this preliminary work is quite promising, these compounds are not yet clinically available.

ANTIPLATELET DRUGS
Mechanism of Action

Another site of action for inhibition of the normal blood coagulation cascade is at the level of the platelets (39). This is accomplished through either reducing the formation or inhibiting the action of chemical signals that promote platelet aggregation (Fig. 26.10). Several chemical messengers are important in platelet aggregation. For example, thrombin production releases adenosine diphosphate (ADP). ADP is a potent inducer of platelet aggregation and stimulates prostaglandin synthesis from arachidonic acid in the platelet membrane. The prostaglandins synthesized, prostacyclin (PGI$_2$) and thromboxane A$_2$ (TXA$_2$), have opposite effects on thrombogenesis. PGI$_2$ is synthesized in the walls of the vasculature and inhibits thrombus formation. Conversely, TXA$_2$, which is synthesized in the platelets, induces vasoconstriction and thrombogenesis. Serotonin (5-HT), also released from the platelets, has similar and additive effects to those of TXA$_2$. Numerous drugs affect platelet secondary aggregation including salicylates, dipyridamole, ticlopidine and sulfinpyrazone. These drugs are categorized as antiplatelet drugs. Many physiological processes including inflammation, wound healing, allergy and thrombosis are mediated by the oxidative metabolism of arachidonic

acid and other eicosanoids (3,6). Because eicosanoids are the products of many of the listed physiological processes, interference with their production has been the source of numerous therapeutic agents including analgesics, antiinflammatory drugs and antithrombotics.

Aspirin

Specific Drugs
Aspirin

The enzyme cyclooxygenase is present in platelets. The major product of this enzyme's actions on arachidonic acid is a cyclic endoperoxide precursor of thromboxane A$_2$. Thromboxane A$_2$ is a potent vasoconstrictor as well as a labile platelet aggregation inducer. The production of thromboxane A$_2$ is effectively blocked by aspirin, which permanently inactivates cyclooxygenase through covalent acylation of a serine residue in close proximity to the active site. A cumulative inactivation effect occurs on platelets with long-term therapy as platelets do not synthesize new cyclooxygenase. Therefore, the effects of aspirin last for the lifetime of the platelet (7–10 days). A once daily dose of 160 mg of aspirin is sufficient to completely inactivate platelet cyclooxygenase. Despite its also being an NSAID, inactivation of platelet function by ibuprofen is reversible upon withdrawal of the drug. This property has been exploited therapeutically (40).

Dipyridamole

Dipyridamole

Dipyridamole is an adenosine uptake antagonist typically used for its vasodilatory effects. Platelet function is interrupted by dipyridamole through the drug's effect of increasing cellular concentrations of cAMP by inhibiting cyclic nucleotide phosphodiesterase or blocking adenosine uptake (which acts at A2 adenosine receptors to stimulate platelet adenyl cyclase). Less common uses for this drug include inhibition of embolization from prosthetic heart valves when used in combination with warfarin (the only current recommended use) and reduction of thrombosis in patients with thrombotic disease when used in combination with aspirin. Alone, dipyridamole has little, if any, benefit in the treatment of thrombotic conditions (41).

Ticlopidine   (S)-Clopidogrel

Ticlopidine and Clopidogrel

Ticlopidine and clopidogrel are thienopyridines used in thrombosis prevention in cerebrovascular and coronary artery disease in patients who cannot tolerate aspirin. These drugs are thought to induce a thromboasthenic-like state by interacting with glycoprotein IIb/IIIa (a fibrinogen receptor) resulting in an inhibition of the binding of fibrinogen to activated platelets. This blockade prevents fibrinogen from individual platelets from crosslinking to form an aggregated plug. It is also known that drugs of the thienopyridine class exhibit selective inhibition of adenosine diphosphate (ADP)-induced platelet aggregation. The exact mechanism(s) by which the thienopyridines exert their total anticoagulant activity remain unknown.

Despite the fact that the elimination half-life of ticlopidine is 24–36 hours after a single dose, abnormal platelet function continues for several days after discontinuation of the drug (14). One hypothesis to explain this observation is that a long-lived metabolite of ticlopidine is the active antithrombotic agent. Support of this theory is provided by the observation that ticlopidine is not effective in blocking platelet aggregation in vitro when compared to the effect of the drug on the platelets of people taking ticlopidine. The exact identity of the "active metabolite" is not known. It is well established that extensive hepatic metabolism of ticlopidine does take place and a total of 13 metabolites

have thus far been identified in humans. Of these, only the 2-keto metabolite is more potent at inhibiting ADP-induced platelet aggregation. An additional kinetic concern with ticlopidine use in unstable angina is that there is no apparent protection exerted by the drug for the first two weeks of therapy. Therefore, it is not a good therapeutic choice if rapid antiplatelet activity is required.

Clopidogrel is not active in vitro as a platelet inhibitor. The ester form of the drug is absorbed very rapidly and extensively metabolized in the liver. The hepatic metabolism produces a short-lived platelet inhibitor whose structure has not yet been determined. The principal systemic metabolite (though not the active one) is the carboxylic acid, SR 26334 ($t_{1/2}$ = 8 hrs).

Ticlopidine has no effect on eicosanoid metabolism and is thought to exert its anticoagulant effects via a mechanism different than that of aspirin. Additive antiplatelet effects of ticlodipine:aspirin combinations have been documented in both rats and humans.

Sulfinpyrazone

Sulfinpyrazone

Sulfinpyrazone is a structural derivative of the anti-inflammatory drug phenylbutazone. Unlike phenylbutazone, however, sulfinpyrazone does not have significant anti-inflammatory activity. It does have potent uricosuric effects and is frequently used in the treatment of gout. Sulfinpyrazone is also a potent but reversible cyclooxygenase inhibitor that does not affect PGI$_2$ synthesis in endothelial cells. Like NSAID's such as aspirin, this action inhibits the aggregation of platelets into thrombi. At least four metabolites of sulfinpyrazone have been identified including the sulfide, sulfone, *p*-hydroxysulfide and *p*-hydroxysulfinpyrazone derivatives (14). However, only the parent sulfinpyrazone and its reduced sulfide metabolite (Fig. 26.11) are active as cyclooxygenase inhibitors (42). Since these compounds are reversible inhibitors, the antithrombotic activity lasts only as long as blood levels of the drug and metabolite persist ($t_{1/2}$ = 4–6 hrs for parent sulfinpyrazone; 11–14 hours for the sulfide metabolite). Sulfinpyrazone is not yet approved in the United States for use in AMI or for TIA prophylaxis.

Citric acid

Citric Acid

Citric acid is found in high concentrations in citrus fruits such as oranges and lemons as well as in many animal tis-

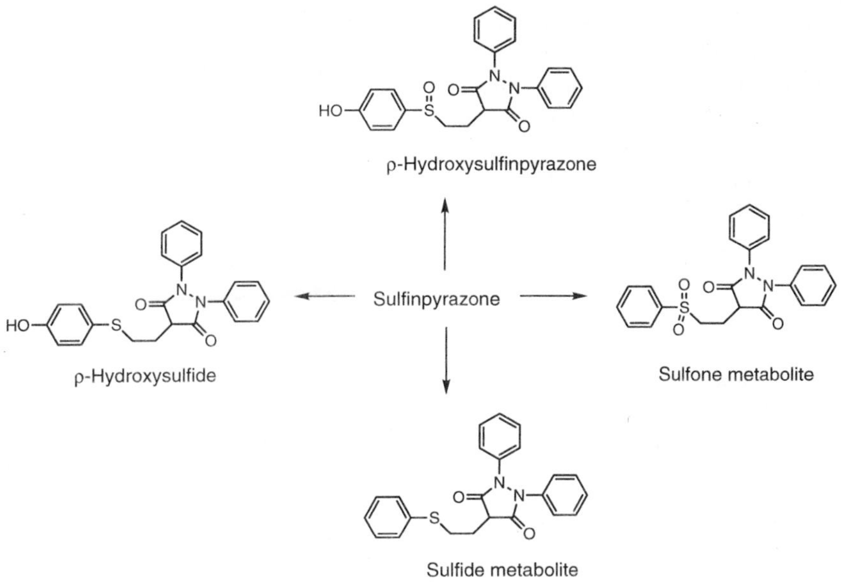

Fig. 26.11. Metabolism of sulfinpyrazone.

sues. This naturally occurring tricarboxylic acid is also used in many soft drinks and candies as well as in pharmaceutical syrups, elixirs, tablets and effervescent powders (7). Trisodium citrate is used therapeutically to treat acidosis. This therapy is not nearly as backward as it sounds. Citrate is metabolically converted into bicarbonate (HCO_3^-) which is an effective buffer useful in the treatment of acidosis. With respect to blood coagulation, trisodium citrate is used as an in vitro anticoagulant in blood collection tubes and units of packed cells for transfusion. The anticoagulant mechanism of action is through the formation of the water soluble chelate of free calcium and citrate anion. Calcium sequestration affects coagulation because calcium ion is one of the necessary components in the conversion of prothrombin to thrombin. Citric acid will not likely ever be useful as an in vivo anticoagulant because the necessary calcium chelation would have significant noncoagulation biological consequences.

Glycoprotein Inhibitors

One of the newest groups of antithrombotic agents is the platelet receptor glycoprotein (GP) IIb/IIIa antagonists (3). This novel class of compounds has been shown to provide more comprehensive inhibition of platelet aggregation than the usual combination of aspirin and heparin. The final common pathway in platelet aggregation is the expression of functional GPIIb/IIIa (integrin $\alpha_{IIb}\beta_3$) receptors. These protein receptors are expressed regardless of the origin of the stimulus initiating the clotting cascade. The normal substrate for the GPIIb/IIIa receptor is fibrinogen. One fibrinogen molecule acts to crosslink two platelets via binding to the GPIIb/IIIa receptors on the platelet surfaces (Fig. 26.10). If the platelet surface receptors are occupied by another substrate that prevents fibrinogen binding and crosslinking, platelet aggregation will

not occur. To this end, a number of novel compounds representing diverse structural groups have been prepared as GPIIb/IIIa receptor antagonists. Included in this list of antagonists are monoclonal antibodies against the natural GPIIb/IIIa receptor, naturally occurring peptides isolated from snake venom that contain the Arg-Gly-Asp (RGD) sequence, synthetic peptides containing either the RGD or KGD (Lys-Gly-Asp) sequences and peptidomimetic and nonpeptide RGD mimetics that compete with fibrinogen and other ligands for occupancy of the receptor.

Snake Venom Induced Coagulopathy

The venom of snakes of the *Crotalinae* family, which includes rattlesnakes, produces a state of impaired coagulation (21). This can lead to both local and systemic hemorrhagic events. Venom consists of many components including phospholipases and hemolysins, which cause cell lysis by disrupting platelet and red cell membranes. The venoms also contain pro-coagulant components that induce the formation of intravascular clots as well as hemorrhagins that destroy vascular integrity. Typically, both PT and aPTT are elevated with total fibrin levels being lowered and fibrin degradation products increased. All of the findings are consistent with a consumptive coagulopathy. Because of the multiple mechanisms affecting coagulation, coagulopathies caused by snake venom are best managed using antivenin.

The initial antibodies against the GPIIb/IIIa receptor were murine in origin. Because of concerns about the antigenicity of a pure murine antibody, a chimeric human-mouse 7E3 Fab was developed (3). This chimera, marketed as abciximab, is the clinically available form of the antibody (43). For an adult patient, the usual dosing scheme is 0.25 mg/kg as an intravenous bolus given 10–60 minutes prior to percutaneous coronary intervention followed by the continuous infusion of 0.125 μg/kg/min for 12 hours to a maximum of 10 μg/kg. Elimination of abciximab is biphasic. The initial phase has a $t_{1/2}$ of 10 minutes while the half-life of the second phase is approximately 30 minutes and is due to platelet binding. Platelet function returns to normal within 48 hours after infusion though abciximab is bound to circulating platelets for about 2 weeks (26).

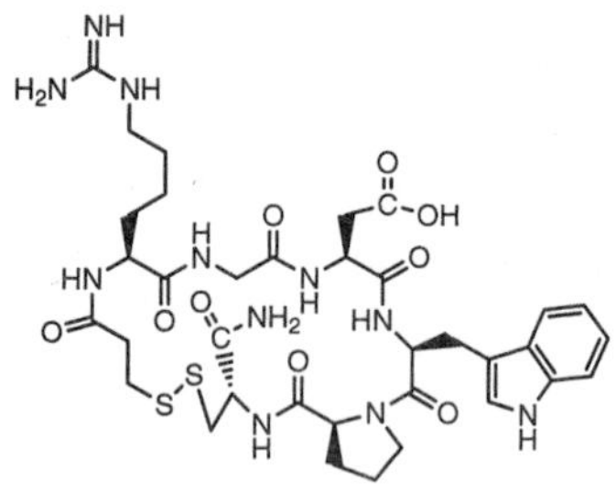

Eptifibatide

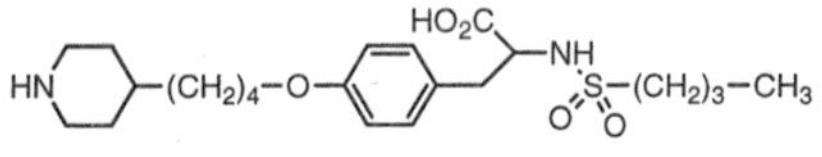

Tirofiban

Other GPII$_b$/III$_a$ antagonists include eptifibatide and tirofiban. Eptifibatide is a cyclic heptapeptide composed of six amino acids and one mercaptopropionyl residue. The cyclization is completed via a disulfide linkage between the cysteine and the mercaptopropionyl moieties. Eptifibatide and its major metabolite, the deamidated eptifibatide, are both excreted renally. The elimination half-life of eptifibatide is approximately 2.5 hours. Tirofiban is a nonpeptide GPII$_b$/III$_a$ antagonist, though it does contain a single L-tyrosine residue. Tirofiban has a half-life of 2 hours and is renally excreted (26).

The GPIIb/IIIa antagonists are indicated for therapy of unstable angina, non-Q-wave myocardial infarction and percutaneous coronary procedures. Like other antithrombotic agents, the main concern associated with GPIIb/IIIa antagonists is bleeding. There has also been suggestion that these drugs may increase the risk of thrombocytopenia.

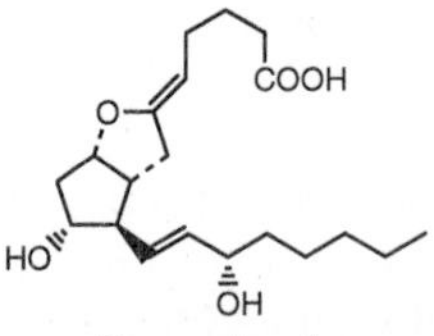

Epoprostenol 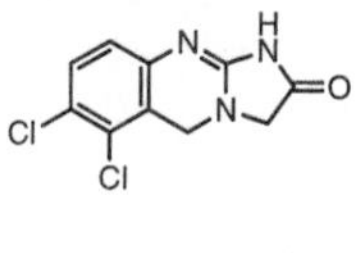   Anagrelide

Miscellaneous Antiplatelet Drugs

Two commercially available but less commonly used platelet aggregation inhibitors are epoprostenol and anagrelide. Epoprostenol (prostacyclin, PGI$_2$, PGX) is a bicyclic oxidative prostaglandin metabolite of arachidonic acid with potent vasodilatory and antiplatelet aggregation properties. This drug is extensively metabolized and is subject to rapid degradation at neutral pH. Rapid spontaneous hydrolysis results in the formation of 6-keto-PGF$_{1\alpha}$ while enzymatic metabolism produces 6,15-diketo-13,14-dihydro PGF$_{1\alpha}$ (26) (Fig. 26.12).

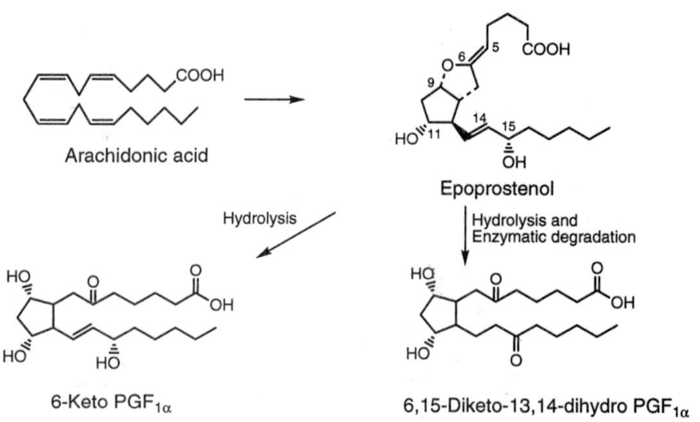

Fig. 26.12. Metabolic production and degradation of epoprostenol.

Both of these compounds are slightly pharmacologically active (although significantly less than the parent drug). At least 14 additional minor metabolites of epoprostenol have also been identified. The elimination half-life of epoprostenol is only 3–6 minutes and the metabolites are renally excreted (26). Because of its very short half-life, epoprostenol is administered intravenously.

Anagrelide is a dichlorinated dihydroimidazoquinazolinone. This compound is also extensively metabolized and excreted through the kidneys. The elimination half-life of anagrelide is approximately 1.3 hours (26).

New Developments in Antiplatelet Drugs

Several newer approaches to antiplatelet drug development have been recently discovered. Indobufin, an isoindolinylphenylacetic acid, inhibits platelet aggregation by blocking collagen induced thrombus formation. Indobufen is currently only available for routine clinical use in Europe. Other approaches to platelet inhibition include the use of serotonin antagonists (as serotonin induces platelet aggregation), phosphodiesterase inhibitors and inducers of adenyl cyclase.

Specific inhibitors of thromboxane synthetase have been tested for their ability to block this enzyme without inhibiting the entire arachidonic acid cascade. This allows for an accumulation of PGG$_2$ and PGH$_2$ which can then be channeled into an increased production of prostacyclin, which also has antithrombotic activity.

Another class of compounds with antiplatelet activity is made up of a series of 7-hydroxycoumarins substituted on the C7 oxygen by an α-methylene-γ-butyrolactone (Fig. 26.13) (44). This conjugate addition acceptor portion of the molecule has been proven in vivo to be integral to the antiplatelet activity of these compounds. Within the series of compounds assayed for their in vitro inhibition of aggregation of washed rabbit platelets, the compounds with the greatest activity had a single aromatic ring attached to the lactone and no alkyl substituent at C3, C4 or C8 of the coumarin nucleus. The compound with the greatest activity against both platelet activating factor (PAF) and arachidonic acid (AA) is sub-

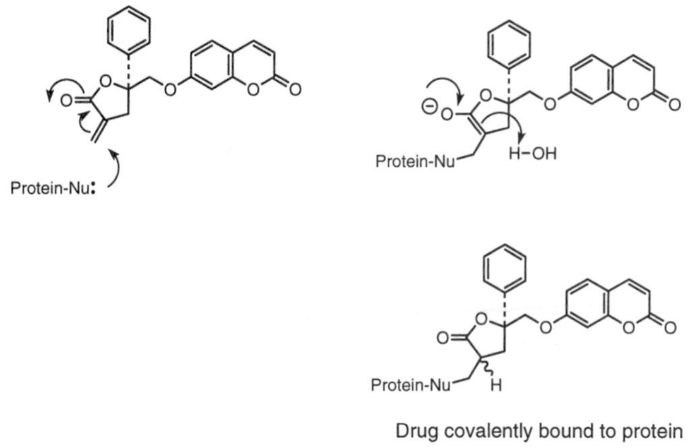

Fig. 26.13. Mechanistic scheme detailing the conjugate addition of necessary coagulation protein (Protein-Nu) to a coumarin α-methylene-γ-butyrolactone derivative γ-butyrolactone as described by Chen (21). The drug binds covalently to the protein causing a structural modification of the protein that renders it inactive in the coagulation cascade.

stituted with a phenyl ring on the 2 position of the lactone. The IC_{50} values for this compound are 3.6 and 16.4 μM against PAF and AA, respectively (44). These compounds are still investigational and not yet commercially available.

THROMBOLYTIC DRUGS
Mechanism of Action

Previously mentioned anticoagulants are designed to prevent thrombus formation. If a thrombus has already been formed, as in conditions such as deep venous thrombosis, acute pulmonary embolus or acute myocardial infarction, certain medications can be used to break down the existing clot. Blood clots are dissolved by the actions of the fibrinolytic system whose purpose is the removal of unwanted clots without damaging the integrity of the vascular system. This system works via a relatively nonspecific protease enzyme called plasmin, the function of which is to digest fibrin. The lack of substrate specificity of plasmin is illustrated by the fact that it degrades fibrin clots as well as some plasma proteins and coagulation factors. Plasmin is released from the inactive "proenzyme" plasminogen following the cleavage of a single peptide bond by a group of "plasminogen activators." The principal activator, tissue plasminogen activator (t-PA), is released from the vascular endothelium. Thrombolytic medications act with plasminogen to convert this proenzyme to the active plasmin. Endogenously, plasmin activity is regulated by two specific inactivators known as tissue plasminogen activator inhibitors 1 and 2 (t-PAI-1 & t-PAI-2).

Specific Drugs
Streptokinase (Streptose)

Streptokinase is a protein purified from culture broths of Group C β-hemolytic streptococci bacteria. Alone, it has no intrinsic enzymatic activity. To be active, it must form a 1:1 complex with the proactivator plasminogen. This complex then acts to convert uncomplexed plasminogen to the active fibrinolytic enzyme, plasmin. The streptokinase:plasminogen complex not only degrades fibrin clots, it also catalyzes the breakdown of fibrinogen and factors V and VII. Streptokinase is typically used in the management of deep venous thrombosis, arterial thrombosis, occluded access shunts and acute pulmonary embolism or myocardial infarction. Unfortunately, the $t_{1/2}$ of streptokinase is less than 30 minutes which is frequently too short to completely lyse a thrombus. Because it is a foreign protein, streptokinase is associated with significant hypersensitivity reactions. Most people have, at some point in their lives, had a streptococcal infection and therefore have developed circulating antistreptococcal antibodies. These antibodies are frequently also active against streptokinase. The response of the streptokinase to these antibodies can vary widely from inactivation of the fibrinolytic properties of the protein to rash, fever and rarely, anaphylaxis. Significant allergic reactions to streptokinase occur in approximately 3% of patients.

Anistreplase (Eminase)

Anistreplase is a pro-drug of the streptokinase:plasminogen complex used to improve the streptokinase pharmacokinetic profile. In vitro alteration of the chemical structure of the complex through acylation with an anisoyl group of a lysine in the active site of plasminogen blocks any fibrinolytic activity until after it has bound to fibrin. Acylation of the lysine residue does not affect fibrin binding. Once the complex is bound, the anisole group is slowly cleaved through spontaneous hydrolysis opening the plasminogen active site. Because of the necessity of fibrin binding to the clot prior to removal of the anisole moiety, anistreplase is semi-selective for lysis only at the clot site. The inactivity of the circulating anistreplase also allows this drug to be given as a very rapid IV infusion (typically, 30 units over 3–5 minutes). Tissue reperfusion following anistreplase therapy compares favorably to streptokinase due to the extended $t_{1/2}$ (90 minutes) of anistreplase.

Urokinase (Abbokinase)

Urokinase is an enzyme with the ability to directly degrade fibrin and fibrinogen. It is isolated from cultures of human fetal kidney cells. This method of isolation is much more efficient than the original isolation of urokinase from human urine. Because of its source, the human body does not see urokinase as a foreign protein. Therefore, it lacks the antigenicity associated with streptokinase and is frequently used for patients with a known hypersensitivity to streptokinase. Plasmin cannot be used directly because of the presence of naturally occurring plasmin antagonists in plasma. However, no such inhibitors of urokinase exist in the plasma allowing this enzyme to have clinical utility. Urokinase is, however, much more expensive than streptokinase and has an even shorter half-life ($t_{1/2} = 15$ minutes).

Alteplase (Activase), Reteplase (Retavase)

Alteplase (tissue-type plasminogen activator, tPA) is a serine protease with a low affinity for free plasminogen but a very high affinity for the plasminogen bound to fibrin in a thrombus. Both streptokinase and urokinase lack this specificity and act on free plasminogen inducing a generalized thrombolytic state. Alteplase also has a greater specificity for older clots over newer clots relative to streptokinase and urokinase. Alteplase was originally isolated from cultures of human melanoma cells but is now produced commercially using recombinant DNA technology. Alteplase is unmodified human tPA while reteplase is human tPA that has had several specific amino acid sequences removed. At low doses, alteplase is quite selective for degrading fibrin without concomitant lysis of other proteins such as fibrinogen. However, at the higher doses currently used therapeutically, alteplase activates free plasminogen to some extent and therefore can cause hemorrhage. Many of the therapeutic indications for the other thrombolytic agents are also indications for alteplase (i.e., myocardial infarction, massive pulmonary embolism and acute ischemic stroke). The $t_{1/2}$ of alteplase is very short (~5 minutes) necessitating its administration as a 15 mg IV bolus followed by a 85 mg IV infusion over 90 minutes or as 60 mg infused over the first hour with the remaining 40 mg given at a rate of 20 mg/hr.

Toxicity of Antithrombotics and Thrombolytics

Antithrombotic Toxicity

Recall that warfarin exhibits its anticoagulation effects by preventing γ-carboxylation of specific glutamate residues necessary for vitamin K dependent coagulation. However, γ-carboxyglutamate proteins are not isolated to coagulation factors. These types of proteins are also synthesized in bone. As would be expected, warfarin also interferes with the carboxylation of these proteins resulting in an inhibition of the effects of vitamin K on osteoblast development. It has been suggested that this is the mechanism responsible for bone abnormalities in neonates born to mothers who were treated with warfarin while pregnant (21). There is no evidence that bone metabolism or development is affected by warfarin when the drug is administered to children or adults. Due to the mechanism of action of the warfarin-like drugs, the management of their toxicity is largely based upon vitamin K therapy. This agent is discussed in greater detail in the Coagulants section of this chapter.

Unlike warfarin, heparin is safe for anticoagulant therapy in pregnancy (34). Though warfarin is known to cause serious fetal malformations when used in pregnancy, heparin does not cross the placental barrier and has shown no tendency to induce fetal damage. Furthermore, heparin does not increase fetal mortality or prematurity. In order to minimize the risk of postpartum hemorrhage, it is recommended that heparin therapy be withdrawn 24 hours before delivery.

Despite its safety in pregnancy, there exist several potential problems associated with heparin therapy. Since heparins (HMWH and LMWH) are isolated from animal sources, the chance of antigenic hypersensitivity exists, though it is rarely observed. Heparin competitively binds many other plasma proteins (i.e., vitronectin and PF4) in addition to the antithrombin resulting in inactivation of the heparin as an anticoagulant. This is a possible cause of heparin resistance. One of the most serious heparin-induced complications is thrombocytopenia. Typically, this condition occurs 7–14 days after initiation of heparin therapy, though it may occur earlier in patients with previous exposures to heparin. In these cases, heparin-induced platelet aggregation occurs and may result in the production of antiplatelet antibodies. Development of this condition necessitates termination of heparin therapy and institution of antiplatelet compounds, oral anticoagulants, heparinoid Org 10172 or ancrod (a defibrination enzyme isolated from snake venom). Upon withdrawal of heparin, the thrombocytopenia is usually reversible. Mild increases in liver function tests are frequently associated with heparin therapy. Long term use of full therapeutic doses of heparin (>20,000 U/day for 3–6 months) has been associated with osteoporosis and spontaneous vertebral fractures have been infrequently reported.

Hemorrhagic complications of heparin therapy are managed, in part, with the specific antagonist protamine sulfate. This agent is discussed in greater detail in the Coagulants section of this chapter.

The structural and mechanistic diversity of the antiplatelet drugs disallows a cohesive description of their toxicities. Although hemorrhage is certainly a concern, other more drug-specific toxicities may be of greater immediate concern. It is suggested that toxicity information for antiplatelet medications be obtained from appropriate references for the specific agent in question.

Thrombolytic Toxicities

The lack of specificity of the enzyme plasmin as a thrombolytic results in action not only on fibrin but also on many other plasma proteins including several coagulation factors. As is expected, thrombolytic drugs not only attack pathologic clots but also exert their actions upon any other site of compromised vascular integrity. The dissolution of necessary clots results in the principal side effect of thrombolytic therapy, hemorrhage.

Multiple studies have examined the incidence of life-threatening hemorrhage (i.e., intracranial hemorrhage) with the various thrombolytic medications. These studies indicate that the rate of significant hemorrhagic complication is essentially the same (0.1–0.7%) regardless of the specific therapeutic agent used. Supportive care is indicated in cases of thrombolytic toxicity. Though no specific antagonist exists to manage thrombolytic medication-induced hemorrhage, antifibrinolytic drugs such as aminocaproic acid and tranexamic acid are often used. These compounds are described in detail in the Coagulants section of this chapter.

COAGULANTS

A variety of pathologic and toxicologic conditions can result in excessive bleeding from inadequate coagulation. Depending upon the etiology and severity of the hemorrhagic episode, several possible blood coagulation inducers can be therapeutically employed.

Vitamin K₁

Vitamin K₃

Vitamin K₄

Vitamin K

Because the orally active anticoagulants such as warfarin and the indandiones act through interruption of the normal actions of vitamin K, it stands to reason that vitamin K should be effective in treating bleeding induced by these agents (21). Vitamin K_1 (phytonadione) is the form of vitamin K most often used therapeutically. Vitamin K_1 is safe for use in infants, pregnant women and patients with glucose-6-phosphate (G6P) deficiency. Furthermore, phytonadione works more rapidly than other vitamin K preparations (6 versus 12 hours) and requires smaller doses than vitamin K_3 (menadione) or vitamin K_4 (menadiol sodium diphosphate). Both vitamins K_3 and K_4 may produce hyperbilirubinemia and kernicterus in neonates as well as hemolysis in neonates and G6P deficient patients. In fact, the only advantage of vitamin K_3 and K_4 over K_1 is that while absorption of K_1 requires the presence of bile absorption of K_3 and K_4 does not as they are absorbed via a passive process directly from the intestine (21). This may be of slight advantage for patients with cholestasis or severe pancreatic dysfunction. However, only vitamin K_1 is appropriate therapy for bleeding associated with warfarin and superwarfarin anticoagulation. Vitamin K_2 is not used therapeutically.

Vitamin K_1 is effective at inducing coagulation when administered orally, subcutaneously, intramuscularly or intravenously. Though the oral route is preferred, it is not always practical in a critically hemorrhaging patient. The other routes of administration, though used clinically, all have significant potential drawbacks. Larger doses (e.g., a volume >5 mL) are not appropriate for subcutaneous administration. Intramuscular injection is generally avoided in patients at risk for significant hematoma formation (e.g., hemophiliacs). Intravenous vitamin K dosing has been associated with severe ana-

phylactoid reactions (including death) presumably secondary to colloidal formulation.

The half-life of vitamin K_1 is somewhat dependent upon the route of administration, being quite short with IV 1.7 hours and 3–5 hours orally. When given orally, vitamin K_1 is absorbed directly from the proximal small intestine in an energy dependent and saturable process that requires the presence of bile salts. These kinetic features argue for administration in divided doses rather than larger single daily doses. The typical starting point for adults with drug-induced hypoprothrombinemia is 2.5–10 mg of vitamin K_1 orally repeating in 12–48 hours, if needed. However, in cases of ingestion of long acting superwarfarin rodenticides (e.g., brodifacoum) therapy may be 125 mg per day for weeks or months. Practically speaking, since vitamin K_1 is dispensed as 5 mg tablets, superwarfarin-poisoned patients may require 10–30 tablets every 6 hours.

Due to the short half-life of vitamin K_1, dosing must be repeated 2–4 times per day for the duration of treatment. Furthermore, regardless of the route of administration, coagulant effects are not evident for up to 24 hours. Because of this delay in onset, severe acute hemorrhage is better managed initially with intravenous infusion of fresh frozen plasma followed by vitamin K therapy.

Protamine
Mechanism of Action

Protamine sulfate has been approved in the U.S. as a specific antagonist to heparin since 1968 (21). Protamines are an arginine rich highly basic group of simple proteins derived from salmon sperm. The highly acidic heparin polysaccharides exhibit their anticoagulant activity through binding to antithrombin III. Due to the basicity of protamine, heparin has an increased affinity for protamine relative to antithrombin III. In fact, its binding affinity for protamine is so much greater than antithrombin III, that protamine will actually induce dissociation of the heparin:antithrombin III complex. If protamine is administered in the absence of heparin, it can have marked effects on coagulation. Protamine is not completely selective for heparin and in vivo also interacts with fibrinogen, platelets and other plasma proteins causing *anti*coagulation. For this reason, use of the minimal amount of protamine necessary to antagonize heparin associated bleeding should be employed (usually 1 mg of protamine intravenously for every 100 U of heparin remaining in the patient).

Side Effects

Anaphylaxis has also been associated with the use of protamine. Though development of protamine anaphylaxis is not limited to diabetics, those patients with diabetes that have used protamine containing insulin (NPH or protamine zinc) do have a slightly increased risk of anaphylaxis. Some less common reactions to protamine include pulmonary vasoconstriction, hypotension and thrombus formation.

H$_2$N–CH$_2$-CH$_2$-CH$_2$-CH$_2$-CH$_2$-COOH

Aminocaproic acid

CH$_3$–N–⬡–COOH
　　H

Tranexamic acid

H$_2$N–CH$_2$-CH$_2$-CH$_2$-CH$_2$-CH-COOH
　　　　　　　　　　　　　　NH$_2$

Lysine

Aminocaproic Acid (Amicine) and Tranexamic Acid (Cyklokapron)

Mechanism of Action

Control of a variety of fibrinolytic states can be achieved using a number of compounds. Drugs such as tranexamic acid and aminocaproic acid are synthetic agents that completely inhibit plasminogen activation. Plasmin binds to fibrin through a lysine binding site to activate the final stages of fibrinolysis. Aminocaproic acid is a lysine analog that binds at the lysine receptors on plasminogen and plasmin preventing the binding of plasmin to fibrin.

Pharmacokinetics

Both aminocaproic acid and tranexamic acid are readily absorbed when administered orally. They can also be given intravenously although significant hypotension can result if the infusion is run too fast. Elimination of the drugs is primarily renal with little metabolism taking place. The half-lives of aminocaproic acid and tranexamic acid are each approximately 2 hours.

These drugs find clinical utility in settings such as prevention of rebleeding in intracranial hemorrhages, as adjunctive therapy in hemophilia and, of course, treating bleeding associated with fibrinolytic therapy. However in most bleeding conditions aminocaproic acid therapy has not been shown to be of definitive benefit. The major risk associated with aminocaproic or tranexamic acid therapy is intravascular thrombosis as a direct result of the inhibition of plasminogen activator. Thrombi that form during therapy are not easily lysed and can therefore have additional ischemic consequences. Additional possible complications include hypotension, abdominal discomfort and, rarely, myopathy and muscle necrosis.

Aprotinin (Traysylol)

Operative procedures such as heart valve replacement frequently have effects on platelet function and endogenous coagulation factors. These effects may result in significant peri- or postoperative bleeding. Aprotinin is a serine protease inhibitor that blocks kallikrein and plasmin and also provides some protection to platelets from mechanical injury. The inhibition of fibrinolysis results in profound antihemorrhagic effects. Side effects of aprotinin therapy are usually minor though anaphylaxis has possibly been implicated in a small population ($<0.5\%$). For this reason, it is suggested that a small test dose be given prior to initiation of the therapeutic infusion.

Plasma Fractions

Spontaneous bleeding can result from dysfunction or deficiencies of specific coagulation factors. A list of coagulation factors and deficiency states is given in Table 26.2.

This usually happens when the activity of coagulation factors falls below 5% of normal. Typically, these deficiencies are the result of a chronic disease state such as von Willebrand's Disease or hemophilia. Management of an acute hemorrhagic event in a coagulation factor deficient patient includes administration of the appropriate factors in concentrated form. The most common inherited clotting factor deficiencies involve factor VIII (classic hemophilia A) and factor IX (hemophilia B or Christmas Disease).

Two forms of factor VIII concentrate are clinically available: cryoprecipitate and lyophilized factor VIII concentrate. Cryoprecipitate is a factor VIII rich plasma protein fraction prepared from whole blood that also contains approximately 300 mg of fibrinogen per unit. Immediately before infusion, the required number of cryoprecipitate units are thawed in a sterile saline/citrate solution and pooled. The lyophilized factor VIII concentrates are prepared from large plasma pools and are also rich in fibrinogen. Lyophilized factor VIII concentrates are not useful in therapy for von Willebrand's Disease. This is because during the extraction and lyophilization process the polymeric structure of factor VIII in the von Willebrand protein that supports platelet adhesion is destroyed rendering the preparation inactive. Because of the pooling of blood from multiple donors in the preparation of lyophilized factor VIII concentrates, it is generally held that cryoprecipitate, which is isolated from a single donor, is safer.

The major concern associated with the use of concentrated clotting factors is the risk of viral transmission (primarily HIV and hepatitis B). This fear has somewhat attenuated the use of concentrated plasma fractions, even in diseases such as hemophilia. Ultrapure factor VIII concentrates produced using recombinant DNA technology have been approved for use. However, the expense of these recombinant agents is frequently the reason that the more traditional plasma isolates are used, despite the possibility of viral transmission.

Lyophilized preparations of prothrombin, factor IX and factor X are also available. The manufacturing process involves plasma extraction with solvents and detergents that renders the preparations virally inactive but can activate clotting factors. In order to prevent excessive thrombus formation in these situations, heparin is often added to the therapeutic regimen.

There are times when a hemorrhagic event is possible but the patient does not require immediate coagulation therapy. For example, if a patient with mild hemophilia A needs to have a dental extraction performed, the potential for hemorrhage exists. In these cases, it is possible to increase the activity of the endogenous factor VIII through pretreatment with desmopressin acetate. This preoperative measure may alleviate the need for clotting factor replacement.

Table 26.2. Clotting Factors

Factor	Common Name	Deficiency State	Source	$t_{1/2}$ (Days) of Infused Factor	Target for Action of:
I	Fibrinogen	Afibrinogenemia, defibrination syndrome	Liver	4	
II	Prothrombin	Prothrombin deficiency	Liver (requires vitamin K)	3	Heparin (IIa); warfarin (synthesis)
III	Tissue thromboplastin, thrombokinase, tisse factor		Liver (may require vitamin K)		
IV	Calcium (Ca²⁺)				
V	Proaccelerin, labile factor	Factor V deficiency	Liver	1	
VI	Deleted factor				
VII	Proconvertin, stable factor	Factor VII deficiency	Liver (requires vitamin K)	0.25	Heparin (VIIa); warfarin (synthesis)
VIII	Antihemophilic A factor (AHF), antihemophilic globulin (AHG)	Hemophilia A (classic) Von Willebrand's disease	Liver	0.5 Unknown	
IX	Antihemophilic B factor, plasma thromboplastin component (PTC), Christmas factor	Hemophilia B (Christmas disease)	Liver (requires vitamin K)	1	Heparin (IXa); warfarin (synthesis)
X	Stuart or Stuart-Prower factor	Stuart-Prower defect	Liver (requires vitamin K)	1.5	Heparin (IXa); warfarin (synthesis)
XI	Plasma thromboplastin antecedent (PTA)	PTA deficiency	Unknown	3	
XII	Hageman factor, contact factor	Hageman defect	Unknown	Unknown	
XIII	Fibrin stabilizing factor, fibrinase	Fibrin-stabilizing factor deficiency	Unknown	6	
	Fletcher factor, prekallikrein factor		Liver		
	Fitzgerald factor, high-molecular-weight kininogen		Liver		
AT III		Antithrombin III deficiency		3	
Proteins C & S					Warfarin (synthesis)
Plasminogen					Thrombolytic enzymes, aminocaproic acid

PLASMA EXTENDERS AND BLOOD SUBSTITUTES

Maintenance of circulation is secondary only to airway and breathing in the American Heart Association chain of survival (45). Circulation is governed by the three components of the Fick Principle: 1) On-loading of oxygen onto the erythrocytes (red blood cells); 2) Delivery of oxygen-laden erythrocytes to the various cells and tissues; 3) Off-loading of the oxygen from the erythrocytes to the tissue cells (46). Interruption of any of these three components results in physiologic compromise. Inadequate blood volume (specifically, a loss of red blood cells) will disallow the transport of oxygen to tissues.

Severe anemia, such as that secondary to major hemorrhage, is a complicated condition to manage. Simply replacing lost blood with new blood may not always be practical or even beneficial to the patient. Numerous approaches and theories exist attempting to define the best method of emergently managing severe blood loss. Two basic types of fluid infusion are used for the resuscitation of severely anemic patients. These are sanguinous (blood containing) in which fluids such as whole blood and fractionated blood products are used and asanguinous (non-blood containing) in which various crystalloids, colloids, blood substitutes and plasma expanders are employed.

Sanguinous Resuscitation

It seems intuitive that resuscitation following severe blood loss would be best accomplished by replacing lost blood with fresh blood (i.e., sanguinous resuscitation).

This is not always in the best interest of the resuscitation. Nonetheless, infusion of blood and blood products is recommended in certain hypovolemic circumstances. Generally, if hemodynamic instability exists in a hypovolemic adult following the infusion of 2 liters of crystalloid (three successive 20 mL/kg body weight infusions in a child) addition of blood to the resuscitative regimen is recommended (47). The most significant advantage of sanguinous resuscitation is that infusion of red blood cells can replace both volume and oxygen carrying capacity. Significant disadvantages of sanguinous resuscitation include limited supply, risk of transfusion reaction, expense and possible transmission of blood borne diseases.

At one time, a significant controversy existed over whether survivability was increased with the use of whole blood transfusion or infusion of packed red blood cells (known as "component therapy"). The decision made traditionally was based on cost and the fact that few hospitals actually stored whole blood. Fortunately, scientists reached the same decision as the fiscal experts (47). The three major conclusions drawn from the scientific community are: 1) "Whole blood out" does not require "whole blood in." Banked whole blood stored at 4°C lacks functional platelets and also suffers a progressive deterioration in the activities of various clotting factors. There is little difference in these parameters between banked whole blood and packed red blood cells. Since trauma patients require red blood cells, clotting factors and platelets to varying degrees, it makes more sense to use functional components to replace what is specifically needed at that time. 2) Whole blood is not infused more rapidly than packed red blood cells. In fact, infusion technology exists that allows replacement of packed red blood cells suspended in normal saline as fast as 1600 mL/min. 3) The overall risk of antigenic hypersensitivity reactions is greatly increased when using whole blood as opposed to specific components. The standard of care at this time is judicious use of the individual components with crystalloid infusion to maintain volume while the defect resulting in the blood loss is repaired.

Asanguinous Resuscitation

Crystalloids are aqueous electrolyte containing solutions without proteins or large molecules. Examples of crystalloids are normal saline (0.9% NaCl) and lactated Ringers solution. Colloids are aqueous solutions that contain various proteins or other larger molecules as well as electrolytes. Protein containing colloids include albumin and plasma protein fraction (PPF). Nonprotein colloids include the dextrans and hetastarch. A list detailing the compositions of several common crystalloids and colloids is given in Table 26.3.

Crystalloids

Crystalloids have several advantages including being inexpensive and free of risk of transferring blood borne pathogens or inducing anaphylaxis. Furthermore, they are largely compatible with drugs and undergo rapid renal clearance. However, the crystalloids have a very short resident time in the intravascular space—only 30% remains in the vasculature within a few minutes following infusion. These fluids rapidly leak out of the vasculature into the interstitial space and can result in significant extravascular fluid accumulations ("third spacing"). Furthermore, crystalloids do not have any oxygen carrying capacity.

Attempts at lengthening intravascular resident time of the solution and limit third spacing have resulted in the development of "hypertonic" crystalloid solutions. An example of a hypertonic solution is 3% NaCl ("hypertonic saline"). It has been suggested that the increased electrolyte concentration will result in an osmotic gradient pulling fluid from the interstitial and intracellular spaces into the vasculature. These fluid shifts would therefore require less total volume to be infused. As expected the possibility of severe hypernatremia and hyperchloremia, among other electrolyte disturbances, exists.

Protein Colloids

Protein colloids contain larger molecules and have a longer intravascular resident time than crystalloids though eventual fluid loss to the extravascular space does occur. Protein colloids such as albumin and PPF are prepared from pooled human blood and therefore carry with them a risk of transmission of viral infection or induction of anaphylaxis. PPF is a 5% mixture (5g protein in 100ml NaCl 0.9% solution) of proteins that is osmotically equivalent to human plasma. The composition of the protein mixture is 83–90% albumin. Albumin is typically administered as either a 5% or 25% solution. By definition, albumin preparations must be composed of a protein mixture that is >90% albumin. PPF is generally favored over albumin for fluid resuscitation, as albumin appears to cause more interstitial edema.

Dextran polymer

Nonproteinaceous Colloids

Dextrans. Nonproteinaceous colloids are also used in fluid resuscitation. These compounds are generally complex mixtures of sugar polymers. Dextrans are glucose polymers produced by bacteria linked in an α-1,6 chain and having an α-1,3 or α-1,4 branch about every fifth residue. The specific positioning of the branching varies by the bacterium producing it. The molecular weights of these chains are generally 40 or 70 kD (Dextran-40 and Dextran-70, respectively), and the compounds work via an osmotic

Table 26.3. Composition of Common Intravenous Fluids

Solution	Common/ Trade Name	Concentration Solute	Ionic Concentration g/dL	mEq/L	Indications	Contraindications
CRYSTALLOIDS 0.9% Saline	Normal Saline	NaCl	0.90	Na+ 154 Cl− 154	Hypovolemia Heat-related emergencies Freshwater drowning Diabetic ketoacidosis	CHF
0.45% Saline	Half-Normal Saline	NaCl	0.45	Na+ 77 Cl− 77	Compromised cardiac function	Emergent rehydration
3% Saline	Hypertonic Saline	NaCl	3.0	Na2+ 513 Cl− 513	Hypovolemia, hyponatremia, TCA OD	Hypernatremia Hyperchloremia
5% Dextrose in Water	D₅W	Glucose	5.0		Intravenous drug route. Dilution of concentrated drugs for intravenous infusion	Volume replacement
Lactated Ringer's	Hartman's Solution	NaCl KCl CaCl₂ Na Lactate	0.86 0.03 0.02 0.31	Na+ 130 K+ 4 Ca2+ 3 Cl− 109 Lactate 28	Hypovolemic shock Obstetric emergencies	CHF Renal failure Lactic Acidosis
COLLOIDS Plasma Protein Fraction	Plasmanate	Albumin Globulin	4.4 0.6	Na+ 130−160 Cl− 130−160	Hypovolemic shock	Coagulopathy (relative)
Albumin		Albumin	5 25	Na+ 130−160 Cl− 130−160	Hypovolemic shock	Coagulopathy (relative)
Hetastarch	Hespan	Hydroxyethyl Starch	6 (in saline)	Na+ 154 Cl− 154	Hypovolemic shock.	Factor VIII deficiency

gradient similar to the colloids and hypertonic crystalloid solutions. Dextran-70 is a 4% solution while dextran-40 is a 10% preparation. Dextrans have a longer intravascular resident time than albumin which limits interstitial edema. As with the crystalloids and other colloids, the dextrans have no oxygen carrying capacity. Further, since they are bacterial products, the dextrans have the potential to be potent antigens and induce anaphylaxis. The incidence of serious antigenic response seems to increase if the dextran used has a significant fraction of components with molecular weight > 100 kD. In these cases, administration of dextran-1 (MW = 1 kD) prior to the higher dextrans minimizes formulation of the very large immunogenic complexes. This approach has been shown to decrease sensitivity responses to high molecular weight dextrans by as much as 15–20-fold. This is particularly important in a number of European countries where dextran-150 (MW ~ 150 kD) is routinely used.

Hetastarch.   Hetastarch, another nonprotein colloid, is a complex mixture of ethoxylated amylopectins, ranging in molecular weight from 10–1000 kD (average MW ~ 450 kD). When infused as a 6% solution, hetastarch approximates the activity of human albumin. However, the larger molecular weight increases its intravascular resident time as well as its plasma expansion effects relative to albumin. Hetastarch is synthetically produced so it is degraded more slowly and is less antigenic than other colloids. Despite these advantages, hetastarch is quite expensive and has no oxygen carrying capacity.

Plasma substitutes such as dextrans and hetastarch have some additional unusual disadvantages specific to the various classes. High molecular weight (MW 70 kD) dextran coats erthyrocytes making subsequent blood typing and crossmatching difficult. On the other hand, low molecular weight (MW 40 kD) dextran coats platelets which can induce a bleeding disorder. Hetastarch has a dilutional effect on factor VIII and should therefore not be used to treat patients with factor VIII deficiency (e.g., hemophilia) related hemorrhage.

Combination use of hypertonic crystalloids with nonprotein colloids has been investigated. For example, 7.5% NaCl in 6% dextran-70 (hypertonic saline-dextrose, HSD) has been studied in a variety of animal models and in human trauma patients with some success. Particularly promising are animal studies of closed head injury, which suggest not only a hemodynamic benefit but also a sustained decrease in intracranial pressure. Studies in this system as well as in burn and trauma patients are ongoing.

Blood Substitutes/"Synthetic Blood"

Some religious groups, such as Jehovah's Witnesses, frequently refuse blood and blood product administration even under dire circumstances (47). This healthcare dilemma as well as cost and ease of collection was largely

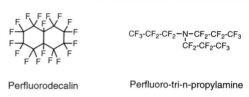

Perfluorodecalin   Perfluoro-tri-n-propylamine

Fig. 26.14. Chemical structures of perfluorochemical blood substitutes.

responsible for the development of synthetic blood substitutes. Two common components of the synthetic blood substitutes are perfluorodecalin and perfluoro-tri-n-propylamine (Fig. 26.14) (14). These compounds are referred to as perfluorochemicals or "PFC's."

The most significant benefit of PFC's is their ability to transport oxygen to the body tissues via the circulatory system. This ability is due to the high solubility of gases such as oxygen and carbon dioxide in the PFC preparations. Red blood cells with fully functional hemoglobin have an oxygen solubility of 17–20 mL/dL. Red blood cells without hemoglobin can only dissolve about 0.3 mL of oxygen per dL. The oxygen solubility of PFC preparations is about 7 mL/dL.

The PFC's are formulated as stable aqueous emulsions with dextrose, egg yolk phospholipids and physiologic electrolytes. These emulsions are somewhat less viscous than whole blood at 37°C. The PFC's have a dose-dependent $t_{1/2}$ of 8–24 hours. Normal doses are ~10 mL/kg, though short-term doses of up to 30 mL/kg have been reported. The PFC's are not metabolized and are eliminated unchanged in expired respiratory gases. Because they are highly lipophilic, multiple doses can cause PFC accumulation in the liver and spleen. Therefore, it is recommended that these compounds not be administered more than once in a 6-month period.

During the early 1980s, PFC emulsions were used to treat trauma victims in battlefield hospitals in the Yunan Province during the Sino-Vietnam border conflict (37). The Chinese investigators reported good success and no complications with this therapeutic approach. A 1993 American report presents a case of a 40-year-old Jehovah's Witnesses female with postpartum hemorrhage who had refused blood products and was treated with Fluosol (a 20% emulsion of perfluorodecalin and perfluoro-tri-n-propylamine). The PFC therapy was ineffective in this case and the patient died (48).

Another use for PFC emulsions is decreasing or preventing myocardial ischemia during PTCA in high-risk patients. The emulsion is preoxygenated and injected transluminally through the coronary angioplasty balloon to deliver the oxygenated emulsion to areas distal to the point of balloon inflation. Less common but also investigated uses of PFC emulsions include therapy for carbon monoxide intoxication, oxygenation in cases of cerebral hypoxia, autoimmune hemolytic anemic and nonavailability of compatible blood products.

Genetically Engineered and Chimeric Hemoglobins

Stroma-free hemoglobin appears to hold significant promise as a potential acellular oxygen transporter. These preparations have no effect on colloid osmotic pressure and are not effective as plasma expanders. A number of potential advantages exist with this technology. For example, stroma-free hemoglobin can be prepared from bovine or outdated human erythrocytes, no crossmatch is necessary, it is lyophilized for convenient and space efficient storage and it is reconstituted in normal saline (49).

Two major problems that are currently being addressed are large-scale production of the material and the fact that stroma-free hemoglobin does not readily release oxygen to the tissues at normal oxygen tensions. Recombinant DNA technology has allowed for the production of large amounts of hemoglobin through synthetic gene expression in *E. coli* and *Saccharomyces cerevisiae*. New developments in hemoglobin polymerization also show promise (49).

Another approach to stroma-free hemoglobin technology is the development of chimeric hemoglobins. Human hemoglobin stripped from red blood cells is not functional. Diphosphoglycerate (DPG) is required for oxygen release from hemoglobin and there is insufficient DPG available outside the red cell to induce oxygen release (i.e., oxygen affinity for hemoglobin is too high in the absence of DPG). Tetrameric human hemoglobin decomposes into dimers when infused into the bloodstream. These dimers precipitate in the kidneys potentially causing severe renal damage. In native red cell bound hemoglobin, this decomposition is prevented by the high concentration of proteins inside the red blood cells. Interestingly, not all species require ATP and DPG to diminish oxygen affinity for hemoglobin. The crocodile is one such animal in which red blood cells do not contain DPG and this phosphate has no effect on oxygen affinity to their hemoglobin. Crocodile hemoglobin cannot be used directly in humans as certain features of human hemoglobin are necessary for recognition and signaling. Genetic engineering technology has allowed the creation of a chimeric hemoglobin that is part human and part crocodile which is useful in humans (49). It has the advantage of providing hemoglobin oxygen carrying capacity without transmitting human blood borne diseases. One major disadvantage is the chimeric hemoglobins are not endogenous proteins and therefore may be potent antigens. A great deal of investigation is still necessary before chimeric hemoglobins will see any clinical utility.

NEW DIRECTIONS IN COAGULATION-BASED THERAPEUTICS

A number of exciting possibilities for coagulation therapy are currently under investigation (50). These newer approaches tend to attempt exploitation of parts of the coagulation cascade not traditionally used. Some examples of these newer therapeutic modalities include inhibiting platelet recruitment, enhancing endogenous anticoagulant activity and fibrinolysis, and blocking the initiation of both the intrinsic and extrinsic pathways of the coagulation cascade. Though still investigational at this time, many of the proposed ideas are quite promising.

Victoria F. Roche, S. William Zito, and Robert B. Palmer

LV, a 65-year-old male, ingested what was described as a "large quantity" of D-con Mouse Prufe-II rodenticide (0.005% brodifacoum) in a suicidal gesture. He told his wife of the ingestion six hours later and she immediately called 911. Police and paramedics arrived and the man was transported by ambulance to the local emergency department (ED). On arrival in the ED, the patient was alert, oriented and tearful. His vital signs on presentation were: HR 100, BP 140/86 mmHg, RR 16 and non-labored. His past medical history is significant only for an appendectomy at age 35 and a myocardial infarction (MI) at age 59. LV has been on daily aspirin therapy since his MI and he has no known medical allergies. The attending ED physician asks you, the pharmacist at the local poison control center, to review the toxicity of brodifacoum and to suggest a course for initial management for this case. You are aware that the hospital from which the physician is calling has on its formulary compounds 1-4, which should be considered when making the recommendations.

1. Identify the therapeutic problem(s) where the pharmacist's intervention may benefit the patient.

2. Identify and prioritize the patient specific factors that must be considered to achieve the desired therapeutic outcomes.

3. Conduct a thorough and mechanistically oriented structure-activity analysis of all therapeutic alternatives provided in the case.

4. Evaluate the SAR findings against the patient specific factors and desired therapeutic outcomes and make a therapeutic decision.

5. Counsel your patient.

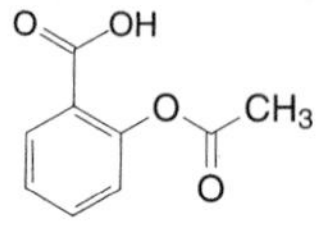

Aspirin

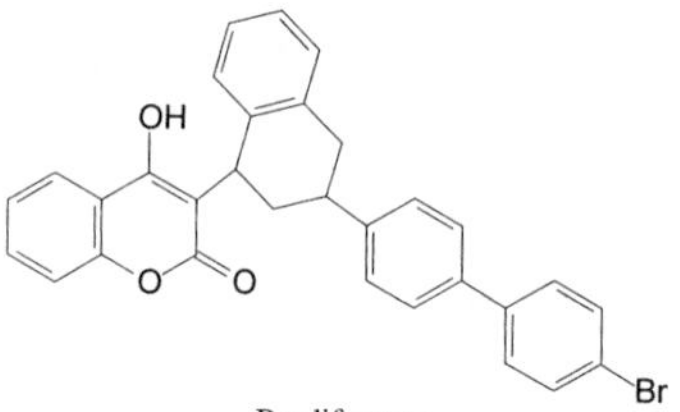

Brodifacoum

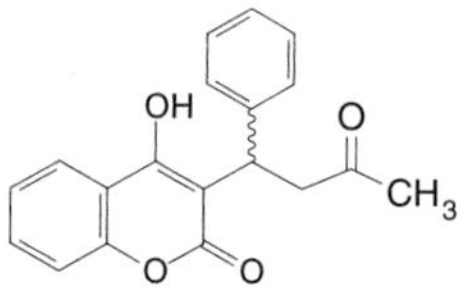

1

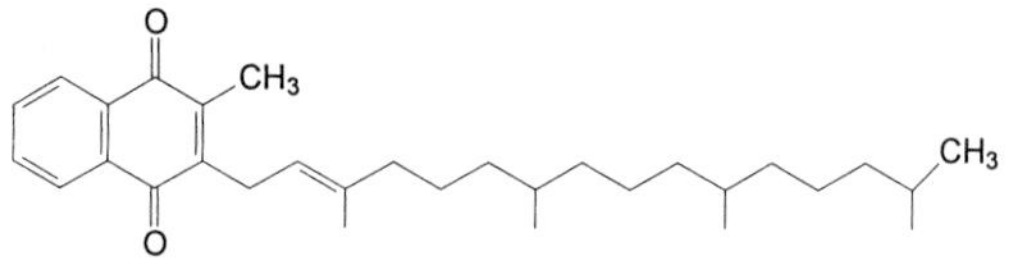

2

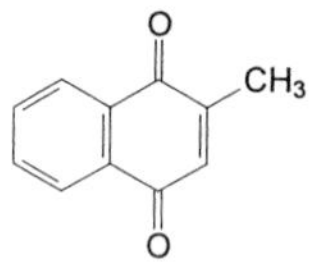

3

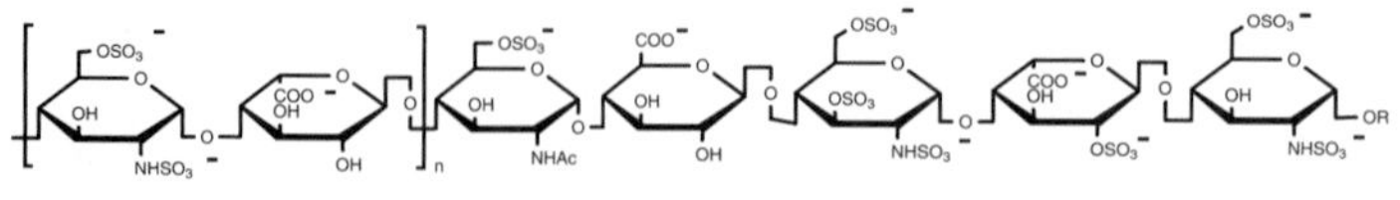

4

R =

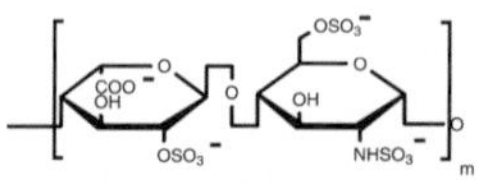

REFERENCES

1. Wright IS. The discovery and early development of anticoagulants: A historical perspective. Circulation 1959; 19:73–134.
2. Stryer L. Biochemistry. 3rd ed. New York :W. H. Freeman and Company, 1988.
3. O'Reilly RO. Drugs Used in Disorders of Coagulation. In: Katzung BG, ed. Basic and Clinical Pharmacology, 7th ed. Stamford, CT: Appleton & Lange, 1998.
4. Fevig JM, Wexler RR. Anticoagulants: thrombin and factor Xa inhibitors, In: Doherty AM, ed. Ann Rep in Med Chem; San Diego: Academic Press, 1999; 34:81–100.
5. Brookoff D. Hematologic Evaluation. In: Flomenbaum N, Goldfrank L, Jacobson S, eds. Emergency Diagnostic Testing, 2nd ed. St. Louis, MO: Mosby, 1995.
6. Majerus PW, Broze GJ Jr, Miletich JP, et al. Anticoagulant, thrombolytic and antiplatelet drugs. In: Hardman JG, Limbird LE, Molinoff PB, et al, eds. Goodman and Gilman's The Pharmacological Basis of Therapeutics. 9th ed. New York : McGraw-Hill, 1996; 1341 – 1359.
7. Hammer RH. Anticoagulants, Coagulants and Plasma Extenders. In: Foye WO, Lemke TL, Williams DA, eds. Principles of Medicinal Chemistry. 4th ed. Philadelphia: Williams and Wilkins, 1995; 388–404.
8. Arora RB, Mathur CN. Relationship between structure and anticoagulant activity of coumarin derivatives. Br J Pharmacol 1963; 20:29–35.
9. Valente EJ, Lingafelter EC, Porter WR, et al. Structure of warfarin in solution. J Med Chem 1977; 20:1489–1493.
10. Awni LM, Hussein Z, Granneman GR, et al. Pharmacodynamic and stereoselective pharmacokinetic interactions between zileuton and warfarin in humans. Clin Pharmacokinet 1995; 29 Suppl 2:67–76.
11. O'Reilly RO, Goulart DA, Kunze KL, et al. Mechanisms of the stereoselective interaction between miconazole and racemic warfarin in human subjects. Clin Pharmacol Ther 1992; 51: 656–667.
12. Niopas I, Toon S, Rowland M. Further insight into the stereoselective interaction between warfarin and cimetidine in man. Br J Clin Pharmacol 1991; 32:508–511.
13. Baselt RC, ed. Disposition of Toxic Drugs and Chemicals in Man, 5th ed. Foster City, CA: Chemical Toxicology Institute, 2000.
14. USPDI Drug Information for the Health Care Professional, 16th ed. Rockville, MD: United States Pharmacopeial Convention, Inc., 1996: 236–246.
15. Fanelli O. Some pharmacological properties of 2-aryl-1,3-indandione derivatives. Drug Res 1975; 25:873–877.
16. Hollinger BR, Pastoor TP. Case management and plasma half-life in a case of brodifacoum poisoning. Arch Intern Med 1993; 153:1925–1928.
17. Palmer RB, Alakija P, Cde Baca, JE, et al. Fatal brodifacoum rodenticide poisoning: autopsy and toxicologic findings. J Forensic Sci 1999; 44:851–855.
18. Redfern R, Gill JE, Hadler MR. Laboratory evaluation of WBA8119 (brodifacoum) as a rodenticide for use against warfarin-resistant and non-resistant rats and mice. J Hygiene 1976; 77:419–426.
19. Bachmann KA, Sullivan TJ. Dispositional and pharmacodynamic characteristics of brodifacoum in warfarin-sensitive rats. Pharmacol 1983; 27:281–288.
20. Slattery J, Yacobi A, Levy G. Comparative pharmacokinetics of coumarin anticoagulants, XXV: warfarin-ibuprofen interaction in rats, J Pharm Sci 1977; 66:943–947.
21. Hoffman RS. Anticoagulants. In: Goldfrank LR, Flomenbaum NE, Lewin NA, et al, eds. Goldfrank's Toxicologic Emergencies, 6th ed. Stamford, CT: Appleton & Lange, 1998.
22. Budavari S, ed. Merck Index, 11th ed. Rahway, NJ: Merck and Company, 1989.
23. Hirsh J. Warkentin TE, Raschke R, et al. Heparin and low-molecular-weight heparin: Mechanisms of action, pharmacokinetics, dosing, considerations, monitoring, efficacy and safety. Chest 1998; 114:489S-510S.
24. Hovanessian HC. New Generation Anticoagulants: The low molecular weight heparins. Ann Emerg Med 1999; 34:768–779.
25. Rosenberg RD. Biochemistry and pharmacology of low molecular weight heparin. Sem in Hematol 1997; 4(Suppl 4):2–8.
26. Physician's Desk Reference, 53rd ed., Montvale, NJ: Medical Economics Company, 1999.
27. Petitou M, Herault J, Bernat A, et al. Synthesis of thrombin-inhibiting heparin mimetics without side effects. Nature 1999; 398:417–422.
28. Leone-Bay A, Paton DR, Freeman J, et al. Synthesis and evaluation of compounds that facilitate the gastrointestinal absorption of heparin. J Med Chem 1998; 41:1163–1171.
29. Zoppetti G, Caramazza I, Murakami Y, et al. Structural requirements for duodenal permeability of heparin-diamine complexes. Biochim et Biophys Acta 1992; 1156:92–98.
30. Andriuoli G, Caramazza I, Galimberti G, et al. Intraduodenal absorption in the rabbit of a novel heparin salt. Haemostasis 1992; 22:113–116.
31. Engel RH, Riggi SJ. Intestinal absorption of heparin facilitated by sulfated or sulfonated surfactants. Proc Soc Exp Biol Med 1969; 130:706–710.
32. Guarini S, Ferrari W. Olive oil-provoked, bile-dependent absorption of heparin from the gastrointestinal tract in rats. Pharm Res Commun 1986; 17:685–694.
33. Ueno M, Nakasake T, Horikoshi I, et al. Oral administration of liposomally entrapped heparin to beagle dogs. Chem Pharm Bull 1982; 30:2245–2247.
34. Steiner S, Rosen R. Delivery systems for pharmacological agents encapsulated with proteinoids. U.S. Patent 4,925,673 (1990).
35. Leone-Bay A, Leipold H, Agarwal R, et al. The evolution of an oral heparin dosing solution. Drugs Future 1997; 22: 885–891.
36. Johnson PH. Hirudin: Clinical potential of a thrombin inhibitor. Annu Rev Med 1994; 45:165–177.
37. Krstenansky JL, Owen TJ, Yates MT, et al. Design, synthesis and antithrombin activity for conformationally restricted analogs of peptide anticoagulants based on the C-terminal region of the leech peptide, hirudin. Biochim Biophys Acta 1988; 957:53–59.
38. Maraganore JM, Bourdon P, Jablonski J, et al. Design and characterization of hirulogs: A novel class of bivalent peptide inhibitors of thrombin. Biochemistry 1990; 29:7095–7101.
39. Patrano C, Collar B, Dalen JE, et al. Platelet-active drugs: The relationships among dose, effectiveness and side effects. Chest 1998; 114:470S-488S.
40. Parks WM, Hoak JC, Czervionke RL. Comparative effect of ibuprofen on endothelial and platelet postaglandin synthesis. J Pharmacol Exp 1981; 219: 415–419.
41. Harvey RA, Champe PC, Mycek MJ, eds. Drugs affecting the blood. In: Lippincott's Illustrated Review in Pharmacology, 2nd ed. Philadelphia, PA: Lippincott-Raven Publishers, 1997.
42. Kuo BS, Ritschel WA. Correlation between inhibitory effect on platelet aggregation and disposition of sulfinpyrazone and its metabolites in rabbits. Part II: Multiple dose study. Biopharm Drug Dispos 1987; 8:11–21.
43. Genetta TB, Mauro VF. ABCIXIMAB: A new antiaggregant used in angioplasty. Ann Pharmacother 1996; 30:251–257.

44. Chen Y, Wang T, Liang S, et al. Synthesis and evaluation of coumarin α-methylene-γ-butyrolactones: a new class of platelet aggregation inhibitors. Chem Pharm Bull 1996; 44:1591–1595.

45. Cummins RO, ed. Textbook of Advanced Cardiac Life Support, 1997–1999 ed. Dallas, TX: American Heart Association, 1997.

46. McSwain NE, Frame S, Paturas, JL, eds. Shock and fluid resuscitation in basic and advanced prehospital trauma life support, 4th ed., St. Louis, MO: Mosby, 1999.

47. Pollack C. Prehospital fluid resuscitation of the trauma patient. Emerg Med Clin of North America 1993; 11:61–70.

48. Kale PB, Sklar GE, Wesolowicz LA, et al. Fluosol: therapeutic failure in severe anemia. Ann Pharmacother 1993; 27:1452–1454.

49. Komiyama N, Tame J, Nagai K. A hemoglobin-based blood substitute: transplanting a novel allosteric effect of crocodile Hgb. Biol Chem 1996; 377:543–548.

50. Weitz JI, Hirsh J. New antithrombotic agents. Chest 1998; 114:715S-727S.

27. Insulin and Oral Hypoglycemic Drugs

ROBERT A. WILEY

DIABETES MELLITUS
History and Epidemiology

The word diabetes is Greek for siphon, applied to this condition because one of its symptoms is excessive thirst. The other symptoms of diabetes mellitus (weight loss, excessive hunger, and the presence of glucose in the urine as determined by tasting) were described in the Ebers Papyrus nearly 3500 years ago. In 1869 Paul Langerhans observed that the pancreas consists of two types of cells, the acinar cells which secrete digestive enzymes and cells clustered like islets which had an unknown function. Serum glucose levels were associated with the pancreas in 1889 (1). Banting and Best, in a landmark 1921 paper, showed that a pancreatic extract could reduce serum glucose levels in pancreatectomized dogs (2). In 1922 a pancreatic extract was administered to a 14-year-old patient exhibiting a serum glucose level of 500 mg/dL, who survived 15 years on insulin obtained from animal sources. This success led many to conclude, erroneously, that diabetes is a disease of elevated blood sugar, easily corrected by exogenous insulin. We now know that such is far from the case. Diabetes is a generalized degenerative disorder, probably involving several peptide hormones, which causes highly significant morbidity and mortality in its victims, often in spite of our best hypoglycemic therapy.

There are about 8.3 million diabetics in the United States, of which about 600,000 suffer from type 1 (insulin dependent) diabetes. The incidence is far higher among some ethnic groups. For example, 50% of Pima Indians over 40 years of age have diabetes. Diabetes is the fifth leading cause of death in the U.S. as well as the leading cause of adult blindness, and is responsible for 50% of heart attacks, 75% of strokes, and 85% of gangrenous leg amputations. It is therefore a force to be reckoned with, and the high level of research interest resulted in the publication in 1998 of 6100 papers on diabetes, of which about 100 dealt only with the etiology of the disease.

Definitions

Clinical diabetes mellitus occurs in two forms, with different causes and methods of therapy.

Type 1 Diabetes

Formerly known as insulin-dependent diabetes mellitus (IDDM), this condition occurs when the β-cells of the pancreatic islets of Langerhans are destroyed, probably by an autoimmune process, such that insulin production is grossly deficient. This is accompanied by significant metabolic derangement; victims of type 1 diabetes are therefore prone to develop diabetic β-ketoacidosis and other manifestations of severe diabetes. There exists only a weak genetic link in the etiology of this form of diabetes. Type 1 diabetes is invariably treated with insulin.

Type 2 Diabetes

Formerly known as noninsulin-dependent diabetes mellitus (NIDDM), type 2 diabetes is very frequently associated with obesity in its mainly adult victims. Serum insulin levels are normal or elevated, so in essence this is a disease of insulin resistance. The disease is generally milder, rarely progressing to β-ketoacidosis although other degenerative processes do occur. There is a strong genetic link in the etiology of the condition, and insulin therapy is not always required.

Etiology of Diabetes
Type 1 Diabetes Mellitus

Interleukin 1 (IL-1) is a protein cytokine which is the principal trigger of all immune responses. This substance is produced by macrophages as a result of antigen processing; it mobilizes B and T cells and stimulates T-helper cells to produce IL-2, another cytokine important to the immune response. Most significantly, the pancreatic islets of animals with spontaneous diabetes have been shown to contain inflammatory cells incorporating IL-1, and incubation of islets with IL-1 selectively destroys β-cells. Moreover, development of type 1 diabetes normally occurs over a period of a few weeks, and in a few instances where this was spotted very early and the patients treated with immunosuppressants such as cyclosporine, the diabetic process was ameliorated. These facts indicate that type 1 diabetes probably results from an autoimmune process involving IL-1, but the question then remaining is what causes the production of this cytokine. The short answer is that we don't know. There are a handful of cases in which viruses have been implicated in development of type 1 diabetes. One of the most convincing involves a previously healthy young boy who suddenly developed very severe diabetes and died after 7 days. Coxsackie B4 viruses were cultured from his body, which produced diabetes when injected into animals.

There is a weak concordance (36%) among identical twins for type 1 diabetes mellitus (3). Much work has been done searching for genetic correlations between diabetes and the cell recognition proteins known as human leucocyte antigens (HLA), which govern recognition in cell-mediated immune reactions. About 95% of patients with type 1 diabetes are positive for HLA-Dr3 or Dr4, whereas only 40% of nondiabetics exhibit these proteins (4). On the other hand, the haplotype HLA-Dr2 appears negatively associated with type 1 diabetes incidence. The nature of the residue at position 57 of the HLA-DQβ chain correlates even more closely with type 1 diabetes. If the residue is alanine, valine, or serine, the susceptibility to diabetes is high, whereas if aspartate is found at this position there is a negative correlation (5). Substitution of glutamate with its side chain carboxyl group for the nonpolar residues mentioned would be expected to change the shape of the antigen binding site dramatically. In this case, it has been suggested that this alters binding of antibodies such as islet cell autoantibody. Another promising lead is the observation that a key protein target of autoimmune attack is the enzyme glutamic acid decarboxylase (GAD). This enzyme produces γ-aminobutyric acid, a neurotransmitter intimately involved in intercellular signalling (6, 7). It was possible to block β-cell destruction in mice by "tolerizing" the young immune system to GAD, so that the enzyme is not erroneously recognized as foreign, thereby triggering an autoimmune process.

Type 2 Diabetes Mellitus

In type 2 diabetes mellitus, serum insulin measurements indicate normal or elevated serum insulin concentrations, although there is some confusion about exactly what is being measured using currently available technology (see below). The problem, then, is probably not insulin availability, but insulin resistance. There is a much stronger genetic link in this condition than in type 1 diabetes, for studies with identical twins point to a concordance rate in identical twins of 90–100% (3). There is also a most intriguing suggestion that mutations in the gene for the enzyme glucokinase represent the genetic defect in a form of type 2 diabetes known as maturity onset diabetes of the young (MODY). This type 2-like condition is quite rare, but very strongly genetically linked in affected families. In a recent study, 18 of 32 families with MODY exhibited mutations of the hexokinase gene, whereas only 1 of 14 disease-free families did. Several of the mutations were studied in detail and one, in codon 300 of exon 8 of the glucokinase gene was found in all 41 affected members of one family and in none of their disease-free relatives.

This mutation causes a change of GAG (Guanine-Adenine-Guanine) to CAG (Cytosine-Adenine-Guanine) and results in substitution of Gln for Glu; the resulting protein fails to function as an enzyme. This is important, because glucokinase is found only in pancreas and liver and the rates of glucokinase function, the rate-controlling step in the glycolytic cycle, and insulin secretion are linked. β-cells and hepatocytes also contain GLUT-2, a high-capacity glucose transporter (one of five glucose transporter molecules abbreviated as GLUT 1–5), so plasma glucose

changes are quickly mirrored intracellularly, and insulin secretion is stimulated. Thus, glucokinase can be regarded as the "glucose sensor" in the body. If ineffective glucokinase is produced, the rate of metabolism at any given serum insulin level is reduced. A new steady state is reached, in which insulin functions more or less normally, but at a higher serum glucose level than is normally found. Therefore, the patient with a defective glucokinase gene is diabetic (8). Other proposals have been made, such as one involving the gene for the enzyme glycogen synthase (9). In this study, 70% of type 2 diabetes patients were homozygous for glycogen synthase allele A₁ whereas 92% of normal controls were (or, four times as many diabetics were not homozygous for A₁ as were normal subjects). Moreover, the presence of the A₂ allele was associated with a strong history of diabetes and with a profound defect in insulin-mediated glucose storage as glycogen. Thus, glycogen synthase is a serious candidate for a genetic mutation in type 2 diabetes, but remember that only a minority of diabetics had the A₂ allele, and that many normal subjects also had it.

There is also evidence that diet *per se* can cause type 2 diabetes. A detailed study among Hispanics in Colorado revealed that addition of 40 grams of fat per day to a carefully studied basal diet increased the diabetes odds ratio for type 2 diabetes 1.51-fold, and the odds ratio for impaired fasting glucose 1.62-fold (10). Also, a study among Australian aboriginal people revealed that when exposed to a Western diet the incidence of diabetes increased from zero to about 25% in the 35–65 age group (11). When returned to their normal diet, the diabetes essentially disappeared. It appears that a genetic predisposition to insulin resistance may be a survival adaptation. Aboriginals may eat 2–3 kg of meat at one time if it is available, then fast for some days. Insulin essentially encourages cells to burn glucose, and lack of effective insulin encourages nutrient storage. Persons with this adaptation will fare better on a starvation diet, and not so well when food, especially fat, is plentiful.

Knowledge is also accumulating concerning how body weight is regulated generally (12). It seems that we can now add insulin to the list of hormones which exhibit CNS effects. For some time, it has been known that the hormone leptin, produced by adipose cells, is involved in obesity. Now, it has been shown that postprandial secretion of both leptin and insulin is exactly proportional to how much fat the body contains—the more fat, the more insulin. The highest density of central leptin and insulin receptors is found in the arcuate nucleus of the hypothalamus, an area long known to be involved in obesity. In addition, at least eight other peptide hormones have been shown to be involved in eating behavior.

With increasing knowledge of the causes of the two main forms of diabetes, one hopes that more effective counter therapies will be developed, which may attack the disease at its genetic roots. At the present time, all therapy is meant to ameliorate the symptoms.

Biochemistry and Pathogenesis of Diabetes
Glucose Uptake into Liver, Fat, and Muscle Cells

Role of Insulin. Insulin is secreted, in response to elevated serum glucose levels, by the β-cells of the pancreatic islets of Langerhans. It is interesting that islet α-cells secrete glucagon, a hormone with actions nearly opposite those of insulin, the δ-cells secrete somatostatin, and the F-cells secrete pancreatic polypeptide. All of these substances may also play a role in diabetes. The role of insulin is to stimulate the GLUT-4 glucose transporter. GLUT-4 is the most important of the glucose transporter molecules and by insertion into the muscle and adipose cell membranes serves to facilitate glucose delivery into these cells. This is the only mechanism by which glucose can be delivered to fat, muscle, and also liver cells (Fig. 27.1). No matter how high the serum glucose level, glucose can access these types of cells only if a functioning insulin system is present. Under normal circumstances, liver and muscle cells take up glucose and convert any excess to the storage form glycogen. Fat cells store energy as fat. If insulin is absent, these three types of cells will undergo "starvation in the midst of plenty," and have to resort to last-ditch methods, once glycogen is exhausted, to obtain glucose, which is required as an energy source by all cells. Insulin is also involved in uptake of amino acids by muscle cells.

In diabetic fat cells, it is possible to obtain glucose from fatty acids *via* production of glycerol, but the first step in the synthesis is the conversion of fatty acids to β-keto acids, which can then be converted to acetyl-CoA. The problem is that β-keto acids are produced in excess, and spill into the blood. β-keto acids are very acidic, and are capable of producing β-ketoacidosis, a life-threatening complication of diabetes. Moreover, in this acidic milieu the β-keto acids can undergo spontaneous decarboxylation to produce ketone bodies, including acetone. The presence of acetone in urine is a diagnostic feature of ketoacidosis. Muscle cells attempt to use amino acids to synthesize glucose, but this process is inefficient and releases quantities of ammonia into the serum, which in itself presents disposal problems.

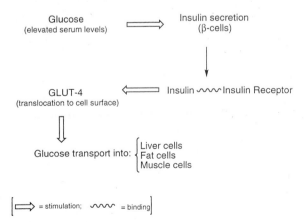

Fig. 27.1. Diagrammatic representation of the roles of glucose and insulin in the stimulation of cellular glucose absorption.

Liver cells attempt to use both fatty acids and amino acids as glucose sources, with the same undesirable consequences noted for fat and muscle cells. It is very important to emphasize that in liver, fat, and muscle cells glucose transport is absolutely under the control of insulin, whereas in other cells it is not.

Other Glucose Transporters. Among the glucose transporters, GLUT-1 transporter governs basal glucose uptake into all cells, but especially brain and red cells, whereas GLUT-2 and 3 regulate insulin release and insulin uptake mostly into neurons and kidney cells, respectively. GLUT-4, as we have seen, is the principal insulin-sensitive glucose transporter. GLUT-2 and GLUT-3 are not governed by insulin, and GLUT-3 has a Michaelis constant value (<1mM) lower than that for GLUT-4 (5mM), so that it is available at low serum insulin levels (13). As a practical matter, then, when serum glucose levels are high, intracellular glucose concentration in neurons, kidney cells, and other types of cells is also high.

Insulin Levels in Diabetes/Insulin Resistance

Diabetes has been known since antiquity, and for many years it was assumed that all diabetics were deficient in insulin. With the invention of radioimmunoassay by R. Yalow in the 1960s, however, it became possible to measure serum insulin levels for the first time and to everyone's amazement it was shown that insulin levels in type 2 diabetes were normal or elevated. The problem in this condition, then, is not insulin deficiency but rather insulin resistance. However, current clinical assays for serum insulin cannot differentiate between insulin and insulin-like materials, such as proinsulin. When specific assays are carried out, it is observed that proinsulin rises from about 6% of total insulin in normal subjects to at least 20% in type 2 diabetics (14). Thus, it could be that more type 2 diabetics than we suspect are actually hypoinsulinemic. It has also been shown that elevated concentration of a partially cleaved proinsulin known as 32, 33 split proinsulin is strongly predictive for development of type 2 diabetes, to a much greater degree than concentrations of either glucose or intact proinsulin (15).

Insulin resistance is not a well-understood phenomenon. As noted above, it appears to be induced in many obese patients. It is unlikely to involve morphologic changes in the insulin receptor, but rather a possible postreceptor defect in the intracellular glucose transporter activating system. One noteworthy recent observation is that serum insulin levels in type 2 diabetic patients rise with increasing serum glucose up to glucose levels of about 140 mg/dL, whereupon the serum insulin level begins to fall. Moreover, this level of serum glucose seems paradoxically to increase gluconeogenesis and lipogenesis, thereby exacerbating an already bad situation.

Insulin resistance can also occur in the absence of hyperglycemia. Patients with hypertension and hypercholesterolemia sometimes develop severe insulin resistance in a condition known as Syndrome X. Such patients frequently display increased VLDL lipoprotein and decreased HDL lipoprotein. They constitute a large fraction of patients likely to develop premature arteriosclerosis.

Complications of Diabetes

It has been emphasized previously that when serum glucose spikes to very high levels, the intracellular concentration of glucose in many types of cells, notably nerve, epithelial, and kidney cells, also rises greatly. This so-called "spiking" of intracellular glucose levels is believed to cause most of the serious complications of diabetes. It appears that controlling serum glucose concentrations as closely as possible (so-called "strict control") reduces the incidence of diabetic complications; this is shown in Table 27.1. At abnormally high levels of glucose, the enzyme aldose reductase is activated. This enzyme converts the excess glucose into the corresponding sugar alcohol, known as sorbitol. Sorbitol, like all sugar alcohols, is so polar it is unable to cross any biological membrane, and is metabolized to fructose only very inefficiently (recall also that mannitol, another sugar alcohol, given parenterally is a diuretic, whereas if given orally it is a laxative). Thus, sorbitol concentration in affected cells rises a little with each glucose spike, until finally the cell osmolality becomes so high that the cell ceases to function, or ruptures. Almost all the difficulties encountered in diabetes arise from this phenomenon, and this explains why prevention of these glucose spikes occupies such a prominent place in modern diabetes treatment. It has been suggested that there may be a glycemic threshold for diabetes complications. According to this proposal, hyperosmotic complications are unlikely if hemoglobin HbA$_{1c}$ levels (see below) remain below 8.1% (16).

Complications of diabetes might be prevented if one had drugs which inhibited aldose reductase. A large-scale effort to identify such drugs was mounted in the 1980s but the only clinical candidate drug, known as sorbinil, had unacceptable toxicity. Recently, however, at least two new second generation aldose reductase inhibitors have been identified, which do not share the nerve damage potential and other problems of first generation drugs. These

Zenarestat   Zopolrestat

drugs, known as zenarestat and zopolrestat, have been studied clinically. The former remains under evaluation, but development of the latter for nerve damage has been suspended due to disappointing clinical results. It may remain viable in treatment of aldose reductase-initiated kidney and heart damage.

Ocular Problems. In diabetic retinopathy, the epithelial cells undergo hyperplasia, so that the basement membrane may become three times as thick as normal. This produces vascular lesions which in turn promote the growth of small, fragile blood vessels in the retina. These are easily ruptured, producing retinopathy, for which the only treatment is laser photocoagulation. Sorbitol can also cause cataracts by producing an osmotic overhydration of eye tissue; diabetes is a leading cause of cataract formation.

Diabetic Nephropathy. This condition was probably the most life-threatening of all the diabetes complications.

Excess sorbitol causes lesions in small blood vessels similar to those seen in the eye. Hypertension appears to exacerbate the condition, and recently it has been shown that angiotensin converting enzyme inhibitors not only prevent development of diabetic nephropathy but alleviate this condition, even if systemic hypertension is not present (17). The proposal is that ACE inhibitors reduce possible renal hypertension. Recent work has also suggested a reduction of the incidence of diabetic nephropathy. Among 25-year diabetics, mortality results mostly from nephropathy (25–30%). In a large study, it was observed that nephropathy occurred in 30% of patients newly diagnosed in 1961–1965, 8% in patients diagnosed in 1966–1970, and was not found in patients diagnosed in 1971–1975 (18). Thus, this feared condition seems to occur less frequently, possibly because diabetes is being diagnosed earlier, and an effective treatment for nephropathy may have been found.

Atherosclerosis and Other Vascular Complications. Hardening of the arteries is very apparent in diabetics, and is associated with an increased risk of stroke, heart attack, and other conditions. Blood vessel deterioration is associated with sorbitol production as described earlier. Compromised circulation in the legs can lead to nonhealing leg ulcers with gangrene, sometimes requiring amputation of the affected limbs. Skin infections, especially those due to *Candida albicans*, are also commonly observed in diabetics.

Table 27.1. Strict vs. Loose Serum Glucose Control

Diabetes Complication	Strict Control	Loose Control	No Treatment
HbA$_{1c}$ level (glycosylated hemoglobin)	7.1%	8.5%	9.5%
Loss of visual acuity	14%	35%	Not measured
Retinopathy	27%	52%	Not measured
Nephropathy	0%	6%	Not measured

Reichard P, Nilsson BY, Rosenqvist U. The effect of long-term intensified insulin treatment on the development of microvascular complications of diabetes mellitus. N Engl J Med 1993; 329: 304–309.

Signs and Symptoms of Diabetes

The classic triad of symptoms in diabetes is polyphagia (hunger), polydypsia (thirst), and polyuria (excess urine). All three result directly from excessive serum glucose levels. Clinical type 1 diabetes usually develops in an acute manner, although the destructive autoimmune process may have been underway for some time. In addition to the symptoms listed above, precipitous weight loss is commonly observed, and glucose can be detected in the urine. Type 2 diabetes has a more insidious, often asymptomatic onset, and its presence is usually detected by routine medical examinations.

Diagnosis of Diabetes

Serum Glucose Levels

Current ADA guidelines provide that a fasting plasma glucose (FPG) test level of 126 mg/dL or higher constitutes presumptive diagnosis of diabetes (19). Alternatively, a casual serum glucose level in excess of 200 mg/dL taken without regard to timing of caloric intake is also diagnostic for diabetes. If the FPG test yields a result between 110 and 126, the patient is said to suffer from impaired fasting glucose (IFG) disorder, often a precursor condition to diabetes.

Although not used commonly today, it is also possible to carry out an oral glucose tolerance test, in which 75 g of glucose is taken orally and glucose serum levels followed for a few hours. If the serum glucose is 200 mg/dL or greater 2 hours after ingesting the glucose, the patient is said to have diabetes.

Hemoglobin HbA$_{1c}$

Hemoglobin HbA$_{1c}$ is a glycosylated hemoglobin, normally found in the body. It is formed when serum glucose level is high, and has a half-life of about 120 days in erythrocytes. Thus, the serum level of this hemoglobin gives a useful history of serum glucose spikes over the last eight weeks or so. HbA$_{1c}$ levels are expressed as a percentage of total hemoglobin, and there is a direct correlation between serum glucose and HbA$_{1c}$ levels, which is given in Table 27.2.

The normal level of HbA$_{1c}$ in nondiabetics is 5–8%, while the maximum observed in severe diabetics is about 12% (20). Although the ADA does not at this time recommend use of HbA$_{1c}$ levels as a diagnostic test, a level of 10% or higher would indicate frank diabetes. HbA$_{1c}$ levels can also be used as an index of success in diabetes therapy.

Role of Hormones Other Than Insulin in Diabetes

Insulin-like Growth Factors

Insulin-like growth factor 1 (IGF-1) appears to be a principal mediator of the actions of growth hormone, and also displays insulin-like activity. There are several other IGF's, the functions of which are not well defined. Insulin appears weakly active at IGF receptors, and conversely. However, proinsulin, which exhibits only 2% of

Table 27.2. Serum Glucose-Glycosylated Hemoglobin Relationship (20)

HbA$_{1c}$ Level %	Ave. 2-hr Postprandial Serum Glucose (mg/dl)
<6	93
6–7	124
7–8	166
8–9	183
9–10	221
>11	241

the metabolic potency of insulin, contains half of insulin's mitogenic potency. Since the mitogenic effect of insulin may contribute to an increased risk of atherosclerosis, it will be important to assess the mitogenic effect of any insulin analogues considered for use in diabetes therapy.

Glucagon

Glucagon is a 29-residue peptide, produced by the α-cells of the pancreas. The role of glucagon is to prevent hypoglycemia. It interacts with specific receptors in liver to trigger glycogenolysis and an increase in gluconeogenesis through cAMP related events. Serum levels of glucagon are always elevated in diabetic patients, even those with high serum glucose levels. This aberrant effect has yet to receive a satisfactory explanation. It is thought that glucagon antagonists may be helpful in reducing serum glucose levels in type 2 diabetes, and both peptide and nonpeptide glucagon antagonists have been studied for this purpose (21). There is also a related hormone, glucagon-like peptide 1 (GLP-1), which increases secretion of insulin (this effect was falsely ascribed to glucagon). GLP-1 agonists might therefore be useful in type 2 diabetes, and several materials, mostly peptides, are under study for this purpose (21).

Somatostatin

Somatostatin, produced by the δ-cells of the pancreas and originally discovered as a growth hormone inhibitor, is now known to affect the release of other pancreatic hormones. It inhibits the release of both insulin and glucagon, and when administered to untreated diabetic patients ameliorates elevation in both the postprandial and fasting serum glucose levels. Moreover, when given to type 1 diabetic patients suddenly deprived of insulin, the severity of the resulting hyperglycemia is much reduced and ketoacidosis is not encountered. It has also been shown that administration of somatostatin causes a reduction in the dose of insulin necessary to maintain type 1 diabetic patients. Recently, using a lead obtained through molecular modeling and a database search, a combinatorial library was prepared, which yielded a number of interesting nonpeptide somatostatin agonists, especially L-779,976 and L-803,087 (22,23).

L-779,976

L-803,087

Pancreatic Polypeptide

These small peptides, also produced by the pancreas, appear to have a role in the control of insulin secretion and possibly of glucose metabolism. Both avian and beef pancreatic polypeptide appear to normalize the hyperinsulinemia, hyperglycemia, and weight gain seen in obese mice.

Proinsulin C-peptide

This connecting peptide is released when proinsulin is converted to insulin (Fig. 27.2). It was long thought that the C-(connecting) peptide did not have any specific role. Recently, however, Ido has reported that in pharmacologic (not physiologic) doses the C-peptide does exhibit antidiabetic activity (24). Specifically, it reduces the diabetes-induced increase in ATPase, impaired nerve conduction, and increase in vascular permeability which usually accompany hyperglycemia. Remarkably, the usual rules of peptide hormone selectivity are flagrantly abused here. While the sequence of amino acids in the C-peptide is essential, the stereochemistry of the amino acids is not (D-amino

acids work just as well as the usual L-amino acids), and activity is retained when the amino acid sequence is in reverse order (the so-called retro peptide) (24).

Amylin and Amylin Analogues

The presence of amyloid plaques in the pancreas was noted at the beginning of the 20th century, but it was not until 1987 that the structure of the precursor peptide amylin (also known as islet-amyloid polypeptide) was elucidated. This 37-residue peptide, which exhibits a 20% sequence homology with calcitonin and a strong resemblance to a portion of the insulin B-chain, is co-secreted with insulin in response to a nutrient stimulus. It is deficient in type 1 diabetes and elevated in the type 2 disease (25). Elevation of amylin has also been noted in patients with the impaired serum glucose syndrome, obese subjects, and pregnant women, both those with normal glucose metabolism and those suffering from gestational diabetes mellitus. However, there is now doubt that amylin elevation and diabetic symptoms are temporally correlated. Also, although amylin was found to be elevated in a Japanese study of type 2 diabetic men, there was no correlation between amylin levels and clinical features of their disease (26). Early experimental studies suggested that amylin inhibits basal insulin secretion and induces insulin resistance in skeletal muscle. The current view is that amylin works with insulin and glucagon to maintain glucose homeostasis, and that the primary roles of amylin are to regulate gastric emptying time, thereby controlling the

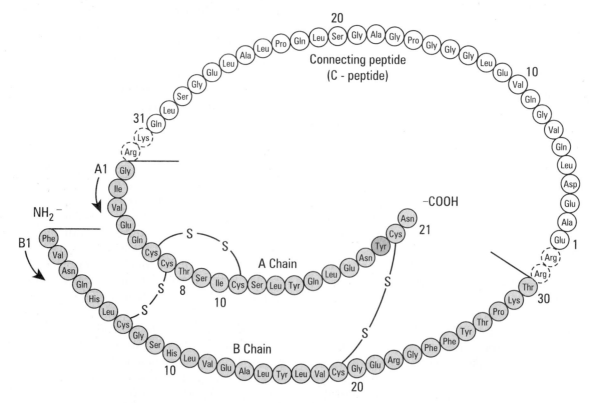

Fig. 27.2. Primary structure of proinsulin, showing cleavage sites to produce insulin.

rate of entry of glucose into the system, and to inhibit hepatic gluconeogenesis.

If amylin does possess the essentially anti-insulin properties suggested, it is possible that amylin antagonists might serve to control postprandial serum glucose levels in type 2 diabetes. Pramlintide (AC 127, or 25, 28, 29-triprolyl amylin) has been extensively examined for this purpose. Several studies showed encouraging effects on fasting and postprandial serum glucose levels as well as HbA$_{1c}$ levels. However, in a large multicenter trial statistically significant reductions in mean 24-hour glucose profiles at 30 mg/kg subcutaneous dose levels were found, but the results at 100 mg/kg did not rise to statistical significance. This was regarded as a disappointment, but further tests are underway (27).

Structural similarity between amylin and calcitonin has been noted above. It is therefore interesting that the 8–32 fragment of salmon calcitonin (see Chapter 6) has been shown to inhibit the amylin-induced decrease in insulin secretion when co-administered with amylin (28).

INSULIN
Physical-Chemical Properties
Primary Structure

The primary structure of insulin was determined by Sanger in the 1950s. As Figure 27.2 shows, the immediate precursor to insulin is the single chain peptide known as proinsulin. Like all biologically relevant peptides, proinsulin folds to afford the correct orientation of disulfide bonds and all other necessary conformational constraints by virtue of its primary structure only. Actually, proinsulin itself has a precursor, a peptide known as preproinsulin, which consists of hundreds of additional residues. When a need is presented, insulin is liberated from proinsulin by cleaving proinsulin at the two points indicated. This affords insulin, which consists of a 21-residue A chain connected with two disulfide bonds to a 30-residue B chain. These are always correctly oriented due to the predictable nature of proinsulin folding.

The primary structure of insulin from at least 28 species of animals has been determined. In general, they are similar but in a few cases as few as 50% of the residues are identical. The animal insulins of greatest interest are those of the pig and the cow, which represent the only animal insulins used to treat diabetes. As indicated in Table 27.3, porcine insulin differs from the human variety by a single residue at the B-chain C-terminal residue.

Bovine insulin incorporates two additional variations in the A-chain, at positions 8 and 10. The apparent closer similarity of porcine insulin to human insulin than that of the cow has led to the assertion that porcine insulin produces fewer side effects in humans but this seems to lack experimental verification.

Solution Structure of Insulin

Details concerning the solution structure of insulin have emerged slowly over many years, and have consider-

Table 27.3. Animal and Human Insulins

Species	Location:	A Chain 8	A Chain 10	B Chain 30
Human		Thr	Ile	Thr
Porcine		Thr	Ile	Ala
Bovine		Ala	Val	Ala

ably enhanced our understanding of its behavior. The secondary and tertiary structure has been extensively studied, and is essentially the same for all insulins regardless of differences in primary structure found in various species. The A-chain has two α-helices, whereas the B-chain forms an α-helix and a β-turn, with the B21 to B30 region present as a β-strand. This conformation serves to bury a number of hydrophobic A-chain residues in the interior of the peptide, thereby improving water solubility and stability. Interestingly, phenol and cresol, frequently used as preservatives in insulin formulations, produce profound changes in insulin conformation. Phenol, in the presence of zinc, causes formation of a B1-B8 helix which involves movement of more than 25 Å in the B1 residue (29). Thus, addition of these preservatives may have serendipitously enhanced the activity of insulin.

Only the insulin monomer is able to interact with insulin receptors, and native insulin exists as a monomer only at low, physiologic concentrations (<0.1μM). A careful 2D-NMR study of the conformation of an insulin analogue which remains monomeric at neutral pH has been reported, and in general this solution conformation is very similar to that in the crystal (30). Insulin dimerizes at the higher concentrations (0.6 mM) found in pharmaceutical preparations, and at neutral pH in the presence of zinc, hexamers form (31). These zinc-associated hexamers are also the storage form of insulin in man. At concentrations above 0.2 mM, hexamers form even in the absence of zinc.

Nominal changes in insulin concentration can profoundly affect its absorption following subcutaneous administration (32). Insulin given at a concentration of 40 Units/mL (formerly used commercially) is absorbed nearly as rapidly as lispro insulin (see below), whereas 100 Units/mL insulin (almost always used now) is absorbed significantly more slowly. This apparently reflects decreasing concentration of insulin monomer, the only absorbable form, as the concentration of insulin increases. The pharmacokinetics of NPH insulin are also markedly distorted if it is diluted to 15 Units/mL prior to injection. It has been suggested that insulin injected at 8° C is more slowly absorbed than if material at 37° C is used, but this was found not to be the case. Temperature of the injection solution does not affect absorption rate.

X-ray, 2D-NMR, and other studies have identified intermolecular interactions responsible for dimer and hexamer formation (33–35). Briefly, hydrogen bonds between B24 and B26 residues are important, as are β-sheet associations between the B-chain C-terminal sequences. (This explains why efforts to produce monomeric insulins which would not enter into intermolecular associations frequently involve modifications of the C-terminal region of the B-chain.) Dimers then associate more loosely to form hexamers.

The importance of zinc in stabilizing insulin preparations has been known since Scott carried out an early crystallization of insulin in the presence of zinc in 1934 (36). Suspensions of zinc insulin were used clinically at that time. Presently, all pharmaceutical preparations are either solutions of zinc insulin or suspensions of insoluble forms of zinc insulin. A search for longer acting and more stable forms of insulin first yielded protamine zinc insulin, prepared by precipitating insulin in the presence of zinc and protamine, a basic protein. This precipitate is now known to contain two zinc atoms per insulin hexamer. A somewhat shorter-acting and more acceptable preparation is NPH (neutral protein Hagedorn) insulin, which includes m-cresol as a preservative. This preparation is also known as isophane (equal or nearly equal proportions of insulin and protamine) insulin. Six m-cresol molecules occupy cavities in the hexamer involving, *inter alia*, the B1–B8 helix formed as a result of the presence of the m-cresol. Later, it was found that when small extra amounts of zinc were added to hexameric 2-zinc insulin in neutral media (acetate buffer), insulin could be made to crystallize in several forms with varying rates of dissolution in water. It is now thought that the rapidly soluble amorphous semilente insulin is a 2-zinc insulin, whereas the crystalline, more slowly soluble ultralente insulin is a 4-zinc form (37,38).

One further associated form of insulin is known. Partially unfolded insulin molecules can form a viscous gel or insoluble precipitates known as fibrils. Shielding of hydrophobic domains is the principal driving force for this phenomenon. Recent crystal analysis and molecular modeling have revealed that when the exposed hydrophobic domain (A2, A3, B11, B15) interacts with the aliphatic residues A13, B6, B14, and B18, normally buried in the hexameric structure, fibrils form (39). Fibrils have also been studied by electron microscopy, and packing considerations in the crystal lattice explain why fibril formation is accelerated when insulin is in the monomeric state (40). Insulin fibrils do not resuspend on shaking, and are pharmaceutically useless.

Insulin Stability

Insulin fibril formation, a physical instability discussed above, is particularly important with the advent of infusion pumps to deliver insulin, because in these devices insulin is exposed to elevated temperatures, the presence of hydrophobic surfaces, and shear forces, all factors increasing insulin's tendency to self-associate. These problems are ameliorated if the insulin is prepared with phosphate buffer or other additives. Actually, synthetic insulin analogues dominate the market of insulin to be administered by pump, as will be noted below. One other physical sta-

bility problem associated with insulin is adsorption to tubing and other surfaces. This normally occurs if the insulin concentration is less than 5 Units/mL (0.03 mM), and can be prevented by adding albumin to the dosage form if use of dilute insulin solutions is essential (31).

There are also chemical instability issues associated with insulin. For 40 years the only rapid acting form of insulin was a solution of zinc insulin, whose pH was 2–3. If this insulin is stored at 4° C, deamidation of the asparagine at A21 occurs at a rate of 1–2% per month. C-terminal asparagine, under acidic conditions, undergoes cyclization to the anhydride which in turn may react with water leading to deamidation. The anhydride may also react with the N-terminal Phe of another chain to yield a crosslinked molecule. If stored at 25° C the inactive deamidated derivative constitutes 90% of the total protein after six months (31). These reactions are illustrated in Figure 27.3.

If stored at neutral pH, entirely different reactions occur. Here the deamidation occurs on the Asn residue at B3, and the products, the aspartate and isoaspartate-containing insulins, are equiactive with native insulin. Deamidation is virtually undetectable in insulin zinc suspensions prepared from bovine sources (37). More deleterious transformations are also possible, including chain cleavage between Thr (A8) and Ser (A9) and covalent crosslinking, either to another insulin chain or to protamine, if present. These processes are relatively slow compared to the deamidations, but have the potential to cause allergic reactions. Specific antibodies against insulin dimers have been found in 30% of diabetic patients receiving insulin (41).

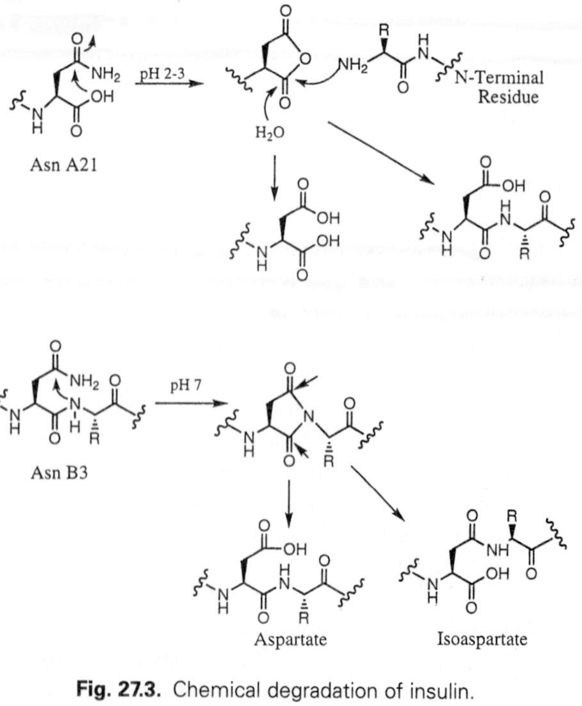

Fig. 27.3. Chemical degradation of insulin.

Production of Insulin

Natural Sources

For many years, porcine and bovine insulin were obtained from abattoir-derived pancreas glands. The initial preparations were very crude by modern standards; among other materials, they contained 4% glucagon, essentially an anti-insulin hormone. Until 1972, the proinsulin content of commercial insulin was 10,000–40,000 parts per million (ppm), when a gel-exclusion chromatography process reduced proinsulin content to 50 ppm. This product, originally known as "single peak" insulin, is still on the market (Iletin I-Lilly). In 1980, "purified" insulins, containing less than 10 ppm of proinsulin (prepared by an ion exchange process) were introduced. These are sold by Lilly as Iletin II products. What one should realize is that all insulin products on the market today are highly purified compared to earlier materials.

Biosynthetic Sources

Beginning in the 1960s concerns were expressed that the worldwide supply of bovine and porcine insulin would be insufficient to meet the demand for insulin by growing numbers of diabetic patients. Fortunately, the techniques of biotechnology became available, and a serious effort was made to produce human insulin using these techniques (see Chapter 41 for a discussion of gene cloning). Initially, synthetic genes for the A and B chains of insulin were constructed and inserted into a *lacZ'* reading frame in *E. coli*. The insulin genes were controlled by a strong *lac* promoter, and are expressed as a fusion protein between insulin and a few residues of glucosidase. The system was designed so that these two peptides would be connected by methionine, the only such residue present in the product. Due to the unique chemistry of the sulfur-containing Met, selective cleavage to release insulin could be carried out using cyanogen bromide (CNBr). Following this procedure, the insulin A and B chains were obtained separately and combined randomly to afford human insulin (42). Unfortunately, the final disulfide bond forming step is quite inefficient. A much improved synthesis was therefore devised, which involved the synthesis of proinsulin. This material, as noted elsewhere, folds to give the correct disulfide configuration almost every time. Enzymatic cleavage of human proinsulin yields human insulin in good yield at 97% purity. This is the process used today to produce commercial insulin. An alternative process in *Saccharomyes cerevisiae* has also been described. The A and B chain are cloned together with only a few amino acids between them, yielding a modified proinsulin, correctly folded, which is exported from the cell so that it can be easily isolated. Insulin at 99.9% purity can be obtained from this process (43).

It is also possible to obtain human insulin chemically from porcine material, since they differ by only one amino acid. To do this, one removes the Ala residue at B30 of porcine insulin using a carboxypeptidase enzyme, after which the required Thr can be attached chemically to afford human insulin. This is possible in large measure because B30 is the C-terminal residue on the B chain, so reasonable enzyme selectivity is obtained. This process was used by Novo-Nordisk for several years to obtain commercial human insulin, but recently the company has switched to the biotechnology-based synthesis described earlier.

Insulin Analogs

Although the literature of chemical modifications to the primary structure of insulin is not large, interesting work has been published, and these efforts have recently led to marketed drugs. One of the first reports of a chemically modified insulin is that of Hallas-Møller, who chemically linked insulin with phenyl isocyanate to afford a long-acting insulin derivative (44). Removal of amino acids from the A and B chains have been reported. Hengesh has noted that insulin can tolerate removal of a few residues from the C-terminus of the B chain; removal of eight residues, however, abolishes activity (45). Removal of the N-terminal Phe from the B chain produces a compound with activity while loss of the N-terminal Gly from the A chain significantly diminishes activity. An early review summarizes work on insulin analogues (46).

More recently, work has focused on the C-terminal region of the B-chain; as noted, this is the region important for dimer formation. If dimer formation can be inhibited, rapidly acting insulins may be obtained. Balschmidt has reported that single residue deletions at positions B24 through B26 provide analogs about twice as potent as insulin (47). Activity can also be completely lost, however, as Svoboda found when he prepared B24, B25-bis Phe insulin. In the same study, B24 (p-ethyl-D-Phe) insulin retains about 50% of insulin's activity (48). Interestingly, in a series where the natural B26 Tyr was replaced with Phe and the B24 or B25 Phe replaced with D-Tyr, substitution at 24 provided a compound twice as potent as insulin. The corresponding B25 D-Tyr compound was inactive (49). Several authors have reported that active compounds can be obtained by removing the B27–B30 tetrapeptide (50), even when the B26 residue is modified (51). For example, the B26-D-Tyr amide was about three times as potent as native insulin.

Chemists at Novo-Nordisk also used X-ray data to ascertain which residues were involved in dimer-hexamer formation. The identified amino acids are mutated to achieve rapidly acting nonassociating insulins. Success was obtained when B9-Ser and B27-Thr were mutated to Asp and Glu, respectively. The resulting product, Actrapid HM, has been marketed in Europe as a short-acting insulin analogue (52). The Lilly approach to compounds of this type stems from the observation that the hormone insulin-like growth factor (IGF-1) has a reasonable structural homology with insulin, particularly in the C-terminal region of the B-chain. It was also noted that in IGF-1 a Lys residue occupies the B28 position and a Pro is found at B29, whereas in insulin these are reversed. Preparation of B28 Lys-B29 Pro insulin (lispro insulin) afforded a potent short acting insulin, now marketed as Humalog (53). This insulin is also being developed as a crystalline protamine suspension, NPL (neutral protamine lispro), which has a pharmacokinetic pattern similar to NPH insulin, and as a mixture of the two lispro insulins. It is not surprising that shifting the position of Pro in the chain would affect conformation and therefore dimerization, since Pro, unique among all the amino acids, exhibits very little preference for trans over cis amide bond formation (all others strongly prefer trans). Since Pro can facilely enter into cis-amide bonds, it easily forms β-turns, the location of which are an important factor governing peptide conformation in solution.

Novo-Nordisk has also begun clinical trials on Insulin Aspart, in which the B28 proline of insulin has been replaced by aspartic acid (54). This material, like lispro insulin, is absorbed quite rapidly.

Other B-chain modifications can produce long-, rather than short-acting insulins. Novo-Nordisk has shown, for example, that B27-Arg-B30-Thr-NH2 insulin is soluble in acid but crystallizes at the higher plasma pH because the Arg shifts the compound's isoelectric point. This results in a quite long-acting drug.

Interesting structural modifications not involving the B-chain C-terminal region have also been carried out. The Hoechst group has noted that mutation of the C-terminal A21 from Asn to Arg also shifts the isoelectric point and makes the resulting insulin quite long-acting, and that this effect is magnified by adding two Arg residues to B31 and B32 (55). Arg residues are found at these positions in proinsulin.

Addition of nonpeptide elements also has interesting effects on insulin action. Baudys, for example, has shown that glycosylation of insulin is consistent with potent glycolytic potency. Several p-succinamidophenyl glucopyranoside insulin conjugates (SAPG-insulin) were prepared; nearly all were as potent as insulin and exhibited improved physical stability (56). Another long lasting insulin emerged when the B29 residue was mutated to Lys in which the ε-amino group was esterified with palmitic acid (a very lipophilic moiety). The resulting insulin was twice as potent as native insulin, and had a half-life seven times as long as insulin, most likely because it strongly binds to serum albumin (57). Finally, the insulin receptor interactions of HOE 901, a long-lasting human insulin also bearing the unusual B31 and B32 Arg residues (A2-Gly B31-Arg B32-Arg) have been carefully studied. It has been determined that HOE 901 behaves like native insulin in every respect, whereas B10-Asp insulin differs qualitatively in phosphorylation characteristics on insulin receptor proteins (58). Thus, one is reminded again of the need to characterize carefully the biological properties of drug analogs of all types.

Diabetes Treatment with Insulin
Mechanism of Action

The major effect of insulin is to activate the GLUT-4 glucose transporter system in liver, fat, and muscle cells. These cells are entirely dependent on the transporter for their glucose supply. The receptor has been cloned, and is known to be a heterodimeric transmembrane receptor which provides tyrosine kinase activity to activate an intramolecular kinase cascade and other signaling events via a series of phosphorylation reactions involving phosphoinositol pyrophosphate and diacylglycerol. These in turn cause translocation of glucose transporters from an intracellular compartment to the plasma membrane, where they facilitate glucose uptake. It is important to recall that other types of cells use other glucose transporters which are not under insulin control. In these cells (nerve, epithelial, kidney) the transporters are sensitive to serum glucose concentration; the higher the serum glucose, the higher the intracellular glucose level. This has profound consequences in diabetic patients, as we have seen. It is worth noting parenthetically that scientists have been able to incorporate human GLUT-4 genes into Type II diabetic mice to increase GLUT-4 activity, thereby markedly alleviating the diabetes (59).

Pharmacokinetics

Two broad categories of insulin are used in therapy (Table 27.4). It should be noted that Lilly has announced its intention to discontinue marketing of all Iletin I preparations. Regular insulins consist of solutions of zinc insulin; only preservatives are added. These exhibit activity 30–45 minutes after injection and remain active for about 6 hours. In the other type of insulin, exemplified by the NPH and lente preparations, additives are present which slow insulin's activity, usually by retarding the rate of dissolution of the insulin. Depending on the preparation, onset of activity can occur in 1–2 hours, peak activity occurs at 3–7 hours and the duration of activity is from 8–24 hours (although ultralente insulin can last up to 36 hours). Lispro insulin is much shorter-lived. Its onset occurs in about 15 minutes and the duration of action is about 2–4 hours.

All commercial insulin preparations now have a concentration of 100 Units/mL, except a 500 Units/mL preparation of regular insulin is available for emergency use in diabetic coma.

Figure 27.4 shows the diurnal variation in insulin levels in a nondiabetic person, together with approximate insulin levels achieved by various insulin dosage schedules in a type 1 diabetic patient. In a normal person there is a baseline concentration of insulin around the clock, with sharp but short-lived postprandial increases in serum insulin levels. In order to produce a pattern similar to this in diabetic patients it has become popular to administer mixtures of long- and short-acting insulins, such as isophane and regular insulin. When such mixtures are prepared in a single syringe,

Table 27.4. Commercially Available Insulins

General Type	Products
Animal insulins—single peak (beef and pork)	
Insulin (single peak)	Regular Iletin I <20 ppm PI*
Isophane (NPH)	NPH Iletin I
Insulin zinc susp. (Lente)	Lente Iletin I
Insulin zinc rapid (Semilente)	Semilente Iletin I
Insulin zinc extended (Ultralente)	Ultralente Iletin II
Animal insulins—purified	
Insulin (purified)	Regular purified pork insulin (pork <1ppm PI)
	Regular Iletin II (pork <10 ppm PI)
	Regular Iletin II (500 U/ml, concentrated)
Isophane (NPH)	NPH Iletin II
	NPH purified pork Isophane Insulin susp.
Insulin Zinc (Lente)	Lente Iletin II (MPB)
	Lente Purified pork insulin
Human insulin	
Human regular	Humulin R
	Novolin R
	Novolin R penfill
	Novolin R prefilled
Parenteral injection (buffered)	Velosulin BR Human
Isophane (NPH)	Humulin N
	Novolin N (NPH)
	Novolin N penfill
Isophane (70%) +	Humulin 70/30
	Novolin 70/30 penfill
Human reg. (30%)	Novolin 70/30
Isophane (50%) +	Humulin 50/50
Human reg. (50%)	
Human zinc	Humulin L
	Novolin L (MPB)
Human zinc extended	Humulin U
Lys—Prol Insulin	
Lispro Insulin	Humalog

*PI = Proinsulin.

it is important to draw the regular insulin into the syringe first so that the regular insulin vial will not become contaminated with the long-lasting insulin; such contamination can alter the properties of the remaining regular insulin.

Until now it has been difficult to mimic the natural insulin concentration pattern using available preparations. One major difficulty is that insulin levels fall to near zero as the patient sleeps (see NPH+regular serum insulin levels in Fig. 27.4). To combat this difficulty, patients are sometimes given more insulin with the evening meal or at bedtime, but this undesirably raises insulin levels in the early evening. Another problem is that insulin level increases achieved with regular insulins last significantly longer than postprandial insulin level increases seen in nondiabetic persons. There is therefore the danger of inducing hypoglycemia both in these patients and in patients given insulin at bedtime.

Ideally, one would administer a long-lasting insulin once daily to maintain baseline serum insulin levels around the clock, and supplement this with a very short acting insulin at mealtimes. Lispro insulin seems to have almost exactly the characteristics required for mealtime administration, especially if it could be given by a nonparenteral route. Work on the requisite long lasting insulins is also proceed-

ing, as described in an earlier section in this chapter. Nonparenteral administration of insulin by almost any imaginable route, has long been a research goal. These studies, sometimes using absorption "enhancers" which generally injure endothelial tissue, have been reviewed (37). Recently, very promising clinical studies in which insulin was inhaled into the lungs as a micronized powder have produced clinically useful serum levels of insulin without evidence of pulmonary irritation. Use of nonaggregating long- and short-acting insulins by a nonparenteral route could provide the most "natural" variations in artificial diurnal insulin levels yet attainable.

A number of so-called insulin pumps which administer insulin on a pre-set schedule have been made commercially available (37). Either continuous subcutaneous insulin infusion or implantable intraperitoneal pumps are available. These have not achieved great popularity, because they are expensive and generally do not improve the effectiveness of insulin therapy. Formerly, a buffered insulin product designed exclusively for pumps was available, but at the present time lispro insulin is almost invariably used in insulin pumps because it is nonaggregating and exhibits improved stability. Pen and jet injectors are also available, in which insulin is administered transdermally (37).

DIURNAL INSULIN LEVELS

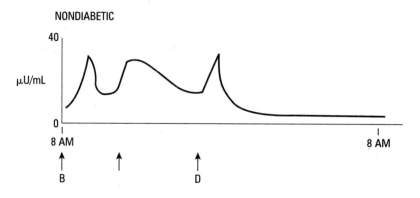

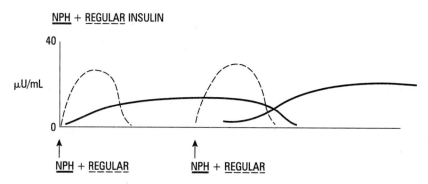

Fig. 27.4. Diurnal serum glucose variation.

It is customary to refrigerate, but not freeze, insulin preparations. All commercial insulin preparations now have a pH between 6 and 8, and are therefore much more stable than the older acidic solutions. The monthly rate of activity loss at 25° C varies between 0.2 and 2%, so patients can be advised that their insulin, even if kept outside the refrigerator for a few months, will be quite active (31).

Insulin Dose Setting

There are several paradigms for setting insulin doses. One thought is that each unit of insulin can "cover" about 2 g of glucose, and the amount of glucose excreted can be determined by following urine glucose levels. The other approach is to administer 10–20 units of insulin and observe the result. Regardless of the method used, it is important to follow serum glucose levels carefully for several weeks in newly diagnosed patients. Normally there is a "honeymoon" period during which insulin works very well, but this is invariably followed by a need to increase insulin dosage levels.

A discussion has recently arisen concerning insulin therapy regardless of the dose employed, and that is whether it is worthwhile to control serum glucose levels "tightly" or "loosely." The former method requires measuring serum glucose several times daily and using insulin at least twice daily, whereas the latter is not so demanding.

The Diabetes Control and Complications Trial has recently examined this question, and reported that tight control seemed to reduce diabetes complications, improve the well being of patients, and lower serum hemoglobin HbA_{1c}. These results are illustrated in Table 27.1. There is some suggestion that tight control leads to an increased incidence of hypoglycemia. The reader will also recall that normal serum HbA_{1c} levels are 5–8%; if one tries to lower the level in diabetics to 7.5%, there appears to be an increased risk of developing hypoglycemia in the patients. Rather, reduction of serum HbA_{1c} to a level of about 9% is taken as an indication of successful therapy of diabetes.

Human Versus Animal Insulin

Almost all newly diagnosed diabetic patients are being placed on human insulin. For some time there was reluctance to switch patients from animal to human insulin due to fear of hypoglycemia, but recently many patients have been transferred to human insulin, which now controls most of the market.

Adverse Reactions
Diabetic Coma (β-ketoacidosis)

When insulin-mediated glucose uptake into fat and liver cells is inadequate, these cells attempt to obtain energy by oxidizing fatty acids. This results in overproduction of β-keto acids, which spill into the blood. The β-keto acids are much more acidic than normal fatty acids, such that the buffer capacity of the blood is overwhelmed, and life-threatening acidosis is produced. The only treatment aside from emergency electrolyte manipulation is very large doses of insulin.

Insulin Shock

The only systemic difficulty with insulin therapy is hypoglycemia, in which an excess of insulin causes an excessive fall in serum glucose levels. This results in bizarre behavior, confusion, and coma. Normally, autonomic warning signs occur, including tachycardia, sweating, and hunger. These signs are less frequently observed in patients taking human insulin. This may explain why patients taking human insulin seem more prone to develop severe hypoglycemia than those using animal insulins, especially if they are practicing strict diabetes control. The symptoms of hypoglycemia are promptly relieved by administration of sugars; this is why many diabetics carry hard candy.

Lipodystrophy and Lipohypertrophy

Repeated injection into the same site, especially in females using older acidic insulin products, has caused atrophy of subcutaneous fatty tissue. This produces unsightly depressions in the tissue. Surprisingly, injection of newer neutral preparations into such sites seems to alleviate the problem. In males, one sometimes sees lipohypertrophy, the converse condition in which subcutaneous lumps of adipose tissue form. This seems to occur regardless of the type of insulin used. In any event, it is helpful to use as many different injection sites as possible.

Drug Interactions

The most important drug interactions observed with insulin are that stress of any kind, including febrile illness, increases the insulin requirement, because under these conditions the body is producing more glucose. It is usually thought that during illness the patient eats less and therefore needs less insulin, but in fact the reverse is true. Some drugs, such as oral contraceptives, glucocorticoids, and sympathomimetic amines, also increase the insulin requirement in diabetic patients.

ORAL HYPOGLYCEMIC AGENTS
History

The hypoglycemic effect of salicylates has been known for 100 years. The mechanism was never established with certainty, although it appears that salicylates enhance insulin secretion. Clinical use of salicylates was not feasible, since the very large doses required produced intolerable side effects. The hypoglycemic effects of the thiadiazole sulfonamide known as IPTD, used to treat typhoid fever in the 1940s, were also noted. This drug produced many deaths which were subsequently attributed to prolonged drug-induced hypoglycemia. At about the same time these

effects were noted, the synthesis of sulfonylureas such as carbutamide, far more active as hypoglycemic agents, was reported. Since then, about 12,000 sulfonylureas have been tested, and about 10 are currently on the market. The hypoglycemic effects of guanidine were noted in 1918, but toxic effects prevented its use. The guanidine derivatives synthalin A and synthalin B were introduced into therapy in the 1920s, but chronic toxicity forced their abandonment in the 1930s. The widely used biguanides phenformin and metformin were prepared in the 1950s, and the latter is still in widespread use. Other classes of hypoglycemic agents, notably the thiazolidinediones, have been introduced more recently.

First and Second Generation Sulfonylureas

The classic first- and second-generation sulfonylureas share many attributes; the newer third-generation materials are notably different. Structures of the 1st and 2nd generation sulfonylureas are shown in Table 27.5.

Mechanism of Action

The principal effect of these drugs is to stimulate the release of insulin; the mechanism by which this was carried out was unknown until recently. Sulfonylureas interact with receptors on pancreatic β-cells to block ATP-sensitive potassium channels. This in turn leads to opening of voltage-sensitive calcium channels which produces an influx of calcium; the influx of calcium results in β-cells production of insulin (60). There is a direct correlation between receptor binding affinity and hypoglycemic effect among these drugs (61). The pattern of insulin secretion induced by sulfonylureas is similar, but not the same, as that induced by glucose. Thus, the drugs are still effective in type 2 diabetics, whose insulin-secreting capacity is intact but who have lost the ability to produce adequate insulin despite the presence of elevated serum glucose levels. Interestingly, however, the drug effect on insulin secretion is transient; although serum insulin levels initially rise, they generally fall back to normal within a short time (glipizide is an exception; hyperinsulinemia can persist for up to two years). Nevertheless, serum glucose levels remain lowered. Although the precise reasons for this remain to be elucidated, it has been suggested that the drug improves the responsiveness of the pancreatic cells to insulin (61). Eliason has reported cloning of a second, high-affinity sulfonylurea receptor, which may be mediated by protein kinase C and have additional cellular functions.

An additional effect of sulfonylureas is suppression of gluconeogenesis in the liver (62). The reader will recall that increased gluconeogenesis is a major cause of hyperglycemia among type 2 diabetics with elevated glucose levels.

Physical-Chemical Properties

Sulfonylureas are weak acids due to the marked delocalization of the nitrogen lone electron pair by the sulfonyl group (Fig. 27.5). Their pKa's cluster around 5.0 and

Table 27.5. First and Second Generation Sulfonylureas

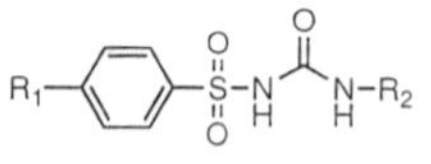

Generic Name	Trade Name	R₁	R₂
1st Generation			
Tolbutamide	Orinase	CH_3-	$-CH_2CH_2CH_2CH_3$
Chlorpropamide	Diabinese	$Cl-$	$-CH_2CH_2CH_3$
Tolazamide	Tolinase	CH_3-	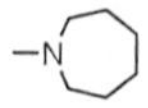
Acetohexamide	Dymelor	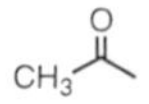	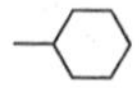
2nd Generation			
Glyburide (Glibenclamide)	Diabeta Micronase Glynase PresTab	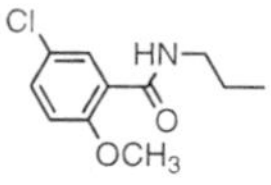	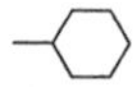
Glipizide	Glucotrol	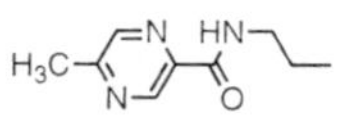	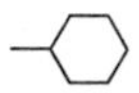

they, like other weak acids, are strongly protein bound. As such, sulfonylureas compete with other weak acids for protein binding sites, which may result in elevated levels of free drug in the presence of other protein binding drugs. While this does not usually represent a long-term problem if doses are adjusted correctly, short-term dislocations could occur if, for example, tolbutamide were given to a patient also taking dicoumarol; sharp increases in prothrombin time, possibly leading to hemorrhaging, could be observed.

Other side effects of these drugs are few; only about 5% of patients experience side effects, and only 2% discontinue therapy as a result. Such side effects include nausea, vomiting, diarrhea, and skin reactions. Chlorpropamide causes water retention by increasing antidiuretic hormone output, whereas acetohexamide, tolazamide, and glyburide are diuretics. Other, more serious side effects such as blood dyscrasias are very rare.

As with insulin, compounds with hyperglycemic effects (glucocorticoids, oral contraceptives, sympathomimetic agents) will antagonize the effects of sulfonylureas.

Pharmacokinetics

The pharmacokinetic characteristics of sulfonylureas are listed in Table 27.6. Here it is seen that the duration of

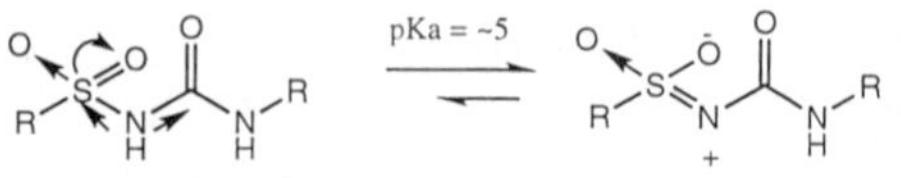

Fig. 27.5. Sulfonylureas as weak acids.

action of chlorpropamide is considerably longer than most other compounds. The second-generation compounds are inherently more active, but of short duration, and are strongly protein bound. Apparently, because of their potency, once daily dosing is suggested. Among the first generation agents, tolbutamide is normally given in divided doses, chlorpropamide in one daily dose, and the others in one or two doses daily, depending on how much drug is to be given.

Both second-generation drugs, glyburide and glipizide, are available in micronized versions (Prestab and Glucotrol XL, respectively) which contain smaller particles of the drug than those found in conventional formulations. These evidently produce a quicker onset of action, and they are not bioequivalent with conventional formulations. Whereas the nonmicronized dosage form is usually given at 1.25–20 mg daily, the micronized product requires doses of 0.75–12 mg daily.

Metabolism

Metabolism plays an important role in the biological properties of sulfonylureas. Tolbutamide is metabolized in the liver to p-hydroxy tolbutamide (Fig. 27.6). Although this metabolite retains about 35% of the activity of the parent compound, it is converted very rapidly to the inactive tolbutamide 4-carboxylic acid, so that tolbutamide is the least potent of the sulfonylureas.

Tolazamide is also oxidized to a carboxylic acid by the same two-stage process, and can in addition yield 4'-hydroxy tolazamide (Fig. 27.6). These hydroxylated materi-

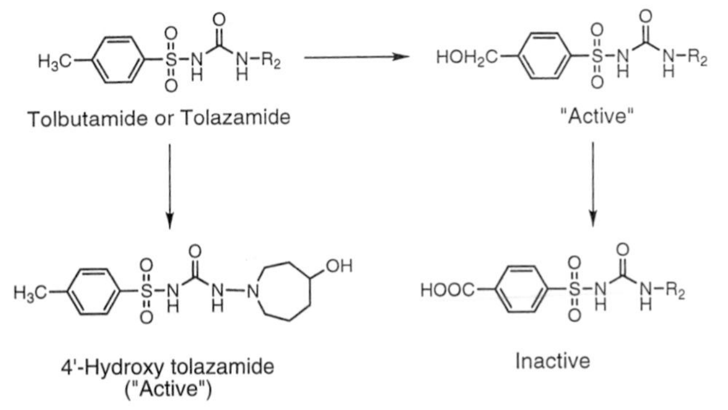

Fig. 27.6. Metabolism of tolbutamide and tolazamide.

als are less potent than tolazamide, but more so than tolbutamide. Consequently, tolazamide exhibits both increased potency and increased duration of action when compared with tolbutamide.

The acetyl carbonyl group of acetohexamide is rapidly reduced to yield 4-(1-hydroxyethyl) acetohexamide, which has 2.5 times the hypoglycemic activity of acetohexamide and also accounts for the long duration of action of acetohexamide. Acetohexamide can also afford a small amount of 4'-hydroxyacetohexamide, an inactive metabolite.

Chlorpropamide undergoes relatively slow hydroxylation on the propyl chain to afford 2'- and 3'-hydroxychlorpropamide. Because these processes are slow, chlorpropamide is a long-lasting drug.

The second-generation agents glyburide and glipizide undergo similar and interesting biotransformations. As shown in Figure 27.7, glyburide affords *trans*-4'-hydroxyglyburide as the major product, accompanied by some *cis*-3'-hydroxy material. The 4'-hydroxy metabolite retains about 15% of the activity of the parent compound. Glipizide undergoes the same transformations, as depicted in Figure 27.7. In addition, it undergoes an interesting cleavage of the pyrazine ring to afford the N-acetyl derivative shown. None of these metabolites exhibits useful therapeutic activity.

Structure-activity Relationships

There must be reasonable bulk on the urea nitrogen; methyl and ethyl compounds are not active. Usually, there

is only one (normally substituent para) on the sulfonyl aromatic ring. Many simple substituents are active, and the *p*-(β-arylcarboxamidoethyl) grouping seen in second generation compounds is consistent with high potency. Among these compounds, it is thought that the spatial relationship between the amide nitrogen of the substituent and the sulfonamide nitrogen is important.

Therapeutic Application

In general, the effects of the first- and second-generation sulfonylureas are similar, although their pharmacokinetic properties vary widely (see above). All produce reliable hypoglycemia in type 2 diabetics, and in recalcitrant cases combination sulfonylurea-insulin therapy may be considered (63). These agents work best in patients whose type 2 diabetes is relatively mild (fasting serum glucose less than 200 mg/dL or who can be controlled on 20 units or less of insulin daily). Frequency of administration varies among the compounds.

The only major difficulty with sulfonylureas arose with the observation of the University Group Diabetes Program (UGDP) that cardiovascular deaths in three treatment groups were 12.7%, 6.2%, and 4.9% for tolbutamide, insulin, and placebo groups, respectively. Based on these results, consideration was given to the withdrawal of sulfonylureas from the market. At present, the sulfonylureas have a supplemental warning label, but are still prescribed. Since then, the UGDP has reported that tolbutamide plus

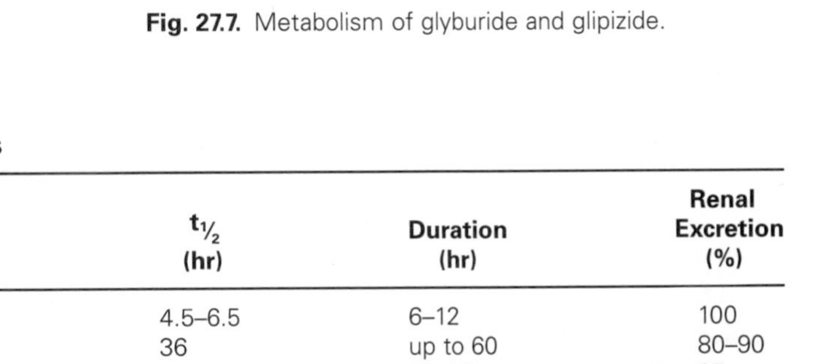

Fig. 27.7. Metabolism of glyburide and glipizide.

Table 27.6. Pharmacokinetic Properties of the Sulfonylureas

Drug (Sulfonylureas)	Equivalent Dose (mg)	Serum Protein Binding (%)	$t_{1/2}$ (hr)	Duration (hr)	Renal Excretion (%)
Tolbutamide	1000	95–97	4.5–6.5	6–12	100
Chlorpropamide	250	88–96	36	up to 60	80–90
Tolazamide	250	94	7	12–14	85
Acetohexamide	500	65–88	6–8	12–18	60
Glyburide	5	99	1.5–3.0	up to 24	50
Glipizide	5	92–97	4	up to 24	68
Glimepiride	2	99	2–3	up to 24	40

diet was no more effective than diet alone in prolonging life, and that insulin was no more effective than diet in reducing diabetic cardiovascular complications (64). There has been criticism of the design of the UGDP, and many prospective studies have been undertaken to validate or disprove the UGDP findings. Results will be most useful.

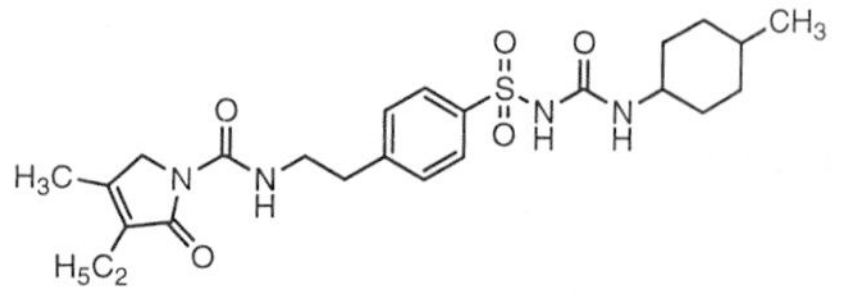

Glimepiride

Third-generation Sulfonamides and Related Compounds
Glimepiride

Glimepiride, a sulfonylurea with a quick onset of action and a long duration of action, may bind to a different protein in the putative sulfonylurea receptor than earlier drugs, and may exert its hypoglycemic effect with less secretion of insulin (65). In hyperinsulinemic KK-A mice, glimepiride reduced serum glucose by 40%, plasma insulin by 50%, and HbA$_{1c}$ by 33%, whereas glyburide had no effect on these parameters (66). In the dog, glimepiride exhibits a lower ratio of insulin-increasing to glucose-lowering activity than do other sulfonylureas, including glyburide, which is thought to represent the most unusual of the earlier sulfonamides. It has also been suggested that glimepiride may cause translocation of the GLUT-4 glucose transporter from the cytoplasm to an active position in the cell membrane. Thus, while all sulfonylureas exhibit both insulin-secreting and extrapancreatic activities, glimepiride relies upon extrapancreatic effects for a greater portion of its hypoglycemic effect. Perhaps for this reason it is said to be less likely to produce unwanted hypoglycemia. Glimepiride is metabolized, primarily in liver, as shown in Figure 27.8. The M-1 metabolite appears to be formed by Cytochrome P-450 enzymes (mostly CYP-2C9) in liver microsomes. Further metabolism catalyzed by cytosolic dehydrogenases affords the carboxylic acid metabolite M-2 (67). Metabolite M-1 exhibits

significant hypoglycemic activity in man, whereas metabolite M-2 is inactive.

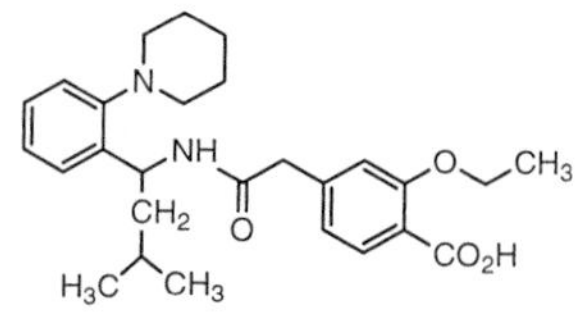

Repaglinide

Repaglinide

Repaglinide, a nonsulfonylurea (but still an acidic molecule), was approved in 1998 for use in the treatment of type 2 diabetes mellitus. This drug is even more rapid- and short-acting than other hypoglycemic drugs. It is not associated with the prolonged hyperinsulinemia seen with the sulfonylureas, and possibly for this reason produces fewer side effects including weight gain and possibly dangerous hypoglycemia. Some authors, however, dispute the last assertion (68). Regardless, it is beyond doubt that replaglinide is at least 5 times more potent than glyburide on intravenous administration; the difference on oral administration is about 10-fold.

In an interesting conformational study, it was shown that repaglinide and several other active nonsulfonylurea hypoglycemics, as well as the sulfonylureas glyburide and glimepiride, displayed a comparable U-shaped conformation when analyzed by molecular modeling. In this conformation, hydrophobic cycles were placed at the end of each branch and a peptidic bond was at the bottom of the U. Several inactive analogues of repaglinide and the poorly active drug meglitinide displayed a different conformation, with a greater distance between the hydrophobic cycles (69).

Biguanides

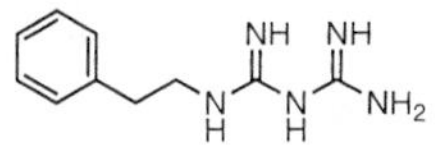

Phenformin 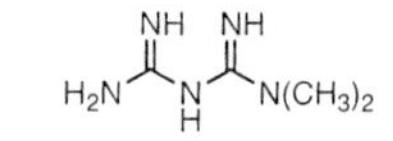   Metformin (Glucophage)

Several guanidine derivatives are active as antihyperglycemic agents, of which metformin and phenformin are of most interest. Phenformin was introduced to the U.S.

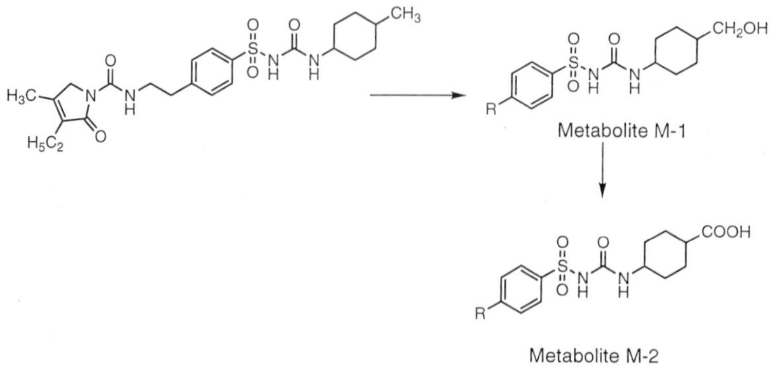

Fig. 27.8. Metabolism of glimepiride.

market in 1957. Shortly thereafter, it was found to produce increased serum lactic acid levels, which sometimes progressed to lactic acidosis. This condition was observed in about 2 cases per 1000 users, and was associated with 50% mortality. Phenformin was therefore withdrawn from the U.S. market in 1977.

Metformin has been in use throughout the world, with the exception of the U.S., for decades. It produces 0–0.084 cases of lactic acidosis per 1000 users, of which 30% are fatal. Studies have shown, however, that almost all cases of lactic acidosis occurred in patients for whom metformin was contraindicated. The drug has been in use in Canada for more than 20 years and is estimated to comprise about 25% of all orders for hypoglycemic drugs; not a single case of drug-associated lactic acidosis has been reported (70). Metformin was approved for use in the U.S. in 1995.

Mechanism of Action

The mechanism of action of metformin is not altogether clear, although it is sometimes classified as an inhibitor of hepatic glucose production. Its effect does not depend on the presence of functioning β cells nor on the secretion of insulin; moreover, the drug does not induce hypoglycemia at any reasonable dose. For that reason, metformin is usually said to be an antihyperglycemic (or euglycemic) rather than a hypoglycemic agent. Overall, the drug appears to increase glucose utilization (71). It has no effect on the secretion of glucagon, cortisol, or somatostatin. Inhibition of gluconeogenesis appears to be an important component of the drug's activity, as is increased anaerobic glucose utilization in the small intestine. Aerobic metabolism in other tissues is also enhanced, and effects on glucose transporter proteins have also been suggested (72).

Therapeutic Application

Metformin is absorbed mainly from the small intestine with a bioavailability of about 60%. Unlike sulfonylureas, it is not protein bound, is not metabolized, and is rapidly eliminated by the kidney. It is widely used as monotherapy or in combination with a sulfonylurea in type 2 diabetes, particularly when the patient is obese and insulin-resistant. Weight loss is sometimes noted. Patients with compromised kidney or liver function should not receive the drug; other contraindications include cardiac failure, history of lactic acidosis, or chronic hypoxic lung disease. All these predispose to increased lactate production.

Acute side effects include diarrhea, abdominal discomfort, nausea, and anorexia. These can be minimized by increasing drug dosage slowly and by taking it with meals.

Thiazolidinediones

The thiazolidinediones (Fig. 27.9), also known as the "glitazones," are sometimes referred to as insulin enhancers. They are exemplified by ciglitazone, the first of the glitazones. Ciglitazone's antihyperglycemic effects were discovered serendipitously. The first drug in this class to be

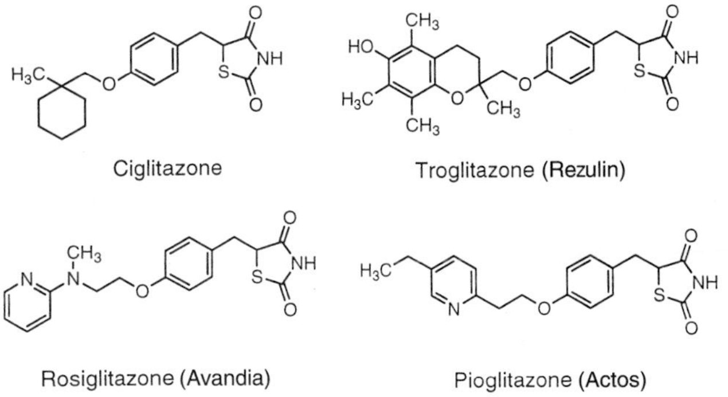

Fig. 27.9. Thiazolidinedione hypoglycemic agents ("glitazones").

marketed is the drug troglitazone, introduced in the United States in 1997. While clinical studies did indicate hepatic and cardiac toxicity the toxicities were not considered severe and it was felt that the drug could be used if liver function were closely monitored. In a 96 week study in type 2 diabetics, little or no cardiac toxicity was noted (73). Unfortunately, rare cases of liver failure, liver transplants, and deaths were reported during postmarketing use and the drug was voluntarily withdrawn on March 21, 2000 (74). More recently two new glitazones have been approved and marketed. These include rosiglitazone and pioglitazone. Both drugs have been approved for monotherapy and combination therapy with metformin, sulfonylureas or insulin. The glitazones lower blood glucose concentrations by improving sensitivity to insulin in target tissue which includes adipose tissue, skeletal muscle, and liver. These agents are dependent upon insulin for their activity.

Mechanism of Action

The thiazolidinediones are beneficial in type 2 diabetics through a unique set of pharmacologic effects. In a six month study of type 2 diabetes, a 600 mg daily dose of troglitazone lowered fasted serum glucose by 60 mg/dL, HbA$_{1c}$ by 1.1%, insulin by 2.4 μU/mL, and triglycerides by 72 mg/dL versus placebo (75). The drugs appear to enhance insulin action, especially in liver, muscle and fat tissue where insulin-dependent glucose transport is essential.

An interesting effect of these antihyperglycemic drugs is on the peroxisome-proliferator activated receptor γ (PPARγ). These drugs act as agonists upon binding to PPARγ which preferentially binds to DNA activating transcription of a wide variety of metabolic regulators. The regulators increase expression of a number of genes involved in the regulation of glucose and lipid metabolism. Studies have shown that there is a good correlation between PPARγ-affinity and antihyperglycemic effects (76,77).

Metabolism

The thiazolidinediones differ by the nature of the groups attached to the 2,4-thiazolidinedione nucleus (Fig. 27.9). These agents are extensively metabolized with all metabolic changes occurring on or adjacent to the aryl

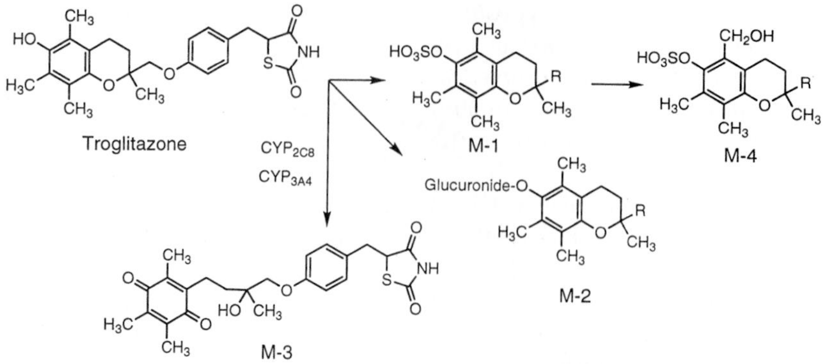

Fig. 27.10. Metabolic pathway of troglitazone.

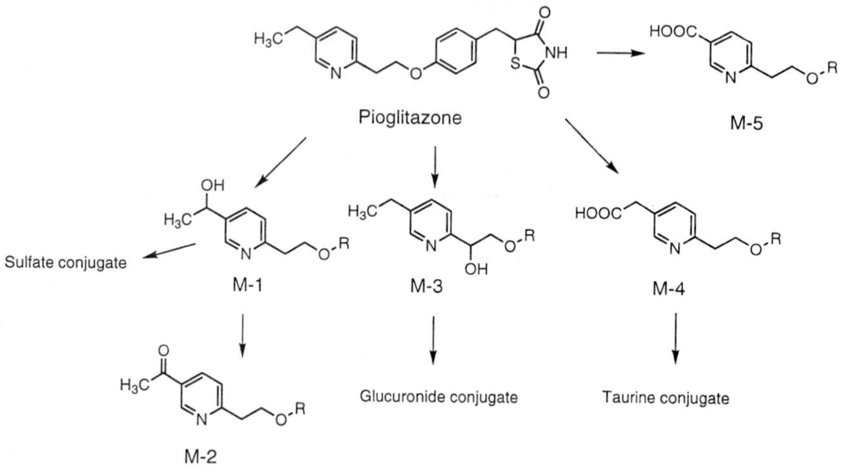

Fig. 27.11. Metabolic pathway of pioglitazone.

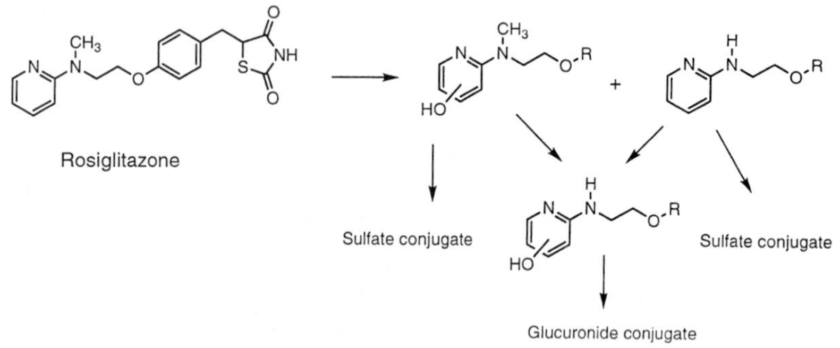

Fig. 27.12. Metabolic pathway of rosiglitazone.

group found in the side chain. Considerable interest in the metabolism of troglitazone exists since the hepatic toxicity may be associated with a metabolite of troglitazone. Metabolic studies in rats, mice, dogs, monkeys, and humans report the presence of the four metabolites shown in Figure 27.10, with sulfate conjugation (M-1) being the primary metabolite found in man (78,79). The more interesting metabolite is the quinone product M-3 which is thought to arise by a cytochrome P-450 catalyzed reaction involving isoenzymes CYP2C8 and CYP3A4. Quinone-type metabolites are considered to be active intermediates which may induce hepatic toxicity.

The metabolism of pioglitazone has been studied in rats and dogs and has led to the discovery of up to eight metabolic products. These products result from oxidation at either carbon adjacent to the pyridine ring and are found as various conjugates in the urine and bile (Fig. 27.11) (80,81). Metabolites M-1, M-2, and M-3 appear to contribute to the biologic activity of pioglitazone.

The metabolism of rosiglitazone has been reported in humans and in excess of 14 metabolites have been identified (82). The primary metabolites consist of sulfate and glucuronic acid conjugates of hydroxylation and N-demethylation products (Fig. 27.12). It is unlikely that these metabolites contribute to the biologic activity of rosiglitazone.

α-Glucosidase Inhibitors

To be absorbed from the gastrointestinal tract into the bloodstream, the complex carbohydrates we ingest as part of our diet, primarily starch and sucrose, must first be hydrolyzed to monosaccharides (Fig. 27.13). The rationale for the α-glucosidase inhibitor class of drugs is that by preventing the hydrolysis of carbohydrates their absorption could be reduced. Starch is normally digested by salivary and pancreatic α-amylases to yield disaccharides (maltose), trisaccharides (maltotriose), and oligosaccharides (dextrin). The oligosaccharidases responsible for final hydrolysis of these materials are all located in the brush border of the small intestine, and consist of two classes. The β-galactosidases hydrolyze β-disaccharides such as lactose, whereas the α-glucosidases act on α-sugars such as maltose, isomaltose, and sucrose (83).

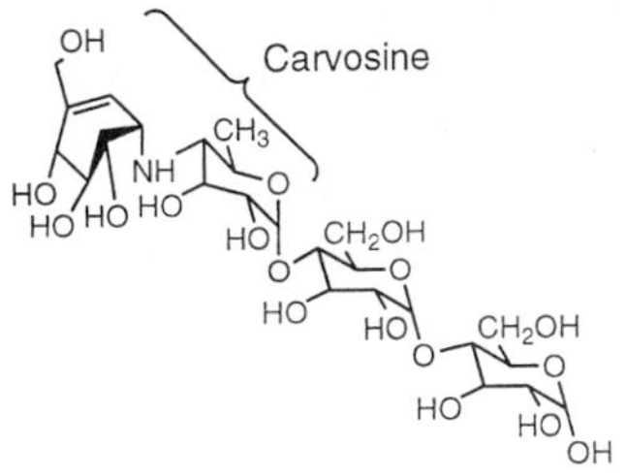

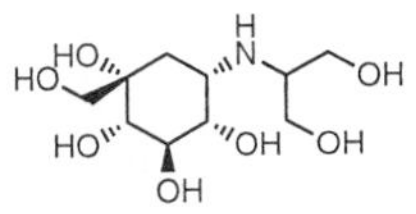

Voglibose (Basen)   Miglitol (Diastabol)

Acarbose (Precose)

Mechanism of Action

An extensive search for α-glucosidase inhibitors from microbial cultures led to the isolation of acarbose from an actinomycete (84). Extensive structure-activity investigations revealed that active inhibitors had a common active site comprising a substituted cyclohexane ring and a 4,6-dideoxy-4-amino-D-glucose unit known as carvosine. It appears the secondary amino group of this core structure prevents an essential carboxyl group of the α-glucosidase from protonating the glycosidic oxygen bonds of the substrate (85).

More recently, screening programs of small molecules have yielded several other α-glucosidase inhibitors, of which miglitol has been introduced to the market. Most of the substances tested resemble simple amino sugars.

Clinical Studies

Clinical studies on these molecules reveal that disaccharide hydrolysis is not blocked, but rather delayed. However, since acarbose impacts end-stage hydrolysis of both starch and sucrose, it affects all primary dietary sources of glucose. Type 2 diabetic patients have an insulin response which is slow as well as inadequate; therefore, slowing the rate of absorption of glucose following a meal should be helpful in preventing the large postprandial increases in serum glucose which are associated with degenerative complications of diabetes. Treatment with acarbose in insulin requiring type 2 diabetes patients was associated with significantly decreased levels of HbA_{1c} (0.4%) and in total daily insulin dose (8.3%) (86). There were also significant decreases in fasting glucose and in area under the glucose-time curves following a meal. Overall, 45% of patients in the Coiff study showed a good clinical response to acarbose therapy. Acarbose is only minimally absorbed (0.5–1.7%) into the bloodstream, and is not associated with any significant systemic toxicity at normal doses. Because doses in excess of 100 mg three times daily are associated with increased serum transaminase levels indicative of liver damage, doses above 100 mg are not recommended. Acarbose is also not recommended in patients with significant renal dysfunction, or who suffer from inflammatory bowel disease, colonic ulceration, or partial intestinal obstruction. The drug does cause annoying flatulence and bloating in about 60% of the patients who use it, and it is suggested that this may be overcome by using a low dose of the drug, then titrating the dose upward. Acarbose (50–100 mg) is taken with the first bite of each meal.

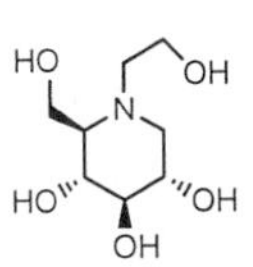

Other α-glucosidase inhibitors are also available. Voglibose, unlike acarbose a small molecule, was marketed in Japan in 1994. It also slows the release of monosaccharides from polymeric materials, and thereby lowers postprandial glucose levels. The drug also maintains low levels of glucose, triglycerides, and insulin in genetically obese rats, indicating possible effectiveness in conditions, such as obesity, other than diabetes.

Miglitol, introduced in 1998, seems to produce therapeutic results similar to acarbose. It causes significant lowering of HbA_{1c} and of postprandial and fasting serum glucose. Unlike acarbose, however, miglitol is rapidly and completely absorbed into the bloodstream following oral

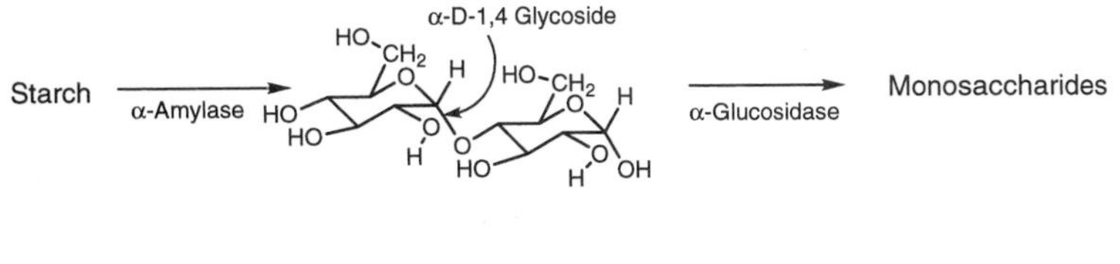

Maltose (also Dextrin, Maltotriose)

Fig. 27.13. Metabolism of complex carbohydrates.

administration. It is distributed primarily to the extracellular space, and is rapidly cleared through the kidney without evidence of hepatic metabolism. It is not transferred into the central nervous system (87,88).

Insulinmimetics

Although some drug types currently effective in treating diabetes may have multiple mechanisms of action, all are believed to act primarily in one way or another by influencing the effects of insulin itself. Until now no small molecule capable of interacting with insulin receptors to mimic the effects of insulin has been discovered. In 1999, however, Zhang reported the isolation of a compound known as L-783,281 which may have these effects (89). This complex five-ring quinone, isolated from the

L-783,281

African fungus *Pseudomassaria*, was a selective activator of protein phosphorylation due to the insulin receptor system from Chinese hamster ovary cells. The compound was at least 100 times more potent than other substances tested. It did not affect phosphorylation due to insulin-like growth factor, platelet-derived growth factor, or epidermal growth factor. In two mouse models of type 2 diabetes, the material seemed to reduce serum glucose and ameliorate the insulin resistance commonly seen in type 2 diabetes.

Summary

The oral antihyperglycemic agents have greatly expanded the therapeutic options for successful management of diabetes mellitus. Therapy for mildly hyperglycemic individuals should begin with metformin, acarbose, or thiazolidinediones because these agents pose very little risk of hypoglycemia. Patients with more severe hyperglycemia should receive a sulfonylurea. In cases of moderate hyperglycemia, sulfonylureas would be used in nonobese individuals, while metformin or troglitazone would be preferred in type 2 obese insulin-resistant patients. Acarbose is used primarily to reduce postprandial serum glycose fluctuations and improve glycemic stability.

CASE STUDY

Victoria F. Roche and S. William Zito

HP is a 23-year-old woman who works as a toll taker at the Bay-Bridge tunnel. She complains of constant thirst, frequent urination and the loss of almost 30 lbs in the last month in spite of her continued good appetite. She likes to bake cookies and shares them daily with her fellow toll takers. HP has been obese from adolescence, suffers from Crohn's disease and her mild hypertension is being controlled with propranolol (Betachron E-R, 80mg QD; structure #1). A random serum glucose determination yielded a value of 150 mg/dl (normal 70–110 mg/dl). Her serum insulin was 67 μU/ml (normal 5–15 μU/ml). A 7-unit insulin challenge produced no effect on serum glucose levels. All clinical signs are indicative of Type 2 Diabetes Mellitus. Evaluate the drawn structures and select an appropriate therapy for HP.

1. Identify the therapeutic problem(s) where the pharmacist's intervention may benefit the patient.

2. Identify and prioritize the patient specific factors that must be considered to achieve the desired therapeutic outcomes.

3. Conduct a thorough and mechanistically oriented structure-activity analysis of all therapeutic alternatives provided in the case.

4. Evaluate the SAR findings against the patient specific factors and desired therapeutic outcomes and make a therapeutic decision.

5. Counsel your patient.

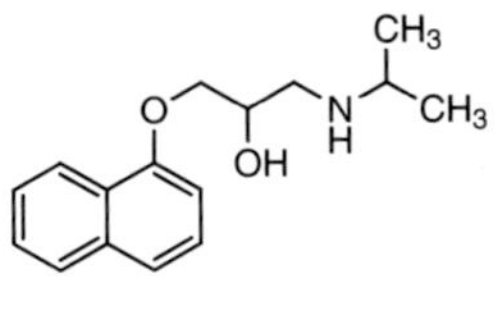

1

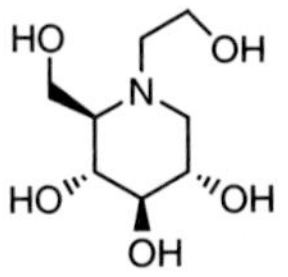

2

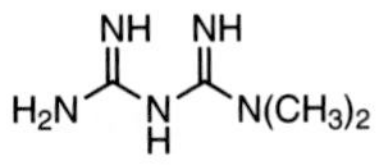

3

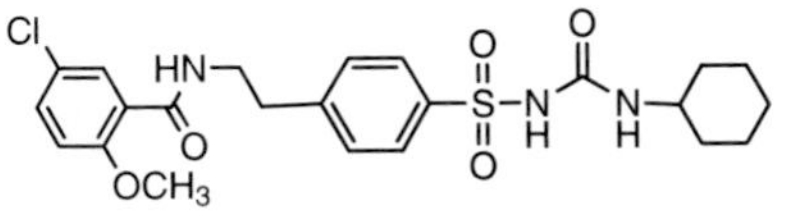

4

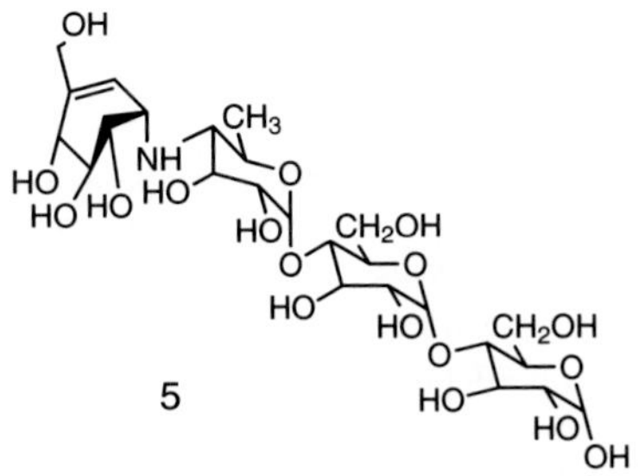

5

REFERENCES

1. Luft R, Minkowski O. Discovery of the pancreatic origin of diabetes. Diabetologia. 1989;32:399–401.
2. Tattersall RB, Pyke DA. Diabetes in identical twins. Lancet 1972;2:1120–5.
3. Lo S, et al. Diabetes Metab Rev 1991:7: 223.
4. Nerup J, Plaz MP, Ryder LF, et al. Aspects of the Genetics of Insulin-dependent Diabetes Mellitus. In: Adreani D, Dimario R, Federlin KF, Hedings LG, eds. Immunology in Diabetes. London: Kimpton Medical Pub, 1984;63–70.
5. Todd JA, Bell JI, McDevitt HO. HLA-DQ beta gene contributes to susceptibility and resistance to insulin -dependent diabetes mellitus. Nature. 1987;329:599–604.
6. Tisch R, Yang XD, Singer SM, et al. Immune response to glutamic acid decarboxylase correlates with insulitis in non-obese diabetic mice. Nature. 1993;366:72–75.
7. Kaufman DL, Clare-Salzler M, Tian J, et al. Spontaneous loss of T-cell tolerance to glutamic acid decarboxylase in murine insulin-dependent diabetes. Nature 1993;366:69–72.
8. Froguel P, Zouali H, Vionnet N, et al. Familial hyperglycemia due to mutations in glucokinase. Definition of a subtype of diabetes mellitus. New Engl J Med 1993;328:697–702.
9. Groop LC, Kankuri M, Schalin-Jantti C, et al. Genome Association between polymorphism of the glycogen synthase gene and non-insulin-dependent diabetes mellitus. N Engl J Med 1993; 328:10–14.
10. Marshall JA, Hamman RF, Baxter J. High-fat, low-carbohydrate diet and the etiology of non-insulin-dependent diabetes mellitus: the San Luis Valley Diabetes Study. Am J Epidemiol 1991;134:590–603.
11. O'Dea K. Diabetes in Australian aborigines: impact of the western diet and life style. J Intern Med 1992;232:103–17.
12. Rawls RL. Weighing In On Obesity. Chem. Eng News, 1999; 77(25):35–44.
13. Karam JH. Pancreatic Hormones & Antidiabetic Drugs. In: Katzung BG, ed. Basic and Clinical Pharmacology 7th ed. Stamford CT: Appleton and Lange, 1999:684–705.
14. Davis SN, Butler PC, Brown M, et al. The effects of human proinsulin on glucose turnover and intermediary metabolism. Metabolism 1991;40:953–961.
15. Wareham NJ, Byrne CD, Williams R, et al. Fasting proinsulin concentrations predict the development of type 2 diabetes. Diabetes Care 1999;22:262–270.
16. Viberti GC. A Glycemic Threshold for Diabetic Complications? N Engl J Med 1995;332:1293–1294.
17. Lewis EJ, Hunsicker LG, Bain RP, et al. The effect of angiotensin-converting enzyme inhibition on diabetic nephropathy. The Collaborative Study Group. N Engl J Med 1993;329: 1456–1462.
18. Bojestig M, Arnqvist HJ, Hermansson G, et al. Declining incidence of nephropathy in insulin-dependent diabetes mellitus. N Engl J Med 1994;330:15–18.
19. Gavin JHI, et al. Report of the Expert Committee on the Diagnosis and Classification of Diabetes Mellitus. Diabetes Care. 1997;20:1183–1197.
20. Jovanovic L, Peterson CM. The clinical utility of glycosylated hemoglobin. Am J Med 1981;70:331–338.
21. Livingston JN, Schoen WR. Glucagon and Glucagon-Like Peptide-1. In Ann Reports Med Chem 1999;34:189–198.
22. Bunin BA, Dener JM, Livingston DA. Application of combinatorial and Paralled Synthesis to medicinal Chemistry. In Ann reports Med Chem 1999;34:267–286.
23. Rohrer SP, Birzin ET, Mosley RT, et al. Rapid identification of subtype-selective agonists of the somatostatin receptor through combinatorial chemistry. Science 1998;282:737–740.
24. Ido Y, Vindigni A, Chang K, et al. Prevention of vascular and neural dysfunction in diabetic rats by C-peptide. Science 1997;277:563–566.
25. Ludik B, Kautzky-Willer A, Prager R, et al. Amylin: history and overview. Diabet Med 1997:14 Suppl 2:S9–13.
26. Tasaka Y, Nakaya F, Matsumoto H, et al. Pancreatic amylin content in human diabetic subjects and its relation to diabetes. Pancreas 1995;11:303–308.
27. Thompson RG, Peterson J, Gottlieb A, et al. Effects of pramlintide, an analog of human amylin, on plasma glucose profiles in patients with IDDM: results of a multicenter trial. Diabetes 1997;46:632–636.
28. Silvestre RA, Salas M, Rodriquez-Gallardo J, et al. Effect of (8-32) salmon calcitonin, an amylin antagonist, on insulin, glucagon and somatostatin release; study in the perfused pancreas of the rat. Br J Pharmacol 1996;117:347–350.
29. Wollmer A, Rannefeld B, Johansen BR, et al. Phenolpromoted structural transformation of insulin in solution. Biol Chem Hopper Seyler 1987;368:903–911.
30. Olsen HB, Ludvigsen S, Kaarsholm NC. Protein. Structure. Solution structure of an engineered insulin monomer at neutral pH. Biochemistry 1996;35:8836–8845.
31. Brange J, Langkjaer. Insulin Structure and Stability. In: Stability and Characterization of Protein and Peptide Drugs. Wang YL, Pearlman, eds. New York Plenum Press, 1993: 315–350.
32. Polaschegg E. Effect of physiochemical variables of regular insulin formulations on their absorption from the subcutaneous tissue. Diabetes Res Clin Pract 1998;40:39–44.
33. Dodson EJ, Dodson GG, Hubbard RE, et al. Insulin Assembly: Its Modification by Protein Engineering and Ligand Binding. Phil. Trans. of the Royal Society (London) 1993; 345:153–164.
34. Weiss MA, Nguyen DT, Khait I, et al. Two-dimensional NMR and photo-CIDNP studies of the insulin monomer: assignment of aromatic resonances with application to protein folding, structure, and dynamics. Biochemistry 1989;28: 9855–9873.
35. Kline AD, Justice RM Jr. Complete sequence-specific 1H NMR assignments for human insulin. Biochemistry 1990;29: 2906–2913.
36. Scott DA. Crystalline Insulin. Biochem. J. 1934;28:1592–1602.
37. Constantino HR, Liauw S, Mitragotri S, et al, eds, Washington DC, American Chemical Society, 1997, p. 29–66.
38. Smith GD, Swenson DC, Dodson EJ, et al. Structural stability in the 4-zinc human insulin hexamer. Proc Natl Acad Sci U S A 1984;81:7093–7097.
39. Brange J, Andersen L, Laursen ED, et al. Toward understanding insulin fibrillation. J Pharm Sci 1997;86:517–525.
40. Brange J, Whittingham J, Edwards D. Insulin Structure and Diabetes Treatment. Current Science India 1997;72:470–476.
41. Maislos M, Mead PM, Gaynor DH, et al. The source of the circulating aggregate of insulin in type I diabetic patients is therapeutic insulin. J Clin Invest 1986;77:717–723.
42. Brown, TA. Gene Cloning in Medicine, London: Chapman and Hall, 1986;248–249.
43. Thim L, Hansen MT, Norris K, et al. Secretion and processing of insulin precursors in yeast. Proc Natl Acad Sci U S A 1986; 83:6766–6770.

44. Halles-Moller K. Chemical and Biological Insulin Studies I and II. PhD Dissertation, University of Copenhagen, Copenhagen, 1945.

45. Hengesh EJ. In: Foye WO, Lemke TL, Williams DA, eds. Principles of Medicinal Chemistry, 4th Ed. Baltimore, Williams & Wilkins,1995;581–600.

46. Brange J. Owens DR, Kang S, et al. Monomeric insulins and their experimental and clinical implications. Diabetes Care 1990;13:923–954.

47. Balaschmidt P, Brange J. Fast Acting Human Insulin Analogues With a Single Amino Acid Deletion in the B-Chain. Diabetologia 1992;35:B4.

48. Svoboda I, Brandenburg D, Barth T, et al. Semisynthetic insulin analogues modified in positions B24, B25 and B29. Biol Chem Hoppe Seyler 1994;375:373–378.

49. Mirmia RG, Nakagawa SH, Tager HS. Importance of the character and configuration of residues B24, B25, and B26 in insulin-receptor interactions. J Biol Chem 1991;266:1428–1436.

50. Hartmann H, Korf J, Ottmers U, et al. Acute metabolic actions of des-(B27–B30)-insulin and related analogues in adult rats. Acta Diabetol 1993;30:108–114.

51. Lenz V, Gattner HG, Sievert D, et al. Semisynthetic des-(B27–B30)-insulins with modified B26-tyrosine. Biol Chem Hoppe Seyler 1991;372:495–504.

52. Brange J, Ribel U, Hansen JF, et al. Monomeric insulins obtained by protein engineering and their medical implications. Nature 1988:333:679–682.

53. DiMarchi RD, Mayer JP, Fan L, et al. Synthesis of a Fast-Acting Insulin Based on Structural Homology With Insulin-Like Growth Factor I. In: Smith JA, Rivier JE, eds. Peptides-Chemistry and Biology; Proceedings of the 12th American Peptide Symposium. Leiden: Escom. 1992:26–28.

54. Mudaliar SR, Lindberg FA, Joyce M, et al. Insulin aspart (B28 asp-insulin): a fast-acting analog of human insulin: absorption kinetics and action profile compared with regular human insulin in healthy nondiabetic subjects. Diabetes Care 1999; 22:1501–1506.

55. Seipke G, Gelsen K, Neubauer H-P, et al. New Insulin Preparations with Prolonged Action Peptides. Diabetologica 1992; 35:A4.

56. Baudys M, Uchio T, Mix D, et al. Physical Stabilization of insulin by glycosylation. J Pharm Sci 1995;84:28–33.

57. Myers SR, Yakubu-Madus FE, Johnson WT, et al. Acylation of human insulin with palmitic acid extends the time action of human insulin in diabetic dogs. Diabetes 1997;46:637–642.

58. Berti L, Kellerer M, Bossenmaier B, et al. The long acting human insulin analog HOE 901: characteristics of insulin signalling in comparison to Asp(GB10) and regular insulin. Horm Metab Res 1998;30:123–129.

59. Gibbs EM, Stock JL, McCoid SC, et al. Glycemic improvement in diabetic db/db mice by overexpression of the human insulin-regulatable glucose transporter (GLUT4). J Clin Invest 1995;95:1512–1518.

60. Malaisse WJ, Lebrun P. Mechanisms of sulfonylurea-induced insulin release. Diabetes Care 1990;13 Suppl 3:9–17.

61. Groop LC. Sulfonylureas in NIDDM. Diabetes Care 1992; 15:737–754.

62. DeFronzo RA, Bonadonna RC Ferrannini E. Pathogenesis of NIDDM. A balanced overview. Diabetes Care 1992;15:318–368.

63. Bailey TS, Mezitis NH. Combination therapy with insulin and sulonfylureas for type II diabetes. Diabetes Care 1990;13:687–695.

64. Annonymous. Effects of hypoglycemic agents on vascular complications in patients with adult-onset diabetes. VIII. Evaluation of insulin therapy: final report. Diabetes 1982;31 Suppl 5:1–81.

65. Wolffenbuttel BH, Graal MB. New treatments for patients with type 2 diabetes mellitus. Postgrad Med J 1996;72:657–662.

66. Muller G, Satoh Y, Geisen K. Extrapancreatic effects of sulfonylureas—a comparison between glimepiride and conventional sulfonylureas. Diabetes Res Clin Pract 1995;28 Suppl: S115–137.

67. Langtry HD, Balfour JA. Glimepiride. A review of its use in the management of type 2 diabetes mellitus. Drugs 1998;55:563–584.

68. Anonymous. F-D-C Reports (The Pink Sheet). 1998:15.

69. Lins L, Brasseur R, Malaisse WJ. Conformational analysis of non-sulfonylurea hypoglycemic agents of the meglitinide family. Biochem Pharmacol 1995;50:1879–1884.

70. Vigneri R, Goldfine ID. Role of metformin in treatment of diabetes mellitus. Diabetes Care 1987;10:118–22.

71. Bailey CJ. Biguanides and NIDDM. Diabetes Care 1992;15:755–772.

72. Matthaei S, Hamann A, Klein HH, et al. Association of Metformin's effect to increase insulin-stimulated glucose transport with potentiation of insulin-induced translocation of glucose transporters from intracellular pool to plasma membrane in rat adiopocytes. Diabetes 1991;40:850–857.

73. Driscoll J, Ghazzi M, Perez J, et al. 96-Week Follow Up on Cardiac Safety in Patients with Type II Diabetes Treated with Troglitazone. Diabetes 1997;46 Suppl 1:149A.

74. Valiquett T, Huang S, Whitcomb R. Effects of Troglitazone Monotherapy in Patients with NIDDM: A 6-Month Multicenter Study. Diabetes 1997; 46 Suppl 1:43A.

75. Anonymous. Substituting for Troglitazone (Rezulin). Med Letters 2000;42:36.

76. Spiegelman BM. PPAR-gamma: adipogenic regulator and thiazolidinedione receptor. Diabetes 1998;47:507–514.

77. Staels B, Auwerx J. Role of PPAR in the Pharmacological Regulation of Lipoprotein Metabolism by Fibrates and Thiazolidinediones. Curr Pharmaceutical Design 1997;3:1–14.

78. Kawai K, Kawasaki-Tokui Y, Odaka T, et al. Disposition and metabolism of the new oral antidiabetic drug troglitazone in rats, mice and dogs. Arzneimittelforschung 1997;47:356–368.

79. Yamazaki H, Shibata A. Suzuki M. et al. Oxidation of troglitazone to a quinone-type metabolite catalyzed by cytochrome P-450 2C8 and P-450 3A4 in human liver microsomes. Drug Metab Dispos 1999;27:1260-1266.

80. Krieter PA, Colletti AE, Doss GA, et al. Disposition and metabolism of the hypoglycemic agent pioglitazone in rats. Drug Metab Dispos 1994;22:625–630.

81. Tanis SP, Parker TT, Colca JR, et al. Synthesis and biological activity of metabolites of the antidiabetic, antihyperglycemic agent pioglitazone. J Med Chem. 1996;39:5053–63.

82. Cox PJ, Ryan DA, Hollis FJ, et al. Absorption, disposition, and metabolism of rosiglitazone, a potent thiazolidinedione insulin sensitizer, in humans. Drug Metab Dispos 2000;28:772–780.

83. Clissold SP, Edwards C. Acarbose. A preliminary review of its pharmacodynamic and pharmacokinetic properties, and therapeutic potential. Drugs 1988;35:214–43.

84. Schmidt DD, Frommer W, Junge B, et al. alpha-Glucosidase inhibitors. New complex oligosaccharides of microbial origin. Naturwissenschaften. 1977 Oct;64(10):535–6.

85. Heiker FR, Boeshagen H, Junge B, et al. Studies designed to localize the essential structureal unit of glycoside-hydrolase inhibitors of the carbose type. In: Crutzfeld W, ed. Proceedings of the First International Symposium on Acarbose. Montreux: Excerpta Medica, 1981:137–141.

86. Coniff RF, Shapiro JA, Seaton TB, et al. A double-blind placebo-controlled trial evaluating the safety and efficacy of acarbose for the treatment of patients with insulin-requiring type II diabetes. Diabetes Care 1995;18:928–932.

87. Segal P, Feig PU, Schernthaner G, et al. The efficacy and safety of miglitol therapy compared with glibenclamide in patients with NIDDM inadequately controlled by diet alone. Diabetes Care 1997;20:687–691.

88. Ahr HJ, Boberg M, Brendel E, et al. Pharmacokinetics of miglitol. Absorption, distribution, metabolism, and excretion following administration to rats, dogs, and man. Arzneimittelforschung 1997;47:734–745.

89. Zhang B, Salituro G, Szalkowski D, et al. Discovery of a small molecule insulin mimetic with antidiabetic activity in mice. Science 1999;284:974–977.

28. Adrenocorticoids

DUANE D. MILLER, ROBERT W. BRUEGGEMEIER, AND JAMES T. DALTON

INTRODUCTION

The adrenocorticoids and sex hormones (Chapter 29) have much in common. All are steroids, and consequently the rules that define their structures, chemistry, and nomenclature are the same. The rings of these biochemically dynamic and physiologically active compounds have a similar stereochemical relationship. Changes in the geometry of the ring junctures generally result in inactive compounds regardless of the biologic category of the steroid. Similar chemical groups are used to render some of these agents water soluble or active when taken orally or to modify their absorption.

In addition, the adrenocorticoids and the sex hormones, which include the estrogens, progestins, and androgens, are mainly biosynthesized from cholesterol, which, in turn, is synthesized from acetyl-CoA. Cholesterol and steroid hormone catabolism take place primarily in the liver. Although the products found in the urine and feces depend upon the hormone undergoing catabolism, many of the metabolic reactions are similar for these compounds. For example, reduction of double bonds at positions 4 and 5 or 5 and 6, epimerization of 3α-hydroxyl groups, reduction of 3-keto groups to the 3α-hydroxyl function, and oxidative removal of side chains are transformations common to these agents.

Despite their similarities in chemical structures and stereochemistry, each class of steroids demonstrates unique and distinctively different biologic activities. Adrenocorticoids are composed of two classes of steroids, the glucocorticoids, which regulate carbohydrate, lipid, and protein metabolism and the mineralocorticoids, which influence salt balance and water retention. The sex hormones include the female sex hormones, progestins and estrogens, and the male sex hormones, androgens. Minor structural modifications to the steroid nucleus, such as changes in or insertion of functional groups at different positions, cause marked changes in physiologic activity. The first part of this chapter focuses on the similarities among the steroids and reviews steroid nomenclature, stereochemistry, and the general mechanism of action. The second portion of the chapter focuses on the adrenocorticoids and discusses the biosynthesis, metabolism, medicinal chemistry, pharmacology and pharmacokinetics of endogenous steroid hormones, synthetic agonists, and synthetic antagonists.

STEROID NOMENCLATURE AND STRUCTURE

Steroids consist of four fused rings (A, B, C, and D) (Fig. 28.1). Chemically, these hydrocarbons are cyclopentanoperhydrophenanthrenes; they contain a five-membered cyclopentane (D) ring plus the three rings of phenanthrene. A perhydrophenanthrene (rings A, B, and C) is the completely saturated derivative of phenanthrene. The polycyclic hydrocarbon known as cholestane will be used to illustrate the numbering system for a steroid (Fig. 28.1). The term cholestane refers to a steroid with 27 carbons that includes a side chain of eight carbons at position 17. Numbering begins in ring A at C1 and proceeds around rings A and B to C10, then into ring C beginning with C11 and snakes around rings C and D to C17. The angular methyl groups are numbered 18 (attached to C13) and 19 (attached to C10). The 17 side chain begins with C20 and numbering finishes in sequential order. Using the planar representation for drawing the steroid structure (Fig. 28.2), the basic steroid structure becomes a plane with two surfaces; a top or β surface is pointing out towards the reader, and the bottom or α surface away from the reader. Hydrogens or functional groups on the β side of the molecule are denoted by solid lines; those on the α side are designated by dotted lines. The 5α notation is used to denote the configuration of the hydrogen atom at C5, which is opposite from the C19 angular methyl group, making the A/B ring juncture *trans*. The C19 angular methyl group is assigned the β side of the molecule. Simi-

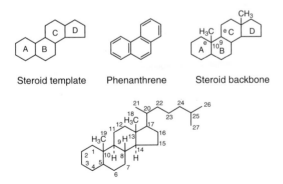

Fig. 28.1. Basic steroid structure and numbering system.

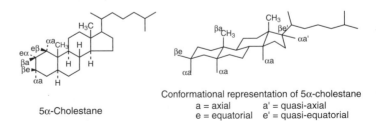

Conformational representation of 5α-cholestane
a = axial   a' = quasi-axial
e = equatorial   e' = quasi-equatorial

5α-Cholestane

Fig. 28.2. Planar and conformational structures of 5α-cholestane.

653

larly, the configuration for the 8β and 9α hydrogens, and 14α hydrogen and C18 angular methyl group, denote *trans* fusion for rings B/C and C/D. The side chains at C17 are always β unless indicated by dotted lines or in the nomenclature of the steroid (e.g., 17β or 17α).

Just as cyclohexane can be drawn in a chair conformation, the three-dimensional conformational representation of the planar structure for 5α-cholestane is shown in Figure 28.2. Although cyclohexane may easily undergo a flip in conformation, steroids are rigid structures because they generally have at least one *trans* fused ring system, and these rings must be diequatorial to each other.

If one is aware that the C18 and C19 angular methyl groups always have a β-axial orientation (i.e., perpendicular to the plane of the rings) the conformational orientation of the remaining bonds of a steroid can be assigned easily. For example, in 5α-cholestane the two bonds at C3 must be β-equatorial and α-axial, as indicated in Figure 28.2. The orientation of the remaining bonds on a steroid may be determined if one recalls that groups on a cyclohexane ring that are positioned on adjacent carbon atoms (vicinal, $-C_1H-C_2H-$) of the ring (i.e., 1, 2 to each other) are *trans* if their relationship is 1,2-diaxial or 1,2-diequatorial and are *cis* if their relationship is 1,2-equatorial-axial.

Steroid chemists often refer to the series of carbon-carbon bonds shown with heavy lines as the backbone of the steroid (Fig. 28.1). The *cis* or *trans* relationship of the four rings may be expressed in terms of the backbone. 5α-Cholestane is said to have a trans-trans-trans (all *trans*) backbone; all the fused rings have *trans* stereochemistry, i.e., the A/B fused ring, the B/C fused ring, and the C/D fused ring are all *trans*. 5β-cholestane on the other hand, has a cis-trans-trans backbone, in which the A/B rings are *cis* fused with B/C and C/D, *trans* (Fig. 28.3). Thus, the conventional drawing for the steroid nucleus is the natural *trans* configuration for rings B/C and C/D and therefore the hydrogens at 8β, 9α, or 14β positions are not shown. If the C5 is saturated, the hydrogen is shown either as 5α (*trans*) or 5β (*cis*) to denote type of ring fusion between rings A and B. Also, the conventional drawing of a steroid molecule has the C18 and C19 methyl groups shown only as solid lines (no CH_3).

The stereochemistry of the rings markedly affects the biologic activity of a given class of steroids. Nearly all biolog-

ically active hormonal steroids have the cholestane-type backbone, except for the cardiac glycosides (Chapter 21), which have a cis-trans-cis ring fusions. The metabolites for many of the hormonal steroids have a 5β configuration making them inactive. In most of the important steroids discussed in this chapter, a double bond is present between positions 4 and 5 or 5 and 6, and consequently there is no *cis* or *trans* relationship between rings A and B. The symbol Δ is often used to designate a carbon carbon double bond (C=C) in a steroid. If the C=C is between the 4 and 5 position, the compound is referred to as a $Δ^4$-steroid; if the C=C is between positions 5 and 10, the compound is designated a $Δ^{5(10)}$-steroid.

Cholesterol (cholest-5-en-3β-ol) is a $Δ^5$ steroid or, more specifically, a $Δ^5$-sterol because it is an unsaturated alcohol.

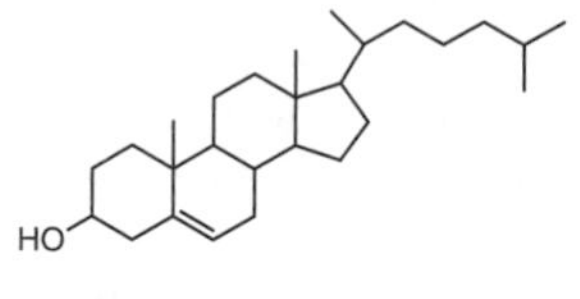

Cholesterol

Three other hormone steroid hydrocarbons having the 5α-cholestane configuration are discussed in Chapter 29. These biologically active steroids include members of the 5α-pregnane, 5α-androstane, and 5α-estrane steroid classes (Fig. 28.4). Pregnanes are steroids with 21 carbon atoms with a 17β side chain (C20 and C21); androstanes have 19 carbon atoms; and estranes have 18 carbon atoms, with the C19 angular methyl group at C10 replaced by hydrogen. Numbering is the same as in 5α-cholestane.

The adrenocorticoids (adrenal cortex hormones) are pregnanes (Fig. 28.4) and are exemplified by hydrocortisone (cortisol), which is a 11β, 17α,21-trihydroxypregn-4-ene-3,20-dione. Its acetate ester is named hydrocortisone

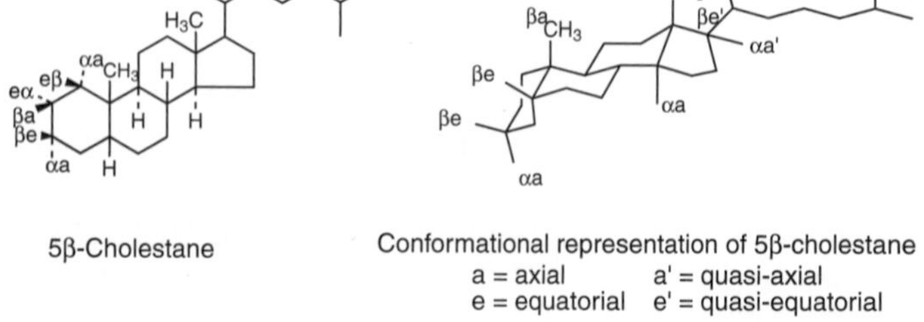

Fig. 28.3. Planar and conformational structures for 5β-cholestane.

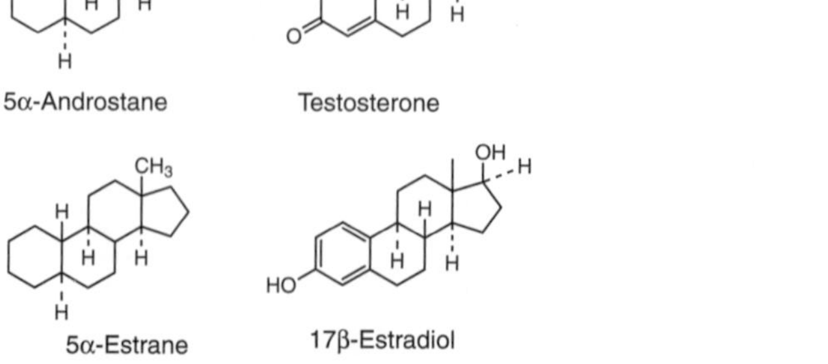

Fig. 28.4. Steroid classes and corresponding natural hormones.

21-acetate. Progesterone (pregn-4-ene-3,20-dione), a female sex hormone synthesized by the corpus luteum, is also a pregnane analog. The male sex hormones (androgens) are based on the structure of 5α-androstane. Testosterone, an important naturally occurring androgen, is named 17β-hydroxy-4-androsten-3-one. The estrogens, which are female sex hormones synthesized by the graafian follicle of the ovaries, are estrane analogs containing an aromatic A ring. Although the A ring does not contain isolated C=C groups, these analogs are named as if the bonds were in the positions shown in 17β-estradiol. Hence, 17β-estradiol, a typical member of this class of drugs, is named estra-1,3,5,(10)-triene-3,17β-diol. Other examples of steroid nomenclature are found throughout this chapter.

Aliphatic side chains at position 17 are always assumed to be β when cholestane or pregnane nomenclature is employed; hence, the notation 17β need not be used when naming these compounds. If a pregnane has a 17α chain, however, this should be indicated in the nomenclature. Finally, the final e in the name for the parent steroid hydrocarbon is always dropped when it precedes a vowel, regardless of whether a number appears between the two parts of the word. Note the nomenclature for cholesterol and testosterone versus that for hydrocortisone, for example. For a more extensive discussion of steroid nomenclature, consult the literature (1).

MECHANISM OF STEROID HORMONE ACTION

In addition to their structural similarities, adrenocorticoids, estrogens, progestins, and androgens share a common mode of action. They are present in the body only in extremely low concentrations (e.g., 0.1–1.0 nM), where they exert potent physiologic effects on sensitive tissues. They bind with high affinity to intracellular receptors. Extensive research activities directed at elucidation of the general mechanism of steroid hormone action have been performed for several decades, and many reviews have appeared (2–7).

The steroid hormones act on target cells to regulate gene expression and protein biosynthesis via the formation of steroid-receptor complexes, as outlined in Figure 28.5. The lipophilic steroid hormones are carried in the bloodstream, with the majority of the hormones reversibly bound to serum carrier proteins. The free steroids can diffuse through the cell membrane and enter cells. Those cells sensitive to the particular steroid hormone (referred to as target cells) contain steroid receptors capable of high-affinity binding with the steroid. These receptors are soluble intracellular proteins that can both bind steroid ligands with high affinity and act as transcriptional factors via interaction with specific deoxyribonucleic acid (DNA) sites. Early studies suggested that the unoccupied steroid receptors were located solely in the cytosol of target cells (8). However recent investigations on estrogen, progestin, and androgen action indicate that active, unoccupied receptors are also present in the nucleus of the cell (2,7,9). Prior to the binding of the steroid, the steroid receptor is complexed with heat shock proteins (HSP). In the current model, the steroid enters the cell and binds to the steroid receptor in the cytoplasm or nucleus. This binding initiates a conformational change and dissociation of the HSP allowing steroid receptor dimerization and translocation to the nucleus. The receptor dimer interacts with particular regions of the cellular DNA, referred to as hormone-responsive elements (HRE), and with various nuclear transcriptional factors. Binding of the nuclear steroid-receptor complex to DNA initiates transcription of the DNA sequence to produce messenger ribonucleic acid (mRNA). Finally, the elevated levels of mRNA lead to an increase in protein synthesis in the endoplasmic reticulum. These proteins include enzymes, receptors, and secreted factors that subsequently result in the steroid hormonal response regulating cell function, growth, differentiation and playing central roles in normal physiological processes as well as in many important diseases.

The primary amino acid sequences of the various steroid hormone receptors have been deduced from cloned complementary DNA (cDNA) (3,5). The steroid receptor proteins are part of a larger family of nuclear receptor proteins that also include receptors for vitamin D, thyroid hormones, and retinoids. The overall structures of the receptors have strong similarities (Fig. 28.6). A high degree of homology (sequence similarities) in the steroid receptors is found in the DNA binding region that interacts with the HRE. The DNA binding region has critically placed cysteine amino acids that chelate zinc ions, forming finger-like projections called zinc fingers that bind to the DNA. Structure-function studies of cloned receptor proteins also identify regions of the molecules that are important for interactions with nuclear transcriptional factors, activation of gene transcription, and protein to protein interactions. Recent evidence suggests that the protein-protein interactions with AP-1 and NFκB (other known transcriptional proteins) work to titrate out the effects of the steroid receptors on DNA. This may be critical for cross talk between signaling pathways within the cell and may play an important role in feedback systems. Additional evidence suggests that steroid receptors may activate transcription in the absence of hormone; an effect that appears to depend on the phosphorylation of the receptor via a cross-talk with membrane bound adrenergic and growth factor receptors (10). The interactions necessary for formation of the steroid-receptor complexes and subsequent activation of gene transcription are complicated, involve multi-stage processes, and leave many unanswered questions.

The basic mechanism of steroid hormone action on target cells is similar for the various classes of agents. Differences in the actions of adrenocorticoids, estrogens, progestins, and androgens arise from the specificity of the particular receptor proteins, the particular genetic processes initiated, and the specific cellular proteins produced.

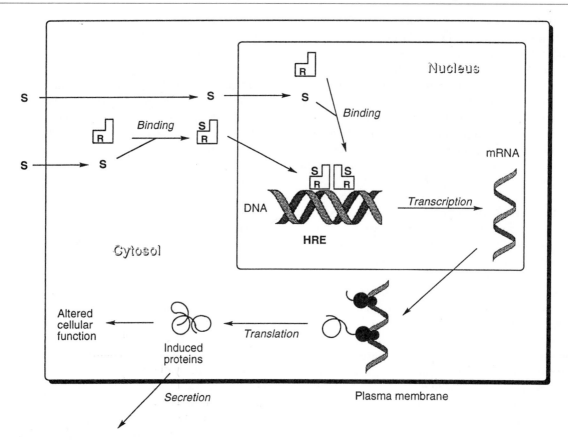

Fig. 28.5. Mechanism of steroid hormone action.

Receptor Structures:

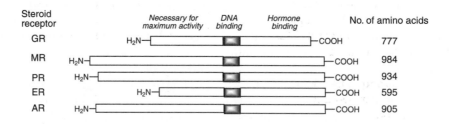

Steroid receptor	Necessary for maximum activity	DNA binding	Hormone binding	No. of amino acids
GR				777
MR				984
PR				934
ER				595
AR				905

Hormone responsive element (HRE):

nucleotide sequence

GRE	G G T A C A n n n T G T T C T
MRE	G G T A C A n n n T G T T C T
PRE	G G T A C A n n n T G T T C T
ERE	G G T A C A n n n T G T T C T
ARE	A G G T C A n n n T G A C C T

Fig. 28.6. Structural features of steroid hormone receptors and hormone responsive elements. Schematic comparison of the amino acid sequences of steroid receptors (GR, glucocorticoid; MR, mineralocorticoid; PR, progesterone; ER, estrogen; AR, androgen) with high homology in the DNA binding region. HRE sequences are also compared (GRE, glucocorticoid; MRE, mineralocorticoid; PRE, progesterone; ERE, estrogen; ARE, androgen).

ADRENOCORTICOSTEROIDS—HISTORY AND DISEASE STATES

The adrenal glands are flattened, caplike structures located above the kidneys. The inner core (medulla) of the gland secretes catecholamines, while the shell (cortex) of the gland synthesizes steroids known as the adrenocorticoids. The adrenocorticoids are divided according to their biochemical mechanism of action into glucocorticoids (hydrocortisone) and mineralocorticoids (aldosterone).

The importance of the adrenal glands was recognized long ago. Addison's disease, Cushing's disease, and Conn's syndrome are pathologic conditions related to the adrenal cortex and the hormones produced by the gland.

Addison's disease was named after Thomas Addison. In 1855, Addison described a syndrome in which the physiologic significance of the adrenal cortex was emphasized (11). This disease is characterized by extreme weakness, anorexia, anemia, nausea and vomiting, low blood pressure, hyperpigmentation of the skin, and mental depression caused by decreased secretion of steroid hormones by the adrenal cortex. Addison's disease is a rare affliction which affects roughly 1 in 100,000 people and is seen equally in both sexes and all age groups.

Conditions of this type, generally referred to as hypoadrenalism, may result from several causes, including destruction of the cortex by tuberculosis or atrophy or decreased secretion of adrenocorticotropin (ACTH) because of diseases of the adenohypophysis (anterior pituitary). Cushing's disease, or hyperadrenalism, on the other hand, may result from adrenal cortex tumors or increased production of ACTH caused by pituitary carcinoma. Cushing's syndrome is also rare, occurring in only 2–5 people for every one million people each year. About 10% of newly diagnosed cases are observed in children and teenagers.

Conn's syndrome is apparently due to an inability of the adrenal cortex to carry out 17α-hydroxylation during the biosynthesis of the hormones from cholesterol. Consequently, the disease is characterized by a high secretory level of aldosterone which lacks a 17α-hydroxyl functional group. In addition, hypernatremia, polyuria, alkalosis, and hypertension are observed (12).

The importance of the adrenocorticoids is most dramatically observed in adrenalectomized animals. There is an increase of urea in the blood, muscle weakness (asthenia), decreased liver glycogen and decreased resistance to insulin, lowered resistance to trauma, such as cold and mechanical or chemical shock, and electrolyte disturbances. Potassium ions are retained, and excretion of Na^+, Cl^-, and water is increased. Adrenalectomy in small animals causes death in a few days.

After Addison's observations in 1855, physiologists, pharmacologists, and chemists from many countries contributed to our understanding of adrenocorticoids. It was not until 1927, however, that Rogoff and Stewart found that extracts of adrenal glands, administered by intravenous injection, kept adrenalectomized dogs alive.

Since this discovery, similar experiments have been repeated many times. Originally, it was thought that the biologic activity of the extract was due to a single compound. Later, 47 compounds were isolated from such extracts, and some were highly active. Among the biologically active corticoids isolated, hydrocortisone, corticosterone, aldosterone, cortisone, 11-desoxycorticosterone, 11-dehydrocorticosterone, and 17α-hydroxy-11-desoxycorticosterone, were found to be most potent (13). The biosynthesis of these steroids is described next.

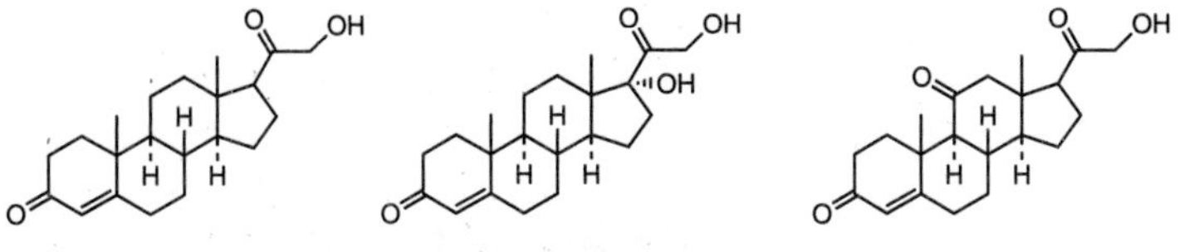

11-Desoxycorticosterone   17α-Hydroxy-11-desoxy-corticosterone   11-Dehydrocorticosterone

BIOSYNTHESIS
Pregnenolone Formation

In the adrenal glands cholesterol is converted by enzymatic cleavage of its side chain to pregnenolone, which serves as the biosynthetic precursor of the adrenocorticoids (Fig. 28.7). This biotransformation is performed by a mitochondrial cytochrome P450 enzyme complex. This enzyme complex found in the mitochondrial membrane consists of three proteins—CYP11A1, adrenodoxin, and adrenodoxin reductase (14). Defects in CYP11A1 lead to a lack of glucocorticoids, feminization and hypertension. Three oxidation steps are involved in the conversion, and three moles of NADPH and molecular oxygen are consumed for each mole of cholesterol converted to pregnenolone. The first oxidation results in the formation of cholest-5-ene-3β,22R-diol (step a), followed by the second oxidation yielding cholest-5-ene-3β,20R,22R-triol (step b). The third oxidation step catalyzes the cleavage of the C20-C22 bond to release pregnenolone and isocaproic aldehyde (step c).

Pregnenolone serves as the common precursor in the formation of the adrenocorticoids and other steroid hor-

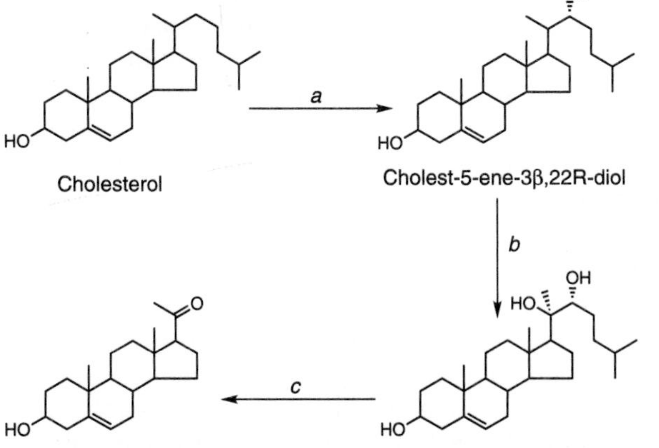

Fig. 28.7. Biosynthesis of pregnenolone from cholesterol.

mones. This C21 steroid is converted via enzymatic oxidations and isomerization of the double bond to a number of physiologically active C21 pregnane steroids, including the female sex hormone progesterone and the adrenocorticoids hydrocortisone (cortisol), corticosterone, and aldosterone. Oxidative cleavage of the two carbon side chain of pregnenolone and subsequent enzymatic oxidations and isomerization lead to C19 steroids, including the androgens testosterone and dihydrotestosterone. The final group of steroids, the C18 female sex hormones, are derived from oxidative aromatization of the A ring of androgens to produce estrogens. More detailed information on these biosynthetic pathways are described in this and in Chapter 29 under the particular class of steroid hormones.

Pregnenolone to Glucocorticoids and Mineralocorticoids

Hydrocortisone and aldosterone are regulated by independent mechanisms. The glucocorticoids are biosynthesized and released under the influence of peptide hormones secreted by the hypothalamus and adenohypophysis (anterior pituitary gland) to activate the adrenal cortex (HPA axis). On the other hand, the secretion of the mineralocorticoids, aldosterone and corticosterone, are under the influence of the octapeptide, angiotensin II. Angiotensin II is the active metabolite resulting from the renin catalyzed proteolytic hydrolysis of plasma angiotensinogen to angiotensin I in the blood. Removal of the pituitary gland results in atrophy of the adrenal cortex and a marked decrease in the rate of glucocorticoid formation and secretion. However, in hypophysectomized animals, the rate of secretion of aldosterone is only slightly decreased or remains unchanged. Consequently, the electrolyte balance remains nearly normal.

The peptide hormone in the adenohypophysis that influences glucocorticoid biosynthesis in the adrenal cortex is adrenocorticotropic hormone (ACTH; corticotropin), whereas the peptide hormone in the hypothalamus is corticotropin-releasing factor (CRF). The production of both ACTH and CRF is regulated by the central nervous system (CNS) and by a negative corticoid feedback mechanism. CRF is released by the hypothalamus and is transported to the adenohypophysis, where it stimulates the release of ACTH into the bloodstream where it is transported to the adrenal glands. There it stimulates the biosynthesis and secretion of the glucocorticoids. The circulating levels of glucocorticoids act on the hypothalamus and adenohypophysis by negative feedback to regulate the release of both CRF and ACTH. As the levels of glucocorticoids rise, smaller amounts of CRF and ACTH are secreted and a negative feedback is observed (HPA suppression). A variety of stimuli, including pain, noise, environmental conditions, and emotional reactions, increase the secretion of CRF, ACTH, and consequently, the glucocorticoids. Once the stimulus is alleviated or removed, the negative feedback mechanism inhibits further production and helps return the body to a normal hormonal balance (15,16).

ACTH acts at the adrenal gland by binding to a receptor protein on the surface of the adrenal cortex cell to stimulate the biosynthesis and secretion of glucocorticoids. The only steroid stored in the adrenal gland is cholesterol, found in the form of cholesterol esters stored in lipid droplets. ACTH stimulates the conversion of cholesterol esters to glucocorticoids by initiating a series of biochemical events through its surface receptor. The ACTH receptor protein is coupled to a G protein and to adenyl cyclase. Binding of ACTH to its receptor leads to activation of adenyl cyclase via the G protein. The result is an increase in intracellular cyclic adenosine monophosphate (cAMP) levels. One of the processes influenced by elevated cAMP levels is the activation of cholesterol esterase, which cleaves cholesterol esters and liberates free cholesterol.

Free cholesterol is then converted within mitochondria to pregnenolone via the side-chain cleavage reaction described earlier in Figure 28.7. Pregnenolone is converted to adrenocorticoids by a series of enzymatic oxidations and double bond isomerization (Fig. 28.8). The next several enzymatic steps in the biosynthesis of glucocorticoids occur in the endoplasmic reticulum of the adrenal cortex cell. Hydroxylation of pregnenolone at position 17 by the enzyme 17α-hydroxylase (CYP17) produces 17α-hydroxypregnenolone (step b). The 17α-hydroxyl group is important for adrenocorticoid hormone action. In one step, 17α-hydroxypregnenolone is oxidized to a 3-keto intermediate by the action of the enzyme 5-ene-3β-hydroxysteroid dehydrogenase and isomerized to 17α-hydroxyprogesterone by the enzyme 3-oxosteroid-4,5-isomerase (step c,d). Another hydroxylation occurs by the action of 21-hydroxylase (CYP21) to give 11-deoxycortisol, which contains the physiologically important 17β ketol ($-CO-CH_2OH$) side chain (step e). A lack of CYP21 prevents cortisol synthesis, diverting excess 17α-hydroxyprogesterone into overproduction of testosterone biosynthesis. The final step in the biosynthesis is catalyzed by the enzyme 11β-hydroxylase, mitochondrial CYP11B1. This results in the formation of hydrocortisone (cortisol), the most potent endogenous glucocorticoid secreted by the adrenal cortex. Cortisone, the inactive metabolite, is formed by oxidation of the 11β-hydroxy group of hydrocortisone by 11β-hydroxysteroid dehydrogenase, thus making hydrocortisone and cortisone metabolically interconvertible, just as estradiol and estrone are interconvertible. Approximately 15–20 mg of hydrocortisone is synthesized daily. Several reviews (15,17–20) provide more detailed discussions about the enzymology and regulation of adrenal steroidogenesis.

The pathway for the formation of the potent mineralocorticoid molecule, aldosterone, is similar to that for hydrocortisone and uses several of the same enzymes (Fig. 28.8). Aldosterone is biosynthesized in the zona glomerulosa which is the outer layer of the adrenal cortex. The preferred pathway involves the conversion of pregnenolone to progesterone by 5-ene-3β-hydroxysteroid dehydrogenase and 3-oxosteroid-4,5-isomerase (step c,d), followed by hydroxylation at C21 of progesterone by 21-hydroxylase re-

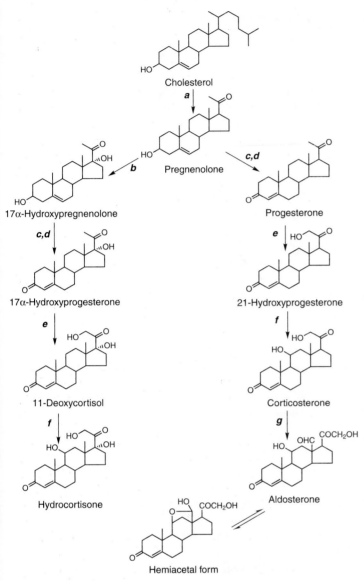

Fig. 28.8. Biosynthesis of the adrenocorticoids from cholesterol.

sulting in formation of 21-hydroxyprogesterone (deoxycorticosterone) (step e). Again, these first conversions occur in the endoplasmic reticulum of the cell, whereas the next enzymatic steps occur in the mitochondria. 11β-hydroxylase (CYP11B2) catalyzes the conversion of deoxycorticosterone to corticosterone (step f), which exhibits about 1/20 the mineralocorticoid activity of aldosterone (Table 28.1). The final two oxidations involve hydroxylations at the C18 methyl group and are catalyzed by 18-hydroxylase (step g). These reactions produce first 18-hydroxycorticosterone (not shown) and then aldosterone, the most powerful endogenous mineralocorticoid secretion of the adrenal cortex. The aldehyde at C18 of aldosterone exists in equilibrium with its hemiacetal form.

METABOLISM

Hydrocortisone and cortisone are biochemically interconvertible by the enzyme 11β-hydroxysteroid dehydroge-

nase, with the reaction equilibrium towards hydrocortisone (Fig. 28.9). Hydrocortisone is metabolized by the liver following administration by any route with a half-life of about 1–1.5 hours (21). Hydrocortisone is mainly excreted in the urine as inactive O-glucuronide conjugates and minor O-sulfate conjugates of urocortisol, 5β-dihydrocortisol, and urocortisone (Fig. 28.9). The tetrahydro metabolite urocortisol, is the major metabolite formed and has the 5β-pregnane geometry and 3α-hydroxyl function. The 5β-configuration is similar to the ring geometry for the nonhormonal bile acids. Several compounds of this type have been isolated (22,23). All of the biologically active adrenocorticoids contain a ketone at the 3-position and a double bond in the 4,5-position. The formation of 5β-metabolites from hydrocortisone is characterized by reduction of the 4,5-double bond to a 5β geometry for rings A and B (a *cis* configuration) by 5α- or 5β-reductase or reduction of the 3-ketone by 3α-hydroxysteroid dehydrogenase (3α-hydroxyl configuration) or 3β-hydroxysteroid dehydrogenase (3β-hydroxyl configuration). These reactions represent the major pathways of metabolism for the glucocorticoids and their endogenous counterparts. Urocortisol and urocortisone are named after cortisol (hydrocortisone) and cortisone. Reversible oxidation of the 11β-hydroxyl group of many glucocorticoids (e.g. hydrocortisone, prednisolone and methylprednisolone, but not dexamethasone and other 9α-fluorinated glucocorticoids) by 11β-hydroxysteroid dehydrogenase inactivates these drugs and limits their mineralocorticoid activity in the kidneys. Other routes of metabolism include 6β-hydroxylation (CYP3A4) and reduction of the 20-ketone (e.g. prednisolone) to form 20-hydroxyl analogs, oxidation of the 17-ketol side chain to 17β-carboxylic acids and loss of the 17-ketol side chain resulting in 11β-hydroxy-17-keto-C19 steroids with the geometry of either 5α-androstane or 5β-androstane (17–20). In addition, some ring A aromatic adrenocorticoid metabolites that resemble the estrogens have been isolated (24). Biliary and fecal excretion contribute little to the elimination of the adrenocorticoids. The rate of formation of 6β-hydroxyhydrocortisone is a biomarker for determining the level of HPA suppression and adrenal insufficiency.

DEVELOPMENT OF ADRENOCORTICOID DRUGS
Systemic Corticosteroids
Overview

The clinically available adrenocorticoids may be administered by intravenous injection, oral tablets or solutions, topical formulations, intra-articular administration, and by oral or nasal inhalation (Table 28.2). The route of administration depends on the disease being treated and the physicochemical, pharmacologic, and pharmacokinetic properties of the drug (Table 28.1). Only a handful of corticosteroids are used clinically by the oral route, including hydrocortisone, prednisone, prednisolone, methylprednisolone, and dexamethasone (Fig. 28.10). These corticosteroids are often described as short-acting, intermediate-

Table 28.1. Pharmacologic and Pharmacokinetic Properties for Some Adrenocorticoids

| Adrenocorticoid | Oral Gluco-corticoid Dose (mg)[1] | Potency Relative to Hydrocortisone | | Protein Binding (%)[5] | Half-life (hr) | | Duration of Action (days) |
		Gluco-corticoid Activity[2]	Mineralo-corticoid Activity[3]		Plasma	Biologic (tissue)	
Short-Acting							
Hydrocortisone	20	1	2+	>90	1.5–2	8–12	1–1.5
Cortisone	25	0.8	2+	>90	0.5	8–12	1–1.5
Intermediate-Acting							
Prednisone	5	3.5	1+	>90	3.4–3.8	18–36	1–1.5
Prednisolone	5	4	1+	>90	2.1–3.5	18–36	1–1.5
Methylprednisolone	5	5	0[4]		>3.5	18–36	1–1.5
Triamcinolone	5	5	0[4]	>90	2–5	18–36	1–1.5
Long-Acting							
Dexamethasone	0.75	20–30	0[4]	>90	3–4.5	36–54	2.8–3
Betamethasone	0.6	20–30	0[4]	>90	3–5	36–54	2.8–3
Fludrocortisone	Not employed	10	10	<90	3.5	18–36	1–2
Fluprednisolone	1.6	10	0[4]				
Aldosterone	Not employed	0.2	800				
11-Desoxycorticosterone	Not employed	0	40				
Corticosterone	IM	0.5	5				

[1]Based on the oral dose of an anti-inflammatory agent in rheumatoic arthritis.
[2]Anti-inflammatory, immunosuppressant, metabolic effects.
[3]Sodium and water retention, potassium depletion effects.
[4]Although these glucocorticoids are considered not to have significant mineralocorticoid activity, hypokalemia and/or sodium and fluid retention may occur, depending upon the dosage, duration of use and patient predisposition.
[5]Hydrocortisone binds to transcortin (Corticosteroid binding globulin; CBG) and to albumin. Prednisone also binds to CBG, but not betamethasone, dexamethasone or triamcinolone.

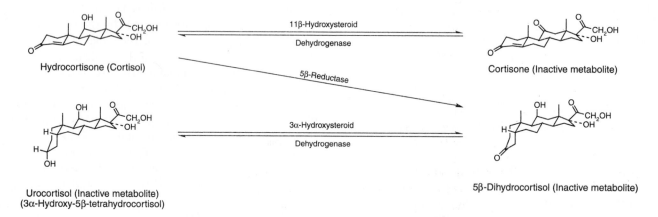

Fig. 28.9. Major routes of metabolism for hydrocortisone.

acting or long-acting according to their biologic half-life and duration of action (Table 28.1). They are well-absorbed, undergo little first pass metabolism in the liver, and demonstrate oral bioavailabilities (F) of 70–80%, except for triamcinolone (Table 28.3). The larger volume of distribution for methylprednisolone compared to prednisolone is thought to result from a combination of increased lipophilicity, decrease in metabolism and better tissue penetration. Glucocorticoids vary in the extent to which they are bound to the plasma proteins, albumin and corticosteroid-binding globulin (transcortin) (Table 28.1) (25).

Hydrocortisone is extensively bound to the plasma proteins, primarily to transcortin (corticosteroid-binding globulin) with only 5–10% of plasma hydrocortisone unbound. Prednisolone and methylprednisolone, but not the 9α-fluoro analogs betamethasone, dexamethasone, or triamcinolone, have a high affinity for transcortin and thus compete with hydrocortisone for this binding protein. The 9α-halo analogs bind primarily to albumin. Only the unbound fraction of hydrocortisone and the synthetic corticosteroids are biologically active. Generally, the amount of transcortin in the plasma determines the distribution of

Table 28.2. Adrenocorticoids, Their Trade Names and Their Routes of Administration

Adrenocorticoid	Trade Name	PO	IV	IM	Inhaled/Intransal	Topical
Alclomethasone dipropionate	Alclovate					•
Amcinonide	Cyclocort					•
Beclomethasone dipropionate	Beclovent, Vanceril, Beconase				•	
Beclomethasone dipropionate Monohydrate	Beconase AQ, Vancenase AQ				•	
Betamethasone	Celestone	•				
Betamethasone dipropionate	Diprosone, Maxivate					•
Betamethasone sod phosphate	Celestone Phosphate			•		
Betamethasone valerate	BetaVal, Valisone,					•
Budesonide	Pulmicort, Rhinocort				•	
Clobetasol propionate	Temovate					•
Clocortolone pivalate	Cloderm					•
Cortisone acetate		•		•		
Desonide	Tridesolone					•
Dexamethasone	Decadron	•				•a
Dexamethasone acetate	Decadron-LA, Dalalone, Dexasone			•		
Dexamethasone sod phosphate	Decadron Phosphate		•	•	•	
Desoximetasone	Topicort					•
Diflorasone Diacetate	Maxiflor, Florone, Psorcon					•
Fludrocortisone acetate	Florinef	•				
Flumethasone pivalate	Flocort					•
Flunisolide	Aerobid, Nasalide, Nasarel				•	
Fluocinolone acetonide	Synalar, Flurosyn					•
Fluocinonide	Lidex, Fluonex					•
Fluoromethalone	FML, Fluor-Op					•a
Fluoromethalone acetate	Flarex					•a
Flurandenolide	Cordran					•
Fluticasone propionate	Cutivate, Flovent, Flonase				•	•
Halcinonide	Halog					•
Halobetasol propionate	Ultravate					•
Hydrocortisone	Hydrocortone	•				•b
Hydrocortisone acetate	Hydrocortone Acetate			•		•c
Hydrocortisone buteprate	Pandel					•
Hydrocortisone butyrate	Locoid					•
Hydrocortisone cypionate	Cortef	•				
Hydrocortisone sod phosphate	Hydrocortone Phosphate		•	•		
Hydrocortisone sod succinate	Solu-Cortef		•	•		
Hydrocortisone valerate						•
Methylprednisolone	Medrol	•				
Methylprednisolone acetate	Depo-Medrol, Depopred			•		•
Methylprednisolone sod succinate	Solu-Medrol		•	•		
Mometasone furoate	Elocon					•
Mometasone furoate monohydrate	Nasonex				•	
Prednicarbate	Dermatop					•
Prednisolone	Deltacortef	•				
Prednisolone acetate	Pred-Mild, Pred-Forte					•a
Prednisolone acetate	Precor, Predalone, Key Pred	•				
Prednisolone sod phosphate	Pediapred, Inflamase, Hydeltrasol, AK-Pred	•		•		•a
Prednisolone tebutate				•		
Prednisone	Deltasone, Meticorten, Orasone	•				•
Triamcinolone	Aristocort, Kenacort,	•				
Triamcinolone acetonide	Kenalog, Triderm, Delta-Tritex, Flutex					•
Triamcinolone acetonide	Azmacort, Nasacort, Nasacort AQ				•	
Triamcinolone diacetate	Aristocort Forte, Triam Forte			•		
Triamcinolone hexacetonide	Aristospan			•		

aOphthalmic formulations.
bAlso in otic, ophthalmic, and rectal formulations (Cortenema).
cAlso in intrarectal foam (Cortifoam).

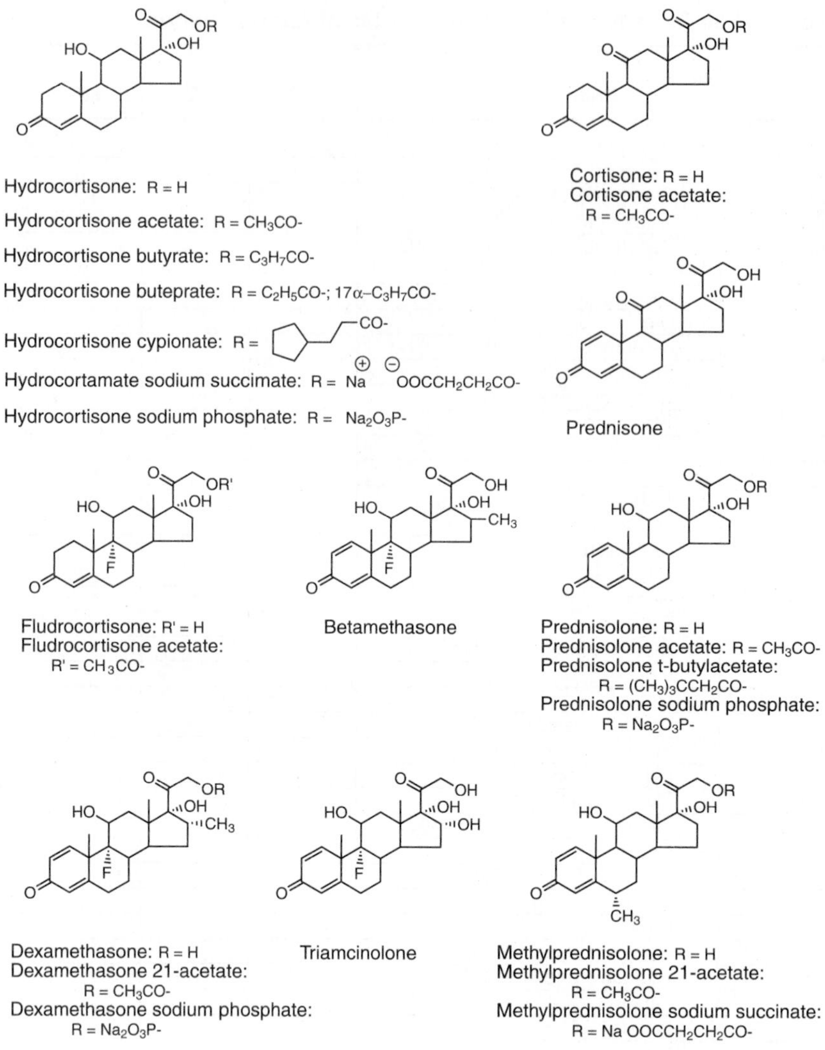

Hydrocortisone: R = H

Hydrocortisone acetate: R = CH₃CO-

Hydrocortisone butyrate: R = C₃H₇CO-

Hydrocortisone buteprate: R = C₂H₅CO-; 17α–C₃H₇CO-

Hydrocortisone cypionate: R =

Hydrocortamate sodium succimate: R = Na⁺ ⁻OOCCH₂CH₂CO-

Hydrocortisone sodium phosphate: R = Na₂O₃P-

Cortisone: R = H
Cortisone acetate:
R = CH₃CO-

Prednisone

Fludrocortisone: R' = H
Fludrocortisone acetate:
R' = CH₃CO-

Betamethasone

Prednisolone: R = H
Prednisolone acetate: R = CH₃CO-
Prednisolone t-butylacetate:
R = (CH₃)₃CCH₂CO-
Prednisolone sodium phosphate:
R = Na₂O₃P-

Dexamethasone: R = H
Dexamethasone 21-acetate:
R = CH₃CO-
Dexamethasone sodium phosphate:
R = Na₂O₃P-

Triamcinolone

Methylprednisolone: R = H
Methylprednisolone 21-acetate:
R = CH₃CO-
Methylprednisolone sodium succinate:
R = Na OOCCH₂CH₂CO-

Fig. 28.10. Systemic corticosteroids.

Table 28.3. Pharmacokinetics of Commonly Used Oral Adrenocorticoids

Adrenocorticoid	F (%)	Half-Life (hr)	Volume (L/kg)	Clearance (ml/min/70 kg)
Dexamethasone	78	3.0	0.8	260
Hydrocortisone	96	1.7	0.5	400
Methylprednisolone	90	2.3	1.2	430
Prednisone	80	3.6	1.0	250
Prednisolone	82	2.8	0.7	60
Triamcinolone	23	2.6	1.3	61

glucocorticoids between free and bound forms, and free glucocorticoid concentrations determine the drug's half-life. Glucocorticoids cross the placenta and may be distributed into milk.

The degree of systemic side effects is dose-dependent, related to the half-life of the drug, frequency administration, time of day when administered, and route of administration; i.e., the higher the plasma corticosteroid concentration and longer the half-life, the greater will be the systemic side effects (Table 28.3).

Regardless of the route of administration, all of the synthetic adrenocorticoids are excreted from the body in a manner similar to the endogenous adrenocorticoids (i.e., they are metabolized in the liver and excreted into the urine primarily as glucuronide conjugates, but also as sulfate conjugates) (26). In fact, hepatic oxidative metabolism rapidly converts many of the systemic and topical corticosteroids to inactive metabolites, and thus serves to protect patients from the HPA suppressive effects of these drugs on endogenous steroid production. The corticosteroids are metabolized in many tissues, including the liver, muscles, and red blood cells (18,19,27). However, the liver metabolizes them most rapidly. The fact that many of the endogenous corticosteroids are rapidly metabolized by the liver precludes their administration by the oral route. Catabolic products can be isolated from the urine and bile and can be formed in tissue preparations in vitro (28,29).

Specific Drugs

11-Desoxycorticosterone was the first naturally occurring corticoid to be synthesized. It was prepared, before its isolation from the adrenal cortex, by Steiger and Reichstein (30). Because of his synthesis of 11-desoxycorticosterone and other early work with corticoids, Reichstein later shared the Nobel Prize with Kendall, another chemist who was instrumental in carrying out early steroid syntheses, and with Hench, a rheumatologist who in 1929 discovered that cortisone is effective in the treatment of rheumatoid arthritis. Kendall's basic research ultimately led to the synthesis of cortisone from naturally occurring bile acids (31).

Cortisone, Hydrocortisone and Their Derivatives. After the synthesis of 11-desoxycorticosterone in 1937, all the corticoids were synthesized and their structures confirmed. The first synthesis of cortisone from methyl 3α-hydroxy-11-ketobisnorcholanate was reported by Sarett in 1946 (32). Earlier work of Kendall and co-workers involving its preparation from the methyl ester of desoxycholic acid was used in his research (33). Later, several chemists, including Sarett (34), Kendall, and Tishler, found ways to improve the yields and to decrease the labor involved in the multistep conversion of bile acids to cortisone acetate. In 1949 Merck sold limited quantities of this glucocorticoid to physicians at $200 per gram for treating rheumatoid arthritis. Subsequent improvements in the methods of synthesis reduced the price to $10 per gram by 1951. In 1955 Upjohn used an efficient process involving the synthesis of cortisone acetate from progesterone, the latter steroid being prepared from diosgenin. This further reduced the price to $3.50 per gram (31). In 1998 the cost was $11 per gram. Other pharmaceutical companies also began to sell cortisone synthesized from bile acids by a well-developed but lengthy procedure, and by 1958 sales of this and other corticoids reached $100 million per year in the United States (31).

Cortisone is administered orally or IM injection as its 21-acetate (cortisone acetate). Cortisone acetate or hydrocortisone are usually the corticosteroid of choice for replacement therapy in patients with adrenocortical insufficiency, because these drugs have both glucocorticoid and mineralocorticoid properties. Following oral administration cortisone acetate and hydrocortisone acetate are completely and rapidly deacetylated by first pass metabolism (35). However, much of the oral cortisone is inactivated by oxidative metabolism (Figure 28.9) before it can be converted to hydrocortisone in the liver. The pharmacokinetics for hydrocortisone acetate is indistinguishable from that of orally administered hydrocortisone. Oral hydrocortisone is completely absorbed with a bioavailability >95% and a half-life of 1–2 hours (21). The metabolism of hydrocortisone (Fig. 28.9) has been previously described. Cortisone acetate is slowly absorbed from IM injection sites over a period of 24–48 hours, and is reserved for patients who are unable to take the drug orally. The acetate ester derivative demonstrates increased stability and has a longer duration of action when administered by IM injection. Thus, smaller doses can be used. Similarly, hydrocortisone may be dispensed as its 21-acetate (hydrocortisone acetate), which is superior to cortisone acetate when injected intra-articularly. Systemic absorption of hydrocortisone acetate from intra-articular injection sites is usually complete within 24–48 hours. When administered intrarectally, hydrocortisone is poorly absorbed (36,37).

The usual oral or intramuscular dose for cortisone acetate is between 10 and 400 mg daily; usually 25 mg four times daily, administered orally. The usual intra-articular dose of hydrocortisone acetate is 25 mg; as a topical anti-inflammatory agent, the drug is used in 0.5 and 2.5% lotions, creams and ointments.

Other ester derivatives that are available include hydrocortisone cypionate [21-(3-cyclopentylpropionate) ester], hydrocortisone butyrate (17α-butyrate ester), hydrocortisone buteprate (17α-butyrate, 21-propionate esters), hydrocortisone valerate (17α-valerate ester), hydrocortisone sodium succinate (21-sodium succinate ester), and hydrocortisone sodium phosphate (the 21-sodium phosphate ester) (Fig. 28.10). The water-insoluble hydrocortisone cypionate is used orally in doses expressed in terms of hydrocortisone for slower absorption from the gastrointestinal tract. The extremely water-soluble 21-sodium succinate and 21-sodium phosphate esters are used for intravenous or intramuscular injection in the management of emergency conditions that can be treated with anti-inflammatory steroids. The phosphate ester is completely and rapidly metabolized by phosphatases, with a half-life of less than 5 minutes (38). Peak hydrocortisone levels are reached in about 10 minutes. The sodium succinate ester is slowly and incompletely hydrolyzed and peak hydrocortisone levels attained in 30–45 minutes (38). The usual intramuscular dosage ranges from 100–500 mg daily. Hydrocortisone butyrate, hydrocortisone buteprate, and hydrocortisone valerate are used topically.

After the introduction of cortisone (1948) and later hydrocortisone (1951) for the treatment of rheumatoid arthritis, many investigators began to search for superior agents having fewer side effects. When these drugs are used in doses necessary to suppress symptoms of rheumatoid arthritis, they also affect other metabolic processes. Side effects such as excessive sodium retention and potassium excretion, negative nitrogen balance, increased gastric acidity, edema, and psychosis are exaggerated manifestations of the normal metabolic functions of the hormones.

It was hoped that a compound with high glucocorticoid and low mineralocorticoid activity could be synthesized. Because it was recognized early that a carbonyl group at C3, a double bond between carbons 4 and 5, an oxygen (C=O or β-OH) at carbon 11, and a β-ketol side chain at position 17 are necessary for superior glucocorticoid activity, investigators began to synthesize analogs containing these functional groups. Additional groups were inserted into other positions of the basic steroid structure with the expectation that these new substituents might modify the glucocorticoid and mineralocorticoid activities of the parent drugs.

The first potent analogs discovered, however, did not result from a concentrated effort to find a better drug, but rather from basic chemical research concerned with the preparation of hydrocortisone from 11-epicortisol (11α hydrocortisone).

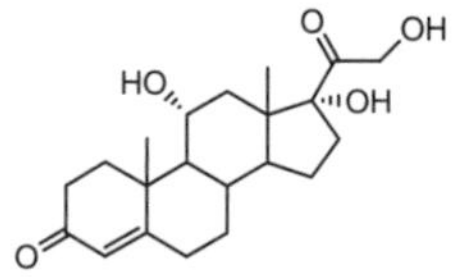

11-Epicortisol

Fludrocortisone. A 9α-bromo analog that had one-third the glucocorticoid activity of cortisone acetate was prepared in these investigations (39). Other halogens were introduced into the 9α-position, and it was soon observed that glucocorticoid activity is inversely proportional to the size of the halogen at carbon 9. The 9α-fluoro analog (fludrocortisone) is approximately 11 times more potent than cortisone acetate (Fig. 28.10). Fludrocortisone is orally administered as its 21-acetate derivative. When tested clinically in patients with rheumatoid arthritis, it was found to be effective at about one-tenth the dose of cortisone acetate. Although glucocorticoid activity is increased 11-fold by insertion of the 9α-fluoro-substituent, mineralocorticoid activity is increased 300–800 times (25,41). Because of its intense sodium-retaining activity, fludrocortisone is contraindicated in all conditions except those which require a high degree of mineralocorticoid activity because it leads to edema. Fludrocortisone acetate is used orally for mineralocorticoid replacement therapy in patients with adrenocortical insufficiency, such as Addison's disease. This drug, introduced in 1954, helped to provide the impetus for the synthesis and biologic evaluation of newer halogenated analogs.

Prednisone, Prednisolone and its Derivatives. One year after the introduction of fludrocortisone, the Δ-corticoids were brought forth into clinical medicine. Investigators at Schering observed that the 1-dehydro derivatives of cortisone and hydrocortisone, namely prednisone and prednisolone, are more potent anti-rheumatic and anti-allergenic agents than hydrocortisone and produced fewer undesirable side effects. These compounds are known as Δ¹-corticoids because they contain an additional double bond between positions 1 and 2 (Fig. 28.10).

The Δ¹-corticoids, which can be prepared by microbial dehydrogenation of cortisone or hydrocortisone with Corynebacterium simplex (42) and by several synthetic methods (31), represent the first chemical innovation leading to the creation of a modified compound that could be prescribed for rheumatoid arthritis. One high-yield route involves oxidation of 5α-pregnane or 5β-pregnane precursors that have appropriate oxygen substitutions with selenium dioxide (43,44).

Both prednisone and prednisolone were found to have adrenocortical activity (measured by eosinopenic response, liver glycogen decomposition, and thymus involution in adrenalectomized mice). In these tests, prednisone and prednisolone were found to be three or four times more potent than cortisone or hydrocortisone (Table 28.2). Antiphlogistic strengths in human subjects were similarly augmented, but their electrolyte activities were not proportionately increased.

The increased potency reflects the effect in the change in geometry for ring A caused by the introduction of the additional C1=C2 function on glucocorticoid receptor affinity and altered pharmacokinetics (primarily metabolism). The 5β-function inhibits reduction of ring A to Δ¹-metabolites. Although the remaining portions of the steroid structure are essentially unchanged (except for less easily visualized molecular perturbations), the conformation of ring A changes from a chair, as in 5α-pregnan-3-one, to a half-chair (pregn-4-en-3-one) and to a flattened boat (pregna-1,4-dien-3-one) upon introduction of unsaturation (Fig. 28.11). The order of glucocorticoid receptor affinity is dexamethasone (10×) > triamcinolone (5×) > methylprednisolone (4×) > prednisolone (2×) > hydrocortisone (1) (45).

When orally administered, prednisone and prednisolone are almost completely absorbed with a bioavailability of >80% (Table 28.3) (46,47a). As with the relationship between cortisone and hydrocortisone, prednisone and prednisolone are interconvertible by 11β-hydroxysteroid dehydrogenase in the liver. For all practical purposes, prednisone and prednisolone are equally potent and may be used interchangeably. When prednisone or prednisolone is used in the treatment of rheumatoid arthritis, smaller doses are required than for hydrocortisone; the usual dose is 5 mg two to four times a day. Prednisolone is metabolized into a number of hydrophilic and less active metabolites as shown in Figure 28.12, except there is no reduction of ring A as with hydrocortisone. The major metabolites (6β- and 16β-hydroxy) are primarily ex-

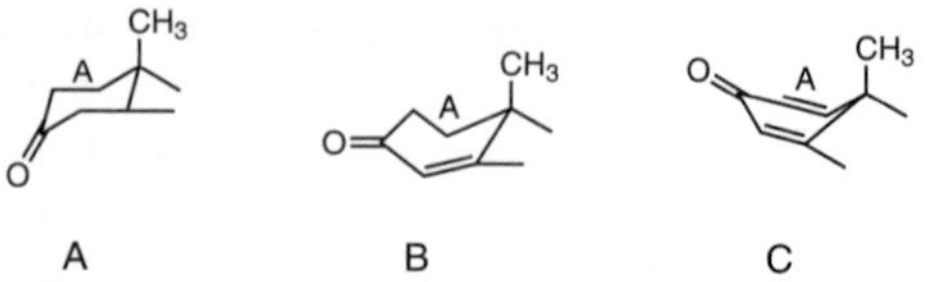

Fig. 28.11. Ring A conformations for 5α-pregnan-3-one **(A)**, for pregn-4-en-3-one **(B)**, and for pregna-1,4-dien-3-one **(C)**.

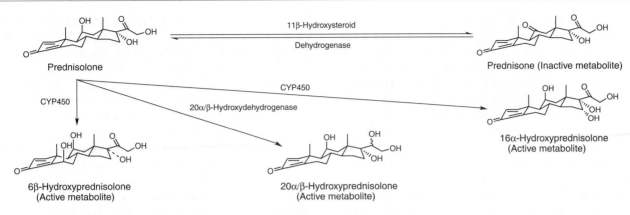

Fig. 28.12. Major routes of metabolism for prednisolone.

creted as glucuronide conjugates in the urine. Prednisolone acetate is available in suspension and ointment forms for use externally. As with hydrocortisone, several other 21-esters of prednisolone are available. Prednisolone tert-butylacetate (3,3-dimethylbutyrate) is used in suspension form and by injection for the same reasons the 21-ester derivatives of hydrocortisone are employed. The butylacetate ester, which is suitable only for use by IM or intra-articular injection, has a long duration of action owing to poor water solubility and a slow rate of hydrolysis. The drug is administered in doses of 4–20 mg.

Prednisolone sodium phosphate is the water-soluble sodium salt of the 21-phosphate ester having a half-life of < 5 minutes because of rapid hydrolysis by phosphatases (48). Peak plasma levels for prednisolone are attained in about 10 minutes following its administration by injection (usual dose of 20 mg intravenously or intramuscularly). Topically, 1 or 2 drops of a 0.5% solution may be used four to six times daily for its anti-inflammatory action in the eye.

When doses of equivalent antirheumatic potency are given to patients not treated with steroids, the Δ^1-corticoids promote the same pattern of initial improvement as hydrocortisone. Statistical results of the improvement status during the first few months of therapy have been similar with prednisolone, prednisone, and hydrocortisone. The results of longer-term therapy have been significantly better with the modified compounds. Studies indicate that the Δ^1-corticoids may be used continuously in patients with rheumatoid arthritis without undue gastrointestinal hazard. Although the Δ^1-corticoids are considered not to have significant mineralocorticoid activity, hypokalemia and sodium and fluid retention may occur, depending upon the dosage, duration of use.

Methylprednisolone. Between 1953 and 1962, many derivatives of the Δ^1-corticoids and the halogen-containing analogs (especially fluorinated compounds) were synthesized, and some became useful clinical agents. Studies with methylcorticoids revealed 2α-methyl derivatives to be inactive, whereas the 2α-methyl-9α-fluoro analogs had potent mineralocorticoid activity. Methylprednisolone (6α-methyl analog of prednisolone) was synthesized in 1956 and introduced into clinical medicine (Fig. 28.10). Methylprednisolone is extensively metabolized with about 10% recovered unchanged in urine (47b). The metabolic pathways include reduction of C20 ketone, oxidation of 17β-ketol group to C21-COOH and C20-COOH, and 6β-hydroxylation. These compounds potentiated glucocorticoid activity with negligible salt retention for short term therapy (Table 28.1) (49).

In human subjects, its metabolic effects did not differ appreciably from those of prednisolone. Its activities with respect to nitrogen excretion, ACTH suppression, and reduction of circulating eosinophils were similar to those of prednisolone. The sodium retention and potassium loss were slightly less than with prednisolone (50). Methylprednisolone dosage ranges from 2–60 mg. Generally, 4 mg are administered four times daily in the treatment of rheumatoid arthritis.

Methylprednisolone is administered intravenously as its water-soluble sodium salt of the 21-succinate ester. The succinate ester is slowly and incompletely hydrolyzed; peak plasma levels for methylprednisolone is attained in about 30–60 minutes following its IV administration and approximately 15% of its IV dose is recovered unchanged in the urine (47,51a).

Triamcinolone. A natural extension of Δ^1-corticoid research involved synthesis and examination of compounds containing both a 9α-fluoro group and a double bond between positions 1 and 2. Triamcinolone introduced in 1958, combines the structural features of a Δ^1-corticoid and 9α-fluoro corticoid (Fig. 28.10). As mentioned previously, the 9α-fluoro group increases the anti-inflammatory potency, but it also markedly increases the mineralocorticoid potency. This is undesirable if the drug is to be used internally for the treatment of rheumatoid arthritis.

The original interest in synthesizing 16α-hydroxycorticosteroids stemmed from their isolation from the urine of a boy with an adrenal tumor. The desire of chemists was to synthesize these corticoids, with the hope that such analogs might have potent biologic activity furthered their development (52–54). Therefore, by inserting a 16α-hydroxy group into 9α-fluoroprednisolone resulted in triamcinolone with glucocorticoid activity equivalent to prednisolone but with decreased mineralocorticoid activity. In fact, 16α-hydroxy analogs of natural corticoids retain glucocorticoid activity and have a considerably reduced mineralocorticoid activity. The lower than expected oral anti-inflammatory potency for triamcinolone (Table 28.1) has been attributed to its low oral bioavailability (Table 28.3) due in part to increased hydrophilicity from the 16α-hydroxy group and first pass metabolism primarily to its 6β-hydroxy metabolite. These glucocorticoids may actually cause sodium excretion rather than sodium retention. Triamcinolone diacetate (17,21-diacetate) and its hexacetonide [16α, 17α-methylenedioxy-21-(3,3-dimethylbutyrate)] esters are administered IM or intra-articularly for a prolonged release of triamcinolone. Triamcinolone diacetate has a duration of action depending upon its route of administration from 1–8 weeks and triamcinolone hexacetonide, a duration of action of 3–4 weeks (55,56).

On a weight-for-weight basis, the antirheumatic potency of triamcinolone is greater than that of prednisolone (about 20%) and about the same as that of methylprednisolone. Initial improvement following administration of triamcinolone is similar to that noted with other compounds. Reports in the literature, however, indicate that the percentage of patients maintained satisfactorily for long periods has been distinctly smaller than with prednisolone.

Even though triamcinolone has an apparent decreased tendency to cause salt and water retention and edema and may induce sodium and water diuresis, it causes other unwanted side effects, including anorexia, weight loss, muscle weakness, leg cramps, nausea, dizziness, and a general toxic feeling (57). Intramuscular triamcinolone is reportedly effective and safe in the treatment of dermatoses, and in combination with folic acid antagonists, it is effective in the treatment of psoriasis (58,59).

Dexamethasone. Research with 16-methyl substituted corticoids was initiated in part because investigators hoped to stabilize the 17β-ketol side chain to metabolism in vivo and improve bioavailability (Fig. 28.10). These studies led to the development of dexamethasone (9-fluoro-16α-methyl analog), which was introduced for clinical trial. A 16α-methyl group increases the stability of the steroid to metabolism in human plasma in vitro (60,61). Unlike 16α-hydroxylation, a methyl group increases the anti-inflammatory activity by increasing lipophilicity and consequently receptor affinity. Like the 16α-hydroxyl group, the methyl group appears to reduce markedly the salt-retaining properties of the corticosteroid (Table 28.1). The data from these investigations were published in 1958 (62–65). The activity of dexamethasone, as measured by glycogen deposition, is 20 times greater than that of hydrocortisone. Clinical data indicate that dexamethasone has 5–7 times the antirheumatic potency of prednisolone. It is roughly 30 times more potent than hydrocortisone. Its pharmacokinetics are presented in Table 28.3. Routes of metabolism for dexamethasone are similar to those for prednisolone with its primary 6β-hydroxy metabolite being recovered in urine (66). Dexamethasone sodium phosphate is the water-soluble

sodium salt of the 21-phosphate ester having a IV half-life of <10 minutes because of rapid hydrolysis by plasma phosphatases (67). Peak plasma levels for dexamethasone are usually attained in about 10–20 minutes following its IV administered dose. A similar reaction occurs when the phosphate ester is applied topically or by inhalation.

In practical management, 0.75 mg of dexamethasone promotes a therapeutic response equivalent to that from 4 mg of triamcinolone or methylprednisolone, 5 mg of prednisolone, and 20 mg of hydrocortisone (Table 28.1). Clinical investigations with small groups of patients indicate that dexamethasone could control patients who did not respond well to prednisolone. Over long periods, the improved status of some patients deteriorated.

In summarizing the biologic properties of this drug, it seems clear that, with doses of corresponding antirheumatic strength, this steroid has approximately the same tendency as prednisolone to produce facial mooning, acne, and nervous excitation. Peripheral edema is uncommon (7%) and mild. The more common and most objectionable side effects are excessive appetite and weight gain, abdominal bloating, and distention. The frequency and severity of these symptoms vary with the dose (1 mg maximum for females and 1.5 mg maximum for males). The longer biologic half-life for dexamethasone significantly increases the potential for glucocorticoid-induced adrenal insufficiency (see Adverse Effects).

The striking increase in potency does not confer a general therapeutic index on dexamethasone that is higher than that of prednisolone. Again, this drug is probably best employed as a special-purpose corticoid for short term use. It may be useful when other steroids are no longer effective or when increased appetite and weight gain are desirable (68,69–74). Its efficacy may be increased when it is used in combination with cyproheptadine as an antiallergenic, antipyretic, and anti-inflammatory agent (62,63).

Betamethasone. Shortly after the introduction of dexamethasone, betamethasone, which differs from dexamethasone only in configuration of the 16-methyl group (Fig. 28.10), was made available for the treatment of rheumatic diseases and dermatologic disorders. This analog, which contains a 16β-methyl group, is as effective as dexamethasone or perhaps slightly more active (Table 28.1). Although this drug has been reported to be less toxic than other corticosteroids, some clinical investigators suggest it is best used for short-term therapy. Toxic side effects, such as increased appetite, weight gain and facial mooning, occur with prolonged use. Generally, a 0.5-mg tablet of betamethasone is equivalent to a 5.0-mg tablet of prednisolone, and except for isolated instances, this drug is apparently on a par with dexamethasone (75,76).

Discontinued Oral Glucocorticoids. Paramethasone acetate (formerly administered as Haldrone) synthesized in 1960, retains the 16α-methyl group of dexamethasone except that the 9α-fluoro substituent has been moved to the 6α position. It was thought that this manipulation would reduce the electrolyte loss associated with dexamethasone. Reports in the literature indicate that paramethasone causes a slight loss of sodium and chloride with little or no loss of potassium (with doses as large as 15 mg). However, an analysis of continuous therapy over 9 months showed that the therapeutic efficacy of paramethasone did not differ greatly from that of fluprednisolone (77).

Fluprednisolone (6α-fluoro) is the 16-desmethyl analog of paramethasone. Its activity is similar to that of paramethasone, and it has about 2 1/2 times the antirheumatic potency of prednisolone. With doses of 2–7 mg, evidence of salt and water retention has not been noted. The therapeutic index, however, is probably the same or only a little greater than that for prednisolone, and appears on a short-term basis that a 6α-fluoro group does not deleteriously affect the activity of prednisolone (50,78).

Topical Glucocorticoids

Topically applied glucocorticoids are also capable of being systemically absorbed, although to a much smaller extent. The extent of absorption of topical adrenocorticoids is determined by several factors, including the type of cream or ointment, the condition of the skin to which it is being applied, and the use of occlusive dressings. Previous studies with halobetasol propionate showed that about 6% of the drug was systemically absorbed after topical application. Although this is a small fraction of the dose, the very high potency of halobetasol propionate contributed to its ability to cause mild adrenal suppression in some patients. The relative potency of the topical glucocorticoids is commonly determined using topical vasoconstriction assays, and is dependent on the intrinsic activity of the drug, its concentration in the formulation, and the vehicle in which it is applied (Table 28.4).

Table 28.4. Potency Ranking for Topical Corticosteroids

Drug Name	Dosage Form	Strength (%)
I. Very High Potency		
Augmented Betamethasone dipropionate	ointment	0.05
Clobetasol propionate	cream, ointment	0.05
Diflorasone diacetate	ointment	0.05
Halobetasol propionate	cream, ointment	0.05
II. High Potency		
Amcinonide	cream, ointment, lotion	0.1
Augmented Betamethasone dipropionate	cream	0.05
Betamethasone dipropionate	cream, ointment	0.05
Betamethasone valerate	ointment	0.1
Desoximetasone	cream, ointment, gel	0.05–0.25
Diflorasone diacetate	cream, ointment	0.05
Fluocinolone acetonide	cream	0.2
Fluocinonide	cream, ointment, gel	0.05
Halcinonide	cream, ointment	0.1
Triamcinolone acetonide	cream, ointment	0.5
III. Medium Potency		
Betamethasone benzoate	cream, gel, lotion	0.025
Betamethasone dipropionate	lotion	0.05
Betamethasone valerate	cream	0.1
Clocortolone pivalate	cream	0.1
Desoximetasone	cream	0.05
Fluocinolone acetonide	cream, ointment, topical solution	0.025–0.2
Flurandrenolide	cream, ointment, lotion	0.025–0.05
	tape	4 mcg/cm
Fluticasone propionate	cream, ointment	0.005–0.05
Hydrocortisone butyrate	cream, ointment	0.1
Hydrocortisone valerate	cream, ointment	0.2
Mometasone fluroate	cream, ointment, lotion	0.1
Triamcinolone acetonide	cream, ointment, lotion	0.025–0.1
IV. Low Potency		
Alclometasone dipropionate	cream, ointment	0.05
Desonide	cream	0.5
Dexamethasone	gel, topical aerosol	0.01–0.04
Dexamethasone sodium phosphate	cream	0.1
Fluocinolone acetonide	cream, topical solution	0.025–0.2
Hydrocortisone	cream, ointment, lotion topical aerosol solution, topical solution	0.25–2.5
Hydrocortizone acetate	cream, ointment, lotion topical aerosol foam	0.5–1
Prednicarbate	cream	0.1

The relative potency is based on the drug concentration, type of vehicle used, and the vasoconstrictor assay as a measure of topical anti-inflammatory activity.

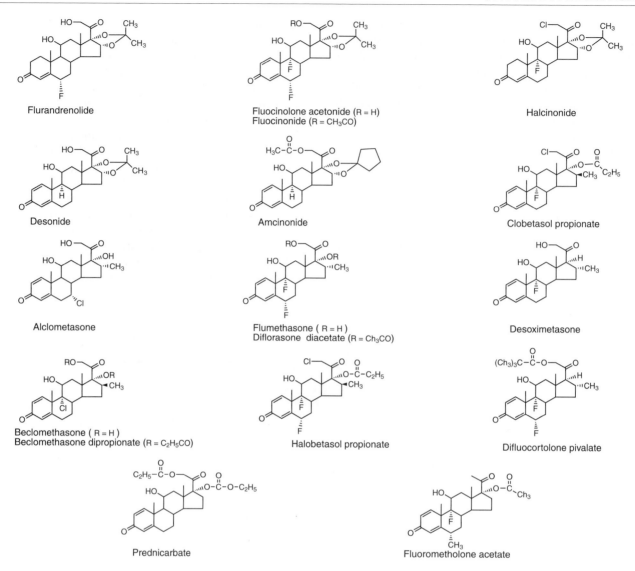

Fig. 28.13. Topical corticosteroids.

Once absorbed through the skin, topical corticosteroids are handled through metabolic pathways similar to the systemically administered corticosteroids. They are metabolized, primarily in the liver, and are then excreted into the urine or in the bile (79). The fact that circulating levels of the topical glucocorticoids are often well below the level of detection doesn't reduce the risk for potential adverse effects from systemic exposure of topical corticosteroids. The structures for the glucocorticoids applied topically are shown in Figure 28.13, and their relative potencies in Table 28.4. Topical dermatological products with a low potency ranking have a modest anti-inflammatory effect and are safest for chronic application; those products with a medium potency ranking are used in moderate inflammatory dermatoses of limited duration; high potency preparations are used in more severe inflammatory dermatoses but only for a short treatment duration; very high potency products are used primarily as an alternative to systemic corticosteroid therapy when local areas are involved and used for only a short duration of therapy and on small surface areas.

Triamcinolone to be used topically is generally dispensed as its more potent and lipophilic acetonide, a $16\alpha,17\alpha$-methylenedioxy cyclic ketal or isopropylidene derivative (Fig. 28.14) (to be discussed in more detail in the section on Inhaled and Intranasal Glucocorticoids). It is effective in the treatment of psoriasis and other corticoid-sensitive dermatologic conditions. Topically, triamcinolone acetonide is a more potent derivative of triamcinolone and is about 8 times more active than prednisolone. The side effects of the drug, however, have occurred with sufficient frequency to discourage its routine use for rheumatoid patients requiring steroid therapy. The drug may be employed advantageously as a special-purpose steroid in instances in which salt and water retention (due to other corticoids, hypertension, or cardiac compensation) or excessive appetite and weight gain are problems in management.

Newer synthetic glucocorticoids have incorporated chlorine atoms onto the steroid molecule as fluorine substitutes. Beclomethasone, a 9α-chloro analog of betamethasone, is a potent glucocorticoid with about 1/2 the potency of its fluoro analog. It is used topically as its dipropionate derivative in inhalation aerosol therapy for asthma and rhinitis (see section for inhaled and intranasal glucocorticoids) but not for treatment of steroid-responsive dermatoses (80). The topical anti-inflammatory potency for beclomethasone dipropionate is about 5000 times greater than hydrocortisone; 500 times greater than betamethasone, or dexamethasone; and about 5 times greater than fluocinolone acetonide or triamcinolone acetonide, as measured by vasoconstrictor assay. Another potent topical glucocorticoid that contains a 7α-chloro group is alclometasone (81).

Additional mono and difluorinated analogs for topical application include fluorometholone (6α-methyl-9α-fluoro) (ophthalmic use), flurandrenolide (6α-fluoro, 16α,17α-acetonide), fluocinolone acetonide (a 6α,9α-difluoro-16α,17α-acetonide) and fluocinonide (21-acetate ester of fluocinolone acetonide) (Fig. 28.13). These compounds are classified as high to medium potent anti-inflammatory agents depending upon concentration and vehicle used (Table 28.4). The acetonides (ketals) derivatives at the 16,17-position enhance lipophilicity to provide potent topical anti-inflammatory agents (Table 28.4).

Psoriasis is one of the few inflammatory dermatoses that has not responded to routine topical steroid therapy, but these more potent steroids appear to work if a special occlusive dressing is used. In this technique, a thin layer of cream or ointment containing flurandrenolide is applied to the individual patch of psoriasis. The area is then covered with plastic food wrap or a similar pliable plastic film.

Clinical investigations generally show flurandrenolide (0.05%) to be more effective than 1% hydrocortisone acetate and about the same in activity as 0.1% triamcinolone acetonide. Some investigators believe its greater activity is due to an increased biologic half-life. In other words, these analogs are not metabolized as readily. Fluocinolone acetonide has about the same anti-inflammatory activity as fluorometholone.

Clobetasol propionate, halcinonide, halobetasol propionate, and mometasone furoate are examples of 21-chlorocorticoids, where the 21-chloro group replaces the 21-hydroxyl group (82–85). (Figs. 28.13 and 28.14). Clobetasol propionate, the 21-chloro analog of betamethasone 17-propionate, is about eight times more active as topical anti-inflammatory agent than betamethasone 17α-valerate, the standard of comparison for topical vasoconstrictor/anti-inflammatory activity. Mometasone furoate, a 9α, 21-dichloro derivative (to be discussed in more detail in the section on Inhaled and Intranasal Glucocorticoids), is also about eight times more active than betamethasone 17α-valerate as a topical anti-inflammatory agent. Thus, substitution of a chlorine (or a fluorine) atom for the 21-hydroxyl group on the glucocorticoids greatly enhances topical anti-inflammatory activity (83). Clobetasol propionate and halobetasol propionate are classified as very high potency topical corticosteroid preparations currently available (Table 28.4). HPA suppression has occurred following the topical application of 2 g of the 0.05% clobetasol propionate oint-

ment or cream (1 mg of clobetasol propionate total) daily. Because of its high potency and potential for causing adverse systemic effects during topical therapy, the usual dosage for very high potency topical steroids should not be exceeded. Fluticasone propionate is similar to the 21-chloro steroids, except that it has a 17α-fluoromethylcarbothioate group instead of the 17-ketol group derivative (to be discussed in more detail in the section on Inhaled and Intranasal Glucocorticoids) (Fig. 28.14). Although mometasone furoate and fluticasone propionate are very lipophilic and have the highest binding affinity for the glucocorticoid receptor (see section on Inhaled and Intranasal Glucocorticoids) when compared to triamcinolone acetonide and dexamethasone, their topical potency are listed as medium is due in part to their insolubility and poor dissolution into inflamed tissue.

Several nonfluorinated analogs of triamcinolone acetonide with the potency enhancing cyclic ketal moiety are marketed, suggesting that halogens are not always necessary for topical activity. These nonfluorinated cyclic ketals include desonide and amcinonide (Fig. 28.13). Amcinonide's potency is greatly enhanced by the more lipophilic cyclopentanone ketal and 21-acetate. A recent addition to the nonhalogenated prednisolone derivatives is prednicarbate, a 17,21-diester (17α-ethylcarbonate-21-propionate) derivative of prednisolone (Fig. 28.13), which is used for the local treatment of corticoid-sensitive skin diseases (87). Any prednicarbate that is absorbed systemically is readily metabolized by hydrolysis of the 21-ester to its primary and pharmacologically active metabolite, prednisolone-17-ethylcarbonate. This metabolite has a half-life of about 1–2 hours and is further metabolized by the liver to prednisolone. In vitro binding studies with the glucocorticoid receptor suggest that the ethyl carbonate metabolite has a receptor binding affinity comparable to that of dexamethasone. The low systemic bioavailability for prednicarbate after dermal application has been attributed to its metabolism to less active prednisolone which may be a factor for prednicarbate's low systemic side effects.

Inhaled and Intranasal Glucocorticoids
Overview

It is generally accepted that the anti-inflammatory effect of glucocorticosteroids cannot be separated from their adverse effects at the receptor level. Therefore, pulmonary and nasal pharmacokinetics become important determinants for the potential of an inhaled or nasally applied corticosteroid to cause systemic effects, because the lung and nasal tissue provide an enormous surface area from which drug absorption can occur into the systemic circulation (88,89). The main areas of concern with regard to drug-induced systemic effects include HPA axis suppression, change in bone mineral density and growth retardation in children, cataracts and glaucoma. The degree of systemic side effects is dose-dependent, related to the half-life of the drug, frequency of administration, time of day when administered, and route of administration; i.e., the higher the plasma corticosteroid concentration and longer the half-life, the greater will be the systemic side effects (90). Thus, the search is to develop inhaled/intranasal corticosteroids with the following desirable pharmacokinetic qualities: they would exhibit fast systemic clearance following gastrointestinal absorption (high degree of first pass intestinal/hepatic metabolism); a short half-life; lack of active metabolites; and high affinity for the corticosteroid receptor. These qualities determine the proportion of the drug that reaches the target cells as well as the fraction of the dose that reaches the systemic circulation to produce side effects.

Modification of the pharmacokinetics through structural alterations has provided several new steroids with a better glucocorticoid receptor affinity and therapeutic index and lower bioavailability than the older drugs (Fig. 28.14). The new inhaled/intranasal glucocorticosteroids like mometasone furoate, budesonide and fluticasone propionate are more lipophilic than those used in oral and systemic therapy and have greater affinity for the glucocorticoid receptor than does dexamethasone as a consequence of their greater lipophilicity (45). Several of the topical corticosteroids such as mometasone furoate, beclomethasone dipropionate, triamcinolone acetonide and flunisolide, were reintroduced as inhalation and intranasal dosage forms for treatment of respiratory diseases, e.g., asthma or rhinitis. Inhaled budesonide and flunisolide are readily absorbed from the airway mucosa into the blood and are rapidly biotransformed in the liver into inactive metabolites. Mometasone furoate and fluticasone propionate are very potent anti-inflammatory steroids with an oral bioavailability of less than 1%. Obviously, the risk of systemic side effects for these newer corticosteroids is greatly reduced when compared with the older glucocorticosteroids, e.g. dexamethasone. Beclomethasone dipropionate was discovered to be a pro-drug, and this discovery lead to the re-examination of other 17α-monoesters

as the active form of the corticosteroid esters. The absorption of budesonide, fluticasone propionate and beclomethasone dipropionate into the airway tissue was 25–130 times greater than that for dexamethasone and hydrocortisone (90). The glucocorticoid receptor affinity and the pharmacokinetic properties for the inhaled and intranasal corticosteroids are listed in Table 28.5.

It is generally recognized that when administered by oral inhalation, 10–30% of a dose of the corticosteroid is deposited in the respiratory tract depending upon type of inhaler (metered dose inhaler, MDI; or dry powder inhaler, DPI) and spacer used (91,92). The remainder of the dose is primarily deposited in the mouth and throat, to be swallowed into the GI tract where the drug may be absorbed, metabolized and eliminated unchanged in the feces. Thus, systemic bioavailability of the inhaled/intranasal steroids is determined by the fraction of the dose absorbed from the lungs/nasal mucosa and the GI tract into systemic circulation and the degree of first-pass metabolism. Although these corticosteroids are very lipid soluble they display variable degrees of absorption from respiratory and gastrointestinal tissues in part due to dissolution problems. When systemically absorbed, they are capable of suppressing the HPA and adrenal function with high and chronic dosing regimens (92,93). Although as much as 40% of the dose for the high potency adrenocorticoids, flunisolide, mometasone furoate or fluticasone propionate is absorbed into airway and nasal tissues during oral inhalation, the remainder of the drug is swallowed to undergo extensive first-pass metabolism in the liver to essentially inactive metabolites with no apparent suppression effects on adrenal function with long-term therapy.

Lipophilicity can positively or negatively alter the pharmacokinetic and pharmacodynamic actions of the inhaled/intranasal steroids (94). The lipophilic substituents attached to the corticosteroid nucleus may improve receptor affinity (Table 28.5), or they can affect pharmacokinetic properties such as absorption, protein and tissue binding, distribution and excretion. The inhaled/intranasal corticosteroids are inhaled as microcrystals, and need sufficient water solubility in order to be dissolved in the nasal or lung epithelial tissue for local anti-inflammatory activity to occur. However, lipophilicity can delay their rate of dissolution into these tissues, which may be advantageous by prolonging their retention within these tissues affecting their onset and duration of action, or a disadvantage by facilitating their transport away from these tissues by mucociliary clearance before full dissolution can occur. The systemic steroids prednisolone and hydrocortisone are less effective as inhaled/intranasal steroids because of their higher water solubility and lower lipophilicity. For the inhaled/intranasal steroids, there is a sharp drop in water solubility when the lipophilicity is ≥log P 4.5 (P = 30,000), which is the case for fluticasone propionate, mometasone furoate and BDP. High lipophilicity correlates well with low oral bioavailability (Table 28.5).

The use of dexamethasone sodium phosphate inhalation aerosol is not recommended because of the potential for ex-

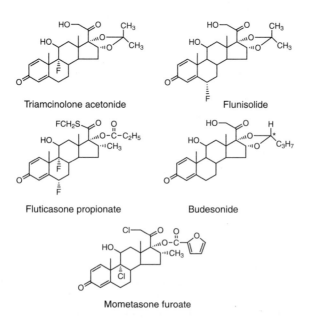

Triamcinolone acetonide

Flunisolide

Fluticasone propionate

Budesonide

Mometasone furoate

Fig. 28.14. Inhaled and intranasal corticosteroids.

Table 28.5. Pharmacokinetics of Inhaled and Intranasal Corticosteroids*

Parameters	Beclomethasone Dipropionate	Budesonide	Flunisolide[4]	Triamcinolone Acetonide	Fluticasone Propionate	Mometasone Furoate[4]
Receptor binding affinity[1]	0.4 13.5[2]	9.4 22R 11.2 22S 4.2	1.8	3.6	18	25–27
Relative Lipophilicity[7]	79432 25120 BMP	3980	2512	2512	31622	50120[8]
Pulmonary bioavailability	~20%[3]	~39%	40%	25%[5]	~30% (aerosol)	<1% (aerosol)
Nasal bioavailability	~20%[3]	<20%	50%	25%[5]	13–16% (powder)	not detectable (powder)
Oral bioavailability (systemic)	15–20%	~10%, oral	6–10%	23%	<2%	<1%
Protein binding	87% (transcortin & albumin)	85 to 90% (albumin)	Moderate (transcortin & albumin)	68%[5] (albumin)	91% (albumin)	90%
Half-life	30 min IV 10 min inhaled 6.5 h BMP IV 2–7 h BMP inhaled	2–3 hr IV	1–2 hr IV	1–2 hr IV 1–7 hr nasal 3.1 hr solution	~7.8 hr IV ~14 hr inhaled	4–6 h IV aerosol (not detectable) inhaled (not detectable)
Metabolism	Lung and liver esterase, liver (CYP3A4) first pass	Liver (CYP3A) first pass	Liver first pass	Liver first pass	liver (CYP3A4) first pass	Liver
Onset of Action	3–7 d	2–3 d	3–7 d	4–7 d	2–3 d	7 h
Excretion	Feces, urine 12–15%	Urine ~60% Feces ~30%	Renal ~50% Feces ~40%	urine ~40% feces ~60%	80–90% feces <5% urine	50–90% feces 6–10% urine

*Data from McEvoy GK ed. AHFS 2001 Drug Information, Bethesda, MD American Society of Health-System Pharmacists 2001.
[1]Binding affinity to human glucocorticoid receptors in vitro; relative to dexamethasone. Kelly HW. J Allergy Clin Immunol 1998;102:S36–51.
[2]Beclomethasone diproprionate is converted in the liver to the more active beclomethasone monopropionate.
[3]Estimated for inhaled beclomethasone aerosol.
[4]Nasarel and Nasalide are not bioequivalent. Total absorption of Nasarel was 25% less and the peak plasma concentration was 30% lower than Nasalide. The clinical significance of this is likely to be small because clinical efficacy is dependent on local effects on the nasal mucosa.
[5]Data from oral inhalation administration.
[6]Data from oral dose.
[7]Measured from RP-HPLC technique; Log k' data from Brattsand R Eur. Respir Rev 1997; 7: 356–361., was converted to antilogs. k' for water = 1. Hydrocortisone = 794; prednisolone = 316; dexamethasone = 400.
[8]Calculated log P for mometasone furoate 4.7.

tensive systemic absorption and the long metabolic half-life for dexamethasone after absorption resulting in an increased risk of adverse effects with usual inhalation doses (25). Following the oral inhalation of dexamethasone sodium phosphate, a cumulative dose of 1200 mcg per day will result in the systemic absorption of 400–600 mcg of dexamethasone, which is sufficient to cause HPA suppression. Dexamethasone sodium phosphate nasal aerosol delivers 100 mcg per metered spray. The total daily adult nasal dose is 1200 mcg.

Specific Drugs

Triamcinolone Acetonide. Triamcinolone acetonide is frequently used by inhalation for the treatment of lung diseases, e.g., asthma. After inhalation, triamcinolone acetonide can become systemically available when the inhaled formulation is swallowed and absorbed unchanged from the GI tract, causing undesirable systemic effects (95–97). Triamcinolone acetonide that is swallowed is metabolized to 6β-hydroxytriamcinolone acetonide, 21-carboxytriamcinolone acetonide, and 21-carboxy-6β-hydroxytriamcinolone acetonide, all of which are more hydrophilic than their parent drug. Only about 1% of the dose was recovered from the urine as triamcinolone

acetonide (97). Triamcinolone is not a major metabolite of triamcinolone acetonide in humans suggesting that acetonide is resistant to hydrolytic cleavage. Triamcinolone acetonide is about 8 times more potent than prednisolone.

Triamcinolone acetonide inhalation aerosol for pulmonary delivery is a microcrystalline suspension in a chlorofluorocarbon propellant that delivers 200 mcg per metered spray, which is equivalent to 100 mcg delivered at the mouthpiece. The total daily adult nasal dose for triamcinolone acetonide is 1.6 mg. Triamcinolone acetonide nasal aerosol is a microcrystalline suspension in a chlorofluorocarbon propellant that delivers 55 mcg per metered spray. The total daily dose for triamcinolone acetonide is 440 mcg.

Beclomethasone 17,21-dipropionate. Beclomethasone dipropionate (BDP) is primarily utilized as an inhalation aerosol therapy for asthma and rhinitis (80). A breakthrough in the discovery of new inhalation corticosteroids with reduced risks from systemic absorption was that the 17α-monopropionate ester of beclomethasone (17-BMP) was more active than BDP and 21-monopropionate (21-BMP) esters (98). Thus, BDP is a prodrug which is rapidly metabolized by esterases in the lung, liver and other tissues to its more active metabolite, 17-BMP, which has 30 times greater affinity for the glucocorticoid receptor than does BDP and about 14 times dexamethasone (Table 28.5) (45).

Orally administered or BDP that is swallowed from inhalation undergoes rapid first-pass metabolism of the unhindered 21-ester via enzymatic hydrolysis in the liver or GI tract primarily to 17-BMP, but more slowly to 21-BMP and to beclomethasone, and to other unidentified metabolites and polar conjugates (99,100). The terminal half-life for 17-BMP is 6.5 hours. The portion of the inhaled dose of BDP that enters the lung is rapidly metabolized to 17-BMP in the respiratory tract before reaching systemic circulation, where it can be further metabolized by the liver. Following oral administration, BDP and its metabolites are excreted mainly in feces via biliary elimination and 12–15% of a 4-mg dose of BDP is excreted in urine as free and conjugated metabolites. The usual therapeutic dose (less than 1200 mcg/day) for beclomethasone dipropionate oral inhalation does not produce systemic glucocorticoid effects, probably because the drug is rapidly metabolized to less active metabolites. At doses >1200 mcg/day HPA suppression has been observed (25).

BDP monohydrate nasal suspension is available as an aqueous microcrystalline suspension of BDP which delivers 42 mcg per metered spray. The BDP nasal aerosol or inhalation aerosol consists of microcrystalline suspension of BDP in chlorofluorocarbon propellant, both of which delivers 42, 50 or 84 mcg per metered spray. The total daily adult dose for BDP from the nasal spray or nasal inhaler is 600 mcg, and for the aerosol inhaler, 336–1000 mcg. Doses exceeding 2000 mcg/day need to be monitored for HPA suppression.

Flunisolide. When administered intranasally or by inhalation, flunisolide (Fig. 28.14) is rapidly absorbed from nasal or lung tissue (Table 28.5) (101). This corticosteroid is efficiently metabolized by the liver to inactive metabolites with no apparent effects on adrenal function with long-term therapy. Flunisolide that is swallowed undergoes extensive first-pass metabolism in the liver, and that which is absorbed directly from the nasopharyngeal mucosa or lung bypasses this initial metabolism (102). It is not known if the drug undergoes metabolism in the GI tract. Flunisolide is rapidly hydroxylated by CYP3A4 at the 6β position followed by elimination of the 6α-fluoro group to its more polar 6β-hydroxy metabolite, which attains plasma concentrations that are usually greater than those for flunisolide (101,102).

Following IV administration of flunisolide, the 6β-hydroxy metabolite has 1/100 potency of flunisolide and a plasma half-life of 3.9–4.6 hours. Flunisolide and its 6β-hydroxy metabolite are conjugated in the liver to inactive glucuronides and sulfates. After intranasal administrations of 100 mcg, the plasma levels for flunisolide were undetectable within 4 hours. The duration of its systemic effects are short because of its short half-life.

Flunisolide nasal solution is available in an aqueous solubilized form which delivers 25 mcg per spray. The total daily adult dose for flunisolide from the nasal spray is 200–400 mcg. Flunisolide inhalation aerosol for pulmonary delivery is a microcrystalline suspension in a chlorofluorocarbon propellant that delivers 250 mcg per metered spray. The total daily adult inhalation dose for flunisolide is 1000 mcg. Doses exceeding 2000 mcg/day need to be monitored for HPA suppression.

Budesonide. Budesonide is a highly potent nonhalogenated glucocorticoid intended for the local treatment of lung disease and rhinitis. It was designed to have a high ratio between local and systemic effects. Budesonide is composed of a 1:1 mixture of epimers of the 16,17-butylacetal creating a chiral center (Fig. 28.14) (103). The 22R-epimer binds to the glucocorticoid receptor with higher affinity than does the 22S-epimer (Table 28.5) (45). The butyl acetal chain provided the highest potency for the homologous acetal chains. Its rate of topical uptake into epithelial tissue is more than 100 times faster than that for hydrocortisone and dexamethasone. Approximately 85% of the IV administered dose of budesonide undergoes extensive first-pass hepatic metabolism by CYP3A4 to its primary metabolites, 6β-hydroxybudesonide and 16α-hydroxyprednisolone, which have about 1/100 the potency of budesonide (104,105); an important inactivation step in limiting budesonide's systemic effect on adrenal suppression. Budesonide was metabolized 3–6 times more rapidly than is triamcinolone acetonide. The pharmacokinetics of budesonide after inhalation, oral and intravenous administration displayed a mean plasma half-life of 2.8 hours and a systemic bioavailability of about 10% after oral administration (Table 28.5) (105). Pulmonary bioavailability is <40% after inhalation (70–75% after correction for the amounts of budesonide deposited in the inhalation device and oral cavity.) No oxidative metabolism was observed in the lung. When given by inhalation, 32% of the dose is excreted in the urine as metabolites, 15% in the feces and 41% of the dose remained in the mouthpiece of the inhaler. Following intranasal administration, very little of intranasal budesonide is absorbed from the nasal mucosa. However, much of the intranasal dose (approximately 60%) was swallowed and remained in the GI tract to be excreted unchanged in the feces, while that fraction of the intranasal dose which was absorbed was extensively metablized.

Inhaled budesonide, in spite of its lower lipophilicity, exhibits greater retention within the airways than does other inhaled corticosteroids (104,105). This unusual behavior for inhaled budesonide has been attributed to the subsequent formation of intracellular fatty acid esters of the 21-hydroxy group of budesonide in the airway and lung tissue (106). Following inhalation, approximately 70–80% of budesonide was reversibly esterified by free fatty acids in the airway tissue. These inactive esters behave like an intracellular depot drug by slowly regenerating free budesonide. Thus, this reversible esterification prolongs the local anti-inflammatory action of budesonide in the airways and may contribute to the high efficacy and safety of budesonide in the treatment of mild asthma when inhaled once daily.

The systemic availability of budesonide in children was estimated to be 6.1% of the nominal dose and the terminal half-life was 2.3 hours (108,109). Approximately 6% of the nominal dose reached the systemic circulation of young children after inhalation of nebulized budesonide. This is about half the systemic availability found in healthy adults using the same nebulizer.

Budesonide nasal aerosol is supplied as a micronized suspension using a chlorofluorocarbon propellant, which delivers 32 mcg from the nasal adapter supplied per metered spray. The total daily adult dose for budesonide is 256 mcg. Budesonide powder for pulmonary inhalation uses micronized dry powder in a turboinhaler (DPI) that delivers 200 mcg per meter sprayed. The total daily adult dose for budesonide from the DPI is 200–800 mcg. Full benefit is attained in about 1–2 weeks.

Mometasone Furoate. The development of mometasone furoate resulted from re-examination of the effect of 17α ester functionalities on topical anti-inflammatory potency relative to the potent 17-benzoate ester of betamethasone. The SAR study involved substitution of the 17-benzoate ester with heteroaromatic furoic, thienoic and pyrrolic esters (110). Of the numerous 17α-heteroaryl esters studied, the 2-furoate ester displayed the greatest increase in potency. Therefore, combining the 17α (2-furoate) ester with the potency enhancing effect of the 21-chloro group, the resultant glucocorticoid (mometasone furoate) (Fig. 28.14) was 5–10 times more potent than the betamethasone benzoate ester, with a more rapid onset of action. Mometasone furoate was originally marketed as a topically applied corticosteroid, but because of its low systemic bioavailability, it was found to be more useful in the treatment of allergic disorders and lung diseases (111). It has the greatest binding affinity for the glucocorticoid receptor (Table 28.5) followed by fluticasone propionate, budesonide, triamcinolone acetonide, and dexamethasone (45). Mometasone furoate has strong local anti-inflammatory activity equivalent to that of fluticasone propionate. It has a quick onset of action relative to the other inhaled/intra nasal steroids with the least systemic availability and, consequently, the fewest systemic side effects.

Following IV suspension or inhalation administration, mometasone furoate was detected in the plasma for up to 8 hours, with a half-life of 4–6 hours (Table 28.5) and an oral bioavailability of less than 1%. It is extensively metabolized with less than 10% of the administered dose recovered in the urine unchanged (112). Among the polar metabolites (~80%) and their conjugates (42%) recovered were 6β-hydroxymometasone furoate and its 21-hydroxy metabolite. In contrast, following intranasal administration, its plasma concentrations were below the limit of quantification and the systemic bioavailability by this route was estimated to be less than 1%. The majority of the intranasal dose for mometasone furoate is deposited in the nasal mucosa and swallowed without absorption in the GI tract until eliminated in the feces (about 50–90% of the intranasal dose is recovered in the feces). That portion of the intranasal dose which was absorbed was extensively metabolized. These results indicate that inhaled mometasone furoate has negligible systemic bioavailability and is extensively metabolized with reduced risk for causing systemic adrenal suppression effects.

Mometasone furoate nasal suspension is supplied as an aqueous suspension with an atomizing pump that dispenses 50 mcg per metered spray. The total daily dose for mometasone furoate is 200 mcg.

Androstane-17β-carboxylates (R = OCH₂F)
Androstane-17β-carbothioates (R = SCH₂F)
(X = acetate or propionate)

Androstane 17β-carboxylates and 17β-carbothioates. The androstane 17β-hydroxyl-17β carboxylates and 17β-carbothioates were designed to be metabolically susceptible to hydrolysis and to have a low systemic bioavailability to minimize systemic glucocorticoid-induced adrenal suppression. The androstane 17α-hydroxyl-17β carboxylates lacked the 17-ketol group found in most of the systemic corticosteroids. However, when these 17β carboxylates were esterified to their 17α/β diesters, they proved to be extremely potent anti-inflammatory corticosteroids, while the parent carboxylic acids were inactive (113). Thus, enzymic hydrolysis of the 17-carboxylate ester function by intestinal or liver esterases would lead to formation of inactive metabolites. The greatest anti-inflammatory activity was observed with 17α-acetoxy and 17α-propionoxy groups and simple alkyl carboxylate esters, although the fluoromethyl esters showed the highest activity. Superseding the androstane 17β-carboxylates where the corresponding 17β-carbothioates (thioesters) derived from flumethasone. The 17β-fluoromethylcarbothioate when combined with the 17α-propionoxy group, yielded fluticasone (Fig. 28.14) (114). The androstane 17β-carbothioates proved not only to be very potent anti-inflammatory agents, but to exhibit weak HPA suppression in the rat. Both the androstane 17β-carboxylates and the androstane 17β-carbothioates are very lipophilic and exhibit minimal oral bioavailability and very low systemic activity after inhalation due to intestinal and hepatic enzymic hydrolysis to inactive metabolites which have 1/2000 the activity of the parent molecule (115).

Fluticasone Propionate. Fluticasone propionate, a trifluorinated glucocorticoid based on the androstane 17β-carbothioate nucleus (Fig. 28.14), was designed to be metabolically susceptible to hydrolysis and to have a low systemic bioavailability, in order to minimize the systemic effects on plasma hydrocortisone levels. Its susceptibility to metabolic hydrolysis is doubly enhanced by the combination of a thioester and the high electronegativity of the fluorine group. Fluticasone propionate is about 1/2 times more lipophilic than BDP, 8 times budesonide, and 13 times triamcinolone acetonide (Table 28.5) (94). It also displays high in vitro selectivity for the glucocorticoid receptor and a relative receptor affinity 1.5 times 17-BMP and mometasone furoate, 3 times budesonide, 18 times dexamethasone and 20 times flunisolide and triamcinolone acetonide (45). The rate of association for fluticasone dipropionate with the receptor is faster and the rate of dissociation slower than the other corticosteroids. The half-life of the fluticasone propionate active steroid-receptor complex is >10 hours, compared with approximately 5 hours for budesonide, 7.5 hours for 17-BMP, and 4 hours triamcinolone acetonide (45).

Following topical application to the nasal mucosa or after inhalation, fluticasone propionate produces potent anti-inflammatory effects with an onset of action of about 2–3 days. The topical anti-inflammatory potency for fluticasone propionate is about equal to mometasone furoate, 13 times greater than triamcinolone acetonide, 9 times fluocinolone acetonide, 3 times betamethasone 17-valerate, and 2 times BDP (115). Because of its low systemic bioavailability when administered intranasally or by inhalation and nondetectability in plasma, most pharmacokinetic data for fluticasone propionate are based on IV or oral administration (Table 28.5). Its rate of topical uptake into epithelial tissue is more than 100 times faster than that for hydrocortisone and dexamethasone, but similar to BDP and budesonide.

As a consequence of its high lipophilicity (Table 28.5), fluticasone propionate is very insoluble and is therefore poorly absorbed from the respiratory (10–13%) and GI tract following nasal inhalation of the drug (116–118). The majority of the intranasal dose for fluticasone propionate is deposited in the nasal mucosa and swallowed into the GI tract until eliminated in the feces (about 80–90% of the intranasal dose is recovered metabolized and unchanged in the feces). After administration of an IV suspension, fluticasone propionate displayed a systemic bioavailability less than 2% and underwent extensive hydrolysis and CYP3A4 first-pass metabolism in the liver with an elimination half-life of approximately 3 hours. Its primary hydrolysis product is 17β-carboxylate metabolite, which has 1/2000 the affinity for the glucocorticoid receptor, can be recovered from the urine along with other unidentified hydroxy metabolites and their conjugates. Following oral administration of 1–40 mg, fluticasone propionate is poorly absorbed from the GI tract because of hydrolysis and its insolubility with an oral bioavailability of less than 1%. Less than 5% of the oral dose

was excreted unchanged in the urine. Fluticasone propionate was not detected in plasma for up to 6 hours after IV or oral administration (117). Approximately 80–90% of the oral dose is excreted unchanged in the feces of which about 3–40% is the hydrolyzed 17β-carboxylate metabolite. Pulmonary bioavailability ranges between 16–30% depending upon inhalation device used with an elimination half-life of about 14 hours, increasing its potential for drug accumulation with repeated dosing (118). The long elimination half-life for fluticasone propionate is due in part to its very high lipophilicity and very poor water solubility, and consequently slow dissolution into lung tissue. Some suppression of overnight hydrocortisone levels has been reported with inhaled fluticasone propionate at higher dosages (indicative of HPA axis suppression) (119).

Fluticasone propionate nasal suspension and inhalation aerosol are both available as micronized suspensions in a chlorofluorocarbon propellant that delivers 50 mcg per metered spray. The total daily adult dose for fluticasone propionate from the nasal suspension is 200 mcg, and 880 mcg for the inhalation aerosol.

SUMMARY OF THE STRUCTURE-ACTIVITY RELATIONSHIPS FOR GLUCOCORTICOIDS AND MINERALOCORTICOID ACTIVITY

The structure in Figure 28.15 depicts the ring conformation and absolute configuration for hydrocortisone and prednisolone. The all *trans* (B/C and C/D) backbone that is necessary for activity is very evident.

As previously pointed out, the adrenocorticoids are generally classified as either glucocorticoids, which affect intermediary metabolism and are associated with inhibition of the inflammatory process, or mineralocorticoids. In fact, most naturally occurring and semisynthetic analogs exhibit both of these actions. The 17β-ketol ($-COCH_2OH$) side chain and the Δ^4-3-ketone functions are found in clinically used adrenocorticoids, and these groups do contribute to the potency of the agents. Modifications of these groups may result in derivatives that retain biologic activity. For example, replacement of the 21-OH group with fluorine increases glucocorticoid and sodium-retaining activities, whereas, substitution with chlorine or bromine abolishes activity. Some compounds that do not contain the Δ^4-3-ketone system have appreciable activity. It has been suggested that this group makes only a minor contribution to the specificity of action of these drugs or to the steroid-receptor association constant (120).

Based on structure-activity studies, the C and D rings, involving positions 11, 12, 13, 16, 17, 18, 20, and 21, are more important for receptor binding than are the A and B rings.

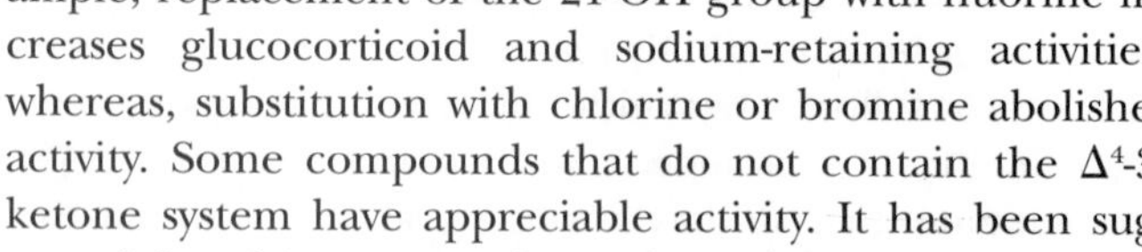

Fig. 28.15. Conformations of hydrocortisone and prednisolone.

Table 28.6. Biologic Potencies of Modified Adrenocorticoids in the Rat and Humans*

| | | Potency Relative to Hydrocortisone (Cortisol) | | | |
| | | Rat | | Humans | |
Adrenocorticoid	Thymus Involution	Liver Glycogen Deposition	Eosinopenic Potency	Hyperglycemic Potency	Antirheumatic Potency
Corticosterone	—	0.8	0.06	0.06	<0.1
Prednisone	—	3	—	4	4
Prednisolone	2	3.9	4	4	4
Methylprednisolone	10	11	5	5	5
Triamcinolone	4	47	5	5	5
Paramethasone	—	150	12	12	11
Dexamethasone	56	265	28	28	29
Fludrocortisone acetate	6	9	8	8	10
Fluprednisolone	6	81	9	9	10
Triamcinolone acetonide	33	242	3	3	3
Flurandrenoione	4	—	1	—	2
Fluorometholone	25	115	10	10	—
Fluocinolone	19	112	5	6	9

Data from I. Ringler, in Methods of Hormone Research, Vol.3. Part A, R.I. Dorfman, New York, Academic Press, 1964.

Generally, insertion of bulky substituents on the β-side of the molecule abolishes glycogenic activity, while insertion on the α-side does not. It has been suggested that association of these steroids with receptors involves β-surfaces of rings C and D and the 17β-ketol side chain (120). It is possible, however, that association with the α-surface of rings A, C, and D, as well as with the ketol side chain, is essential for sodium-retaining activity. Many functional groups, such as 17α-OH, 17α-CH$_3$, 16α-CH$_3$ and 16β-CH$_3$, 16α-CH$_3$O and 16α-OH substituents, abolish or reverse this activity in 11-desoxycorticosterone and 11-oxygenated steroids. Discussions of exceptions of these generalities are found in the literature (120).

Although some steroids cause sodium retention, many have glucocorticoid and either sodium-retaining or sodium-excreting action. Difficulties in correlating the structures of adrenocorticoids with biologic action are compounded because of differences in assay methods, species variation, and the mode of drug administration. For example, whereas liver glycogen and anti-inflammatory assays in the rat correlate well, some drugs show high anti-inflammatory action in the rat but little or no antirheumatic activity in humans (121). The 9α-F analog, fludrocortisone acetate, is more active than the 9α-Cl analog in terms of sodium retention in the dog; the reverse is true in the rat. While 16α-methylation or 16β-methylation enhance glucocorticoid activity, anti-inflammatory action is increased disproportionately to glycogenic action in both series.

In humans, eosinopenic and hyperglycemic potencies are essentially the same. There is a close correlation in efficacy ratios derived from these tests and antirheumatic potency (Table 28.6). Because the eosinopenic-hyperglycemic activity and antirheumatic potency show excellent agreement, it has been suggested that these assays afford advantages in the preliminary estimation of anti-inflammatory potency (121).

Structure-activity studies of glucocorticoids have mainly been carried out in animals and are not necessarily applicable to clinical efficacy in man. Relative activity and dose correlations for the clinically useful drugs are found in Table 28.1.

Several other compounds have been studied in animals and used to derive structure-activity relationships. For example, insertion of a double bond between positions 1 and 2 in hydrocortisone increases glucocorticoid activity. Δ^1-corticoids have a much longer half-life in the blood than hydrocortisone; ring A is resistant to metabolism to its 5β-metabolite. But it is oxidatively metabolized at other positions especially the 6β position and the 17β-ketol (Fig. 28.12) (121). If, however, a double bond is inserted between positions 9 and 11 (no oxygen function at 11), a decrease in glucocorticoid activity is observed. Except for cortisone, which results in an analog with decreased glucocorticoid activity when a double bond is inserted between position 6 and 7, such modification of other glucocorticoids generally produces no change in activity (121).

Insertion of α-CH$_3$ groups at positions 2 (in 11β-OH analogs), 6, and 16 increases glucocorticoid activity in animals. Again, insertion of a 2α-CH$_3$ group into the glucocorticoid almost completely prevents reduction of the Δ^4-3-ketone system in vivo and in vitro, however, 16α/β-methyl blocks hydroxylation enhancing potency. Substitution at positions 4α, 7α, 9α, 11α, and 21 decreases activity (121).

Although some analogs, such as 16α, 17α-acetonides and the 1,2-dihydro derivative, are 11-desoxysteroids and are biologically active, the 11β-OH group of hydrocortisone is essential for the drug-receptor interaction (120). Cortisone, which contains an 11-keto function, is reduced in vivo to hydrocortisone. The drug 2α-methylhydrocortisone exhibits high glucocorticoid activity. This is probably because of steric hindrance to reduction (i.e., C=O → C-β-OH) by the methyl group, thus rendering the analog inactive (39,123,124). Insertion of α-OH groups into most other positions (1, 6, 7, 9, 14, and 16) or reduction of the 20-ketone, however, decreases glucocorticoid activity, due in part to increased hydrophilicity.

The 9α-F group increases glucocorticoid activity and nearly prevents metabolic oxidation of the 11β-OH group to a ketone (120). Redox metabolism of Δ⁴-steroids is mainly restricted to the Δ⁴-3-ketone, 6 and 16 positions and the 17β-ketol side chain whereas for the Δ¹-corticoids it is only the 6 and 16 positions and 17β-ketol side chain. The 9α-F group may increase activity by an inductive effect, which increases the acidic dissociation constant of the 11β-OH group and thereby increases the ability of the drug to hydrogen bond to the glucocorticoid receptor.

A 6α-F group also increases glucocorticoid activity, but it has less effect than the 9α-F function on sodium retention. Insertion of 2α-, 11α- (no OH group at 11), or 21-F groups decreases glucocorticoid activity. Of particular interest is a 12α-F group. When this function is inserted into corticosterone, which has no 17α-OH group, it potentiates activity to the same extent as a 9α-F group. Insertion of a 12α-F group into a 16α,17α-dihydroxy steroid, however, renders the compound inactive. A 9α-F group potentiates activity in such analogs.

It has been proposed that hydrogen bonding between the 12α-F and 17α-OH groups renders the analog inactive (Fig. 28.16). Conversion to the 16α,17α-isopropylidine-dioxy(acetonide) derivative, which cannot hydrogen bond, restores biologic activity (125).

The mineralocorticoid activity of the adrenocorticoids is another action of major significance. Many toxic side effects, making it necessary to withdraw steroid therapy in rheumatoid patients, are a result of this action. Highly active naturally occurring mineralocorticoids have no OH function in positions 11 and 17. In fact, OH groups in any position reduce the sodium-retaining activity of the adrenocorticoid.

Generally, 9α-F, 9α-Cl, and 9α-Br substitution causes increased retention of urinary sodium with an order of activity in which F > Cl > Br, but species differences do exist. For these reasons, such compounds are not used internally in the treatment of diseases such as rheumatoid arthritis. Insertion of a 16α-OH group into the molecule affects the sodium retention activity so markedly that it not only negates the effect of the 9α-F atom, but also causes sodium excretion.

A double bond between positions 1 and 2 (Δ¹-corticoids) also reduces the sodium retention activity of the parent drug. This functional group, however, contributes to the parent drug only about one-fifth the sodium-excreting tendency of a 16α-OH group (126).

12α-F, 2α-CH₃, and 9α-Cl substitution contribute equally to sodium retention. A 21-OH group, found in all these drugs, contributes to this action to the same degree. Because 21-OH groups also contribute to glucocorticoid activity, it is easy to understand why it is difficult to develop compounds with only one major action.

A 2α-CH₃ group is about three times and a 21-F substituent two times as effective as unsaturation between positions 1 and 2 in reducing sodium retention. Other substituents reported to inhibit sodium retention include 16α-CH₃ and 16β-CH₃, 16α-CH₃O, and 6α-Cl functions. A 17α-OH group, present in naturally occurring and semisynthetic analogs, reduces sodium retention to about the same extent as does unsaturation between positions 1 and 2.

Conversion of the 17α-hydroxy to either a 17α-ester or an ether as with 16α,17α-isopropylidinedioxy (acetonide), greatly enhances the anti-inflammatory potency and glucocorticoid receptor affinity (Table 28.5). However, as evidenced with beclomethasone dipropionate, esterifying the 21-hydroxy group reduces activity and receptor affinity. On the other hand, 21-halogens or 21-halomethylene groups greatly increase topical anti-inflammatory activity with no change or a decrease in mineralocorticoid activity. Perhaps, a hydrogen bonding group at 21 enhances or retains mineralocorticoid receptor affinity.

ADRENOCORTICOID ANTAGONISTS

Antagonists of adrenocorticoids include agents that compete for binding to steroid receptors (antiglucocorticoids or antimineralocorticoids) and inhibitors of adrenosteroid biosynthesis. The action of adrenal steroids can be blocked by antagonists that compete with the endogenous steroids for binding sites on their respective cytosolic receptor proteins. The antagonist-receptor complexes are unable to stimulate the production of new mRNA and protein in the target tissues and are thus unable to elicit the biologic responses of the hormone agonist. Spironolactone and related analogs bind to the mineralocorticoid receptor in the kidney and result in the diuretic response of increased Na⁺ excretion and K⁺ retention. The 3-keto-4-ene A-ring is essential for this antagonistic activity and the opening of the lactone ring dramatically reduces activity. The 7α-substituent increases both intrinsic activity and oral activity (127,128). Progesterone also has shown antimineralocorticoid activity at 10^{-4} molar concentrations.

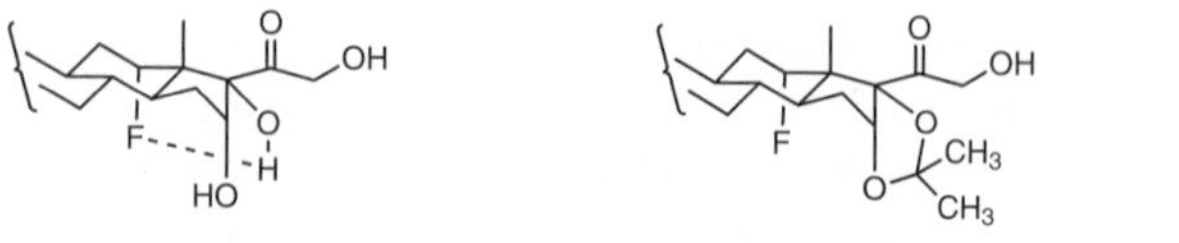

16α, 17α-Dihydroxy steroid   16α, 17α-Isopropylidenedioxy steroid

Fig. 28.16. Hydrogen bonding between 17α-hydroxyl and 12α-fluoro groups.

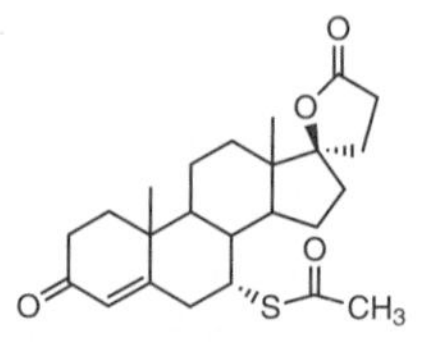

Spironolactone

Receptor antagonists of glucocorticoids have been described; they are derivatives of 19-nortestosterone (129,130). Mifepristone (RU 486) was originally developed as an antiprogestin and is described in more detail in Chapter 29. Mifepristone also exhibits very effective antagonism of glucocorticoids.

Several inhibitors of adrenocorticoid biosynthesis have been described, with the majority of nonsteroidal agents inhibiting one or more of the cytochrome P450 enzyme complexes involved in adrenosteroid biosynthesis. Metyrapone reduces cortisol biosynthesis by primarily inhibiting mitochondrial 11β-hydroxylase. It also inhibits to a lesser degree 18-hydroxylase and side chain cleavage. This agent is used to test pituitary-adrenal function and the ability of the pituitary to secrete ACTH (131). Aminoglutethimide inhibits side chain cleavage (132) and has been utilized as a medical adrenalectomy. Several azole antifungal drugs inhibit adrenocorticoid biosynthesis; ketoconazole is one example. It inhibits fungal sterol biosynthesis at low concentrations; however, at higher doses, ketoconazole inhibits several cytochrome P450 enzymes in adrenosteroid biosynthesis (133). Trilostane is a steroidal inhibitor of 3β-hydroxysteroid dehydrogenase (134) and has been used to treat Cushing's syndrome.

MECHANISMS OF ADRENOCORTICOID ACTION
Molecular Interaction

Glucocorticoid action is mediated through the glucocorticoid receptor, which is found primarily in the cytosol of the cell when not bound to glucocorticoids. The glucocorticoid receptor is stabilized in the cytosol by complexation with phosphorylated proteins, including a 90 Kd protein referred to as a heat-shock protein (hsp90) (135). The steroid molecule binds to the glucocorticoid receptor, resulting in a conformational change of the receptor to dissociate the other proteins and initiate translocation of the steroid-receptor complex into the nucleus. The steroid-nuclear glucocorticoid receptor complex interacts with particular HRE regions of the cellular DNA, referred to as glucocorticoid responsive elements (GREs), and initiates transcription of the DNA sequence to produce mRNA. Finally, the elevated levels of mRNA lead to an increase in protein synthesis in the endoplasmic reticulum; these proteins then mediate glucocorticoid effects on carbohydrate, lipid and protein metabolism. An alternative isoform of the glucocorticoid receptor has been identified. This isoform of the receptor does not bind known glucocorticoids and its function remains to be determined (136,137). Some of the specific proteins induced by glucocorticoids have been identified and are discussed later. Mineralocorticoid effects are observed in several tissues and specific mineralocorticoid receptors have been characterized that mediate mineralocorticoid functions (138).

Physiologic Effects
Glucocorticoid

Corticosteroids influence all tissues of the body and produce numerous and varying effects in cells. These steroids regulate carbohydrate, lipid, and protein biosynthesis and metabolism (glucocorticoid effects), and they influence water and electrolyte balance (mineralocorticoid effects). Cortisol (endogenous hydrocortisone) is the most potent glucocorticoid secreted by the adrenal gland, and aldosterone is the most potent endogenous mineralocorticoid. Both naturally occurring glucocorticoids and related semi-synthetic analogs can be evaluated in terms of their ability to sustain life, (139,140) to stimulate an increase in blood glucose concentrations and a deposition of liver glycogen, (141) to decrease circulating eosinophils, (142) and to cause thymus involution in adrenalectomized animals (143,144). In addition, corticosteroids can affect immune system functions, inflammatory responses, and cell growth.

The primary physiologic function of glucocorticoids is to maintain blood glucose levels and thus ensure glucose-dependent processes critical to life, particularly brain functions. Cortisol and related steroids accomplish this by stimulating the formation of glucose, by diminishing glucose use by peripheral tissues, and by promoting glycogen synthesis in the liver in order to increase carbohydrate stores for later release of glucose. For glucose formation, glucocorticoids mobilize amino acids and promote amino acid metabolism and gluconeogenesis. These steroids, acting via the glucocorticoid receptor mechanism, induce the production of a variety of enzymes important for glucose formation. The synthesis of tyrosine aminotransferase increases within 30 minutes of glucocorticoid exposure (145–148). This enzyme promotes the transfer of amino groups from tyrosine to α-ketoglutarate to form glutamate and hydroxyphenylpyruvate. Another amino-acid metabolizing enzyme induced rapidly by glucocorticoids is tryptophan oxidase (150). This enzyme oxidizes tryptophan to formylkynurenine, which is subsequently converted to alanine. Alanine transaminase is also induced by glucocorticoids (151,152). Alanine and, to a lesser extent, glutamate are important for gluconeogenesis in the liver.

Several other enzymes important in gluconeogenesis and glycogen formation are elevated for several hours following glucocorticoid administration, including glycogen synthetase, pyruvate kinase, phosphoenol pyruvate carboxykinase, and glucose-6-phosphate kinase (16,153,154). The delayed increases in these enzymes suggest their biosyntheses are not regulated directly by glucocorticoids (16). In peripheral tissues, glucocorticoid-induced inhibition of phosphofructokinase is observed. This enzyme catalyzes the formation of D-fructose-1,6-diphosphate from D-fructose-6-phosphate during glycolysis. Inhibition of this enzyme decreases glucose utilization by peripheral tissues and results in maintaining blood glucose levels. Reviews of the multiple effects of glucocorticoids on carbohydrate metabolism have been published (16,154).

Additional effects of glucocorticoids in the body are preventing or minimizing inflammatory reactions and suppressing immune responses. These steroids interfere with both early events in inflammation (such as release of mediators, edema, and cellular infiltration) and later stages (capillary infiltration and collagen formation). Only a few of the mechanisms involved in glucocorticoid suppression of inflammation are known. Cortisol will induce the production of lipocortin and related proteins by increasing gene expression through the glucocorticoid receptor mechanism (155). Lipocortin inhibits the activity of phospholipase A_2, which liberates arachidonic acid and leads to the biosynthesis of eicosanoids (such as prostaglandins and leukotrienes). Lipocortin also mediates the decreased production and release of platelet activating factor (156). Glucocorticoids can also suppress the expression of interleukin-1 (IL-1), tumor necrosis factor (TNF) and inducible nitric oxide synthase (iNOS) (157–159). These eicosanoids and peptide factors are important as mediators in the inflammatory response. Some of these factors also play important roles in cellular infiltration and capillary permeability in the inflamed region. Suppression of the immune responses are also mediated by inhibition of the synthesis and release of important mediators. In macrophages, glucocorticoids inhibit IL-1 synthesis and thus interfere with proliferation of B-lymphocytes, important for antibody production (160). IL-1 is also important for activation of resting T-lymphocytes, important for cell-mediated immunity. The activated T-cells produce interleukin-2 (IL-2); its biosynthesis is also reduced by glucocorticoids (161).

Mineralocorticoid

The primary physiologic function of mineralocorticoids is to maintain electrolyte balances in the body by enhancing Na^+ reabsorption and increasing K^+ and H^+ secretion in the kidney. Similar effects on cation transport are observed in a variety of secretory tissues, including the salivary glands, sweat glands, and mucosal tissues of the gastrointestinal tract and the bladder. Aldosterone is the most potent endogenous mineralocorticoid. Deoxycorticosterone is approximately 20–40 times less potent than aldosterone. Cortisol exhibits weak mineralocorticoid activity in vivo due to rapid metabolism of cortisol to cortisone by 11β-hydroxysteroid dehydrogenase. The mechanism of action of aldosterone involves binding of the steroid to the mineralocorticoid receptor and initiation of gene transcription, mRNA biosynthesis, and protein production. A protein referred to as aldosterone-induced protein (AIP) is produced through this mechanism and is thought to aid in Na^+ retention. One possible mode of action of AIP is to act as a permease to increase the permeability of the cell membrane to Na^+ (162). This results in an accelerated rate of Na^+ influx and elevated activity of Na^+, K^+-ATPase to pump Na^+ into extracellular space (163).

Pharmacologic Effects and Clinical Applications

In addition to their natural hormonal actions, the adrenocorticoids have many clinical uses. Glucocorticoids and mineralocorticoids may be used for the treatment of adrenal insufficiency (hypoadrenalism), which results from failure of the adrenal glands to synthesize adequate amounts of the hormones. Adrenocorticoids are also used to maintain patients who have had partial or complete removal of their adrenal glands or adenohypophysis (adrenalectomy and hypophysectomy, respectively). Glucocorticoids can cross the placenta and may be distributed into milk.

Two major uses of glucocorticoids are in the treatment of rheumatoid diseases and allergic manifestations. Their use in the treatment of severe asthma is well documented (164). Their utility in sepsis and acute respiratory distress syndrome are now being investigated (165,166). They are effective in the treatment of rheumatoid arthritis, acute rheumatic fever, bursitis, spontaneous hypoglycemia in children, gout, rheumatoid carditis, sprue, allergy, including contact dermatitis, and other conditions. The treatment of chronic rheumatic diseases and allergic conditions with glucocorticoids is symptomatic and continuous; symptoms return after withdrawal of the drug.

In addition, these drugs are moderately effective in the treatment of ulcerative colitis, dermatomyositis, periarteritis nodosa, idiopathic pulmonary fibrosis, idiopathic thrombocytopenic purpura, regional ileitis, acquired hemolytic anemia, nephrosis, cirrhotic ascites, neurodermatitis, and temporal arteritis. The newer analogs with medium to high potency rankings (Table 28.4), such as diflorasone diacetate, desoximetasone, flurandrenolide, or fluocinonide (Fig. 28.12), are effective topically in the treatment of psoriasis. Glucocorticoids may be combined with antibiotics to treat pneumonia, peritonitis, typhoid fever, and meningococcemia (167).

When dosages with equivalent antirheumatic potency are given to patients not treated with steroids, the Δ^1-corticoids (prednisone and prednisolone) promote the same pattern of initial improvement as hydrocortisone. Statistical results of improvement during the first few months of therapy have been similar with prednisone, prednisolone, and hydrocortisone; the results of longer term therapy have been significantly better with the modified compounds.

Satisfactory rheumatic control, lost after prolonged cortisone or hydrocortisone therapy, may be regained in an appreciable number of patients by changing to prednisone, prednisolone, or other modified drugs. Of patients whose conditions deteriorate below adequate levels during hydrocortisone administration, nearly half reach their previous level of improvement after Δ^1-corticoids (in doses slightly larger in terms of antirheumatic strength) are used. With further prolongation of steroid therapy, improvement again wanes in some patients. In other patients such management is successful for longer than 2 years. In some instances, the improvement is attributed to increased effectiveness of the drug due to correction of salt and water retention; in other instances, there is no adequate explanation.

When these drugs are administered in doses that have similar antirheumatic strengths, the general incidence of adverse reactions with prednisone and prednisolone is about the same as with hydrocortisone. The compounds differ, however, in their tendencies to induce individual side effects. The incidence and degree of salt and water retention and blood pressure elevation are less with the Δ^1-corticoids. Conversely, these analogs are more likely to promote digestive complaints, peptic ulcer, vasomotor symptoms, and cutaneous ecchymosis.

Although these analogs have unwanted side effects, most clinical investigators prefer the Δ^1-corticoids to hydrocortisone for rheumatoid patients who require steroid therapy. The reasons are that these drugs have less tendency to cause salt and water retention and potassium loss, and that they restore improvement in a significant percentage of patients whose therapeutic control has been lost during cortisone and hydrocortisone therapy.

It seems desirable to administer prednisone and prednisolone in conjunction with nonabsorbable antacids. This affords improvement of long-term therapy. It appears that the therapeutic indices of these two analogs, especially when used in conjunction with nonabsorbable antacids, are higher than for the naturally occurring glucocorticoids.

Most important, glucocorticoids should not be withdrawn abruptly in cases of acute infections or severe stress, such as surgery or trauma. Myasthenia gravis, peptic ulcer, diabetes mellitus, hyperthyroidism, hypertension, psychological disturbances, pregnancy (first trimester), and infections may be aggravated by glucocorticoid administration. Hormone therapy is contraindicated in these conditions and should be used only with the utmost precaution.

Semisynthetic analogs exhibiting high mineralocorticoid activity are not employed in the treatment of rheumatic disorders because of toxic side effects resulting from a disturbance of electrolyte and water balance. Some newer synthetic steroids (Table 28.1) are relatively free of sodium-retaining activity; they may show other toxic manifestations, however, and eventually have to be withdrawn.

Glucocorticoids are sometimes used in the treatment of scleroderma, discoid lupus, acute nephritis, osteoarthritis, acute hepatitis, hepatic coma, Hodgkin's disease, multiple myeloma, lymphoid tumors, acute leukemia, metastatic carcinoma of the breast, and chronic lymphatic leukemia (167). Glucocorticoids may be more or less effective in these diseases depending on the clinical condition.

Some modified compounds have been recommended for use when other analogs are no longer effective or when it is desirable to promote increased appetite and weight gain. Triamcinolone may be used advantageously when salt and water retention (from other glucocorticoids, hypertension, or cardiac compensation) or excessive appetite and weight gain are problems in management.

One factor that must not be overlooked when applying potent anti-inflammatory agents with high potency rankings is percutaneous absorption. The relative rate of percutaneous absorption, administered as a cream in rats, was triamcinolone acetonide > hydrocortisone > dexamethasone, but dexamethasone was deposited in skin longer than the other two drugs; hydrocortisone disappeared most rapidly (168).

Topical Applications

Topical dermatological products with a low potency ranking have a modest anti-inflammatory effect and are safest for chronic application (Table 28.4). These products are also the safest products for use on the face with occlusion, and in infants and young children. Those products with a medium potency ranking are used in moderate inflammatory dermatoses, such as chronic hand eczema and atopic eczema, and may be used on the face and intertriginous areas for a limited duration. High potency preparations are used in more severe inflammatory dermatoses such as severe eczema and psoriasis. They may be used for a limited duration and for longer periods in areas with thickened skin due to chronic conditions. High potency preparations may also be used on the face and intertriginous areas but only for a short treatment duration. Very high potency products are used primarily as an alternative to systemic corticosteroid therapy when local areas are involved. Examples of conditions for which very high potency products are frequently used include thick, chronic lesions caused by psoriasis, lichen simplex chronicus, and discoid lupus erythematosus. They may be used for only a short duration of therapy and on small surface areas. Occlusive dressings should not be used with these products. It has been suggested that patients using a lotion or ointment containing these drugs be instructed to apply them sparingly and to spread them lightly over the affected areas. The extent and frequency of applications should be carefully considered. Apparently, a lotion vehicle is more effective when treating a dermatitis, but a greater degree of percutaneous absorption occurs than when ointments are used (169,170).

Intranasal and Inhaled Applications

The pulmonary and nasal bioavailability are important determinants for the potential of an inhaled or nasally applied corticosteroid to cause systemic effects, because the lung and nasal tissue provide an enormous surface area from which drug absorption can occur into the systemic circulation. The main areas of concern with regard to systemic effects include HPA axis suppression, change in bone mineral density and growth retardation in children, cataracts and glaucoma. The degree of systemic side effects is dose-dependent, related to the half-life of the drug, frequency administration, time of day when administered, and route of administration; i.e., the higher the plasma corticosteroid concentration and longer the half-life, the greater will be the systemic side effects (Table 28.5) (25). The amount of an inhaled or nasal corticosteroid reaching the systemic circulation is the sum of the drug concentration available following absorption from the lungs/nasal mucosa and from the gastrointestinal tract. The fraction deposited in the mouth will be swallowed and the systemic availability will be determined by its absorption from the GI tract and the degree of first-pass metabolism.

Delivery devices can produce clinically significant differences in activity by altering the dose deposited in the lung (10–25%) and, for orally absorbed drugs, the amount deposited in the oropharynx and swallowed (75–90%). Clinical studies have shown the following relative potency differences: mometasone furoate> fluticasone propionate > budesonide = beclomethasone dipropionate > triamcinolone acetonide = flunisolide. Potency differences can be overcome by giving larger doses of the less potent drug, which increases risks from systemic effects. Adrenal suppression may be associated with high doses of inhaled corticosteroids above 1.5 mg/d (0.75 mg/d for fluticasone propionate), although there is a considerable degree of interindividual susceptibility.

All currently used inhaled corticosteroids are rapidly cleared from the body, but show varying levels of oral bioavailability, with fluticasone propionate having the lowest (Table 28.5). Following inhalation, there is also considerable variability in the rate of absorption from the lung, and pulmonary residence times are greatest for fluticasone propionate and triamcinolone acetonide, and shortest for budesonide and flunisolide. Adrenal suppression has not been observed when intranasal fluticasone propionate was administered in dosages of 200–4000 mcg daily for up to 12 months.

Adverse Effects (25)

Although short-term administration of corticosteroids are unlikely to produce harmful effects, when these drugs are used for longer than brief periods, however, they can produce a variety of devastating effects, including glucocorticoid-induced adrenocortical insufficiency, glucocorticoid-induced osteoporosis and generalized protein depletion. The duration of anti-inflammatory activity of glucocorticoids approximately equals the duration of HPA-axis suppression. In one study, the duration of HPA-axis suppression after a single oral dose of glucocorticoids is shown in Table 28. 7. When given for prolonged periods, glucocorticoids suppress the HPA axis thereby decreasing secretion of endogenous corticosteroids and adrenal atrophy. Glucocorticoids inhibit ACTH production by the adenohypophysis and this, in turn, reduces endogenous glucocorticoid production. With time, atrophy of the adrenal glands takes place. The degree and duration of adrenocortical insufficiency produced by the synthetic glucocorticoids is highly variable among patients and depends on the dose, frequency and time of administration, and duration

Table 28.7. Effect of an Oral Single Dose on the Duration of HPA Suppression*

Adrenocorticoid	Duration of Suppression (days)
Hydrocortisone (250 mg)	1.25–1.5
Cortisone (250 mg)	1.25–1.5
Methylprednisolone (40 mg)	1.25–1.5
Prednisone (50 mg)	1.25–1.5
Prednisolone (50 mg)	1.25–1.5
Triamcinolone (40 mg)	2.25
Dexamethasone (5 mg)	2.75
Betamethasone (6 mg)	3.25

*Modified from McEvoy GK ed. AHFS 2001 Drug Information, Bethesda MD, American Society Health-System Pharmacist 2001.

of glucocorticoid therapy. This effect may be minimized by use of alternate-day therapy.

Patients who develop drug-induced adrenocortical insufficiency may require higher corticosteroid dosage when they are subjected to stress (e.g., infection, surgery, trauma). In addition, acute adrenal insufficiency (even death) may occur if the drugs are withdrawn abruptly or if patients are transferred from systemic glucocorticoid therapy to oral inhalation therapy. Therefore, the drugs should be withdrawn very gradually following long-term therapy with pharmacologic dosages. Adrenal suppression may persist up to 12 months in patients who receive large dosages for prolonged periods. Until recovery occurs, patients may show signs and symptoms of adrenal insufficiency when they are subjected to stress and replacement therapy may be required. Since mineralocorticoid secretion may be impaired, sodium chloride or a mineralocorticoid should also be administered.

Although side effects and toxicities vary with the drug and sometimes with the patient, facial mooning, flushing, sweating, acne, thinning of the scalp hair, abdominal distention, and weight gain are observed with most glucocorticoids. Protein depletion (with osteoporosis and spontaneous fractures), myopathy (with weakness of muscles of the thighs, pelvis, and lower back), and aseptic necrosis of the hip and humerus are other side effects. These drugs may cause psychological disturbances, headache, vertigo, and peptic ulcer, and may suppress growth in children.

Patients with well-controlled diabetes must be closely monitored and their insulin dosage increased if glycosuria or hyperglycemia ensues during or following glucocorticoid administration. Patients should also be watched for signs of adrenocorticoid insufficiency after discontinuation of glucocorticoid therapy. Individuals with a history of tuberculosis should receive prophylactic doses of antituberculosis drugs.

Osteoporosis is one of the most serious adverse effects of long-term glucocorticoid therapy. Moderate- to high-dose glucocorticoid therapy is associated with loss of bone and an increased risk of fracture that is most rapid during the initial 6 months of therapy. These adverse effects of glucocorticoids appear to be both dose and duration dependent, with oral prednisone dosages of 7.5 mg or more daily for 6 months or longer often resulting in clinically important bone loss and increased fracture risk. Bone loss has even been associated with oral inhalation of glucocorticoids and is of great concern in children. Most patients receiving long-term glucocorticoid therapy will develop some degree of bone loss, and more than 25% will develop osteoporotic fractures. Vertebral fractures have been reported in 11% of asthmatic patients receiving systemic glucocorticoids for at least 1 year, and glucocorticoid-treated patients with rheumatoid arthritis are at increased risk of fractures of the hip, rib, spine, leg, ankle, and foot. Muscle wasting or weakness and atrophy of the protein matrix of the bone resulting in osteoporosis are manifestations of protein catabolism which may occur during prolonged therapy with glucocorticoids. These adverse effects may be especially serious in geriatric or debilitated patients. Post-menopausal women, the fact that they are especially prone to osteoporosis.

To minimize the risk of glucocorticoid-induced bone loss (osteoporosis) and those with low mineral bone density, the smallest possible effective dosage and duration should be used. Topical and inhaled preparations should be used whenever possible. The immunosuppressive effects of glucocorticoids increases the susceptibility to and mask symptoms of infections, and may result in activation of latent infection or exacerbation of intercurrent infections. The most common adverse effect of oral inhalation therapy with glucocorticoids is fungal infections of the mouth, pharynx, and occasionally the larynx. The mineralocorticoid effects are less frequent with synthetic glucocorticoids (except fludrocortisone) than with hydrocortisone or cortisone, but may occur, especially when synthetic glucocorticoids are given in high dosage for prolonged periods.

CASE STUDY

Victoria F. Roche and S. William Zito

AF is a 64-year-old, retired school teacher who has been battling debilitating rheumatoid arthritis for several years. She has been through several different NSAIDs including the COX-2 selective ones and, while they really helped her arthritis, she experienced significant gastric bleeding with these agents. Her physician then tried her on oral methotrexate, but she developed renal dysfunction and methotrexate-induced lung disease and had to discontinue therapy. She is now in the clinic for re-evaluation, and a decision is made to cautiously initiate corticosteroid therapy. AF is an insulin-dependent diabetic, and takes enalapril for high blood pressure.

1. Identify the therapeutic problem(s) where the pharmacist's intervention may benefit the patient.

2. Identify and prioritize the patient specific factors that must be considered to achieve the desired therapeutic outcomes.

3. Conduct a thorough and mechanistically oriented structure-activity analysis of all therapeutic alternatives provided in the case.

4. Evaluate the SAR findings against the patient specific factors and desired therapeutic outcomes and make a therapeutic decision.

5. Counsel your patient.

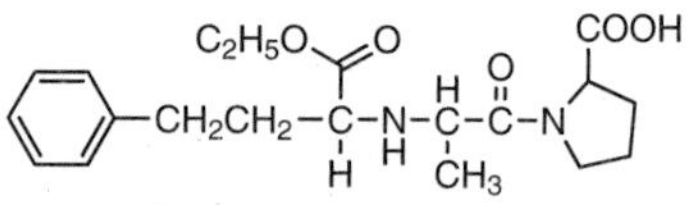

Enalapril

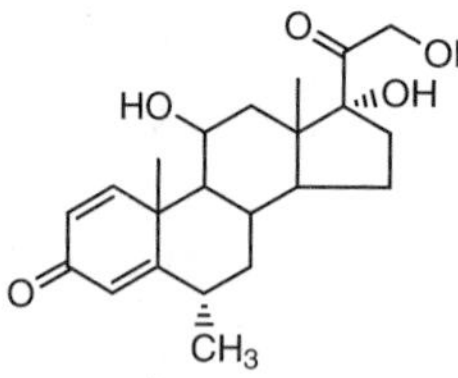

1 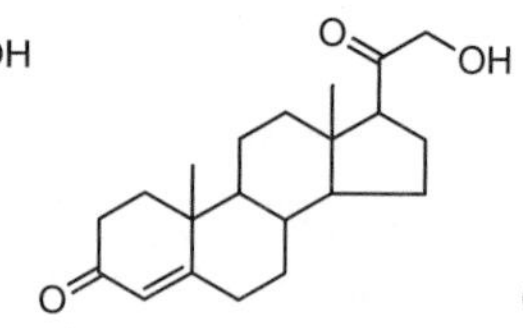   2 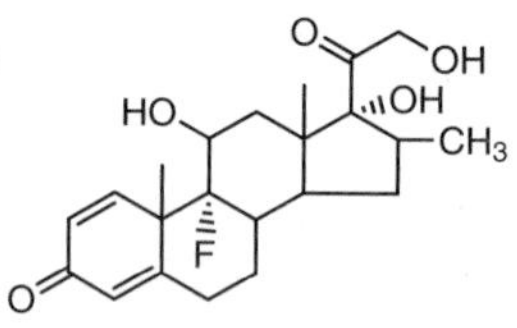   3

REFERENCES

1. Eur. J. Biochem. 1989: 186; 429.
2. Gustaffson JA et al. Endocr. Rev. 1987: 8; 185.
3. Evans RM. Science 1988: 240; 889.
4. Ringold E. Steroid Hormone Action New York: Liss, 1988.
5. Beato M. Cell 1989: 56; 335.
6. O'Malley B. Mol. Endocrinol. 1990: 4;363.
7. Carson-Jurica MA, et al. Endocr. Rev. 1990: 11; 201.
8. Jacobsen EV, et al. Recent Prog. Horm. Res. 1962: 18; 387.
9. Gorski J et al. Rec. Prog. Horm. Res. 1986: 42; 297.
10. Eickelberg O, et al. J. Biol. Chem. 1999: 274; 1005.
11. Addison T. On the Constitutional and Local Effects of Disease of the Suprarenal Capsules. London: Samuel Higley, 1855.
12. Murison PJ. Med. Clin. North Am. 1967: 51; 883.
13. Shoppee CW. Chemistry of Steroids; 2nd ed. London: 1964.
14. Simpson ER. Mol. Cell. Endocrinol. 1979: 13; 213.
15. Nelson LT, et al. Handbook of Physiology 1975: 6; 55.
16. Haynes RC. Goodman and Gilman's The Pharmacological Basis of Therapeutics; 8th ed. New York: Pergamon Press, 1990.
17. Kremers PJ. Steroid Biochem. Mol. Biol. 1976: 7; 571.
18. Makin HLJ. Biochemistry of Steroid Hormones, Second Edition Blackwell Scientific, Oxford: 1984.
19. Waterman ER, et al. Annu. Rev. Physiol. 1988: 50; 427.
20. Miller WL. Endocrine Rev. 1988: 9; 295.
21. Derendorf H Mollmann H, Barth J, et al. J Clin Pharmacol 1991; 31:473-476.
22. Romanoff LP, et al. J. Clin. Endocrinol. 1961: 21; 1413.
23. Fukushima DK, et al. J. Biol. Chem. 1955: 212; 449.
24. Dao, E. C. a. T. I. Biochim. Biophys. Acta 1962: 57; 609.
25. McEvoy GK, ed. AHFS 2000 Drug Information. Bethesda, MD: American Society of Health-System Pharmacists; 2000: 2738-2766.
26. Lunnon CH. G. a. J. B. J. Endocrinol. 1956: 3; 19.
27. Robbins ED, et al. J. Clin. Endocrinol. 1957: 17; 111.
28. Stevens W, et al. Endocrinology 1961: 68; 875.
29. Glick JH. Endocrinology 1957: 60; 368.
30. Reichstein MS. a. T. Helv. Chim. Acta 1937: 20; 1164.
31. Fieser LF. F. a. M. Steroids: New York, 1959.
32. Sarett LH. J. Biol. Chem. 1946: 162; 601.
33. McKenzie BF, et al. J. Biol. Chem. 1948: 173; 271.
34. Sarett LH. J. Am. Chem. Soc. 1949: 71; 2443.
35. Heazelwood VJ, Galligan JP, Cannell GR, et al. Br J Clin Pharmacol 1984;17:55-9.
36. Lima JJ, Jusko WJ. Clin Pharmacol Ther 1980;28:262-9.
37. Mollmann H, Barth J, Mollmann C, et al. J Pharm Sci 199; 80:835-6.
38. Derendorf H, Rohdewald P, Mollmann H, et. al. Biopharm Drug Dispos 1985;6:423-32.
39. Mahesh IE. et. al. Biochem. J. 1959: 71; 718.
40. Robinson HM. Bull. Sch. Med. Univ. Maryland 1955: 40; 72.
41. Stuart D. Pharmindex 1959: 1; 6.
42. Nobile A et al. J. Am. Chem. Soc. 1955: 77; 4184.
43. Myestre C et al. Helv. Chim. Acta 1956: 39; 734.
44. Szpilfogel SA et al. Rec. Trav. Chim. 1956: 75; 402.
45. Smith CL, Kreutner W. Arzneimittelforschung 1998;48:956-60.
46. Barth J, Damoiseaux M, Mollmann H, et al. Int J Clin Pharmacol Ther Toxicol 1992;30:317-24n.
47a. Rohatagi S, Barth J, Mollmann H, et al. J Clin Pharmacol 1997;37:916-25.
47b. Vree TB, Verwey-van Wissen CP, Lagerwerf AJ, et al. Isolation and identification of the C6-hydroxy and C20-hydroxy metabolites and glucuronide conjugate of methylprednisolone by preparative high-performance liquid chromatography from urine of patients receiving high-dose pulse therapy. J Chromatogr B Biomed Sci Appl 1999;726:157-168.
48. Mollmann H, Rohdewald P, Barth J, et al. Biopharm Drug Dispos 1989;10:453-64.
49. Spero GB, et al. J. Am. Chem. Soc. 1957: 79; 1515.
50. Boland E. W. Ann. Rheum. Dis 1962: 21; 176.
51. Derendorf H, Mollmann H, Rohdewald P, et al. Clin Pharmacol Ther 1985;37:502-7.
52. Hirshmann H, et al. J. Am. Chem. Soc. 1953: 75; 4862.
53. Ellis B, et al. J. Chem. Soc. 1955: 77; 4383.
54. Bernstein, WS. J. Am. Chem. Soc. 1955: 77; 1028.
55 Bernstein, WS. J. Am. Chem. Soc. 1956: 78; 1909.
56.a. Hochhaus G, Portner M; Barth J, et al. Pharm Res 1990; 7:558-60.
56.b. Portner M, Mollmann H, Barth J, Rohdewald P. Arzneimittelforschung 1988;38:1838-40.
57. Boland EW. Ann. N.Y. Acad. Sci. 1959: 82; 887.
58. Weiner AL. Antibiot. Chemother. 1962: 12; 360.
59. Dobes WL. South. Med. J. 1963: 56; 187.
60. Arth GE et al. J. Am. Chem. Soc. 1958: 80, 3160.
61. Oliveto EP, et al. J. Am. Chem. Soc. 1958: 80; 4428.
62. Sperber PA. Curr. Ther. Res. 1962: 4; 70.
63. Ede AL. W. a. M. J. New Drugs 1962: 2; 223.
64. Silber RH. Ann. N.Y. Acad. Sci. 1959: 82; 821.
65. Tolksdorf S. Ann. N.Y. Acad. Sci. 1959: 82; 829.
66. Loew D, Schuster O, Graul EH. Eur J Clin Pharmacol 1986; 30:225-30.
67. Rohdewald P, Mollmann H, Barth J, et al. Biopharm Drug Dispos 1987;8:205-12.
68. Nierman MM. Clin. Med. 1962: 69; 1311.
69. Coldman AC. a. J. Penn. Med. J. 1962: 65; 347.
70. Cohen AI. Antibiot. Chemother. 1962: 12; 91.
71. Bartolomei DLU. Ann. Allerg. 1961: 19; 1312.
72. Fox J, et. al. Br. Med. J. 1961: 1; 876.
73. Fox JH, et al. Br. Med. J. 1961: 2; 650.
74. Wilkinson D. S. Br. Med. J. 1961: 1; 1319.
75. Irwin GW, et al. Metabolism 1961: 10; 852.
76. Simon SW. Ann. Allerg. 1962: 20; 460.
77. Stritzler C, et al. Arch. Derm. 1962: 85; 505.
78. Feinberg SM, et al. J. New Drugs 1961: 1; 268.
79. Andersson P, Lihne M, Thalen A, et al. Xenobiotica 1987; 17:35-44.
80. Brogden RN, et al. Drugs 1984: 28; 99.
81. Green MJ, et al. J. Steroid Biochem. 1979: 11; 61.
82. Asche H, et al. Pharm. Acta Helv. 1985: 60; 232.
83. Bodor N, et al. J. Med. Chem. 1983: 26; 318.
84 Popper TL, et al. J. Steroid Biochem. Mol. Biol. 1987: 27; 837.
85. Shapiro WL, et al. J. Med. Chem. 1987: 30; 1581.
87. Barth J, Lehr KH, Derendorf H, et al. Skin Pharmacol 1993; 6:179-86.
88.a. Kelly HW. J Allergy Clin Immunol 1998; 102:S36-51.
88.b. Kelly HW Ann. Pharmacother 1998; 32:220-32.
89. Derendorf H. Respir Med 1997; 91(SUPPL. A): 22-28.
90. Derendorf H. Hochhaus G. Meibohm B. et al. J Allergy Clin Immunol 1998; 101:S440-6.
91. Wales D, Makker H, Kane J, et al. Chest 1999;115:1278-84.
92. Shaw RJ. Respir Med 1999; 93:149-60.
93. Lipworth BJ. Arch Int Med 1999; 159:941-55.
94. Brattsand R. Eur Respir Rev; 1997; 7 : 356-361.
95. Rohatagi S, Hochhaus G, Mollmann H, et al. J Clin Pharmacol 1995; 35:1187-93.
96. Argenti D, Shah B, Heald D. J Clin Pharmacol 1999; 39: 695-702.
97. Derendorf H, Hochhaus G, Rohatagi S, et al. J Clin Pharmacol 1995; 35:302-5.
98. Seale JP, Harrison LI. Respir Med 1998; 92 Suppl A:9-15.
99. Lipworth BJ, Jackson CM. Br J Clin Pharmacol 1999; 48:866-8.

100. Harrison LI, Soria I, Cline AC, et al. J Pharm Pharmacol 1999; 51:1235–40.

101. Mollmann H, Derendorf H, Barth J, et al. J Clin Pharmacol 1997; 37:893–903.

102. Dickens GR, Wermeling DP, Matheny CJ, et al. Ann Allergy Asthma Immunol 2000; 84:528–32.

103. Thalen BA, Axelsson BI, Andersson PH, et al. Steroids 1998; 63:37–43.

104. Ryrfeldt A, Andersson P, Edsbacker S, et al. Eur J Respir Dis 1982; 122(Supplement):86–95.

105. Szefler SJ. J Allergy Clin Immunol 1999; 104:175–83.

106. Miller-Larsson A, Mattsson H, Hjertberg E, et al. Drug Metab Dispos 1998;26:623–30.

107. Miller-Larsson A, Jansson P, Runstrom A, et al. Am J Respir Crit Care Med 2000;162:1455–61.

108. Pedersen S, Steffensen G, Ekman I, et al. Eur J Clin Pharmacol 1987; 31:579–82.

109. Agertoft L, Andersen A, Weibull E, et al. Arch Dis Child 1999; 80:241–7.

110.a. Popper TL, Gentles MJ, Kung TT, et al. J Steroid Biochem 1987;27:837-43.

110.b. Shapiro EL, Gentles MJ, Tiberi RL, et al. J Med Chem 1987;30:1068–73.

111. Onrust SV, Lamb HM. Drugs 1998; 56:725–45.

112. Afrime MB, et al. J Clin Pharmacol 2000; 40:1227–1236.

113. Phillipps GH. Respir Med 1990; 84(SUPPL. A):19–23; Phillipps GH, Bailey EJ, Bain BM, et al. J Med Chem 1994;37: 3717–29.

114. Harding SM. Respir Med 1990; 84(SUPPL. A):25–29.

115. Johnson M. J Allergy Clin Immunol 1998;101:S434–9.

116. Mollmann H. Wagner M. Meibohm B. et. al. Eur J Clin Pharmacol 1998; 53:459–67.

117. Mackie AE, Ventresca GP, Fuller RW, et al. Br J Clin Pharmacol 1996; 41:539–42.

118. Thorsson L, Dahlstrom K, Edsbacker S, et al. Br J Clin Pharmacol 1997; 43:155-61.

119. Rohatagi S, Bye A, Falcoz C, et al. J Clin Pharmacol 1996; 36:938-41.

120 Bush IE. Pharmacol. Rev. 1962: 14; 317.

121. Ringler I. Methods of Hormone Research; New York: Academic Press, 1964; Vol. 3.

122. Glenn EM, et al. Endocrinology 1957: 61; 128.

123. Dulin WE, et al. Proc. Soc. Exp. Biol. Med. 1957: 94, 303.

124. Fried J. Inflammation and Diseases of Connective Tissue: Philadelphia, 1961.

125. Borman JF, et al Vitam. Horm. 1958: 16; 303.

126. Funder IW, et al. Biochem. Pharmacol. 1974: 23; 1493.

127. Peterfalvi M, et al. Biochem. Pharmacol. 1980: 29, 353.

128. Duval D, et al. J. Steroid Biochem. 1984: 20; 283.

129. Agarwal MK, et al. FEBS Lett. 1987: 217; 221.

130. Counsell J. N. et. al. J. Med. Chem. 1977: 20; 762.

131. Shaw MA, et al. J. Steroid Biochem. Mol. Biol. 1988: 31, 1988.

132. Sonino, N. N. Engl. J. Med. 1987: 317; 812.

133. Potts GO, et al. Steroids 1978: 32.

134. Pratt W. B. J. Cell Biochem 1987: 35; 51.

135. de Castro M, et al. Molecular Medicine 1996: 25.; 597–607.

136. Bamberger CM, et al. J. Clinical Investigation 1995: 956.; 2435–2441.

137. Marver D. Vitam. Horm. 1980: 38; 57.

138. Dorfman R. I. Hormone Assay; New York: Academic Press, 1950.

139. Junkman K. Arch. Exp. Pathol. 1955: 227; 212.

140. Kendall RM, et al. Endocrinology 1942: 31; 573.

141. Meyer R. S. et. al. Endocrinology 1951: 48; 316.

142. Brownfield I. et al. Endocrinology 1960: 66; 900.

143. Dorfman, RI.et al. Endocrinology 1961: 69; 283.

144. Sereni F, et al. J. Biol. Chem. 1959: 234; 609.

145. Kupfer, D. Arch. Biochem. Biophys. 1968: 127; 200.

146. Tomkins GM, et al.. Proc. Natl. Acad. Sci. U.S.A. 1970: 65; 701.

147. Lee KL, et al. J. Biol. Chem. 1970: 245; 5806.

148. Feigelson P, et al. Recent Prog. Horm. Res. 1975: 31; 213.

149. Felig P, et al. Science 1970: 167 1003.

150. Kenney K L, et al. Biochem. Biophys. Res. Commun. 1970: 40; 469.

151. Ballard, P. L. Glucocorticoid Hormone Action; Springer: New York; 1979.

152. McMahon M, et al. Diabetes Metab. Rev. 1988: 4; 17.

153. DiRosa M, et al. Agents Actions 1985: 17; 284.

154. Flower LP, et al.. 1985: Life Sci. 1225.

155. Mier, CAD, et. al. N. Engl. J. Med. 1987: 317; 940.

156. Cerami, B. B. et al N. Engl. J. Med. 1987: 316; 379.

157. Radomski MW, et al. Proc. Natl. Acad. Sci. USA 1990: 87; 10043–10047.

158. Lew W, et al. J. Immunol. 1988: 140; 1895.

159. Goodwin JS, et al. J. Clin. Invest. 1986: 77; 1244.

160. Leaf G. W. et. al. A. Recent Prog. Horm. Res. 1966: 22; 431.

161. Koeppen BM, et al. Am. J. Physiol. 1983: 244; F35.

162. Wilson A. F. Fortschritte de Arzneimittelforschung; Basel-Boston-Stuttgart: Birkhauser-Verlag, 1968; Vol. 28.

163. Meduri GU, et al. Critical Care Medicine 1998: 264.; 630–633.

164. Meudri GU, et al. J. Amer. Med. Assoc. 1998: 2805.; 159–165.

165. Sciuchetti L. A. Pharmindex 1963: 5; 7.

166. Suzuki M. 1982: 92; 757.

167. Fitzpatrick TB, et al. J. Am. Chem. Soc. 1955: 158; 1149.

168. Livingood CS, et al. Arch Dermatol. 1955: 72; 313.

169. Vichyanond P, al. J. Allergy and Clinical Immunology 1989: 866; 867–873.

29. Estrogen, Progestins and Androgens

ROBERT W. BRUEGGEMEIER, DUANE D. MILLER, AND JAMES T. DALTON

INTRODUCTION

The sex steroid hormones are steroid molecules that are necessary for reproduction in females and males and affect the development of secondary sex characteristics of both sexes. The sex steroids are comprised of three classes—estrogens, progestins, and androgens. The two principal classes of female sex steroid hormones are estrogens and progestins. Chemically, the naturally occurring estrogens are C_{18} steroids and have in common an unsaturated A ring (which is planar) with a resulting phenolic function in the 3 position that aids in separation and purification from nonphenolic substances. The most potent endogenous estrogen is estradiol. The naturally occurring progestins are C_{21} steroids and have in common a 3-keto-4-ene structure in the A ring and a ketone at the C_{21} position. The most potent endogenous progestin is progesterone. The principal class of the male sex steroid hormone is the androgens. The naturally occurring androgens are C_{19} steroids and have in common oxygen atoms (as either hydroxyl or ketone groups) at both the C_3 and C_{17} positions. The androgen found in the blood is testosterone, with the more potent metabolite 5α-dihydrotestosterone formed in certain androgen target tissues. All three classes of endogenous steroids are present in both males and females, but the production and circulating plasma levels of estrogens and progestins are higher in females whereas the production and circulating plasma levels of androgens are higher in males.

FEMALE SEX HORMONES
Reproductive Cycle

Among the key events in the female reproductive process is ovulation, which is regulated by the endocrine and central nervous systems (1,2). The female reproductive cycle is controlled through an integrated system involving the hypothalamus, adenohypophysis (anterior pituitary gland), ovary, and reproductive tract (Fig. 29.1). The hypothalamus exerts its action on the adenohypophysis through a decapeptide called luteinizing hormone-releasing hormone (LHRH), also referred to as gonadotropin-releasing hormone (GnRH), which is released by the hypothalamus and stimulates the release of gonadotropins, follicle stimulating hormone (FSH) and luteinizing hormone (LH).

The two main gonadotropins, FSH and LH, regulate the ovary and its production of sex hormones. As the name implies, FSH promotes the initial development of the immature graafian follicle in the ovary. This hormone cannot induce ovulation but must work in conjunction with LH. The combined effect is to promote follicle growth and increase secretion of estrogens. Through a negative feedback system the estrogens inhibit production of FSH and stimulate output of LH. The level of LH rises to a sharp peak at midpoint in the menstrual cycle and acts on the mature follicle to bring about ovulation; LH levels are low during the menses. In contrast, FSH reaches its high level during menses, falls to a low level during and after ovulation, and then increases again toward the onset of menses.

Once ovulation has taken place, LH induces luteinization of the ruptured follicle, which leads to corpus luteum formation. After luteinization has been initiated, there is an increase in progesterone from the developing corpus luteum, which in turn suppresses production of LH. Once the corpus luteum is complete, it begins to degenerate toward menses, and the levels of progesterone and estrogen decline. The major events of the ovarian cycle are summarized in Figure 29.2.

The endometrium, a component of the genital tract, passes through different phases, which depend on the steroid hormones secreted by the ovary. During the development of the follicle, which takes approximately 10 days and is referred to as the follicular phase, the endometrium undergoes proliferation owing to estrogenic stimulation. The luteal phase follows ovulation, lasts about 14 days, and ends at menses. During the luteal phase, the endometrium shows secretory activity, and cell proliferation declines.

In the absence of pregnancy, the levels of estrogen and progesterone decline; this leads to sloughing of the endometrium. This, together with the flow of interstitial blood through the vagina, is called menses and lasts for 4–6 days. Because the estrogen and progesterone levels are now low, without feedback control from these hormones the hypothalamus releases more LHRH, and the

Estradiol	Progesterone	Testosterone	5α-Dihydrotestosterone

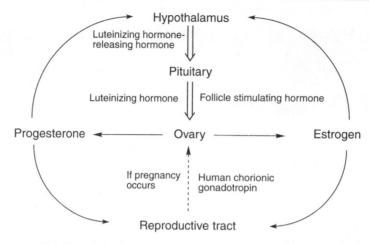

Fig. 29.1. Hypothalamic, ovarian, and reproductive tract interrelationships.

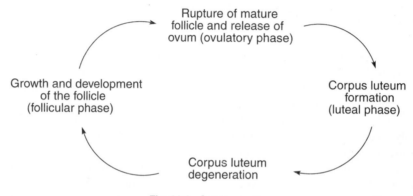

Fig. 29.2. Ovarian cycle.

cycle begins again. The reproductive cycle in the female extends from the onset of menses to the next period of menses, with a regular interval varying from 20–35 days; the average length is 28 days.

If pregnancy occurs, the menstrual cycle is interrupted because of the release of a fourth gonadotropin. In human pregnancy, the gonadotropin produced by the placenta is referred to as human chorionic gonadotropin (hCG). hCG maintains and prolongs the life of the corpus luteum. The hCG level in the urine rises to the point where it can be detected after 14 days and reaches a maximum around the seventh week of pregnancy. After this peak, the hCG concentration falls to a constant level, which is maintained throughout pregnancy.

The corpus luteum, because of hCG stimulation, provides an adequate level of the steroidal hormones to maintain pregnancy during the first nine weeks. After this period, the placenta can secrete the required level of estrogen and progestational hormones to maintain pregnancy. The levels of estrogen and progesterone increase during pregnancy and finally reach their maximal concentrations a few days before parturition. Because the level of hCG in the urine rises rapidly after conception, it has served as the basis for many pregnancy tests.

Sexual maturation, or the period in which cyclic menstrual bleeding begins to occur, is reached between the ages of 8 and 17; the average age is 11. The period of irregular menstrual cycles before the cessation of menses (menopause) (usually between the ages of 40 and 50) is commonly known as perimenopause.

Estrogens

Allen and Doisy (3) showed in 1923 that an extract of ovaries can produce estrus. Soon thereafter, it was found that a good source of estrogens is the urine of pregnant women. Estrone was the first crystalline estrogen to be isolated from such a source. Two other C_{18} estrogen steroids, 17β-estradiol and estriol, were later isolated and characterized to round out what are considered to be the three classic estrogens (4,5).

Estrone   Estriol

Biosynthesis

Estrogens are biosynthesized from cholesterol, primarily in the ovary in mature, premenopausal women. During pregnancy, the placenta is the main source of estrogen biosynthesis and pathways for production change (4,7). Small amounts of these hormones are also synthesized by the testes in the male and by the adrenal cortex, the hypothalamus, and the adenohypophysis in both sexes. The major source of estrogens in both postmenopausal women and men occurs in extraglandular sites, particularly in adipose tissue (8).

In endocrine tissues, cholesterol is the steroid that is stored and is converted to estrogen, progesterone, or androgen when the tissue is stimulated by a gonadotropic hormone. The major pathways for the biosynthesis of sex

steroid hormones are summarized in Figure 29.3. In the ovary, FSH acts on the preovulatory follicle to stimulate the biosynthesis of estrogens. The thecal cells of the preovulatory follicle convert cholesterol into androgens, whereas the granulosa cells convert androgens to estrogens. After ovulation, LH acts on the corpus luteum to stimulate both estrogen and progesterone biosynthesis and secretion.

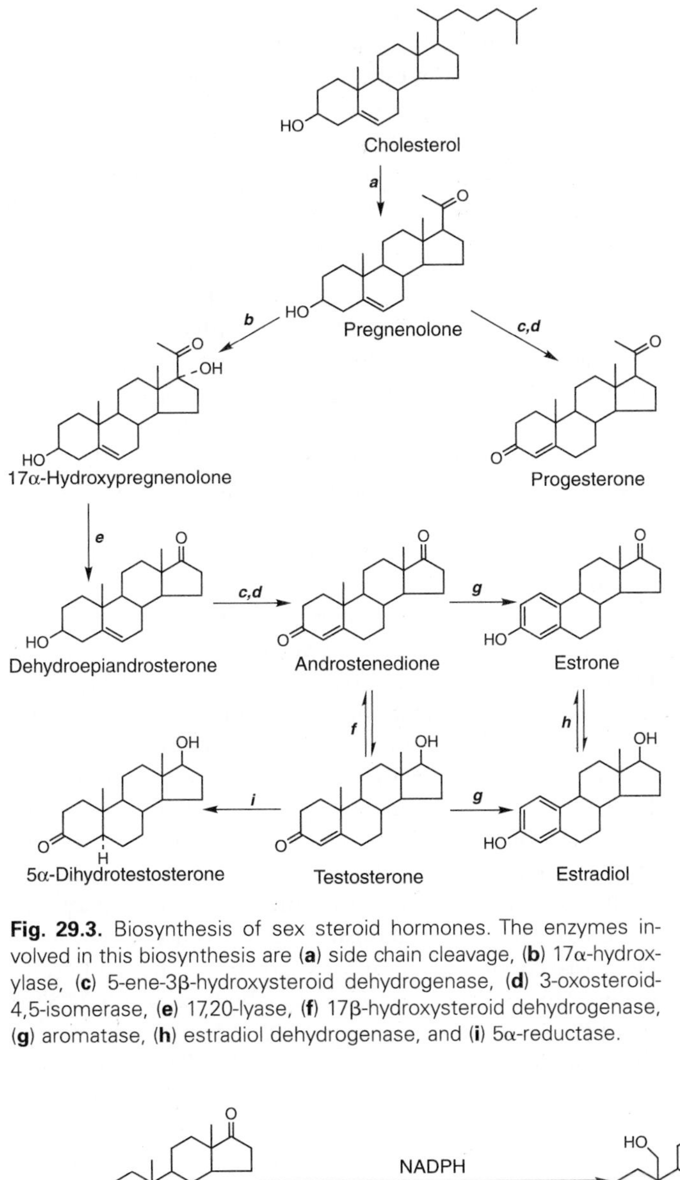

Cholesterol is converted by side chain cleavage into pregnenolone (step a), which can be converted to progesterone or by several steps to the ring A aromatic system found in estrogens (Fig. 29.3) (178). Pregnenolone is converted by 17α-hydroxylase (CYP17 isoform, a CYP450 monooxygenase) to 17α-hydroxypregnenolone (step b). The next biosynthetic step involves cleavage of the C_{17}–C_{20} carbon-carbon bond, or loss of the 17α-acetyl group from 17α-hydroxypregnenolone to yield the C_{19} intermediate dehydroepiandrosterone (DHEA) (step e). Step e is referred to as the 17,20-lyase reaction, and is catalyzed by the same CYP17 (10) which is expressed by the gene *CYP17* found on chromosome 10 in humans. DHEA is converted by 5-ene-3β-hydroxysteroid dehydrogenase and 3-oxosteroid-4,5-isomerase to the 17-ketosteroid, androstenedione (step c,d). This compound is interconvertible with the reduced 17β-hydroxy intermediate (testosterone) by 17β-hydroxysteroid dehydrogenase (step f). The final step in the biosynthesis is the conversion of the C_{19} androgens to the C_{18} estrogens. The loss of the C_{19} angular methyl group and aromatization of ring A of testosterone or androstenedione to form 17β-estradiol or estrone (step g) is catalyzed by the CYP19 isoform, aromatase. 17β-Estradiol and estrone are metabolically interconvertible, catalyzed by estradiol dehydrogenase (step h).

Research interests in the aromatization reaction continue to expand from basic endocrinology and reproductive biology studies to aromatase inhibition for the treatment of estrogen-dependent cancers, as illustrated in several conferences and reviews (11–15). Androstenedione is the preferred substrate for aromatization and three molecules of NADPH and three molecules of oxygen are necessary for conversion of one molecule of androgen to estrogen (16,17). Aromatization (Fig. 29.4) proceeds via three successive steps catalyzed by the CYP450 isoform CYP19 present in the endoplasmic reticulum of the cell. The gene *CYP19*

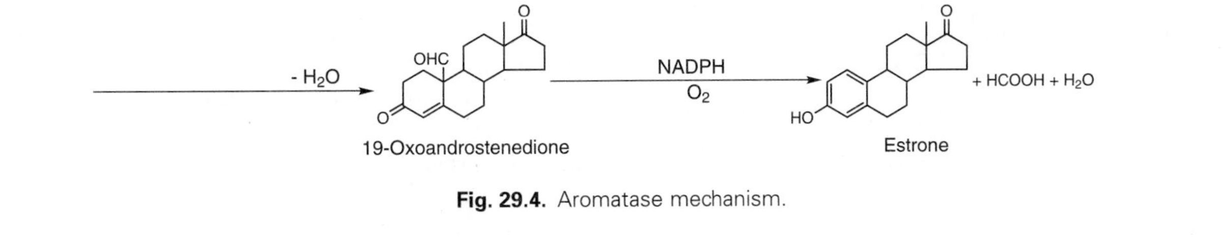

Fig. 29.3. Biosynthesis of sex steroid hormones. The enzymes involved in this biosynthesis are (**a**) side chain cleavage, (**b**) 17α-hydroxylase, (**c**) 5-ene-3β-hydroxysteroid dehydrogenase, (**d**) 3-oxosteroid-4,5-isomerase, (**e**) 17,20-lyase, (**f**) 17β-hydroxysteroid dehydrogenase, (**g**) aromatase, (**h**) estradiol dehydrogenase, and (**i**) 5α-reductase.

Fig. 29.4. Aromatase mechanism.

expresses CYP19 which is located on chromosome 15 in humans; lack of this enzyme causes an estrogen deficiency and failure of females to develop at puberty. The first step involves oxidation of the angular C_{19} methyl group to provide 19-hydroxyandrostenedione. 19,19-Dihydroxyandrostenedione, isolated as 19-oxoandrostenedione, is formed by the second oxidation step. The exact mechanism of the last oxidation remains to be fully determined (18–20). Following the last oxidation, the C_{10}–C_{19} bond is cleaved and aromatization of the A ring occurs. In this last step, the C_{19} carbon atom is lost as formic acid and oxygens from the first and last step are incorporated into the formic acid. The 1β-hydrogen and 2β-hydrogen atoms are also lost during aromatization. A summary of the proposed mechanisms and the biochemistry of aromatase has been reviewed (21).

Metabolism

The endogenous estrogens, estrone and 17β-estradiol, are biochemically interconvertible by the enzyme estradiol dehydrogenase and yield the same metabolic products (Fig.

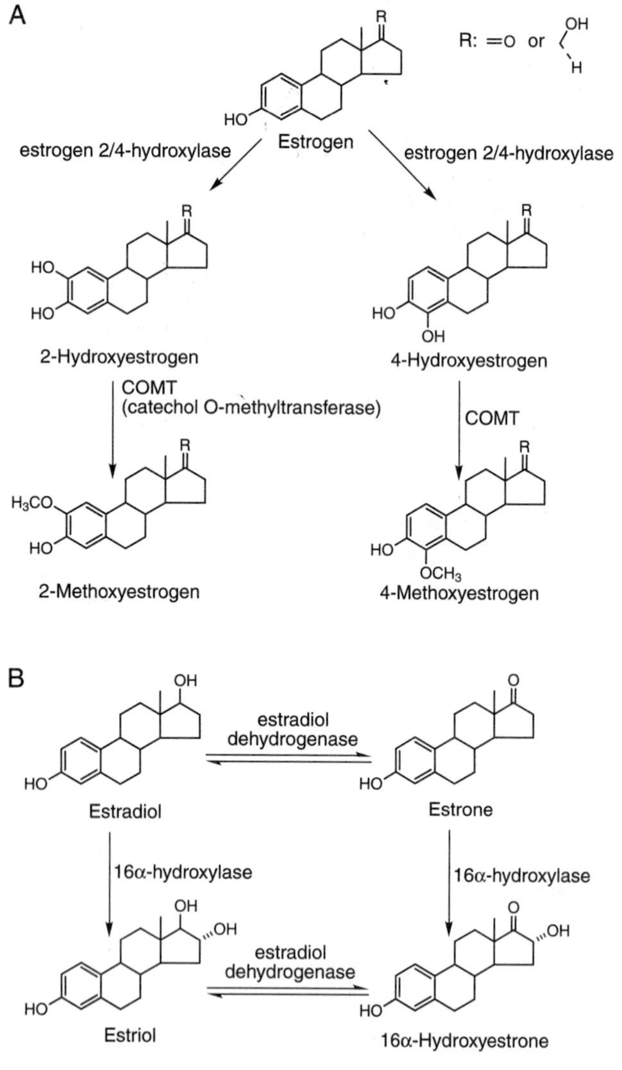

Fig. 29.5. Estrogen metabolism.

29.5A) (22–24). Estradiol dehydrogenase is one member of a family of closely related enzymes called 17β-hydroxysteroid dehydrogenases. These hormones are metabolized mainly in the liver and largely excreted as water-soluble glucuronide and sulfate conjugates. The sulfotransferase isoform SULT1E1 (formerly known as estrogen sulfotransferase, EST) preferentially sulfates estradiol in the nanomolar range and SULT2A1 (formerly known as DHEA-ST or dehydroepiandrosterone sulfotransferase) conjugates DHEA, estradiol in the micromolar range, the synthetic estrogens and other estrogen metabolites. During hepatic metabolism estrogens are desulfated and resulfated to create a drug reservoir of estrogen. Other tissues, such as those in the kidneys and intestines, may also be involved, but unlike the liver, they apparently contain no steroid sulfokinases (25). Renal and intestinal preparations affect sulfate conjugation with low-molecular-weight phenols, but not with estrogens (26). Estrogens exhibit moderate (estriol 50%) to high (estradiol 90%) protein binding to sex hormone-binding globulin (SHBG) and albumin. Estradiol is capable of inducing the synthesis of SHBG.

Most of the accountable metabolites for estradiol appear in the urine, even though 50% of a dose of 17β-estradiol first goes to the kidney through the liver, and the remaining 50% from the liver is found in bile fluid (22). The reason is that much of the material found in bile subsequently enters the intestine, is reabsorbed there, and is returned to the liver; only 10% of the administered dose is found in the feces (4).

Many metabolites have been isolated from urine, but to date no one has been able to account for all the radioactivity of an administered dose of (14) C-labeled 17β-estradiol. The major metabolites are shown in Figure 29.5. Both 17β-estradiol and estrone are converted by the CYP450 enzyme complex 16α-hydroxylase to yield estriol. Estriol is found in the urine as the glucuronide conjugate. The naturally occurring estrogens exhibit poor bioavailability and are thus only weakly active when administered orally because of first pass intestinal (conjugation) and hepatic (oxidation) metabolism. Estrogens are metabolized by hydroxylation at positions ortho to the 3-phenolic group. Metabolism by estrogen 2/4-hydroxylase (CYP3A4) provides the catechol estrogens, 2-hydroxyestrogens and the 4-hydroxyestrogens (Fig. 29.5B). These phenolic metabolites are unstable in vivo and are rapidly converted to their 2-methoxyestrogens and 4-methoxyestrogen metabolites and also to their glucuronide, sulfate, and glutathione conjugates. These metabolites are also found in comparatively large amounts in the urine (22–24). The catechol estrogens will bind to estrogen receptors and produce weak to moderate estrogenic effects. Estrogens have also been shown to be produced in certain CNS tissues such as those in the pituitary and hypothalamus, suggesting possible neuroendocrine functions. The formation, metabolism, and biologic effects of catechol estrogens have been reviewed (30).

Steroidal Estrogens

Estradiol. Estradiol is the most potent endogenous estrogen, exhibiting high affinity for the estrogen receptor and potency when administered parenterally. When administered orally, estradiol is promptly conjugated in the intestine and oxidatively metabolized by the liver, resulting in its low oral bioavailability and therapeutic effectiveness. Its primary metabolite is 2-hydroxyestradiol which is excreted primarily as its sulfate, but also as glucuronide conjugates. Estradiol exhibits high protein binding, especially to sex hormone-binding globulin (SHBG), whose synthesis estradiol is capable of inducing. Comparative dosage ranges for estradiol, estrone, and estriol and their synthetic preparations are shown in Table 29.1 and its pharmacokinetic properties in Table 29.2.

A formulation of estradiol utilized for the treatment of menopause symptoms is a patch which is placed on the abdomen for local release of estradiol. This estrogen patch provides sufficient estradiol concentrations for physiologic effects on the uterus, whereas the systemic levels of estradiol are low because of rapid liver metabolism of the hormone once it enters the circulatory system (35,36). Transdermal estradiol patch with a fixed combination with norethindrone acetate is CombiPatch. Estradiol also is commercially available as a vaginal ring. Estradiol is also formulated in a micronized preparation for the treatment of menopause symptoms.

Ethinyl Estradiol and Mestranol. One successful method for overcoming this rapid oxidative inactivation of 17β-estradiol to estrone by 17β-hydroxysteroid dehydrogenase in the liver has been to block the alcoholic function at C_{17} with an appropriate substituent. Treatment of estrone with potassium acetylide in liquid ammonia results in ethinyl estradiol, an estrogenic substance that is about 15–20 times more potent than estradiol when taken orally (31) (Fig. 29.6). The presence of the 17α-ethinyl or other alkyl group results in an orally effective compound by preventing its conversion to estrone. Following oral administration, ethinyl estradiol is rapidly and almost completely absorbed with an oral bioavailability of approximately 40% and an elimination half-life of 26 hours (pharmacokinetics Table 29.2). Ethinyl estradiol displays linear pharmacokinetics. Ethinyl estradiol undergoes extensive first-pass metabolism to its 3-O-glucuronide and 3-O-sulfate metabolites and by first pass aromatic hydroxylation to its major hydroxylated metabolite, 2–hydroxyethinylestradiol and its O-methyl metabolites. This metabolite is thought to contribute to some of the adverse cardiovascular effects of the drug. Ethinyl estradiol undergoes extensive enterohepatic circulation as glucuronide and sulfate conjugates involving the bacteria in the GI tract which hydrolyze these conjugates that are excreted into the GI tract via bile, allowing reabsorption of ethinyl estradiol. Another semisynthetic estrogen, synthesized by a similar route, is mestranol, the 3-O-methyl ether of ethinyl estradiol (Fig. 29.6). Mestranol is a pro-drug and is rapidly metabolized mainly to ethinyl estradiol by hepatic O-demethylation following its oral administration. Mestranol and ethynylestradiol are used primarily in oral contraceptives (32).

Esters of Estradiol. Whenever long-term estrogenic therapy is needed, esters of 17β-estradiol and other estrogens are preferred and are usually given intramuscularly in contrast to the ethinyl derivatives, which are given orally. Among the esters of estradiol being used include the 17β-valerate and the 17β-cyclopentylpropionate

Table 29.1 Dosages for Estrogens[*]

Estrogen	Trade Name	Route of Administration	Frequency of Administration	Usual Dosage Range (mg)
Estradiol	Estrace	Oral	Daily	0.5–2
	Estrace	Vaginal	Biweekly	0.1–0.2
Estrone		Intramuscular	Daily	0.1–3
Ethinyl estradiol	Estinyl	Oral	1–3 times daily	0.02–2
Estradiol valerate	Delestrogen, Gynogen Valergen	Intramuscular	Monthly	10–20
Estradiol cypionate	depoGynogen, Deopgen	Intramuscular	Biweekly	0.5–5
Estradiol trandermal system	Alora, Climare, Estraderm, Fempatch, Vivelle, Villelle-Dot	Topical/patch	Biweekly	0.25–0.1/24h.
Estradiol ring	Estring	Vaginal	3 months	2/3mo.
Conjugated Estrogens	Premarin, Premphase, Prempro	Oral	Daily	0.3–2.5
	Premarin Intravenous	Parenteral	Twice daily	25
	Premarin Vaginal Cream	Vaginal	Daily	0.3–1.25
Synthetic Conjugated Estrogens A	Cenestin	Oral	Daily	0.625–0.9
Esterified Estrogens	Estratest	Oral, Vaginal	Daily	0.3–2.5
Estropipate (piperazine estrone sulfate)	Ogen Orth-Est	Vaginal	Daily	3–6

[*]Abstracted from McEvoy GK, ed. AHFS 2000 Drug Information, Bethesda, MD; American Society of Health-System Pharmacists.

Table 29.2. Pharmacokinetic Properties for Some Estrogenic and Progestional Agents[1]

Drug	Protein[2] Binding	Oral Bioavailability	Biotransformation	Elimination Half-life (Hrs)	Time to Peak Conc. (Hrs)	Peak Serum Conc. (ng/mL)	Elimination (%)
Estradiol	50–80%	Poor	Hepatic first pass metabolism	20 min		0.1–0.2	Renal: 90[4]
Ethinyl estradiol	98%	40%		26 (6–20)	1–2	33	
Progesterone[3]							
Oral 200 mg micronized	>90%	<10%	Hepatic first pass metabolism	<5 min	2–4	24.3	Renal: 50–60[4]
IM 45 mg			Hepatic	10 wks	28	39.1	Fecal: 10
IM 90 mg				19.6	9.2	53.8	
Vaginal gel 45 mg				34.8	6.8	14.9	
Medroxyprogesterone acetate: Oral 10 mg	>90%	high	Hepatic	30	2–4	19–35	Renal: 15–22[4]
IM 150 mg/mL every 3 months			No first-pass hepatic metabolism	50 days	3 weeks	1–7	Fecal: 45–80
Megestrol acetate							
Oral 160 mg	>90%	ND	Hepatic	38 (13–104)	2–3	200	Renal: 66[4]
Oral 600 mg					2–3	753	Fecal: 20
Norgestrel	.90%	60%	Hepatic	20	24	ND	Renal: 45 Fecal: 32
Levonorgestrel 3/12/60 months implants 216 mg loading dose[3]	>90%	60	No first-pass Hepatic metabolism	16 (8–30)	24	1.6 first week, then 0.26–0.4	Renal: 45[4] Fecal: 32
Desogestrel (Desogen) (as 3-keto-desgestrel)	>90%	76	First pass to 3-ketodesogestrel active metabolite	12–58	1–2	2–6	Renal:[4] Fecal
Norethindrone	>80%	65	Hepatic first pass metabolism	8 (5–14)	0.5–4	5–10	Renal: 50[4] Fecal: 20–40
Norethindrone acetate	>80%	65	Hepatic first pass metabolism	8 (5–14)	0.5–4	5–10	Renal: 50[4] Fecal: 20–40
Norgestimate (as desacetylnorgestimate	>50–60% >90%	60	First pass to Desacetylnorgestimate	37	1–2	0.5–0.7	Renal[4] fecal

[1]USP Drug Information 2000
[2]Sex hormone binding globulin (SHBG) synthesis is stimulated by estrogens and inhibited by androgens; levels are twice as high in women as in men. Progesterone binds strongly to cortisol binding globulin (CBG) 17.7%, SHBG 0.6%, and weakly to albumin 79.3%. Absorption is the rate-limiting step for the elimination half-life. Levonorgestrel: Free, 1.1–1.7%; SHBG 92–62%; albumin 37.56%, but suppresses SHBG by 33%. Norethindrone: Free 3.5%; SHBG 35.5%; albumin 61%. Medroxyprogesterone does not bind SHBG. 3-Keto-desgestrel 64% albumin, 32% SHBG. Norgestimate >90% protein bound; not SHBG
[3]A mean dose of 35 mcg levonorgestrel is released daily. ND = no data available
[4]renal metabolites are primarily conjugates

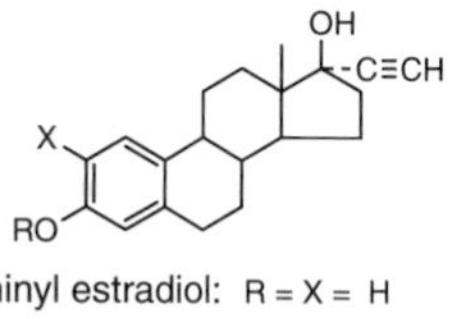

Ethinyl estradiol: R = X = H
Mestranol: R = CH$_3$; X = H
  2-Hydroxyethinylestradiol: R = H; X = OH

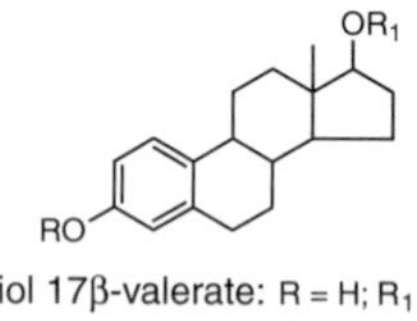

Estradiol 17β-valerate: R = H; R$_1$ = CH$_3$(CH$_2$)$_3$CO
Estradiol 17β-cyclopentylpropionate:

R = H
R$_1$ = cyclopentyl–CH$_2$CH$_2$CO

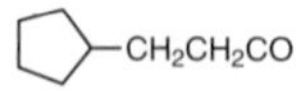

Fig. 29.6. 17α-Ethinyl estrogens, and Estradiol Esters.

(cypionate) (Fig. 29.6). Estradiol cypionate is formed by esterification of the 17β-hydroxy group of estradiol with cyclopentanepropionic acid and is available as a sterile solution of the drug in a suitable oil (e.g., cottonseed oil). Estradiol valerate is the 17β-valerate ester of estradiol and

its injection is available as a sterile solution in a suitable vegetable oil (e.g., sesame oil, castor oil). These esters may be thought of as pro-drugs, because when they are administered intramuscularly, slow hydrolysis of the ester in vivo releases the free estradiol over a prolonged period of time. Estradiol valerate has a duration of action of 14–21 days, and estradiol cypionate has a duration of action of 14–28 days.

Conjugated Estrogens

Conjugated water-soluble metabolites of naturally occurring estrogens obtained from the urine of pregnant mares are also utilized as estrogen preparations, referred to as conjugated estrogenic substances (Fig. 29.7). Conjugated Estrogens USP is a mixture of the sodium salts of the water-soluble sulfate esters of estradiol metabolites derived wholly or in part from equine urine or prepared synthetically from estrone and equilin blended to represent the composition of estrogens derived from pregnant mare urine; primarily a mixture of sodium estrone sulfate (52.5–61.5%) and sodium equilin sulfate (22.5–30.5%) as well as the lesser metabolites, 17α-dihydroequilenin, 17α-estradiol, 17β-dihydroequilenin, 17β-dihydroequilenin, δ8,9-dehydroestrone, and 17β-estradiol as sodium sulfate conjugates. Pregnant mares produce two unique estrogenic compounds, equilenin and equilin which are not found in humans, and are secreted in the urine as their sodium sulfate conjugates. Because the conjugated estrogens are the sodium sulfate conjugates of equilin and estrone, the preparation is incompatible with acidic solutions. Another sulfate conjugate that is soluble in warm water and orally effective is estropipate (piperazine estrone sulfate). This derivative has the same actions and uses as the conjugated naturally occurring estrogens. Esterified Estrogens USP is a blend of estrone sodium sulfate (75–85%) and sodium equilin sulfate (6–15%) which are synthetically derived from plant sterols.

Synthetic Conjugated Estrogens A is a mixture of conjugated estrogens prepared synthetically from plant sources (i.e., soy and yams) containing a mixture of 9 of the 10 known conjugated estrogenic substances present in Conjugated Estrogens USP. Synthetic Conjugated Estrogens A is mixture of the sodium salts of water-soluble estrogen sulfates including primarily estrone sulfate and sodium equilin sulfate, but also 17α-dihydroequilin, 17α-estradiol, 17β-dihydroequilenin, equilenin, and 17β-estradiol as sodium sulfate conjugates.

Nonsteroidal Estrogens

Stilbene Derivatives. The steroid nucleus is not required for estrogenic activity. Many derivatives of stilbene (diphenylethylene), which is considerably more stable as the *trans* isomer, are potent estrogenic substances that were used therapeutically (Fig. 29.8). One of the most important synthetic estrogens was diethylstilbestrol (*trans* α,α′-diethyl-4,4′-stilbenediol, DES). This drug was significantly cheaper than naturally occurring estrogens and yet can produce all the same effects. DES has 10 times the estrogenic potency of its *cis* isomer because the *trans* isomer resembles more closely estradiol (38). However, DES when taken during pregnancy, is believed to be the cause of neoplasias in the offspring. Also, a higher incidence of uterine cancers has been linked to clinical use of estrogens as replacement therapy in menopausal women. For these reasons DES and its diphosphate ester are no longer used as an estrogen in women, but are used to treat prostatic cancer in men.

Hexestrol is the meso form of 3,4-bis(p-hydroxyphenyl)-n-hexane which has the greatest estrogenic potency of the three stereoisomers of the dihydro analog of DES. However, it is less potent than DES.

Another estrogenic substance related to DES is dienestrol which is structurally similar to DES but differs structurally from DES in the substitution of two unsaturated ethylidene groups for the two diethyl groups of DES (Fig. 29.8). Although primarily used intravaginally in the management of

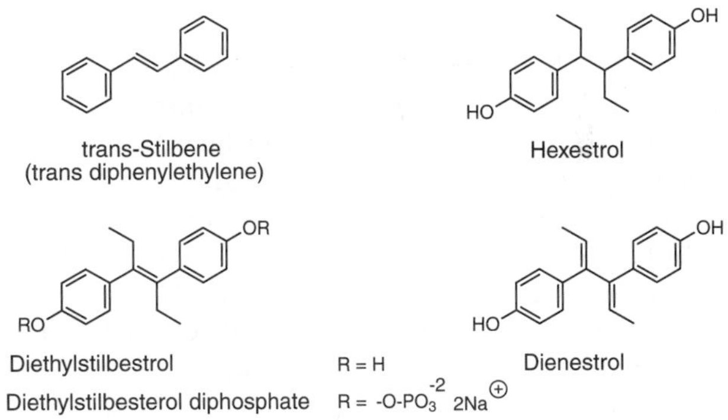

trans-Stilbene
(trans diphenylethylene)

Hexestrol

Diethylstilbestrol — R = H

Diethylstilbesterol diphosphate — R = -O-PO$_3^{-2}$ 2Na$^{\oplus}$

Dienestrol

Fig. 29.8. Nonsteroidal estrogens.

Equilenin

Equilin — R = H
Equilin sodium sulfate — R = SO$_3^-$ Na$^+$

Estrone — R = H
Estrone sodium sulfate — R = SO$_3^-$ Na$^+$
Piperazine estrone sulfate — R = SO$_3^-$

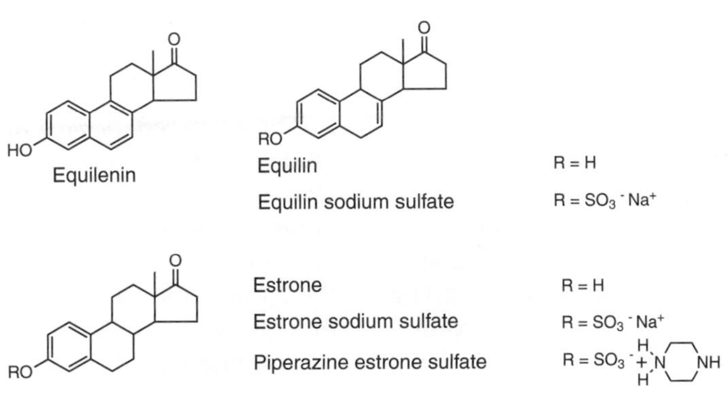

Fig. 29.7. Conjugated and esterified estrogens.

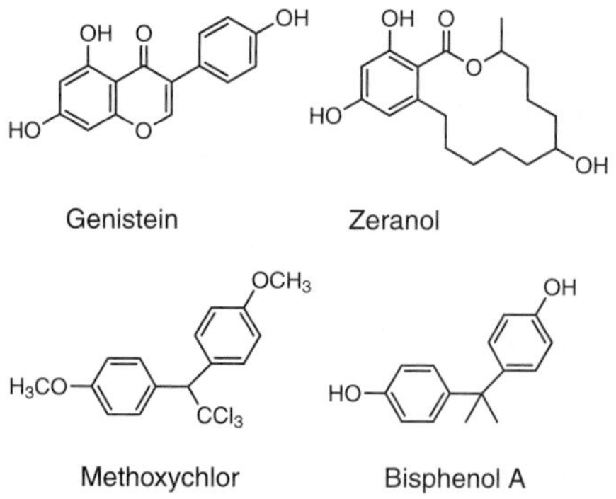

Fig. 29.9. Xenoestrogens.

vaginal and urethral atrophy (atrophic vaginitis), dienestrol shares the pharmacologic and toxic effects of other estrogens, and the usual cautions, precautions, and contraindications associated with estrogen therapy should be observed.

Xenoestrogens. One final group of nonsteroidal agents that have weak estrogenic activity but have received a significant amount of attention in recent years is the xenoestrogens, also referred to as the environmental estrogens (Fig. 29.9) (39). This class is comprised of widely varied structures, including isoflavanoid phytoestrogens such as genistein, the mycotoxin zeranol, pesticides such as methoxychlor, and industrial chemicals such as bisphenol A. All of these compounds have significantly weaker estrogenic activities (less than 1.0% of estradiol).

Structure-activity Relationships. Analysis of the biological activities of both steroidal and nonsteroidal estrogens, *in vitro* investigations with subcellular fractions containing estrogen receptors, and recent X-ray crystallography studies on the ligand binding domain of the estrogen receptor have resulted in an extensive knowledge of the structure-activity relationships for estrogens (40–43). These studies demonstrated the high affinity and specificity of the most potent endogenous estrogen, estradiol. The aromatic A-ring and the hydroxyl substituent at C_3 of the steroid nucleus are structural features essential for estrogenic activity, with the hydroxyl group being involved in hydrogen bonding. The 17β-hydroxyl functional group, the distance between the two hydroxyl groups, and a planar hydrophobic molecule are also important for imparting full estrogenic activity to the molecule.

For optimal estrogenic activity, the distance between the oxygen atoms of the two hydroxyl groups ranges from 10.3 Å–12.1 Å. Two models are proposed for the distance range. In the first model, the region of the estrogen receptor that binds the D-ring is flexible and can conform to ligands with different distances (e.g., 10.9 Å for estradiol and 12.1 Å for DES). The second model proposes that a water molecule present with estradiol bridges the difference in the O-O distances. Many other potent steroidal and nonsteroidal estrogens conform to this hypothesis.

Substituents on the estrogen nucleus significantly modify estrogenic activity. On the A-ring, any functionality at the C_1 position greatly reduces activity and only small groups can be accommodated at the 2 and 4 positions. Insertion of hydroxyl groups at positions 6, 7, and 11 reduces activity. Removal of the oxygen function from position 3 or 17 or epimerization of the 17β-hydroxyl group of estradiol to the α-configuration results in a less active estrogenic substance (44). Introduction of unsaturation into the B ring similarly reduces potency. Substituents at the 11β position can be well tolerated; for example, 11β-methoxy or 11β-ethyl have significantly greater affinity for estrogen receptor compared to estradiol.

Modifications at the 17α and 16 positions can lead to enhanced activity. 17α-ethinyl or 17α-vinyl groups provide the greatest activity, while highly polar groups are poorly tolerated. At the 16 position, moderate size and polarity are tolerated. Enlargement of the D ring of both estradiol and estrone (i.e., D-homoestradiol,) greatly reduces estrogenic activity. On the other hand, an intact D ring is not required for estrogenic activity in rats; doisynolic acid, obtained from cleavage of estrone by a strong base, retains a high degree of hormonal activity.

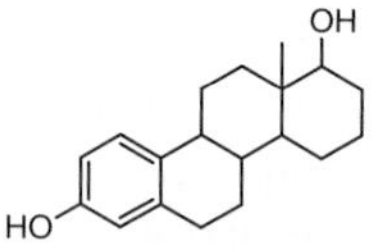

D-Homoestradiol 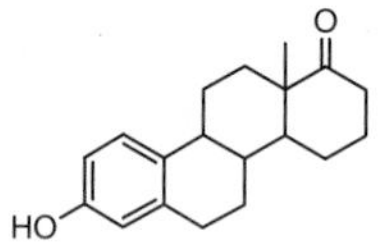   D-Homoestrone 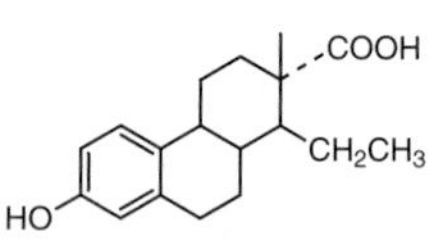   Doisynolic acid

Many compounds have estrogenic activity; this includes substances that do not have the estrane steroid nucleus (45). Estrogenic activity is unique in that it does not require a strict structural configuration as do the other sex hormones and the adrenocorticoids. The constituents of many plants have estrogenic activity, and one of these xenoestrogens, genistein, found in both soy products and subterranean clover, causes infertility in Australian sheep when eaten (Fig. 29.9). Another naturally occurring xenoestrogen found in a number of legumes is coumestrol, which is even more potent than genistein (46).

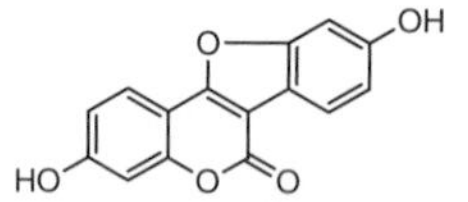

Coumestrol

The observed *in vivo* biologic activity varies with the mode of administration of the estrogens. The order of activity of the three naturally occurring steroids when administered subcutaneously is estradiol > estrone > estriol. The order changes to estriol > estradiol > estrone, however, when the drugs are administered orally (47). Although the naturally occurring steroids have activity when administered orally, chemical modifications have led to better orally effective estrogens.

Therapeutically, ethinyl estradiol is a more effective oral estrogen than many others because of its resistance to metabolism in the gastrointestinal tract and in the liver. Also, metabolic conjugation may produce estrogens that retain some of their activity; it has been reported that estrone sulfate is actually more active than the original hormone when administered orally to rats. The modified drug also retains some activity in humans (48,49).

Ester derivatives (valerates and cypionates) of the naturally occurring and synthetic estrogens have a prolonged action. The free hormone is released slowly because of hydrolysis of the ester in vivo. Another attempt to prepare highly active estrogens has led to the development of labile ethers of various estrogens (50). Two potent derivatives of estradiol are the 3-(2-tetrahydropyranyl) and 17β-(2-tetrahydropyranyl) derivatives. These drugs proved to be 12 and 15 times as active, respectively, as estradiol. The estrogenic activity was greatest when these drugs were administered orally. The remarkably high ratio of oral to subcutaneous potency of 403 observed with 17β-estradiol-3-(2-tetrahydropyranyl) ether may be contrasted with the 3,17β-bis-(2-tetrahydropyranyl) derivative, which is less active than estradiol.

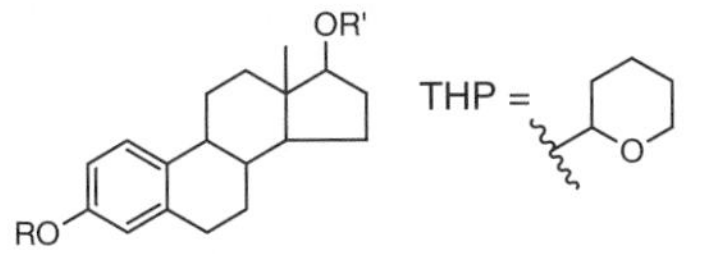

3-(2-Tetrahydropyranyl) derivative   R = THP; R' = H
17β-(2-tetrahydropyranyl) derivative   R = H; R' = THP
3,17β-bis-(2-Tetrahydropyranyl) derivative   R = R' = THP

When estrogens were first obtained, the scarcity of the natural hormones led chemists to prepare synthetic materials that could be used as substitutes. DES, prepared in 1939, was one of the most active and commercially successful nonsteroidal estrogens (51–53). Although many stilbene estrogen derivatives have been prepared, they are not commonly used today. The synthetic estrogens have the same spectrum of effects as the natural steroidal estrogens.

Estrogen Antagonists

Agents that antagonize the actions of estrogens are of particular interest for their ability to modify reproductive processes and for the treatment of estrogen-dependent breast cancer. Three groups of agents are identified as estrogen antagonists—impeded estrogens, triphenylethylene antiestrogens, and aromatase inhibitors.

The impeded estrogens interact with the estrogen receptor in target tissues but dissociate from the receptor too rapidly to produce any strong estrogenic effect. If, however, the impeded estrogens are present in a high local concentration, these agents compete with or impede the access of estradiol to the receptor site, thus decreasing the estradiol's effect on the cell (54,4). The classical impeded estrogen is estriol.

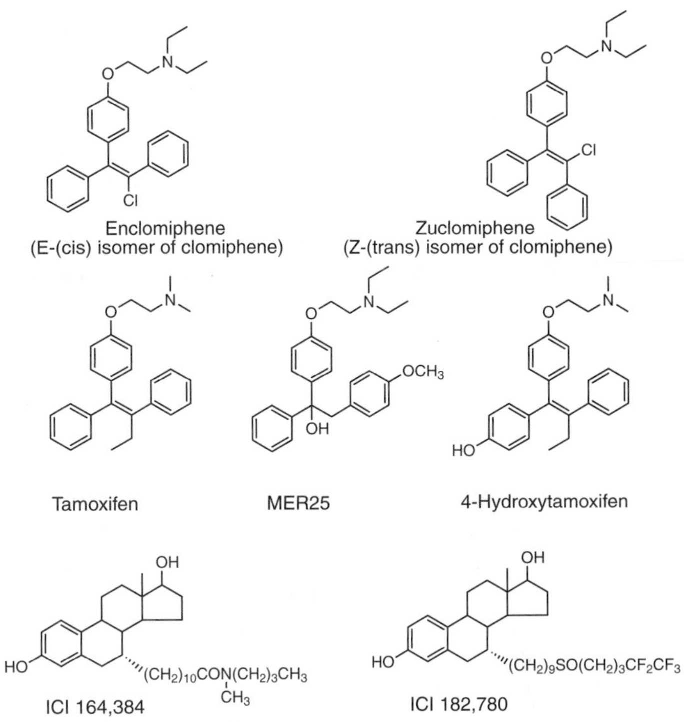

Antiestrogens—Triphenylethylene Analogs. A search for more potent antiestrogens related to MER25, a weak

Fig. 29.10. Antiestrogens.

antiestrogen, lead to the discovery of a number of triphenylethylene antiestrogens (Fig. 29.10), which are also structurally related to the stilbene (diphenylethylene) family of nonsteroidal estrogens and to the antilipidemic agent, triparanol. They exhibit a strong and persistent binding to the estrogen receptor, producing antiestrogen-receptor complexes that are either unable to translocate into the nucleus of target cells or, if translocated, do not bind properly to the acceptor site of the chromatin to produce an estrogenic response (55,56).

Clomiphene citrate (Clomid) has both estrogenic and antiestrogenic properties (partial agonist) and is used to induce ovulation for the treatment of infertility. Clomiphene is orally administered as a mixture of two geometric isomers; the Z (cis, also called zuclomiphene) diastereomer displays estrogenic activity and the E (trans, also called enclomiphene) diastereomer, antiestrogenic activity. Collectively, these geometric isomers are responsible for clomiphene's estrogenic and antiestrogenic properties. It produces an increase in the secretion of the pituitary gonadotropins, follicle-stimulating hormone (FSH), and luteinizing hormone (LH). This effect results in development and maturation of the ovarian follicle, ovulation, and subsequent development and function of the corpus luteum (4). This effect is the result of the binding of clomiphene to estrogen receptors in the hypothalamus, leading to a blockade of the feedback inhibition exhibited by estrogens. Clomiphene is readily absorbed from the GI tract following oral administration with a half-life of about 5 days. It is metabolized in the liver, and its metabolites are excreted principally in the feces via enterohepatic recirculation.

Tamoxifen (Nolvadex) is an estrogen agonist-antagonist (partial agonist) that is used as an antiestrogen in the treatment of estrogen-dependent breast cancer (see Chapter 43 for more discussion), but with weak estrogen-like (agonist) effects at several sites, including endometrium, bone, and lipids. Tamoxifen is orally administered as the Z-diastereomer which undergoes rapid N-demethylation to its major metabolite N-demethyltamoxifen by CYP3A4, and primarily by CYP2D6 to its minor metabolite, 4-hydroxytamoxifen. Evidence suggests that 4-hydroxytamoxifen is the active metabolite of tamoxifen (57,58). The aminoethyl ether side chain of the triphenylethylene antiestrogens is critical for the antiestrogenic activity of these agents. Tamoxifen produces antagonist effects in breast tissue, whereas it produces agonist effects in other estrogen responsive tissues such as uterus and bone.

Toremifene (chlorotamoxifen, Fareston) is structurally and pharmacologically related to tamoxifen, but differs from tamoxifen by chlorination of the ethyl side chain, which reduces its antiestrogenic potency (Fig. 29.10). Toremifene, like tamoxifen undergoes rapid N-demethylation to its active metabolite N-demethyltoremifene, by CYP3A4 and <10% is excreted in the urine. As with any of these triphenylethylene antiestrogens because they are extensively metabolized in the liver, they should be used with caution in patients with hepatic impairment since their elimination can be prolonged in these patients.

Recently, steroidal derivatives ICI 164,384 and ICI 182,780 have been described and are referred to as pure antiestrogens because they bind tightly to estrogen receptors, effectively block estradiol binding, and are completely devoid of estrogenic activity (59,60).

Selective Estrogen Receptor Modulators. Recent advances in the molecular pharmacology of estrogen and estrogen receptors have resulted in the development of substances that function as selective estrogen receptor modulators (called SERMs) that activate the estrogen receptor but that also exhibit tissue-specific estrogen-agonist or -antagonist activity (partial agonists) (see Chapter 43 for more discussion) (61). A search for antiestrogens that

are rigid analogs of the triphenylethylene series without the problems of geometric isomers, lead to the development of 3,4-dihydronaphthalene and benzothiophene analogs as SERMs. The first SERM marketed is the benzothiophene, raloxifene (Evista), which was introduced to maintain bone density in controlling osteoporosis postmenopausal women (an estrogen effect).

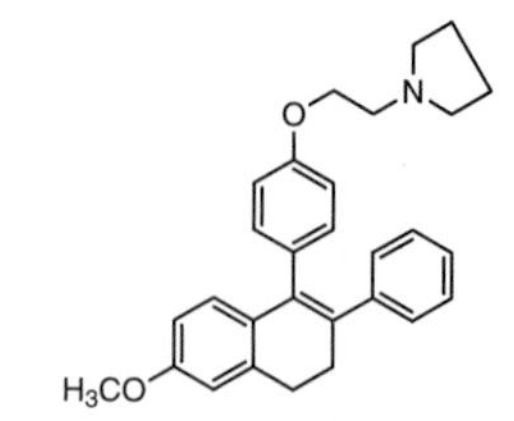

Nafoxidine
(a 3,4-Dihydronaphthalene analog)

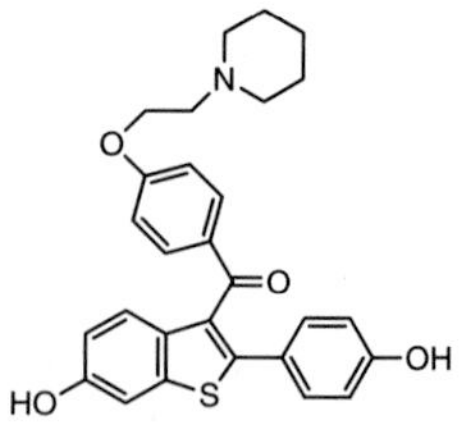

Raloxifene
(a benzothiophene analog)

Furthermore, raloxifene produces antiestrogenic effects in breast tissue and does not exhibit estrogenic effects in the uterus (62). Following oral administration, raloxifene undergoes rapid first pass metabolism to form its glucuronide conjugates, and thus has an oral bioavailability of less than 5%. Any CYP450 oxidation is minimal.

Aromatase Inhibitors

Androstenedione Derivatives. Inhibitors of aromatase (CYP19) block the conversion of androgens to estrogens and thus have therapeutic potential in the control of reproductive functions and in the treatment of estrogen-dependent cancers such as breast cancer. Steroidal agents under investigation include 4-hydroxyandrostenedione (63), various 7α-substituted androst-4-ene-3,17-diones (64) and androsta-1,4-diene-3,17-diones (65), 10β-propynylestr-4-ene-3,17–dione (66), 1-methylandrost-4-ene-3,17-dione (67), and 6-methyleneandrost-4-ene-3,17-dione (Fig. 29.11) (68). These steroidal agents compete with androstenedione for binding to the active site of the aromatase enzyme. In addition, 4-hydroxyandrostenedione, several androsta-1,4-diene3,17-diones, and 10β-propynylestr-4-ene-3,17-dione act as enzyme-

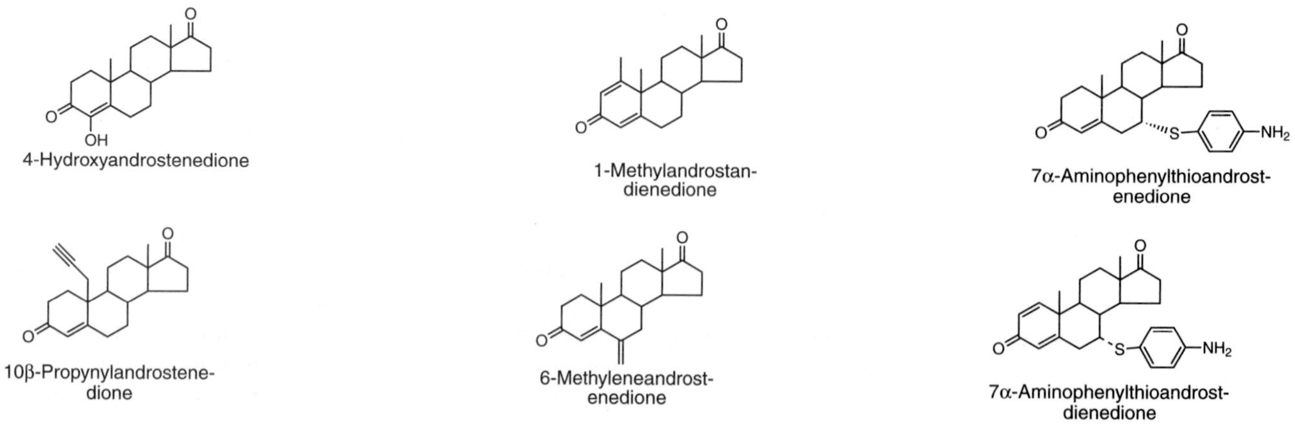

4-Hydroxyandrostenedione

1-Methylandrostan-dienedione

7α-Aminophenylthioandrost-enedione

10β-Propynylandrostene-dione

6-Methyleneandrost-enedione

7α-Aminophenylthioandrost-dienedione

Fig. 29.11. Androstenedione aromatase inhibitors.

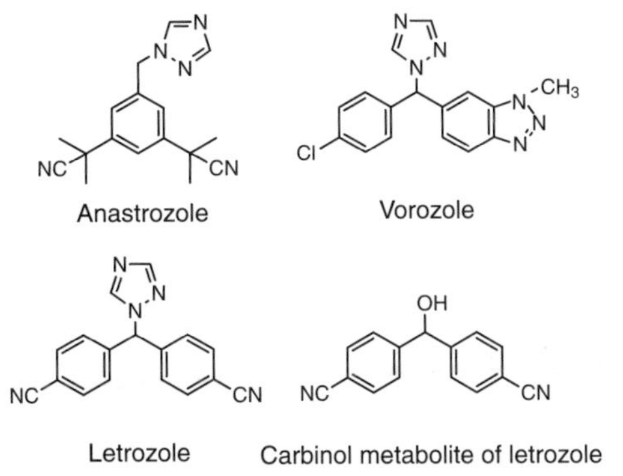

Fig. 29.12. Triazole aromatase inhibitors.

activated irreversible inhibitors (suicide substrates) *in vitro*. The structure-activity relationships of steroidal aromatase inhibitors indicate that the best inhibitors are analogs of the substrate, with only small structural changes made on the A-ring and at C_{19}. Incorporation of aryl functionalities at the 7α-position results in inhibitors with enhanced affinity for the enzyme.

Triazole Derivatives. The development of the triazole nonsteroidal inhibitors of aromatase were based on the aromatase inhibitor, aminoglutethimide (69,70). These drugs include the clinically available anastrazole (Arimidex) (72) and letrozole (Femara) (73) (Fig. 29.12) (71). Anastrazole and letrozole are competitive inhibitors of aromatase that selectively inhibit the conversion of testosterone to estrogens in all tissues reducing serum concentrations of circulating estrone, estradiol, and estrone sulfate, but do not affect the synthesis of adrenocorticosteroids, aldosterone, or thyroid hormone. Because estrogen acts as a growth factor for hormone-dependent breast cancer cells, reduction of serum and tumor concentrations of estrogen inhibits tumor growth and delays disease progression. In postmenopausal women, ovarian secretion of estrogen declines and conversion of androstenedione and testosterone to estrone and estradiol in peripheral tissues (adipose, muscle, and liver). Anastrazole and the other triazoles inhibit the aromatase enzyme by binding of the N-4 nitrogen of the triazole ring with the heme iron atom of the CYP19 enzyme complex. Competitive aromatase inhibitors also have been referred to as type II inhibitors of the enzyme. The structure-activity relationships of these inhibitors has been reviewed (21,74,77). Anastrazole, a benzyltriazole derivative, differs structurally from aminoglutethimide but shares the pharmacologic activity of competitive aromatase inhibition, although anastrazole is more potent and selective on a molar basis. Anastrazole is well absorbed with biliary elimination as its primary route (85%) and about 11% renal, with an elimination half-life of about 50 hours. About 60% of an oral dose is metabolized in the liver by N-dealkylation, hydroxylation, and glucuronidation to inactive triazole metabolites. A 70% reduction of serum estradiol usually occurs within 24 hours, with an 80%

reduction in serum estradiol occurring after 14 days. Peak concentration is reached in about 7 days with a duration of action of up to 6 days following its discontinuation. Letrozole is rapidly absorbed with an elimination half-life of 2 days, exhibiting nonlinear pharmacokinetics. About 85% of an oral dose is metabolized by CYP3A4 and CYP2A6 to its carbinol metabolite (4,4'-methanolbisbenzonitrile) (Fig. 29.12) which is eliminated in the urine as its glucuronide conjugate, with <10% unchanged. Anastrazole and letrozole are used for the treatment of advanced breast cancer in postmenopausal women with disease progression following tamoxifen therapy.

Mechanism of Estrogen Action

Molecular Interactions. The search for a biochemical mechanism of action of estradiol focused on the female reproductive tissues, since estrogens localize and produce dramatic and selective responses in these female tissues. Using labeled estradiol, Jensen and Jacobson (78) showed that uptake of estradiol is rapid; the estradiol is retained to a high degree in the uterus and vagina.

The biochemical mechanism of estrogen action is the regulation of gene expression and subsequent induction of protein biosynthesis via specific, high affinity estrogen receptors, as described in general terms in Chapter 28 and illustrated in Figure 29.13. Receptor binding sites for estradiol are located in the nucleus of target cells (79,80) and exhibit both high affinity ($K_D = 10^{-11}$ to 10^{-10} M) and low capacity. Binding to the estrogen receptor is specific. The uptake of $[2,4,6,7-^3H]$-17β-estradiol by the receptors can be inhibited by pretreatment with unlabeled 17β-estradiol or diethylstilbestrol. Pretreatment with testosterone, cortisol, or progesterone does not inhibit binding of radiolabeled estradiol. The binding is stereospecific because 17α-estradiol, an epimer of 17β-estradiol which differs in the configuration of the 17-hydroxyl group, does not prevent the binding of 17β-estradiol to the estrogen receptor (81).

Recently, a second estrogen receptor has been identified, (82) and the two estrogen receptors are now referred to as ERα (representing the classical ER, the first ER studied) and ERβ (the second ER identified). The two receptors differ in size, with ERα having 595 amino acids and ERβ having 485 amino acids. The predominant estrogen receptor in the female reproductive tract and mammary glands is ERα, whereas ERβ is the primary estrogen receptor in vascular endothelial cells, bone, and male prostate tissues. Estradiol has similar affinities for both ERα and ERβ, whereas certain nonsteroidal estrogenic compounds and antiestrogens have differing affinities between ERα and ERβ, with slightly higher affinities for ERβ (83).

When estradiol binds to the estrogen receptor, a conformational change of the estradiol-receptor complex occurs and results in interactions of the estradiol-receptor complex with particular HRE regions of the cellular DNA, referred to as estrogen responsive elements (EREs). Bind-

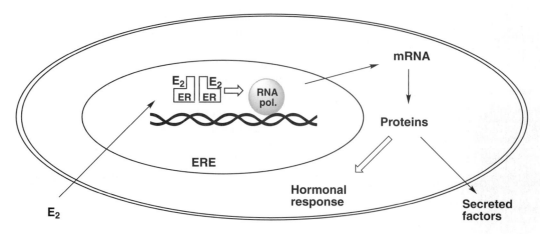

Fig. 29.13. Mechanism of estrogen action.

ing of the complex to ERE elements results in initiation of transcription of the DNA sequence to produce mRNA. Finally, the elevated levels of mRNA lead to an increase in protein synthesis in the endoplasmic reticulum.

Estrogens produce their effects upon the mammalian uterus by increasing synthesis of RNA in the target cells. Within 24 hours after administration of estradiol to mice, there is an increase in uterine RNA concentrations without a similar increase in DNA. The stimulatory effect on nuclear RNA synthesis occurs within 2 minutes after administration of estrogens (80). It has been observed that RNA synthesized by estrogen-stimulated nuclei differs from that produced by nonstimulated nuclei (80,84,85). Estradiol, for example, increases the frequency of the consecutive pairs guanine and uracil (GpU) and adenine and uracil (ApU) and decreases frequency of the consecutive pairs uracil and uracil (UpU) and cytosine and uracil (CpU) in nearest-neighbor nucleotide analysis of RNA synthesized by rat uterine nuclei.

Metabolic inhibitors have been used to delineate the role of estrogens in the activation of RNA synthesis. Actinomycin D, an inhibitor of DNA-dependent RNA synthesis, prevents the acceleration of protein and phospholipid synthesis induced by estradiol (86). Puromycin, an inhibitor of protein synthesis, blocks the response of administered estrogen (87). The RNA extracted from a uterus that has been stimulated by estrogens appears to produce several uterine effects seen with normal estrogen stimulation. When the RNA extract obtained from estrogenized uterine tissue is treated with RNAase or diphosphoesterase, it loses most estrogenic activity. In addition, RNA taken from other tissues, such as from the liver, treated with estrogens has no estrogenic effect on the uterus. The increased RNA synthesis eventually leads to an increase in the synthesis of proteins. Several proteins produced in target cells by the action of estrogens have been identified. In the chick oviduct the transport protein ovalbumin is induced by estrogen (80). One protein initially termed IP (Induced Protein) and later identified as the brain-type creatine kinase (88,89) is pro-

duced in rat uterine tissue on E_2 stimulation. Also, levels of progesterone receptors increase in uterine tissue, thus preparing the tissue for the actions of progesterone on the uterus during the later half of the reproductive cycle (90).

Estrogens affect the activity of various enzyme systems. The activity of enzyme systems increases with the proper concentration of estrogens (91) including lactic dehydrogenase, β-glucuronidase, alkaline phosphatase (from the uterus), peroxidase, (92,93) glucose-6-phosphate dehydrogenase, cathepsin D, and plasminogen activator (90).

Physiologic Effects.   Estrogens act on many tissues, such as those of the reproductive tract, breast, and CNS. The primary physiologic action of estrogens is to stimulate the development of secondary sex tissues. The growth and development of tissues in the reproductive tract of animals, in terms of actual weight gained, are not seen for as long as 16 hours after administration of the estrogen, although some biochemical processes in the cell are affected immediately. The growth response produced in the uterus by estrogens is temporary, and the maintenance of such growth requires the hormone to be available almost continuously. The initial growth induced by the estrogen is therefore of limited duration, and atrophy of the uterus occurs if the hormone is withdrawn.

Another physiologic effect of estrogens, observed 1 hour after their administration, is edema in the uterus. During this period, vasodilation of the uterine pre- and postcapillary arterioles occurs, and there is an increase in permeability to plasma proteins. These effects appear to occur predominantly in the endometrium and not to any great extent in the myometrium (94).

Another target of estrogens is breast tissue. Estrogens can stimulate the proliferation of breast cells and promote the growth of hormone-dependent mammary carcinoma. Because the breast is the primary site for cancer in women, considerable research has been focused on understanding breast cancer and the factors that influence its growth. Estradiol will stimulate gene expression and the production of several proteins in breast cancer cells via the estrogen receptor mechanism. These proteins include both intracellular proteins important for breast cell function and growth, and secreted proteins that can influence tumor growth and metastasis. Intracellular proteins include enzymes needed for DNA synthesis, such as DNA polymerase, thymidine kinase, thymidylate synthetase, and dihydrofolate reductase (95,96). Progesterone receptors are induced in breast cells by estrogens, (97) and the content of both estrogen receptors and progesterone receptors is utilized clinically as markers for hormone responsiveness of the breast cancer in determining hormonal therapy (98). Another prominent protein made in breast cells is a 7-kd protein, whose function is yet unknown, and is derived from estrogen-induced mRNA referred to as pS2 (99). Several secreted proteins induced via the estrogen receptor are potential cellular growth factors (100). Stimulatory growth factors induced by estrogen treatment include transforming growth factor-α (TGFα) (101,103) and insulin-like growth factor I (IGF-I) (104). A secreted 52-kd glycoprotein, a cathepsin D protein that exhibits protease activity, is also induced by estrogens and is thought to be important in breast cancer cell metastasis (105). The levels of another growth factor protein, transforming growth factor-β (TGFβ), are decreased in breast cancer cells by estrogen treatment and are induced by antiestrogens, (106) suggesting that it may exert a negative effect on cell growth and serve as an endogenous regulator.

Pharmacology, Side Effects, and Clinical Applications.

Administration of estrogens to immature animals can increase the rate of sexual maturity. One of the principal actions of estrogens is to promote the development of secondary sex characteristics in the female. The feminizing characteristics include growth of hair, softening of skin, growth of breasts, and accretion of fat in the thighs, hips, and buttocks. Estrogens also stimulate the growth and development of the female reproductive tract, including the uterine oviduct, cervix, and vagina. The proliferative changes that occur in the endometrium and myometrium on estrogen administration resemble those that take place naturally. Bleeding often follows withdrawal of the estrogens.

These hormones appear to prevent coronary atherosclerosis in women before menopause because of an alteration in the composition of circulating lipids (107). Because of feminizing effects, estrogen therapy in males is limited. One of the primary therapeutic uses is in the treatment of menopausal symptoms such as hot flashes, chilly sensations, dizziness, fatigue, irritability, and sweating. For many women, menopause does not cause much discomfort; in some, however, both physical and mental discomfort may occur and can usually be prevented through estrogen therapy.

Oral and transdermal estrogens are used in a wide variety of menstrual disturbances, such as the management of moderate to severe vasomotor symptoms associated with menopause; management of vulvar and vaginal atrophy

(atrophic vaginitis, kraurosis vulvae) female hypoestrogenism due to hypogonadism, castration, or primary ovarian failure, as well as amenorrhea, dysmenorrhea, and oligomenorrhea. They are also effective in failure of ovarian development, acne, and senile vaginitis. After childbirth, estrogens have been used to suppress lactation. In nonresectable prostate carcinoma, the treatment of choice is combined estrogen therapy and castration. One of the most widespread uses of estrogens is in birth control. These hormones are used in postmenopausal osteoporosis because it is thought that an estrogen deficiency in postmenopausal women can lead to this serious disorder of the bone.

Oral conjugated estrogens USP and synthetic conjugated estrogens A are used in women for the management of moderate to severe vasomotor symptoms associated with menopause and share the usual cautions, precautions, and contraindications associated with estrogen therapy.

Nausea appears to be the main side effect; other adverse effects include vomiting, anorexia, and diarrhea. If small doses are used to initiate therapy, and the dose is gradually increased, most of the side effects can be avoided. Excessive doses of estrogens inhibit the development of bones in young patients by accelerating epiphyseal closure.

When estrogens are given in large doses over long periods of time, they can inhibit ovulation because of their feedback inhibition of the release of FSH from the adenohypophysis resulting in inhibition of ovulation. Administration of these drugs may promote sodium chloride retention; the result is retention of water and subsequent edema. This effect, however, is less pronounced than with glucocorticoids. More detailed information on the pharmacology and toxicology of estrogens can be found in published reviews (4,5,40).

Progestins

Once ovulation has taken place, the tissue remaining from the ruptured follicle forms the corpus luteum, which has the important function of preparing for and maintaining pregnancy if it occurs. Fraenkel (108) first observed in 1903 that removal of the corpus luteum shortly after conception results in termination of the pregnancy. In 1914, Pearl and Surface (109) showed that the corpus luteum can prevent ovulation in animals. In 1929, Corner and Allen (110) developed a method of assay for progestational activity.

By 1934, the progestational hormone progesterone had been isolated by several research groups (111). It was shown in 1937 that pure progesterone alone can maintain pregnancy in animals (112). Besides performing important functions in the reproductive system, this hormone serves as a precursor to androgens, estrogens, and adrenocorticoids (Fig. 29.3).

The most abundant pregnane steroid found in the urine during pregnancy is 5β-pregnanediol (cis A/B ring juncture) (Fig. 29.14), present as its glucuronide, which is

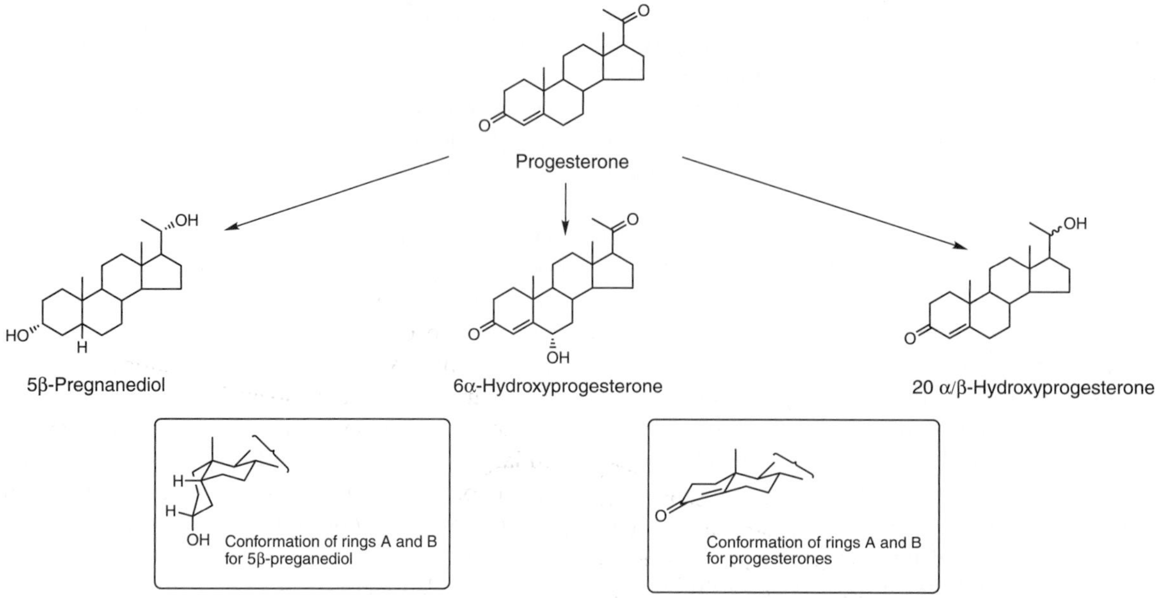

Fig. 29.14. Metabolism of progesterone.

also the main metabolite of exogenous progesterone. This conjugated substance can serve as an index of the corpus luteum placenta activity and a premature drop in its level in the urine may be a warning of possible miscarriage. 5β-pregnanediol appears to have no progestational activity, but it apparently can antagonize the action of progesterone in certain animals (113).

Biosynthesis

Progesterone is biosynthesized and secreted by the corpus luteum of the ovary during the luteal phase of the reproductive cycle. Luteinizing hormone (LH), the adenohypophysis glycoprotein hormone, binds to the LH receptor on the surface of the cells to initiate progesterone biosynthesis. As in other endocrine cells such as adrenal cortical cells, the binding of LH results in an increase in intracellular cAMP levels via activation of a G protein and adenylyl cyclase. One of the processes influenced by elevated cAMP levels is the activation of cholesterol esterase, which cleaves cholesterol esters and liberates free cholesterol. The free cholesterol is then converted in mitochondria to pregnenolone via the side-chain cleavage reaction described earlier, and progesterone is formed from pregnenolone by the action of 5-ene-3β-hydroxysteroid dehydrogenase and 3-oxosteroid-4,5-isomerase (steps c,d; Fig. 29.3).

Metabolism

Progesterone, the female sex hormone synthesized by the corpus luteum, is rapidly metabolized by the liver following administration by any route with a half-life of 5–10 minutes (Fig. 29.14). Progesterone is mainly excreted as glucuronide and sulfate conjugates of 5β-pregnanediol. Other routes of metabolism include 6α-hydroxylation (CYP3A4) and reduction of the 20-ketone to an alcohol by a dehydrogenase. The

formation of 5β-pregnanediol from progesterone is characterized by reduction of the 4,5-double bond to a 5β geometry for rings A and B (a *cis* configuration) and reduction of the 3-ketone to the 3α configuration. Minor pathways of metabolism in the liver can occur with the elimination of the 17 acetyl side-chain and pathways similar to those for the metabolism of androgens have been observed.

Synthetic Progestins
Pregnanes

Progesterone and Its Derivatives. Progesterone, being an important hormone for maintaining pregnancy and normal menstrual bleeding, was used to correct disorders in these areas. The naturally occurring hormone was recognized for its ability to prevent ovulation during pregnancy; it can be considered a natural contraceptive (114). A good source of progesterone was therefore desired.

Sequences were devised for the synthesis of progesterone from naturally occurring steroids, including diosgenin, ergosterol, and bile acids. Progesterone, however, has many drawbacks, including a relatively low bioavailability when orally administered; because of this, the hormone is administered parenterally for therapeutic effects. Because progesterone had to be injected repeatedly over relatively short periods for best results and because in some instances this method of administration produced local irritation and pain, orally active derivatives were desired. The pharmacokinetics for progesterone and its derivatives are listed in Table 29.2.

Medroxyprogesterone Acetate (Provera, Depo-Provera, Amen). Although many of the early structural modifications of progesterone led to weakly active or inactive progestational agents (Fig. 29.15), it was eventually shown that 17α-acetoxyprogesterone had some activity when administered orally even though the parent compound, 17α-hydroxyprogesterone, was inactive (115). A second derivative of 17α-hydroxyprogesterone, the 17-caproate ester, is used extensively in therapeutics and because of its long duration of action, the drug is administered parenterally for locating problems related to deficiency of natural progesterone (116). Further structural modifications of 17α-acetoxyprogesterone have enhanced its oral contraceptive action. In most instances, these modifications are carried out at the carbon 6, which is the site of metabolic hydroxylation. Substituents in the C_6 position hinder 6-hydroxylation of the progestins and increase their lipid solubility; the result is an enhanced biologic effect (117). Among the first of these interesting analogs of 17α-acetoxyprogesterone to be used in progestational therapy was medroxyprogesterone acetate (6α-methyl analog) (118). The 6α-methyl group blocks 6-hydroxylation and thus is 25 times more active than the norandrogen ethisterone, with low estrogenic and no androgenic activity. Medroxyprogesterone acetate is completely and rapidly deacetylated by first pass metabolism to medroxyprogesterone following oral administration. Plasma protein binding for medroxyprogesterone is approximately 86%, with binding primarily to serum albumin and no binding with SHBG. It is extensively metabolized via pathways similar to that for progesterone, except for 6α-hydroxylation. Most medroxyprogesterone acetate metabolites are excreted in the urine as glucuronide conjugates with only small amounts excreted as sulfates.

Megestrol Acetate (Megace). Progestational activity is further enhanced with 6-substituted 17α-acetoxyprogesterones when a double bond is introduced between positions 6 and

7. Megestrol acetate and chlormadinone acetate are typical examples of clinically useful progestins. Less than 10% of an oral dose of megestrol is metabolized. Major metabolites recovered in the urine include 2-hydroxy and 6-hydroxymethyl megestrol and their glucuronide conjugates. Megestrol is primarily used in the treatment of breast and endometrial carcinoma and in postmenopausal women with advanced hormonally dependent carcinoma.

Progestational activity of a steroid does not have to be related to its antiovulatory or antigonadotropic activity. Dydrogesterone (Fig. 29.15), which has a *cis* juncture between rings B and C is a progestational agent that can maintain pregnancy in spayed rats when administered subcutaneously. This isomer does not inhibit ovulation (even in large doses). However, it exhibits no androgenic, estrogenic, or masculinizing effects on the female fetus, as well as no thermogenetic activity.

19-Norandrostanes

Ethisterone and Its Analogs. The first synthetic progestin to be used to any extent is ethisterone (the 17α-ethynyl derivative of testosterone) which was synthesized from male sex hormones (androstanes) in 1937 in an attempt to find an orally active androgen (119). The substance later proved to be an effective oral progestin and became useful in the treatment of menstrual dysfunctions (120). Several molecular modifications of ethisterone have enhanced progestational activity; introduction of methyl groups in the $C_{6α}$ and C_{21} positions, as in dimethisterone, provided active analogs (Fig. 29.16) (5). Ethisterone, therefore, paved the way for the synthesis of other progestins that did not have a typical progesterone-type C_{17} side chain.

A second breakthrough was made in 1944 when Ehrenstein (121) discovered that the C_{19} methyl group on steroids

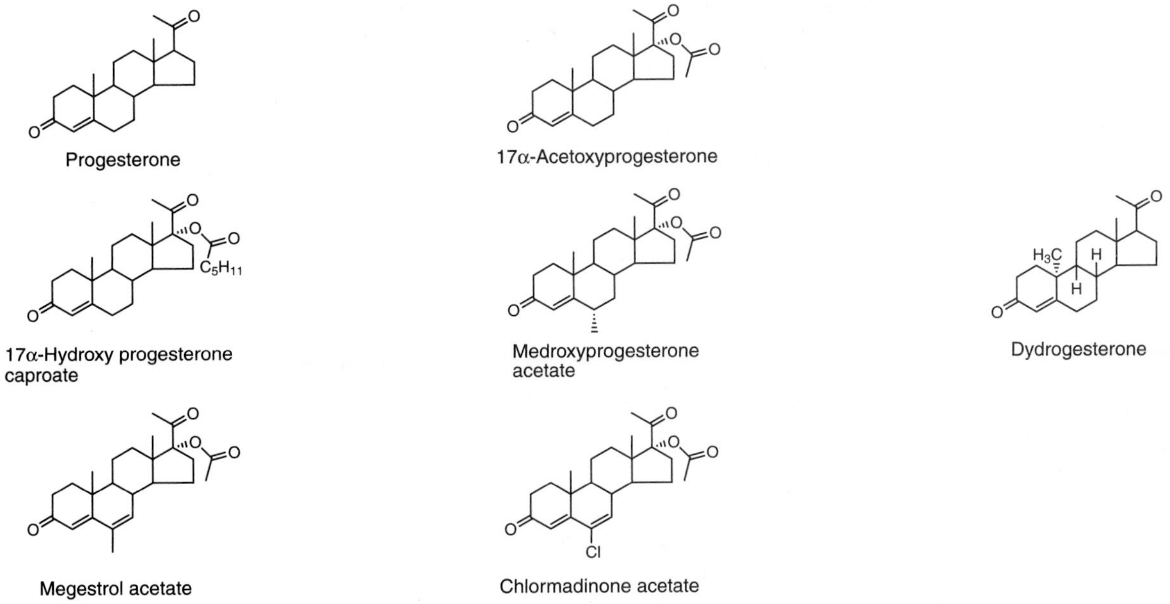

Progesterone

17α-Acetoxyprogesterone

17α-Hydroxy progesterone caproate

Medroxyprogesterone acetate

Dydrogesterone

Megestrol acetate

Chlormadinone acetate

Fig. 29.15. Progesterone and its derivatives.

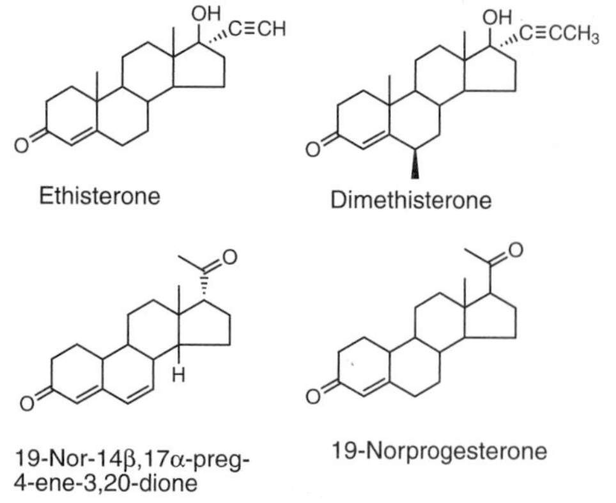

Fig. 29.16. Progestins and 19-norandrostane.

is not necessary for progestational activity. In fact, his work showed that loss of the C_{19} methyl (from a compound he thought was progesterone, but later turned out to be a stereoisomer of progesterone, namely, 19-nor-14β,17α-pregn-4-ene-3,20-dione), results in activity equal to or greater than that of parenterally administered progesterone. Ehrenstein's procedure for converting strophanthidin (a cardiac aglycone) to a stereoisomer of 19-norprogesterone using a 12-step process was too complicated and unsuited for further preparations of C_{19} nor steroids. This work, however, did lead to intensive attempts to prepare orally active progestins that were devoid of estrogenic and androgenic activities. Eventually, in 1953, Djerassi and co-workers (122) did synthesize 19-norprogesterone. This drug differed from the natural hormone only in replacement of the C_{19} angular methyl group by hydrogen. This analog was 8 times more active than progesterone when administered parenterally (Clauberg's test) and was the most potent progestin known.

Norethindrone and Norethynodrel. This research on 19-nor-steroids as potential progestins culminated in the synthesis of two potent, orally active progestins, namely, norethindrone and norethynodrel (2). Because the progestational activity of norethynodrel is about one-tenth that of norethindrone, it is no longer used in oral contraceptives. Both compounds appear to have weak estrogenic activity. These two substances were among the first 19-nor steroids to be used clinically for progesterone hormonal disorders. They also afforded a method, when used with estrogens such as ethinyl estradiol or mestranol, for control of conception. The first oral contraceptive, Enovid, is a combination of mestranol and norethynodrel introduced in 1960, but is no longer clinically available. Following oral administration norethindrone acetate is completely and rapidly deacetylated by first pass metabolism to norethindrone with an oral bioavailability of about 64%. The pharmacokinetics for norethindrone acetate is indistinguishable from that of orally administered norethindrone. The usefulness of norethynodrel and norethindrone for therapy of irregular menses and as contraceptive agents provided the impetus to continue research in the area of 19-nor steroids. Another 19-nor steroid reported to be effective and exhibit few side

effects is ethynodiol diacetate. This drug has been used as an oral progestin (123).

Other Progestins. The progestinic component of the commercially available oral contraceptive combinations is desogestrel, ethynodiol diacetate, levonorgestrel, norethindrone, norethindrone acetate, norgestimate, or norgestrel, derivatives of 19-nortestosterone (Fig. 29.17) (Table 29.3). Their pharmacokinetic data are listed in Table 29.2. Norgestrel is a racemic mixture with its levo isomer, levonorgestrel, as the pharmacologically active isomer. In terms of oral progestational activity, desogestrel, levonorgestrel, norgestimate and norgestrel are the most potent of these progestins and norethindrone is the least potent. Levonorgestrel and norgestrel have the greatest androgenic activity while norgestimate, desogestrel, ethnyodiol and norethindrone have the weakest androgenic activity. Desogestrel and norgestimate appear to have a substantially higher selectivity for progesterone receptors than for androgen receptors when compared to the conventional progestins (e.g., levonorgestrel, norethindrone).

The oral contraceptive steroids are almost completely absorbed and may be either metabolized in the GI mucosa during absorption or on first pass through the liver. For example, when orally administered, the pro-progestin, desogestrel is rapidly metabolized in the intestinal mucosa and on first pass through the liver to its progestin metabolite 3-ketodesogestrel (Recently, 3-ketodesogestrel (etonogestrel) in combination with ethinyl estradiol has been approved by the FDA for use as a vaginal insert ring providing month-long contraceptive protection under the trade name of NuvaRing.). Following oral administration, the relative bioavailability for desogestrel, as measured by serum levels of

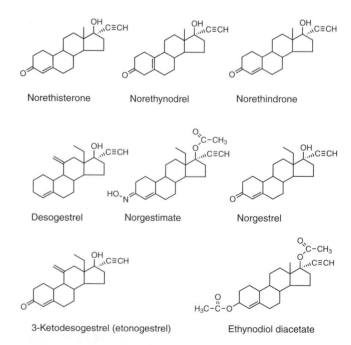

Fig. 29.17. 19-Norandrostanes used clinically in oral contraceptives.

Table 29.3. Oral Contraceptives

Trade Name	Progestin	mg	Estrogen	mcg
Monophasic				
Alesse	Levonorgestrel	0.1	Ethinyl estradiol	20
Brevicon	Norethindrone	0.5	Ethinyl estradiol	35
Demulen 1/35	Ethynodiol diacetate	1.0	Ethinyl estradiol	35
Demulen 1/50	Ethynodiol diacetate	1.0	Ethinyl estradiol	50
Desogen	Desogestrel	0.15	Ethinyl estradiol	30
Levien	Levonorgestrel	0.15	Ethinyl estradiol	30
Levlite	Levonorgestrel	0.1	Ethinyl estradiol	20
Levora 0.15/30	Levonorgestrel	0.15	Ethinyl estradiol	30
Loestrin 21 1/20	Norethindrone acetate	1.0	Ethinyl estradiol	20
Loestrin 1.5/30	Norethindrone acetate	1.5	Ethinyl estradiol	30
Lo/Ovral	Norgestrel	0.3	Ethinyl estradiol	30
Modicon	Norethindrone	0.5	Ethinyl estradiol	35
Nelova 0.5/35E	Norethindrone	0.5	Ethinyl estradiol	35
Nelova 1/35E	Norethindrone	1.0	Ethinyl estradiol	35
Nelova 1/50M	Norethindrone	1.0	Mestranol	50
Nordette	Levonorgestrel	0.15	Ethinyl estradiol	30
Norinyl 1 + 35	Norethindrone	1.0	Ethinyl estradiol	35
Norinyl 1 + 50	Norethindrone	1.0	Mestranol	50
Ortho-Cept	Desogestrel	0.15	Ethinyl estradiol	30
Ortho-Cyclen	Norgestimate	0.25	Ethinyl estradiol	35
Ortho-Novum 1/35	Norethindrone	1.0	Ethinyl estradiol	35
Ortho-Novum 1/50	Norethindrone	1.0	Mestranol	50
Ovcon-35	Norethindrone	0.4	Ethinyl estradiol	35
Ovcon-50	Norethindrone	1.0	Ethinyl estradiol	50
Ovral-28	Norgestrel	0.5	Ethinyl estradiol	50
Biphasic Oral Contraceptives:				
Jenest	Norethindrone	0.5	Ethinyl estradiol	35
	Norethindrone	1	Ethinyl estradiol	35
Mircette	Desgestrel	0.15	Ethinyl estradiol	20
	Desgestrel	0.0	Ethinyl estradiol	10
Necon 10/11	Norethindrone	0.5	Ethinyl estradiol	35
	Norethindrone	1	Ethinyl estradiol	35
Nelova 10/11	Norethindrone	0.500	Ethinyl estradiol	35
	Norethindrone	1.000	Ethinyl estradiol	35
Ortho-Novum 10/11	Norethindrone	0.500	Ethinyl estradiol	35
	Norethindrone	1.000	Ethinyl estradiol	35
Triphasic Oral Contraceptives:				
Estrocept-21	Norethindrone acetate	1	Ethinyl estradiol	20
	Norethindrone acetate	1	Ethinyl estradiol	30
	Norethindrone acetate	1	Ethinyl estradiol	35
Ortho-Novum 7/7/7/	Norethindrone	0.5	Ethinyl estradiol	35
	Norethindrone	0.75	Ethinyl estradiol	35
	Norethindrone	1	Ethinyl estradiol	35
Ortho Tricyclen	Norgestimate	0.18	Ethinyl estradiol	35
	Norgestimate	0.215	Ethinyl estradiol	35
	Norgestimate	0.25	Ethinyl estradiol	35
Tri-Levien	Levonorgestrel	0.050	Ethinyl estradiol	30
	Levonorgestrel	0.075	Ethinyl estradiol	40
	Levonorgestrel	0.125	Ethinyl estradiol	30
Tri-Norinyl	Norethindrone	0.500	Ethinyl estradiol	35
	Norethindrone	1.000	Ethinyl estradiol	35
	Norethindrone	0.500	Ethinyl estradiol	35
Triphasil	Levonorgestrel	0.050	Ethinyl estradiol	30
	Levonorgestrel	0.075	Ethinyl estradiol	40
	Levonorgestrel	0.125	Ethinyl estradiol	30
Trivora-28	Levonorgestrel	0.05	Ethinyl estradiol	30
	Levonorgestrel	0.075	Ethinyl estradiol	40
	Levonorgestrel	0.125	Ethinyl estradiol	30
Progestin Oral Contraceptives:				
Micronor	Norethindrone	0.35		
Nor-Q.D.	Norethindrone	0.35		
Ovrette	Norgestrel	0.075		

3-ketodesogestrel, is approximately 84%. The other inactive metabolites for desogestrel recovered in the urine as glucuronide and sulfate conjugates include 3α-OH-desogestrel, 3β-OH-desogestrel, and 3α-OH-5α-desogestrel. Similarly, norgestimate may also be considered as a pro-progestin, because it is also metabolized by first pass metabolism to its active metabolite, 17-desacetylnorgestimate. Unlike some of the other progestins, 3-desacetylnorgestimate is strongly protein bound, but not to SHBG. The progestins are strongly protein bound mainly to albumin, but also to sex hormone binding globulin (SHBG). Plasma concentrations for desogestrel, norethindrone, levonorgestrel and 3-keto-desogestrel display nonlinear pharmacokinetics because of increased SHBG binding of the progestins as a result of its induction by the daily administration of ethinyl estradiol. Generally, the amount of SHBG in plasma determines the distribution of progestins between free and bound forms, and free progestin concentrations determine the drug's half-life. The binding capacity of SHBG for progestins is not only enhanced by ethinyl estradiol, but by other enzyme-inducing drugs such as carbamazepine, phenobarbital or rifampin. Only the unbound fraction of oral contraceptive steroids is biologically active.

Oral contraceptive steroids may be distributed into bile. Small amounts of oral contraceptive steroids are also distributed into breast milk with plasma-to-breast milk ratios for levonorgestrel (100:20) and norethindrone (100:10). It has been estimated that about 0.02% of a 50-μg dose of ethinyl estradiol is distributed into breast milk.

Structure-activity Relationships

Progestational activity appears to be restricted to molecules with a steroid nucleus. Klimstra has pointed out that it is difficult to compare progestins on the basis of studies reported in the literature because there are many ways to do so (124). Two of the most common methods of measuring uterine glandular development are Clauberg's and McGinty's tests. Other biologic evaluations of the progestins include their effect on uterine carbonic anhydrase, inhibition of gonadotropin hormones, and delay of parturition, and their ability to maintain pregnancy in a spayed female animal. Substances should be evaluated in the same laboratory; the resulting data are more informative.

The synthetic progestins can generally be divided into two classes of compounds, namely, the androgens (19-norandrostane or estrane derivatives) and the 17α-hydroxyprogesterones (2,91,117,124). In the androgen series, a 17α-substituent, such as ethynyl, methyl, ethyl, and variations of these, renders the molecule active when administered orally.

Ethisterone, the first androgenic compound found to be effective, has about one-third the activity of progesterone in women when taken subcutaneously but is 15 times more active when taken orally. Because this analog is closely related to testosterone, it has androgenic activity. Removal of the CH₃ group at position 19 leads to norethindrone (norethisterone), which has five to ten times more progestational activity. The activity of norethindrone may be increased fur-

ther by substituting a chlorine atom at position 21 which blocks metabolic hydroxylation at this point, or by adding a methyl group at carbon 18 (norgestrel). Ethynodiol acetate is an extremely potent oral progestin; it is more active orally than parenterally and is effective as an oral contraceptive when combined with an estrogen.

Further unsaturation of the B or C ring of 19-androstane derivatives usually enhances progestational activity. Introduction of halogen or methyl substituents in the 6α-position or 7α-position generally increases hormonal activity. Acetylation of the 17β-OH of norethindrone results in a longer duration of action. Removal of the keto function of norethindrone at carbon 3 gives lynestrenol, which retains potent progestational activity and is free of androgenic effects. This hormone is used in combination with an estrogen as a contraceptive agent.

Lynestrenol

Activity of 17α-hydroxyprogesterones is enhanced by unsaturation at positions 6 and 7 and substitution of a methyl group or a halogen at position 6. This activity may be further increased by introducing a CH₃ group at position 11. These substitutions on the progesterone molecule probably prevent metabolic reduction of the two carbonyl groups and metabolic oxidation at position 6. Substitution of a fluoro group at position 21 apparently prevents metabolic hydroxylation at this point and enhances the oral effectiveness. Some of the potent orally administered progestins belong to this series of compounds.

A progestin with a prolonged duration of action is 16α,17-dihydroxyprogesterone acetophenide. When given parenterally, this agent appears to be devoid of both androgenic and estrogenic activities.

16α,17α-Dihydroxyprogesterone
acetophenide

Inversion of the configuration at positions 9 and 10 in progesterone leads to retroprogesterone, which is more active parenterally and orally than progesterone. Further unsaturation at positions 6 and 7 of retroprogesterone gives dydrogesterone, which has previously been discussed. The adrenocortical hormone 21-hydroxyprogesterone and the precursor of progesterone, pregnenolone, have minimal or no progestational activity.

Progestin Antagonists
Mefepristone (Mifeprex)

An antiprogestin, a compound that antagonizes the actions of progesterone by competing for its receptor, would be an important agent for interfering with the early phases of pregnancy. This area of research has received considerable attention but few results. In 1982, the first antiprogestin, mifepristone

Mifepristrone   Onapristrone

(RU 38,486 or abbreviated RU 486), was reported (125). Following oral administration, mifepristone is rapidly absorbed with a peak plasma concentration occurring in approximately 90 minutes, with an oral bioavailability of about 70% and exhibits a terminal elimination half-life of 18 hours. It is 98% bound primarily to albumin and α_1-acid glycoprotein. Mifepristone displays nonlinear pharmacokinetics with respect to plasma concentration and clearance. Mifepristone is primarily metabolized via CYP3A4 pathways involving mono- and di-N-demethylation and terminal hydroxylation of the 17-propynyl chain. The fact that about 83% of the drug is recovered in the feces and 9% in the urine, suggests biliary as the principal route of elimination. Mifepristone blocked implantation of fertilized eggs in rats and was shown to interrupt early stages of implantation and pregnancy in humans (126). Mifepristone also demonstrates antiglucocorticoid activity (127). Additional antiprogestin analogs, such as onapristone (ZK 98,299), have been developed that exhibit lowered antiglucocorticoid activity (128). These antiprogestins have also demonstrated therapeutic potential for the treatment of hormone-dependent breast cancer (129).

Mechanism of Progestin Action—Molecular Interactions

The uterus is the primary site of progesterone action in the female. Once the endometrium proliferates and becomes dense under the influence of estrogens, the levels of progesterone rise. This hormone inhibits the proliferation of, and initiates a secretory phase of, the reproductive cycle. During this stage, the endometrium becomes edematous and glycogen increases in the epithelium of the endometrium.

In an attempt to understand the cellular transformations induced by progesterone that involve gene expression, O'Malley, Shrader, and colleagues studied the effects of progesterone on the chick oviduct, a particularly useful biologic system for the examination of the mechanism of action of progesterone (130). These studies on progesterone receptors extend into mammalian systems as well (131). The progesterone receptor consists of two hormone binding proteins, receptors A and B (132,133). Biologically active progesterone receptors are present in the nucleus of target cells, whereas inactive receptors have been found in the cytosol as a complex with hsp90, (134) similar to inactive glucocorticoid complexes. The nuclear progesterone receptor heterodimer binds progesterone with high affinity, resulting in a conformational change in the complex. The steroid-receptor complex interacts with particular HRE regions of the cellular DNA, referred to as progesterone responsive elements (PRE), and initiates transcription of the DNA sequence to produce mRNA. Finally, the elevated levels of mRNA lead to an increase in protein synthesis in the endoplasmic reticulum. Administration of progesterone to estrogen-stimulated chicks resulted in the synthesis of the specific oviduct protein, avidin. In mammals, uteroglobin (a small secretory protein of the uterus) and the enzyme estradiol dehydrogenase have been identified as proteins induced by progesterone.

Physiologic Effects. Progesterone has many biologic functions. The primary site of the physiologic action of progesterone is the uterus. The hormone acts on both the endometrium (inner mucous lining) and the myometrium (muscle mass) of the uterus. It acts on the endometrium, which has been primed by the estrogens, to induce the secretory phase, during which the endometrial glands grow and secrete large amounts of carbohydrates that will possibly be used by the fertilized ovum as a source of energy.

The primary function of progesterone with respect to the myometrium is to stop the spontaneous rhythmic contractions of the uterus. The effects of progesterone on the uterus are to prepare the endometrium for reception, implantation, and maintenance of the fertilized ovum and to suppress the myometrial contractions so that the embryo is not dislodged from the uterus.

The corpus luteum is the primary source of progesterone for the first third of pregnancy; subsequently, the developing placenta is the major source of progesterone and estrogens. Both hormones are secreted continually in large amounts until parturition. The high levels of progesterone produced by the corpus luteum and placenta during pregnancy act upon the hypothalamus through the negative feedback system to prevent the formation of new ova. Additionally, this steroid hormone is important for maintenance of pregnancy. Thus, progesterone is often referred to as the "hormone of pregnancy."

Extragenital effects of progesterone, except when secreted in large amounts, are slight. Progesterone is natriuretic, probably because of antagonism of aldosterone. Subsequently, increased sodium excretion stimulates secretion of aldosterone, which affects sodium retention. Progesterone is also catabolic, because it increases the total nitrogen excretion brought about by catabolism of amino acids (135).

The main feedback effects of progesterone in the central nervous system are thought to occur in the hypothalamus; this causes inhibition of pituitary secretion (136). Progesterone receptors have been identified in the hypothalamus and are involved in this feedback inhibition. Prior administration of estrogens or progestins does not appear to inhibit ovulation induced by exogenous gonadotropins. Progesterone appears to have a biphasic feedback effect on ovulation. During the first few hours after administration of this hormone, ovulation is produced and the effects are inhibited. It appears that the effects of progesterone are reversed as time passes.

Development of the alveolar sacs in the mammary gland during pregnancy is stimulated by progesterone and estrogens, but lactation does not occur until after the levels of these hormones fall at parturition. Progesterone also increases the basal temperature and decreases the motility of the fallopian tubes. In large doses, progesterone can produce weak analgesia and general anesthesia.

Recent investigations have identified additional actions of progesterone and progesterone metabolites in the central nervous system. The identification of various C_{21} and C_{19} steroids and enzymatic processes for their production in brain tissues led investigators to suggest that these steroids have a possible function in the CNS (137). Two 5α-reduced metabolites of progesterone, 3α-hydroxy-5α-pregnan-20-one and its hydroxy derivative (3α,21-dihydroxy-5α-pregnan-20-one), have been shown to bind to the gamma amino butyric acid A (GABA$_A$) receptor complex at 10^{-8} M concentrations and potentiate GABA responses (138,139). Another C_{21} metabolite found in CNS tissues is pregnenolone sulfate, which demonstrates an inhibitory activity on the GABA$_A$ receptor complex (140). The physiologic relevance of these progestin metabolites in CNS function remains to be determined.

It has been suggested that the temperature-raising effect of progesterone may be due to increased body heat resulting from reduced sweating. This effect is not unique to progesterone; other steroids in the pregnane and androstane series can also produce it (141).

Pharmacology, Side Effects, and Clinical Applications. The mechanism controlling ovarian secretion of progesterone involves the release of LH from the adenohypophysis during ovulation. The LH induces progesterone secretion from the corpus luteum during the second half of the menstrual cycle. As stated earlier, the high levels of progesterone produced by the corpus luteum and placenta during pregnancy act upon the hypothalamus through the negative feedback system to prevent the formation of new ova. This information led to studies involving progesterone and its analogs as contraceptives (4,142). If conception does not occur, the corpus luteum regresses and progesterone production decreases. This finally leads to sloughing of part of the endometrium during menstruation.

Progesterone, and more recently its synthetic analogs, has been used to treat dysmenorrhea, endometriosis, functional uterine bleeding, and amenorrhea. Progesterone and its derivatives have been used to treat habitual abortions, although not always successfully (143). This seems to be a reasonable use because progesterone is considered a pregnancy-supporting hormone. Because abortion is not always due to a hormonal deficiency, however, progestin treatment has not been as successful as predicted.

An early pregnancy can be diagnosed by giving the combination of an estrogen and a progestin for several days and then withdrawing it. If bleeding occurs in a few days, the patient is not pregnant. Progesterone has also been used in the treatment of carcinoma of the endometrium. The major use of progestins is in combination with estrogens as a contraceptive.

Among the side effects seen with progestins are nausea and vomiting, drowsiness, spotting and irregular bleeding; these may occur when these drugs are taken for a short time. With prolonged therapy, a greater incidence of side effects may be seen, including edema and weight gain, breast discomfort, breakthrough bleeding, decreased libido, and masculinization of the female fetus.

Female Oral Contraceptives and Abortifacients

Pincus and his colleagues initiated the use of steroidal hormones in oral contraception in the early 1950s (144). Early findings in animals were extended to human subjects in Haiti and Puerto Rico; such investigations showed that a combination of an estrogen and a progestin prevents conception (145). At about the same time, Greenblatt and Goldzieher developed a sequential method of contraception (146). At present, the combination estrogen-progestin pill is used in various forms, but the sequential method is no longer being used. A summary of oral contraceptive preparations available is given in Table 29.3.

In the monophasic method, both an estrogen and a progestin are administered for 20 or 21 days and then stopped for 7 or 8 days (including the 5-day menstrual period); administration is then repeated. In some instances, a 28-day regimen is given that includes 6 or 7 inert tablets or 7 tablets of 75 mg of ferrous fumarate. In the obsolete sequential method, the estrogen was first administered alone, and then a progestin was added toward the end of each cycle. In some cases a placebo was administered (in the sequential method) between the estrogen-progestin sequence and the starting estrogen. The discontinuation of sequential agents was due to an increased complication rate, linkage to endometrial cancer, and decreased efficiency in preventing pregnancies (147). The new biphasic and triphasic formulations are designed to simulate more closely the normal menstrual cycle and minimize breakthrough bleeding (148).

A third method of contraception is to administer continuously a small dose of a progestin (Table 29.3). In what is referred to in some instances as the mini pill, no estrogen is given at any time. This is thought to reduce some of the risks associated with the use of higher doses of estrogens. A major disadvantage is that irregular bleeding is usually observed during the first 18 months of therapy. After this period, it has been reported, abnormal bleeding does not occur (149). Progestin contraceptive therapy is thought to cause less interference with the endocrine system. There is no pituitary inhibition, and this method does not produce the thromboembolic episodes reported with the regular combination and sequential methods.

Various long-term steroidal contraceptives such as once-a-week and once-a-month preparations are being investigated. One of these longer-term products uses an injectable form of medroxyprogesterone acetate every 3 months. Prolonged infertility or permanent infertility, however, may occur after the use of such a depot contraceptive. Norplant is another product that has been developed as a long-term steroidal contraceptive. It consists of slender Silastic tubes containing 36 mg of the synthetic progestin, levonorgestrel, in a powdered form. Six of these tubes (total dose 216 mg) are implanted under the skin and release the progestin over a period of 3–5 years (150).

Approximately 55 million women use oral contraceptives, the most popular form of contraception used in the world today (151). The oral contraceptive steroids appear to be superior to any other method of preventing pregnancies. The failure rate of oral contraceptives is 0.2–0.6 per 100 woman-years; these data include absorption abnormalities, e.g., those produced by diarrhea. The more recent contraceptive steroid combination or progestin-only products produce fewer side effects than the original agents. The safety of the oral contraceptives has been a subject of keen interest. One of the more studied uses of estrogens has been the treatment of postmenopausal women, and reports have concentrated on the increased risk of cancer of the endometrium in such therapy (152,153). Among the side effects more commonly encountered are nausea, vomiting, menstrual disturbances, breakthrough bleeding, decreased hepatic function, breast tenderness, weight gain, changes in libido, and headaches.

Evidence indicates an increased risk of a more serious nature—thromboembolic and vascular problems in women using oral contraceptives. Other serious conditions are increased risk of myocardial infarction, hepatic adenomas, hypertension, gallbladder disease, breast cancer, and altered carbohydrate metabolism (149,151,154,156). Most of these studies were done with oral contraceptives containing relatively high doses of estrogen and the trend has been toward lowering the estrogen component. Apparently, the estrogenic substance is the prime component in oral contraceptives that is responsible for producing thromboembolisms, and lowering the dose of the estrogen has provided a lower incidence of this problem (155).

Other toxic effects that may be induced by the estrogen include altered carbohydrate metabolism and cancer (149,156). Oral contraceptives are contraindicated in pregnancy because of the possibility of masculinization of the fetus (157). The effects of prolonged use of these agents are still under investigation.

The mode of action for the combination oral contraceptives involves suppression of gonadotropins through a sex steroid feedback mechanism. Although the primary mechanism of this action is inhibition of ovulation, other alterations include changes in the cervical mucus, which increase the difficulty of sperm entry into the uterus, and changes in the endometrium which reduce the likelihood of implantation.

PGE$_2$ PGF$_{2\alpha}$

In recent years, two prostaglandins, PGE$_2$ and PGF$_{2\alpha}$, have been used as abortifacients. PGF$_{2\alpha}$ is injected into the amniotic sac, whereas PGE$_2$ is given by vaginal suppository to induce abortion. Saline-induced abortions have also been used previously. The oral combination of mifepristone and the prostaglandin, misoprostol, have been recommended for inducing an abortion.

ANDROGENS

The primary testicular androgen, testosterone, has important sexual and metabolic activities. It controls the development and maintenance of the sex organs, including the vas deferens, prostate, seminal vesicles, and penis. Spermatogenesis also depends on testosterone. Functional sperm, therefore, depends on both the gonadotropins and testosterone.

This androgen is also needed for the development of secondary sex characteristics. The male voice deepens because of thickening of the laryngeal mucosa and lengthening of the vocal cords. It plays a role first in stimulating the growth of hair on the face, arms, legs, and pubic areas and later in the recession of the male hairline. The fructose content of human semen and the size and secretory capacity of the sebaceous glands also depend on the levels of testosterone.

Testosterone causes nitrogen retention by increasing the rate of protein synthesis while decreasing the rate of protein catabolism. The positive nitrogen balance therefore results from both decreased catabolism and increased anabolism of proteins that are used in male sex accessory apparatus and muscle. The thickness and linear growth of bones are stimulated and later limited by testosterone because of closure of the epiphyses.

Most of the androgens and anabolic steroid products are subject to controlled by the U.S. Federal Control Substances Act as amended by the Anabolic Steroid Control Act of 1990 as Schedule III (CIII) drugs.

Biosynthesis

The mechanisms controlling growth and development of the male gonads are similar to those in the female. The hypothalamus controls the adenohypophysis through the same releasing factor as for females, namely, LHRH. This substance then brings about the release of follicle-stimulating hormone (FSH) and luteinizing hormone (LH), or, as the latter is more commonly called in the male, interstitial cell-stimulating hormone (ICSH), from the adenohypophysis. The two gonadotropins appear to have separate functions. FSH promotes sperm development, or spermatogenesis, by stimulating the seminiferous tubules. The primary action of ICSH, on the other hand, is to stimulate the interstitial Leydig's cells to secrete androgens.

The feedback system between the testes and hypothalamus is not well understood. If the androgens, primarily testosterone, reach a certain level, they cause a decrease in LHRH released from the hypothalamus with a resultant decrease in FSH secretion from the adenohypophysis. Castration causes a deficiency of endogenous testosterone; the result is an increase in secretion of the gonadotropins from the adenohypophysis along with an increase in urinary excretion.

Androgens (male sex hormones) are synthesized from cholesterol in the testes and adrenal cortex. The major pathway for the biosynthesis of testosterone, the most important androgen, is shown in Figure 29.3 (158–160). In the liver, androgens are formed from C_{21} steroids. Small amounts are also secreted by the ovary. This is not surprising because androgens are intermediates in the biosynthesis of estrogens. Testosterone is the major circulating androgen in males; the primary source of testosterone are the Leydig's cells of the testes. LH binds to its receptor on the surface of the Leydig's cells to initiate testosterone biosynthesis. As in other endocrine cells, the binding of the go-

nadotropin results in an increase in intracellular cAMP levels via activation of a G protein and adenylyl cyclase.

One of the processes influenced by elevated cAMP levels is the activation of cholesterol esterase, which cleaves cholesterol esters and liberates free cholesterol. The free cholesterol is then converted in mitochondria to pregnenolone via the side-chain cleavage reaction (Fig. 29.3). Testosterone is formed by reduction of the 17-ketone of androstenedione by 17β-hydroxysteroid dehydrogenase (step f), thus making testosterone and androstenedione metabolically interconvertible, just as estradiol and estrone are interconvertible (161,162). These androgens are precursors for 17β-estradiol and estrone (steps g and h). This interconversion is important in the ovary and testes, but of minor significance in the adrenal glands. Testosterone is secreted by the Leydig's cells and can act in a negative feedback fashion in the hypothalamus and pituitary to decrease the release of gonadotropins.

Metabolism

The metabolism of testosterone, can lead either to physiologically active steroids or to inactive molecules, as shown in Figure 29.18 (158–160). Both reductive and oxidative pathways of metabolism of testosterone can produce important, physiologically active androgens. In androgen target tissues such as the prostate gland, testosterone is converted by 5α-reductase to 5α-dihydrotestosterone (5α-DHT) (Fig. 29.18), the most potent endogenous androgen metabolite of testos-

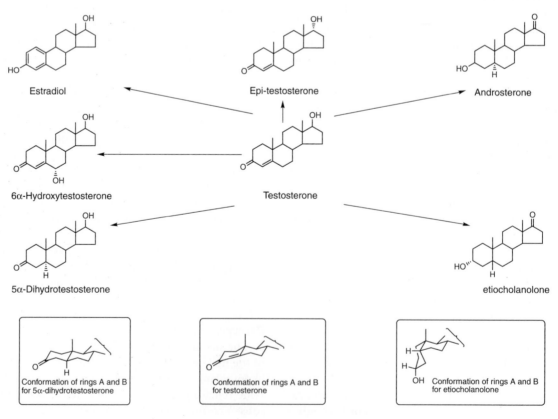

Fig. 29.18. Metabolism of testosterone.

terone. 5α-Reductase is located in both the microsomal fraction and the nuclear membrane of homogenized target tissues. The 5α-reductase enzyme catalyzes an irreversible reaction and requires NADPH as a cofactor, which provides the hydrogen at C_5 (163,164). In ovarian and adipose tissues, the angular C_{19} methyl group of testosterone or androstenedione is oxidized by aromatase to lead to the cleavage of the methyl group, aromatization of the A ring, and the production of estradiol (step g, Fig. 29.3). In CNS tissues, both pathways are active, and research suggests that these biotransformations influence brain differentiation and function (165,166). Testosterone is highly protein bound; 80% to SHBG, 19% to albumin, and 1% free. The metabolite DHT has greater affinity for SHBG than does testosterone.

As with cholesterol and the other physiologically active steroids, the liver is a major site for the metabolic inactivation of androgens (158–160). In the urine, metabolites of the major androgenic agent, testosterone, are found as their more water-soluble glucuronide conjugates and to a lesser extent as sulfate conjugates or in the free form (167). Androsterone and its 5β-diastereoisomer etiocholanolone (cis A/B ring juncture) are the predominant inactive metabolites of testosterone (Fig. 29.18). A number of minor metabolites of testosterone have also been isolated from urine and identified as 5α-androstanes and 5β-androstanes with a 3α-hydroxyl function. Most 17-ketosteroids isolated from the urine result from catabolism of the adrenocorticoids rather than from metabolism of androgens. Epitestosterone is a unnatural metabolite found in the urine of those athletes abusing testosterone for its anabolic properties.

Naturally Occurring Androgens

One of the early and unusual experiments with testicular extracts was carried out in 1889 by the French physiologist Brown-Séquard. He administered such an extract to himself and reported that he felt an increased vigor and capacity for work (168). In 1911, Pézard (169) showed that extracts of testicular tissue increase comb growth in capons. Early attempts to isolate pure male hormones from the testes failed because only small amounts are present in this tissue. The earliest report of an isolated androgen was presented by Butenandt in 1931 (170). He isolated 15 mg of crystalline androsterone from 15,000 liters of human male urine. A second crystalline compound, dehydroepiandrosterone (DHEA), which has weak androgenic activity, was isolated by Butenandt and Dannenberg in 1934 (171). In the following year, testosterone was isolated from bull testes by David and associates (172). This hormone was shown to be 6–10 times as active as androsterone.

Testosterone

Shortly after testosterone was isolated, Butenandt and Hanisch (173) reported its synthesis. In the same year, extracts of urine from males were shown to cause nitrogen retention as well as the expected androgenic effects (174). Many steroids with androgenic activity have subsequently been synthesized. Steroid hormones may have many potent effects on various tissues, and slight chemical alterations of androgenic steroids may increase some of these effects without altering others (175).

Testosterone was the first androgen to be used clinically for its anabolic activity, but new sources of the hormone were needed because only 270 mg could be isolated from a ton of bull testes (176). Commercially, testosterone is prepared from various steroids, including sarsasapogenin, diosgenin, and certain androgens found in stallion urine. Owing to its androgenic action, testosterone is limited in its use in humans as an anabolic steroid. Many steroids were synthesized in an attempt to separate the androgenic and the anabolic actions. Because testosterone had to be given parenterally, it was also desirable to find orally active agents.

Following the oral administration of testosterone, only small amounts of the drug reach the systemic circulation unchanged because of rapid first pass metabolism primarily to inactive 17-ketosteroid, etiocholanolone and androsterone, and androstanediol metabolites in the GI mucosa during absorption and in the liver (Fig. 29.18). The plasma half-life of testosterone is less than 30 minutes. Approximately 90% of a dose of testosterone is metabolized and its metabolites are excreted in the urine primarily as glucuronide conjugates with approximately 6% of a dose excreted in the feces as unconjugated testosterone. Generally, the amount of SHBG in plasma determines the distribution of testosterone between free and bound forms, and free testosterone concentrations determine the drug's half-life. Unlike oral testosterone, both intramuscular and transdermal testosterone administration avoid first-pass metabolism with a half-life of 10–100 minutes. Comparative dosage ranges for testosterone and its synthetic preparations are shown in Table 29.4.

Derivatives of Testosterone

Among the esters of testosterone available include the 17β-propionate, 17β-enanthate and the cypionate (17β-cyclopentylpropionate) (Fig. 29.19). Testosterone enanthate is formed by esterification of the 17β-hydroxy group of testosterone with heptanoic acid and testosterone cypionate with cyclopentanepropionic acid. Sterile solutions of these esters are available in a suitable oil (e.g., cottonseed oil). These esters may be thought of as prodrugs when administered intramuscularly because slow hydrolysis of the ester in vivo releases free testosterone over a prolonged period. The cypionate and enanthate esters of testosterone have a duration of action of up to 2–4 weeks. Testosterone propionate has a shorter duration of action than the other esters following IM administration. Because IM injection of testosterone or its esters causes local irritation, the rate of absorption may be erratic. The duration of action of subcutaneous testosterone pellets is usually 3–4 months following subcutaneous implantation of such pellets.

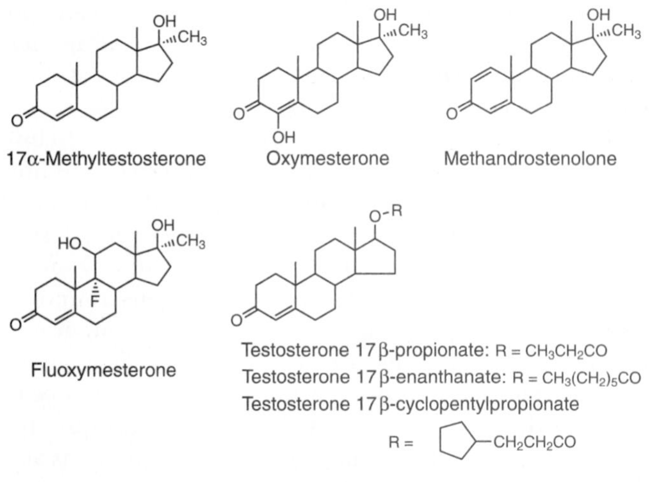

17α-Methyltestosterone   Oxymesterone   Methandrostenolone

Fluoxymesterone

Testosterone 17β-propionate: R = CH_3CH_2CO
Testosterone 17β-enanthanate: R = $CH_3(CH_2)_5CO$
Testosterone 17β-cyclopentylpropionate

R = ◯—CH_2CH_2CO

Fig. 29.19. Androgenic derivatives of testosterone.

In addition to the esters, testosterone transdermal systems are also available and include a reservoir-type transdermal systems.

Synthetic Androgens and Anabolic Agents
Specific Androgens
17α-Methyltestosterone. Some of the early studies with androgens included structural modifications of the naturally occurring hormones. As with estradiol, blocking the metabolism of the 17β-hydroxy group with substituents in the 17α-position resulted in androgens with an increased duration of action when given orally. The synthetic androgens include methyltestosterone and fluoxymesterone (Fig. 29.19).

The synthesis of 17α-methyltestosterone made available a compound that was orally active (177) in daily doses between 10 and 50 mg, which is equivalent to a 400 mg oral dose of testosterone. The presence of 17α alkyl group reduces susceptibility to hepatic oxidative metabolism, thereby increasing oral bioavailability by slowing metabolism. Following oral administration, methyltestos-

terone is well absorbed from the GI tract with a half-life of about 3 hours. This drug has the androgenic and anabolic activities of testosterone. Although orally active, it is more effective when administered sublingually.

Increasing the length of the alkyl side chain at the 17α-position, however, resulted in decreased activity, and the incorporation of other substituents, such as the 17α-ethynyl group, produced compounds with useful progestational activity. Several modifications of 17α-methyltestosterone lead to potent, orally active anabolic agents. Two hydroxylated analogs include oxymesterone (Fig. 29.19) and oxymetholone (Fig. 29.20). These drugs have at least three times the anabolic and half the androgenic activity of the parent compound (158–160).

Selenium dioxide dehydrogenation of 17α-methyltestosterone yields the 1,4-diene analog, methandrostenolone (Fig. 29.19) which has several times the anabolic activity of the starting material. It has low androgenic activity but can apparently produce mammogenic effects in men. These effects are thought to result from estrogenic metabolites.

Fluoxymesterone. By substituting a 9α-fluoro group onto an analog of 17α-methyltestosterone, fluoxymesterone has 20 times the anabolic and 10 times the androgenic activity of 17α-methyltestosterone (177). It has a mean half-life of 9 hours and less than 5% of the drug excreted unchanged. An adverse effect of fluoxymesterone is sodium and water retention that could lead to edema.

Anabolic Steroids
Androgens, having no methyl group in the 10 position of the steroid nucleus, are an important class of anabolic agents often referred to as the 19-norandrogens, and as such have androgenic properties (Fig. 29.20). The removal of the 19-CH$_3$ group of the androgen results in reduction of its androgenic properties but retention of its anabolic, tissue-building properties. Since complete dissociation of anabolic and androgenic effects is not possible,

Table 29.4. Dosages for Androgens and Anabolic Steroids*

Androgen/Anabolic	Trade Name	Route of administration	Frequency of Administration	Usual Dosage Range (mg)
Testosterone aqueous		Intramuscular	2–3 x weekly	25–50
Testosterone propionate		Intramuscular	2–3 x weekly	25–50
Testosterone enanthate	DelaTestryl, Andro LA	Intramuscular	2–4 weeks	50–400
Testosterone cypionate	DuraTest, DepoTest, Andro-Cyp	Intramuscular	2–4 weeks	50–400
Testosterone transdermal system	Androderm, TestoDerm	Topical/patch	daily	2.5–5/24 h
Testosterone pellets	Testopel	Subcutaneous	3–6 mo	150–450
Methyltestosterone	Android, Testred, Oreton-Methyl	Oral	daily	10–50
	Oreton-Methyl	Buccal	daily	5–25
Fluoxymestrone	Halo-Testin, Ora-Testyl	Oral	daily	5–40
Oxymetholone	Androl-50	Oral	daily	1–5/kg
Oxandrolone	Oxandrin	Oral	daily	5–10
Nandrolone phenpropionate	Durabolin, Hybolin	Intramuscular	weekly	50–100
Nandrolone decanoate	Deca-Durabolin, Neo-Durabolic	Intramuscular	weekly	50–100
Stanozolol	Wintrol	Oral	daily	6

*Abstracted from McEvoy GK, ed. AHFS 2000 Drug Information, Bethesda, MD; American Society of Health-System Pharmacists.

many of the actions of anabolic steroids are similar to those of androgens. Comparative dosage ranges for the anabolic steroids are shown in Table 29.4.

Specific Anabolic Steroids. The 17-alpha alkylated anabolic steroids in clinical use are oxandrolone, oxymetholone, stanozolol, and nandrolone decanoate and phenpropionate. These steroids can be synthesized by the Birch reduction of the aromatic A ring of a 3-methoxy estrogen to a 2,5(10)-estradiene. Cleavage of the enol ether with HCl results in a 19-nortestosterone derivative. In animal assays, 19-nortestosterone has about the same anabolic activity as the propionate ester of testosterone, but its androgenic activity is much lower. Because 19-nortestosterone showed some separation of anabolic and androgenic activities, related analogues were synthesized and biologically investigated. Two of the more potent members of the series are norethandrolone, a 17α-ethyl analog, and ethylestrenol.

Norethandrolone has a better ratio of anabolic to androgenic activity than does either 19-nortestosterone or 17α-methyl-19-nortestosterone. The usual dose of norethandrolone is 30–50 mg per day administered orally or parenterally. Both androgenic and progestational side effects have been observed with this agent. Ethylestrenol is more potent than norethandrolone as an anabolic agent and is used in a dosage of 4 mg per day orally.

Klimstra (177) reported that alkylation in the 1, 2, 7, and 18 positions of the androstane molecule generally increases anabolic activity. One of these derivatives, methenolone acetate is an example of a potent anabolic agent that does not have an alkyl substituent at the 17α-position. This compound is administered parenterally in a dose of 20 mg per week for its anabolic action. A halo-genated anabolic agent used in about the same dosage is chlortestosterone acetate.

A 2-oxasteroid analog of 17α-methyltestosterone is oxandrolone which contains a lactone in the A ring (oxygen bioisostere of ring A) and is therefore susceptible to in vivo hydrolysis. It has three times the anabolic activity of 17α-methyltestosterone, but exhibits slight androgenic activity. Another heterocyclic compound used for its anabolic effects is the pyrazole derivative, stanozolol.

The anabolic steroid oxymetholone is used primarily to stimulate production of erythropoietin in the treatment of anemias resulting from bone marrow failure.

Nandrolone phenpropionate and nandrolone decanoate are esters of 19-nortestosterone that when administered intramuscularly, slow hydrolysis of the ester in vivo releases free 19-nortestosterone over a prolonged period. Nandrolone decanoate is the longer acting ester intended for deep intramuscular injection preferably into the gluteal muscle, in the treatment of anemia associated with renal insufficiency. Nandrolone phenpropionate has a shorter duration of action than the decanoate and is used in the treatment of metastatic breast cancer in women.

Testolactone (Teslac), a 18-oxasteroid, is a D-homo-oxoandrostandienedione analog with ring D being a 6-membered lactone ring. Although testolactone possesses some anabolic activity with weak androgenic effects, it is used primarily in the treatment of breast cancer as a non-competitive irreversible inhibitor of aromatase to reduce the level of estrogens that would stimulate the growth of breast tissue. It is primarily excreted in the urine unchanged, but is metabolized in the liver by partial reduction of the 4-ene double bond in ring A to the 5β-metabolite (*cis* A/B ring juncture). Testolactone is available in both parenteral and oral forms.

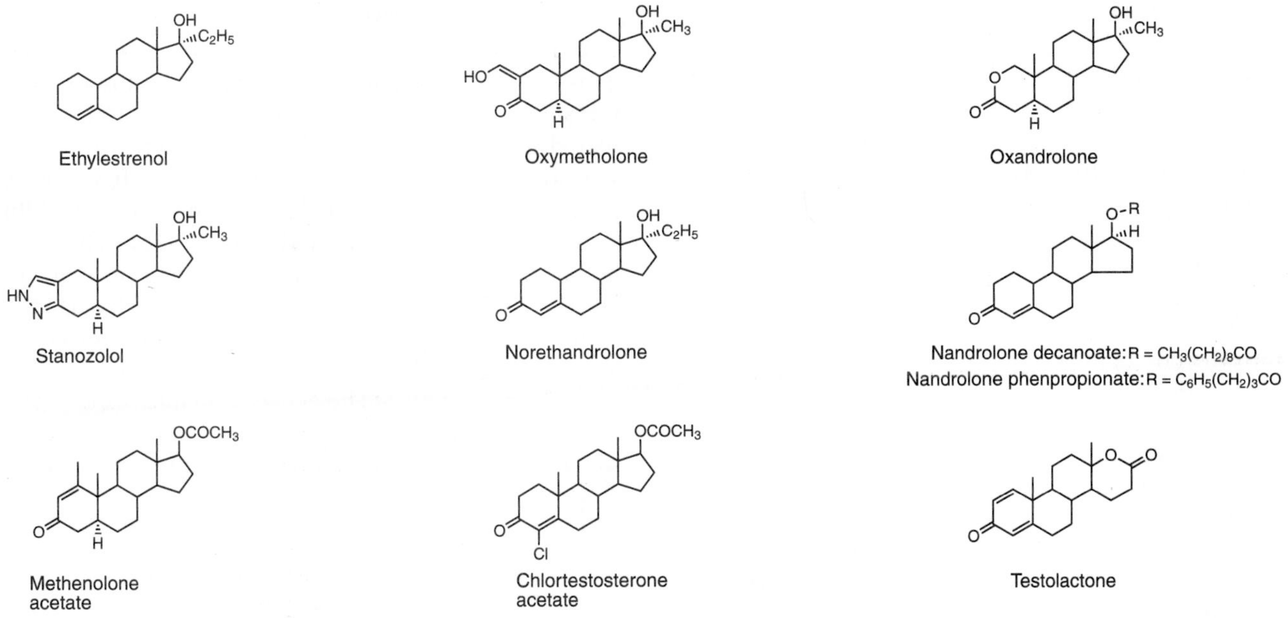

Ethylestrenol

Oxymetholone

Oxandrolone

Stanozolol

Norethandrolone

Nandrolone decanoate: R = $CH_3(CH_2)_8CO$
Nandrolone phenpropionate: R = $C_6H_5(CH_2)_3CO$

Methenolone acetate

Chlortestosterone acetate

Testolactone

Fig. 29.20. Anabolic steroids.

Danazol

2-Hydroxymethylethisterone
(Danazol metabolite)

Gonadotropin Inhibitor

Danazol (Danocrine), an isoxazole derivative of ethisterone, is a gonadotropin inhibitor for use in the treatment of endometriosis. Previous treatment of endometriosis had been surgical or with progestins or a combination of estrogen and progestin. Danazol reportedly suppresses the pituitary-ovarian axis by inhibiting output of pituitary and hypothalamic gonadotropins and may inhibit the synthesis of sex steroids (178). It binds to sex steroid receptors in the cytoplasm of target tissues and may thereby exhibit antiestrogen, anabolic, and weakly androgenic effects. The drug possesses weak androgenic and anabolic properties but exerts no estrogenic or progestogenic activity. Bioavailability studies indicate nonlinear pharmacokinetics for danazol; danazol concentrations do not increase proportionally with increases in dose. Danazol is metabolized to 2-hydroxymethylethisterone, which appears in the plasma in a concentration 5–10 times greater than that of the unchanged drug. Danazol is used for the palliative treatment of endometriosis in patients in whom alternative hormonal therapy is ineffective, intolerable, or contraindicated.

Structure-activity Relationships

For a substance to have androgenic activity, it must contain a n androstane steroid skeleton (217). Oxygen functional groups normally occurring at positions 3 and 17 are not essential because the basic nucleus, 5α-androstane, has androgenic activity. This appears to be the minimal structural requirement for hormonal activity. For derivatives of etiocholane, in which the hydrogen is in the 5β-position, thereby affording a *cis*-A/B ring juncture, no active androgens and anabolic agents are known (180). The *cis* A/B ring juncture prevents any affinity for the androgen receptor. Generally, both ring expansion (to form homo derivatives by inserting a methylene group into one of the rings in the steroid nucleus) or ring contraction (by removing a methylene group) significantly reduces or destroys the androgenic and anabolic activities.

Introduction of a 3-keto function or a 3α-OH group enhances androgenic activity, but the 17-keto eliminates androgenic activity. A hydroxyl group in the 17α-position of androstane contributes no androgenic or anabolic activity; no known substituent can approach the effectiveness of a 17β-OH group. Evidence indicates that the longer-acting esters of the 17β-OH compounds are hydrolyzed in vivo to the free alcohol, which is the active species (181). It is thought that the 17β-oxygen atom is important for attachment to the receptor site (180) and that 17α-alkyl groups are important for preventing metabolic changes at this po-

sition. Such 17α-substituents render the compounds orally active.

Ordinarily, halogen substitution produces compounds with decreased activity except when inserted into positions 4 or 9. Replacement of a carbon atom in position 2 by oxygen has produced the only clinically successful heterocyclic steroid among a number of azasteroids and oxasteroids. Some of the 2-oxasteroids are potent anabolic agents.

Introduction of an sp² hybridized carbon atom into the A ring renders the ring more planar, and this in turn may be responsible for greater anabolic activity. The 19-norsteroids are of interest because these agents seem to produce a more favorable ratio of anabolic to androgenic activity. Vida (180) has extensively reviewed the replacement of various hydrogens on the androgen steroid skeleton by other functional groups. It appears that certain substitutions at positions 1, 2, 7, 17, and 18 may result in compounds with favorable activities that will be of clinical importance (177).

Bioassays used in determining the androgenic activity of these hormones include measurements of capon comb growth (in terms of size and weight), increased weight of seminal vesicles, and increased weight of the ventral part of the prostate of castrated rats. Measurements of anabolic activity are based on an increase in nitrogen retention or an increase in mass of specific muscles in animals.

Although much effort has concentrated on the development of female contraception, some work has been carried out in males (182). A surgical method of male contraception, vasectomy, is reported to be the most effective method and to be widely used. It is a rather simple surgical procedure that disrupts spermatozoal exit and produces few side effects. The irreversible nature of vasectomy and the subsequent psychologic barrier raised in some men has prompted a continuing search for reversible approaches to vasectomy and drugs (183).

It has been shown that androgens, progestins, estrogens, and many chemically nonrelated substances have the ability to interfere with the formation of mature ejaculated spermatozoa (367). Unfortunately, none of the steroid preparations is without side effects. It has been reported that, in a village in China, not a single childbirth occurred over a 10-year period from 1930 to 1940, whereas before and after this period, fertility was normal (184). During those years, it was noted that the villagers had switched from soybean oil to cottonseed oil for cooking. Tests in animals showed that cottonseed oil had an antispermatogenic effect. The active principle responsible for the infertility effect is gossypol, the main side effects of which are fatigue, gastrointestinal upsets, weakness, hy-

Gossypol

pokalemia, low libido, and carcinogenic effects in the skin of mice. The finding of the activity of gossypol is an important milestone in the search for male antifertility agents (185). Gossypol has been tested in men in China as a male contraceptive.

Androgen Antagonists

Antagonists of androgens include agents that block androgen receptors (antiandrogens) and inhibitors of androgen biosynthesis.

Antiandrogens

Overview. An antiandrogen is a substance that antagonizes the actions of 5α-dihydrotestosterone at the androgen receptor and, when administered with an androgen, blocks or diminishes the effectiveness of androgens in androgensensitive tissues. Such compounds have shown potential therapeutic use in the treatment of acne, virilization in women, and hyperplasia and neoplasia of the prostate (186). Several steroidal and nonsteroidal agents have demonstrated antiandrogenic activity (Figs. 29.21 and 29.22). Cyproterone acetate suppresses gonadotropin release (187) and binds with high affinity to the androgen receptor (188). Oxendolone also acts by competing for the receptor binding sites (189). A novel androgen receptor antagonist, WIN 49,596, was described (190); this agent contains a fused pyrazole ring at carbons 2 and 3 of the steroid nucleus that is similar to stanozolol, but without anabolic properties.

Nonsteroidal Antiandrogens. The search for nonsteroidal antiandrogens lead to the development of the substituted toluidides, flutamide (Eulexin), bicalutamide (Casodex), and nilutamide (Nilandron) (Fig. 29.22). These toluidides are pure antiandrogens and compete with DHT for the human prostate androgen receptor. They are used in combination with other drugs in the treatment of metastatic prostate cancer. Although these compounds possess no intrinsic hormonal activity, their antiandrogenic mechanism of action is via competitive blockade of androgen receptors for DHT in the hormone-sensitive tumor cells of the prostate (191). As a result of this antagonism,

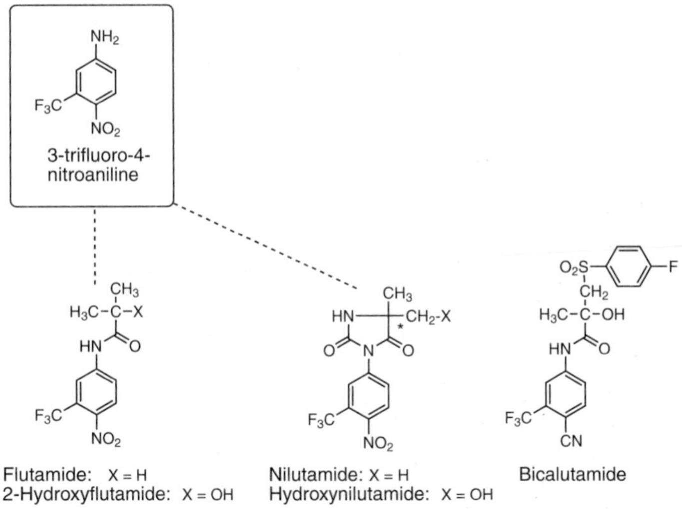

Fig. 29.22. Nonsteroidal androgens.

androgen-dependent DNA and protein synthesis is inhibited causing arrest or regression of the prostatic tumor. Since these nonsteroidal antiandrogens are metabolized extensively in the liver, they should be used with caution in patients with liver function abnormalities.

Specific Drugs. Following oral administration, flutamide is completely absorbed from the GI tract and undergoes extensive first pass metabolism by CYP1A2 to its major metabolite, 2-hydroxyflutamide and its hydrolysis product, 3-trifluoromethyl-4-nitroaniline (Fig. 29.22). 2-Hydroxyflutamide is a more powerful antiandrogen in vivo, with higher affinity for the receptor than flutamide (192). 2-Hydroxyflutamide has an elimination half-life of about 8 hours. Bicalutamide is administered as a racemate, but its R-enantiomer is the active antiandrogenic stereoisomer, which has approximately a 4-fold higher affinity for the prostate androgen receptor than does hydroxyflutamide. Following oral administration, the racemate displays stereoselective oxidative metabolism of its R-enantiomer with an elimination half-life of about 6 days. The inactive S-enantiomer forms only a glucuronide conjugate metabolite. Nilutamide is a hydantoin analog of flutamide that is completely absorbed after oral administration with a mean elimination half-life of 50 hours (38–60 hours). One of the methyl groups attached to the hydantoin ring is stereoselectively hydroxylated to a chiral metabolite, which is subsequently oxidized to its carboxylic acid metabolite. Less than 2% of nilutamide is excreted unchanged in the urine.

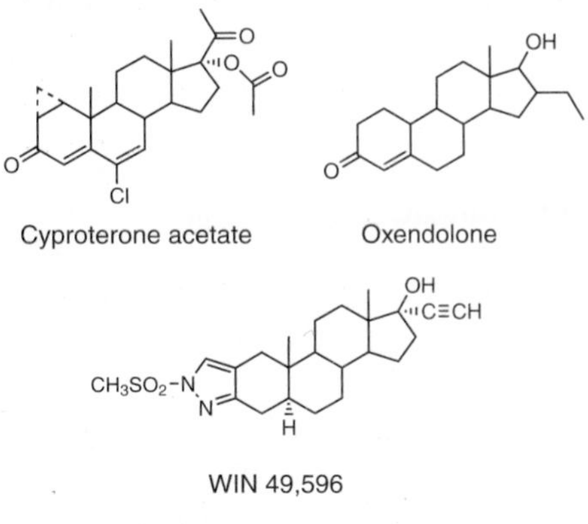

5α-Reductase Inhibitors

Inhibitors of androgen biosynthesis result in a decrease in active androgen concentrations in target tissues and thus antagonize androgen action. The critical enzyme targeted for inhibition is 5α-reductase, which converts testosterone to the most potent endogenous androgen, 5α-dihydrotestosterone.

Fig. 29.21. Steroid antiandrogens.

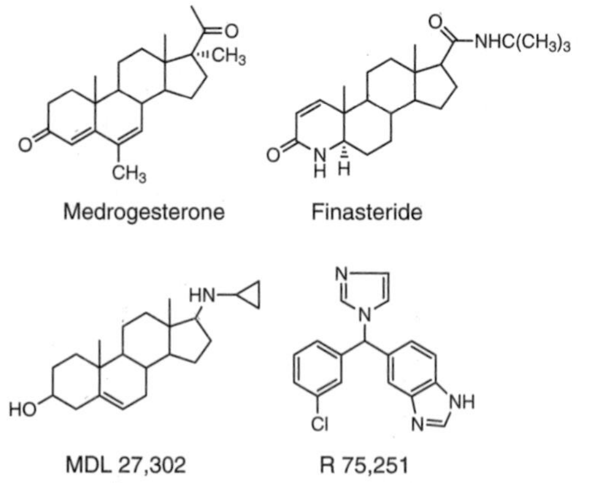

Fig. 29.23. 5α-Reductase and 17α-hydroxylase inhibitors.

The first agent to demonstrate 5α-reductase inhibition was a progestin analog, medrogesterone (Fig. 29.23) (193). The 4-azasteroid finasteride (Proscar, Propecia) is a potent inhibitor of 5α-reductase (194,195) and effectively decreases 5α-DHT concentrations in both plasma and in prostate tissues (195–197). Since finasteride is metabolized extensively in the liver, it should be used with caution in patients with liver function abnormalities. Its elimination rate of the drug is decreased in males 70 years of age or older with a mean terminal half-life of approximately 8 hours (range: 6–15 hours) compared with 6 hours (range: 4–12 hours) in males 45–60 years of age. This drug is approved for treatment of symptomatic benign prostatic hyperplasia and management of alopecia in males. A second enzyme system targeted for inhibition is 17α-hydroxylase and 17,20-lyase, which converts pregnenolone to DHA and subsequently testosterone. Since testosterone has significant androgenic activity by itself, inhibition of its biosynthesis would be useful in treating androgen-dependent diseases such as prostate cancer. The antifungal agent, ketoconazole, inhibits 17α-hydroxylase at high concentrations and demonstrated clinical activity in metastatic prostate cancer patients (198). The steroidal compound, MDL 27,302 (199) and the nonsteroidal agent, R 75,251 (198) are under development as potentially more selective inhibitors of 17α-hydroxylase and 17,20–lyase.

Mechanism of Androgen Action
Molecular Interactions

Androgens produce various physiologic effects. Nevertheless, research has shown the mechanism of action of androgens to be through regulation of protein synthesis in target cells by the formation of a steroid-receptor complex. Extensive reviews on the mechanism of androgen action have appeared (80,158,200–203). The current concept of this mechanism of action has evolved from studies using androgen-sensitive rat ventral prostate. Testosterone was found to be rapidly converted to 5α-dihydrotestosterone (DHT) in the prostate, and this reduced metabolite was selectively retained (163,204). Thus, the mechanism of action for the prohormone, testosterone, in the

prostate begins with the conversion of testosterone to DHT by 5α-reductase. DHT binds to proteins present in the nucleus of prostate cells with extremely high affinity and specificity for DHT (205). This DHT-receptor complex then undergoes a conformational change and the steroid-receptor complex then interacts with the chromatin present in the target cell and results in the increased production of messenger RNA (mRNA) (205–208). These elevated levels of mRNA result in increased protein synthesis and subsequent stimulation of cell growth and differentiation.

Androgen receptors have been identified in other tissues, such as seminal vesicles, (209,210) testis, (211,212) epididymis, (211,213) kidney, (214) brain, (215–217) liver, (218) and androgen-sensitive tumors (219,220). DHT, however, is not the only functioning form of androgen in other androgen-sensitive tissues. DHT is rapidly biosynthesized in tissues such as those of the prostate, but is not readily formed in tissues such as those of the kidney. The mechanism of anabolic action of the androgens also appears to involve the formation of a steroid-receptor complex. Testosterone has greater activity than DHT in the androgen-mediated growth of muscle both in vivo and in tissue culture (221–223). Receptor proteins specific for testosterone have been identified in muscle tissues (224–230). Thus, the involvement of specific receptor proteins and the resulting increase in protein synthesis are the common mechanism of action of the androgens in various target tissues.

Pharmacology, Side Effects, and Clinical Applications

The male sex hormones are responsible for normal growth and development of the male sex organs and for the retention of nitrogen and certain inorganic substances, such as potassium, calcium, chloride, phosphorus, and sodium. The anabolic effect of androgens is responsible for the fast growth of males at puberty.

Among the important therapeutic applications of the androgenic hormones is replacement therapy in patients with deficient endogenous androgen production. Various preparations of testosterone and its congeners include aqueous suspensions and oil solutions for parenteral administration, tablets for oral administration, tablets for buccal and sublingual absorption, and transdermal patches. Solid pellets are also available for implantation under the skin.

The various androgen preparations can be used in the treatment of eunuchism and eunuchoidism to restore or maintain secondary sexual characteristics. Gonadotropins may be administered when hypogonadism exists to determine if the testes are capable of producing the needed hormones. Androgens have been used alone and in combination with gonadotropins for cryptorchidism (failure of the testes to descend), and are also used for the treatment of faulty spermatogenesis, benign prostatic hypertrophy, and impotency.

In older men who are undergoing the male climacteric, which is analogous to menopause in women, androgens may be beneficial. In women the androgens are used for breast engorgement, inoperable mammary carcinoma, hypolibido, and chronic cystic mastitis. At one time, the androgens were used in menstrual disorders, but this treatment has been supplanted by the progestins and estrogens. In small amounts, androgens, along with estrogens, are used in the treatment of menopause.

The androgens have been used in both sexes as anabolic agents, to increase weight in both adults and children, and to reverse the loss of protein resulting from trauma, prolonged immobilization, and wasting diseases. Because androgens retain calcium, they are used in the treatment of osteoporosis, which often occurs in the elderly.

The use of androgens is limited because of the side effects they can produce in humans. In women, masculinization may occur, particularly during long-term therapy. This leads to growth of hair on the face, voice changes, and the development of a more muscular body. In both sexes, there may be increased retention of electrolytes and water during extended periods of androgen therapy, leading to edema.

Hepatic dysfunction may occur in patients taking the 17α-alkylated androgens, but this appears to be a transitory effect because hepatic function returns to normal on cessation of therapy. Premature epiphyseal closure and virilization limit the use of anabolic agents in children. Caution must also be exercised when using androgens in conjunction with other drugs. The anticoagulant response of coumarin-type anticoagulants can be increased by norethandrolone (231).

Use and Abuse of Anabolic Steroids for Performance Enhancement

The stimulatory effects of anabolics on tissue and muscle growth (referred to as myotrophic effects) have also led to the use and the abuse of these agents by athletes (232–235). This nonmedical use of anabolics has resulted in significant concern and debate. Conflicting reports on the effectiveness of anabolics to increase strength and power in healthy males have resulted from clinical trials. Several groups reported no significance differences between groups of male college-age students receiving anabolics and weight training and those groups receiving placebo plus the weight training in double blind studies (236–239). Other reports cited only minor improvement in strength and power, but these studies utilized small numbers of subjects or were only single blind studies (240–243). A recent study on "supraphysiologic" doses of anabolics has demonstrated enhancement of muscle size and strength (244). Anabolic steroids also exhibit an anticatabolic effect, i.e., reversing the catabolic effects of glucocorticoids released in response to stress. Such effects would enable individuals to recover more quickly following strenuous workouts. The nonmedical uses of anabolics in women and adolescents clearly demonstrate increases in muscle size and strength; however, no scientific studies have been performed to fully evaluate effects of anabolics in healthy populations.

An alarming percentage of amateur and professional athletes utilize anabolic steroids that are readily available "on the street" (245). The use of these steroids for increasing strength and power is banned in intercollegiate and international sports, and very sensitive assays (RIA, GC-MS) have been developed for measuring anabolic levels in urine and blood (233). The most serious toxicities resulting from the use of anabolic steroids are liver damage, virilization, stunted height, and lower HDL-cholesterol levels. Liver damage including jaundice and cholestasis can occur after use of the 17α-alkylated C_{19} steroids (246–249). Also, individuals who have received anabolic agents over an extended period have developed hepatic adenocarcinomas. Virilization and stunted height due to premature epiphesial closure are significant side effects in women and adolescents (233–250). The effects of anabolics on lowering HDL-cholesterol may increase risks to coronary artery disease later in life. Such clinical reports serve to underscore the inherent risks associated with anabolic steroid use in athletes.

CASE STUDY

Victoria F. Roche and S. William Zito

NS is a 52-year-old, female anthropology professor who has been on estrogen replacement therapy for two years after undergoing a complete hysterectomy and oophorectomy to remove fibroid tumors. Her doctor placed her on p.o. Estinyl® (ethinyl estradiol) and she is doing well. An active adventurer and South American scholar, she is taking her graduate students on a five week trip to the Amazon to study an obscure tribe of hunter-gatherers known as the Chemophilongi. She will be traveling light, and would rather not have to worry about taking medication on the trip. She asks you, her trusted community pharmacist, for advice on how she can conveniently keep up with her therapy. She is taking no other medication except the estrogen replacement therapy.

1. Identify the therapeutic problem(s) where the pharmacist's intervention may benefit the patient.

2. Identify and prioritize the patient specific factors that must be considered to achieve the desired therapeutic outcomes.

3. Conduct a thorough and mechanistically oriented structure-activity analysis of all therapeutic alternatives provided in the case.

4. Evaluate the SAR findings against the patient specific factors and desired therapeutic outcomes and make a therapeutic decision.

5. Counsel your patient.

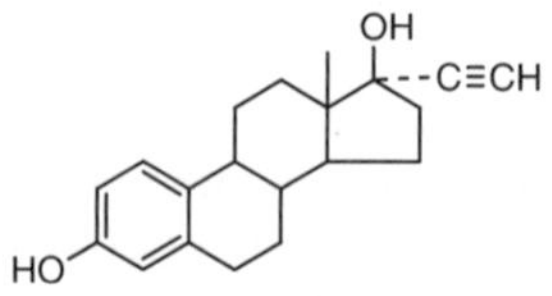

Ethinyl estradiol

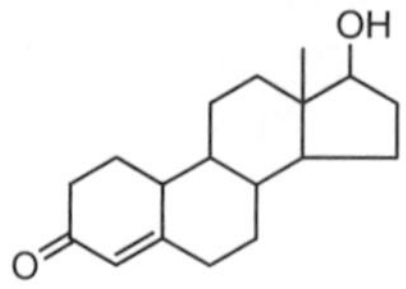

1

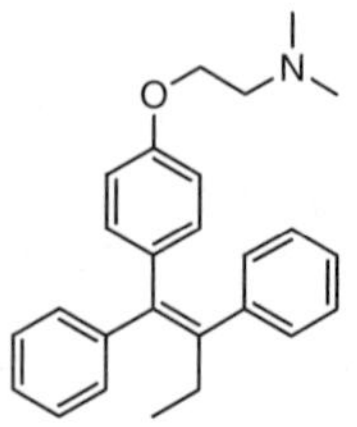

2

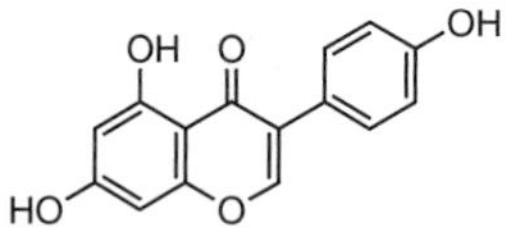

3

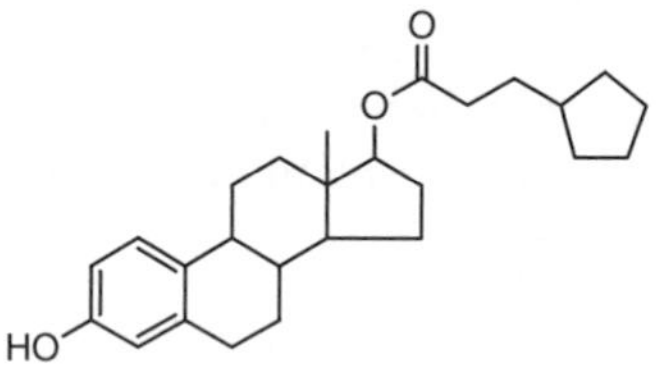

4

714

REFERENCES

1. GW Harris and F Naftolin, Br Med Bull, 26, 1(1970).
2. RB Jaffe, et al., Chapter 1, in Contraception: The Chemical Control of Fertility, D Lednicer, Ed. New York, Marcel Dekker, 1969.
3. E Allen and EA Doisy, JAMA, 81, 819(1923).
4. C Williams and GM Stancel, Chapter 57, in Goodman and Gilman's The Pharmacological Basis of Therapeutics, 9th ed., JG Hardman, et al., Eds., New York, Pergamon Press, 1996, pp. 1411–1440.
5. PC Ruentiz, Chapter 57, in Burger's Medicinal Chemistry, Volume 4, 5th Ed., ME Wolff, Ed., NY, Wiley, 1997, pp. 553–588.
6. J Fishman, et al., J Biol Chem, 237, 1487(1962).
7. E Gurpide, et al., J Clin Endocrinol, 22, 935(1962).
8. E R. Simpson, et al., Endocr Rev, 10, 136(1989).
9. KJ Ryan and OW Smith, Recent Prog Horm Res, 21, 367(1965).
10. S Najakin and PF Hall, J Biol Chem, 256, 3871(1981).
11. HA Harvey, et al., Eds., Cancer Res, 42, 3267s-3468 (1982).
12. RJ Santen, Ed., Steroids, 50, 1–655(1985).
13. RJ Santen and AMH Brodie, Eds., Third International Aromatase Conference, J Steroid Biochem Mol Biol, 44 321–696 (1993).
14. A Bhatnagar, AMH Brodie, RW Brueggemeier, et al., Eds., Fourth International Aromatase Conference, J. Steroid Biochem Mol Biol, 61 107–426 (1997).
15. AMH Brodie, Ed., J. Enzyme Inhib, 4, 75–200(1990).
16. KJ Ryan, J Biol Chem, 234, 268(1959).
17. EA Thompson and PK Siiteri, J Biol Chem, 249, 5364(1974).
18. J Goto and J Fishman, Science, 195, 80(1977).
19. M Akhtar, et al., Biochem J, 201, 569(1982).
20. PA Cole and CH Robinson, J Am Chem Soc, 110, 1284(1988).
21. RW Brueggemeier, J. Enzyme Inhibition, 4, 101(1990).
22. JB Brown, Adv Clin Chem, 3, 157(1960).
23. H Breuer, Vitam Horm, 20, 285(1962).
24. E Diczfalusy and C Lauritzen, Oestrogen bein Menschen., Berlin, Springer, 1961.
25. Y Nose and F. Lipmann, J Biol Chem, 233, 1348(1958).
26. CH Gray and JB Lunnon, J Endocrinol, 3, 19(1956).
27. CJ Migeon, et al., J Clin Invest, 38, 619(1959).
28. BT Brown, et al., Nature, 182, 50(1958).
29. J Fishman, et al., J Biol Chem, 235, 3104(1960).
30. GR Merriam and MB Lipsett, Catechol Estrogens, New York, Raven Press, 1983.
31. HH Inhoffen and W Hohlweg, Naturwissenschaften, 29, 96(1938).
32. LB Colton, et al., J Am Chem Soc., 79, 1123(1957).
33. A Ercoli and R. Gardi, Chem Ind (Lond), 1037(1961).
34. FR Zuleski, et al., J Pharm Sci, 67, 1138(1978).
35. RJ Chetkowski, et al., N Engl J Med, 314, 1615(1986).
36. H Judd, Am J Obstet Gyneco., 156, 1326(1987).
37. RE Vanderlinde, et al., J Am Chem Soc, 77, 4176(1955).
38. UV Solmssen, Chem Rev, 37, 481(1945).
39. Adlercreutz H Environ Health Perspect., 103 (Suppl. 7), 103–112 (1995).
40. PJ Bentley, Endocrine Pharmacology, Cambridge, Cambridge University Press, 1980.
41. GM Anstead, KE Carlson and JA Katzenellenbogen, Steroids, 62, 268–303 (1997).
42. AM Brzozowski, ACW Pike, A Dauter, et al. Nature, 389, 753–758 (1997).
43. AK Shiau, D Barstad, PM Loria, et al. Cell, 95, 927–937 (1998).
44. JS Baran, J Med Chem, 10, 1188(1967).
45. AA Albanese, et al., NY State J Med, 65, 2116(1965).
46. E Heftmann, Steroid Biosynthesis. New York, Academic Press, 1970, p. 141.
47. LF Fieser and M Fieser, in Steroids. New York, Reinhold, 1959, p. 477.
48. GA Grant and D Beall, Recent Prog Horm Res, 5, 307(1950).
49. HS Kupperman, et al., J Clin Endocrinol, 13, 688(1953).
50. AD Cross, et al., Steroids, 4, 423(1964).
51. M Rubin and H Wiskinsky, J Am Chem Soc, 66, 1948(1944).
52. EC Dodds, Nature, 142, 34(1938).
53. GW Harris and F Naftolin, Br Med Bull, 26, 197(1970).
54. IW Funder, et al., Biochem Pharmacol, 23, 1493(1974).
55. BS Katzenellenbogen and ER Ferguson, Endocrinology, 97, 1(1975).
56. JH Clark, et al., Nature, 251, 446(1974).
57. VC Jordan, et al., J Endocrinol, 75, 305(1977).
58. VC Jordan and CS Murphy, Endocrine Rev, 11, 578(1990).
59. AE Wakeling and J Bowler, J Steroid Biochem, 30, 141(1988).
60. AE Wakeling, et al., Cancer Res., 51, 3867(1991).
61. Jordan VC. Selective Estrogen Receptor Modulators. In Foye's Principles of Medicinal Chemistry 5th Lemke T, Willimas DA. Eds. Chapter 43. Baltimore, Lippincott Williams Wilkins, 2002.
62. TA Grese, JP Sluka, HW Bryant, et al. Proc Natl Acad Sci, 94, 14105–14110 (1997).
63. AMH Brodie, et al., Cancer Res, 42, 3360s(1982).
64. RW Brueggemeier, et al., Cancer Res, 42, 3334s(1982).
65. RW Brueggemeier, et al., J Steroid Biochem Mol Biol, 37, 379(1990).
66. JO Johnston, et al., Endocrinology, 115, 776(1984).
67. D Henderson, et al, Endocrinology, 115, 776(1986).
68. D Giudici, et al., J Steroid Biochem Mol Biol, 30, 391(1988).
69. HA Salhanick, Cancer Res., 42, 3315s(1982).
70. AS Bhatnagar, et al., J Steroid Biochem Mol Biol, 37, 363(1990).
71. R De Coster, et al., J Steroid Biochem Mol Biol, 37, 335(1990).
72. AU Budzar, W Jonat, A Howell, et al. J Steroid Biochem Mol Biol, 61, 145–150 (1997).
73. AS Bhatnagar, A Hausler, K Schieweck, et al. J. Steroid Biochem Mol Biol, 37, 1021–1027 (1990).
74. JA Johnston and BW Metcalf, in Novel Approaches to Cancer Chemotherapy, P. Sunkara, Ed., New York, Academic Press, 1984, p. 307.
75. L Banting, et al., J. Enzyme Inhib, 2, 215(1988).
76. DF Covey, in Sterol Biosynthesis Inhibitors, D Berg and M. Plempel, Eds., Chichester, UK, Ellis Horwood, 1988, p. 534.
77. L Banting, et al., Prog Med Chem, 26, 253(1989).
78. EV Jensen and HI Jacobsen, Recent Prog Horm Res, 18, 387(1962).
79. J Gorski, et al., Rec Prog Horm Res, 42, 297(1986).
80. L Chan and B W O'Malley, N Engl J Med, 294, 1322–1328, 1372–1381, 1430–1437(1976).
81. WP Noteboom and J Gorski, Arch Biochem Biophys, 111, 559(1965).
82. GGJM Kuiper, E Envark, M Pelto-Huikko, et al. Proc Natl Acad Sci, 93, 5925–5930 (1996).
83. GGJM Kuiper, B Carlson, K Grandien, et al. Endocrinology, 138, 863–870 (1997).
84. S Liao and AH Lin, Proc Natl Acad Sci USA, 57, 379(1967).
85. BW O'Malley, et al., Recent Prog Horm Res, 25, 121(1969).
86. H Wi and GC Mueller, Proc Natl Acad Sci USA, 50, 256(1963).
87. GC Mueller, et al., Proc Natl Acad Sci USA, 47, 164(1961).
88. BS Katzenellenbogen and J Gorski, J Biol Chem, 247, 1299(1972).
89. AM Kaye, J Steroid Biochem, 19, 33(1983).
90. SJ Segal and SS Koide, in Pharmacology of Estrogens, International Encyclopedia of Pharmacology and Therapeutics, Section 106, Pergamon Press, Oxford, 1981, pp. 113–150.

91. E Heftmann, Steroid Biochemistry. New York, Academic Press, 1970, p. 140.
92. PH Jellinck and AM Newcombe, J Endocrinol, 74, 147(1977).
93. CR Lyttle and ER DeSombre, Nature, 268, 337(1977).
94. O Hechter and IDK. Halkerston, Hormones, 5, 799(1964).
95. SC Aitken and ME Lippman, Cancer Res, 43, 4681(1983).
96. SC Aitken and ME Lippman, Cancer Res, 45, 1611(1985).
97. KB Horwitz and WL McGuire, J Biol Chem, 253, 2223(1978).
98. ME. Lippman, in Williams' Textbook of Endocrinology, 9th ed., JD Wilson, DW Foster, HM Kronenberg, et al. Eds., Philadelphia, WB Saunders, 1998, pp. 1675–1692.
99. SB Jakolew, et al., Nucleic Acids Res, 12, 2861(1984).
100. RB Dickson and M. E. Lippman, Endocr Rev, 8, 29(1987).
101. SE Bates, et al., Cancer Res, 46, 1707(1986).
102. RB Dickson, et al., Science, 232, 1540(1986).
103. RB Dickson, et al., Endocrinology, 118, 138(1986).
104. KK Huff, et al., Cancer Res, 46, 4613(1986).
105. F Vignon, et al., CR Acad Sci III, 296, 151(1983).
106. D Bronzert, et al., Cancer Res, 47, 1234(1987).
107. RW Brueggemeier and P-K Li, in Antilipidemic Drugs, Medicinal, Chemical and Biological Aspects, DL Witiak, HAI Newman, and DF Feller, Eds, Amsterdam, Elsevier Science Publishers, 1992, pp. 493–526.
108. S Fraenkel, Arch. Gynaek, 68, 438(1903).
109. R Pearl and FM Surface, J Biol Chem, 19, 263(1914).
110. GW Corner and WM Allen, Am J Physiol, 88, 326(1929).
111. LF Fieser and M Fieser, Chapter 19, in Steroids. New York, Reinhold, 1959.
112. AW Makepace, et al., Am J Physiol, 119, 512(1937).
113. E Heftmann and E. Mosetlig, in Biochemistry of Steroids. New York, Reinhold, 1960, p. 106.
114. C Djerassi, Science, 151, 1055(1966).
115. ME Davis and GL Wied, J Clin Endocrinol, 15, 923(1955).
116. I Siegel, Obstet Gynecol, 21, 666(1963).
117. A Klopper, Br. Med. Bull., 26, 39(1970).
118. JC Babcock, et al., J Am Chem Soc, 80, 2904(1958).
119. L Ruzicka and K Hofmann, Helv Chim Acta, 20, 1280(1937).
120. PD Klimstra, Am J Pharm 34, 630(1970).
121. M Ehrenstein, J Org Chem, 9, 435(1944).
122. C Djerassi, et al., J Am Chem Soc, 75, 4440(1953).
123. G Pincus, Science, 138, 439(1962).
124. PD Klimstra, Am. J Pharm Ed, 34, 630(1970).
125. D Philibert, R Deraedt, et al., 64th Annual Meeting of The Endocrine Society, San Francisco, June 1982, Abstract No. 668.
126. EE Baulieu, Science, 245, 1351(1989).
127. MK Agarwal, et al., FEBS Lett, 217, 221(1987).
128. W Elger, et al., J Steroid Biochem Mol Biol, 25, 835(1986).
129. KB Horwitz, Endocr Rev, 13, 146(1992).
130. BW O'Malley, et al., Recent Prog Horm Res, 25, 105(1969).
131. MA Carson-Jurica, et al., Endocr Rev, 11, 201(1990).
132. H Gronemeyer, et al., EMBO J, 6, 3985(1987).
133. M Misrahi, et al., Biochem Biophys Res Commun, 143, 740(1987).
134. MA Carson-Jurica, et al., J Steroid Biochem Mol Biol, 34, 1(1989).
135. K Fotherby, Vitam Horm, 22, 153(1964).
136. GW Harris and OF Naftolin, Br Med Bull, 26, 3(1970).
137. EE Baulieu, in Steroid Hormone Regulation of the Brain, K. Fuxe, et al., Eds., Oxford, Pergamon Press, 1981, pp. 3–14.
138. MD Majewska, et al., Science, 222, 1004(1986).
139. MD Morrow, et al., Eur J Pharmacol, 142, 483(1987).
140. EE Baulieu and P Robel, J Steroid Biochem Mol Biol, 37, 395(1990).
141. I Rothchild, in Metabolic Effects of Gonadal Hormones and Contraceptive Steroids, HA Salhanick, et al., Eds., New York, Plenum Press, 1969, p. 668.
142. VA Drill, Oral Contraceptives. New York, McGraw-Hill, 1966, p. 3.
143. J Crossland, Chapter 38, in Lewis's Pharmacology, London, E & S Livingstone, 1970.
144. G Pincus, Science, 153, 493(1966).
145. G Pincus, et al., Science, 130, 81(1959).
146. V Petrow, Chem Rev, 70, 713(1970).
147. HW Berendes, in Pharmacology of Steroid Contraceptive Drugs, S Garattini and HW Berendes, Eds., New York, Raven Press, 1977, p. 223.
148. GV Upton, Int J Fertil, 28, 121(1983).
149. C Dodds, Clin Pharmacol Ther, 10, 147(1969).
150. D Shoupe and DR Mishell, Am J Obstet Gynecol, 60, 1286(1989).
151. R Wiechert, Angew, Chem Int Ed Engl, 16, 506(1977).
152. FDA Consumer, Women and Estrogens, April 1976, p. 4.
153. FDA Drug Bulletin, Estrogens and Endometrial Cancer, 6, 18(1976).
154. Facts and Comparison, Sex Hormones, St. Louis, Mo., Facts and Comparison Inc., 1975, p. 107d.
155. Med Lett, 18, 21(1976).
156. A Klopper, Br Med J, 26, 39(1970).
157. MM Grumbach and JR Ducharme, Fertil. Steril., 11, 157(1960).
158. RW Brueggemeier, Burger's Medicinal Chemistry, Fifth Edition, Volume 3, ME Wolff, Ed., N.Y., John Wiley & Sons, 1996, pp. 445–510.
159. RW Brueggemeier, Handbook of Hormones, Vitamins, and Radiopaques, M. Verderame, Ed., Boca Raton, FL, CRC Press, 1986, pp. 1–49.
160. RI Dorfman and F Ungar, Metabolism of Steroid Hormones. New York, Academic Press, 1965, p. 123.
161. JM Rosner, et al., Endocrinology, 75, 299(1964).
162. EE Baulieu, et al., Steroids, 2, 429(1963).
163. N Bruckovsky and JD Wilson, J Biol Chem, 243, 2012(1968).
164. P Ofner, Vit. Horm., 26, 237(1968).
165. L Martini, in Subcellular Mechanisms in Reproductive Endocrinology, F Naftolin, et al., Eds., Amsterdam, Elsevier, 1976, p. 327.
166. F Naftolin, et al., in Subcellular Mechanisms in Reproductive Endocrinology, F Naftolin, et al., Eds., Amsterdam, Elsevier, 1976, p. 347.
167. AE Kellie and ER Smith, Biochem J, 66, 490(1957).
168. CE Brown-Séquard, CR Seanc. Soc Biol, 1, 420(1889).
169. A Pézard, CRH Acad Sci, 153, 1027(1911).
170. A Butenandt, Angew. Chem, 44, 905(1931).
171. A Butenandt and H Dannenberg, Z Physiol Chem, 229, 192(1934).
172. K David, et al., Z Physiol Chem, 233, 281(1935).
173. A Butenandt and G Hanisch, Chem Ber, 68B, 1859(1935).
174. CD Kochakian and JR Murlin, J Nutr, 10, 437(1935).
175. JA Vida, Chapter 1, in Androgens and Anabolic Agents. New York, Academic Press, 1969.
176. FC Kock, Bull. N Y Acad. Med, 14, 655(1938).
177. PD Klimstra, Chapter 8, in The Chemistry and Biochemistry of Steroids, Vol. 3. Los Altos, Calif., Geron-X, 1969.
178. BW O'Malley and AR Means, Receptors for Reproductive Hormones, New York, Plenum Press, 1974.
179. A Segaloff and RB Grabbard, Endocrinology, 67, 887(1960).
180. JA Vida, Chapter 3, in Androgens and Anabolic Agents. New York, Academic Press, 1969.
181. J Van der View, Acta Endocrinol, 49, 271(1965).
182. RI Dorfman, Chapter 30, in Burger's Medicinal Chemistry, Part II, 4th ed., ME Wolff, Ed., New York, Wiley, 1979.
183. S Grombe, East Afr Med J, 60, 203(1983).
184. S Qian and Z Wang, Annu. Rev. Pharmacol Toxicol, 24, 329(1984).

185. MRN Prasad and E Siczfalusy, Int J Androl, Suppl. 5, 53(1982).
186. L Martini and M Motta, Eds., Androgens and Antiandrogens. New York, Raven Press, 1977.
187. RO Neri, Adv Sex Horm Res, 2, 233(1976).
188. S Fang and S Liao, Mol Pharmacol, 5, 240(1969).
189. G Goto, et al., Chem Pharm Bull, 13, 1294(1965).
190. BW Snyder, et al., J Steroid Biochem Mol Biol, 33, 1127(1989).
191. S Laio, et al., Endocrinology, 94, 1205(1974).
192. AE Wakeling, et al., J Steroid Biochem, 15, 355(1981).
193. SY Tan, et al., J Clin Endocrinol Metab, 39, 936(1974).
194. GH Rasmussen, et al., J Med Chem, 29, 2298(1986).
195. T Liang, et al., Endocrinology, 117, 571(1985).
196. A Vermeulen, et al., Prostate, 14, 45(1989).
197. JD McConnell, et al., J Urol, 141, 239A(1989).
198. JP Van Wauwe and PAJ Janssen, J Med Chem, 32, 2231(1989).
199. MR Angelastro, et al., Biochem Biophys Res Commun, 162, 1571(1989).
200. RJB King and WP Mainwaring, Steroid-Cell Interactions, Baltimore, University Park Press, 1974.
201. S Liao, Int Rev Cytol, 41, 87(1975).
202. HG Williams-Ashman and AH Reddi, in Biochemical Actions of Hormones, Vol. 2, G. Litwack, Ed., New York, Academic Press, 1972, 257.
203. WIP Mainwaring, The Mechanism of Action of Androgens, New York, Springer-Verlag, 1977.
204. WIP Mainwaring, J Endocrinol, 44, 323(1969).
205. S Fang and S Liao, J Biol Chem, 246, 16(1971).
206. WIP Mainwaring and BM Peterken, Biochem J, 125, 285(1971).
207. JL Tymoczko and S Liao, Biochem Biophys Acta, 252, 607(1971).
208. WIP. Mainwaring, et al., Biochem J, 137, 513(1974).
209. KJ Tvter and O Unhjem, Endocrinology, 84, 963(1969).
210. JM Stern and AJ Eisenfeld, Science, 166, 233(1969).
211. WIP Mainwaring and FR Mangan, J Endocrinol, 59, 121(1973).
212. V Hansson, et al., Steroids, 23, 823(1974).
213. DJ Tindall, et al., Biochem Biophys Res Commun, 49, 1391(1972).
214. EM Ritzin, et al., Endocrinology, 19, 116(1972).
215. P Jovan, et al., J. Steroid Biochem, 4, 65(1973).
216. M Sar and WE Stumpf, Endocrinology, 92, 251(1973).
217. DP Cardinali, et al., Endocrinology, 95, 179(1974).
218. AK Roy, et al., Biochem Biophys. Acta, 354, 213(1974).
219. N Bruchovsky and JW Meakin. Cancer Res., 33, 1689(1973).
220. N Bruchovsky, et al., Biochem Biophys Acta, 381, 61(1975).
221. RL Gloyna and JD Wilson, J. Clin. Endocrinol, 29, 970(1969).
222. V Hansson, et al., J Steroid Biochem, 3, 427(1972).
223. G Giannopoulos, J Biol Chem, 248, 1004(1973).
224. ML Powers and JR Florini, Endocrinology, 90, 1043(1975).
225. I Jung and EE Baulieu, Nature [New Biol.], 237, 24(1972).
226. G Michel and EE Baulieu, CR Acad Sci III, 279, 421(1974).
227. M Krieg, Steroids, 28, 261(1976).
228. M Krieg and KD Voigl, Acta Endocrinol. (Copenh), Suppl., 214, 43(1977).
229. M Snochowski, et al., Eur J Biochem., 111, 603(1980).
230. M Snochowski, et al., J Steroid Biochem, 14, 765(1981).
231. JJ Schrozie and HM Solomon, Clin Pharmacol Ther, 8, 797(1967).
232. AJ Ryan, Athletics, in Anabolic-Androgenic Steroids, C.D. Kochakian, ed., New York, Springer-Verlag, 1976, p. 516.
233. JD Wilson, Endocrine Rev, 9, 181 (1988).
234. GC Lin and L Erinoff, ed., Anabolic Steroid Abuse, NIDA Research Monograph, 102, 29 (1990).
235. SE Lukas, Trends Pharmacol Sci, 14, 61 (1993).
236. S Casner, R Early, and BR Carlson, J Sports Med Phys Fit, 11, 98 (1971).
237. TD Fahey and CH Brown, Med Sci Sports, 5, 272 (1973).
238. LA Golding, JE Freydinger, and SS Fishel, Physician and Sports-Medicine, 2, 39 (1974).
239. SB Strömme, H.D. Meen, and A Aakvaag, Med Sci Sports, 6, 203 (1974).
240. G Ariel and W Saville, J Appl Physiol, 32, 795 (1972).
241. G Ariel, J Sports Med Phys Fit, 13, 187 (1973).
242. LC Johnson, G Fisher, LJ Silvester, et al. Med Sci Sports, 4, 43 (1972).
243. M Steinbach, Sportarzt und Sportmedizin, 11, 485 (1968).
244. S Bashin, TW Storer, N Berman, et al., N Engl J Med, 335, 1–7 (1996).
245. N Wade, Science, 176, 1399 (1972).
246. AA de Lorimier, GS Gordan, RC Lowe, et al. Arch. Intern Med, 116, 289 (1965).
247. IM Arias, in Influence of Growth Hormone, Anabolic Steroids, and Nutrition iii Health and Disease, F. Gross, ed., Berlin, Springer-Verlag, 1962. p. 434.
248. HA Kaupp and FW Preston, J Am Med Assoc, 180, 411 (1962).
249. D Westaby, SJ Ogle, FJ Paradinas, et al. Lancet, 2, 261, (1977).
250. FCW Wu, Clinical Chem, 43, 1289–1292 (1997).

SELECTED READINGS

M Beato, Cell, 56, 335(1989).

PJ Bentley, Endocrine Pharmacology, Cambridge, Cambridge University Press, 1980.

RW Brueggemeier, in Handbook of Hormones, Vitamins, and Radiopaques, M. Verderame, Ed., Boca Raton, FL, CRC Press, 1986, pp. 1–49.

RW Brueggemeier, Burger's Medicinal Chemistry, Fifth Edition, Volume 3, ME Wolff, Ed., John Wiley & Sons, N.Y., 1996, pp. 445–510.

MA Carson-Jurica, WT Schrader, and BW O'Malley, Endocrine Rev., 11, 201–220 (1990).

RM Evans, Science, 240, 889(1988).

DW Fullerton, Chapter 18 in Wilson and Gisvold's Textbook of Organic Medicinal and Pharmaceutical Chemistry, Ninth Edition, J. N Delgado and WA Remers, Eds., Philadephia, JB Lippincott Co., 1991, pp. 675–765.

RA Magarian, et al., in Handbook of Hormones, Vitamins, and Radiopaques, M Verderame, Ed., Boca Raton, FL, CRC Press, 1986, pp. 51–92.

HJL Makin, Ed., Biochemistry of Steroid Hormones, Second Edition, Oxford, UK, Blackwell Scientific Publications, 1984.

PC Ruentiz, Chapter 57, in Burger's Medicinal Chemistry, Volume 4, 5th Ed., ME Wolff, Ed., NY, Wiley, 1997, pp. 553–588.

JD Wilson, Chapter 58 in Goodman and Gilman's The Pharmacological Basis of Therapeutics, 9th ed., AG Gilman, et al., Eds., New York, Pergamon Press, 1996, pp. 1441–1458.

RF Witzman, Steroids: Keys to Life, New York, Van Nostrand-Reinhold, 1981.

C Williams and GM Stancel, Chapter 57, in Goodman and Gilman's The Pharmacological Basis of Therapeutics, 9th ed., J. G. Hardman, et al., Eds., New York, Pergamon Press, 1996, pp. 1411–1440.

FJ Zeelen, Medicinal Chemistry of Steroids, Amsterdam, Elsevier, 1990.

30. Thyroid Function and Thyroid Drugs

ALI R. BANIJAMALI

INTRODUCTION

The thyroid gland is a highly vascular, flat structure located at the upper portion of the trachea, just below the larynx. It is composed of two lateral lobes joined by an isthmus across the ventral surface of the trachea. The gland is the source of two fundamentally different types of hormones, thyroxine (T_4) and triiodothyronine (T_3). Both are vital for normal growth and development and control essential functions, such as energy metabolism and protein synthesis.

The word thyroid, meaning shield-shaped, was introduced by Wharton in his description of the gland (1). Like many before him, he attributed a solely cosmetic function to it because of the more frequent presence of enlarged glands in women, giving the throat region a more beautiful roundness. Later it was observed, however, that some characteristic symptoms for diseases always were accompanied by an obvious change in the size of the thyroid. This change was correctly interpreted as evidence that this structure plays a major role in normal body function.

An important step in the understanding of thyroid function was taken by Baumann (2) who discovered that the thyroid gland was the only organ in mammals that had the capability to incorporate iodine into organic substances. That discovery was important in research on the phylogeny of the thyroid.

Major clues to the physiologic roles of thyroid hormones were provided when normal and abnormal thyroid function were related to oxygen uptake (3) and when thyroid hormones were found to induce metamorphosis in tadpoles (4). The first discovery led to investigations into the role of thyroid hormone in metabolism and calorigenesis, and the second inspired research into specific receptors as points of initiation of thyroid hormone expression. A patient lacking thyroid hormones may be treated with synthetic hormones or natural preparations. Better agents to treat hyperthyroidism are still being sought. Presently available drugs, other compounds affecting thyroid function, and present approaches in the search of new drugs are presented in this chapter within the context of thyroid biochemistry and physiology.

NORMAL BIOCHEMISTRY AND PHYSIOLOGY
Thyroid Follicular Cells

All vertebrates have a thyroid gland consisting of functional units, the follicles. The morphologic and functional characteristics of the follicles are essentially similar in all vertebrate groups.

The follicle is a spherical, cystlike structure about 300 μ in diameter and consists of a luminal cavity surrounded by a one-cell-deep layer of cells called follicular or acinar cells. The center of the follicles is filled with a gelatinous colloid, the main component of which is a glycoprotein called thyroglobulin. The follicular cells contain an extensive network of rough endoplasmic reticulum, a well-developed Golgi apparatus, and lysosomes of various sizes (5). Thyroglobulin is synthesized in the rough endoplasmic reticulum of the follicle cells and transported by way of the Golgi complex to the exocytic vesicles, which empty the thyroglobulin into the follicle lumen.

The follicle cell contains two major assembly lines operating in opposite directions (6). One line moves in an apical direction and produces thyroglobulin that is delivered to the follicle lumen; the other line begins at the apical cell surface with endocytosis of thyroglobulin and ends by delivering hormones at the basolateral cell surface. The follicle cell seems, therefore, to fulfill the functions of typically secretory and typically absorptive cells simultaneously. In addition to the functions associated with these two lines, the follicle has the specific ability to metabolize iodine, comprising the accumulation of iodide, iodination of tryosyl residues in thyroglobulin, and coupling of iodinated tyrosyls to form thyroid hormones.

Parafollicular cells, also called light cells or C cells, are located individually or in clusters between follicular cells but do not border on the colloid. These cells produce thyrocalcitonin, a peptide hormone involved in calcium homeostasis. The extrafollicular space of the gland is occupied by blood vessels, capillaries, lymphatic vessels, and connective tissue.

Hormones of the Thyroid Gland

Thyroid hormones are iodinated amino acids derived from L-tyrosine, synthesized in the thyroid gland and stored as amino acid residues of thyroglobulin. The thyroid hormones, tetraiodo-L-thyronine and triiodo-L-thyronine play numerous, profound roles in regulating metabolism, growth, and development and in the maintenance of homeostasis. It is generally believed that these actions result from effects of thyroid hormones on protein synthesis.

The first biologically active iodine-containing compound of the thyroid gland was isolated from thyroid extracts by Kendall (7) and named L-thyroxine (T_4). Later its structure was established by Harington (8) as the 3,5,3',5'-tetraiodo-L-thyronine (T_4) (Fig. 30.1), and its synthesis was accomplished by Harington and Bargar (9). Twenty-five

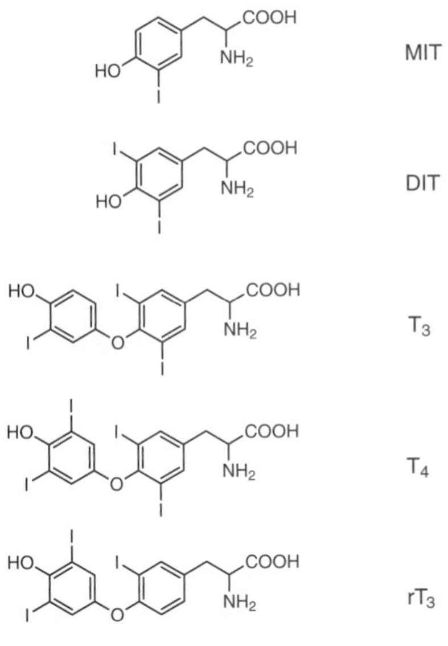

Fig. 30.1. Structure of the iodinated compounds of the thyroid glands.

years later, with the availability of chromatographic techniques and radioactive iodine, another thyroid hormone was characterized and identified as 3,5,3'-triiodo-L-thyronine (T₃) (Fig. 30.1) simultaneously by Gross and Pitt-Rivers (10) and Roch and co-workers (11). The thyroid gland also contains two quantitatively important iodinated amino acids; diiodo-L-tyrosine (DIT) was isolated from thyroid tissues by Harington and Randall (12), and monoiodo-L-tyrosine (MIT) was discovered by Fink and Fink (13). In addition, there are small amounts of other iodothyronines, such as 3,3'-diiodo-L-thyronine (T₂) and 3,3',5'-triiodo-L-thyronine (reverse T₃, rT₃). None of the latter compounds possess any significant hormonal activity.

Chemically, MIT is 3-iodo-L-tyrosine and DIT is 3,5-diiodo-L-tyrosine. The coupling of two DIT residues or of one DIT with one MIT residue (each with the net loss of alanine) leads to the formation of the two major thyroid hormones, T₄ and T₃, respectively.

It has been estimated that thyroglobulin, which has a molecular weight of 660,000, accounts for one-third of the weight of the thyroid gland and carries an average of 6 tyrosyl residues as monoiodo-L-tyrosine, 5 residues as diiodo-L-tyrosine, 0.3 residues as T₃, and 1 residue as T₄ (14). From these values, it can be estimated that a 20-g gland stores roughly 10 μmol (7.8 mg) of T₄ and 3 μmol (2.0 mg) of T₃ and that the normal human thyroid gland contains enough potential T₄ to maintain a euthyroid state for 2 months without new synthesis (15). The structures of the iodinated compounds of the thyroid gland are shown in Figure 30.1.

Biosynthesis of Thyroid Hormones

The thyroid hormones T₃ and T₄ are formed in a giant prohormone molecule, thyroglobulin, the major component of the thyroid and more precisely of the colloid. Thyroglobulin is an iodinated glycoprotein made up of two identical subunits, each with a molecular weight of 330,000 daltons. It is of special importance because it is necessary for the synthesis of thyroid hormones and represents their form of storage.

The formation of the thyroid hormones depends on an exogenous supply of iodide. The thyroid gland is unique in that it is the only tissue of the body able to accumulate iodine in large quantities and incorporate it into hormones. The iodine atoms play a unique role in the conformational preferences for T₃ and T₄ because of their large steric bulkiness. The metabolism of iodine is so closely related to thyroid function that the two must be considered together. The formation of thyroid hormones involves the following complex sequence of events: (1) active uptake of iodide by the follicular cells, (2) oxidation of iodide and formation of iodotyrosyl residues of thyroglobulin, (3) formation of iodothyronines from iodotyrosines, (4) proteolysis of thyroglobulin and release of T₄ and T₃ into blood, and (5) conversion of T₄ to T₃. These processes are summarized in Figure 30.2 (16).

Active Uptake of Iodide by Follicular Cells.

The first step in the synthesis of the thyroid hormones is the uptake of iodide from the blood by the thyroid gland. An adequate intake of iodide is essential for the synthesis of sufficient thyroid hormone. Dietary iodine is converted to iodide and almost completely absorbed from the gastrointestinal tract. Blood iodine is present in a steady state in which dietary iodide, iodide "leaked" from the thyroid gland, and reclaimed hormonal iodide provide the input, which thyroidal uptake, renal clearance, and a small biliary excretion providing the output. The thyroid gland regulates both the fraction of circulating iodide it takes up and the amount of iodide that it leaks back into the circulation. A simplified scheme of iodide metabolism is present in Figure 30.3.

The mechanism enabling the thyroid gland to concentrate blood iodide against a gradient into the follicular cell is the iodide pump, which is regulated by thyroid stimulating hormone. Decreased stores of thyroid iodine enhance iodide uptake, conversely, dietary iodide can reverse this process. It brings about a ratio of thyroid iodide to serum iodide (T/S ratio) of 20:1 under basal conditions but of more than 100:1 in hyperactive gland. The iodide pump is also found in the placenta and mammary tissue to enable the fetal thyroid and the natal thyroid glands to develop properly.

Iodide uptake may be blocked by several inorganic ions, such as thiocyanate and perchlorate. Because iodide uptake involves concurrent uptake of potassium, it can also be blocked by cardiac glycosides that inhibit potassium accumulation.

Oxidation of Iodide and Formation of Iodotyrosines

The second step in the process is a concerted reaction in which iodide is oxidized to an active iodine species that,

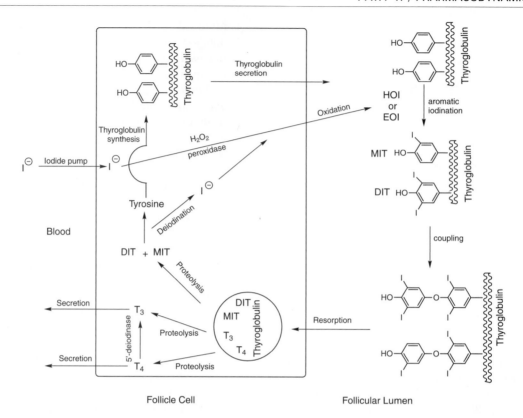

Fig. 30.2. Schematic representation of thyroid hormone biosynthesis and secretion. Thyroglobulin is synthesized on the rough endoplasmic reticulum of the follicle cell, and carbohydrate moieties are added by the Golgi apparatus. Thyroglobulin migrates to the surface of the follicle cell, where it fuses with the cell membrane to be discharged into the follicular lumen. Iodide enters the follicle cell by the iodide pump and is oxidized by thyroid peroxidase and hydrogen peroxide at the follicular membrane to form hypoiodate (OI^-) or an enzyme hypoiodate complex (E-OI), which in turn iodinates the tyrosine residues in thyroglobulin to form diiodotyrosyl (DIT), and monoiodotyrosyl (MIT) residues. Two iodinated tyrosyl groups couple in ether linkage via peroxidase to form T4 and T3, both of which are still attached to thyroglobulin. The iodinated thyroglobulin is resorbed into the follicular cell where complete proteolysis occurs by lysosomal protease to the amino acids, T4, T3, diiodotyrosine (DIT), and monoiodotyrosine (MIT). T4 and T3 are secreted by the cell into the blood; T4 is deiodinated to T3. DIT and MIT are deiodinated to free tyrosine and iodide, both of which are recycled back into iodinated thyroglobulin. (From H. M. Goodman and L. Van Middlesworth, The thyroid gland, in Medical Physiology, Vol 2, V. B. Mooncastle, Ed., St. Louis, C. V. Mosby, 1980, p. 1500.)

in turn, iodinates the tyrosyl residues of thyroglobulin. Consistent with the conditions necessary for aromatic halogenation, the iodination of the tyrosyl residues requires the iodinating species to be in a higher oxidation state than is the iodide anion. The iodinating species is thought to be hypoiodate (OI^-) (as hypoiodous acid HOI) or an enzyme-linked hypoiodate complex (E-OI). The oxidation of iodide to its reactive species is accomplished by thyroid peroxidase, a membrane bound heme-enzyme that utilizes hydrogen peroxide as the oxidant. The reaction takes place at the surface of the lumen using iodide concentrated within the follicle. Although the diiodotyrosyl residues constitute the major products, some MIT peptides are also produced. The generation of hydrogen peroxide apparently stimulates thyroid stimulating hormone and thus, the process of iodination.

In the thyroid follicle cell, intracellular iodide taken up from blood is bound in organic form in a few minutes so <1% of the total iodine of the gland is found as iodide. Therefore, inhibition of the iodide transport system requires blockade of organic binding. This can be achieved by the use of antithyroid drugs, of which n-propyl-6-thiouracil and 1-methyl-2-mercaptoimidazole (methimazole) are the most potent.

Coupling of Iodotyrosine Residues.

This reaction takes place at thyroglobulin and involves the coupling of two DIT residues or one DIT with one MIT residue (each with the net loss of alanine) to produce peptide-containing residues of the two major thyroid hormones T_4 and T_3. It is also believed that these reactions are catalyzed by the same peroxidase that effects the iodination and, therefore, can be blocked by compounds such as thiourea, thiouracils, and sulfonamides.

Proteolysis of Thyroglobulin and Release of Iodothyronines

The release of thyroid hormones from thyroglobulin begins with the resorption of thyroglobulin via endocytosis into the follicular epithelial cells and its subsequent complete proteolysis by the lysosomal digestive enzymes of the follicular cells. Thyroglobulin proteolysis yields MIT,

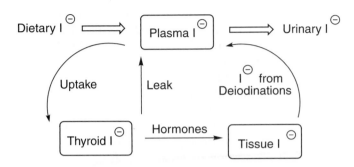

Fig. 30.3. Simplified scheme of iodide metabolism.

DIT, T_3, and T_4. Although MIT and DIT are formed, they do not leave the thyroid, but instead, are selectively deiodinated to tyrosine. The tyrosine is recycled into new thyroglobulin and the iodide is recycled into hypoiodate for subsequent iodination; conservation of essential nutrients for the thyroid gland. T_3 and T_4 are secreted by the cell into the circulation.

Conversion of Thyroxine to Triiodothyronine

Although T_4 is by far the major thyroid hormone secreted by the thyroid (about 8–10 times the rate of T_3), it is usually considered to be a prohormone. Because T_4 has a longer half-life, much higher levels of T_4 than T_3 are in the circulation. The enzymatic conversion of T_4 to T_3 is an obligate step in the physiologic action of thyroid hormones in most extrathyroidal tissues. In the peripheral tissues, about 33% of the T_4 secreted undergoes 5'-deiodination to give T_3, and another 40% undergoes deiodination of the inner ring to yield the inactive material rT_3 (17). The deiodination of T_4 is a reductive process catalyzed by a group of enzymes named iodothyronine deiodinases referred to as deiodinases and symbolized by D, found in a variety of cells. About 80% of the T_3 is derived from circulating T_4.

Three types of deiodinases are currently known and are distinguished from each other primarily based on their location, substrate preference, and susceptibility to inhibitors. Type I deiodinase is found in liver and kidney and catalyzes both inner ring and outer ring deiodination (i.e., T_4 to T_3 and rT_3 to $3,3'$-T_2). Type II deiodinase catalyzes mainly outer ring deiodination (i.e., T_4 to T_3 and T_3 to $3,3'$-T_2) and is found in brain and the pituitary. Type III deiodinase is the principal source of rT_3 and is present in brain, skin, and placenta (18).

Transport of Thyroid Hormones in Blood

The iodothyronines secreted by the thyroid gland into thyroid vein blood are of limited solubility. They equilibrate rapidly, however, through noncovalent association with three major binding proteins: thyroid binding globulin (TBG), transthyretin (TTR, formerly called T_4 binding pre-albumin, TBPA) and albumin. TBG is the primary serum binding protein because of its higher affinity for T_4. Under normal conditions, 75% of T_4 is bound to TBG,

10–15% to TTR, and 5–15% to albumin. When bound, T_4 is not physiologically active but provides a storage pool of thyroid hormone which can last 2–3 months (mean half-life of T_4 = 6.7 days in adults). The plasma proteins involved in thyroid hormone transport and their approximate association constants (K_a) for T_3 and T_4 are shown in Table 30.1. This table indicates that TBG has a high affinity for T_4 (K_a about 10^{10} M) and lower affinity for T_3. TTR and albumin also transport thyroid hormones in the blood; transthyretin has K_a values of about 10^7 and 10^6 M for T_4 and T_3. The equilibrium between the free hormone and that which is protein bound determines the accessibility of the free thyroid hormone for the tissue receptors as well as to peripheral sites where biotransformations take place. The lower binding affinity for T_3 to plasma proteins may be an important factor in the more rapid onset of action and in the shorter biologic half-life for T_3.

Thyroid hormones are taken into cells by facilitated diffusion or by active transport secondary to a sodium gradient (15). Once in the cell, thyroid hormones bind to cytosolic binding proteins and are not readily available for exchange with plasma hormones (19). T_3 and T_4 are not evenly distributed in body cells; a great part of T_4 is stored in liver and kidney, whereas most T_3 appears in muscle and brain (15).

Metabolism and Excretion

As discussed earlier, T_4 is considered to be a prohormone, and its peripheral metabolism occurs in two ways: outer ring deiodination by the enzyme 5'-D, which yields T_3, and inner ring deiodination by the enzyme 5-D, which yields rT_3, for which there is no known biologic function (Fig. 30.4). In humans, deiodination is the most important metabolic pathway of the hormone, not only because of its dual role in the activation and inactivation of T_4, but also in quantitative terms.

Degradative metabolism of the thyroid hormones, apart from peripheral deiodination, occurs mainly in the liver, where both T_3 and T_4 are conjugated to form either glucuronide (mainly T_4) or sulfate (mainly T_3) through the phenolic hydroxyl group. The resulting iodothyronine conjugates are excreted via the bile into the intestine, where a portion is hydrolyzed by bacteria. It also undergoes marginal enterohepatic circulation and is excreted unconjugated in feces.

Table 30.1. Plasma Proteins Involved in Thyroid Hormone Transport

Protein	Concentr. mg/dl	Binding of T_4		Binding of T_3	
		K_a	% Bound	K_a	% Bound
TBG	1.5	10^{10}	75	10^9	70
TTR	25	10^7	15	10^6	
Albumin	4000	10^6	10	10^5	30

TBG = Thyroxine-binding globulin; TTR = transthyretin.

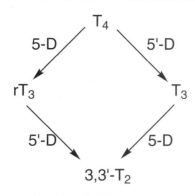

Fig. 30.4. Deiodination of T_4.

T_4 is conjugated with sulfate in kidney and liver, and the T_4'-O-sulfate, an excellent substrate for 5'-D (20), is believed to play a role in the regulation of T_4 metabolism.

Additional metabolism, involving side-chain degradation, proceeds by transamination, oxidative deamination, and decarboxylation to yield thyroacetic acid (21) and thyroethanediol (22); also, cleavage of the diphenyl ether linkage (23) has been detected both in vitro and in vivo. The reactions through which thyroid hormone is metabolized are summarized in Figure 30.5.

Physiologic Actions of Thyroid Hormones— Oxygen Consumption and Calorigenesis

The two most important actions of thyroid hormone are those related to oxygen consumption and those related to protein synthesis. Most effects of thyroid hormones can be related to the activation of genes following the binding of the hormone to high-affinity receptors of cell nuclei, but direct interactions of thyroid hormones with other cellular receptors cannot be excluded (24).

A respiratory component of the action of thyroid hormones was first observed almost a century ago. Respiratory exchange was depressed in patients diagnosed as hypothyroid and increased in patients diagnosed as hyperthyroid (3). The increase in respiration that follows the administration of thyroid hormone reflects an increase in metabolic rate thyroid function has indeed long been assessed by measuring the basal or resting metabolic rate (BMR), a test in which the oxygen consumed, measured in an individual at rest, is used to calculate total body energy production. The BMR of a hyperthyroid individual is above the normal range, or positive, and that of a hypothyroid individual below the normal range, or negative.

Thyroid hormones increase the oxygen consumption of most isolated tissues but not of isolated adult brain. This suggests that the behavioral changes seen in abnormal thyroid states (anxiety and nervousness in hyperthyroidism and impaired memory in hypothyroidism) in the adult are not directly linked to overall changes in brain oxygen consumption.

Because most of the energy produced by cellular respiration eventually appears as heat, an increase in cellular respiration leads necessarily to an increase in heat production, i.e., to a thermogenic or calorigenic effect. Thus, to the degree that thyroid hormones control BMR, they also control thermogenesis (25).

Clinically the inability to adjust to environmental temperature is symptomatic of departure from the euthyroid status. Patients with myxedema frequently have subnormal body temperature, have cold and dry skin, and tolerate cold poorly; the thyrotoxic patient, who compensates for excess heat production by sweating (warm, moist hands) does not easily tolerate a warm environment.

Thyroid hormones regulate the turnover of carbohydrates, lipids, and proteins. They promote glucose absorption, hepatic and renal gluconeogenesis, hepatic glycogenolysis, and glucose utilization in muscle and adipose tissue (26). They increase de novo cholesterol synthesis but even more increase low-density lipoprotein (LDL) degradation and cholesterol disposal, leading to a net decrease in total and in LDL cholesterol plasma levels (27). Thyroid hormones are anabolic when present at normal concentrations; they then stimulate the expression of many key enzymes of metabolism. Thyroid hormones at the levels present in hyperthyroidism are catabolic; they lead to the mobilization of tissue protein and especially of muscle tissue protein for gluconeogenetic processes (28). Thus, the depletion of liver glycogen, the increased breakdown of lipids, and the negative nitrogen balance observed in hyperthyroidism represent toxic effects. The metabolic processes of hypermetabolism are wasteful. In hyperthyroidism, a smaller than normal amount of liberated energy is available for useful work, and an excessive amount is wasted as heat.

Because of the role of mitochondria in cellular respiration and energy production, efforts to elucidate the mechanism of thyroid hormone action on metabolism and calorigenesis have focused on mitochondrial studies. Thyroid hormones in vitro are known to uncouple oxidative phosphorylation in isolated mitochondria, but these effects occur at unphysiologic doses of T_4; in physiologic concentrations, T_4 increases ATP formation and the number and inner membrane surface area of mitochondria (29) but does not reduce the efficiency of oxidative phosphorylation. Further 2,4-dinitrophenol, a classic uncou-

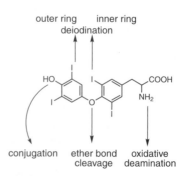

Fig. 30.5. Metabolic pathways for thyroxine.

pler of oxidative phosphorylation, can neither relieve hypothyroidism nor duplicate other physiologic effects of thyroid hormones.

Because in most physiologic circumstances oxygen consumption is controlled by energy metabolism, Ismail-Beigi and Edelman (30) proposed that the primary effect of thyroid hormones is to increase the amount of energy expended in translocating cations across cell membranes, probably as a response to an increased passive leak of sodium into, and potassium out of, cells. The extent to which this transport contributes to heat production and ATP utilization is uncertain. The stimulation of futile cycles by thyroid hormones (26) has been suggested to be an additional component of ATP disposal.

The effectiveness of β-blocking agents in treating the symptoms of thyrotoxicosis has led to investigations that have indicated that thyroid hormones modulate adrenergic effects by increasing the number of β-adrenergic receptors (31) and, at least in cardiac tissue (32), by increasing adenylyl adrenergic receptors are seen as coupled with a membrane-bound adenyl cyclase (33), both observations appear mutually consistent. The role of thyroid hormones in adaptive thermogenesis (25) could be effected by stimulating an increase in brown adipose tissue β-adrenergic receptors, catecholamines, which are known to activate the β receptor-linked adenylyl cyclase in that tissue (34), would then start the lipolysis cascade resulting in heat production.

Differentiation and Protein Synthesis

Stimulation of amphibian metamorphosis by thyroid hormones has been known for a long time (4). Changes in amphibian morphogenesis, such as involution of the tail of Xenopus (toads) and metamorphosis of the axolotl (salamanders) and of rana (frogs) species, have been repeatedly used as end points for the bioassay of thyroid analogs. In young mammals, thyroid hormone is necessary not only for general growth, but also for proper differentiation of the central nervous system. The counterpart of amphibian metamorphosis in the developing mammalian brain is myelogenesis and the formation of axons and dendrites (35). Behavioral studies in neonate hypothyroid mammals show that impairment in learning capacity (35) paralleled the impairment of proper anatomic development in the brain. A deficiency of thyroid hormone during the critical period when the developing human brain is sensitive to thyroid hormone results in an irreversible clinical entity termed cretinism, which is characterized by stunted growth and mental retardation.

A great deal of attention has been devoted to the events taking place in the roughly 48-hour interval between the administration of thyroid hormone and the manifestation of certain effects caused by that administration. After Tata (36) had observed that the anabolic effects observed in rats given T_4 could be blocked by inhibitors of protein synthesis, further investigations led Tata and Widnell (37) to the conclusion that thyroid hormones were activating protein synthesis at the ribosomal level. Subsequently, Dillmann and co-workers (38) showed that the T_3-induced formation of α-glycerophosphate dehydrogenase (E.C. 1.1.99.5) could be blocked by α-amanitin, an inhibitor of RNA polymerase II, inferring that thyroid hormones affected the transcription process. In 1972, when the partition of thyroid hormones between plasma and a number of tissues was investigated, Schadlow and associates (39) demonstrated that the uptake of T_3 by unfractionated pituitary tissue was inverse to the dose, suggesting that the pituitary was limited in its capacity to bind T_3. This finding prompted efforts to find the subcellular location of the binding sites and to search for the presence of specific binding sites in other tissues (40). The research revealed that the binding sites were located in cell nuclei and were present also in liver and kidney (40). Eventually, receptors were located in all mammalian tissues and eventually also in tadpole erythrocytes (41). In cultured pituitary cells, the receptor was described as an acidic, nonhistone 50,000-dalton protein (42) with an equilibrium dissociation (Kd) constant of 2.9×10^{-11} for T_3 and of 2.6×10^{-10} for T_4, indicating that T_3 had a 10-fold greater affinity than T_4 for the receptor. There were 6000 nuclear binding sites in the pituitary, 4000 in the liver, but only 16 in the testis, a tissue that is not responsive to thyroid hormone (43). Tata's findings of the activation of one RNA polymerase (37) were extended to all RNA polymerases, suggesting that thyroid hormones were involved in all phases of gene activation.

Receptors located on the plasma membrane, in the cytoplasm, and in mitochondria have also been described (44). Plasma membrane receptors are believed to mediate the transport of hormone into the cell and possibly to mediate nonnuclear, immediate effects of thyroid hormone (44). The presence of a large number of low-affinity cytosol binding proteins has been known for some time (45), but these proteins have not been assigned a specific physiologic role; it has been proposed that the cytosolic binding proteins merely serve as a large intracellular thyroid hormone reservoir delaying the metabolic disposition of thyroid hormone.

Because thyroid hormones immediately increase oxygen uptake and ATP formation and eventually lead to an increase in the number, size, and inner-membrane surface area of mitochondria as well as to the induction of many mitochondrial enzymes (46–48), many efforts to characterize mitochondrial thyroid hormone receptors have been made. Sterling and co-workers (49) have reported the presence of very high affinity receptors in mitochondria but their work has not been duplicated, and many authors believe that most mitochondrial enzymes are synthesized on cytoplasmic ribosomes and then transferred into mitochondria (50).

Control of Thyroid Hormone Biosynthesis

The primary role of thyroid is to produce thyroid hormones. The primary regulator of thyroid, both its function and growth, is the pituitary hormone, thyrotropin (thyroid-stimulating hormone [TSH]). Thyrotropin is a glycoprotein with a molecular weight of about 28,000, which can dissociate into two equally large polypeptide chains, an α-chain, which is also present in other pituitary peptides, and a β-chain, which is present in TSH only. TSH is produced by and released from the anterior pituitary gland causing the thyroid hormone to initiate new thyroid hormone synthesis. Increases in iodide uptake, the iodination of thyroglobulin, and endocytosis of colloid are all observed in response to stimulation of TSH. The effects of TSH on the thyroid appear to be the consequence of binding to high-affinity receptors on the capillary membrane of follicular cells and activation of adenylyl cyclase and protein kinase enzymes, found on the inner side of the membrane, with subsequent phosphorylation of cellular proteins. It is believed that most, if not all, effects of TSH are mediated through the cyclic adenosine monophosphate (cAMP) formed by the adenylyl cyclase and possibly also by cAMP-activated intracellular phosphokinases.

The amount of thyroid hormone circulating in body fluids and present in tissues remains fairly constant. Accounting for this constancy are the relatively long biologic half-life of the thyroid hormones, the regulation of gland activity by the pituitary-hypothalamic system, and the availability of iodide. Thyroid hormone research points to T_3 as the thyroid hormone, and therefore factors affecting peripheral T_3 formation by the 5′-D enzymes are highly relevant.

The relation of biologic half-life to protein binding has already been alluded to. T_4 firmly bound to plasma proteins; only 0.05% of T_4 is not protein bound, and T_4 had a biologic half-life of 1 week as compared to 1 day for the less firmly bound T_3.

The biosynthesis and secretion of TSH is, in turn, regulated by thyrotropin-releasing hormone (TRH) and the quantity of thyroid hormone in circulation through feedback control. TRH, the tripeptide pyroglutamylhistidylprolylamide, is formed in the hypothalamus, reaches the thyrotrophs (i.e., the TSH-producing pituitary cells) by way of the hypophyseal portal system, and stimulates TSH release by binding to the TRH receptors of the thyrotrophs (51). The ability of thyroid hormones to prevent the release of TSH is referred to as feedback regulation. It is believed that T_3 prevents the TRH stimulated release of TSH by stimulating the synthesis of a peptide that would compete with TRH for the TRH receptor sites on the thyrotroph (52). Inhibition of the transcription of the α and β subunits of TSH by thyroid hormone (53) may also contribute to the feedback effect.

The amount of iodide available to the gland for hormone synthesis is also an important regulator of thyroid function. The efficiency of the thyroid pump mechanism and the rate of thyroglobulin and thyroid peroxidase (TPO) synthesis are all TSH-dependent. In cases of iodide deficiency, the production of thyroid hormone is lowered, and TSH rises through the pituitary feedback mechanism described previously. The effect of the increased TSH is to produce more thyroid hormone by increasing efficiency of the iodide pump and increasing thyroglobulin and TPO synthesis. Thus, in iodide deficiency, there is an increased uptake of iodide and (54) larger MIT-to-DIT ratios, which leads to larger T_3-to-T_4 ratio. T_3 is the more rapidly acting hormone, mitigating the effect of iodide deficiency. When iodide deficiency is severe, a persistent rise in TSH is observed. This then results in thyroid growth.

In the presence of an excess of circulating iodide, the absolute amount of iodide taken up remains approximately constant. There is a decrease in the fraction of the total iodide taken up and an increase in the amount of iodide leaked from the thyroid gland. In addition, there may be a decrease in organification (i.e., in the formation of iodinated TG residues) and in the release of hormones from the gland. The decrease in organification that occurs at excessive physiologic doses of iodide has been called the Wolff-Chaikoff block (55). The block may be caused by an interaction of iodide with NADPH (56), which depletes follicular NADPH and, in turn, depletes the H_2O_2 necessary for TPO activity. The decrease in hormone release occurs when iodide is given in pharmacologic (mg) quantities; it may last for a few weeks.

The activity of deiodinases reflects thyroid status, general health, and food intake. In hypothyroidism, there is a decrease in hepatic 5′ D-I but an increase in 5′ D-II activity (57). There is a decrease in T_3 and an increase in rT_3 after hepatic disease (58) renal damage (59), chronic illness (60), and starvation (61), indicating a decrease in the activity of the quantitatively more important 5′ D-I. An increase in deiodinase activity has been observed after overfeeding subjects or after the administration of a high-carbohydrate or high-fat diet (62) to experimental animals. The mechanism of deiodinase control is presumably intricate, but the inhibiting effects of propranolol (63) on 5′ D-I and of prazosin on the 5′ D-II of BAT (64) infer the involvement of adrenergic components in the regulation. In addition, the rapid change in activity observed after asphyxia (65) points to a rapid, possibly cAMP-related control (65).

DISEASES INVOLVING THE THYROID GLAND
Hypothyroidism
Goiter

An enlarged, palpable thyroid gland is referred to as a goiter. When insufficient thyroid hormone is liberated from the thyroid gland, the breakdown of the thyroid-pituitary-hypothalamic feedback mechanism results in the release of excess TSH and in the formation of a thyroid

TRH

hypertrophy referred to as a nontoxic goiter. The increase in size of a nontoxic goiter is a compensatory mechanism, which may lead to a normal thyroid hormone output.

Endemic goiters are those that occur in a significant segment of a given population. Goiters are most frequently caused by inadequate intake of dietary iodide in regions not reached by iodide-providing sea mists and occasionally by the prolonged intake of goitrogens derived from plant sources or aquifers.

A characteristic sign of hypothyroidism is a decrease in metabolic rate, with a reduction in calorigenic effect and defective thermoregulation. The elevated serum cholesterol level seen in hypothyroidism is the result of a decrease in cholesterol degradation that exceeds the decrease in cholesterol biosynthesis; it reflects a general slowdown in catabolic processes. The slurred speech and lethargy of adult myxedema are symptomatic of a depressed central nervous system and indicate that the adult brain, which does not respond to thyroid administration by an increase in oxygen uptake, is sensitive to thyroid hormone (66).

Cretinism

Cretinism, the irreversible clinical entity characterized by defective physical and mental development, appears when thyroid hormone is not available in early childhood for normal bone formation and normal brain growth and differentiation.

Myxedema

Myxedema is used either as a specific term to describe the infiltration of the intercellular spaces of skin and muscle with mucopolysaccharide or as a general term, as in adult myxedema or pituitary myxedema, to denote hypothyroid status.

Hyperthyroidism

The increased metabolic rate of hyperthyroidism results in symptoms opposite to those seen in hypothyroidism. The increased oxygen demand in hyperthyroidism leads to an increased heart rate and increased cardiac output and thereby places strain on the heart. Exaggerated catabolic processes lead to decreased serum cholesterol and possibly also to poor glucose tolerance and glucosuria, and the excessive calorigenic effect produced by catabolic processes causes anorexia and poor thermoregulation. Excessive hormone function is expressed by the word toxic, as in toxic goiter, toxic adenoma, and thyrotoxicosis. Thyrotoxic crisis or thyroid storm is an emergency caused by a stress-triggered augmentation of the symptoms of thyrotoxicosis (67).

Graves' Disease

Graves' disease is the most frequently encountered form of hyperthyroidism caused by a generalized overactivity of the entire thyroid gland. Named after the physi-

cian who first described it, Graves' disease is an autoimmune condition in which the body's immune system tricks the thyroid into producing too much thyroid hormone. It is also called "diffuse toxic goiter": "diffuse" because the entire thyroid gland is involved in the disease process; "toxic" because the patient appears hot and flushed, as if feverish due to an infection; and "goiter" because the thyroid gland enlarges in this condition. Signs of this disease may include goiter, a protrusion of the eyeballs called exophthalmos, and pretibial myxedema. Hyperthyroidism due to graves' disease is, in general, easily controlled and safely treated.

In the serum of most patients suffering from Graves' disease, an immunoglobulin (IgC) is present that, after a slow onset, elicits a long-lasting stimulation of the thyroid gland. Because the release of the long-acting thyroid stimulator (LATS) is not controlled by thyroid hormone levels as is TSH, patients with LATS have a hyperplastic, hypertrophied gland, which produces and releases an excessive amount of hormone.

The indications are that the exophthalmos is caused by a substance produced by a distinct autoimmune system (70), possibly in response to a modified TSH of pituitary origin.

Hashimoto's Disease

Hashimoto's disease (68) is the most frequently encountered form of hypothyroidism in the United States. Named after the physician who first described it, Hashimoto's disease is an autoimmune condition in which plasma cells, lymphocytes, and fibrous tissue attack and destroy the thyroid gland. Pitt-Rivers and Tata (69) suggested that the sequence of events in Hashimoto's disease was initiated by injury to some thyroid structure, following which the normally sequestered thyroglobulin would be released and exposed to immunologic mechanisms, thus setting into motion a progressive interaction between thyroglobulin and circulating autoantibodies. Hashimoto antibodies are present in adult-onset myxedema and in most persons with Graves' disease, but it is recognized that other antigenic factors are involved in these and in other autoimmune diseases of the thyroid. Hypothyroidism resulting from Hashimoto's disease requires lifelong treatment with thyroid hormone replacement.

Thyroid Cancer

Thyroid cancer is a disease in which malignant cells are found in the tissues of the thyroid gland. There are four main types of cancer of the thyroid, based on how the cancer cells look under a microscope: papillary, follicular, medullary, and anaplastic. Each year in the United States, about 20,000 people are diagnosed with thyroid cancer and it is more common in women than in men. A study from National Cancer Institute predicts that these numbers may rise as individuals who were exposed to radioactive iodine from nuclear testing in western states in the

1950s and 1960s reach 40, the average age at diagnosis. Fortunately, treatment is straightforward and effective, but follow-up testing can be uncomfortable because it requires a hypothyroid state. Follow-up takes two forms: serum thyroglobulin measurement and a radioiodine whole-body scan, as described later (Section IV C).

THERAPEUTIC AGENTS
Thyroid Replacement Therapy

A large number of organic and some inorganic compounds stimulate or prevent thyroid hormone formation by interfering with iodide uptake into follicular cells, inhibiting TPO, preventing thyroid hormone binding to plasma proteins, or acting as effectors of thyroid deiodinases. Some of the agents described in this section are of therapeutic or diagnostic value, some illustrate potential side effects of drugs, and some are experimental compounds designed to achieve unmet therapeutic goals or to define structural parameters necessary for thyroid hormone actions.

Thyroid hormone replacement appears to be the established therapy in the hypothyroidism represented by myxedema, cretinism and simple goiter. The choice in replacement therapy is between a biologic preparation, such as desiccated thyroid or partially purified thyroglobulin, and synthetic, crystalline T_4.

Natural Thyroid Hormone Preparations

Hormone replacement appears to be the established therapy in the treatment of various forms of hypothyroidism, from the complete absence of thyroid function seen in myxedema to the simple goiter and cretinism. Formerly, desiccated, defatted porcine or bovine thyroid glands designated thyroid, USP, and partially purified thyroglobulin designated Proloid have been used orally. The hormones were released from the proteolytic activity of gut enzymes. Potency is based on total iodine content or bioassay and is somewhat variable with different preparations.

Desiccated thyroid preparations (Thyroid USP) are essentially acetone powders of bovine or porcine thyroid glands compressed into oral tablets. A diluent is usually present because the preparations (especially those of porcine origin) commonly exceed the 0.17–0.23% iodine content required by the United States Pharmacopeia. Because the iodine of desiccated thyroid is in the form of the iodinated tyrosyl and thyronyl residues of the precipitated thyroglobulin, the preparation owes its efficacy to the hormones that are eventually liberated by intestinal proteases. In desiccated preparations, T_3 and T_4 may be present in a ratio approximately that found in humans. Desiccated preparations are less expensive than synthetic hormones but have been shown to produce variable T_4/T_3 blood levels because of inconsistencies between and within animal sources of the thyroid gland. Most comments regarding desiccated thyroid apply to partially purified thyroglobulin because the two preparations differ in their total as well as in their relative amounts of T_4 and T_3.

Synthetic Thyroid Hormones

Synthetic, crystalline thyroid hormones are more uniformly absorbed than biologic preparations and contain more precisely measured amounts of active ingredient in their dosage forms. Of present interest are T_4 (levothyroxine), T_3 (liothyronine), dT_4 (dextrothyroxine), and T_4-T_3 mixtures referred to as liotrix (71).

Levothyroxine. Because of its firmer binding to carrier proteins, synthetic crystalline (levothyroxine sodium, Synthtoid, Euthyrox) has a slower onset of action than has crystalline T_3 or than a desiccated thyroid preparation. Its administration leads to greater increase in serum T_4 but to a lesser increase in serum T_3 than that of thyroid, USP (72). The availability of 11 different tablet strengths, ranging from 25–300 mcg, allows for individual dosing.

Liothyronine. Crystalline T_3 (liothyronine sodium, Cytomel) has a rapid onset and short duration and is the therapy of choice in circumstances in which it is desirable to have rapid onset or cessation of activity, such as in patients with heart disease.

Liotrix. A mixture of the sodium salts of T_4 and T_3 in a 4:1 ratio by weight is distributed as liotrix.

Dextrothyroxine. Dextrothyroxine, the synthetic D(+) stereoisomer isomer of L(−)-T_4, was introduced in hypocholesteremic-hypolipidemic therapy with the premise that it would be void of calorigenic effects. The possibility of trace contamination with and metabolic conversion to T_4 and congeners has restricted its use, however, especially in patients with coronary heart disease (71).

Thyroid Imaging Agents
Radioiodine

All isotopes of iodine are rapidly taken up in thyroid follicles. So far, only the isotopes ^{131}I and ^{125}I have been used consistently. The isotope ^{131}I, which decays to ^{131}Xe mainly with the emission of 0.6 meV β-particle and of approximatively 0.3 meV γ-rays, has a half-life of 8 days. The isotope ^{125}I, with a half-life of 60 days, decays to ^{125}Te by electron capture. The major component of its decay is a 27 keV X-ray, and the minor component is a 35.5 keV γ-ray.

The γ-radiation emitted by ^{131}I can be detected by a suitably placed scintillation crystal. This is the basis for the diagnostic use of this isotope in iodine uptake and in thyroid-scanning procedures.

The absorption of ^{131}I β-radiation, which leads to the highly localized destruction of the thyroid follicles in which the isotope is taken up, has promoted radioiodine as a therapeutic alternative to surgical removal of the gland. Advantages of radioiodine therapy over surgery include the simplicity of the procedure, its applicability to patients who are poor surgical risks, and the avoidance of surgical complications such as hypoparathyroidism. The development of late hypothyroidism (75) and the fear of chromosomal damage are arguments against the use of radioiodine in patients under age 20 years and during pregnancy.

A review of the use of ^{125}I in thyrotoxicosis has indicated that the potential advantages of the ^{125}I isotope, which are based on its lower penetrability and more localized action, have not been realized in practice (76).

Radioiodine whole body scan and serum thyroglobulin measurement are commonly used as the follow-up testing in thyroid cancer patients. Both follow-up tests have limitations and are uncomfortable because it requires a hypothyroid state. In order for thyroid cells to take up the labeled iodine, thyrotropin must be available and in order for pituitary to supply it, the body must be free of T_3 and T_4. This means patients must completely stop taking medication for several weeks before the scan day. This results in a severe hypothyroidism and also about 25% of patients produce antibodies against thyroglobulin, rendering the immunoassay useless. To make the follow up tests easier Food and Drug Administration recently approved the use of Thyrogen (thyrotropin alfa for injection), a recombinant human thyrotropin produced in Chinese hamster ovary cells. Thyrogen has been shown to significantly enhance the sensitivity of thyroglubulin testing in patients maintained on thyroid hormone therapy and allows thyroid cancer patients to avoid the debilitating effects of hypothyroidism when undergoing radioiodine imaging scans.

Perchlorate and Pertechnetate

The ability of large anions to be taken up into the thyroid by way of the iodide pump is linearly related to molar volume (77). The affinity of iodide for the iodide pump was equal to that of thiocyanate but much smaller than that of the larger perchlorate and pertechnetate ions.

In contrast to iodide and SCN^-, TcO_4^- and ClO_4^- do not undergo intrathyroidal metabolism after they are trapped. This property has made TcO_4^- labeled with the short-lived technetium-99^m, a widely used radioisotope for thyroid trapping and for thyroid imaging.

Perchlorate, which competitively inhibits the uptake of iodide, has been used in both diagnosis and treatment of thyroid disease. In continental Europe, perchlorate has been used for surgical preparation and in the long-term treatment of thyrotoxicosis. In the United States, the use of perchlorate was drastically curtailed after aplastic anemia and severe renal damage were reported following its use.

Diagnostically, perchlorate is used to assess the intrathyroidal organification of iodine. When perchlorate is administered after a dose of radioactive iodine, perchlorate washes out or discharges intrathyroidal inorganic iodide but does not affect covalently bound organic iodide. When organification is inadequate, there is a sharp decrease in intrathyroidal radioactive iodine after perchlorate administration.

Antithyroid Drugs for the Treatment of Hyperthyroidism
Iodide

Inhibition of the release of thyroid hormone by iodide is the basis for its use in hyperthyroidism. Iodide decreases the vascularity of the enlarged thyroid gland and also lowers the elevated BMR. It has also been suggested that excess iodide might change the conformation of thyroglobulin, making the protein less susceptible to thyroidal proteolysis (73).

With the use of antithyroid drugs, the role of iodide in hyperthyroidism has been relegated to that of preparation for thyroid surgery. Iodide, as Lugol's solution (strong iodine solution, USP) or as saturated potassium iodide solution, is administered for about 2 weeks to ensure decreased vascularity and firming of the gland. Iodism, a side effect of iodine administration, is apparently an allergic reaction, characterized by dermatologic and common cold-like symptoms (74).

Methimazole, Propylthiouracil, and Related Compounds

Thionamides are the most important class of antithyroid compounds in clinical practice used in nondestructive therapy of hyperthyroidism. These agents are potent inhibitors of the thyroid peroxidase enzymes (TPO) responsible for iodination of tyrosine residues of thyroglobulin and the coupling of iodotyrosine residues to form iodothyronines. These drugs have no effect on iodide trap or on thyroid hormone release. The most clinically useful thionamides are thioureylenes, which are five- or six-membered heterocyclic derivatives of thiourea and include the thiouracil, 6-n-propyl-2-thiouracil (PTU), and the thioimidazole, 1-methyl-2-mercaptoimidazole (methimazole, Tapazole, MMI).

Thiouracil; R = H
Methylthiouracil; R = CH$_3$
Propylthiouracil (PTU); R = n-C$_3$H$_7$

Methimazole(MMI), R = H
Carbimazole (R = C$_2$H$_5$CO)

Chemically the grouping R-CS-N- been referred to as thioamide, thionamide, thiocarbamide, or if R is N as it is in thiouracil, PTU and MMI, it is called a thioureylene. This structure may exist in either the thioketo or thioenol tautomeric forms.

Thioamide

Thioketo   Thioenol (SH form)

Thioureylene tautomers

The study of 6-alkylthiouracil showed maximal antithyroid activity with 6-propylthiouracil. 6-Methylthiouracil has less than one-tenth the activity of PTU.

The ability of PTU to inhibit the enzyme 5' D-I, i.e., the peripheral deiodination of T_4 to T_3 (in addition to its intrathyroidal inhibition of thyroid hormone formation) has made PTU the drug of choice in the treatment of emergency of thyroid storm (78). Single doses of PTU in excess of 300 mg are capable of almost total blockage of peripheral T_3 production (79).

A number of studies have defined the structure-activity relations of thiouracils and other related compounds as inhibitors of outer-ring deiodinase (80). The C_2 thioketo/thioenol group and an unsubstituted N_1 position are essential for activity. The enolic hydroxyl group at C_4 in PTU and the presence of alkyl group at C_5 and C_6 enhance the inhibitory potency.

Methimazole has more thyroid peroxidase inhibitory activity and is longer-acting than PTU but, in contrast to PTU, is not able to inhibit the peripheral deiodination of T_4 presumably because of the presence of the methyl group at N_1 position. The suggested maintenance dosages listed in USP DI 1986 are 50–800 mg daily for PTU and 5–30 mg daily for MMI.

Efforts to improve the taste and decrease the rate of release of MMI led to the development of 1-carbethoxy-3-methylthioimidazole (carbimazole, see page 727). Carbimazole, the pro-drug derivative of methimazole, gives rise to methimazole in vivo and is used in the same dosage.

The side effects of thioamides include diarrhea, vomiting, jaundice, skin rashes, and, at times, sudden onset of agranulocytosis. There does not appear to be a great difference in toxicity among the compounds currently in use.

PTU and MMI are extensively taken up by the thyroid gland and act as substrates for and inhibitors of thyroid peroxidase (TPO). Taurog described the thioureylenes as potent inhibitors of thyroidal iodination and suggested that a thioureylene such as propylthiouracil (PTU-SH) would prevent the formation of a TPO-iodine complex when the thioureylene-to-iodide ratio was high and compete with thyroglobulin tyrosyl residues (TG-Tyr) when the PTU-SH-to-iodide ratio was low (81). In the course of the reaction, the thioureylene PTU-SH would be oxidized (82), possibly to a dimer such as PTU-SS-PTU. Because of the rapid reaction of sulfenyl iodide with thioureylenes, a TPO sulfenyl iodide intermediate (TPO-SI) has been proposed to be a part of the reaction:

$$\text{TPO-SI} + \text{PTU-SH} \longrightarrow \text{TPO-SH} + \text{PTU-SI}$$
$$\text{PTU-SI} + \text{PTU-SH} \longrightarrow \text{PTU-S-S-PTU} + \text{HI}$$

Thioureylene drugs also effectively prevent the coupling of thyroglobulin residues, which yields iodinated thyronines. This effect has been related to an alteration of the conformation of TG brought on by the binding of the thioureylene to TG (i.e., by the formation of a compound such as TPO-S-S-PTU) (83).

After the observation that PTU inhibited the peripheral deiodination of T_4 (78,84), attempts to relate deiodinase inhibitory activity to structural parameters were undertaken (84). These studies emphasized the need for tautomerization to a thiol form and for the presence of a polar hydrogen on the nitrogen adjacent to the sulfur-bearing carbon. A study of the relation of chemical structure to 5' D-I inhibitory activity related to similar studies of structural requirements for TPO inhibition could prove fruitful in the design of improved antithyroid drugs.

Thyrotoxicosis

Because symptoms of thyrotoxicosis resemble those of adrenergic overstimulation, attempts to decrease such symptoms by adrenergic blockade have been undertaken. Reserpine and guanethidine, both depletors of catecholamines, and propranolol, a β-blocking agent, have been used effectively to decrease the tachycardia, tremor, and anxiety of thyrotoxicosis. Because of its less serious side effects, propranolol has become the drug of choice in this adjunctive therapy. Reports of decreased T_3 plasma levels during propranolol treatment suggest that blocking of the peripheral deiodination of T_4 may contribute to the beneficial effects of propranolol. The use of propranolol as a preventive drug in acute thyrotoxicosis has been found to be beneficial by some but not by others.

Goitrogens and Drugs Affecting Thyroid Function

The presence of environmental goitrogens was suggested by the resistance of endemic goiters to iodine prophylaxis and iodide treatment in Italy and Colombia. In the past, endemic outbreaks of hypothyroidism have pointed to calcium as a source of water-borne goitrogenicity, and it is presently believed that calcium is a weak goitrogen able to cause latent hypothyroidism to come to the surface.

Lithium salts have been used as safe adjuncts in the initial treatment of thyrotoxicosis (85). Lithium is concentrated by the thyroid gland (86) with a thyroid-to-serum ratio of more than 2:1, suggesting active transport. Lithium ion inhibits adenylyl cyclase, which forms cAMP. cAMP is formed in response to TSH and is a stimulator of the processes involved in thyroid hormone release from the gland. Inhibition of hormone secretion by lithium has proved a useful adjunct in treatment of hyperthyroidism (87).

In view of the role of cysteine residues in the conformation of thyroglobulin, the mode of action of TPO, and the deiodination of T_4, the effect of sulfur-containing compounds on thyroid hormone formation is hardly surprising. Most naturally occurring sulfur compounds are derived from glucosinolates (88) (formerly referred to as thioglucosides), present in foods such as cabbage, turnip, mustard seed, salad greens, and radishes (most of these are from the genus *Brassica* or *Cruciferae*) as well as in the milk of cows grazing in areas containing *Brassica* weeds. Chemically, glucosinolates can give rise to many components, including thiocyanate (CNS^-), isothiocyanate (SCN^-), nitriles (RCN), and thiooxazolidones. Thiocyanate is a large anion that competes with iodide for uptake by the thyroid gland; its goitrogenic effect can be reversed by iodide intake. Goitrin, 5-R-vinyloxazolidine-2-thione, is a potent thyroid peroxidase inhibitor (89), claimed to be more effective than PTU in humans (90) and held to be the cause of a mild goiter endemia in Finland. In rats, goitrin is actively taken up by the thyroid gland and appears to inhibit the coupling of TG diiodotyrosyl residues (91). Many workers believe, however, that the goitrogenic effects of *Brassica* are due to the additive effects of all goitrogenic components present.

Goitrin

Other compounds affecting thyroid function include sulfonamides, anticoagulants, and oxygenated and iodinated aromatic compounds. The hypoglycemic agent carbutamide and the diuretic Diamox are examples of sulfonamides. Of the anticoagulants, heparin appears to interfere with the binding of T_4 to plasma transport proteins (92), but warfarin and dicoumarol are competitive inhibitors of the substrate T_4 or rT_3 in the 5'D reaction, with a K_i in the micromolar range (93). Other oxygenated compounds affecting the 5'D include resorcinol, long known to be a goitrogen, and phloretin, a dihydrochalocone with an I_{50} of 4 M.

Warfarin

Phloretin

Carbutamide

The ability of oxidation products of 3,4-dihydroxycinnamic acid to prevent the binding of TSH to human thyroid membranes (94) suggests that other oxygenated phenols may interfere with thyroid hormone function in more than one way. Examples of iodinated drugs affecting thyroid function are the antiarrhythmic agent amiodarone and the radiocontrasting agents iopanoic acid and ipodoic acid. All of these compounds interfere with the peripheral deiodination of T_4 and are being tested as adjuncts in the treatment of hyperthyroidism.

Amiodarone

Iopanoic acid

The binding of thyroid hormones to plasma carrier proteins is affected by endogenous agents or by drugs that can change the concentration of these proteins or compete with thyroid hormones for binding sites. Examples of the first group are testosterone (and related anabolic agents) that are able to decrease and estrogens (and related contraceptive agents) that are able to increase the concentration of T_4-binding globulin. Salicylates, diphenylhydantoin, and heparin are members of the large group competing with thyroid hormones for binding sites. Alterations in the binding of T_3 and T_4 are of no large physiologic consequence because the steady-state concentrations of free hormone are rapidly restored by homeostatic mechanisms. Knowledge of the presence of agents affecting thyroid hormone binding is, however, important for the interpretation of diagnostic tests assessing the presence of free or total hormone in plasma.

THYROID HORMONE ANALOGS

The search for thyroid hormone analogs was prompted by the desire to establish structure-activity relationships for the hormone and by the need for a safe, specific antagonist able to block thyroid action without delay at a peripheral site. The reader will recall that TPO inhibitors such as PTU do not affect the extensive amount of hormone stored in thyroidal thyroglobulin.

Some early analogs designed as antagonists were butyl-3,5-diiodo-4-hydroxybenzoate (BHDB), which was designed as a deiodinase inhibitor and is to a degree effective as such, and 2'6'-diiodothyronine, which has a small antithyroid effect.

DHDB

2',6'-Diiodothyronine

When the activity of T_3 was discovered in 1955, and when none of the many analogs tabulated by Selenkow and Asper (95) demonstrated significant antithyroid activity, efforts were made to redefine the structural requirements for thyroid-like activity to provide a better rationale for the design of a peripheral thyroid antagonist. The biologic assay methods used to assay the newer compounds included measurements of in vivo oxygen uptake, of hepatic lipogenic enzyme activity, of goiter formation, of the rate of amphibian metamorphosis, and, more recently, of the binding to nuclear receptors.

The measurement of oxygen uptake provides a direct index of metabolic rate; this measurement can be done simply by placing experimental animals in a calibrated vessel maintained at constant temperature and connected to an oxygen analyzer (96). Repeatedly used as an index of thyromimetic activity have been the in vitro assay of oxygen uptake (48) by suspended mitochondria and the spectrophotometric assays of rat liver mitochondrial α-glycerophosphate dehydrogenase (97) and of cytoplasmic malic enzyme (98).

In the "goiter" or "antigoiter" assay, goiter formation is induced by the administration of a TPO inhibitor, such as thiouracil. The inhibitor is blended with the food or added to the drinking water and given to experimental animals for 10–14 days. The increase in gland weight caused by the TPO inhibitor can be reversed by T_4 or by a test compound with thyromimetic activity. The effect of a given dose of thyromimetic agent compared with that of a given dose of T_4 yields the "antigoitrogenic effect" of the compound. Further, when both a test compound and T_4 are given to an animal receiving a TPO inhibitor, the ability of the test compound to antagonize T_4, the "antithyroid effect" of the test compound, can be assessed.

Discrepancies have been seen between the results obtained with amphibian metamorphosis and those obtained with other assays. These discrepancies have been attributed to the ability of test animals such as tadpoles to concentrate test compounds, and especially lipophilic test compounds, from the medium (99). The binding affinity of thyroid analogs to nuclear receptors correlates well with the effectiveness of these analogs in the antigoiter assay, provided that the metabolism of the analogs is taken into consideration (99).

Structure-activity Relationships of Thyroid Analogs

The synthesis and biologic evaluation of a wide variety of T_4 and T_3 analogs allowed a significant correlation of structural features with their relative importance in the production of hormonal responses. The key findings are summarized in Table 30.2. In general, only compounds with the appropriately substituted phenyl-X-phenyl nucleus (as shown on top of Table 30.2) have shown significant thyroid hormonal activities. Both single ring compounds such as DIT and a variety of its aliphatic and alicyclic ether derivatives showed no T_4-like activity in the rat antigoiter test (100), the method most often used in determining thyromimetic activity in vivo (101). Structure-activity relationships are discussed in terms of single structural variations of T_4 in the (1) alanine side chain, (2) 3- and 5-positions of the inner ring, (3) the bridging atom, (4) 3'- and 5'-positions of the outer ring, and (5) the 4'-phenolic hydroxyl group.

Aliphatic Side Chain

The naturally occurring hormones are biosynthesized from L-tyrosine and possess the L-alanine side chain. The L-isomers of T_4 and T_3 (Compounds 1, 3) are more active than the D-isomers (Compounds 2, 4) (Table 30.2). The carboxylate ion and the number of atoms connecting it to the ring are more important for activity than is the intact zwitterionic alanine side chain. In the carboxylate series, the activity is maximum with the two-carbon acetic acid side chain (Compounds 7, 8) but decreases with either the shorter formic acid (Compounds 5, 6) or the longer pro-

pionic and butyric acid analogs (Compounds 9 through 12). The ethylamine side chain analogs of T_4 and T_3 (Compounds 13, 14) are less active than the corresponding carboxylic acid analogs. In addition, isomers of T_3 in which the alanine side chain is transposed with the 3-iodine or occupies the 2-position were inactive in the rat antigoiter test (102), indicating a critical location for the side chain in the 1-position of the inner ring.

Alanine Bearing Ring

The phenyl ring bearing the alanine side chain, called the inner ring or α-ring, is substituted with iodine in the 3 and 5 positions in T_4 and T_3. As shown in Table 30.2, removal of both iodine atoms from the inner ring to form $3',5'-T_2$ (Compound 15) or $3'-T_1$ (Compound 16) produces analogs devoid of T_4-like activity primarily owing to the loss of the diphenyl ether conformation. Retention of activity observed on replacement of the 3 and 5 iodine atoms with bromine (Compounds 17, 18) implies that iodine does not play a unique role in thyroid hormone activity. Moreover, a broad range of hormone activity found with halogen free analogs (Compounds 19, 20) indicates that a halogen atom is not essential for activity. In contrast to T_3, 3'-isopropyl-3,6-dimethyl-L-thyronine (Compound 20) has the capacity to cross the placental membrane and exerts thyromimetic effects in the fetus after administration to the mother. This could prove useful in treating fetal thyroid hormone deficiencies or in stimulating lung development (by stimulating lung to synthesize special phospholipids [surfactant], which ensure sufficient functioning of the infant's lungs at birth) immediately before premature birth (103). Substitution in the 3- and 5-positions by alkyl groups significantly larger and less symmetric than methyl groups, such as isopropyl and secondary butyl moieties, produces inactive analogs (Compounds 21, 22). These results show that 3,5-disubstitution by symmetric, lipophilic groups, not exceeding the size of iodine, is required for activity.

Bridging Atom

Several analogs have been synthesized in which the ether oxygen bridge has been removed or replaced by other atoms. The biphenyl analog of T_4 (Compound 23), formed by removal of the oxygen bridge, is inactive in the rat antigoiter test. The linear biphenyl structure is a drastic change from the normal diphenyl ether conformation found in the naturally occurring hormones. Replacement of the bridging oxygen atom by sulfur (Compound 24) or by a methylene group (Compound 25) produces highly active analogs. This provides evidence against the Niemann quinoid theory, which postulates that the ability of a compound to form a quinoid structure in the phenolic ring is essential for thyromimetic activity, and emphasizes the importance of the three-dimensional structure and receptor fit of the hormones. Attempts to prepare amino and carbonyl-bridged analogs of T_3 and T_4 have been unsuccessful (104–105).

Table 30.2. Relative Rat Antigoiter Activity of Thyroxine Derivatives

No.	R₁	R₃	R₅	X	R₃'	R₅'	R₄'	Antigoiter Activity*
1. L-T₄	L-Ala	I	I	O	I	I	OH	100
2. D-T₄	D-Ala	I	I	O	I	I	OH	17
3. L-T₃	L-Ala	I	I	O	I	H	OH	550
4. D-T₃	D-Ala	I	I	O	I	H	OH	41
5.	COOH	I	I	O	I	I	OH	0.1
6.	COOH	I	I	O	I	H	OH	0.4
7.	CH₂COOH	I	I	O	I	I	OH	50
8.	CH₂COOH	I	I	O	I	H	OH	36
9.	(CH₂)₂COOH	I	I	O	I	I	OH	15
10.	(CH₂)₂COOH	I	I	O	I	H	OH	20
11.	(CH₂)₃COOH	I	I	O	I	I	OH	4
12.	(CH₂)₃COOH	I	I	O	I	H	OH	5
13.	(CH₂)₂NH₂	I	I	O	I	I	OH	0.6
14.	(CH₂)₂NH₂	I	I	O	I	H	OH	6
15.	L-Ala	H	H	O	I	I	OH	<0.01
16.	L-Ala	H	H	O	I	H	OH	<0.01
17.	DL-Ala	Br	Br	O	I	H	OH	93
18.	L-Ala	Br	Br	O	iPr	H	OH	166
19.	L-Ala	Me	Me	O	Me	H	OH	3
20.	L-Ala	Me	Me	O	iPr	H	OH	20
21.	DL-Ala	iPr	iPr	O	I	H	OH	0
22.	DL-Ala	sBu	sBU	O	I	H	OH	0
23.	DL-Ala	I	I	—	I	I	OH	0
24.	DL-Ala	I	I	S	I	H	OH	132
25.	DL-Ala	I	I	CH₂	I	H	OH	300
26.	L-Ala	I	I	O	H	H	OH	5
27.	L-Ala	I	I	O	OH	H	OH	1.5
28.	L-Ala	I	I	O	NO₂	H	OH	<1
29.	DL-Ala	I	I	O	F	H	OH	6
30.	L-Ala	I	I	O	Cl	H	OH	27
31.	DL-Ala	I	I	O	Br	H	OH	132
32.	L-Ala	I	I	O	Me	H	Oh	80
33.	L-Ala	I	I	O	Et	H	OH	517
34.	L-Ala	I	I	O	iPr	H	OH	786
35.	L-Ala	I	I	O	nPr	H	OH	200
36.	DL-Ala	I	I	O	Phe	H	OH	11
37.	DL-Ala	I	I	O	F	F	OH	2.3
38.	L-Ala	I	I	O	Cl	Cl	OH	21
39.	L-Ala	I	I	O	I	H	NH₂	<1.5
40.	DL-Ala	I	I	O	I	H	H	>150
41.	DL-Ala	I	I	O	CH₃	H	CH₃	0
42.	L-Ala	I	I	O	I	H	CH₃O	225

*See Refs. 107, 108. In vivo activity in rats relative to L-T₄ = 100% or DL-T₄ = 100% for goiter prevention.

Phenolic Ring

The phenolic ring, also called the outer or β-ring, of the thyronine nucleus is required for hormonal activity. Variations in 3′ or 3,′5′ substituents on the phenolic ring have dramatic effects on biologic activity and the affinity for the nuclear receptor. The unsubstituted parent structure of this series L-T₂ (Compound 26) possesses low activity. Substitution at 3′-position by polar hydroxyl or nitro groups (Compounds 27, 28) causes decrease in activity as a consequence of both lowered lipophilicity and intramolecular hydrogen bonding with the 4′-hydroxyl (106). Conversely, substitution by nonpolar halogen or alkyl groups results in an increase in activity in direct relation to bulk and lipophilicity of the substituent, e.g., F < Cl < Br < I (Compounds 29 through 31) and CH₃ < CH₂CH₃ < CH(CH₃)₂ (Compounds 32 through 34). Although 3′-isopropylthyronine (Compound 34) is the most potent analog known, being about 1.4 times as active as L-T₃, n-propylthyronine (Compound 35) is only about one-fourth as active as isopropyl, apparently because of its less compact structure. As the series is further ascended, activity decreases with a further reduction for the more bulky 3′-phenyl substituent (Compound 36). Substi-

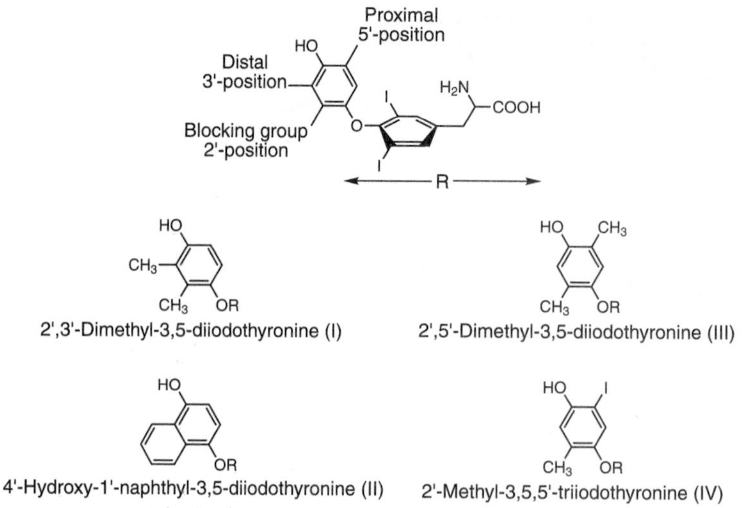

Fig. 30.6. Structures of representative distal and proximal compounds.

tution in both 3'- and 5'-positions by the same halogen produces less active hormones (Compounds 37, 38) than the corresponding 3'-monosubstituted analogs (Compounds 29, 30). The decrease in activity has been explained as due to the increase in phenolic hydroxyl ionization and the resulting increase in binding to TBG (107) (the primary carrier of thyroid hormones in human plasma). In general, a second substituent adjacent to the phenolic hydroxyl (5'-position) reduces activity in direct proportion to its size.

Phenolic Hydroxyl Group

A weakly ionized phenolic hydroxyl group at the 4'-position is essential for optimum hormonal activity. Replacement of the 4'-hydroxyl with an amino group (Compound 39) results in a substantial decrease in activity, presumably as a result of the weak hydrogen bonding ability of the latter group. The retention of activity observed with the 4'-unsubstituted compound (Compound 40) provides direct evidence for metabolic 4'-hydroxylation as an activating step. Introduction of a 4'-substituent that cannot mimic the functional role of a hydroxyl group, such as a methyl group (Compound 41), and that is not metabolically converted into a functional residue results in complete loss of hormonal activity. The thyromimetic activity of the 4'-methyl ether (Compound 42) was ascribed to the ready metabolic cleavage to form an active 4'-hydroxyl analog. The pK_a of 4'-phenolic hydroxyl group for T_4 is 6.7 (90% ionized at pH 7.4) and for T_3 is 8.5 (approximately 10% ionized). The greater acidity for T_4 is reflective of its stronger affinity for plasma proteins and consequently its longer plasma half-life.

Conformational Properties of Thyroid Hormones and Analogs

The importance of the diphenyl ether conformation for biologic activity was first proposed by Zenker and

Jorgensen (108–109). Through molecular models, they showed that a perpendicular orientation of the planes of the aromatic rings of 3,5-diiodothyronines would be favored, to minimize interactions between the bulky 3,5 iodines and the 2',6' hydrogens. In this orientation, the 3'- and 5'-positions of the ring are not conformationally equivalent, and the 3' iodine of T_3 could be oriented either distal (away from) or 5' proximal (closer) to the side chain-bearing ring (Fig. 30.6). Because the activity of compounds such as 3',5'-dimethyl-3,5-diiodothyronine had demonstrated that alkyl groups could replace the 3'- and 5'-iodine substituents, model compounds bearing alkyl groups in the 3'-position and alkyl or iodine substituents in the 5'-position (in addition to the blocking 2'-methyl group) were synthesized for biologic evaluation (109).

Biologic evaluation of 2',3'- and 2',5'-substituted diiodothyronines (110) revealed that 3'-substitution was favorable for thyromimetic activity but that 5'-substitution was not. The structures of representative distal analogs, 2',3'-dimethyl-3,5-DL-diiodothyronine (I) and O-(4'-hydroxy-1'-naphthyl)-3,5-DL-diiodotyrosine (II), and of the proximal analogs, 2',5'-dimethyl-3,5-DL-diiodothyronine (III) and 2'-methyl-3,5,5'-DL-triiodothyronine (IV), are given in Figure 30.6. The effectiveness of these compounds in rat antigoiter assay (111) is presented in Table 30.3. These results clearly indicate that in 2' blocked analogs, a distal 3' substitution is favorable for thyromimetic activity, but a proximal 5' substitution is not.

The perpendicular orientation of the rings of 3,5-diiodothyronines, which was postulated from molecular models, has been confirmed by X-ray crystallographic studies (112), molecular orbital calculations (113), and nuclear magnetic resonance studies (114–115).

In addition to being perpendicular to the inner ring, the outer phenolic ring can adopt conformations relative to the alanine side chain, which would be *cis* or *trans.* In other words, the cisoid and transoid conformations result from the methine group in the alanine side chain being either *cis* or *trans* to the phenolic ring (Fig. 30.7). Although the bioactive conformation of the alanine side chain in thyroid hormone analogs has not yet been defined, these conformations appear to be similar in energy because both are found in thyroactive structures determined by X-ray crystallography (116). The synthesis of conformationally fixed cyclic or unsaturated analogs may allow evaluation of the bioactivity of the two conformers.

Transthyretin Receptor Model

An additional tool in structural analysis and analog design has been transthyretin (TTR, formerly called T$_4$ binding pre-albumin-TBPA), a plasma protein that binds as much as 27% of plasma T$_3$ (117). The amino acid sequence of the TTR T$_3$ binding site is known, and the protein has therefore served as a model, although admittedly an approximate model, for the T$_3$ receptor. The TTR model portrays the T$_3$ molecule as placed in an envelope near the axis of symmetry of the TTR dimer. In this envelope, hydrophobic residues, such as those of leucine, lysine, and alanine, are near pockets accommodating the 3,5,3'- and 5'-positions of T$_3$, whereas the hydrophilic groups of serine and threonine, hydrogen bonded to water, are between the 3' substituent and 4' phenolic group. Taking this model into account, Ahmad suggested that 3'-acetyl-3,5-di-iodothyronine might be a good analog or a good inhibitor of T$_3$ because the carbonyl group of the 3' acetyl substituent would form a strong hydrogen bond with the 4' phenolic hydrogen, preventing thereby its bonding with the hydrated residue of the putative receptor (118).

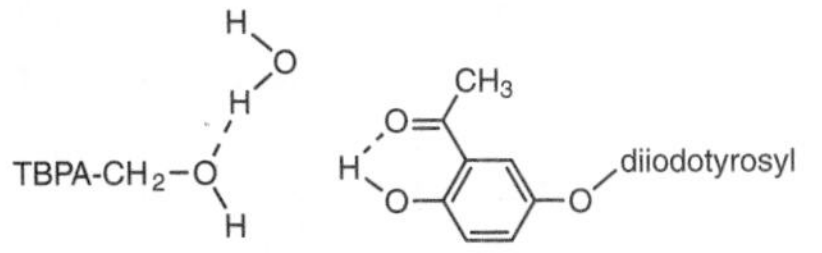

The compound, prepared by Benson and co-workers (119), was found to be indistinguishable from T$_3$ in oxygen uptake and glycerophosphate activity tests and to be half as active as T$_3$ in displacing labeled T$_3$ from rat liver nuclei in specific in vivo conditions.

Table 30.3. Effectiveness of Distal and Proximal Compounds

| Compound | Antigoiter Assay | |
	Dose*	% T$_4$ act.
I	0.025	50
II	0.013	>100
III	2.3	<1
IV	0.5	2

*mg/kg/day.

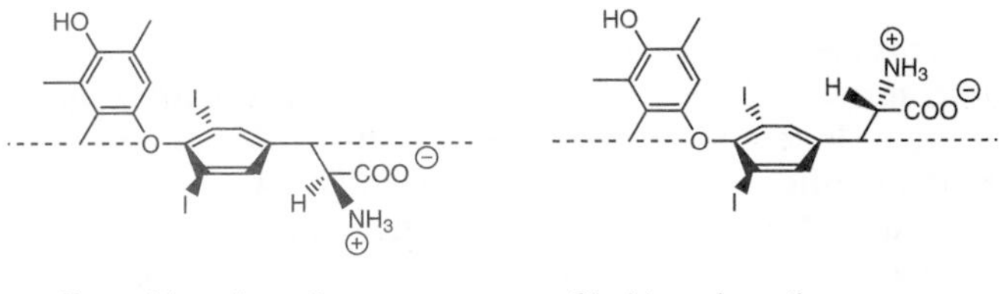

Fig. 30.7. Side-chain conformations of thyroid hormones; transoid (left) and cisoid (right).

Review Questions

What organs and functions of the body are regulated by thyroid hormones?

Thyroid hormones regulate the body's metabolism and organ function, affecting heart rate, cholesterol level, body weight, energy level, muscle strength, skin condition, menstrual regularity, memory and many other conditions.

List classes of drugs that interact (interfere) with thyroid hormones therapy.

- Oral Anticoagulants—Thyroid hormones increase catabolism of vitamin K-dependent clotting factors.
- Insulin or Oral Hypoglycemics—Initiating thyroid replacement therapy cause increases in insulin or oral hypoglycemic requirements. The effects seen are poorly understood and depend upon a variety of factors such as endocrine status of the patient and type of thyroid preparations.
- Cholestyramine—Cholestyramine binds both T$_4$ and T$_3$ in the intestine, thus impairing absorption of these thyroid hormones.
- Estrogen, Oral Contraceptives—Estrogens tend to increase serum thyroxine-binding globulin (TBG), thus increasing thyroid requirements.
- Antidepressant drugs

Why the use of thyroid hormones in therapy of obesity is unjustified?

Drugs with thyroid hormone activity, alone or together with other therapeutic agents, have been used for treatment of obesity. In euthyroid patients, doses within the range of daily hormonal requirements are ineffective for weight reduction. Larger doses may produce serious or even life threatening manifestation of toxicity, particularly when given in association with sympathomimetic amines such as those used for their anorectic effects.

What is the purpose of prescribing beta-blockers along with thyroid drugs in treatment of hyperthyroidism?

Because beta-adrenergic blocking agents such as atenolol, nadolol, metoprolol, or propranolol block the action of circulating thyroid hormone on the body tissues, slowing heart rate and lessening nervousness. These drugs may be extremely helpful in reducing symptoms until one of the other forms of treatment has a chance to take effect. They are not used, however, in patients who have asthma or heart failure which may be worsened with these drugs.

Patients with hypothyroidism and organic depression may need both levothyroxine and antidepressant drug therapy. In levothyroxine-treated patients with hypothyroidism who were treated with sertraline, there was an elevated serum thyrotropin concentration, indicative of a decrease in the efficacy of levothyroxine. What is the possible mechanism of interaction between the two drugs?

Sertraline may interfere by increasing the clearance of thyroxine.

REFERENCES

McCowen K, Garber J, and Spark R. Elevated Serum Thyrotropin in Thyroxine-Treated Patients with Hypothyroidism Given Sertraline. N Engl J Med, 1997; 337, 1010–1011.

Harel Z, Biro FM, Tedford WL. Effect of long term treatment with sertraline (Zoloft) simulating hypothyroidism in an adolescent. J Adolesc Health 1995;16:232–4.

Shelton RC, Winn S, Ekhatore N, et al. The effects of antidepressants on the thyroid axis in depression. Biol Psychiatry 1993;33:120–6.

What are the tests for checking the thyroid function?

1. Total serum T_4. This includes both bound and free T_4 concentration.
2. T_3 resin uptake (T_3RU). The T_3 resin uptake test measures the amount of unsaturated binding sites on the thyroid hormone transport proteins. A proportion of the labeled T_3 will bind to available sites on the serum TBG; any excess will bind to the resin. Resin uptake is inversely proportional to the number of vacant binding sites, and therefore inversely proportional to the total TBG.

    In thyrotoxicosis, there are fewer vacant binding sites available on thyroxine binding globulin due to the high circulating levels of thyroid hormone. This means less radioactive T_3 will be able to bind to TBG and more will bind to the resin. Hence, resin uptake is higher in hyperthyroid patients than it is in normals. The converse is true in hypothyroid states. In high TBG states, such as pregnancy or estrogen therapy, the T_3RU will be low. However the physiologically active free T_4 level will still be normal.

3. Free thyroxine Index (FT_4I). FT_4I is a reflection of the amount of free T_4 in most situations. It is a calculated value and corrects for changes in TBG concentrations by using the following formula:

    FTI = (Total T_4) X (T_3 Resin Uptake / T_3RU control).

    Mean normal T_3RU for the particular assay (i.e., normal range 25–35%, mean normal is 30%). With extreme changes in TBG concentrations, acute medical illness, heparin therapy or low protein states secondary to nephrotic syndrome, the FT_4I may not accurately reflect the amount of free T_4 concentrations.

4. TSH Test. Measuring the serum TSH has become the screen test of choice for thyroid disease. Primary hypothyroidism produces elevated TSH levels whereas patients with primary hyperthyroidism (i.e., Graves) should have undetectable TSH values. This relationship is true only in individuals with an intact hypo-

thalamic-pituitary-thyroid axis. Patients who present with a normal or detectable TSH level and elevated thyroid hormone concentrations require further evaluation to exclude central causes of hyperthyroidism.

5. TRH Test. The administration of thyrotropin releasing hormone (TRH) causes a rise in TSH concentration in normal subjects (TSH = 2–30 mU/L.) An exaggerated response occurs in primary hypothyroid subjects (TSH often > 30 mU/L, depending on the baseline TSH elevation.) Hyperthyroid patients have a mild or absent TSH response (TSH < 2 mU/L) since the suppressed TSH cannot be stimulated by exogenous TRH. The introduction of sensitive TSH assays that can detect low suppressed TSH levels, identifying patients with primary hyperthyroidism, has virtually made the TRH stimulation test obsolete.

6. Iodine Test. Plasma iodine in the form of iodide is concentrated (trapped) in the thyroid cells by an energy requiring active transport mechanism where it is incorporated into T_3 and T_4 via organification. Therefore, iodine measures both trapping and organification by the thyroid gland.

List the conditions associated with decrease and increase levels of TBG?

TBG is synthesized by the liver under the influence of estrogen. An increase in TBG concentration in response to higher estrogen levels may result in higher measured total T_4 concentration. However, the amount of free T_4 concentration remains constant and the patient remains clinically euthyroid.

Conditions associated with increased levels of TBG:
- Estrogen Effects—pregnancy, oral contraceptives
- Infectious Hepatitis
- Biliary Cirrhosis
- Genetic Determination

In contrast, factors that cause a decrease in TBG concentration or lower affinity for T_4 binding to TBG may result in low measured total T_4 concentration without affecting free T_4 levels.

Conditions associated with decreased binding of T_4 by TBG:
- Androgens and Anabolic Steroids
- Large doses of Glucocorticoids
- Nephrotic Syndrome
- Major Systemic Nonthyroidal Illness
- Active Acromegaly
- Chronic Liver Disease
- Drugs—dilantin, tegretol
- Genetic Determination

Considering T_3 does not cross the placental membrane and therefore can not be useful in treating fetal thyroid hormone deficiencies or in stimulating lung development immediately before premature birth, what would be your solution to overcome this problem?

(Refer to QSAR Section)

3'-isopropyl-3,6-dimethyl-L-thyronine has the capacity to cross the placental membrane and exerts thyromimetic effects in the fetus after administration to the mother.

CASE STUDY

Victoria F. Roche and S. William Zito

Dr. IG is an endocrinologist with a 27-year-old, female patient who has just become pregnant. The patient was diagnosed with Grave's disease about 6 months ago and is currently undergoing anti-thyroid therapy with methimazole (1). The physician doesn't want to discontinue therapy because he believes that to do so at this stage would jeopardize the patient's ability to carry the baby to term. Concerned about the serious effect that anti-thyroid drugs may have on the developing fetus, he consults you about the relative merits of the 4 drugs drawn below. Evaluate them in this case and make a recommendation.

1. *Identify the therapeutic problem(s) where the pharmacist's intervention may benefit the patient.*

2. *Identify and prioritize the patient specific factors that must be considered to achieve the desired therapeutic outcomes.*

3. *Conduct a thorough and mechanistically oriented structure-activity analysis of all therapeutic alternatives provided in the case.*

4. *Evaluate the SAR findings against the patient specific factors and desired therapeutic outcomes and make a therapeutic decision.*

5. *Counsel your patient.*

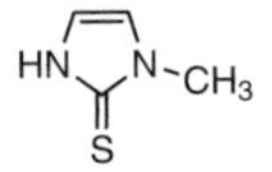

Methimazole (1) 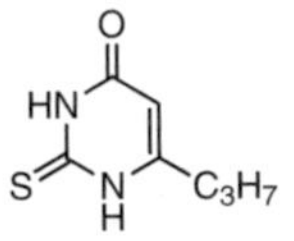   2   3   4

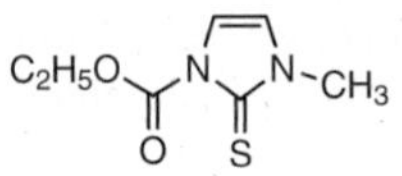

REFERENCES

1. Harington CR. Biochemical Basis of Thyroid Function. Lancet 1935;1:1199–1204;1261–1266.
2. Baumann EJ. Z Physiol Chem 1896;21:319.
3. Magnus-Levy A. Berl Klin Wocheschr 1895;32:650.
4. Gudernatsch JF. Arch Entwicklungsmech Organ 1912;35:457.
5. Nadler NJ. In: Greer MA, Solomon DH, eds. Handbook of Physiology. Washington, DC. Sec. 7, Vol. III, Ch. 4, Am Physiol Soc 1974.
6. Ekholm R, Bjorkman U. In: Martini L, ed. The Thyroid Gland. New York: Raven Press, 1990;38–39.
7. Kendall EC JAMA 1915;64:2042.
8. Harington CR. Chemistry of Thyroxine II Constitution and synthesis of desiodothyroxine. Biochem J 1926;20:300.
9. Harington CR, Chemistry of Thyroxine. III. Constitution and synthesis of Thyroxine. Barger C. Biochem J 1927;21:169.
10. Gross J, Pitt-Rivers R. 3:5:3'-Triiodothyroxine.1. Isolation from the Thyroid Gland. Biochem J 1953;53:645.
11. Roche J, C R Acad Sci (Paris) 1952;234:1228.
12. Harington CR, Randall SS. Observations on the Iodine-containing compounds of the thyroid gland. Isolation of DL-3:5-diiodotyrosine. Biochem J 1929;23:373.
13. Fink K, Fink RM. Science 1948;108:358.
14. Sawin CT. The Hormones. Boston: Little & Brown, 1969;98.
15. de Groot LJ, et al. The Thyroid and its Diseases. New York: Wiley, 1984;5th ed.
16. Goodman HM, Van Middlesworth L. The thyroid gland. In: Mouncastle VB, ed. Medical Physiology. St. Louis: Mosby 1980; 2:1500.
17. Chopra IJ, Solomon DH, Chopra U, et al. Pathways of metabolism of thyroid hormones. Rec Prog Horm Res 1978;34:521–567.
18. Visser TJ, Docter R, Krenning EP, Hennemann G. Regulation of thyroid hormone bioactivity. Endocrinol Invest 1986;9 (Suppl 4):17–26.
19. Obregon MJ, Roelfsema F, Morreale de Escobar G, et al. Exchange of triiodothyronine derived from thyroxine with circulating triiodothyronine as studied in the rat. Clin Endocrinol 1979;10:305–315.
20. Visser TJ, Mol JA, Otten MH. Rapid deiodination of triiodothyronine sulfate by rat liver microsomal fraction. Endocrinology 1983;122:1547–1549.
21. Pitt-Rivers R. Physiological Activity of acetic acid analogs of some iodinated thyronines. Lancet 1953;2:234.
22. Han S, Gordon JT, Bhat K, et al. Synthesis of side chain-modified iodothyronines. Int J Peptide Protein Res 1987; 30:652–656.
23. Wynn J, Gibbs R. Thyroxine degradation. II. Products of thyroxine degradation by rat liver microsomes. J Biol Chem 1962;237:3499.
24. Muller MJ, Seitz HJ. Pleiotypic action of thyroid hormones at the target cell level. Biochem Pharmacol 1984;33:1579–1584.
25. Himms-Hagen J. Cellular thermogenesis. Annu Rev Physiol 1976;38:315–51.
26. Muller MJ, Seitz HJ. Thyroid hormone action on intermediary metabolism. Part I: respiration, thermogenesis and carbohydrate metabolism. Klin Wochenschr 1984;62:11–18.
27. Muller MJ, Seitz HJ. Thyroid hormone action on intermediary metabolism. Part II: Lipid metabolism in hypo- and hyperthyroidism. Klin Wochenschr 1984;62:49–55.
28. Muller MJ, Seitz HJ. Thyroid hormone action on intermediary metabolism. Part III. Protein metabolism in hyper- and hypothyroidism. Klin Wochenschr 1984;62:97–102.
29. Sterling K. The mitochondrial route of thyroid hormone action. Bull N Y Acad Med. New York 1977;53:260–266.
30. Ismail-Beigi F, Edelman IS. Mechanism of thyroid calorigenesis: role of active sodium transport. Proc Natl Acad Sci USA 1970;67:1071–1078.
31. Williams LT, Lefkowitz RJ, Watanabe AM, et al. Thyroid hormone regulation of beta-adrenergic receptor number. J Biol Chem 1977;252:2787–2789.
32. Levey GS, Epstein SE. Myocardial adenyl cyclase: activation by thyroid hormones and evidence for two adenyl cyclase systems. J Clin Invest 1969;48:1663–9.
33. Stryer L. Biochemistry 2nd ed. San Francisco: Freeman, 1981:843.
34. Sutherland EW, Robinson GA. The role of cyclic-3,'5'-AMP in responses to catecholamines and other hormones. Pharmacol Rev 1966;18:145–161.
35. Eayrs JT, Lishman WA. The mutation of behavior in hypothyroidism and salvation. Br J Anim Behav 1955;3:17.
36. Tata JR. Inhibition of the biological action of thyroid hormones by actinomycin D and puromycin. Nature 1963;197:1167.
37. Tata JR, Widnell CC. Ribonucleic acid synthesis during the early action of thyroid hormones. Biochem J 1966;98:604–620.
38. Dillmann WH, Schwartz HL, Silva E, et al. Alpha-amanitin administration results in a temporary inhibition of hepatic enzyme induction by triiodothyronine: further evidence favoring a long-lived mediator of thyroid hormone action. Endocrinology 1977;100:1621–1627.
39. Schadlow AR, Surks MI, Schwartz HL, Oppenheimer JH. Specific triiodothyronine binding sites in the anterior pituitary of the rat. Science 1972;176:1252–1254.
40. Oppenheimer JH, Koerner D, Schwartz HL, Surks MI. Specific nuclear triiodothyronine binding sites in rat liver and kidney. J Clin Endocrinol Metab 1972;35:330–333.
41. Galton VA. Putative nuclear triiodothyronine receptors in tadpole erythrocytes: regulation of receptor number by thyroid hormone. Endocrinology 1984;114:735–742.
42. Samuels HH. In: Oppenheimer JH, Samuels HH, eds. Molecular Basis of Thyroid Hormone Action. New York: Academic Press, 1983;35–65.
43. Oppenheimer JH. In: Oppenheimer JH, Samuels HH, eds. Molecular Basis of Thyroid Hormone Action. New York: Academic Press, 1983;1–34.
44. Barsano CP, DeGroot LJ. In: Oppenheimer JH, Samuels HH, eds. Molecular Basis of Thyroid Hormone Action. New York: Academic Press, 1983;139–177.
45. Robbins J, Rall JE. Physiol Rev 1960;40: 415.
46. Lee YP et al. Enhanced oxidation of α-glycerophosphate by mitochondria of thyroid-fed rats. J Biol Chem 1959;234:3051.
47. Westerfeld WW, Richert DA, Ruegamer WR. New assay procedure for thyroxine analogs. Endocrinology 1965;77:802–811.
48. Lutsky BN, Zenker N, Hanker JS, Morizono Y, et al. Carcinogens 3,4-benzpyrene and 3-methylcholanthrene: induction of mitochondrial oxidative enzymes. Science 1968;159:1102–1103.
49. Sterling K, Milch PO, Brenner MA, Lazarus JH. Thyroid hormone action: the mitochondrial pathway. Science 1977; 197:996–999.
50. Schwartz HL, Oppenheimer JH. Physiologic and biochemical actions of thyroid hormone, Pharmacol Ther 1978;B 3:349–376.
51. Barden N, Labrie F. J Receptor for thyrotropin-releasing hormone in plasma membranes of bovine anterior pituitary gland. Role of lipids. Biol Chem 1973;248:7601–7606.
52. Sterling K, Lazarus JH. The thyroid and its control. Annu Rev Physiol 1977;39:349–371.

53. Carr FE, Ridgeway EC, Chin WW. Regulation of the alpha and thyrotropin beta-subunit messenger ribonucleic acids by thyroid hormones. Endocrinology 1985;116:873–878.

54. Greenspan FS, Forsham PH. Basic and Clinical Endocrinology. Los Altos: Lange Medical, 1983:141.

55. Wolff J, Chaikoff IL. Plasma inorganic iodide as homeostatic regulator of thyroid function. J Biol Chem 1948;174:555.

56. Virion A, Michot JL, Deme D, Pommier J. NADPH oxidation catalyzed by the peroxidase/H2O2 system. Iodide-mediated oxidation of NADPH to iodinated NADP. Eur J Biochem 1985;148:239–248.

57. Leonard JL, Kaplan MM, Visser TJ, et al. Cerebral cortex responds rapidly to thyroid hormones. Science 1981;214:571–573.

58. McConnon J, Row VV, Volpe R. The influence of liver damage in man on the distribution and disposal rates of thyroxine and triiodothyronine. J Clin Endocrinol Metab 1972;34:144–153.

59. Lim VS, Fang VS, Katz AI, Refetoff S. Thyroid dysfunction in chronic renal failure. A study of the pituitary-thyroid axis and peripheral turnover kinetics of thyroxine and triiodothyronine. J Clin Invest 1977;60:522–534.

60. Carter JN, Eastmen CJ, Corcoran JM, Lazarus L. Inhibition of conversion of thyroxine to triiodothyronine in patients with severe chronic illness. Clin Endocrinol 1976;5:587–594.

61. Spaulding SW, Chopra IJ, Sherwin RS, Lyall SS. Effect of caloric restriction and dietary composition of serum T3 and reverse T3 in man. J Clin Endocrinol Metab 1976;42:197–200.

62. Chacon MA, Tildon JT. Mode of death and post-mortem time effects on 3,3',5-triiodothyronine levels—relevance to elevated post-mortem T3 levels in SIDS. Fed Proc 1984;43:866.

63. Heyma P, Larkins RG, Campbell DG. Inhibition by propranolol of 3,5,3'-triiodothyronine formation from thyroxine in isolated rat renal tubules: an effect independent of beta-adrenergic blockade. Endocrinology 1980;106:1437–1441.

64. Silva JE, Larsen PR. Abstract, Am Thyr Assoc 59th Meeting 1983.

65. Zenker N, Chacon MA, Tildon JT. Mode of death effect on rat liver iodothyronine 5' deiodinase activity: role of adenosine 3',5' monophosphate. Life Sci 1984;35:2213–2217.

66. Eberhardt NL, Valcana T, Timiras PS. Triiodothyronine nuclear receptors: an in vitro comparison of the binding of triiodothyronine to nuclei of adult rat liver, cerebral hemisphere, and anterior pituitary. Endocrinology 1978;102:556–561.

67. Rosenberg IN. Thyroid storm. N Engl J Med 1970;283:1052–3.

68. Hashimoto H, Arch J. Klin Chir 1912;97:219.

69. Pitt-Rivers R, Tata JR. In: Thomas Charles C, The Chemistry of Thyroid Disease. Springfield, Ill, 1960;38.

70. Mahaux JE, Chamla-Soumenkoff J, Delcourt R, Nagel N, Levin S. The effect of triiodothyronine on cervical lymphoid structures, thyroid activity, IgG and IgM immunoglobulin level and exophthalmos in Graves' disease. Acta Endocrinol 1969;61:400–406.

71. Selenkow HA, Rose LI. Pharmacol Ther C 1976;1:331.

72. Jackson IM, Cobb WE. Why does anyone still use desiccated thyroid USP?. Am J Med 1978;64:284–288

73. Lamas L, Ingbar SH. In: Robbins J, Braverman LE, eds. Thyroid Research. Amsterdam: Excerpta Medica, 1976:213.

74. Pittman JA, Jr. Diagnosis and Treatment of Thyroid Disease. Philadelphia: F. A. Davis, 1963:48.

75. Pittman JA, Jr. In: Selenkow HA, Hoffman F, eds. Diagnosis and Treatment of Common Thyroid Disease. Amsterdam: Excerpta Medica 1971:72–73.

76. Bremner WF, Spencer CA, Ratcliffe WA, et al. The assessment of 125I treatment of thyrotoxicosis. Clin Endocrinol 1976;5:225.

77. Wolff J, Maurey JR. Thyroidal iodide transport. IV. The role of ion size. Biochem Biophys Acta 1963;69:58.

78. Morreale de Escobar G, Escobar del Rey R. Extrathyroid effects of some antithyroid drugs and their metabolic consequences. Rec Prog Horm Res 1967;23:87–137.

79. Cooper DS, Saxe VC, Meskell M, et al. Acute effects of propylthiouracil (PTU) on thyroidal iodide organification and peripheral iodothyronine deiodination: correlation with serum PTU levels measured by radioimmunoassay. J Clin Endocrinol Metab 1982;54:101–7.

80. Visser TJ, van Overmeeren E, Fekkes D, et al. Inhibition of iodothyronine 5'-deiodinase by thioureylenes; structure–activity relationship. FEBS Lett. 1979;103:314–318.

81. Taurog A. The mechanism of action of the thioureylene antithyroid drugs. Endocrinology 1976;98:1031–1046.

82. Nakashima T, Taurog A, Riesco G. Mechanism of action of thioureylene antithyroid drugs: factors affecting intrathyroidal metabolism of propylthiouracil and methimazole in rats. Endocrinology 1978;103:2187–2197.

83. Papapetrou PD, Mothon S, Alexander WD. Binding of the 35-S of 35-S-propylthiouracil by follicular thyroglobulin in vivo and in vitro. Acta Endocrinol 1975;79:248–258.

84. Chopra IJ, Chua Teco GN, Eisenberg JB, et al. Structure-activity relationships of inhibition of hepatic monodeiodination of thyroxine to 3,5,3'-triiodothyronine by thiouracil and related compounds. Endocrinology 1982;110:163–168.

85. Turner JG, Brownlie BE, Sadler WA, Jensen CH. An evaluation of lithium as an adjunct to carbimazole treatment in acute thyrotoxicosis. Acta Endocrinol 1976;83:86–92.

86. Berens SC, Wolff J, Murphy DL. Lithium concentration by the thyroid. Endocrinology 1970;87:1085–1087.

87. Temple R, Berman M, Robbins J, Wolff J. The use of lithium in the treatment of thyrotoxicosis. J Clin Invest 1972;51:2746–56.

88. Tookey HL et al. In: Liener IE, ed. Toxic Constituents of Foodstuffs. New York: Academic Press, 1980;103–142.

89. Langer P, Michajlovskij N. Effect of naturally occurring goitrogens on thyroid peroxidase and influence of some compounds on iodide formation during the estimation. Endocrinol Exp 1972;6:97–103.

90. Greer MA. Rec Prog Horm Res 1962;18:187.

91. Elfving S. Studies on the naturally occurring goitrogen 5-vinyl-2-thiooxazolidone. Metabolism and antithyroid effect in the rat. Ann Clin Res 1980;12(Suppl 28):7–47

92. Tabachnick M, Hao YL, Korcek L. Effect of oleate, diphenylhydantoin and heparin on the binding of 125 I-thyroxine to purified thyroxine-binding globulin. J Clin Endocrinol Metab 1973;36:392.

93. Goswami A, Leonard JL, Rosenberg IN. Inhibition by coumadin anticoagulants of enzymatic outer ring monodeiodination of iodothyronine. Biochem Biophys Res Comm 1982;104:1231–1238.

94. Auf'mkolk M, Amir SM, Kubota K, Ingbar SH. The active principles of plant extracts with antithyrotropic activity: oxidation products of derivatives of 3,4-dihydroxycinnamic acid. Endocrinology 1985;116:1677.

95. Selenkow HA, Asper SP, Jr. Physiol Rev 1955;35:426.

96. Zenker N, Goudonnet H, Truchot R. Effect of thyroid status and cold stress on tyrosine hydroxylase activity in adrenal gland and brown adipose tissue. Life Sci 1976;18:183–188.

97. Zenker N, Truchot R, Goudonnet H, Chaillot B, Michel R. Isopropyldiiodothyronine and alpha-methylthyroxine: com-

parison of their in vitro and in vivo effects with those of thyroid hormones. Biochem Pharmacol 1976;25:1757–1762.

98. Tarentino AL, Richert DA, Westerfeld WW. The concurrent induction of hepatic alpha-glycerophosphate dehydrogenase and malate dehydrogenase by thyroid hormone. Biochim Biophys Acta 1966;124:295–309.

99. Jorgensen EC. Structure activity relationships of thyroxine analogs. Pharmacol Ther 1976;B 2:661–682.

100. Jorgensen EC, Lehman PA. Thyroxine Analogs. IV. Synthesis of aliphatric and alicyclic ethers of 3,5-Diiodo-DL-tyrosine. J Org Chem 1961;26:894.

101. Mussett MV, Pitt-Rivers R. Metab Clin Exp 1957;6:18.

102. Jorgensen EC, Reid J AW. Thyroxine Analogs. XI. Structural isomers of 3,5,3′-triiodo-DL-thyronine. J Med Chem 1964;7:701.

103. Ballard PL, et al. Prolactin in umbilical cord blood and the respiratory distress syndrome. Pediatr Res 1978;12:1164.

104. Tripp SL, Block FB, Barile G. Synthesis of Methylene- and Carbonyl-Bridged Analogs of Iodothyronine and Iodothyroacetic acids. J Med Chem 1973;236:2891.

105. Mukherjee R, Block P, Jr. Thyroxine analogues: synthesis and nuclear magnetic resonance spectral studies of diphenylamines. J Chem Soc (C) 1971:1596–600.

106. Leeson PD, Ellis D, Emmett JC, et al. Thyroid hormone analogues. Synthesis of 3′-substituted 3,5-diiodo-L-thyronines and quantitative structure-activity studies of in vitro and in vivo thyromimetic activities in rat liver and heart. J Med Chem 1988;31:37–54.

107. Jorgensen EC. Thyroid Hormones. In: Li CH, ed. Hormonal Proteins and Peptides. Vol. 6, New York: Academic Press, 1978;108.

108. Jorgensen EC. Thyroid Hormones. In: Wolff ME, ed. Burger's Medicinal Chemistry, Part 3, 4th ed. New York: Wiley, 1981;103.

109. Zenker N, Jorgensen EC. Thyroxine analogs. I. Synthesis of 3,5-Diiodi-4-(2′alkylphenoxy)-DL-phenylalanine. J Am Chem Soc 1959;81:4643.

110. Jorgensen EC, et al. Thyroxine analogs. III. Antigoitrogenic and calorigenic activity of some alkyl substituted analogs of thyroxine. J Biol Chem 1960;235:1732.

111. Jorgensen EC, et al. Thyroxine analogs. VII. Antigoitrogenic, calorigenic and hypocholesteremic activities of same aliphatic, alicyclic and aromatic ethers of 3,5-diiodotyrosine in the rat. J Biol Chem 1962;237:3832.

112. Cody V, Hazel J, Langs DA, et al. Molecular structure of thyroxine analogues. Crystal structure of 3,5,3′-triiodothyroacetic and 3,5,3′,5′-tetraoiodothyroacetic acid N-diethanolamine (1:1) complexes. J Med Chem 1977;20:1628–1631.

113. Kollman PA, Murray WJ, Nuss ME, et al. Molecular orbital studies of thyroid hormone analogs. J Am Chem Soc 1973;95: 8518–8525.

114. Lehman PA, Jorgensen EC. Thyroxine analogs. XIII. NMR evidence for hindered rotation in diphenyl ethers. Tetrahedron 1965;21:363.

115. Duggan BM, Craik DJ. 1H and 13C NMR relaxation studies of molecular dynamics of the thyroid hormones thyroxine, 3,5,3′-triiodothyronine, and 3,5-diiodothyronine. J Med Chem 1996;39:4007–4016.

116. Cody V. Thyroid hormones: crystal structure, molecular conformation, binding, and structure-function relationships. Rec Prog Horm Res 1978;34:437–475.

117. Ekins R, et al. Free Thyroid Hormones. Amsterdam: Excerpta Medica, 1979; 7.

118. Ahmad P. Fyfe CA, Mellors A. Parachors in drug design. Biochem Pharmacol 1975;24:1103–1110.

119. Benson MG, Ellis D, Emmett JC, et al. 3′-Acetyl-3,5-diiodo-L-thyronine: a novel highly active thyromimetic with low receptor affinity. Biochem Pharmacol 1984;33:3143–3149.

SUGGESTED READINGS

E.S. Gilbert, et.al., Thyroid cancer rates and I-131 doses from Nevada atmospheric nuclear bomb tests. J Na Cancer Ins, 90:1654, 1998.

P.W. Ladenson, et.al., Comparison of administration of recombinant human thyrotropin with withdrawal of thyroid hormone for radioactive iodine scanning in patients with thyroid carcinoma. N Engl J Med, 337, 888, 1997.

R. Lewis, New tests monitor thyroid cancer. The Scientist, January 18, 1999.

K.C. McCowen, J.R. Garber, and R. Spark. Elevated Serum Thyrotropin in Thyroxine-Treated Patients with Hypothyroidism Given Sertraline. N Engl J Med, 337, Number 14, 1997.

31. Calcium Homeostasis

ROBIN M. ZAVOD

INTRODUCTION

Three primary hormones, calcitonin, parathyroid hormone, and vitamin D control the homeostatic regulation of calcium and its principle counter ion, inorganic phosphate. Homeostatic control of these ions is essential not only for the moderation of longitudinal bone growth and bone remodeling, but also for blood coagulation, neuromuscular excitability, plasma membrane structure and function, muscle contraction, glycogen and ATP metabolism, neurotransmitter/hormone secretion, and enzyme catalysis (1). Approximately 1 kg of calcium is found in an average 70 kg adult, 99% of which is located in the bone. The principle calcium salt contained in the hydroxyapatite crystalline lattice of teeth and bones is $Ca_{10}(PO_4)_6(OH)_2$. Similarly, about 500–600 g of phosphate is present, 85% of which is found in the bone. The normal plasma concentration of calcium is about 4.5–5.7 mEq/L, 50% of which is protein bound. The remainder of the calcium is either complexed to corresponding counter ions (46%) or exists in its ionized form (4%). It is only the ionized form of calcium that is tightly hormonally regulated (varies less than 5–10%) (1,2). As serum calcium concentrations fluctuate so do the plasma levels of the hormones associated with calcium homeostasis. Serum phosphorous levels vary with age, diet and hormonal status. The most common form of phosphate in the blood (pH=7.4) is HPO_4^{2-}.

The bone is composed of two distinct tissue structures: cortical (compact) bone and trabecular (cancellous) bone (3). Eighty percent of the skeleton is composed of cortical bone (e.g., long bones such as the humerus, radius and ulna) (4,5), which is a relatively dense tissue (80–90% calcified) (4) that provides structure and support (3). Bone marrow cavities, flat bones and the ends of long bones are all composed of trabecular bone, which is considerably more porous (5–20% calcified) (4,5). In order to maintain healthy, well mineralized bone, a continuous process of bone resorption (loss of ionic calcium from bone) and formation occurs along the bone surface. Cortical bone is remodeled at the rate of 3% per year, whereas 25% of trabecular bone, which has considerably higher surface area, is remodeled annually (3).

Inorganic and organic components are both present in the bone. The highly crystalline inorganic component is hydroxyapatite; the collagen matrix comprises the major portion (90%) of the organic component. The collagen matrix serves as the foundation for hydroxyapatite mineralization. Osteocalcin and osteonectin are minor organic constituents that serve to promote binding of hydroxyapatite and calcium to the collagen matrix and regulate the rate of bone mineralization respectively (5).

In general, peak bone mass occurs between 30–40 years of age (3,6) and is dependent upon genetic factors as well as proper intake of calcium, maintenance of quality nutrition, and participation in weight bearing exercise (6). Thereafter, peak bone mass progressively declines at the rate of 0.3–0.5% of cortical bone/year (3). After menopause bone loss is accelerated (2%/year in the spine) (6) for a period of 5–10 years due to the loss of estrogen. This can result in up to a 30% decrease in bone mineral density.

HORMONAL REGULATION OF SERUM CALCIUM LEVELS

Arnaud (7) has developed a "butterfly model" that provides a diagrammatic view of the complex interrelationships among the three hormones, parathyroid, calcitonin and Vitamin D, that control calcium homeostasis (serum concentrations of ionic calcium) and their target organs (bone, kidney, and intestine) (Fig. 31.1). The right side (B loops) of the butterfly model describes the processes that serve to increase the serum calcium concentration in response to hypocalcemia, while the left side (A loops) depicts the events that occur in response to hypercalcemia.

Calcitonin

Human calcitonin

Human calcitonin is a 32 amino acid peptide (MW 3527) biosynthesized in the parafollicular "C" cells found within the thyroid gland. This hormone contains a critical disulfide bridge between residues 1 and 7, with the entire amino acid sequence required for biologic activity. The amino terminal residue is a proline amide (8). "Pro-calcitonin," a precursor peptide, has been identified and is proposed to facilitate intracellular transport and secretion. Calcitonin is secreted in response to elevated serum calcium concentrations (>9mg/100mL) and serves to oppose the hormonal effects of parathyroid hormone. In response to a hypercalcemic state (Fig. 31.1 loops B), increased calcitonin secretion drives serum calcium concentrations down *via* stimu-

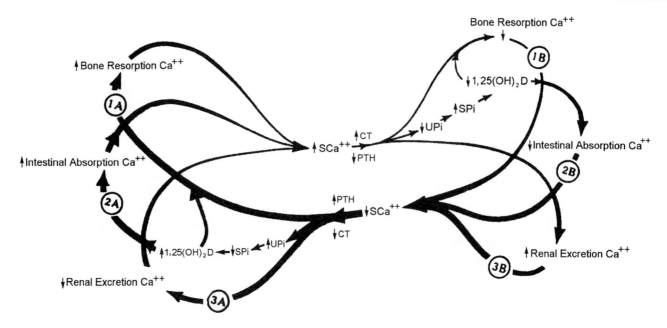

Fig. 31.1. The Arnaud's butterfly model for regulating calcium homeostasis consists of three overlapping loops that interlock and relate to one another through the serum concentrations of ionic calcium (SCa), parathyroid hormone (PTH), and calcitonin (CT). The right side (B loops) of the model describes the physiologic processes that serve to increase the serum calcium concentration in response to hypocalcemia, while the left side (A loops) depicts the events to decrease the serum calcium concentration in response to hypercalcemia. The letters of the loops refer to the tissues affected; loop 1 for bone resorption; loop 2 for intestinal absorption and loop 3 for renal excretion. SPi is serum inorganic phosphate, and UPi is urinary inorganic phosphate. (Modified from reference 7.)

lation of urinary excretion of both calcium and phosphate (loop 3B), prevention of calcium resorption from the bone *via* inhibition of osteoclast activity (loop 1B), and inhibition of intestinal absorption of calcium (loop 2B). When serum calcium concentrations are low (hypocalcemia), the release of calcitonin is slowed, thereby activating loops 1A, 2A and 3A.

Parathyroid Hormone

```
          H₂N—Met—Met—Ser—Ala—Lys—Asp—Met—Val—Lys—Val
                                                      \
                                                      Met
      Ser—Arg-Ala—Leu—Phe—Cys—Ile—Ala—Leu—Met—Val—Ile
  Asp
      Gly—Lys—Ser—Val—Lys—Lys—Arg—Ser—Val—Ser—Glu—Ile—Gln
                                                         \
                                                         Leu
      Arg—Glu—Met—Ser—Asn—Leu—His—Lys—Gly—Leu—Asn—His—Met
  Val
      Glu-Trp-Leu—Arg—Lys—Lys—Leu—Gln—Asp—Val
                                                \
                                                His
  HO₂C—Gln—Ser—Lys—Ala—Lys—[₇₉·····₃₅]—Phe—Asn
```

Human preproparathyroid hormone

Parathyroid hormone (PTH) is biosynthesized as a 115 amino acid pre-prohormone in the rough endoplasmic reticulum of the parathyroid gland and is cleaved to the prohormone (84 amino acids) in the cisternal space of the reticulum. The active hormone is finally produced (34 amino acids, ~MW 9500) in the Golgi complex and is stored in secretory granules in the parathyroid gland. Unlike calcitonin, the biologic activity of PTH resides solely in residues 1-34 in the amino terminus. The relatively short acting PTH is secreted primarily in response to a hypocalcemic state and serves to oppose the hormonal

effects of calcitonin (1). PTH decreases renal excretion of calcium (Fig. 31.1 loop 3A), indirectly stimulates intestinal absorption of calcium (Fig. 31.1 loop 2A), and in combination with active vitamin D promotes bone resorption (Fig. 31.1 loop 1A) by a complex unknown mechanism, thereby elevating serum calcium concentrations. In addition, the secretion of PTH stimulates the biosynthesis and release of the third hormone associated with calcium homeostasis, vitamin D. When serum calcium concentrations are high, the release of PTH is inhibited.

Vitamin D

Derived from cholesterol, vitamin D is biosynthesized from its prohormone cholecalciferol (D_3), the product of solar ultraviolet irradiation of 7-dehydrocholesterol in the skin (2). In 1966, it was first recognized that vitamin D must undergo activation *via* two oxidative metabolic steps (Fig. 31.2). The first oxidation to 25-hydroxycholecalciferol ($25(OH)D_3$:calcifediol; Calderol) occurs in the endoplasmic reticulum of the liver and is catalyzed by vitamin D 25-hydroxylase. This activation step is not regulated by plasma calcium concentrations. $25(OH)D_3$ is the major circulating form (10–80 µg/mL), as well as the primary storage form of vitamin D (2). In response to a hypocalcemic state and the secretion of PTH, a second oxidation step is activated in the mitochondria of the kidney, catalyzed by vitamin D 1α-hydroxylase (2,9,10). The product of this reaction, 1,25-dihydroxycholecalciferol ($1,25(OH)_2D_3$: 1,25-calcitriol; Rocaltrol, Calcijex) is the active form of vitamin D. Its concentration in the blood is 1/500 that of its mono-

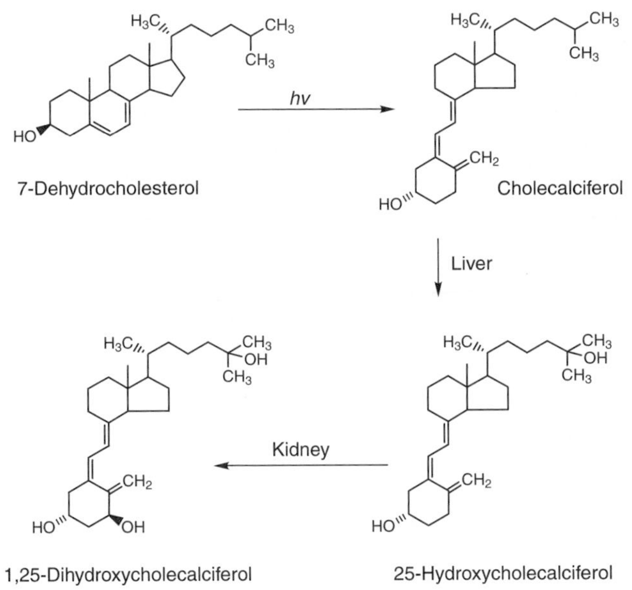

Fig. 31.2. Bioactivation of vitamin D.

hydroxylated precursor. The biosynthesis of vitamin D is tightly regulated based on the serum concentrations of calcium, phosphate, PTH and active vitamin D (2).

Sterol specific cytoplasmic receptor proteins (VDR; vitamin D receptor) mediate the biologic action of vitamin D (9). The active hormone is transported from the cytoplasm to the nucleus *via* the VDR and, as a result of the interaction of the hormone with target genes, a variety of proteins are produced that stimulate the transport of calcium in each of the target tissues. Active vitamin D works in concert with parathyroid hormone to enhance active intestinal absorption of calcium, to stimulate bone resorption and to prohibit renal excretion of calcium (2,9). If serum calcium or 1,25-calcitriol concentrations are elevated, then vitamin D 24-hydroxylase (in renal mitochondria) is activated to oxidize 25(OH)D_3 to inactive 24,25-dihydroxycholecalciferol, as well as to further oxidize active vitamin D to the inactive 1,24,25-trihydroxylated derivative. Both the 1,24,25-trihydroxylated and the 24,25-dihydroxylated products have also been found to suppress parathyroid hormone secretion. Several factors have been identified in the regulation of the biosynthesis of vitamin D including low phosphate concentrations (stimulatory) and pregnancy and lactation (stimulatory).

Other Hormones

Other systemic hormones that can be given in high doses over a long period of time, such as thyroid hormone and the glucocorticoids, also alter the process of bone remodeling and have been linked to enhanced incidence of osteoporosis (3).

NORMAL PHYSIOLOGY

During growth periods in childhood and early adulthood bone formation characteristically exceeds bone loss. In young adulthood bone formation and bone resorption

are nearly equal. After the age of 40 however, bone resorption is slightly greater than bone formation and this results in a gradual decline in skeletal mass. Osteoblasts, osteoclasts and osteocytes are the three types of cells that make up the bone remodeling unit (3) or bone metabolizing unit (4) and are therefore largely responsible for the bone remodeling process.

Osteoblasts, which are of mesenchymal origin and are formed in the bone marrow, stimulate bone formation (6). In the maturation process, osteoblasts undergo multiple cell divisions and, in so doing, express the gene products that are needed to form the bone matrix or osteoid (3), as well as those products responsible for mineralization of that tissue (6). Multiple endogenous substances are involved in osteoblast maturation, including many cytokines (interleukins and granulocyte-macrophage colony stimulating-factor (GM-CSF) (3), hormones and growth factors (6). It is in the rough endoplasmic reticulum that the biosynthesis of the bone matrix protein occurs (4).

Osteoclasts are the large multinucleated cells of hemopoietic origin (6) that are responsible for carrying out the bone resorption or destroying process. Cytokines, PTH and the active form of vitamin D activate these cells. Bone lining flat cells, derived from "retired" osteoclasts and osteoblasts, are located on the bone surface (3). The function of these flat cells is thought to serve to identify areas of the bone that have become weakened or misshapen and to send a signal to the bone remodeling unit to prepare the bone. Lining cells then digest the outer layer of the bone matrix in preparation for bone remodeling. The osteoclast membrane then comes into contact with the bone surface and forms an impermeable "sealing zone" of approximately 500–1000μm (2) in size (6). The H$^+$ ATPase rich osteoclast membrane that is in contact with the bone surface forms a ruffled border, the sealing zone becomes acidified and ultimately the bone minerals dissolve (6). Several types of lysosomal enzymes have been proposed to then digest the collagen matrix (3), thereby pitting the bone surface to a depth of 50 μm (4–6). Only calcitonin acts directly on the osteoclast to prevent bone resorption.

There is yet another type of cell that is found deep within the bone matrix, the osteocyte. While the role of this type of cell has yet to be elucidated, it has been proposed that it may be responsible for maintaining bone integrity (3) and providing nutrition to the bone.

PTH stimulates bone resorption by several mechanisms: 1) transformation of osteoprogenitor cells into osteoclasts is stimulated in the presence of PTH; 2) PTH promotes the deep osteocytes to mobilize calcium from perilacunar bone; 3) surface osteocytes are stimulated by PTH to increase the flow of calcium out of the bone.

Quantification of bone mineral density (BMD) can be measured by noninvasive radiographic tests such as single (3) or dual photon absorptiometry (DPA; spine, hip, total body) (11), dual energy X-ray absorptiometry (3,12) (DEXA; spine, hip, total body) (11), quantitative com-

Table 31.1. Classification of Osteoporosis (13)

Etiology	Type I (Postmenopausal) Increased Osteoclast Activity and Bone Resorption	Type II (senile) Decreased Osteoblast Activity and Bone Formation; Decreased GI Ca Absorption		Type III (Secondary) Drug Therapies; Disease States
Typical age at diagnosis	50–75	>70		any age
Gender ratio	6:1 women/men	2:1 women/men		1:1 women to men
Typical fracture site	vertebrae, distal radius	femoral, neck, hip		vertebrae, hip, extremities
Bone morphology	decreased trabecular	decreased trabecular and normal cortical bone		decreased cortical bone
Rate of bone loss	2–3%/year	0.3–0.5%/year		variable

puted tomography (QCT) (spine) and peripheral QCT (pQCT; wrist) (11). DEXA is considered the gold standard for measuring bone density and has an accuracy that exceeds 95% (4). These techniques measure the attenuation of X-rays or gamma rays as they cross the spine, hip or radius before they reach the detector (6). Other methods under development that measure BMD include ultrasound, traditional X-rays, and blood/urine tests (6). While the traditional X-rays can identify the site of fracture, they cannot measure bone mineral density (3). Blood/urine tests can identify if the patient is suffering from a medical condition (3) that is contributing to the loss of bone mineral density and can identify important biochemical markers that can assess the rate of bone resorption and bone turnover. The measurement of serum calcium, phosphorous and Vitamin D levels may also provide insight into the cause of decreased bone mineral density (3). Often patients suffer from multiple vertebral compression fractures (3) without seeking treatment other than an OTC analgesic and the diagnosis of osteoporosis occurs only after the patient has already lost significant (as much as 30%) bone mass.

DISEASE STATES ASSOCIATED WITH ABNORMAL CALCIUM HOMEOSTASIS
Osteoporosis

Osteoporosis is a skeletal disease that is characterized by loss of bone mass as well as microarchitectural deterioration of the bone tissue. This disease is associated with increased bone fragility and susceptibility to fracture. It is a condition that is characterized not by inadequate bone formation, but rather as a deficiency in the production of well mineralized bone mass. Whereas there typically is no medical cause (3) evident in primary osteoporosis, secondary osteoporosis classically stems from medical illness or medication use. There are two types of primary adult osteoporosis, type I or postmenopausal and type II or senile (Table 31.1). In type I osteoporosis there is an accelerated rate of bone loss *via* enhanced resorption at the onset of menopause. In this form of the disease the loss of trabecular bone is three times greater than cortical bone. This disproportionate loss of bone mass is the primary cause of the vertebral crush fractures, and wrist and ankle fractures experienced by postmenopausal women. In type II osteoporosis, associated with aging, the degree

of bone loss is similar in both trabecular and cortical bone (5) and is caused by decreased bone formation by the osteoblasts (13).

Drug or disease induced osteoporosis (type III) (Table 31.2) accounts for up to 30% of the cases of vertebral fractures reported annually. It can be caused by a variety of factors including long term suppression of osteoblast function, an inhibition of calcium absorption from the gut or excessive loss of calcium in the urine, as a result of estrogen deficiency, hyperparathyroidism (6,12), hyperthyroidism (6,12), hypogonadism (12,14), renal disease (6), depression (15), and treatment with glucocorticoids (14), thyroid hormone, anticonvulsants, methotrexate (14), cyclosporin (14), warfarin, lithium or immunosuppressive therapy (6). Warfarin impairs the vitamin K dependent biosynthesis of osteocalcin (14), it prevents the recycling of oxidized vitamin K to its active reduced form *via* inhibition of vitamin K epoxide reductase and vitamin K reductase. Long term therapy with glucocorticoids has been shown to directly suppress osteoblast function and reduce calcium absorption from the gut (14). Vitamin D deficiency, as the cause of pseudohyperparathyroidism, is a common cause of osteoporosis in the elderly who are institutionalized and lack adequate sunlight exposure (2).

Osteoporosis is the cause of nearly 1.5 million fractures annually in the United States (3), including 250,000 hip fractures and 550,000 vertebral fractures. Caucasian women in the United States who reach the age of 50 have a 50% chance of incurring an osteoporetic fracture. It has been predicted that one in every three women who live to

Table 31.2. Causes of Secondary (Type III) Osteoporosis (14)

Alcohol	Hypopituitarism
Algodystrophy	Mastocytosis
Anorexia nervosa	Mylenoma
Coeliac disease	Organ transplant
Crohn's disease	Osteogenesis imperfecta
Diabetes mellitus	Primary biliary cirrhosis
Drug-induced	Pregnancy
(corticosteroids,	Rheumatic diseases
heparin, warfarin)	Thyrotoxicosis/thyroid replacement
Exercise induced amenorrhea	Turner's syndrome
Gastrectomy	Ulcerative colitis
Hyperparathyroidism	
Hypogonadism	

Table 31.3. Risk Factors for Osteoporosis (3)

Lifestyle Factors	Genetic Factors	Medical Disorders	Drugs
Smoking	White or Asian	Cushing's syndrome	Glucocorticoids
Sedentary Lifestyle	Female	Hyperthyroidism	Thyroid hormone
Calcium intake	Family history	Congenital hypogonadism	Phenytoin
Milk intolerance	Small frame	Primary biliary cirrhosis	Carbamazepine
Excessive caffeine	Early menopause	Malabsorption syndromes	Heparin
Excessive alcohol		Gastrointestinal resection	Aluminum antacids
Nulliparity		Primary hyperparathyroidism	GnRH agonists
High protein intake		Anorexia nervosa	Furosemide
		Multiple myeloma	
		Depression	

the age of 90 will experience a hip fracture (3,13). It has been estimated that 15–35% of hip fracture patients will require long term nursing home care. A surprising 60% of hip fracture patients do not regain full function and within 3–4 months of hip fracture as many as 25% die as a result of secondary complications (pneumonia, infection, etc.). Mortality is also increased 17% after both femoral and vertebral fractures. The risk factors associated with osteoporosis are presented in Table 31.3. Given these statistics, osteoporosis should be considered a significant health problem that only stands to worsen unless appropriate interventions are pursued.

Hypocalcemia

A state of hypocalcemia (Table 31.4) will inhibit calcitonin release. This results in an elevation of PTH biosynthesis and release and indirectly causes an increase in the production of Vitamin D. The left wing of Arnaud's butterfly model (Fig. 31.1) would be activated to increase serum calcium concentrations. In the absence of calcitonin, osteoclast activity is unregulated and therefore bone resorption is accelerated. In acute cases of hypocalcemia, specifically in the case of hypocalcemic tetany, PTH is administered to correct the hormonal imbalance.

Hypercalcemia

A state of hypercalcemia (Table 31.4) will promote calcitonin biosynthesis and release. As a result, PTH biosyn-

thesis and its secretion is inhibited, as is the production of Vitamin D. The right wings of Arnaud's butterfly model (loops B) (Fig. 31.1) would be activated to decrease serum calcium concentrations. In the presence of calcitonin, osteoclast activity is inhibited and so bone resorption is slowed. In acute cases of hypercalcemia, calcitonin is administered to reestablish calcium homeostasis. Hypercalcemia can also be treated with sulfate, EDTA, furosemide, ethacrynic acid, glucocorticoids and plicamycin.

Hypoparathyroidism

Hypoparathyroidism is characterized by hypocalcemia, hyperphosphatemia and reduced levels of circulating vitamin D as a result of decreased serum PTH concentrations. The right wings of Arnaud's butterfly model is predominant (Fig. 31.1) and serum calcium concentrations precipitously decrease. Administration of IV calcium gluconate and PTH serves to acutely correct plasma calcium levels. Chronic oral administration of active vitamin D as well as calcium supplements has been effective in maintaining appropriate serum calcium concentrations.

Pseudohypoparathyroidism

In this disease state, levels of PTH are normal or even elevated, however serum calcium concentrations are low. End organ insensitivity to PTH has been proposed to be the cause of the hypocalcemic state. Treatment of this condition with calcium and vitamin D has proven to be successful.

Table 31.4. Calcium Homeostasis-Related Disorders

Type of Disorder	Treatment	Examples
Disorders leading to Hypocalcemia	Vitamin D analogs and calcium	Inadequate dietary Ca and/or vitamin D Malabsorption due to defective activation of vitamin D Malabsorption due to end organ resistance to vit. D Hypoparathyroidism Pseudohypoparathyroidism
Disorders leading to Hypercalcemia	Fluids, low calcium diet, sulfate, loop diuretics, glucocorticoids, calcitonin, EDTA	Hyperparathyroidism Hypervitaminosis D Sarcoidosis Neoplasia Hyperthyroidism Immobilization
Disorders of bone remodeling	Bisphosphonates, calcitonin, Estrogen, calcitonin, calcium, fluoride, PTH + vitamin D	Paget's disease of the bone Osteoporosis

Hyperparathyroidism

Increased levels of PTH leads to moderately to severely elevated serum calcium concentrations (2) and, as a result, a significant loss of calcium from the bone. Deposits of calcium salts in soft tissue, as well as formation of renal calculi can also result from this hormonal imbalance. Treatment of this condition with salmon calcitonin, loop diuretics or other classical treatments for hypercalcemia has been favorable. The intravenous vitamin D analog paricalcitol (Zemplar), used for both the prevention and treatment of hyperparathyroidism secondary to chronic renal failure, has been shown to reduce parathyroid levels an average of 30% after 6 weeks of treatment.

Paricalcitol

RICKETS AND OSTEOMALACIA

During the industrial revolution there was widespread incidence of rickets in children and adults, as inadequate exposure to sunlight prevented the biosynthesis of active vitamin D in the skin. Both rickets and osteomalacia are metabolic bone diseases that are characterized by poor bone mineralization. Without adequate plasma levels of vitamin D and calcium, deposition of the calcium salts in the bone markedly decreases. Vitamin D supplementation, to improve intestinal absorption of calcium and mineralization of the bone, as well as oral calcium supplementation are required to treat these diseases once established. Today the incidence of rickets in the United States has dropped dramatically through vitamin D supplemented food programs, however it is still considered a world wide health problem.

In addition to the classical environmental or nutritional cause of these diseases, both osteomalacia and rickets can have a pharmacologic origin *via* chronic treatment with anticonvulsants (phenobarbital and phenytoin) or glucocorticoids. These agents interfere with intestinal absorption of calcium and thereby cause pseudohyperparathyroidism. As a result, an increase in bone turnover and a decrease in the formation of appropriately mineralized bone is observed. In these patients, treatment with vitamin D improves calcium absorption, ultimately enhancing mineralization of the bone.

PAGET'S DISEASE

Paget's disease (Table 31.4) is characterized by excessive bone resorption followed by replacement of the normally mineralized bone with soft, poorly mineralized tissue (16). It has been determined that the osteoclasts have an abnormal structure, are hyperactive and are present at elevated levels (16). Patients afflicted with this painful condition often suffer from multiple compression fractures. Administration of calcitonin and oral calcium and phosphate supplements had been the treatment of choice until the bisphosphonate risedronate was approved by the FDA. Daily administration of risedronate results in a decreased rate of bone turnover and a decrease in the levels of serum alkaline phosphatase and urinary hydroxyproline, two biochemical markers of bone turnover (4,16). A significant advantage to treatment with the bisphosphonates is long term suppression of the disease (16). Calcium supplementation, which is often necessary in these patients, must be dosed separately from the risedronate, as calcium and aluminum or magnesium containing antacids interfere with absorption of the bisphosphonates.

Risedronate

DRUG THERAPIES USED TO TREAT OSTEOPOROSIS

Agents used in the treatment and prevention of osteoporosis are categorized as either antiresorptive agents or bone restorative agents depending upon the primary mechanism of action (17). For most effective therapies, bone mass increases for the first few years of treatment, however, eventually all of the pits or lacunae will be filled in with new bone and no additional increase in bone mass will occur. Antiresorptive agents have been shown to increase bone mass by as much as 8–9% at the lumbar spine and 3–6% in the femoral neck.

Estrogen Analogs—Estrogen Replacement Therapy (ERT)

The precise mechanism by which estrogen prevents bone resorption has not been elucidated, however it has been proposed to be associated with inhibition of osteoclast activity. A limited amount of evidence exists to support the presence of estrogen specific receptors (present on osteoclasts) having a biochemical role in the regulation of bone remodeling (13). Estrogen improves calcium absorption, promotes calcitonin biosynthesis and increases the vitamin D receptors on osteoclasts. While the primary mechanism of action is unclear, hormone replacement therapy (HRT) is widely heralded as the treatment of choice for osteoporosis, as it provides the most significant beneficial effects on bone of all therapies. ERT (e.g., 17β-estradiol, estrone sodium sulfate, or 17-ethinyl estradiol) (17) is classified as antiresorptive therapy in the treatment of osteoporosis. Fractures of the spine, wrist and hips decrease by 50–70% and spinal bone density increases by 5% (18) in those women treated with estrogen within three years of the onset of menopause and for 5–10 years thereafter (5,12,19). The minimum dose required and that which is considered standard therapy is 0.625mg/day of conjugated estrogens (Premarin) however, a 0.3 mg/day dose of esterified estrogen (Estratab) has recently been shown to be adequate for the prevention of osteoporosis (5). Estrogen replacement therapy is available in several types of formulations including transdermal patches (Climera, Estraderm, or Vivelle).

Initiated at the onset of menopause and continued indefinitely, this therapy also has favorable effects on serum cholesterol levels (reduces LDL and elevates HDL levels) and has been shown to decrease the risk of cardiovascular disease and death by 50% (3,13,14,17). Women taking ERT have found relief from hot flashes, vaginal dryness, and urinary stress incontinence (17). It is recommended that the estrogen be combined with a progestin for those women with an intact uterus so as to decrease the risk of endometrial cancer (13). HRT is not necessarily the treatment of choice for all women, as some women are intolerant to this type of therapy or have a disease state in which ERT is contraindicated (e.g., breast cancer, liver disease and active thromboembolic disease) (3).

Selective Estrogen Receptor Modulators (SERMs)

The triarylethylene antiestrogen tamoxifen citrate (Nolvadex) and raloxifene hydrochloride (Evista) possess agonist activity in certain tissues (e.g., bone and cardiovascular) and antagonist activity in others (e.g., breast and uterus) (6,17) (Chapter 43). Raloxifene, the first selective estrogen receptor modulator (SERM), has been approved for the prevention of osteoporosis in postmenopausal women. Raloxifene, a benzothiophene derivative (18), acts as an estrogen agonist on receptors in osteoblasts and osteoclasts, but acts as an antagonist at breast and uterine estrogen receptors. This selective action means that this agent does not increase the risk of endometrial or breast cancer, as is the case with estrogen therapy. Since this agent does not have a stimulatory effect at its receptors on most tissues, it does not prevent the hot flashes and other symptoms of menopause as estrogen does (5). Clinical trials have shown that raloxifene, in combination with oral calcium supplementation, prevents bone loss in the spine and hip and promotes bone formation, albeit to a lesser extent than estrogen. Raloxifene has been shown to have a beneficial effect on lipid profiles (12). Raloxifene should not be administered in combination with cholestyramine (decreased absorption), coumadin (prothrombin times and INRs must be monitored more closely), and those drugs that are highly protein bound such as clofibrate, diazepam, ibuprofen, indomethacin and naproxen.

From a structural perspective, the only pure antiestrogens are 7α-substituted estrogens (17). In the triarylethylene class of agents the A ring phenol is critical for binding to the estrogen receptor, as it mimics the essential 3-phenolic group in estrogens (17). The orientation of the three aryl rings in a propeller type of arrangement is

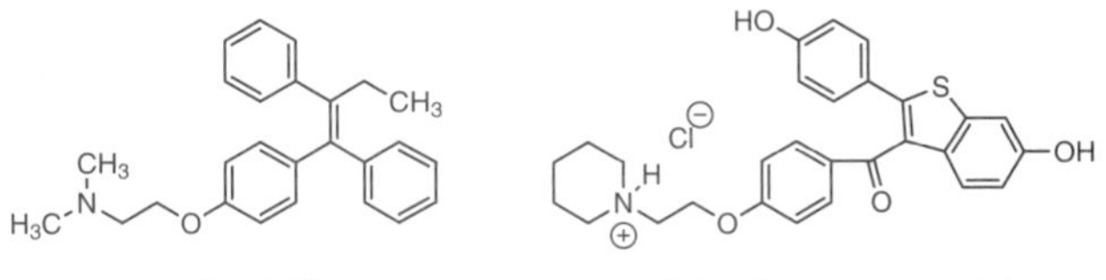

Tamoxifen

Raloxifene hydrochloride

also important for tight receptor binding and biological activity (17).

Bisphosphonates

The bisphosphonates are synthetic in origin and are designed to mimic pyrophosphate, where the oxygen in P-O-P is replaced with a carbon atom to create a nonhydrolyzable backbone (18,19) (Fig. 31.3). Since pyrophosphate is a normal constituent of bone, these analogs selectively bind to the hydroxyapatite portion of the bone (19,20). The bisphosphonates (Fig. 31.4 and Fig. 31.5) effectively inhibit osteoclast proliferation, decrease osteoclast activity, reduce osteoclast lifespan and, as a result, decrease the number of sites along the bone surface where bone resorption occurs (19). By these three mechanisms the bisphosphonates are able to limit bone turnover and allow the osteoblasts to form well-mineralized bone without opposition (3). The precise mechanism(s) of action of these antiresorptive agents has not been elucidated; it is equally uncertain whether all of the bisphosphonates act by a similar mechanism (19). To date, cell surface receptors have not been identified nor has a second messenger system(s) been detected.

Structure-activity Relationships for the Bisphosphonates

From a structural perspective the bisphosphonates have been proposed to have specific molecular interactions with their biologic target for drug action even though precise structure-activity relationships (SAR) have not been elucidated. In fact the exact molecular target is still under investigation. The central carbon of the geminal phosphonate has been substituted with a variety of functional groups to yield a large family of compounds with differing physicochemical and biologic properties (19). SAR studies (Fig. 31.3) have concluded that a hydroxyl substituent (R_1) maximizes the affinity of the agent for the hydroxyapatite, as well as improves the antiresorptive character of the agent (17,21). The character of the R_2 substituent varies widely and clearly has a significant influence on the potency of this class of compounds (Fig. 31.4, Fig. 31.5).

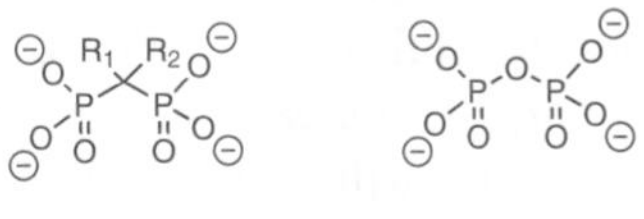

Bisphosphonate
R_1 = hydroxy
R_2 = varies

Pyrophosphate

Fig. 31.3. Bisphosphonate structure-activity relationships.

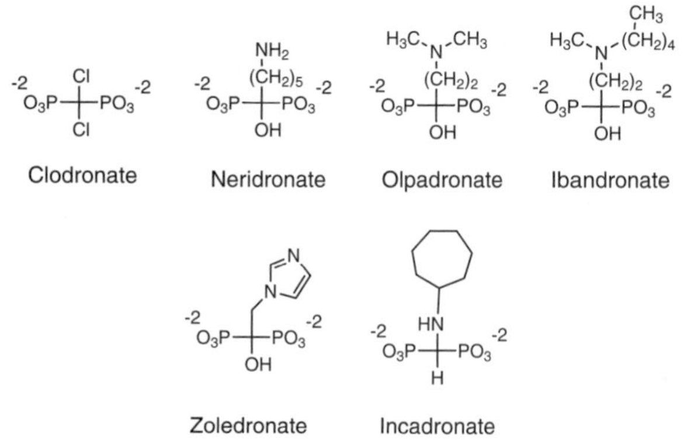

Fig. 31.4. Bisphosphonate analogs.

The R_2 amino substituted bisphosphonates (pamidronate, alendronate, and neridronate) are more potent than etidronate and clodronate (not available in the United States). The R_2 four carbon amino linear chain for alendronate is more potent than the R_2 three carbon derivative pamidronate and the R_2 six carbon analog neridronate (17). Alkylation of the amine functional group improves potency is demonstrated by compounds with branched amine substitutents at R_2 (e.g., olpadronate and ibandronate) and those that contain rings at R_2 (e.g., risedronate, incadronate, tiludronate, and zoledronate). The third generation of analogs contain a basic heterocyclic side chain at R_2 tethered to the central carbon by a variety of linkages (potency $NH>CH_2>S>O$) (17,21). Since structural variation of R_2 has a significant effect on potency, it can be surmised that R_2 interacts at an "active site" and participates in a specific molecular interaction. The bisphosphonate itself as well as the hydroxyl group at R_1 should also be included as critical SAR features (17).

Pharmacokinetics for the Bisphosphonates

To date four generations of bisphosphonates have been developed for the treatment of osteoporosis (Fig. 31.5). Absorption of these agents from the gut is quite poor (1–5%) (12) due to their polar nature and, as a therapeutic class, they have limited cellular penetration. Up to 50% of the actual absorbed dose is taken up specifically by the bone within 4–6 hours and the rest is exclusively excreted by the kidney (6,18). Uptake of these agents in the bone is concentrated in areas of the bone that are actively undergoing remodeling (20). Between the selective uptake and the rapid rate of clearance, the bisphosphonates enjoy a short circulating half-life and very limited drug exposure to nontarget tissues (19). Since the bisphosphonates are only released from the bone when the bone is resorbed they have a tissue half-life of 1–10 years, however these agents remain pharmacologically active only while they are exposed on bone resorption surfaces (20).

Etidronate Disodium, Tiludronate

Agents in the first generation, e.g., etidronate disodium (Didronel), that were dosed continuously, produced poorly mineralized bone (3,15), as there was no interval for appropriate bone mineralization to occur. Subsequent studies that utilized a cyclic dosing schedule (400 mg/day for 2 weeks followed by 2.5 months of calcium supplementation only) showed improvement in bone mineralization (12,21). Etidronate has been approved for treatment of Paget's disease of the bone, but not osteoporosis (5). Tiludronate (6), another analog of the first generation, is approximately 10 times more potent than etidronate and when given orally for 6 months (200, 400 or 800 mg/day) increases bone mineral density by 2%. No further bone loss was detected in patients 6 months after cessation of therapy.

Alendronate Sodium; Pamidronate Disodium

The second-generation agent alendronate sodium (Fosamax) (6) was the first bisphosphonate agent approved by the U.S. Food and Drug Administration (FDA) for the prevention and treatment of osteoporosis and Paget's disease of the bone (20,22) and is 1000 times more potent than etidronate (6). This derivative, when dosed continuously (5–10 mg/day for osteoporosis; 40 mg/day for Paget's disease) and given with oral calcium supplements (500 mg/day), produced well-mineralized bone and significantly improved bone mineral density (7% in the spine and 4% in the hip) within 18 months (6). In addition, the vertebral fracture rate was shown to decrease by 47%. A side effect associated with alendronate, chemical esophagitis (2,3,12,18), has been attributed to inadequate intake of water and lying down after taking the medication. Specific patient instructions were developed to limit the incidence of upper gastrointestinal problems and include: 1) taking the medication with 6–8 ounces of water upon arising in the morning; 2) remaining in an upright position for at least 30 minutes after taking the medication; 3) delaying drinking other liquids/eating for at least 30 minutes, if not 1–2 hours, to allow for maximal absorption of the agent (3). To enhance absorption, calcium supplements and any aluminum or magnesium containing antacids should be dosed separately from the agents in this class. These agents are not recommended in patients with renal impairment (serum creatinine <2.5 mg/dL), a history of

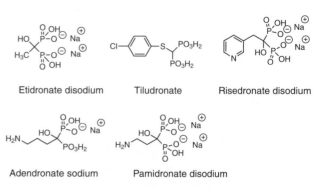

Fig. 31.5. Clinically used bisphosphonates.

esophageal disease, gastritis, or peptic ulcer (5). Pamidronate (Aredia), a second generation agent, is 100 times more potent than etidronate (6). It has been approved in other countries for the treatment of hypercalcemia of mailgnancy and has been shown to increase bone mass in patients with steris induced osteoporosis. Erosive esophagitis has been reported with the use of pamidronate sodium.

Risedronate Disodium

The third generation agent risedronate disodium (Actonel) (6) has been approved not only for the treatment of osteoporosis, but also for the treatment of Paget's disease of the bone. Risedronate is 1000–5000 times more potent than etidronate. At the end of an 18-month study, 53% of those patients that took risedronate for 2 months remained in remission as compared to 14% of the patients that took etidronate for 6 months, an earlier generation bisphosphonate. Oral administration of this agent suffers from the same problems as other bisphosphonate agents. Risedronate should not be given to patients with creatinine clearance less than 30 mL/min.

Calcitonin

Calcitonin has been approved for the treatment of postmenopausal osteoporosis, hypercalcemia of malignancy and Paget's disease of the bone. There are several sources available (e.g., eel, human, salmon, and porcine). The calcitonin isolated from salmon is the preferred source since it has greater receptor affinity and a longer half-life than the human hormone (3,7). Calcitonin is commercially available as synthetic calcitonin-salmon which contains the same linear sequence of 32 amino acids as occurs in natural calcitonin-salmon. Calcitonin salmon differs structurally from human calcitonin at amino acids 2, 8, 11–13, 15–17, 19, 20, 22, 24, 26, 27, 29, and 31 (see Fig. 6.13, p. 136 for primary structure differences between human and salmon calcitonin). The pharmacologic activity of these calcitonins is the same, but calcitonin salmon is approximately 50 times more potent on a weight bases then human calcitonin with a longer duration of action. The duration of action for calcitonin salmon is 8–24 hours following IM or subcutaneous administration and 30 minutes to 12 hours following IV administration. The parenteral dose required for the treatment of osteoporosis is 100 IU per day (21). Initially only available by intramuscular or subcutaneous injection (Calcimar), the peptide hormone calcitonin salmon is now available as a nasal spray (Miacalcin) and as a rectal suppository (6). The bioavailability of calcitonin-salmon nasal spray shows great variability (range 0.3%–30.6% of IM dose). It is absorbed rapidly from the nasal mucosa with peak plasma concentrations appearing 30–40 minutes after nasal administration compared to 16–25 minutes following parental dosing. Calcitonin-salmon is readily metabolized in the kidney with an elimination half-life calculated to be 43 minutes. As a result, the intranasal dose required is 200 IU per day (3). Once the Miacalcin nasal pump has been activated, the bottle may be kept at room temperature until the medication is finished (2 weeks). This type of therapy also requires the concomitant oral administration of elemental calcium (500 mg/day). Clinical studies have shown that the combination of intranasal calcitonin salmon (200 IU/day), oral calcium supplementation (>1000 mg/day elemental calcium) and vitamin D (400 IU/day) (27) has decreased the rate of new fractures by over 75% and has improved vertebral bone mineral density by as much as 3% annually (3). Calcitonin prevents the abnormal bone turnover characteristic of Paget's disease of the bone and has antiresorptive activity. In the presence of calcitonin the osteoclast brush borders disappear and the osteoclasts move away from the bone surface undergoing remodeling (23). Side effects are significantly more pronounced when calcitonin salmon is administered by injection and can include nausea, vomiting, anorexia and flushing. Because calcitonin-salmon is protein in nature, the possibility of a systemic allergic reaction should be considered, and appropriate measures for treatment of hypersensitivity reaction should be readily available. Although calcitonin-salmon does not cross the placenta, it may pass into breast milk. Calcitonin salmon is a possible alternative to ERT, however, there is only limited evidence that it has efficacy in women who already have fractures. Resistance to calcitonin salmon can result from the development of neutralizing antibodies (24).

In addition to its antiresorptive action *via* suppression of osteoclast activity, calcitonin salmon exhibits a potent analgesic effect and has provided considerable relief to those patients suffering from the pain associated with Paget's disease and osteoporosis. This analgesic effect is a result of calcitonin-stimulated endogenous opioid release. The potency of this analgesic effect has been demonstrated to be 30–50 times that of morphine in selected patients. Calcitonin is preferred over estrogen and the bisphosphonates when treatment of both osteoporosis and related bone pain is warranted.

Inorganic Calcium Salts

Appropriate intake of calcium in childhood, adolescence and early adulthood serves to increase peak bone mineral density and may reduce the overall risk of developing osteoporosis. For those who are at low risk for developing osteoporosis and have adequate bone mineral density, consumption of the recommended amounts of calcium is typically sufficient to prevent bone loss (1200–1500 mg of elemental calcium per day for teenagers; 1000 mg/day for premenopausal women and men; up to 1500 mg/day for postmenopausal women not taking ERT; 1000 mg/day for postmenopausal women taking ERT) (13). This can often be accomplished by eating a well-balanced diet. For those patients with established osteoporosis or areas of poorly mineralized bone, calcium supplementation alone is not sufficient to reverse the bone loss or to significantly improve mineralization of the bone (12).

Table 31.5. Percent of Elemental Calcium Content in Various Salts (3)

Salt	Calcium (%)	mg Elemental Calcium/Tablet
Calcium carbonate	40	
Tums (500 mg chewable)		200 mg
Titrilac (1 g/5 mL suspension)		400 mg/ 5 mL
Alka-Mints (850 mg chewable)		340 mg
Os-Cal 500 (1250 mg table)		500 mg
Tricalcium Phosphate	39	
Calcium chloride	27	
Tribasic calcium phosphate	23	
Posture (1565.2 mg tablets)		600 mg
Calcium citrate	21	
Citrical (950 mg tablets)		200 mg
Citrical Liquitab (2376 mg effervescent tabs)		500 mg
Calcium lactate	13	
Generics (325 mg tablets)		42 mg
Generics (650 mg tablets)		84 mg
Calcium gluconate	9	
Neo-Calglucon (1.8 g/5 mL syrup)		115 mg/5 mL

Patient Based Case

During a recent annual exam, Vera Stanow, a 52-year-old postmenopausal woman, is diagnosed with hyper-parathyroidism. She is not currently on any prescription medications and occasionally uses aspirin for headaches and antihistamines for seasonal allergies.

A. What do you expect to find if you measure Vera's plasma calcium levels? According to the "Butterfly Model" for calcitonin and parathyroid hormones, what are the three relevant physiological reasons for this patient to have the plasma calcium levels that you have proposed?

B. Why might this patient potentially be at risk for osteoporosis? Without knowing her X-ray results, describe a type of drug therapy that prevents osteoporosis. Be sure to include a mechanism of action in your answer.

An X-ray determining bone mineral density indicates that Vera already has significant loss of bone density. Describe a different type of drug therapy for the treatment of osteoporosis. Be sure to include a mechanism of action in your answer.

The actual amount of elemental calcium that is present in the available calcium salts varies considerably, however no one particular salt has been identified as an exceptional source of elemental calcium (Table 31.5). Absorption of calcium from the gastrointestinal tract (25–40%) improves under acidic conditions (3) and therefore those medications that change the acidic environment of the stomach (e.g., H_2 antagonists, proton pump inhibitors) have an adverse effect on calcium absorption (3). Total daily doses of elemental calcium that exceed 500 mg should be spaced out over the day to improve absorption (5,13). The more water soluble and therefore more easily absorbed salts (e.g., citrate, lactate and gluconate) are less dependent on the acidic environment for appropriate absorption and would be appropriate alternatives for patients who produce low levels of acid. While calcium carbonate is a poorly soluble form of calcium, it is inexpensive and only requires the patient to take a few tablets per day with acidic food or beverages like citrus juice (13).

Sodium Fluoride

Sodium fluoride (NaF) promotes the proliferation and activity of osteoblasts and is classified as a nonhormonal bone-forming agent. Since treatment with NaF induces bone formation, it is essential that this therapy be coupled with oral calcium supplementation (1000 mg/day). NaF also exhibits moderate antiresorptive activity, as it inhibits osteoclastic activity when it is absorbed into the bone matrix. In the treatment of osteoporosis the therapeutic window for this agent is fairly narrow, as doses less than 45 mg/day are subtherapeutic and doses in excess of 75 mg/day impair bone mineralization. In addition, the bone that is formed in the presence of NaF is neither as well mineralized or as strong as normal bone tissue. In fact, some studies have demonstrated that patients taking sodium fluoride have increased bone fragility despite the increase in bone mass and,

as a result, have an increased nonvertebral fracture rate as compared to the placebo group (5,21,17). As a result, its use in the treatment of osteoporosis has not been approved and is considered somewhat controversial. Several studies have examined the benefits of continuous vs. cyclic dosing of NaF in the treatment of osteoporosis. Intermittent dosing (25 mg BID for 12 months followed by 2 months of calcium supplementation alone) of a slow release formulation of sodium fluoride (SR-NaF, Neosten) with 400 mg of calcium citrate was shown to effectively improve bone mass (5%/year vertebral and 2%/year femoral neck) as well as decrease the number of vertebral fractures (25,26).

Miscellaneous Therapies

The thiazide diuretics, which reduce urinary calcium excretion, may also reduce the rate of bone loss (21). Elevated concentrations of proton pump inhibitors such as omeprazole have been shown to inhibit bone resorption via inhibition of H^+/K^+ ATPase, a potential energy pump located in the osteoclast ruffled border (21). Androgens such as stanozolol (12), nandrolone (12), methandrostenolone, and the testosterone patch have been shown to increase bone mass by 5–10% and may be appropriate for men with a deficiency in testosterone. While an increase in trabecular bone mass by as much as 50% has been demonstrated in patients treated with low doses of PTH, it comes at the expense of the cortical bone (1,12,19). Treatment with high doses of PTH is correlated with stimulation of bone resorption (16). Cyclical therapy with PTH and calcitonin has been shown to improve bone mineral density in the spine without adverse effects in the cortical bone (12). When given in combination with estrogen, PTH promoted the formation of well-mineralized trabecular bone. Gallium nitrate (Ganite) has been approved for the treatment of hypercalcemia of malignancy (21).

CASE STUDY

Victoria F. Roche and S. William Zito

OP is a 72-year-old, white female who is recovering from a hip fracture sustained during a square dance lesson at the assisted living facility where you are the consultant pharmacist. OP has Type II (senile) osteoporosis and her bone mass density is >2.5 standard deviations below the mean bone mass density of a young adult women. A heavy smoker who enjoys her cigarettes and coffee throughout the day, OP was not a candidate for post-menopausal estrogen therapy because of a strong family history of breast cancer. OP has Stage I hypertension controlled with a loop diuretic, furosemide. Her physician wants to treat the osteoporosis with the hope of preventing continued bone loss (0.3–0.5%/year) and any further fractures. In addition to calcium carbonate (500mg TID) supplementation and Vitamin D (400 units qd), she wants to initiate calcium anti-resorp-

tive therapy and asks your opinion of the following 4 possible therapeutic candidates.

1. Identify the therapeutic problem(s) where the pharmacist's intervention may benefit the patient.

2. Identify and prioritize the patient specific factors that must be considered to achieve the desired therapeutic outcomes.

3. Conduct a thorough and mechanistically oriented structure-activity analysis of all therapeutic alternatives provided in the case.

4. Evaluate the SAR findings against the patient specific factors and desired therapeutic outcomes and make a therapeutic decision.

5. Counsel your patient.

749

REFERENCES

1. Copp DH. Calcitonin: discovery, development, and clinical application. Clin Invest Med, 1994 17(3): 268–277.
2. Bouillon R, Carmeliet G, Boonen S. Aging and Calcium Metabolism. Bailliere's Clin Endocrinol Metab 1997:11;341–365. [For a review of how aging effects calcium homeostasis]
3. Haines ST, Caceres B, Yancey L. Alternatives to Estrogen Replacement Therapy for Preventing Osteoporosis. J Amer Pharm Assoc NS36:1996; 707–715.
4. Christenson RH. Biochemical Markers of Bone Metabolism: An Overview. Clin Biochem 1997:30;573–593.
5. Miller DR, Hanel HJ. Prevention and Treatment of Osteoporosis. US Pharmacist. 1999:24;81–90.
6. Rodan GA. Emerging Therapies in Osteoporosis. Ann Rpts Med Chem. Vol. 29. 1994, Academic Press, 275–285.
7. Arnaud CD. Calcium homeostasis: Regulatory elements and their integration. Fed Proc. 1978:37;2557.
8. Potts JT. Chemistry of the Calcitonins. Bone and Mineral, 1992: 16;169–173.
9. DeLuca HF, Zierold C. Mechanisms and Functions of Vitamin D. Nutrition Reviews 1998:56;S4–S10.
10. Friedlander G, Amiel C. Cellular Mode of Action of Parathyroid Hormone. Adv Nephrol Necker Hosp. 1994:23;265–279.
11. Schaefer B, Cone S. Increasing Awareness of Osteoporosis: A Community Pharmacy's Experience. US Pharmacist. 1998: 23;72–85.
12. Francis RM. Management of established osteoporosis. Br J Clin Pharmacol. 1998:45;95–99.
13. American Pharmaceutical Association, Special Report, "Therapeutic Options for Osteoporosis" 1993, Washington, DC.
14. Reid DM, Harvie J. Secondary Oseteoporosis. Bailliere's Clin Endocrin Metab 1997:11;83–99. [For a review of the causes of secondary osteoporosis]
15. Michelson, D, Stratakis C, Hill L, et al. Bone mineral density in women with depression. N Engl J Med 1996:335;1176–1181. [Study about particular patient population]
16. Reginster J-YL, LeCart M-P. Efficacy and Safety of Drugs for Paget's Disease of Bone. Bone 1995:17;485S–488S.
17. De Silva Jardine P, Thompson D. Anti-osteoporosis Agents. Ann Rpts Med Chem, Vol. 31, 1996, Academic Press, pp 211–220.
18. Francis RM. Bisphosphonates in the Treatment of Osteoporosis in 1997: A review. Curr Therap Res. 1997:58;656–678.
19. Yates AJ, Rodan GA. Alendronate and osteoporosis. Drug Discovery Today 1998:3;69–78. [Excellent review of bisphosphonates]
20. Diener KM. Bisphosphonates for controlling pain from metastatic bone disease. Am J Health-Syst Pharm 1996:53;1917–1927.
21. Caggiano TJ, Zask A, Bex F. Recent Advances in Bone Metabolism and Osteoporosis Research. Ann Rpts Med Chem, Vol. 26, 1991, Academic Press,
22. Ashworth L. Focus on Alendronate. Formulary 1996:31;23–30.
23. Reginster J. Calcitonin for Prevention and Treatment of Osteoporosis. Amer J Med, 1993:95[Suppl. 5A];5A-44S to 5A-47S.
24. Gennari C, Agnusdei D, Camporeale A. Long Term Treatment With Calcitonin in Osteoporosis. Horm. Metab. Res. 1993 25:484–485.
25. Pak CYC, Sakhaee K, Rubin C, et al. Update of Fluoride in the Treatment of Osteoporosis. The Endocrinologist 1998:8;15–20.
26. Pak CY, Sakhaee K, Rubin C, et al. Treatment of Postmenopausal Osteoporosis with Slow-Release Sodium Fluoride. Ann Intern Med 1995:123;401–408.
27. American Pharmaceutical Association, New Product Bulletin, "Miacalcin Nasal Spray," 1996, Washington, DC.

SUGGESTED READINGS

Civitelli, R Parathyroid Hormone Control of Intracellular Calcium. J Endocrin Investig 1992 15[Suppl. 6];35–41.

de Groen PC, Lubbe DF, Hirsch LJ, et al. Esophagitis associated with the use of alendronate. N E J Med 1996:335;1016–1021.

Gennari C, Agnusdei D. Calcitonins and Osteoporosis. Brit J Clin Pract 1994:48;196–200.

Patel S, Lyons AR, Hosking DJ. Drugs Used in the Treatment of Metabolic Bone Disease. Drugs 1993:46;594–617.

Raisz LG. Closer to the Bone. Odyssey 1995:1;8–15.

Riggs BL. Formation-Stimulating Regimens Other Than Sodium Fluoride. Amer J Med 1993:95[Suppl 5A];5A-62S -67S.

Silver J, Moallem E, Epstein E, et al. New aspects in the control of parathyroid hormone secretion. Curr Opin Nephrol Hyperten, 1994:3;379–385.

Whitfield JF, Morley P. Small bone-building fragments of parathyroid hormone: new therapeutic agents for osteoporosis. Trends Pharmacol Sci 1995:16;382–386.

32. Nonsteroidal Anti-inflammatory Agents

RONALD F. BORNE

INTRODUCTION

Nonsteroidal anti-inflammatory agents continue to be one of the more widely used groups of therapeutic agents. The classification of drugs covered in this chapter as nonsteroidal anti-inflammatory agents (NSAIAs) is somewhat misleading since many of these entities possess antipyretic and analgetic properties in addition to anti-inflammatory properties which are useful in the treatment of a number of rheumatic disorders. On the other hand, there are agents that possess analgetic-antipyretic properties but are essentially devoid of anti-inflammatory activity. Additionally, agents that possess uricosuric properties useful in the treatment of gout will also be covered here. The prototype agent of this class is acetylsalicylic acid, aspirin, which has therapeutically useful analgetic, antipyretic and anti-inflammatory actions; other agents to be covered may possess only one or two of these properties. Steroids that are useful anti-inflammatory agents are covered separately.

The medicinal agents covered in this chapter represent a major market in both prescription and nonprescription drugs. Other than caffeine or ethyl alcohol, aspirin may be the most widely used drug in the world (1). An estimated 70–100 million prescriptions are written annually for NSAIAs with over-the-counter use accounting for an additional use which may be up to seven times higher. Rheumatic diseases, which have been classified by the American Rheumatism Association (Table 32.1) (2), are inflammatory disorders affecting more individuals than any chronic illness. Approximately 15% of the U.S. population suffer from a rheumatoid disease with females being affected about twice as much as males. Approximately 7 million Americans suffer from arthritis in its most debilitating forms (3). Rheumatoid arthritis is thought to affect 2.5 million Americans, 1.8 million of whom are females, while juvenile arthritis affects 71,000 children under 16 years of age, 61,000 of whom are females. In addition, nonrheumatoid osteoporosis affects 24 million females (half of all women over the age of 45 and 90% of all women over the age of 75) and 16 million males (3). Because more than 80% of the U.S. population over the age of 55 have joint abnormalities detectable radiographically, the use of NSAIAs will increase as Americans experience a greater life expectancy (4). It is not surprising, therefore, that the development of new NSAIAs continues at a rapid pace.

DISEASE STATES

The diseases mentioned are considered to be host defense mechanisms. Inflammation is a normal and essential response to any noxious stimulus that threatens the host and may vary from a localized response to a generalized response (5). The inflammation can be summarized as follows: 1) initial injury causing release of inflammatory mediators (e.g., histamine, serotonin, leukokinins, SRS-A, lysosomal enzymes, lymphokinins, prostaglandins); 2) vasodilation; 3) increased vascular permeability and exudation; 4) leukocyte migration, chemotaxis and phagocytosis; and 5) proliferation of connective tissue cells. The most common sources of chemical mediators include neutrophils, basophils, mast cells, platelets, macrophages and lymphocytes (5). The etiology of inflammatory and arthritic diseases has received a great deal of recent attention but remains, for the most part, unresolved, hindering the development of new agents which are curative in nature. Currently available agents relieve the symptoms of the disease but are not curative.

Table 32.1. Classification of Rheumatic Diseases

I. Polyarthritis of Unknown Etiology
A. Rheumatoid arthritis
B. Juvenile rheumatoid arthritis
C. Ankylosing spondylitis
D. Reiter's syndrome
E. Others
II. Connective Tissue Disorders
A. Systemic lupus erythematosus
B. Progressive scleroderma
C. Polymyositis and dermatomyositis
D. Mixed connective disease
E. Necrotizing arteritis and other forms of vasculitis
F. Others
III. Acute Rheumatic Fever
IV. Degenerative Joint Disease (Osteoarthritis)
V. Nonarticular Rheumatism
VI. Diseases with Which Arthritis is Frequently Associated
A. Sjögren's syndrome
B. Others
VII. Associated with Known Infectious Agents
A. Bacterial
B. Rickettsial
C. Viral
D. Fungal
E. Parasitic
VIII. Traumatic Neurogenic Disorders
IX. Associated with Known Biochemical or Endocrine Abnormalities
A. Gout
B. Others
X. Neoplasma
XI. Allergy and Drug reactions
XII. Inherited and Congenital Disorders
XIII. Miscellaneous Disorders

Modified from Primer on the Rheumatic Diseases, ninth Edition, copyright 1968. Used by permission of the Arthritis Foundation.

Pathogenesis

The currently accepted pathogenesis of these disorders can be summarized as follows: an unknown antigen gains access to the patient's tissues and combines with an antibody in the joint activating the complement sequence. An antigen-complement-antibody immune complex then precipitates in the synovium and joint fluid generating the release of chemical mediators that then cause the migration of numerous polymorphonuclear leukocytes phagocytizing the immune complexes. Lysosomal membranes become unstable and discharge hydrolytic enzymes (proteases, collagenases, etc.) from the leukocytes and synovial cells. Tissue damage ensues with continuing inflammation, tissue destruction, collagen depolymerization and loss of physical properties of the connective tissue and joints. Anti-inflammatory agents may thus act by interfering with any one of several mechanisms including immunological mechanisms such as antibody production or antigen-antibody complexation, activation of complement, cellular activities such as phagocytosis, interference with the formation and release of the chemical mediators of inflammation, or stabilization of lysosomal membranes.

Role of Complement

The role of complement in inflammation is of considerable interest (6–8). The complement system is one component of the host defense system that aids in the elimination of various microorganisms and antigens from blood and tissues. Although complement normally plays a functional role in the development of disease states, by promoting inflammation locally, excessive complement activation is detrimental. Individuals with a deficiency of individual complement proteins, either acquired or hereditary, are more susceptible to infections caused by pyrogenic bacteria and diseases resulting from the generation of autoantibodies and immune complexes. Complement proteins are numbered C1-C9 and their cleavage products indicated by suffixes a, b, etc. The complement system consists of two activating pathways (an antibody-mediated classical pathway and a nonimmunologically activated alternate pathway), a single termination pathway, regulatory proteins and complement receptors and involves approximately 30 membrane and plasma proteins (7). A major function of complement is to mark antigens and microorganisms with C3 fragments that direct them to cells containing C3 receptors, such as phagocytic cells (7). Complement has been implicated in numerous diseases including allergic, hematologic, dermatologic, infectious, renal, hepatic, inflammatory (rheumatoid arthritis and systemic lupus erythematosus), pulmonary and others (e.g., multiple sclerosis, myasthenia gravis). Complement activation can induce the synthesis or release of inflammatory mediators such as interleukin-1 (a potent pro-inflammatory cytokine) and prostaglandins (PGE_2). Leukotrienes (LTB_4) and thromboxanes are also released. Complement also aids the immigration of phagocytes associated with inflammation. Thus, inhibition of the complement system by controlling its activation or inhibiting those active fragments that are produced should be beneficial in reducing or eliminating tissue damage associated with inflammatory diseases.

Connective Tissue Diseases

Connective tissue diseases include the following states: RA, ankylosing spondylitis, systemic lupus erythematosus, polyarteritis nodosa, gout, rheumatic fever and osteoarthritis. The most common forms of connective tissue diseases are RA, osteoporosis and gout. Rheumatoid arthritis (RA) is a subacute or chronic, inflammatory disease of unknown cause affecting primarily peripheral synovial joints. The onset is usually insidious with immunologic reactions playing a major role. The pathogenesis of RA has been summarized as follows: 1) an unknown initiation factor causes the production of antigenic IgG which stimulates the synthesis of the rheumatoid factors IgM and IgG forming immune complexes; 2) IgG aggregates activating the complement system leading to the generation of chemotactic factors which attract polymorphonuclear leukocytes into the articular cavity; and 3) the polymorphonuclear leukocytes ingest immune complexes to become RA cells which discharge hydrolases from lysosomal granules which, in turn, degrade extracellular tissue components, polysaccharides, and collagens in cartilage, thus provoking an inflammatory response in rheumatoid joints (9). Clinical symptoms characteristically include symmetric swelling of joints accompanied by tenderness, erythema, stiffness and pain. The joints primarily involved are those of the extremities and the patient oftentimes suffers a low grade fever accompanied by malaise, anorexia and fatigue. Serum protein irregularities are common. It is often difficult to distinguish RA from other connective tissue diseases. Treatment usually involves a program of rest, exercise, and a balanced diet with the initial use of salicylates. If conservative management fails, drug therapy, including NSAIAs, corticosteroids and the antirheumatic gold salts are employed.

Osteoarthritis, also known as degenerative joint disease, is the most common form of arthritis and is characterized by degeneration of cartilage and hypertrophy of bone at the articular margin. Secondary inflammation of synovial tissue is common. The most common symptoms involve joint pain associated with movement and, sometimes, bone enlargement. Weight-bearing joints and joints of the hands and fingers are generally involved. Abnormalities in laboratory tests are generally not observed. Treatment usually involves exercise and salicylates. Aspirin is considered first-choice therapy with NSAIAs being employed in patients who do not tolerate salicylates.

Gout is a metabolic disease characterized by recurrent episodes of acute arthritis, usually monoarticular, and is associated with abnormal levels of uric acid in the body, particularly the presence of monosodium urate crystals in synovial fluid. Primary gout is a hereditary disease in which hyperuricemia is due to an error in uric acid metabolism—either overproduction or an inability to excrete uric acid. Secondary gout refers to those cases in which hyperuricemia is due to an acquired disease or disorder such as chronic renal disease, lead poisoning or myeloproliferative disorders. Gout generally occurs in mid-life and affects males significantly more than females (9:1). Treatment usually involves the use of uricosuric agents, colchicine, NSAIAs or corticosteroids.

Drug Screening Methods

The search for new and effective treatment modalities requires the availability of adequate screening tests. Although no model adequately reflects the events that occur in human arthritic conditions, several *in vivo* and *in vitro* assays are used. The most common *in vivo* animal assays measure the ability of anti-inflammatory agents to inhibit edema induced in the rat paw by carrageenan (a mucopolysaccharide derived from a sea moss of the *Chondrus* species), to inhibit adjuvant arthritis in rats induced by *Mycobacterium butyricum* or *M. tuberculosis,* to inhibit granuloma formation usually induced by the implantation of a cotton pellet beneath the abdominal skin of rats, or to in-

hibit erythema of guinea pig skin as a result of exposure to UV radiation. *In vitro* techniques include the ability of NSAIAs to stabilize erythrocyte membranes or, more commonly, to inhibit the biosynthesis of prostaglandins, particularly in cultured human synoviocytes and chondrocytes, and monocyte culture fluid stimulated bovine synoviocytes and chondrocytes.

Role of Chemical Mediators in Inflammation
Overview

As indicated previously, a number of chemical mediators have been postulated to play important roles in the inflammatory process. Prior to 1971, the proposal by Shen that the NSAIAs exert their effects by interacting with a hypothetical anti-inflammatory receptor was widely accepted (10–11). The topography of the proposed receptor was based upon known structure-activity relationships primarily within the series of indole acetic acid derivatives of which indomethacin was the prototype. Most NSAIAs, whether they be salicylates, arylalkanoic acids, oxicams or anthranilic acid derivatives, possess the common structural features of an acidic center, an aromatic or heteroaromatic ring and an

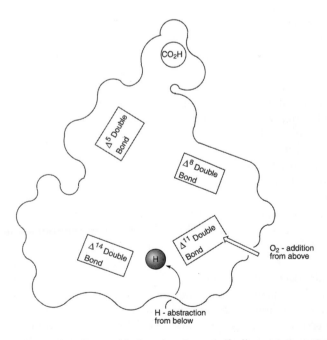

Fig. 32.1. Shen's proposed model of the fatty acid substrate binding site of prostaglandin synthetase. (Modified with permission from ref. 13, Copyright 1977 American Chemical Society.)

additional center of lipophilicity in the form of either an alkyl chain or an additional aromatic ring. The proposed receptor to which indomethacin was postulated to bind consisted of a cationic site to which the carboxylate anion would bind, a flat area to which the indole ring would bind through Van der Waals forces, and an out-of-the-plane trough to which the benzene ring of the *p*-chlorobenzoyl group would bind through hydrophobic or charge-transfer interactions. Additional binding sites for the methoxy and carbonyl groups were also suggested. In 1971, Vane published a classic paper in which he reported that indomethacin, aspirin, and salicylate, in this descending order of potency, inhibited the biosynthesis of prostaglandins from arachidonic acid using cell-free preparations of guinea pig lung and further suggested that the clinical actions of these agents were due to this inhibition (12). This theory has become the most widely accepted mechanism of action of NSAIAs. Shen subsequently modified his hypothesis and proposed that his earlier anti-inflammatory receptor model actually described the active site of the key enzyme in prostaglandin biosynthesis, viz., prostaglandin cyclooxygenase (Fig. 32.1) (13).

Prostaglandins, Thromboxanes, Prostacyclin and Leukotrienes

Prostaglandins are naturally occurring 20-carbon cyclopentano-fatty acid derivatives produced in mammalian tissue from polyunsaturated fatty acids. They belong to the class of eicosanoids, a member of the group of autocoids derived from membrane phospholipids. The eicosanoids are derived from unsaturated fatty acids and include the following groups of compounds: prostaglandins, thromboxanes, prostacyclin and leukotrienes. They have been found in essentially every compartment of the body. In 1931 Kurzrok and Lieb reported that human seminal fluid possessed potent contractile and relaxant effects on uterine smooth muscle (14). Shortly thereafter, Goldblatt (15) in England and von Euler (16) in Sweden independently reported vasodepressor and smooth muscle contracting properties in seminal fluid; von Euler identified the active constituent as a lipophilic acidic substance which he termed prostaglandin. These observations attracted little attention during World War II, but shortly thereafter, primarily through the efforts of Samuelsson and Bergstrom (17) it was realized that von Euler's prostaglandin was actually a mixture of a number of structurally-related fatty acids. The first report of the structure of the prostaglandins in 1962 stimulated several studies relating to the chemical and biological properties of these potent substances.

The general structure of the prostaglandins (PGs) is shown in Figure 32.2. All naturally occurring PGs possess this substitution pattern, a 15α-hydroxy group and a *trans* double bond at C-13. Unless a double bond occurs at the C-8, C-12 positions, the two side chains (the carboxyl-bearing chain termed the α-chain and the hydroxyl-bearing chain termed the β-chain) are of the *trans* stereochemistry depicted. The PGs are classified by the capital letters

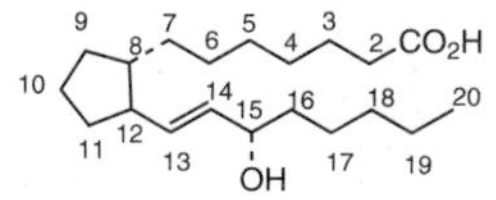

Fig. 32.2. General structure of the prostaglandins.

A, B, C. D, E, F, G, H and I depending on the nature and stereochemistry of oxygen substituents at the 9-and 11-positions. For example, members of the PGE series possess a keto function at C-9 and an α-hydroxyl group at C-11, whereas members of the PGF series possess α-hydroxyl groups at both of these positions. Members of the PGG and PGH series are cycloendoperoxide intermediates in the biosynthesis of prostaglandins as depicted in Figure 32.3. The number of double bonds in the side chains connected to the cyclopentane ring is designated by subscripts 1, 2 or 3, indicative of the nature of the fatty acid precursor. The subscript 2 indicates an additional *cis* double bond at the C-5, C-6 positions while the subscript 3 indicates a third double bond of *cis* stereochemistry at the C-17, C-18 positions.

Prostaglandins are derived biosynthetically from unsaturated fatty acid precursors. The number of double bonds contained in the naturally occurring PGs reflects the nature of the biosynthetic precursors. Those containing one double bond are derived from 8,11,14-eicosatrienoic acid, those with two double bonds from arachidonic acid (5,8,11,14-eicosatetraenoic acid), and those with three double bonds from 5,8,11,14,17-eicosapentenoic acid. The most common of these fatty acids in humans is arachidonic acid and hence PGs of the 2 series play an important biological role. Arachidonic acid is derived from dietary linoleic acid or is ingested from the diet and esterified to phospholipids (primarily phosphatidylethanolamine or phosphatidylcholine) in cell membranes (18). Various initiating factors interact with membrane receptors coupled to G proteins (guanine nucleotide-binding regulatory proteins) activating phospholipase A_2 which, in turn, hydrolyzes membrane phospholipids resulting in the release of arachidonic acid. Other phospholipases (e.g., phospholipase C) are also involved. Phospholipase C differs from phospholipase A_2 by inducing the formation of 1,2-diglycerides from phospholipids with the subsequent release of arachidonic acid by the actions of mono- and diglyceride lipases on the diglyceride (16). A polypeptide produced by leukocytes, interleukin-1, which mediates inflammation, increases phospholipase activity and thus PG biosynthesis. The steroidal anti-inflammatory agents (corticosteroids) appear to act, in part, by inhibiting these phospholipases. The liberated arachidonic acid may then be acted on by two major enzyme systems: arachidonic acid cyclooxygenase (prostaglandin endoperoxide synthetase or COX) to produce prostaglandins, thromboxanes and prostacyclin, or by lipoxygenases to produce leukotrienes.

Interaction of arachidonic acid with COX in the presence of oxygen and heme produces first the cyclic en-

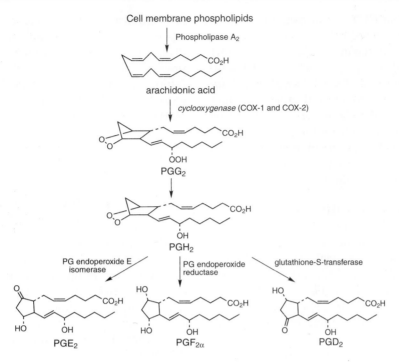

Fig. 32.3. Biosynthesis of prostaglandins from arachidonic acid.

doperoxide, PGG_2 and thence, through its peroxidase activity, to PGH_2, both of which are chemically unstable and decompose rapidly ($t_{1/2}$ ~ five minutes). PGE_2 is formed by the action of PGE isomerase and PGD_2 by the actions of isomerases or glutathione-S-transferase on PGH_2 while $PGF_{2\alpha}$ is formed from PGH_2 via an endoperoxide reductase system (Fig. 32.3). It is at the cyclooxygenase step at which the NSAIAs inhibit PG biosynthesis preventing inflammation. Since PGG_2 and PGH_2 themselves may possess the ability to mediate the pain responses and produce vasoconstriction, and since PGG_2 may mediate the inflammatory response, cyclooxygenase inhibition would have a profound effect on the reduction of inflammation.

COX was first purified in 1976 and first cloned in 1988. Among the more significant advances of the past decade was the isolation of a second form of the COX enzyme, named COX-2, whose expression is inducible by cytokines and growth factors (19–23). COX-1 and COX-2 are very similar in structure and are almost identical in length varying from 599 (human) to 602 (mice) amino acids in COX-1 and 603 (mice) to 604 (human) for COX-2. Both isoforms possess molecular masses of 70–74 Kda and contain just over 600 amino acids with an approximately 60% homology within the same species (24–25). COX-2 contains an 18 amino acid insert near the C-terminal end of the enzyme that is not present in COX-1, but all other residues that have been previously identified as being essential to the catalytic activity of COX-1 are present in COX-2. Both isoforms have been cloned from various species including human and are heme-containing membrane proteins that exist as dimers (24). The three-dimensional X-ray crystal structure of COX-2 derived from human or murine sources

can be superimposed on that of COX-1. Residues that form the substrate binding channel, the catalytic sites and those residues immediately adjacent are essentially identical with the exception of two minor differences. The isoleucine at positions 434 and 523 in COX-1 is exchanged for valine in COX-2. The smaller size of Val 523 in COX-2 allows inhibitor access to a side pocket off the main substrate channel while the longer side chain of Ile in COX-1 sterically blocks inhibitor access. A major difference between COX-1 and COX-2 is that COX-2 lacks a sequence of 17 amino acids from the N-terminus but contains a sequence of 18 amino acids at the C-terminus compared to COX-1. This difference causes a difference in the numbering systems of the two isoforms such that the serine residue acetylated by aspirin in COX-1 is numbered Ser 530 while in COX-2 the serine residue acetylated is Ser 516. Yet the amino acid residues which are thought to be responsible for providing the catalytic role are the same with both isoforms displaying similar ability to convert arachidonic acid to PGH_2. COX-1 appears to be more specific for fatty acid substrates than COX-2 since COX-2 accepts a wider range of fatty acid substrates than COX-1. COX-1 primarily metabolizes arachidonic acid while COX-2 metabolizes C-18 and C-20 fatty acid substrates. Selective inhibitors of COX-2 do not bind to Arg 120 that is used by the –COOH of arachidonic acid and the carboxylic acid selective or nonselective COX-1 inhibitors.

From a therapeutic viewpoint, the major difference between COX-1 and COX-2 lies in physiological function rather than structure. Little COX-2 is present in resting cells but its expression can be induced by cytokines in vascular smooth muscle, fibroblasts and epithelial cells leading to the suggestion that COX-1 functions to produce PGs that are involved in normal cellular activity (protection of gastric mucosa, maintenance of kidney function) while COX-2 is responsible for the production of PGs at inflammatory sites (26). Inducible COX-2 linked to inflammatory cell types and tissues are believed to be the target enzyme in the treatment of inflammatory disorders by NSAIAs. Until recently, most NSAIAs inhibited both COX-1 and COX-2 but with varying degrees of selectivity. Selective COX-2 inhibitors may eliminate side effects associated with NSAIAs due to COX-1 inhibition, such as gastric and renal effects.

Prostaglandins are rapidly metabolized and inactivated by various oxidative and reductive pathways. The initial step involves rapid oxidation of the 15α-OH to the corresponding ketone by the prostaglandin specific enzyme prostaglandin 15-OH dehydrogenase. This is followed by reduction of the C-13, C-14 double bond by prostaglandin Δ^{13}-reductase to the corresponding dihydro ketone, which for PGE_2 represents the major metabolite in plasma. Subsequently, enzymes normally involved in β- and ω-oxidation of fatty acids more slowly cleave the α-chain and oxidize the C-20 terminal methyl group to the carboxylic acid derivative, respectively. Hence, dicarboxylic acid derivatives containing only 16 carbon atoms are the major metabolites of PGE_1 and PGE_2 that are excreted.

The pharmacologic actions of the various PGs are quite diverse (Table 32.2). When administered intravaginally, PGE_2 will stimulate the endometrium of the gravid uterus to contract in a manner similar to uterine contractions observed during labor. Thus, PGE_2 is therapeutically used as an abortifacient at 12–20 weeks gestation and for evacuation of uterine content in missed abortion or intrauterine fetal death up to 28 weeks gestation. PGE_2 is also a potent stimulator of smooth muscle of the GI tract and can elevate body temperature in addition to possessing potent vasodilating properties in most vascular tissue while possessing constrictor effects at certain sites. PGEs in general cause pain when administered via the intradermal route. Many of these properties are shared by $PGF_{2\alpha}$ and the synthetic 15-methyl derivative of $PGF_{2\alpha}$ which are available as tromethamine salts (see Table 32.2). $PGF_{2\alpha}$ differs from PGE_2, however, in that it does

not significantly alter blood pressure in humans. PGD_2 causes both vasodilation and vasoconstriction. While the PGEs produce a relaxation of bronchial and tracheal smooth muscle, PGFs and PGD_2 cause contraction. PGE_1 (alprostadil) is used to maintain patency of the ductus arteriosus in neonates until surgery can be performed to correct congenital heart defects.

Carboprost tromethamine   Alprostadil

The effects of prostaglandins on the GI tract deserve special mention. PGEs and PGI_2 inhibit gastric secretion that may be induced by gastrin or histamine. PGs appear to play a major cytoprotective role in maintaining the integrity of gastric mucosa. PGE_1 exerts a protective effect on gastroduodenal mucosa by stimulating secretion of an alkaline mucus and bicarbonate ion and also by maintaining or increasing mucosal blood flow. Thus, inhibition of PG formation in joints produces favorable results as indicated by a reduction in fever, pain and swelling but inhibition of PG biosynthesis in the GI tract is unfavorable since it may cause disruption of mucosal integrity resulting in peptic ulcer disease which, as will be discussed later, is commonly associated with the use of NSAIAs and aspirin.

Alternatively, nonprostanoids can also be formed from PGH_2 as illustrated in Figure 32.4. Thromboxane synthetase acts on PGH_2 to produce thromboxane A_2 (TxA_2) while prostacyclin synthetase converts PGH_2 to prostacyclin (PGI_2), both of which possess short biologic half-lives. TxA_2, a potent vasoconstrictor and inducer of platelet aggregation, has a biologic half-life of about 30 seconds, being rapidly nonenzymatically converted to the more stable, but inactive, TxB_2 (Table 32.2). Prostacyclin, a potent hypotensive and inhibitor of platelet aggregation, has a half-life of about three minutes and is nonenzymatically converted to 6-keto-$PGF_{1\alpha}$. Platelets contain primarily thromboxane synthetase while endothelial cells contain primarily prostacyclin synthetase. Considerable research efforts are being expended in the development of stable prostacyclin analogues and thromboxane antagonists as cardiovascular agents.

Table 32.2. Pharmacologic Properties of Prostaglandins, Thromboxane, and Prostacyclin

Chemical Abbreviation	Generic Name	Trade Name	Abortifacient	Bronchial Smooth Muscle	Platelets	Blood Vessels
PGE_2	Dinoprostone	Prostin E_2	12–20 wks	Dilation		Dilation
$PGF_{2\alpha}$	Dinoprost	Prostin F2 alpha	16–20 wks	Constriction		Constriction
15-methyl$PGF_{2\alpha}$	Carboprost	Prostin 15/M	13–20 wks			
PGE_1	Alprotadil	Prostin VR		Dilation		
PGI_2	Epoprostenol	Flolan			Inhibit aggregation	Dilation
TxA_2	Tromboxane A_2				Aggregation	Constriction

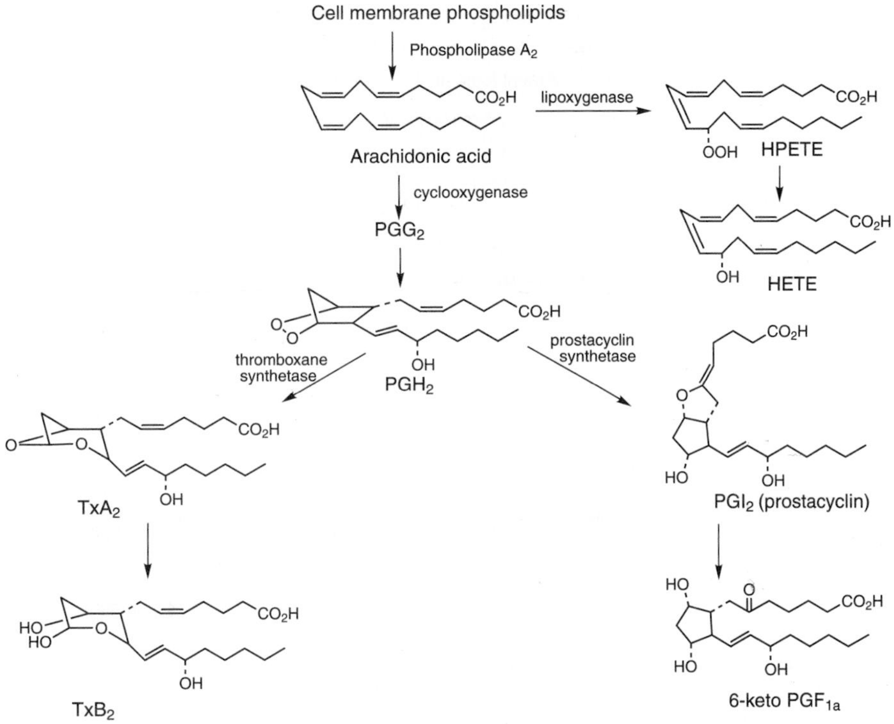

Fig. 32.4. Biosynthesis of thromboxanes, prostacyclin and leukotrienes.

The existence of distinct prostaglandin receptors may explain the broad spectrum of action displayed by the prostaglandins. The nomenclature of these receptors is based on the affinity displayed by natural prostaglandins, prostacyclin or thromboxanes at each receptor type. Thus, EP receptors are those receptors for which the PGEs have high affinity, FP receptors for PGFs, DP receptors for PGDs, IP receptors for PGI_2 and TP receptors for TxA_2. These receptors are coupled through G proteins to effector mechanisms that include stimulation of adenyl cyclase, and hence increased cAMP levels, and phospholipase C that results in increased levels of IP_3 (inositol 1,4,5-triphosphate). Three distinct receptors for leukotrienes have also been identified.

Lipoxygenases are a group of enzymes which oxidize polyunsaturated fatty acids possessing two *cis* double bonds separated by a methylene group to produce lipid hydroperoxides (18). Arachidonic acid is thus metabolized to a number of hydroperoxy-eicosatetraenoic acid derivatives (HPETEs). These enzymes differ in the position at which they peroxidize arachidonic acid and in their tissue specificity. For example, platelets possess only a 12-lipoxygenase while leukocytes possess both a 12-lipoxygenase and a 5-lipoxygenase (27). The HPETE derivatives are not stable, being rapidly converted to a number of metabolites. Leukotrienes are products of the 5-lipoxygenase pathway and are divided into two major classes: hydroxylated eicosatetraenoic acids (LTs) represented by LTB_4 and peptidoleukotrienes (pLTs) such as LTC_4, LTD_4 and LTE_4. 5-Lipoxygenase will produce leukotrienes from 5-HPETE as

shown in Figure 32.5. LTA synthetase converts 5-HPETE to an unstable epoxide termed LTA_4 that may be converted by the enzyme LTA hydrolase to the leukotriene LTB_4 or by glutathione-S-transferase to LTC_4. Other leukotrienes (e.g., LTD_4, LTE_4, LTF_4) can then be formed from LTC_4 by the removal of glutamic acid and glycine and then reconjugation with glutamic acid, respectively. One mediator of inflammation, known as SRS-A (slow-reacting substance of anaphylaxis), is primarily a mixture of two leukotrienes, LTC_4 and LTD_4. The physiologic roles of the various leukotrienes are becoming better understood. LTB_4 is a potent chemotactic agent for polymorphonuclear leukocytes and causes the accumulation of leukocytes at inflammation sites and leads to the development of symptoms characteristic of inflammatory disorders. LTC_4 and LTD_4 are potent hypotensives and bronchoconstrictors. Because of the role played by LTs and pLTs in inflammatory conditions and asthma, it is not surprising that intensive research is being conducted in the area of inhibitors of leukotriene biosynthesis.

THERAPEUTIC APPROACH TO ARTHRITIC DISORDERS

The management of arthritic disorders involves a stepwise approach to the use of therapeutic agents currently available. Relief of pain and reduction of inflammation are immediate goals because of the severity of symptoms most frequently encountered in arthritics. Longer-term goals would be to halt the progression of the disease and preserve the functions of muscles and joints in order to permit the patient to lead a productive life. Fortunately, a large

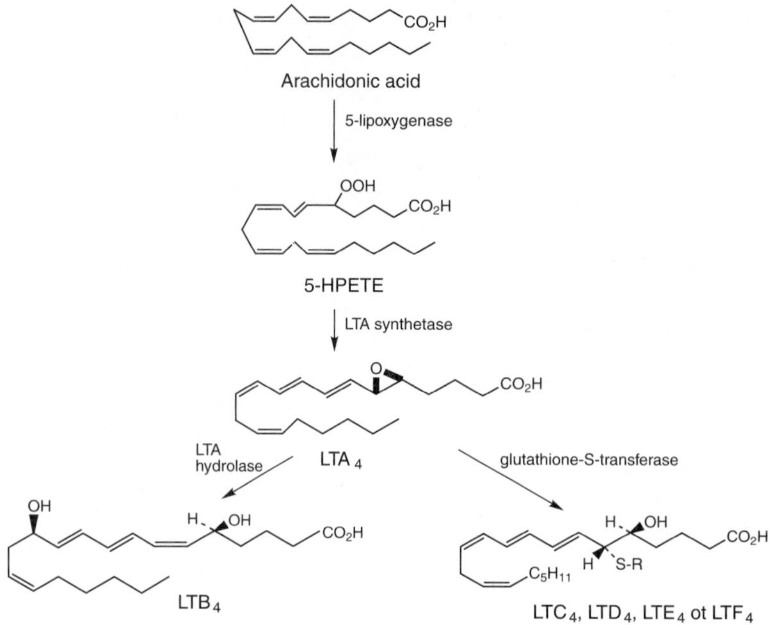

Fig. 32.5. Biosynthesis of leukotrienes.

number of NSAIAs are therapeutically available, differing in efficacy, but perhaps more importantly, differing also in overall toxicity. As a group, NSAIAs can cause GI toxicity such as dyspepsia, abdominal pain, heartburn, gastric erosion, peptic ulcer formation, bleeding, diarrhea, renal disorders such as acute renal failure, tubular necrosis, and analgesic nephropathy, and other effects such as tinnitus and headache. A recent report of the Arthritis, Rheumatism, and Aging Medical Information System Post-Marketing Surveillance Program, prior to the introduction of COX-2 selective agents, ranked the overall toxicity of NSAIAs in the following decreasing order: indomethacin > tolmetic > meclofenamate > ketoprofen > fenoprofen > salsalate > aspirin. If these agents prove ineffective, alternate treatments should be considered. These include the use of disease-modifying antirheumatic agents, corticosteroids and immunosuppressive agents.

A generally accepted stepwise approach to treatment is:

Step 1. Physical Therapy, Rest, Patient Education and Counseling
Step 2. Salicylates (aspirin)
Step 3. Nonsteroidal Anti-inflammatory Agents (NSAIAs)
Step 4. Disease-Modifying Antirheumatic Drugs (DMARDs)
Step 5. Corticosteroids
Step 6. Immunosuppressive Agents

THERAPEUTIC CLASSIFICATIONS
Antipyretic Analgesics
Mechanism of Action

Agents are included in this class which possess analgesic and antipyretic actions but lack anti-inflammatory effects. Antipyretics interfere with those processes by which pyrogenic factors produce fever, but do not appear to lower body temperature in afebrile subjects. It had been historically accepted that the antipyretics exert their actions within the CNS, primarily at the hypothalamic thermoregulatory center but more recent evidence suggests that peripheral actions may also contribute. Endogenous leukocytic pyrogens may be released from cells which have been activated by various stimuli and antipyretics may act by inhibiting the activation of these cells by an exogenous pyrogen. Or the antipyretics may act by inhibiting the release of endogenous leukocytic pyrogens from the cells once they have been activated by the exogenous pyrogen. Substantial evidence exists suggesting a central antipyretic mechanism: an antagonism which may result from either a direct competition of a pyrogen and the antipyretic agent at CNS receptors or an inhibition of prostaglandin synthesis in the CNS (28). Despite its extensive use, the mechanism of action of acetaminophen has not been fully elucidated. Acetaminophen may inhibit pain impulses by exerting a depressant effect on peripheral receptors; an antagonistic effect on the actions of bradykinin may play a role. The antipyretic effects may not result from inhibition of release of endogenous pyrogen from leukocytes but by inhibiting the action of released endogenous pyrogen on hypothalamic thermoregulatory centers. The fact that acetaminophen is an effective antipyretic-analgesic but an ineffective anti-inflammatory agent may be due to its greater inhibition of prostaglandin biosynthesis in the CNS than in the periphery.

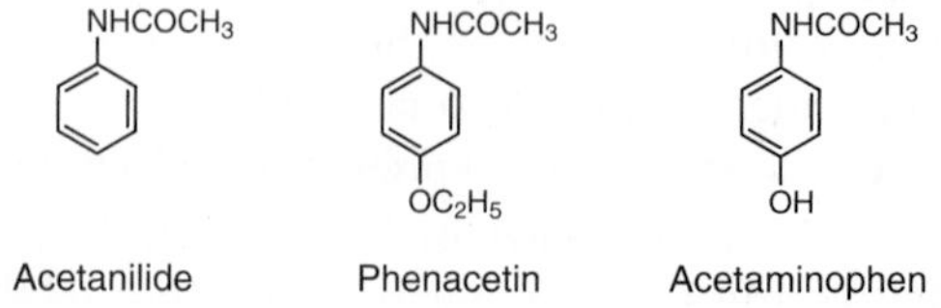

Acetanilide   Phenacetin   Acetaminophen

Historical Background

Acetanilide was introduced into therapy in 1886 under the name antifebrin as an antipyretic-analgetic agent but was subsequently found to be too toxic (methemoglobinemia and jaundice), particularly at high doses, to be useful. Phenacetin was introduced the following year and remained in use until recently when reports of nephrotoxicity resulted in its removal from the market. Phenacetin is longer acting than acetaminophen despite the fact that it is metabolized to acetaminophen but is a weaker antipyretic. Acetaminophen (paracetamol) was introduced in 1893 but remained unpopular for over 50 years until it was observed that it is a metabolite of both acetanilide and phenacetin. It remains the only useful agent of this group and is widely used as a nonprescription antipyretic-analgesic under a variety of trade names (Tylenol, Patrol, and Tempera). While the analgesic activity of acetaminophen is comparable to aspirin, it lacks useful anti-inflammatory activity. However, its advantage over aspirin as an analgetic is that individuals who are hypersensitive to salicylates generally respond well to acetaminophen.

Structure-activity Relationships

The structure-activity relationships of *p*-aminophenol derivatives have been widely studied. Based on the comparative toxicity of acetanilide and acetaminophen, aminophenols are less toxic than the corresponding aniline derivatives, although *p*-aminophenol itself is too toxic for therapeutic purposes. Etherification of the phenolic function with methyl or propyl groups produces derivatives with greater side effects than with ethyl. Substituents on the nitrogen atom which reduce basicity reduce activity unless that substituent is metabolically labile, e.g., acetyl. Amides derived from aromatic acids, e.g., N-phenylbenzamide, are less active or inactive.

Acetaminophen, U.S.P.

Acetaminophen is a weakly acidic, colorless powder which can be synthesized by the acetylation of *p*-aminophenol. Acetaminophen is indicated for use as an antipyretic-analgesic, particularly in individuals displaying an allergy or sensitivity to aspirin. While it does not possess anti-inflammatory activity, it will produce analgesia in a wide variety of arthritic and musculoskeletal disorders. It is weakly bound to plasma proteins and is available in various formulations (Table 32.3). Acetaminophen, unlike aspirin, is stable in aqueous solution making liquid formulations readily available, a particular advantage in pediatric cases.

Metabolism and Toxicity. The metabolism of acetanilide, acetaminophen and phenacetin is illustrated in Figure 32.6 (29). As indicated earlier, both acetanilide and phenacetin are metabolized to acetaminophen. Additionally, both undergo hydrolysis to yield aniline derivatives that produce directly, or through their conversion to hydroxylamine derivatives, significant methemoglobinemia and hemolytic anemia which resulted in their removal from the U.S. market. On the other hand, acetaminophen is metabolized primarily by conjugation reactions, the O-sulfate conjugate being the primary metabolite in children and the O-glucuronide being the primary metabolite in adults. A minor, but significant product of both acetaminophen and phenacetin is the N-hydroxyamide produced by a cytochrome P450 (CYP450) mixed function oxidase system. The hydroxyamide is then converted to a reactive toxic metabolite, an acetimidoquinone, which has been suggested to produce the nephrotoxicity and hepatotoxicity associated with acetaminophen and phenacetin (30). Normally this quinone is detoxified by conjugation with hepatic glutathione. However, in cases of ingestion of large doses or overdoses of acetaminophen, hepatic stores of glutathione may be depleted by more than 70% allowing the reactive quinone to interact with nucleophilic functions, primarily -SH groups, on hepatic proteins resulting in the formation of covalent adducts which produce hepatic necrosis. Overdoses of acetaminophen can produce potentially fatal hepatic necrosis, renal tubular necrosis and hypoglycemic coma. Various sulfhydryl-containing compounds were found to be useful as antidotes to acetaminophen overdoses. The most useful of these, N-acetylcysteine, serves as a substitute for the depleted glutathione, by enhancing hepatic glutathione stores, or by enhancing disposition by nontoxic sulfate conjugation (31). N-Acetylcysteine may also inhibit the formation of

Table 32.3. Indications, Doses, and Dosage Forms of Acetaminophen and Salicylates

Drug	Indication	Dose	pKa	Plasma Binding (%)	Dosage Form
Acetaminophen	Analgesic/Antipyretic	325–650 mg q 4–6 h	9.54	18–25	Tab, Cap, S₁, S₂, Gran
Aspirin	Analgesic	325–650 mg q 4 h	3.5	90	Tab, Cap, S₂, Buffered Tab, Enteric Tab
	Antiinflammatory	3.2–6 g/day			
	TIA	1.3 g/day			
	MI	300–325 mg/day			
Salicylamide	Analgesic/Antipyretic	300–650 mg q 6–8 h	8.2	40–55	Tab
Salsalate	Analgesic/Antipyretic	3000 mg/day	3.5/9.8		Cap, Tab
Diflunisal	Analgesic/Antiinflammatory	250–500 mg q 8–12 h	3.3	99	Tab

Tab = Tablet; Cap = Capsule; S₁ = Solution; S₂ = Suppositories; Gran = Granules.

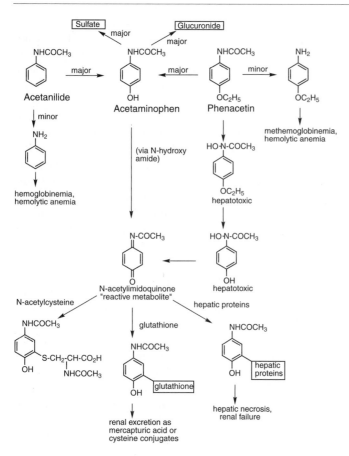

Fig. 32.6. Metabolism of acetaminophen (modified from ref. 28).

the toxic imidoquinone metabolite (32). In cases of overdoses, N-acetylcysteine is administered as a 5% solution in water, soda or juice. The recommended dose is 140 mg/kg followed by 17 maintenance doses of 70 mg/kg every 5 hours.

Drug Interactions. Hepatic necrosis develops at much lower doses of acetaminophen in some heavy drinkers than would be expected due, perhaps, to the induction of the CYP450 system, depletion of glutathione stores, or by aberrations in the primary sulfate and glucuronide conjugation pathways (29). Acetaminophen has been reported to potentiate the response to oral anticoagulants although the effect on prothrombin time is not clear. Interactions with warfarin, dicumarol, anisindione and diphenadione have been suggested. The mechanism of these interactions has not been fully elucidated but may be associated with competition for plasma protein binding sites because acetaminophen is a weak acid and is weakly bound, but may also be due to the induction of hepatic microsomal enzymes. The effects of acetaminophen are reduced in the presence of microsomal enzyme inducers such as barbiturates and are enhanced by metoclopramide and salicylamide. The absorption of acetaminophen is enhanced by polysorbate and sorbitol and is reduced by anticholinergics and narcotic analgesics. Chemical incompatibilities have also been

reported based on hydrolysis by strong acids or bases or phenolic oxidation in the presence of oxidizing agents. Acetaminophen forms "sticky" mixtures with diphenhydramine HCl and discolors under humid conditions in the presence of caffeine or codeine phosphate.

Anti-inflammatory Agents

Salicylates

The use of salicylates dates back to the 19th century. Salicylic acid itself was first obtained in 1838 from salicin, a glycoside that is present in most willow and poplar bark. Interestingly, Hippocrates prescribed chewing willow bark for pain relief in the fifth century. In 1860 Kolbe synthesized salicylic acid from sodium phenoxide and carbon dioxide, a method which produced large quantities inexpensively. Derivatives of salicylic acid began to receive medical attention shortly thereafter. Sodium salicylate was employed as an antipyretic-antirheumatic agent in 1875 and the phenyl ester was used in 1886. Acetylsalicylic acid was prepared in 1853 but was not used medicinally until 1899. The name aspirin was given to acetylsalicylic acid by Dreser, director of pharmacology at Frederich Bayer and Company in Germany as a contraction of the letter *a* from acetyl and *spirin,* an older name given to salicylic acid (spiric acid) which was derived from a natural source in spirea plants. Since then, numerous derivatives of salicylic acid have been synthesized and evaluated pharmacologically, yet only a relatively few derivatives have achieved therapeutic utility.

In addition to possessing antipyretic, analgesic and anti-inflammatory properties, salicylates possess other actions that have been proven to be therapeutically beneficial. Because salicylates promote the excretion of uric acid they are useful in the treatment of gouty arthritis. More recent attention has been given to the ability of salicylates to inhibit platelet aggregation, which may contribute to heart attacks and stroke. Aspirin appear to inhibit prostaglandin cyclooxygenase in platelet membranes thus blocking formation of the potent platelet aggregating factor thromboxane A$_2$ in a manner that is irreversible. The Physicians Health Study concluded that in a group of 22,071 participants there was a 44% reduction in the risk of myocardial infarction in the group taking a single 325 mg aspirin tablet taken every other day vs. the placebo group (33). The role of aspirin in reducing cardiac mortality has been reviewed (34). An additional study suggested that aspirin and other NSAIAs might be protective against colon cancer (35). Thus the therapeutic utility of aspirin continues to increase. Unfortunately, a number of side effects are associated with the use of salicylates, most notable GI disturbances such as dyspepsia, gastroduodenal bleeding, gastric ulcerations and gastritis.

Mechanism of Action. A number of possible mechanisms of action have been proposed for salicylates over the years. Among those that have been suggested are inhibition of the biosynthesis of histamine, antagonism of the actions of various kinins, inhibition of mucopolysaccharide biosynthesis, inhibition of lysosomal enzyme release and inhibition of leukocyte accumulation. The most widely accepted mechanism of action currently is the ability of salicylites to inhibit the biosynthesis of prostaglandins at the cyclooxygenase stage discussed earlier. Aspirin is the only NSAIA that covalently modifies COX by acetylating Ser-530 of COX-1 and Ser-516 of COX-2. However, aspirin is 10–100 times more potent against COX-1 than COX-2 (36). Aspirin's actions on COX-1 prevent both endoperoxide and 15-peroxidation of arachidonic acid but its action on COX-2 does not prevent formation of 15-OOH arachidonic acid (24).

Structure-activity Relationships. Despite the vast effort which has been expended in the search to find a "better" aspirin, that is, one possessing: fewer gastrointestinal side effects, increased potency, longer duration of action, inexpensive, with antipyretic, analgesic and anti-inflammatory activity, none has been discovered. The following structure-activity relationships have been established.

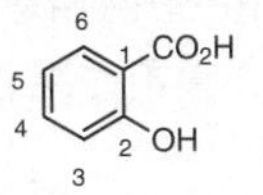

Salicylic acid

The active moiety appears to be the salicylate anion. Side effects of aspirin, particularly the GI effects, appear to be associated with the carboxylic acid functional group. Reducing acidity of this group (converting to an amide, salicylamide) maintains the analgesic actions of salicylic acid derivatives but eliminates the anti-inflammatory properties. Substitution on either the carboxyl or phenolic hydroxyl groups may affect potency and toxicity. Benzoic acid itself has only weak activity. Placing the phenolic hydroxyl group meta- or para- to the carboxyl group abolishes activity. Substitution of halogen atoms on the aromatic ring enhances potency and toxicity. Substitution of aromatic rings at the 5-position of salicylic acid increases anti-inflammatory activity (e.g., diflunisal).

Absorption and Metabolism. Most salicylates are rapidly and effectively absorbed on oral administration with the rate of absorption and bioavailability being dependent on a number of factors including the dosage formulation, gastric pH, food contents in the stomach, gastric emptying time, the presence of buffering agents or antacids, and particle size. Since salicylates are weak acids absorption generally takes place primarily from the small intestine and to a lesser extent from the stomach by the process of passive diffusion of unionized molecules across the epithelial membranes of the GI tract. Thus, gastric pH is an important factor in the rate of absorption of salicylates. Any factor that increases gastric pH, e.g., buffering agents, will slow the rate of absorption since more of the salicylate

will be in the ionized form. This may be counteracted by an increased solubility of salicylates which enhances absorption. The differences in the rates of absorption of aspirin, salicylate salts and the numerous buffered preparations of salicylates are actually quite small with absorption half-times in humans ranging from approximately 20 minutes for buffered preparations to 30 minutes for aspirin itself. The presence of food in the stomach slows the rate of absorption. Formulation factors may contribute to the differences in absorption rates of the various brands of plain and buffered salicylate preparations. Tablet formulations consisting of small particles are absorbed faster than those of larger particle size. The bioavailability of salicylate from enteric-coated preparations may be inconsistent. Absorption of salicylate from rectal suppositories is slower and incomplete and is not recommended when high salicylate levels are required. Topical preparations of salicylic acid are effective in that the rate of salicylate absorption from the skin is rapid.

Salicylates are highly bound to plasma protein albumin with binding being concentration dependent. At low therapeutic concentrations of 100 mcg/ml approximately 90% is plasma protein bound while at higher concentrations, >400 mcg/ml, only 76% binding is observed. Plasma protein binding is a major factor in the drug interactions observed for salicylates.

The major metabolic routes of esters and salts of salicylic acid are illustrated in Figure 32.7. The initial route of metabolism of these derivatives is their conversion to salicylic acid which may be excreted in the urine as the free acid (10%) or undergo conjugation with either glycine, to produce the major metabolite salicyluric acid (75%), or with glucuronic acid to form the glucuronide ether and ester (15%). In addition, small amounts of metabolites resulting from microsomal aromatic hydroxylation are found. The major hydroxylation metabolite, gentisic acid, was once

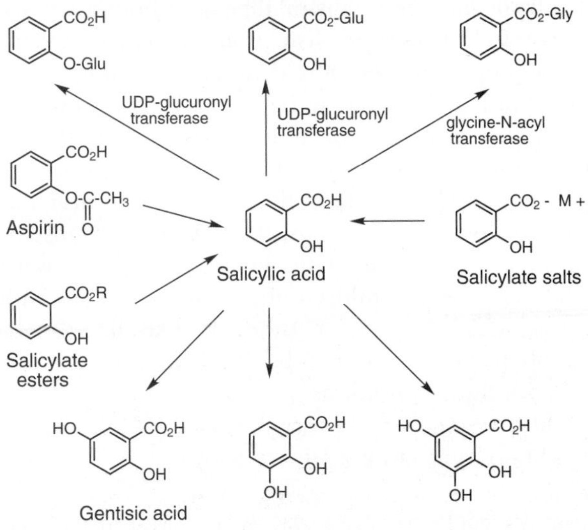

Fig. 32.7. Metabolism of salicylic acid derivatives. (Glu = glucuronide conjugate, Gly = glycine conjugate.)

thought to be responsible for the anti-inflammatory actions of the salicylates but its presence in trace quantities would rule out a major role for gentisic acid, or the other hydroxylation metabolites, in the pharmacologic action of salicylates. The metabolism of pharmacokinetic properties of salicylates has been extensively reviewed (37).

Side Effects. The most commonly observed side effects associated with the use of salicylates relate to disturbances of the gastrointestinal tract. Nausea, vomiting, epigastric discomfort, intensification of symptoms of peptic ulcer disease such as dyspepsia and heartburn, gastric ulcerations, erosive gastritis, and gastrointestinal hemorrhage occur in individuals on high doses of aspirin. The incidence of these side effects is rarer at low doses but a single dose of aspirin can cause GI distress in 5% of individuals. Gastric bleeding induced by salicylates is generally painless but can lead to fecal blood loss and may cause a persistent iron deficiency anemia. At dosages that generally are useful in anti-inflammatory therapy, aspirin may lead to a loss of 3–8 ml of blood per day. The mechanism by which salicylates cause gastric mucosal cell damage may be due to a number of factors, including gastric acidity, the ability of salicylates to damage the normal mucosal barrier which protects against the back diffusion of hydrogen ions, the ability of salicylates to inhibit the formation of prostaglandins, particularly those of the PGE series which normally inhibit gastric acid secretion, and inhibition of platelet aggregation leading to an increased tendency toward bleeding. Thus, salicylate use prior to surgery or tooth extraction is contraindicated.

Reye's Syndrome is an acute condition that may follow influenza and chicken pox infections in children from infancy to their late teens with the majority of cases seen between the ages of 4 and 12 years. It is characterized by symptoms including sudden vomiting, violent headaches and unusual behavior in children who appear to be recovering from an often mild viral illness. Although a rare condition (60–120 cases per year or an incidence of 0.15 per 100,000 population of 18 years of age or younger), it can be fatal with a death rate of between 20–30%. Fortunately, the number of cases is declining, partly due to the observations that over 90% of children with Reye's Syndrome were on salicylate therapy during a recent viral illness. Based on these observations, the FDA has proposed that aspirin and other salicylates be labeled with a warning against their use in children under 16 years of age with influenza, chicken pox or other flu-like illness. Acetaminophen would appear to be the drug of choice in children with these conditions.

Salicylates account for approximately 25% of all accidental poisonings in the United States.

Drug Interactions. Because of the widespread use of salicylates, it is not surprising that interactions with many other drugs used in therapeutic combinations have been observed, several of which are clinically significant. More data is available for aspirin than any other specific salicylate product. As mentioned previously, acetylsalicylic acid is a weak acid highly bound to plasma proteins (50–80%) and will compete for these plasma protein binding sites with other drugs which are highly bound to these sites. The interaction that results from the combination of salicylates with oral anticoagulants represents one of the most widely documented clinically significant drug interactions reported to date. The plasma concentration of free anticoagulant increases in the presence of salicylates, necessitating a possible decrease in the dosage of anticoagulant required to produce a beneficial therapeutic effect. The ability of salicylates to produce GI ulcerations and bleeding coupled with the inhibition of the clotting mechanism results in a clinically significant drug interaction. In addition, salicylates may inhibit the synthesis of prothrombin by antagonizing the actions of vitamin K. NSAIAs can also produce these interactions. The competition for plasma protein binding sites can also lead to an increase in free methotrexate levels (thus enhancing the toxicity of methotrexate), enhanced toxicity of long-acting sulfonamides, and a hypoglycemic effect resulting from displacement of oral hypoglycemic agents. In large doses, salicylates given concomitant with uricosuric agents such as probenecid and sulfinpyrazone may lead to a retention of uric acid and thus antagonize the uricosuric effect, despite the fact that salicylates when used alone increases urinary excretion of uric acid. The diuretic activity of aldosterone antagonists, such as spironolactone, may be antagonized by salicylates. Corticosteroids may decrease blood levels of salicylates because of their ability to increase the glomerular filtration rate. The incidence and severity of GI ulcerations may be increased if corticosteroids, salicylates and NSAIAs are administered together. The GI bleeding induced by salicylates may be enhanced by the ingestion of ethanol. Numerous other interactions have been reported but their clinical significance has not been fully established.

Salicylate hypersensitivity, particularly to aspirin, is relatively uncommon but must be recognized since severe and potentially fatal reactions may occur. Signs of aspirin hypersensitivity appear soon within administration and include skin rashes, watery secretions, urticaria, vasomotor rhinitis, edema, bronchoconstriction and anaphylaxis. Less than 1% of the U.S. population may experience aspirin hypersensitivity; this group consists primarily of middle-aged individuals. Females are more likely to experience aspirin intolerance or hypersensitivity. Aspirin-sensitive asthmatics are especially at high risk. Mild salicylism may occur after repeated administration of large doses. Symptoms include dizziness, tinnitus, nausea, vomiting, diarrhea and mental confusion. Doses of 10–30 g have been known to cause death in adults but some individuals have ingested up to 130 g without fatality. Over 10,000 cases of serious salicylate toxicity occur in the United States each year.

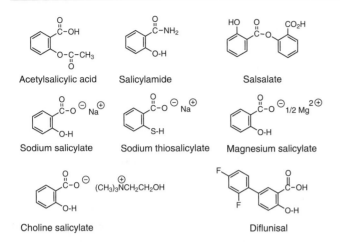

Fig. 32.8. Structures of marketed derivatives of salicyclic acid.

Preparations Available (Table 32.3)

The structures of the marketed preparations of salicylic acid are presented in Figure 32.8.

Aspirin, U.S.P. Acetylsalicylic acid, or aspirin, is a white powder that is stable in a dry environment but which is hydrolyzed to salicylic acid and acetic acid under humid or moist conditions. Hydrolysis can also occur when aspirin is combined with alkaline salts or with salts containing water of hydration. Stable aqueous solutions of aspirin are thus unobtainable despite the addition of modifying agents that tend to decrease hydrolysis. Aspirin is rapidly absorbed from the stomach and upper small intestine upon oral administration largely intact but is rapidly hydrolyzed by plasma esterases. Peak plasma levels are usually achieved within 2 hours after administration. Increasing the pH of the stomach by the addition of buffering agents may affect absorption since the degree of ionization would be increased.

Aspirin is indicated for the relief of minor aches and mild to moderate pain, for arthritis and related arthritic conditions, to reduce the risk of transient ischemic attacks in men, and for myocardial infarction prophylaxis (Table 32.3).

Salicylamide. Salicylamide is a white crystalline powder which is much less acidic than other salicylic acid derivatives. Although poorly soluble in water, stable solutions can be formed at pH 9. It is absorbed from the GI tract on oral administration and is rapidly metabolized to inactive metabolites by intestinal mucosa, but not by hydrolysis. Activity appears to reside in the intact molecule. It is approximately 40–55% plasma protein bound. Salicylamide competes with other salicylates and acetaminophen for glucuronide conjugation decreasing the extent of conjugation of these other agents. Excretion occurs rapidly, primarily in the urine. The major advantages of salicylamide are its general lack of gastric irritation, relative to aspirin, and its use in individuals who are hypersensitive to aspirin. Salicylamide enters the CNS more rapidly than other salicylates and will cause sedation and drowsiness when administered in large doses. Whereas salicylamide is reported to be as effective as aspirin as an analgesic-antipyretic and is effective in relieving pain associated with arthritic conditions, it does not appear to possess useful anti-inflammatory activity (38). Thus indications for the treatment of arthritic disease states are unwarranted and its use is restricted to the relief of minor aches and pain (Table 32.3). Its effects in humans are not reliable however, and its use is not widely recommended.

Salicylate Salts. Several salts of salicylic acid, sodium salicylate, U.S.P., choline salicylate, U.S.P., and magnesium salicylate, U.S.P., and one salt of thiosalicylic acid, sodium thiosalicylate, U.S.P., are available. These salts are used primarily to decrease GI disturbances or because they form stable aqueous solutions. Sodium salicylate is half as potent, on a weight basis, as aspirin as an analgesic and antipyretic but produces less GI irritation and equivalent blood levels, and is useful in patients exhibiting hypersensitivity to aspirin. It generates salicylic acid in the GI tract accounting for some gastrointestinal irritation and sodium bicarbonate is sometimes given concomitantly to reduce acidity. Sodium salicylate, unlike aspirin, does not affect platelet function although prothrombin times are increased. It is available as tablets, enteric-coated tablets, and as a solution for injection.

Choline salicylate has lower GI side effects than aspirin and has been shown to be particularly useful in treating juvenile rheumatoid arthritis where aspirin was ineffective. It is absorbed more rapidly than aspirin and produces higher salicylate plasma levels. It is available as a mint-flavored liquid.

Magnesium salicylate has a low incidence of GI side effects. Both sodium salicylate and magnesium salicylate should be used cautiously in individuals in whom excessive amounts of these electrolytes might be detrimental. The possibility of magnesium toxicity in individuals with renal insufficiency exists. It is available as tablets but its safety in children under 12 years of age has not been fully determined.

Sodium thiosalicylate is indicated for rheumatic fever, muscular pain and acute gout and is available as a solution for intramuscular injection.

Salsalate (Disalcid). Salsalate, salicylsalicylic acid, is a dimer of salicylic acid (Fig. 32.8). It is insoluble in gastric juice but is soluble in the small intestine where it is partially hydrolyzed to two molecules of salicylic acid and absorbed. On a molar basis it produces 15% less salicylic acid than aspirin. It does not cause GI blood loss and can be given to aspirin-sensitive patients. Salsalate is available as capsules and tablets.

Diflunisal (Dolobid). Diflunisal was introduced in the United States in 1982 and has gained considerable acceptance as an analgesic and to treat rheumatoid arthritis and osteoarthritis. It is a white, odorless crystalline powder which is practically insoluble in water at neutral or acidic pH but is soluble in most organic solvents and aqueous alkaline solutions and is stable to both heat and light. Diflunisal is metabolized primarily to ether and ester glucuronide conjugates. No metabolism involving changes in ring substituents has been reported. It is more potent than aspirin but produces fewer side effects, and has a biologic half-life 3–4 times greater than that of aspirin. It is rapidly and completely absorbed on oral administration with peak plasma levels being achieved within 2–3 hours of administration. It is highly bound (99%) to plasma proteins after absorption. Side effects most frequently reported include disturbances of the GI system (nausea, dyspepsia and diarrhea), dermatologic reactions and CNS effects such as dizziness and headache.

Diflunisal is a moderately potent inhibitor of prostaglandin biosynthesis but differs from the manner in which aspirin inhibits the cyclooxygenase system in that the inhibition is competitive and reversible in nature. Diflunisal does not have an appreciable effect on platelet aggregation, however, and does not significantly produce gastric or intestinal bleeding.

$$\underset{\substack{\text{R} \\ | \\ \text{AR--CH--C--OH}}}{\overset{\substack{\text{O} \\ || }}{}}$$

R = H, CH$_3$ or alkyl
AR = aryl or heteroaryl

Arylalkanoic Acids

The largest group of nonsteroidal anti-inflammatory agents is the arylalkanoic acid class of drugs. Several factors have caused this group of drugs to be the most active areas of drug development in recent years. The impact that the introduction of phenylbutazone in the 1950s had on arthritis therapy was more than matched by the interest generated by the introduction of indomethacin in the mid-1960s. As a result of a study designed to investigate the anti-inflammatory activity of 350 indole acetic acid derivatives related structurally to serotonin and metabolites of serotonin, the Merck group, led by Shen reported the synthesis and antipyretic and anti-inflammatory activity of the most potent compound in the series, indomethacin (39). The observation that indomethacin possessed 1085 times the anti-inflammatory activity and 20 times the antipyretic activity of phenylbutazone (and 10 times the antipyretic activity of aminopyrine) generated considerable interest in the development of other aryl and heteroaryl acetic acid and propionic acid derivatives. The marketplace was ripe for new anti-inflammatory agents and most pharmaceutical companies joined in the search for new arylalkanoic acids. The introduction of ibuprofen in the 1970s by Upjohn was quickly followed by the appearance of fenoprofen calcium, naproxen and tolmetin. Sulindac, an analog of indomethacin, was introduced in the late 1970s. The 1980s produced zomepirac, benoxaprofen, ketoprofen, flurbiprofen, suprofen and diclofenac sodium. The 1990s produced ketorolac, etodolac, nabumetone and,

most significantly, the development of selective COX-2 inhibitors, two of which, celecoxib and rofecoxib, reached the marketplace at the end of the decade. This rapid development has been accompanied by some set-backs, however. Zomepirac, introduced in 1980 as an analgesic was withdrawn in 1983 because of severe anaphylactoid reactions, particularly in patients sensitive to aspirin. Benoxaprofen was withdrawn within six months of its introduction in 1982 because of several deaths caused by cholestatic jaundice in Europe and the U.S. In addition, benoxaprofen produced photosensitivity reactions in patients when they were exposed to sunlight and onycholysis (loosening of the fingernails) in some patients. Suprofen, introduced as an analgesic in 1985 was removed from the market two years later because of flank pain and transient renal failure. It was re-introduced in 1989 for ophthalmic use. Numerous other arylalkanoic acids are currently being evaluated in various stages of clinical trials.

As discussed earlier, most NSAIAs possess a number of biochemical and pharmacologic actions. As was the case for the salicylates, the arylalkanoic acids, to various extents, share the property of inhibition of prostaglandin biosynthesis by inhibiting COX-1 and COX-2 with varying degrees of selectivity.

General Structure-activity Relationships. Agents of this class share a number of common structural features. These general structure-activity relationships will be discussed here as they pertain to the proposed mechanism of action. Specific structure-activity relationships for each drug or drug class will be presented separately, where appropriate.

All nonselective COX inhibitors possess a center of acidity which can be represented by a carboxylic acid function, an enolic function, a hydroxamic acid function, a sulfonamide, or a tetrazole ring. The relationship of this acid center to the carboxylic acid function of arachidonic acid is obvious. The activity of ester and amide derivatives of carboxylic acids is generally attributed to the metabolic hydrolysis products. One nonacidic drug, nabumetone, has been recently introduced in the U.S. but, as will be discussed later, its activity is attributed to its bioactivation to an active acid metabolite. The center of acidity is generally located one carbon atom adjacent to a flat surface represented by an aromatic or heteroaromatic ring. The distance between these centers is crucial since increasing this distance to two or three carbons generally diminishes activity. Derivatives of aryl or heteroaryl acetic or propionic acids are most common. This aromatic system appears to correlate with the double bonds at the 5- and 8-positions of arachidonic acid (Fig. 32.1). Substitution of a methyl group on the carbon atom separating the acid center from the aromatic ring tends to increase anti-inflammatory activity. The resulting α-methyl acetic acid, or 2-substituted propionic acid, analogs have been given the class name "profens" by the U.S. Adopted Name Council. Groups larger than methyl decrease activity, but incorporation of this methyl group as part of an alicyclic ring system does not drastically affect activity. Introduction of a methyl group creates a center of chirality. Anti-inflammatory activity in those cases where the enantiomers have been separated and evaluated, whether determined in vivo or in vitro by cyclooxygenase assays, is associated with the (S)-(+)-enantiomer. Interestingly, in those cases where the propionic acid is administered as a racemic mixture, in vivo conversion of the R-enantiomer to the biologically active S-enantiomer is observed to varying degrees. A second area of lipophilicity that is generally noncoplanar with the aromatic or heteroaromatic ring generally enhances activity. This second lipophilic area may correspond to the area of the double bond in the 11-position of arachidonic acid. This lipophilic function may consist of an additional aromatic ring or alkyl groups either attached to or fused to the aromatic center.

General Metabolism. Essentially all of the arylalkanoic acid derivatives that are therapeutically available are extensively metabolized. Metabolism occurs primarily through hepatic microsomal enzyme systems and may lead to deactivation or bioactivation of the parent molecules. Metabolism of each drug will be treated separately.

Drug Interactions. All of the arylalkanoic acids are highly bound to plasma proteins and may thus displace other drugs from protein binding sites resulting in an enhanced activity and toxicity of the displaced drugs. Interestingly, despite the high degree of plasma protein binding, indomethacin does not display this characteristic drug interaction. The most commonly observed interaction is that between the arylalkanoic acid and oral anticoagulants, particularly warfarin. Coadministration may prolong prothrombin time. Potential interactions with other acidic drugs, such as hydantoins, sulfonamides, and sulfonylureas should be monitored. Concomitant administration of aspirin decreases plasma levels of arylalkanoic acids by as much as 20%. Probenecid, on the other hand, tends to increase these plasma levels. Interactions with drugs that may induce hepatic microsomal enzyme systems (such as phenobarbital) may enhance or diminish anti-inflammatory activity depending on whether the arylalkanoic acid is metabolically bioactivated or inactivated by this enzyme system. Certain diuretics, such as furosemide, inhibit the metabolism of prostaglandins by 15-hydroxy-prostaglandin dehydrogenase and the resulting increase in PGE_2 levels induces plasma renin activity. Because the arylalkanoic acids block the biosynthesis of prostaglandins, the effects of furosemide can be antagonized, in part, offering a potentially significant drug interaction.

Aryl- and Heteroarylacetic Acids. The structures of the aryl- and heteroarylacetic acid derivatives are presented in Figure 32.9.

Indomethacin. Indomethacin (Fig. 32.9) is a yellow-tan crystalline powder that is odorless, possesses a bitter taste

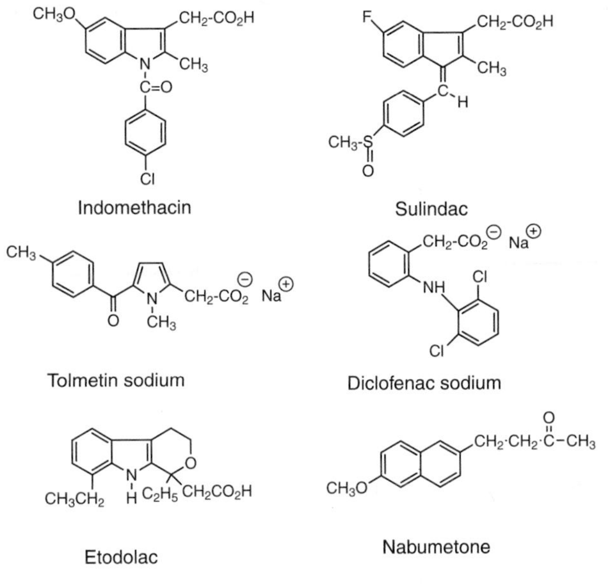

Fig. 32.9. Structures of aryl- and heteroarylacetic acid derivatives.

and is light sensitive. It is water soluble and although soluble in base, alkaline solutions are not stable due to the ease of hydrolysis of the *p*-chlorobenzoyl group. The synthesis of indomethacin was reported by Shen in 1963 and the drug was introduced onto the U.S. market in 1965. It is still one of the most potent NSAIAs in use. It is also a more potent antipyretic than either aspirin or acetaminophen and possesses about 10 times the analgesic potency of aspirin, although the analgesic effect is widely overshadowed by concern over the frequency of side effects.

Structure-activity Relationships. Replacement of the carboxyl group with other acidic functionalities decreases activity. Anti-inflammatory activity generally increases as the acidity of the carboxyl group increases and decreases as the acidity is decreased. Amide analogues are inactive. Acylation of the indole nitrogen with aliphatic carboxylic acids or aralkylcarboxylic acids results in amide derivatives that are less active than those derived from benzoic acid. N-Benzoyl derivatives substituted in the *para*-position with fluoro, chloro, trifluoromethyl or thiomethyl groups are the most active. The 5-position of the indole ring is most flexible with regard to the nature of substituents that enhance activity. Substituents such as methoxy, fluoro, dimethylamino, methyl, allyloxy, acetyl are more active than the unsubstituted indole ring. The presence of an indole ring nitrogen is not essential for activity because the corresponding 1-benzylidenylindene analogs (e.g., sulindac) are active. Alkyl groups, especially methyl, at the α-position are more active than aryl substituents. Substitution of a methyl group at the α-position of the acetic acid side chain (to give the corresponding propionic acid derivative) leads to equiactive analogs. The resulting chirality introduced in the molecules is important. Anti-inflammatory activity is displayed only by the (S)(+)-enantiomer. The conformation of indomethacin appears to play a crucial role in its anti-inflammatory actions. The acetic acid side chain is flexible and can assume a large number of different conformations. The preferred conformation of the N-*p*-chlorobenzoyl group is one in which the chlorophenyl ring is oriented away from the 2-methyl group (or *cis* to the methoxyphenyl ring of the indole nucleus) and is non-coplanar with the indole ring because of steric hindrance produced by the 2-methyl group and the hydrogen atom at the 7-position. This conformation may be represented as follows:

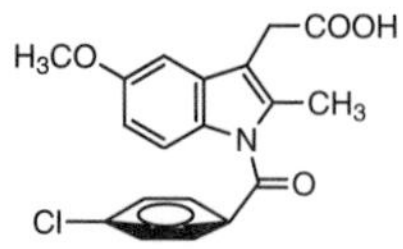

Absorption and Metabolism. Absorption of indomethacin occurs rapidly on oral administration and peak plasma levels are obtained within 2–3 hours (See Table 32.4). Being an acidic substance, it is highly bound to plasma proteins. Indomethacin is converted to inactive metabolites, approximately 50% of a single dose being converted to the O-demethylated metabolite and 10% conjugated with glucuronic acid. Nonhepatic enzyme systems hydrolyze indomethacin to N-deacylated metabolites. The metabolism of indomethacin is illustrated in Figure 32.10.

The ability of indomethacin to potently inhibit prostaglandin biosynthesis may account for its anti-inflammatory, antipyretic and analgesic actions. Pronounced side effects are frequently observed at antirheumatic doses. A large number of individuals taking indomethacin experience undesirable effects of the GI tract (nausea, dyspepsia and diarrhea), the CNS (headache, dizziness and vertigo) and the ears (tinnitus) and many must discontinue its use. As with other arylalkanoic acids, administration of indomethacin with food or milk decreases GI side effects.

Indomethacin is available for the treatment of rheumatoid and acute gouty arthritis, ankylosing spondylitis, and moderate to severe osteoarthritis in a number of dosage forms, Table 32.4. An injectable form is available as the sodium trihydrate salt for intravenous use in premature infants with patent ductus arteriosus. Because of its ability to suppress uterine activity by inhibiting prostaglandin biosynthesis, indomethacin also has an unlabeled use to prevent premature labor.

Sulindac. Sulindac (Fig. 32.9) is a yellow crystalline powder that is soluble in water only at alkaline pH. It is stable in alkaline aqueous solutions and in air at 100°C. It was introduced in the U.S. in 1978 by the same company as indomethacin as a result of chemical studies designed to produce an analog free of the side effects commonly associated with the use of indomethacin, particularly GI irritation. It achieved wide popularity and remains one of the more widely used NSAIAs. Its synthesis was also reported by Shen's group (40). Sulindac is a "pro-drug" and is converted to a metabolite that appears to inhibit the cyclooxygenase system about eight times as effectively as aspirin. In anti-inflammatory and antipyretic assays it is only about one-half as potent as indomethacin but is equipotent in analgesic assays.

Structure-activity Relationships. The use of classical bioisosteric changes in medicinal chemistry drug design was invoked in the design of sulindac. The isosteric replacement of the indole ring with the indene ring system resulted in a derivative with therapeutically useful anti-inflammatory activity and less CNS and GI side effects but which possessed other undesirable effects, particularly poor water solubility and resulting crystalluria. The replacement of the N-*p*-chlorobenzoyl substituent with a benzylidiene function resulted in active derivatives. However, when the 5-methoxy group of the indene isostere was replaced with a fluorine atom, enhanced analgesic effects were observed. The decreased water solubility of the indene isostere was alleviated by replacing the chlorine atom of the phenyl substituent with a sulfinyl group. The importance of stereochemical features in the action of sulindac, introduced by the benzylidene double bond, is evidenced by the observation that the (Z)-isomer is a much more potent anti-inflammatory agent than the corresponding (E)-isomer. This cis-relationship of the phenyl substituent to the aromatic ring bearing the fluoro substituent (see Fig. 32.9) is similar to the proposed conformation of indomethacin suggesting that both indomethacin and sulindac assume similar conformations at the active site of arachidonic acid cyclooxygenase.

Absorption and Metabolism. Sulindac is well absorbed on oral administration, reaches peak plasma levels within 2–4 hours and, being acidic, is highly bound to serum proteins (Table 32.4). The metabolism of

Table 32.4. Pharmacokinetic Properties of Aryl- and Heteroaryl Acetic Acids

Drug	Trade Name	Peakblood Level (hr)	Plasma Binding (%)	pKa	Anti-inflammatory Dose (mg/day)	Dosage Forms (mg/unit)
Indomethacin	Indocin	2–3	97	4.5	75–150	Cap (25, 50, 75); S$_2$ (50); S$_3$ (25 mg/5 ml)
Sulindac	Clinoril	2–4	93	4.5	400	Tab (150, 200)
Tolmetin	Tolectin	<1	99	3.5	1200	Tab (200, 600); Cap (400)
Diclofenac	Voltarin	1.5–2.5	99.5	4.0	100–200	Enteric Tab (25, 50, 75)
Etodolac	Lodine	1–2	99	—	800–1200	Cap (200, 300)
Nabumetone	Relafen	—		7.0	1000–2000	Tab (500, 750)

Tab = Tablet; Cap = Capsule; S$_2$ = Suppositories; S$_3$ = Suspension.

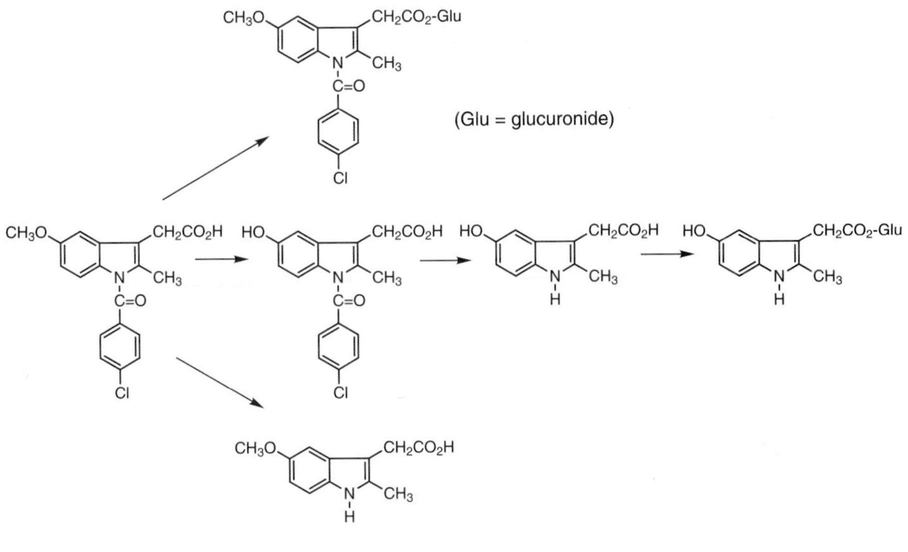

Fig. 32.10. Metabolism of indomethacin.

sulindac plays a major role in its actions since all of the pharmacologic activity is associated with its major metabolite. Sulindac is, in fact, a pro-drug, the sulfoxide function being reduced to the active sulfide metabolite (Fig. 32.11). Sulindac is absorbed as the sulfoxide that is not an inhibitor of prostaglandin biosynthesis in the GI tract. As discussed earlier, prostaglandins exert a protective effect in the GI tract and inhibition of their synthesis here leads to many of the gastrointestinal side effects noted for most NSAIAs. Once sulindac enters the circulatory system it is reduced to the sulfide which is an inhibitor of prostaglandin biosynthesis in the joints. Thus, sulindac produces less GI side effects, such as bleeding, ulcerations, etc. than indomethacin and many other NSAIAs. In addition, the active metabolite has a plasma half-life approximately twice that of the parent compound (~16 hours vs. 8 hours), which favorably affects the dosing schedule. In addition to the sulfide metabolite, sulindac is oxidized to the corresponding sulfone, which is inactive. A minor product results from hydroxylation of the benzylidene function and the methyl group at the 2-position. Glucuronides of several metabolites are also found. Sulindac, the sulfide and the sulfone metabolites are all highly protein-bound. Despite the fact that the sulfide metabolite is a major activation product and is found in high concentration in human plasma, it is not found in human urine, perhaps because of its high degree of protein binding. The major excretion product is the sulfone metabolite and its glucuronide conjugate.

Whereas the toxicity of sulindac is lower than that observed for indomethacin and other NSAIAs, the spectrum of adverse reactions is very similar. The most frequent side effects reported are associated with irritation of the GI tract (nausea, dyspepsia, diarrhea), although these effects are generally mild. Effects on the CNS (dizziness and headache) are less common. Dermatologic effects are less frequently encountered.

Sulindac is indicated for long-term use in the treatment of rheumatoid arthritis, osteoarthritis, ankylosing spondylitis and acute gouty arthritis. Dose and dosage forms are shown in Table 32.4. It is recommended that sulindac be administered with food.

Tolmetin Sodium. Tolmetin sodium (Fig. 32.9) is a light yellow crystalline solid that is very water soluble. The free acid form, however, is virtually water insoluble. Tolmetin is synthesized straightforwardly from 1-methylpyrrole (41). It was introduced in the U.S. in 1976, and like other NSAIAs, inhibits prostaglandin biosynthesis. Tolmetin also inhibits polymorph migration and decreases capillary permeability, however. Its anti-inflammatory activity, as measured in the carrageenan-induced rat paw edema and cotton pellet granuloma assays, is intermediate between that of phenylbutazone and indomethacin.

Structure-activity Relationships. The relationship of tolmetin to indomethacin is clear, each containing a noncoplanar *p*-chlorobenzoyl group and an acetic acid function. Tolmetin possesses a pyrrole ring instead of the indole ring in indomethacin. Replacement of the 5-*p*-toluoyl group with a *p*-chlorobenzoyl moiety produced little effect on activity while introduction of a methyl group in the 4-position of the pyrrole ring produced interesting results. The 4-methyl-5-*p*-chlorobenzoyl analog is approximately four times as potent as tolmetin. McNeil marketed this compound in 1980 as zomepirac, an analgesic that was removed from the market in 1983 because of severe anaphylactic reactions particularly in patients sensitive to aspirin. Unlike the previous structure-activity relationships discussed for arylalkanoic acids, the propionic acid analogue is slightly less potent than tolmetin.

Absorption and Metabolism. Tolmetin sodium is rapidly and almost completely absorbed on oral administration with peak plasma levels being attained within the first hour of administration. It has a relatively short plasma half-life (~1 hour) and is highly bound to plasma protein (Table 32.4). Excretion of tolmetin and its metabolites occurs primarily in the urine. Tolmetin is extensively metabolized with approximately 70% of the drug being metabolized to the dicarboxylic acid shown below.

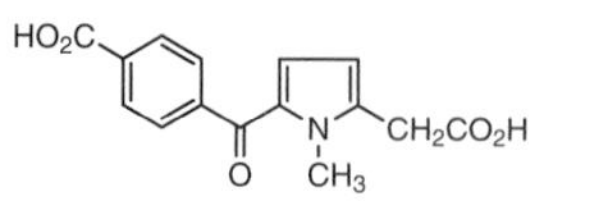

This metabolite is inactive in standard in vivo anti-inflammatory assays. Approximately 15–20% of an administered dose is excreted unchanged and 10% as the glucuronide conjugate of the parent drug. Conjugates of the dicarboxylic acid metabolite account for the majority of the remaining administered drug.

The most frequently observed adverse reactions are those involving the GI tract (abdominal pain, discomfort, nausea) but appear to be less than those observed with aspirin. CNS effects (dizziness and drowsiness) are also observed. Few cases of overdosage have been reported but in such cases recommended treatment includes elimination of the drug from the GI tract by emesis or gastric lavage and elimination of the acidic drug from the circulatory system by enhancing alkalinization of the urine with sodium bicarbonate.

Tolmetin sodium is indicated for the treatment of rheumatoid arthritis, juvenile rheumatoid arthritis and osteoarthritis. The recommended dosage and dosage forms are shown in Table 32.4.

Diclofenac Sodium. Diclofenac sodium (Fig. 32.9) is a faintly yellow-white to light beige, odorless, slightly hygro-scopic crystalline powder which is sparingly soluble in water (42). It is available in 120 different countries and is perhaps the most widely used NSAIA in the world. It was introduced in the U.S. in 1989 but was first marketed in Japan in 1974. It ranks among the top prescription drugs in the U.S. Diclofenac possesses structural characteristics of both arylalkanoic acid and the anthranilic acid classes of anti-inflammatory agents and displays anti-inflammatory, analgesic and antipyretic properties. In the carrageenan-induced rat paw edema assay it is twice as potent as indomethacin and 450 times as potent as aspirin. As an analgesic, it is 6 times more potent than indomethacin and 40 times as potent as aspirin in the phenyl-benzoquinone-induced writhing assay in mice. As an antipyretic it is twice as potent as indomethacin and over 350 times as potent as aspirin in the yeast-induced fever assay in rats. Diclofenac is unique among the NSAIAs in that it possesses three possible mechanisms of action: 1) inhibition of the arachidonic acid cyclooxygenase system (3–1000 times more potent than other NSAIAs on a molar basis) resulting in a decreased production of prostaglandins and thromboxanes; 2) inhibition of the lipoxygenase pathway resulting in decreased production of leukotrienes, particularly the pro-inflammatory leukotriene B_4; and 3) inhibition of arachidonic acid release and stimulation of its re-uptake resulting in a reduction of arachidonic acid availability.

Structure-activity Relationships. Structure-activity relationships in this series have not been extensively studied. It does appear that the function of the two *o*-chloro groups is to force the anilino-phenyl ring out of the plane of the phenylacetic acid portion, this twisting effect being important in the binding of NSAIAs to the active site of the cyclooxygenase enzyme, as previously discussed.

Absorption and Metabolism. It is rapidly and completely absorbed on oral administration with peak plasma levels being reached within 1.5–2.5 hours (Table 32.4). The free acid is highly bound to serum proteins,

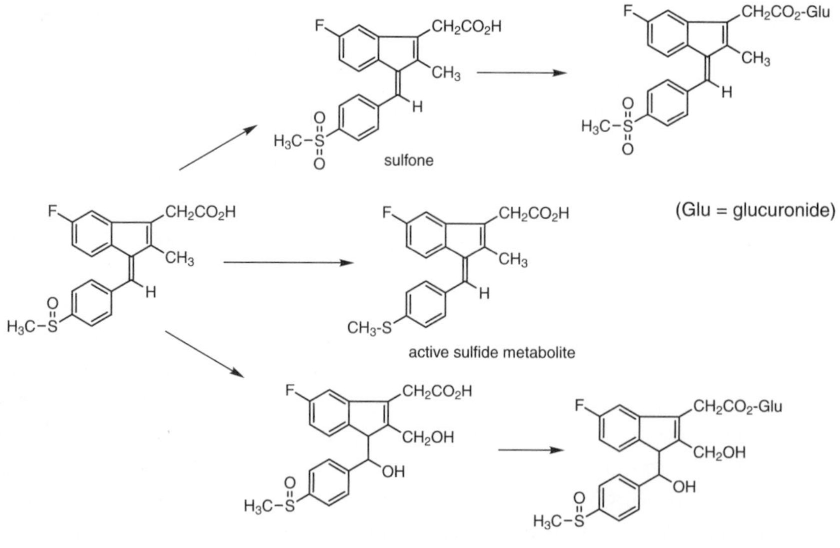

Fig. 32.11. Metabolism of sulindac.

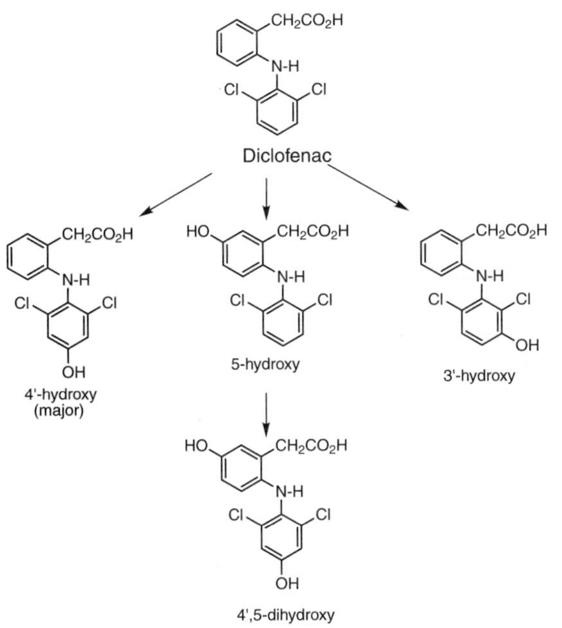

Fig. 32.12. Metabolism of diclofenac.

primarily albumin. Only 50–60% of an oral dose is bioavailable due to extensive hepatic metabolism. Four major metabolites resulting from aromatic hydroxylation have been identified. The major metabolite, the 4′-hydroxy derivative accounts for 20–30% of the dose excreted while the three others, the 5-hydroxy, the 3′-hydroxy and the 4′,5-dihydroxy metabolites each account for 10–20% of the excreted dose. The remaining drug is excreted in the form of sulfate conjugates. Although the major metabolite is much less active than the parent compound, it may exhibit significant biologic activity since it accounts for 30–40% of all of the metabolic products. The metabolism of diclofenac is illustrated in Figure 32.12.

Diclofenac sodium is indicated for the treatment of rheumatoid arthritis, osteoarthritis and ankylosing spondylitis. Recommended doses and dosage forms are shown in Table 32.4.

Etodolac. Etodolac (Fig. 32.9) is a white, crystalline compound which is insoluble in water but soluble in most organic solvents. It is promoted as the first of a new chemical class of anti-inflammatory agents, the pyranocarboxylic acids. Although not strictly an arylacetic acid derivative (because there is a two-carbon atom separation between the carboxylic acid function and the hetero-aromatic ring), it still possesses structural characteristics similar to the heteroarylacetic acids and is classified here. It was introduced in the U.S. in 1991 for acute and long-term use in the management of osteoarthritis and as an analgesic. It is registered in several other countries around the world. It also possesses antipyretic activity. Etodolac is marketed as a racemic mixture although only the (S)(+)-enantiomer possesses anti-inflammatory activity in animal models. Etodolac also displays a high degree of enantioselectivity in its inhibitory

effects on the arachidonic acid cyclooxygenase system. With regard to its anti-inflammatory actions, etodolac was about 50 times more active than aspirin, 3 times more potent than sulindac, and one-third as active as indomethacin. The ratio of the anti-inflammatory activity to the ED50 for gastric ulceration or erosion was more favorable for etodolac (ID50/ED50 = 10) than for aspirin, naproxen, sulindac or indomethacin (ID50/ED50 = 4). At 2.5–3.5 times the effective anti-inflammatory dose, etodolac was reported to produce less GI bleeding than indomethacin, ibuprofen or naproxen. The primary mechanism of action appears to be inhibition of the biosynthesis of prostaglandins at the cyclooxygenase step, with no inhibition of the lipoxygenase system. Etodolac, however, possesses a more favorable ratio of inhibition of prostaglandin biosynthesis in human rheumatoid synoviocytes and chondrocytes than by cultured human gastric mucosal cells compared to ibuprofen, indomethacin, naproxen, diclofenac and piroxicam. Thus, although etodolac is no more potent an NSAIA than many others, the lower incidence of GI side effects represents a potential therapeutic advantage.

Structure-activity Relationships. During a search for newer, more effective antiarthritic agents in the 1970s, the Ayerst group led by Humber, investigated a series of pyranocarboxylic acids of the general structure shown

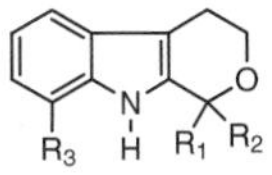

below (43). Structure-activity relationship studies indicated that alkyl groups at R_1 and an acetic acid function at R_2 enhanced anti-inflammatory activity. Lengthening the acid chain, or ester or amide derivatives gave inactive compounds. The corresponding α-methylacetic acid derivatives were also inactive. Increasing the chain length of the R_1 substituent to ethyl or n-propyl gave derivatives that were 20 times more potent than methyl. A number of substituents on the aromatic ring were evaluated and substituents at the 8-position (R_3) were most beneficial. Among the most active were the 8-ethyl, 8-n-propyl, and 7-fluoro-8-methyl derivatives. Etodolac was found to possess the most favorable anti-inflammatory to gastric distress properties among these analogs.

Absorption and Metabolism. Etodolac is rapidly absorbed following oral administration with maximum serum levels being achieved within 1–2 hours and is highly bound to plasma proteins (Table 32.4). The penetration of etodolac into synovial fluid is greater than or equal to tolmetin, piroxicam or ibuprofen. Only diclofenac appears to provide greater penetration. Etodolac is metabolized to three hydroxylated metabolites and to glucuronide conjugates, none of which possess important pharmacologic activity. Metabolism appears to be the same in the elderly as in the general population so no dosage adjustment appears necessary.

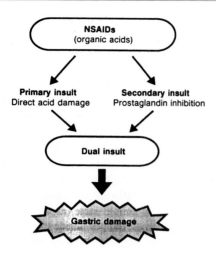

Fig. 32.13. NSAIA-induced production of gastric damage by a dual insult mechanism. (Reprinted with permission from Goudie A, et al. J Med Chem 1978; 21:1260.)

Etodolac is indicated for the management of the signs and symptoms of osteoarthritis and for the management of pain (See Table 32.4 for dose and dosage forms).

Nabumetone. Nabumetone (Fig. 32.9) is a nonacidic, white to off-white crystalline compound which is insoluble in water but soluble in most organic solvents. It is unique among the NSAIAs in that it represents a new class of nonacidic pro-drugs, being rapidly metabolized after absorption to form a major active metabolite. It was synthesized in 1978 and introduced in the U.S. in 1992 (44). Gastric damage produced by NSAIAs generally involves a dual insult mechanism (Fig. 32.13).

Most NSAIAs are acidic substances which produce a primary insult due to direct acid damage, an indirect contact effect and a back diffusion of hydrogen ions. The secondary insult results from inhibition of prostaglandin biosynthesis in the GI tract where prostaglandins exert a cytoprotective effect. The dual insult leads to gastric damage. Nabumetone, being nonacidic, does not produce a significant primary insult and is an ineffectual inhibitor of prostaglandin cyclooxygenase in gastric mucosa thus producing minimum secondary insult. The result is that gastric side effects of nabumetone appear to be minimized. Once the parent drug enters the circulatory system, however, it is metabolized to an active metabolite, 6-methoxy-naphthalene-2-acetic acid (6MNA) (Fig. 32.14), which is an effective inhibitor of prostaglandin synthesis in joints. Nabumetone thus represents a classic example of the prodrug approach in drug design.

In the carrageenan-induced rat paw assay, nabumetone is approximately 13 times more potent than aspirin, one-third as active as indomethacin and half as active as diclofenac. It is only one-half as active as aspirin as an analgesic as measured by the phenylquinone-induced writhing assay in mice. Despite its lower potency, advantages to nabumetone may reside in the favorable gastric irritancy profile. The ratio of gastric irritancy in rats (GTD$_{50}$) to anti-inflammatory activity in rats (ED$_{50}$) for nabumetone is 21.25 while this ratio is 0.41 for aspirin, 0.55 for indomethacin, 0.72 for diclofenac, 3.00 for tolmetin, and 7.85 for zomepirac.

Structure-activity Relationships. Introduction of methyl or ethyl groups on the butanone side chain greatly reduced anti-inflammatory activity. The ketone function can be converted to a dioxolane with retention of activity while converting the ketone to an oxime reduced activity. Removal of the methoxy group at the 6-position reduced activity, but replacement of the methoxy with a methyl or chloro group gave active compounds. Replacement of the methoxy with hydroxyl, acetoxy or N-methylcarbamoyl groups, or positional isomers of the methoxy group at the 2- or 4-positions greatly reduced activity. The active metabolite, 6MNA, is closely related structurally to naproxen, differing only by the lack of an α-methyl group. The ketone precursor [4-(6-methoxy-2-naphthyl)pentan-2-one] that would be expected to produce naproxen as a metabolite, was inactive in chronic models of inflammation.

Absorption and Metabolism Nabumetone is absorbed primarily from the duodenum. Milk and food increase the rate of absorption and the bioavailability of the active

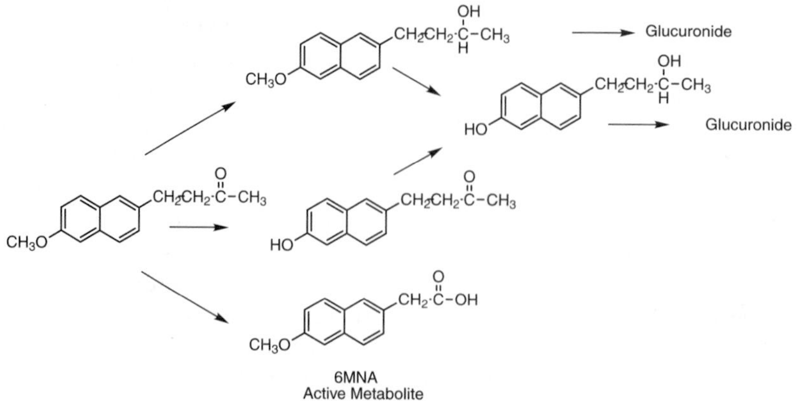

Fig. 32.14. The metabolism of nabumetone.

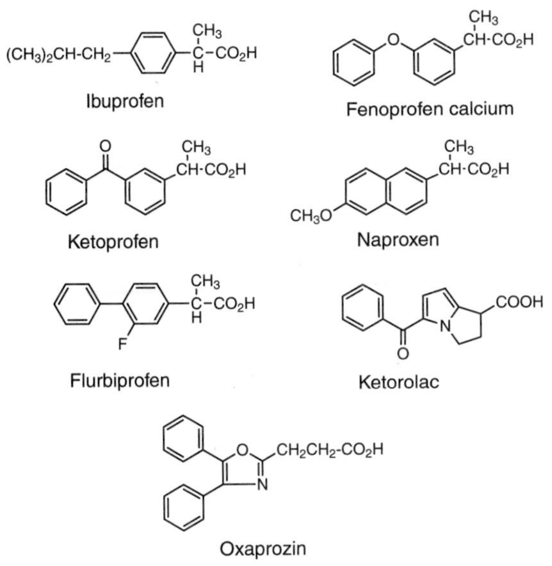

Fig. 32.15. Structures of Aryl- and Heteroarylpropionic Acid Derivatives.

metabolite. Plasma concentrations of unchanged drug are too low to be detected in most subjects after oral administration so most pharmacokinetic studies have involved the disposition of the active metabolite. Pharmacokinetic properties are altered in elderly patients with higher plasma levels of the active metabolite having been noted. Nabumetone undergoes rapid and extensive metabolism in the liver with a mean absolute bioavailability of the active metabolite of 38%. The metabolism of nabumetone is illustrated in Figure 32.14. The major, most active metabolite is 6MNA but the initial alcohol metabolite, a minor product, and its esters also possess significant anti-inflammatory properties.

Nabumetone is indicated for the acute and chronic treatment of the signs and symptoms of osteoarthritis and rheumatoid arthritis. The recommended starting dosage is 1000 mg as a single dose with or without food. More symptomatic relief of severe or persistent symptoms may be obtained at doses of 1500 mg or 2000 mg per day (Table 32.4).

Aryl- and Heteroarylpropionic Acids. The structures of the aryl- and heteroaryl propionic acid derivatives are presented in Figure 32.15.

Ibuprofen. Ibuprofen (Fig. 32.15) is a colorless, crystalline solid that is only very slightly soluble in water, but is soluble in most organic solvents. The synthesis of ibuprofen was originally reported in 1964 but the drug was not marketed in the U.S. until 1974 despite the fact that it had been available for several years in Europe (45). It was the first NSAIA since indomethacin and the first arylpropionic acid derivative to be marketed in the U.S. Its success precipitated the introduction of many new agents in the 1970s. This chemical class currently comprises the largest group of NSAIAs under investigation with as many as 25 derivatives in various stages of development. Ibuprofen became the first prescription NSAIA to become available as an over-the-counter analgesic in almost 30 years and is available under a number of trade names. The continuing popularity of ibuprofen is evidenced by the appearance of proprietary and nonproprietary forms in the list of Top 200 prescription drugs in the U.S. It is marketed as the racemic mixture although biologic activity resides almost exclusively in the (S)(+)-isomer. Ibuprofen is more potent than aspirin but less potent than indomethacin in anti-inflammatory and prostaglandin biosynthesis inhibition assays and produces moderate degrees of gastric irritation.

Structure-activity Relationships. The substitution of an α-methyl group on the alkanoic acid portion of acetic acid derivatives enhances anti-inflammatory actions and reduces many side effects. For example, the acetic acid analogue of ibuprofen, ibufenac (*p*-isobutylphenylacetic acid), is less potent and more hepatotoxic than ibuprofen. The stereochemistry associated with the chiral center in the arylpropionic acids, but lacking in the acetic acid derivatives, plays an important role in both the in vivo and in vitro activities of these agents. As indicated earlier, although marketed as a racemic mixture, the (+)-enantiomer of ibuprofen possess greater activity in vitro than the (−)-isomer. The eudismic (S/R) ratio for the inhibition of bovine prostaglandin synthesis is approximately 160, but in vivo, the two enantiomers are equiactive (see section on metabolism). The (+)-enantiomer of ibuprofen, and of most of the arylpropionic acids under investigation, has been shown to possess the (S)-absolute configuration.

Absorption and Metabolism. Ibuprofen is rapidly absorbed on oral administration with peak plasma levels being generally attained within 2 hours (Table 32.5). As with most of these acidic NSAIAs, ibuprofen is extensively bound to plasma proteins and will interact with other acidic drugs which are protein bound. Metabolism occurs rapidly and the drug is nearly completely excreted in the urine as unchanged drug and oxidative metabolites within 24 hours following administration. Metabolism involves primarily ω-, ω-1 and ω-2 oxidation of the *p*-isobutyl side chain, followed by alcohol oxidation of the primary alcohol resulting from ω-oxidation to the corresponding carboxylic acid. All metabolites are inactive. When ibuprofen is administered as the individual enantiomers, the major metabolites isolated are the (+)-isomers whatever the configuration of the starting enantiomer. Interestingly, the (R)(−)-enantiomer is inverted to the (S)(+)-enantiomer in vivo, accounting for the observation that the two enantiomers are bioequivalent in vivo. This is a metabolic phenomenon that has also been observed for other arylpropionic acids such as ketoprofen, benoxaprofen, fenoprofen and naproxen (46). The metabolism of ibuprofen is shown in Figure 32.16.

Table 32.5. Pharmacokinetic Properties of Aryl- and Heteroanyl Propionic Acids

Drug	Trade Name	Peakblood Level (hr)	Plasma Binding (%)	pKa	Anti-inflammatory (Analgesic) Dose (mg/day)	Dosage Forms (mg/unit)
Ibuprofen	Motrin, Advil, Nuprin	2	99	4.43	1200–3200 (1200–2400)	Tab (200, 300, 400, 600, 800) S$_3$ (100 mg/5ml)
Fenoprofen calcium	Nalfon	2	99	4.5	1200–2400	Tab (600), Cap (200, 300)
Ketoprofen	Orudis	0.5–2	99	5.94	150–300 (75–200)	Cap (25, 50, 75)
Naproxen(+)	Naprosyn	2–4	99.6	4.15	500–1000 (750–1000)	Tab (250, 375, 500), S3 (125 mg/5ml)
Naproxen sodium(−)	Anaprox	2–4	99.6	4.15	550–1100 (825–1100)	Tab (275, 550)
Flurbiprofen	Ansaid Ocufen	1.5	99	4.22	200–300 (1 drop/30 min)	Tab (50, 100) OS (0.03%)
Ketorolac tromethamine	Toradol Acular	—	99	3.54	(60–120) (40–60)	Inj (15 mg/ml, 30 mg/ml) Tab (10)
Oxaprozin	Daypro	3–5	99.9	4.3	1200	Caplets (600)

Tab = Tablet; Cap = Capsule; S$_3$ = Suspension; OS = Opthalmic solution; Inj = Injectable.

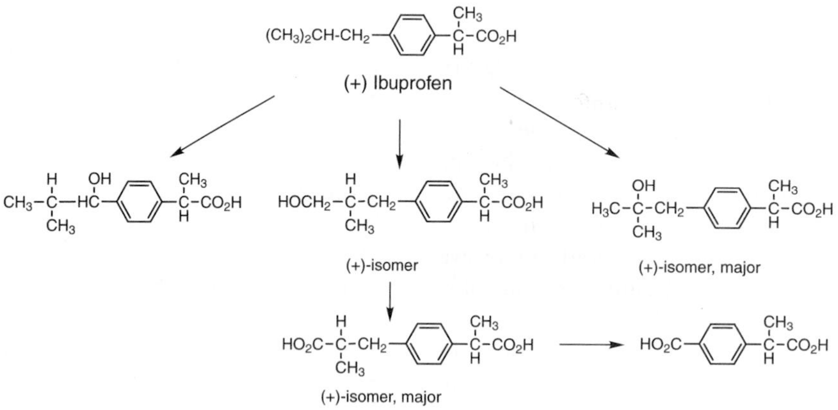

Fig. 32.16. Metabolism of ibuprofen.

Ibuprofen is indicated for the relief of the signs and symptoms of rheumatoid arthritis and osteoarthritis, the relief of mild to moderate pain, the reduction of fever, and the treatment of dysmenorrhea. The recommended antiarthritic and analgesic doses are shown in Table 32.5.

Fenoprofen Calcium. Fenoprofen calcium (Fig. 32.15) is a white crystalline powder that is slightly soluble in water. The calcium and sodium salts of fenoprofen possess similar bioavailability, distribution and elimination characteristics, however, it is the calcium salt that is marketed because it has the advantage of being less hygroscopic. Its original synthesis was reported in 1970 and it was marketed in the U.S. in 1976 (47). Fenoprofen is less potent in anti-inflammatory assays than ibuprofen, indomethacin, ketoprofen or naproxen. As an inhibitor of prostaglandin biosynthesis it is much less potent than indomethacin more potent than aspirin and about equipotent as ibuprofen. It also possesses analgesic and antipyretic activity. It possesses other pharmacologic properties such as inhibition of phagocytic and complement functions and stabilization of lysosomal membranes. Fenoprofen is marketed as a racemic mixture because no differences have been observed in the in vivo anti-inflammatory or analgesic properties of the individual enantiomers. The ability of (R)(−)-arylpropionic acids to undergo inversion to the (S)(+)-enantiomers may be involved, however. Like other NSAIAs, in vitro prostaglandin synthesis assays indicate that the (S)(+)-enantiomer is more potent than the (R)(−)-isomer.

Structure-activity Relationships. Placing the phenoxy group in the ortho- or para-position of the arylpropionic acid ring markedly decreases activity. Replacement of the oxygen bridge between the two aromatic rings with a carbonyl group yields an analog (ketoprofen) which is also marketed.

Absorption and Metabolism. Fenoprofen is readily absorbed (85%) upon oral administration and is highly bound to plasma proteins. Additional pharmacokinetic parameters are shown in Table 32.5. Fenoprofen is rather extensively metabolized, primarily through glucuronide conjugation with the parent drug and the 4′-hydroxy metabolite.

Fenoprofen calcium is indicated for treatment of rheumatoid and osteoarthritis and the relief of mild to moderate pain. Dose and dosage forms are shown in Table 32.5.

Ketoprofen. Ketoprofen (Fig. 32.15) is a white or off-white, odorless fine to granular powder that is practically insoluble in water but is soluble in most organic solvents. It was synthesized in 1968 but not introduced into the market until 1986 (48). Ketoprofen, unlike many NSAIAs, inhibits the synthesis of leukotrienes and leukocyte migration into inflamed joints in addition to inhibiting the biosynthesis of prostaglandins. It stabilizes the lysosomal membrane during inflammation resulting in decreased tissue destruction. Antibradykinin activity has also been observed. Bradykinin is released during inflammation and can activate peripheral pain receptors. In addition to anti-inflammatory activity, ketoprofen also possesses antipyretic and analgesic properties. Although it is less potent than indomethacin as an anti-inflammatory agent and as an analgesic, its ability to produce gastric lesions is about the same (49).

Absorption and Metabolism. Ketoprofen is rapidly and nearly completely absorbed on oral administration, reaching peak plasma levels within 0.5–2 hours. It is highly plasma protein-bound despite a lower acidity than some other NSAIAs (Table 32.5). Wide variation in plasma half-lives has been reported. It is metabolized by glucuronidation of the carboxylic acid, hydroxylation of the benzoyl ring, and reduction of the keto function.

Ketoprofen is indicated for the long-term management of rheumatoid arthritis and osteoarthritis, for mild to moderate pain, and for primary dysmenorrhea. The usual recommended dosage for arthritic indications and primary dysmenorrhea (analgesic) are shown in Table 32.5.

Naproxen. Naproxen (Fig. 32.15) is a white to off-white crystalline powder possessing a slightly bitter taste. Solubility in water is attained only at alkaline pH. The racemic mixture is synthesized from 2-methoxynaphthalene and the (+)-isomer obtained by resolution with cinchonidine (50). It was introduced in the U.S. in 1976 and has consistently been among the more popular NSAIAs. It is marketed as the (S)(+)-enantiomer but, interestingly, the sodium salt of the (−)-isomer is also on the market as Anaprox. As an inhibitor of prostaglandin biosynthesis the (+)-isomer is 12 times more potent than aspirin, 10 times more potent than phenylbutazone, 3–4 times more potent than ibuprofen and 4 times more potent than fenoprofen but is about 300 times less potent than indomethacin. In vivo anti-inflammatory assays are consistent with this relative order of potency. In the carrageenan rat paw edema assay it is 11 times more potent than phenylbutazone and 55 times as potent as aspirin but 0.7 times as potent as indomethacin. In the phenylquinone writhing assay for analgesia it is 9 times as potent as phenylbutazone and 7 times

as potent as aspirin but only 10% as potent as indomethacin. In the yeast-induced pyrexia assay for antipyretic activity it is 7 times as potent as phenylbutazone, 22 times as potent as aspirin, and 1.2 times as potent as indomethacin. The order of gastric ulcerogenic activity is sulindac < naproxen < aspirin, indomethacin, ketoprofen and tolmetin.

Structure-activity Relationships. In a series of substituted 2-naphthylacetic acids, substitution in the 6-position led to maximum anti-inflammatory activity. Small lipophilic groups such as Cl, CH_3S, and CHF_2O were active analogues with CH_3O being the most potent. Larger groups were found to be less active. Derivatives of 2-naphthylpropionic acids are more potent than the corresponding acetic acid analogues. Replacing the carboxyl group with functional groups capable of being metabolized to the carboxyl function (e.g., $-CO_2CH_3$, $-CHO$ or $-CH_2OH$) led to a retention of activity. The (S)(+)-isomer is the more potent enantiomer. Naproxen is the only arylalkanoic acid NSAIA marketed as optically active isomers.

Absorption and Metabolism Naproxen is almost completely absorbed following oral administration. Peak plasma levels are achieved within 2–4 hours following administration. Like most of the acidic NSAIAs it is highly bound to plasma proteins. Approximately 70% of an administered dose is eliminated as either unchanged drug (60%) or as conjugates of unchanged drug (10%). The remainder is converted to the 6-desmethyl metabolite (5%) and the glucuronide conjugate of the demethylated metabolite (22%). The 6-desmethyl metabolite lacks anti-inflammatory activity. Like most of the arylalkanoic acids the most common side effect associated with the use of naproxen is irritation to the GI tract. The most common other adverse reactions are associated with CNS disturbances such as nausea and dizziness.

Naproxen is indicated for the treatment of rheumatoid arthritis, osteoarthritis, juvenile arthritis, ankylosing spondylitis, tendinitis, bursitis, acute gout, primary dysmenorrhea and for the relief of mild to moderate pain. The recommended dose for arthritic indications is shown in Table 32.5 (juvenile arthritis the total daily dose is 10 mg/kg in 2 divided doses). The maximum adult antiinflammatory dose is 1.5 g/day for limited periods while analgesic doses should not exceed 1.25 g daily.

As stated, the sodium salt of the (−)-enantiomer is available as Anaprox which generally has the same indications and dosage regimens. Anaprox is not indicated in juvenile arthritis and daily doses should not exceed 1.375 grams.

Flurbiprofen. Flurbiprofen (Fig. 32.15) is a white or slightly yellow, crystalline powder that is soluble in water at pH 7.0 and readily soluble in most polar organic solvents. Its synthesis was originally reported in 1973 (51). During a study of the pharmacologic properties of a large number of substituted phenylalkanoic acids, including ibuprofen and ibufenac, the most potent were found to be substituted 2-(4-biphenylyl)propionic acids. Further toxicologic and pharmacologic studies indicated that flurbiprofen possessed the most favorable therapeutic profile so it was selected for further clinical development. It was not marketed until 1987 when it was introduced as the sodium salt as Ocufen as the first topical NSAIA indicated for ophthalmic use in the U.S. The indication of Ocufen is to inhibit intraoperative miosis induced by prostaglandins in cataract surgery. Thus, flurbiprofen is an inhibitor of prostaglandin synthesis. The oral form was introduced in 1988 as Ansaid (another nonsteroidal anti-inflammatory drug) and gained immediate acceptance. In acute inflammation assays in adrenalectomized rats, flurbiprofen was found to be 536 times more potent than aspirin and 100 times more potent than phenylbutazone. Orally it was one-half as potent as methylprednisolone. As an antipyretic it was 403 times as potent as aspirin in the yeast-induced fever assay in rats and was 26 times more potent than ibuprofen as an antinociceptive.

Absorption and Metabolism. Flurbiprofen is well absorbed after oral administration. Although food alters the rate of absorption it does not alter the extent of its bioavailability. Flurbiprofen is extensively bound to plasma proteins and has a plasma half-life of 2–4 hours (Table 32.5). Metabolism is extensive with 60–70% of flurbiprofen and its metabolites being excreted as sulfate and glucuronide conjugates and 20–25% of the drug being excreted unchanged. None of these metabolites demonstrates significant anti-inflammatory activity. The metabolism of flurbiprofen is presented in Figure 32.17.

Flurbiprofen is indicated as an oral formulation for the acute or long-term treatment of rheumatoid arthritis and osteoarthritis and as an ophthalmic solution for the inhibition of intraoperative miosis. The recommended oral dose and the ophthalmic dose and dosage forms are shown in Table 32.5.

Ketorolac Tromethamine. Ketorolac (Fig. 32.15) represents a cyclized heteroarylpropionic acid derivative with the α-methyl group being fused to the pyrrole ring. It was

Suprofen

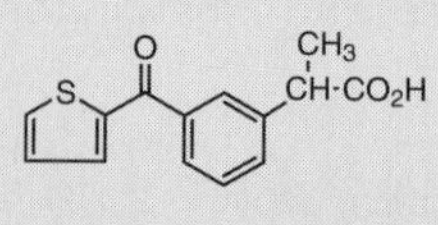

Suprofen (Profenal)

Suprofen is a white, microcrystalline powder that is slightly soluble in water. It was originally introduced in the U.S. in 1985 for the treatment of dysmenorrhea and as an analgesic for mild to moderate pain (52). Reports of severe flank pain and transient renal failure appeared abruptly within several hours after one or two doses and suprofen was removed from the U.S. market in 1987. Suprofen was re-introduced in the U.S. in 1990 as a 1% ophthalmic solution for the prevention of surgically-induced miosis during cataract extraction. Miosis complicates the removal of lens material and implantation of a posterior chamber intraocular lens that thus increases the risk of ocular trauma. The mechanism of action also involves inhibition of prostaglandin synthesis because prostaglandins constrict the iris sphincter independent of a cholinergic mechanism. Additionally, prostaglandins also break down the blood-aqueous barrier allowing the influx of plasma proteins into aqueous humor resulting in an increase in intraocular pressure.

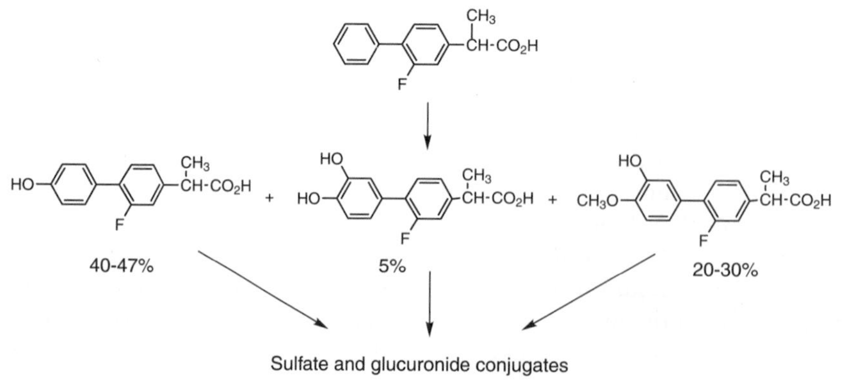

introduced in 1990 and is indicated as a peripheral analgesic for short-term use and for the relief of ocular itching caused by seasonal allergic conjunctivitis, although it exhibits anti-inflammatory and antipyretic activity as well. It was initially introduced only in an injectable form but recently an oral formulation has been made available. Its analgesic activity resembles that of the centrally acting analgesics with 15–30 mg of ketorolac producing equivalent analgesia as a 12 mg dose of morphine and it has become a widely accepted alternative to narcotic analgesia. Ketorolac inhibits prostaglandin synthesis. Although the analgesic effect is achieved within 10 minutes of injection, peak analgesia lags behind peak plasma levels by 45–90 minutes. The free acid has a pKa of 3.54 and is highly

Fig. 32.17. Metabolism of flurbiprofen.

plasma protein bound (Table 32.5). Ketorolac is metabolized to the *p*-hydroxy derivative and to conjugates that are excreted primarily in the urine.

Ketorolac tromethamine is available as an injectable solution and as tablets for analgesia and as a 0.5% solution for ocular use. The recommended intramuscular dose is 30–60 mg as a loading dose followed by one-half the loading dose every 6 hours. The oral dose is shown in Table 32.5. The recommended dose for ocular itching is 1 drop (0.25 mg) 4 times a day.

Oxaprozin. Oxaprozin (Fig. 32.15) is a white to off-white powder that is insoluble in water and slightly soluble in alcohol. It was marketed in 1993 for acute and long-term use in the management of signs and symptoms of osteoarthritis and rheumatoid arthritis. oavailability. The recommended dose and dosage forms are shown in Table 32.5.

N-Arylanthranilic Acids (Fenamic Acids)

The anthranilic acid class of NSAIAs is the result of the application of classical medicinal chemistry bioisosteric drug design concepts since these derivatives are nitrogen isosteres of salicylic acid. In the early 1960s, the Parke-Davis research group reported the development of a series of N-substituted anthranilic acids that have been since given the chemical class name of fenamic acids. The fact that this class of compounds possesses little advantage over the salicylates with respect to their anti-inflammatory and analgesic properties has diminished interest in their large scale development relative to the arylalkanoic acids. Mefenamic acid was introduced in the U.S. in 1967 as an analgesic and this remains the primary indication despite the fact that it possesses modest anti-inflammatory activity. Flufenamic acid has been available in Europe as an antirheumatic agent but there are no apparent plans to introduce this drug in the U.S. With regard to anti-inflammatory activity, mefenamic acid is approximately 1.5 times as potent as phenylbutazone and one-half as potent as flufenamic acid. Meclofenamic acid was introduced in the U.S. as its sodium salt in 1980 primarily as an antirheumatic agent and analgesic. The structures of these fenamic acids are shown in Figure 32.18.

The fenamic acids share a number of pharmacologic properties with the other NSAIAs. Since these agents are potent inhibitors of prostaglandin biosynthesis, it is tempting to speculate that this represents their primary mechanism of action. Scherrer, like Shen, had proposed a hypothetical receptor for NSAIAs and later modified the receptor to represent the active site of arachidonic acid cyclooxygenase (53a). Structurally, the fenamic acids fit the proposed active site of arachidonic acid cyclooxygenase proposed by Shen (Fig. 32.1) since they possess an acidic function connected to an aromatic ring along with an additional lipophilic binding site, in this case the N-aryl substituent (11). The greater anti-inflammatory activity of meclofenamic acid compared to that of mefenamic acid

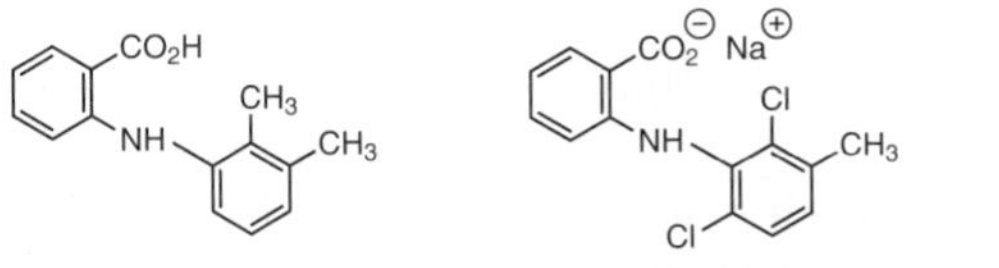

Fig. 32.18. Structures of N-arylanthranilic acids (fenamic acids).

correlates well with the ability to inhibit prostaglandin synthesis. Scherrer (53b) compared the in vivo anti-inflammatory activities, clinical anti-inflammatory doses in humans, and the in vitro inhibition of prostaglandin synthesis activities of mefenamic acid, meclofenamic acid, phenylbutazone, indomethacin and aspirin and suggested an important role of prostaglandin synthesis inhibition in the production of therapeutic effects of the fenamic acids.

Side effects are those primarily associated with GI disturbances (dyspepsia, discomfort, and especially diarrhea), some CNS effects (dizziness, headache, drowsiness), skin rashes and transient hepatic and renal abnormalities. Isolated cases of hemolytic anemia have been reported.

General Structure-activity Relationships. Substitution on the anthranilic acid ring generally reduces activity while substitution of the N-aryl ring can lead to conflicting results. In the UV erythema assay for anti-inflammatory activity, the order of activity is generally $3' > 2' >> 4'$ for monosubstitution with the $3'$-CF_3 derivative (flufenamic acid) being particularly potent. The opposite order of activity was observed, however, in the rat paw edema assay with the $2'$-Cl derivative being more potent than the $3'$-Cl analogue. In disubstituted derivatives, where the nature of the two substituents is the same, $2,'3'$-disubstitution appears to be the most effective. A plausible explanation may be found in an examination of the proposed topography of the active sites of arachidonic acid cyclooxygenase using either the Shen or Sherrer models. Proposed binding sites include a hydrophobic trough to which a lipophilic group, non-coplanar with the ring bearing the carboxylic acid function, binds. Substituents on the N-aryl ring which force this ring to be non-coplanar with the anthranilic acid ring should enhance binding at this site and thus enhance activity. This may account for the enhanced anti-inflammatory activity of meclofenamic acid (which has two ortho-substituents forcing this ring out of the plane of the anthranilic acid ring) over flufenamic acid (no ortho-substituents) and mefenamic acid (one ortho-substituent). Meclofenamic acid possesses 25 times greater anti-inflammatory activity than mefenamic acid. The NH-moiety of anthranilic acid appears to be essential for activity since replacement of the NH function with O, CH_2, S, SO_2, N-CH_3 or N-$COCH_3$ functionalities significantly reduces activity. Finally, the position, rather than the nature, of the acidic function is critical for activity. Anthranilic acid derivatives are active whereas the *m*- and *p*-aminobenzoic acid analogs are not. Replacement of the carboxylic acid function with the isosteric tetrazole moiety has little effect on activity.

Drug Interactions.   The pKa's of the N-arylanthranilic acids (4.0–4.2) resemble those of the arylalkanoic acids, thus it is not surprising that they are strongly bound to plasma proteins with interactions with other drugs which are highly protein bound being very probable. The most common interactions reported are those of mefenamic acid and meclofenamic acid with oral anticoagulants. Concurrent administration of aspirin results in a reduction of plasma levels of meclofenamic acid.

Mefenamic Acid—Absorption and Metabolism.   Mefenamic acid (Fig. 32.18) is a white to off-white crystalline solid that possesses a bitter aftertaste. It will darken if exposed to light for long periods of time but is otherwise stable at room temperature. It is virtually water insoluble except at alkaline pH. It was first reported in 1962 (54). Mefenamic acid is the only fenamic acid derivative that produces analgesia centrally and peripherally.

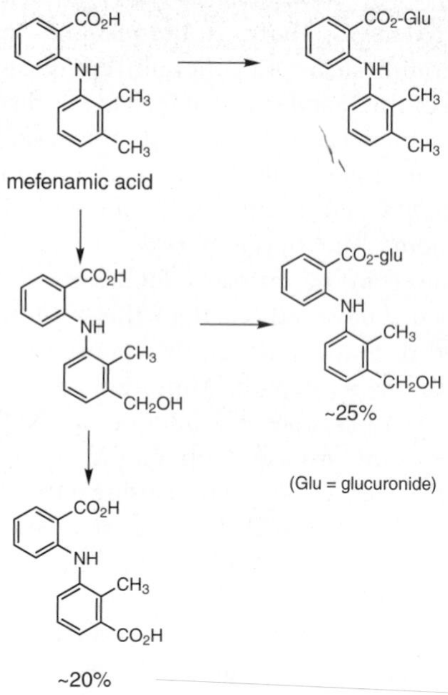

Fig. 32.19. Metabolism of mefenamic acid.

Mefenamic acid is absorbed rapidly following oral administration with peak plasma levels being attained within 2–4 hours. It is highly bound to plasma proteins and has a plasma half-life of 2–4 hours (Table 32.6). Metabolism occurs through regioselective oxidation of the 3'-methyl group and glucuronidation of mefenamic acid and its metabolites. Urinary excretion accounts for approximately 50–55% of an administered dose with unchanged drug accounting for 6%, the 3'-hydroxymethyl metabolite (primarily as the glucuronide) accounting for 25% and the remaining 20% as the dicarboxylic acid (of which 30% is the glucuronide conjugate) (Fig. 32.19). These metabolites are essentially inactive.

Mefenamic acid is indicated for the short term relief of moderate pain and for primary dysmenorrhea. The recommended dose and dosage forms are shown in Table 32.6.

Meclofenamate Sodium—Absorption and Metabolism. Meclofenamate sodium (Fig. 32.18) is a white powder which is highly water soluble. The pH of the aqueous solution is 8.7 (55).

Meclofenamate sodium is rapidly and almost completely absorbed following oral administration. It is highly bound to plasma proteins and has a plasma half-life of 2–4 hours (Table 32.6). Metabolism involves oxidation of the methyl group, aromatic hydroxylation, monodehalogenation and conjugation. Urinary excretion accounts for approximately 75% of the administered dose. The major metabolite is the product of methyl oxidation and has been shown possess anti-inflammatory activity. The metabolism of meclofenamic acid is illustrated in Figure 32.20.

Meclofenamate sodium is indicated for the relief of mild to moderate pain, the acute and chronic treatment of rheumatoid arthritis and osteoarthritis, treatment of primary dysmenorrhea, and treatment of idiopathic heavy menstrual blood loss. The analgesic and arthritic dose and dosage forms are shown in Table 32.6

Oxicams

The new enolic acid class of NSAIAs has been termed "oxicams" by the USAN Council to describe the series of 4-hydroxy-1,2-benzothiazine carboxamides that possess anti-inflammatory and analgesic properties. These structurally distinct agents resulted from extensive studies by the Pfizer

Table 32.6. Pharmacokinetic Properties of N-arylanthranilic Acids and Oxicams

Drug	Trade Name	Peakblood Level (hr)	Plasma Binding (%)	pKa	Analgesic Dose (mg/day)	Dosage Forms (mg/unit)
Mefenamic acid	Ponstel	2–4	78.5	4.2	1000	Cap (250)
Meclofenamide sodium	(Generic)	2	99.8	4.0	200–400	Cap (50, 100)
Piroxicam	Feldene	2	99.3	6.3	20	Cap (10, 20)
Meloxicam	Mobic	5–11	99.1–99.7	—	7.5–15	Tab

Tab = Tablet; Cap = Capsule.

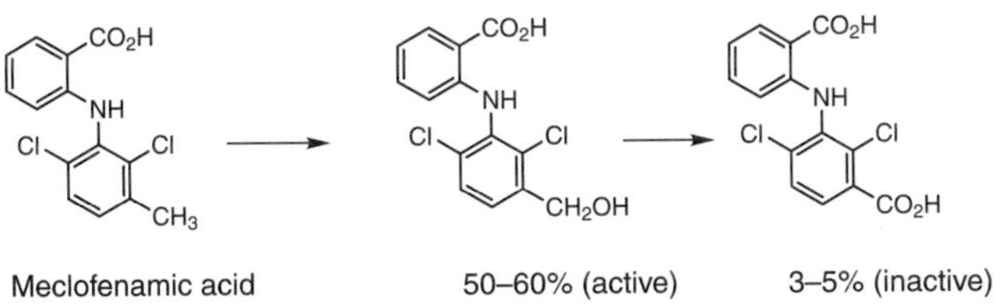

Fig. 32.20. Metabolism of meclofenamic acid.

group in an effort to produce non-carboxylic acid, potent, and well-tolerated anti-inflammatory agents. Several series were prepared and evaluated including 2-aryl-1,3-indanediones, 2-arylbenzothiophen-3-(2H)-one 1,1-dioxides, dioxoquinoline-4-carboxamides and 3-oxa-2H-1,2-benzothiazine-4-carboxamide 1,1-dioxides. These results, combined with the previously known activity of 1,3-dicarbonyl derivatives such as phenylbutazone, led to the development of the oxicams. The first member of this class, piroxicam, was introduced in the U.S. in 1982 as Feldene and gained immediate acceptance, ranking among the top 50 prescription drugs in the U.S. for several years. Although piroxicam remains the only agent of this class in therapeutic use today, several other members of this class are being clinically evaluated and represent a potentially important class of NSAIAs.

Piroxicam is potent in standard in vivo assays, being 200 times more potent than aspirin and at least 10 times as potent as any other standard agent in the UV erythema assay, as potent as indomethacin and more potent than phenylbutazone or naproxen in the carrageenan rat paw edema assay, and equipotent with indomethacin and 15 times more potent than phenylbutazone in the rat adjuvant arthritis assay. It is less potent than indomethacin, equipotent with aspirin, and more potent than fenoprofen, ibuprofen, naproxen and phenylbutazone as an analgetic in the phenylquinone writhing assay. Piroxicam inhibits the migration of polymorphonuclear cells into inflammatory sites and inhibits the release of lysosomal enzymes from these cells. It also inhibits collagen-induced platelet aggregation. It is an effective inhibitor of arachidonic acid cyclooxygenase, being almost equipotent with indomethacin and more potent than ibuprofen, tolmetin, naproxen, fenoprofen, phenylbutazone and aspirin in the inhibition of prostaglandin biosynthesis by methylcholanthrene-transformed mouse fibroblasts (MC-5) assay. A template for designing anti-inflammatory agents based upon CPK space filling models of the peroxy radical precursor of PGG and inhibitors of cyclooxygenase was proposed and the ability of oxicams, particularly piroxicam, to inhibit this enzyme was subsequently rationalized on the ability of oxicams to assume a conformation resembling that of the peroxy radical precursor (56,57).

Approximately 20% of individuals on piroxicam report adverse reactions. Not unexpectedly, the greatest incidence of side effects are those resulting from GI disturbances. The incidence of peptic ulcers reported is less than 1%, however.

As will be discussed later, a new oxicam derivative, meloxicam, has been approved as an selective COX-2 inhibitor for the treatment of osteoarthritis.

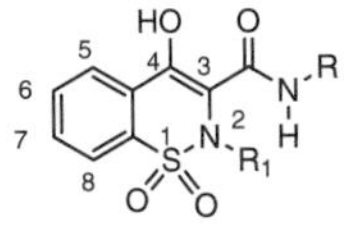

General Structure-activity Relationships. Within the series of 4-hydroxy-1,2-benzothiazine carboxamides represented by the general structure shown above, optimum activity was observed when R1 was a methyl substituent. The carboxamide substituent, R, is generally an aryl or heteroaryl substituent since alkyl substituents are less active. Oxicams are acidic compounds with pKa's in the range of 4–6. N-Heterocyclic carboxamides are generally more acidic than the corresponding N-aryl carboxamides and this enhanced acidity was attributed to stabilization of the enolate anion by the pyridine nitrogen atom as illustrated in tautomer A and additional stabilization by tautomer B (58):

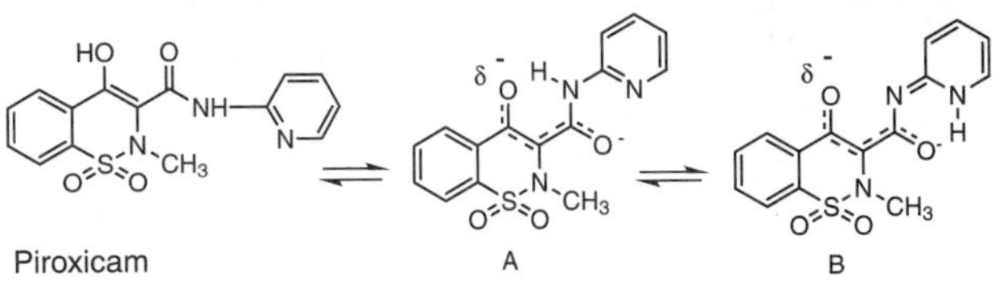

This explains the observation that primary carboxamides are more potent than the corresponding secondary derivatives since no N-H bond would be available to enhance the stabilization of the enolate anion. When the aryl group is o-substituted, variable results were obtained while m-substituted derivatives are generally more potent than the corresponding p-isomers. In the aryl series, maximum activity is observed with a m-Cl substituent. No direct correlations were observed between acidity and activity, partition coefficient, electronic or spatial properties in this series. However, two major differences are observed when R = heteroaryl rather than aryl: pKa's are generally 2–4 units lower and anti-inflammatory activity increased as much as 7-fold. The greatest activity is associated with the 2-pyridyl (as in piroxicam), 2-thiazolyl, or 3-(5-methyl)isoxazolyl ring systems, the latter derivative (isoxicam) having been withdrawn from the European market in 1985 following several reports of severe skin reactions. In addition to possessing activity equal to or greater than indomethacin in the carrageenan rat paw edema assay, the heteroaryl carboxamides also possess longer plasma half-lives providing an improvement in dosing scheduling regimens.

General Metabolism. Although the metabolism of piroxicam varies quantitatively from species to species, qualitative similarities are found in the metabolic pathways found in humans, rats, dogs, and rhesus monkeys. It is extensively metabolized in humans with less than 5% of an administered dose being excreted unchanged. The major metabolites in humans result from hydroxylation of the pyridine ring and subsequent glucuronidation, other metabolites being of lesser importance. Aromatic hydroxylation at several positions of the aromatic benzothiazine ring also occurs; two hydroxylated metabolites have been extracted from rat urine. On the basis of NMR deuterium-exchange studies, hydroxylation at the 8-position was ruled out indicating that hydroxylation occurs at two of the remaining positions. Other novel metabolic reactions occur. Cyclodehydration gave a tetracyclic metabolite (the major metabolite in dogs) while ring contraction following amide hydrolysis and decarboxylation eventually yields saccharin (Fig. 32.21). All of the known metabolites of piroxicam lack anti-inflammatory activity. Related oxicams undergo different routes of metabolism. For example, sudoxicam (the N-2–thiazolyl analogue) undergoes primarily hydroxylation of the thiazole ring following by ring-opening while isoxicam undergoes primarily cleavage reactions of the benzothiazine ring.

Drug Interactions. Few reports of therapeutically significant interactions of oxicams with other drugs have appeared. Concurrent administration of aspirin has been shown to reduce piroxicam plasma levels by about 20% while the anticoagulant effect of acenocoumarin is potentiated presumably as a result of plasma protein displacement.

Piroxicam. Piroxicam is a white crystalline solid which is sparingly soluble in water. The parent ring system is synthesized by ring expansion reactions of saccharin derivatives (59). Piroxicam is readily absorbed on oral administration reaching peak plasma levels in about 2 hours (Table 32.6). Food does not markedly affect bioavailability of piroxicam, but may effect peak plasma levels when administered at low doses (30 mg) but not at higher doses (60 mg). Being acidic (pKa = 6.3) it is highly bound to plasma proteins (99.3%). Piroxicam possesses an extended plasma half-life (38 hours) making single daily dosing possible.

Piroxicam is indicated for long-term use in rheumatoid arthritis and osteoarthritis. The initial recommended maintenance dose is a single 20 mg dose that may be divided.

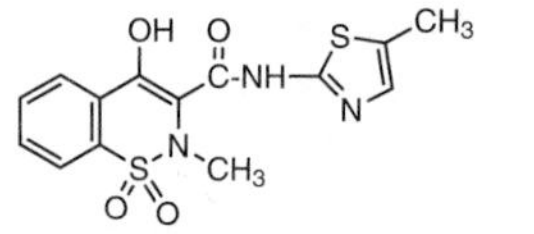

Meloxicam

Meloxicam. In April, 2000, the FDA approved meloxicam for the treatment of osteoarthritis. When meloxicam was initially introduced in the United Kingdom it was advertised and promoted as a selective COX-2 inhibitor. However, meloxicam is less selective than either of the two COX-2 inhibitors (celecoxib and rofecoxib- see Selective cycloxygenase-2 inhibitors) in vitro studies. Meloxicam is readily absorbed when administered orally and highly bound to plasma protein (Table 32.6). Meloxicam is extensive metabolized in the liver primarily by CYP2C and to a lesser extent by CYP3A4.

Gastroenteropathy Induced by Non-COX Selective NSAIAs

The effectiveness and popularity of the NSAIAs in the U.S. and Europe make this class one of the most commonly used classes of therapeutic entities. Over 75 million prescriptions are written annually for the NSAIAs, including aspirin. Unfortunately, until the recent introduction of the COX-2 selective inhibitors, almost all of the current agents, which are nonselective COX-1 and COX-2 inhibitors, share the undesirable property of producing damaging effects to gastric and intestinal mucosa resulting in erosion, ulcers, and gastrointestinal bleeding and these represent the major adverse reactions to the use of NSAIAs. As many as 20,000 deaths and 100,000 hospitalizations a year have been associated with GI complications resulting from the use of NSAIAs. Approximately 30–40% of patients taking NSAIAs report some type of gastric injury and about 10% discontinue therapy because of these effects. These acute and chronic injuries to gastric mucosa result in a variety of lesions referred to as NSAIA "gastropathy" which differs from peptic ulcer disease by their localization more frequently in the stomach rather than in the duodenum. NSAIA-induced lesions also occur more frequently in the

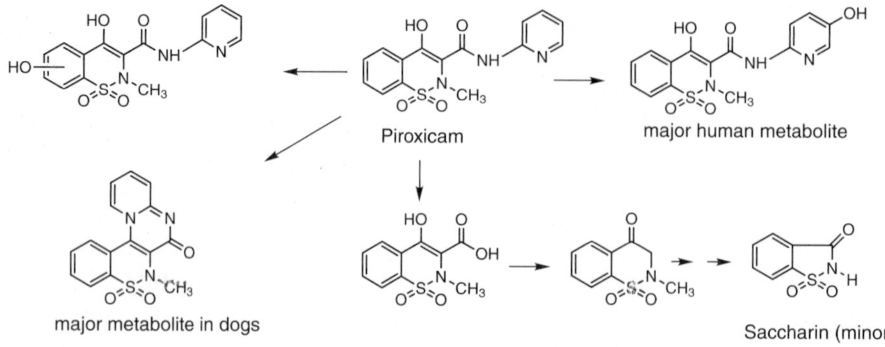

Fig. 32.21. Metabolism of piroxicam.

elderly than typical peptic ulcers. Normally the stomach protects itself from the harmful effects of hydrochloric acid and pepsin by a number of protective mechanisms referred to as the "gastric mucosal barrier" which consists of epithelial cells, the mucus and bicarbonate layer and mucosal blood flow. Gastric mucosa is actually a gel consisting of polymers of glycoprotein which limit the diffusion of hydrogen ions. These polymers reduce the rate at which hydrogen ions (produced in the lumen) and bicarbonate ions (secreted by the mucosa) mix and thus a pH gradient is created across the mucus layer. Normally, gastric mucosal cells are rapidly repaired when they are damaged by factors such as food, ethanol or acute ingestion of NSAIAs. Among the cytoprotective mechanisms is the ability of prostaglandins of the PGE series, particularly PGE_1, to increase the secretion of bicarbonate ion and mucus and to maintain mucosal blood flow. PGs also decrease acid secretion permitting the gastric mucosal barrier to remain intact.

As mentioned earlier, Figure 32.13 illustrates the ability of aspirin and NSAIAs to induce gastric damage by a dual insult mechanism. Aspirin and the NSAIAs are acidic substances which can damage the GI tract, even in the absence of hydrochloric acid, by changing the permeability of cell membranes allowing a back diffusion of hydrogen ions. These weak acids remain unionized in the stomach but the resulting lipophilic nature of these agents allows an accumulation or concentration in gastric mucosal cells. Once inside these cells, however, the higher pH of the intracellular environment causes the acids to dissociate and become "trapped" within the cells. The permeability of the mucosal cell membrane is thus altered and the accumulation of hydrogen ions causes mucosal cell damage. This gastric damage is a result, therefore, of the primary insult of acidic substances. As detailed earlier in this chapter, the primary mechanism of action of the NSAIAs is to inhibit the biosynthesis of PGs at the cyclooxygenase step. The resulting nonselective inhibition of PG biosynthesis in the GI tract prevents the PGs from exerting their protective mechanism on gastric mucosa and thus the NSAIAs induce gastric damage through this secondary insult mechanism.

Misoprostol

The use of PGE_1 to reduce NSAIA-induced gastric damage is limited by the fact that it is ineffective orally and degrades rapidly on parenteral administration, primarily by oxidation of the 15-hydroxy group. To overcome these limitations, misoprostol was synthesized as a PG pro-drug analogue. The orally active methyl ester is hydrolyzed to the active acid following absorption. Oxidation of the 15-hydroxy group was overcome by moving the hydroxy group to the 16-position thus "fooling" the enzyme prostaglandin 15-

OH dehydrogenase. Oxidation was further limited by the introduction of a methyl group at the 16-position producing a tertiary alcohol that is more difficult to oxidize than the secondary alcohol present in the PGs. Misoprostol was introduced in 1989 as a mixture of stereoisomers at the 16-position for the prevention of NSAIA-induced gastric ulcers (but not duodenal ulcers) in patients at high risk of complications from a gastric ulcer, particularly the elderly and patients with concomitant debilitating disease and in individuals with a history of gastric ulcers.

Selective Cycloxygenase-2 Inhibitors

Background. As discussed earlier, the most notable achievement in the development of NSAIAs has been in the area of selective COX-2 inhibitors. Classical NSAIAs share similar side effect profiles, particularly on the GI tract, many of which have been attributed to the inhibition of cyclooxygenase, the rate-limiting step in prostaglandin biosynthesis. With the discovery of two isoforms of cyclooxygenase, COX-1 and COX-2, and the realization that COX-1 is beneficial in maintaining normal processes in the GI tract by stimulating bicarbonate secretion and mucus and producing an overall reduction in acid secretion, the search for agents which selectively inhibit the COX-2 isoform has received much attention. The traditional NSAIAs inhibit COX-1, COX-2 and thromboxane synthetase with a varying degrees of selectivity. Decreased gastric mucosal protection (resulting in an enhanced risk of ulceration) and stress-induced decreased renal perfusion result from nonselective inhibition of COX. Inhibition of thromboxane synthesis results in increased prostaglandin synthesis, reduction in platelet aggregation, and an increased bleeding tendency. Those NSAIAs that have a greater selectivity for COX-1 generally cause greater gastrointestinal bleeding and renal toxicity than those with greater selectivity for COX-2.

NS-398   DuP 697

These early studies led to extensive efforts by many laboratories to develop selective inhibitors of the COX-2 isoform with the goal of developing NSAIAs that selectively inhibits COX-2, reducing the inflammatory response, but not interfering with the GI protective functions of COX-1. Two early lead compounds were developed, NS-398 and DuP 697, that have served as the basis of the development of two widely explored chemical classes. NS-398 is the prototype of compounds known as "sulides" while DuP 697 is the prototype of a class of COX-2 inhibitors named "coxibs." These efforts have led to the recent introduction of two selective COX-2 inhibitors in the U.S. market, celecoxib and rofecoxib while a number of other selective inhibitors are currently under investigation (Fig. 32.22). An excellent review of the various chemical classes of selective COX-2 inhibitors has recently appeared (60). Selective COX-2 inhibitors have been designed to take advantages of the much larger NSAIA binding site on COX-2 compared to the NSAIA binding site on COX-1 resulting from the substitution of the smaller amino acid valine in COX-2 for isoleucine at position 523 in COX-2 (see earlier discussion). In COX-1, the larger isoleucine residue near the active site restricts access by larger, relatively rigid side chain substituents, such as sulfamoyl or sulfonyl side chains usually seen in the selective COX-2 inhibitors.

A comparison of the selectivity of several NSAIAs, and selective COX-2 inhibitors was recently presented (Fig.

32.23) (61). In another study regarding the pharmacologic and biochemical profile of rofecoxib, the comparison shown in Table 32.7 of COX-1/COX-2 selectivity for rofecoxib, celecoxib, meloxicam, diclofenac and indomethacin was reported (62).

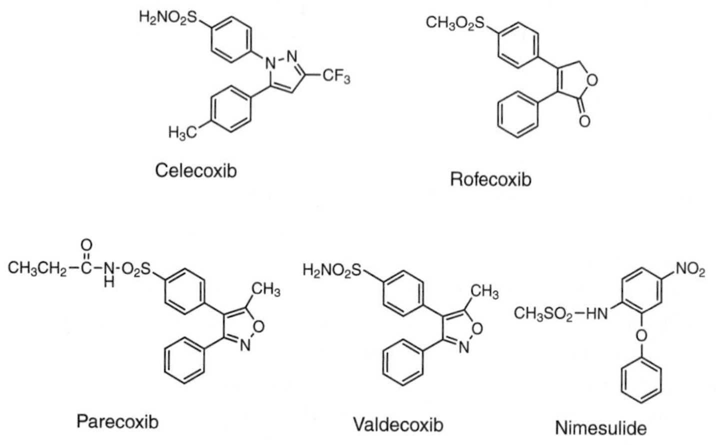

Among the NSAIAs, aspirin, indomethacin, diclofenac, piroxicam and 6–MNA (the active metabolite of nabumetone) are generally considered nonselective COX inhibitors, while celecoxib, rofecoxib, etodolac, meloxicam and numesulide are considered to be COX-2 selective.

Perhaps as interesting as the role that COX-2 selective inhibitors play in reducing the incidence of GI side effects among NSAIAs are the reports of other potential therapeutic uses for this new class of drugs including potential use in the treatment of Alzheimer's disease and various carcinomas. COX-2 appears to be induced in inflammatory plaques that are evident in the CNS in Alzheimer's disease. Several reports have appeared indicating that patients taking NSAIAs have a lower incidence and a decreased rate of progression of Alzheimer's disease. Epidemiological studies suggest a significant reduction in the risk for colon cancer in patients regularly taking aspirin. NSAIAs have also been reported to reduce the growth rate of polyps in the colon in humans as well as the incidence of tumors of the colon in animals. The expression of COX-2 appears to be significantly upregulated in carcinoma of the colon. The effectiveness of NSAIAs in the prevention and treatment of other cancers such as prostate cancer and mammary carcinoma has also been reported. This effectiveness is more noticeable among COX-2 selective agents.

Fig. 32.22. Structures of selective COX-2 inhibitors.

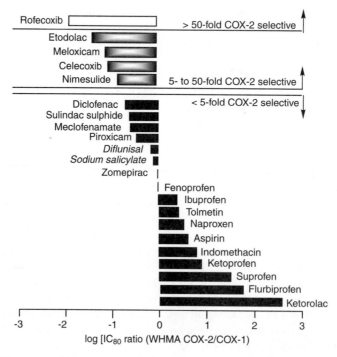

Fig. 32.23. Selectivity of COX-2 inhibitors and NSAIAs given as log inhibitory concentration (IC_{80}) ratio. The '0' line indicates equipotency. (Modified with permission from Warner TD, et al) (61).

Table 32.7. Selective vs. Nonselective COX Inhibitors

Drugs	COX-1/COX-2 Ratio
Rofecoxib	35.5
Celecoxib	6.6
Meloxicam	2.0
Diclofenac	3.0
Indomethacin	0.4

Preparations Available

Celecoxib. Celecoxib (Fig. 32.22) is an odorless, white to off-white crystalline powder that is very slightly soluble in water. Solubility increases in strongly basic solutions. The synthesis of celecoxib was reported in 1997 (63). It was the first NSAIA marketed as a selective COX-2 inhibitor. Celecoxib is well absorbed from the GI tract with peak plasma concentrations being generally attained within 3 hours of administration (Table 32.8). Peak plasma levels in geriatric patients may be increased but dosage adjustments in elderly patients are not generally required unless the patient weighs less than 50 kg. Celecoxib is excreted in the urine and feces primarily as inactive metabolites with less than 3% of an administered dose being excreted as unchanged drug. Metabolism occurs primarily in the liver by the cytochrome CYP2C9 and involves hyrdoxylation of the 4-methyl group to the primary alcohol which is further oxidized to the corresponding carboxylic acid, the major metabolite (73% of the administered dose) (Fig. 32.24).

The carboxylic acid is conjugated to a slight extent with glucuronic acid to form the corresponding glucuronide. None of the isolated metabolites have been shown to exhibit pharmacologic activity as inhibitors of either COX-1 or COX-2. Celecoxib also inhibits CYP2D6, thus the potential of celecoxib to alter the pharmacokinetic profiles of other drugs inhibited by this isoenzyme exists. However, celecoxib does not appear to inhibit other isoenzymes. Other drug interactions related to the metabolic profile of celecoxib have been noted particularly with other drugs that inhibit CYP2C. For example, co-administraiton of celecoxib with fluconazole can significantly increase plasma concentration of celecoxib since fluconazole inhibits CYP2C9.

Celecoxib is currently indicated for the relief of signs and symptoms of osteoarthritis and rheumatoid arthritis,

and to reduce the number of adenomatous colorectal polyps in familial adenomatous polyposis as an adjunct to usual care. Celecoxib is at least as effective as naproxen in the symptomatic management of osetoarthritis and at least as effective as naproxen and diclofenac in the symptomatic treatment of rheumatoid arthritis, and is less likely to cause adverse G.I. effects. Celecoxib appears to be effective in the management of pain associated with both of these arthritic conditions, but effectiveness in acute or chronic pain has not been fully demonstrated. Unlike aspirin, celecoxib does not exhibit antiplatelet activity. Concomitant administration of aspirin and celecoxib may increase the incidence of GI side effects. Another notable potential drug interaction with celecoxib is its ability, like other NSAIAs, to reduce the blood pressure response to angiotensin-converting enzyme inhibitors. A more detailed discussion of the chemical, pharmacologic, pharmacokinetic and clinical aspects of celecoxib is available (64).

The recommended dose and dosage forms are shown in Table 32.8.

Rofecoxib. Rofecoxib (Fig. 32.22) is a white to off-white to light yellow powder that is only slightly soluble in water. Rofecoxib has been synthesized by a number of synthetic routes that have been summarized (65). It was the second selective COX-2 inhibitor to be marketed. Rofecoxib is well absorbed from the GI tract on oral administration with peak plasma levels being generally attained within

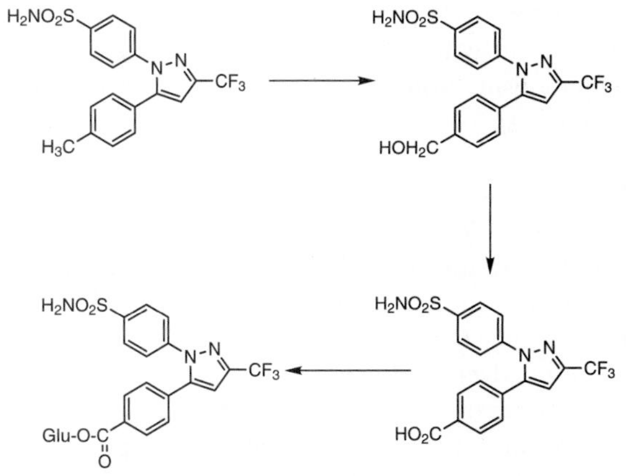

Fig. 32.24. Metabolism of celecoxib.

Table 32.8. Properties of COX-2 Inhibitors

Drugs	Trade Name	Peak Blood Level (hr)	Utility	Dose (mg/day)	Dosage Form (mg/unit)
Celecoxib	Celebrex	3	Osteoarthritis	200	Cap (100, 200)
			Rheumatous arthritis	100–200	
			Adenomatous colorectal polyps	—	
Rofecoxib	Vioxx	2–3	Osteoarthritis	12.5–25	Tab (12.5, 25),
			Postoperative dental pain	50	Susp (12.5,
			Dysmennorhea	50	25/5ml)

Tab = Tablets; Cap = capsule; Susp = suspension.

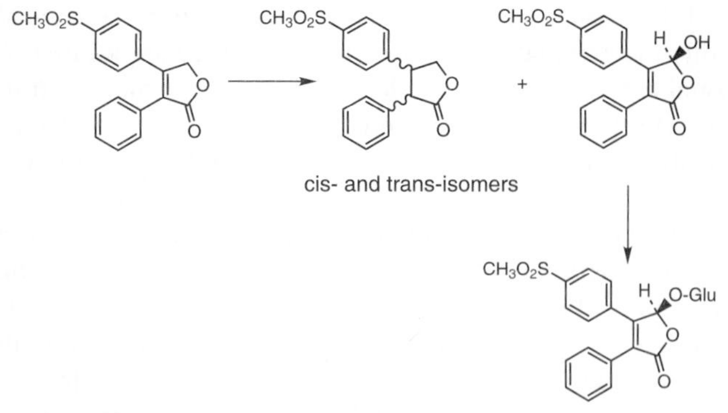

Fig. 32.25. Metabolism of rofecoxib.

2–3 hours of dosing (Table 32.8). Bioavailability averages 93% following administration of a single dose. The area under the plasma concentration time curve (AUC) is increased in patients over the age of 65 compared to younger adults and is increased slightly in black and Hispanic patients compared with white individuals but the difference is not considered to be clinically significant.

Rofecoxib is excreted primarily in the urine (72%) as metabolites. Less than 1% is excreted in the urine as unchanged drug while about 14% is excreted in the feces as unchanged drug. Although the metabolism of rofecoxib has not been fully determined, the microsomal CYP450 system appears to play only a minor role—a major difference in the metabolic routes of rofecoxib and celecoxib. The major metabolic route appears to lead to the *cis* and *trans* γ-lactone (Fig. 32.25). Also isolated is the glucuronide of a hydroxy derivative that results from oxidative metabolism. None of the isolated metabolites of rofecoxib possess pharmacological activity as COX-1 or COX-2 inhibitors.

Rofecoxib is indicated for the relief of the signs and symptoms of osteoarthritis, for the management of acute pain in adults, and for the treatment of primary dysmenorhea. Rofecoxib, diclofenac and ibuprofen possess comparable efficacy in the treatment of osteoarthritis but serious GI tract adverse effects are observed with rofecoxib. In the treatment of pain, 50 mg of rofecoxib, 550 mg of naproxen sodium and 400 mg of ibuprofen possess similar effects. Similar ratios of effectiveness are seen between rofecoxib, naproxen sodium, and ibuprofen for treatment of postoperative dental pain and between rofecoxib and naproxen sodium for the treatment of primary dysmenorhea in female adults (Table 32.8). Like celecoxib, rofecoxib does not affect platelet aggregation or bleeding and should not be used as a substitute for aspirin in the prevention of cardiovascular events. A more detailed discussion of the chemical, pharmacologic, pharmacokinetic and clinical aspects of rofecoxib is available (66).

The recommended dose and dosage forms of rofecoxib are shown in Table 32.8. The bioavailability of rofecoxib following administration of tablets and suspensions appears to be the same.

Disease-modifying Antirheumatic Drugs (DMARDs)

The agents previously discussed as NSAIAs, both the non-selective COX and selective COX-2 inhibitors, have proven to be beneficial in the symptomatic treatment of arthritic disorders and have proven to be a popular therapeutic regimen. Despite their effectiveness and popularity, however, it should be remembered that none of these agents are effective in preventing or inhibiting the underlying pathogenic, chronic inflammatory processes. Recent interest has been generated by agents which are effective in the treatment of arthritic disorders yet fail to demonstrate significant activity in the standard screening assays for anti-arthritic agents. Disease-modifying antirheumatic drugs (DMARDs) differ from the previously discussed drugs in that they are agents which retard or halt the underlying progression of arthritis while lacking anti-inflammatory and analgesic effects observed for the NSAIAs. They are much slower acting, taking as long as three months for measurable clinical benefits to be observed. These agents also possess potentially dangerous adverse side effects, which, in many cases, limit their long-term use. Yet DMARDs are effective in reducing joint destruction and the progression of arthritic disorders in patients. The group of drugs which comprise the DMARDs include the gold compounds, some 4-aminoquinolines, and immunosuppressive agents (Fig. 32.26).

Gold Compounds

Historical Background. At the end of the 19th century the chemotherapeutic applications of heavy metal derivatives were gaining considerable interest. Among those metals receiving the greatest attention were gold compounds (or gold salts). The first of these, gold cyanide, was effective in vitro against *Mycobacterium tuberculosis*. This discovery prompted others to extend the use of gold compounds in other disease states thought to be tubercular in origin. Early clinical observations had suggested similarities in the symptoms of tuberculosis and rheumatoid arthritis and some thought rheumatoid arthritis to be an atypical form of tuberculosis. In 1927, aurothioglucose was found to relieve joint pain when used to treat bacterial endocarditis. The area of chrysotherapy had begun. Subsequent investigations led to an extensive study of gold compounds in Great Britain by the Empire Rheumatism Council which reported in 1961 that sodium aurothiomalate was effective in slowing the development of progressive joint diseases. Both aurothioglucose and sodium aurothiomalate are orally ineffective and have to be administered by injection. In 1985 the first orally effective gold compound for arthritis, auranofin, was introduced in the U.S. Several other gold compounds have been evaluated clinically but do not appear to offer efficacy or toxicity advantages.

Mechanism of Action. The biochemical and pharmacologic properties shared by gold compounds are quite di-

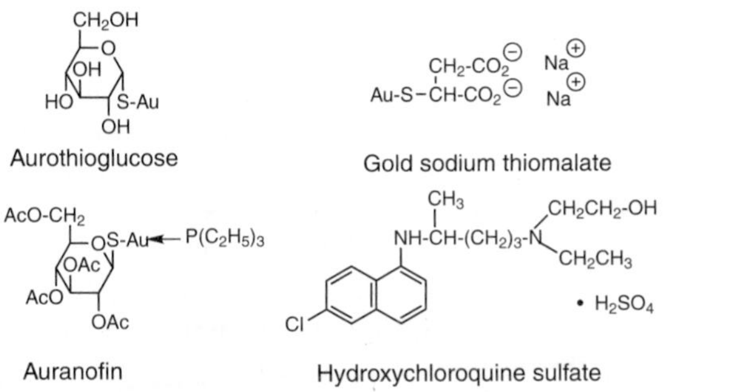

Fig. 32.26. Structures of Disease-Modifying Antirheumatic Drugs (DMARDs)

verse. The mechanism by which they produce their antirheumatic actions has not been totally determined. The following observations and mechanisms have been proposed: 1) the earlier observations that gold compounds were effective in preventing arthritis induced by hemolytic streptococci and by pleuropneumonia-like organisms led to the postulation that they acted through an antimicrobial mechanism. The inability of gold compounds to consistently inhibit mycoplasma growth in vitro while still inhibiting the arthritic process independent of microbial origins, however, argued against this mechanism. 2) The involvement of immunologic processes in the pathogenesis of arthritis suggested that a direct suppression of the immunologic response by gold compounds was involved. While enzymatic mediators released as a result of the immune response may be inhibited by gold compounds, no direct effect on either immediate or delayed cellular responses is evident to support an immunosuppressive mechanism. 3) Suggestions have been made that through protein denaturation and macroglobulin formation, proteins become antigenic and thus initiate an immune response producing biochemical changes in connective tissue which ultimately leads to rheumatoid arthritis. The possibility that gold compounds inhibit the aggregation of macroglobulins and in turn inhibit the formation of immune complexes may account for their ability to slow connective tissue degradation. Interaction with collagen fibrils and thus reduction of collagen reactivity that alters the course of the arthritic process has been also postulated. 4) Perhaps the most widely accepted mechanism of action is related to the ability of gold compounds to inhibit lysosomal enzymes, the release of which promotes the inflammatory response. The lysosomal enzymes glucuronidase, acid phosphatase, collagenase and acid hydrolases are inhibited presumable through a reversible interaction of gold with sulfhydryl groups on the enzymes. Other enzmyes inhibited by gold compounds include: Gold thiomalate inhibition of glucosamine-6-phosphate synthetase, a rate-limiting step in mucopolysaccharide biosynthesis, a property shared to a lesser extent by several NSAIAs; gold sodium thiosulfate a potent uncoupler of oxidative phosphorylation; and gold sodium thiomalate a fairly effective inhibitor of pro-

staglandin biosynthesis in vitro. The relationship of the latter inhibition to the antiarthritic actions of gold compounds has not been clarified.

Side Effects. Toxic side effects have been associated with the use of gold compounds with the incidence of reported adverse reactions in patients on chrysotherapy being as high as 55%. Serious toxicity occurs in 5–10% of reported cases. The most common adverse reactions include dermatitis (erythema, papular, vesicular and exfoliative dermatitis), mouth lesions (stomatitis preceded by a metallic taste and gingivitis), pulmonary disorders (interstitial pneumonitis), nephritis (albuminuria and glomerulitis) and hematologic disorders (thrombocytopenic purpura, hypoplastic and aplastic anemia, and eosinophilia; blood dyscrasias are rare in incidence but can be severe). Less commonly reported reactions are GI disturbances (nausea, anorexia and diarrhea), ocular toxicity (keratitis with inflammation and ulceration of the cornea and subepithelial deposition of gold in the cornea), and hepatitis. In those cases in which severe toxicity occurs, excretion of gold can be markedly enhanced by the administration of chelating agents, the two most common of which are dimercaprol (British Anti-Lewisite, BAL) and penicillamine. Corticoids also suppress the symptoms of gold toxicity and the concomitant administration of dimercaprol and corticosteroids has been recommended in cases of severe gold intoxication.

General Structure-activity Relationships. Structure-activity relationships of gold compounds have not received a great amount of attention. Two important relationships have been established, however: 1) monovalent gold (aurous ion, Au$^+$) is more effective than trivalent gold (auric ion, Au^{3+}) or colloidal gold and 2) only those compounds in which aurous ion is attached to a sulfur-containing ligand are active (Fig 36.26). The nature of the ligands affects tissue distribution and excretion properties and are usually highly polar, water-soluble functions. Aurous ion has only a brief existence in solution and is rapidly converted to metallic gold or to auric ion. Aqueous solutions decompose on standing at room temperature posing a stability problem for the two injectable gold compounds therapeutically available (aurothioglucose and gold sodium thiomalate). Complexation of Au$^+$ with phosphine ligands stabilizes the reduced valence state and results in nonionic complexes that are soluble in organic solvents and an enhancement of oral bioavailability. Other changes also occur. In the phosphine-Au-S compounds gold has a coordination number of 2 and the molecules are nonconducting monomers in solution. The injectable gold compounds are monocoordinated. Whereas nongold phosphine compounds are ineffective in arthritic assays, the nature of the phosphine ligand in the gold coordination complexes appears to play a greater role in antiarthritic activity than the other groups bound to gold. Within a homologous series, the triethylphosphine gold derivatives provide greatest activity.

Absorption and Metabolism. Gold compounds are generally rapidly absorbed following intramuscular injection and the gold is widely distributed in body tissues with highest concentrations found in the reticuloendothelial system and in adrenal and renal cortices. Binding of gold from orally administered gold to red blood cells is higher than in injectable gold. Gold accumulates in inflamed joints where high levels persist for at least 20 days following injection. Although gold is excreted primarily in the urine, the bulk of injected gold is retained.

Drug Interactions. The only significant drug interactions reported are the concurrent administration of drugs that also produce blood dyscrasias (most notably phenylbutazone and the antimalarial and immunosuppressive drugs) and one report suggesting that phenytoin blood levels may be increased when auranofin and phenytoin are co-administered.

Preparations Available

Gold Sodium Thiomalate. Gold sodium thiomalate (Fig. 32.26)—actually a mixture of mono- and disodium salts of gold thiomalic acid—is a white to yellow-white odorless powder that is very water soluble. It is available as a light sensitive, aqueous solution of pH 5.8–6.5. The gold content is approximately 50%. It is administered intramuscularly because it is not absorbed on oral administion and is highly bound to plasma proteins (Table 32.9).

Gold sodium thiomalate is indicated in the treatment of active adult and juvenile rheumatoid arthritis as one part of a complete therapy program. It is recommended that injections be given to patients only when they are in a supine position. They must remain so for 10 minutes following injection. The recommended dosage schedule is 10 mg initially followed by gradual increases in weekly injections to 25–50 mg until either toxic symptoms or signs of clinical improvement appear. If neither appear, weekly injections should continue until the cumulative administered reaches 1000 mg.

Aurothioglucose. Aurothioglucose (Fig. 32.26) is a nearly odorless, yellow powder. Although highly water soluble, aqueous solutions decompose on long standing. It is therefore available as a suspension in sesame oil. Gold content is approximately 50%. Following intramuscular injection it is highly bound to plasma protein and peak plasma levels are achieved within 2–6 hours. Following single 50-mg dose the biologic half-life ranges from 3–27 days but following successive weekly doses the half-life increases to 14–40 days after the third dose. The therapeutic effect does not correlate with serum plasma gold levels but appears to depend on total accumulated gold.

Aurothioglucose is indicated for the adjunctive treatment of adult and juvenile rheumatoid arthritis. See Table 32.9 for dose and dosage forms.

Auranofin. Auranofin (Fig. 32.26) is a crystalline substance that is essentially insoluble in water but is soluble in organic solvents. Gold content is approximately 29%. The carbohydrate portion assumes a chair conformation with all substituents occupying the equatorial position. It is the first orally effective gold compound used to treat rheumatoid arthritis. On a mg gold/kg basis, it is reported to be as effective in the rat adjuvant arthritis assay as the parenterally effective agents. Daily oral doses produce a rapid increase in kidney and blood gold levels for the first 3 days of treatment with a more gradual increase on subsequent administration. Plasma gold levels are lower than those attained with parenteral gold compounds. The major route of excretion is via the urine. Auranofin may produce fewer adverse reactions than parenteral gold compounds but its therapeutic efficacy may also be less.

Auranofin is indicated in adults with active rheumatoid arthritis who have not responded sufficiently to one or more NSAIAs. The usual dose and dosage form are shown in Table 32.9.

Aminoquinolines

Background. The 4-aminoquinolines class, used as antimalarial agents, has been known to possess pharmacologic actions that are beneficial in the treatment of rheumatoid arthritis. Two of these agents, chloroquine and hydroxy-

Table 32.9. Disease-modifying Antirheumatic Drugs (DMARDs)

Drugs	Trade Name	Gold Content (%)	Plasma Binding (%)	Dose (mg)	Dosage Forms (mg/unit)
Gold sodium thiomalate	Aurolate	50%	95	25–50/wk (cum 1000)	Inj sol (25, 50/ml) (1 and 10 ml vials)
Aurothioglucose	Solganal	50	95	10–50/wk (cum 800–1000)	Inj susp (50/ml) (10 ml vial)
Auranofin	Ridaura	29	—	6–9/day	Cap (3)
Hydroxychloroquine sulfate	Plaquenil	—	—	400–600/day	Tab (200)

Tab = Tablets; Cap = capsule; Inj sol = injectable solution; Inj susp = injectable suspension; cum = maximum cumulative administered dose.

chloroquine, have been used as antirheumatics since the early 1950s. However, the corneal and renal toxicity of chloroquine has resulted in its discontinuance for this purpose, however, although it is still indicated as an antimalarial agent and as an amebicide. Whereas hydroxychloroquine is less toxic, it is also less effective than chloroquine as an antirheumatic. The mechanism of action of these agents as an antirheumatic remains unresolved. Interestingly, most of the data available relates to chloroquine rather than hydroxychloroquine but is assumed applicable to the latter. The spectrum of action of the 4-aminoquinolines differs from the NSAIAs in that chloroquine appears to be an antagonist of certain preformed prostaglandins. This effect, however, would indicate an acute, rather than a chronic, antirheumatic effect while chloroquine has been shown to be similar to gold compounds in that it possesses a slow onset of action—beneficial effects are noted only after 1–2 months of administration. Chloroquine inhibits chemotaxis of polymorphonuclear leukocytes in vitro but not in vivo. Its effects on collagen metabolism in connective tissue are also unclear. The most widely accepted mechanism of action of chloroquine, and presumably hydroxychloroquine, is related to its ability to accumulate in lysosomes. Although evidence indicating stabilization of lysosomal membranes is not convincing, it may inhibit the activity of certain lysosomal enzymes such as cartilage chondromucoprotease and cartilage cathepsin B. There does not appear to be a correlation of the antirheumatic effects of 4-aminoquinolines with their antimalarial activity.

Hydroxychloroquine Sulfate.   Hydroxychloroquine sulfate (Fig. 32.26) is a white to off-white, odorless, bitter tasting crystalline powder. The sulfate salt is highly water soluble and exists in two different forms with different melting points. It is readily absorbed on oral administration reaching peak plasma levels within 1–3 hours. It concentrates in organs such as the liver, spleen, kidneys, heart, lung and brain, thereby prolonging elimination. Hydroxychloroquine is metabolized by N-dealkylation of the tertiary amines followed by oxidative deamination of the resulting primary amine to the carboxylic acid derivative. In addition to possessing corneal and renal toxicity, hydroxychloroquine may also cause CNS, neuromuscular, GI and hematologic side effects.

Hydroxychloroquine sulfate is indicated for the treatment of rheumatoid arthritis, lupus erythematosus and malaria. Dose and dosage forms are shown in Table 32.9.

Immunosuppressive agents
Background.   The area of drugs that modify the immune response, whether as immunoregulatory, immunostimulatory or immunosuppressive agents, has been the focus of much recent research activity. Several agents that suppress the immune system have been explored as antirheumatic agents because the etiology of rheumatoid arthritis may involve a destructive immune response. Thus, unlike agents previously discussed, immunosuppressive agents may act at the steps involved in the pathogenesis of rheumatic disorders, an attractive approach to antirheumatic drugs. These agents are quite cytotoxic and as a group were initially developed as anticancer drugs. Among the more widely employed immunosuppressives are azathioprine, methotrexate, leflunomide, and cyclophosphamide. Because of the high potential for toxicity they are indicated for rheumatoid arthritis only in those patients with severe, active disease who have not responded to full dose NSAIA therapy and at least one DMARD. Interestingly, while aspirin and NSAIAs are effective in only one-third of children with juvenile arthritis, methotrexate, given in low doses to minimize side effects, appears to offer promise. More recently, cyclosporine has been investigated in rheumatoid arthritis and appears to offer short-term benefits although its toxic effects limit its long-term use. Cyclosporine appears to inhibit activation of T-helper/inducer lymphocytes involved in the etiology of rheumatoid arthritis.

Pathophysiology.   As discussed earlier in this chapter, there is considerable expression of the cytokines interleukin (IL)-1, IL-6 and tumor necrosis factor-α (TNFα) by the rheumatoid synovium. TNFα is a proinflammatory cytokine that plays a major role in the pathologic inflammatory process of rheumatoid arthritis. TNF is an important mediator of local inflammation and the release of TNFα produces increased vascular permeability, release of nitric oxide with vasodilation, local activation of vascular endothelium, increased expression of adhesion molecules on endothelial blood vessels, and increased platelet activation and adhesion. Rheumatoid arthritis patients display elevated levels of macrophage products such as TNFα, IL-1 and IL-6 in synovial fluid and tissue and there appears to be a correlation between the amount of these products present and the severity of the disease. A significant advance in the treatment of arthritic diseases was the observation that therapy directed toward diminishing the effects of TNFα appeared to improve the symptoms of the disease. Two different approaches have been developed to decrease TNF activity that has resulted in marketable drugs: administration of soluble TNF receptors (etanercept) and treatment with anti-TNFα antibodies (infliximab). Infliximab is the more specific of the two since etanercept binds to both TNFα and TNFβ while infliximab is an antibody that binds only to TNFα. Because TNF is an important host defense against infections, the effects of long-term use on toxicity require further study. Substantial improvements in the course of the disease have been noted with both therapeutic approaches. Several other immunosuppressive agents are being explored and future developments in this area appear promising.

Etanercept (Enbrel). Etanercept is produced by recombinant DNA technology in a Chinese hamster ovary cell line and is the first biotechnology-derived drug to be introduced for the treatment of rheumatoid arthritis. It is a dimeric soluble form of the p75 TNF receptor capable of binding to two TNF molecules. It was recently introduced for the reduction of the signs and symptoms of moderately to severely active rheumatoid arthritis in patients who have not adequately responded to one or more DMARDs. It consists of the extracellular ligand binding portion of the 75 kd human tumor necrosis factor receptor (TNFR) fused with the Fc portion of human IgG1. Two TNFRs have been identified, a 75 kd protein and a 55 kd protein, that occur as monomeric molecules on cell surfaces and in soluble forms. The biologic activity of TNF requires binding to either of the two cell surface TNFRs. Etanercept can bind specifically to two molecules of TNFα or TNFβ. By binding specifically to a naturally occurring cytokine, tumor necrosis factor (TNF), etanercept blocks its interaction with cell surface TNFRs. Etanercept in its dimeric form has greater affinity for recombinant TNFα and has a longer elimination half-life than monomeric sTNFR. It can be used as monotherapy or in combination with methotrexate. Some concern exists because of reports that etanercept may cause serious infections in some cases and may have contributed to the deaths of several patients using the drug. An excellent review of the properties and use of etanercept has recently appeared (67).

Etanercept is available as a powder for injection in single-use vials containing 25 mg of the drug. Injectable solutions are prepared by reconstituting with 1 ml of Bacteriostatic Water for Injection that is supplied. The reconstituted solution should be clear and colorless. It is administered as a 25-mg dose twice weekly as a subcutaneous injection.

Infliximab (Remicade). Infliximab is a chimerical IgG1κ monoclonal antibody to human TNFα which binds to both the transmembrane and soluble forms of TNFα and thus neutralizes the biologic activity of TNFα. It does not bind to TNFβ (lymphotoxin α). Infliximab is produced by recombinant technology. It is indicated for the treatment of rheumatoid arthritis in combination with methotrexate and for Crohn's disease. Long-term use may be associated with the development of anti-infliximab antibodies, an effect that does not appear when it is used with methotrexate. Warnings associated with the use of infliximab include risks of autoimmunity, infections, and hypersensitivity reactions. An excellent review of the properties and use of infliximab has recently appeared (68).

Infliximab is available as a powder for injection in 20-ml single use vials containing 100 mg of the drug. The vials do not contain antibacterial preservatives so the solution should be used immediately after reconstitution. Reconstitution of each vial is achieved by adding 10 ml of Sterile water for Injection. The reconstituted solution should be colorless to light yellow and opalescent.

AGENTS USED TO TREAT GOUT
Pathophysiology

Gout is an inflammatory disease characterized by elevated levels of uric acid (as urate ion) in the plasma and urine and may take two forms, acute and chronic. Acute gouty arthritis results from the accumulation of needlelike crystals of monosodium urate monohydrate within the joints, synovial fluid, and periarticular tissue and usually appears without warning. Initiating factors may be minor trauma, fatigue, emotional stress, infection, overindulgence in alcohol or food, or by specific drugs such as penicillin or insulin. Chronic gout symptoms develop as permanent erosive joint deformity appears. The increase in extracellular urate may be due to increased uric acid biosynthesis, decreased urinary excretion of uric acid, or perhaps a combination of both. The formation of uric acid from adenine and guanine is illustrated in Figure 32.27. Deamination of adenine by adenine deaminase followed by oxidation leads to xanthine a direct metabolic product of guanine deamination. Oxidation of xanthine by xanthine oxidase gives rise to uric acid. Thus, uric acid is an excretory product of purine metabolism in humans. In mammals, uric acid is hydrolyzed to allantoin by the enzyme uricase that is then subsequently hydrolyzed by allantoinase to allantoic acid. Hydrolysis of allantoic acid by allantoicase yields the final products urea and glyoxylic acid.

Normal levels of uric acid are approximately 1000–1200 mg in males and one-half that in females. In patients suffering from gout, these levels may be as high as two or three times the normal levels. Uric acid is a weak acid (pKa = 5.7 and 10.3) with very low water solubility. At physiologic pH it exists primarily as the monosodium salt which is somewhat more soluble in aqueous media than the free acid. In humans, uric acid is reabsorbed primarily via renal tubular absorption. When levels of uric acid in the body increase either as a result of decreased excretion or increased formation, the solubility limits of sodium urate are exceeded and precipitation of the salt from the resulting

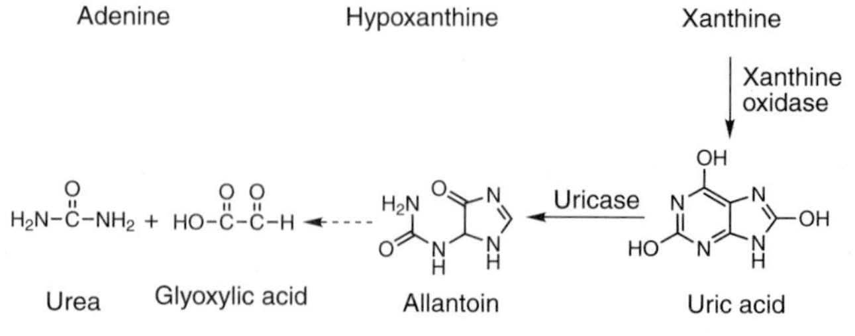

Fig. 32.27. Formation of uric acid, urea and glyoxylic acid from purines.

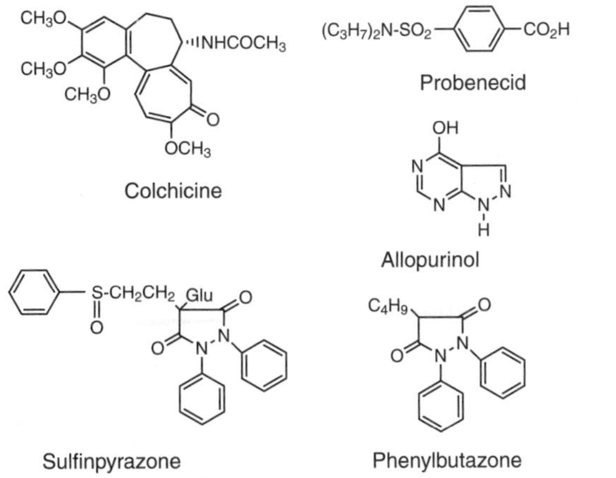

Fig. 32.28. Structures of agents used to control gout.

supersaturated solution causes deposits of urate crystals to form. It is the formation of these urate crystals in joints and connective tissue that initiate attacks of gouty arthritis.

Treatment of Acute Attacks of Gout

The control of gout has been approached with the following therapeutic strategies: a) control of acute attacks with drugs that reduce inflammation caused by the deposition of urate crystals; b) increasing the rate of uric acid excretion (by definition these drugs are termed uricosuric agents); and c) inhibiting the biosynthesis of uric acid by inhibiting the enzyme xanthine oxidase.

Colchicine

Colchicine (Fig. 32.28) is a pale yellow, odorless powder that is obtained from various species of *Colchicum*, primarily *Colchicum autumnale L.* Its total chemical synthesis has been achieved but the primary source of colchicine currently remains alcohol extraction of the alkaloid from the corm and seed of *C. autumnale L.* It darkens on exposure to light and possesses moderate water solubility. Colchicine has a pKa of 12.35. Its use in the treatment of gout dates back to the 6th century A.D. Unlike those agents that will be discussed next, colchicine does not alter serum levels of uric acid. It does appear to retard the inflammation process initiated by the deposition of urate crystals. Acting on polymorphonuclear leukocytes and diminishing phagocytosis, colchicine inhibits the production of lactic acid causing an increase in the pH of synovial tissue. At an elevated pH uric acid solubility is increased. Additionally, colchicine inhibits the release of lysosomal enzymes during phagocytosis that also contributes to the reduction of inflammation. Since colchicine does not lower serum urate levels it has been found beneficial to combine colchicine with a uricosuric agent, particularly probenecid.

Absorption and Metabolism. Colchicine is absorbed upon oral administration with peak plasma levels being attained within 0.5–2 hours after dosing. The drug is weakly bound to plasma protein (Table 32.10). It concentrates primarily in the intestinal tract, liver, kidney and spleen and is excreted primarily in the feces with only 20% of an oral dose being excreted in the urine. Colchicine is retained in the body for considerable periods and may be detected in the urine and leukocytes for up to 10 days following a single dose. Metabolism occurs primarily in the liver, the major metabolite being the amine resulting from amide hydrolysis.

Side Effects. Colchicine may produce bone marrow depression with long-term therapy resulting in thrombocytopenia or aplastic anemia. At maximum dose levels GI disturbances (nausea, diarrhea, and abdominal pain) may occur. Acute toxicity is characterized by GI distress, which includes severe diarrhea resulting and excessive fluid loss, respiratory depression, and kidney damage. Treatment normally involves measures that prevent shock and diminish abdominal pain. A number of potential drug interactions have also been reported. In general, the actions of colchicine are potentiated by alkalinizing agents and inhibited by acidifying drugs. Responses to CNS depressants and to sympathomimetic agents appear to be enhanced. Clinical tests may be affected, most notably elevated alkaline phosphatase and SGOT values and decreased thrombocyte values may be obtained.

Dosing. Colchicine is indicated for the treatment of acute attacks of gout. The usual dose is 1.0–1.2 mg followed by maintenance doses of 0.5–1.2 mg every 1–2 hours until either pain relief is observed or symptoms of GI distress are observed. When a rapid response is required, or if GI reactions warrant discontinuance of oral administration, I.V. administration is used. Dose and dosage forms are shown in Table 32.10. Colchicine is often given in combination with probenecid and combination products of the two are available in tablets containing 500 mg of probenecid and 0.5 mg of colchicine.

Probenecid

Probenecid (Fig. 32.28) is a white, practically odorless, crystalline powder which possesses a slightly bitter taste, but pleasant aftertaste. It is insoluble in water and acidic solutions but soluble in alkaline solutions buffered to pH 7.4. Probenecid was initially synthesized as a result of studies in the 1940s on sulfonamides that indicated that the sulfonamides decreased the renal clearance of penicillin thus extending the half-life of penicillin. Probenecid was thus initially used, and is still indicated, for that purpose. Probenecid promotes the excretion of uric acid by decreasing the reabsorption of uric acid in the proximal tubules (uricosuric agent). The overall effect is to decrease plasma uric acid concentrations thus decreasing the rate and extent of urate crystal deposition in joints and synovial fluids. Probenecid is completely absorbed from the GI tract on oral administration with peak plasma levels observed within 2–4 hours and is extensively plasma protein bound

Table 32.10. Properties of Agents Used to Treat Gout

Drugs	Trade Name	Peak Blood Level (hr)	pKa	Plasma Binding (%)	Dose (mg)	Dosage Forms (mg/unit)
Colchicine	(Generic)	0.5–2	12.35	31	0.5–1.2 mg every 1–2 hr	Tab (0.5–0.6) Inj (1/2ml)
Probenecid	(Generic)	2–4	3.4	93–99	500–1000	Tab (500)
Sulfinpyrazone	Anturane	1–2	2.8	98–99	200–800	Tab (100) Cap (200)
Allopurinal	Zyloprim	1	9.4	—	200–600	Tab (100, 300)

Tab = Tablets; Cap = capsule; Inj = injection.

(Table 32.10). The primary route of elimination of probenecid and its metabolites is the urine. It is extensively metabolized in humans with only 5–10% being excreted unchanged. The major metabolites detected result from glucuronide conjugation of the carboxylic acid, ω-oxidation of the n-propyl side chain and subsequent oxidation of the resulting alcohol to the carboxylic acid derivative, ω-1 oxidation of the n-propyl group, and N-dealkylation. Those metabolites possessing a free carboxylic acid function generally possess some uricosuric activity. Probenecid appears to be generally well tolerated with few adverse reactions. The major side effect is GI distress (nausea, vomiting, anorexia) but these occur in only 2% of patients at low doses. Other effects include headache, dizziness, urinary frequency, hypersensitivity reactions, sore gums, and anemia. Overdosing does not appear to present major difficulties. Should overdosage occur, treatment consists of emesis or gastric lavage, short-acting barbiturates (if CNS excitation occurs) and epinephrine (for anaphylactic reactions). A number of drug interactions have been reported. Despite the high degree of plasma protein binding, displacement interactions with other drugs bound to plasma proteins does not appear to occur to any significant extent. Salicylates counteract the uricosuric effects of probenecid. Increased plasma levels of the following drugs may be observed since probenecid inhibits their renal excretion: aminosalicylic acid, methotrexate, sulfonamides, dapsone, sulfonylureas, naproxen, indomethacin, rifampin, and sulfinpyrazone. The effects on penicillin plasma levels were discussed previously.

Probenecid is indicated for the treatment of hyperuricemia associated with gout and gouty arthritis and for the elevation and prolongation of plasma levels of penicillins and cephalosporins. In gout, treatment should not begin until an acute attack has subsided. It is not recommended in individuals with known uric acid kidney stones or blood dyscrasias or for children under 2 years of age. The recommended dose and dosage forms are shown in Table 32.10.

Sulfinpyrazone

Sulfinpyrazone (Fig. 32.28) is a white crystalline powder which is only slightly soluble in water but soluble in most organic solvents and alkaline solutions (69). It produces its uricosuric effect in a manner similar to that of probenecid. A dose of 35 mg produces a uricosuric effect equivalent to

that produced by 100 mg of probenecid while 400 mg/day of sulfinpyrazone produces an effect comparable to that obtained with doses of 1.5–2 grams of probenecid. It also possesses, not surprisingly, some of the properties of phenylbutazone. It is an inhibitor of human platelet prostaglandin synthesis at the cyclooxygenase step resulting in a decrease in platelet release and a reduction in platelet aggregation. This antiplatelet effect suggests a role for sulfinpyrazone in reducing the incidence of sudden death which can occur in the first year following a myocardial infarction. However, it lacks the analgesic and anti-inflammatory effects of phenylbutazone.

Sulfinpyrazone is a strong acid, a factor which is important in the production of the uricosuric effect since within a series of pyrazolidinedione derivatives, the stronger the acid the more potent the uricosuric effect. Polar substitution on the side chain also influences uricosuric activity as discussed previously with regard to the pyrazolidinediones.

Oral administration results in rapid and essentially complete absorption, peak plasma levels being attained within 1–2 hours of administration. It is highly bound to plasma proteins and it is excreted in the urine primarily (50%) as unchanged drug.

Metabolites produced result from sulfoxide reduction, sulfur and aromatic oxidation and C-glucuronidation of the heterocyclic ring in a manner similar to that for phenylbutazone. The metabolite resulting from p-hydroxylation of the aromatic ring possesses uricosuric effects in humans. The sulfide metabolite, a major metabolic product, may contribute to the antiplatelet effects of sulfinpyrazone but not the uricosuric effects. The most frequent adverse reactions are GI disturbances, however, the incidence is relatively low. It has been suggested that sulfinpyrazone is a much weaker inhibitor of prostaglandin synthesis in bovine stomach microsomes than either aspirin or indomethacin, a factor which may account for its gastric tolerance. There are much rarer reports of blood dyscrasias and rash. Overdosage produces symptoms that are primarily gastrointestinal in nature (nausea, diarrhea and vomiting) but may also involve impaired respiration and convulsions. Treatment of overdoses consists of emesis or gastric lavage and supportive treatment. Like probenecid, its uricosuric effects are antagonized by salicylates and probenecid markedly inhibits the renal tubular secretion of sulfinpyrazone. It potentiates the actions of other drugs which are highly plasma-protein bound such as coumarin-type oral anticoagulants, antibacterial sulfonamides and hypoglycemic sulfonylureas.

Sulfinpyrazone is indicated for the treatment of chronic and intermittent gouty arthritis. Dose and dosage forms are shown in Table 32.10.

Allopurinol

Mechanism of Action. The biosynthesis of uric acid from the immediate purine precursors is illustrated in Figure 32.27. The enzyme xanthine oxidase is involved in two steps, the conversion of hypoxanthine to xanthine, and the conversion of xanthine to uric acid. Allopurinol was originally designed as an antineoplastic antimetabolite to antagonize the actions of key purines. It is an isomer of hypoxanthine (Figs. 32.27 and 32.28), in that the nitrogen and carbon atoms at the 7- and 8-position of the purine are inverted. It was subsequently found that allopurinol serves as a substrate for xanthine oxidase (15–20 times greater the affinity of xanthine) and reversibly inhibits that enzyme. Normally, uric acid is a major metabolic end product in humans but when allopurinol is administered, xanthine and hypoxanthine are elevated in the urine and uric acid levels decrease. When the synthesis of uric acid is inhibited, plasma urate levels decrease, supersaturated solutions of urate are no longer present and urate crystal deposits dissolve, eliminating the primary cause of gout. The increased plasma levels of hypoxanthine and xanthine pose no real problem since they are more soluble than uric acid and are readily excreted.

Absorption and Metabolism. Allopurinol is a white fluffy powder possessing a slight odor but no taste. It is only very slightly soluble in water but is soluble in polar organic solvents and alkaline aqueous solutions. It was synthesized in 1956 as part of a study of purine antagonists (70). It is well absorbed on oral administration with peak plasma concentrations appearing within 1 hour. Decreases of uric acid can be observed within 24–48 hours. Excretion of allopurinol and its metabolite occurs primarily in the urine with about 20% of a dose being excreted in the feces. Allopurinol is rapidly metabolized via oxidation and the formation of numerous ribonucleoside derivatives. The major metabolite of allopurinol is the oxidation product alloxanthine or oxypurinol.

Allopurinol

Alloxanthine
(oxypurinol)

Allopurinol has a much longer half-life (18–30 hours vs. 2–3 hours) than the parent drug and is an effective, al-

though less potent, inhibitor of xanthine oxidase. The longer plasma half-life of alloxanthine results in an accumulation in the body during chronic administration thus contributing significantly to the overall therapeutic effects of allopurinol. The major adverse effects are primarily dermatologic in nature (skin rash and exfoliative lesions). Other effects such as GI distress (nausea, vomiting, and diarrhea), hematopoietic effects (aplastic anemia, bone marrow depression and transient leukopenia), neurologic disorders (headache, neuritis and dizziness) and ophthalmologic effects (cataracts) are less commonly encountered. Allopurinol may also initiate attacks of acute gouty arthritis in the early stages of therapy and may require the concomitant administration of colchicine. Drug interactions include those drugs which are normally also metabolized by xanthine oxidase. Allopurinol also has an inhibitory effect on liver microsomal enzymes thus prolonging the half-lives of drugs such as oral anticoagulants that are normally metabolized and inactivated by these enzymes, although this effect is quite variable. The incidence of ampicillin-related skin rashes increases with the concurrent administration of allopurinol.

Allopurinol is indicated for the treatment of primary and secondary gout, for malignancies such as leukemia and lymphoma, and the management of patients with recurrent calcium oxalate calculi. The dose and dosage forms are shown in Table 32.10.

FUTURE DEVELOPMENTS

The future for the development of new approaches and agents to treat arthritic processes is promising. Among the research areas receiving considerable attention are:

- The continued exploration of selective COX-2 inhibitors with minimal GI effects. Additionally, the continued exploration of the use of these agents for nonarthritic conditions such as various cancers and for cognitive disorders such as Alzheimer's disease should increase. A third isoform of cyclooxygenase, COX-3, has been proposed that would represent a new therapeutic approach to the development of the next generation anti-inflammatory agents (71).
- Interleukins play an important role in the immune response and are also receiving a great deal of attention. Interleukin-1 (IL-1) is one of a class of pro-inflammatory proteins (cytokines) produced by stimulated mononuclear phagocytes which plays a major role in inflammatory and immunologic processes of infection and tissue damage. It has been implicated in various chronic inflammatory disorders including rheumatoid arthritis. Thus, inhibitors of interleukin synthesis, release or inhibition of the interaction of interleukins such as IL-1 with their "receptors" represent potential approaches to the control of inflammatory diseases.
- Continued exploration of anti-TNF therapies with a goal of balancing efficacy, toxicity, and cost. Also, the role of nuclear factor κB (NF-κB) regulation by NF-κB-inducing kinae (NIK) in affecting signal transduction in disease states such as inflammation, cancer and immunology should receive increased attention (72). Activation of NF-κB appears to in-

duce proteins that increase a cells' resistance to TNF cytotoxicity. Also of potential interest is the earlier observation that inhibitors of the serine/threonine p38 MAP kinase have been shown to block both IL-1 and TNF (73).

- The role of naturally occurring compounds continues to be of potential interest in the development of new drugs. For example, parthenolide, the predominant sesquiterpene lactone in European feverfew (*Tanacetum parthenium*), has been shown to inhibit the expression of COX-2 and TNFα and IL-1 in lipopolysaccharide-stimulated macrophages (74).

- Activation of matrix metalloproteinases (MMP) can destroy all components of cartilage. MMPs are found in rheumatoid and osteoarthritic synovial fluid, among other places. New drugs which specifically inhibit active MMPs may represent a new approach to therapy (75).

- The investigation of inhibitors of leukotrienes as anti-inflammatory agents. Both leukotrienes and prostaglandins are involved in the inflammatory processes. Currently available NSAIAs all appear to act through the same mechanism of action, viz., inhibition of prostaglandin biosynthesis at the cyclooxygenase stage. This results in a buildup of arachidonic acid which permits the other major arachidonic acid pathway, the biosynthesis of leukotrienes, to function more significantly and produce leukotrienes that play a major role in inflammation as a pro-inflammatory agent while LTC_4

and LTD_4 are potent hypotensives and bronchoconstrictors. The enzyme 5-lipoxygenase is the key enzyme in the process specific for the biosynthesis of leukotrienes and its inhibition would block their biosynthesis. Thus, continued development of anti-inflammatory agents as novel dual inhibitors of the cyclooxygenase and leukotriene pathways may lead to the development of "safer" NSAIAs, agents which possess a lower side effect profile than currently available agents. Agents which inhibit the activation of 5-lipoxygenase, rather than inhibitors of the enzyme, are also being investigated as are mixed 5-lipoxygenase/leukotriene antagonists.

- The role of complement and complement receptors in the immune response is also an intense area of research. Complement is one of the major mediators of the acute inflammatory response therefore the control of the activation of complement or the inhibition of active complement fragments are potential ways of reducing tissue damage in inflammatory diseases. Several approaches are being explored including the use of endogenous inhibitors of the complement system prepared by recombinant DNA technology and complement receptor inhibitors.

Acknowledgment: The invaluable assistance of Mark S. Levi, graduate student in the Department of Medicinal Chemistry, The University of Mississippi, is deeply appreciated.

CASE STUDY

Victoria F. Roche and S. William Zito

JM is a 56-year-old hairdresser who suffers from rheumatoid arthritis. Early in the course of her disease her symptoms were well controlled with aspirin, but lately she has been experiencing salicylate-resistant stiffness, swelling and pain. Her hands, wrists, shoulders and ankles are predominantly affected, and she is finding it difficult to work. JM has been fairly healthy but does have mildly elevated blood pressure, which she keeps under control with a low-salt diet, low-dose hydrochlorothiazide therapy and, until recently, walking the three miles to and from work. She now has to take the bus, and this has become problematic as she can no longer pick up a few groceries or stop for a quick visit with her best friend on her way home. Her busy day doesn't allow time for much exercise, but her joints hurt too much for that anyway.

JM is in the clinic to investigate "next step" therapy. She's quite worried about her condition, as she lives alone and has no family close by; she must work to support herself. Her medical work-up shows a normal urinalysis and blood profile, but occult blood is found in her stool. There is cancer and heart disease in her family history, but she has not experienced anything beyond her hypertension. Your advice as to appropriate NSAIA therapy is sought.

1. *Identify the therapeutic problem(s) where the pharmacist's intervention may benefit the patient.*

2. *Identify and prioritize the patient specific factors that must be considered to achieve the desired therapeutic outcomes.*

3. *Conduct a thorough and mechanistically oriented structure-activity analysis of all therapeutic alternatives provided in the case.*

4. *Evaluate the SAR findings against the patient specific factors and desired therapeutic outcomes and make a therapeutic decision.*

5. *Counsel your patient.*

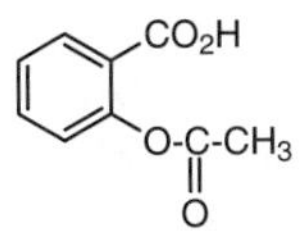

Aspirin

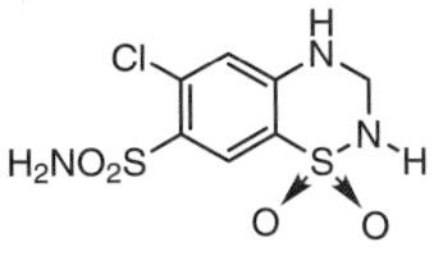

Hydrochlorothiazide

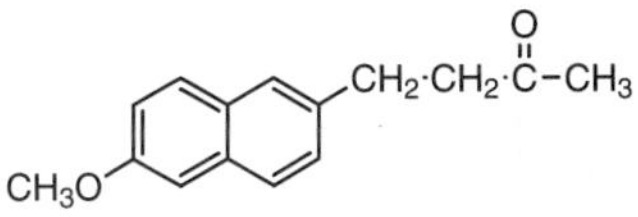

1

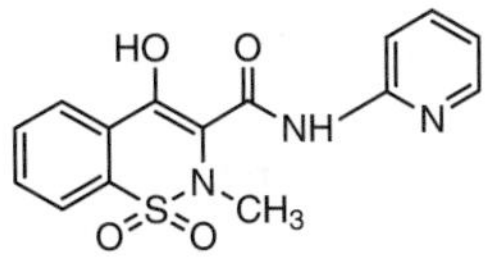

2

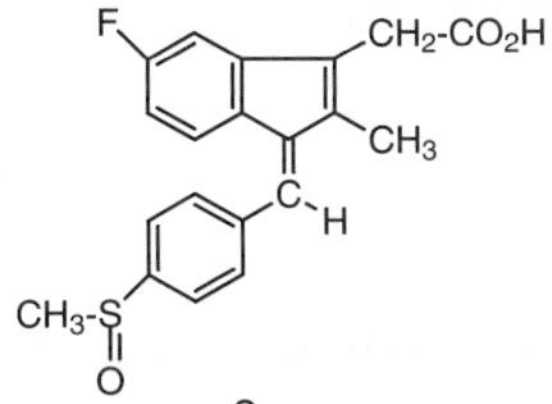

3

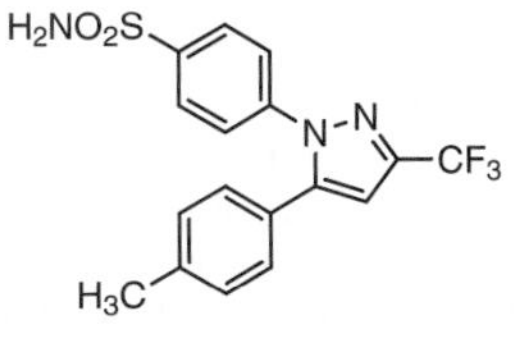

4

REFERENCES

1. Borne RF. Non-steroidal anti-inflammatory agents, antipyretics, and uricosuric agents. In: Verderame M, ed. Handbook of cardiovascular and anti-inflammatory agents. Boca Raton: CRC Press, 1986;27–104.

2. Rodman GP, Schumacher HR, eds. Primer on the Rheumatic Diseases. 8th ed. Atlanta: Arthritis Foundation, 1983.

3. A. Schwartz, In a World of New Diseases, Arthritis Is Still the #1 Crippler. U.S. Pharmacist 1990; 15(6):8.

4. Bennett RW. Treatment Strategies for Osteo- and Rheumatoid Arthritis. U.S. Pharmacist 1990; 15(6):30.

5. Hamor GH. Non-steroidal anti-inflammatory drugs. In: Foye WO, ed. Principles of Medicinal Chemistry. 3rd ed. Philadelphia: Lea & Febiger, 1989; 503–530.

6. Walport M. Complement. In: Roitt IM, Brostoff J, Male DK, eds. Immunology. 2nd ed. St. Louis: C.V. Mosby Co., 1989; Ch. 13.

7. Kinoshita T. Biology of complement: the overture. Immunol Today 1991; 12:291–295.

8. Frank MM, Fries LF. The role of complement in inflammation and phagocytosis. Immunol Today 1991; 12:322–326.

9. Shen TY. Non-steroidal anti-inflammatory agents. In: Wolff M, ed. Burger's Medicinal Chemistry Part III. 4th ed. New York: John Wiley & Sons, 1981; 1205–1272.

10. Shen TY. Proc. Int. Symp. Milan, 1964. In: Grattini S, Dukes MNG, eds. Excerpta Medica, Amsterdam, 1965; 18.

11. Shen TY. Anti-Inflammatory Agents. Top Med Chem 1967, 1: 29.

12. Vane JR Inhibition of prostaglandin synthesis as a mechanism of action for aspirin-like drugs. Nat New Biol 1971; 231: 232–235.

13. Gund P, Shen TY. A model for the prostaglandin synthetase cyclooxygenation site and its inhibition by antiinflammatory arylacetic acids. J Med Chem 1977; 20:1146–1152.

14. Kurzrok R, Lieb C. Biochemical studies of human semen II the action of semen on the human uterus. Proc Soc Exptl Biol N.Y. 1931; 28:268.

15. Goldblatt MW. Properties of human seminal plasma. J Physiol (London) 1935; 84:208–218.

16. Euler U.S. v. The Specific vasodilating and plain muscle-stimulating substances from accessory genital glands in man and certain animals (prostaglandin and vesiglandin). J Physiol (London) 1936; 88:213–234.

17. Bergstrom S, Samuelsson B. The prostaglandins. Endeavour 1968; 27:109–113.

18. Campbell WB. Lipid-derived autacoids: Eicosanoids and platelet-activating factor. In: Gilman, AG, Rall TW, Nies AS, et al, eds. Goodman and Gilman's The Pharmacological Basis of Therapeutics. 8th ed. New York: Pergamon Press, 1990; 600–601.

19. Hla T, Nielson K. Human cyclooxygenase-2 cDNA. Proc. Natl. Acad. Sci. USA. 1992; 89:7384–7388.

20. Jones DA, Carlton DP, McIntyre TM, et al. Molecular cloning of human prostaglandin endoperoxide synthase type II and demonstration of expression in response to cytokines. J Biol Chem 1993; 268:9049–9054.

21. Kennedy B, Chan C-C, Culp S, et al. Cloning expression of rat prostaglandin endoperoxide synthase (cyclooxygenase)-2 cDNA. Biochem Biophys Res Commun 1993; 197:494–500.

22. Kujubu DA, Fletcher BS, Varnum C, et al. TIS10, a phorbol ester tumor promoter-inducible mRNA from Swiss 3T3 cells, encodes a novel prostaglandin synthase/cyclooxygenase homologue. J Biol Chem 1991; 266:12866–12872.

23. Xie W, Chipman JG, Robertson DL, et al. Expression of a mitogen-responsive gene encoding prostaglandin synthase is regulated by mRNA splicing. Proc Natl Acad Sci, USA. 1991; 88:2692–2696.

24. Chang HW, Jahng Y. Selective cyclooxygenase-2 inhibitors as anti-inflammatory agents. Korean J Med Chem, 1998; 8:48–79.

25. Vane JR, Bakhle YS, Botting YM. Cyclooxygenases 1 and 2. Ann Rev Pharmacol Toxicol 1998; 38:97–120.

26. Botting JH. Nonsteroidal anti-inflammatory agents. Drugs Today 1999; 35:225–235.

27. Okazaki T, Sagawa N, Okita JR, et al. Diacylglycerol metabolism and arachidonic acid release in human fetal membranes and decidua vera. J Biol Chem 1981; 256:7316–7321.

28. Clark WG. Mechanisms of antipyretic action. Gen Pharmacol 1979; 10:71–77.

29. Kunkel DB. Emergency medicine. Geigy Pharmaceuticals, July 15, 1985.

30. Calder IC, Creek MJ, Williams PJ, et al. N-hydroxylation of p-acetophenetidide as a factor in nephrotoxicity. J Med Chem 1973; 16:499–502.

31. Smilkstein MJ, Knapp GL, Kulig KW, et al. Efficacy of oral N-acetylcysteine in the treatment of acetaminophen overdose. Analysis of the national multicenter study (1976 to 1985). New Engl J Med, 1988; 319:1557–1562.

32. Buckpitt AR, Rollins DE, Mitchell JR. Varying effects of sulfhydryl nucleophiles on acetaminophen oxidation and sulfhydryl adduct formation. Biochem Pharmacol 1979; 28:2941–2946.

33. Hennekens CH, et al. Final report on the aspirin component of the ongoing physicians' health study. New Engl J Med 1989; 321:129–135.

34. Gossel TA. Aspirin's role in reducing cardiac mortality. U.S. Pharmacist 1988, 13(2):34.

35. Thun MJ, Namboodiri MM, Heath CW. Unsuccessful emergency medical resuscitation-are continued efforts in the emergency department justified? New Engl J Med 1991; 325:1393–1398.

36. Kalgutkar AS, Crews BC, Rowlinson SW, et al. Aspirin-like molecules that covalently inactivate cyclooxygenase-2. Science 1998; 280:1268–1270.

37. Davison C. Salicylate metabolism in man. Ann NY Acad Sci 1971; 179:249–268.

38. Paulus HE, Whitehouse MW. Some relevant clinical conditions and the available therapy. In: Rubin AA, ed. Search for New Drugs. vol. 6. New York: Marcel Dekker, 1972; 11–40.

39. Shen TY, Ellis RL, Windholz TB, et al. Non-steroid anti-inflammatory agents. JACS 1963; 85:488–489.

40. Shen TY, Witzel BE, Jones H, et al. U.S. Patent 3,654,349, 971. Chem Abstr 1971; 74:141379v.

41. Carson JR, McKinstry DN, Wong S. 5-Benzoyl-1-methylpyrrol-2-acetic acids as antinflammatory agents. J Med Chem 1971; 14:646–647.

42. Sallman A, Pfister R. Ger. Patent 1,815,802. 1969. Chem Abstr 1970; 72:12385d.

43. Demerson CA, Humber LG, Dobson TA, et al. Chemistry and anti-inflammatory activities of prodolic acid and related 1,3,4,9-tetrahydropyrano[3,4,-b]indole-1-alkanoic acids. J Med Chem 1975; 18:189–191. Demerson CA, Humber LG, Phillip AH, et al. Etodolic acid and related compounds. Chemistry and anti-inflammatory actions of some potent di- and trisubstituted 1,3,4,9-tetrahydropyrano [3,4-b]indole-1-acetic acids. J Med Chem 1976; 19:391–395.

44. Goudie AC, Gaster LM, Lake AW, et al. 4-(6-Methoxy-2-naphthyl)butan-2-one and related analogues, a novel structural class of anti-inflammatory compounds. J Med Chem, 1978; 21:1260–1264.

45. Nicholson JS, Adams SS. Brit. Patent. 971,700, Chem Abstr 1964; 61:14591d.

46. Hutt AJ, Caldwell J. The metabolic chiral inversion of 2–arylpropionic acids—a novel route with pharmacological consequences. J Pharm Pharmacol 1983; 35:693–704.

47. Marshall WS. French Patent 2,015,728. 1970. Chem Abstr 1971; 75:48707m.

48. Farge D, Messer MN, Moutonnier C. U.S. Patent 3,641,127. 1972. Chem Abst 1974; 81:50040f.

49. Ueno K, Kubo S, Tagawa H, et al. 6,11-Dihydro-11-oxodibenz [b,e] oxepinacetic acids with potent antiinflammatory activity J Med Chem, 1976; 19:941–946.

50. Harrison IT, Lewis B, Nelson P, et al. Nonsteroidal antiinflammatory agents. I. 6-substituted 2-naphthylacetic acids. J Med Chem, 1970; 13:203–205.

51. Adams SS, Bernard J, Nicholson JS, et al. U.S. Patent 3,755,427. 1975. Chem Abst 1973; 79:104952j.

52. Janssen PAJ, Van Deale GHP, Boey JM. Ger. Patent 2,353,375. 1974. Chem Abst 1974; 81: 49433e.

53. (a) Scherrer RA. Introduction to the Chemistry of Anti-inflammatory and Anti-arthritic Agents. In: Scherrer RA, Whitehouse MW, eds. Anti-Inflammatory Agents, vol. 1. New York: Academic Press, 1974; 35; (b) Scherrer RA. Aryl- and Heteroarylcarboxylic Acids. In: Scherrer RA. Whitehouse MW, eds. Anti-Inflammatory Agents, vol. 1. New York: Academic Press, 1974; 56.

54. Winder CV, Wax J, Scotti L, et al. Anti-inflammatory, antipyretic and antinociceptive properties of N-(2,3-xylyl) anthranilic acid (mefenamic acid). J Pharmacol Exp Ther. 1962; 138:405–413.

55. Juby PF, Hudyma TW, Brown M. Preparation and anti-inflammatory properties of some 5-(2-anilinophenyl)tetrazoles. J Med Chem 1968; 11:111–117.

56. Appleton RA, Brown K. Conformational requirements at the prostaglandin cyclooxygenase receptor site: a template for designing non-steroidal anti-inflammatory drugs. Prostaglandins 1979; 18:29–34.

57. Carty TJ, Stevens JS, Lombardino JG, et al. Piroxicam, a structurally novel antiinflammatory compound. Mode of prostaglandin synthesis inhibition. Prostaglandins 1980; 19:671–682.

58. Lombardino JG, Wiseman EH. Piroxicam and other antiinflammatory oxicams. Med Res Rev 1982; 2:127–152.

59. Lombardino JG, Wiseman EH, Chiaini J. Potent anti-inflammatory N-heterocyclic 3-carboxamides of 4-hydroxy-2-methyl-2H-1,2-benzothiazine 1,1-dioxide. J Med Chem 1973; 16: 493–496.

60. Prasit P, Riendeau D. Selective cyclooxygenase-2 inhibitors. Ann Rep Med Chem, 1997; 32:211–220.

61. Warner TD, Giuliano F, Vojnovic I, et al. Nonsteroid drug selectivities for cyclo-oxygenase-1 rather than cyclo-oxygenase-2 are associated with human gastrointestinal toxicity: a full in vitro analysis. Proc Natl Acad Sci U.S.A. 1999; 96:7563–7568.

62. Chan CC, Boyce S, Brideau C, et al. Rofecoxib [Vioxx, MK-0966; 4-(4'-methylsulfonylphenyl)-3-phenyl-2-(5H)-furanone]: a potent and orally active cyclooxygenase-2 inhibitor. Pharmacological and biochemical profiles. J Pharmacol Exp Ther 1999; 290:551–560.

63. Penning TD, Talley JJ, Bertenshaw SR, et al. Synthesis and biological evaluation of the 1,5-diarylpyrazole class of cyclooxygenase-2 inhibitors: identification of 4-[5-(4-methylphenyl)-3-(trifluoromethyl)-1H-pyrazol-1-yl]benzenesulfonamide (SC-58635, celecoxib). J Med Chem, 1997; 40:1347–1365.

64. McEvoy GK, ed. American Hospital Formularly Service Drug Information 2000; 1872–1879.

65. Sorbera LA, Leeson PA, Castaner J Rofecoxib Drugs Fut 1998; 23:1287–1296.

66. McEvoy GK, ed. American Hospital Formularly Service Drug Information 2000; 1879–1883.

67. Jarvis B, Faulds D. Lamivudine. A review of its therapeutic potential in chronic hepatitis B. Drugs 1999; 57:945–966.

68. Markham A, Lamb HM. Infliximab: a review of its use in the management of rheumatoid arthritis. Drugs 2000; 59:1341–1359.

69. Pfister R, Häflinger F. Über derivate und analoġe de phenylbutazoins IV analoġe mit schwefelhaltiġen seitenkitten. Helv Chim Acta 1961; 44:232–237.

70. Robins RK. Potential Purine Antagonist. I. Synthesis of some 4,6-substituted pyrazolo[3,4-d] pyrimidines. JACS. 1956; 78:784–90.

71. Willoughby DA, Moore AR, Colville-Nash PR. COX-1, COX-2, and COX-3 and the future treatment of chronic inflammatory disease. Lancet 2000; 355:646–648.

72. Malinin NL, Boldin MP, Kovalenko AV, et al. MAP3K-related kinase involved in NF-κB induction by TNF, CD95 and IL-1. Nature 1997; 385:540–4.

73. Lee JC, Laydon JT, McDonnell PC, et al. A protein kinase involved in the regulation of inflammatory cytokine biosynthesis, Nature 1994; 372:739–746.

74. Hwang D, Fischer NH, Jang BC, et al. Inhibition of the expression of inducible cyclooxygenase and proinflammatory cytokines by sesquiterpene lactones in macrophages correlates with the inhibition of MAP kinases. Biochem Biophys Res Comm 1996; 226:810–818.

75. Cawston T. Matrix metalloproteinases and TIMPs: properties and implications for the rheumatic diseases. Mol Med Today 1998; 4:130–137.

33. Antihistamines and Related Antiallergic and Antiulcer Agents

WENDEL L. NELSON

INTRODUCTION

Histamine [2-(imidazol-4-yl)ethylamine] was synthesized and its effects in model biological systems were studied before it was found in tissues. Early hypotheses about its physiologic function were based on the observed effects in guinea pigs that are dramatic, and include massive bronchial spasm and effects on smooth muscle and the vasculature resembling anaphylactic shock. Marked species differences in the observed effects occur however, and these dramatic effects are not observed in humans.

Histamine is located in many tissues and upon release its effects are principally local ones, as it functions as an autocoid or paracrine (1). Its physiologic function is complex and not completely understood. Histamine is one of the many mediators involved in allergic responses, and it has an important role in the regulation of the secretion of gastric acid. These observations have led to development of important drugs that antagonize its effects and which are useful in treatment of allergic disorders (H_1 antagonists) and in the treatment of gastric hypersecretory disorders (H_2 antagonists).

CHEMISTRY

Histamine has pKas of 9.40 (aliphatic primary amine) and 5.80 (imidazole). Thus it exists as an equilibrium mixture of tautomeric cations at physiologic pH, with the monocation making up more than 96% of the total, and the dication about 3%, with only a very small amount of the nonprotonated species. At lower pHs, e.g., the pH of acidic lipids, a much larger proportion of the dication exists (2). The two protonated species (mono and dication) are often considered the biologically active forms. Penetration of membranes would be expected to occur *via* the nonprotonated species, and the unprotonated imidazole group would be expected to participate readily in proton transfer processes physiologically. Several aromatic ring

congeners of histamine with weakly and very weakly basic heteroaromatic rings (e.g., 4-chloroimidazole, 1,2,4-triazole, thiazole, and pyridine) exhibit histamine agonist activity (Table 33.1) (3), although they are less potent than histamine. These data suggest that the monocation (protonated aliphatic amine) is sufficient for agonist activity, and that protonation of the heterocyclic ring is not an absolute requirement.

In aqueous solutions, the tautomeric equilibrium of the imidazole ring apparently favors the N^τ-H tautomer by about 4:1 (4). The free base also prefers the N^τ-H tautomer (5). However, in the crystal of the mono-hydrochloride salt of histamine, a situation where intermolecular packing forces are important, the N^π-H tautomer is preferred (6). Changes in tautomeric composition of analogs

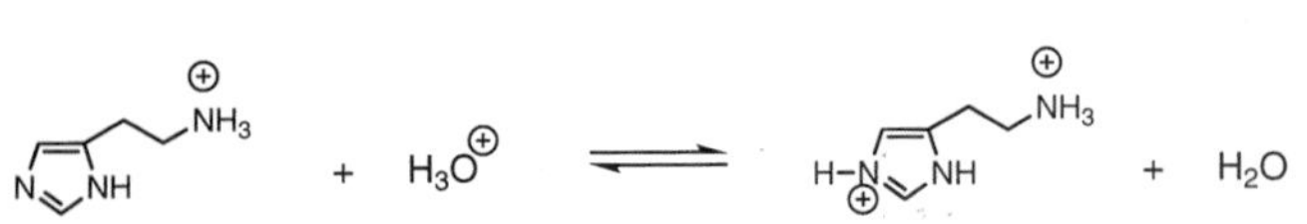

Table 33.1. Histamine-related Agonists*

	Relative H_1 Activity vs. Histamine	Relative H_2 Activity vs. Histamine	Relative H_3 Activity vs. Histamine
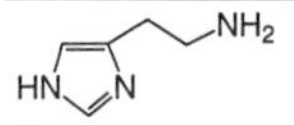	100	100	100
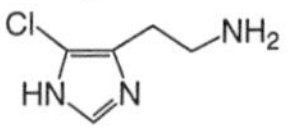	1.7	12	ND[†]
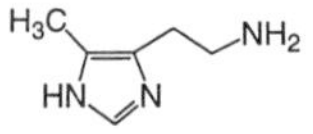	0.23	39	<0.008
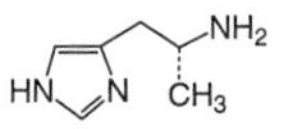	0.49	1.0	1550
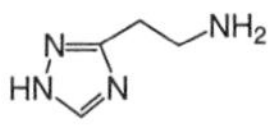	12.7	13.7	ND
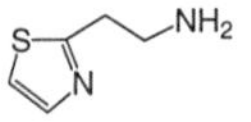	26	~0.3	<0.008
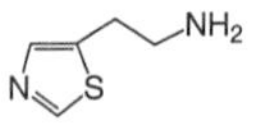	0.01	~0.1	ND
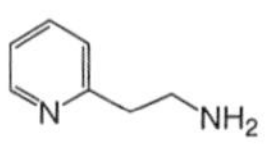	5.6	2.5	<0.06
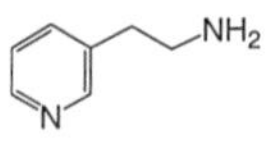	Inactive	Inactive	ND
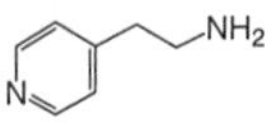	~0	~0.4	ND

* Activity expressed relative to histamine = 100, determined in vitro on guinea pig ileum (H_1), guinea pig atrium (H_2) and rat cerebral cortex (H_3). Ref. 3, p. 504.
† ND = not determined.

pKa 9.40   pKa 5.80

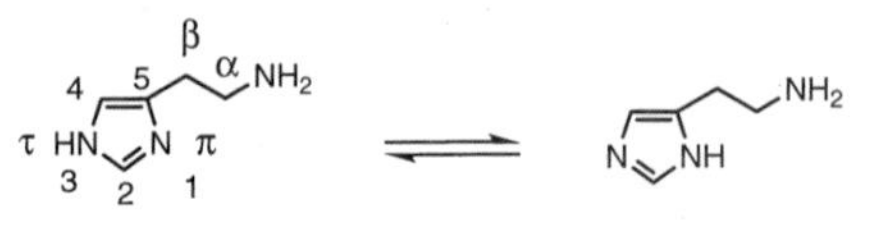

Tautomers of histamine

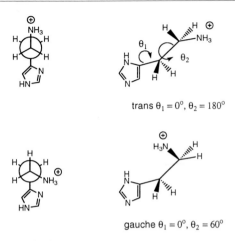

trans $\theta_1 = 0°$, $\theta_2 = 180°$

gauche $\theta_1 = 0°$, $\theta_2 = 60°$

Fig. 33.1. Conformers of histamine.

occur with changes in the 4-substituent, e.g., Me vs. Cl where the proportion of N$^\tau$-H tautomer is decreased in the chlorine-substituted congener to 12% vs. 70% for 4-methylhistamine, and decreased agonist potency is observed (Table 33.1) (7). An interpretation of these results is that tautomeric composition might be important in the agonist-receptor interaction.

Results of conformational studies performed on histamine and its congeners indicate both *trans* and gauche conformations exist in solution (Fig. 33.1) (7,8). However, the *trans* conformation of 4-methylhistamine, which is a selective H$_2$ agonist, cannot readily adopt the fully extended *trans* conformation because of interaction of the 4-methyl group with the aliphatic two-carbon chain (9). Since α- and β-methylhistamine exist predominantly as gauche conformers (7,10), and both are very weak H$_1$ and H$_2$ agonists, it has been suggested that *trans* conformation of histamine is preferred at both H$_1$ and H$_2$ receptors. A gauche conformation has been suggested for histamine at the H$_3$ receptor because α-methylhistamine and some other more conformationally restricted analogs are potent H$_3$-agonists.

Addition of other alkyl substituents onto the histamine molecule generally produces compounds with decreased potency at H$_1$ and H$_2$ receptors. 2-Methylhistamine is a selective H$_1$ agonist (vs. 4-methylhistamine, a selective H$_2$ agonist), but imidazole N-substitution (N^1 or N^3) with methyl groups results in nearly inactive agents. Similarly, aliphatic amine nitrogen substitution results in decreasing activity NH$_2$ > NHMe > NMe$_2$ > N$^+$Me$_3$ (quaternary ammonium salt) at both H$_1$ and H$_2$ receptors (11).

PHYSIOLOGIC CHARACTERISTICS OF HISTAMINE
Synthesis and Metabolism of Histamine

Histamine is synthesized in the Golgi apparatus of mast cells and basophils by enzymatic decarboxylation of histidine. This conversion is catalyzed by L-histidine decarboxylase, with pyridoxal phosphate serving as a cofactor for this

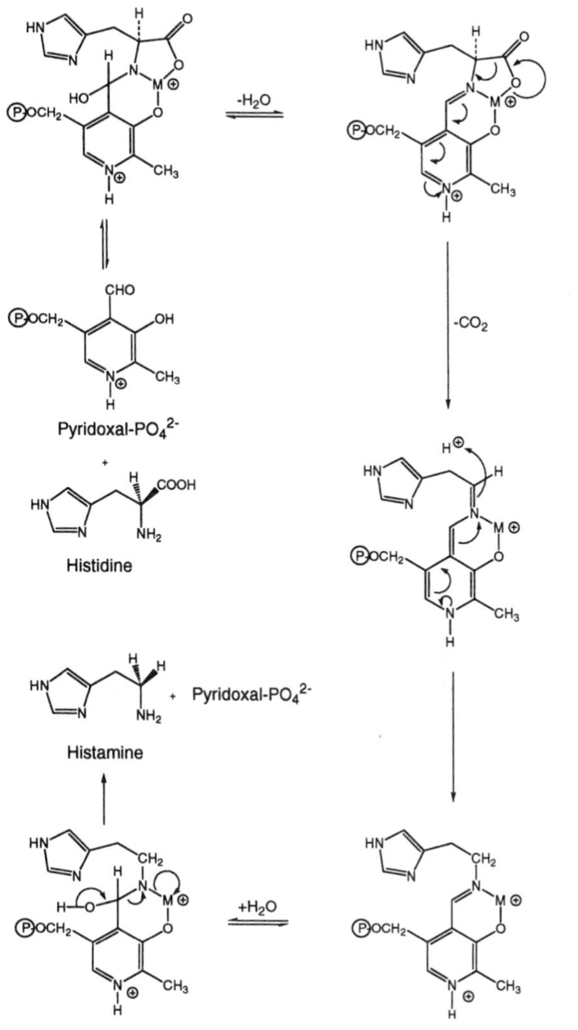

Fig. 33.2. Formation of histamine by decarboxylation of histidine.

process. The reaction mechanism for this decarboxylation probably involves the formation of a Schiff base (imine) intermediate followed by the loss of carbon dioxide, a mechanism demonstrated to occur for decarboxylation of many α-amino acids (Fig. 33.2). Pyridoxal phosphate provides an important catalytic function, and in the final step, the product is released by hydrolysis of the enzyme-bound Schiff base of histamine. Mechanism-based inhibitors of this process such as α-fluoromethylhistidine (12,13) have been evaluated for their ability to decrease the rate of synthesis of histamine, and as such to deplete cells of histamine as a process to treat allergic symptoms, peptic ulcers, and motion sickness. These agents have not been successful therapeutically. α-Fluoromethylhistidine is primarily a pharmacologic tool.

Once released, histamine is rapidly metabolized in vivo (based on products from radiolabeled histamine administered intradermally) to nearly inactive metabolites by two major pathways: N-methylation and oxidation (Fig. 33.3). Methylation (S-adenosylmethionine) which is catalyzed by the intracellular enzyme N-methyltransferase yields an inactive metabolite. A portion of the N-methylated metabo-

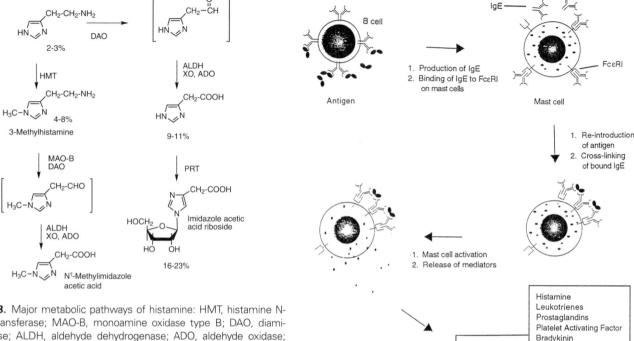

Fig. 33.3. Major metabolic pathways of histamine: HMT, histamine N-methyltransferase; MAO-B, monoamine oxidase type B; DAO, diamineoxidase; ALDH, aldehyde dehydrogenase; ADO, aldehyde oxidase; XO, xanthine oxidase; PRT, phosphoribosyl transferase. From intradermal histamine as measured in the urine in 12 hours in human males (14).

Fig. 33.4. Sequence of events in immediate hypersensitivity. Initial contact with an antigen leads to specific IgE synthesis by B cells. Secreted IgE binds to mast cells or basophils through high-affinity Fcε receptors (FcεRI). Upon subsequent exposure to the antigen, an immediate hypersensitivity reaction is triggered by cross-linking the IgE molecules.

lite is oxidized sequentially by monoamine oxidase and then aldehyde oxidase to the corresponding N-methylimidazole acetic acid. Histamine is also oxidized to imidazole acetic acid by diamine oxidase (histaminase). A small amount of this acid intermediate is converted to the corresponding ribotide, an unusual metabolite (14).

Storage and Release of Histamine

In mast cells, histamine is stored in secretory granules as a complex with acidic residues of the proteoglycan heparin, and in basophils as a complex with chondroitin sulfate (15,16). Although histamine is secreted at low levels from mast cells and basophils, the primary mechanism of release is associated with cell activation by IgE-mediated hypersensitivity processes (Fig. 33.4). Immediate hypersensitivity is initiated when allergen molecules crosslink to Fab components of adjacent IgE antibody molecules bound to high-affinity FcεRI receptors on the surface of these cells. Dimerization of occupied IgE-Fc receptors results in several membrane and cytosolic events. These include release of preformed mediators from secretory granules by exocytosis, the synthesis and release of newly formed lipid mediators, and stimulation of synthesis of cytokines and their subsequent release. Other cell activation stimuli for the release of histamine include concanavalin A, substance P, polyamines, opiates and several lymphokines and cytokines. There are different subpopulations of cells that respond differently to these stimuli. With the exocytotic response, histamine rapidly dissociates from the partially solubilized granule matrix. From basophils, the release process may be slightly different, occurring without degranulation occurring. Other cell types,

including lymphocytes, platelets, neutrophils, monocytes and some macrophages, secrete histamine releasing factors. These cells also have distinct low-affinity receptors for IgE which when occupied result in secretion of mediators that selectively recruit and activate secondary effector cells in the inflammatory process.

Mast cells play an important role in the early response to allergens and they provide mediators that lead to initial and late stages of the process and subsequently to chronic inflammatory reactions (17,18). Early stages appear to be related to degranulation and the release of many mediators, including histamine, PGD$_2$ and LTC$_4$, platelet activating factor, ATP, kinins and some enzymes, e.g., tryptase and chymase. Thus, additional important mediators other than histamine have very significant roles. These mediators include platelet activation factor, substance P, neurokinin A, and others. Besides processes of vasodilation and edema, activation of secondary inflammatory cells occurs and adherence of neutrophils, eosinophils and T cells to postcapillary venule endothelial cells occurs, this later process is mediated by specific cell adhesion molecules. A further array of mediators and cellular responses follows. A series of interleukins are generated and secreted by subtypes of T cells. Important cytokines are liberated, including TNF-α, IL-4 and IL-5, IL-1 and IL-6, which are involved in chemokine secretion and regulation of cell maturation and proliferation processes, changes that occur in late stage reactions. Thus the inflammatory cascade is a complex and very intricate one, and the effects of histamine are only a small part of these processes.

As a result of occupation of H_1 receptors by histamine, constriction of bronchial and gastrointestinal smooth muscle occurs. Spasm of the bronchi to inhaled histamine at one time was a test for airway reactivity. Intradermal injection of histamine produces vasodilation of arterioles, as the first step in the "triple response," mediated at H_1 and H_2 receptors. A flare response follows this stimulation resulting in release of substance P and other neuropeptides. Edema from exudation of plasma fluids follows due to contraction of endothelial cells of postcapillary venules. The wheal and flare responses are mostly H_1 receptor mediated.

Histamine Receptors—Molecular and Mechanistic Aspects

Histamine has a number of physiologic effects mediated through activation of specific cell surface receptors. The discovery of antagonists that incompletely blocked all of the effects of histamine, and subsequently of selective agonists and very selective antagonists, has led to designations of different classes of histamine receptors: H_1, H_2 and subsequently H_3 (principally an autoreceptor).

Histamine receptors are found in various tissues. Among these are the H_1 receptors in smooth muscle of the bronchi, gut and uterus. Contraction of the bronchi facilitated by histamine leads to restriction of air flow in the lungs. Histamine increases the permeability of capillary walls. Plasma constitutents flow into extracellular spaces due to contraction of endothelial cells; this process leads to edema. In the stomach, parietal cell stimulation increases production and secretion of acid, mediated through H_2 receptors. At the level of the central nervous system, histamine secretion appears to be associated in wakefulness, as H_1 receptor blockade is associated with drowsiness.

The human H_1 receptor gene encodes for a 487 amino acid protein which has the structure features of a G protein-coupled receptor (seven transmembrane domains, N-terminal glycosylation sites, phosphorylation sites for protein kinase A and C, and a large intracellular loop with several serine and threonine residues) (19,20). Receptors from several species are similar. The structural features fit well with known coupling of receptor to phosphatidyl inositol turnover as the second messenger system. This receptor shows 40% homology with the muscarinic M_1 receptor and the M_2 receptor. An aspartic acid in the third transmembrane domain is highly conserved in several species, and it is suggested as a recognition site for the protonated aliphatic amine function of histamine, at both H_1 and H_2 receptors. Based on mutation studies and homologous positions to α-adrenergic receptors, suggestions for sites of binding of the imidazole portion of histamine to amino acids threonine or asparagine in the fifth transmembrane have been made (21-24).

Signal transduction processes begin with the hydrolysis of phosphatidylinositol-4,5-bisphosphonate to IP_3 (inositol-

1,4,5-triphosphate) and 1,2-diacylglycerol, which occurs via activation of phospholipase C. Evidence exists that a Gq-like protein, a pertussis toxin insensitive G protein, is involved in activation of phospholipase C. Elevation of intracellular calcium ion from intracellular stores occurs. Voltage gated calcium channels may be opened by activation of ion channels permeable to Na^+ and K^+ ions. Calcium channel antagonists block some effects of histamine on intestinal smooth muscle (25).

The gene for the H_2 receptor, which has been cloned from several sources, shows some species differences (26–28). The receptor is smaller (359 amino acids in humans), but it has some features similar to the H_1 protein, e.g., N-terminal glycosylation sites, and phosphorylation sites in the C-terminal (29). An aspartic acid residue in the third transmembrane loop appears to be critical to agonist and antagonist binding, and threonine or aspartate in the fifth transmembrane domain appear to be important for binding of the imidazole part of the histamine molecule (27,30,31).

The structural features are characteristic with receptors positively coupled through cAMP as second messenger, and it is generally accepted that H_2 receptors are coupled to the adenylate cyclase system (32). Activation occurs through a guanyl nucleotide process and the model is usually written in a fashion analogous to that of the well-studied β-adrenergic receptor mediated events, although no direct evidence is available for a Gs protein. Yet, it appears that in some cells, other processes like breakdown of phosphoinositides, control of intracellular calcium ion levels and phospholipase A_2 activity can be regulated by other cAMP-independent pathways.

Much less is known about the molecular characteristics and functions of the H_3 receptor.

INHIBITORS OF HISTAMINE RELEASE
Mechanism of Action

The bronchodilatory activity of khellin, a chromone obtained from a plant source (*Ammi visnaga*) used by ancient Egyptians for spasmolytic activity, stimulated the search for related compounds with similar pharmacologic properties (33). From a study of many bischromones, cromolyn sodium was developed and marketed (Fig. 33.5). Though

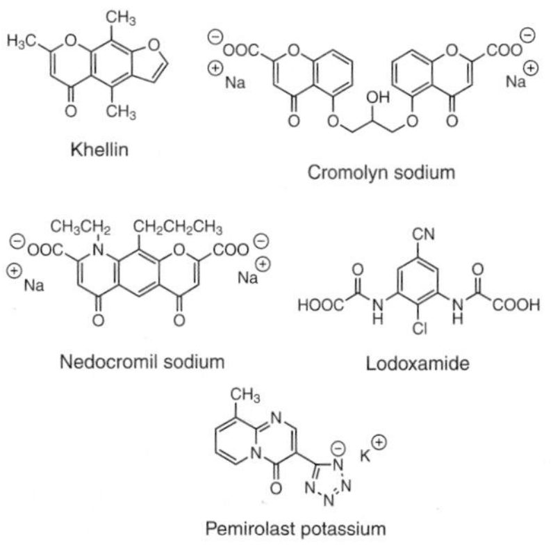

Fig. 33.5. Mast cell degranulation inhibitors.

it prevents bronchospasm, it does not reverse antigen-induced bronchiolar constriction. Thus it and other agents like it that followed prevent the release of histamine and do not block the effects of histamine at its receptors.

Until recently, the view was very well accepted that cromolyn inhibits degranulation of sensitized mast cells after exposure to specific antigens, thus inhibiting the release of transmitters including histamine, LTC_4, LTD_4, and PDE_2. Cromolyn and nedocromil (vide infra) apparently inhibit function of cells other than mast cells; these effects may occur in later stages of inflammatory responses (34). Cromolyn does not have intrinsic antihistaminic or antiinflammatory activity.

Therapeutic Applications of Specific Drugs
Cromolyn (Intal, Nasalcrom)

Cromolyn is usually used prophylactically for bronchial asthma (as an inhaled powder), prevention of exercise-induced bronchospasm, and for seasonal and perennial allergic rhinitis (nasal solution) (35–37). Topically, it is also used as eye drops for allergic conjunctivitis and keratitis. In the management of asthmatic conditions, it is administered using a power-operated nebulizer. The bioavailability is very low on oral administration because of poor absorption. By inhalation, the powder is irritating to some patients. After inhalation, less than 10% of the dose reaches the systemic circulation. An oral dosage form is used for mastocytosis, and it is being evaluated for treatment of food allergies and in other situations.

Nedocromil (Alocril Tilade)

Nedocromil is a chromone analog also used by inhalation as an aerosol primarily in the prophylaxis of asthma and reversible obstructive airway disease (38,39). It inhibits release of allergic mediators, and it is effective in a broad range of patients. Other structurally related compounds are available in other markets, but are not currently available in the U.S. An ophthalmic solution is available and a nasal solution is under investigation.

Lodoxamide (Alomide)

Lodoxamide, which shows some structural similarities to cromolyn and nedocromil, is also a mast cell stabilizer that inhibits the immediate hypersensitivity reaction, preventing increases in vascular permeability associated with antigen-IgE mediated responses. Its precise mechanism(s) of action is(are) not completely understood. It is used topically in the eye principally for conjunctivitis and keratitis associated with vernal allergens (40).

Pemirolast (Alamast)

Pemirolast, with an acidic tetrazole as an isoteric replacement for a carboxylic acid, was recently approved as a topical agent for use in the eye to prevent itching associated with allergic conjunctivitis. It is an inhibitor of release of histamine and other inflammatory mediators, including leukotrienes. Significant use as a systemic agent has been reported, and it has been shown to be useful in preventing restenosis after percutaneous coronary angiopathy (41).

INHIBITORS OF RELEASED HISTAMINE
Historical Background

The first antihistamine was discovered by Forneau and Bovet, who observed that piperoxan protected guinea pigs against histamine-induced bronchospasm (42). The sensitivity of the guinea pig was initially thought to make it a good model for anaphylaxis. Piperoxan also has important effects related to antagonism of norepinephrine at α-adrenergic receptors.

Piperoxan

Antihistamines, specifically H_1 antagonists (3), are useful in the treatment of allergy and inflammatory disorders, where many effects are mediated via histamine, but not others. Compounds that had antagonistic effects in these assays did not antagonize the effects of histamine on the stomach (acid secretion) and heart (positive chronotropic and inotropic effects). These differences suggested the presence of H_1 and H_2 receptors, and ultimately to the development of selective H_2 antagonists to diminish the secretion of gastric acid. Subsequently, a third class of histamine receptors, designated H_3 receptors, was designated on the basis of activity of some additional selective agonists and antagonists. H_3 receptors appear primarily to be autoreceptors that control the synthesis and release of histamine presynaptically and heteroreceptors that control the release of other transmitters, primarily in the CNS.

The first-generation antihistamines are useful and effective in the treatment of allergic responses, e.g., hay fever, rhinitis, urticaria and food allergy. These agents also have effects at cholinergic, dopaminergic and serotonergic receptors. Adverse central effects include sedation, drowsiness, decreased cognitive ability, and somnolence. Peripheral side effects associated with cholinergic blockade include blurred vision, dry mouth, urinary retention and constipation. Other effects observed have included appetite stimulation, muscle spasm, anxiety, confusion, and occasionally irritability, tremor and tachycardia. Of all the side effects, CNS depression is most common and can be so pronounced that some of these agents with short durations of action make them useful as OTC sleep aids. The separation of CNS depressant and anticholinergic effects from peripheral antihistaminic effects in later agents led to the second-generation antihistamines (vide infra).

Structural classes of H_1 classical receptor antagonists can be represented by a general structure of two aromatic groups linked through at short chain to a tertiary aliphatic amine (Fig. 33.6). The aromatic groups (Ar_1, Ar_2) are usu-

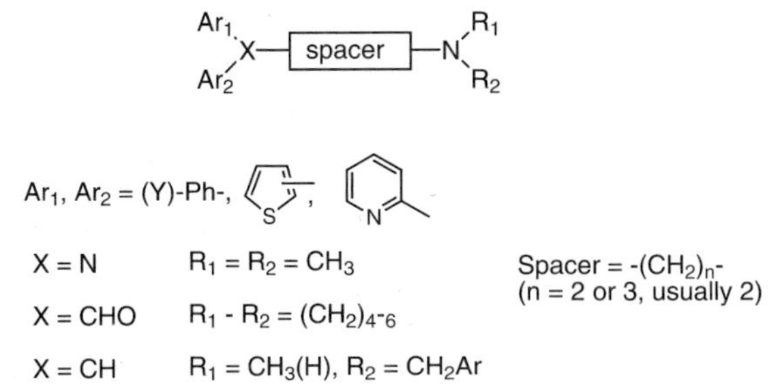

Fig. 33.6. General structure of first generation antihistamines.

ally phenyl or substituted phenyl, thienyl, or pyridyl. These substituents are attached to the X group, which is a nitrogen atom in the ethylenediamines, a carbon attached to an ether oxygen atom in the ethanolamine ether series, or a carbon atom in the alkyl amines. The spacer is usually two or three carbons in length, and it may be in a ring, it may be branched, and it may be saturated or unsaturated. The R groups attached to the aliphatic amine are usually simple alkyl groups, usually methyl, or occasionally aralkyl groups.

First Generation H₁ Antihistamines

Ethylenediamines

The earliest series of H_1 antagonist agents are the ethylenediamines. Two, two-carbon spacers may appear between the two nitrogen atoms in the piperazine series (vide infra). Examples of agents in the ethylenediamine class, of which phenbenzamine was the first of these agents, appear in Table 33.2. Compounds with several different but closely related

Table 33.2. Examples of Ethylenediamine Antihistamines

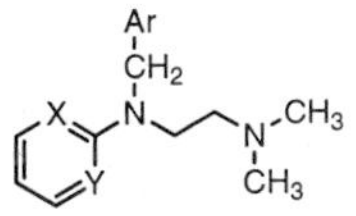

Drugs	X	Y	Ar
Phenbenzamine	CH	CH	phenyl
Pyrilamine (mepyramine)	N	CH	CH₃O-phenyl
Tripelennamine (pyribenzamine)	N	CH	phenyl
Methapyrilene	N	CH	thienyl
Thonzylamine	N	N	CH₃O-phenyl

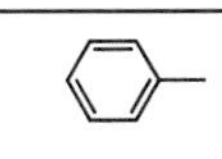

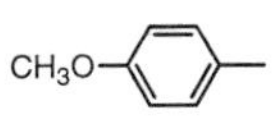

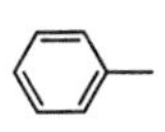

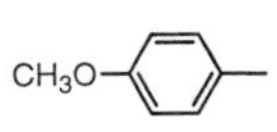

Related compound:

Antazoline

aromatic rings are useful, e.g., phenyl, 2-pyridyl, halogen- and methoxy-substituted phenyl, or pyrimidyl. Thiazole, furanyl and thiophene-ring congeners had also been available in the past. The small substituents on basic nitrogen are usually methyl groups. A number of these agents are still used. With the exception of antazoline, all have the ethylenediamine spacer. In antazoline, the alkyl tertiary amine in phenbenzamine is replaced with an imidazoline group. CNS effects, usually sedation, are very common among agents in this class.

Information on pharmacokinetic and metabolic disposition is limited as this early group of compounds was not studied in depth. Only later, with second-generation compounds, or where issues of potential toxicity have arisen concerning some of the early compounds, has metabolic disposition been examined more completely. Thus, the available information on the metabolism on these early antihistamines is sparse. From some of the ethylenediamines, predictable products of N-demethylation and subsequent deamination have been reported. In addition, some produce quaternary N-glucuronides as urinary metabolites, a process that occurs to some extent in many relatively unhindered tertiary aliphatic amines among the antihistamines and also in other lipophilic aliphatic tertiary amine drug classes (43).

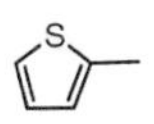

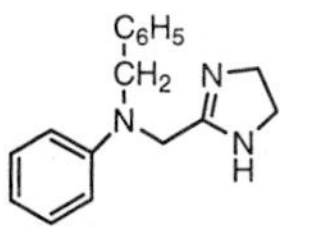

Ethanolamine Ethers

Structure-activity Relationships. The prototype of the aminoalkyl ethers is diphenhydramine, a benzhydryl ether still widely used for allergic conditions, more than a half-century after its introduction. Structural analogs with various ring substituents (Me, OMe, Cl, Br) in one of the aromatic rings have also been developed, as have compounds with a 2-pyridyl group replacing one of the phenyl groups (Table 33.3).

Table 33.3. Ethanolamine Ether Antihistamines

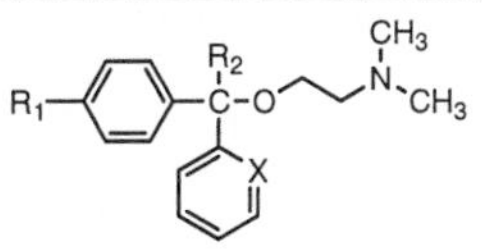

Drugs	Trade Name	R₁	R₂	X
Diphenhydramine	Benadryl	H	H	CH
Dimenhydrinate	Dramamine			
Bromodiphenhydramine		Br	H	CH
Chlorodiphenhydramine		Cl	H	CH
Carbinoxamine	Colistin	Cl	H	N
Doxylamine	Decapryn, Unisom	H	CH₃	N

Related compounds:

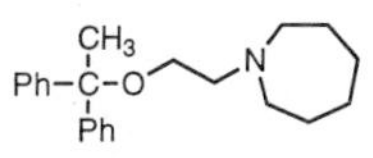

Setastine (Loderix)   Clemastine (Tavist)

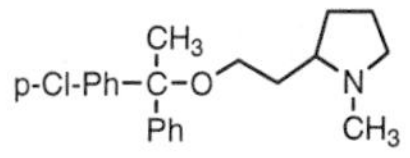

Significant anticholinergic side effects are observed among members of the group (dry mouth, blurred vision, tachycardia, urinary retention, constipation, etc.). Sedative properties are also very common among members of this group. Sedation, accompanied with a relatively short half-life and a wide margin of safety, allows some of these compounds to be used as OTC sleep aids. The 8-chlorotheophyllinate salt of diphenhydramine is marketed as dimenhydrinate for use in the treatment of motion sickness. The compound with the aryl groups *p*-Cl-Ph and 2-pyridyl is carbinoxamine, a potent antihistamine. Substitution of a methyl group at the carbon α to the ether function affords the related compound doxylamine, in which the aryl groups are phenyl and 2-pyridyl. Clemastine, a homolog with an additional carbon atom between the oxygen and the basic nitrogen which is incorporated into a ring, is a recent addition to the group, with less sedative properties. Other analogs are used elsewhere. For example, setastine, a compound with the alkyl amine substituent being incorporated into a seven-membered hexahydroazepine ring, is available in Europe (44).

Antihistaminic vs. Anticholinergic Activity. Besides the structural analogs in Table 33.3 that possess increased selectivity for histamine H_1 receptors over muscarinic receptors, introduction of alkyl substituents at C-2′ or C-4′ of one aromatic ring results in significant changes in selectivity in tissue-based assays for antihistaminic vs. anticholinergic activity. With increasing alkyl group size (Me, Et, iPr, tBu) at C-2′, large decreases in antihistaminic activity and increases in anticholinergic activity are observed (45–47). With larger alkyl groups, the possible spatial orientations of the two aromatic rings with regard to each other are limited due to increasing rotameric restrictions. Introduction of these alkyl sub-

stituents at C-4′ decreases anticholinergic activity and yields small increases in antihistaminic activity. A chiral center is introduced with these changes, and differences in pharmacologic properties of the enantiomers of each compound are observed; two examples are shown in Table 33.4.

Stereochemical and Structural Effects. The change in receptor selectivity (histamininergic vs. cholinergic) stimulated the synthesis of a large number of related homologs. For example, orphenadine, the C-2′ methyl-substituted analog of diphenhydramine, is marketed for use in treatment of parkinsonism because of its central anticholinergic properties. Other anticholinergic agents that are structurally related to the benzhydryl ether antihistamines are also used in the treatment of parkinsonism. Compounds with central anticholinergic and antihistaminic effects have been used as one approach to the treatment of parkinsonism (see Chapter 20).

The observed differences in potency of enantiomers in tissue-based assays suggest significant stereoselective interactions of antagonists at the receptor level. Differences in affinity of 60–200-fold are noted between enantiomers in several analogs where the chiral center results because of differences in the two aromatic rings, e.g., Ph and 2-pyridyl, or Ph and *p*-Br-Ph (47,48). Enantiomers with the S-absolute configuration are usually more potent. Clemastine, a more complex homolog is marketed as the R,R-enantiomer, which is the more potent of R,R and S,S enantiomeric pair, and more potent than either the R,S- and S,R-enantiomers of the other diastereomer (49). Consistent with results from related compounds, the chiral center at the benhydryl carbon has a significant influence on potency, while the chiral center in the pyrrolidine ring is of lesser importance (Table 33.5).

Very small changes in the arrangement of aromatic groups in the members of the ethanolamine ether series alter the scope of their pharmacologic properties significantly. Previous work has shown that the two aromatic rings in diphenhydramine can be located slightly differently with

Table 33.4. Antihistamine and Anticholinergic Activity of Enantiomers of Ring Substituted Ethanolamine Ethers (44–46)

		Antihistaminic Activity			Anticholinergic Activity	
$R_{2'}$	$R_{4'}$	pD_2	Ratio of Potency of (+)- to (−)-Isomer	pD_2	Ratio of Potency of (+)- to (−)-Isomer
$(CH_3)_3C$	H	(+) 8.76*	78	(+) 6.14	1.9
		(−) 6.87		(−) 5.89	
H	CH_3	(+) 6.36	2.3	(+) 6.03	
		(−) 6.00		(−) 8.12*	0.008†

* Most potent enantiomer in each assay.
† (−)-Enantiomer is ~125 times as potent as the (+)-enantiomer.

Table 33.5. Antihistamine Activity of Stereoisomers of Clemastine (41,48)

Drug		pA_2	ED_{50}*
Clemastine	(R,R)	9.45	0.04 mg/kg
	(S,S)	7.99	5.0
	(R,S)	9.40	0.28
	(S,R)	8.57	11.0

*ED_{50} vs. lethal dose of histamine in guinea pigs (48).

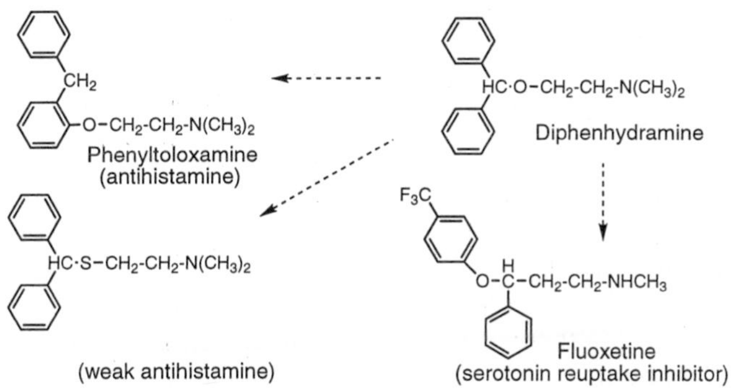

Fig. 33.7. Structural similarities among diphenhydramine-related structures.

R = H   Pheniramine

R = Cl   Chlorpheniramine (Chlortrimeton)
Dexchlorpheniramine (Polaramine)

R = Br   Brompheniramine (Dimetane)
Dexbrompheniramine (Disomer)

E - Pyrrobutamine (Pyronil)

Triprolidine (Actidil)   Dimethindene (Forhistal)   Phenindamine (Nolahist)

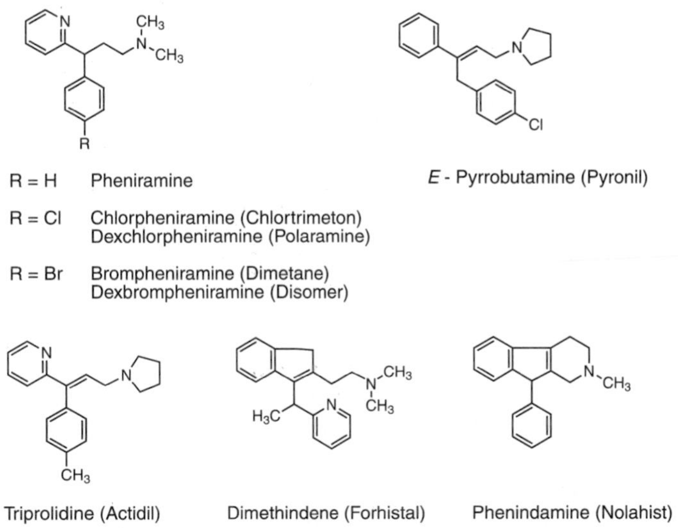

Fig. 33.9. Examples of alkane and alkene antihistamines.

respect to each other as in phenyltoloxamine, a potent antihistamine. However, an "inverted rearrangement" of carbon and oxygen atoms, prepared in an attempt to investigate structural requirements for antihistamines, afforded significantly different pharmacologic properties and ultimately led to a series of very important selective serotonin reuptake inhibitors, like fluoxetine (Fig. 33.7). Unlike the bioisosteric oxygen to nitrogen atom replacement, conversion of the oxygen atom to a sulfur atom in the diphenhydramine series results in a compound with significantly decreased antihistaminic activity (50).

Metabolism. Only limited metabolic disposition information is available on this group of compounds. As expected, N-demethylation (formation of the corresponding secondary amine) and subsequent deamination (formation of the carboxylic acid metabolite) is a major pathway for diphenhydramine (Fig. 33.8) and some of its analogs. Although the early experiments are relatively incomplete, it appears that the N-demethylation products have shorter half-lives than the corresponding parent drugs, and they probably contribute very little to the observed antihistaminic properties. Minor metabolites that are conjugates of the carboxylic acid products of deamination or of ether cleavage products have been found in some animal species. Compounds with short half-lives, like diphenhydramine, when used as antihistamines, require repeated administration, but the short half-life is an advantage when the same drugs are used as sleep aids (51,52).

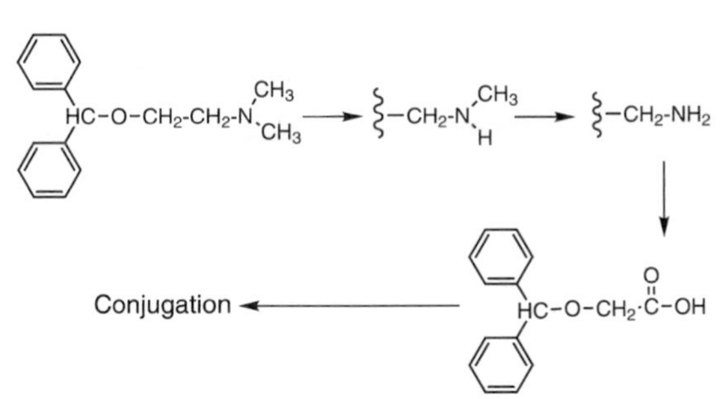

Alkyl Amines

A third class of analogs is one in which a carbon atom replaces the heteroatom spacer in the general structure. Examples are pheniramine, chlorpheniramine and brompheniramine, and the E-isomers of olefinic homologs (Fig. 33.9). The ring halogen-substituted compounds are widely used OTC antihistamines for mild seasonal allergies. These agents are characterized by a long duration of antihistaminic action and by a decreased incidence of central sedative side effects, when compared to the ethylenediamines and ethanolamine ether series. This structural change introduces a chiral carbon when the two aromatic rings are different (e.g., Ph and 2-pyridyl). These were the most extensively used antihistamines until the more selective second-generation antihistamines appeared.

Structural and Stereochemical Effects. E- and Z-isomers of the alkenes in this series show very large differences in potency in tissue-based assays, e.g., E-pyrrobutamine is more potent than its Z-isomer by 165-fold (53) and E-triprolidine (Fig. 33.9) is more potent than its Z-isomer by about 1000-fold (54). Dimethidene has many of the structural features of both of these two agents in a more complex cyclized structure. The observed difference in potency between the E- and Z-isomers shows that the two aromatic rings probably have quite different binding environments at the receptor (55). These observations provide evidence suggesting a 5–6Å distance between the tertiary aliphatic amine and one of the aromatic rings is required at the site of receptor binding (Fig. 33.10) (56).

Differences in potency between the enantiomers of the conformationally mobile amino-alkanes have also been observed. The S-enantiomers have greater affinity for H_1 histamine receptors, occasionally by very large amounts, e.g., by 200–1000-fold in radioligand displacement assays and in tissue-based assays for

Conjugation

Fig. 33.8. Metabolism of diphenhydramine.

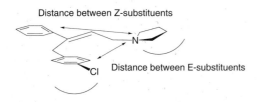

Fig. 33.10. Potential binding sites based upon E/Z configurations.

(+)-S- vs. (−)-R-chlorpheniramine, with the (+)-enantiomer being more potent (Ar = X-Ph, 2-pyridyl). Greater selectivity for H₁ receptors vs. muscarinic and adrenergic receptors is also observed. For members of the series, the chiral center of the more potent enantiomers correlates stereochemically with the more active enantiomer of the oxygen congener carbinoxamine (Ar = Ph, Ar = *p*-Br-Ph) (Table 33.3) (51,57). Single enantiomers of these agents are available, e.g., dexchlorpheniramine and dexbrompheniramine.

Half-life and Metabolism. The alkyl amines have significantly less CNS depressant effects than benzhydryl ethers of ethanolamines. Additionally, these compounds have long half-lives and extended durations of action. These agents have decreased anti-emetic effects and decreased anticholinergic properties compared to ethanolamine ethers. Many are available in OTC preparations for hay fever and other mild allergic conditions, sometimes in combination with adrenergic decongestants. Most are suitable for once-a-day dosing because of their long half-lives, up to 24 hours, although they are routinely administered more frequently (51).

Information on the metabolic disposition of some these agents has been reported. As expected, N-dealkylation is a major pathway with the corresponding secondary and primary amines being found in the plasma, as well as the parent drug (58,59). In cases where O-methyl aryl ethers are

present, O-demethylation products have been reported, as expected.

Piperazines

Members of the piperazine class of agents are structurally related to both the ethylenediamines and the benzhydryl ethers of ethanolamines. Their structures include the two-carbon separation between nitrogen atoms, which is incorporated into the piperazine ring (Table 33.6).

Diarylmethylene groups (benzhydryl substituents, like in diphenhydramine) are attached to one of the nitrogen atoms and an alkyl or aralkyl substituent is attached to the other nitrogen. Early compounds, like cyclizine, chlorcyclizine, meclizine, buclizine and hydroxyzine, have been widely used as antihistamines and as agents for treatment of motion sickness, as they have useful central anti-emetic effects.

These agents also have significant anticholinergic and antihistaminic properties. Anticholinergic side effects and drowsiness are common. The primary use of these compounds remains as treatment of motion sickness, vertigo and suppression of nausea and vomiting. Although teratogenic effects of cyclizine and meclizine have been observed in rodents, large studies have not demonstrated adverse fetal effects in humans. However, these agents are used cautiously in pregnant women and children. Hydroxyzine is used in treatment of pruritis, and at higher dosages, it is used in the management of anxiety and emotional stress. Its acid metabolite, cetirizine, which is formed from oxidation of the terminal primary alcohol to the corresponding carboxylic acid, is usually classified with the second-generation nonsedating antihistamines. The amphoteric nature of cetirizine, having both the tertiary aliphatic amine and carboxylic acid functional group, appears to be associated with decreased, but not absent, sedative side effects.

Tricyclic H₁ Antihistamines

The two aromatic groups noted in several of the classes of antihistamines can be connected to each other through additional atoms, e.g., heteroatoms like sulfur or oxygen, or through a short one or two carbon chain. They have a general structure shown in Figure 33.11. The earliest potent tricyclic antihistamines (Table 33.7) were phenothiazines (Y = S, X = N).

The phenothiazine antihistamines contain a two or three-carbon branched alkyl chain between the nonbasic phenothiazine nitrogen and the aliphatic amine. They dif-

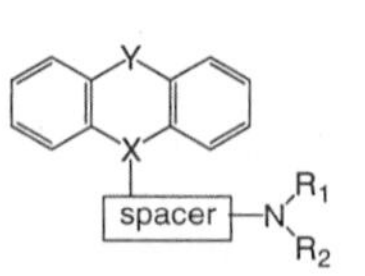

Table 33.6. Examples of Piperazine Antihistamines

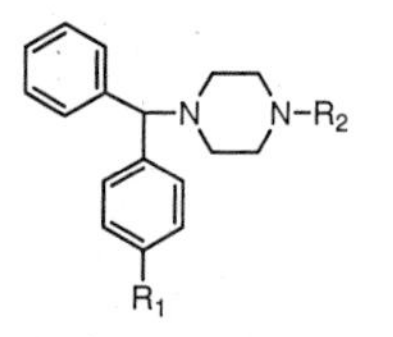

Drugs	Trade Name	R₁	R₂
Cyclizine	Marezine	H	CH₃
Chlorcyclizine	Mantadil	Cl	CH₃
Meclizine	Bonine	Cl	H₂C— (3-CH₃-phenyl)
Buclizine	Softram	Cl	H₂C— (phenyl) —C(CH₃)₃
Hydroxyzine	Atarax	Cl	CH₂CH₂OCH₂CH₂OH
Cetirizine	Zyrtec	Cl	CH₂CH₂OCH₂COOH

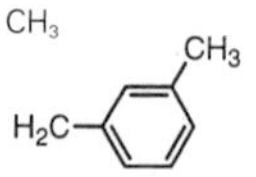

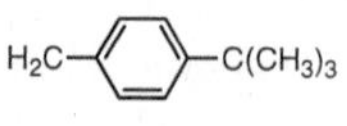

X = C, CH, N, etc.
Y = CH₂, S, O, NH, CH₂O, CH₂CH₂, CH=CH, etc.
spacer = two or three carbons
R₁, R₂ = Me, or five membered ring

Fig. 33.11. General structure of tricyclic antihistamines.

Table 33.7. Examples of Tricyclic Antihistamines

Drugs	Trade Name	Y	Z
Promethazine	Phenergan	S	N with CH3, N(CH3)2, CH3 side chain
Pyrathiazine		S	N with CH2CH2-pyrrolidine side chain
Trimeprazine	Temaril	S	N with CH3, N(CH3)2, CH3 side chain
Methdilazine	Tacaryl	S	N with CH2-N-CH3 pyrrolidine side chain

Cyproheptadine (Periactin)   Azatadine (Optimine)

fer from the antipsychotic phenothiazine derivatives in which the chain is usually three carbons long and un-branched, and lack of substitution in the aromatic ring. Besides useful antihistaminic effects, most have pronounced sedative effects and long durations of action. Other uses include the treatment of nausea and vomiting associated with anesthesia and for the treatment of motion sickness.

Conformational and Stereochemical Effects. In the active agents, the steric restrictions and decreased degrees of conformational freedom resulting from the connection of the two aromatic rings together suggests that certain spatial relationships between these two rings are acceptable in the drug receptor interaction for H_1 antagonism. These ring systems are not flat, but are somewhat puckered with the

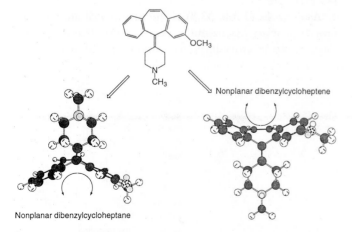

Nonplanar dibenzylcycloheptane

Nonplanar dibenzylcycloheptene

Fig. 33.12. Enantiomers (atropisomers) of 3-methoxycyproheptadine.

two aromatic rings not in the same plane. However, the conformations usually undergo rapid intraconversion. In some closely related systems, where this intraconversion is very slow, conformational enantiomers (atropisomers) have been obtained and studied, including cyproheptadine, doxepine and hydroxylated metabolites of loratadine (60,61). The enantiomers of 3-methoxycyproheptadine have significantly different pharmacologic potency as antihistamines, antiserotonin and anticholinergic agents (Fig. 33.12) (62). The ($-$)-isomer retained antihistaminic, antiserotonin and appetite-stimulating effects similar to cyproheptadine, while the ($+$)-enantiomer had greater anticholinerigic potency. Differences of 9–60-fold were observed in the reported assays.

Promethazine, an early agent in the series has many useful pharmacologic affects other than being an antihistamine. It has significant anti-emetic and anticholinergic properties. It is has sedative-hypnotic properties and has been used to potentiate the effects of analgesic drugs. Subsequent analogs like trimeprazine and methdilazine are used primarily as antipruritic agents in the treatment of urticaria.

Compounds in which the sulfur atom is replaced with another bridge, e.g., two methylene groups, etc. are also available. Some have a pyridine ring replacing one of the benzenoid systems. Cyproheptadine, with a two-carbon spacer between the aromatic rings, also has anticholinergic, antiserotonergic and appetite-stimulating properties, which are useful in treatment of anorexic nervosa and in cachexia. The pyridine analog apparently lacks most of these qualities. Doxepine, an oxygen congener of cyproheptadine, also has significant affinity for other receptors, and it has CNS depressant qualities. It exists as a mixture of Z- and E-isomers (15:85) in its olefenic non-piperidine side chain. In tissue-based assays, the Z-isomer is more potent than the E-isomer by more than 3-fold (60). Most widely used among the group is loratadine, which is considered in the group of nonsedating, second-generation antihistamines (vide infra).

Metabolism. Information on the metabolic disposition and pharmacokinetic properties of agents in this group is limited, including incomplete identification of primary metabolic pathways, results of liver microsomal metabolic experiments, and only occasionally pharmacokinetic information. Products from the phenothiazines include products of N-demethylation, aromatic hydroxylation and occasionally sulfoxidation in man. From tricyclic analogs metabolites resulting from N-demethylation, aromatic hydroxylation and formation of N-quaternary glucuronides have been reported.

Second-generation Nonsedating H_1 Antihistamines
Background

Agents reaching the market in the last 20 years that have improved H_1 selectivity, little or no sedative qualities, and

Table 33.8. Second-generation Nonsedating Antihistamines

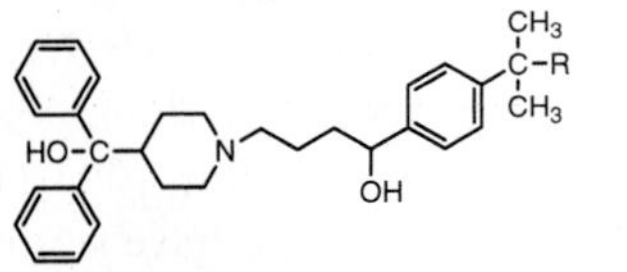

Terfenadine (R = CH₃)
Fexofenadine (R = COOH)

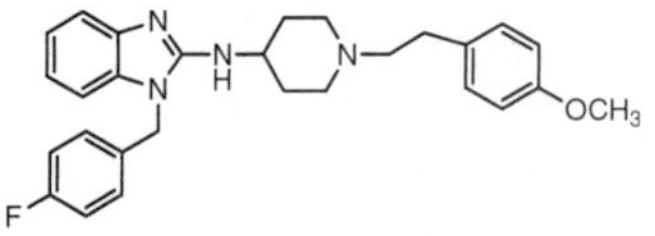

Astemizole

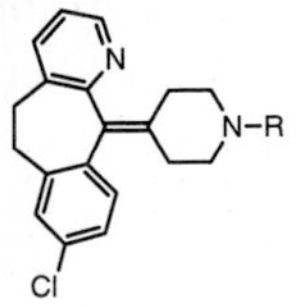

Loratadine (R = —COOCH₂CH₃)
Desloratadine (R = H)

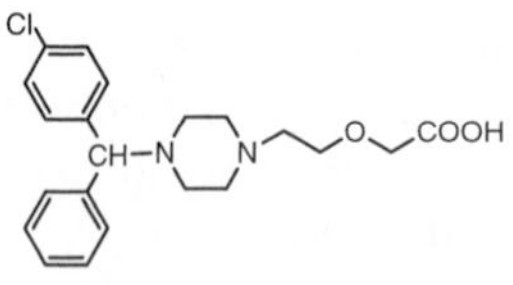

Cetirizine

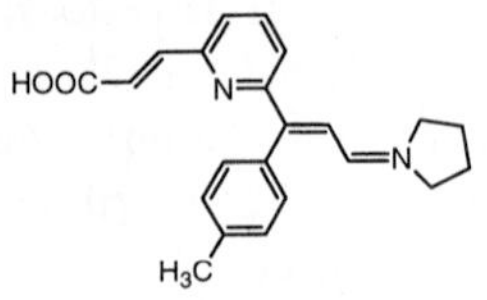

Acrivastine

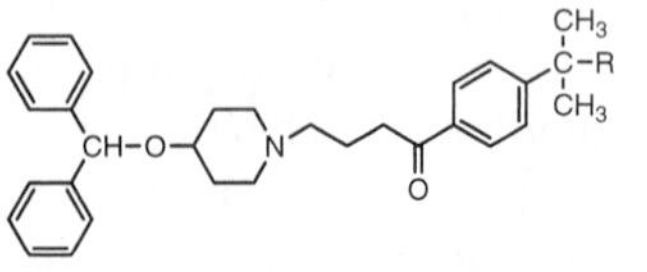

Ebastine (R = CH₃)
Carebastine (R = COOH)

which may have antiallergic effects apart from antihistaminic activity have been called second generation antihistamines. They vary widely in structure (Table 33.8), but less so in pharmacologic properties, having effects principally in the periphery. Structural resemblance to the first generation H₁ antagonists is not always obvious as some of these agents were discovered while investigating other pharmacologic targets. These agents possess selective peripheral H₁ antagonism effects, and they usually have less anticholinergic activity. Furthermore, they also have decreased affinity for adrenergic and serotonergic receptors, and have limited CNS effects. The active agents apparently do not penetrate the blood-brain barrier significantly, perhaps because of their amphoteric nature (most are zwitterionic at physiologic pH) and partitioning characteristics or because they are substrates for the drug efflux P-glycoprotein transporter or organic anion transporter protein (63). A slow rate of dissociation from H₁ receptors is also reported for some of the agents. Several have antiallergic properties that are separate from their antihistaminic properties, which are not thoroughly understood. In most cases, the parent drug or its important metabolites have half-lives sufficiently long to account for the extended duration of action. Most are administered once daily. Comparative reviews have appeared recently (64,65).

Terfenadine and Fexofenadine (Allegra)

Pharmacologic Effects. Terfenadine was the first agent of this group of non-sedating antihistamines, which is commonly thought to include, astemizole, cetirizine and loratadine. The acid metabolite of terfenadine, fexo-

fenadine, is also included in this group, as are some newer agents. Terfenadine was synthesized as an analog of azacyclanol, in a search for antipsychotic agents. The initial reports of its antihistaminic properties included the observation of similar effects of it acid metabolite fexofenadine (66–68). Although terfenadine was once a very widely used nonsedating antihistamine (seldene), extensive clinical experience resulted in the reports of dangerous cardiac arrhythmias occurring occasionally when certain other drugs were taken concomitantly. These cardiac arrhythmias included prolongation of the QT interval and torsades de pointes, a life-threatening ventricular arrhythmia. These effects are associated with blockade of delayed rectifier potassium channels in cardiac tissue, and are associated only with the parent molecule. The side effects occur primarily at high concentrations of the agent, and usually in the presence of other CYP3A4 substrates like ketoconazole or macrolide antibiotics, e.g., oleandomycin (69,70). In the presence of competing CYP3A4 substrates, high plasma concentrations of the parent agent result. Terfenadine is no longer available in the U.S.

Metabolism. Rapid oxidation of terfenadine in vivo ultimately results primarily in formation of the carboxylic acid metabolite (Fig. 33.13) (71), now available as fexofenadine. The acid metabolite probably accounts for the antihistaminic properties of terfenadine in man as the parent compound is very rapidly metabolized via CYP3A4 catalyzed processes. Members of the family of organic anion transporter protein family and the drug efflux transporter P-glycoprotein are involved in the disposition of fexofenadine (63). Fexofenadine is a safer alternative, without the antiarrhymic side effects of terfenadine. The initial hydroxylation of terfenadine is catalyzed by CYP3A4 (72), and further metabolic oxidation of the intermediate alcohol affords the acid. Azacyclanol, the original antipsychotic agent on which terfenadine was based, is a minor product of N-dealkylation of terfenadine.

Astemizole

Astemizole (Table 33.8) is the product of an extensive search of several benzimidazoles (73–75). These benzimidazoles can be considered as 4-aminopiperidines in which

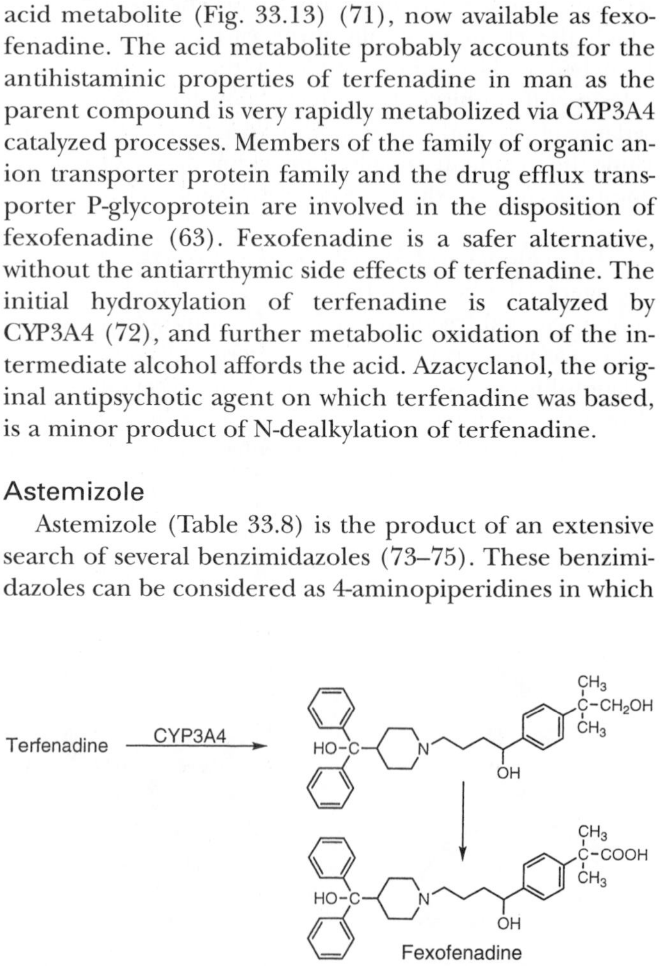

Fig. 33.13. Metabolism of terfenadine leading to fexofenadine.

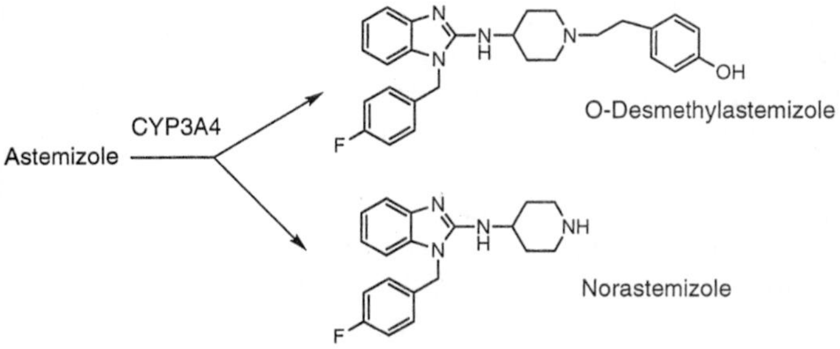

Fig. 33.14. Metabolism of astemizole.

the 4-amino group bears the two aromatic rings, one in the benzimidazole structure, and the other as 4-fluorophenyl group attached at one of the nitrogens. The parent molecule also has untoward effects on myocardial conduction, like terfenadine. In the presence of other CYP3A4 substrates and inhibitor(s), toxicity has been reported. Restrictions and warnings associated with the use of astemizole have been put into place. A long list of competing substrates for CYP3A4 is included in these warnings, as is grapefruit juice [an hydroxylated bergamottin appears to be a significant inhibitor (76)] and the presence of liver disease. Potential adverse drug-drug interactions include azole antifungals, clarithromycin, quinidine, HIV protease inhibitors, zileuton and some selective serotonin reuptake inhibitors (See Chapter 8).

The duration of action of astemizole is extremely long and its onset of action is slow (metabolism dependent). There are at least two active metabolites, the O-demethyl compound, which has a half-life of about 10–20 days, and norastemizole resulting from N-dealkylation (Fig. 33.14). A third metabolite may also contribute to its effects (77). Administration of the astemizole for several days is needed to reach steady state plasma concentrations of the O-demethyl metabolite (78). There is some evidence that this phenolic product has some cardiovascular toxicologic potential similar to terfenadine (79,80). The active metabolite norastemizole is currently under study as a potential safer alternative. With removal of astemizole (Hismanal) from the market in the U.S., it is unclear whether these potential alternatives will be developed further.

Loratadine (Claritin) and Desloratadine (Clarinex)
Pharmacologic Effects. Loratadine (Table 33.8) is related to the first generation tricyclic antihistamines and to

antidepressants. It is nonsedating, and neither it nor its major metabolite, descarboethoxyloratadine (desloratadine), is associated with the potentially cardiotoxic effects reported for terfenadine and astemizole. Upon chronic dosing, the AUC (plasma concentration vs. time curve) for the metabolite is greater than for the parent drug and its half-life is longer (81). Desloratadine is reported to be a more potent H_1 antagonist and a more potent inhibitor of histamine release (81,82). This metabolite, which contributes very significantly to the therapeutic antihistaminic properties of loratadine, has been marketed in Europe and is expected soon in the U.S. Metabolism of desloratadine to ring-hydroxylated products may contribute to its pharmacologic effects (83,84).

Metabolism. The metabolic conversion of loratadine to descarboethoxyloratadine occurs via an oxidative process and not via direct hydrolysis (Fig. 33.15). CYP2D6 and 3A4 appear to be the CYP450 isozymes catalyzing this oxidative metabolic process (85,86). Apparently, the metabolite does not reach the CNS in significant concentrations. Among the nonsedating second-generation antihistamines, this metabolite appears to be the only nonzwitterionic species. While the failure of zwitterionic molecules to reach CNS sites in significant concentrations can be rationalized readily, a similar explanation is not apparent for loratadine or its metabolite (65). Competitive substrates for CYP3A4 do not produce a significant drug-drug interaction, as they have with astemizole and terfenadine (69) because the parent molecule lacks effects on potassium rectifying channels in cardiac tissue.

Cetirizine (Zyrtec)
Cetirizine, the acid metabolite from oxidation of the primary alcohol of the antihistamine hydroxyzine (Fig. 33.16, see also Table 33.6) was widely used in Europe before its introduction in the U.S. It has a long duration of action and is highly selective for H_1-receptors. No cardiotoxicity has been reported (87), but some drowsiness occurs. Some interest currently exists in possible development of a single enantiomer of the agent to induce less CNS sedation (88–90).

Acrivastine (Semprex)
Acrivastine (Table 33.8), an acidic congener of triprolidine in which a carboxylic acid-substituted chain has been attached, is also a second-generation nonsedating antihistamine. Penetration of the blood-brain barrier is limited,

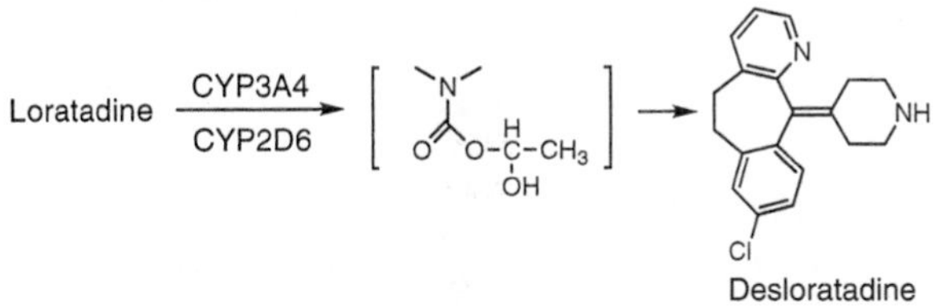

Fig. 33.15. Metabolism of loratadine.

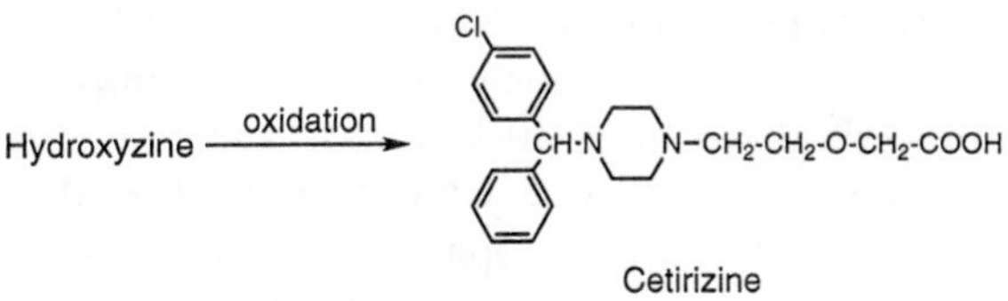

Fig. 33.16. Metabolism of hydroxyzine to cetirizine.

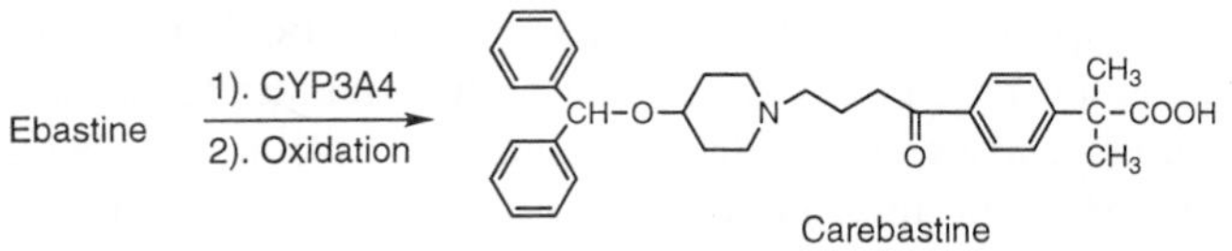

Fig. 33.17. Metabolism of ebastine to carebastine.

and it is less sedating than is triprolidine (91). It is used principally in a combination with a decongestant (92).

Ebastine and Carebastine

Benzhydryl ethers of piperidinols are also useful antihistamines. Those with large N-substituents, like those in terfenadine and other nonsedating antihistamines, are most successful. Ebastine (Table 33.8), structurally similar to terfenadine, has a potent selective H_1 antagonist as measured in radioligand displacement assays. In these assays, its acid metabolite is significantly higher affinity than the parent molecule. It is nonsedating and apparently free of anticholinergic effects (93). Ebastine, like some other second generation antihistamines, blocks release of PGD_2 and leukotriene C_4/D_4 in cellular assays (94). Pharmacokinetic data indicate that its acid metabolite carebastine is responsible for its antihistaminic properties (65), as the parent drug has a very short half-life and the active metabolite a much longer one (Fig. 33.17). In an animal model of torsades de pointes, ebastine, at a high dose, produced significant cardiac conduction abnormalities, e.g., prolongation of the QT interval, while the metabolite did not (95). At lower doses, these effects occurred only in the presence of competitive CYP3A4 substrates. However, some in vitro data suggest CYP450 isozymes other than CYP3A4 may be important in the initial hydroxylation (96). The pharmacologically active acid metabolite carebastine is metabolically analogous to fexofenadine (oxidation of a *t*-butyl group), the acid metabolite of terfenadine. Ebastine is marketed in several countries outside the U.S.

Topical H_1 Antihistamines

Therapeutic Applications

Topical application of H_1 receptor antagonists to the eye relieves itching, congestion of the conjunctiva, and erythema (97). The density of mast cells in the conjunctiva is high, and the histamine concentrations in tear film are significant in the ocular allergic response (98,99). Topical application of H_1 antagonists to the eye relieves pruritis, conjunctivial effects and erythema when volunteers are challenged with eye drops of allergens (100). From eye drops, only small amounts of the antihistamine (1–5%) penetrate the cornea. More of the compound is absorbed via the conjunctiva and nasal mucosa, and still more ends up swallowed from tear duct and nasal drainage. Until recently, topical ocular antihistamines were limited to two classical agents: antazoline (Table

33.2) from the ethylenediamine series and pheniramine (Fig. 33.9) from the alkylamine series. Both are used in combination with sympathomimetic vasoconstictors.

A slow rate of receptor dissociation of H_1 antagonists is associated with long duration of action systemically, which occurs with the more recently available ocular antihistamines. Based on correlations of pKas and lipophilicity data, it appears that compounds with a log D (the sum of the partition coefficients of both the ionized and unionized species) near 1.0 ± 0.5 at pH 7.4 are most efficacious and their water-soluble salts also show a low incidence of ocular irritation. Relationships between partitioning characteristics of these and other antihistamines, indicate receptor affinity (moderate at least) and a particular range of lipophilicity is optimum for topical ocular antihistamines with minimal of ocular irritation (96,99). Some of these compounds, as discussed below, are currently available or are being evaluated as nasal sprays, while some of the topical agents are also occasionally used as systemic antihistamines.

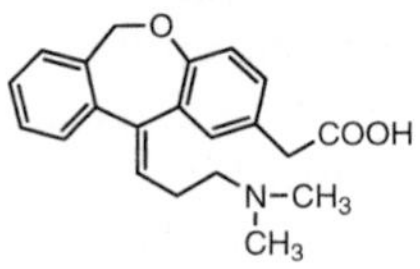

Olopatadine

Olopatadine (Patanol)

A relatively new agent olopatadine is available in the U.S. It is structurally related to the tricyclic antihistamines. It has a long duration of action when applied topically, and it appears to also inhibit the release of inflammatory mediators (histamine, tryptase, PGD_2, etc.) from mast cells. Its selectivity for H_1 receptors in tissue assays (over H_2 and H_3 receptors) is very high, and its selectivity for H_1 receptor blockade over α-adrenergic, dopaminergic, serotonergic, and muscarinic receptors is also very high. Olopatadine is reported to have a rapid onset of action and a long duration of action, consistent with high receptor affinity and a slow rate of receptor dissociation (101–103). The presence of the carboxylic acid side chain is apparently responsible for the observed lack of muscarinic receptor affinity. This feature may also be responsible for limited penetration.

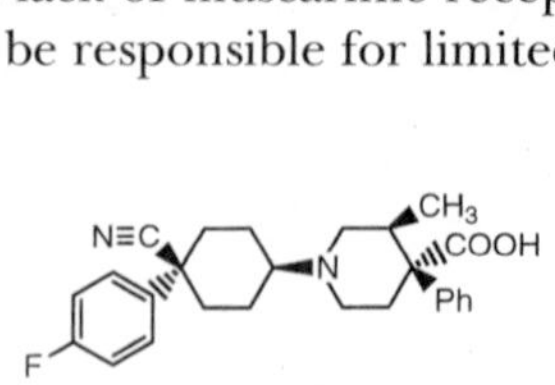

Levocabastine

Levocabastine (Livostin)

Levocabastine is a potent selective H_1 receptor antagonist used topically in eye drops for seasonal allergic conjunctivitis. A small amount of systemic absorption of the compound is reported. The agent also prevents release of transmitters from mast cells (104,105). A nasal spray used for allergic rhinitis is available outside the U.S.

Emedastine

Emedastine (Emadine)

Emedastine is also a newer antihistamine used topically in the eye for conjunctivitis (106–108). It has very high H_1 receptor selectivity characteristics and it is structurally related to the benzimidazoles such as astemizole. Inhibition of mast cell release of inflammatory mediators has been noted (109).

Azelastine

Azelastine (Astelin, Optivar)

Azelastine, although not a close structural analog to the benzimidazoles, has some structural similarities to them. It is used as a nasal spray for allergic rhinitis, and the agent is available in Europe for systemic use for the treatment of asthma and seasonal allergies. Besides antihistaminic effects, it may also block mediator release from mast cells (110–113). When administered orally, the N-dealkylated metabolite appears to contribute significantly to its pharmacological effects (114).

Ketotifen

Ketotifen (Zaditor)

Ketotifen is a potent selective H_1 receptor antagonist that also prevents release of transmitters from mast cells. Although recently approved in the U.S. for topical use to prevent itching of the eye due to allergic conjunctivitis, it is used as a systemic anti-allergy agent in several other countries for the treatment of seasonal allergic rhinitis, hay fever and for asthma (115). Being structurally analogous to the cyproheptadine-like antihistamines, differences in activity of the two enantiomers (atropisomers) has been noted, being about 6–7-fold in ligand displacement and rodent-based assays (116).

Antiulcer Agents
Background

The secretion of gastric acid occurs at the level of parietal cells of the oxyntic gland in the gastric mucosa (Fig. 33.18) producing 2–3 liters of gastric juice per day, pH 1 in hydrochloric acid. Ultimately, this secretory process occurs via an H^+/K^+-ATPase that exchanges hydronium ion (H_3O^+) with uptake of a potassium ion. Several mediators regulate this secretion by way of receptor systems on the basolateral membrane. The H_2 histaminergic pathway is cAMP dependent. Gastrin and muscarinic receptors also regulate the secretion of gastric acid through calcium ion dependent pathways. In parietal cells, E series prostaglandins work in opposition to the histaminergic pathway, inhibiting histamine-stimulated adenylate cyclase activity. Other epithelial cells in the mucosal lining under the influence of prostaglandin mediated pathways secrete bicarbonate and mucus, both of which are important in protecting the gastric lining from the effects of acid secretion. In many cases, hypersecretion of gastric acid appears to be associated with *Helicobacter pylori* infection, which may contribute to defects in mucosal protective defenses. There is evidence that some H_2 antagonists, particularly cimetidine and ranitidine, have regulatory effects on T-cell lymphocyte proliferation by augmenting cytokine production and immunoglobulin production. These effects may not be associated with histamine receptors and may not be shared by nizatidine and famotidine.

Therapeutic Applications of H_2 Antihistamines

H_2 antagonists are used in the treatment of duodenal ulcers, gastric ulcers, gastroesophageal reflux disease (GERD), pathological hypersensitivity disorders, upper GI bleeding in critically ill patients, and are sold OTC for acid indigestion (117). They are also included in multi-drug treatment protocols for eradication of *H. pylori* in treatment of peptic ulcers and prior to surgery to prevent aspiration pneumonitis. Combinations of H_1 and H_2 antagonists are useful in idiopathic urticaria not responding to H_1 antagonists alone, and to itching and flushing of anaphylaxis, pruritis and contact dermatitis.

Structural Requirements. H_2 antagonists specifically designed to decrease the secretion of gastric acid are based on an extensive investigative approach to drug design that began from the structures of partial agonist molecules very closely related to histamine. This process has been well documented (118,119). Ultimately, this work resulted in the development of cimetidine (Table 33.9), in

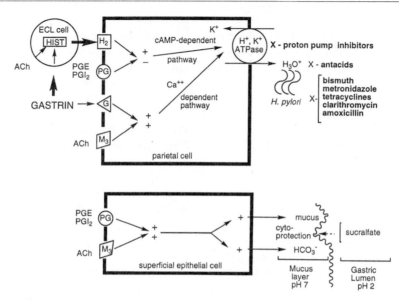

Fig. 33.18. Secretion of gastric acid and peptic ulcer disease. Histamine is secreted from an ECL cell (endochromaffin-like cell) which is inner-vated by muscarinic receptors (M) via the enteric nervous system and by gastrin receptors (G). Agonist occupation of histamine H_2 receptors in parietal cells leads to gastric secretion. Other input at parietal cells includes the prostaglandins (PG), gastrin, and muscarinic receptors. Adapted from Brunton LL. Agents for the control of gastric acidity and treatment of peptic ulcers. Chapter 37, In: Hardman JG, Limbird LE, Mollinoff PB, Ruddon RW, editors. Goodman and Gilman's The Pharmacological Basis of Therapeutics. 9th ed. New York: McGraw-Hill; 1995: 902.

which the imidazole ring like that of histamine is maintained. The imidazole ring is substituted with a C-4 methyl group, which in histamine agonists affords H_2 selectivity, a four-atom side chain which includes one sulfur atom (the sulfur atom increases potency compared to carbon and oxygen congeners) and a terminal polar nonbasic unit, in this case an N-cyanoguanidine substituent (119). Guanidines substituted with electron withdrawing groups have

significantly decreased basicity compared to guanidine, and they are neutral (nonprotonated) at physiologic pH. Thus, these are logical substituents to replace the terminal thiourea feature in unsuccessful earlier homologous candidates, burimamide and metiamide. The former agent was not marketed due to untoward effects, including agranulocytosis, and the latter one lacked significant oral bioavailability. Subsequently, the nitromethylene unit was a replacement of the aminocyano group in the substituted guanidine analogs affording compounds of increased potency. Replacement for the imidazole ring with other heteroaromatic rings resulted in other useful analogs.

Metabolism. Cimetidine, ranitidine and famotidine are subject to first pass metabolism and each has oral bioavailability of about 50%. The oral bioavailability of nizatidine is about 90%. All have half-lives of 1.5–4 hours, with that of nizatidine being the shortest. Significant amounts of each of these H_2-antagonists are excreted unchanged, with small amounts of urinary products of sulfoxidation being a common metabolic feature. As expected, hydroxylation of the imidazole C-4 methyl groups occurs in cimetidine. Ranitidine is excreted largely unchanged, but minor metabolic pathways include N-demethylation, and N- and S-oxidation (120,121). The metabolites are not thought to contribute to the therapeutic properties of the parent drugs, with the exception of nizatidine from which the N-desmethyl metabolite retains H_2-antagonist activity (122,123).

Side Effects and Drug Interactions. Cimetidine, the earliest of these agents, shows the greatest number of drug interactions (124). Among these are somnolence and

Table 33.9. H_2 Receptor Antihistamines

Drug	Trade Name	R	X	Y
Burimamide		H	CH_2	S
Cimetidine	Tagamet	CH_3	S	N–C≡N
Metiamide		CH_3	S	S

Drug	Trade Name	Ar
Ranitidine	Zantac	
Nizatidine	Axid	
Famotidine	Pepcid	

confusion in elderly patients with decreased renal function. Gynecomastia, presumably related to increased prolactin secretion, has been reported. Cimetidine inhibits CYP450-dependent metabolic processes affording increased concentration of several agents, the most important being those having narrow therapeutic concentration windows, e.g., phenytoin, theophylline, some benzodiazepines, warfarin, quinidine, etc. Inhibition of several CYP450 oxidative processes is associated with the presence of imidazole ring of cimetidine, which apparently replaces the histidine that serves as a ligand to the porphyrin iron in CYP450 enzymes. Other agents in this group contain heterocyclic rings other than imidazole, and do not show this effect. Cimetidine also inhibits renal tubular secretion of some drugs, e.g., procainamide (125). These tubular secretion effects are also less prevalent or absent with other agents in this class. The other agents in the group show significant differences in potency; being more potent than cimetidine. Of these, ranitidine is the most widely used. The agents have reached OTC status and are thus widely available for gastric hyperacidity (126).

Proton Pump Inhibitors

The final step in acid secretion in parietal cells of the gastric mucosa is mediated by H$^+$/K$^+$-ATPase, the gastric proton pump, an enzyme with significant homology to Na$^+$/K$^+$-ATPase. This H$^+$/K$^+$-ATPase has some similarities to the H$^+$/K$^+$-ATPase in osteoclasts, which is involved in bone resorption. Gastric acid secretion can be inhibited in many ways. These include by antagonists at muscarinic, gastrin or histamine H$_2$ receptors, by agonists at inhibitory receptors for prostaglandins and somatostatin, by proton pump inhibitors, or by carbonic anhydrase inhibitors.

Mechanism of Action. Omeprazole, lansoprazole and related analogs (Table 33.10), produce inhibition of stimulated gastric acid secretion irrespective of the receptor stimulation process. Nearly all of the compounds are close structural relatives, being weakly basic 2-pyridymethyl-sulfinylbenzimidazoles. Only a few successful changes of the heterocyclic rings are possible (127,128). These agents have irreversible effects on the secretion of gastric acid because the molecule rearranges in the strongly acidic environment of the parietal cell. Covalent binding of the rearranged inhibitor to the H$^+$/K$^+$-ATPase results in inactivation of the catalytic function of the proton pump. There is evidence that two molecules of the intermediate from omeprazole are bound to the active site of the cysteine-rich H$^+$/K$^+$-ATPase, one of these sites has been identified as cysteine-813 (and probably cysteine-822) of the H$^+$/K$^+$-ATPase (129, 130). In the covalent binding, a disulfide bond to the receptor is formed. Similar results are reported for lansoprazole, pantoprazole and rabeprazole (131). A chemical mechanism for the process is shown in Figure 33.19. Because the initial rearrangement only occurs at a strongly acidic pH, acid-stable oral dosage

Table 33.10. H$^+$/K$^+$-ATPase Proton Pump Inhibitors

Drugs	Trade Name	R$_1$	R$_2$	R$_3$	R$_4$
Omeprazole	Prilosec	OCH$_3$	CH$_3$	CH$_3$	CH$_3$
Esomeprozole (S-enantiomer)	Nexium	OCH$_3$	CH$_3$	CH$_3$	CH$_3$
Lansoprazole	Prevacid	H	CH$_3$	CH$_2$CF$_3$	H
Rabeprazole	Aciphex	H	CH$_3$	(CH$_2$)$_3$OCH$_3$	H
Pantoprazole	Protonix	OCHF$_2$	OCH$_3$	CH$_3$	H

forms are used that allow for dissolution, release and absorption of drug in the intestine, e.g., enteric coated granules in capsules or enteric coated tablets. Subsequent acid-catalyzed rearrangement of absorbed drug then occurs selectively in the acidic environment of the parietal cells. Some differences may occur in the sites of binding of the agents, and differences have been noted in recovery times, with rabeprazole having a shorter duration of action (132,133).

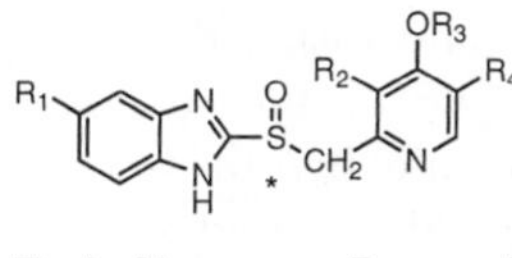

Metabolism. Omeprazole is rapidly oxidized during and after intestinal absorption. The sulfone, sulfide and hydroxylated metabolites have been reported. Omeprazole is a substrate for CYP2C19 and may elevate concentrations of other substrates for this enzyme, e.g., diazepam, when given concurrently. Further oxidation of the sulfone affords additional metabolites, which are excreted in the feces. The analog lansoprazole is metabolized by analogous routes (134). Fewer drug interactions with lansoprazole have been reported, although it is also a substrate for CYP2C19. Rabeprazole and pantoprazole were recently marketed in the U.S. (135,136).

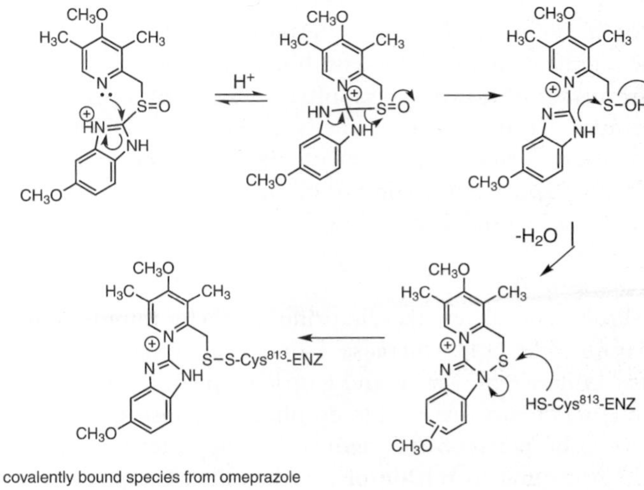

covalently bound species from omeprazole

Fig. 33.19. Acid catalyzed activation of omeprazole to reactive sulfenamide. At the parietal cell H$^+$/K$^+$-ATPase, a cysteine residue reacts to form disulfide-attached enzyme-inhibitor.

These sulfoxides have a chiral sulfur atom, and recent work has been reported on the effects of stereochemistry on pharmacologic and dispositional characteristics. Substrate stereoselectivity in the metabolism of the enantiomers of omeprazole has been observed with R-(+)-omeprazole being hydroxylated at the C-5 methyl group by CYP2C19 and the S-(−)-enantiomer being preferentially metabolized by CYP3A4 (137). Esomeprazole, the S-(−)-enantiomer of omeprazole, has recently been marketed in the U.S. A single enantiomer might avoid interactions based on competitive CYP2C19 substrates (138,139). Differences in the dispositional characteristics and protein binding of the enantiomers of lansoprazole have been noted when a single dose of racemic compound is administered orally (140). Only small differences in inhibitory effects on the H^+/K^+-ATPase in isolated canine parietal cells have been reported (141). Some initial work on disposition of the pantoprazole enantiomers in humans has been reported (142).

Combination Therapy in *Helicobacter pylori* Infections. The majority of peptic ulcers are related to *H. pylori* infections and NSAID therapy. *H. pylori,* apparently penetrates the layer of gastric mucus by producing ammonia and carbon dioxide (urease catalyzed hydrolysis of urea) to withstand the acidic environment of the stomach. More than 90% of duodenal ulcer patients, excluding those with gastrinoma or taking NSAIDs, show the presence of *H. pylori*. Determination of *H. pylori* infection is routinely performed by measuring production of carbon dioxide (breath) or bicarbonate (blood) after oral administration of ^{13}C- or ^{14}C-labeled urea. Endoscopic examination and antigen-based serological tests may be used as confirmation (143). Eradication of *H. pylori* markedly decreases the incidence of ulcer recurrence. Several regimens of antibiotic therapy, widely used with proton pump inhibitors or less commonly with H$_2$-antagonists, are effective. Combination antimicrobial regimens appear to be more effective than single agents. Among the combinations used are clarithromycin for two weeks plus concurrent ranitidine bismuth citrate for four weeks, a regimen of bismuth subsalicylate and metronidazole and tetracycline, and a recently approved regimen of omeprazole, clarithromycin and amoxicillin.

Prokinetic Agents

Prokinetic drugs like cisapride, metaclopramide, and levosulpiride (144) increase esophageal sphincter pressure, enhance peristalsis and gastric emptying, thus counteracting factors that lead to esophagitis. These agents appear to be partial 5-HT$_4$ agonists in the enteric nervous system leading to release of acetylcholine. Cisapride was preferred over metaclopramide in the U.S. because of fewer side effects (145). It was removed from the prescrip-

tion market because of metabolism based interactions. In the presence of competing CYP3A4 substrates, high concentrations of the parent molecule lead to serious cardiac arrhythmias, similar to the H$_1$ antagonists terfenadine and astemizole (146). It is available only through an investigational limited access program. Levosulpiride is available in Europe.

Cisapride

Prostaglandins

Misoprostol   Prostaglandin E$_1$

Prostaglandins have antisecretory effects on gastric acid (Fig. 33.16). Besides inhibiting adenylcyclase activity in parietal cells which results in secretion of gastric acid, prostaglandins stimulate secretion of mucus and bicarbonate in adjacent superficial cells. Cytoprotective effects of endogenous E series prostaglandins and of other more-stable synthetic congeners are observed (Fig. 33.18). The only available oral prostaglandin in the U.S. is misoprostol. The orally administered ester is hydrolyzed to the pharmacologically active carboxylic acid. It is a synthetic analog of prostaglandin E$_1$, in which structural changes at C-13,14,15,16 are made to prevent rapid metabolic conversion to inactive products. The presence of the tertiary alcohol one-carbon removed to C-16 obviates the usual conversion of the allylic secondary alcohol ($\Delta^{13,14}$-15-alcohol) of prostaglandins to the corresponding saturated ketones. A mixture of diastereomers is used, with most of the activity residing in the 11R,16S-isomer (147). Misoprostol reduces basal levels of gastric acid secretion, but it has considerable smooth muscle contraction effects.

Therapeutic Applications and Side Effects. In the U.S., misoprostol is administered with some current nonsteroidal anti-inflammatory agents (NSAIA) to reduce the risk of complications of gastric ulceration and bleeding. A primary mechanism of action of NSAIAs is derived from their inhibition of formation of prostaglandins from arachidonic acid. A prostaglandin may be added for the duration of NSAIA therapy. A combination product of diclofenac (an NSAIA) and misoprostol is available. Unlabelled uses of misoprostol include treatment of duodenal ulcers, for which it appears effective, and in the treatment of duodenal ulcers unresponsive to H₂ antagonists. In other countries it has been used in the treatment of duodenal ulcers (148).

Significant side effects are those associated with abortifacient properties and other smooth muscle contractural effects, e.g., diarrhea, and abdominal pain. Results of several studies show that misoprostol is an effective and low cost cervical ripening agent useful by vaginal application in the induction of labor (149,150). Its use with methotrexate to induce medical abortions is under study (151,152), and it has been used with RU-486 as an abortifacient in other countries (153–155).

Sucralfate and Insoluble Bismuth Preparations

Sucralfate   R = SO₃[Al₂(OH)₅]

Sucralfate is a complex of the sulfuric acid ester of sucrose and aluminum hydroxide. Secondary polymerization with aluminum hydroxide forms intermolecular bridges between molecules of sulfate esters with aluminum (156). Limited dissociation of the complex occurs in gastric acid, but the anionic sulfate esters form insoluble adherent complexes with the proteinaceous exudate at the abraded surface of a crater of the ulcerated area in the stomach. This physical complex protects the ulcer from the erosive action of pepsin and bile salts. Sucralfate also stimulates synthesis and release of prostaglandins, bicarbonate, and epidermal and fibroblast growth factors (157). Significant ulcer healing effects are noted in placebo controlled trials. Only small amounts of sucralfate are absorbed systemically. In renal impairment, there is a risk of accumulation of absorbed aluminum from the drug (143). Sucralfate reduces absorption of other drugs including, H₂-antagonists, quinolone antibiotics, phenytoin, and perhaps warfarin (158,159).

Bismuth-containing preparations, e.g., those containing colloidal bismuth subcitrate have effects similar to sucralfate apparently due to their similar physical properties and coating effects. A combination of ranitidine-bismuth citrate is used with clarithromycin for eradication of *H. pylori* in the treatment and prevention of recurrence of duodenal ulcers. Combinations of bismuth subcitrate with other antibiotics are also used, with H₂-receptor antagonists. Bismuth subsalicylate is used in this way also.

H₃ RECEPTOR AGONISTS AND ANTAGONISTS
Physiologic Role of H₃ Receptors

The H₃ receptor has been described as an autoreceptor that regulates the release of histamine, and it appears also

Table 33.11. Examples of H₃ Agonists and Antagonists

to be a heteroreceptor on neurons in the CNS, which have been shown to be involved in the regulation of other transmitters. In addition, H₃ heteroreceptors have been identified in peripheral tissues, including the airway and GI tract (28,160,161). Thus far, the sequence of the H₃ receptor has not been reported, and the corresponding signal transduction system is unclear.

Selected H₃ Agonists and Antagonists

Several H₃ agonists and antagonists have been studied (Table 33.11). R-α-Methylhistamine is a more potent agonist than is histamine, as determined by effects on [³H]-histamine release in rat cortex (162). The addition of methyl groups to the side chain of histamine usually results in potent H₃ agonists, e.g., α,α-dimethylhistamine and β-methylhistamine (163), unlike the deleterious effect of these changes on H₁ and H₂ agonist activity. Other selective agonists are the isothioureas imetit and SKF 91606, and immepip, a substituted piperidine. All retain the imidazole portion of histamine.

H₃ Antagonists, like clobenpropit, impromidine, thioperamide and GT2016(164) are pharmacologic tools. These agents show some structural resemblance to H₂ antagonists like burimamide, an early H₂ antagonist agent related to cimetidine. As with the H₃ agonists, these agents retain the imidazole group but possess widely varying substituents.

Therapeutic Potential for H₃ Agonists and Antagonists

So far no H₃ agonists have been introduced, however several applications for these agents are being examined. H₃ agonists may have potential use in asthma by reducing nonadrenergic-non-cholinergic and cholinergic neurotransmission to reduce microvascular leakage, and by producing relaxation of the airway, and in myocardial ischemia by reducing excessive norepinephrine release (165). Other potential uses appear to be as antidiarrheals or for the treatment of ulcers to decrease acid secretion. H_3 Antagonists that reach the CNS would appear to be theoretically useful to regulate wakefulness. Other therapeutic possibilities include the treatment of epilepsy where higher densities of H_1 receptors have been observed, and other CNS disorders where histamine regulates other transmitter release (166).

CASE STUDY

Victoria F. Roche and S. William Zito

It's a typically cold and wintry Thanksgiving week in Omaha, Nebraska and CJ, an executive with the Union Pacific railroad and a single mom, is about to head out across the state to Grandma's house in Scottsbluff with her 30-month-old daughter KJ. KJ is actually CJ's second child, but her first-born was lost tragically at 2 months to sudden infant death syndrome (SIDS). Fortunately, KJ has been a healthy child, although she did experience prolonged jaundice when she was first born.

As if the trip across the flat and seemingly endless Platte River valley wasn't going to be long enough, KJ has developed a pruritic rash on her arms and legs from wearing pajamas that were exposed to perfume from the new brand of dryer sheet that CJ used when doing yesterday's laundry. The itching kept KJ and her mom from getting a full night's sleep last night. CJ purchased a tube of 1% hydrocortisone cream in the morning, and it has helped a bit, but KJ is still scratching and acting cranky. If the weather doesn't close in, the trip to Grandma's should take a full 8 hours, and CJ is worried that her daughter will be uncomfortable and fussy the whole time. She called the pediatrician, who has recommended that KJ be given an antihistamine and seeks your advice. The four H_1 receptor antagonists shown below have been mentioned as possible therapeutic alternatives.

1. *Identify the therapeutic problem(s) where the pharmacist's intervention may benefit the patient.*

2. *Identify and prioritize the patient specific factors that must be considered to achieve the desired therapeutic outcomes.*

3. *Conduct a thorough and mechanistically oriented structure-activity analysis of all therapeutic alternatives provided in the case.*

4. *Evaluate the SAR findings against the patient specific factors and desired therapeutic outcomes and make a therapeutic decision.*

5. *Counsel your patient.*

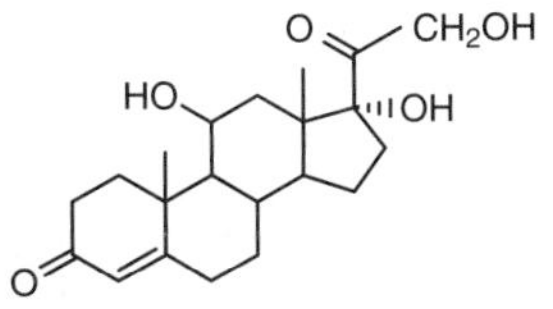

Hydrocortisone

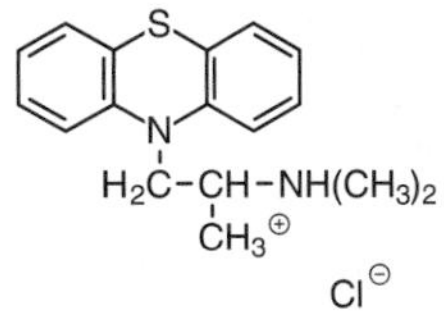

1

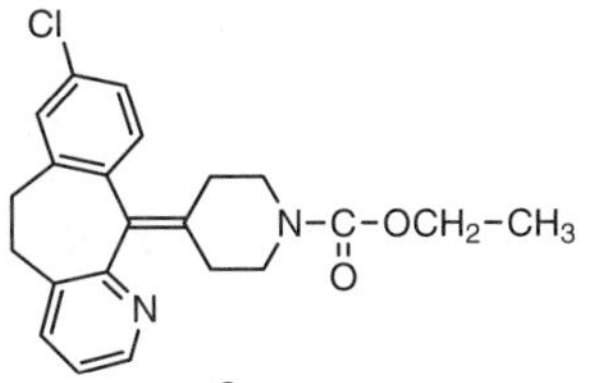

2

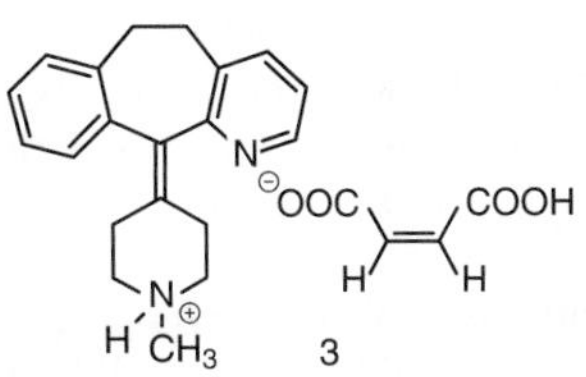

3

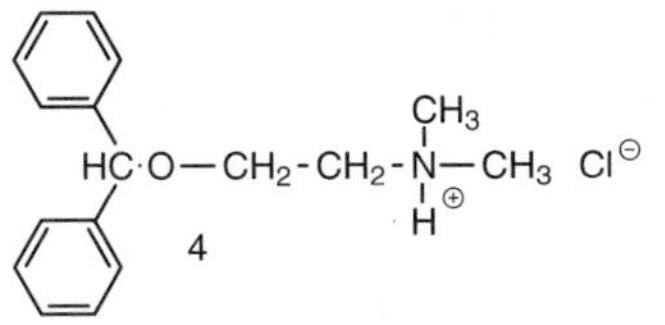

4

REFERENCES

1. Babe KSJ, Serafin WE. Histamine, bradykinin, and their antagonists. In: Hardman JG, Limbird LE, Mollinoff PB, et al, editors. Goodman and Gilman's The Pharmacological Basis of Therapeutics. 9th ed. New York: McGraw-Hill; 1995. p. 581–600.
2. Cooper DG, Young RC, Durant GJ, et al. 5 Histamine receptors. In: Emmett JC, editor. Comprehensive Medicinal Chemistry. The Rational Design, Mechanistic Study, and Therapeutic Application of Chemical Compounds, Vol. 3: Membranes and Receptors. Oxford: Pergamon Press; 1990. p. 343–421.
3. Zhang M-Q, Leurs R., Timmerman H. Histamine H_1-receptor antagonists. In: Wolff ME, editor. Burger's Medicinal Chemistry and Drug Discovery. 5th ed. New York: John Wiley & Sons, Inc.; 1997. p. 495–559.
4. Durant GJ, Ganellin CR, Parsons ME. Chemical differentiation of histamine H_1- and H_2-receptor agonists. J Med Chem 1975;18(9):905–9.
5. Wasylishen RE, Tomlinson G. Application of long-range $^{13}C,^1H$ nuclear spin-spin coupling constants in the study of imidazole tautomerism in L-histidine, and related compounds. Can J Biochem 1977;55:579–82.
6. Cole LB, Holt EM. Histamine complexation: structural studies of [$CaCl_4(H_2O)_2CaCl_2(H_2O)_2$(histamine)$_2$] and histamine hydrobromide. J Chem Soc, Perkin Trans 1 1986:151–4.
7. Ganellin CR, Pepper ES, Port GN, et al. Conformation of histamine derivatives. 1. Application of molecular orbital calculations and nuclear magnetic resonance spectroscopy. J Med Chem 1973;16:610–6.
8. Ham NS, Casy AF, Ison RR. Solution conformations of histamine and some related derivatives. J Med Chem 1973;16:470–5.
9. Ganellin CR, Port GN, Richards WG. Conformation of histamine derivatives. 2. Molecular orbital calculations of preferred conformations in relation to dual receptor activity. J Med Chem 1973;16:616–20.
10. Durant GJ, Emmett JC, Ganellin CR, et al. Potential histamine H_2-receptor antagonists. 3. Methylhistamines. J Med Chem 1976;19:923–8.
11. Black JW, Duncan WA, Durant CJ, et al. Definition and antagonism of histamine H_2-receptors. Nature 1972;236:385–90.
12. Kollonitsch J, Perkins LM, Patchett AA, et al. Selective inhibitors of biosynthesis of aminergic neurotransmitters. Nature 1978;274:906–4.
13. Abeles RH, Maycock AL. Suicide enzyme inactivators. Acc Chem Res 1976;9:313–19.
14. Schayer RC, Cooper JAD. Metabolism of ^{14}C histamine in man. J Appl Physiol 1956;9:481–483.
15. Du Buske LM. Clinical comparison of histamine H_1-receptor antagonist drugs. J Allergy Clin Immunol 1996;98:S307–18.
16. Abbas AK, Lichtman AH, Pober JS. Effector mechanisms of immunoglobulin E-initiated immune reactions. In: Cellular and Molecular Immunology. 3rd ed. Philadelphia: Saunders; 1997. p. 297–312.
17. Church MK, Holgate ST, Shute JK, et al. Mast cell-derived mediators. In: Middleton E, Jr. et al., editor. Allergy. Principles and Practice. 5th ed. St. Louis: Mosby; 1998. p. 146–167.
18. Holgate ST, Robinson C, Church MK. Mediators of immediate hypersensitivity. In: Middleton E, Jr. et al., editor. Allergy: Principles and Practice. 4th ed. St. Louis: Mosby; 1993. p. 267–302.
19. Fukui H, Fujimoto K, Mizuguchi H, et al. Molecular cloning of the human histamine H_1 receptor gene. Biochem Biophys Res Commun 1994;201:894–901.

20. Yamashita M, Fukui H, Sugama K, et al. Expression cloning of a cDNA encoding the bovine histamine H_1 receptor. Proc Natl Acad Sci U S A 1991;88:11515–9.
21. Birdsall NJ. Cloning and structure-function of the H_2 histamine receptor. Trends Pharmacol Sci 1991;12:9–10.
22. Timmerman H. Cloning of the H_1 histamine receptor. Trends Pharmacol Sci 1992;13:6–7.
23. Leurs R, Smit MJ, Tensen CP, et al. Site-directed mutagenesis of the histamine H_1-receptor reveals a selective interaction of asparagine-207 with subclasses of H_1-receptor agonists. Biochem Biophys Res Commun 1994;201:295–301.
24. Smit MJ, Hoffmann M, Timmerman H, et al. Molecular properties and signalling pathways of the histamine H_1 receptor. Clin. Exp. Allergy 1999;29(Suppl. 3):19–28.
25. Leurs R, Smit MJ, Timmerman H. Molecular pharmacological aspects of histamine receptors. Pharmacol Ther 1995;66:413–63.
26. Gantz I, Munzert G, Tashiro T, et al. Molecular cloning of the human histamine H_2 receptor. Biochem Biophys Res Commun 1991;178:1386–92.
27. Gantz I, DelValle J, Wang LD, et al. Molecular basis for the interaction of histamine with the histamine H_2 receptor. J Biol Chem 1992;267:20840–3.
28. Ruat M, Traiffort E, Arrang JM, et al. Cloning and tissue expression of a rat histamine H_2-receptor gene. Biochem Biophys Res Commun 1991;179:1470–8.
29. Morel N, Hardy JP, Godfraind T. Histamine-operated calcium channels in intestinal smooth muscle of the guinea-pig. Eur J Pharmacol 1987;135:69–75.
30. Nederkoorn PH, van Gelder EM, Donne-Op den Kelder GM, et al. The agonistic binding site at the histamine H_2 receptor. II. Theoretical investigations of histamine binding to receptor models of the seven α-helical transmembrane domain. J Comput Aided Mol Design 1996;10:479–89.
31. Nederkoorn PH, van Lenthe JH, van der Goot H, et al. The agonistic binding site at the histamine H_2 receptor. I. Theoretical investigations of histamine binding to an oligopeptide mimicking a part of the fifth transmembrane α-helix. J Comput Aided Mol Design 1996;10:461–78.
32. Johnson CL. Histamine receptors and cyclic nucleotides. In: Schwartz J-C, Haas HL, editors. The Histamine Receptor: Receptor Biochemistry and Methodology. New York: Wiley-Liss; 1992. p. 129–143.
33. Shapiro GG, Konig P. Cromolyn sodium: a review. Pharmacotherapy 1985;5:156–70.
34. Pelikan Z, Knottnerus I. Inhibition of the late asthmatic response by nedocromil sodium administered more than two hours after allergen challenge. J Allergy Clin Immunol 1993;92:19–28.
35. Berman BA, Ross RN. Cromolyn. Clin Rev Allergy 1983;1:105–21.
36. Church MK, Warner JO. Sodium cromoglycate and related drugs. Clin Allergy 1985;15:311–20.
37. Murphy S, Kelly HW. Cromolyn sodium: a review of mechanisms and clinical use in asthma. Drug Intell Clin Pharm 1987;21:22–35.
38. Parish RC, Miller LJ. Nedocromil sodium. Ann Pharmacother 1993;27:599–606.
39. Brogden RN, Sorkin EM. Nedocromil sodium. An updated review of its pharmacological properties and therapeutic efficacy in asthma. Drugs 1993;45:693–715.
40. Caldwell DR, Verin P, Hartwich-Young R, et al. Efficacy and safety of lodoxamide 0.1% vs cromolyn sodium 4% in patients with vernal keratoconjunctivitis. Am J Ophthalmol 1992;113:632–7.

41. Yoshinuma M. Preventive mechanisms and effects of pemirolast potassium on restenosis after percutaneous transluminal coronary angioplasty: serial coronary angiography and intravascular ultrasound studies. J Cardiol 1999;33:81–8.

42. Forneau E, Bovet D. Recherches sur l'action sypmathicolytique d'un nouveau derive du dioxane. Arch Int Pharmacodyn 1933;46:178–191.

43. Hawes EM. N^+-Glucuronidation, a common pathway in human metabolism of drugs with a tertiary amine group. Drug Metab Dispos 1998;26:830–7.

44. Lantos A, Toth A, Zsiray M. Loderix (setastine) tablets in the treatment of allergic rhinoconjunctivitis. Ther Hung 1991; 39:22–4.

45. Harms AF, Nauta WT. The effects of alkyl substitution in drugs—I. Substituted dimethylaminoethyl benzhydryl ethers. J Med Pharm Chem 1960;2:57–77.

46. Ariens EJ. Stereoselectivity of bioactive agents: general aspects. In: Ariens EJ, Soudijn W, Timmermans PBM, editors. Stereochemistry and Biological Activity. Oxford: Blackwell Scientific Publications; 1983. p. 11–32.

47. Rekker RF, Timmerman H, Harms AF, et al. Antihistaminic and anticholinergic activities of optically active diphenhydramine derivatives. Concept of complementarity. Arzneim-Forsch 1971;21:688–91.

48. Casy AF, Drake AF, Ganellin CR, et al. Stereochemical studies of chiral H-1 antagonists of histamine: the resolution, chiral analysis, and biological evaluation of four antipodal pairs. Chirality 1992;4:356–66.

49. Ebnoether A, Weber HP. Synthesis and absolute configuration of clemastine and its isomers. Helv Chim Acta 1976;59:2462–8.

50. Timmerman H, Rekker RF, Harms AF, et al. Effect of alkyl substitution in drugs. XXII. Antihistaminic and anticholinergic activity of a series of thio ether analogs of substituted diphenhydramines. Arzneim-Forsch 1970;20:1258–9.

51. Paton DM, Webster DR. Clinical pharmacokinetics of H_1-receptor antagonists (the antihistamines). Clin Pharmacokinet 1985;10:477–97.

52. Simons KJ, Simons FER. H_1-receptor antagonists: Pharmacokinetics and clinical pharmacology. Clin Allergy Immunol 1996;7(Histamine and H_1-Receptor Antagonists in Allergic Disease):175–213.

53. Casy AF, Ison RR. Stereochemical influences upon antihistamine activity. Further studies of isomeric 4-amino-1,2-diarylbutenes. J Pharm Pharmacol 1970;22:270–8.

54. Ison RR, Franks FM, Soh KS. The binding of conformationally restricted antihistamines to histamine receptors. J Pharm Pharmacol 1973;25:887–94.

55. Towart R, Sautel M, Moret E, et al. Investigation of the antihistaminic action of dimethindene maleate (Fenistil) and its optical isomers. Agents Actions Suppl. 1991;33(New Perspect Histamine Res):403–8.

56. Hanna PE, Ahmed AE. Conformationally restricted analogs of histamine H_1 receptor antagonists. *trans-* and *cis*-1,5-Diphenyl-3-dimethylaminopyrrolidine. J Med Chem 1973;16:963–8.

57. Shafi'ee A, Hite G. The absolute configurations of the pheniramines, methyl phenidates, and pipradrols. J Med Chem 1969;12:266–70.

58. Rumore MM. Clinical pharmacokinetics of chlorpheniramine. Drug Intell Clin Pharm 1984;18:701–7.

59. Yasuda SU, Wellstein A, Likhari P, et al. Chlorpheniramine plasma concentration and histamine H_1-receptor occupancy. Clin Pharmacol Ther 1995;58:210–20.

60. Otsuki I, Ishiko J, Sakai M, et al. Pharmacological activities of doxepin hydrochloride in relation to its geometrical isomers. Oyo Yakuri 1972;6:973–84.

61. Piwinski JJ, Wong JK, Chan TM, et al. Hydroxylated metabolites of loratadine: an example of conformational diastereomers due to atropisomerism. J Org Chem 1990;55:3341–50.

62. Remy DC, Rittle KE, Hunt CA, et al. (+)- and (−)-3-Methoxycyproheptadine. A comparative evaluation of the antiserotonin, antihistaminic, anticholinergic, and orexigenic properties with cyproheptadine. J Med Chem 1977;20:1681–4.

63. Cvetkovic M, Leake B, Fromm MF, et al. OATP and P-glycoprotein transporters mediate the cellular uptake and excretion of fexofenadine. Drug Metab Dispos 1999;27:866–871.

64. Walsh GM, Annunziato L, Frossard N, et al. New insights into the second generation antihistamines. Drugs 2001;61:207–236.

65. Simons FE, Simons KJ. Clinical pharmacology of new histamine H_1 receptor antagonists. Clinical Pharmacokinetics 1999;36:329–52.

66. Woodward JK, Munro NL. Terfenadine, the first non-sedating antihistamine. Arzneim-Forsch 1982;32:1154–6.

67. Carr AA, Meyer DR. Synthesis of terfenadine. Arzneim-Forsch 1982;32:1157–9.

68. Garteiz DA, Hook RH, Walker BJ, et al. Pharmacokinetics and biotransformation studies of terfenadine in man. Arzneim-Forsch 1982;32:1185–90.

69. Smith SJ. Cardiovascular toxicity of antihistamines. Otolaryngol Head Neck Surg 1994;111:348–54.

70. Woosley RL. Cardiac actions of antihistamines. Ann Rev Pharmacol Toxicol 1996;36:233–52.

71. Lalonde RL, Lessard D, Gaudreault J. Population pharmacokinetics of terfenadine. Pharm Res 1996;13:832–8.

72. Jurima-Romet M, Crawford K, Cyr T, et al. Terfenadine metabolism in human liver. In vitro inhibition by macrolide antibiotics and azole antifungals. Drug Metab Dispos 1994;22:849–57.

73. Janssens F, Torremans J, Janssen M, et al. New antihistaminic N-heterocyclic 4-piperidinamines. 1. Synthesis and antihistaminic activity of N-(4-piperidinyl)-1H-benzimidazol-2-amines. J Med Chem 1985;28:1925–33.

74. Janssens F, Torremans J, Janssen M, et al. New antihistaminic N-heterocyclic 4-piperidinamines. 2. Synthesis and antihistaminic activity of 1-[(4-fluorophenyl)methyl]-N-(4-piperidinyl)-1H-benzimidazol-2-amines. J Med Chem 1985;28:1934–43.

75. Janssens F, Torremans J, Janssen M, et al. New antihistaminic N-heterocyclic 4-piperidinamines. 3. Synthesis and antihistaminic activity of N-(4-piperidinyl)-3H-imidazo[4,5-b]pyridin-2-amines. J Med Chem 1985;28:1943–7.

76. Edwards DJ, Bellevue FH, 3rd, Woster PM. Identification of 6,′7′-dihydroxybergamottin, a cytochrome P450 inhibitor, in grapefruit juice. Drug Metab Dispos 1996;24:1287–90.

77. Kamei C, Mio M, Izushi K, et al. Antiallergic effects of major metabolites of astemizole in rats and guinea pigs. Arzneim-Forsch 1991;41:932–6.

78. Levron JC, Gillardin JM, Sabbah A. Astemizole: its pharmacokinetics and pharmacologic properties. Allerg Immunol (Paris) 1990;22:233–41.

79. Vorperian VR, Zhou Z, Mohammad S, et al. Torsade de pointes with an antihistamine metabolite: potassium channel blockade with desmethylastemizole. J Am Coll Cardiol 1996;28:1556–61.

80. Hey JA, del Prado M, Sherwood J, et al. Comparative analysis of the cardiotoxicity proclivities of second generation antihistamines in an experimental model predictive of adverse clinical ECG effects. Arzneim-Forsch 1996;46:153–8.

81. Norman P, Dihlmann A, Rabasseda X. Desloratadine: A preclinical and clinical overview. Drugs Today 2001;37:215–227.

82. McClellan K, Jarvis B. Desloratadine. Drugs 2001;61:789–796.

83. Barecki ME, Casciano CN, Johnson WW, Clement RP. In vitro characterization of the inhibition profile of loratadine, desloratadine, and 3-OH-desloratadine for five human cytochrome P-450 enzymes. Drug Metab Dispos 2001;29:1173–1175.

84. Gupta S, Banfield C, Kantesaria B, Marino M, Clement R, Affrime M, Batra V. Pharmacokinetic and safety profile of desloratadine and fexofenadine when coadministered with azithromycin: A randomized, placebo-controlled, parallel-group study. Clin Ther 2001;23:451–466.

85. Yumibe N, Huie K, Chen KJ, et al. Identification of human liver cytochrome P450 enzymes that metabolize the nonsedating antihistamine loratadine. Formation of descarboethoxyloratadine by CYP3A4 and CYP2D6. Biochem Pharmacol 1996;51:165–72.

86. Yumibe N, Huie K, Chen KJ, et al. Identification of human liver cytochrome P450s involved in the microsomal metabolism of the antihistaminic drug loratadine. Int Arch Allergy Immunol 1995;107:420.

87. Spencer CM, Faulds D, Peters DH. Cetirizine. A reappraisal of its pharmacological properties and therapeutic use in selected allergic disorders. Drugs 1993;46:1055–80.

88. Gray NM, inventor Sepracor, Inc., assignee. Methods for treating allergic disorders using optically pure (−)-cetirizine. U.S. patent 5,698,558. 1998.

89. Carmeliet E. Effects of cetirizine on the delayed K⁺ currents in cardiac cells: comparison with terfenadine. Br J Pharmacol 1998;124:663–668.

90. Cossement E, Bodson G, Gobert J, inventors; UCB SA, Belg., assignee. Enantiomers of 1-[(4-chlorophenyl)phenylmethyl]-4-[(4-methylphenyl)sulfonyl]piperazine and their preparation and use as intermediates for antihistaminics. EP 617028. 1994.

91. Brogden RN, McTavish D. Acrivastine. A review of its pharmacological properties and therapeutic efficacy in allergic rhinitis, urticaria and related disorders. Drugs 1991;41:927–40.

92. Williams BO, Hull H, McSorley P, et al. Efficacy of acrivastine plus pseudoephedrine for symptomatic relief of seasonal allergic rhinitis due to mountain cedar. Ann Allergy Asthma Immunol 1996;76:432–8.

93. Hurst M, Spencer CM. Ebastine: an update of its use in allergic disorders. Drugs 2000;59:981–1006.

94. Campbell A, Michel FB, Bremard-Oury C, et al. Overview of allergic mechanisms. Ebastine has more than an antihistamine effect. Drugs 1996;52(Suppl 1):15–9.

95. Ki I, Inui A, Ito T. Effects of histamine H₁ receptor antagonists on action potentials in guinea-pig isolated papillary muscles. Arch Int Pharmacodyn Ther 1996;331:59–73.

96. Hashizume T, Mise M, Terauchi Y, et al. N-Dealkylation and hydroxylation of ebastine by human liver cytochrome P450. Drug Metab Dispos 1998;26:566–71.

97. Sharif NA, Hellberg MR, Yanni JM. Antihistamines, topical ocular. In: Wolff ME, editor. Burger's Medicinal Chemistry and Drug Discovery. 5th ed. New York: John Wiley & Sons, Inc.; 1997. p. 255–279.

98. Proud D, Sweet J, Stein P, et al. Inflammatory mediator release on conjunctival provocation of allergic subjects with allergen. J Allergy Clin Immunol 1990;85:896–905.

99. Irani AM, Butrus SI, Tabbara KF, et al. Human conjunctival mast cells: distribution of MCT and MCTC in vernal conjunctivitis and giant papillary conjunctivitis. J Allergy Clin Immunol 1990;86:34–40.

100. Berdy GJ, Abelson MB, George MA, et al. Allergic conjunctivitis: a survey of new antihistamines. J Ocul Pharmacol 1991;7:313–24.

101. Sharif NA, Xu SX, Miller ST, et al. Characterization of the ocular antiallergic and antihistaminic effects of olopatadine (AL-4943A), a novel drug for treating ocular allergic diseases. J Pharmacol Exp Ther 1996;278:1252–61.

102. Sharif NA, Xu SX, Yanni JM. Olopatadine (AL-4943A): ligand binding and functional studies on a novel, long acting H₁-selective histamine antagonist and anti-allergic agent for use in allergic conjunctivitis. J Ocul Pharmacol Ther 1996;12:401–7.

103. Yanni JM, Stephens DJ, Miller ST, et al. The in vitro and in vivo ocular pharmacology of olopatadine (AL-4943A), an effective anti-allergic/antihistaminic agent. J Ocul Pharmacol Ther 1996;12:389–400.

104. Noble S, McTavish D. Levocabastine. An update of its pharmacology, clinical efficacy and tolerability in the topical treatment of allergic rhinitis and conjunctivitis. Drugs 1995;50:1032–49.

105. Dechant KL, Goa KL. Levocabastine. A review of its pharmacological properties and therapeutic potential as a topical antihistamine in allergic rhinitis and conjunctivitis. Drugs 1991;41:202–24.

106. Sharif NA, Su SX, Yanni JM. Emedastine: a potent, high affinity histamine H₁-receptor-selective antagonist for ocular use: receptor binding and second messenger studies. J Ocul Pharmacol 1994;10:653–64.

107. Sharif NA, Xu SX, Magnino PE, et al. Human conjunctival epithelial cells express histamine-1 receptors coupled to phosphoinositide turnover and intracellular calcium mobilization: role in ocular allergic and inflammatory diseases. Exp Eye Res 1996;63:169–78.

108. Yanni JM, Stephens DJ, Parnell DW, et al. Preclinical efficacy of emedastine, a potent, selective histamine H₁ antagonist for topical ocular use. J Ocul Pharmacol 1994;10:665–75.

109. Saito T, Hagihara A, Igarashi N, et al. Inhibitory effects of emedastine difumarate on histamine release. Jpn J Pharmacol 1993;62:137–43.

110. McNeely W, Wiseman LR. Intranasal azelastine. A review of its efficacy in the management of allergic rhinitis. Drugs 1998;56:91–114.

111. Richards IS, Miller L, Solomon D, et al. Azelastine and desmethylazelastine suppress acetylcholine-induced contraction and depolarization in human airway smooth muscle. Eur J Pharmacol 1990;186:331–4.

112. Adusumalli VE, Wichmann JK, Wong KK, et al. Pharmacokinetics of the new antiasthma and antiallergy drug, azelastine, in pediatric and adult beagle dogs. Biopharm Drug Dispos 1993;14:233–44.

113. Hoshino M, Nakamura Y. The effect of azelastine on the infiltration of inflammatory cells into the bronchial mucosa and clinical changes in patients with bronchial asthma. Int Arch Allergy Immunol 1997;114:285–92.

114. McTavish D, Sorkin EM. Azelastine. A review of its pharmacodynamic and pharmacokinetic properties, and therapeutic potential. Drugs 1989;38:778–800.

115. Grant SM, Goa KL, Fitton A, et al. Ketotifen. A review of its pharmacodynamic and pharmacokinetic properties, and therapeutic use in asthma and allergic disorders. Drugs 1990;40:412–48.

116. Polivka Z, Budesinsky M, Holubek J, et al. 4H-Benzo[4,5-cyclohepta[1,2-b]thiophenes and 9,10-dihydro derivatives. Sulfonium analogs of pizotifen and ketotifen. Chirality of ketotifen. Synthesis of the 2-bromo derivative of ketotifen. Collect Czech Chem Commun 1989;54:2443–69.

117. Hatlebakk JG, Berstad A. Pharmacokinetic optimisation in the treatment of gastro-oesophageal reflux disease. Clin Pharmacokinet 1996;31:386–406.

118. Ganellin R. 1980 Award in medicinal chemistry: Medicinal chemistry and dynamic structure-activity analysis in the discovery of drugs acting at histamine H_2 receptors. J Med Chem 1981;24:913–20.

119. Ganellin CR. Discovery of Cimetidine. In: Roberts SM, Price BJ, editors. Medicinal Chemsitry, The Role of Organic Chemistry in Drug Research. London: Academic Press; 1985. p. 93–118.

120. Smith IL, Ziemniak JA, Bernhard H, et al. Ranitidine disposition and systemic availability in hepatic cirrhosis. Clin Pharmacol Ther 1984;35:487–94.

121. Roberts CJ. Clinical pharmacokinetics of ranitidine. Clin Pharmacokinet 1984;9:211–21.

122. Saima S, Echizen H, Yoshimoto K, et al. Hemofiltrability of histamine H_2-receptor antagonist, nizatidine, and its metabolites in patients with renal failure. J Clin Pharmacol 1993;33:324–9.

123. Price AH, Brogden RN. Nizatidine. A preliminary review of its pharmacodynamic and pharmacokinetic properties, and its therapeutic use in peptic ulcer disease. Drugs 1988;36:521–39.

124. Feldman M, Burton ME. Histamine₂-receptor antagonists. Standard therapy for acid-peptic diseases. 1. N Engl J Med 1990;323:1672–80.

125. Somogyi A, Muirhead M. Pharmacokinetic interactions of cimetidine. Clin Pharmacokinet 1987;12:321–66.

126. Holt S. Over-the-counter histamine H_2-receptor antagonists. How will they affect the treatment of acid-related diseases? Drugs 1994;47:1–11.

127. Herling AW, Weidmann K. Gastric proton pump inhibitors. In: Wolff ME, editor. Burger's Medicinal Chemistry and Drug Discovery. 5th ed. New York: John Wiley & Sons, Inc.; 1996. p. 119–151.

128. Lindberg P, Brandstrom A, Wallmark B, et al. Omeprazole: the first proton pump inhibitor. Med Res Rev 1990;10:1–54.

129. Shin JM, Besancon M, Bamberg K, et al. Structural aspects of the gastric H^+,K^+-ATPase. Ann N Y Acad Sci 1997;834:65–76.

130. Richardson P, Hawkey CJ, Stack WA. Proton pump inhibitors. Pharmacology and rationale for use in gastrointestinal disorders. Drugs 1998;56:307–35.

131. Besancon M, Simon A, Sachs G, et al. Sites of reaction of the gastric H,K-ATPase with extracytoplasmic thiol reagents. J Biol Chem 1997;272:22438–46.

132. Morii M, Takeguchi N. Different biochemical modes of action of two irreversible H^+,K^+- ATPase inhibitors, omeprazole and E3810. J Biol Chem 1993;268:21553–9.

133. Morii M, Hamatani K, Takeguchi N. The proton pump inhibitor E3810 binds to the N-terminal half of the alpha-subunit of gastric H^+,K^+-ATPase. Biochem Pharmacol 1995;49:1729–34.

134. Andersson T. Pharmacokinetics, metabolism and interactions of acid pump inhibitors. Focus on omeprazole, lansoprazole and pantoprazole. Clin Pharmacokinet 1996;31:9–28.

135. Prakash A, Faulds D. Rabeprazole. Drugs 1998;55:261–8.

136. Fitton A, Wiseman L. Pantoprazole: A review of its pharmacological properties and therapeutic use in acid-related disorders. Drugs 1996;51:460–82.

137. Äbelö A, Andersson TB, Antonsson M, et al. Stereoselective metabolism of omeprazole by human cytochrome P450 enzymes. Drug Metab Dispos 2000;28:966–72.

138. Spencer CM, Fawlds D. Esomeprazole. Drugs 2000;60:321–329.

139. Andersson T, Hassan-Alin M, Hasselgren G, Rohss K. Drug interaction studies with esomeprazole, the (S)-isomer of omeprazole. Clin Pharmacokinet 2001;40:523–537.

140. Katsuki H, Yagi H, Arimori K, et al. Determination of R(+)- and S(−)-lansoprazole using chiral stationary-phase liquid chromatography and their enantioselective pharmacokinetics in humans. Pharm Res 1996;13:611–5.

141. Nagaya H, Inatomi N, Nohara A, et al. Effects of the enantiomers of lansoprazole (AG-1749) on (H_1/K+)-ATPase activity in canine gastric microsomes and acid formation in isolated canine parietal cells. Biochem Pharmacol 1991;42:1875–8.

142. Tanaka M, Ohkubo T, Otani K, Suzuki A, Kaneko S, Sugawara K, Ryokawa Y, Ishizaki T. Stereoselective pharmacokinetics of pantoprazole, a proton pump inhibitor, in extensive and poor metabolizers of S-mephenytoin. Clin Pharmacol Ther 2001; 69:108–113.

143. Chisholm MA. Pharmacotherapy of duodenal and gastric ulcerations. Am J Pharm Ed 1998;62:196–203.

144. Corazza GR, Tonini M. Levosulpiride for dyspepsia and emesis: A review of its pharmacology, efficacy and tolerability. Clin Drug Invest. 2000;19:151–162.

145. Kahrilas PJ. Gastroesophageal reflux disease. J Am Med Assn 1996;276:983–8.

146. Tonini M, De Ponti F, Di Nucci A, et al. Review article: cardiac adverse effects of gastrointestinal prokinetics. Aliment Pharmacol Ther 1999;13:1585–91.

147. Won-Kim S, Kachur JF, Gaginella TS. Stereospecific actions of misoprostol on rat colonic electrolyte transport. Prostaglandins 1993;46:221–31.

148. Walt RP. Misoprostol for the treatment of peptic ulcer and antiinflammatory drug-induced gastroduodenal ulceration. N Engl J Med 1992;327:1575–80.

149. Bauer TA, Brown DL, Chai LK. Vaginal misoprostol for term labor induction. Ann Pharmacother 1997;31:1391–3.

150. Vengalil SR, Guinn DA, Olabi NF, et al. A randomized trial of misoprostol and extra-amniotic saline infusion for cervical ripening and labor induction. Obstet Gynecol 1998;91:774–9.

151. Grimes DA. Medical abortion in early pregnancy: a review of the evidence. Obstet Gynecol 1997;89(5 Pt 1):790–6.

152. Gold M, Luks D, Anderson MR. Medical options for early pregnancy termination. Am Fam Physician 1997;56:533–8.

153. Aubeny E. Trends since 1989, in France, of induced abortions by mifepristone (RU486) combined with a prostaglandin analogue. Contracept Fertil Sex 1997;25:777–81.

154. Ulmann A, Silvestre L. RU486: the French experience. Hum Reprod 1994;9(Suppl 1):126–30.

155. Schaff EA, Stadalius LS, Eisinger SH, et al. Vaginal misoprostol administered at home after mifepristone (RU486) for abortion. J Fam Pract 1997;44:353–60.

156. Nagashima R, Yoshida N. Sucralfate, a basic aluminum salt of sucrose sulfate. I. Behaviors in gastroduodenal pH. Arzneim-Forsch 1979;29:1668–76.

157. Tarnawski A. Cellular and molecular mechanisms of ulcer healing. Drugs Today 1997;33:697–706.

158. Brogden RN, Heel RC, Speight TM, et al. Sucralfate. A review of its pharmacodynamic properties and therapeutic use in peptic ulcer disease. Drugs 1984;27:194–209.

159. Marks IN. Sucralfate: worldwide experience in recurrence therapy. J Clin Gastroenterol 1987;9(Suppl 1):18–22.

160. Leurs R, Timmerman H, editors. The histamine H_3 receptor: a target for new drugs. 1st ed. Amsterdam: Elsevier; 1998.

161. Leurs R, Vollinga RC, Timmerman H. The medicinal chemistry and therapeutic potentials of ligands of the histamine H_3 receptor. Prog Drug Res 1995;45:107–65.

162. van der Werf JF, Bijloo GJ, van der Vliet A, et al. H_3 receptor assay in electrically-stimulated superfused slices of rat brain cortex; effects of N a-alkylated histamines and impromidine analogues. Agents Actions 1987;20:239–43.

163. Lipp R, Arrang JM, Garbarg M, et al. Synthesis, absolute configuration, stereoselectivity, and receptor selectivity of

(αR,βS)-α,β-dimethylhistamine, a novel high potent histamine H_3 receptor agonist. J Med Chem 1992;35:4434–41.

164. Tedford CE, Yates SL, Pawlowski GP, et al. Pharmacological characterization of GT-2016, a non-thiourea-containing histamine H_3 receptor antagonist: in vitro and in vivo studies. J Pharmacol Exp Ther 1995; 275:598–604.

165. Levi R, Smith NC. Histamine H_3-receptors: a new frontier in myocardial ischemia. J Pharmacol Exp Ther 2000;292: 825–30.

166. Simons FER. Antihistamines. In: Middleton E, Jr. et al., editor. Allergy: Principles and Practice. 5th ed. St. Louis: Mosby; 1998. p. 612–637.

34. Antibiotics and Antimicrobial Agents

LESTER A. MITSCHER

INTRODUCTION

Antibiotics are microbial metabolites or synthetic analogs inspired by them that, in small doses, inhibit the growth and survival of microorganisms without serious toxicity to the host. Selective toxicity is the key concept. Examples are the penicillins and the tetracyclines. Antibiotics are among the most frequently prescribed medications today although microbial resistance due to evolutionary pressures and misuse threatens their continued efficacy. In many cases the clinical utility of natural antibiotics has been enhanced through medicinal chemical manipulation of the original structure leading to broader antimicrobial spectrum, greater potency, lesser toxicity, more convenient administration, etc. Examples of such semisynthetic antibiotics are amoxicillin and doxycycline. Through customary usage, the many synthetic substances that are unrelated to natural products but still inhibit or kill microorganisms are referred to as antimicrobial agents instead. Examples are sulfisoxazole and ciprofloxacin.

Our environment, body surfaces, and cavities support a rich and characteristic microbial flora. These cause us no significant illness or inconvenience as long as our neighbors or we do not indulge in behavior that exposes us to exceptional quantities or unusual strains of microbes or introduces bacteria into parts of the body where they are not normally resident. Protection against this happening is obtained primarily through public health measures, healthful habits, intact skin and mucosal barriers, and a properly functioning immune system. All of the parts of our bodies that are in contact with the environment support microbial life. All of our internal fluids, organs, and body structures are sterile under normal circumstances and the presence of bacteria, fungi, viruses, etc., in these places is diagnostic evidence of infection. When mild microbial disease occurs, the otherwise healthy patient will often recover without requiring treatment. Here an intact, functioning immune system is called upon to kill invasive microorganisms. When this is insufficient to protect us, appropriate therapeutic intervention is indicated.

The chronicle of civilization before the discovery of bacteria and their role in infectious disease and, subsequently, of the discovery of antibiotics and antimicrobial agents is punctuated by the outbreak of recurrent devastating pandemics. An example is the successive waves of bubonic plague which dramatically decreased the population of Europe in the Middle Ages. Mankind was mystified as to the cause of infectious disease and what one might constructively do for prevention and cure. In warfare, infections often disabled or killed more individuals than did the action of generals. Our own family histories record the premature loss of loved ones, particularly small children, to one infection or another and in the third world this pattern is all too common today. This depressing picture has been altered dramatically in this century by the discovery and application of the powerful therapeutic agents described in this chapter. It is fortunately no longer common for persons to live short lives and it is now rare for parents to bury their children. Public health measures such as purification of water supplies, routine preventive vaccination, Pasteurization of milk, personal cleanliness and avoidance of unhealthy behavior (such as spitting in public places) have also greatly diminished our exposure to infection.

Considering that the first truly effective antimicrobial agents date from the mid 1930s (the sulfonamides) and the first antibiotics came into use in the 1940s (the penicillins), it is amazing that we have already grown complacent. Diseases which very recently seemed on their way to extinction, such as tuberculosis and gonorrhea, are once again becoming serious public health problems because of societal changes and resistance emergence by pathogens. It is disturbing to consider that previously unknown infectious diseases, such as acquired immunodeficiency syndrome (AIDS), Ebola virus infections, and Legionnaires' disease, are an increasing feature of modern life. Unfortunately, we cannot any longer confidently depend upon the discovery of increasing numbers of novel antibiotics and antimicrobial agents to keep infectious diseases under control but must increasingly pay attention to neglected public health measures and concentrate upon using antibiotics safely and effectively only when these measures fail.

HISTORY

Humankind has been subject to infection by microorganisms since before the dawn of recorded history. One presumes that mankind has been searching for suitable therapy for nearly as long. This was a desperately difficult enterprise given the acute nature of most infections and the nearly total lack of understanding of their origins prevalent until the last century. Although one can find indications in old medical writings of folkloric use of plant and animal preparations, soybean curd, moldy bread and cheese, counter infection with other microbes, the slow development of public health measures, and an understanding of the desirability of personal cleanliness, these factors were erratically and inefficiently applied and they often failed. Until after the discovery of bacteria 300 years ago, and subsequent understanding of their role in infection about 150 years ago, there was no hope for rational therapy.

In Germany, in the last century, Robert Koch showed that specific microorganisms could always be isolated from the excreta and tissues of people with particular infectious diseases and that these same microorganisms were usually absent in healthy individuals. They could then be grown on culture media and be used to reproduce in healthy individuals all of the classic symptoms of the same disease following inoculation. Finally, the identical microorganism could then be isolated from this deliberately infected person. Following these rules, at long last, a chain of cause and effect was forged between certain microorganisms and specific infectious diseases.

Louis Pasteur reported in 1877 that when what he termed "common bacteria" were introduced into a pure culture of anthrax bacilli, the bacilli died, and that an injection of deadly anthrax bacillus into a laboratory animal was harmless if "common bacteria" were injected along with it. This did not always work but led to the appreciation of antibiosis wherein two or more microorganisms competed with one another for survival. It was more than a half century later that the underlying mechanisms by which this phenomenon was achieved began to be appreciated and applied to routinely successful therapy.

The modern anti-infective era opened with the discovery of the sulfonamides in France and Germany in 1936 as an offshoot of Paul Ehrlich's earlier achievements in treating infections with organometallics and his theories of vital staining. The discovery of the utility of sulfanilamide was acknowledged by the awarding of a Nobel Prize in 1938. The well known observation of a clear zone of inhibition (lysis) in a bacterial colony surrounding a colony of contaminating air-borne Penicillium mold by Robert Fleming in England in 1929 and the subsequent purification of penicillin from it in the late 1930s and early 1940s by Florey, Chain, Abraham and Heatley, provided important additional impetus. With the first successful clinical trial of crude penicillin on February 12, 1941, and the requirements of war times, an explosion of successful activity ensued which continues over 50 years later. In rapid succession, deliberate searches of the metabolic products of a wide variety of soil microbes led to discovery of tyrothricin (1939), streptomycin (1943), chloramphenicol (1947), chlortetracycline (1948), neomycin (1949), erythromycin (1952), and more, and this ushered in the age of the miracle drugs.

Microbes of soil origin remain to this day the most fruitful sources of antibiotics, although the specific means employed for their discovery are infinitely more sophisticated today than those employed 50 years ago. Initially, extracts of fermentations were screened simply for their ability to kill pathogenic microorganisms in vitro. Those that did were pushed along through ever more complex pharmacologic and toxicologic tests in attempts to discover clinically useful agents. Today many thousands of such extracts of increasingly exotic microbes are tested each week and the tests now include sophisticated assays for agents operating through particular biochemical mechanisms or possessing particular desirable properties. The impact of genomics is expected to have very substantial impact on this effort. As a consequence of this work mankind now has many choices for powerful, effective and specific therapy for some of its most ancient and common bacterial infections.

In the year 2000 worldwide commerce in antibiotics is measured in multiple tons and is valued in excess of $10 billion. About half of this is associated with β-lactam antibiotics alone. More than 20% of the most frequently prescribed outpatient medications in the U.S. are anti-infective agents. Approximately 100 antibiotics have seen substantial clinical use, although more than 20,000 other natural antibiotics have been described in the literature and an order of magnitude more semi- and totally synthetic antimicrobial agents has been prepared. These agents have had a major impact on the practice of medicine and of pharmacy, and on the lives of persons still living who well remember the perils and uncertainties of life before antibiotics became available.

This salubrious picture has an increasing dark side, however, because of the increasing impact of bacterial resistance. Intrinsic resistance to antimicrobial agents (resistance present before exposure to antibiotics) was recognized from the beginning. Some bacteria are immune to treatment from the outset because they do not take up the antibiotic or lack a susceptible target. Already starting in the 1940s, however, and encountered with increasing frequency to this day, bacteria which were previously expected to respond were found to be resistant and many, alarmingly, became resistant during the course of chemotherapy and others were simultaneously resistant to several different antibiotics. The latter were found to be capable of passing this trait on to other bacteria, even to those belonging to different genera. Similar findings are now encountered with fungi, viruses and even tumors indicating that this is a general biologic phenomenon. The spread of this phenomenon is abetted by their short generation time and genetic versatility, as well as by poor antibiotic prescribing and utilization practices. Some authorities are sufficiently upset about this as to predict an impending return to the defenseless days of the preantibiotic era. An understanding of these phenomena and the devising of appropriate practical response measures is an important contemporary priority.

GENERAL PRINCIPLES
Drug Nomenclature

The names given to antimicrobials and antibiotics are as varied as their inventor's taste, and yet some helpful unifying conventions are followed. For example, the penicillins are produced by fermentation of fungi and their names most commonly end in the suffix -cillin as in the term ampicillin. The cephalosporins are likewise fungal products, although their names mostly begin with the prefix cef- (or sometimes, following the English practice, spelled ceph-). The synthetic fluoroquinolones mostly end in the suffix -floxacin. Although helpful in many respects, this nomenclature does result in many related substances possessing quite similar names. This can make remembering them a burden. Most of the remaining antibiotics are produced by fermentation of soil microorganisms belonging to various *Streptomyces* species. By convention these have names ending in the suffix -mycin as in streptomycin. Some prominent antibiotics are produced by fermentation of various *Micromonospora* sp. These antibiotics have names ending in -micin, e.g., gentamicin. The student has to take considerable care to avoid confusing them in written communication. Whereas pronunciation is essentially identical, they are spelled differently.

In earlier times, the terms broad- and narrow-spectrum had specific clinical meaning. The widespread emergence of single-agent and multiple-agent resistant microbial strains has made these terms much less meaningful. It is, nonetheless, still valuable to remember that some antimicrobial families have the potential of inhibiting a wide range of bacterial genera belonging to both Gram (+) and Gram (−) cultures and so are called broad spectrum (such as the tetracyclines). Others inhibit only a few bacterial genera and are termed narrow-spectrum (such as the glycopeptides, typified by vancomycin, which are used almost exclusively for a few Gram (+) and anaerobic microorganisms).

The Importance of Identification of the Pathogen
Empiric Based Therapy

Fundamental to appropriate antimicrobial therapy is an appreciation that individual species of bacteria are associated with particular infective diseases and that specific antibiotics are more likely to be useful than others for killing them. Sometimes this can be used as the basis for successful empiric therapy. For example, first course community acquired urinary tract infections in otherwise healthy individuals are most commonly caused by Gram (−) *Escherichia coli* of fecal origin. Even just knowing this much can give

Gram Stain

The Gram stains were developed in the last century by Hans Christian Gram, a Danish microbiologist, in order to visualize bacteria more easily under the microscope. The basis of these differential stains lies in the chemistry of the bacterial cell walls, which causes certain bacteria to react differently with the stains employed. Gram (+) microbes stain blue. Gram (−) do not retain the blue dye when washed with alcohol and are counterstained red upon treatment with a different dye. It is a convenient fact for the study of antibiotics that Gram (+) bacteria are generally more sensitive to comparatively nontoxic antibiotics than are Gram (−) ones. Thus it is useful for the student of antibiotics to be familiar with the Gram staining characteristics of given pathogens. The student should also exercise care not to lapse into convenient jargon by referring to a Gram (+) infection when what is really meant is an infection caused by a Gram (+) microorganism.

the physician several convenient choices for useful therapy. Likewise, skin infections, such as boils, are commonly the result of infection with Gram (+) *Staphyloccus aureus.* In most other cases, the cause of the disease is less obvious and so is the agent that might be useful against it. It is important to determine the specific disease one is dealing with in these cases and what susceptibility patterns are exhibited by the causative microorganism. Knowing these factors enables the clinician to narrow the range of therapeutic choices. The only certainty, however, is that inability of a given antibiotic to kill or inhibit a given pathogen in vitro is a virtual guarantee that the drug will fail in vivo. Unfortunately, activity in vitro all too often also results in failure to cure in vivo but here, at least, there is a significant possibility of success. Before the emergence of widespread bacterial resistance, identification of the causative microorganism often was sufficient for selecting a useful antibiotic. Now this is only a useful first step and much more detailed laboratory studies are needed.

Experimentally Based Therapy

The modern clinical application of Koch's discoveries to the selection of an appropriate antibiotic involves sampling infectious material from a patient before instituting anti-infective chemotherapy, culturing the microorganism on suitable growth media, and identifying its genus and species. The bacterium in question is then grown in the presence of a variety of antibiotics to see which of them will inhibit its growth or survival and what concentrations will be needed to achieve this result. This is expressed in minimum inhibitory concentration units (m.i.c.). The term m.i.c. refers to that concentration which will inhibit 99% or more of the microbe in question and represents the minimum quantity which must reach the site of the infection in order to be useful. It is usually desirable to have several multiples of the m.i.c. at the site of infection. This brings into play an understanding of pharmacokinetic and pharmacodynamic considerations as well as the results of accumulated clinical experience. The choice of anti-infective agent is made from among those that are active. One of the most convenient experimental procedures is that of Kirby and Bauer. With this technique, sterile filter paper disks impregnated with fixed doses of commercially available antibiotics are placed upon the seeded Petri dish. The dish is then incubated at 37° C for 12–24 hours. If the antibiotic is active against the particular strain of bacterium isolated from the particular patient, a clear zone of inhibition will be seen around the disk. If a given antimicrobial agent is ineffective, the bacterium may even grow right up to the edge of the disk. The diameter of the inhibition zone is directly proportional to the degree of sensitivity of the bacterial strain and the concentration of the antibiotic in question. Currently, a given zone size in millimeters is dictated above which the bacterium is sensitive, and below which it is resistant. When the zone size obtained is near this break point the drug is regarded as intermediate in sensitivity and clinical failure can occur. This powerful methodology gives the clinician a choice of possible antibiotics to use in the particular patient. The widespread occurrence of resistance of individual strains of bacteria to given antibiotics reinforces the need to perform Kirby-Bauer susceptibility disk testing. Other laboratory methods can be employed for similar purposes. For example, broth and agar dilution studies utilize media in which fixed concentrations of the antibiotic are dissolved or suspended and bacterial growth is measured after an appropriate period of incubation.

Bactericidal vs. Bacteriostatic

Almost all antibiotics have the capacity to be bactericidal in vitro; that is to say they will kill bacteria, if the concentration or dose is sufficiently high. In the laboratory, it is almost always possible to use such doses. Subsequent inoculation of fresh, antibiotic free, media with a culture that has been so treated will not produce growth of the culture as the cells are dead. When such doses are achievable in live patients, such drugs are clinically bactericidal. At somewhat lower concentrations, bacterial multiplication is prevented even though the microorganism remains viable.

The smallest concentration that will prevent visible growth is the minimum inhibitory concentration (m.i.c.). The spread between a bactericidal dose (m.b.c.) and a bacteriostatic dose (m.i.c.) is characteristic of given families of antibiotics. With gentamicin, for example, doubling or quadrupling the dose changes the effect on bacteria from bacteriostatic to bactericidal. Such doses are usually achievable in the clinic. The difference between bactericidal and bacteriostatic doses with tetracycline is approximately 40-fold. It is not possible to achieve such doses safely in patients so tetracycline is referred to as clinically bacteriostatic. If a bacteriostatic antibiotic is withdrawn prematurely from a patient, the microorganism can resume growth and the infection can reestablish itself because the culture is still alive. Subsequent inoculation of fresh laboratory media not containing the antibiotic with a culture so treated will result in colony development. Obviously, in immunocompromised patients who are unable to contribute natural body defenses to fight their own disease, having the drug kill the bacteria is essential for recovery. When a patient is immunocompetent or the infection is not severe, however, a bacteriostatic concentration will break the fulminating stage of the infection (when bacterial cell numbers are increasing at a logarithmic rate). With *E. coli*, for example, the number of cells doubles every two hours. A bacteriostatic agent will interrupt this rapid growth and give the immune system a chance to deal with the disease. Cure usually follows if the numbers of live bacteria are not excessive at this time. Thus, whereas it is preferred that an antibiotic be bactericidal, bacteriostatic antibiotics are widely used and are usually satisfactory. Obviously though, patients should not skip doses or prematurely stop treatment!

Microbial Susceptibility
Resistance

Resistance is the failure of microorganisms to be killed or inhibited by antimicrobial treatment. Resistance can either be intrinsic (be present before exposure to drug) or acquired (develop subsequent to exposure to a drug). Resistance of bacteria to the toxic effects of antimicrobial agents and to antibiotics develops fairly easily both in the laboratory and in the clinic and is an ever-increasing public health hazard. Challenging a culture in the laboratory with sublethal quantities of an antibiotic kills the most intrinsically sensitive percentage of the strains in the colony. Those not killed or seriously inhibited continue to grow and have access to the remainder of the nutrients. A mutation to lower sensitivity also enables individual bacteria to survive against the selecting pressure of the antimicrobial agent. If the culture is treated several times in succession with sublethal doses in this manner, the concentration of antibiotic required to prevent growth becomes ever higher. When the origin of this form of resistance is explored, it is almost always found to be due to an alteration in the biochemistry of the colony so that the molecular target of the antibiotic has become less sensitive, or it can lead alternatively to decreased uptake of antibiotic into the cells. This is genomically preserved and passes to the next generation by binary fission. The altered progeny may be weaker than the wild strain so that they die out if the antibiotic is not present to give them a competitive advantage. In some cases additional compensatory mutations can occur which restore the vigor of the resistant organism. Resistance of this type is usually expressed toward other antibiotics with the same mode of action so is a familial characteristic—most tetracyclines, for example, show extensive cross resistance with other tetracyclines. This is very enlightening with respect to discovery of the molecular mode of action but is not very relevant to the clinical situation.

In the clinic, resistance more commonly takes place by Resistance-(R) factor mechanisms. In the more lurid examples, enzymes are elaborated that attack the antibiotic and inactivate it. Mutations to resistance occur by many mechanisms. They can result from point mutations, insertions, deletions, inversions, duplications, transpositions of segments of genes or by acquisition of foreign DNA from plasmids, bacteriophages and transposable genetic elements. The genetic material coding for this form of resistance is very often carried on extrachromosomic elements consisting of small circular DNA molecules known as plasmids. A bacterial cell may have many plasmids or none. The plasmid may carry DNA for several different enzymes capable of destroying structurally dissimilar antibiotics. Such plasmid DNA may migrate within the cell from plasmid to plasmid or from plasmid to chromosome by a process known as transposition. Such plasmids may migrate from cell to cell by conjugation (passage through a sexual pilus), transduction (carriage by a virus vector), or by transformation (excretion of DNA from cell A and its subsequent uptake by cell B). These mechanisms can convert an antibiotic-sensitive cell to an antibiotic-resistant cell. This can take place many times in a bacterium's already short generation time. The positive selecting pressure of inadequate levels of antibiotic favors explosive spread of R-factor resistance. This provides a rationale for conservative but aggressive application of appropriate antimicrobial chemotherapy. Bacterial resistance is generally mediated through one of three mechanisms: failure of the drug to penetrate into or stay in the cell; destruction of the drug by defensive enzymes; or alterations in the cellular target of the enzymes. It is also rarely an all or nothing effect. In many cases a resistant microorganism can still be controlled by achievable, though higher, doses.

Persistance

Sensitive bacteria may not all be killed. Survivors are thought to have been resting (not metabolizing) during the drug treatment time and, therefore, still viable when tested subsequently. These bacteria are still sensitive to the drug even though they survived an otherwise toxic dose. Some bacteria also can aggregate in films. The cells laying deep within such a film may not be reached by a poorly penetrating antibiotic. Such cells, although intrinsically sensitive, may survive antibiotic treatment.

Postantibiotic Effect

Some antibiotics exert a significant toxicity to certain microorganisms that persists for a time after the drug is withdrawn. A constant multiple of the minimum inhibitory concentration of drug may not be essential for therapeutic success when a postantibiotic effect (PAE) is operating because the microbe is still affected for a time after the drug is withdrawn. The PAE is defined by the time required for a 10-fold increase in viable bacterial colonies to occur after exposure to a single dose of the antimicrobial agent. The pharmacologic basis for this effect is not clear. It is speculated that adherence to the intercellular target prevents some significant quantity of the antimicrobial agent from being washed away for a time. Others believe that there are other drug-related effects that injure the bacterium and that it is only slowly able to repair. Some as yet undiscovered cause may be at play. Under some conditions a PAE can be detected for days in the chemotherapy of mycobacterial infections. The PAE has been observed for a variety of antibiotics and its duration varies with the drug, the organism, the concentration of drug and the duration of treatment. This phenomenon can be used to assist in patient compliance by decreasing the frequency and the length of chemotherapy, however it may also lead to drug resistance and should be employed conservatively.

Biphasic ("Eagle") Effect

The biphasic effect is associated primarily with β-lactam antibiotics. It is a curious phenomenon in which low doses in vitro against certain bacteria (*staphylococci* and *streptococci*) produce lysis whereas higher doses do not. This is believed to be due to the differential sensitivity of the penicillin binding proteins (see below for an explanation of this term) in that higher doses of β-lactams inhibit the autolysins (this term will also be defined later) which enzymes also contribute to bacterial lysis.

Inoculum Effect

In a number of cases microbial resistance is mediated by the production of bacterial enzymes that attack the antibiotic molecule changing its structure to an inactive form. This can lead to a so called inoculum effect in which a susceptible antibiotic is apparently less potent when larger numbers of bacteria are present in the medium than when fewer cells are employed. The more bacteria taken, the more antibiotic-destroying enzyme is present and the more antibiotic is required to overcome this to achieve the desired response. An antibiotic which is not enzyme modified is comparatively free from inoculum effects. These circumstances, when present, make quantitative comparisons of the likely effectiveness of a susceptible agent with a resistant agent tricky to interpret. Inoculum effects are comparatively frequently encountered in testing β-lactam antibiotics, for example.

Antimicrobial Dosing
Use of Antibiotics in Fixed Dose Combinations

The student may suppose that use of combinations of antibiotics would be superior to the use of individual antibiotics because this would broaden the antimicrobial spectrum and make less critical the accurate identification of the pathogen. It has been found, however, by experiment, that all too often such combinations are antagonistic. A useful generalization, but one which is not always correct, is that one may often successfully combine two bactericidal antibiotics, particularly if their molecular mode of action is different. A common example is the use of a β-lactam antibiotic, and an aminoglycoside for first day empiric therapy of overwhelming sepsis of unknown etiology. Therapy must be instituted as soon after a specimen is obtained as is humanly possible, or the patient may die. This often does not allow the microbiological laboratory sufficient time to identify the offending microorganism nor to determine its antibiotic susceptibility. An emergency resort is therefore made to what is called shotgun therapy. Both of the antibiotic families applied in this example are bactericidal in readily achievable parenteral doses. As will be detailed later in this chapter, the β-lactams inhibit bacterial cell wall formation and the aminoglycosides interfere with protein biosynthesis and membrane function. Their modes of action are supplementary. Because of toxicity considerations and the potential for untoward side effects, this empiric therapy is replaced by suitable specific monotherapy at the first opportunity after the sensitivity of the offending bacterium is experimentally established.

One may also often successfully combine two bacteriostatic antibiotics for special purposes, for example, a macrolide and a sulfonamide. These are occasionally used in combination for the treatment of an upper respiratory tract infection caused by *Hemophilus influenzae* as the combination of a protein biosynthesis inhibitor and an inhibitor of DNA biosynthesis gives fewer relapses than the use of either agent alone. The use of a bacteriostatic agent, such as tetracycline, in combination with a bactericidal agent, such as a β-lactam, is usually discouraged. The β-lactam antibiotics are much more effective when used against growing cultures and a bacteriostatic agent interferes with bacterial growth, often giving an indifferent or antagonistic response when such agents are combined. Additional possible disadvantages of combination chemotherapy are higher cost, greater likelihood of side effects, and difficulties in demonstrating synergism in humans. The rising tide of antibiotic resistance may overcome these reservations and make combination therapy more popular.

Serum Protein Binding

The influence of serum protein binding upon antibiotic effectiveness is fairly straightforward. It is considered in most instances that the percentage of antibiotic so bound is not available at that moment for the treatment of infections so must be subtracted from the total blood level in order to get the effective blood level. The tightness of the binding is also a consideration. Thus a heavily and firmly serum protein bound antibiotic would not generally be a good choice for the treatment of septicemias or infections in deep tissue, even though the microorganism involved is susceptible in in vitro tests. If the antibiotic is rapidly released from bondage, however, this factor decreases in importance and the binding becomes a depot source. Distinguishing between these two types of protein binding is accomplished by comparing the percentages of binding to the excretion half-life. A highly bound but readily released antibiotic will have a comparatively short half-life and work well for systemic infections. An antibiotic that is not significantly protein-bound will normally be rapidly excreted and have a short half-life. Thus, some protein binding of poorly water-soluble agents is normally regarded as helpful. The student will recall that under most circumstances the urine is a protein-free filtrate so that proportion of an antibiotic that is firmly bound to serum proteins will be retained in the blood. Thus, a highly and firmly protein bound antibiotic could be satisfactory for mild urinary tract infections.

Preferred Means of Dosing

Under ideal circumstances it is desirable for an antibiotic to be available in both parenteral and oral forms. Whereas there is no question that the convenience of oral medication makes this ideal for outpatient and community use, very ill patients often require parenteral therapy. It would be consistent with today's practice of discharging patients "quicker and sicker" to send them home from the hospital with an efficacious oral version of the same antibiotic that led to the possibility of discharge in the first place. In that way, the patient would not have to come back to the hospital at intervals for drug administration nor would one have to risk treatment failure by starting therapy with a new drug. For drugs with significant toxicities, the physician will prefer the injection form. The physician using this method is certain that the whole dose has been taken at the appropriate time. If the local pharmacist is adept at administration of parenteral medication, these considerations become less important. Developing this capability would also avoid many aspects of noncompliance by employing directly observed chemotherapy (DOT).

Initiation of Therapy

As bacteria multiply rapidly—populations often double in 2 or 3 hours—it is important to institute antibiotic therapy as soon as possible. It is thus often desirable to initiate therapy with a double (loading) dose and then to follow this with smaller (maintenance) doses. To prevent relapse the patient must be instructed not to skip doses and to take all of the medication provided even though the presenting symptoms, e.g., diarrhea or fever, resolve before the entire drug is taken. Treatment failure and the emergence of resistance is probably all too often caused by poor compliance or premature cessation of therapy by the patient.

Prophylactic Use of Antibiotics

Antibiotics are often used prophylactically, for example in preoperative bowel sanitization and orally for treatment of viral sore throats. These are not sound practices because the patient is exposed to the possibility both of drug-associated side effects and a suprainfection by drug resistant microorganisms; moreover the therapeutic gain from such practices is often marginal. However, frustrating as this may be to the infectious diseases specialist, these are common medical practices and hence difficult to stop.

Agricultural Use of Antibiotics

It is estimated that half of the antibiotics of commerce are used for agricultural purposes. Their use for treatment of infections of plants and animals is not to be discouraged so long as drug residues from the treatment do not contaminate foods. In contamination, problems such as penicillin allergy or subsequent infection higher up the food chain by drug resistant microbes can occur. Several instances of death in humans have been recorded in the 1990s from such incidents. Animals demonstrably grow more rapidly to marketable size when antibiotics are added to their feed even though the animals have no apparent infection. This is believed to be due in large part to suppression of subclinical infections that would consequently divert protein biosynthesis from muscle and tissue growth into proteins needed to combat the infection. Under appropriate conditions antibiotic feed supplementation is partly responsible for the comparative wholesomeness and cheapness of our food supplies. This practice has the potential, however, to contaminate the food we consume or to provide reservoirs of drug-resistant enteric microorganisms. Occasionally, infections are traced to this cause and

Cost

Antibiotics are often expensive, but so is morbidity and mortality. For many patients, nonetheless, cost is a significant consideration. The pharmacist is in an ideal position to guide the physician and the patient on the question of possible alternative equivalent treatments that might be more affordable. The most frequent comparisons are based on the cost of the usual dose of a given agent for a single course of therapy (usually the wholesale cost to the pharmacist for ten days worth of drug).

resistance genes can originate in this manner and pass from strain to strain and even to other species. It might be better to use antibiotics for such purposes which are not systemically absorbed and which are not cross-resistant with antibiotics used in clinical practice in humans. This is, in fact, the practice in England and some other countries.

The use of antibiotic resistance genes as insertionally inactivatable markers for development of genetically altered plant foods has raised fears that these genes could also provide a reservoir of antibiotic resistance genes as they enter the food chain. It is posited that this may result in a subtle contribution to the antibiotic resistance problem.

In summary, when antibiotics are used intelligently they are remarkably effective and the population explosion and the increased life span that has characterized recent generations can be traced in part to them. When used carelessly or inappropriately they can lead to complex ecological problems such as infection with multidrug resistant microorganisms. This phenomenon is increasingly troublesome and pessimists forecast a return to the comparative vulnerability of the preantibiotic era.

SYNTHETIC ANTIMICROBIAL AGENTS

Synthetic antimicrobial agents have not been modeled after any natural product so they may not properly be called "antibiotics." Some synthetics are extremely effective for treatment of infections and are widely used. Very few antibiotics are known to work in precisely the same way as these agents in killing bacteria. Also curious is the fact that those agents whose molecular mode of action is known are at present nearly all effective against key enzymes needed for the biosynthesis of nucleic acids. Because they interrupt the biosynthesis of nucleic acids rather than attacking the finished products or substituting for them in nucleic acids they are not genotoxic but are comparatively safe to use.

Prontosil Rubrum   Sulfanilamide

Sulfonamides
History

Sulfonamides were discovered in the mid 1930s following an incorrect hypothesis, but by observing the results carefully and drawing correct conclusions. Prontosil rubrum, a red dye, was one of a series of dyes examined by Gerhard Domagk of Bayer of Germany in the belief that it might be taken up selectively by certain pathogenic bacteria and not by human cells, in a manner analogous to the way that the Gram-stain works, and so serve as a selective poison to kill these cells. If this were true, this would be a useful validation and extension of theories elaborated by Paul Ehrlich at the turn of the century. The dye, indeed, proved active in vivo against streptococcal infections in mice. Curiously, it was not active in vitro. Trefouel and Bovet in France soon showed that the urine of prontosil rubrum-treated animals was bioactive in vitro. Fractionation led to identification of the active substance as p-aminobenzenesulfonic acid amide (sulfanilamide), a colorless cleavage product formed by reductive liver metabolism of the administered dye. Today we would call prontosil rubrum a pro-drug. The discovery of sulfanilamide's in vivo antibacterial properties ushered in the modern anti-infective era, and these investigators shared the award of a Nobel Prize for medicine in 1938. As poor as the potency of sulfanilamide is when compared with that of the modern agents that began to succeed it shortly thereafter, its impact on medicine was enormous. For the first time in the long and weary chronicle of human struggle against infectious disease, physicians now had a comparatively safe and responsive oral drug to use. Anxious friends and family at long last had hope that loved ones would not succumb to bacterial disease at an early age. Taken along with the use of penicillin only five or so years later the era of the so-called wonder drugs had dawned. It is one of life's great ironies to consider that although sulfanilamide had been synthesized in 1908, it had not been tested before as an anti-infective because there was no reason at that time to suppose that it would be useful to do so.

Once mainstays of antimicrobial chemotherapy, the sulfonamides have decreased enormously in popularity and are now comparatively minor drugs. The comparative cheapness of the sulfonamides is one of their most attractive features and accounts for much of their persistence on the market.

Mechanism of Action

The sulfonamides are bacteriostatic when administered in achievable doses. They inhibit the enzyme dihydropteroate synthase, an important enzyme needed for the biosynthesis of folic acid derivatives and, ultimately, DNA. They do this by competing at the active site with p-aminobenzoic acid (PABA), a normal structural component of folic acid derivatives. PABA is otherwise incorporated into the developing tetrahydrofolic acid molecule by condensation with a dihydropteroate diphosphate precursor under the influence of dihydropteroate synthetase. Thus sulfonamides may also be classified as antimetabolites (Fig. 34.1). Indeed, the antimicrobial efficacy of sulfonamides can be reversed by adding significant quantities of PABA into the diet (in some multivitamin preparations and certain local anesthetics), or into the culture medium.

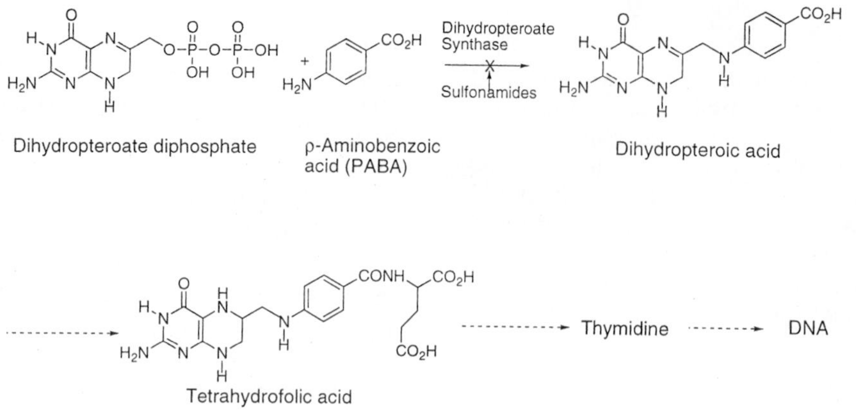

Fig. 34.1. Biosynthetic site of action of sulfonamides.

Most susceptible bacteria are unable to take up preformed folic acid from their environment and convert it to a tetrahydrofolic acid but, instead, synthesize their own folates de novo. As folates are essential intermediates for the preparation of certain DNA bases, without which bacteria cannot multiply, this inhibition is strongly bacteriostatic and ultimately bactericidal. Humans are unable to synthesize folates from component parts, lacking the necessary enzymes (including dihydropteroate synthase), and folic acid is consumed as a dietary. Sulfonamides have no lethal effect upon human cell growth. The basis for the selective toxicity of sulfonamides is, thus, clear.

In a few strains of bacteria, however, the picture is somewhat more complex. Here, sulfonamides are attached to the dihydropteroate diphosphate in the place of the normal PABA. The resulting product, however, is not capable of undergoing the next necessary reaction, condensation with glutamic acid. This false metabolite is also an enzyme inhibitor and the net result is inability of the bacteria to multiply as soon as the preformed folic acid in their cells is used up and further nucleic acid biosynthesis becomes impossible. The net result is the same, but the molecular basis of the effect is somewhat different in these strains (Fig. 34.2). Bacteria which are able to take up preformed folic acid into their cells are intrinsically resistant to sulfonamides.

Structure-activity Relationships

The basis of the structural resemblance of sulfonamides to PABA that is so devastating to these bacteria is clear. The functional group that differs in the two molecules is the carboxyl of PABA and the sulfonamide moiety of sulfanilamide. The strongly electron withdrawing character of the aromatic SO_2 group makes the nitrogen atom to which it is directly attached partially electropositive. This, in turn, increases the acidity of the hydrogen atoms attached to the nitrogen so that this functional group is slightly acidic (pKa 10.4). The pKa of the carboxyl group of PABA is approximately 6.5. It was soon found, following a crash synthetic program, that replacement of one of the NH_2 hydrogens by an electron withdrawing heteroaromatic ring was not only consistent with antimicrobial activity but also greatly acidified the remaining hydrogen and dramatically enhanced potency. With suitable groups in place, the pKa came down to the same range as that of PABA itself. Not only did this markedly increase the antibacterial potency of the product but dramatically increased the water solubility under physiologic conditions. The pKa of sulfisoxazole, one of the most popular of the sulfonamides in present use, is approximately 5.0. The poor water solubility of the earliest sulfonamides led to occasional crystallization in the urine (crystalluria) and resulted in kidney damage because the molecules were un-ionized at urine pH values. It is still recommended to drink increased quantities of water to avoid crystalluria when taking certain sulfonamides but this form of toxicity is now comparatively uncommon with the more important agents used today because they are at least partly ionized and hence reasonably water soluble at urinary pH values.

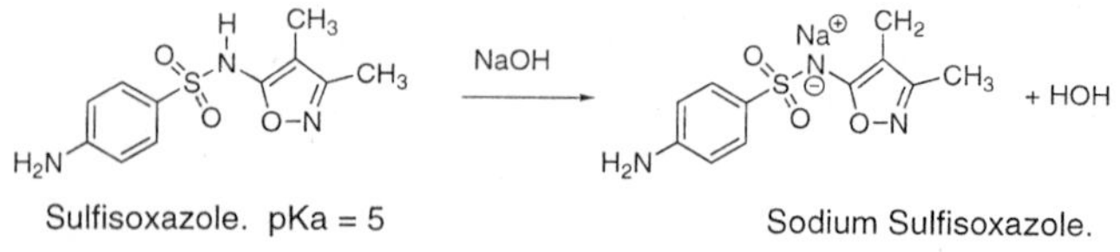

Sulfisoxazole. pKa = 5   Sodium Sulfisoxazole.

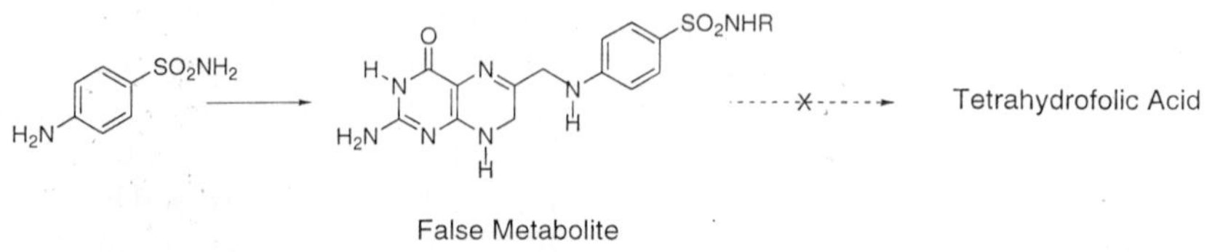

False Metabolite

Fig. 34.2. False metabolite formation by sulfanilamide.

Therapeutic Applications

Of the thousands of sulfonamides that have been evaluated, sulfisoxazole is currently the most popular. Along with the surviving sulfonamides (Table 34.1) it has a comparatively broad antimicrobial spectrum in vitro but its clinical use is generally restricted to the treatment of primary uncomplicated urinary tract infections and occasionally as a back up to other normally more preferred agents in special situations. Resistance is common and usually involves alternations in dihydropteroate synthase so that it discriminates better between PABA and the sulfonamides.

Sulfisoxazole is well absorbed following oral administration, distributes fairly widely and is excreted by the kidneys. Protein binding is intermediate (30–70%) and the more lipophilic sulfonamides are the more metabolized examples. Plasmid-mediated resistance development is common, particularly among Gram-(−) microorganisms and usually takes the form of decreased sensitivity of dihydropteroate synthase or increased production of PABA. A popular pro-drug is acetyl sulfisoxazole. Sulfonamides are partly deactivated by acetylation at N-4 and glucuronidation of the anilino nitrogen in the liver. In addition to frequent resistance, another drawback of the sulfonamides which decreases their use is the frequency of some severe side effects. Allergic reactions are the most common and take the form of rash, photosensitivity and drug fever. Less common problems are kidney and liver damage, hemolytic anemia and other blood problems. The most severe side effect is the Stevens-Johnson syndrome characterized by sometimes-fatal erythrema multiforme and ulceration of mucous membranes of the eye, mouth and urethra. Fortunately these effects are comparatively rare.

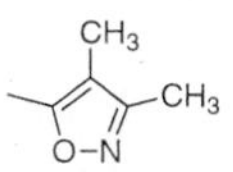

Other sulfonamides still in use include sulfadiazine, sulfamethizole, sulfamethoxazole and sulfasalazine. Multiple (or triple) sulfas are a 1:1:1 combination of sulfabenzamide, sulfacetamide, and sulfathiazole. The combination is primarily used as a creme for *Gardnerella vaginalis* vaginal infections.

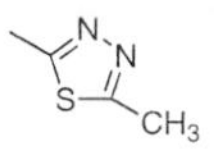

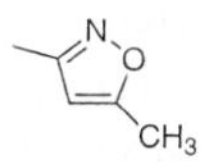

Of the group of less commonly employed sulfonamides, sulfasalazine stands out for other reasons. It is a pro-drug in that the absence of a free para-amino moiety makes it intrinsically inactive. Sulfasalazine is a red azo dye given orally and is largely not absorbed in the gut so the majority of the dose is delivered to the distal bowel. Reductive metabolism by gut bacteria converts the drug to sulfapyridine and 5-aminosalicylic acid (Fig. 34.3), the active component. The liberation of 5–aminosalicylic acid (mesalamine), an antiinflammatory agent, is the purpose for administering this drug. This agent is used to treat ulcerative colitis and Crohns disease. Direct administration of salicylates is otherwise irritating to the gastric mucosa.

Following the intensive effort of half a century ago that produced many thousands of analogs, the sulfonamide area has progressively fallen out of fashion and the field is quiescent today.

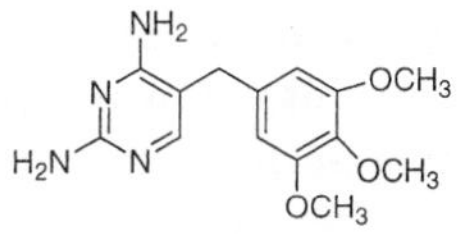

Trimethoprim (Proloprim, Trimpex)

Trimethoprim
Mechanism of Action

A further step in the pathway leading from the pteroates to folic acid and on to DNA bases requires the enzyme dihydrofolate reductase. Exogenous folic acid must be reduced stepwise to dihydrofolic acid and then to tetrahydrofolic acid an important cofactor essential for purine biosynthesis and ultimately for DNA synthesis (Fig. 34.4). Endogenously produced dihydrofolate must also be reduced by the same enzyme in order to enter the pathway involved in DNA synthesis. Inhibition of this key enzyme had been widely studied in attempts to find anticancer

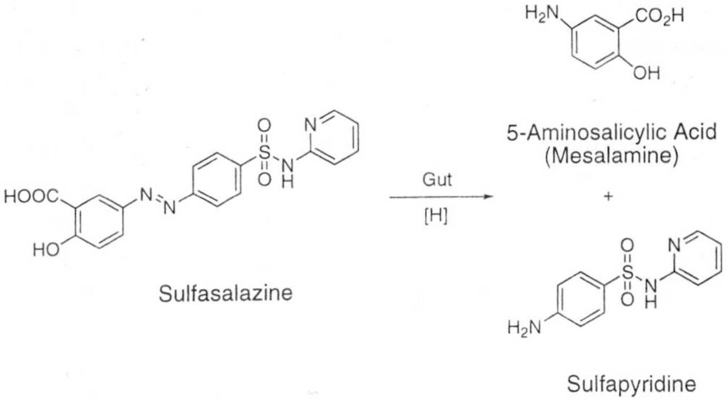

Table 34.1 Clinically Relevent Sulfonamides

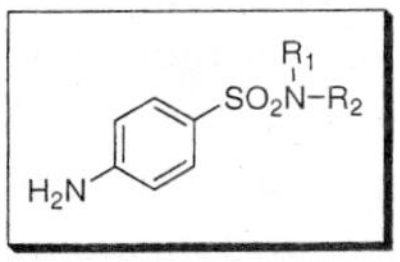

Generic Name	R₁	R₂
Sulfacetamide	H	COCH₃
Sulfabenzamide	H	COPh
Sulfadiazine	H	(2-pyrimidinyl)
Sulfamethizole	H	(5-methyl-1,3,4-thiadiazol-2-yl)
Sulfamethoxazole	H	(5-methylisoxazol-3-yl)
Sulfathiazole	H	(2-thiazolyl)
Acetyl Sulfisoxazole	—C(O)—CH₃	(3,4-dimethylisoxazol-5-yl)

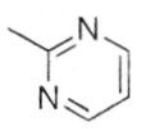

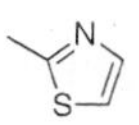

Fig. 34.3. Activation of sulfasalazine to PAS.

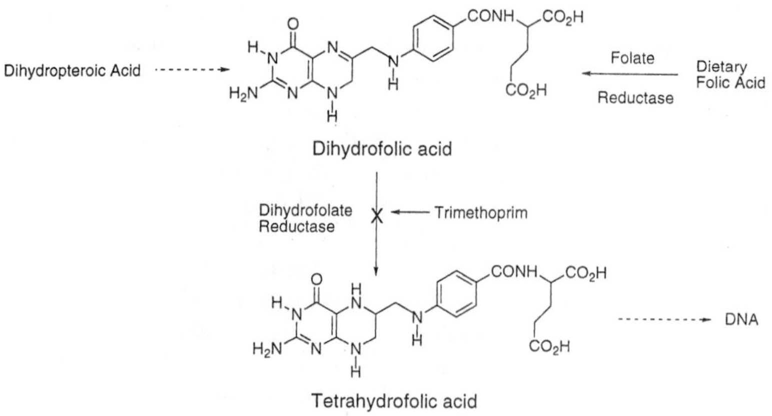

Fig. 34.4. Site of action of trimethoprim.

agents by starving rapidly dividing cancer cells of needed DNA precursors. The student will recall that methotrexate and its analogs came from such studies. Methotrexate is, however, much too toxic to be used as an antibiotic. Subsequently, however, trimethoprim was developed by George Hitchings and Gertrude Elion (who shared a Nobel Prize for this and other contributions to chemotherapy in the 1980s). This inhibitor prevents tetrahydrofolic acid synthesis and results in bacteriostasis. The student may wonder at first how this can work, because it is clear that mammals must also perform this enzymatic step. The basis for the favorable selectivity comes from subtle but significant architectural differences between the bacterial and the mammalian dihydrofolate reductases away from the active site. Whereas the bacterial enzyme and the mammalian enzyme both efficiently catalyze the conversion of dihydrofolic acid to tetrahydrofolic acid, the bacterial enzyme is sensitive to inhibition by trimethoprim by up to 40,000 times lower concentrations than is the mouse enzyme. This difference explains the useful selective toxicity of trimethoprim.

Therapeutic Application

Trimethoprim is frequently used as a single agent clinically for the oral treatment of uncomplicated urinary tract infections caused by susceptible bacteria (predominantly community acquired *E. coli* and other Gram-(−) rods). It is, however, most commonly used in a 1:5 fixed ratio with the sulfonamide sulfamethoxazole (Bactrim, Septra). This combination is not only synergistic in vitro but is less likely to induce bacterial resistance than either agent alone. It is rationalized that microorganisms not completely inhibited by sulfamethoxazole at the pteroate condensation step will not likely be able to push substrates past a subsequent blockade of dihydrofolate reductase. Thus these agents block sequentially at two different steps in the same essential pathway, and this combination is extremely difficult for a naive microorganism to survive. It is also comparatively uncommon that a microorganism will successfully mutate

to resistance at both enzymes during the course of therapy. Of course, if the organism is already resistant to either drug at the outset of therapy, which happens more and more often, much of the advantage of the combination is lost.

Pairing these two particular antibacterial agents was based upon pharmacokinetic factors and convenient availability. For such a combination to be useful in vivo the two agents must arrive at the necessary tissue compartment where the infection is at the correct time and in the right ratio. In this context, the optimum ratio of these two agents in vitro is 1:20. Of all of the combinations tried, sulfamethoxazole came closest to being optimal for trimethoprim and it was already on the market so did not have to be approved specially by the FDA for this purpose.

It is easier to demonstrate synergy in vitro than in vivo and concerns about the toxic contribution of the sulfonamide (and doubtless commercial considerations also) have led to a recent vogue for use of trimethoprim alone. Trimethoprim is broad-spectrum in vitro so it is potentially useful against many microorganisms. Combined with sulfamethoxazole, it is used for oral treatment of urinary tract infections, shigellosis, otitis media, traveler's diarrhea, MRSA, legionella, and bronchitis.

Among the opportunistic pathogens that afflict AIDS patients is the pneumonia causing protozoan *Pneumocystis carinii*. Immunocompetent individuals rarely become infected with *P. carinii* but it is a frequent pathogen in AIDS patients, and it is nearly 100% fatal in such immunocompromised individuals. The combination of sulfamethoxazole-trimethoprim has proven to be useful and comparatively nontoxic for these patients. A form for injection is available for use in severe infections and is particularly used in AIDS patients. This treatment form leads to more frequent toxic reactions, however. The most frequent side effects of trimethoprim-sulfamethoxazole are rash, nausea and vomiting. Blood dyscrasias are less common as is pseudomembranous colitis (caused by non-antibiotic sensitive opportunistic gut anaerobes, often *Clostridium difficile*). Many broad-spectrum antimicrobials can lead to such severe drug-related diarrhea and this side effect must be monitored carefully. Severe, nonresolving diarrhea can be fatal. It is, therefore, a justification for withdrawing existing therapy in favor of antianaerobic antibiotic. Despite a significant effort, no structurally related analog has emerged to compete with trimethoprim.

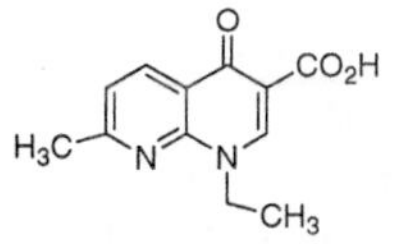

Nalidixic Acid

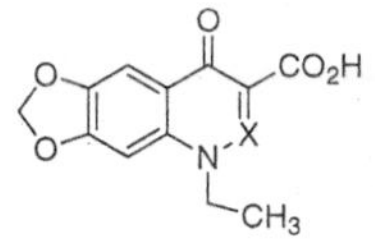

Oxolinic Acid, X = CH
Cinoxacin, X = N

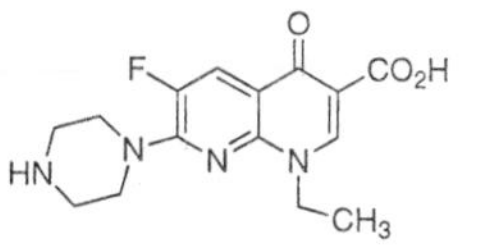

Enoxacin

Quinolones
First-generation Quinolones

The quinolone antimicrobials comprise a group of synthetic substances possessing in common an N-1-alkylated 3-carboxypyrid-4-one ring fused to another aromatic ring, which itself carries other substituents. The first quinolone to be marketed (in 1965) was nalidixic acid.

Nalidixic acid is still available and is primarily effective against Gram (−) bacteria. It is primarily reserved for oral treatment of uncomplicated urinary tract infections caused by susceptible microorganisms, usually *E. coli*. Over the following years the remaining first generation quinolones were introduced. These compounds consist of more potent and somewhat broader spectrum agents such as oxolinic acid, cinoxacin and enoxacin but they are not very popular today and are classified only as urinary tract disinfectants. The quinolones are often well absorbed following oral administration and are highly serum-protein bound. This leads to a comparatively long half-life but restricts their use mainly to protein free compartments such as the urinary tract. The tendency, because of their comparatively low potency, is to use them in fairly high doses to achieve coverage, and this leads to a frequent incidence of side effects, notably gastrointestinal upset, rash and visual disturbances. These drugs are proconvulsant and photosensitizing in susceptible individuals.

Second-generation Quinolones

The quinolones remained a small group of not very widely used agents until the discovery of the fluoroquinolones, of which norfloxacin was the first to become important. Norfloxacin (1986) is broad spectrum and equivalent in potency to many of the fermentation-derived antibiotics. Following its introduction, intense competition ensued and over a thousand of these second-generation analogs have now been made. Ciprofloxacin, ofloxacin, levofloxacin, sparfloxacin, trovafloxacin, norfloxacin, enoxacin, lomefloxacin and gatifloxacin are currently marketed in the USA (Fig. 34.5).

The properties of ciprofloxacin, the market leader, are typical of those of the group. It is rapidly and nearly completely absorbed on oral administration and is not highly protein bound. Lomefloxacin has a comparatively long half-life and it is conveniently administered less frequently than the other quinolones. Levofloxacin is the optically active version of ofloxacin and is roughly twice as active and somewhat more water-soluble. It has become very popular recently. Sparfloxacin and trovafloxacin have rather better anti Gram (+) activity than the classical quinolones which preceded them.

Mechanism of Action

The quinolones are rapidly bactericidal largely as a consequence of inhibition of DNA gyrase and topoisomerase IV key bacterial enzymes that dictate the conformation of DNA so that it can be stored properly, unwound, replicated, repaired, and transcribed on demand. These enzymes alter the conformation of DNA by catalyzing transient double strand cuts staggered by four base pairs, passing the uncut portion of the molecule through the gap and resealing the molecule back together. This alters the degree of twisting of DNA and releases torsional stress

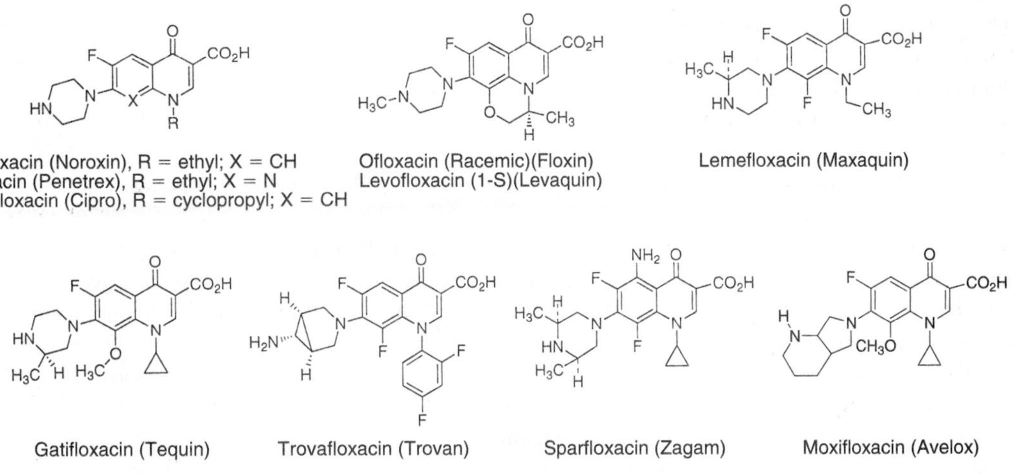

Norfloxacin (Noroxin), R = ethyl; X = CH
Enoxacin (Penetrex), R = ethyl; X = N
Ciprofloxacin (Cipro), R = cyclopropyl; X = CH

Ofloxacin (Racemic)(Floxin)
Levofloxacin (1-S)(Levaquin)

Lemefloxacin (Maxaquin)

Gatifloxacin (Tequin)

Trovafloxacin (Trovan)

Sparfloxacin (Zagam)

Moxifloxacin (Avelox)

Fig. 34.5. Second-generation quinolones.

in the molecule. Inhibition of DNA gyrase and topoisomerase IV makes a cell's DNA inaccessible and leads to cell death, particularly if the cell must deal with other toxic effects at the same time. Different quinolones inhibit these essential enzymes to different extents. Topoisomerase IV seems more important to some Gram (+) and DNA gyrase to some Gram (−) organisms. Topoisomerase IV is involved in decatenation.

Humans shape their DNA with a topoisomerase II, an analogous enzyme that, however, does not bind quinolones at normally achievable doses so the quinolones of commerce do not kill host cells.

Resistance to the quinolones is becoming more frequent taking the form of reduced cellular uptake or, more commonly, mutation to lesser sensitivity of the enzymes. Resistance by plasmid mediated mechanisms does not seem to take place.

Chemical Incompatabilities

The quinolones chelate polyvalent metal ions (Ca^{2+}, Mg^{2+}, Al^{3+}, and Fe^{2+} to form less water-soluble complexes and thereby lose considerable potency. Thus co-administration of certain antacids, hematinics, tonics and consumption of dairy products soon after quinolone administration is contraindicated.

Side Effects

Among the toxicities associated with quinolones is a proconvulsant action, especially in epileptics, but this is mainly associated with the first generation agents. Other CNS problems include hallucinations, insomnia, visual disturbances. Some patients also experience diarrhea, vomiting, abdominal pain and anorexia. The second-generation (fluoroquinolone) drugs are generally much better tolerated. The quinolones are associated with erosion of the load bearing joints of young animals. As a precaution, these drugs are not used casually before puberty or in sexually active females of childbearing age. They are also potentially damaging in the first trimester of pregnancy because of a risk of severe metabolic acidosis and of hemolytic anemia. Co-administration with theophylline potentiates the action of the latter and should be monitored closely. Although it takes much higher concentrations of fluoroquinolones to inhibit human topoisomerase II than either DNA gyrase or bacterial topoisomerase IV, some agents have a narrower safety margin. Temafloxacin, for example, was removed from the market because of hemolysis, renal failure and thrombocytopenia even though structurally closely related molecules appear relatively free of this problem.

Quite recently, severe liver toxicity has also led to the removal from the market of trovafloxacin except for severe infections involving institutional care where the patient can be closely monitored. Grepafloxacin was introduced on the market in late 1997 as a broad spectrum fluoroqinolone and withdrawn from the market in 1999 based upon cardiovascular toxicity. The drug was reported to cause a prolonged QTc interval. These drugs were well on the way to great popularity when these untoward events were detected. These phenomenon were not apparently revealed during extensive prior animal and clinical studies.

Therapeutic Applications

The second-generation quinolones are more widely used than the first. Whereas norfloxacin is mainly used for urinary tract infections (*enterobacter, enterococcus* or *Pseudomonas aeruginosa*) the others, particularly ciprofloxacin, are also used for prostatitis, upper respiratory tract infections, bone infections, septicemia, staphylococcal and pseudomonal endocarditis, meningitis, sexually transmitted diseases (gonorrhea and chlamydial), chronic ear infections, and purulent osteoarthritis. Anaerobes, staphylococci and pseudomonads must be watched carefully for emergence of resistance. Lomefloxacin is used once daily for urinary tract and upper respiratory tract infections due to susceptible microorganisms.

In summary, the first quinolones had relatively narrow antiGram negative spectra. These were followed by significantly broad-spectrum agents that found widespread office use. The more modern quinolones are intended to fill in the gaps in coverage left by the second generation by being directed primarily against Gram positive microorganisms, anaerobes, and bacteria resistant to present quinolones. The quinolones are still under very active investigation and newer agents are expected to appear at regular intervals. In particular, an isomeric series, called the 2-pyridones, look very promising at this time.

Nitrofurantoin
(Furadantin, Macrodantin)

Miscellaneous Agents
Nitrofurans

Nitrofurantoin a widely used oral antibacterial substance has been available since World War II. It is used for prophylaxis or treatment of urinary tract infections when kidney function is not impaired, and it inhibits kidney stone growth. Nausea and vomiting are common side effects. This is avoided in part by slowing the rate of absorption of the drug through use of wax-coated large particles (Macrodantin). Nitrofurantoin inhibits DNA and RNA functions through mechanisms that are not well understood. Resistance is not commonly encountered.

Metronidazole (Flagyl)

Metronidazole

Initially introduced for the treatment of vaginal infections caused by amoeba, it is also useful for the treatment of trichomoniasis, giardiasis and *Gardnerella vaginalis* infections. It has found increasing use of late in the parenteral treatment of anaerobic infections and for treatment of pseudomembranous enterocolitis due to *Clostridium difficile*. *C. difficile* is an opportunistic pathogen which occasionally flourishes as a consequence of broad-spectrum antibiotic therapy and its infections can be life threatening. The drug is believed to be metabolically activated by reduction of its nitro group to produce reactive oxygen species (See Chapter 35). Metronidazole is also a component of a multidrug cocktail used to treat *Helicobacter pylori* infections associated with gastric ulcers.

$$\xrightarrow{H_3O^+} \quad 4\ NH_3 + 6\ CH_2O$$

Methenamine

Methenamine

A venerable drug used for the disinfection of acidic urine, structurally methenamine is a low molecular weight polymer of ammonia and formaldehyde which reverts to its components under mildly acid conditions. Formaldehyde is the active antimicrobial component. Methenamine is used for recurrent urinary tract infections.

Phosphomycin (Monurol)

Phosphomycin

Phosphomycin inhibits enolpyruvial transferase, an enzyme catalyzing an early step in bacterial cell wall biosynthesis. Inhibition results in reduced synthesis of peptidoglycan an important component in the bacterial cell wall. Phosphomycin is bactericidal against *E. coli* and *Enterobacter faecalis* infections.

Antibiotics: Inhibitors of Bacterial Cell Wall Biosynthesis

Bacterial Cell Wall

The bacterial cell wall differs dramatically in structure and function compared to the outer layers of mammalian cells and thus provides a number of potentially attractive targets for selective chemotherapy of bacterial infections. For one thing, the bacterial cell wall is chemically distinct from mammalian cell walls and so is constructed by enzymes that often have no direct counterpart in mammalian cell construction. Three of the main functions of the bacterial cell wall are: (1)

to provide a semi-permeable barrier interfacing with the environment through which only desirable substances may pass; (2) to provide a sufficiently strong barrier so that the bacterial cell is protected from changes in the osmotic pressure of its environment; and (3) to prevent digestion by host enzymes. The initial units of the cell wall are constructed within the cell, but soon the growing and increasingly complex structure must be extruded; final assembly takes place outside of the inner membrane. This circumstance makes the enzymes involved later in the process more vulnerable to inhibition. Whereas individual bacterial species differ in specific details, the following generalized picture of the process is sufficiently accurate to illustrate the process.

Gram (+) Bacteria. The cell wall of Gram (+) bacteria, although complex enough, is simpler than that of Gram (−) organisms. A schematic representation is shown in Figure 34.6. On the very outside of the cell is a set of characteristic carbohydrates and proteins that together make up the antigenic determinants that differ from species to species and that also cause adherence to particular target cells. The next barrier that the wall presents is the peptidoglycan layer. This is a spongy, gel-forming layer consisting of a series of alternating sugars (N-acetylglucosamine [NAG] and N-acetylmuramic acid [NAM]) linked (1,4)-β in a long chain (Fig. 34.7). To the free lactic acid carboxyl moieties of the N-acetylmuramic acid units is attached, through an amide linkage, a series of amino acids of which L-ala-D-glu-L-lys-D-ala is typical. One notes the D-stereochemistry of the glutamate and the terminal alanine. This feature is presumably important in protecting the peptidoglycan from hydrolysis by host peptidases, particularly in the GI tract. This unusual structural feature enables successful parasitism. The terminal D-alanyl unit is bonded to the lysyl unit of an adjacent tetrapeptide strand through a pentaglycyl unit. This last step in the biosynthesis is a transamidation wherein the terminal amino moiety on the last glycine of the A strand displaces the terminal D-ala unit on the nearby B strand. This step is catalyzed by a cell wall transamidase (one of the penicillin-binding proteins, PBP) which forms a transient covalent bond during the synthesis phase with a particular serine hydroxyl on the enzyme. Completion of the catalytic cycle by cross linking through displacement of the enzyme and substitution by a glycine residue regenerates the enzyme and produces a thickened three-dimensional cell wall. This process gives the structure strength

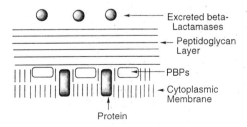

Fig. 34.6. Schematic of some features of the Gram (+) bacterial cell wall.

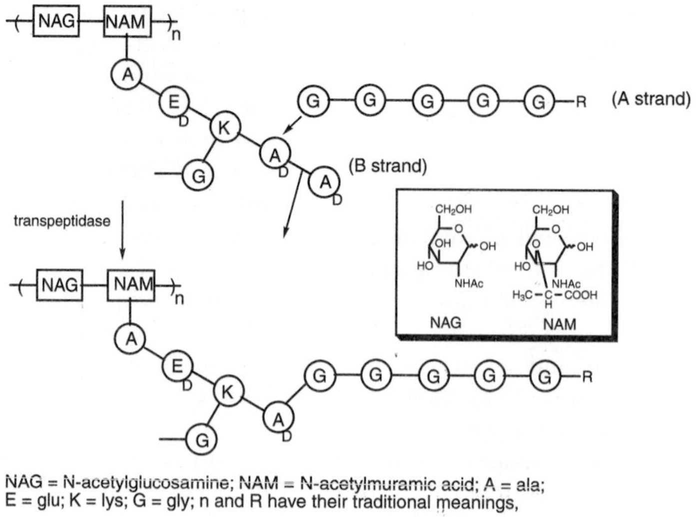

Fig. 34.7. Schematic of cell wall cross-linking. Pentaglycyl group displaces terminal D-ala.

NAG = N-acetylglucosamine; NAM = N-acetylmuramic acid; A = ala;
E = glu; K = lys; G = gly; n and R have their traditional meanings,

through adding the third dimension, much as would be achieved by gluing the pages of a book together. This provides the strong barrier needed against osmotic stress and accounts for the retention of characteristic morphological shape of Gram (+) bacteria (globes and rods, for example). This step is highly sensitive to inhibition of β-lactam antibiotics. The peptidoglycan layer is traversed by teichoic and teichuronic acids. Beneath this layer is the lipoidal cytoplasmic cell membrane in which a number of important protein molecules float in a lipid bilayer. Among these are the β-lactam receptors, known as the penicillin binding proteins (PBPs). In Gram-(+) bacteria the outer layers are relatively ineffective in keeping antibiotics out. It is this inner membrane which provides the principal barrier to uptake of antibiotics. There are at least seven types of PBPs. Those of *E. coli* are classified in Table 34.2. The functions of all of these are not entirely known but they are important in construction and repair of the cell wall. β-lactam antibiotics bind to these agents and kill bacteria by preventing the biosynthesis of a functional cell wall. Various β-lactam antibiotics display different patterns of binding to these proteins. These proteins must alternate in a controlled and systematic way between their active and inert states so that bacterial cells can grow and multiply in an orderly manner. Selective interference by β-lactam antibiotics with their functioning prevents normal growth and repair and creates serious problems for bacteria, particularly young cells needing to grow and mature cells needing to repair damage or to divide. The rapid bactericidal effect of penicillins on such cells can readily be imagined. The cell wall not only protects the bacterium from its environment but also provides a confining case that must be repaired when damaged or be remodeled and expanded so that the cell can grow. Inhibition of the PBPs creates serious problems for growing bacterial cells. The β-lactamases are secreted outside the Gram (+) cell and must be replenished frequently.

Gram (−) Bacteria. With the Gram (−) bacteria, the cell wall is more complex and more lipoidal (Fig. 34.8). These cells usually contain an additional, outer, membrane. The outer layer contains complex lipopolysaccharides that encode antigenic responses, cause septic shock, provide the serotype, and influence morphology. This exterior layer also contains a number of enzymes and exclusionary proteins. Important among these is the porins. These are transmembranal super molecules made up of two or three monomeric proteins. The center of this array is a transmembranal pore of various dimensions. Some allow many kinds of small molecules to pass and others contain specific receptors that allow only certain molecules to come in. The size, shape and lipophilicity are important considerations controlling porin passage. Antibiotics have greater difficulty in penetrating into Gram (−) bacterial cells as a consequence. Below this lies a somewhat less impressive, as compared to Gram (+) organisms, layer of peptidoglycan. Next comes a periplasmic space in which the β-lactamases are found. This is followed by a phospholipid rich cytoplasmic membrane in which floats a series of characteristic proteins with various functions. The β-lactam receptors (PBPs) are found here. Binding of β-lactam antibiotics to PBP-1A and B (transpeptidase)

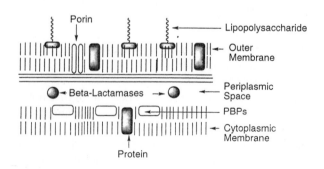

Fig. 34.8. Schematic of some features of the Gram (−) bacterial cell wall.

Table 34.2. Penicillin Binding Proteins (PBP) of *E. coli*

PBP	Function	Lethality?
1A	Cell elongation (peripheral wall extension)	Yes
1B	Cell elongation (peripheral wall extension)	Yes
2	Maintenance of rod shape	Yes
3	Septum formation	No
4	Limit the amount of cross linking of the peptidoglycan	No
5	Limit the amount of cross linking of the peptidoglycan	No
6	Limit the amount of cross linking of the peptidoglycan	No

V. Lorian, Ed., Antibiotics in Laboratory Medicine, Williams & Wilkins, Baltimore (1986).

of *E. coli* leads to cell lysis; to PBP-2 (transpeptidase) leads to oval cells deficient in rigidity and to inhibition of cell division; to PBP-3 (transpeptidase) gives abnormally long, filamentous shapes by failure to produce a septum; and to PBP-4-6 (carboxypeptidases) leads to no lethal effects. Approximately 8% of a dose of benzyl penicillin binds to PCP-1; 0.7% to PCP-2; 2% to PBP-3; 4% to PBP-4; 65% to PBP-5 and 21% to PBP-6. Thus the majority of the dose bonds to PBP's whose function remains obscure. Binding to PBP-1 is lethal. Other β-lactam antibiotics display different binding patterns. Amoxicillin and the cephalosporins bind more avidly to PBP-1; methicillin and cefotaxime to PBP-2, and mezlocillin and cefuroxime to PBP-3.

Since the β-lactamases lie in the periplasmic space they remain within the cell so need not be produced in the quantities characteristic of Gram (+) bacteria. Other inner membrane proteins are involved in transport, energy and biosynthesis. In many such cells there are proteins that actively pump out antibiotics and other substances at the expense of energy and which may require the simultaneous entrance of oppositely charged materials to maintain an electrostatic balance.

beta-lactam
azetidinone

β-Lactam Antibiotics

The name lactam is given to cyclic amides and is analogous to the name lactone given to cyclic esters. In an older nomenclature, the second carbon in an aliphatic carboxylic acid was designated alpha, the third beta, and so on. Thus a β-lactam is a cyclic amide with four atoms in its ring. The contemporary name for this ring system is azetidinone. This structural feature was very rare when it was found to be a feature of the structure of the penicillins so the name β-lactam came to be a generic descriptor for the whole family. It is fortunate that this ring ultimately proved to be the main component of the pharmacophore so the term possesses medicinal as well as chemical significance. The penicillin subclass of β-lactam antibiotics is characterized by the presence of a substituted 5-membered thiazoldine ring fused to the β-lactam ring. This fusion and the chirality of the β-lactam ring results in the molecule possessing a "V" shape. This drasti-

cally interferes with the planarity of the lactam bond and resonance of the lactam nitrogen with its carbonyl group. Consequently the β-lactam ring is much more sensitive to hydrolysis as compared with normal planar amides.

History. The general outlines of the story of the discovery of the penicillins are widely known. In 1929, Alexander Fleming, a physician and a clinical microbiologist, was preserving a culture of a pathogen and the plate became contaminated with an airborne fungus, *Penicillium notatum* (now named *P. chrysogenum*), which not only grew but also produced a clear zone of inhibition around its colony. Recognizing the potential significance of this antibiotic effect, he preserved the fungus and tried to identify its active constituent. The state of development of the art and his background and training were insufficient for the task at hand at that time. It was not until a decade later that a group of English chemists including Abraham, Chain, Florey and Heatley succeeded in purifying the unstable antibiotic. Finally, on February 12, 1941, following heroic efforts necessitated by war time conditions and lack of suitable equipment and technology, enough material was available for clinical examination and the demonstration that penicillin actually worked in humans. Much new technology had to be developed before large-scale use of penicillin could take place. The efforts of an international team solved, for example, the problems of large-scale sterile aerobic submerged fermentation, directed fermentation, strain improvement and many other vexing problems. By 1943 penicillin was being produced in very large quantities for the use of the armed forces. The penicillin field gradually expanded to include orally active penicillins, broad-spectrum and enzymatically stable penicillins, and then the cephalosporins of three generations, the monobactams, carbapenems, β-lactamase stable penicillins and cephalosporins, β-lactamase inhibitors, and so on. In 1993 about half of the money spent worldwide on antibiotics was for β-lactams. Over a hundred thousand of these compounds have been prepared by partial or total chemical synthesis.

Penicillins. The medicinal classifications, chemical structures, and generic names of the penicillins currently available are set forth in Table 34.3.

Preparation of Penicillins. The original fermentation-derived penicillins were produced by uncontrolled fermen-

Table 34.3. Commercially Significant Penicillins and Related Molecules

Generic Name	Trade Name	R₁	X	Y
Fermentation-Derived Penicillins				
6-Aminopenicillanic acid		H	—	—
Benzylpenicillin (Penicillin G)	Generic	$C_6H_5\text{-}CH_2\text{-}$	—	—
Phenoxymethylpenicillin (Penicillin V)	Generic	$C_6H_5\text{-}OCH_2\text{-}$	—	—
Semi-Synthetic Penicillinase-Resistant Parenteral Penicillins				
Methicillin			—	—
Nafcillin	Nallpen, Unipen		—	—
Semi-Synthetic Penicillinase-Resistant Oral Penicillins				
Oxacillin	Bactocill		H	H
Cloxacillin	Cloxapen		H	Cl
Dicloxacillin	Dycil, Pathocil		Cl	Cl
Semi-Synthetic Penicillinase-Sensitive, Broad Spectrum, Parenteral Penicillins				
Carbenizillin (R₂ = H)			—	—
Carbenicillin phenyl (R₂ = C₆H₅)			—	—
Carbenicillin indanyl (R₂ =)	Geocillin		—	—
Ticarcillin	Ticar		—	—
Azlocillin			H	—
Mezolcillin	Mezlin		$CH_3SO_2\text{-}$	—
Piperacillin	Pipracil		—	—
Semi-Synthetic Penicillinase-Sensitive, Broad-Spectrum, Oral Penicillins				
Ampicillin	Principen, Omnipen		H	—
Amoxicillin	Amoxil, Trimox, Wymox		HO	—

tation of the fungus *Penicillium chrysogenum* with the result that they were mixtures differing from one another in the identity of the side chain moiety. When a sufficient supply of phenylacetic acid is present in the medium, this is preferentially incorporated into the molecule to produce mainly benzylpenicillin (penicillin G in the old nomenclature). Use of phenoxyacetic acid instead leads to phenoxymethyl penicillin (penicillin V). More than two dozen different penicillins have been made in this way, but these two are the only ones which remain in clinical use. The bicyclic penicillin nucleus itself is prepared biosynthetically via a complex process from an acylated cysteinyl valyl peptide. The complete exclusion of side chain precursor acids from the medium produces the fundamental penicillin nucleus, 6-aminopenicillanic acid (6-APA), but in poor yield. By itself, 6-APA has only very weak antibiotic activity but when substituted on its primary amino group with a suitable amide side chain, its potency and antibacterial spectrum are profoundly enhanced. With this key precursor isolated, limitations caused by enzyme specificities in

biosynthesis could be overcome by use of partial chemical synthesis. A more practical modern process for making 6-APA employs naturally occurring fungal enzymes that selectively hydrolyze away the side chain of natural penicillins without cleaving the β-lactam bond. These enzymes are found in Gram (−) bacteria but appear to be of negligible importance with respect to bacterial resistance to β-lactam antibiotics. More recently, ingeniously selective chemical processes have been devised for accomplishing removal of less interesting side chains from biosynthetic penicillins. The operational chemical freedom resulting from the availability of 6-APA has led to partial synthesis of many thousands of analogs.

The sodium and potassium salts of penicillins are crystalline, hydroscopic, and water-soluble; they are employed orally or parentally. When dry, they are stable for long periods, but hydrolyze rapidly when in solution. Their best stability is noted at pH values between 5.5–8, especially at pH 6.0–7.2. The procaine and benzathine salts of benzylpenicillin, on the other hand, are water insoluble. They are used for repository purposes following injection when long-term blood levels are required.

Procaine

Benzathine

Nomenclature. The nomenclature of the penicillins, as with most antibiotics, is complex. The Chemical Abstracts system is definitive and unambiguous but too complex for ordinary use (Fig. 34.9). For example, the chemical name for benzylpenicillin sodium is monosodium (2S,5R,6R)-3,3-dimethyl-7-oxo)-6-(2-phenylacetamido)-4-thia-1azabicyclo-[3.2.0]heptane-2-carboxylate. Confusingly, the United States Pharmacopoeia uses a different system which results in the atoms being numbered differently. The simplest system has stood the test of time and involves taking the repeating radical, carbonyl-6-aminopenicillanic acid, and using the chemical trivial name for the radical that completes the structure. Thus use of the names benzylpenicillin and phenoxymethylpenicillin makes practical sense. There are three asymmetric centers in the benzylpenicillin molecule as indicated by the asterisk in Table 34.3.

Clinically Relevant Degradation Reactions of Penicillins. The most unstable bond in the penicillin molecule is the highly strained and reactive β-lactam amide bond. This bond cleaves only moderately slowly in water unless heated, but much more rapidly in alkaline solutions to produce penicilloic acid which readily decarboxylates to produce penilloic acid (Fig. 34.10). Penicilloic acid has a negligible tendency to reclose to the corresponding penicillin so this reaction is essentially irreversible under physiologic conditions. Because the β-lactam ring is an essential portion of the pharmacophore, this reaction deactivates the antibiotic. A fairly significant degree of hydrolysis also takes place in the liver. The bacterial enzyme, β-lactamase, catalyzes this reaction also and is a principal cause of bacterial re-

sistance in the clinic. Alcohols and amines bring about the same cleavage reaction but the products are the corresponding esters and amides. A reaction with a specific primary amino group of aminoglycoside antibiotics is of clinical relevance as it inactivates penicillins and cephalosporins. It will be discussed later. When proteins serve as the nucleophiles in this reaction, the antigenic conjugates which cause many penicillin allergies are produced. Small molecules that are not inherently antigenic but react with proteins to produce antigens in this manner are called haptens. Commercially available penicillin salts may be contaminated with small amounts of these antigenic penicilloyl proteins derived from reaction with proteins encountered in their fermentative production or by high molecular weight self-condensation derived polymers resulting when penicillins are concentrated and react with themselves. Both of these classes of impurities are antigenic and may sensitize some patients.

Solutions of penicillins for parenteral use should be refrigerated, used promptly, and not stored. In acidic solutions, the hydrolysis of penicillins is much more complex. Hydrolysis of the β-lactam bond can be shown through kinetic analysis to involve participation of the side chain amide oxygen because the rate of this reaction differs widely depending upon the nature of R. The main end products of the acidic degradation are penicillamine, penilloic acid and penilloaldehyde (Fig. 34.11). The intermediate penicillenic acid is highly unstable and undergoes subsequent hydrolysis to the corresponding penicilloic acid. An alternate pathway involves sulfur ejection to a product which in turn fragments to liberate penicilloic acid also. Penicilloic acid readily decarboxylates to penilloic acid. The latter hydrolyzes to produce penilloaldehyde and penicillamine (itself used clinically as a chelating agent). Several related fragmentations to a variety of other products take place. None of these products has antibacterial activity. At gastric pH (ca. 2.0) and temperature of 37° C, benzyl penicillin has a half-life measured in minutes. The less water soluble amine salts are more stable.

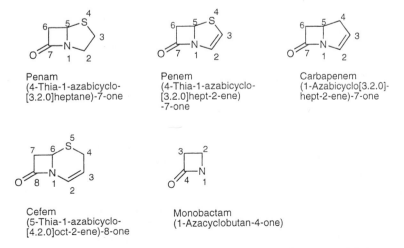

Penam
(4-Thia-1-azabicyclo-
[3.2.0]heptane)-7-one

Penem
(4-Thia-1-azabicyclo-
[3.2.0]hept-2-ene)
-7-one

Carbapenem
(1-Azabicyclo[3.2.0]-
hept-2-ene)-7-one

Cefem
(5-Thia-1-azabicyclo-
[4.2.0]oct-2-ene)-8-one

Monobactam
(1-Azacyclobutan-4-one)

Fig. 34.9. Ring and numbering systems of clinically available β-lactam antibiotic types.

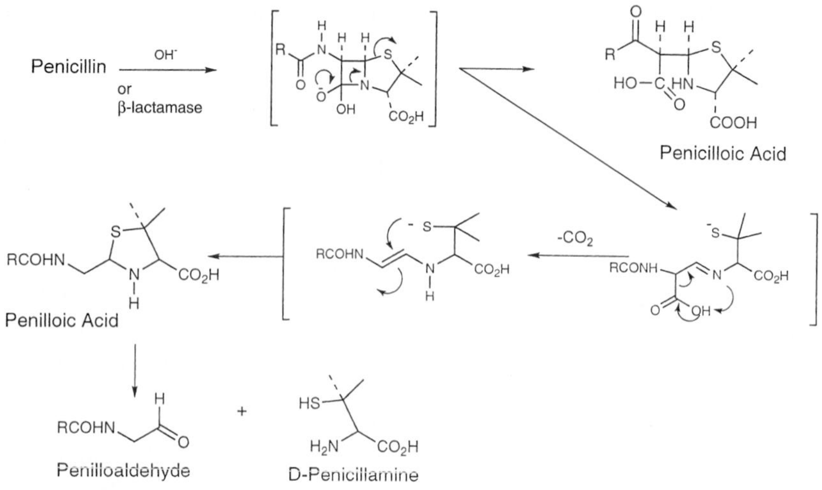

Fig. 34.10. Instability of β-lactams to nucleophiles.

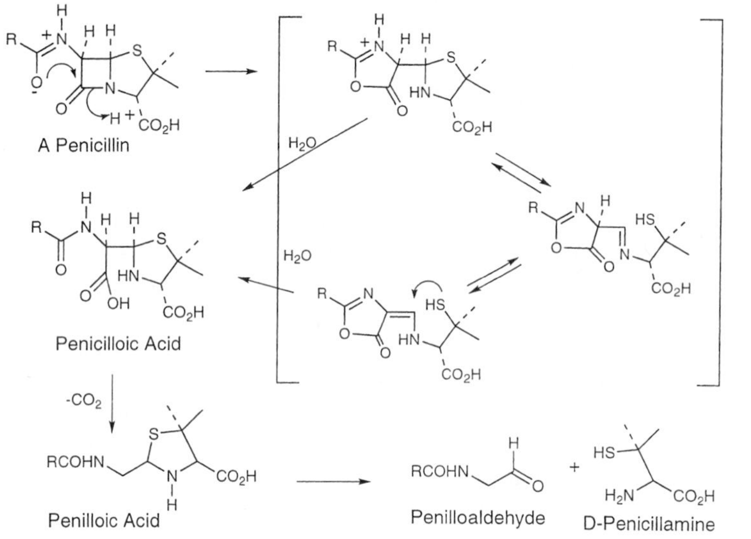

Fig. 34.11. Instability of penicillins to acid. Hydrolysis involves the C-6 side chain.

The installation of a side chain R group which is electron withdrawing decreases the electron density on the side chain carbonyl and protects these penicillins in part from acid degradation. This property has clinical implications as these compounds survive passage through the stomach better and many can be given orally for systemic purposes. It is estimated that 15–30% of an oral dose of benzylpenicillin survives passage through the stomach under fasting conditions whereas 60–73% of an oral dose of phenoxymethyl penicillin survives under these conditions. The blood concentration peaks in 1/2–1 hour. Phenoxymethyl penicillin has a half-life of about 5 hours under simulated gastric conditions.

In vitro degradation reactions of penicillins can be retarded for clinical purposes by keeping the pH of solutions between 6.0 and 6.8 and by refrigerating them. Metal ions such as mercury, zinc, and copper catalyze the degradation of penicillins so they should be kept from contact with penicillin solutions. The lids of containers used today are routinely made of inert plastics in part to minimize such problems.

Protein Binding. The more lipophilic the side chain of a penicillin, the more serum protein bound is the antibiotic (Table 34.4). While this has some advantages in terms of protection from degradation, it does reduce the effective bactericidal concentration of the drug. Contrary to popular assumption, the degree of serum protein binding of the penicillins has comparatively little influence upon their half-lives. The penicillins are actively excreted into the urine via an active transport system for negatively charged ions and the rate of release from their bound form is sufficiently rapid that the controlling rate is the

Table 34.4. Protein Binding of Penicillins

Penicillin	% Protein Binding
Benzyl penicillin	45–68
Phenoxymethyl penicillin	75–89
Methicillin	35–80
Ampicillin	25–30
Amxoicillin	25–30
Carbenicillin	~50
Oxacillin	>90
Cloxacillin	>90

kidney secretion rate. The serum half-life of penicillin G is about 0.4–0.9 hours and phenoxymethyl penicillin is about 0.5 hours. Both are excreted into the urine by tubular excretion.

Mechanism of Action. The generally accepted molecular mode of action of the β-lactam antibiotics is a selective and irreversible inhibition of the enzymes processing the developing peptidoglycan layer (Fig. 34.12). Just before cross-linking occurs, the peptide pendant from the lactate carboxyl of a muramic acid unit terminates in a D-ala-D-ala unit. This is cleaved between these two amino acids by hydrolysis catalyzed by a cell wall transamidase. This is one of the penicillin-binding proteins (carboxypeptidases, endopeptidases, and transpeptidases) that normally reside in the bacterial inner membrane and perform construction, repair, and housekeeping functions maintaining cell wall integrity and playing a vital role in cell growth and division. They differ significantly from bacterium to bacterium and this is used to rationalize different potency and morphologic outcomes following β-lactam attack on the different bacteria. The cell wall transamidase uses a serine hydroxyl group to attack the penultimate D-ala unit forming a covalent bond and the terminal D-ala, which is released by this action, diffuses away. The enzyme-peptidoglycan complex is attacked by the free amino end of a pentaglycyl unit of an adjacent strand regenerating the transpeptidase's active site for further catalytic action and producing a new amide bond, which glues two adjacent strands together.

The three-dimensional geometry of the active site of the enzyme perfectly accommodates to the shape and separation of the amino acids of its substrate. Because the substrate has unnatural stereochemistry at the critical residues, this enzyme is not expected to attack host peptides or even other bacterial peptides composed of natural amino acids.

The present belief is that the penicillins and the other β-lactam antibiotics resemble closely the geometry of acylated D-ala-D-ala and that the enzyme mistakenly accepts it as its normal substrate. The highly strained β-lactam ring is much more reactive than a normal amide, particularly when fused into the appropriate bicyclic system. The intermediate acyl-enzyme complex, however, is rather different structurally from the normal intermediate in that the hydrolysis does not break penicillins into two pieces as it does with its normal substrate. In the penicillins, a heterocyclic residue is still covalently bonded and cannot diffuse away as the natural terminal D-ala unit does. This presents a steric barrier to approach by the pentaglycyl unit and keeps the enzyme's active site from being regenerated and the cell wall precursors from being cross-linked. The resulting cell wall is structurally weak and subject to osmotic stress. Cell lysis can result and the cell rapidly dies (the later process is assisted by another class of bacterial enzymes, the autolysins, which are peptidoglycan hydrolases that clean up cellular debris.) The result is a defective cell wall and an inactivated enzyme. The relief of strain that is obtained upon enzymatic β-lactam bond cleavage is so pronounced that there is virtually no tendency for the reaction to reverse. Water is also an insufficiently effective nucleophile and cannot hydrolyze the complex either. Thus, the cell wall transamidase is stoichiometrically inac-

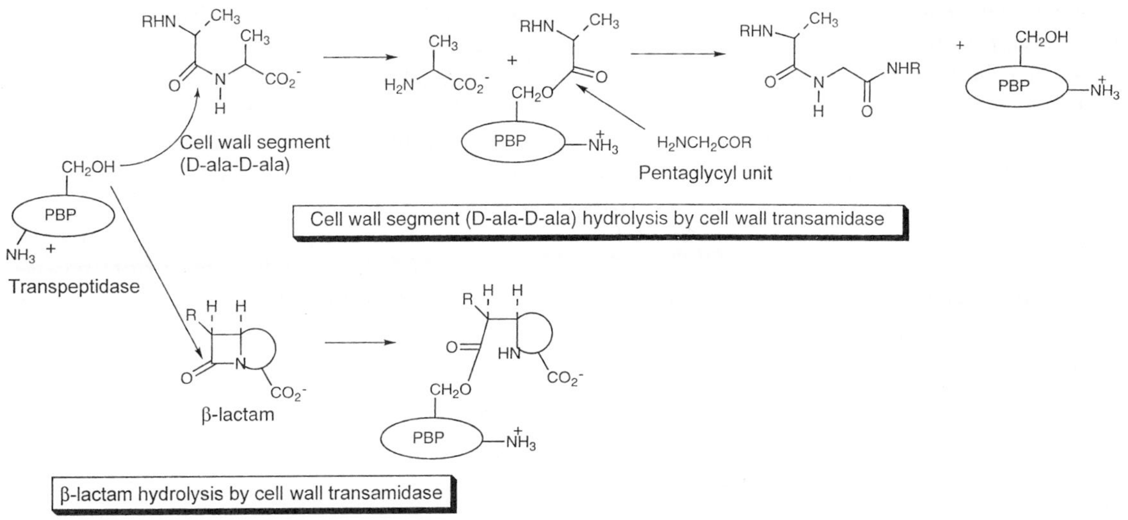

Fig. 34.12. Cell wall cross-linking and MOA of β-lactams.

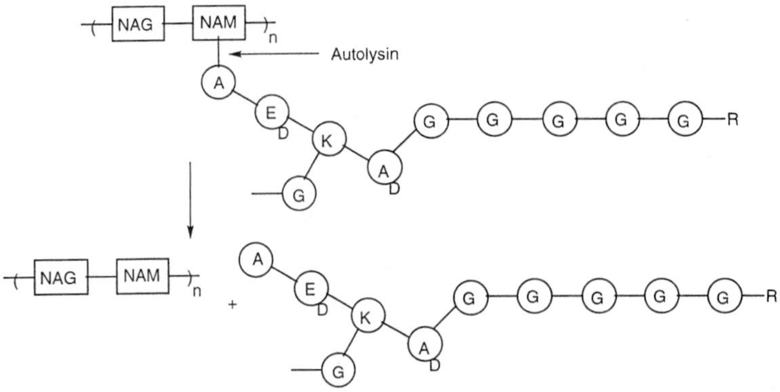

Fig. 34.13. Autolysin cleavage of cell wall segment.

tivated. More details of the putative drug-enzyme interaction will be discussed with the other classes of β-lactams.

Another important class of enzymes exists whose action enhances the bactericidal action of β-lactams. These are the autolysins (Fig. 34.13). The autolysins cleave the N-acetylmuramic acid-peptide bond to L-ala. The result of this is that the whole amino acid side chain falls away with effects quite lethal to the bacterium.

Resistance. Resistance to β-lactam antibiotics is unfortunately increasingly common. It can be intrinsic and involve decreased cellular uptake of drug, or involve lower binding affinity to the PBPs. This is particularly the case with methicillin-resistant *Staphylococcus aureus* (MRSA) whose PBP-2 has been mutated so that it does not bind methicillin efficiently any longer. Much more common, however, is the elaboration of a β-lactamase. β-lactamases are enzymes (serine proteases) elaborated by microorganisms that catalyze hydrolysis of the β-lactam bond and inactivate β-lactam antibiotics to penicilloic acids before they can reach the PCPs (Fig. 34.14). In this they resemble somewhat the cell wall transamidase but they are released distally from the inner membrane. Hydrolytic regeneration of the β-lactamase's active site is dramatically more facile than is the case with cell wall transamidase so that the enzyme can turn over many times and a comparatively small amount of enzyme can destroy a large amount of drug. With Gram (+) bacteria, such as staphylococci, the β-lactamases are usually shed continuously into the medium and meet the drug outside the cell wall. With Gram (−) bacteria, a more conservative course is followed. Here the β-lactamases are secreted into the periplasmic space between the inner and outer membrane

so, while still distal to the PBPs, they do not readily escape into the medium and need not be resynthesized as often. Numerous β-lactamases with various antibiotic substrate specificities are now known, Table 34.5–34.7. Elaboration of β-lactamases is often R-factor mediated and, in some cases, is even induced by the presence of β-lactam antibiotics. The normal function of β-lactamases in the absence of antibiotic is not readily apparent.

Allergenicity. About 6–8% of the U.S. population is allergic to β-lactam antibiotics. Most commonly this is expressed as drug rash or itching and is of delayed onset but occasionally the reaction is immediate and profound. In the latter cases, cardiovascular collapse and shock can result in death. This is most common with injections. Sometimes penicillin allergy can be anticipated by taking a medication history and often patients likely to be allergic are those with a history of hypersensitivity to a wide variety of allergens, e.g., foods and pollens. A prior history of allergy to penicillins is a contraindicating factor to their use. Topical wheal and flare tests are available when there is doubt. When an allergic reaction develops, the drug must be discontinued and, because cross sensitivity is common, other β-lactam drugs should generally be avoided. Considering all therapeutic categories, penicillins, especially the ones most commonly employed (benzylpenicillin and ampicillin/amoxicillin), are probably the drugs most associated with allergy. Erythromycin and clindamycin are useful alternate choices in many cases of penicillin allergy.

In some cases the patient may have become sensitized without knowing it due to prior passive exposure through contaminated foodstuffs or cross-contaminated

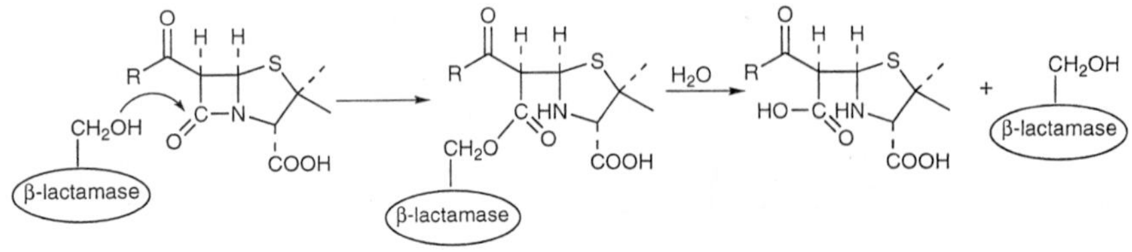

Fig. 34.14. β-lactamase catalyzed hydrolysis of penicillins.

Table 34.5. β-Lactamase Classifications According to Sykes and Matthew

Type	Substrate Preferences	Gene Location	Inducibility
Gram +/−	Penicillins mainly	r-Plasmid	Mostly
I	Cephalosporins mainly	Chromosome	Mainly
II	Penicillins mainly	Chromosome	Constituitive
III	Broad-spectrum	r-Plasmid	Constituitive
IV	Broad-spectrum	Chromosome	Constituitive
V	Methicillin, oxacillin, cloxacillin	r-Plasmid	Constituitive

Sykes RB, Matthew M. J Antimicrob Chemother 1976;2: 115–117.

Table 34.7. β-Lactamase Classifications According to Bush-Jacoby-Medeiros

Group	Characteristics
1	Cephalosporinases that are not inhibited by clavulanic acid
2	β-lactamases inhibited by β-lactamase inhibitors
3	Metallo-β-lactamases that are poorly inhibited by all classical β-lactamase inhibitors
4	Penicillinases that are not inhibited by clavulanic acid

Bush K, Jacoby GA, Medeiros AA. Antimicrob Agts Chemother 1995; 39: 1211–1233.

medications. For some time it has been required that penicillins be manufactured in facilities separate from those used to prepare other drugs in order to prevent cross contamination and possible sensitization. Animals treated with penicillins are required to be drug free for a significant time before products prepared from them can be consumed. The number of pharmacists who unknowingly override these protective measures by failing to cleanse their pill counters properly between prescriptions is unknown.

Because the origin of the allergy is a haptenic reaction with host proteins and the responsible bond in the drug is the β-lactam moiety, this side effect is caused by the pharmacophore of the drug and is unlikely to be overcome by molecular manipulation.

Specific Penicillins

Benzylpenicillin. With the exception of *Neisseria gonorrhoeae* and *Haemophilus influenza,* and a few bacteria encountered less frequently, the useful antimicrobial spectrum of benzyl penicillin is primarily against Gram (+) cocci. Because of its cheapness, efficacy, and lack of toxicity (except for acutely allergic patients), benzylpenicillin remains a remarkably useful agent for treatment of diseases caused by susceptible microorganisms. It is the drug of choice for more infections than any other antibiotic. This justifies the screener's lament, "first is best!" As with most antibiotics, susceptibility tests must be performed as many formerly highly sensitive microorganisms are now comparatively resistant. Infections of the upper and lower respiratory tract and the genitourinary tract are the particular province of benzylpenicillin. Infections

Table 34.6. β-Lactamase Classifications According to Ambler

Class	Characteristics
A	Penicillinases and TEM-type broad spectrum enzymes
B	Increased activity against cephalosporins
C	Chromosomal cephalosporinases of Gram (−) bacteria
D	Oxacillin hydrolyzing enzymes

Ambler RP. Phil Trans Royal Soc London B 1980; 289: 321–331.

caused by group A β-hemolytic streptococci (pharyngitis, scarlet fever, cellulitis, pelvic infections, and septicemia) are commonly responsive. Group B hemolytic streptococcus infections, especially of neonates (acute respiratory distress, pneumonia, meningitis, septic shock, and septicemia.) usually respond. *Pneumococcal* pneumonia, *H. influenza* pneumonia of children, *S. pneumoniae* and *S. pyogenes*-caused otitis media and sinusitis, meningococcal meningitis and brain abscess, meningococcal and pneumococcal septicemia, streptococcal endocarditis (often by *S. viridans*), pelvic inflammatory disease (often by *N. gonorrhoeae* and *S. pyogenes*), uncomplicated gonorrhea (*N. gonorrhoeae*), meningitis (*N. meningitidis*), syphilis (*Treponema pallidum*), Lyme disease (*Borrelia burgdorferi*), gas gangrene (*Cl. perfringens*), and tetanus (*Cl. tetani*) are among the diseases that commonly respond to benzylpenicillin therapy, either alone or sometimes with other drugs used in combination. Nonpenicillinase producing *Staph. aureus* and *Staph. epidermidis* are quite sensitive but are all too rare today. Other, less common, bacterial diseases also respond such as those cased by *Bacillus anthracis* (anthrax) and *C. diphtheriae* (diptheria).

Because of its cheapness, mild infections with susceptible microorganisms can be treated with comparatively large oral doses, although the most effective route of administration is parenteral because five times the blood level can be regularly achieved in this manner.

The need to improve defects in benzylpenicillin stimulated an intense research effort that persists to this day. Overcoming such negative features as comparative instability (particularly to acid), comparatively poor oral absorption, allergenicity, sensitivity to β-lactamases, and relatively narrow antimicrobial spectrum, have been objectives of this work. Only antigenicity has failed to respond significantly to this effort.

Phenoxymethyl Penicillin. Penicillin V is produced by fermentation where the medium is enriched in phenoxyacetic acid. It is considerably more acid stable than benzylpenicillin. This is rationalized as being due to the electronegative oxygen atom in the C-7 amide side chain inhibiting participation in β-lactam bond hydrolysis. In any case, penicillin V was the first of the so-called oral penicillins giving higher and more prolonged blood levels than penicillin G itself. Its antimicrobial and clinical spectrum is roughly the same as that of benzylpenicillin, although it is somewhat less potent and is not, as a rule, used for acutely serious infections. Penicillin V has approximately the same sensitivity to β-lactamases and allergenicity as penicillin G.

Penicillinase-resistant Parenteral Penicillins. Fortunately β-lactamases are much less tolerant to the presence of steric hindrance near the side-chain amide bond than are the penicillin binding proteins. When the aromatic ring is attached directly to the side chain carbonyl and both ortho-positions are substituted by methoxy groups, β-lactamase stable methicillin results (Fig. 34.15). Methicillin is unstable to gastric acid having a half-life of 5 minutes at pH 2 so it must be administer via injection. Movement of one of the methoxy groups to the para position or replacing one of them by a hydrogen results in an analog sensitive to β-lactamases. Putting in a methylene between the aromatic ring and 6-APA likewise produces a β-lactamase-sensitive agent (Fig. 34.15). These findings provide strong support for the hypothesis that resistance to enzyme degradation is based on differential steric hindrance. Methicillin is significantly narrower in antimicrobial spectrum and less potent so it is restricted to clinical use primarily for parenteral use in infections due to β-lactamase producing *Staph. aureus*. Nosocomial (treatment related) staphylococcal cellulitis is the primary indication. When the strain is sensitive to penicillin G or V, these are greatly to be preferred. Lately, an increasing number of infections are being found that are caused by methicillin-resistant *Staphylococcus aureus* (MRSA). The mode of resistance in these cultures appears to be reduced uptake and alterations in the PBPs. In particular, an altered PBP-II is formed which has a very low affinity for β-lactams, including methicillin. Vancomycin is the current favorite for treatment of infections by MRSA with co-trimoxazole and rifampin often of value as well. Methicillin is an efficient inducer of penicillinases so it should be restricted for use in infections that uniquely require it.

Nafcillin (Table 34.3) has a fused benzene ring on one flank and an ethoxy moiety on the other of the side chain amide linkage. Although slightly more acid stable than methicillin, it is clinically virtually identical to it.

Penicillinase-Resistant Oral Penicillins. Using an isoxazolyl ring as a bioisosteric replacement for the benzene ring and a methyl on one flank and a substituted benzene ring on the other in place of the methoxyls of methicillin produces the isoxazolyl penicillins. These are oxacillin, cloxacillin and dicloxacillin (Table 34.3). Chemically, they differ from one another in the number of chlorine substituents on the benzene ring. Like methicillin, these are

generally less potent than benzylpenicillin against Gram (+) microorganisms (generally staphylococci and streptococci) that do not produce a β-lactamase but retain their potency against those that do. An added bonus exists in their being somewhat more acid stable, thus they may be taken orally, and they are more potent as well. Because they are highly serum protein bound (more than 90%), they are not good choices for treatment of septicemia. Microorganisms resistant against methicillin are generally also resistant to the isoxazolyl group of penicillins.

Like methicillin and nafcillin, the isoxazoyl group of penicillins is primarily used against *Staph. aureus* in osteomyelitis, septicemia, endocarditis, and CNS infections.

Penicillinase-sensitive, Broad-Spectrum, Oral Penicillins. The important first member of this group, ampicillin, is a benzylpenicillin analog in which one of the hydrogen atoms of the side chain methylene has been replaced with a primary amino group to produce an R-phenylglycine moiety (Table 34.3). In addition to significant acid stability and, therefore, its successful oral use, the antimicrobial spectrum is shifted so that many common Gram (−) pathogens are sensitive to ampicillin. This is believed to be due to greater penetration of ampicillin into Gram (−) bacteria. The acid stability is generally believed to be caused by the electron-withdrawing character of the protonated primary amine group reducing participation in hydrolysis of the β-lactam bond as well as to the comparative difficulty of bringing another positively charged species (H_3O^+) into the vicinity of the protonated amino group. In any case, ampicillin has an apparent half-life of about 15–20 hours at pH 2.0 and 35° C. Ampicillin is very widely prescribed by general practitioners. It unfortunately lacks stability towards β-lactamases and resistance is an ever-increasing phenomenon. To assist in dealing with this, several additives for coadministration have been developed.

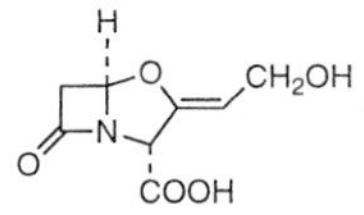

Clavulanic acid

Clavulanic acid, for example, is a mold product that has only weak intrinsic antibacterial activity but it is an excellent irreversible inhibitor of most β-lactamases. It is believed to acylate the active site serine by mimicking the normal substrate. While hydrolysis occurs with some β-lactamases, in many cases subsequent reactions occur which inhibit the enzyme irreversibly. This leads to its classification as a mech-

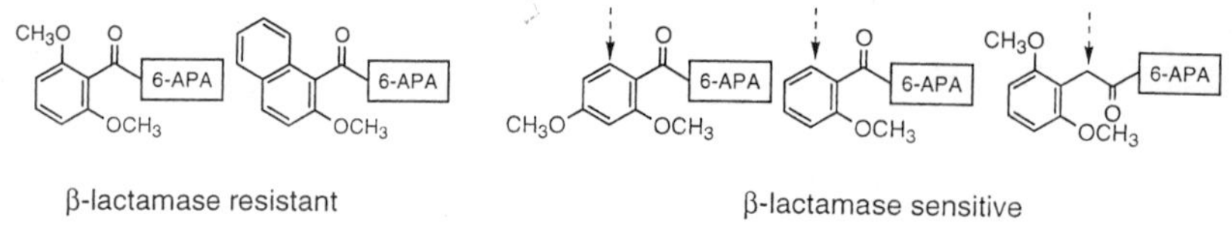

β-lactamase resistant   β-lactamase sensitive

Fig. 34.15. β-lactamase resistant/sensitive structural features.

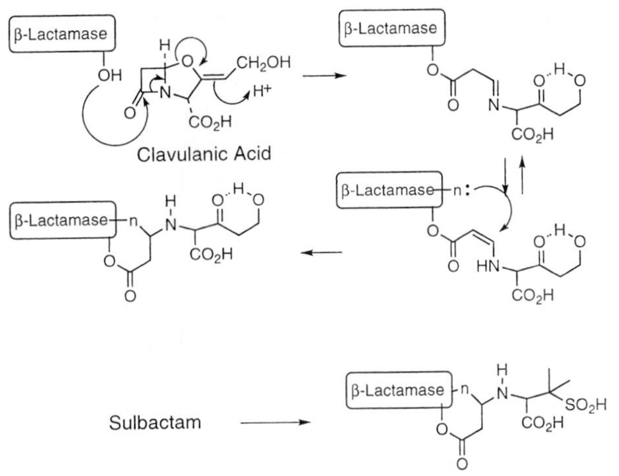

Fig. 34.16. Speculative mechanism for irreversible inactivation of β-lactamase by clavulanic acid and sulbactam.

anism-based inhibitor (or so-called suicide substrate). The precise chemistry is not well understood (Fig. 34.16) but when clavulanic acid is added to ampicillin preparations, the potency against β-lactamase producing strains is markedly enhanced.

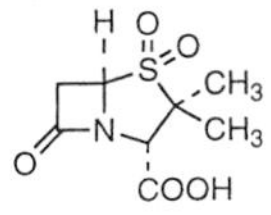

Sulbactam

Another such β-lactamase disabling agent is sulbactam. Sulbactam is prepared by partial chemical synthesis from penicillins. The oxidation of the sulfur atom to a sulfone greatly enhances the potency of sulbactam.

If a penetration barrier is responsible for resistance, clavulanic acid and sulbactam are not able to overcome this so synergy is not seen. Chromosomal mediated β-lactamases are generally not sensitive to clavulanic acid or to sulbactam.

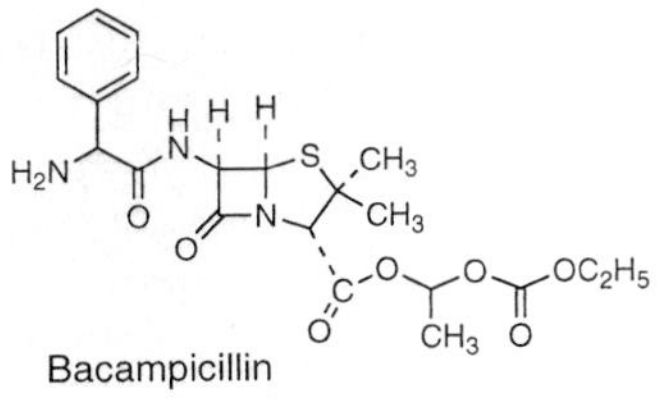

Bacampicillin

Although comparatively well absorbed (30–55%), ampicillin's oral efficacy for systemic infections can be enhanced significantly through the preparation of prodrugs. In contrast to ampicillin itself, which is amphoteric, bacampicillin is a weak base and is very well absorbed in the duodenum (80–98%). Enzymatic ester hydrolysis in the gut wall liberates carbon dioxide and ethanol followed by spontaneous loss of acetaldehyde and production of ampicillin. The acetaldehyde is metabolized oxidatively by alcohol dehydrogenase to produce acetic acid, which joins the normal metabolic pool.

In addition to the usual mode of penicillin allergenicity, concentrated preparations of ampicillin can self condense to form high molecular weight aggregates through reaction of its primary amino group with the β-lactam bond of another molecule. These aggregates are thought to be antigenic and to be responsible for ampicillin allergenicity—a form of hypersensitivity that differs in some details from the usual penicillin allergenicity which ampicillin also possesses. Ampicillin and amoxicillin are the penicillins most commonly associated with drug induced rash. Avoiding use of old preparations is a somewhat effective means of dealing with this potential problem.

Ampicillin is essentially equivalent to benzyl penicillin for pneumococcal, streptococcal and meningococcal infections and many strains of Gram (−) *Salmonella*, *Shigella*, *Proteus mirabilis*, and *Escherichia coli*, as well as many strains of *Haemophilis influenzae* and *N. gonorrhoeae* respond well to oral treatment with ampicillin. It is particularly widely used for out-patient therapy of uncomplicated community-acquired urinary tract infections.

Amoxicillin is a close analog of ampicillin in which a para-phenolic hydroxyl group has been introduced into the side chain phenyl moiety. This adjusts the isoelectric point of the drug to a more acidic value and this is believed by many to be responsible for the enhanced blood levels obtained with amoxicillin as compared to ampicillin itself. Better oral absorption (74–92%) leads to less disturbance of the normal GI flora and, therefore, less drug-induced diarrhea. The antimicrobial spectrum and clinical uses of amoxicillin are approximately the same as those of ampicillin itself and it is presently one of the most popular drugs in North America. The addition of clavulanic acid (Augmentin) serves to protect it to a considerable extent against β-lactamases.

Penicillinase-sensitive, Broad-Spectrum, Parenteral Penicillins. Azlocillin, mezlocillin and piperacillin are ampicillin derivatives in which the D-side chain amino group has been converted by chemical processes to a variety of ureas (Table 34.3). They are collectively known as acylureidopenicillins. They preserve the useful antiGram (+) activity of ampicillin but have higher antiGram (−) potency. Some strains of *Pseudomonas aeruginosa*, for example, are sensitive to these agents. It is speculated that the added side chain moiety mimics a longer segment of the peptidoglycan chain than ampicillin does. This would give more points of attachment to the penicillin-binding proteins and perhaps these features are responsible for their enhanced antibacterial properties. These agents are used parenterally with particular emphasis on Gram (−) bacteria, especially *Klebsiella pneumoniae* and the anaerobe, *Bacteroides fragilis*. Resistance due to β-lactamases is a prominent feature of their use so disk testing and incorporation of additional agents (such as an aminoglycoside) for the treatment of severe infections is advisable.

Tazobactam is often co-administered with piperacillin (Zosyn) because of tazobactam's ability to inhibit β-lactamases.

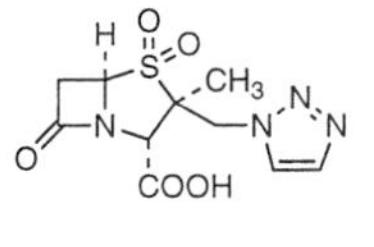

Tazobactam

Carbenicillin and Ticarcillin. Carbenicillin is a benzyl penicillin analog in which one of the methylene hydrogens of the side chain has been substituted with a carboxylic acid moiety (Table 34.3). The specific stereochemistry of this change is not very important as both diastereoisomers are configurationally unstable and mutarotate with time to produce the same mixture of epimers. The introduction of the side chain carboxyl produces enhanced antiGram (−) activity. In fact, carbenicillin is intrinsically one of the broadest-spectrum penicillins. The clinical use of carbenicillin is nonetheless restricted primarily to high dose therapy of *P. aeruginosa* and *Proteus vulgaris* as well as some enterobacter and Serratia infections. Carbenicillin is an order of magnitude less potent than the acylureidopenicillins. The drug is susceptible to β-lactamases and is acid unstable and so must be given by injection. To enhance the likelihood of clinical success with carbenicillin, it is often administered in conjunction with an aminoglycoside antibiotic. When used in this manner, the antibiotics are chemically incompatible so should not be administered in the same solution.

Being a malonic acid hemiamide with a carbonyl (amide) moiety beta to the carboxyl group, carbenicillin can decarboxylate readily to produce benzyl penicillin (Fig. 34.17). While still an antibiotic, this degradation product has no activity against the organisms for which carbenicillin is indicated so this is still considered a degradation. In addition, the large doses of carbenicillin sodium employed (multigrams per day) results in ingestion of a significant amount of sodium ion, which could be a consideration with heart patients. Many of these problems are avoided with the oral use of the pro-drug indanyl ester carbenicillin. Unfortunately, the potency of this preparation does not allow it to be used as a full substitute for carbenicillin but it is instead primarily used for oral treatment of urinary tract infections. Ticarcillin is a sulfur-based bioisostere of carbenicillin that cannot decarboxylate as carbenicillin does. This agent is somewhat more potent against pseudomonads, especially when laced with sulbactam.

Cephalosporins

History. In contrast to the discovery of the penicillins, in which the first agent had such outstanding biologic antibiotic

properties that it entered clinical use with comparatively little change, the cephalosporins are remarkable for the level of persistence required before their initial discovery yielded economic returns. The original cephalosporin-producing culture, *Cephalosporium acremonium*, was discovered in a sewage outfall off the Sardinian coast by Brotsu. In England, Abraham and Newton pursued it because one of the constituents had the useful property of activity against penicillin-resistant cultures due to its stability to β-lactamases. Cephalosporin C, the component of special interest, is not potent enough to be a useful antibiotic but removal, through chemical means, of the natural side chain produced 7-aminocephalosporanic acid (7-ACA) which, analogous to 6-aminopenicillanic acid, could be fitted with unnatural side chains by chemists (Fig. 34.18). Many of the compounds produced in this way are remarkably useful antibiotics. They differ from one another in antimicrobial spectrum, β-lactamase stability, absorption from the GI tract, metabolism, stability, and side effects as detailed below. Exploitation of sulfenic acid chemistry by Robert Morin, then at Eli Lilly and Company, resulted in the conversion of penicillins to cephalosporins, including 3-desacetoxy-7-aminocephalosporanic acid (7-ADCA). This process is practical because the penicillin fermentation is much more efficient than cephalosporin fermentations making the transformation financially rewarding. Unfortunately, the chemistry involved is too complex to be covered in the space available here. Intensive investigation of the chemistry of 7-ACA and 7-ADCA has resulted in the subsequent preparation of many thousands of analogs from these two starting materials.

Chemical Properties. The cephalosporins have their β-lactam ring annealed to a 6-membered dihydrothiazine ring in contrast to the penicillins wherein the β-lactam ring is fused to a 5-membered thiazolidine ring. As a consequence the cephalosporins should be less strained and less reactive/potent. Much of the reactivity loss is, however, made up by possession of an olefinic linkage at C-2,3 and a methyleneacetoxy group at C-3. When the β-lactam ring is opened by hydrolysis, the acetoxy group can be ejected carrying away the developing negative charge. This greatly re-

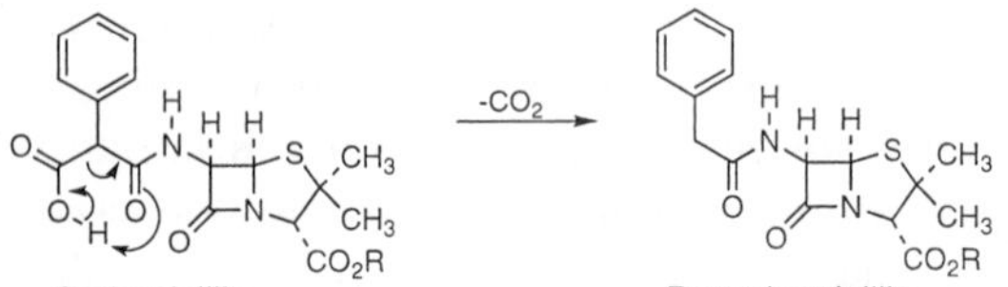

Fig. 34.17. Decarboxylation of carbenicillin to benzylpenicillin.

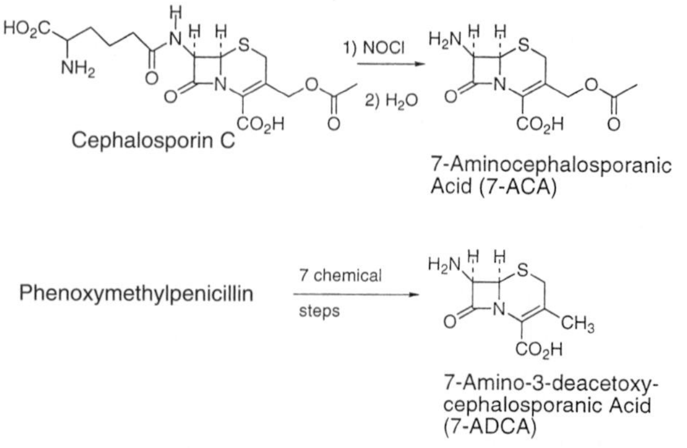

Fig. 34.18. Chemical preparation of 7-ACA and 7-ADCA.

duces the energy required for the process. Thus the facility with which the β-lactam bond of the cephalosporins is broken is modulated both by the nature of the C-7 substituent (analogous to the penicillins) as well as the nature of the C-3 substituent and its ability to carry away a negative charge. Considerable support for this hypothesis comes from the finding that isomerization of the olefinic linkage to C-3,4 leads to great losses in antibiotic activity. In practice, most cephalosporins are comparatively unstable in aqueous solutions and the pharmacist is often directed to keep injectable preparations frozen before use. Being carboxylic acids, they form water soluble sodium salts whereas the free acids are comparatively water insoluble. In many cases where the free acids are supplied, the injectable forms contain sodium bicarbonate to facilitate solution.

Mechanism of Action. The cephalosporins are believed to act in a manner analogous to that of the penicillins by binding to the penicillin-binding proteins followed by cell lysis. The full details of the manner in which bacterial cells are killed are obscure as yet. Cephalosporins are bactericidal in clinical terms.

Resistance. Analogous to the penicillins, susceptible cephalosporins can be hydrolyzed by β-lactamases before they reach the penicillin-binding proteins. Many β-lactamases are known. Some are more efficient at hydrolysis of penicillins, some of cephalosporins and some are indiscriminate. Certain β-lactamases are constitutive (chromosomally encoded) in certain strains of Gram (−) bacteria (*Citrobacter, Enterobacter, Pseudomonas* and *Serratia*) and are normally repressed. These are induced (or derepressed) by certain β-lactam antibiotics, e.g., imipenem, cefotetam, and cefoxitin. As with the penicillins, specific examples will be seen below wherein resistance to β-lactamase hydrolysis is conveyed by strategic steric bulk near the side-chain amide linkage. Recently an increasing number of metallo-β-lactamases have been discovered. The mechanism of these enzymes is dependent upon divalent metal ions, commonly zinc. These are both chromosomally and plasmid derived and are as yet confined to the Gram (−) rods. Commonly these enzymes attack penicillins, some cephalosporins and carbapenems. Penetration barriers to the cephalosporins are also well known.

Allergenicity. Allergenicity is less commonly experienced and is less severe with cephalosporins than with penicillins. Cephalosporins are frequently administered to patients who have had a mild or delayed penicillin reaction, however cross allergenicity is comparatively common and this should be done with caution for patients with a history of allergies. Patients who have had a rapid and severe reaction to penicillins should not be treated with cephalosporins.

Nomenclature and Classification. Most cephalosporins have generic names beginning with cef- or ceph-. This is convenient for classification but makes discriminating between individual members a true memory test. The cephalosporins are classified by a trivial nomenclature system loosely derived from the chronology of their introduction but more closely related to their antimicrobial spectrum. The first generation cephalosporins are primarily active in vitro against Gram (+) cocci (penicillinase positive and negative *Staph. aureus* and *S. epidermis*), group A β-hemolytic streptococci (*Strep. pyogenes*), group B streptococci (*Strep. agalactiae*), and *Strep. pneumoniae*. They are not effective against methicillin-resistant *Staph. aureus*. They are not significantly active against Gram (−) bacteria although some strains of *E. coli, Kl. pneumoniae, P. mirabilis* and *Shigella sp.* may be sensitive. The second-generation cephalosporins generally retain the antiGram (+) activity of the first but include *H. influenzae* as well and add to this better antiGram (−) activity so that some strains of *Acinetobacter, Citrobacter, Enterobacter, E. coli, Klebsiella, Neisseria, Proteus, Providencia,* and *Serratia* are also sensitive. Cefotetan, cefmetazole, and cefoxitin also have some antianaerobic activity as well. The third-generation cephalosporins are less active against staphylococci than the first-generation agents but are much more active against Gram (−) bacteria than either the first or the second-generation drugs. They are frequently particularly useful against nosocomial multidrug-resistant hospital-acquired strains. One adds also *Morganella, Bacteroides fragilis* and *Pseudomonas aeruginosa* to the list of species that are often sensitive. Unfortunately, the third-generation agents are more expensive. The fourth-generation cephalosporins have an antibacterial spectrum like the third-generation drugs but add *Pseudomonas aeruginosa* and some enterobacteria that are resistant to the third-generation cephalosporins. They are also more active against some Gram (+) organisms.

Therapeutic Application. The incidence of cephalosporin resistance is such that it is usually preferable to do disk testing before instituting therapy. Infections of the upper and lower respiratory tract, skin and related soft tissue, urinary tract, bones and joints, as well as septicemias and endocarditis and intra-abdominal and bile tract infections caused by susceptible Gram (+) organisms are usually responsive to cephalosporins. When a Gram (+) bacteria is involved, a first-generation agent is preferable. When the pathogen is Gram (−) and the infection is serious, parenteral use of a third-generation agent is recommended. For pelvic inflammatory disease (PID), the number one cause of sterility in sexually active young women, a combination with doxycycline is preferred. This infection is often mixed and frequently includes *Chlamydia trachomitis,* anaerobes, and other microorganisms that are not cephalosporin sensitive, along with *Neisseria gonorrheae* and penicillinase which are producing N. gonorrheae.

Side Effects. Aside from mild or severe allergic reaction, the most commonly experienced cephalosporin toxicities are mild and temporary nausea, vomiting, and diarrhea associated with disturbance of the normal flora. Rarely, a life-threatening pseudomembranous colitis diarrhea is associated with the opportunistic and toxin-producing anaerobic pathogen, *Clostridium difficile*, can be experienced. Rare blood dyscrasias, which can even include aplastic anemia, are also seen. Certain structural types (details below) are associated with prolonged bleeding times and an antabuse-like acute alcohol intolerance.

Clinically Relevant Degradation Reactions. The principal chemical instability of the cephalosporins is associated with β-lactam bond hydrolysis. The role of the C-7 and C-3 side chains in these reactions was discussed previously. Ejection of the C3 substituent following β-lactam-bond cleavage is usually drawn for convenience as though this is an unbroken (concerted) process. Evidence on this point being equivocal, ejection of the side chain may at certain times and with specific cephalosporins involve a discrete intermediate with the β-lactam bond broken, but the C-3 substituent not yet eliminated, while other cephalosporins have nonejectable C-3 substituents. The tetrazolethiomethyl

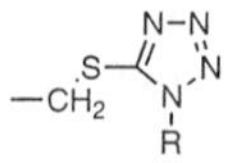

$$-CH_2-S-\overset{N-N}{\underset{\underset{R}{N}}{\underset{\|}{N}}}$$

group, found in a number of cephalosporins, is capable of elimination. In addition, this moiety is believed to be responsible in part for clotting difficulties and acute alcohol intolerance in certain patients. The role of the C-7 side chain in all of these processes is clearly important, but active participation of the amide moiety in a manner analogous to the penicillins is rarely specifically invoked. The same considerations that modulate the chemical stability of cephalosporins are also involved in dictating β-lactamase sensitivity, potency, and allergenicity as well.

Metabolism. Those cephalosporins that have an acetyl group in the side chain are subject to enzymatic hydrolysis in the body. The result is molecules with a hydroxymethyl moiety at C-3. A hydroxy moiety is a poor leaving group so this change is considerably deactivating with respect to breakage of the β-lactam bond. In addition, the particular geometry of this part of the molecule leads to facile lac-

tonization with the carboxyl group attached to C-2. (Fig. 34.19). In principle this should result in formation of a different but reasonable leaving group. The result is, instead, inactivation of the drugs involved. The penicillin binding proteins have an absolute requirement for a free carboxyl group to mimic that of the terminal carboxyl of the D-ala-D-ala moiety in their normal substrate. Lactonization masks this docking functional group and as a result blocks affinity of the inhibitor for the enzyme.

Specific Agents—First Generation (Table 34.8)

Cephapirin. Cephapirin has a pyridylthiomethylene containing side chain at C-7. It is comparatively resistant to staphylococcal β-lactamase although it is sensitive to many other β-lactamases. Cephapirin is sensitive also to host deacetylation in the liver, kidneys and plasma, which reduces potency by about half. Nonetheless it finds significant use in the parenteral treatment of infections due to susceptible bacteria. It is a substitute for methicillin and the isoxazolyl subgroup of penicillins. It is not orally active. It is comparatively painful on intramuscular injection and its doses must be reduced in the presence of renal impairment. Following injection, it is excreted primarily in the urine, partly by glomerular filtration and partly by tubular secretion.

Cefazolin. Cefazolin has the natural acetyl side chain at C-3 replaced by a thio-linked thiadiazole ring. While this group is an activating leaving group, the moiety is not subject to the inactivating host hydrolysis reaction that characterizes cephapirin. At C-7 it possesses a tetrazoylmethylene unit. Cefazolin is less irritating on injection than its cohort in this generation of drugs and has a longer half-life than cephapirin. Its dosing should be reduced in the presence of kidney damage. It is comparatively unstable and should be protected from heat and light.

Cephalexin. Use of the ampicillin-type side chain conveys oral activity to cephalexin. Whereas it no longer has an activating side chain at C-3, and as a consequence is somewhat less potent, it does not undergo metabolic deactivation and thus maintains potency. It is rapidly and completely absorbed from the GI tract and has become quite popular. Somewhat puzzling is the fact that the use of the ampicillin side chain in the cephalosporins does not result in a comparable shift in antimicrobial spectrum. Cephalexin, like the other first-generation cephalosporins is active against many Gram (+) aerobic cocci but is limited against Gram (−) bacteria. It is a widely used drug, particularly against Gram (−) bacteria causing urinary tract infections, Gram (+) infections of soft tissues

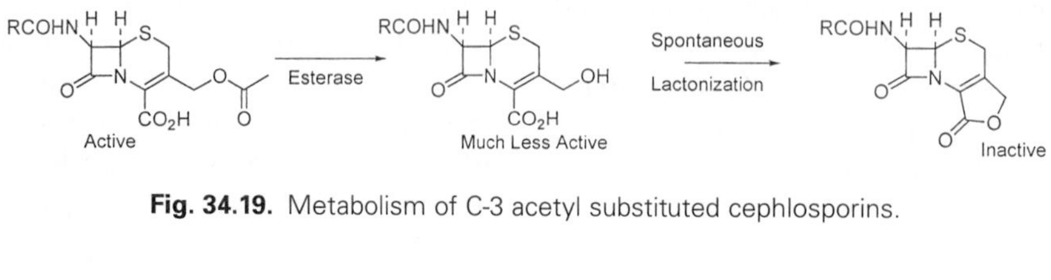

Fig. 34.19. Metabolism of C-3 acetyl substituted cephlosporins.

Table 34.8. First-generation Cephalosporins

Generic Names	Trade Names	R	X	Salt
Parenteral Agents:				
Cephapirin	Cefadyl	(pyridine)-SCH₂-	OAc	Na
Cefazolin	Ancef, Kefzol, Zolicef	(tetrazole)N-CH₂-	(thiadiazole-CH₃)	Na
Oral Agents:				
Cephalexin	Keflex, Biocef Keftab	(phenyl-CH, NH₂)	H	HCl
Cefadroxil	Duricef	(HO-phenyl-CH, NH₂)	H	—
Oral and Parenteral Agents:				
Cephradine	Velosef	(cyclohexadiene-CH, NH₂)	H	—

(*S. aureus*, *S. pneumoniae* and *S. pyogenes*), pharyngitis, and minor wounds.

Cefadroxil. Cefadroxil has an amoxicillin-like side chain at C-7 so its oral activity is not surprising. There are some indications that cefadroxil has some immunostimulant properties mediated through T-cell activation and that this is of material assistance to patients in fighting infections. The prolonged biologic half-life of cefadroxil allows for one-a-day dosage.

Cephradine. In cephradine an interesting drug design device has been used. The aromatic ring in the ampicillin side chain has been partially hydrogenated by a Birch reduction, such that the resulting molecule is still planar and pi-electron excessive, but has no conjugated olefinic linkages. It is comparatively acid stable so is rapidly and nearly completely absorbed from the GI tract. Cephradine has the useful characteristic that it can be used both orally and IM, so that parenteral therapy can be started in an institutional setting and then, the patient can be sent home with the oral form, avoiding the risk of having to establish a different antibiotic. This is consistent with the present economics requiring sending patients home earlier than some physicians prefer. Unfortunately, however, for other reasons the IM and IV versions of cephradine are no longer available in the U.S.

Specific Agents—Second Generation (Table 34.9)
Cefamandole Nafate. Cefamandole nafate has a C-7 side chain formate ester derived from D-mandelic acid. The formate ester is cleaved rapidly in the host to release the more active cefamandole. The esterification apparently also overcomes instability of cefamandole

when it is stored in dry form. This agent has increased activity against *Haemophilus influenzae* and some Gram (−) bacilli as compared with the first-generation cephalosporins. Loss of the 5-thio-l-methyl-l-H-tetrazole moiety (referred to sometimes by the acronym, NMTT) from C-3 is associated with prothrombin deficiency and bleeding problems as well as with an antabuse-like acute alcohol intolerance. On the other hand, this grouping enhances potency and prevents metabolism by deacetylation. Like the other second-generation cephalosporins, cefamandole is more active against Gram (−) bacteria. The principle clinical use is for lower respiratory tract, skin and skin structures, and bone and joint infections as well as septicemia and urinary tract infections when the organisms are sensitive.

Cefonicid. Cefonicid has an unesterified D-mandelic acid moiety at C-7 and a methylsulfothiotetrazole group at C-3. The latter is related to the NMTT moiety mentioned above under cefamandole nafate, however the clotting problems and antabuse-like side effects associated with NMTT have not been reported with cefonicid. The extra acid group in the C-7 side chain leads to this molecule being sold as an injectable disodium salt. Pain and discomfort at I.M. sites is experienced by some patients as is a burning sensation and phlebitis with I.V. cefonicid. Cefonicid has a longer half-life than the other members of its group but achieves this at the price of somewhat lower potency against Gram (+) bacteria and aerobes. The drug is somewhat unstable and needs to be protected from light and heat and may yellow or darken. This, however, if modest does not necessarily mean that the potency has decreased significantly. Overt pre-

Table 34.9. Second-generation Cephalosporins

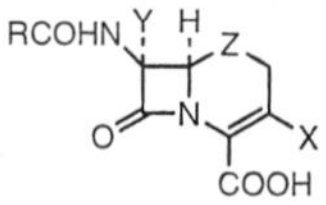

Generic Name	Trade Name	R	X	Y	Z	Salt
Parenteral Agents						
Cefamandole nafate	Mandol	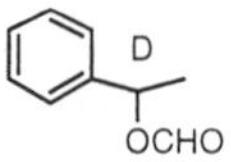 (phenyl-CH(OCHO)-)	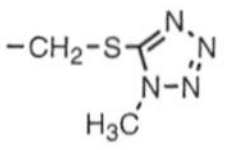 $-CH_2-S-$(N-methyltetrazole)	H	S	—
Cefonicid	Monocid	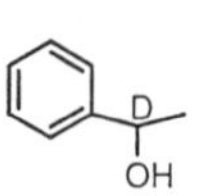 (phenyl-CH(OH)-)	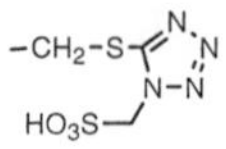 $-CH_2-S-$(tetrazole, HO_3S-CH_2)	H	S	diNa
Cefuroxime	Ceftin, Kefurox, Zinacef	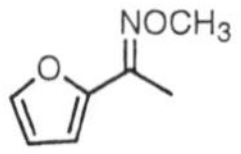 (furyl-C(=NOCH$_3$)-)	$-CH_2OCONH_2$	H	S	Na
Cefoxitin	Mefoxin	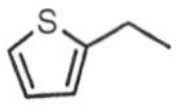 (thienyl-CH$_2$-)	$-CH_2OCONH_2$	OCH$_3$	S	Na
Cefotetan	Cefotan	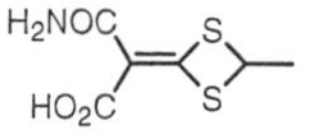 (H$_2$NOC, HO$_2$C substituted dithietane)	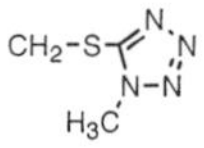 CH_2-S-(N-methyltetrazole)	OCH$_3$	S	diNa
Oral Agents						
Cefaclor	Ceclor	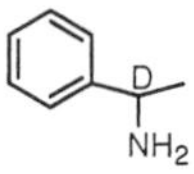 (phenyl-CH(NH$_2$)-)	Cl	H	S	—
Loracarbacef	Lorabid	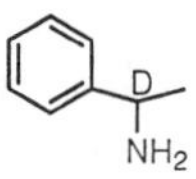 (phenyl-CH(NH$_2$)-)	Cl	H	CH$_2$	—
Cefprozil	Cefzil	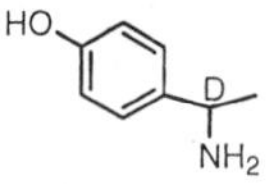 (HO-phenyl-CH(NH$_2$)-)	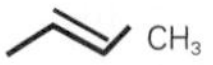 (CH=CH-CH$_3$)	H	S	—

cipitation, on the other hand, does. Kirby-Bauer disk testing may overestimate the sensitivity of β-lactamase producing bacteria to this agent so some extra caution in interpretation of laboratory results is called for.

Cefuroxime. Cefuroxime has a syn-oriented methoxy-imino moiety as part of its C-7 side chain (Fig. 34.20). This conveys considerable resistance to attack by many β-lactamases but not by all. This is believed to result from the steric demands of this group. This hypothesis is supported by the finding that the anti-analog is attacked by β-lactamases. Resistance by *Pseudomonas aeruginosa*, on the other hand, is attributed to lack of penetration of the drug rather than to enzymatic hydrolysis. The carbamoyl moiety at C-3 is intermediate in metabolic stability between the classic acetyl moieties and the thiotetrazoles. Cefuroxime penetrates comparatively well into cerebral spinal fluid and is used in cases of H. influenzae meningitis.

In the form of its axetil ester (1-[acetyloxy]ethyl ester) pro-drug, cefuroxime axetil, a more lipophilic drug is produced which gives satisfactory blood levels on oral administration. The ester bond is cleaved metabolically and the resulting intermediate form loses acetaldehyde spontaneously to produce cefuroxime itself. Conveniently for the patient, cefuroxime axetil is stable for about 24 hours when it is dissolved in apple juice.

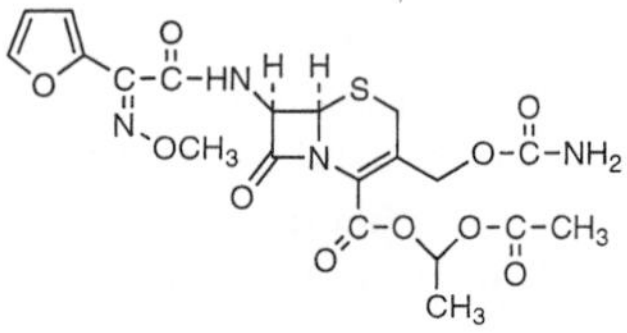

Cefuroxime axetil

Cefoxitin. Cefoxitin contains the same C-7 side chain as cephalothin and the same C-3 side chain as cefuroxime. The most novel chemical feature of cefoxitin is the possession of an α-oriented methoxyl group in place of the normal H-atom at C-7. This increased steric bulk conveys very significant stability against β-lactamases. The inspiration for these functional groups was provided by the discovery of the naturally occurring antibiotic cephamycin C derived from fermentation of *Streptomyces*

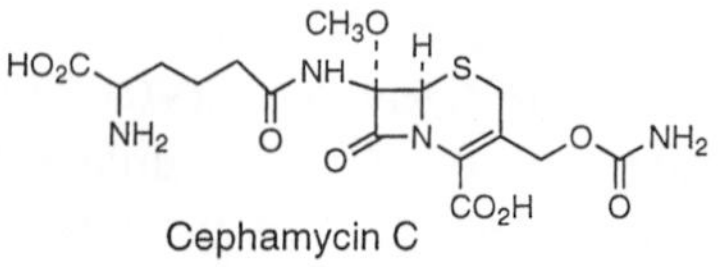

Cephamycin C

lactamdurans. Cephamycin C itself has not seen clinical use but provided the structural clue that led to useful agents such as cefoxitin. Ingenious chemical transformations now

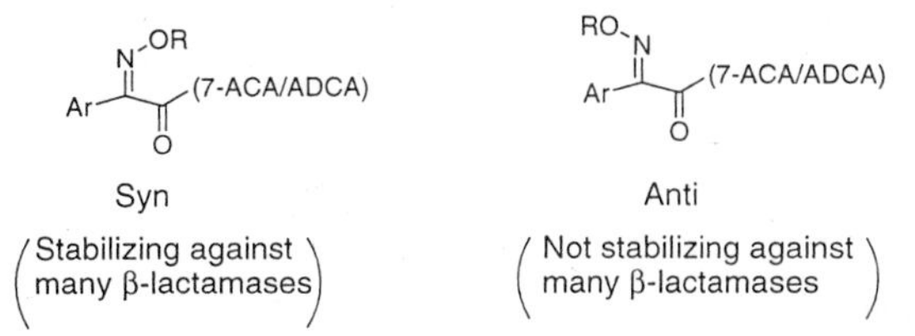

Fig. 34.20. Syn and anti oxime configuration and effect on β-lactamse stability.

enable synthetic introduction of such a methoxy group into cephalosporins lacking this feature.

Cefoxitin has useful activity against gonorrhea and against some anaerobic infections as compared with its second-generation relatives. On the negative side, cefoxitin has the capacity to induce certain broad-spectrum β-lactamases but the clinical meaning of this is unclear.

Cefotetan. Cefotetan is clearly also cephamycin C inspired but has a rather unusual sulfur containing C-7 side chain amide. Possession of two carboxyl groups leads to its marketing as a disodium salt. The C-3 NMTT side chain suggests caution in monitoring prothrombin levels and bleeding times as well as care in ingesting alcohol when using this agent. Like cefoxitin, cefotetan has better activity against anaerobes than the rest of this group. Cefotetan is comparatively stable lasting for about 24 hours at room temperature when reconstituted. Slight yellowing and slight darkening produces materials that are still acceptable for therapy. Cefotetan is chemically incompatible with tetracycline, aminoglycosides and with heparin, often forming precipitates with them. With respect to its molecular mode of action, it has a special affinity for PBP 3 of Gram (−) bacteria consequently producing filamentous forms. It also binds well with PBPs 1A and 1B therefore leading to cell lysis and death. Whereas it is stable to a wide range (but not all) of β-lactamases, it is also a potent inducer in some bacteria.

Cefaclor. Cefaclor differs from cephalexin primarily in the bioisosteric replacement of methyl by chlorine at C-3 and is quite acid stable allowing for oral administration. It is also quite stable to metabolism. It is less active against Gram (−) bacteria than the other second generation cephalosporins but is more active against Gram (−) bacteria than the first-generation drugs.

Loracarbef. Loracarbef is a synthetic C-5 "carba" analog of cefaclor. The smaller methylene moiety (as compared to sulfur) would be expected to make loracarbef more reactive/potent and this seems to be the case. It is more stable chemically, however, and this adds to its virtues. Diarrhea is the most common adverse effect with loracarbef and this, and certain other side effects, are more frequently seen with children so this lessens enthusiasm for this drug in patients under the age of about twelve.

Cefprozil. Cefprozil has an amoxicillin-like side chain at C-7 but at C-3 there is now a l-propenyl group conjugated with the double bond in the six-membered ring. The double bond is present in its two geometric isomeric forms

both of which are antibacterially active. Fortunately, the predominant trans form (illustrated in Table 34.9) is much more active against Gram (−) organisms. Cefprozil most closely resembles cefaclor in its properties but is a little more potent. It is about 90% bioavailable following oral administration and peak levels are not significantly smaller when taken with food. The oral suspension of cefprozil is sweetened with aspartame so phenylketonuric patients should be wary of this formulation.

Specific Agents—Third Generation (Table 34.10)

Cefotaxime. Cefotaxime, like cefuroxime, has a syn-methoxyimino moiety at C-7 which conveys significant β-lactamase resistance. Microorganisms that produce chromosomal mediated β-lactamases are usually resistant following mutation to derepression of these enzymes. Cefoxitin, cefotetan and imipenems are quite effective inducers of these enzymes. The enzymes that result either hydrolyze the drug in the usual way or bind tightly to them preventing them from attaching to the PBPs. The clinical importance of this phenomenon is unclear.

The oxime moiety of cefotaxime is connected to an aminothiazole ring. Like other third-generation cephalosporins, it has excellent antiGram (−) activity and is useful institutionally. It has a metabolically vulnerable acetoxy group attached to C-3 and loses about 90% of its activity when this is hydrolyzed. This metabolic feature also complicates the pharmacokinetic data as both active forms are present and have different properties. Cefotaxime should be protected from heat and light and may color slightly without significant loss of potency. Like other third-generation cephalosporins, cefotaxime has less activity against staphylococci but has greater activity against Gram (−) organisms.

Ceftizoxime. In ceftizoxime the whole C-3 side chain has been omitted to prevent deactivation by hydrolytic metabolism. It rather resembles cefotaxime in its properties however not being subject to metabolism its pharmacokinetic properties are much less complex.

Ceftriaxone. Ceftriaxone has the same C-7 side chain moiety as cefotaxime and ceftizoxime, but the C-3 side chain consists of a metabolically stable and activating thiotriazinedione in place of the normal acetyl group. The C-3 side chain is sufficiently acidic that at normal pH it forms an enolic sodium salt and thus the commercial product is a disodium salt. It is useful for many severe infections and notably in the treatment of some meningitis infections caused by Gram (−) bacteria. It is quite stable to many β-lactamases but is sensitive to some inducible chromosomal β-lactamases.

Ceftazidime. In ceftazidime the oxime moiety is more complex, containing two methyl groups and a carboxylic acid. This assemblage conveys even more pronounced β-lactamase stability, greater anti *Pseudomonas aeruginosa* and increased activity against Gram (+) organisms. The C-3 side chain has been replaced by a charged pyridinium moiety. The latter considerably enhances water-solubility and also highly activates the β-lactam bond towards

Table 34.10. Third-generation Cephalosporins

Generic Name	Trade Name	R	X	Salt
Parenteral Agents Cefotaxime	Claforan		CH₂OAc	Na
Ceftizoxime	Cefizox		H	Na
Ceftriaxone	Rocephin			diNa
Ceftazidime	Fortaz Ceptax Tazidime Tazicef			H or Na
Cefoperazone	Cefobid			Na
Oral Agents Cefixime	Suprax		—HC=CH₂	—
Ceftibuten	Cedax		H	—
Cefpodoxime proxetil (2-carboxyester=)	Vantin		-CH₂OCH₃	—
Cefdinir	Omnicef		—HC=CH₂	—

cleavage. The drug must be protected against heat and light and may darken without significant loss of potency. It is not stable under some conditions such as the presence of aminoglycosides and vancomycin. It is also attacked readily in sodium bicarbonate solutions. Resistance is mediated by chromosomally mediated β-lactamases and also by lack of penetration into target bacteria. Otherwise, it has a very broad antibacterial spectrum.

Cefoperazone. Cefoperazone has a C-7 side chain reminiscent of piperacillin's and also possesses the C-3 side chain (NMTT) that is often associated with the bleeding and alcohol intolerance problems among patients taking cephalosporins. Its useful activity against pseudomonads partly compensates for this although it is not potent enough to be used as a single agent against this difficult pathogen. The C-7 side chain does not convey sufficient resistance to many β-lactamases although the addition of clavulanic acid or sulbactam would presumably help.

There are comparatively few orally active third-generation agents. This group is currently represented by ceftibuten, cefixime, cefdinir and cefpodoxime proxetil.

Cefixime. In cefixime, in addition to the β-lactamase stabilizing syn-oximino acidic ether at C-7, the C-3 side chain is a vinyl group analogous to the propenyl group of cefprozil. This is believed to contribute strongly to the oral activity of the drug. Cefixime has antiGram (−) activity intermediate between that of the second-generation and third-generation agents described previously. It is poorly active against staphylococci as it does not bind satisfactorily to PBP 2.

Ceftibuten. Ceftibuten has a *cis* ethylidinecarboxyl group at C-7 instead of the syn-oximino ether linkages seen previously. This conveys enhanced β-lactamase stability and may contribute to oral activity as well. Ceftibuten has no C-3 side chain so is not measurably metabolized. It is highly (75–90%) absorbed on oral administration but this is decreased significantly by food. Being lipophilic and acidic, it is significantly serum protein bound (65%). Some isomerization of the geometry of the olefinic linkage appears to take place in vivo before excretion. It is mainly used for respiratory tract infections, otitis media, pharyngitis and tonsilitis, as well as urinary tract infections by susceptible microorganisms.

Cefpodoxime Proxetil. Cefpodoxime proxetil is a pro-drug. It is cleaved enzymically to isopropanol, carbon dioxide, acetaldehyde, and to cefpodoxime in the gut wall. It has better anti-*Staphylococcus aureus* activity than cefixime and is used to treat pharyngitis, urinary tract infections, upper and lower respiratory tract infections, otitis media, skin and soft tissue infections, and gonorrhea.

Cefdinir. Cefdinir has an unsubstituted syn-oxime in its C-7 side chain the consequence of which is attributed its somewhat enhanced antiGram (+) activity—its main distinguishing feature. It has a vinyl moiety attached to C-3 which is associated with its oral activity. It has reasonable but not spectacular resistance to β-lactamases, and is 20–25% absorbed on oral administration unless taken with fatty foods which significantly diminishes blood levels.

Cefepime (Maxipime)

Specific Agents—Fourth Generation. Cefepime is a semi-synthetic agent containing a syn-methoxyimine moiety and an aminothiazolyl group at C-7 broadening its spectrum and increasing its β-lactamase stability as well as increasing its antistaphylococcus activity. The quaternary N-

methylpyrrolidine group at C-3 seems to help penetration into Gram (−) bacteria. The fourth-generation cephalosporins are characterized by enhanced antistaphylococcal activity and broader antiGram (−) activity than the third-generation group. Cefepime is used IM and IV against urinary tract infections, skin and skin structure infections, pneumonia and intra abdominal infections.

Because the cephalosporin field is being very actively pursued, the student can expect continual developments into the foreseeable future.

Thienamycin

Imipenem

Cilastatin sodium

Carbapenems

Thienamycin and Imipenem. Thienamycin was isolated from *Streptomyces cattleya*. Because of its extremely intense and broad-spectrum antimicrobial activity and its ability to inactivate β-lactamases, it combines in one molecule the functional features of the best of the β-lactam antibiotics as well as the β-lactamase inhibitors. It differs structurally in several important respects from the penicillins and cephalosporins. The sulfur atom is not part of the five-membered ring but rather has been replaced by a methylene moiety at that position. Carbon is roughly half the molecular size of sulfur. Consequently, the carbapenem ring system is highly strained and very susceptible to reactions cleaving the β-lactam bond. The sulfur atom is now attached to C-3 as part of a functionalized side chain. The endocyclic olefinic linkage also enhances the reactivity of the β-lactam ring. Both make thienamycin unstable and this caused great difficulties in the original isolation studies. The terminal amino group in the side chain attached to C-3 is nucleophilic and attacks the β-lactam bond of nearby molecules, so that the drug became less stable as it was purified and became more concentrated. Ultimately, this problem was overcome by changing the amino group to a less nucleophilic N-formiminoyl moiety by a semisynthetic process to produce imipenem. At C6 there is a 2-hydroxyethyl group attached with α-stereochemistry. Thus the absolute stereochemistry of the molecule is 5R,6S,8S. With these striking differences from the penicillins and cephalosporins, it is not surprising that thienamycin binds differently to the penicillin-binding proteins (especially strongly to PBP 2) but it is gratifying that the result is very potent broad-spectrum activity. Thienamycin and imipenem penetrate very well through porins and are very stable, even inhibitory, to many β-lactamases. Imipenem is not, however, orally active. Unfortunately, when used in urinary tract infections, renal dehydropeptidase-l hydrolyzes imipenem and deactivates it. An inhibitor for this enzyme, cilastatin, is co-administered with imipenem to protect it. Inhibition of human dehydropeptidase does not seem to have deleterious consequences to the patient, making this combination highly efficacious.

The combination of imipenem and cilastatin (Primaxin) is about 25% serum-protein bound. On injection it penetrates well into most tissues, but not cerebrospinal fluid, and it is subsequently excreted in the urine. It is broader in its spectrum than any other antibiotic presently available in the United States. This very potent combination is especially useful for treatment of serious infections by aerobic Gram (−) bacilli, anaerobes, and *Staph. aureus*. It is used clinically for severe infections of the gut in adults as well as GU tract, bone, skin and endocardia, with allergic reactions as its main risk factor; imipenem also has the unfortunate property of being a good β-lactamase inducer. Because of these features, imipenem-cilastatin is rarely a drug of first choice, but is reserved for use in special circumstances.

Meropenem (Merrem)

Meropenem.   Meropenem is a synthetic carbapenem possessing a more complex side chain at C-3. It also has a chiral methyl group at C-5. This methyl group conveys intrinsic resistance to hydrolysis by dehydropeptidase-1. As a consequence, it can be administered as a single agent for the treatment of severe bacterial infections.

Aztreonam disodium (Azactam)

Monobactams

Aztreonam.   Fermentation of unusual microorganisms led to the discovery of a class of monocyclic β-lactam antibiotics, named monobactams. None of these molecules have proven to be important but the group served as the inspiration for the synthesis of aztreonam. Aztreonam is a totally synthetic parenteral antibiotic whose antimicrobial spectrum is devoted almost exclusively to Gram (−) microorganisms, and it is capable of inactivating some β-lactamases. Its molecular mode of action is closely similar to that of the penicillins, cephalosporins and carbapenems, the action being characterized by strong affinity for PBP 3 producing filamentous cells as a consequence. Whereas the principal side chain closely resembles that of ceftazidime, the sulfamic acid moiety attached to the β-lactam ring was unprecedented.

Remembering the comparatively large size of sulfur atoms, this assembly may sufficiently spatially resemble the corresponding C-2 carboxyl group of the precedent β-lactam antibiotics to confuse the penicillin binding protons. The strongly electron withdrawing character of the sulfamic acid group probably also makes the β-lactam bond more vulnerable to hydrolysis. In any case, the monobactams demonstrate that a fused ring is not essential for antibiotic activity. The α-oriented methyl group at C-2 is associated with the stability of aztreonam towards β-lactamases.

The protein binding is moderate (about 50%) and the drug is nearly unchanged by metabolism. Aztreonam is given by injection and is primarily excreted in the urine. The primary clinical use of aztreonam is against severe infections caused by Gram (−) microorganisms, especially those acquired in the hospital. These are mainly urinary tract, upper respiratory tract, bone, cartilage, abdominal, obstetric, and gynecologic infections and septicemias. The drug is well tolerated and side effects are infrequent. Interestingly, allergy would not be unexpected, but cross allergenicity with penicillins and cephalosporins has not often been reported.

Antibiotics: Inhibitors of Protein Biosynthesis
Basis for Selectivity

Some antibiotic families exert their lethal effects on bacteria by inhibiting ribosomally mediated protein biosynthesis. At first glimpse this may seem anomalous because eukaryotic organisms also construct their essential proteins on ribosomal organelles and the sequence of biochemical steps in both biologic classes is closely analogous to that in prokaryotic microorganisms. At a molecular level, however, the apparent anomaly resolves itself. In *E. coli*, for example, the 70S ribosomal particle is composed not only of RNA but also of 55 different structural and functional proteins (21 on the 30S and 34 on the 50S subparticle). These proteins differ in structure from those in the eukaryotic 80S ribosome. The binding sites for the important antibiotics lie on the proteins or the ribosomal DNA of the bacterial 70S ribosome. The aminoglycosides, for example, bind to a site on the mRNAs of the 30S subparticle associated with the presence of a specific protein, whereas the macrolides, lincosaminides and chloramphenicol bind to a different site on the 50S subparticle. There is evidence that the tetracyclines bind to both subparticles. At normal doses, these antibiotics do not bind to nor interfere with the function of 80S ribosomal particles. The basis for the selective toxicity of these antibiotics is then apparent. Interference with bacterial protein biosynthesis prevents repair, cellular growth, and reproduction and the effect, in clinically achievable doses, is bacteriostatic or bactericidal.

Aminoglycosides and Aminocyclitols

General Properties.   The aminoglycoside/aminocyclitol class of antibiotics contains a pharmacophoric 1,3-di-

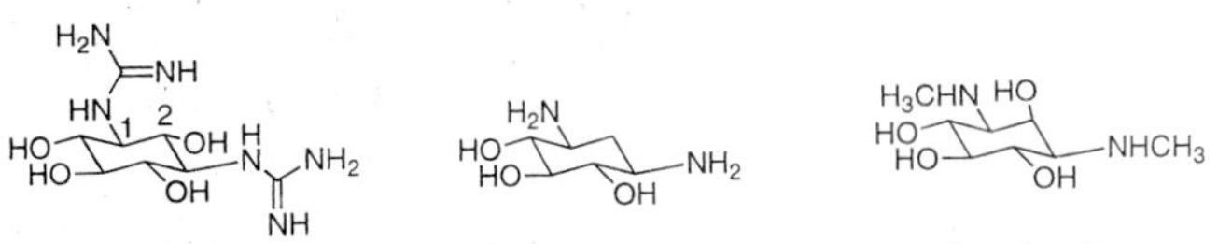

Fig. 34.21. 1,3-Diaminoinositol moieties present in aminoglycosides.

aminoinositol moiety: either streptamine, 2-deoxystreptamine, or spectinamine (Fig. 34.21). Several of the alcoholic functions of the 1,3-diaminoinositol are substituted through glycosidic bonds with characteristic aminosugars to form pseudo-oligosaccharides. The chemistry, spectrum, potency, toxicity, and pharmacokinetics of these agents are a function of the specific identity of the diaminoinositol unit and the arrangement and identity of the attachments. The various aminoglycoside antibiotics are freely water soluble at all achievable pHs, are basic and form acid addition salts, are not absorbed in significant amounts from the gastrointestinal tract, and are excreted in active form in fairly high concentrations in the urine following injection. When the kidneys are not functioning efficiently, the concentrations injected must be reduced to prevent accumulation to toxic levels. When given orally, their action is primarily confined to the gastrointestinal tract. They are more commonly given intramuscularly or by perfusion. Recently, tobramycin has been sprayed into the lungs successfully to treat *Pseudomonas aeruginosa* infections in cystic fibrosis patients. This results in significantly reduced toxicity to the patient. These agents have intrinsically broad antimicrobial spectra but their toxicity potential limits their clinical use to severe infections by Gram (−) bacteria. These toxicities involve ototoxicity to functions mediated by the eighth cranial nerve, such as hearing loss and vertigo. Their use can also lead to kidney tubular necrosis producing decreases in glomerular function. These toxic effects are related to blood levels and are apparently mediated by the special affinity of these aminoglycosides to kidney cells and to the sensory cells of the inner ear. The effects may have a delayed onset, making them all the more treacherous as the patient can be injured significantly before symptoms appear. Less common is a curare-like neuromuscular blockade believed to be caused by competitive inhibition of calcium-ion-dependent acetylcholine release at the neuromuscular junction. This side effect can exaggerate the muscle weakness of myasthenia gravis and Parkinsonian patients. In current practice all of these toxic phenomena are well known, therefore creatinine function is determined and the dose is adjusted downward accordingly so that these side effects are less common and less severe than previously. The aminoglycoside antibiotics are widely distributed (mainly in extracellular fluids) and have low levels of protein binding.

Mechanism of Action. The aminoglycosides are bactericidal due to a combination of toxic effects. At less than toxic doses, they bind to the 16S-ribosomal DNA portion of the 30S ribosomal subparticle impairing the proofreading function of the ribosome. This leads to mistranslation of RNA templates and the consequent selection of wrong amino acids and formation of so-called nonsense proteins. The most relevant of these unnatural proteins are involved in upsetting bacterial membrane function. Their presence destroys the semipermeability of the membrane and this damage cannot be repaired without de novo programmed protein biosynthesis. Among the substances that are admitted by the damaged membrane are large additional quantities of aminoglycoside. At these increased concentrations, protein biosynthesis ceases altogether. These combined effects are devastating to the target bacterial cells. Given their highly polar properties, the student may wonder how these agents can enter bacterial cells at all. Aminoglycosides apparently bind initially to external lipopolysacchardes and diffuse into the cells in small amounts. The uptake process is inhibited by Ca^{2+} and Mg^{2+} ions. These ions are, then, partially incompatible therapeutically. Passage through the cytoplasmic membrane is dependent on electron transport and energy generation. At high concentrations eukaryotic protein biosynthesis can also be inhibited by aminoglycoside/aminocyclitol antibiotics.

Bacterial Resistance. Bacterial resistance to aminoglycoside antibiotics in the clinic is most commonly due to bacterial elaboration of R-factor mediated enzymes that N-acetylate (AAC-aminoglycoside acetylase), O-phosphorylate (APH-aminoglycoside phosphorylase), and O-adenylate (ANT-aminoglycoside nucleotide transferase) specific functional groups, preventing subsequent ribosomal binding. In some cases, chemical deletion of the functional groups transformed by these enzymes leaves a molecule which is still antibiotic but no longer a substrate, thus substances with intrinsically broader-spectrum can be made semisynthetically in this way. In some other cases, novel functional groups can be attached to remote functionality which converts these antibiotics to poorer substrates for these R-factor mediated enzymes and this expands their spectra, as discussed later in this chapter. Resistance due to decreased aminoglycoside/aminocyclitol uptake into bacterial cells is also encountered.

Therapeutic Application. Intrinsically, aminoglycosides have broad antibiotic spectra against aerobic Gram (+) and Gram (−) bacteria but are reserved for serious infections caused by Gram (−) organisms because of serious toxicities which are often delayed in onset. They are active against Gram (−) aerobes such as *Acenetobacter sp.*, *Citrobacter sp.*, *Enterobacter sp.*, *E. coli*, *Klebsiella sp.*, *P. vulgaris*, *Providentia sp.*, *Ps. aeruginosa*, *Salmonella sp.*, *Serratia marscesans*, *Shigella sp.*, and Gram (+) aerobes such as *Staph. epidermidis*.

Streptomycin and spectinomycin differ from the others in their useful antimicrobial spectra.

Streptomycin is most commonly used for the treatment of tuberculosis and spectinomycin for treatment of gonorrhea. The other antibiotics of this class are inferior for these purposes.

These antibiotics have similar clinical spectra to those of the quinolones and are decreasing in popularity as

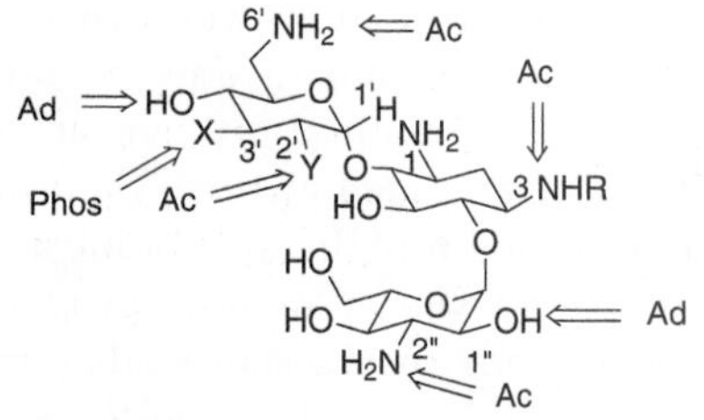

Tobramycin
(X=H, Y= NH₂, R =H)

Kanamycin A
(X=OH, Y = OH, R =H)

Amikacin
(X=Y=OH, R=COCHOHCH₂CH₂NH₂)

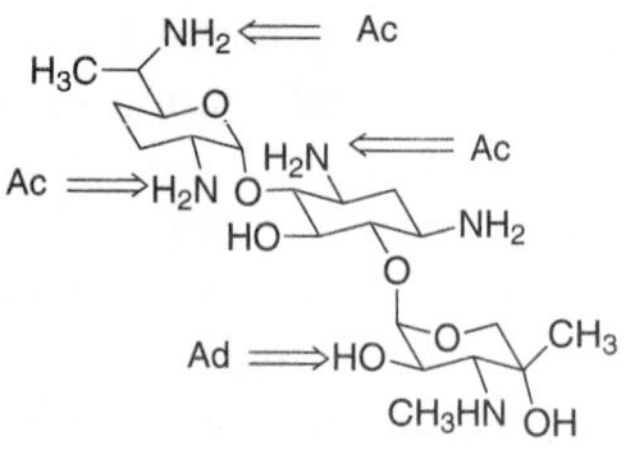

Gentamicin C-2

Fig. 34.22. Commercially important 2-desylstreptamine containing aminoglycosides. Some points of inactivating attack by specific R factor-medicated-enzymes are indicated by the following symbols. Ad → adenylation; Ac → acetylation; Phos → phosphorylation. APH (3′)-1, for example, is an acronym for an enzyme which phosphorylates aminoglycosides at the 3′-OH position.

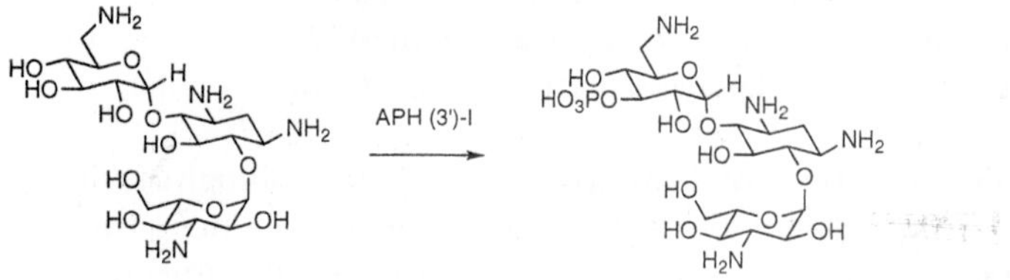

Kanamycin A, active   Kanamycin A 3'-phosphate, inactive

quinolone use increases. Those aminoglycoside antibiotics in present clinical are illustrated in Figure 34.22 along with some of their sites of enzymatic inactivation.

Specific Agents

Kanamycin. Kanamycin is a mixture of at least three components (A, B, and C, with A predominating), isolated from *Streptomyces kanamyceticus.* In addition to typical aminoglycoside antibiotic properties, it, along with gentamicin, neomycin, and paromomycin, is among the

most chemically stable of the common antibiotics. These substances can be heated without loss of activity for astonishing periods in acid or alkaline solutions and can even withstand autoclaving temperatures. Kanamycin is, however, unstable to R-factor enzymes, being O-phosphorylated on the C-3′ hydroxyl by enzymes APH(3′)-I and APH(3′)-II and is also N-acetylated on the C-6′ amino group, among others. These transformation products are antibiotically inactive. Kanamycin is used parenterally against some Gram (−) bacteria, but *Pseudomonas aeruginosa* and anaerobes are usually resistant. Although it can also be used in combination with other agents against certain mycobacteria (*M. kansasii, M. marinum, M. intracellulare*), its popularity for this use is fading. Injections of kanamycin are painful enough to require use of a local anesthetic. Kanamycin is occasionally used in antitubercular admixtures.

Amikacin. Amikacin antibiotic is made semisynthetically from kanamycin A. Interestingly, the L-hydroxlyamino-buteryl amide (HABA) moiety attached to N-3 inhibits adenylation and phosphorylation in the distant amino sugar ring (at C-2′ and C-3′) even though the HABA substituent is not where the enzymatic reaction takes place. This effect is attributed to decreased binding to the R-factor mediated enzymes. With this change, potency and spectrum are strongly enhanced and amikacin is used competitively with gentamicin for the treatment of sensitive strains of *Mycobacterium tuberculosis, Yersinia tularensis* and severe *Pseudomonas aeruginosa* infections resistant to other agents.

Tobramycin. Tobramycin is one (factor 6) of a mixture produced by fermentation of *Streptomyces tenebrarius.* Lacking the C-3′ hydroxyl group, it is not a substrate for APH(3′)-1 and -II so has an intrinsically broader-spectrum than kanamycin. It is a substrate, however, for adenylation at C-2′ by ANT(2′), acetylation at C-3 by AAC(3)-I and -II and at C-2′ by AAC(2′). It is widely used parenterally for difficult infections, especially those by gentamicin resistant *Pseudomonas aeruginosa.* It is believed by some clinicians to be less toxic than gentamicin.

Gentamicin. Gentamicin is a mixture of several antibiotic components produced by fermentation of *Micromonospora purpurea* and other related soil microorganisms (hence its name is spelled with an "i" instead of a "y"). Gentamicins C-1, C-2 and C-1a are most prominent. Gentamicin is the most important of the aminoglycoside antibiotics still in use. Gentamicin was, for example, one of the first antibiotics to have significant activity against *Pseudomonas aeruginosa* infections. This water-loving opportunistic pathogen is frequently encountered in burns, pneumonias and in urinary tract infections. It is highly virulent. As noted above, some of the functional groups that serve as targets for R-factor mediated enzymes are missing in the structure of gentamicins so their antibacterial spectrum is enhanced. They are, however, inactivated through C-2′ adenylation by

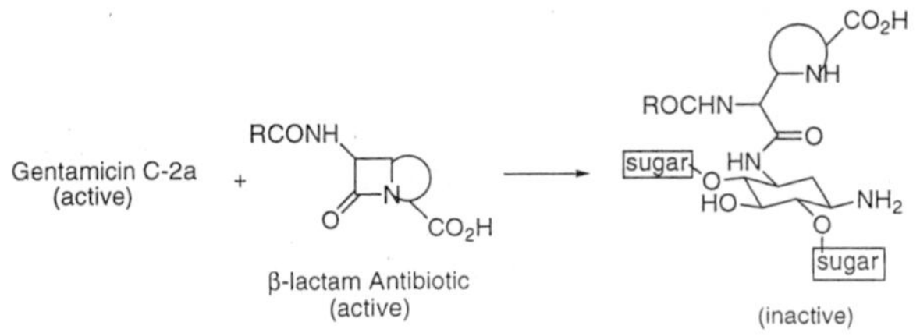

Fig. 34.23. A chemical drug-drug incompatibility between gentamicin C-2a and β-lactams.

enzyme ANT(2′) and acetylation at C-6′ by AAC(6′), at C-l by AAC(1)-I and -II, and at C-2′ by AAC(2′). It is often combined with other anti-infective agents and an interesting incompatibility has been uncovered. With certain β-lactam antibiotics, the two drugs react with each other so that N-acylation on C-l of gentamicin by the β-lactam antibiotic takes place, thus inactivating both antibiotics (Fig. 34.23). The two agents should not, therefore, be mixed in the same solution and should be administered into different tissue compartments (usually one in each arm) to prevent this. This incompatibility is likely to be associated with other aminoglycoside antibiotics as well.

Gentamicin is used for urinary tract infections, burns, some pneumonias, and bone and joint infections caused by susceptible Gram (−) bacteria. It is often used to prevent fouling of soft contact lenses. It is also used in polymer matrices in orthopedic surgery to prevent sealed in sepsis. It is given topically, sometimes in special dressings, to burn patients.

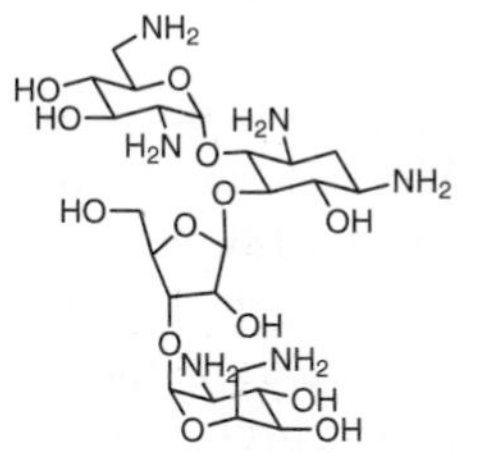

Neomycin B

Neomycin. Neomycin is a mixture of three compounds produced by fermentation of *Streptomyces fradiae* with neomycin B predominating. It is sometimes used in preoperative bowel sanitation and the treatment of enteropathogenic *E. coli* infections. It has also seen some use in lowering serum cholesterol.

Netilmicin. Netilmicin is produced semisynthetically by adding an N-ethyl substituent at C-3 onto sisomicin, a now archaic antibiotic produced by fermentation of *Micromonospora inyoensis* and related soil microorganisms. Netilmicin is similar in its clinical properties to gentamicin and tobramycin, although its antimicrobial spectrum is broader against many R-factor carrying strains. Netilmicin and sisomicin are chemically unusual for this antibiotic class because of the unsaturation in the upper left sugar ring.

Orally Used Aminoglycosides. Kanamycin and two otherwise archaic members of the aminoglycoside antibiotic group, neomycin and paromomycin find some oral use for the suppression of gut flora. Paromomycin is also used for the oral treatment of amoebic dysentery. Ameba are persistent pathogens causing chronic diarrhea and are acquired most frequently by travelers who consume food supplies contaminated with human waste. Suppression of gut flora is otherwise mostly employed prophylactically before gut surgery to decrease the likelihood of post surgical peritonitis. Neomycin is also used as an external ointment. Neomycin is too toxic under most circumstances by today's standards for parenteral use.

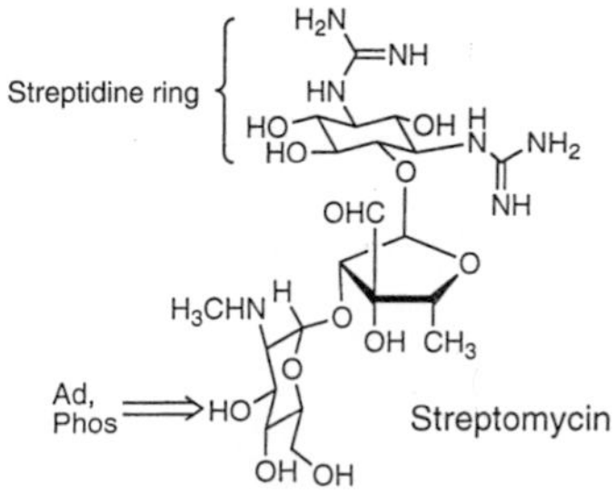

Streptomycin

Streptomycin. With a modified pharmacophore in that the diaminoinositol unit is streptamine, streptomycin has an axial hydroxyl group at C-2 and two highly basic guanido groups at C-l and C-3 in place of the primary amine moieties of 2-deoxystreptamine. Streptomycin is produced by fermentation of *Streptomyces griseus* and several related soil microorganisms. It was introduced in 1943 primarily for the treatment of tuberculosis (Chapter 37). The other aminoglycoside antibiotics are not nearly as useful against tuberculosis as is streptomycin, although kanamycin and amikacin are growing in popularity. Tuberculosis was controlled only by public health measures before the advent of streptomycin. Control of this ancient scourge was greeted with such enthusiasm that Selmon Waksman, the discoverer of streptomycin, received a Nobel Prize in 1952. It is possible that the unusual pharmacophore of streptomycin accounts in large measure for its unusual antibacterial spectrum. Another feature, the α-hydroxy-aldehyde function, is a center of instability such that streptomycin cannot be sterilized by autoclaving, so streptomycin sulfate solutions that need sterilization are made by ultrafiltration. Streptomycin is rarely used today as a single agent.

Resistance to streptomycin takes the now familiar course of N-acetylation, O-phosphorylation and O-adenylation of specific functional groups in the streptomycin molecule. Streptomycin is not very useful against the *M. avium* complex (MAC) and the other unusual mycobacteria which have become more common pathogens among immunosuppressed patients, including AIDS patients. Streptomycin is useful also against bubonic plague, leprosy, and tularemia. *Candida albicans*, an opportunistic yeast, is not inhibited by streptomycin and overgrowth leading to thrush and vaginal candidiasis can be a conse-

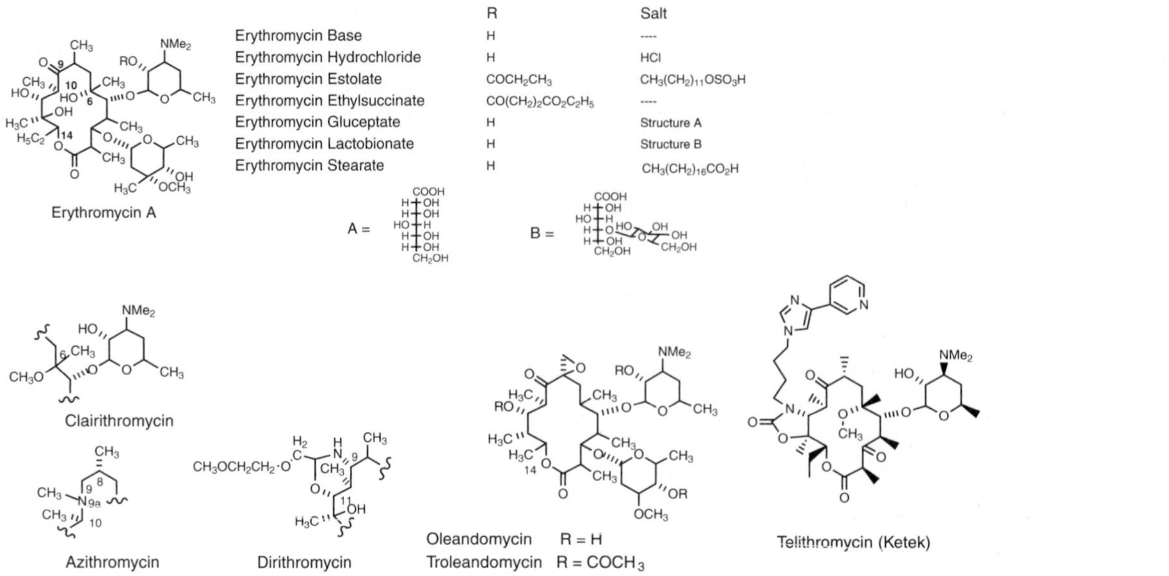

	R	Salt
Erythromycin Base	H	----
Erythromycin Hydrochloride	H	HCl
Erythromycin Estolate	$COCH_2CH_3$	$CH_3(CH_2)_{11}OSO_3H$
Erythromycin Ethylsuccinate	$CO(CH_2)_2CO_2C_2H_5$	----
Erythromycin Gluceptate	H	Structure A
Erythromycin Lactobionate	H	Structure B
Erythromycin Stearate	H	$CH_3(CH_2)_{16}CO_2H$

Fig. 34.24. Clinically important macrolide antibiotics.

quence of its long-term therapeutic use because of its concomitant disturbance of the normal flora.

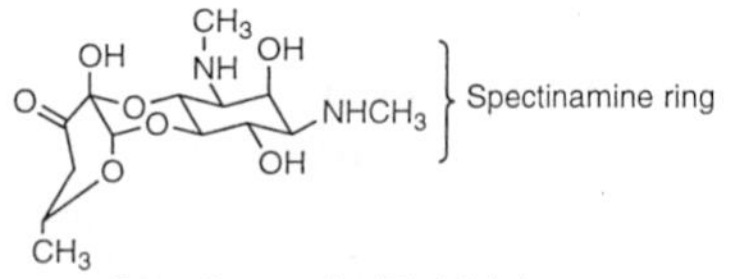

Spectinomycin (Trobicin)

Spectinomycin. Another unusual aminoglycoside antibiotic, spectinomycin is produced by fermentation of *Streptomyces spectabilis* and differs substantially in its clinical properties from the others. The diaminoinositol unit (spectinamine) contains two mono-N-methyl groups and the hydroxyl between them has a stereochemistry opposite to that in streptomycin. The glycosidically attached sugar is also unusual in that it contains three consecutive carbonyl groups, either overt or masked, and is fused by two adjacent linkages to spectinamine to produce an unusual fused three ring structure. Spectinomycin is bacteriostatic as normally employed. It is almost exclusively used in a single bolus injection intramuscularly against *Neisseria gonorrhea*, especially penicillinase-producing strains (PPNG), in cases of urogenital or oral gonorrhea and does not apparently produce any serious oto- or nephrotoxicity when used in this way. It is particularly useful for the treatment of patients allergic to penicillin and patients not likely to comply well with a medication scheme. It would likely be more widely used except that syphilis and chlamydia do not respond to it. It causes significant mistranslation following ribosomal binding but does not cause much inhibition of overall programmed protein biosynthesis. Resistance to spectinomycin is known but the mechanism is unclear as yet.

Macrolide Antibiotics

The term macrolide is derived from the characteristic large lactone (cyclic ester) ring found in these antibiotics. The clinically important members of this antibiotic family (Fig. 34.24) have two or more characteristic sugars attached to the 14-membered ring. One of these sugars usually carries a substituted amino group so their overall chemical character is weakly basic (pKa = 8). They are not very water-soluble as free bases but salt formation with certain acids (glucoheptonic and lactobiononic acids in Fig. 34.24) increase water solubility while other salts decrease solubility (laurylsulfate and stearic). Macrolide antibiotics with 16-membered rings are popular outside the United States but one example, tylosin, finds extensive agricultural use in the United States. The 14-membered ring macrolides are biosynthesized from propionic acid units so that every second carbon of erythromycin, for example, bears a methyl group and the rest of the carbons, with one exception, are oxygen bearing. Two carbons bear so-called "extra" oxygen atoms introduced later in the biosynthesis (not present in a propionic acid unit) and two hydroxyls are glycosylated (Fig. 34.25).

Mechanism of Action. The macrolides inhibit bacteria by interfering with programmed ribosomal protein biosynthesis by inhibiting translocation of aminoacyl t-RNA following binding to the 50S subparticle. More

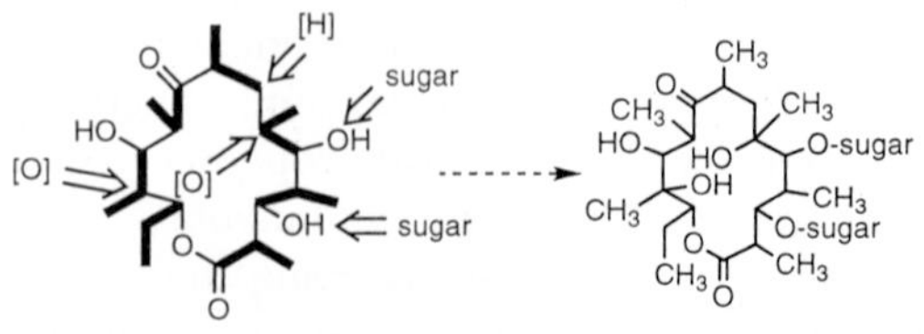

Fig. 34.25. Biosynthetic pathway to erythromycins from propionic acid units. ⇒ refers to modifications to the basic ring skeleton.

recent studies suggest that the macrolides inhibit protein synthesis by binding to domain V of the bacterial 23S rRNA making contact with adenosine 2058 (A2058) and additionally bind to domain II hairpin 35 in the same rRNA. Much of this work related to the newest macrolide-like molecules referred to as the ketolide. An example of a ketolide is the drug Telithromycin (Fig. 34.24). They are bacteriostatic in the clinic in achievable concentrations.

Resistance. Developed bacterial resistance is primarily caused by bacteria possessing R-factor enzymes which methylate a specific guanine residue on their own ribosomal RNA making them somewhat less efficient at protein biosynthesis but comparatively poor binders of macrolides. The erythromycin producing soil organism utilizes the same ribosomal methylation technique to protect itself against the toxic effects of its own metabolite. This leads to the speculation that the origin of some antibiotic resistance genes may lie in the producing organism itself and that this genetic material is acquired by bacteria from this source.

A second mechanism of resistance is associated with the mutation of adenine to guanine which occurs at A2058. This change results in a 10,000 fold reduction of binding capacity of erythromycin and clarithromycin to the 23S rRNA. This mutation is much less likely to occur with the ketolide derivatives.

Some bacterial strains, however, appear to be resistant to macrolides due to the operation of an active efflux process in which the drug is expelled from the cell at the cost of energy. Intrinsic resistance of Gram (−) bacteria is primarily caused by lack of penetration as the isolated ribosomes from these organisms are often susceptible.

Chemical Reactivity. The macrolides of the erythromycin class are chemically unstable in acid due to rapid internal cyclic ketal formation leading to inactivity (Fig. 34.26). This reaction is believed to be clinically important. Many macrolides have an unpleasant taste, which is partially overcome with water-insoluble dosage forms which also reduce acid instability and the gut cramps. Enteric coatings are also beneficial in reducing theses side effects. The free base, the hydrochloride, and the stearate salts are examples of such dosage forms.

Drug-Drug Interactions. Drug-drug interactions with macrolides are comparatively common and usually involve competition for oxidative liver metabolism by a member (CYP3A4) of the P-450 oxidase family. Such drugs as ergotamine, theophylline, carbamazepine, bromocryptine, warfarin, digoxin, oral contraceptives, carbamazepine, cyclosporin, astemizole, terfenadine, midazolam, triazolam, and methylprednisone can be involved. These interactions can have severely negative consequences for the patient. The result of this interaction is a longer half-life and enhanced potential toxicity by increasing the effective dose over time. The interaction with astemizole and terfenadine can lead to very serious cardiovascular effects. The main product of liver metabolism of erythromycin is the N-demethylated analogue.

Therapeutic Application. The macrolides are often used for the treatment of upper and lower respiratory tract and soft tissue infections primarily caused by Gram (+) microorganisms like *Strep. pyogenes* and *Strep. pneumoniae*, in Legionnaire's disease, prophylaxis of bacterial endocarditis by *Strep. viridans*, upper respiratory tract and lower respiratory tract infections and otitis media caused by *Haemophilus influenzae* (with a sulfonamide added), for mycoplasmal pneumonia, in combination with rifabutin in *M. avium* complex infections in AIDS patients, and also find some use for certain sexually transmitted diseases, such as gonorrhea and PID (pelvic inflammatory disease), caused by mixed infections involving cell-wall free organisms such as *Chlamydia trachomitis*. Clarithromycin is also used to treat gastric ulcers due to *H. pylori* infection as a component of multidrug cocktails. Thus, the macrolides have a comparatively narrow antimicrobial spectrum, reminiscent of the medium spectrum penicillins, but the organisms involved include many of the more commonly encountered community-acquired agents and the macrolides are remarkably free of serious toxicity to the host and, of course, do not cause β-lactam allergy. The macrolides are primarily used orally for mild systemic infections of the respiratory tract, liver, kidneys, prostate, and milk gland even though absorption is somewhat irregular, especially when taken with food. Some derivatives are propropulsive through stimulation of gastrin production. The resulting hyperperistalsis causes uncomfortable gastrointestinal cramps in some patients.

Specific Agents

Erythromycin Estolate. One of the two most popular erythromycin pro-drugs, erythromycin estolate, is a C-2″-propi-

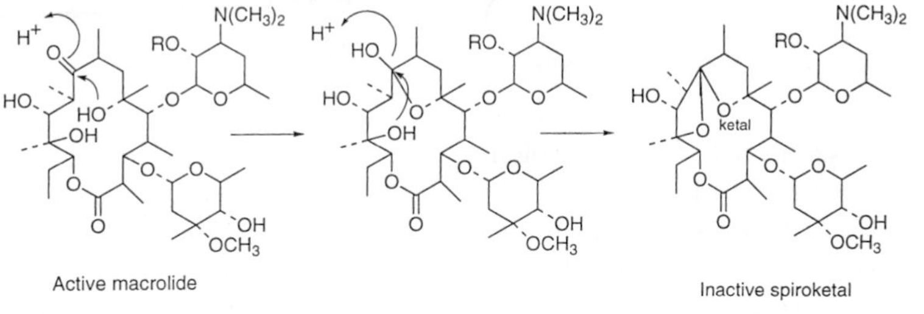

Active macrolide   Inactive spiroketal

Fig. 34.26. Acid catalyzed intramolecular ketal formation with erythromycin.

onyl ester, N-laurylsulfate salt (Fig. 34.24). Administration of erythromycin estolate produces higher blood levels following metabolic regeneration of erythromycin. In a small number of cases, a severe, dose-related, cholestatic jaundice occurs in which the bile becomes granular in the bile duct, impeding flow so that the bile salts back up into the circulation. This seems to be partly allergic and partly dose-related. If the drug causes hepatocyte damage, perhaps this releases antigenic proteins that promote further damage. When cholestatic jaundice occurs, the drug must be replaced by another, nonmacrolide, antibiotic such as one of the penicillins, cephalosporins or clindamycin. It is postulated that the propionyl ester group is transferred to a tissue component which is antigenic although the evidence for this is not compelling.

Erythromycin Ethyl Succinate (EryPed, E.E.S.). Erythromycin ethyl succinate is a mixed double ester pro-drug in which one carboxyl of succinic acid esterifies the C-2″ hydroxyl of erythromycin and the other ethanol (Fig. 34.24). This pro-drug is frequently used in an oral suspension for pediatric use largely to mask the bitter taste of the drug. Film coated tablets are also used to deal with this. Some cholestatic jaundice is beginning to be associated with the use of EES.

Clarithromycin. Recently, new chemical entities have been introduced into the macrolide class. Clarithromycin differs from erythromycin in that the C-6 hydroxy group has been converted semisynthetically to a methyl ether. The C-6 hydroxy group is involved in the process, initiated by protons, leading to internal cyclic ketal formation in erythromycin which results in drug inactivation (Fig. 34.26). This ketal, or one of the products of its subsequent degradation, is also associated with gastrointestinal cramping. Conversion of the molecule to its more lipophilic methyl ether prevents internal ketal formation which not only gives better blood levels through chemical stabilization, but also results in less gastric upset. An extensive saturable first-pass liver metabolism of clarithromycin leads to formation of its C-14 hydroxy analog, which has even greater antimicrobial potency, especially against *Haemophilus influenzae*. The enhanced lipophilicity of clarithromycin also allows for lower and less frequent dosage for mild infections.

Azithromycin. Azithromycin, called an "azalide," has been formed by semisynthetic conversion to a ring-expanded analog in which an N-methyl group has been inserted between carbons 9 and 10 of erythromycin and the carbonyl moiety removed (Fig. 34.24). Azithromycin has a 15-membered lactone ring. This new functionality does not form a cyclic internal ketal. Not only is azithromycin more stable to acid degradation than erythromycin, but it also has a considerably longer half-life, attributed to greater and longer tissue penetration, allowing once-a-day dosage. A popular treatment schedule with azithromycin is to take two tablets on the first day and one a day for the following five days and then to discontinue treatment. This is convenient for patients who comply poorly. The drug should be taken on an empty stomach. It does, however, give a metallic taste. Azithromycin has greater antiGram (−) activity than either erythromycin or clarithromycin. Both these new macrolides are quite similar in usage to erythromycin itself and are cross-resistant with it, but their future impact on medical practice is not yet determined. Azithromycin has a significant postantibiotic effect against a number of pathogens.

Troleandomycin. Troleandomycin is prepared semisynthetically by chemical transformation of oleandomycin, itself produced by fermentation of *Streptomyces antibioticus.* Troleandomycin is a pro-drug requiring metabolic conversion back to oleandomycin in vivo. With a bacteriostatic spectrum similar to that of erythromycin it is significantly less active and frequently cross-resistant with it. It is not commonly used today.

Erythromycyclamine

Dirithromycin. Dirithromycin is a semisynthetic macrolide pro-drug hydrolyzed to erythromycyclamine, an active semisynthetic erythromycin analog, on passage through the gut before absorption. It is much more acid stable than erythromycin but is less active against anaerobes, *Helicobacter, Legionella* and *Haemophilus.* Dirithromycin is not a substrate for P-450 and so has fewer dangerous drug-drug interactions than erythromycin.

Research activity in the macrolide antibiotic class has been intense recently in attempts to reduce side effects and to broaden their antimicrobial spectra. Recent introduction of several new agents attests to this. The most recent of these agents belonging to the semisynthetic ketolide class which is expected to appear on the market in early 2002. Telithromycin, 800 mg tablets used once daily orally, is effective in the treatment of community-acquired pneumonia, acute bacterial exacerbations of chronic bronchitis and acute sinusitis.

Lincomycin (Lincocin)

Clindamycin, R = H (Cleocin)
Clindamycin phosphate, R = PO₃H

Lincosaminides

The lincosamides (lincomycin and clindamycin) contain an unusual 8-carbon sugar, a thiomethyl aminooctoside (O-thio-lincosamide), linked by an amide bond to an n-propyl substituted N-methylpyrrolidylcarboxylic acid (N-methyl-n-propyl-*trans*-hygric acid). Lincosamides are weakly basic and form clinically useful hydrochloric acid salts. They are chemically distinct from the macrolide antibiotics but possess many pharmacologic similarities to them. Lincomycin is a natural product isolated from fermentations of *Streptomyces lincolnensis var. lincolnensis.* It serves as the starting material for the synthesis of clindamycin by a S_N-2 reaction that inverts the R stereochemistry of the C-7 hydroxyl to a C-7 S-chloride. Clindamycin is more bioactive and lipophilic than lincomycin, and is thus better absorbed following oral administration. The lincosamides bind to 50S ribosomal subparticles at a site partly overlapping with the macrolide site and are mutually cross-resistant with macrolides and work through essentially the same molecular mechanism of action. Clindamycin is significantly less painful than erythromycin when injected as a C-2 phosphate ester pro-drug and clindamycin is about 90% absorbed when taken orally. Clindamycin has a clinical spectrum rather like the macrolides although it distributes better into bones. Clindamycin works well for Gram (+) coccal infections, especially in patients allergic to β-lactams, and also has generally better activity against anaerobes. Unfortunately, however, the lincosaminides are associated increasingly with G.I. complaints (nausea, vomiting, cramps, and drug-related diarrheas). The most severe of these is a pseudomembranous colitis caused by release of a glycoproteinaceous endotoxin produced by lysis of *Clostridium difficile,* an opportunistic anaerobe. Its overgrowth results from suppression of the normal flora whose presence otherwise preserves a healthier ecological balance. The popularity of clindamycin in the clinic has decreased even though pseudomembranous colitis is comparatively rare and is now also associated with several other broad-spectrum antibiotics. A less common side effect is exudative erythrema multaform (Stevens-Johnson syndrome). Clindamycin has excellent activity against *Propionobacterium acnes* when applied topically to comedones and because it is white, it can be cosmetically tinted to match flesh tones better than the yellow tetracy-

Table 34.11. Commercially Available Tetracyclines

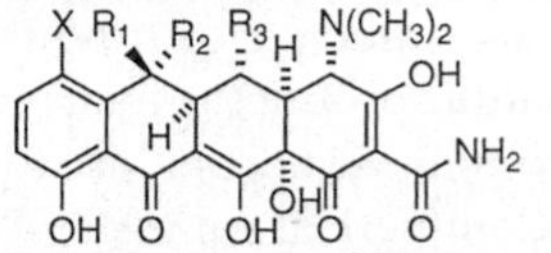

Generic Name	Trade Name	X	R_1	R_2	R_3
Tetracycline	Achromycin Sumycin Tetralan	H	OH	CH_3	H
Demeclocycline	Declomycin	Cl	OH	H	H
Minocycline	Minocin	$N(CH_3)_2$	H	H	H
Sancycline		H	H	H	H
Oxytetracycline	Terramycin	H	OH	CH_3	OH
Methacycline		H		CH_2	OH
Doxycycline	Vibramycin Doryx	H	H	CH_3	OH

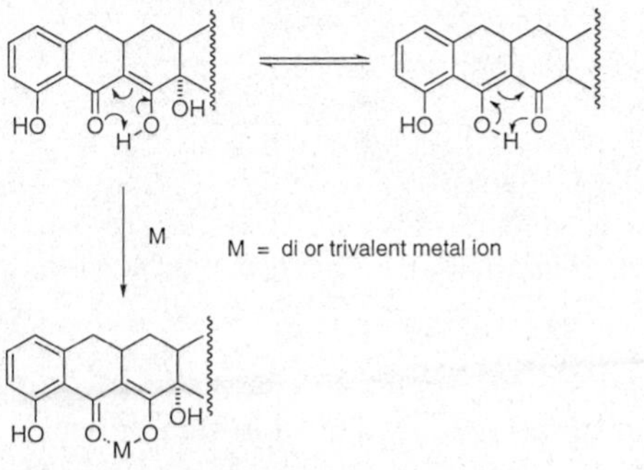

Fig. 34.27. Metal chelation with the tetracyclines.

clines. Clindamycin and lincomycin undergo extensive liver metabolism resulting primarily in N-demethylation. The N-desmethyl analog is biologically active. A very water insoluble palmitate hydrochloride pro-drug of clindamycin is also available (lacks bitter taste).

Tetracyclines

Physical-Chemical Properties. The tetracycline family is widely used in office practice. This family of antibiotics is characterized by a highly functionalized, partially reduced naphthacene (four linearly fused six-membered rings) ring system from which both the family name and numbering system are derived.

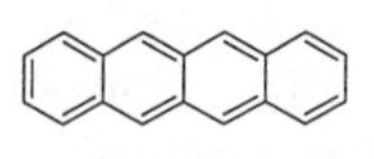

Naphthacene

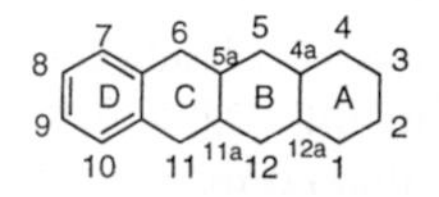

Tetracycline

(1,2,3,4,4a,5,5a,6,11,11a,12,12a-dodecahydronaphthacene)

They are amphoteric substances with three pK values revealed by titration (2.8–3.4, 7.2–7.8, and 9.1–9.7) and have an isoelectric point at about pH 5. The basic function is the C-4-α-dimethylamino moiety. Commercially available tetracyclines are comparatively water-soluble hydrochloride salts (Table 34.11). The conjugated phenolic enone system extending from C-10 to C-12 is associated with the pKa at about 7.5, whereas the conjugated trione system extending from C-1 to C-3 in ring A is nearly as acidic as is acetic acid (pKa about 3). Students who remember the principle of vinylogy will visualize this readily (see later discussion). These resonating systems can be drawn in a number of essentially equivalent ways with the double bonds in alternate positions. The formulae normally given are those settled upon by popular convention.

Chelation is an important feature of the chemical and clinical properties of the tetracyclines. The acidic functions of the tetracyclines are capable of forming salts through chelation with metal ions. The salts of polyvalent metal ions, such as Fe^{2+}, Al^{3+}, Ca^{2+}, Mg^{2+}, are all quite insoluble at neutral pHs, Figure 34.27. This insolubility is not only inconvenient for the preparation of solutions, but also interferes with blood levels on oral administration.

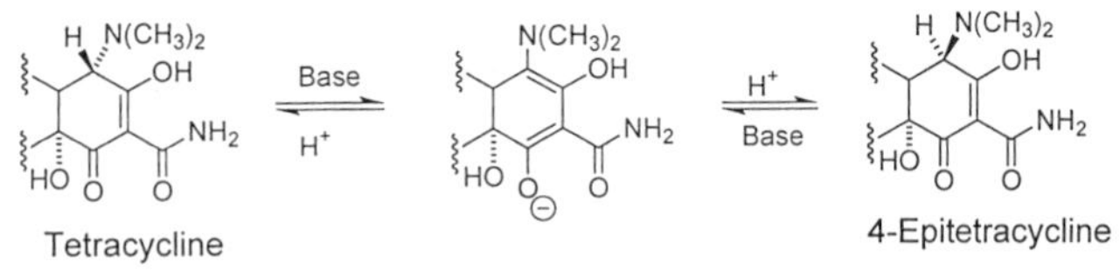

Fig. 34.28. Epimerization of tetracyclines.

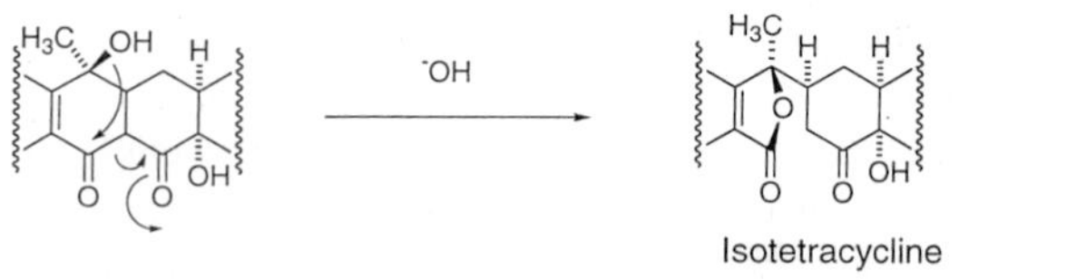

Fig. 34.30. Base catalyzed instability of tetracyclines.

Consequently, the tetracyclines are incompatible with co-administered multivalent ion-rich antacids and with hematinics, and concomitant consumption of daily products rich in calcium ion is also contraindicated. Further, the bones, of which the teeth are the most visible, are calcium-rich structures at nearly neutral pHs and so accumulate tetracyclines in proportion to the amount and duration of therapy when bones and teeth are being formed. As the tetracyclines are yellow, this leads to a progressive and essentially permanent discoloration in which, in advanced cases, the teeth are even brown. The intensification of discoloration with time is said to be a photochemical process. This is cosmetically unattractive but does not seem to be deleterious except in extreme cases where so much antibiotic is taken up that the structure of bone is mechanically weakened. To avoid this, tetracyclines are not normally given to children once they are forming their permanent set of teeth (ages 6–12). Tetracyclines are painful upon intramuscular injection. This has been attributed in part to formation of insoluble calcium complexes. To deal with this, the injectable formulations contain EDTA and are buffered at comparatively acidic pH levels where chelation is less pronounced and water solubility is higher. In severe cases, the teeth can be treated with dilute HCl solution to dissolve away the colored antibiotic. This also significantly erodes the mineral matrix of the teeth and has to be repaired by plastic impregnation. People naturally prefer to avoid this heroic and expensive process. When concomitant oral therapy with tetracyclines and incompatible metal ions must be done, the ions should be given 1 hour before or 2 hours after the tetracyclines.

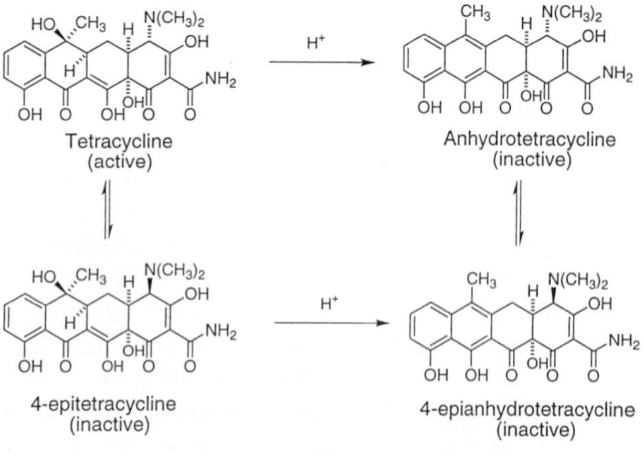

Routes of Administration. Tetracyclines can cause thrombophlebitis upon intravenous injection. The preferred route of administration is oral whereupon they are reasonably well absorbed in the absence of multivalent metal ion-rich gut contents.

Chemical Instability

Epimerization. The α-stereo orientation of the C-4 dimethylamino-moiety of the tetracyclines is essential for their bioactivity. The presence of the tricarbonyl system of ring A allows enolization involving loss of the C-4 hydrogen (Fig. 34.28). Reprotonation can take place from either the top or bottom of the molecule. Reprotonation from the top of the enol regenerates tetracycline. Reprotonation from the bottom, however, produces inactive 4-epitetracycline. At equilibrium the mixture consists of nearly equal amounts of the two diasteromers. Thus, old tetracycline preparations can lose approximately half their potency in this way. The custom is thus to overfill the capsules by about 15% during manufacture to allow for a longer shelf life at or near labeled potency. The epimerization process is most rapid at about pH 4 and is relatively slower in the solid-state.

Dehydration. Most of the natural tetracyclines have a tertiary and benzylic hydroxyl group at C-6. This function has the ideal geometry for acid catalyzed dehydration involving the C-5a α-oriented hydrogen (antiperiplanar *trans*). The resulting product is a naphthalene derivative, so there are energetic reasons for the reaction proceeding in that direction (Fig. 34.29). C-5a,6-anhydrotetracycline is much deeper in color than tetracycline and is biologically inactive.

Discolored old tetracyclines are suspect and should be discarded. Not only can inactive 4-epitetracyclines dehydrate to produce 4-epianhydrotetracyclines, but anhydrotetracycline can epimerize to produce the same product. This degradation product is toxic to the kidneys and produces a Fanconi-like syndrome that, in extreme cases, has been fatal. Commercial samples of tetracyclines are closely monitored for the presence of 4-epidehydrotetracycline and injuries from this cause are now, fortunately, rare. Those tetracyclines, such as minocycline and doxycycline, which have no C-6-hydroxyl groups cannot undergo dehydration and so are completely free of this toxicity.

Cleavage in Base. Another untoward degradation reaction involving a C-6-hydroxyl group is cleavage of the C-ring in alkaline solutions at or above pH 8.5 (Fig. 34.30). The lactonic product, an isotetracycline, is inactive. The

Fig. 34.29. Acid catalyzed instability of tetracyclines.

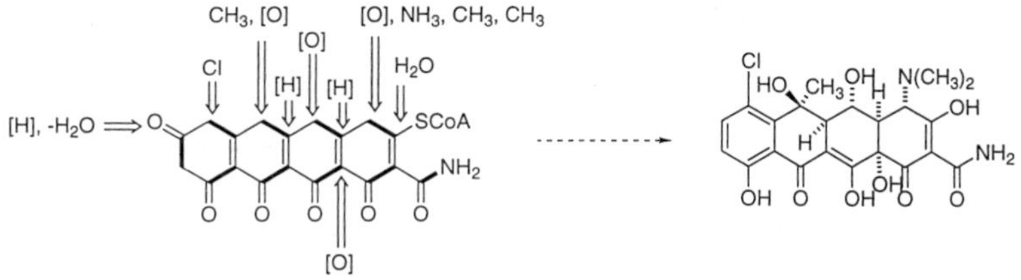

Fig. 34.31. Tetracycline biosynthesis from malonamyl and malonyl coenzyme A units.

clinical impact of this degradation under normal conditions is uncertain.

Phototoxicity. Certain tetracyclines, most notably those with a C-7-chlorine, absorb light in the visible region leading to free radical generation and potentially cause severe erythryma to sensitive patients on exposure to strong sun light. Patients should be advised to be cautious about such exposure for at least their first few doses to avoid potentially severe sunburn. This effect is comparatively rare with most currently popular tetracyclines.

Mechanism of Action. The tetracyclines of clinical importance interfere with protein biosynthesis at the ribosomal level leading to bacteriostasis. Tetracyclines bind to the 30S subparticle with the possible cooperation of a 50S site by a process that remains imprecisely understood despite intensive study. Bound tetracycline inhibits subsequent binding of aminoacyltransfer-RNA to the ribosomes resulting in termination of peptide chain growth. The more lipophilic tetracyclines, typified by minocycline, are also capable of disrupting cytoplasmic membrane function causing leakage of nucleotides and other essential cellular components from the cell and have bactericidal properties. The more lipophilic tetracyclines enter bacterial cells partly by passive diffusion and the more water soluble members partly through water-lined protein porin routes, perhaps assisted by the formation of highly lipophilic calcium and magnesium ion chelates. Deeper passage, however, through the inner cytoplasmic membrane is an energy requiring active process suggesting that the tetracyclines are mistaken by bacteria as food.

Resistance. Resistance results in part from an unusual ribosomal protection process involving elaboration of bacterial proteins TET(M), TET(O), and TET(Q). These proteins associate with the ribosome, thus allowing protein biosynthesis to proceed even in the presence of bound tetracyclines, although exactly how this works is not understood. Another important resistance mechanism involves R-factor-mediated, energy-requiring, active efflux of magnesium-chelated tetracyclines from cells in exchange for protons. This is particularly prominent in Gram (−) cells. Certain other microbes, such as Mycoplasma and Neisseria seem to have modified membranes that either accumulate fewer tetracyclines or have porins through which tetracy-

clines have difficulty in passing. Because resistance is now widespread, these once extremely popular antibiotics are falling into comparative disuse. The tetracyclines distinguish imperfectly between the bacterial 70S ribosomes and the mammalian 80S ribosomes so, in high doses, or in special situations, i.e., intravenous use in pregnancy, these drugs demonstrate a significant antianabolic effect. This can lead to severe liver and kidney damage so tetracyclines are not administered in these situations. Diuretics can enhance tetracycline-associated azotemia so they are contraindicated as are inducers of metabolism such as hydantoins, carbamazepine, and barbiturates.

Biosynthesis. The biosynthesis of the tetracyclines (Fig. 34.31) proceeds by a complex sequence of transformations involving condensation of malonamyl coenzyme A and eight malonate units in a process quite analogous to fatty acid biosynthesis. Tetracycline biosynthesis differs however significantly in that the majority of the carbonyl groups remain in the molecule and self condense in a controlled way to produce the partially reduced naphthacene nucleus. An involved sequence of reductions, oxidations, methylations, aminations and dehydrations completes the biosynthesis. The individual tetracyclines arise from deletions or additions of various individual steps.

Therapeutic Application. The tetracyclines possess very wide bacteriostatic antibacterial activity. Because of the resistance phenomenon, and the comparative frequency of troublesome side effects, they are rarely any longer the drugs of first choice. Nonetheless they are still very popular for office use against susceptible microbes. The differences between the antimicrobial spectra of various tetracyclines are not large. They are popular for low dose oral and topical therapy for acne, first course community acquired urinary tract infections (largely due to *E. coli*), brucellosis, borreliosis, upper respiratory tract infections, ophthalmic infections, sexually transmitted diseases, chancroid, rickettsial infections, mycoplasmal pneumonia, prophylaxis for malaria, prevention of traveler's diarrhea, shigellosis, cholera, *Campylobacter fetus*, bacteroides, *Enterobacter*, *Helicobacter* cocktails, Lyme Disease, Rocky Mountain spotted fever, scrub typhus, and many other less common problems. The tetracyclines are also used in tonnage quantities for agricultural use, often in the form of feed supplements where it can be demonstrated that animals reach market weight more quickly and economically with their use.

Specific Agents (Table 34.11)

Tetracycline. Tetracycline is produced by fermentation of *Streptomyces aureofaciens* and related species, or by catalytic reduction of chlortetracycline. It is classical, typical, generic and comparatively cheap. The blood levels achieved upon oral administration are often irregular. Food and milk lower absorption by about 50%.

Demeclocycline. Demeclocycline lacks the C-6-methyl of tetracycline and is produced by fermentation of a genetically altered strain of *S. aureofaciens*. It is, being a secondary alcohol, more chemically stable than tetracycline against dehydration and has served as the source of numerous semisynthetic analogs as well as enjoying its own clinical vogue. Food and milk co-consumption decrease absorption by half although it is 60–80% absorbed by fasting adults.

Minocycline. An important antibiotic produced by semisynthesis from demeclocycline is minocycline. The C-7-chloro and the C-6-hydroxy groups can both be removed by catalytic reduction to produce sancycline, the chemically simplest tetracycline with characteristic tetracycline properties. Sancycline has not, however, become an important antibiotic. Nitration of sancycline in strongly acidic solutions is possible because of its great chemical stability and is followed by separation of the C-7 and the C-9 nitro analogs produced in the reaction. Reductive amination of the C-7 nitro analog with formaldehyde produces minocycline. Using a rather more involved process, the C-9 nitro analog can be processed to produce more minocycline. Minocycline is much more lipophilic than its precursors, gives excellent blood levels following oral administration (90–100% available), and can be given once a day. Its absorption is lowered by about 20% when taken with food or milk. It is less dependent upon active uptake mechanisms and has a somewhat broader antimicrobial spectrum. It is also, apparently, less painful upon intramuscular or intravenous injection. It has, however, vestibular toxicities (e.g., vertigo, ataxia, and nausea) not shared by other tetracyclines. It is particularly broad-spectrum with emphasis on important Gram (+) pathogens, both staphylococci and streptococci, and so has become a very popular drug in North America.

Oxytetracycline. Oxytetracycline is also one of the classic tetracyclines. It is produced by fermentation of *Streptomyces rimosis* and other soil microorganisms. The most hydrophilic tetracycline on the market, it has largely now been replaced by its semisynthetic descendants. It is about 60% bio-available when taken orally by fasting adults and this is lowered by half when taken with food or milk.

Doxycycline. Methacycline is produced from oxytetracycline by an ingenious process involving blocking of C-lla by a halogen atom, dehydrating with strong acid, which now takes an exocyclic course since the ring can no longer aromatize, and carefully removing the blocking halogen so that the double bond does not move. It serves as the chemical precursor, through further transformations including catalytic reduction processes, of doxycycline, the most important of the present day tetracyclines. The direct catalytic reduction of methacycline (also known as rondomycin) has the capability of producing two isomers. The isomer with the same stereochemistry as the naturally occurring tetracyclines (α-oriented methyl) is significantly more potent. Catalytic reduction of the 11a-halo analog followed by dehalogenation leads to a preponderance of doxycycline.

Doxycycline is well absorbed on oral administration (90–100% when fasting; reduced by 20% by co-consumption with food or milk), has a half-life permitting one a day dosing for mild infections, and is excreted partly in the feces and partly in the urine. Because it causes fewer gastrointestinal disturbances and cannot participate in degradation processes involving a C-6-hydroxyl group, it is the tetracycline of choice for many physicians.

Once very widely used, the popularity of the tetracyclines has faded considerably due to wide spread resistance and the introduction of newer broad spectrum agents such as amoxicillin with clavulanate. Research, however, continues and novel analogs prepared from 9-nitrodemethyldeoxytetracycline and 9-nitrominocycline, known as the glycylcyclines, may be marketed soon for the treatment of certain infections caused by bacteria resistant to previous tetracyclines.

Reserve or Special Purpose Antibiotics

This group of antibiotics consists of a miscellaneous collection of structural types whose toxicities or narrow range of applicability give them a more specialized place in antimicrobial chemotherapy than those covered to this point. They are reserved for special purposes.

R = H   Chloramphenicol (Chloromycetin)
R = COCH$_2$CH$_2$CO$_2$H   Chloramphenicol hemisuccinate
R = CO(CH$_2$)$_{12}$CH$_3$ Chloramphenicol palmitate

Chloramphenicol. Chloramphenicol was originally produced by fermentation of *Streptomyces venezuelae* but its comparatively simple chemical structure soon resulted in several efficient total chemical syntheses. With two asymmetric centers it is one of four diastereomers, only one of which (1R, 2R) is significantly active. As total synthesis produces a mixture of all four, the unwanted isomers must be removed before use. Chloramphenicol is a neutral substance only moderately soluble in water as both nitrogen atoms are nonbasic under physiologic conditions (one is an amide and the other a nitro moiety). It was the first broad-spectrum oral antibiotic used in the United States (1947) and was once very popular. Severe potential blood dyscrasia has greatly decreased its use in North America although its cheapness and efficacy makes it still very popular in much of the rest of the world where it can often be purchased over-the-counter without a prescription.

Metabolism. When given orally, it is rapidly and completely absorbed but has a fairly short half-life. It is mainly excreted in the urine in the form of its metabolites which are a C-3 glucuronide, and to a lesser extent its deamidation product and the product of dehalogenation and reduction. These are all inactive. The aromatic nitro group is also reduced metabolically and this product can also undergo amide hydrolysis. The reduction of the nitro group, however, does not take place efficiently in humans but rather primarily occurs in the gut by the action of the normal flora. Chloramphenicol is also available for parental use. It is about 60% serum protein bound and diffuses well into tissues, especially into inflamed cerebrospinal fluid and is, therefore, of special value in meningitis. It also penetrates well into lymph and mesenteric ganglions rationalizing its particular value in typhoid and paratyphoid fever.

Mechanism of Action. Chloramphenicol is bacteriostatic by virtue of inhibition of protein biosynthesis in both bacterial and to a lesser extent in the host ribosomes. Chloramphenicol binds to the 50S subparticle in a region near where the macrolides bind. Resistance is mediated by several R-factor enzymes that catalyze acetylation of the secondary and, to some extent, the primary hydroxyl groups in the aliphatic side chain. These products no longer bind to the ribosomes so are inactivated. *Escherichia coli* is frequently resistant due to chloramphenicol's lack of intercellular accumulation.

Side Effects. Its toxicities prevent chloramphenicol from being more widely used. Blood dyscrasias are seen in patients predisposed to them. The more serious form is a pancytopenia of the blood that is fatal in about 70% of cases and is believed to be caused by one of the reduction products of the aromatic nitro group. This side effect is known as aplastic anemia, and has even occurred following use of the drug as an ophthalmic ointment. There seems to be a genetic predisposition towards this in a very small percentage of the general population. This devastating side effect is estimated to occur once in every 25,000–40,000 courses of therapy. Less severe, but much more common, is a reversible inhibition of hematopoiesis, seen in aged patients or in those with renal insufficiency. If cell counts are taken, this can be controlled because it is dose-related and marrow function will recover if the drug is withdrawn.

The so-called "gray syndrome," a form of cardiovascular collapse, is encountered when chloramphenicol is given carelessly in the first 48 hours of life when liver glucuronidation is undeveloped and successive doses will lead to rapid accumulation of the drug due to impaired excretion. A dose-related profound anemia accompanied by an ashen gray pallor is seen, as are vomiting, loss of appetite, and cyanosis. Deaths have resulted, often involving cardiovascular collapse.

Pro-drugs. Two pro-drug forms of chloramphenicol are available. The drug is intensively bitter. This can be masked for use as a pediatric oral suspension by use of the C-3 palmitate, which is cleaved in the duodenum to liberate the drug. Chloramphenicol's poor water solubility is largely overcome by conversion to the C-3 hemisuccinoyl ester, which forms a water-soluble sodium salt. This is cleaved in the body by lung, liver, kidney and blood esterases to produce active chloramphenicol. Because cleavage in muscles is too slow, this prodrug is used intravenously rather than intramuscularly.

Chloramphenicol potentiates the activity of some other drugs by inducing liver metabolism. Such agents include anticoagulant coumarins, sulfonamides, oral hypoglycemics, and phenytoin.

Therapeutic Applications. Despite potentially serious limitations, chloramphenicol is an excellent drug when used carefully. Its special value is in typhoid and paratyphoid fevers, Haemophilis infections (especially epiglottitis and meningitis, when given along with ampicillin), pneumococcal and meningococcal meningitis in β-lactam allergic patients, anaerobic infections (especially by Bacteroides), and as a backup to tetracyclines in rickettsial infections. Safer antibiotics should be used whenever possible.

Cyclic Peptides. The usual physiologically significant peptides are linear. Several bacterial species, however, produce antibiotic mixtures of cyclic peptides some with uncommon amino acids and some with common amino acids but with the D absolute stereochemistry. These cyclic substances often have a pendant fatty acid chain as well. One of the consequences of this unusual architecture is that these glycopeptide agents are not readily metabolized. These drugs are usually water soluble and are highly lethal to susceptible bacteria as they attach themselves to the bacterial membranes and interfere with their semipermeability so that essential metabolites leak out and undesirable substances pass in. Unfortunately, they are also highly toxic in humans so their use is reserved for serious situations where there are few alternatives or to topical uses. Bacteria are rarely able to develop significant resistance to this group of antibiotics. They are generally unstable so solutions should be protected from heat, light and extremes of pH.

Vancomycin (Vancocin, Vancoled)   Teicoplanin (Targocid)

Vancomycin and Teicoplanin. Vancomycin is produced by fermentation of *Nocardia orientalis* and is one of two from about 200 known glycopeptide antibiotics that are in clinical use. It has been available for about 40 years but its popularity has increased significantly in the last decade. Its useful spectrum is restricted to Gram (+) pathogens with particular utility against multiply resistant coagulase negative staphylococci and methicillin-resistant *Staphylococcus aureus* (MRSA) which causes septicemias, endocarditis, skin and soft tissue infections, and infections associated with venous catheters. It is used orally against *Clostridium difficile* infections where its use can be life saving. It is usually bactericidal. It does not give useful blood levels following oral administration and is very irritating on intravenous injection. To prevent thrombophlebitis it is slowly instilled rather than pushed. It is only very recently, despite decades of intensive use, that some vancomycin resistant bacteria are emerging. It is alleged that these resistant strains emerged as a consequence of the agricultural use of avoparcin, a structurally related antibiotic which has not found use for human infections in the U.S. The mechanism of resistance appears to be alteration of the target D-ala-D-ala units on the peptidoglycan cell wall precursors to D-ala-D-lactate. This change prevents vancomycin's action for vancomycin has little affinity for the new depsipeptide linkage. It is greatly feared that this form of resistance will become common in the bacteria for which vancomycin is presently the last sure hope for successful chemotherapy. If so, such infection would become untreatable.

These resistant strains are not yet present in clinically relevant strains but most authorities believe that this is only a question of time. Chemically, vancomycin has a glycosylated hexapeptide chain rich in unusual amino acids, many of which contain aromatic rings which are halogenated and cross linked by aryl ether bonds into a rigid molecular framework. The binding site for its target is a peptide-lined cleft having high affinity for acetyl-D-ala-D-ala and related peptides. Thus, vancomycin has a specific peptide receptor and attacks bacterial cell wall biosynthesis at the same step as does the β-lactams but by a different mechanism. By cov-

ering the substrate for cell wall transamidase, it prevents cross-linking resulting in osmotically defective cell walls. Manufactured vancomycin is a mixture of related substances of which vancomycin B predominates. In addition to the danger of thrombophlebitis accompanying rapid administration, higher doses of vancomycin can cause nephrotoxicity and auditory nerve damage. A significant drug rash (the so-called red man syndrome) can occur mediated by histamine release. Other toxic side effects include hearing loss and nephrotoxicity.

Teicoplanin is a mixture of five related fermentation products related to vancomycin. It is more lipid soluble so distributes better into tissues and bacteria. It is also highly protein bound so it can be used IM or IV once daily. It is markedly less irritating than vancomycin upon injection so is better tolerated by patients and does not lead to a significant histamine release on IV administration.

Streptogramins—Quinupristin/Dalfopristin. Very recently a combination of quinupristin and dalfopristin has been approved for IV use in the treatment of infections caused by vancomycin-resistant *Enterococcus faecium* bacteremia as well as skin and skin structure infections caused by methicillin sensitive *Staphylococcus aureus* and *Streptococcus pyogenes*. At this time certain strains of *E. Faecium* are resistant to essentially all other antibiotics. This combination (quinupristin:dalfopristin [30:70]-Synercide) then should find a welcome place in medicine. These particular indications are comparatively rare so this is unlikely to become a major drug. Likely it will be restricted to these uses to prevent the emergence of more resistance.

The two drugs are bacteriostatic when administered individually, but are found to act synergisticly when combined to produce a bactericidal effect. The combination is found to inhibit protein synthesis by binding to the 70S ribosome which is thought to account for the mechanism of action. In vitro tests suggest a strong post-antibiotic effect of from 2.2–18 hours. It has been reported that the combination significantly inhibits CYP3A4 enzyme and could account for a potential drug-drug interaction with other drugs metabolized by this system.

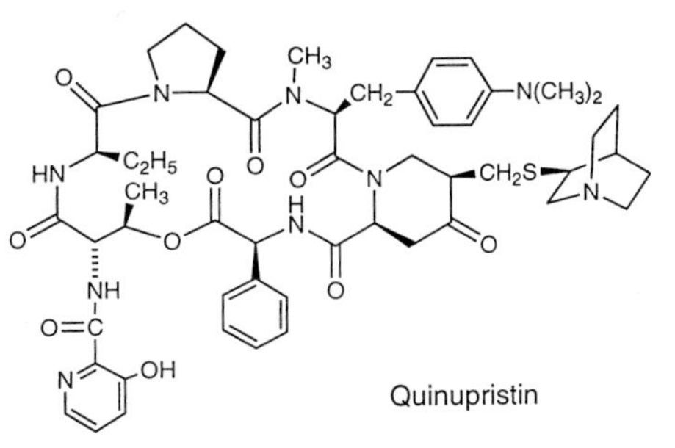

Quinupristin 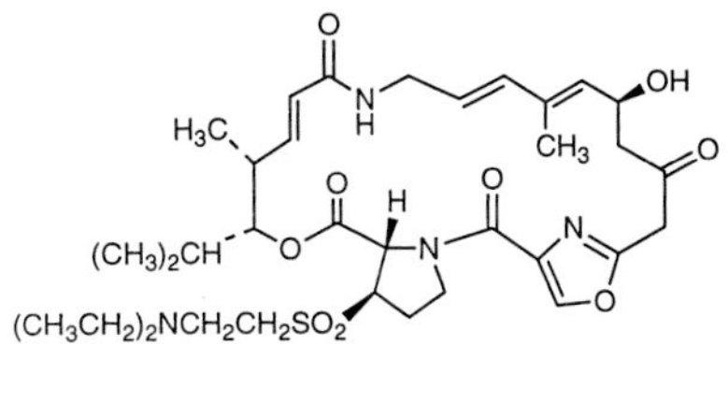   Dalfopristin

Bacitracin. Bacitracin (Fig. 34.32) is a mixture of similar peptides produced by fermentation of the bacterium *Bacillus subtilis.* The A component predominates. Bacitracin got its name from the genus of the producing organism and the family name of the first patient to be treated with it, who was a little girl, named Tracy. It is predominantly active against Gram (+) microorganisms and is used topically or intramuscularly against staphylococci resistant to other agents. It is also used orally for enteropathogenic diarrhea and, especially, against *Clostridium difficile.* It can also be used for preoperative bowel sanitization. It is rather neuro- and nephrotoxic so is employed with caution. Zinc^{2+} ion enhances the activity of bacitracin. Its mode of action is to inhibit both peptidoglycan biosynthesis at a late stage (probably at the dephosphorylation of the phospholipid carrier step) and disruptions of plasma membrane function.

Polymyxin B. Polymyxin B sulfate (Fig. 34.32) is produced by fermentation of *Bacillus polymyxa.* It is separated from a mixture of related cyclic peptides and is primarily active against Gram (−) microorganisms. It apparently binds to phosphate groups in bacterial cytoplasmic membranes and disrupts their integrity. It is used intramuscularly or intravenously to treat serious urinary tract infections, meningitis and septicemia primarily caused by *Pseudomonas aeruginosa* but some other Gram (−) bacteria will also respond. It is also used orally to treat enteropathogenic *E. coli* and *Shigella* sp. diarrheas. Irrigation of the urinary bladder with solutions of polymyxin B sulfate is also employed by some to reduce the incidence of infections subsequent to installation of indwelling catheters. When given parenterally the drug is quite neuro- and nephrotoxic so is employed only after other drugs have failed.

Colistin. Colistin sulfate (Fig. 34.32) is a cyclic polypeptide drug produced by *Bacillus polymyxa var. colistinus.* The A component is the primary article of commerce. It is bactericidal primarily to Gram (−) bacteria following destruction of the integrity of their cytoplasmic membranes. Resistance development is rare. Colistin is used sparingly against severe Gram (−) caused infections because of its nephro- and neurotoxicity. It is also used orally against diarrhea due to *E. coli* and *Shigella* sp. Gramicidin is a mem-

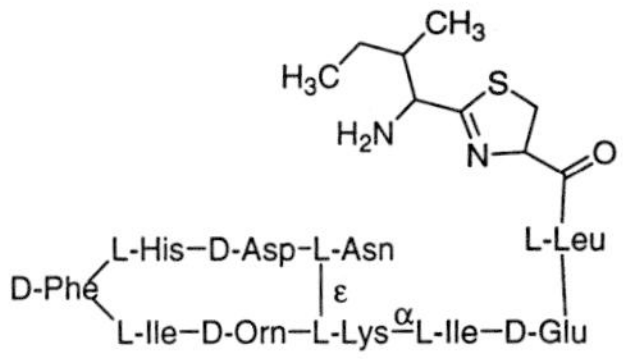

Bacitracin A

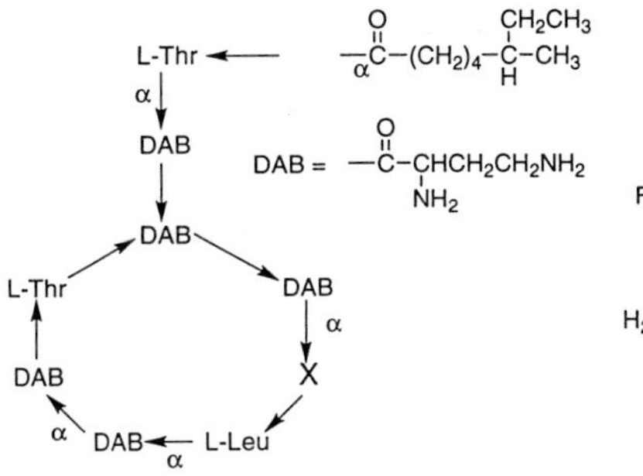

Polymyxin B (X = L-Phe)(Aerosporin)
Colistin (X = D-Leu)(Coly-Mycin S)

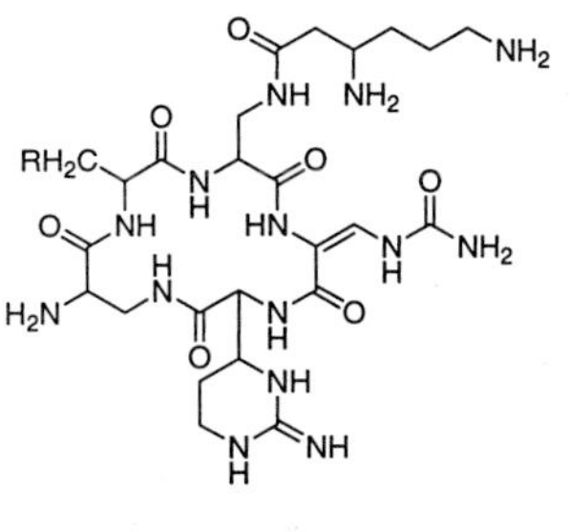

Capreomycin 1A (R = OH) ⎤ (Capastat)
Capreomycin 1B (R = H) ⎦

Fig. 34.32. Cyclic peptides.

ber of the tyrothricin complex and is largely archaic now because of its severe toxicities.

Capreomycin. Capreomycin (Fig. 34.32) is somewhat related structurally. It is produced by fermentation of *Streptomyces capreolus* as a mixture of about four components. It is bacteriostatic against certain mycobacterial strains including *M. tuberculosis, M. bovis, M. kansasii* and *M. avium* by an unknown mechanism. Resistance develops, often during the course of therapy, also by an unknown mechanism. The drug must be employed with caution because of its oto- and nephrotoxicity.

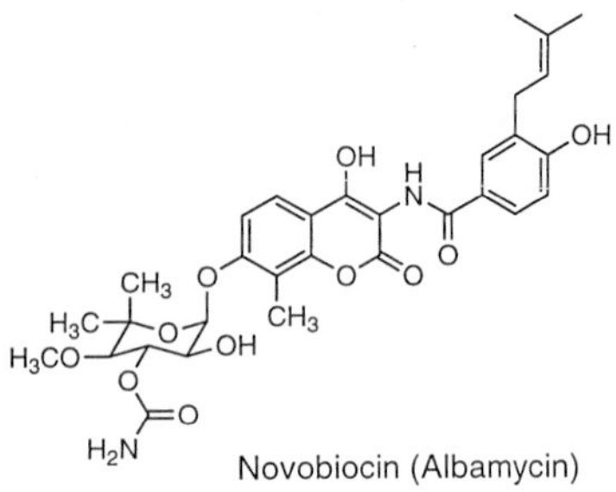

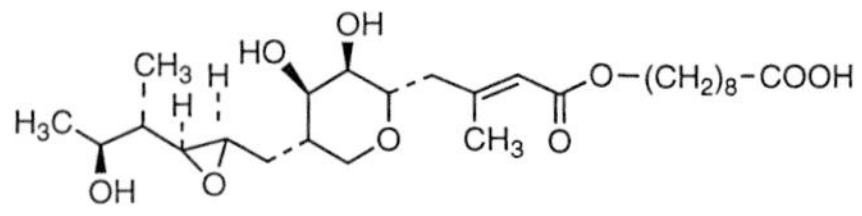

Mupirocin (Bactroban)

It can only be used topically because of hydrolysis in vivo which inactivates the drug. It is intrinsically broad-spectrum but its primary indication is topically against staphylococcal and streptococcal skin infections. Mupirocin binds to bacterial isoleucyl transfer-RNA synthase preventing incorporation of isoleucine into bacterial proteins. Resistance is due to alterations of the synthase target such that the enzyme still functions but does not bind mupirocin.

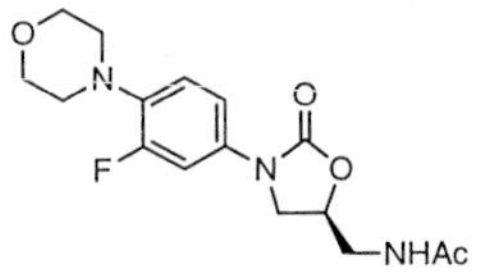

Novobiocin (Albamycin)

Miscellaneous Antibacterial Agents

Novobiocin. Novobiocin is a coumarmycin-family (coumarin containing) antibiotic produced by fermentation of *Streptomyces niveus.* It inhibits the function of DNA gyrase by binding to a different subunit than the fluoroquinolones with which it is synergistic. Novobiocin binding interferes with ATP metabolism which otherwise provides the energy needed for the conformational work of the enzyme. It is orally active and has a fairly broad range of activity against Gram (+) and some Gram (−) organisms but common side effects (rash, blood dyscrasias, and liver damage) and resistance emergence have decreased its utilization significantly. The 4-hydroxy coumarin moiety is vinylogously equivalent to a carboxy group so novobiocin readily forms a sodium and a calcium salt. The sodium salt is used for injections.

Mupirocin. Mupirocin is a member of a group of lipid acids produced by fermentation of *Pseudomonas fluorescens.*

Linezolid (Zyvox)

Oxazolidinones. Linezolid is a recently approved antibacterial agent effective against gram (+) bacteria. This drug is a member of the oxazolidinone class of agents and represents a new synthetic class of antibacterials. The drug, available in injectable, tablet and oral suspension dosage forms, is effective against methicillin-resistant *Staphylococcus aureus* and used to treat nosocomial pneumonia, community-acquired pneumonia, complicated and uncomplicated skin and skin structure infections and vancomycin-resistant *Enterococcus faecium* infections.

The mechanism of action of linezolid is associated with inhibition of protein synthesis, but at a stage different from that of other protein synthesis inhibitors. The oxazolidinones inhibit the initation of protein synthesis by preventing the formation of the ternary complex between N-formylmethionyl-tRNA (tRNA^{fMet})-mRNA-70S (or 30S) subunit. It is believed that the drug distorts the binding site for the initiator-tRNA which overlaps both 30S and 50S ribosomal subunits.

CASE STUDY

Victoria F. Roche and S. William Zito

KC is a 5-year-old female who has been frail and sickly since birth. The only child of two college professors, she attends morning kindergarten at an inner city public school, and spends her afternoons at the University's daycare center. KC's latest health issue was a case of uncomplicated community-acquired streptococcal pneumonia (*S. pneumoniae*) that she picked up from one of her school or daycare playmates. Fortunately, the strain was not penicillinase producing, and KC was starting to respond to oral phenoxybenzylpenicillin (Penicillin VK). KC loves to "help" her mom cook and, on this cold January afternoon, she was standing on a chair, stirring a big pot of homemade chicken soup when the apron she was wearing brushed the burner and caught fire. Although her mom was there and did everything she could to put the fire out, KC suffered second degree burns on her legs and trunk. Now hospitalized, she is receiving PenVK and IV morphine sulfate, but her pneumonia has significantly worsened due to invasion by the opportunistic pathogen *Pseudomonas aeruginosa*. Additional antibiotic therapy is warranted, and you are asked to advise the attending physician on an appropriate parenteral agent. Consider the structural choices drawn below.

1. Identify the therapeutic problem(s) where the pharmacist's intervention may benefit the patient.

2. Identify and prioritize the patient specific factors that must be considered to achieve the desired therapeutic outcomes.

3. Conduct a thorough and mechanistically oriented structure-activity analysis of all therapeutic alternatives provided in the case.

4. Evaluate the SAR findings against the patient specific factors and desired therapeutic outcomes and make a therapeutic decision.

5. Counsel your patient.

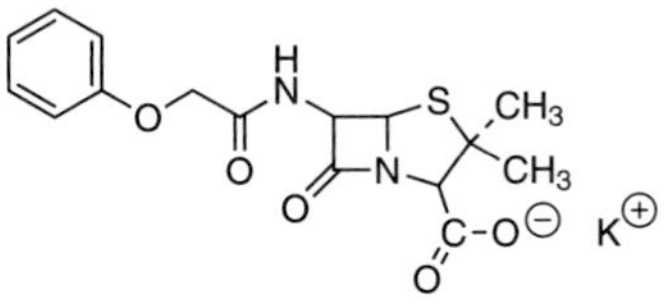

Penicillin VK

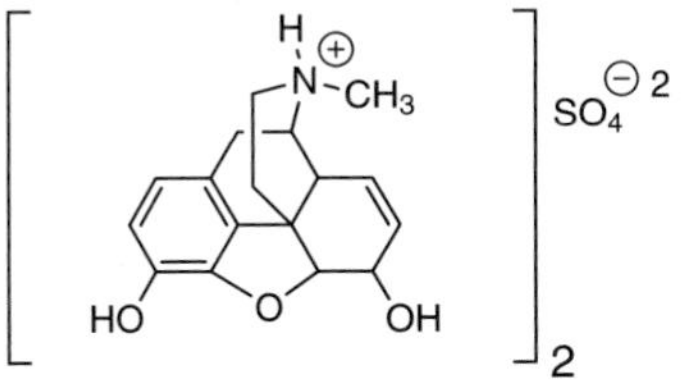

Morphine sulfate

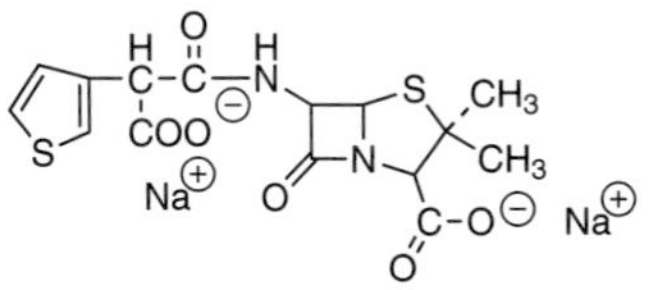

1

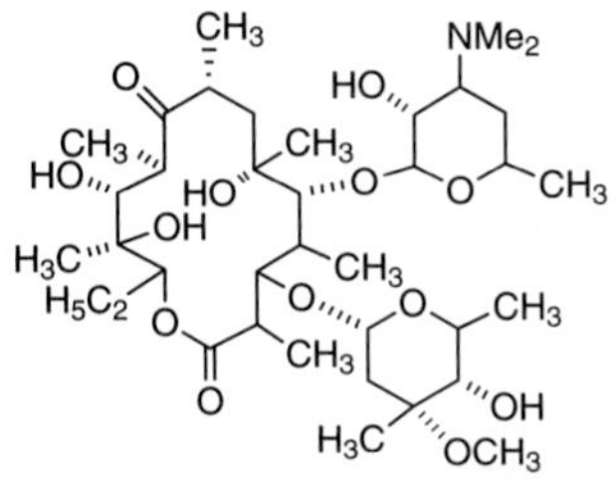

2

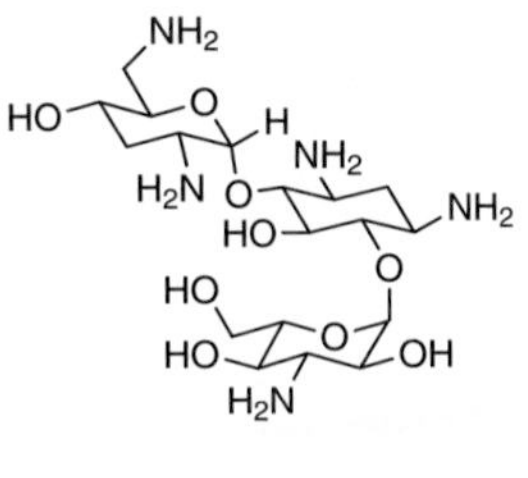

3

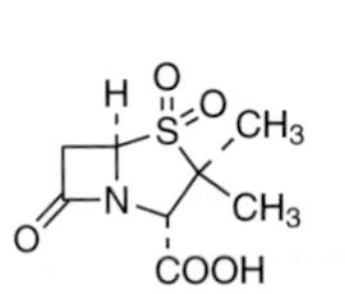

4

SUGGESTED READINGS

Albert A. Selective Toxicity. 6th ed. New York: Chapman and Hall, 1979.

Association Franciaise las Enseignants de Chemie Therapeutique. Medicaments Antibiotiques. Paris: Tec & Doc Lavoisier, 1992:2

Bartmann K. Antitubercular Drugs, Handbook of Experimental Pharmacology. New York: Springer-Verlag, 1988:84.

Burnet M, White DO. Natural History of Infectious Disease 4th ed. New York: Cambridge University Press, 1975.

Dax SL. Antibacterial Chemotherapeutic Agents. New York: Blackie Academic and Professional, 1997.

de Kruif P. Microbe Hunters. New York: Pocket Books, 1965 (Original Edition, New York: Harcourt, Brace, 1926).

Demain AL, Solomon NA, ed. Antibiotics Containing the Beta-lactam Structure, Volumes 1 and 2, Handbook of Experimental Pharmacology, Vol. 67, New York, Springer-Verlag, 1983

Gale EF, Cundliffe E, Reynolds PE, et al. ed. The Molecular Basis of Antibiotic Action. New York: Wiley, 1981:2.

Garrett L. The Coming Plague. New York: Penguin, 1994.

Hitchings GH. Inhibition of folate metabolism in chemotherapy, the Origins and uses of co-trimoxole. In: Hitchings GH, ed. Handbook of Experimental Pharmacology. New York: Springer, 1983:64.

Hlavka JJ, Boothe JH. The Tetracyclines, Handbook of Experimental Pharmacology. New York: Springer-Verlag, 1985:78.

Kuhlmann J, Dalhoff A, Zeiler H-J. Quinolone antibacterials, Handbook of Experimental Pharmacology. New York: Springer, 1998:127.

Kucers A, Bennet N McK. The Use of Antibiotics, 4th Ed., Lippincott, 1987. Philadelphia. Lukacs G and M. Ohno, Eds., Recent Progress in the Chemical Synthesis of Antibiotics, New York, Springer Verlag, 1990.

Levy SB, The Antibiotic Paradox, Plenum Press, New York, 1992.

Mandell GL, et al., Principles and Practice of Infectious Disease, 3rd Ed., New York, Churchill Livingston, 1990.

The Medical Letter on Drugs and Therapeutics, Handbook of Antimicrobial Therapy, New Rochelle, N.Y, The Medical Letter, 1993.

Mitscher LA, The Chemistry of Tetracycline Antibiotics, New York, Decker, 1978.

Mitscher LA, Georg GI and Motohashi N, "Antibiotic and Antimicrobial Drugs," in DF Smith, Ed., Handbook of Stereoisomers: Therapeutic Drugs, Boca Raton, FL., CRC Press, 1989.

Morin RB and Gorman M, Eds., Chemistry and Biology of Beta-lactam Antibiotics, Volumes 1–3., New York, Academic Press, 1982.

Nagarajan R (Ed.), Glycopeptide antibiotics, New York, Marcel Dekker, 1994.

Omura S, Ed., Macrolide Antibiotics, New York, Academic Press, 1984.

Perlman D, Ed., Structure Activity Relationships among the Semisynthetic Antibiotics, New York, Academic Press, 1977.

Plempel M and Otten H, Walter/Heilmeyerís Antibiotika Fibel: Antibiotika und Chemotherapie, 5 th Ed., Stuttgart, Georg Thieme Verlag, 1982.

Pratt WB, Fundamentals of Chemotherapy, New York, Oxford University Press, 1973.

Rosebury T, Microbes and Morals, New York, Balantine Books, 1976.

Ryan F, The Forgotten Plague: How the Battle Against Tuberculosis was Won-and Lost, Boston, Little, Brown and Co., 1993.

Sheehan JC The Enchanted Ring: The Untold Story of Penicillin, Cambridge, MA., MIT Press, 1982. G. W. Stewart, The Penicillin Group of Drugs, Amsterdam, Elsevier, 1965.

Sutcliffe J and Georgopapadakou NH, Eds., Emerging Targets in Antibacterial and Antifungal Chemotherapy, New York, Chapman and Hall, 1992.

Umezawa H, Hooper IR, eds. Aminoglycoside Antibiotics. In: Handbook of Experimental Pharmacology. New York: Springer-Verlag, 1982:62.

Verderame M. ed. Handbook of Chemotherapeutic Agents, Vols. 1, 2, Boca Raton, Fl.: CRC Press, 1986:1–2.

Whelton A, Neu HC, eds. The Aminoglycosides. New York: Dekker, 1982.

Wolfson JS, Hooper DC, eds. Quinolone Antimicrobial Agents. 2nd ed. Washington, D.C.: American Society for Microbiology, 1993.

Zinsser H. Rats, Lice and History. Boston: Little, Brown and Co., 1950.

35. Antiparasitic Agents

THOMAS L. LEMKE

GENERAL CONSIDERATION

An introduction to the topic of parasitic diseases usually emphasize two points. First, parasitic infections affect huge numbers of individuals. It is estimated that well over one billion people are infected worldwide. Secondly, the majority of these parasitic infections are found in developing nations, nations in which the cost of health care is the dominant factor which determines whether the patient is treated or not treated. The incidence of some parasitic diseases may exceed 80% of the population. The high cost of drug discovery and the low incidence of many of the parasitic infections in affluent western countries have combined to reduce the incentive for both the study of the diseases and the development of effective therapy. This may be changing due to global travel, improved communications, and the growth of the developing countries leading to an increased demand for more effective treatments.

The diseases associated with parasitic infections represent a large and diverse number of conditions, some common and some relatively unheard of by the general population. Included under the title of parasitic infections are the numerous types of protozoal infections: amebiasis, giardiasis, babesiosis, Chagas' disease, leishmaniasis, malaria, sleeping sickness, toxoplasmosis, trichomoniasis, and pneumocystosis (also considered a fungal infection). Helminth infections (worms) are also considered parasitic infections and may be caused by any of three classes of helminths: nematode, cestode and trematode infections. Insect infections such as scabies, lice (pediculosis) and chiggers are also considered parasitic infections.

PROTOZOAL DISEASES
Amebiasis

Amebiasis is a disease of the large intestine caused by *Entamoeba histolytica*. The disease occurs mainly in the tropics, but may also be seen in temperate climates. Amebiasis may be carried without significant symptoms or may lead to severe life threatening dysentery. The organism may exist in one of two forms, the motile trophozoite form or the dormant cyst form. The trophozoite form is found in the intestine or wall of the colon and may be expelled from the body with the stools. The cyst form is encased by a chitinous wall which protects the organism from the environment including chlorine used in water purification and thus the organism may be transmitted through contaminated water and foods. It is the cyst form that is responsible for transmission of the disease. The cyst is spread by direct person-to-person contact and is commonly associated with living conditions in which poor personal hygiene, poor sanitation, poverty and ignorance exist. The hosts may be rendered susceptible to infection by preexisting conditions such as protein malnutrition, pregnancy, HIV infection, or high carbohydrate intake. Under these conditions the organism is capable of invading body tissue. The protozoal invasion is not well understood but it does appear to involve the processes indicated in Table 35.1. Symptoms may range from intermittent diarrhea (foul-smelling loose/watery stools) and tenderness and enlargement of the liver (with extraintestinal form) to acute amoebic dysentery. Many patients may experience no symptoms and the organism remains in the bowels as a commensal organism.

Giardiasis

Giardiasis is a disease which shows considerable similarity to amebiasis. It is caused by *Giardia lamblia,* an organism which may be found in the duodenum and jejunum. The organism exists in a motile trophozoite form and an infectious cyst form. The cyst form can be deposited in water (lives up to 2 months) and the contaminated water may then be ingested by the human. The trophozoite, if expelled from the G.I. normally will not survive. *G. lamblia* is the single most common cause of water borne diarrhea in the United States. Giardiasis is a common disease among campers who drink water from contaminated streams. It may also be spread between family members, children in day care centers, and dogs and their masters. The organism can attach to the mucosal wall via a ventral sucking disk and similar to amebiasis the patient may be asymptomatic or develop watery diarrhea, abdominal cramps, distention and flatulence, anorexia, nausea and vomiting. Usually the condition is self limiting in one to four weeks.

Trichomoniasis

Trichomoniasis is a protozoal infection caused by *Trichomonas vaginalis* which exists only in a trophozoite form.

Table 35.1. Entamoeba Histolytica Invasion of Host

Intestinal form	a. Disintegration of cyst wall in small intestine
	b. Movement of trophozoited into the colon
	c. Adhesion of trophozoite to cells of the host which involves a change in composition and production of mucus
Extraintestinal form	d. Penetration of intestinal lining and entrance into portal circulation form
	e. Invasion of liver tissue

Organisms Which Commonly Cause Vaginitis

Vaginitis may also be caused by *Hemophilis vaginalis* (bacteria) or *Candida albicans* (fungus) which are treated differently from the protozoal infection.

The organs most commonly involved in the infection include the vagina, urethra and prostate and thus the disease is considered a venereal infection. The condition is transmitted by sexual contact and it is estimated that trichomoniasis affects 180 million individuals worldwide. Infections in the male may be asymptomatic while in the female the symptoms may consist of: vaginitis; profuse discharge which is foul smelling; burning and soreness upon urination; and vulvar itching. Diagnosis is based upon microscopic identification of the organism in fluids from the vagina, prostate, or urethra.

Leishmaniasis

Leishmaniasis is a disease caused by a number of protozoa in the genus *Leishmania*. The protozoa may be harbored in diseased rodents, canines and various other mammals, transmitted from the infected mammal to man by bites from female sandflies of the genus *Phlehotomus*, and then appearing in one of four major clinical syndromes: visceral leishmaniasis, cutaneous leishmaniasis, mucocutaneous leishmaniasis, or diffuse cutaneous leishmaniasis. The sandfly, the vector involved in spreading the disease, breeds in warm, humid climates and thus the disease is more common in the tropics. As many as 12 million individuals, worldwide are infected by this organism.

The visceral leishmaniasis, also known as Kalaz azar (black fever), is caused by *Leishmania donovani*. This form of the disease is systemic and is characterized in patients by fever, typically nocturnal, diarrhea, cough, and enlarged liver and spleen. Without treatment death may occur in 20 months and is commonly associated with diarrhea, superinfections, or gastrointestinal hemorrhage. The disease is most commonly found in Africa and countries boarding the Mediterranean, but may also be found in China, Latin America and Russia.

The cutaneous and monocutaneous leishmaniasis is characterized by single or multiple localized lesions. These slow-healing and possibly painful ulcers can lead to secondary bacterial infections. The old world cutaneous leishmaniasis is caused by *L. topica* found most commonly in children and young adults, in regions boarding the Mediterranean, the Middle East, Southern Russia and India. *L. major* is endemic to desert areas in Africa, the Middle East and Russia, while *L. aethiopica* is found in Kenyan highlands and Ethiopia. The new world disease caused by *L. peruviana*, *L. braziliensis*, *L. panamensis* is found in South and Central America while *L. mexicana* may be endemic to south-central Texas. The incubation period for cutaneous leishmaniasis ranges from a few weeks to several months. The slow-healing lesions may be seen on the skin in vari-

ous regions of the body depending on the specific strain of organism. Usually these conditions exhibit spontaneous healing, but this may also occur over an extended period of time (1–2 years).

Pneumocystis

The organism responsible for pneumocystis (pneumocystosis, PCP) in humans is *Pneumocystis carinii*. It has the morphologic characteristics of a protozoan (i.e., lack of ergosterol in its cell membrane) but its rRNA and mitochondrial DNA pattern resembles that of fungi. Acute pneumocystis rarely strikes healthy individuals, although the organism is harbored in a wide variety of animals and most humans without any apparent adverse effect. *P. carinii* becomes active only in those individuals who have a serious impairment of their immune systems. Thus, the organism is considered an opportunistic pathogen. More recently, this disease has appeared in AIDS patients, 80% of whom ultimately contract *P. carinii* pneumonia (PCP), as one of the main causes of death. The disease also occurs in those receiving immunosuppressive drugs to prevent rejection following organ transplantation or for the treatment of malignant disease. Pneumocystis is seen in malnourished infants whose immunologic systems are impaired. The disease is thought to be transmitted via an airborne route. The disease is characterized by a severe pneumonia caused by a rapid multiplication of the organisms almost exclusively in lung tissue with the organism lining the walls of the alveoli and gradually filling the alveolar spaces. Untreated, the acute form of the disease is generally fatal. Even patients who recover from pneumocystosis are at risk of recurrent episodes. AIDS patients experience approximately a 50% recurrence rate.

Trypanosomiasis

There are two distinct forms of trypanosomiasis: Chagas' disease and African sleeping sickness.

Chagas' Disease

Chagas' disease, also known as American trypanosomiasis, is caused by the parasitic protozoa *Trypanosoma cruzi* and is found only in the Americas, primarily in Brazil, but may be found in the southern states of the U.S. The protozoa lives in mammals and is spread by the blood sucking insect known as the reduviid bug, assassin bug, or kissing bug. The insect becomes infected by drawing blood from an infected mammal and releases the protozoa with discharged feces. The pathogen then enters the new host through breaks in the skin. Inflammatory lesions are seen at the site of entry. The disease may also be spread through transfusion with contaminated blood. Signs of initial infection may include malaise, fever, anorexia and skin edema at the site where the protozoa entered the host. The disease may ultimately invade the heart where after decades of infection with chronic Chagas' disease the patient may experience an infection associated heart attack.

It is estimated that 5% of the Salvadorian and Nicaraguan immigrants to the U.S. may have chronic Chagas' disease.

African Trypanosomiasis

African trypanosomiasis, sleeping sickness, is caused by several subspecies of *Trypanosoma brucei*. (*T. brucei rhodesiense*—east African sleeping sickness and *T. brucei gambiense*—west African sleeping sickness). In this case the infected animal is bitten by the blood sucking tsetse fly which in turn transmits the protozoa via inoculation during a subsequent biting of a human. The protozoa, initially present in the gut of the vector appears in the salivary gland for inoculation during the subsequent biting of a human. It is estimated that some 50 million people are at risk of African sleeping sickness. The infection progresses through two stages. Stage I may present as fever and high temperatures lasting several days. Hematologic and immunologic changes occur during this stage. Stage II occurs after the organism enters the CNS and may involve symptoms suggesting the disease name—daytime somnolence, as well as loss of spontaneity, halting speech, listless gaze and extrapyramidal signs such as tremors and choreiform movements.

It should be noted that the sole source of energy for the trypanosomal organism is glycolysis which in turn may account for the hypoglycemia seen in the host. In addition, the migration of the organism into the CNS may be associated with the organism's search for a rich source of available glucose.

Malaria

Malaria is transmitted by the infected female Anopheles mosquito. The specific protozoan organisms causing malaria are from the genus *Plasmodium*. Only four of approximately 100 species cause malaria in humans. The remaining species affect birds, monkeys, livestock, rodents, and reptiles. The four species that affect humans are: *Plasmodium falciparum, P. vivax, P. malariae,* and *P. ovale.* Concurrent infections by more than one of these species are seen in endemically affected regions of the world. Such multiple infections further complicate patient management and the choice of treatment regimens.

Malaria affects as many as 300 million humans globally, and causes more than 1 million deaths annually. It is estimated that a third of these fatalities occur in children under 5 years old. Although this disease is found primarily in the tropics and subtropics, it has been observed far beyond these boundaries.

Malaria has essentially been eradicated in most temperate-zone countries. However, more than 1000 cases of malaria were documented recently in United States' citizens returning from travel abroad. Today, malaria is found in most countries in Africa, Central and South America, and Southeast Asia. It is reported to be on the increase in Afghanistan, Bangladesh, Brazil, Burma, Cambodia, Colombia, China, Iran, India, Indonesia, Mexico, the Philippines, Thailand, and Vietnam. Infection from Plasmodia can cause anemia, pulmonary edema, renal failure, jaundice, shock, cerebral malaria, and, if not treated in a timely manner, can result in death.

Types of Malaria

Malarial infections are known according to the species of the parasite involved.

Plasmodium Falciparum. *Plasmodium falciparum* infection has an incubation period (time from mosquito bite to clinical symptoms) of 1–3 weeks (average of 12 days). The *P. falciparum* life cycle in man begins with the bite of an infected female mosquito. The parasites in the sporozoite stage enter the circulatory system through which they can reach the liver in about an hour. These organisms grow and multiply 30,000–40,000-fold by asexual division within liver cells in 5–7 days. Then, as merozoites, they leave the liver to re-enter the blood stream and invade the erythrocytes, red blood cells (RBCs), where they continue to grow and multiply further for 1–3 days. Specific receptors on the surface of the erythrocytes serve as binding sites for the merozoite. These infected RBCs rupture, releasing merozoites in intervals of about 48 hours. Chemicals released by the ruptured cell in turn cause activation and release of additional substances associated with the patients symptoms. The clinical symptom include chills, fever, sweating, headaches, fatigue, anorexia, nausea, vomiting, and diarrhea. Some of the released merozoites are sequestered in vital organs (brain and heart) where they continue to grow. Recurrence of the clinical symptoms on alternate days leads to the terminology of tertian malaria. The *P. falciparum* parasite can also cause RBCs to clump and adhere to the wall of blood vessels. Such a phenomenon has been known to cause partial obstruction and sometimes restriction of the blood flow to vital organs like the brain, liver, and kidneys. Reinfection of RBCs can occur, allowing further multiplication and remanifestation of the malaria symptoms. Some merozoites develop into male and female sexual forms, called gametocytes, which can then be acquired by the female mosquito after biting the infected human. Gametocytes mature in the mosquito's stomach to form zygotes. Growth of the zygotes leads to formation of oocysts (spherical structures located on the outside wall of the stomach). Sporozoites develop from the oocysts, are released into the body cavity of the mosquito, and migrate to the salivary gland of the insect from which they can be transmitted to another human following a mosquito bite. The life cycle of the malaria parasites is shown in the Figure 35.1.

Plasmodium Vivax. *Plasmodium vivax* (benign tertian) is the most prevalent form of malaria. It has an incubation period of 1–4 weeks (2 weeks average). This form of malaria can cause spleen rupture and anemia. Relapses (renewed manifestations of erythrocytic infection) can occur. This

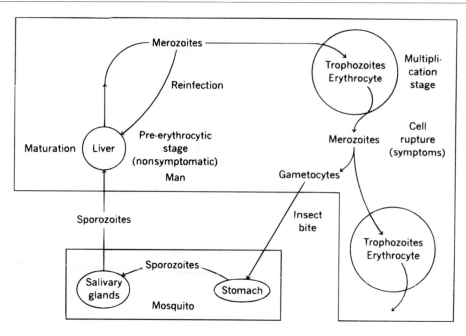

Fig. 35.1. Life cycle of malarial protozoa.

results from the periodic release of dormant parasites (hypnozoites) from the liver cells. The erythrocytic forms are generally considered to be susceptible to treatment.

Plasmodium Malariae. *Plasmodium malariae* is responsible for quartan malaria. It has an incubation period of 2–4 weeks (average of 3 weeks). The asexual cycle occurs every 72 hours. In addition to the usual symptoms, this form also causes nephritis. This is the mildest form of malaria and does not relapse. The RBC infection associated with *P. malariae* can last for many years. The *P. malariae* is quite unlikely to become resistant.

Plasmodium Ovale. *Plasmodium ovale* has an incubation period of 9–18 days (14 days average). Relapses have been known to occur in individuals infected with this plasmodium. The relapse may be indicative of ovale tertian malaria and is associated with the ability of the organism to lie dormant in hepatic tissue for extended periods of time.

Types of Chemotherapy

Tissue Schizonticides. These drugs eradicate the exoerythrocytic liver-tissue stages of the parasite which prevents the parasite's entry into the blood. Drugs of this type are useful for prophylaxis. Some tissue schizonticides can act on the long-lived tissue form (hypnozoites of *P. vivax* and *P. ovale*), and thus can prevent relapses.

Blood Schizonticides. These drugs destroy the erythrocytic stages of parasites and can cure cases of falciparum malaria or suppress relapses. This is the easiest phase to treat because drug delivery into the blood stream can be accomplished rapidly.

Gametocytocides. Agents of this type kill the sexual forms of the plasmodia (gametocytes), which are transmittable to the Anopheles mosquito, thereby preventing transmission of the disease.

Sporontocides (sporozooiticides). These drugs act against sporozoites and are capable of killing these organisms as soon as they enter the bloodstream following a mosquito bite.

It should be noted that antimalarials may operate against more than one form of the organism, and may be effective against one species of plasmodium but lack efficacy against others. In addition, antimalarial drugs may be classified according to their structural types.

GENERAL APPROACHES TO PROTOZOAL THERAPY
Amebiasis and Giardiasis

The most appropriate approach for treatment of this type of protozoal infection is through prevention. Since the infection usually occurs by consumption of contaminated drinking water and food, avoidance is the key to prevention. Drinking bottled water, boiling or disinfecting the water will reduce the risk. Improvement in personal hygiene and general sanitation are also beneficial.

Leishmaniasis, Malaria, and Trypanosomiasis

For these diseases that are spread by insect vectors, the use of insecticides, protective clothing, and insect repellents can greatly reduce the incidence of the disease. Unfortunately, many of these protozoal infections can also infect other hosts beside man and thus even the most successful insect irradiation methods cannot destroy all the reservoirs of the protozoa. While use of insect repellents and protective clothing may be useful for visitors to regions with endemic infections, these procedures may prove ineffective for those living in the area. For such individuals early detection and drug therapy is the method of treatment.

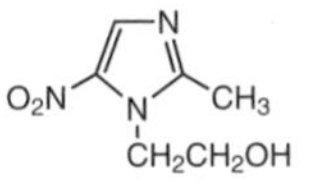

Metronidazole

DRUG THERAPY OF PROTOZOAL INFECTIONS
Treatment of Amebiasis, Giardiasis, and Trichomoniasis
Metronidazole (Flagyl, Metryl, Satric)

Metronidazole was initially introduced for the treatment of vaginal infections caused by *T. vaginalis*, but since has been shown to be effective for treatment of amebiasis, giardiasis, and anaerobic bacterial infections including *Clostridium difficile* .

Mechanism of Action. Despite the availability of metronidazole since the late 1950s, the mechanism of action of the drug is still unknown. It is generally agreed that metronidazole is a pro-drug and that anaerobic organisms reduce the nitro group in metronidazole to a hydroxylamine, as shown in Figure 35.2, during which a reactive derivative or reactive species are produced which cause destructive effects on cell components (DNA, proteins, membranes). Specifically, DoCampo, et al. (1) have reported that nitroaryl compounds (nitroimidazoles—metronidazole; nitrofurans—nifurtomox) are reduced to nitro radical anions which in turn reacts with oxygen to regenerate the nitroaryl and the superoxide radical anion (Fig. 35.3). Further reduction of superoxide radical anion leads to hydrogen peroxide and homolytic cleavage of the latter leads to hydroxyl radical formation. Superoxide radical anion, hydrogen peroxide, and hydroxyl radicals are referred to as reactive oxygen species (ROS) and are the reactive substances which are implicated in damage to critical cellular components of the parasite.

Metabolism. Liver metabolism of metronidazole leads to two major metabolites, hydroxylation of the 2-methyl group to 2-hydroxymethylmetronidazole (HM) and oxidation to metronidazole acetic acid (MAA) (2). Both compounds possess biologic activity. HM is also found in the urine as glucuronide and sulfate conjugates. In addition, a small amount of metronidazole is oxidized to acetamide, a known carcinogen in rats but not in humans, and the oxalate derivative shown in Figure 35.4 (3).

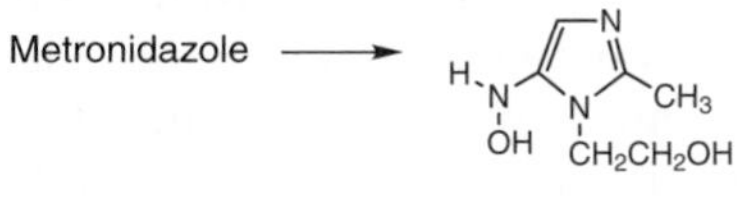

Metronidazole ⟶

Fig. 35.2. Metabolic activation of metronidazole.

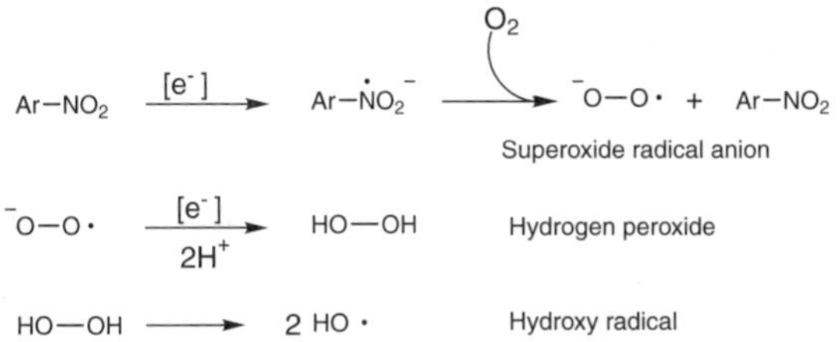

Fig. 35.3. Formation of ROS from nitroaryl compounds.

Pharmacokinetics (2). Metronidazole is available in a variety of dosage forms including IV, PO, rectal, and vaginal suppositories. The bioavailability of metronidazole is nearly 100% when administered orally, but significantly less when administered via the rectal route (67–82%) or vaginal route (19–56%). The drug is not bound to plasma protein. Distribution of the drug is fairly uniform through out the body including mother's milk.

Metronidazole Analog

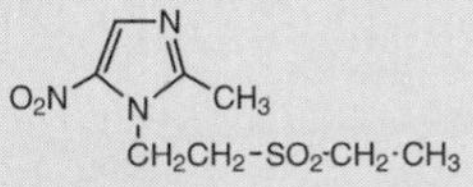

Tinidazole

Although not available in the U.S., tinidazole is an analog of metronidazole which is reported to be effective for treatment of giardiasis and trichomoniasis.

Therapeutic Application. Metronidazole is considered the drug of choice for treatment for the protozoal infections amebiasis, intestinal and extraintestinal, giardiasis, and trichomoniasis (4). It is the drug of choice for treatment of the gram-positive bacilli *Clostridium difficile* and in combination is an alternative therapy for *Helicobacter pylori* infections (5). The common side effects exhibited with metronidazole include abdominal distress, a metallic taste, and a disulfiram-like effect if taken with alcohol. The drug is reported to be carcinogenic in mice, possibly related to the metabolite acetamide, and as a result should not be used during the first trimester of pregnancy.

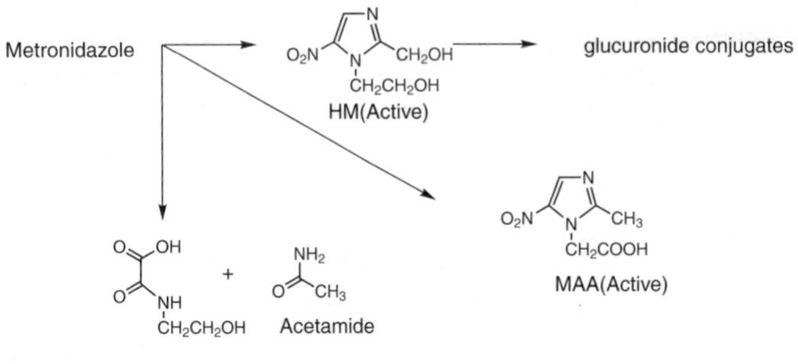

Metronidazole ⟶ HM(Active) ⟶ glucuronide conjugates

Acetamide

MAA(Active)

Fig. 35.4. Metabolism of metronidazole.

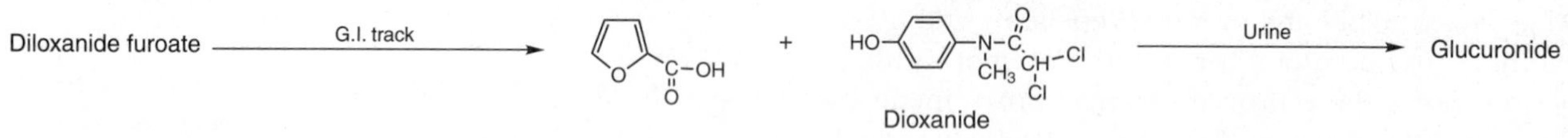

Fig. 35.5. Products formed from diloxanide furoate.

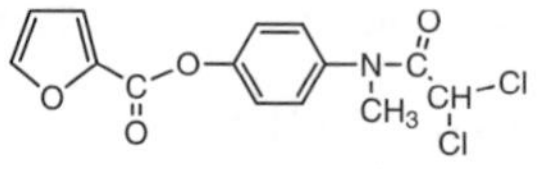

Diloxanide furoate

Diloxanide Furoate

Diloxanide furoate (available from the CDC) is pre-scribed for the treatment of asymptomatic amebiasis, but is ineffective as a single agent for the extraintestinal form of the disease. The drug is administered orally and is hy-drolyzed in the gut to give diloxanide which is considered the active drug. Diloxanide is the only form identified in the blood stream. The drug is found in the urine as the glucuronide (see Fig. 35.5).

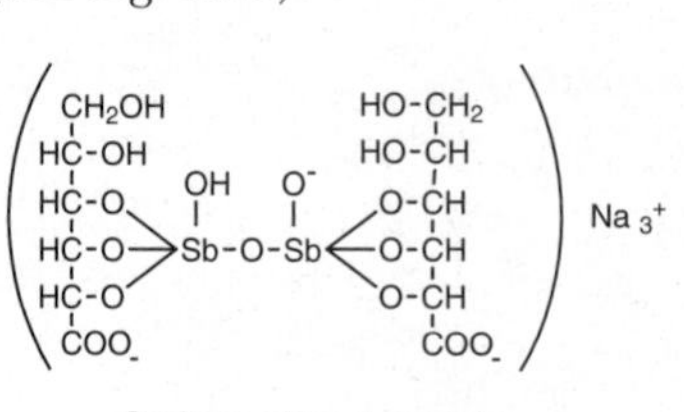

Sodium stibogluconate

Treatment of Leishmaniasis
Sodium Stibogluconate (Pentostam available from the CDC)

Leishmaniasis was first described in the medical litera-ture by deishman and Donovan in 1903 and shortly after that the use of antimony based drugs were introduced as therapeutic agents to treat the condition (6). Although the structure of sodium stibogluconate is commonly drawn as shown the actual compound is probably much more com-plex. The drug is a water soluble preparation which is ad-ministered IM or IV. Pentavalent antimony compounds are thought to inhibit bioenergetic processes in the pathogen with catabolism of glucose and inhibition of glycolytic en-zymes the primary site of action (glucose catabolism is in-hibited by 86–94%). This in turn results in ATP/GTP for-mation inhibition. Sodium sibogluconate is the drug of choice for treatment of most forms of leishmaniasis (or meglumine antimonate another pentavalent antimony agent). The recommended dose is 20 mg/kg of anti-mony/day not to exceed 850 mg of antimony/day. A num-ber of other drugs have been reported to be effective in the treatment of leishmaniasis and these include: pentami-dine, amphotericin B, rifampicin, and ketoconazole (7).

Treatment of Pneumocystis (PCP)(8)
Sulfamethoxazole—Trimethoprim; Co-trimoxazole (Bactrim, Septra, Cotrim)

The combination of sulfamethoxazole-trimethoprim has proven to be the most successful method for treatment and

prophylaxis of pneumocystis in AIDS patients. This combi-nation was first reported as effective in PCP in 1975 and by 1980 had become the preferred method of treatment with a response rate of 65–94%. *P. carinii* appears to be especially susceptible to the sequential blocking action of cotrimazole which inhibits both the incorporation of para aminoben-zoic acid into folic acid as well as the reduction of dihydro-folic acid to tetrahydrofolic acid by dihydrofolate reductase. A detailed discussion of the mechanism of action and struc-ture-activity relationship of these drugs can be found in Chapter 34. Depending on the severity of the infection the combination is administered in doses of 20 mg/kg/day of trimethoprim and 100 mg/kg/day of sulfamethoxazole in four divided doses over a period of 14–21 days.

Orphan Drug Product

Dapsone plus trimethoprim has also been utilized for treatment of pneumocystis with effectiveness nearly equal to cotrimazole.

Pentamidine Isethionate (Pentam 300, Nebupent)

Pentamidine is available as the water soluble isethio-nate salt which is used both intravenously and as an aerosol. The drug has fungicidal and antiprotozoal activ-ity, but today is used primarily for treatment of PCP.

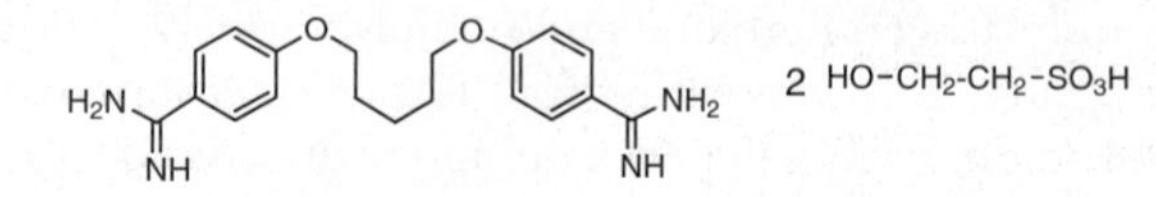

Pentamidine isethionate

Mechanism of Action. While the mechanism of action of pentamidine is not know with certainty, there is strong evidence supporting various mechanisms of action for pentamidine. Pentamidine selectively binds to the DNA in trypanosoma parasite (see below). Pentamidine has been shown to inhibit topoisomerase in *P. carinii* and leading to double strand cleavage of DNA in trypanosoma (9–11). It has been suggested that pentamidine's mechanism of action may be different in different organisms.

Pharmacokinetics. Pentamidine must be adminis-tered IV and after multiple injections daily or on alter-nate days accumulates in body tissue. Plasma concen-trations were measured up to 8 months following a single 2 hour IV infusion. The accumulation aids in treatment as well as prophylaxis. The drug shows poor penetration of the CNS.

Therapeutic Application. Pentamidine is used as a second line agent by itself or in combination for treatment and prophylaxis of PCP. For prophylaxis the aerosol form of the drug is indicated and has minimum toxicity. The limitation of pentamidine, that is the need for IV administration, may be associated with the potential for severe toxicity which includes; breathlessness, tachycardia, dizziness, headache and vomiting. These symptoms may occur in as many as 50% of the patients. These effects are thought to be associated with a too rapid IV administration resulting in the release of histamine.

Atovaquone

Atovaquone (Mepron)

Atovaquone, a chemical with structural similarity to the ubiquinone metabolites, was initially synthesized and investigated as an antimalarial. Although active against Plasmodium, its usefulness is primarily directed toward treatment of PCP.

Mechanism of Action. Atovaquone is thought to produce its antiparasitic action by virtue of its ability to inhibit the mitochondrial respiratory chain. More specifically, atovaquone is an ubiquinone reductase inhibitor, inhibiting at the cytochrome bc₁ complex (12). The compound shows stereospecific inhibition with the *trans* isomer being more active than the *cis* isomer.

Pharmacokinetics. Atovaquone is poorly absorbed from the GI tract due to its poor water solubility and high fat solubility, but the absorption can be significantly increased if taken with a fat rich meal. The drug is highly bound to plasma protein (94%) and does not enter the CNS in significant quantities. It is not significantly metabolized in humans and is exclusively eliminated in feces via the bile.

Therapeutic Applications. With as many as 70% of the AIDS patients developing pneumocystis and of these nearly 60% of the patients on co-trimoxazole developing serious side effects to this combination, atovaquone is an important alternative drug (13). Atovaquone has also been reported to be effective for the treatment of toxoplasmosis caused by *Toxoplasma gondii* although it has not been approved for this use.

Suramin Sodium

Treatment of Trypanosomiasis (14)
Suramin Sodium (Available from the CDC)

Introduced into therapy for the treatment of early trypanosomiasis in the 1920s, suramin, a bis hexasulfonated-naphthylurea is still considered the drug of choice for treatment of non-CNS associated African trypanosomiasis.

Mechanism of Action. The mechanism of action of suramin is unproven, but it is known that the drug has a high affinity for binding to a number of critical enzymes in the pathogen. Among the enzymes to which suramin has been shown to bind are several dehydrogenases and kinases. As a result of binding suramin has been shown to be an inhibitor of dihydrofolate reductase, a crucial enzyme in folate metabolism, and thymidine kinase. In addition, suramin is an inhibitor of glycolytic enzymes in *T. brucei* with binding constants much lower than those seen in mammalian cells. Inhibition of glycolysis would be expected to block energy sources of the pathogen leading to lysis. As to whether one or more of these inhibitor actions represent the toxic action of suramin on the pathogen remains unproven.

Pharmacokinetics. Suramin sodium is a water soluble compound which is poorly absorbed via oral administration and must be administered by IV in multiple injections. Because of it highly ionic nature suramin will not cross the blood-brain barrier and therefore is ineffective for treatment of trypanosomal infections which reach the CNS. In addition, suramin is tightly bound to serum albumin. Despite this binding, the drug is preferentially absorbed by trypanosomes through a receptor-mediated endocytosis of serum protein. Because the drug remains in the blood stream for an extended period of time, suramin has value as a prophylactic drug.

Therapeutic Application. Seramin sodium is effective against east African trypanosomiasis, but has limited value again west African trypanosomiasis. As indicated, since the drug will not enter the CNS the drug is only useful for treatment of early stages of the disease. The drug exhibits a wide variety of side effects which can be severe in debilitated individuals and include nausea, vomiting and fatigue.

Pentamidine, Isethionate (Pentam 300, Nebupent)

First introduced into therapy for treatment of trypanosomiasis in 1937, pentamidine is now used in a variety of protozoal and fungal infections and as such finds use in treatment of trypanosomiasis, leishmaniasis and pneumocystis (PCP). The drug is primarily used for treatment of PCP. When used for trypanosomiasis, pentamidine is only effective against *T. brucei rhodesiense*-east African sleeping sickness and only in the early stage of the disease since it does not readily cross the blood-brain barrier.

Mechanism of Action. As indicated above, several biochemical actions have been reported for pentamidine.

The drug has been shown to bind to DNA through hydrogen bonding of the amidine proton and AT rich regions of DNA. More specifically, pentamidine binds to the N3 of adenine, spans four to five base pairs, and binds to a second adenine to form interstrand cross bonding (9). In addition and possibly separate from this action, pentamidine appears to be a potent inhibitor of type II topoisomerase of mitochondria DNA (kinetoplast-kDNA) of the trypanosoma parasite (10). The mitochondrial DNA is a cyclic DNA. This inhibition leads to double stand breaks in the DNA and linearization of the DNA. The relationship between binding to specific regions of the DNA and inhibition of topoisomerase is unclear.

In the case of *T. Brucei* resistant strains are common. It is thought that resistance develops through an inability of the drug to reach the mitochondrial DNA. Transport into the mitochondria is a carrier-mediated process with the absence of carrier in the resistant strains.

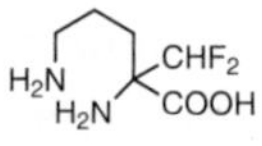

Eflornithine

Eflornithine (Ornidyl)

Metcalf, et al. reported the synthesis of eflornithine (difluoromethyl ornithine, DFMO) in 1978 (15). Their interest arose from the desire to prepare ornithine decarboxylase inhibitors as tools for studying the role of polyamines as regulators of growth processes. Ornithine decarboxylase (ODC) catalyzes the conversion of ornithine to putrescine (1,4-diaminobutane) which in turn leads to the formation of the polyamines, spermine and spermidine. It wasn't until 1980 that Bacchi demonstrated the potential of DFMO in the treatment of trypanosomiasis (16).

Mechanism of Action. DFMO is a suicide inhibitor of ODC, a pyridoxal phosphate dependent enzyme, as shown in Figure 35.6. Evidence suggests that cysteine 360 in ODC is the site of eflornithine alkylation (17). Alkylation of ODC blocks the synthesis of putrescine, the rate determining step in the synthesis of polyamines. Mammalian ODC may also be inhibited, but since the turn-over of ODC is so rapid in mammals, eflornithine does not produce serious side effects.

Pharmacokinetics. Eflornithine may be administered either by IV or PO. IV administration requires large doses and frequent dosing, while poor oral absorption and rapid excretion because of the zwitterionic nature of the drug (an amino acid) has limited this route of administration. The drug does not bind to plasma protein and enters the CNS readily most likely via an amino acid transport system. As a result the drug can be used for both early and late stages of trypanosomiasis.

Therapeutic Application. Eflornithine is indicated for the treatment of west African trypanosomiasis caused by *T. brucei gambiense*, but has proven to be ineffective against east African trypanosomiasis. The cause of this ineffectiveness remains a mystery although there is evidence suggesting that in the resistant organism that endogenous ornithine plus increased activity of S-adenosylmethionine decarboxylase allows for sufficient synthesis of spermidine and spermine to support cell division thus by-passing the need for organism synthesized ornithine (18). Side effects reported for eflornithine consist of anemia, diarrhea, and leukopenia.

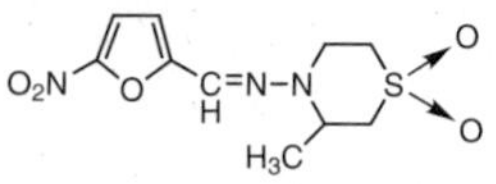

Nifurtimox

Nifurtimox (Available from the CDC)

Another of the nitroaryl compounds, nifurtimox has proven useful as a drug for the treatment of trypanosomiasis.

Mechanism of Action. As discussed for metronidazole, nifurtimox is thought to undergo reduction followed by oxidation and in the process generate ROS such as the superoxide radical anion, hydrogen peroxide, and hydroxyl radical (Fig. 35.1) (1). These species are potent oxidants which may produce damage to DNA and lipids which may affect cellular membranes. In addition, Henderson, et al. have reported that nifurtimox inhibits trypanothione reductase which results in inhibition of trypanothione formation (93% inhibition) (19). Trypanothione is a critical protective enzyme found uniquely in trypanosomal parasites.

Therapeutic Application. Nifurtimox is the drug of choice for treatment of acute Chagas' disease. The drug is

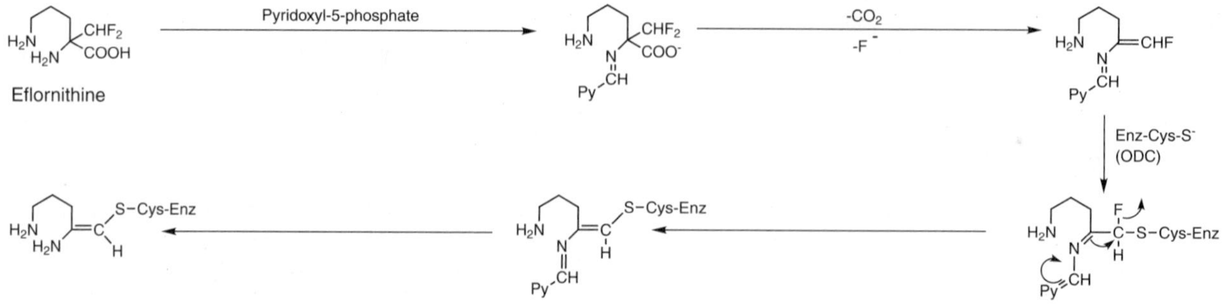

Fig. 35.6. Inhibition of Ornithine decarboxylase (Enz-Cys-SH) by eflornithine.

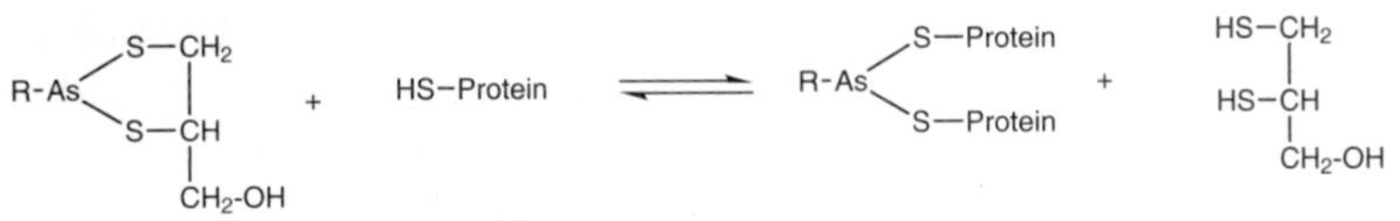

Fig. 35.7. Mechanism of action of trivalent arsenic compounds with trypanosoma organism.

not effective for the chronic stages of the disease. In the acute stage the drug has an 80% cure rate. Side effects of the drug include hypersensitivity reactions, GI complications (nausea and vomiting), myalgia, and weakness.

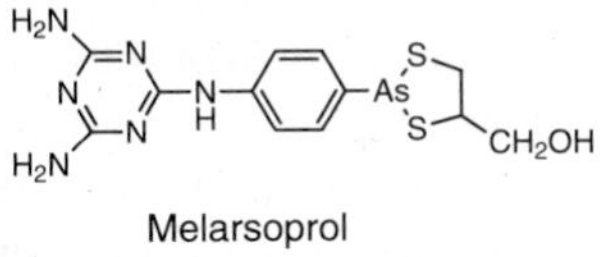

Melarsoprol

Melarsoprol (Available from the CDC)

Knowingly or unknowingly, arsenic containing drugs have been used for treatment of parasitic conditions for thousands of years. In the late 1800s and early 1900s Paul Ehrlich introduced the use of trivalent arsenicals. Melarsoprol, an organoaresenical, came into use in the late 1940s and remains today the first choice drug to treat trypanosomiasis and until 1990 was the only treatment for late stage sleeping sickness.

Mechanism of Action. It is known that trivalent arsenic reacts rapidly and reversibly with sulfhydryl containing proteins as shown in Figure 35.7. It is generally accepted that the enzyme which melarsoprol reacts with is an enzyme involved in glycolysis and as a result inhibition of pyruvate kinase occurs. It is argued though that the inhibition may not occur at pyruvate kinase, but rather at a step prior to the pyruvate kinase. Blockage of glycolysis would be expected to lead to loss of motility and cell lysis. More recently, Fairlamb has proposed a mechanism of action which results in the inhibition of trypanothione reductase through formation of a stable complex between melaroprol and typanothione (20). Melarsoprol reacts with the cysteine sulfhydryl of trypanothione to form the stable adduct shown in Figure 35.8. Supportive of this mechanism is the synergistic action of melarsoprol with eflornithine (DMFO). Two drugs which produce sequential blockage of the synthesis of trypanothione.

Pharmacokinetics. Melarsoprol is administered by IV in multiple doses and multiple sessions. Its major metabolite in humans is the lipophilic melarsen oxide which can penetrate into the CNS. This metabolite apparently is responsible for the protein binding characteristic for melarsoprol.

Therapeutic Application. Melarsoprol is the drug of choice for treatment of late stage meningoencephalitic trypanosomiasis caused by west and east African strains of the disease. Since the drug has the potential for serious nervous system toxicities (convulsions, acute cerebral edema,

coma) the drug is usually administered in a hospital setting with supervision. An additional problem with melarsoprol is the development of resistance by the parasite.

Treatment of Malaria

Quinine (Fig. 35.9), was the first known antimalarial. It is a 4-quinolinemethanol derivative bearing a substituted quinuclidine ring. The use of quinine in Europe began in the 17th century, after the Incas of Peru informed the Spanish Jesuits of the antimalarial properties of the bark of an evergreen mountain tree they called quinquina [later called cinchona after Francisco Henriquez de Ribera (1576–1639), Countess of Chinchona and wife of the Peruvian Viceroy]. The bark, when made into an aqueous solution, was capable of curing most forms of malaria. It was listed in the London Pharmacopeia of 1677. The alkaloid derived from it, quinine, was isolated in the mid-1820s. Quinine, a very bitter substance, has been used by millions of malaria sufferers. Recently it has been employed successfully to treat chloroquine-resistant strains of *P. falciparum* and is considered the drug of choice for these resistant strains.

A second class of chemicals that played a role in the development of synthetic antimalarials were the 9-aminoacridines. 9-Aminoacridine itself was known to exhibit antibacterial activity while a derivative of 9-aminoacridine, quinacrine (Fig. 35.9) synthesized in 1934, was found to possess weak antimalarial activity.

With the beginning of World War II and concern about interruption of the supply of cinchona bark from the East Indies, a massive effort was begun to search for synthetic alternatives to quinine and the development of more effective antimalarial agents than quinacrine. With a basic understanding of the structure-activity-relationship of quinine (see quinine) and the chemical similarities seen with quinacrine, it is easy to visualize the relationship between these agents and the synthetic antimalarials shown in Figure 35.9. The 4-aminoquinoline, chloroquine and hydroxychloroquine

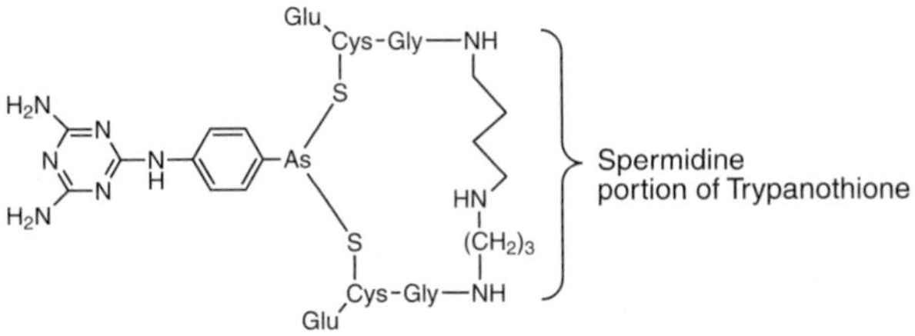

Fig. 35.8. Structure of melarsoprol trypanothione complex.

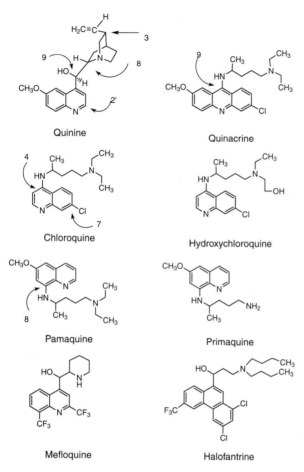

Fig. 35.9. Structures of antimalarial drugs.

intercalated into the DNA of the parasite. This mechanism was soon discarded based upon the fact that the concentration required for inhibition of nucleic acid synthesis is significantly higher than that necessary for inhibition of the plasmodium parasite.

Ferriprotoprophyrin IX. The plasmodium parasite utilizes host hemoglobin as a source of amino acids. As the result of digestion of the hemoglobin a substance referred to as hemozoin is produced as a waste product. A constituent of hemozoin is the chemical substance ferriprotoporphyrin IX (FPIX). FPIX in an unbound form is toxic to host and plasmodium cells leading to lysis of the cells. Normally, the FPIX is bound to an endogenous protein and in this bound form the FPIX is nontoxic. In the presence of 3 (and presumably the other 4-substituted quinolines) FPIX is bound to the drug, but this complex retains its toxicity toward erythrocytes and parasites. Once again there is evidence which argues against this proposed MOA.

Weak Base Hypothesis. The 4-substituted quinolines are weak bases and because of their pKa's, they are thought to accumulate in a location which is acidic (parasites lysosome pH 4.8–5.2). Because the extracellular fluid of the parasite is at pH 7.4 the weak base will move toward a more acidic pH. Once in the lysosome an acid/base reaction occurs elevating the pH in the lysosome which in turn reduces the parasite's ability to digest hemoglobin thus reducing the availability of amino acids. There is evidence to suggest that the movement of the weak bases toward a more acidic media is actually an active process requiring a transport enzyme.

These latter two mechanisms are not necessarily exclusive yet neither of them is entirely satisfactory. It is generally believed that the 4-substituted quinolines disrupt hemoglobin digestion in sensitive organisms.

Mechanism of Resistance. A limiting factor for most of the antimalarial drugs is the development of resistant strains of plasmodium. It should be noted that resistance differs from region to region and in some cases a resistant strain may develop to a particular drug without the drug ever having been introduced to the region (possible cross-resistance). The development of resistance is thought to be a spontaneous gene mutation. The mutation may lead to enhanced drug efflux thus leading to rapid removal of the drug from the organism. Since concentration of the drug within specific regions of the parasite is involved in the postulated mechanisms of action it would appear that increased efflux would reduce the effectiveness of the drugs.

Rapid metabolism of the antimalarials by resistant strains of plasmodium might also be considered to play a significant role in the development of resistance. It has been shown that cyctochrome P-450 activity parallels increased resistant to specific drugs.

(Fig. 35.9), are structurally similar to the right half of quinacrine. The 8-aminoquinoline, pamaquine and primaquine, retain the methoxyquinoline nucleus of quinine and quinacrine (Fig. 35.9). The quinoline-4-methanols, mefloquine and halofantrine, show similarity to the 4-quinolinemethanol portion of quinine (Fig. 35.9).

4-Substituted Quinolines

Five compounds may be considered within this class of drugs: quinine, chloroquine and hydroxychloroquine, mefloquine, and halofantrine (Fig. 35.9). These compounds not only share a structural similarity, but in addition are thought to have similar mechanisms of action, are effective on the same stage of the parasite, and may share similar mechanisms of resistance.

Mechanism of Action. The drug studied in most depth is chloroquine (21), but the other 4-substituted quinolines are thought to act through a similar mechanism of action. Three different mechanisms of actions have been offered at various times to explain the action of this class of drugs.

DNA Intercalation. The earliest proposal for the mechanism of action for quinine was that the drug

Therapeutic Application. The 4-substituted quinolines are referred to as rapidly acting blood schizonticides with activity against plasmodium in the erythrocytic stage. Chloroquine is the drug of choice, but unfortunately the incidence of chloroquine-resistance infections are extremely common today. The spread of chloroquine resistance has reached almost all malarious areas of the world. In addition, multidrug-resistant and cross-resistant strains of plasmodium are now common place. The drug of choice for treatment of malaria caused by *Plasmodium falciparum, P. ovale, P. vivax,* and *P. malariae* in regions infected by chloroquine-resistant *P. falciparum* is quinine with mefloquine and halofantrine as alternative treatment agents.

The 4-substituted quinolines, depending on the specific drug in question, may also be used for prophylaxis of malaria. Two types of prophylaxis are possible, causal prophylaxis and suppressive prophylaxis. The former prevents the establishment of hepatic forms of the parasite, while the latter eradicates the erythrocytic parasites but has no effect on the hepatic forms. Several of the 4-substituted quinolines are effective suppressive prophylactics.

Specific 4-substituted Quinolines

Quinine. Quinine is the most prevalent alkaloid present in the bark extracts (about 5%) of cinchona. Four stereochemical centers exist in the molecule (at C-3, C-4, C-8, and C-9) (Fig. 35-9). Quinine, absolute configuration of 3R:4S:8S:9R, and quinidine, absolute configuration of 3R:4S:8R:9S, and their optical isomers all have antimalarial activity while their C-9 epimers (i.e., the epi-series having either 3R:4S:8R:9R or 3R:4S:8S:9S configurations) are inactive. Modification of the secondary alcohol at C-9, through oxidation, esterification, or similar processes, diminishes activity. The quinuclidine portion is not necessary for activity; however, an alkyl tertiary amine at C-9 is important.

Quinine is metabolized in the liver to the 2′-hydroxy derivative, followed by additional hydroxylation on the quinuclidine ring, with the 2,2′-dihydroxy derivative as the major metabolite. This metabolite has low activity and is rapidly excreted. The metabolizing enzyme of quinine is CYP3A4. With the increased use of quinine and its use in combination with other drugs, the potential for drug interactions based upon the many known substrates for CYP3A4 (see Chapter 8) is of concern (22).

A quinine overdose causes tinnitus and visual disturbances; these side effects disappear on discontinuation of the drug. Quinine can also cause premature contractions in late stages of pregnancy. Although quinine is suitable for parenteral administration, this route is considered hazardous because of its ability to cause hemolysis. Quinidine, the (+) isomer of quinine, has been shown to be more effective in combating the disease, but it has undesirable cardiac side effects.

Chloroquine (Aralen). Chloroquine is the most effective of the hundreds of 4-aminoquinolines synthesized and tested

during World War II as potential antimalarials. Structure-activity relationships demonstrated that the chloro at the eight position increased activity while alkylation at C-3 and C-8 diminished activity. The replacement of one of its N-Ethyl groups with an hydroxyethyl produced hydroxychloroquin, a compound with reduced toxicity, which is rarely used today, except in rheumatoid arthritis.

Chloroquine is commonly administered as the racemic mixture since little is gained by using the individual isomers. The drug is well absorbed from the GI tract and distributed to many tissues where it is tightly bound and slowly eliminated. The drug is metabolized by N-dealkylation by CYP2D6 and CYP3A4 isoforms. It has been reported that the level of metabolism correlates closely with the degree of resistance. The suggestion has been made to co-administer chloroquine with CYP2D6 and CYP3A4 inhibitors to potentiate activity and reduce resistance. While this may be possible it is not commonly practiced.

Chloroquine is an excellent suppressive agent for treating acute attacks of malaria caused by *P. vivax* and *P. ovale.* The drug is also effective for cure and as a suppressive prophylactic for treatment of *P. malariae* and susceptible *P. falciparum.*

Chloroquine is generally a safe drug with toxicity occurring with high doses of medication if the drug is administered too rapidly via parenteral routes. With oral administration the side effects are primarily gastrointestinal, mild headache, visual disturbances, and urticaria.

Additional Therapeutic Indications for Chloroquine

Chloroquine is also prescribed for treatment of rheumatoid arthritis, discoid lupus erythematosus and photosensitivity diseases.

Mefloquine (Lariam) (23). Mefloquine synthesized with the intent of blocking the site of metabolism in quinine with the chemically stable CF_3 group, exists as four optical isomers of nearly equal activity. The drug is active against chloroquine-resistant strains of plasmodium and yet cross-resistance is not uncommon. Metabolism is cited as the possible mechanism of resistance. Mefloquine is slowly metabolized through CYP3A4 oxidation to its major inactive metabolite, carboxymefloquine (Fig. 35.10). Most of the parent drug is excreted unchanged into the urine. Its co-administration with CYP3A4 inhibitors (e.g., ketoconazole) has increased the AUC for mefloquine by inhibiting its metabolism to carboxymefloquine.

Mefloquine is only available in an oral dosage form which is well absorbed. The presence of food in the GI

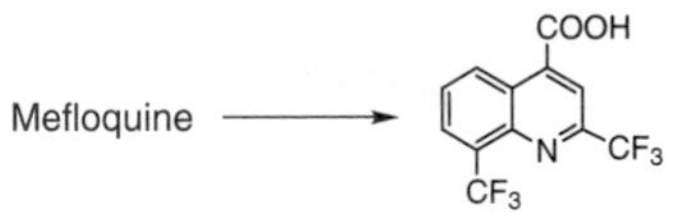

Mefloquine ⟶

COOH

CF_3

CF_3

Fig. 35.10. *P. falciparum* metabolism of mefloquine.

tract affects the pharmacokinetic properties of the drug usually enhancing absorption. The lipophilic nature of the drug accounts for the extensive tissue binding and low clearance of total drug, although the drug does not accumulate after prolonged administration. The drug has a high affinity for erythrocyte membranes.

Mefloquine is an effective suppressive prophylactic agent against *P. falciparum* both in nonimmune populations (travelers coming into regions of malaria) and in resident populations. The drug also has high efficacy against falciparum malaria with a low incidence of recrudescence. The drug is ineffective against sexual forms of the organism.

The incidence of side effects with mefloquine are considered high. The effects are classed as neuropsychiatric, gastrointestinal, dermatologic, and cardiovascular. The neuropsychiatric effects may be serious (suicidal tendencies or seizures) or minor (dizziness, vertigo, ataxia, headaches). Gastrointestinal side effects included nausea, vomiting, and diarrhea, while the dermatologic effects include rash, pruritus, and urticaria. Finally, cardiovascular side effects may include bradycardia, arrhythmias, and extrasystoles.

Halofantrine (Hafan).   Halofantrine (24–25), a member of the 9-phenanthrenemethanol class (Fig. 35.9), originally came out of a synthesis program dating to World War II, but this particular agent was not fully developed until the 1960s. Halofantrine has one chiral center and has been separated into its enantiomers. There appears to be little difference between the enantiomers and thus the drug is used as a racemic mixture.

Halofantrine is considered an alternative drug for treatment of both chloroquine-sensitive and chloroquine-resistant *P. falciparum* malaria, but the efficacy in mefloquine-resistant malaria may be questionable. The drug is metabolized via N-dealkylation to the desbutylhalofantrine by CYP3A4 (Fig. 35.11). The metabolite appears to be several times more active than the administered drug.

Halofantrine is presently only available in a tablet form which has significant implications as it relates to its insolubility and drug absorption (bioavailabililty). Animal studies have shown that following oral administration, the drug is eliminated in feces suggesting poor oral absorption. Its oral suspensions lead to as much as 30% lower plasma levels of the drug in comparison with the tablet. A micronized form of the drug has shown im-

proved bioavailability. Its administration with or without food in the stomach also leads to considerable variation in plasma levels. High-lipid content of a meal taken two hours prior to dosing lead to substantial increases in rate and extent of absorption. Several cases of drug treatment failure appear to be related to poor absorption. Incomplete absorption, and as a result low plasma levels, may play a role in the development of organism resistance. The elimination half-life of halofantrine and desbutylhalofantrine tend to be prolonged which may be another factor in the development of resistance. Low levels of the drug may increase the likelihood of augmenting the emergence of halofantrine resistance.

Absorption problems with halofantrine cannot be solved by increasing the dosage of halofantrine due to significant toxicity problems. Toxicity, while minimal with short term low doses, can be severe with high doses of halofantrine. Gastrointestinal side effects include nausea, vomiting, diarrhea and abdominal pain. Cardiovascular toxicity include orthostatic hypotension and dose-dependent lengthening of QTc intervals.

8-Aminoquinolines

Pamaquine, an 8-aminoquinoline (Fig 35.9), was first introduced for treatment of malaria in 1926 and since has been replaced with primaquine. Primaquine is active against latent tissue forms of *P. vivax* and *P. ovale* and is active against the hepatic stages of *P. falciparum*. The drug is not active against erythrocytic stages of the parasite, but does possess gametocidal activity against all strains of plasmodium.

Mechanism of Action.   While the mechanism of action of the 8-aminoquinolines is unknown it is known that primaquine can generate reactive oxygen species via an autoxidation of the 8-amino group. The formation of a radical anion at the 8-amino group has been proposed by Augusto, et al. (26). As a result cell destructive oxidants such as hydrogen peroxide, superoxide and hydroxyl radical can be formed as shown in Figure 35.3 and discussed above.

Metabolism.   Primaquine is nearly totally metabolized by CYP3A4 (99%) with the primary metabolite being carboxyprimaquine (27) (Fig. 35.12). Trace amounts of N-acetylprimaquine plus aromatic hydroxylation and conjugation metabolites also have been reported.

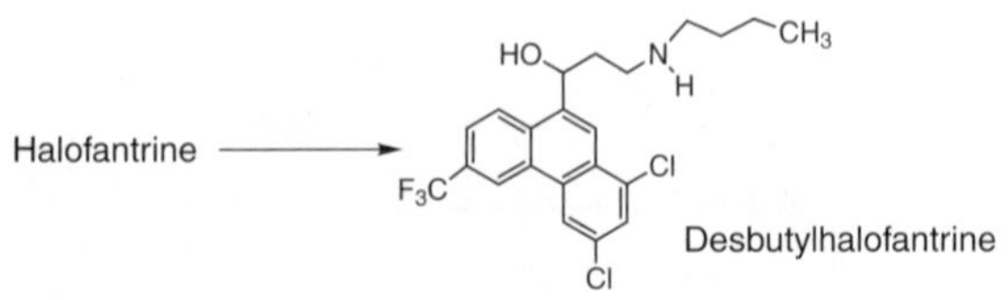

Fig. 35.11. Metabolism of halofantrine.

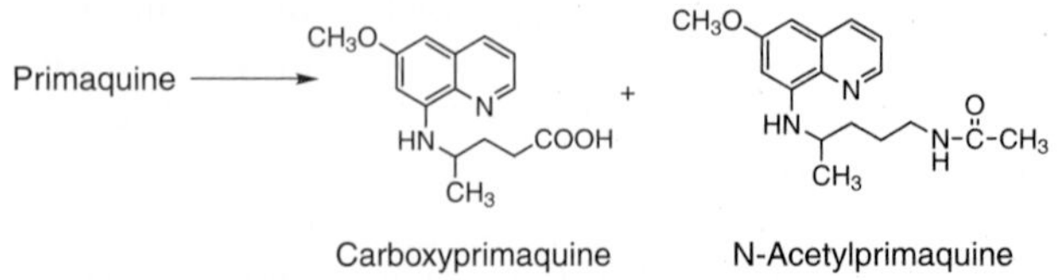

Fig. 35.12. Metabolism of primaquine.

Therapeutic Application. Primaquine is classified as the drug of choice for treatment of relapsing vivax and ovale forms of malaria and will produce a radical cure of the condition. It is recommended that the drug be combined with chloroquine to eradicate the erythrocytic stages of malaria. Primaquine is not given for long-term treatment because of potential toxicity and sensitization. The sensitivity appears most commonly in individuals who have glucose-6-phosphate dehydrogenase deficiency. In these cases hemolytic anemia may develop.

Pyrimethamine   Sulfadoxine

Pyrimethamine

Pyrimethamine (Daraprim) is a potent inhibitor of dihydrofolate reductase (28). The drug has been shown to have a significantly higher affinity for binding to the dihydrofolate reductase of plasmodium than host enzyme (>1000-fold in *P. berghei*) and as a result has been used to selectively treat plasmodium infections. Combined with a long acting sulfonamide, sulfadoxine (Fansidar), which blocks dihydrofolate synthesis, this combination produces sequential blockage of tetrahydrofolate synthesis similar to that reported for treatment of bacterial infections (see Chapter 34). This combination is used with quinine for treatment and prevention of chloroquine-resistant malaria (*Plasmodium falciparum, P. ovale, P. vivax,* and *P. malaria*). Pyrimethamine is a blood schizonticide without effects on the tissue stage of the disease.

Artemisinins (29–32)

The most recent additions to the drug therapy of malaria are artemisinin and derivatives of artemisinins. Isolated from *Artemisia annua* (qinghao), Chinese herbalists have been using this material since 168 BC. Artemisinin and the derivatives, artemether and the synthetic arteflene, are active by virtue of the endoperoxide.

Artemisinin   Artemether (Artenam)   Arteflene

Mechanism of Action. The artemisinins appear to kill the parasite by a free radical mechanism. Not by the generation of reactive oxygen species, but by virtue of a free radical associated with the endoperoxide, possibly involving a carbon radical. The radical in turn produces oxidative damage to the parasites membrane.

Therapeutic Application. The artemisinins are hydrophobic in nature and are partitioned into the membrane of the plasmodium. These compounds have gametocytocidal activity as well as being active against late stage parasites and trophozoites. Little or no cross resistance has been reported with the drugs rapidly clearing the blood of parasites.

HELMINTH INFECTIONS

Helminthiasis, or worm infestation, is one of the most prevalent diseases and one of the most serious public health problems in the world. Many worms are parasitic in humans and cause serious complications. Hundreds of millions if not billions of human infections by helminths exist worldwide and with increased world travel and immigration from the developing countries one might expect to see this pattern of infection continue. It is estimated that one-fourth of the world population may be infected. It is interesting to note that helminths differ from many other parasites in that these organisms multiply outside of the definitive host and have the unique ability to evade host immune defenses for reasons that are not fully understood. As a result helminth infections tend to be chronic, possibly lasting an entire lifetime of the host (for a discussion of the uniqueness of helminth infections see Maizels in Suggested Readings). Helminths that infect human hosts are divided into two categories, or phyla. These are: Platyhelminths (flatworms) and Aschelminths or nematodes (roundworms). The flatworms include the classes Cestode (tapeworms) and Trematode (flukes or schistosomes). The nematode class includes helminths common to the United States: roundworm, hookworm, pinworm, and whipworm. These worms are cylindrical in shape with significant variations in size, proportion, and structure.

Nematode Infections
Ancylostomiasis or Hookworms Infection

The two most widespread types of hookworm in humans are the American hookworm (*Necator americanus*) and the "old world" hookworm (*Ancylostoma doudenale*). The life cycles of both are similar. The larva are found in the soil and are transmitted either by skin penetration or are ingested orally. The circulatory system transports the larva via the respiratory tree to the digestive tract where they mature and live for 9–15 years if left untreated. These worms feed on intestinal tissue and blood. Infestations cause pulmonary lesions, skin reactions, intestinal ulceration, and anemia. The worms are most prevalent in regions of the world with temperatures of 23–33°C, abundant rainfall and well-drained sandy soil.

Enterobiasis or Pinworm Infection
(*Enterobius Vermicularis*)

These worms are widespread in temperate zones, and are a common infestation of households and institutions. The pinworm lives in the lumen of the G-I tract, attaching itself by the mouth to the mucosa of the cecum. Mature worms reach 10 mm in size. The female migrates to the rectum usually at night to deposit her eggs. This event is noted by the symptom of perianal pruritus. The eggs infect fingers, contaminate nightclothes and bed linen where they remain infective for up to three weeks. Eggs resist drying and can be inhaled with household dust to continue the life cycle. Detection of the worm in the perianal region can be accomplished by means of a cellophane tape swabbed in the perianal region in the evening. The worms may be visible with the naked eye. The eggs can be collected in a similar manner but can only be seen under a microscope.

Ascariasis or Roundworm Infections (*Ascaris lumbricoides*)

These roundworms are common in developing countries with the adult roundworm reaching 25–30 cm in length and lodging in the small intestine. Some infections are without symptoms, but abdominal discomfort and pain are common with heavy infestation. Roundworm eggs are released into the soil where they incubate and remain viable for up to six years. When the egg is ingested the larva are released in the small intestine, penetrate the walls of the intestine and are carried via the blood to the lungs. The pulmonary phase of the disease lasts approximately 10 days with the larva passing through the bronchioles, bronchi, trachea, and are swallowed and return to the small intestine. Some patients have reported adult worms exiting the esophagus through the oral cavity. It is not unusual for live ascaris to be expelled with a bowel movement. Poor or lacking sanitary facilities expose the population to infestation through contaminated foods and beverages.

Trichuriasis or Whipworm Infections (*Trichuris trichiura*)

Infections by this parasite are caused by swallowing eggs from contaminated foods and beverages. The eggs are passed with the feces from an infected individual. These eggs may live in the soil for many years. The ingested eggs hatch in the small intestine and the larvae embed in the intestinal wall. The worms then migrate to the large intestine where they mature. Adult worms, which reach about 5 cm, thread their bodies into the epithelium of the colon. They feed on tissue fluids and blood. Infections from this worm cause symptoms of irritation and inflammation of the colonic mucosa, abdominal pain, diarrhea, and distention. Infections can last 5 or more years if not treated. Whipworm infections are commonly seen in individuals returning from visits to the subtropics and are more common in rural areas of the southeastern United States.

Trichinosis or Trichina Infection (*Trichinella spiralis*)

Trichinella Spiralis produces an infection which may be both intestinal and systemic. The worm is found in muscle meat where the organism exists as an encysted larvae. Traditionally, the worm has been associated with domestic pork which feeds on untreated garbage. More recently, outbreaks have occurred in individuals eating infected game such as wild boar, bear, or walrus. Trichinosis infections are more likely to occur after consumption of homemade pork or wild

game sausages. After ingestion the larvae are released from the cyst form and migrate into the intestinal mucosa. After maturation and reproduction the newly released larvae penetrate mucosal lining and are distributed throughout the body where they enter skeletal muscle. During the adult intestinal stage diarrhea, abdominal pain and nausea are the most common symptom, while the muscular form of the disease has symptoms which may include muscle pain and tenderness, edema, conjunctivitis and weakness.

Filariasis

The term filariasis denotes infections with any of the Filarioidea, although it is commonly used to refer to lymphatic-dwelling filaria, such as *Wuchereria bancrofti*, *Brugia malayi*, and *Brugia timori*. Other filarial infections include *Loa Loa* and *Onchocerca volvulus*. The latter two are known as the eyeworm and river blindness worm, respectively. Elephantiasis is the most common disease associated with filariasis. These parasites vary in length from 6 cm for brugia to 50 cm for onchocerca. The incubation periods also vary from 2 months for the brugia to 12 months for the bancroftian filaria. It is estimated that 400 million persons are infected with human filarial parasites. Depending on the specific organism various intermediate hosts are involved in spreading the infection. Mosquitoes are involved with the spread of *Wuchereria bancrofti*, *Brugia malayi*, and *Brugia timori.*, while the female blackfly spreads river blindness. The larvae released by the female filaria are referred to as microfilariae and may commonly be found in lymphatics.

Cestode and Trematode Infections
Cysticercosis or Tapeworm Infection

Helminths of this class that are of concern as potential parasites in humans include:

- Beef Tapeworm (*Taenia saginata*) This worm is found worldwide and infects people who eat undercooked beef. The worm reaches a length of over 5 m and contains about 100 segments/m. Each of these segments contains its own reproductive organs.
- Pork tapeworm (*Taenia solium*) Pork tapeworms are sometimes called bladder worms and are occasionally found in uncooked pork. The worm attaches itself to the intestinal wall of the human host. The adult worm reaches 5 m in length and if untreated, survives in the host for many years.
- Dwarf tapeworm (*Hymenolepis nana*) This infection is transmitted directly from one human to another without an intermediate host. *H. nana* reaches only 3–4 cm in length. It is found in temperate zones, and children are most frequently infected.
- Fish tapeworm (*Diphyllobothrium latum*). The fish tapeworm reaches a length of 10 m and contains about 400 segments/m. These tapeworms attach themselves to the intestinal wall and rob the host of nutrients. They especially absorb vitamin B_{12} and folic acid. Depletion of these critical nutrients, especially vitamin B_{12}, can lead to pernicious anemia. Tapeworm eggs are passed in the patient's feces and contamination of food and drink may result in transmission of the infection.

Schistosomiasis or Blood Flukes

There are three primary trematode species that cause schistosomiasis in man: *Schistosoma hematobium, S. mansoni,* and *S. japonicum*. Infections result from the penetration of the normal skin by living (free-swimming) cercaria (the name given to the infectious stage of the parasite) with the aid of secreted enzymes. The cercaria develop to preadult forms in the lungs and skin. Then these parasites travel in pairs via the bloodstream and invade various tissues. The adult worm reaches approximately 2 cm in length. The female deposits her eggs near the capillary beds, where granulomas form. Some of the eggs will move into the lumen of the intestines, bladder, or ureters and are released into the surrounding where the parasite will seek out the intermediate snail vector. After a period of time the cercaria are again released from the snail to continue the cycle. The patients might experience headache, fatigue, fever, and gastrointestinal disturbances during the early stages of the disease. Hepatic fibrosis and ascites occur in later stages. Untreated patients can harbor as many as 100 pairs of worms. Untreated worms can live 5–10 years within the host. It is estimated that as many as 200 million persons are infected with schistosomes worldwide. Depending on the species of schistosome, the disease is found in parts of South America, the Caribbean Islands, Africa, and the Middle East.

DRUG THERAPY FOR HELMINTH INFECTIONS (33)

Helminths represent a biologically diverse group of parasitic organisms differing in size, life cycle, site of infection (local and systemic), and susceptibility to chemotherapy. With such variation in infectious organisms it is not surprising that the drugs used to control helminth infections also represent a varied group of chemical classes. As indicated in Table 35.2 the drugs may have fairly narrow spectra of activity (pyrantel pamoate) or a broad spectra of activity (benzimidazoles).

Benzimidazoles

The benzimidazoles, Table 35.3, are a broad-spectrum group of drugs discovered in the 1960s with activity against gastrointestinal helminths. Several thousand benzimidazoles have been synthesized and screened for anthelmintic activity with albendazole, mebendazole, and thiabendazole representing the benzimidazole marketed today. The development and chemistry of this class of agents has been reviewed by Townsend and Wise (34).

Table 35.3. Benzimidazole Anethelmintics

Drugs	Trade Name	R$_1$	R$_2$
Thiabendazole	Mintezol	(thiazole ring)	–H
Mebendazole	Vermox	–N(H)–C(=O)–OCH$_3$	–C(=O)–(phenyl)
Albendazole	Zental	–N(H)–C(=O)–OCH$_3$	–SCH$_2$CH$_2$CH$_3$
Oxibendazole		–N(H)–C(=O)–OCH$_3$	–OCH$_2$CH$_2$CH$_3$
Parbendazole		–N(H)–C(=O)–OCH$_3$	–CH$_2$CH$_2$CH$_2$CH$_3$
Ciclobendazole		–N(H)–C(=O)–OCH$_3$	–C(=O)–(cyclopropyl)

Table 35.2. Therapeutic Application of Anthelmintics for Specific Helminth Infections

	Mebendazole	Albendazole	Diethylcarbamazine	Ivermectin	Praziquantel	Pyrantel Pamoate
Nematode Infections						
Necator americanus	√	√				
Ancylostama doudenale	√	√				√
Enterobius vermicularis	√			√		√
Ascaris lumbricoides	√	√		√		√
Trichuris trichiura	√	√		√		
Trichinella spiralis	√	√				
Wuchereria bancrofti			√	√		
Brugia malayi			√	√		
Brugia timori.			√			
Loa Loa		√	√	√		
Onchocerca volvulus		√	√	√		
Cestode Infections						
Taenia saginata	√	√			√	
Taenia solium	√	√			√	
Hymenolepis nana	√				√	
Diphyllobothrium latum					√	
Trematode Infections						
Schistosoma hematobium					√	
S. mansoni					√	
S. japonicum					√	

Mechanism of Action

Two mechanisms have been proposed to account for the action of the benzimidazoles. Fumarate reductase is an important enzyme in helminths which appears to be involved in oxidation of NADH to NAD. The benzimidazoles are capable of inhibiting fumarate reductase (35). Inhibition of fumarate reductase ultimately uncouples oxidative phosphorylation which is important in ATP production.

A second mechanism, and probably the primary action of the benzimidazoles, is associated with the ability of these drugs to bind to the protein tubulin and thus prevent tubulin polymerization to microtubules (36–37). Tubulin is a dimeric protein which is in dynamic equipiblirium with the polymeric microtubules. Binding to the tubulin prevents the self-association of subunits and creats a "capping" of the microtubule at the associating end of the microtubule. The microtubulin continues to dissociate from the opposite end with a net loss of microtubule length. What is interesting is the unique selectivity of the benzimidazoles. It has been shown that benzimidazole can also bind to mammalian tubulin, but when used as anthelmintics these drugs are destructive to the helminth with minimal toxicity to the host. It has been suggested that the selectivity is associated with differing pharmacokinetics between binding to the two different tubulin proteins.

Metabolism

The benzimidazoles have limited water solubility and as a result are poorly absorbed from the GI tract (a fatty meal will increase absorption). Poor absorption may be beneficial since the drugs are used primarily to treat intestinal helminths. To the extent that the drugs are absorbed, they undergo rapid metabolism in the liver and are excreted in the bile (See Fig. 35.13) (38–39). In most cases the parent compound is rapidly and nearly completely metabolized with oxidative and hydrolytic processes predominating. The Phase I oxidative reaction is commonly a cytochrome P-450 catalyzed reaction which may then be followed by a Phase II conjugation.

Albendazole is unique in two ways. First, the presence of a thioether substitutent at the five postion increases the likelihood of sulfur oxidation. Second, the initial metabolite, albendazole sulfoxide, is a potent anthelmintic. This initial oxidation is catalyzed principally (70%) by CYP3A4 and CYP1A2 and flavin-containing monooxygenase (30%) (FMO) giving rise to a compound which is bound to plasma protein. This intermediate has an expanded utility in that it has been shown to be active against the hydatid cyst found in echinococciasis, a tape worm disease (40). Further oxidation by cytochrome P-450 leads to the inactive sulfone. Additional metabolites of the sulfone have been reported which include carbamate hydrolysis to the amine and oxidation of the 5-propyl side chain. These reactions occur only to a minor extent.

Metabolism of mebendazole occurs primarily by reduction of the 5-carbonyl to a secondary alcohol which greatly increases the water solubility of this compound. An additional Phase I metabolite resulting from carbamate hydrolysis has also been reported. Both the secondary alcohol and the amine are readily conjugated, a Phase II metabolism. Evidence would suggest that the anthelmintic activity of mebendazole resides in the parent drug and none of the metabolites.

Thiabendazole is metabolized through aromatic hydroxylation at the five position catalyzed by CYP1A2. The resulting phenol is conjugated to 5-hydroxythiabendazole glucuronide and 5-hydroxythiabendazole sulfate, respectively. The initial metabolite along with minor amount of N_1-methylthiabendazole (from methylation phase 2 reaction) have been reported to be teratogenic in mice and rats.

Therapeutic Application

As indicated in Table 35.2, mebendazole and albendazole have a wide spectrum of activity against intestinal ne-

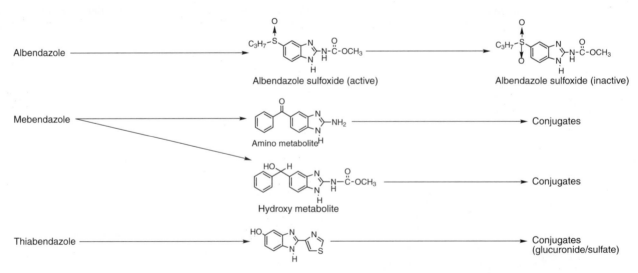

Fig. 35.13. Metabolism of benzimidazoles.

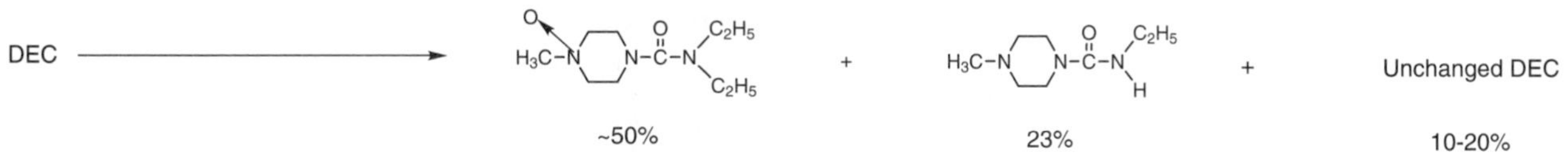

Fig. 35.14. Metabolism of DEC.

matodes. The drugs are useful and effective against mixed infections. The adverse reactions are commonly gastrointestinal in nature (nausea, vomiting, and diarrhea). Both drugs have been reported to be teratogenic in rats and therefore should not be used during the first trimester of pregnancy. A third drug of this class is thiabendazole which remains of some value in treatment of strongyloidiasis, as an alternate drug, and cutaneous larva migrans (creeping eruption) where it is the drug of choice. Thiabendazole is commonly used in veterinary medicine. The drug is less commonly used because of associated toxicity. Thiabendazole has been reported to cause Stevens–Johnson syndrome and has the potential for hepatotoxicity and crystalluria.

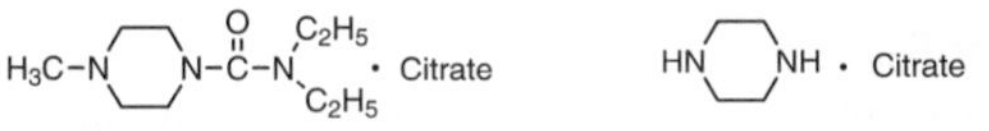

Diethylcarbamazine citrate   Piperazine citrate

Diethylcarbamazine (Hetrazan)

Discovered in the 1940s, diethylcarbamazine (DEC) has proven to be especially effective as a filaricidal agent. The incidence of filariasis among American troops during World War II necessitated a search for drugs with an antifalarial spectrum of activity. The once popular piperazine was also discovered during these initial screenings. While chemically similar the activity again helminths is quite different. Piperazine is active against nematodes while DEC is active against falaria and microfalaria (41).

Mechanism of Action

Although studied extensively the mechanism of action of DEC remains unknown. DEC appears the be the active form of the drug with a very rapid onset of action (within minutes), but of interest is the fact that the drug is inactive in vitro suggesting activation of a cellular component is essential to the filaricidal action. Three mechanisms have been suggested: 1) involvement of blood platelets triggered by the action of filarial excretory antigens. A complex reaction is thought to occur between the drug, the antigen, and platelets (42). The authors were unable to show a direct action of the drug on the microfalaria; 2) inhibition of microtubule polymerization and disruption of preformed microtubules (43); 3) interference with arachadonic acid metabolism (44). DEC is known to have antiinflammatory action which appear to involve blockage at cyclooxygenase and LTA$_4$ synthase (leukotriene synthesis). This action appears to alter vascular and cellular adhesiveness and cell activation. This latter action would suggest a possible relationship between the first and third mechanism.

Metabolism

The metabolism of DEC leads to the compounds shown in Figure 35.14 plus trace amounts of methylpiperazine and piperazine. Nearly all of the metabolites appear in the urine. As indicated by the rapid action of the drug it would appear that none of the metabolites are involved in the therapeutic action of DEC.

Therapeutic Application

DEC citrate is freely soluble in water, is rapidly absorbed, and is effective against microfalariae. The drug does not appear to be effective against the adult worm. In general the drug has mild adverse effects, but under some conditions it may produce serve adverse reactions including anaphylactic reactions, intense pruritus, and ocular complications (45). The severe anaphylactic reaction is known as the Mazzotti reaction and appears to be an immune response related to the presence of dead microfilariae. This reaction is more common in individuals who have a high load microfilarial infection and it may preclude the use of DEC in some patient populations (33).

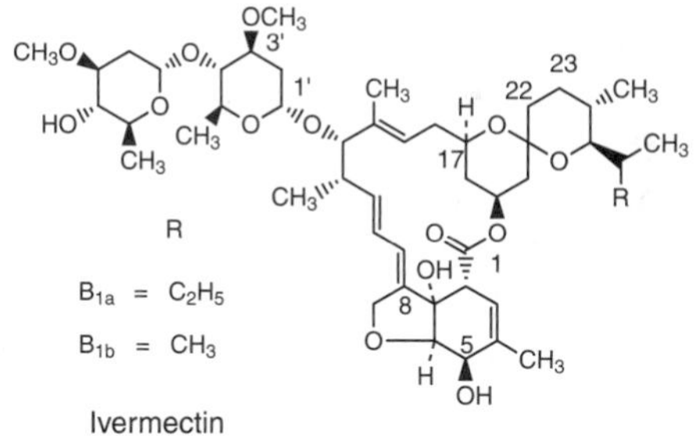

$B_{1a} = C_2H_5$
$B_{1b} = CH_3$

Ivermectin

Ivermectin (Mectizan)

Extracted from the soil actinomycete *Streptomyces avermitilis*, the natural avermectins are 16-membered macrocyclic lactones which upon reduction of the C_{22-23} double bond give rise to ivermectin a 80:20 mixture of dihydroavermectin B_{1a} and B_{1b}, respectively. While the natural avermectins have minimal biologic activity, ivermectin has proven to be quite beneficial for the treatment of various nematode infections.

Mechanism of Action

Two mechanism of action are thought to be involved in the action of ivermectin (33,46). The first is an indirect action in which motility of microfalaria is reduced which in turn allows cytotoxic cells of the host to adhere to the parasite resulting in elimination from the host. This action may occur by virtue of the ability of ivermectin to act either as a GABA agonist or an inducer of chloride ion influx leading to hyperpolarization and muscle paralysis. The chloride ion influx appears to be the more plausible mechanism (47). The result of this action is a rapid decrease in microfilarial concentrations.

A second action of ivermectin leads to the degeneration of microfilaria *in uterio*. This action would result in fewer microfilaria being released from the female worms and occurs over a longer period of time. The presence of degenerated microfilaria *in uterio* prevents further fertilization and production of microfilaria.

Metabolism

Ivermectin is rapidly absorbed, bound to a great extent to plasma protein, and excreted in the urine or feces unchanged or as the 3′-O-demethyl-22,23-dihydroavermectin B_{1a} or as the dihydroavermectin B_{1a} monosaccharide. The absorption of ivermectin is significantly affected by the presence of alcohol. Administration of ivermectin as an alcoholic solution may result in as much as a 100% increase in absorption.

Therapeutic Application

While ivermectin has activity against a variety of microfalaria including *W. bancrofti*, *B. Malayi*, *L. Loa*, and *Mansonella ozzardi*, as well as activity against *S. stercoralis* the drug is used primarily for treatment of onchocerciasis (African river blindness) caused by *O. volvulus*. It is estimated that 20 million people are affected by this condition while an additional 85 million are at risk of the infection. The drug is effective against both the eye worm as well as skin infections of *O. volvulus*. Ivermectin has the distinct advantage over DEC in that ivermectin can be used as a single dose (150 μg/kg) once a year (although there is support for dosing every six months), has far less likelihood of causing the potentially fatal anaphylactic reaction (Mazzotti reaction), and can be used for mass treatment programs.

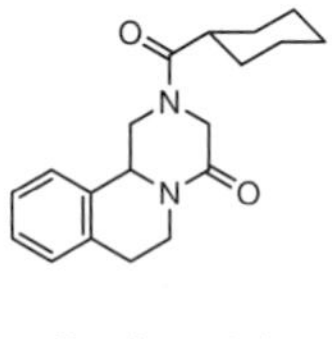

Praziquantel (Biltricide)

Praziquantel (PZQ) is an isoquinoline derivative with most of the biologic activity found in the levo enantiomer. While the compound has no activity against nematodes it is highly effective against cestodes and trematodes.

Mechanism of Action

It would appear that more than one mechanism of action may exist for PZQ possibly dependent upon the type of parasite being treated. In the case of helminths found in the lumen of the host (cestode infection) the drug leads to muscle contraction and paralysis leading to worm expulsion. PZQ has also been shown to inhibit phosphoinositide metabolism which in an undetermined mechanism leads to the the worm paralysis (48). With intravascular dwelling schistosomes, PZQ leads to drug induced damage of the tegument of the worm. As a result, antigens in the helminth are subject to attack by immune antibodies of the host (49–50). An antigen-antibody immunological reaction leads to the death of the parasite.

Metabolism

PZQ is rapidly absorbed and undergoes hepatic first pass metabolism. The metabolites are either less active or inactive and consist of hydroxylated compounds. In the serum the major metabolite appears to be the monohydroxylated 4-hydroxycyclohexylcarboxylate while in the urine 50–60% of the initial PZQ exists as dihydroxylated products (Fig. 35.15) (51). These hydroxylation reactions are catalyzed by CYP2B6 and CYP3A4. The metabolites would be expected to exist in the conjugated form in the urine.

Therapeutic Application

PZQ is the drug of choice for treatment of schistosomiasis and liver flukes (trematode and cestode infections). While an approved drug, PZQ is considered an investigational drug by the FDA for treatment of schistosomiasis and liver flukes. The drug has a bitter taste and therefore should not be chewed. The side effects are usually not severe and consist of abdominal discomfort—pain and diarrhea.

Pyrantel Pamoate (Antiminth)

Pyrantel was first reported for its anthelmintic activity in 1966 (52). While it has activity against most intestinal round worm infections it has not been approved by the FDA for

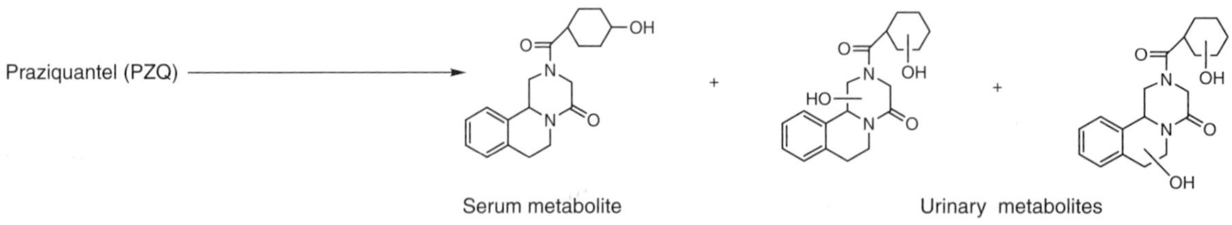

Praziquantel

Fig. 35.15. Metabolism of praziquantel (PZQ).

Pyrantel pamoate

several of these infestations. It is considered the drug of choice for treatment of pinworms. The drug is used as the pamoate salt which is quite insoluble and as a result is not readily absorbed. This property improves the usefulness of the drug for treatment of intestinal helminths. In addition to value in treating enterobiasis, the drug is effective for hookworm and roundworm (ascariasis) infections. Pyrantel acts as a depolarizing neuromuscular blocking agent which activates nicotinic receptors and inhibits cholinesterase ultimately leading to worm paralysis.

ECTOPARASITIC INFECTIONS

Two parasitic organisms which cause common topical infections are *Sarcoptes scabiei* responsible for scabies and *Pediculus humanus* which is responsible for lice infections.

Scabies

Scabies, commonly referred to as the "seven year itch," is a condition caused by *Sarcoptes scabiei* or the itch mite. The condition is commonly spread by direct person to person contact although the organism is capable of living for 2–3 days in clothing, bedding, or house dust. Sharing of clothing is a common means whereby the condition spreads. The organism burrows into the epidermis usually in the folds of the skin of the fingers, the elbows, female breast, penis, scrotum, and buttocks. The female parasite lays eggs in the skin which hatch and mature to adults. The itch mite can live for 30–60 days. The infections are most common in children, but may also be found in adults in institutional settings. The primary symptom of severe itching may foster secondary infections at the site of scratching. Because of the potential for spread to other members of a family it is common to treat all members of the family. This will prevent reinfection from a second family member after successful therapy of the first family member.

Lice

Pediculosis or lice is caused by any of the parasites *Pediculus humanus capitis*, the head louse, *P. humanus corporis*, the body louse, or *Phthirius pubis*, crab louse found in the genital area. Lice are blood sucking insects which live for 30–40 days on the body of the host. The organisms reproduce and the female lays her eggs, the nits, which become attached to hair. The nits are white in color and hatch in 8–10 days. In order for the parasite to live it must feed on blood which it sucks through punctures in the skin. A hypersensitivity reaction occurs at these puncture sites which then leads to pruritus, host scratching, and possible secondary infection.

In addition to the scalp and skin, the eyebrows, eyelids and beard may become sites of infection. The transfer of infection can occur through person to person contact and from infected clothing on which the organism can survive for up to one week. The sharing of clothing is a common means for the spread of body lice. Head lice are quite common among grade school children while crab lice are common among sexually active individuals. Treatment of family members is recommended and clothing and bed linen should be removed and washed in very hot water.

DRUG THERAPY FOR SCABIES AND PEDICULOSIS
Lindane (Kwell)

γ-Benzene hexachloride

Chlorination and reduction of benzene leads to a mixture of hexachlorocyclohexanes. The insecticidal activity resides primarily in the gamma isomer of hexachlorocyclohexane (gamma benzene hexachloride). The compound is thought to produce its insecticidal action by virtue of a CNS stimulatory action which occurs by blockage of GABA. The compound is readily absorbed through the chitinous exoskeleton of the parasite. Unfortunately, lindane is also readily absorbed through intact human skin, especially the scalp, and has the potential for systemic neurotoxicity in the host. Infants and children and possibly the elderly are most prone to the neurotoxic effects of the drug. Since the drug is quite lipophilic and when applied to the scalp as a shampoo if absorbed, it readily enters the CNS of the host and can produce signs of neurotoxicity which consist of convulsions, dizziness, clumsiness, and unsteadiness.

The drug is available in a lotion and shampoo and is recommended for treatment of both pediculosis and scabies. When using the lotion topically it should be applied to dry skin covering the entire surface and left in place for 8 hours. The lindane then should be removed by washing thoroughly. If the shampoo is used for *Pediculosis capitis* the hair should be cleaned of oil and dried prior to application of the lindane shampoo. The shampoo is then worked into the hair and scalp applying in such a way to prevent other parts of the body from coming into contact with the drug. After approximately four minutes the drug is removed by washing with water, the hair dried, and the hair combed with a fine-toothed comb to remove nits.

Pyrethrum and Pyrethroids

The natural occurring pyrethrums have been used as insecticides since the 1800s. These compounds are extracted from the flowering portion of the Chrysanthemum plant. The flowers produced in Kenya have on average of

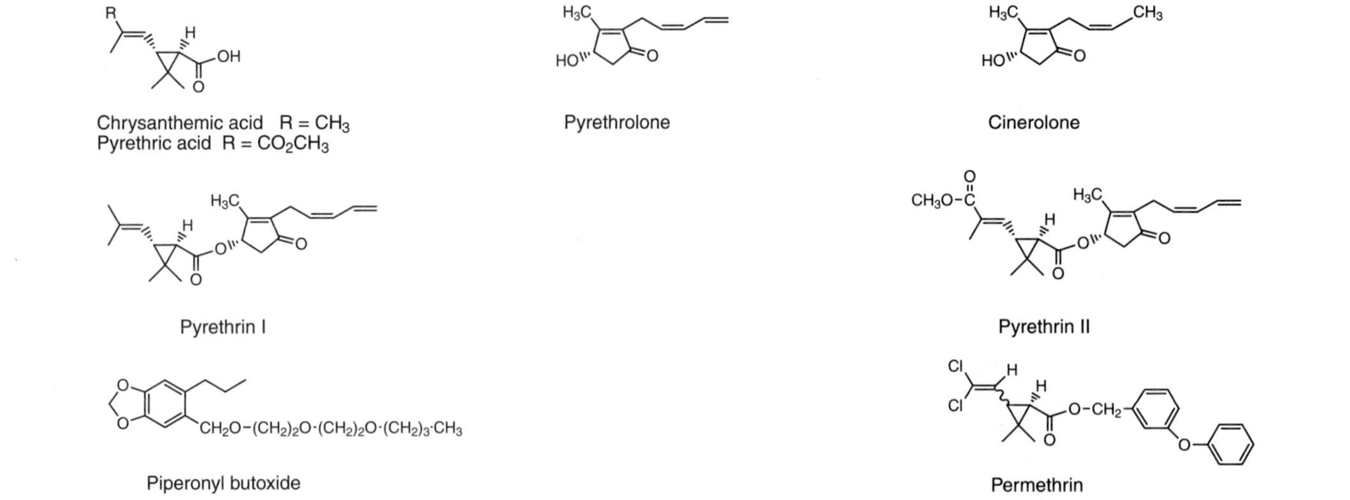

Fig. 35.16. Structures of pyrethrum and pyrethroid.

1.3% pyrethrins. These pyrethrum extracts are a major agricultural product for this country.

Chemistry

The Chrysanthemum extract is a mixture of ester consisting of the acids chrysanthemic and pyrethric and the alcohols pyrethrolone and cinerolone (Fig. 35.16). The esters are prone to hydrolysis and oxidation and as a result should be stored in the cold and protected from light. Because of the high cost, limited availability, and rapid degradation synthetic derivatives have been investigated. The result has been the preparation of pyrethoids, the synthetic derivatives of pyrethrins. The compound used therapeutically is permethrin which exists as a 60:40 mixture of *trans-cis* isomers.

Mechanism of Action (53–56)

The pyrethrins and pyrethroids (permethrin) are nerve membrane sodium channel toxins which do not affect potassium channels. The compounds bind to specific sodium channel proteins and slow the rate of inactivation of the sodium current elicited by membrane depolarization and as a result prolong the open time of the sodium channel. At low concentrations, the pyrethroids produce repetitive action potentials and neuron firing while at high concentrations the nerve membrane is depolarized completely and excitation is blocked.

The receptor interaction of the pyrethrums with the sodium channel complex is stereospecific and dependent on the stereochemistry of the carboxylic acid. In the case of the pyrethroids the most active isomers are the 1R,3-*cis*- and 1R,3-*trans*-cyclopropanecarboxylates. The 1S *cis* and *trans* isomers are inactive and are actually antagonists to the action of the 1R isomers.

Metabolism

A property that enhances the usefulness of the pyrethrums and pyrethroids is that these compounds are highly toxic to the ectoparasites while they are relatively nontoxic to mammals if absorbed. The apparent lack of toxicity is associated with the rapid metabolism of these drugs through hydrolysis and or oxidation (Fig. 35.17) (57–58). The nature of the metabolism, that is hydrolysis verses oxidation, is dependent upon the structure of the pyrethrins or pyrithroids. Oxidation of the *trans* methyl of the isobutylene in the carboxyl moiety initially gives an alcohol which then proceeds to the carboxylic acid, while epoxidation of the terminal alkene of the alcohol portion of pyrethrin I gives either the 1,2-diol or 1,4 diol. No ester hydrolysis is reported. Permethrin is hydroxylated on the terminal aromatic ring either at the 4 or 2 position, oxidized on the methyl group of the dimethylcyclopropane, and hydrolyzed at the ester moiety. The rapid breakdown of these agents also accounts for their low persistence in the environment.

Therapeutic Application

Pyrethrins (A-200, RID).   Because of the high cost and the rapid degradation of the pyrethrins, they are usually combined with piperonyl butoxide, a synergist (Fig. 35.16). Piperonyl butoxide has no insecticidal activity in it own right, but is thought to inhibit the cytochrome P450 enzyme of the insect thus preventing an oxidative inactivation of the pyrethrins by the parasite. The combination is used in a 10:1 ratio of piperonyl butoxide to pyrethrins. The mixture is used for treatment of *Pediculus humanus capitis*, *P. humanus corporis*, and *Phthirius pubis*. Various dosage forms are available including a gel, shampoo, and topical solution.

Permethrin (Nix-1% lotion, Elimite-5% Cream).   Permethrin, due to its increased stability and its availability synthetically, is not used with a synergist. The compound is used in a 1% lotion for treatment of pediculosis capitis and in a 5% cream as a scabicide.

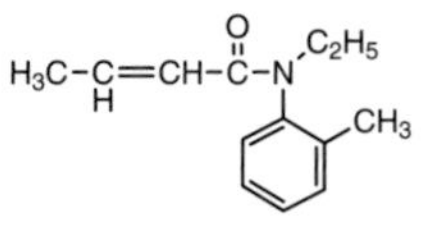

Crotamiton

Crotamiton

Crotamiton is available as a 10% cream for the treatment of scabies although it is less effective than pyrethrins or permethrin (59–60). Since crotamiton may need to be applied a second time for successful treatment of scabies while the pyrethrins or permethrin require a single application, poor patient compliance with crotamiton may reduce its effectiveness. The advantage of crotamiton over lindane comes from the fact that lindane has potential neurotoxicity if absorbed especially in infants and children while crotamiton has less systemic neurotoxicity. The most common side effect reported for crotamiton is skin irritation.

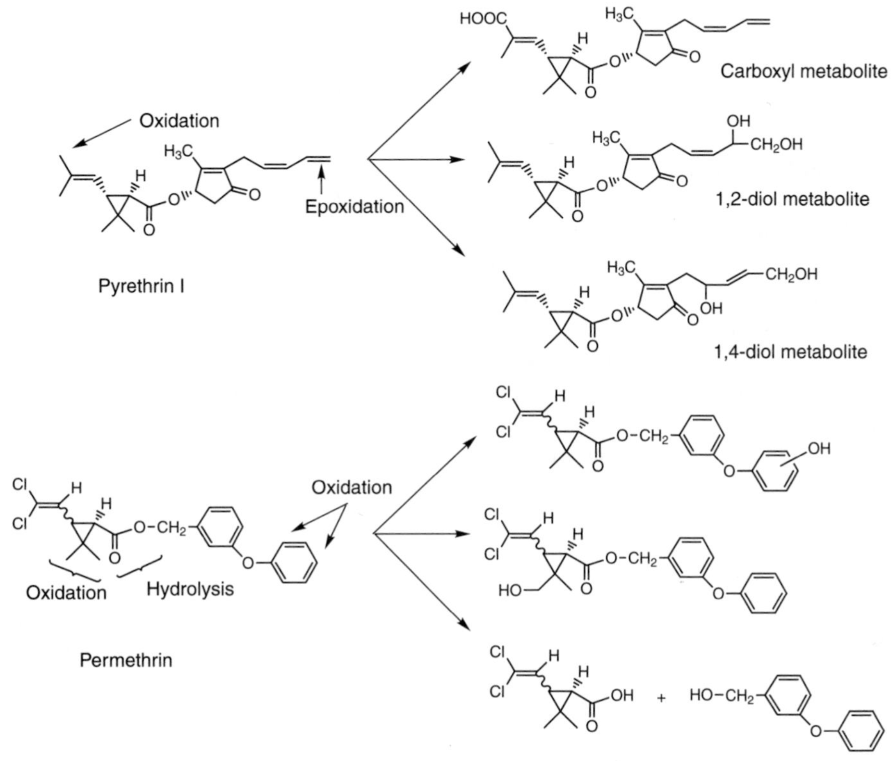

Fig. 35.17. Metabolism of pyrethrin I and permethrin.

CASE STUDY

Victoria F. Roche and S. William Zito

Ms. PU comes to the prescription counter and asks to speak to the pharmacist. She is carrying her 2-year-old son in her arms and appears to be mildly distressed. You ask her what seems to be the problem and she replies that she has just come from picking up her son from his daycare center. The daycare director informed her that the center would be closed tomorrow in order to steam clean the rugs. This was necessary to eradicate an infestation of head lice (pediculus humanis var. capitis). She was also told that her child most likely had head lice and that she should see her pharmacist for advice about the appropriate treatment. You examine the child's fine black hair and observe a few white eggs (nits) but no active lice. Evaluate the 3 pediculocides available (1–3) and choose one that would be best for this situation.

1. *Identify the therapeutic problem(s) where the pharmacist's intervention may benefit the patient.*

2. *Identify and prioritize the patient specific factors that must be considered to achieve the desired therapeutic outcomes.*

3. *Conduct a thorough and mechanistically oriented structure-activity analysis of all therapeutic alternatives provided in the case.*

4. *Evaluate the SAR findings against the patient specific factors and desired therapeutic outcomes and make a therapeutic decision.*

5. *Counsel your patient.*

REFERENCES

1. DoCampo R. Sensitivity of Parasites to Free Radical Damage by Antiparasitic Drugs. Chem-Biol Inter 1990; 73: 1–27.
2. Lau AH, Lam NP, Piscitelli SC, et al. Clinical Pharmacokinetics of Metronidazole Anti-infectives. Clin Pharmcokinet 1992; 23: 328–364.
3. Koch R, Beaulieu BB, Chrystal EJT, et al. Metronidazole Metabolite in Urine and its Risk. Science 1981; 211: 399–400.
4. Drugs for Parasitic Infections. The Medical Letter, 40, The Medical Letter, Inc., New Rochelle, NY, January 2, 1998; 1–12.
5. The Choice of Antibacterial Drugs. The Medical Letter, 40, The Medical Letter, Inc., New Rochelle, NY, March 27, 1998; 33–42.
6. Berman JD. Chemotherapy for Leishmaniasis: Biochemical Mechanisms, Clinical Efficacy, and Future Strategies. Rev Infect Dis 1988; 10: 560–586.
7. Cook GC. Leishmaniasis: Some Recent Developments in Chemotherapy. J Antimicrob Chemo 1993; 31: 327–330.
8. Vohringer H-F, Arasteh K. Pharmacokinetic Optimisation in the Treatment of Pneumocystis carinii pneumonia. Clin. Pharmacokin 1993; 24: 388–412.
9. Edwards KJ, Jenkins T, Neidle S. Crystal Structure of a Pentamidine-Oligonucleotide Complex: Implications for DNA-Binding Properties. Biochem 1992; 31, 7104–7109.
10. Shapiro T, Englund PT. Selective Cleavage of Kinetoplast DNA Minicircles Promoted by Antitrypanosomal Drugs. Proc Natl Acad Sci USA 1990; 87: 950–954.
11. Dykstra CC, Tidwell RR. Inhibition of Topoisomerase from Pneumocystis carinii by Aromatic Dicationic Molecules. J Protozool 1991; 38: 78S-81S.
12. Fry M, Pudney M. Site of Action of the Antimalarial Hydroxymaphthoquinoine, 2-[trans-4-(4'-chlorophenyl)cyclohexyl]-3-hydroxy-1,4-naphthoquinone (566C80). Biochem Pharmacol 1992; 43: 1545–1553.
13. Hughes WT, Gray VL, Gutteridge WE, et al. Efficacy of a Hydroxynaphthoquinone, 566C80, in Experimental Pneumocystis carinii pneumonitis. J Antimicrob Chemotherap 1990; 34: 225–228.
14. Wang CC. Molecular Mechanisms and Therapeutic Approaches to the Treatment of Affician Trypanosomiasis. Annu Rev Pharmacol Toxicol 1995; 35: 93–127.
15. Metcalf BW, Bey P, Danzin C, et al. Catalytic Irreversible Inhibition of Mammalian Ornithine Decarboxylase (E.C. 4.1.1.17) by Substrate and Product Analogues. J Am Chem Soc 1978; 100: 2551–2553.
16. Bacchi CJ, Nathan HC, Hutner SH, et al. Polyamine Metabolism: A Potential Therapeutic Target in Trypanosomes. Science 1980; 210: 332–334.
17. Poulin R, Lu L, Ackermann B, et al. Mechanism of the Irreversible Inactivation of Mouse Ornithine Decarboxylase by α-Difluoromethylornithine. J Biol Chem 1992; 267, 150–158.
18. Bacchi CJ, Garofalo J, Ciminelli M, et al. Resistance to DL α-difluoromethylornithine by Clinical Isolates of Trypanosoma brucei rhodeniense: Role of S-adenosylmethioine. Biochem Pharmacol 1993; 46: 471–481.
19. Henderson GB, Ulrich P, Fairlamb AH, et al. "Subversive" substrates for the enxyme trypanothione disulfide reductase. Alternative Approach to chemotherapy of Chagas' Disease. Proc Natl Acad Sci USA 1988; 85: 5374–5378
20. Fairlamb AH, Henderson GB, Cerami A. Trypanothione is the Primary Target for Ascenical Drugs Against African Trypanosomes. Proc Natl Acad Sci, USA 1989; 86: 2607–2611.
21. Ward SA. Mechanisms of Chloroquine Resistance in Malarial Chemotherapy. Trends in Pharmcol Sci 1988; 9: 241–246.
22. Zhao X-J, Ishizaki T. Metabolic Interactions of Selected antimalarial and Non-antimalarial Drugs with the Major Pathway (3-hydroxylation) of Quinine in Human Liver Microsomes. Br J Clin Pharmacol 1997; 44: 505–511.
23. Palmer KJ, Holliday SM, Brogden RN. Mefloquine: A Review of its Antimalarial Activity, Pharmacokinetic Properties and Therapeutic Efficacy. Drugs 1993; 45: 430–475.
24. Bryson HM, Goa KL. Halofantrine: A Review of tis Antimalarial Activity, Pharmacokinetic Properties and Therapeutic Potential. Drugs 1992; 43: 236–258.
25. Karbwang J, Bangchang KN. Clinical Pharmacokinetics of Halofantrine. Clin Pharmacokinet 1994; 27: 104–119.
26. Augusto O, Schrieber J, Mason RP. Direct ESR Detection of a Free Radical Intermediate Drugin the Peroxidase-Catalyzed Oxidation of the Antimalarial Drug Primaquine. Biochem Pharmacol 1988; 37: 2791–2797.
27. Mihaly GW, Ward SA, Edwards G, et al. Pharmacokinetics of Primaquine in Man: Identification of the Carboxylic Acid Derivative as a Major Plasma Metabolite 1984; Br J Clin Pharmacol 1984; 17:441–446.
28. Ferone R, Burchall JJ, Hitchings GH. Plasmodium berghei Dihydrofolate Reductase Isolation, Properties, and Inhibition by Antifolates. Mol Pharmacol 1969;5:49–59.
29. Cumming JN, Ploypradith P, Posner GH. Antimalial Activity of Artemisinin (Qinghaosu) and Related Trioxanes: Mechanism(s) of Action. Adv Pharmacol 1997; 37: 253–297.
30. Meshnick SR, Taylor TE, Kamchonwongpaisan S. Artemisinin and the Antimalarial Endoperoxides: from Herbal Remedy to Targeted Chemotherapy. Microbiol Rev 1996; 60: 301–315.
31. Posner GH, Cumming JN, Woo S-H, et al. Orally Active Antimalarial 3-Substituted Trioxanes: New Sythnetic Methodology and Biological Evalutaion. J Med Chem 1998; 41: 940–951.
32. Cumming JN, Wang D, Shapiro TA, et al. Design, Synthesis, Derivatization, and Structure-Activity Relationships of Simplified, Tetracyclic, 1,2,4-Trioxane Alcohol Aanalogues of the Antimalarial Artemisinin. J Med Chem 1998; 41: 952–964.
33. deSilva N, Guyatt H, Bundy D. Anthelmintics: A Comparative Review of Their Clinical Pharmacology. Drugs 1997; 53, 769–786.
34. Townsend LB, Wise DS. The Synthesis and Chemistry of Certain Anthelmintic Benzimidazoles. Parasitology Today 1990; 6: 107–112.
35. Prichard RK. Mode of Action of the Anthelmintic Thiabendazole in Haemonchus contortus. Nature 1970; 228: 684–685.
36. Friedman PA, Platzer EG. Interaction of anthelmintic benzimidazoles and benzimidazole derivatives with bovine brain tubulin. Biochim Biophy ACTA 1978; 544, 605–614.
37. Lacey E. Mode of Action of Benzimidazoles. Parasitology Today 1990; 6: 112–115.
38. Braithwaite PA, Roberts MS, Allan RJ, et al. Clinical Pharmacokinetics of High Dose Mebendazole in Patients Treated for Hydatid Disease. Eur J Clin Pharmacol 1982; 22: 161–169.
39. Gottschall DW, Theodorides EJ, Wang R. The Metabolism of Benzimidazole Anthelmintics. Parasitology Today 1990; 6: 115–124.
40. Marriner SE, Morris DL, Dickson B, et al. Pharmacokinetics of Albendazole in Man. Eur J Clin Pharmacol 1986; 30: 705–708.
41. Hawking F. Diethylcarbamazine and New Compounds for the Treatment of Filariasis. Adv Pharmacol Chemo 1979; 16: 129–194.
42. Cesbron J-Y, Capron A, Vargaftig BB, et al. Platelets Mediate the Action of Diethylcarbamazine on Microfilariae. Nature 1987; 325: 533–536.
43. Fujimaki Y, Ehara M, Kimura E, et al. Diethylcarbamazine, Antifilarial Drug, Inhibits Microtubule Polymerization and Disrupts Preformed Microtubules. Biochem Pharmacol 1990; 39: 851–856.

44. Maizels RM, Denham DA. Diethylcarbamazine (DEC): Immuno-pharmacological Interactions of an Anti-filarial Drug. Parasitol 1992; 105: S49–S60.

45. Mackenzie CD. Diethylcarbamazine: A Review of its Action in Onchocerciasis, Lymphatic Filariasis aand Inflammation. Trop Disease Bull 1985; 82: R1–R37.

46. Goa KL, McTavish D, Clissold SP. Ivermectin: A Review of its Antifilarial Activity, Pharmacokinetic Properties and Clinical Efficiacy in Onchocerciasis. Drugs 1991; 42: 640–658.

47. Ottesen EA, Campbell WC. Ivermectin in Human Medicine. J Antimicrob Chemotherap 1994; 34: 195–203.

48. Wiest PM, Li Y, Olds GR, et al. Inhibition of Phosphoinositide Turnover by Praziquantel in Schistosoma mansoni. J Parasitol 1992; 78: 753–755.

49. Xiao S-H, Catto BA, Webster LT, Jr. Effects of Praziquantel on Different Developmental Stages of Schistosoma monsoni in vitro and in vivo. J Infect Dis 1985; 151:1130–1137.

50. Fallon PG, Cooper RO, Probert AJ, et al. Immune-dependent Chemotherapy of Schistosomiasis. Parasitol 1992; 105:S41–S48.

51. Buhring KU, Diekmann HW, Muller H, et al. Eur J Drug Metab Pharmacokinet 1978; 3: 179.

52. Austin WC, Courtney WC, Danilewicz W, et al. Pyrantel Tartrate, a New Anthelmintic Effective Against Infections of Domestic Animals. Nature 1966; 212: 1273–1274.

53. Narahashi T. Nerve Membrane Ionic Channels as the Primary Target of Pyrethroids. NeuroToxicology 1985; 6: 3–22.

54. Vijverberg HPM, deWeille JR. The Interaction of Pyrethroids with Voltage-Dependent Na Channels. NeuroToxicology 1985; 6: 23–34.

55. Grammon DW, Sanders G. Pyrethroid-Receptor Interactions: Stereospecific Binding and Effects on sodium Channels in Mouse Brain Preparartions. NeuroToxicology 1985; 6: 35–46.

56. Lombet A, Mourre C, Lazdunski M. Interaction of Insecticides of the Pyrethroid Family with Specific Binding Sites on the Voltage-dependent Sodium Channel from Mammalian Brain. Brain Res 1988; 459: 44–53.

57. Soderund DM. Metabolic Consideration in Pyrethroid Design. Xenobiotica 1992; 22: 1185–1194.

58. Ruzo LO, Casida JE. Metabolism and Toxicology of Pyrethroids with Dihalovinyl Substituents. Envir Health Perspectives 1977; 21: 285292.

59. Taplin D, Meinkin TL, Joaquin BA, et al. Comparison of Critamiton 10% Cream (Eurax) and Permethrin 5% Cream (Elimite) for the Treatment of Scabies in Children. Ped Dermatol 1990; 7, 67–73.

60. Amer M, El-Ghariband I. Permethrin Versus Crotamiton and Lindane in the Treatment of Scabies. Int J Dernatol 1992; 31: 357–358.

SUGGESTED READINGS

Freeman CD, Klutman EE, Lamp KC. Metronidazole: A Therapeutic Review and Update, Drugs 1997; 54: 679–708.

Maizels RM, Bundy DAP, Selkirk ME, et al. Immunological Modulation and Evasion by Helminth Prarsites in Human Populations Nature 1993; 365: 797–805.

Wilson JD, Braunwald E, Isselbacher KJ, et al, eds. Harrison's Principles of Internal Medicine, 12th ed. New York: McGraw-Hill, 1991:772.

36. Antifungal Drugs

ROBERT GRIFFITH AND TIMOTHY TRACY

INTRODUCTION

Until recently chemotherapy of fungal infections has lagged far behind chemotherapy of bacterial infections. Historically, this lack of progress has been in part because the most common fungal infections in humans have been relatively superficial infections of the skin and mucosal membranes and potentially lethal deep-seated infections were rare. Since most humans with a normally functioning immune system are able to ward off invading fungal pathogens with little difficulty, the demand for improvements in antifungal therapy was small. However, immuno-compromised patients are very susceptible to invasive fungal infections. The onset of the AIDS epidemic combined with increased use of powerful immunosuppressive drugs for organ transplants and cancer chemotherapy has resulted in a greatly increased incidence of life-threatening fungal infections and a corresponding increase in demand for new agents to treat these infections.

Antifungal Drugs in Top 200

Presently, there are three antifungal agents in the Top 200 Drugs in terms of total sales:
  Fluconazole (Diflucan)
  Terbinafine (Lamisil)
  Itraconazole (Sporanox) (Top 200 in dollars of sales)

FUNGAL DISEASES(1)

The fungal kingdom includes yeasts, molds, rusts, and mushrooms. Most fungi are saprophytic, which means they live on dead organic matter in the soil or on decaying leaves or wood. A few of these fungi can cause opportunistic infections if they are introduced into a human through wounds or by inhalation. Some of these infections can be fatal. There are relatively few obligate animal parasites among the fungi, i.e., microorganisms which can only live on mammalian hosts although *Candida albicans* is commonly found as part of the normal flora of the gastrointestinal tract and vagina. The obligatory parasites are limited to dermatophytes that have evolved to live on/in the keratin containing hair and skin of mammals where they cause diseases such as ringworm and athletes foot. (Thus ringworm is not caused by a parasitic worm, but is named for the ring-like appearance of this fungal infection of the skin.)

Fungal infections are caused primarily by various yeasts and molds. Yeasts such as the opportunistic pathogen *Candida albicans* and the bakers' yeast *Saccharomyces cerevisiae* typically grow as single oval cells and reproduce by bud-

ding. *C. albicans* and some other pathogenic yeasts can also grow in multicellular chains called hyphae. Infection sites may contain both yeast and hyphal forms of the microorganism. Molds, such as *Trichophyton rubrum,* one of the causative agents of ringworm, grow in clusters of hyphae called a mycelium. All fungi produce spores which may be transported by direct contact or through the air. A detailed description of fungal disease is outside the scope of this book, but a brief description of some of the more common pathogens and the diseases they cause is given below.

Dermatophytes

Dermatophytes are fungi causing infections of skin, hair, and nails. The dermatophytes obtain nutrients from attacking the cross-linked structural protein keratin which other fungi cannot use as a food source. Dermatophytic infections, known as Tinea, are caused by various species of three genera, *Trichophyton, Microsporium,* and *Epidermophyton* and are named for the site of infection rather than the causative organism. Tinea capitis is a fungal infection of the hair and scalp, tinea pedis—infections of the feet including athlete's foot, tinea manuum—fungal infection of the hands, tinea cruris—infection of the groin (jock itch) and tinea unguium—infection of the fingernails. Athlete's foot in particular may be an infection involving several different fungi including yeasts. Tinea unguium, whether of the fingernails or toenails, can be particularly difficult to treat because the fungi invade the nail itself. Appropriate drug therapy prevents the fungus from spreading to newly formed nail, but penetration of drugs into previously existing nail is problematic and with some drug regimens the infection is not cured until an entirely new, fungus-free nail has grown in. Since this can take months, patient compliance with a lengthy drug regimen can be a problem.

Yeasts

The most common cause of yeast infections is *Candida albicans,* which is part of the normal flora in a significant portion of the population where it resides in the oropharynx, gastrointestinal tract, vagina, and surrounding skin. It is the principal cause of vaginal yeast infections and oral yeast infections (thrush). These commonly occur in mucosal tissue when the normal population of flora has been disturbed by treatment of a bacterial infection with an antibiotic, or when growth conditions are changed by hormonal fluctuations such as occur in pregnancy. *C. albicans* can cause infections of the skin and nails, although the latter are not common. In persons with healthy immune systems, *Candida* infections are limited to superficial infections of the skin and mucosa. However in persons with impaired immune systems, primarily AIDS patients, *C. albicans* may also cause deep-seated systemic infections which can be fatal. There are several other infection causing *Candida* species such as *C. tropicalis, C. krusei, C. parapsilosis, and C. glabrata* (also known as *Torulopsis glabrata*). These organisms are becoming more common and sometimes do not respond to antifungal therapy as readily as *C. albicans.*

Cryptococcus neoformans is a yeast commonly found in bird droppings, particularly pigeon droppings. When dust contaminated with spores is inhaled by persons with a competent immune system, the organism causes a minor, self-limiting, lung infection. Such infections are frequently mistaken for a cold and medical treatment is not sought. However in immunocompromised persons the organism can be carried by the circulatory system from the lungs to many other organs of the body including the central nervous system. Infection of the CNS is uniformly fatal unless treated.

Thermally Dimorphic Fungi

Thermally dimorphic fungi are saprophytes which grow in one form at room temperature and in a different form in a human host at 37°C. The most common infectious agents are *Blastomyces dermatitidus, Paracoccidiodes brasiliensis, Coccidioides immitus,* and *Histoplasma capsulatum,* the causative agents respectively of blastomycosis, paracoccidiomycosis, coccidiomycosis (valley fever), and histoplasmosis. All of these organisms live in soil and cause disease through inhalation of contaminated dust. The resulting lung infections are often mild and self-limiting, but may progress on to a serious lung infection. The circulatory system may transport the organisms to other tissues where the resulting systemic infection may be fatal. *B. dermatitidus* is endemic to south central United States, and *P. brasiliensis* to Central and South America where it is the most common cause of fungal pulmonary infections. *C. immitus* is endemic to the dry areas of the southwestern United States and northern Mexico. It is particularly prevalent in the San Joaquin Valley of California, hence the name valley fever. *H. capsulatum* is endemic to the Mississippi and Ohio River valleys of the United States where nearly 90% of the population tests positive for exposure to the organism.

Molds

Various *Aspergillus* species are found worldwide and are virtually ubiquitous in the environment. The most common organisms causing disease are *A. fumigatus, A. niger,* and *A. flavus.* There are several other *Aspergillus* species known to cause infection and some, such as *A. nidulans* are becoming more common. *Aspergillus* spp. very rarely cause disease in persons with normal immune systems, but are very dangerous to persons with suppressed immune systems. Since *Aspergillus* spores are everywhere, inhalation is the most common route of inoculation but infection through wounds, burns, and implanted devices such as

catheters is also possible. Nosocomial (hospital derived) aspergillosis is a major source of infection in persons with leukemia, receiving organ transplants, and bone marrow transplants. Aspergillosis of the lungs may be contained, but systemic aspergillosis has a high mortality rate.

Zygomycosis (mucormycosis) is a term used to describe infections caused by the genera *Rhizopus, Mucor,* and *Absidia* of the fungal order Mucorales. As with several other opportunistic fungal pathogens, these soil microorganisms are generally harmless to those with a competent immune system but can cause rapidly developing fatal infections in an immunosuppressed patient. These organisms can infect the sinus cavity from which they spread rapidly to the CNS. Blood vessels may also be attacked and ruptured. Zygomycoses spread rapidly and are often fatal.

BIOCHEMICAL TARGETS FOR ANTIFUNGAL CHEMOTHERAPY(2)

Antifungal chemotherapy depends on biochemical differences between fungi and mammals. Unlike bacteria, which are prokaryotes, both fungi and mammals are eukaryotes and the biochemical differences between them are not as great as one might expect. At the cellular level the greatest difference between fungal cells and mammalian cells is that fungal cells have cell walls but mammalian cells do not. Inhibitors of bacterial cell wall biosynthesis, such as penicillins and cephalosporins, have provided powerful antibacterial agents with little toxicity to humans. The fungal cell wall is therefore a logical target for a similar class of drugs which would be expected to be potent antifungals yet have little human toxicity. Unfortunately, although potent inhibitors of fungal cell wall biosynthesis in the laboratory are known, and several have entered clinical trials, such agents have proven very difficult to develop into drugs capable of clearing all the hurdles between the laboratory and the marketplace.

The most therapeutically relevant difference between fungal and mammalian cells is that the cell membranes of fungi and mammals contain different sterols. Sterols are important structural components of fungal and mammalian cell membranes and are critical to the proper functioning of many cell membrane enzymes and ion transport proteins. Mammalian cell membranes contain cholesterol as the sterol component while fungi contain ergosterol.

Cholesterol   Ergosterol

Although the two sterols are quite similar, the side chains are slightly different and when three-dimensional models are constructed, the ring system of ergosterol is slightly flatter because of the additional double bonds in

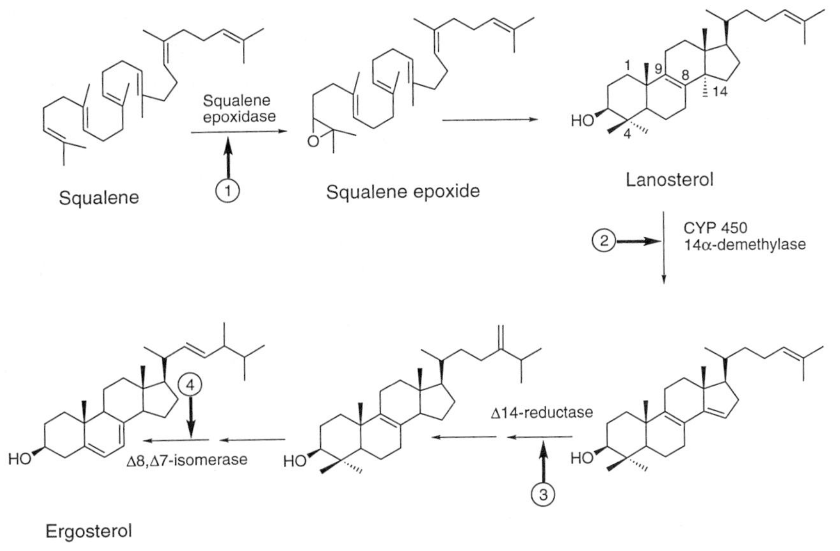

Fig. 36.1. Ergosterol biosynthesis from squalene with key steps shown in this simplified figure. Enzymatic steps known to be the site of action of currently employed antifungal agents are indicated by a heavy black arrow and a number.

the B ring. Nevertheless, with only a few exceptions this difference in sterol components provides the biochemical basis of selective toxicity for most of the currently available antifungal drugs.

A schematic of fungal ergosterol biosynthesis starting from squalene is shown in Figure 36.1. The biosynthetic pathway has been simplified to emphasize steps important to the action of currently employed antifungal drugs. The last nonsteroidal precursor to both ergosterol and cholesterol is the hydrocarbon squalene. Squalene is converted to squalene epoxide by the enzyme squalene epoxidase. Squalene epoxide is then cyclized to lanosterol, the first steroid in the biosynthetic pathway. The steps involved in converting the side chain of lanosterol to the side chain of ergosterol, and the steps in removal of the geminal dimethyl groups on position 4 are not shown since none of these reactions is targeted by clinically employed antifungal agents.

A key step in conversion of lanosterol to both cholesterol and ergosterol is removal of the 14α-methyl group. This reaction is carried out by a cytochrome P450 enzyme, α-demethylase. The mechanism of this reaction involves three successive hydroxylations of the 14α-methyl group converting it from a hydrocarbon through the alcohol, aldehyde, and carboxylic acid oxidation states, (Fig. 36.2). The methyl group is eliminated as formic acid to afford a double bond between C14 and C15 of the D ring. This enzyme is the primary target of the azole antifungal agents discussed below.

Eventually, either before or after modification of the side chain, the Δ14 double bond is reduced by a Δ14–reductase to form a *trans* ring juncture between the C and D rings. Several steps later the double bond between C8 and C9 is isomerized to a Δ7 double bond by the enzyme Δ8–Δ9-isomerase. Many of the steps are identical to those involved in mammalian cholesterol biosynthesis. The basis for selective toxicity to fungal cells will be discussed under the specific agents.

ANTIFUNGAL DRUGS BASED ON AFFECTING THE MEMBRANE ERGOSTEROL
Polyene Membrane Disrupters—Nystatin, Amphotericin B and Congeners (3)

Prior to the mid-1950s effective antifungal therapy was limited to topical applications of undecylenic acid derivatives, mixtures of benzoic acid and salicylic acid, and a few other agents of modest efficacy. There were no reliable treatments for the few cases of deep-seated systemic fungal infections that did occur. The discovery of the polyene antifungal agents provided a breakthrough into both a new class of antifungal agents and the first drug effective against deep-seated fungal infections. The polyenes are macrocyclic lactones with distinct hydrophilic and lipophilic regions. The hydrophilic region contains several alcohols, a carboxylic acid, and usually a sugar. The lipophilic region contains, in part, a chromophore of four to seven conjugated double bonds. The number of conjugated double bonds correlates directly with antifungal activity *in vitro* and inversely with the degree of toxicity to mammalian cells. That is, not only are the compounds with seven conjugated double bonds, such as amphotericin B, approximately 10 times more fungitoxic, but they are the only ones which may be used systemically.

Mechanism of Action

The polyenes have an affinity for sterol containing membranes, insert into the membranes, and disrupt membrane functions. The membranes of cells treated with polyenes become leaky and eventually the cells die because of the loss of essential cell constituents such as ions and small organic molecules. Polyenes have a demonstrably higher affinity for membranes containing ergosterol over cholesterol containing membranes. This is the basis for their greater toxicity to fungal cells. There is some evi-

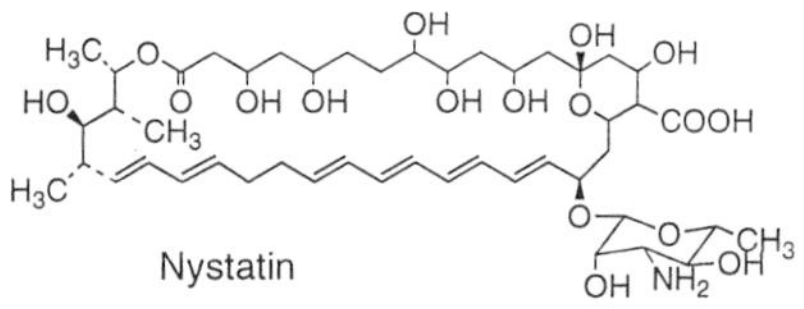

Nystatin

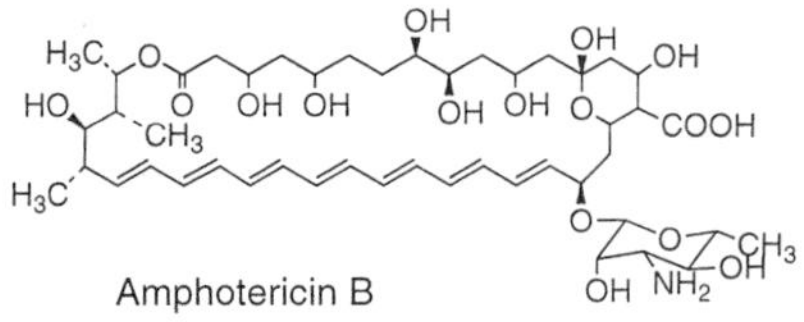

Amphotericin B

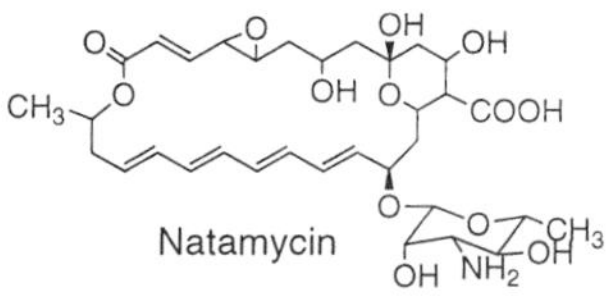

Natamycin

dence that the mechanism of insertion differs between the types of cells. Polyene molecules may insert individually into ergosterol containing membranes, but require prior formation of polyene micelles before inserting into cholesterol containing membranes.

Polyene Drugs

Nystatin. Nystatin, the first clinically useful polyene antifungal antibiotic, is a conjugated tetraene isolated from cultures of the bacterium *Streptomyces noursei* in 1951. Nystatin is an effective topical antifungal against a wide variety of organisms and is available in a variety of creams and ointments. Nystatin is too toxic to be used systemically, but since very little drug is absorbed following oral administration it may be administered by mouth to treat fungal infections of the mouth and gastrointestinal tract (Table 36.1). Although nystatin itself was not a breakthrough in systemic antifungal therapy, the search for other polyenes led to the discovery of a polyene that can be used systemically.

Amphotericin B. Amphotericin B, which as a heptaene has low enough toxicity to mammalian cells to permit in-

travenous administration, was discovered in 1956. Amphotericin B is, nevertheless, a very toxic drug and must be used with caution. Adverse effects include fever, shaking chills, hypotension and severe kidney toxicity. Despite its toxicity, amphotericin B is considered the drug of choice for many systemic, life-threatening fungal infections. The drug cannot cross the blood-brain barrier, and must be administered intrathecally for treatment of fungal infections of the central nervous system. Closely related heptaenes are candicidin, hamycin, and trichomycin.

The nephrotoxicity of amphotericin B has been a serious drawback to the use of this drug since its introduction. Recently, however, the toxicity of the drug has been decreased substantially by changes in formulation (Table 36.1). The polyenes are only sparingly soluble in water, and amphotericin B has long been formulated as a complex with deoxycholic acid for intravenous administration. More recently developed formulations of amphotericin B such as liposomal encapsulation, and lipid complexes have dramatically decreased the toxicity of the drug to humans, which permits higher plasma levels to be employed. The mechanisms by which the new formulations decrease the toxicity are not entirely clear, but altered distribution is clearly a factor. Because the blood vessels at the site of infection are more permeable than those of normal tissue, the large suspended particles of the lipid formulations can penetrate the site of infection more readily than they can penetrate healthy tissue. The result is selective delivery of drug to the site of infection. There is also some evidence that the newer formulations transfer amphotericin B to ergosterol containing fungal cells more efficiently than to cholesterol containing mammalian cells.

Natamycin. Natamycin, a tetraene, is available in the United States as a 5% suspension applied topically for the treatment of fungal infections of the eye (Table 36.1).

Ergosterol biosynthesis Inhibitors—Azoles

Azole antifungal agents are the largest class of antimycotics available today with over 20 drugs on the market.

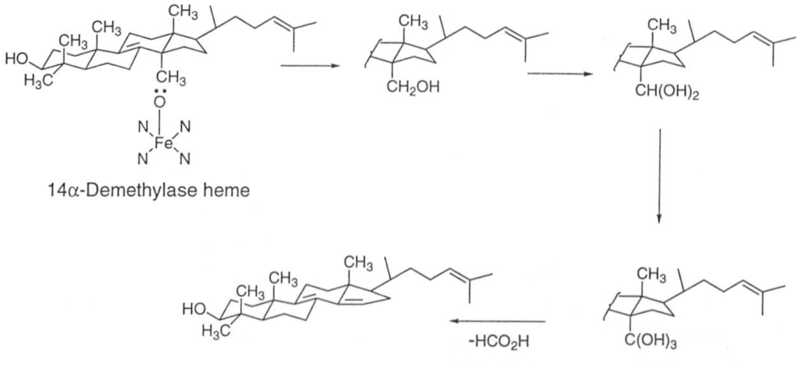

Fig. 36.2. Demethylation of the 14α-methyl group from lanosterol carried out by the cytochrome P450 enzyme sterol 14α-demethylase, CYP51. The mechanism involves three successive heme catalyzed insertions of activated oxygen into the three carbon-hydrogen bonds of the 14α-methyl group which raises the oxidation state of the methyl group to a carboxylic acid. The group is finally eliminated as formic acid to create a double bond between carbons 14 and 15.

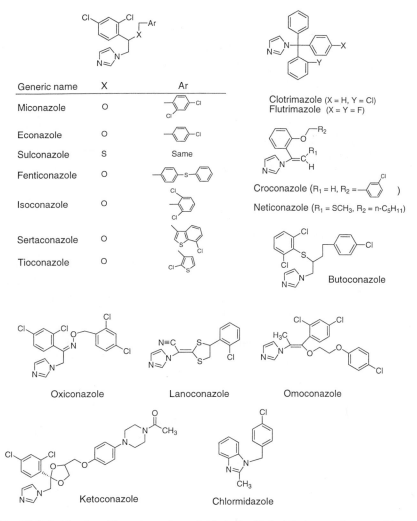

Fig. 36.3. Imidazole antifungal agents available in the United States or other countries.

Some are primarily used topically to treat superficial dermatophytic and yeast infections, while others are administered orally for the treatment of systemic fungal infections (Table 36.1). The oral bioavailability of some azoles, in contrast to amphotericin B, combined with their generally broad-spectrum of activity has led to their widespread use in treating a variety of serious infections. The characteristic chemical feature of azoles from which their name is derived, is the presence of a five-membered aromatic ring containing either two or three nitrogen atoms. Imidazole rings have two nitrogens and triazoles three. In both cases the azole ring is attached through N_1 to a side chain containing at least one aromatic ring. Imidazole containing agents are shown in Figure 36.3 and triazoles in Figure 36.5.

Mechanism of Action

All of the azoles act by inhibiting ergosterol biosynthesis through inhibition of the 14α-demethylase discussed above under ergosterol biosynthesis (Fig. 36.1, Site 2). The basic N_3 atom of the azole forms a bond with the heme iron of the CYP450 prosthetic group in the position normally occupied by the activated oxygen, (Fig. 36.4). The remainder of the azole antifungal forms bonding in-

teractions with the apoprotein in a manner which determines the relative selectivity of the drug for the fungal demethylase versus other CYP450 enzymes.

Inhibition of the 14α-demethylase results in accumulation in the fungal cell membrane of sterols still bearing a 14α-methyl group. These sterols do not have the exact shape and physical properties of the normal membrane sterol ergosterol. This results in permeability changes,

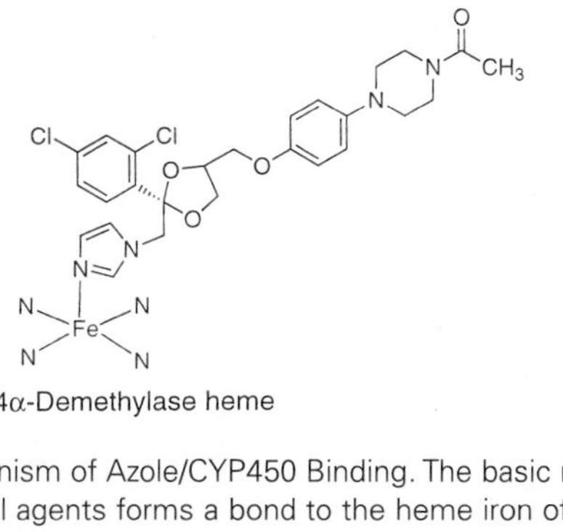

14α-Demethylase heme

Fig. 36.4. Mechanism of Azole/CYP450 Binding. The basic nitrogen of azole antifungal agents forms a bond to the heme iron of CYP450 enzymes, preventing the enzyme from oxidizing its normal substrates. Ketoconazole is representative of the azole antifungals.

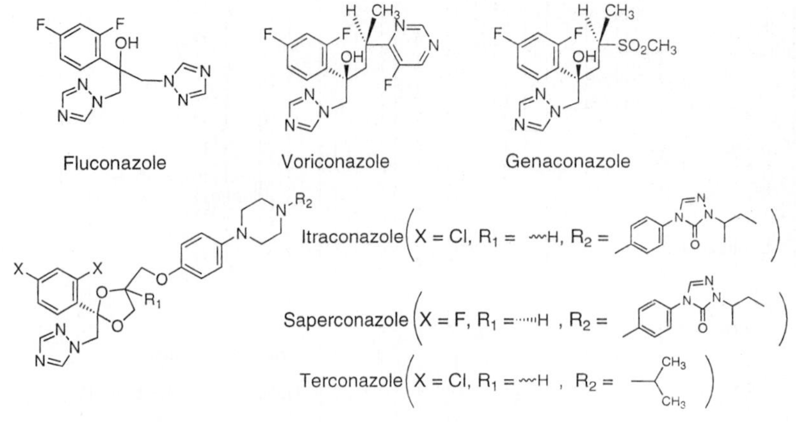

Fig. 36.5. Triazole antifungal agents available in the United States or other countries.

leaky membranes, and malfunction of membrane-imbedded proteins. These effects taken together lead to fungal cell death. Since biosynthesis of the mammalian membrane sterol cholesterol also employs a CYP450 14α-demethylase, why don't 14α-methyl sterols accumulate in human cell membranes? The reason is in the relative strength of inhibition of the same enzyme from different species. The IC_{50} value for ketoconazole against the enzyme from *C. albicans* is approximately $10^{-9}M$ versus approximately $10^{-6}M$ for the human enzyme. This three or-

Table 36.1. Marketed Antifungal Drugs

Chemical Class	Generic Name	Trade Name	Dosage Form and Dosage
Organic Acid	Undecylenate (salts)	Desenex (Zinc) Cruex (Calcium)	Topical, 2–20%
Allylamine	Naftifine	Naftin	Topical, 1%
	Terbinafine	Lamisil	Cream, 1% Tablet, 250 mg/day
	Butenafine	Mentax	Topical cream, 1%
	Tolnaftate (Thiocarbamate)	Tinactin Aftate	Topical, 1% Topical, 1%
Polyene	Amphotericin B	Fungizone (deoxycholic acid)	0.5–0.7 mg/kg
		AmBisome (liposomal)	3–5 mg/kg/day
		Abelcet (lipid complex)	5 mg/kg/day
		Amphotec (cholesteryl)	3–4 mg/kg/day
	Nystatin	Mycostatin	Topical, 100,000 units
		Nilstat	Oral suspension, 100,000–
		Nystex	1 million units/ml
	Natamycin	Natacyn	Topical suspension, 5%
Pyrimidine	5-Fluorocytosine	Ancoban	Capsule, 50–150 mg/kg/day
Azole Imidazole	Butoconazole	Femstat	Topical, 2%
	Clotrimazole	Gyne-Lotrimin	Vaginal tablet, 100–200mg
		Lotrimin	Topical, 1%
		Mycelex	Topical, 1%
	Econoazole	Spectrazole	Topical, 1%
	Ketoconazole	Nizoral	Tablet, 200–400 mg/day
		Nizoral cream, Shampoo	Topical, 2%
	Miconazole	Micatin	Topical, 2%
		Lotrimin	Topical, 2% spray
		Monistat i.v.	I.V., 600 mg–3.6 g/day
	Oxiconazole	Oxistat	Topical, 1%
	Sulconazole	Exelderm	Topical, 1%
		Sulcosyn	Topical, 1%
	Tioconazole	Vagistat-1	Topical, 6.5%
Triazole	Fluconazole	Diflucan	Tablet, 100–200 mg/day
	Itraconazole	Sporanox	Tablet, 100–400 mg/day
	Terconazole	Terazol	Topical, 0.4–0.8%
Misc.	Griseofulvin	Fulvicin: Grifulvin; Grisactin	Microsize 500–1000 mg Ultramicrosize 330–375mg
	Haloprogin	Halotex	Topical, 1%

ders of magnitude difference in strength of inhibition provides the therapeutic index with respect to this particular enzyme. However, as discussed below, many of the azoles are powerful inhibitors of other mammalian cytochrome P450 enzymes.

Metabolism

The azole antifungal drugs are in general extensively and rapidly degraded by first-pass metabolism. As a result, only those drugs with reduced or slow first-pass metabolism (miconazole-IV, ketoconazole-oral, and fluconazole-oral) are used systemically. The other azoles, clotrimazole, tioconazole, terconazole, butoconazole, econazole, oxiconazole, sulconazole, along with miconazole and ketoconazole are available in a variety of creams and ointments for topical use (Table 36.1).

Ketoconazole was the first orally active antifungal azole to be discovered and as a consequence has been more widely studied and employed for the treatment of systemic fungal infections. As with other azoles, it is extensively metabolized, Figure 36.6. All of the metabolites are inactive. Despite the drug's metabolism it was originally thought that ketoconazole was devoid of human CYP450 enzyme activity. However, with time it was discovered that the purported selectivity was not absolute and clinically important drug interactions involving CYP450 in humans receiving ketoconazole began to emerge (see below). In an attempt to prevent ring hydroxylation of ketoconazole and to thus minimize interaction between the imidazole antifungals and human CYP450 enzyme, the triazole class of antifungals were developed. The initial triazoles, fluconazole and itraconazole, were expected to show less affinity for mammalian CYP450, exhibit a broader-spectrum of antifungal activity, and through increased water solubility be more effectively administered. However, clinical experience with fluconazole and itraconazole has shown that these agents also can produce clinically important drug interactions. As a result, one must use caution when administering azole antifungal agents concurrently with drugs having narrow therapeutic indices or a potential for toxicity.

As data continue to emerge, it is becoming increasingly apparent that the primary route of metabolism of the systemic azole antifungals (both imidazoles and triazoles) is via the CYP450 enzyme system. Thus, although their in vitro affinity for human P450s may be lower than for fungal 14α-demethylase, they do have clinically relevant affinity for and are metabolized by human CYP450s. Approximately 95% of a ketoconazole dose undergoes metabolism, primarily by CYP3A4. Likewise, itraconazole is extensively (80–90%) metabolized presumably by CYP3A4. The unique case is that of fluconazole, of which only 10% of the dose is metabolized with the remainder of the drug excreted unchanged. It appears drug-drug interactions between the azoles and an assortment of other drugs occurs via a competitive inhibition of enzymes involved in drug metabolism. However, noncompetitive mechanisms of inhibition may also be possible since, for example, very little of a fluconazole dose is metabolized by human CYP450s and yet it is a potent inhibitor of some of these enzymes.

CYP450 Isoform Inhibition Selectivity

Ketoconazole. As stated above, ketoconazole is a potent inhibitor of the CYP3A4 enzyme and as such has been

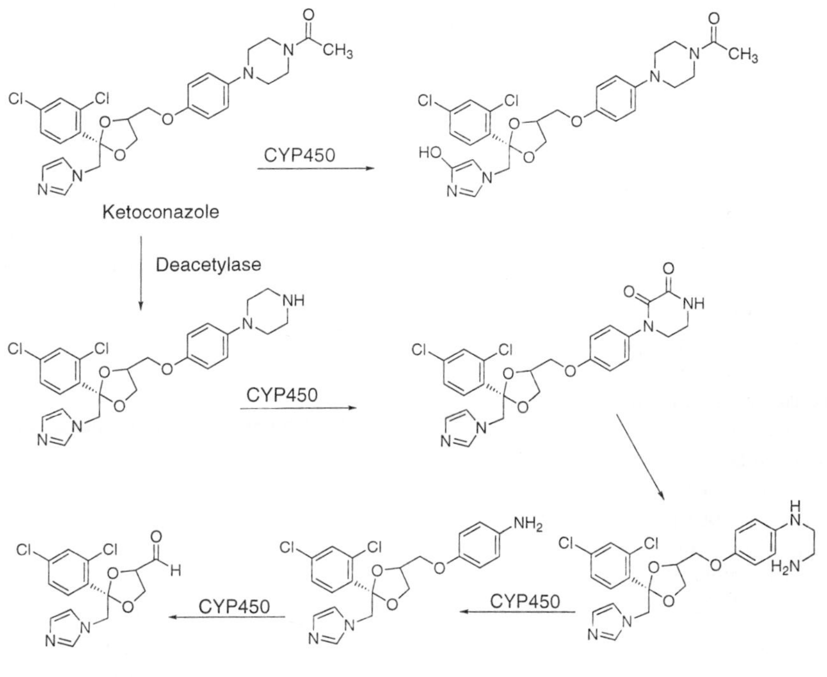

Fig. 36.6. Extensively metabolism of Ketoconazole involving hydrolysis of the N-acetyl by a deacetylase. The oxidation reactions are catalyzed primarily by CYP3A4 and all metabolites are inactive.

demonstrated to cause a number of serious or life-threatening drug interactions when given concomitantly with certain medications also metabolized by this CYP isoform. Ketoconazole was one of the primary drugs shown to inhibit the metabolism of the nonsedating antihistamine terfenadine and thus potentially causing the life-threatening torsade de pointes arrhythmia. Eventually, terfenadine was withdrawn from the market. Ketoconazole, through a similar mechanism, had potentially fatal drug-drug interaction with the prokinetic agent cisapride which led to this drug also being withdrawn from the market. Co-administration of ketoconazole with the hypnotic triazolam results in a 22-fold increase in triazolam's area under the curve (AUC) and a 7-fold increase in half-life. Interestingly, CYP3A4 is also present in the gut and may contribute substantially to the metabolism of many drugs such as the immunosuppressant agent cyclosporine, thus the potential for drug-drug interaction (See Sidebar).

It is of note that ketoconazole is a very weak inhibitor of CYP2C9, which is the enzyme responsible for the metabolism of several narrow therapeutic index drugs such as warfarin and phenytoin (see Fluconazole discussion below). Finally, the coadministration of CYP3A4 inducers such as phenytoin, carbamazepine and rifampin can cause as much as a 50% reduction in levels of ketoconazole due to increased P450 3A4 activity.

Itraconazole. Itraconazole, like ketoconazole, is extensively metabolized by CYP3A4 following oral administration and levels are markedly reduced by co-administration of the CYP450 3A4 inducers phenytoin, carbamazepine and rifampin. With respect to inhibition of drug metabolism by CYP3A4, itraconazole has been demonstrated to cause a 20-fold increase in the area under the curve of the HMG-CoA reductase inhibitors lovastatin and simvastatin. This interaction has proven to be of clinical significance

---

Ketoconazole and Cyclosporine—A Clinically Useful Drug Interaction. (5)

Cyclosporine is an immunosuppressive agent used in transplant patients to help prevent organ rejection. Though effective, cyclosporine therapy is extremely expensive and appears to be only approximately 20% bioavailable following an oral dose. This low bioavailability is due to the metabolism of cyclosporine by the CYP450 system to a number of metabolites. Early reports of co-administration of ketoconazole with cyclosporine described excessive adverse effects attributable to cyclosporine toxicity. From this and knowledge about the effects of ketoconazole on CYP450 mediated metabolism, investigators hypothesized that a much lower dose of cyclosporine could be given concomitantly with ketoconazole producing blood levels of cyclosporine equivalent to those seen with the higher dose at a fraction of the cost. In fact, it appears that ketoconazole given concurrently with cyclosporine may allow up to an 80% reduction in cyclosporine dose.

---

because the risk of developing rhabdomyolysis following lovastatin or simvastatin therapy is increased by co-administration of itraconazole. Itraconazole also appears to interfere with the metabolism of some benzodiazepine sedatives (i.e., triazolam and midazolam) which are metabolized CYP3A4. For example, itraconazole increased the area under the curve of triazolam 27-fold and produced similar effects on midazolam elimination. However, itraconazole appeared to produced little effect on diazepam elimination. Like ketoconazole, itraconazole appears to have little or no effect on CYP2C9 mediated metabolism of warfarin and phenytoin.

Fluconazole. Fluconazole differs from ketoconazole and itraconazole in that it is equally bioavailable when given orally or intravenously. Fluconazole also differs in that its primary inhibition of cytochrome P450 mediated drug metabolism occurs via inhibition of CYP2C9, while exhibiting lesser inhibition of CYP3A4 than the other systemic azoles. For instance, fluconazole doubles the area under the curve of (S)-warfarin (the active enantiomer) and greatly prolongs the prothrombin time in patients receiving warfarin anticoagulant therapy. Since warfarin has such a narrow therapeutic index and excessive anticoagulation can be extremely harmful, this interaction is considered to be of major clinical significance. Fluconazole also decreases the metabolism of the CYP2C9 substrate phenytoin, an anti-epileptic agent also with a narrow therapeutic index. Depending on the dose of fluconazole, co-administration with phenytoin can result in a 75–150% increase in the phenytoin area under the curve and numerous case reports have documented substantial adverse effects following this regimen. Fluconazole will also inhibit CYP3A4, though not to the same degree as ketoconazole and itraconazole. Fluconazole exhibits a dose dependent inhibition of triazolam metabolism (a CYP3A4 reaction) causing as much as a 4-fold increase in triazolam AUC.

Potential of CYP450 Inhibition Following Topical or Intravaginal Administration of Azole Antifungals

Several of the azole antifungals are available in a variety of dosage forms for the treatment of various maladies. For example, ketoconazole is available in both shampoo and cream formulations for treatment of topical fungal infections. Clinical studies have not been able to detect measurable blood levels of ketoconazole following topical administration and no drug interactions have been reported. A great number of the azole antifungals (e.g., miconazole, terconazole and clotrimazole) are also administered vaginally for the treatment of vaginal candidiasis. It would seem plausible that systemic absorption would be more likely following vaginal administration as compared to topical skin administration. Limited data exists on whether clinically significant levels of azole are achieved following vaginal administration and therefore the concerns for drug interactions are unknown.

Azole Antifungals in Agriculture

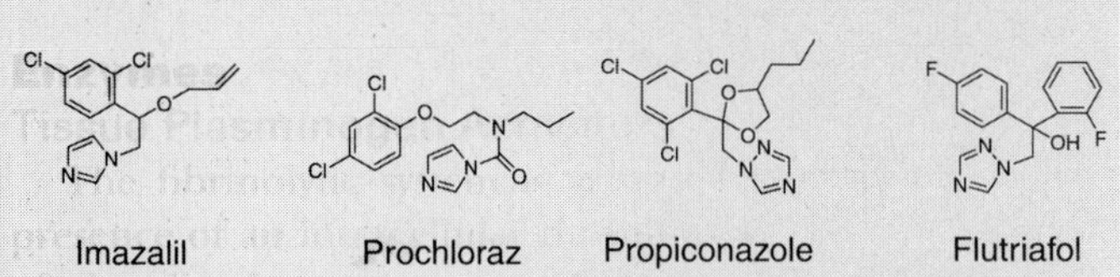

Imazalil   Prochloraz   Propiconazole   Flutriafol

Every year fungal infections of crops causes hundreds of millions of dollars worth of damage to a wide variety of food and other crops. Prior to the development of effective agricultural antifungals crop diseases were the cause of several major famines. The infamous Irish Potato Famine of the 19th Century was caused by a pathogenic fungus *Phytophera infestans*.

Tens of thousands of people starved to death and thousands more emigrated to the United States to escape the famine. Today both imidazole and triazole antifungal agents such as imazalil and propiconazole are among the most effective crop protection agents known. There are over 20 azole antifungals used in crop protection and a representative sample is shown. The mechanism of action of the agricultural antifungals is identical to that of the agents used for mammalian infections. In fact, they bear a remarkable resemblance to antifungal drugs employed in treating human disease.

Ergosterol Biosynthesis Inhibitors—Allyl Amines and Other Squalene Epoxidase Inhibitors

The group of agents generally known as allyl amines strictly includes only naftifine and terbinafine, but since butenafine and tolnaftate function by the same mechanism of action they are included in this class and are shown in Figure 36.7. One can, of course, consider the benzyl group of butenafine to be bioisosteric with the allyl group of naftifine and terbinafine. Tolnaftate, a much older drug, is chemically a thiocarbamate, with the same mechanism of action as the allyl amines. These drugs have a more limited

spectrum of activity than the azoles and are effective only against dermatophytes. Therefore they are employed in the treatment of fungal infections of the skin and nails.

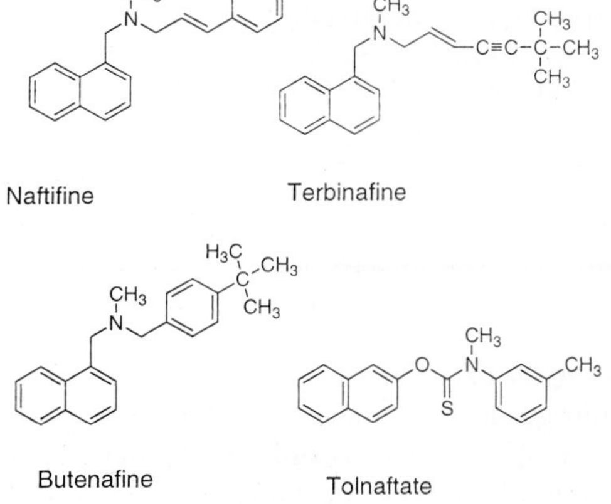

Mechanism of Action

All of the drugs in Figure 36.7 act through inhibition of the enzyme squalene epoxidase, (Fig. 36.1, Site 1). Inhibition of this enzyme has two effects, both of which appear to be involved in the fungitoxic mechanism of this class. First, inhibition of squalene epoxidase results in a decrease in total sterol content of the fungal cell membrane. This decrease alters the physical-chemical properties of the membrane resulting in malfunctions of membrane-imbedded transport proteins involved in nutrient transport and pH balance. Second, inhibition of squalene epoxidase results in a buildup within the fungal cell of the hydrocarbon squalene which is itself toxic when present in abnormally high amounts. Mammals also employ the enzyme squalene epoxidase in the biosynthesis of cholesterol, but a desirable therapeutic index arises from the fact that the fungal squalene epoxidase enzyme is far more sensitive to the drugs than the corresponding mammalian enzyme. Terbinafine has a K_i of 0.03 μM versus squalene epoxidase from *Candida albicans* but only 77 μM versus the same enzyme from rat liver, a 2,500-fold difference(6).

Allyl Amine Drugs

Naftifine. Naftifine was the first allyl amine to be discovered and marketed. It is subject to first-pass metabolism to be orally active, and consequently is only available in topical preparations (Table 36.1). The widest use of naftifine is against various tinea infections of the skin.

Terbinafine. Terbinafine is available in both topical and oral dosage forms (Table 36.1). Although effective against a variety of dermatophytic infections, terbinafine is particularly useful for the treatment of onychomycoses (nail infections). Given orally the drug redistributes from the plasma into the nail where the infection resides.

Butenafine and Tolnaftate. Butenafine and tolnaftate like naftifine, are only available in topical preparation for the treatment of dermatophytic infections (Table 36.1). Tolnaftate has been marketed in a variety of nonprescription drug preparations for decades. Butenafine, more recently discovered, has a somewhat wider spectrum of activity than tolnaftate. For example, butenafine is active against superficial *Candida albicans* infections which are not affected by tolnaftate. Butenafine is available OTC in some countries.

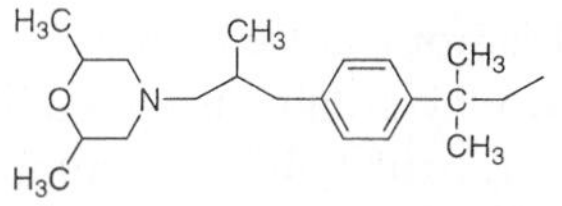

Naftifine   Terbinafine

Butenafine   Tolnaftate

Fig. 36.7. The squalene epoxidase inhibitors, allyl amines. Naftifine was the first drug shown to act by inhibition of squalene epoxidase as does the much older thiocarbamate, tolnaftate.

Amorolfine

Ergosterol Biosynthesis Inhibitors—Morpholines

Amorolfine is the only drug in this class employed clinically in the treatment of human fungal infections. Amorolfine is not currently available in the United States, but it is marketed in Europe and Asia for the topical treatment of dermatophytic infections. There are, however, a number of morpholines employed as agricultural antifungals for the treatment of plant diseases, two of which are shown.

Agricultural Antifungal Orpholines

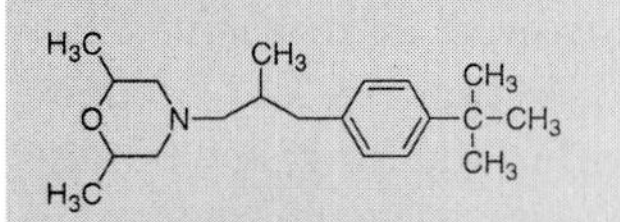

Fenpropimorph 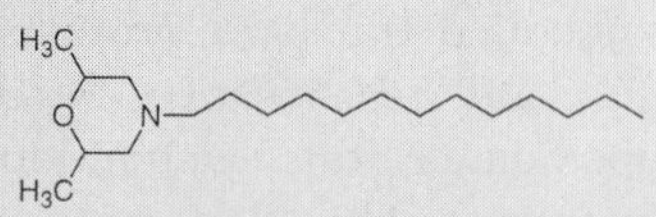　　　　Tridemorph

Just as there are several classes of drugs to treat human fungal infections, there are several classes of "drugs" to treat fungal phytopathogens. The morpholines, fenpropimorph and tridemorph, not used to treat human disease, have wide utility in protecting crops from phytopathogenic fungi.

Mechanism of Action

Morpholine antifungals inhibit ergosterol biosynthesis by acting on the enzymes Δ^{14}-reductase and Δ^8-Δ^7-isomerase, (Fig. 36.1, Site 3 and 4). Inhibition of these enzymes results in incorporation into fungal cell membranes of sterols retaining either a Δ^{14} double bond, a Δ^8 double bond, or both. None of these will have the same overall shape and physical-chemical properties as the preferred sterol ergosterol. As with the antifungals already discussed, this results in membranes with altered properties and malfunctioning of membrane-embedded proteins.

ANTIFUNGAL DRUG NOT AFFECTING MEMBRANE ERGOSTEROL

The vast majority of drugs currently employed in the treatment of fungal infections base their mechanism of action on the differing sterol component of fungal versus mammalian cell membranes. There are, however, several important drugs which do not depend on ergosterol versus cholesterol for their mechanism.

Flucytosine (7)

Flucytosine is a powerful antifungal agent used in the treatment of serious systemic fungal infections such as *Cryptococcus neoformans* and *Candida* spp (Table 36.1). Flucytosine itself is not cytotoxic, but rather is a pro-drug which is taken up by fungi and metabolised to 5-fluorouracil, 5-FU, by fungal cytidine deaminase, Figure 36.8. 5-FU is then converted to 5-fluorodeoxyuridine which as a thymidylate synthase inhibitor interferes with both pro-

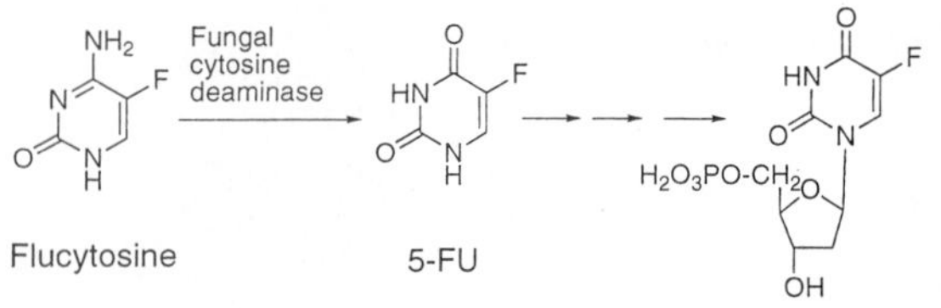

Fig. 36.8. Flucytosine, a pro-drug, is converted by fungal cytosine deaminase to 5-fluorouracil (5-FU). This reaction does not occur in mammalian cells. 5-FU is further transformed to the actual cytotoxic agent 5-fluorodeoxyuridine monophosphate (5-FdUMP).

tein and RNA biosynthesis. 5-FU is cytotoxic and is employed in cancer chemotherapy, (see Chapter 38). Human cells do not contain cytosine deaminase and therefore do not convert flucytosine to 5-FU. However, some intestinal flora do convert the drug to 5-FU so human toxicity does result from this metabolism. Resistance rapidly develops to flucytosine when used alone, so it is almost always used in conjunction with amphotericin B. Use of flucytosine has declined since the discovery of fluconazole.

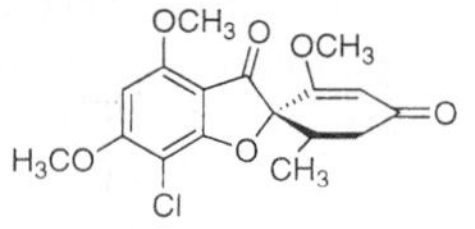

Griseofulvin

Griseofulvin (7)

Griseofulvin is an antifungal antibiotic produced by an unusual strain of *penicillium*. It is used orally to treat superficial fungal infections, primarily fingernail and toenail infections. It does not penetrate skin or nails if used topically. When given orally however, plasma-borne griseofulvin becomes incorporated into keratin precursor cells and ultimately into kearatin which cannot then support fungal growth (Table 36.1). The infection is cured when the diseased tissue is replaced by new, uninfected tissue which can take months. The mechanism of action of griseofulvin is through binding to the protein tubulin which interferes with the function of the mitotic spindle and thereby inhibits cell division. Griseofulvin may also interfere directly with DNA replication. Griseofulvin is gradually being replaced by newer agents.

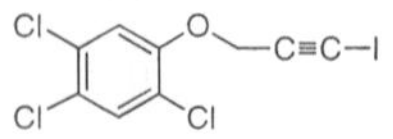

Haloprogin

Haloprogin (7)

Haloprogin is an iodinated acetylene active against dermatophytes. Haloprogin is only used for topical applications (Table 36.1). The mechanism of haloprogin is not clear, but appears to lead to nonspecific metabolic disruption. It has been demonstrated to interfere with DNA biosynthesis and cell respiration.

$$H_2C=CH(CH_2)_8COOH$$

Undecylenic acid

Undecylenic Acid (7)

Undecylenic acid is widely employed, frequently as the zinc salt, in OTC preparations for topical treatment of infections by dermatophytes. Undecylenic acid is fungistatic acting through a nonspecific interaction with components in the cell membrane (Table 36.1).

AGENTS ACTING ON THE CELL WALL (8)

The most notable difference between fungal and mammalian cells is that fungi have a cell wall and mammals do not. Drugs interfering with cell wall biosynthesis would be expected to be relatively nontoxic to mammals. Such drugs have been the foundation of antibacterial therapy since the discovery of penicillin and the development of dozens of effective penicillins and cephalosporins. Interference with fungal cell wall biosynthesis has not been similarly successful. A large number of antibiotic chemicals have been discovered which interfere with various steps in fungal cell wall biosynthesis, and these chemicals are excellent antifungal agents in vitro. Unfortunately, development of these chemicals into useful drugs has proven extremely difficult.

Echinocandins, a group of cyclic peptides with long lipophilic sidechains have been under investigation for a number of years. Echinocandins interfere with cell wall biosynthesis through inhibition of the enzyme β-1,3-glucan synthase. β-glucan is an important polymer component of many fungal cell walls and reduction in the glucan content severely weakens the cell wall leading to rupture of the fungal cell. Several echinocandins have entered clinical trial and made it as far as Phase III only to fail due to formulation problems and limited spectrum of activity in the clinic. Caspofungin, an enchinocandin, has recently been approved by the FDA for treatment of aspergillosis and candida infections, but has proven to be ineffective against *Cryptococcus neoformans*. The drug is administered IV and is highly bound to plasma protein. Caspofungin represents the first class of antifungal agents with a novel mechanism of action to be marketed in over 30 years.

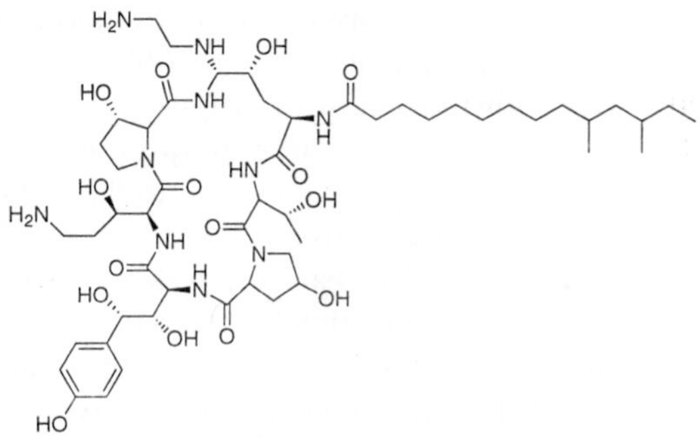

Caspofungin (Cancidas)

Victoria F. Roche and S. William Zito

RO, a 24-year-old accountant, has joined his neighborhood gym to enhance his fitness level and lower his stress. His routine is to swim 30 laps, then take an aerobics class and, if a partner is available, play a little fast-action raquetball. RO does not like to use the shower in the gym because of some very disfiguring scars in his groin area that resulted from burns received when, as a child, he dumped a pot of scalding coffee in his lap. He showers in his swim trunks before entering the pool, but just heads for home after the aerobics and raquetball with the intent of cleaning up there. Oftentimes, however, he is so ravenous when he gets home that he takes time to fix and eat his dinner before showering up.

Because of his barefoot trek across the gym floor and the fact that he keeps his feet trapped in shoes and hot, sweaty socks for a couple of hours after vigorous exercise, he has contracted a rather severe case of athlete's foot. He has been scratching at the fungus, and his skin is now broken and macerated. Other than this dermatophyte infection, RO is healthy and is taking no Rx or OTC medications.

1. *Identify the therapeutic problem(s) where the pharmacist's intervention may benefit the patient.*

2. *Identify and prioritize the patient specific factors that must be considered to achieve the desired therapeutic outcomes.*

3. *Conduct a thorough and mechanistically oriented structure-activity analysis of all therapeutic alternatives provided in the case.*

4. *Evaluate the SAR findings against the patient specific factors and desired therapeutic outcomes and make a therapeutic decision.*

5. *Counsel your patient.*

REFERENCES

1. Crissey JT, Lang H, Parish LC. Manual of Medical Mycology. Cambridge, MA: Blackwell Science, 1995.

2. Koller W. ed. Target Sites of Fungicide Action. Boca Raton, CRC Press: 1992.

3. Koller W. Antifungal agents with target sites in sterol functions and biosynthesis, in Target Sites of Fungicide Action, W. Koller, Ed. 1992, CRC Press: Boca Raton. p. 119–206.

4. Lomaestro BM, Piatek MA. Update on drug interactions with azole antifungal agents. Annals of Pharmacotherapy, 1998; 32: 915–928.

5. Gomez DY, Watcher VJ, Tomlanovich SJ, et al. The effects of ketoconazole on the intestinal metabolism and bioavailability of cyclosporine. Clin Pharmacol Ther. 1995; 58: 15–19.

6. Petranyi G, Stutz A, Ryder NS, et al. Experimental antimycotic activity of naftifine and terbinafine. In: Recent Trends in the Discovery, Development and Evaluation of Antifungal Agents, R.A. Fromtling, Ed. 1987, J.R. Prous Science: Barcelona. p. 441-459.

7. Hunter PA, Darby KG, Russell NJ, Eds. Fifty Years of Antimicrobials: Past Perspectives and Future Trends. Symposia of the Society for General Microbiology, ed. M. Collins. 1995, Cambridge University Press: Cambridge.

8. Balkovec JM. Non-azole antifungal agents. Ann Reports in Med Chem, 1998; 33:173-182.

37. Antimycobacterial Agents

THOMAS L. LEMKE

GENERAL CONSIDERATION

Mycobacteria are a genus of acid-fast bacilli belonging to the Mycobacteriaceae which include the organisms responsible for tuberculosis and leprosy, as well as a number of other less common diseases. Characteristic of mycobacteria is the fact that these organisms tend to be slow growing, difficult to stain, and when they are stained with basic dye can resist decolorization with acid alcohol. The staining characteristics relate to the abnormally high lipid content of the cell wall. In fact, the cell wall or cell envelope of the mycobacterium holds the secrete to many of the characteristics of this genus of organisms. The cell envelope is unique in both structure and complexity. It has been suggested that the cell envelope is responsible for mycobacterium pathogenicity or virulence, multiple drug resistance, cell permeability, immunoreactivity and inhibition of antigen responsiveness, and disease persistence and recrudescence. In addition, several of the successful chemotherapeutic agents are know to inhibit the cell envelope synthesis as their mechanism of action. It is no wonder that significant effort has been put forth to define the chemical structure of the mycobacterium cell envelope. A series of papers were presented and reported in 1991 dealing with the topic of the structure and functions of the cell envelope of mycobacterium (1). As illustrated in Figure 37.1, the mycobacterial cell envelope contains on the interior surface a plasma membrane similar to that found in most bacteria. A conventional peptidoglycan layer affording the organism rigidity appears next. This layer is composed of alternating N-acetyl-D-glucosamines (Glu) linked to N-glycoyl-D-muramic acids (Mur) through 1–4 linkages which in turn is attached to the peptido chain of L-alanine (A), D-glutamine (G), meso-diaminopimelic acid (DP), and L-alanine (A). A novel disaccharde phosphodiester linker made up of N-acetyl-D-glucosamine and rhamnose connects the muramic acid to a polygalactan and polyarabinose chain. The latter polysaccarides are referred to as the arabinogalactan (AG) portion of the cell envelope. The manner in which the arabinosyl and galactosyl resides are arranged is still under investigation. It is known that the arabinosyl chains terminate in mycolic acid residues. The mycolates will be discussed in more detail later in the chapter. Noncovalently bound to the mycolates are a number of free nonpolar and polar lipids, the phthiocerol lipids and the glycopeptidolipids, respectively. Finally, spanning from the interior, embedded in the plasma membrane, to the exterior is the lipoarabinomannan (LAM) polymer. As indicated this unit is composed of polyarabinose, polymannan and various lipids attached through a phosphatidylinositol moiety (for more detail see references 2 and 3).

SPECIFIC DISEASES
Leprosy (Hansen's Disease)

Throughout the Bible one finds reference to the condition of leprosy such as that described in *Leviticus* "is there any flesh in the skin of which there is a burn by fire,

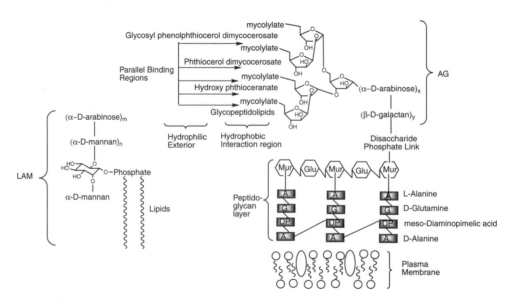

Fig. 37.1. Diagramatic representation of the cell wall/cell envelope of mycobacterium.

and the quick flesh of the burn becomes a bright spot, reddish white or white, ... and if the hair in the bright spot is turned white, and it appears deeper than the skin, it is leprosy broken out in the burn." Associated with the disease was a belief that individuals suffering from this disease were unclean. Today leprosy (Hansen's disease) is recognized as a chronic granulomatous infection caused by *Mycobacterium leprae*. The disease may consist of *lepromatous* leprosy, *tuberculoid* leprosy, or a condition with characteristics between these two poles referred to as *borderline* leprosy. The disease is more common in tropical countries, but is not limited to warm climate regions. It is thought to afflict some 10–20 million individuals. While children appear to be the most susceptible population, the signs and symptoms usually do not occur until much later in life. The incubation period is usually 3–5 years. While the disease is contagious the infectiousness is quite low. Person-to-person contact appears to be the means by which the disease is spread with entrance into the body occurring through the skin or the mucosa of the upper respiratory tract. Skin and peripheral nerves are the regions most susceptible to attack. The first signs of the disease consist of hypopigmented or hyperpigmented macules. Additionally, anesthetic or paresthetic patches may be experienced by the patient. Neural involvement in the extremities will ultimately lead to muscle atrophy, resorption of small bones, and spontaneous amputation. When facial nerves are involved corneal ulceration and blindness may occur. The identification of *Mycobacterium leprae* in skin or blood samples is not always possible, but the detection of the antibody to the organism is an effective diagnostic test especially for the lepromatous form of the disease.

Tuberculosis

Tuberculosis is a disease known to man from the earliest recorded history. It is a disease which is characterized as a chronic bacterial infection caused by the *Mycobacterium tuberculosis*, an acid-fast aerobic bacillus with the previously discussed unusual cell wall. The cell wall has a high lipid content resulting in a high degree of hydrophobicity and resistance to alcohol, acids, alkali, and some disinfectants. The *M. tuberculosis* cell wall after staining with a dye, can not be subsequently decolorized with acid wash and thus the characteristic of being an acid-fast bacillus (AFB). It is estimated that today one-third to one-half of the world population is infected with *M. tuberculosis* leading to approximately 6% of all deaths worldwide (4,5). Tuberculosis is the leading worldwide cause of mortality resulting from an infectious bacterial agent. A steady decline in the reported cases of tuberculosis had been occurring in the United States from the 1950s until 1985. From 1985 until 1988 this decline leveled off, but beginning in 1989 an increase was noted. In 1991 the Center for Disease Control reported 25,701 new cases of tuberculosis. Today the press and professional publications announce the "epidemic" spread of TB. The resurgence has been linked to urban crowding, homelessness, immigration, drug abuse, the disappearance of preventive-medicine health clinics, crowded prisons, and the AIDS epidemic. "Most alarming is the emergence of multidrug-resistant tuberculosis (MDR-TB)" (6). Prior to 1984, only 10% of the organisms isolated from patients with tuberculosis were resistant to any drug. In 1984, 52% of the organisms were resistant to at least one drug and 32% were resistant to more than one drug. MDR-TB may have a fatality rate as high as 50%. As a result of MDR-TB, isolates of *M. tuberculosis* should be tested for antimicrobial susceptibility. In fact, drug resistance is encountered in patients who have never been treated with any of the TB drugs.

M. tuberculosis is transmitted primarily via the respiratory route. The organism appears in water droplets expelled during coughing, sneezing or talking. Either in the droplet form or as the desiccated airborne bacilli, the organism enters the respiratory tract. The infectiousness of an individual will depend on the extent of the disease, the number of organisms in the sputum and the amount of coughing. Usually, within two weeks of beginning therapy the infected individual will no longer be infectious. TB is a disease which mainly affects the lungs (80–85% of the cases), but the *M. tuberculosis* can spread through the bloodstream and the lymphatic system to the brain, bones, eyes and skin (extrapulmonary tuberculosis). In pulmonary tuberculosis, the bacilli reach the alveoli and are ingested by pulmonary macrophages. Substances secreted by the macrophages stimulate surrounding fibroblasts to enclose the infection site leading to formation of granulomas or tubercles. The infection, thus contained locally, may lie dormant encapsulated in a fibrotic lesion for years only to reappear later. The extrapulmonary tuberculosis is much more common in HIV-infected patients (40–75%).

Because of the effect of the AIDS virus on the immune system, all HIV-infected individuals should be screened for tuberculosis and if infected the HIV patient should be treated for TB before an active infections develops. HIV patients with TB are 100 times more likely to develop an active infection than are non-HIV patients. Individuals diagnosed with active TB should be counseled and tested for HIV since the TB may have developed in conjunction with the weakened immune system seen in the HIV patient.

MAC (*Mycobacterium avium—intracellulare* Complex)

Mycobacterium avium and *Mycobacterium intracellulare* are atypical acid-fast bacilli which are ubiquitous in the environment and usually considered nonpathogenic in healthy individuals. Unfortunately, in immune compromised individuals these organisms and possibly other unidentified mycobacteria cause severe life threatening infections. Disseminated *Mycobacterium avium -intracellulare* complex (MAC or MAI) is the most common bacterial opportunistic infection seen in AIDS patients and the third most common opportunistic infection behind *Candida* esophagitis and primary *Pneumocystis carinii* pneumonia reported in AIDS patients. Between 1981 and 1987, and prior to the availability of effective antiretroviral medication, the incidence of MAC was reported as 5%. Today, approximately half of the of the AIDS patients develop an infection caused by MAC. The lungs are the organs most commonly involved in nonAIDS patients but the infection may involve bone marrow, lymph nodes, liver and blood in AIDS patients. CD4 T-lymphocyte count is used as a predictor for risk of disseminated MAC. CD4 T-lymphocyte counts of less than 50 cells/mm^3 in an HIV-infected person (adult or adolescent) is an indication of a potential infection and a recommendation for chemoprophylaxis. MAC grow within macrophages and therefore the drug must be capable of penetration of the macrophage. Treatment of MAC, both prophylactically and for diagnosed infections requires the use of multiple drug therapy and for disseminated MAC this treatment is for the life of the patient.

GENERAL APPROACHES TO DRUG THERAPY

While the mycobacteria have a number of characteristics in common it is important to recognize that the various species vary widely in susceptability to the different drugs and that this in turn may relate to significant differences in the organisms. Some species such as *M. tuberculosis* are very slow-growing with a doubling time of 24 hours while others such as *M. smegmatis* doubles in 2–3 hours. The pathogenic mycobacterial organism can be divided into organisms that are: actively metabolizing and rapidly growing, semi dormant in acidic intracellular environment, semi dormant in a nonacidic intracellular environment, or dormant. The latter characteristic being most problematic and responsible for treatment failures. Thus, successful chemotherapy calls for drugs with bactericidal action against rapidly growing organisms and the ability to destroy semi dormant and dormant populations. The use of combination therapy over an extended period of time is one answer to successful treatment.

DRUG THERAPY—TUBERCULOSIS
First-line Agents
Isoniazid (Isonicotinic Acid Hydrazide, INH)

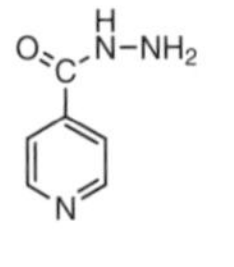

Isoniazid (isonicotinic acid hydrazide, INH) is a synthetic antibacterial agent with bactericidal action against *M. tuberculosis*. The drug was discovered in the 1950s as a beneficial agent orally effective against intracellular and extracellular bacilli and is generally considered the primary drug for treatment of *M. tuberculosis*. Its action is bactericidal against replicating organisms but appears to

be only bacteriostatic at best against semi dormant and dormant populations. After treatment with INH the *M. tuberculosis* loses its acid fastness which may be interpreted as indicating that the drug interferes with cell wall development.

Mechanism of Action. Although extensively investigated the mechanism of action of INH has remained unknown until recently. New investigations into mechanisms of bacterial resistance have shed light on the molecular mechanism of action of INH(7). It is generally recognized that INH is a pro-drug which is activated through an oxidation reaction catalyzed by an endogenous enzyme (8). This enzyme, katG, which exhibits catalase-peroxidase activity converts INH to a reactive species capable of acylation of an enzyme system found exclusively in the *M. tuberculosis*. Evidence in support of the activation of INH reveals that INH-resistant isolates have decreased catalase activity and that the loss of catalase activity is associated with the deletion of the catalase gene, *katG*. Furthermore, reintroduction of the gene into resistance organisms results in restored sensitivity of the organism to the drug. Reaction of INH with catalase-peroxidase results in formation of isonicotinaldehyde, isonicotinic acid, and isonicotinamide which can be accounted for through the reactive intermediate isonicotinoyl radical (I) or perisonicotinic acid (II) as shown in Figure 37.2 (9). Evidence has been offered both for and against the reaction of catalase-peroxidase activated INH with a portion of the enzyme inhA an enzyme involved in the biosynthesis of the mycolic acids (Fig. 37.3) (10–12). The mycolic acids are important constituents of the mycobacterial cell wall in that they provide a permeability barrier to hydrophilic solutes. The enzyme inhA, produced under the control of the gene *inhA*, is a NADH-dependent enoyl reductase protein which is thought to be involved in double bond reduction during fatty acid elongation (Fig. 37.4). INH specifically inhibits long chain fatty acid synthesis (greater

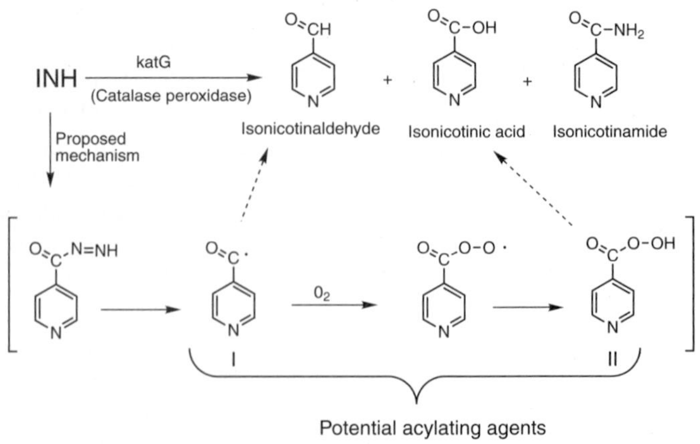

Fig. 37.2. Reaction products formed from catalase-peroxidase reaction with INH.

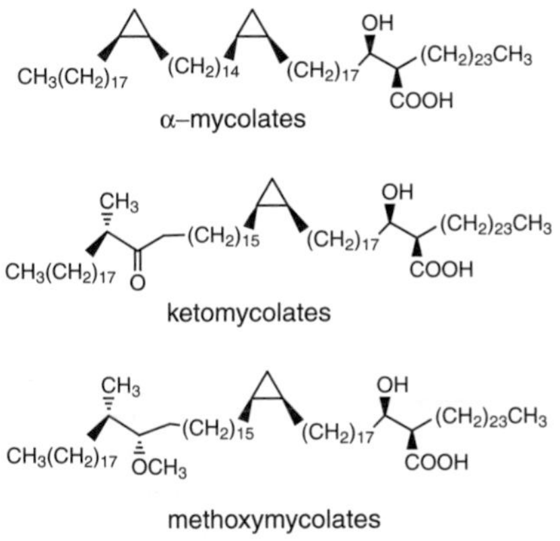

Fig. 37.3. Mycolic acids.

than 26 carbon atoms). It should be noted that the mycolic acids are α-branched lipids having a "short" arm of 20–24 carbons and a "long" arm of 50–60 carbons. It has been proposed that INH is activated to an electrophilic species which acylates the four position of the NADH (Fig. 37.5). The acylated NADH is is no longer capable of catalyzing the reduction of unsaturated fatty acids which are essential for the synthesis of the mycolic acids (13–15).

Structure-activity Relationships. An extensive series of derivatives of nicotinaldehyde, isonicotinaldehyde, and substituted isonicotinic acid hydrazide have been prepared and investigated for their tuberculostatic activity. Isoniazid hydrazones were found to possess activity but these compounds were shown to be unstable in the G.I. tract releasing the active INH. Thus, it would appear that their activity resulted from the INH and not the derivatives (16,17). Substitution of the hydrazine portion of INH with alkyl and aralkyl substituents resulted in a series of active and inactive derivatives (18–21). Substitution on the N2 position re-

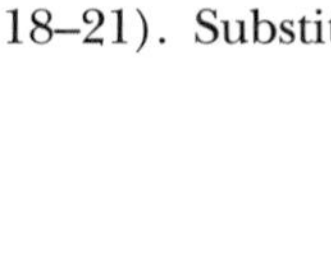

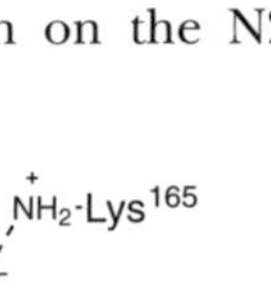

Isoniazid hydrazones   Isonicotinic acid hydrazides

sulted in active compounds (R₁ and R₂ = alkyl; R₃ = H), whereas any substitution of the N1 hydrogen with alkyl groups destroyed the activity (R₁ and R₂ =H; R₃ = alkyl). None of these changes produced compounds with superior activity over INH.

Metabolism. INH is extensively metabolized to inactive metabolites (Fig. 37.6) (22,23). The major metabolite is N-acetylisoniazid. The enzyme responsible for acetylation, cytosolic N-acetyltransferase, is produced under genetic control in an inherited autosomal fashion. Individuals who possess high concentrations of the enzyme are referred to as rapid acetylators while those with low concentrations are slow acetylators. This may result in a need to adjust the dosage for fast acetylators. The N-acetyltransferase is located primarily in the liver and small intestine. Other metabolites include isonicotinic acid, which is found in the urine as a glycine conjugate, and hydrazine. Isonicotinic acid may also result from hydrolysis of acetylisoniazid, but in this case, the second product of hydrolysis is acetylhydrazine. Acetylhydrazine is acetylated by N-acetyltransferase to the inactive diacetyl product. This reaction occurs more rapidly in rapid acetylators. The formation of acetylhydrazine is significant in that this compound has been associated with the hepatotoxicity which may occur during INH therapy. Acetylhydrazine has been postulated to serve as a substrate for CYP450 resulting in the formation of a reactive intermediate which is capable of acetylating liver protein resulting in the liver necrosis (24). It has been suggested that a hydroxylamine intermediate is formed which in turn results in an active acetylating agent (Fig. 37.7). The acetyl radical/cation acylates liver protein.

Pharmacokinetics. INH is readily absorbed following oral administration. Food and various antacids, especially aluminum containing antacids, may interfere or delay the absorption and therefore it is recommended that the drug be taken on an empty stomach. The drug is well distributed to body tissues including infected tissue. A long standing concern about the use of INH during preventive therapy for latent tuberculosis has been the high incidence of hepatotoxicity. Recent studies have concluded that, excluding patients over 35 years of age, if relevant clinical monitoring is employed the rate of hepatotoxicity is quite low (25). The risk of hepatotoxicity is associated

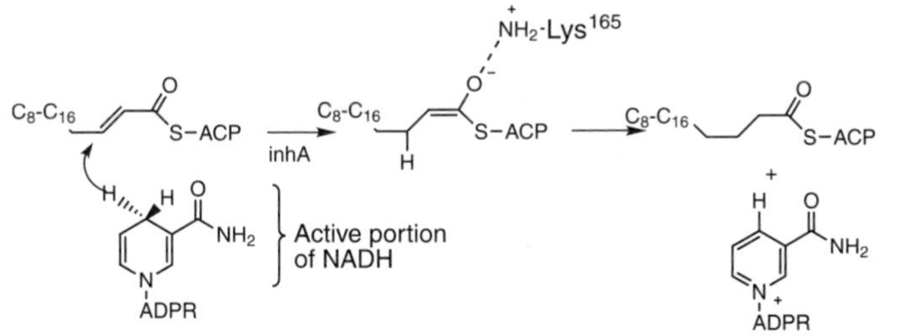

Fig. 37.4. Enoylthioester (ACP = Acyl carrier (protein) reduction catalyzed by NADH and inhA.

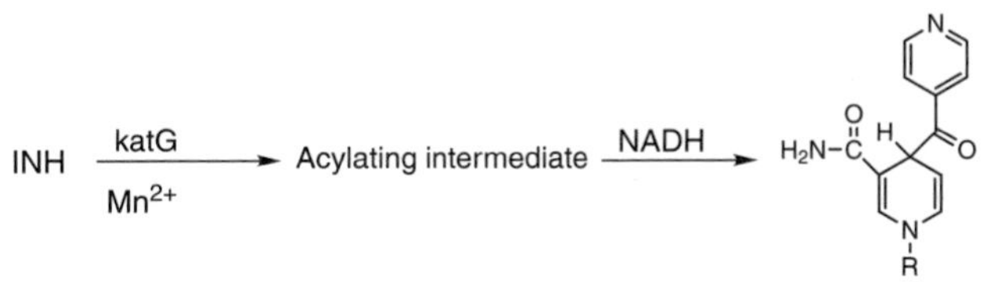

Fig. 37.5. Acylation of NADH and NADH-dependent enoylacyl protein (inhA).

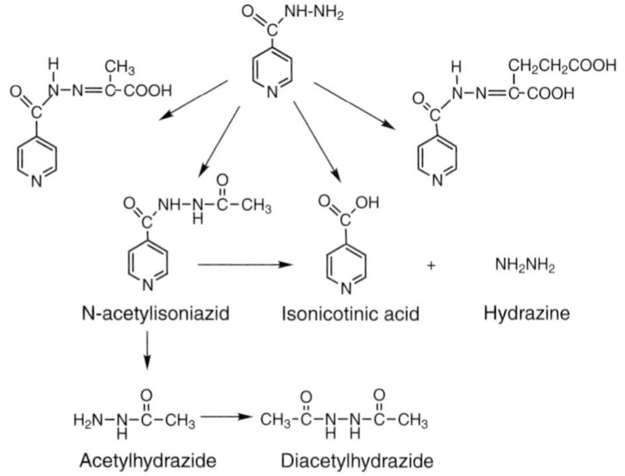

Fig. 37.6. Metabolism of isoniazid.

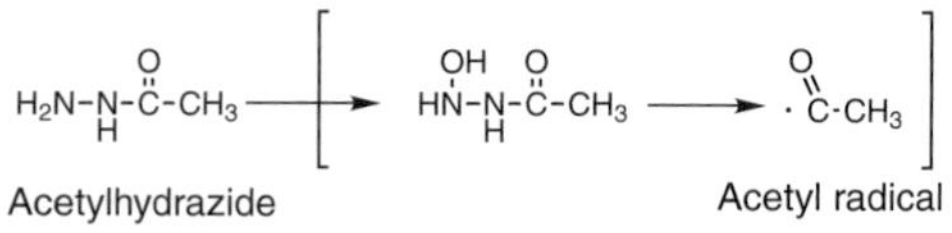

Fig. 37.7. Acylating metabolite of isoniazid.

with increasing age and appears to be higher in women than man.

Rifamycin Antibiotics

The rifamycins are members of the the ansamycin class of natural products produced by *Streptomyces mediterranei*. This chemical class is characterized as molecules with an aliphatic chain forming a bridge between two nonadjacent positions of an aromatic moiety. While investigating the biologic activity of the naturally occurring rifamycins (B, O, and S) a spontaneous reaction gave the biologically active rifamycin SV which was later isolated from natural sources. Rifamycin SV was the original rifamycin antibiotic chosen for clinical development (26). Semisynthetic derivatives are prepared via conversion of the natural rifamycins to 3-formylrifamycin which is derivatized with various hydrazines to give products such as rifampin and rifapentine. Rifampin and the recently FDA approved rifapentine have significant benefit over previously investigated rifamycins in that they are orally active, highly effective against a variety of gram-positive and gram-negative organisms, and have high clinical efficacy in the oral treatment of tuberculosis.

Mechanism of Action. The rifamycins inhibit bacterial DNA-dependent RNA polymerase (DDRP) by binding to the β-subunit of the enzyme and are highly active against rapidly dividing intracellular and extracellular bacilli. Rifampin is active against DDRP from both gram-positive and gram-negative bacteria but due to poor penetration of the cell wall of gram-negative organisms by rifampin, the drug has less value in infections caused by such organisms. Inhibition of DDRP leads to a blocking of the initiation of chain formation in RNA synthesis. It has been suggested that the naphthalene ring of the rifamycins π-π bonds to an aromatic amino acid ring in the DDRP protein (27). DDRP is a metalloenzyme which contains two zinc atoms. It is further postulated that the oxygens at C-1 and C-8 of a rifamycin can chelate to a zinc atom which increases the binding to DDRP and finally, the oxygens at C-21 and C-23 form strong hydrogen bonds to the DDRP. The binding of the rifamycins to DDRP results in the inhibition of RNA synthesis. Specifically, rifampin has been shown to inhibit the elongation of full-length transcripts, but has no effect on transcription initiation (7). Resistance develops when a mutation occurs in the gene responsible for the β-subunit of the RNA polymerase (*rpoB* gene) resulting in an inability of the antibiotic to readily bind to the RNA polymerase (28).

Structure-activity Relationship. A large number of derivatives of the natural occurring rifamycins have been prepared (29). From these compounds the following generalizations can be made concerning the SAR: (1) free -OH groups are required at C-1,8,21 and 23; (2) these groups appear to lie in a plane and appear to be important binding groups for attachment to DDRP, as previously indicated; (3) acetylation of C-21 and C-23 produces inactive compounds; (4) reduction of the double bonds in the macro ring results in a progressive decrease in activity; (5) opening of the macro ring also gives inactive compounds. These latter two changes greatly affect the conformational structure of the rifamycins which in turn decreases binding to DDRP. Substitution at C-3 or C-4 results in compounds with varying degrees of antibacterial activity. The substitution at these positions appear to affect

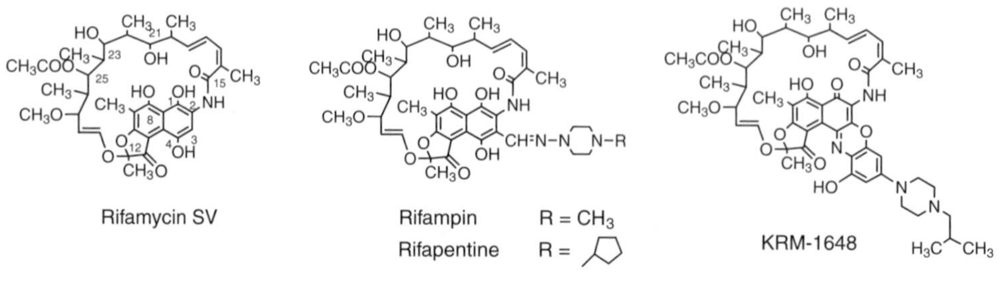

Rifamycin SV

Rifampin   R = CH₃
Rifapentine   R =

KRM-1648

transport across the bacterial cell wall. A compound incorporating such substitution is the benzoxazinorifamycin KRM-1648 which is proceeding through clinical investigation. In vitro studies have shown rapid tissue sterilization and encouraging combination therapy for TB and possibly MAC.

Metabolism. Rifampin and rifapentine are readily absorbed from the intestine although food in the tract may affect absorption. Rifampin's absorption may be reduced by food in the intestine and therefore the drug should be taken on an empty stomach (23), while intestinal absorption of rifapentine has been reported to be enhanced when taken after a meal (30). Neither drug appears to interfere with the absorption of other antituberculin agents, but there are conflicting reports on whether isoniazid affects absorption of rifampin. The major metabolism of rifampin and rifapentine is deacetylation which occurs at the C-25 acetate (Fig. 37.8). The resulting product, desacetylrifampin and desacetylrifapentine, are still active antibacterial agents. While the majority of both desacetyl products are found in the feces, desacetylrifampin glucuronide may also be found in the urine. 3-Formylrifamycin SV has been reported as a second metabolite following both rifampin and rifapentine administration. This product is thought to arise in the gut from an acid catalyzed hydrolysis reaction. Formylrifamycin is reported to possess a broad-spectrum of antibacterial activity (31).

Physical Chemical Properties. Rifampin and rifapentine are red-orange crystalline compounds with zwitterionic properties. The presence of the phenolic groups results in acidic properties, pKa ~ 1.7, while the piperazine moiety gives basic properties, pKa ~ 7.9. These compounds are prone to acid hydrolysis giving rise to 3-formylrifamycin SV, as indicated above. Rifampin and presumably rifapentine, are prone to air oxidation of the para phenolic groups in the naphthalene ring to give the *p*-quinone (C-1,4 quinone) (see Fig. 37.8). Rifampin, rifapentine, and their metabolites are excreted in the urine, feces (biliary excretion), saliva, sweat and tears. Because these agents have dye characteristics one may note the red to orange discoloration of the body fluids containing the drug. Notably, the tears may be discolored and permanent staining of contact lens may occur if worn.

Therapeutic Application

Rifampin (Rifadin, Rimactine). With the introduction of rifampin (RIF) in 1967 the duration of combination therapy for the oral treatment of tuberculosis was significantly reduced from 18 to 9 months. Rifampin is nearly always used in combination with one or more other antituberculin agents. The drug is potentially hepatotoxic and may produce gastrointestinal disturbances, rash and thrombocytopenic purpura. Rifampin is known to induce CYP3A4 and CYP2C isoforms and may decrease the effectiveness of: oral contraceptives, corticosteroids, warfarin, quinidine, methadone, zidovudine, clarithromycin, and the azole antifungal agents (32) (Chapter 8).

Because of the decreased effectiveness of protease inhibitors and non-nucleoside reverse transcriptase inhibitors used in the treatment of HIV, the CDC has recommended avoidance of rifampin in treatment of HIV patients presently on these HIV therapies.

Rifapentine (Priftin). Rifapentine is the first new agent introduced for the treatment of pulmonary tuberculosis in the last 25 years. The drug's major advantage over rifampin is the fact that when used in combination therapy rifapentine can be orally administered twice weekly during the the "intense" phase of therapy followed by once a week during the "continuous" phase of therapy. In contrast, rifampin is normally administered daily during the "in-

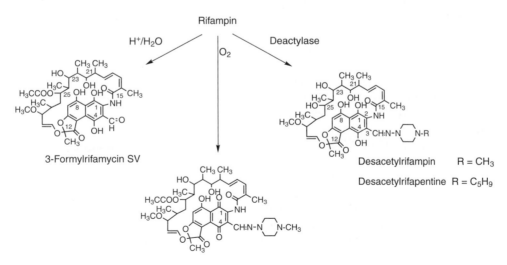

Fig. 37.8. Metabolism and in vitro reactions of rifampin.

tense" phase of therapy followed by twice a week dosing during the "continuous" phase of therapy. Since relapse and the emergence of resistant strains of bacteria are associated with poor patient compliance it is expected that reduced dosing will increase compliance. Initial clinical studies actually showed that the relapse rates in patients treated with rifapentine (10%) were higher than in the patients treated with rifampin (5%). It was found that poor compliance with the nonrifamycin antituberculin agents was responsible for the increased relapse (30).

Rifapentine is readily absorbed following oral administration and is highly bound to plasma protein (97.7% vs. 80% for rifampin). Related to the higher plasma binding, refapentine has a longer mean elimination half-life, 13.2 hours in healthy male volunteers, in comparison with the half-life reported for rifampin of approximately 2–5 hours. Greater than 70% of either drug is excreted in the feces. Rifapentine is generally considered to be more active than rifampin and can be used in patients with varying degrees of hepatic dysfunction without need for dose adjustment (33). This drug, similar to what is seen with rifampin, induces hepatic CYP3A4 and CYP 2C8/9). Rifapentine has been reported to be teratogenic in rats and rabbits (30).

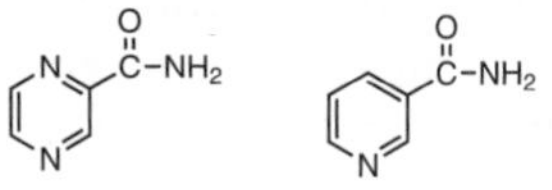

Pyrazinamide   Nicotinamide

Pyrazinamide

Pyrazinamide (PZA, pyrazinecarboxamide) was discovered while investigating analogs of nicotinamide. Pyrazinamide is a bioisostere of nicotinamide and possess bactericidal action against *M. tuberculosis*. Pyrazinamide has become one of the more popular antituberculin agents despite the fact that resistance develops quickly to this agent. Combination therapy has proven an effective means of reducing the rate of resistant strain development. The activity of pyrazinamide is pH dependent with good in vivo activity at pH 5.5 but the compound is nearly inactive at neutral pH.

Mechanism of Action. The mechanism of action of pyrazinamide is unknown, but recent findings suggest that pyrazinamide may be active totally or in part as a pro-drug. Susceptible organisms produce pyrazinamidase which is responsible for hydrolysis of pyrazinamde to pyrazinoic acid intracellularly (7). Mutation in the pyrazinamidase gene (*pncA*) results in resistant strains of *M. tuberculosis* (34). Pyrazinoic acid has been shown to possess biologic activity at a pH of 5.4 or lower, in contrast in vitro tests show pyrazinoic acid is 8–16 times less active than pyrazinamide (35). Pyrazinoic acid may lower the pH in the immediate surroundings of the *M. tuberculosis* to an extent that the organism is unable to grow, but this physicochemical property appears to account for only some of the activity. The obvious structural similarity between pyrazinoic acid and nicotinamide would suggest that the pyrazinoic acid might function as an antimetabolite of nicotinamide and interfere with the synthesis of NAD.

Structure-activity Relationship. Previous structural modification of pyrazinamide has proven ineffective in developing analogs with increased biologic activity. Substitution on the pyrazine ring or the use of alternate heterocyclic aromatic rings have given compounds with reduced activity (36). More recently, using QSAR a series of analogs have been prepared with improved biologic activity. The requirements for successful analogs include: (1) provision for hydrophilicity to allow sufficient plasma concentrations such that the drug can be delivered to the site of infection; (2) lipophilicity to allow penetration into the mycobacterial cell; and (3) susceptibility to hydrolysis such that the pro-drug is unaffected by the "extracellular" enzymes but is readily hydrolyzed at the site of action. Two compounds have been found that meet these criteria and they are *tert*-butyl 5-chloropyrazinamide and 2-(2′-methyldecyl) 5-chloropyrazinamide (37).

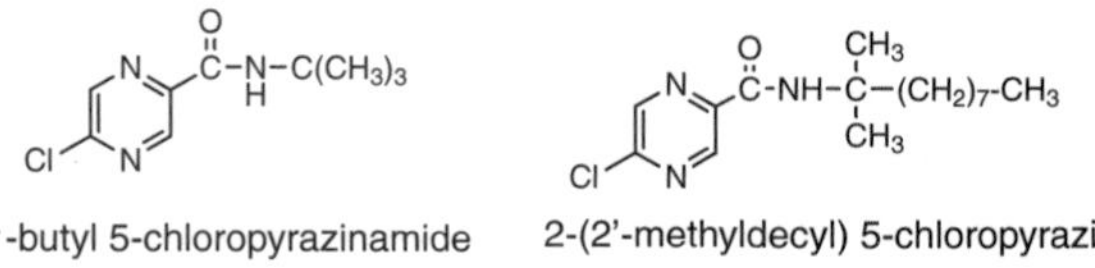

tert-butyl 5-chloropyrazinamide   2-(2'-methyldecyl) 5-chloropyrazinamide

Metabolism. Pyrazinamide is readily absorbed after oral administration but little of the intact molecule is excreted unchanged (Fig. 37.9). The major metabolic route consists of hydrolysis by hepatic microsomal pyrazinamidase to pyrazinoic acid which may then be oxidized by xanthine oxidase to 5-hydroxypyrazinoic acid. The latter compound may appear in the urine either free or as a conjugate with glycine (23).

Therapeutic Application. Pyrazinamide has gained acceptance as an essential component of combination therapy for the oral treatment of tuberculosis (component of Rifater with INH and RIF). The drug is especially beneficial in that it is active against semi dormant intracellular tubercle bacilli that are not affected by other drugs (7,34). The introduction of pyrazinamide combinations has reduced treatment regimens to 6 months from the previous 9 month therapy. The major serious side effect of pyrazinamide is the potential for hepatotoxicity. This effect is associated with dose and length of treatment. Pyrazinamide is not affected by the presence of food in

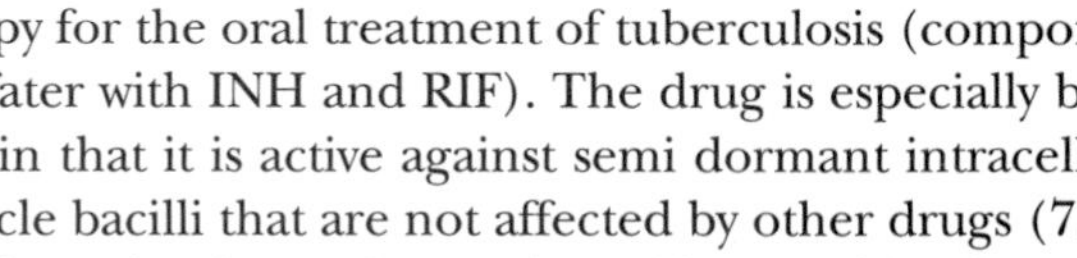

Pyrazinamide   Pyrazinoic acid   5-Hydroxypyrazinoic acid

Fig. 37.9. Metabolism of pyrazinamide.

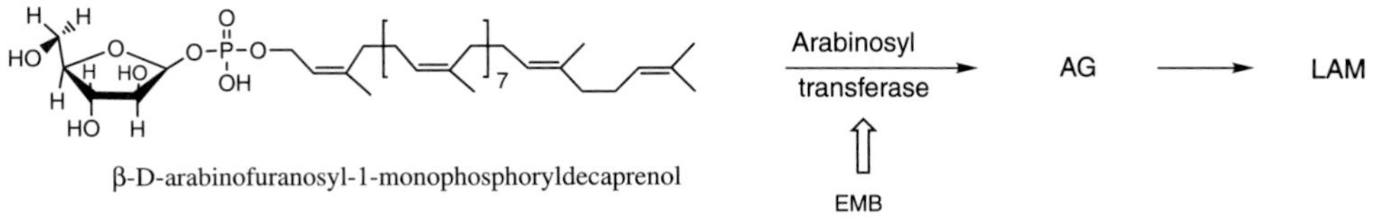

Fig. 37.10. Site of action of Ethambutol (EMB) in cell wall synthesis.

the GI tract nor the use of aluminum-magnesium antacids (38).

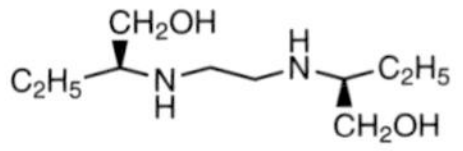

Ethambutol

Ethambutol (Myambutol)

Ethambutol, an ethylenediiminobutanol, (EMB) is administered as its (+)-enantiomer which is 200–500 times more active as a bacteriostatic agent than its (−) enantiomer. The large difference in activity between the two isomers suggests a specific receptor for its site of action. Despite its water solubility, Ethambutol is readily absorbed (75–80%) following oral administration.

Mechanism of Action. The mechanism of action of EMB remains unknown although there is mounting evidence suggesting a specific site of action for EMB. It has been known for sometime that EMB affects mycobacterial cell wall synthesis. The complicated nature of the mycobacterial cell wall has made pinpointing the site of action difficult. In addition to the peptidoglycan portion of the cell wall, the mycobacterium have a unique outer envelop consisting of arabinofuranose and galactose (AG) which is covalently attached to the peptidoglycan and an intercalated framework of lipoarabinomannan (LAM) (Fig. 37.1). The AG portion of the cell wall is highly branched and contains distinct segments of galactan and distinct segments of arabinan. At various locations within the arabinan segments (terminal and penultimate) the mycolic acids are attached to the C5′ position of arabinan (39,40). Initially, Takayama reported that EMB inhibited the synthesis of the AG portion of the cell wall (41). More recently it has been reported that EMB inhibits the enzymes arabinosyl transferase. One action of arabinosyl transferase is to catalyze the polymerization of D-arabinofuranose leading to AG (42,43). EMB mimics arabinan resulting in a build up of the arabinan precursor β-D-arabinofuranosyl-1–monophosphoryldecaprenol and as a result blocks both the synthesis of AG and LAM (Fig. 37.10)(44). The mechanism of resistance to EMB involves a gene over expression of arabinosyl transferase which is controlled by the *embAB* gene (45).

This mechanism of action also accounts for the synergism seen between EMB and intracellular drugs such as rifampin. Damage to the cell wall created by EMB improves the cell penetration of the intracellular drugs resulting in increased biological activity.

Structure-activity Relationship. An extensive number of analogs of ethambutol have been prepared, but none have proven to be superior to ethambutol itself. Extension of the ethylene diamine chain, replacement of either nitrogen, increasing the size of the nitrogen substituents, moving the location of the alcohol groups are all changes that drastically reduce or destroy biologic activity.

Metabolism. The majority of the orally administered ethambutol is excreted unchanged (73%), with no more than 15% appearing in the urine as either Metabolite A, or Metabolite B (Fig. 37.11). Both metabolites are devoid of biologic activity.

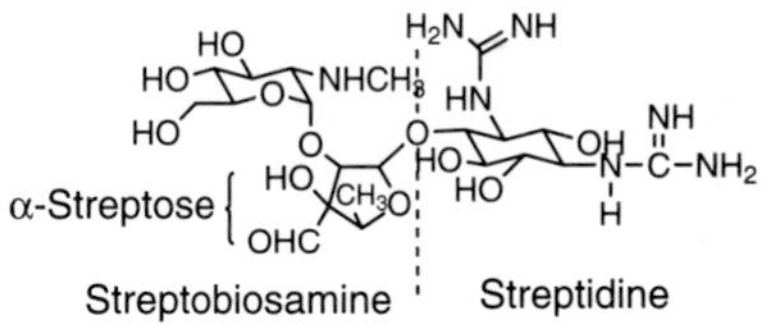

Streptomycin

Streptomycin

Streptomycin (STM) was first isolated by Waksman and coworkers in 1944 and represented the first biologically active aminoglycoside. The material was isolated from a manure-containing soil sample and was ultimately shown to be produced by *Streptomyces griseus*. The structure was proposed and later confirmed by Folkers and co-workers in 1948 (46). STM is water soluble with basic properties. The compound is available as the sesquisulfate salt which is quite soluble in water. The hydrophilic nature of STM results in its very poor absorption from the gastrointestinal tract and therefore STM is commonly administered IM.

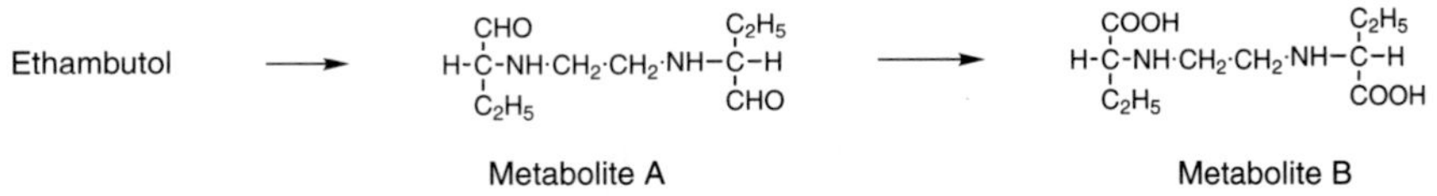

Fig. 37.11. Metabolism of ethambutol.

Orally administered STM is recovered unchanged from the feces indicating that the lack of biologic activity results from poor absorption and not chemical degradation.

Mechanism of Action. The mechanism of action for STM and the aminoglycosides in general has not been fully elucidated. It is known that the STM inhibits protein synthesis, but additional effects on misreading of a m-RNA template and membrane damage may contribute to the bactericidal action of STM. STM is able to diffuse across the outer membrane of *M. tuberculosis* and ultimately penetrate the cytoplasmic membrane through an electron dependent process. Through studies of the mechanism of drug resistance it has been proposed that STM induces a misreading of the genetic code and thus inhibits translational initiation. In STM resistant organisms two changes have been discovered: (1) S12 protein undergoes a change in which the lysine present at amino acid 43 and 88 in ribosomal protein S12 is replaced with arginine or threonine; (2) the pseudoknot conformation of 16S rRNA which results from intramolecular base pairing between GCC bases in regions 524–526 of the rRNA to CGG bases in regions 505–507 is perturbed (47). It is thought that S12 protein stabilizes the pseudoknot which is essential for 16S rRNA function. In some yet to be defined mechanism, STM interferes with one or both of the normal actions of the 16S protein and 16S rRNA.

Structure-activity Relationship. While all of the aminoglycosides have very similar pharmacologic, pharmacodynamic and toxic properties, only STM and to a lesser extent kanamycin are used to treat tuberculosis. This is an indication of the narrow band of structurally allowed modifications which gives rise to active analogs. Modification of the α-streptose portion of STM has been extensively studied. Reduction of the aldehyde to the alcohol results in a compound, dihydrostreptomycin, which has activity similar to STM but with a greater potential for producing delayed severe deafness. Oxidation of the aldehyde to a carboxyl group or conversion to Schiff base derivatives (oxime, semicarbazone, or phenylhydrazone) results in inactive analogs. Oxidation of the methyl group in α-streptose to a methylene hydroxy gives an active analog but with no advantage over STM. Modification of the aminomethyl group in the glucosamine portion of the molecule by demethylation or by replacement with larger alkyl groups reduces activity while removal or modification of either guanidine in the streptidine nucleus results in decreased activity.

Metabolism. No human metabolites of STM have been isolated in the urine of patients who have been administered STM intramuscularly with approximately 50–60% of the dose being recovered as unchanged drug in the urine (23). While metabolism appears insignificant on a large scale, metabolism is implicated as a major

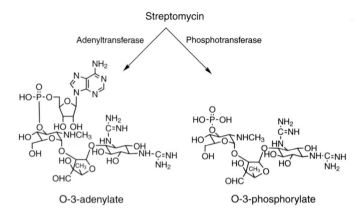

Fig. 37.12. Metabolism of STM as a mechanism of resistance.

mechanism of resistance. An early recognized problem with STM was the development of resistant strains of *M. tuberculosis*. Combination drug therapy was partially successful in reducing this problem but in time resistance has greatly reduced the value of STM as a chemotherapeutic agent for treatment of TB. Various mechanisms may lead to the resistance seen in *M. tuberculosis*. Permeability barriers may result in STM not being transported through the cytoplasmic membrane, but the evidence appears to suggest that enzymatic inactivation of STM represents the major problem. The enzymes responsible for inactivation are adenyltransferase, which catalyzes adenylation of the C-3 hydroxyl group in the N-methylglucosamine moiety to give O-3-adenylate metabolite, and phosphotransferase which phosphorylates the same C-3 hydroxyl to give O-3-phosphorylate metabolite (Fig. 37.12). This latter reaction appears to be clinically the most significant. The result of these chemical modifications is that the resulting metabolites will not bind to ribosomes.

Second-Line Agents

A number of drugs, including ethionamide, para-aminosalicyclic acid, cycloserine, capreomycin, and kanamycin, are considered second-line agents. While these agents are active antibacterial agents, they usually are less well tolerated or have a higher incidence of adverse effects. These agents are utilized in cases of resistance, retreatment or intolerance to the first-line drugs.

Ethionamide (Trecator-SC)

The synthesis of analogs of isonicotinamide resulted in the discovery of ethionamide and a homolog in which the ethyl group is replaced with a propyl (prothionamide). Both compounds have proven to be bactericidal against *M. tuberculosis* and *M. leprae*.

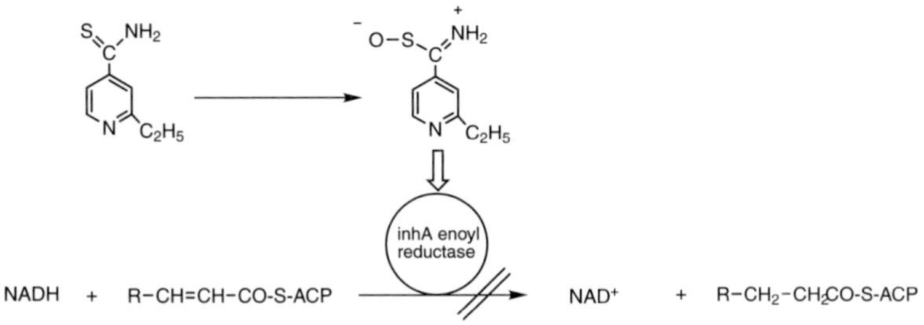

Fig. 37.13. Mechanism of action of ethionamide.

Mechanism of Action. Evidence has been presented which suggests that the mechanism of action for ethionamide is similar to that of INH (see discussion of mechanism of action of INH and references 10,14). Similar to INH, ethionamide is considered to be a pro-drug which is converted via oxidation by catalase-peroxidase to an active acylating agent, ethionamide sulfoxide, which in turn inactivates the inhA enoyl reductase enzyme (Fig. 37.13). In the case of ethionamide it has been proposed that the ethionamide sulfoxide acylates Cys 243 in inhA protein.

Metabolism. Ethionamide is orally active but a single large dose (>500mg) is not well tolerated. The gastrointestinal irritation can be reduced by administration with meals. Additional side effects may include CNS effects, hepatitis and hypersensitivities. Less than 1% of the drug is excreted in the free form with the remainder of the drug appearing as one of six metabolites. Among the metabolites is ethionamide sulfoxide, 2-ethylisonicotinamide, and the N-methylated-6-oxodihydropyridines (Compounds A, B, C) (Fig. 37.14) (48).

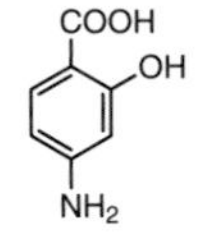

Para-aminosalicylic acid

Para-Aminosalicylic Acid (PAS)

Once a very popular component in TB therapy, PAS is utilized as a second-line agent today. A combination of bacterial resistance and severe side effects has greatly reduced its value. PAS, as a bacteriostatic agent, is used at a dose of up to 12 g/day which causes considerable gastrointestinal irritation, but in addition, hypersensitivity reactions occur in 5–10% of the patients with some of these reactions being life-threatening.

Mechanism of Action. PAS is thought to act as an antimetabolite interfering with the incorporation of para-aminobenzoic acid into folic acid. PAS when co-administered with INH is found to reduce the acetylation of INH, itself being the substrate for acetylation, thus increasing the plasma levels of INH. This action may be especially valuable in rapid acetylators.

Metabolism. PAS is extensively metabolized by acetylation of the amino group, and conjugation with glucuronic acid and glycine at the carboxyl group. PAS is used primarily in cases of resistance, retreatment, and intolerance of other agents. PAS is available from the CDC.

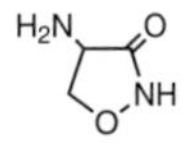

Cycloserine

Cycloserine (Seromycin)

Cycloserine is a natural product from *Streptomyces orchidaceus* as the D (+) enantiomer.

The Mechanism of Action. D-cycloserine (DCS) is considered to be the active form of the drug with its action associated with the ability to inhibit two key enzymes, D-alanine racemase and D-alanine ligase. D-Alanine is an important component of the peptidoglycan portion of the mycobacterial cell wall. Mycobacterium are capable

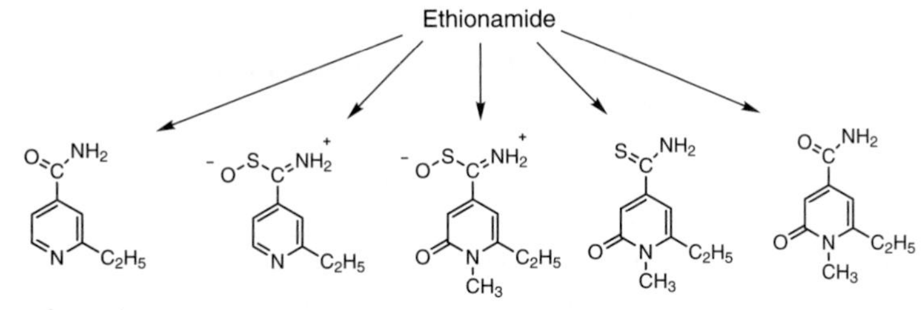

Fig. 37.14. Metabolism of ethionamide.

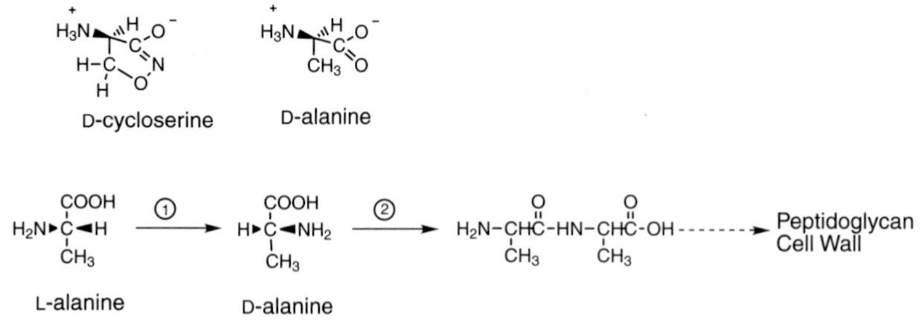

Fig. 37.15. Sites of action of D-cycloserine: ① = D-alanine racemase and ② = D-alanine ligase.

of utilizing natural occurring L-alanine and converting the L-alanine to D-alanine via the enzyme D-alanine racemase. The resulting D-alanine is coupled with itself to form a D-alanine-D-alanine complex under the influence of D-alanine ligase and this complex is incorporated into the peptidoglycan of the mycobacterial cell wall (Fig. 37.15). DCS is a rigid analog of D-alanine and therefore it competitively inhibits the binding of D-alanine to both of these enzymes and its incorporation into the peptidoglycan (Fig. 37.15) (49). Resistance is associated with an over-expression of D-alanine racemase.

Side Effects. Cycloserine is readily absorbed after oral administration and widely distributed, including the CNS. Unfortunately, DCS binds to neuronal N-methylasparate receptors and in addition affects synthesis and metabolism of γ-aminobutyric acid leading to a complex series of CNS effects. As a second-line agent cycloserine should only be used when retreatment is necessary or when the organism is resistant to other drugs. Cycloserine should not be used as a single drug, but must be used in combination with other anti-tuberular drugs.

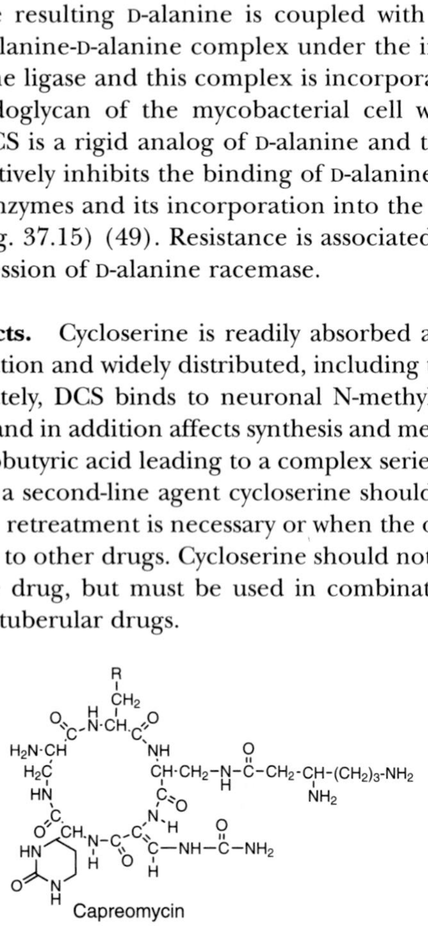

Capreomycin (Capastat)

Capreomycin is a mixture of four cyclic polypeptides of which capreomycin Ia (R=OH) and Ib (R=H) make up 90% of the mixture. Capreomycin is produced by *Streptomyces capreolus* and is quite similar to the antibiotic viomycin. Little if anything is known about its mechanism of action, but if the chemical and pharmacologic similarity to viomycin carries over to mechanism of action, then one might expect a similar action. Viomycin is a potent inhibitor of protein synthesis, particularly that which depends upon m-RNA at the 70S ribosome (50). Viomycin blocks chain elongation by binding to either or both the

50S or 30S ribosomal subunits. As a polypeptide, the drug must be administered parenterally with the preferred route of administration being intramuscularly. As a second-line bacteriostatic antituberculin drug, it is reserved for "resistant" infections and treatment-failure cases. The drug should not be given as a single agent but rather used in combination with ethambutol or INH. Reported toxicity to capreomycin include renal and hepatic damage, hearing loss and allergic reactions.

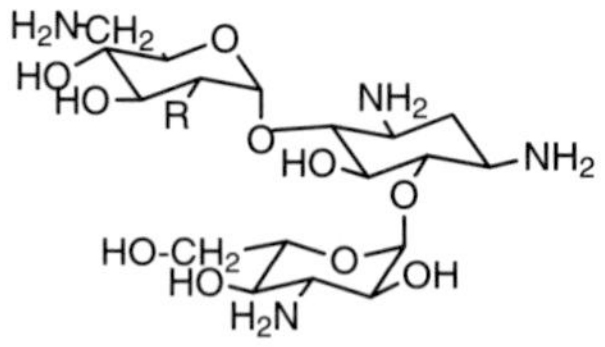

Kanamycin

Kanamycin (Kanamycin A, R = OH; Kanamycin B, R = NH₂; Kantrex)

A member of the aminoglycoside class, kanamycin is a second-line agent with very limited use in the treatment of *M. tuberculosis*. The drug is only utilized to treat resistant organisms and then should be used in combination with other effective agents. The parenteral form of the drug is used, since as an aminoglycoside the drug is poorly absorbed via the oral route. The narrow range of effectiveness and the severe toxicity, especially if the drug is administered over a long period of time, have limited is usefulness. For additional information on kanamycin and aminoglycosides in general you are referred to Chapter 34.

Therapeutic Considerations for Treatment of Tuberculosis
Overview

Various stages of infectious organisms have been identified which may require special consideration for chemotherapy. The organism may be in a dormant stage which is usually not affected by drugs. The continuously growing stage of the organism may find the bacteria either extracellular or intracellular. A stage of the organism, which is classified as the very slowly metabolizing bacteria, exists in a relatively acidic environment. Finally, the organism may exhibit a stage in which it is dormant followed by

6-Fluoro- 4-quinolones

spurts of growth. As noted in the discussion of specific drugs, one stage or another may be more or less susceptible to a particular drug based on the above characteristics. It is also recognized that organisms from some geographic regions may show a low incidence of drug resistance while those from other regions have a high incidence of drug resistance. For tuberculosis patients likely to be infected with organisms suspected of showing low rates of drug resistance, the CDC and the American Thoracic Society currently recommend a 24-week regimen consisting of daily doses of isoniazid (300 mg), rifampin (600 mg), and pyrazinamide (25–35 mg/kg) for eight weeks (induction or sterilization phase). The remaining 16 weeks the therapy consists of isoniazid and rifampin (continuation or maintenance phase). The addition of pyrazinamide to the other two drugs results in a reduction of treatment time from 9–6 months. Individuals on this regimen are considered noninfectious after the first 2 weeks. It is expected that modification of this regimen may be soon recommended in that either streptomycin (15 mg/kg—1 g max. in children too young to be monitored for visual acuity) or ethambutol (15 mg/kg) will be added to the initial three drug therapy. For patients coming from areas which have a high incidence of drug resistance the following regimen is recommended: isoniazid, rifampin, pyrazinamide and ethambutol for 9–12 months or longer. This same group of drugs is recommended for TB patients with AIDS. The "cardinal rules" for all TB regimens is: 1) get drug susceptibility information as soon as possible; 2) always begin therapy with at least three drugs; 3) at all costs avoid a regimen employing only one effective drug; 4) always add at least two drugs to a failing regimen (6,32,51). In addition, it is recommended that consideration be given to treating all patients with directly observed therapy (DOT).

The only proven treatment for prophylaxis of TB (patients with a positive skin test or with a high risk factor) is INH used for 6 or 12 months. High risk factors are considered to be adults and children with HIV infection, close contacts of infectious cases, and those with fibrotic lesions on chest radiograph. Adverse effects when using INH over a long treatment period can be a serious problem. INH may cause severe liver damage and the drug should be removed if serum aminotransferase activity increases to 3–5 times normal or the patient develops symptoms of hepatitis. Peripheral neurophathy may be seen with INH therapy. This condition may be prevented by co-administration of pyridoxine. Persons who are presumed to be infected with INH-resistant organisms should be treated with RIF rather than INH. Hepatitis, thrombocytopenia and nephrotoxicity may be seen with RIF therapy. RIF is thought to potentate the hepatitis caused by INH. Gastrointestinal upset and staining effects caused by RIF are of minor importance.

Fluoroquinolones

The fluoroquinolones are a broad-spectrum class of antibacterials which have been demonstrated to have activity against a wide range of gram-negative as well as gram-positive pathogens including *Mycobacterium tuberculosis*, *M. kansasii*, *M. xenopi*, *M. fortuitum*, *M. avium-intracellulare* (MAC or MAI) complex and *M. leprae*. The quinolones are attractive in that they are active at low concentrations, concentrate within macrophages, and have a low frequency of side effects.

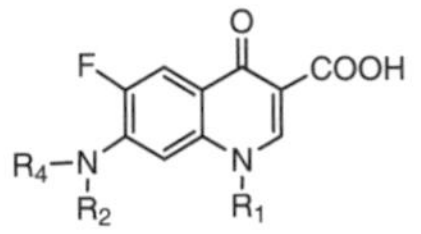

Mechanism of Action. The mechanism of action of the fluoroquinolones is reported in detail in Chapter 34 and basically involves binding to DNA gyrase-DNA complex (GyrA and GyrB) inhibiting bacterial DNA replication and transcription. As a result these drugs exhibit bactericidal activity.

Structure-activity Relationship. The structural requirements for activity against mycobacterium and specifically for activity against the MAC have recently been explored (52,53). It is known that nonfluorinated quinolones are inactive against mycobacteria. In addition, it has been reported that certain fragments or substructures within the quinolones improve activity toward the MAC (biophore) while other fragments deactivate the quinolones (biophobes). The important structural features acting as biophores include: (1) a cyclopropyl ring at the N1 position; (2) fluorine atoms at positions C6 and C8; (3) a C7 heterocyclic substituent. Excessive lipophilicity at N1 can decrease activity (i.e., 2,4-difluorobenzene). The C7 substituents with greatest activity against mycobacteria include the substituted piperazines and pyrrolidines (Fig. 37.16). Two biophobes were also reported and are shown in Figure 37.17.

Recently, several C8 methoxy substituted fluoroquinolones have been reported with superior activity over earlier quinolones (54,55). Moxifloxacin (BAY-12–8039) is reported to be active against *M. tuberculosis* when combined with INH and PD 161148 has been reported to have

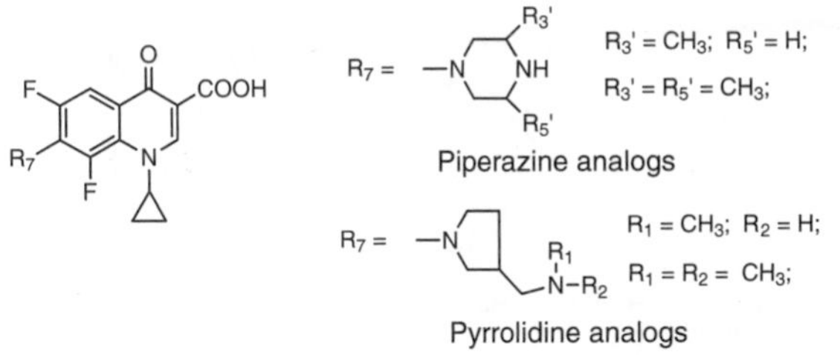

Fig. 37.16. 4-Quinolones demonstrating high activity against mycobacteria.

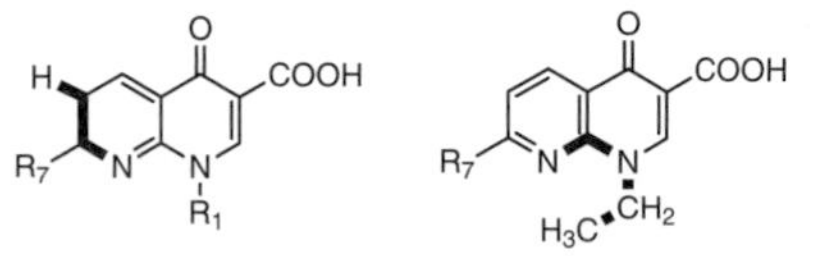

Fig. 37.17. Biophobes (shown in bold) which inactivate 4-quinolones towards mycobacteria.

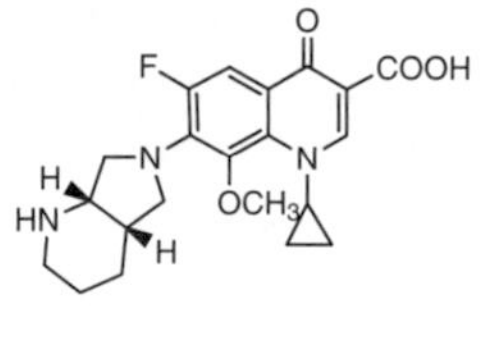

Moxifloxacin 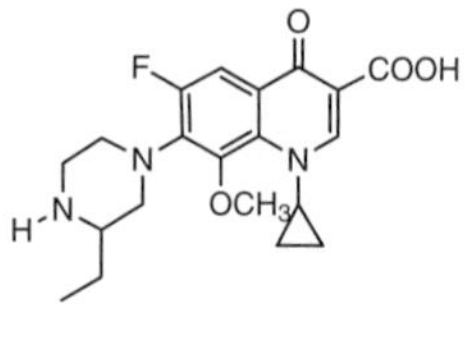   PD 161148

3–4 times the activity of ciprofloxacin and as well as demonstrating active in Gyr A mutated resistant strains.

Therapeutic Application. Fluoroquinolone therapy for tuberculosis is predominantly used in patients infected with multidrug-resistant organisms. Resistance to the quinolones has been reported and appears to be associated with mutations in the *gyrA* and *gyrB* genes leading to single-amino acid substitution in the DNA gyrase protein (7). As a result the use of the fluoroquinolones must be monitored in the treated patient population. The most active floroquinolones available for treatment of tuberculosis are ciprofloxacin (Cipro), sparfloxacin (Zagam) and ofloxacin (Floxin) (Fig. 37.18) (56).

DRUG THERAPY FOR MAC

Drug therapy for the treatment of MAC is complicated and has undergone significant changes over the last few years. Since recommendations for treatment are presently based upon small and in some cases incomplete studies, more changes can be expected in the future. For the most up-to-date information the reader is referred to the CDC's homepage (www.cdc.gov). The 1997 guidelines for prophylaxis of MAC advise that all adults and adolescents with HIV infection with a CD4 lymphocyte count below 50 cells/mm^3 receive clarithromycin 500 mg 2 times/day or azithromycin 1200 mg once/week. This recommendation is considered a standard of care (57–59). For treatment of

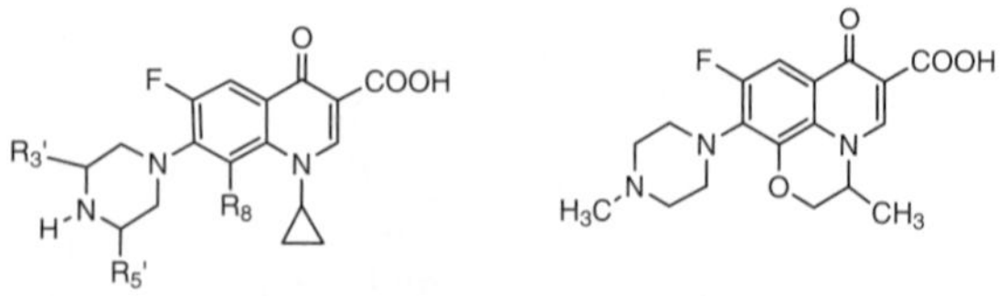

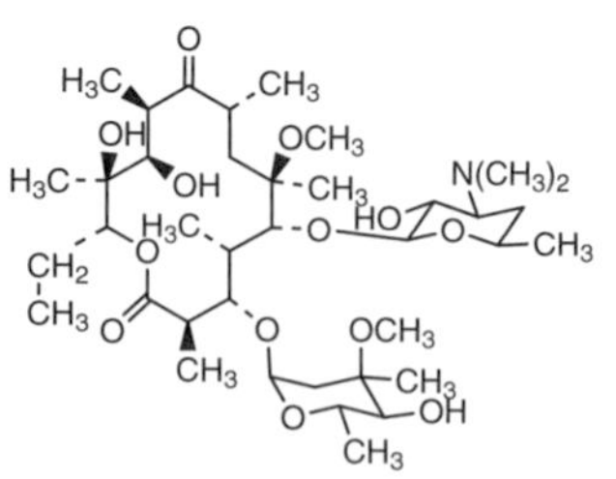

Clarithromycin 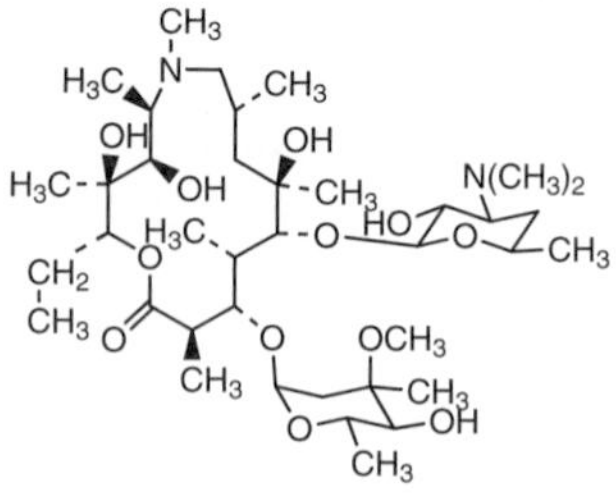   Azithromycin

MAC it is recommended that a combination of drugs be used include at least two drugs (either clarithromycin or azithromycin plus ethambutol for life). Other drugs which can be added to the combination consist of rifabutin, fluoroquinolones, and amikacin. It should be noted that INH and pyrazinamide are ineffective in treating disseminated MAC.

Macrolides

Both clarithromycin or azithromycin are considered first-line agents for the oral prevention and treatment of MAC and have replaced rifabutin. Both macrolides are concentrated in macrophages (clarithromycin concentration is 17.3 times higher in macrophage cells than in extracellular fluid) and appear to be equally effective although clarithromycin has a lower MIC. Azithromycin has an intra-alveolar macrophage half-life of 195 hours compared to a 4 hour half-life for clarithromycin. For prevention, the macrolides may be used orally as single agents although there is a risk of resistant organisms forming and a cross-resistance between clarithromycin and azithromycin. In one study the combination of azithromycin and rifabutin proved more effective than either drug used singlely. For the treatment of MAC, combination therapy is recommended.

Mechanism of Action

The macrolide antibiotics are bacteriostatic agents which inhibit protein synthesis by binding to the 50 S ribosomal units. For a more detailed discussion see Chapter 34.

Metabolism

Clarithromycin is metabolized in the liver to an active metabolite, 14-hydroxyclarithromycin, which is less active than the parent molecule. In addition, the drug is an inhibitor of CYP3A4 which could lead to increased concentrations of some drugs such as rifabutin (see below). Azithromycin is primarily excreted unchanged in the gut and at present there is no evidence of CYP3A4 induction or inhibition.

Rifamycins

Various rifamycin derivatives have been investigated or are under investigation for use in the prevention and treatment of MAC. Up until recently (1997) rifabutin (My-

Ciprofloxacin: $R_8 = R_3' = R_5' = H$ Ofloxacin
Sparfloxacin: $R_8 = F; R_3' = R_5' = CH_3$

Fig. 37.18. Fluoroquinolones active against *Mycobacterium tuberculosis*.

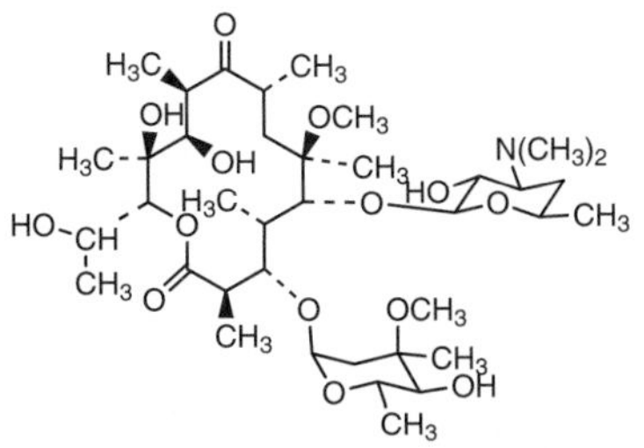

14-Hydroxyclarithromycin

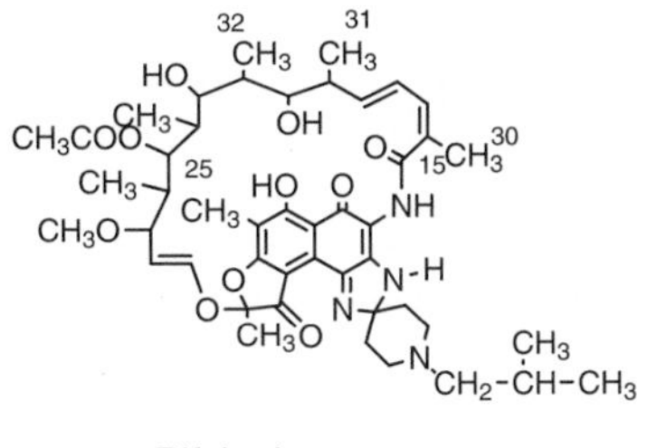

Rifabutin

cobutin)was considered the drug of choice for prophylaxis of MAC patients. Studies since 1995 have suggested that the macrolides are more effective (survival rates), present fewer side effects, and cause fewer drug interactions than rifabutin. Early treatment of MAC bacteremia consists of multidrug regimens usually involving four or five drugs. Drug interactions and in some studies exceptionally high drug doses have given confusing results. It is generally agreed that rifabutin should be used in treatment failures of the macrolides or can be combined with azithromycin for prophylaxis or treatment when clarithromycin is unsuccessful.

Drug Interactions

The most significant drug interaction identified with rifabutin is associated with the fact that this class of drugs are inducers of CYP3A4 and CYP2C family. As a result certain drugs which are substrates for these isoforms will show reduced activity. Rifabutin has been shown to reduce the area under the curve and the maximum concentration of clarithromycin and most HIV protease inhibitors. This action could lead to inactivity or resistance to these agents. In addition, since the HIV protease inhibitors are inhibitors of CYP3A4 a combination of rifabutin plus a HIV protease inhibitor is expected to increase rifabutin area under the curve and maximum concentration increasing the risk of rifabutin side effects. The most serious side effect of rifabutin is uveitis (inflammation of the iris). Under these conditions appropriate changes in dosing are required. If combination therapy is desirable for treatment of MAC the combination of azithromycin and rifabutin is recommended since no significant change in mean serum drug concentration is reported to occur with either agent when used in combination.

Drug Metabolism

The hepatic metabolism of rifabutin is complex with as many as 20 metabolites having been reported. While the structure of most of the metabolites remains unknown several have been identified and include: 25-desacetylrifabutin, 25-desacetylrifabutin-N-oxide, 31-hydroxyrifabutin, 32-hydroxyrifabutin, and 32-hydroxy-25-desacetylrifabutin. The metabolites appear in the urine (50%) and in the feces (30%). Based upon the activity of other rifamycins it might be expected that one or more of the metabolites possess antimycobacterial activity.

Additional Drugs

Various other agents have been combined with the macrolides or rifampins for the prophylaxis and treatment of MAC. As indicated above, the effectiveness of each component in multidrug treatment is not easily defined. The additional drugs utilized include ethambutol, ciprofloxacin, amikacin, and clofazimine. While ethambutol and ciprofloxacin appear to have good activity against MAC, clofazimine has shown unfavorable results. The FDA has advised against using clofazimine in initial therapy of MAC (58).

LEPROSY
Sulfones

The diaryl sulfones represent the major class of agents used to treat leprosy. The initial discovery of the sulfones came about as a result of studies directed at exploring the structure-activity relationship of sulfonamides (Fig. 37.19). A variety of additional chemical modifications have produced several other active agents but none have proved more beneficial than the original lead, 4,4'-diaminodiphenylsulfone (Dapsone). Dapsone was first introduced into the treatment of leprosy in 1943.

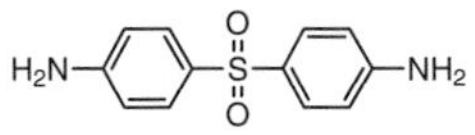

4,4'-Diaminodiphenylsulfone

Dapsone

Dapsone (DDS) is a nearly water insoluble agent which is very weakly basic (pKa 1.0). The lack of solubility may account in part for the occurrence of gastrointestinal irrita-

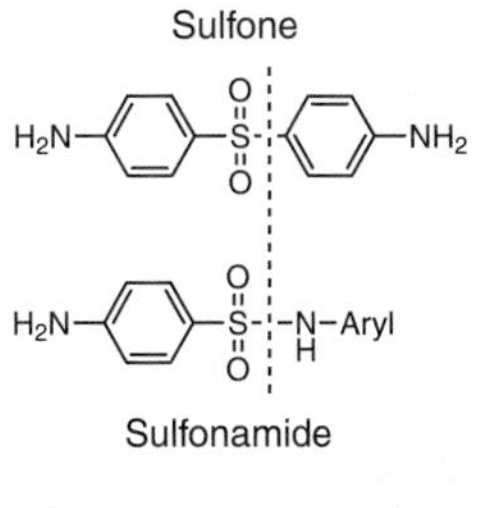

Sulfone

Sulfonamide

Fig. 37.19. Structural comparison of sulfones vs. sulfonamide.

Thiazolsulfone   Acetosulfone   Sulfoxone sodium

tion. Despite the lack of solubility, the drug is efficiently absorbed from the GI tract. Although DDS is bound to plasma protein (at about 70%), it is distributed throughout the body.

Mechanism of Action

Dapsone, a bacteriostatic agent, is thought to act in a manner similar to that of the sulfonamides, namely, through competitive inhibition of *p*-aminobenzoic acid incorporation into folic acid (See Sulfonamide in Chapter 34). Bacteria synthesize folic acid but host cells do not. As a result, co-administration of DDS and PABA will inactivate DDS. DDS and clofazimine have significant anti-inflammatory actions which may or may not play a role in the antimicrobial action. The anti-inflammatory action may also be a beneficial side effect offsetting the complication of erythema nodosum leprosum (ENL) seen in some patients. The anti-inflammatory action may come about by inhibition of myeloperoxidase catalyzed reactions (60).

Structure-activity Relationship

Several derivatives of DDS have been prepared in an attempt to increase the activity of DDS. Isosteric replacement of one benzene ring resulted in the formation of thiazolsulfone. Although still active, it is less effective than DDS. Substitution on the aromatic ring, to produce acetosulfone, reduces activity while increasing water solubility and decreasing GI irritation. A successful substitution consists of adding methanesulfinate to DDS to give sulfoxone sodium. This water soluble form of DDS is hydrolyzed in vivo to produce DDS. Sulfoxone sodium is used in individuals who are unable to tolerate DDS due to GI irritation, but it must be used in a dose three times that of DDS because of inefficient metabolism to DDS. The chemical modification of DDS derivatives continues to be pursued with the intent of finding newer agents useful for the treatment of resistant strains of *M. leprae* (61).

Dapsone

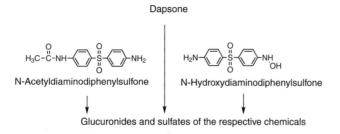

N-Acetyldiaminodiphenylsulfone   N-Hydroxydiaminodiphenylsulfone

Glucuronides and sulfates of the respective chemicals

Fig. 37.20. Metabolites of dapsone.

Additional Uses of Dapsone

Dapsone has a variety of uses in addition to the treatment of leprosy. These include the treatment of dermatitis herpetiformis as well as the unlabeled use in the treatment of brown recluse spider bites, inflammatory bowel disorders, leishmaniasis, malaria prophylaxis, relapsing polychondritis, rheumatic and connective tissue disorders, and the prophylaxis of *Pneumocystis carinii* pneumonia (PCP) in HIV patients and organ transplant patients.

Metabolism

The major metabolic product of DDS results from N-acetylation in the liver by N-acetyltransferase. DDS is also N-hydroxylated to the hydroxylamine derivative. These metabolic reactions are catalyzed by CYP3A4 isoforms. Neither of these compounds possess significant leprostatic activity, although N-acetyldiaminodiphenylsulfone may be deacetylated back to DDS. Products found in the urine consist of small amounts of dapsone, metabolites N-acetyldiaminodiphenylsulfone and N-hydroxydiaminodiphenylsulfone as well as glucuronide and sulfates of each of these substances (Fig. 37.20).

Although the acetylated metabolites of DDS are inactive there is growing concern over the hematologic adverse effects of the hydroxylated metabolite. The specific adverse effected reported for the N-hydroxydiaminodiphenylsulfone metabolite is methemoglobinemia (62).

Clofazimine

Clofazimine (Lamprene)

Although classified as a secondary drug for the oral treatment of leprosy and commonly used as a component of multiple-drug therapy, clofamzimine use appears to be increasing. Clofazimine was first used to treat advanced leprosy unresponsive to DDS or streptomycin in 1966. The chemical, a phenazine derivative, is a water insoluble dye (dark red crystals) which leads to pigmentation of the skin. In addition, discoloration of the feces, lining of the eyelids, sputum, sweat, tears and urine is seen (pink, red or brownish-black discoloration).

Mechanism of Action

The mechanism of action remains unclear at the present time. The molecule possess direct antimycobacterial and immunosuppressive properties. It has been shown that clofazimine increases prostaglandin synthesis and the generation of antimicrobial reactive oxidants from neutrophils, which may play a role in the antileprosy effects. The host cell defense may be stimulated by clofazimine resulting in the generation of oxidants, such as the superoxide anion, which in turn could have a lethal affect on the organism (63,64).

Structure-activity Relationship

Several investigators have reported studies directed toward an understanding of the SAR of clofazimine (65–67). Substituents on the imino group at position 2, *p*-chloro substitution on the phenyls at C-3 and N-10, as well as substituents at position 7, have been investigated. The imino group at C-2 appears essential with activity increased when the imino group is substituted with alkyl and cycloalkyl groups. Halogen substitution on the para position of the two phenyls at C-3 and N-10 enhance activity but are not essential to activity. The following order of activity has been reported: $Br > Cl > CH_3 > EtO > H$ or F. In the analogs studied, the increased activity correlates well with pro-oxidative activities of the molecule e.g., ability to generate superoxide anion, as well as increased lipophilicity.

Metabolism

Various metabolites of clofazimine have been identified, but account for less than 1% of the administered dose. The lack of higher concentrations of the metabolites may, in part, be due to the very slow elimination of clofazimine from the body which has an estimated half-life of from 8.8–69 days. The lipophilic nature of clofazimine results in distribution and storage of the drug in fat tissue. There appears to be some discrepancy as to the structures of the metabolites (67,68). The most recent studies suggest the presence of two conjugates with the possibility of intermediates (Fig. 37.21). Clofazimine is thought to undergo hydroxylic dehalogenation on the 3-chloroaniline followed by sulfate conjugation and 4-hydroxylation followed by glucuronic acid conjugation.

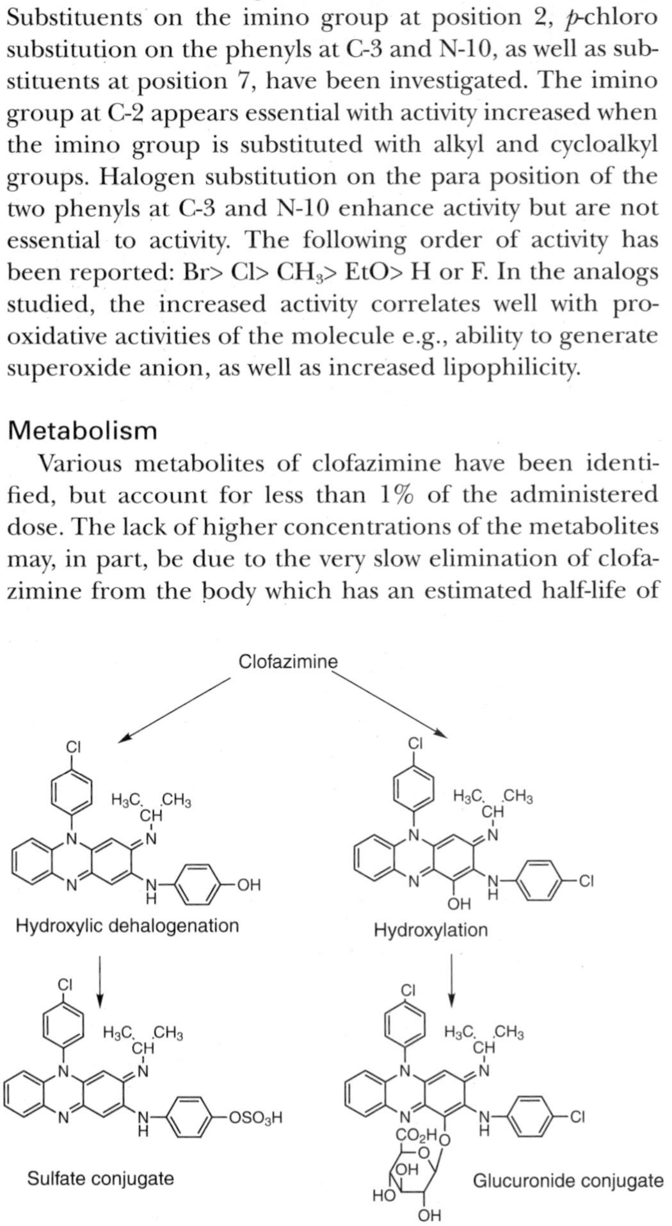

Rifampin (Rifadin, Rimactane)

Rifampin (RIF), an antituberculin drug, has already been discussed. Its actions against *M. leprae* parallels those effects reported for *M. tuberculosis*. Today rifampin is considered an effective antileprosy agent when used in combination with the sulfones.

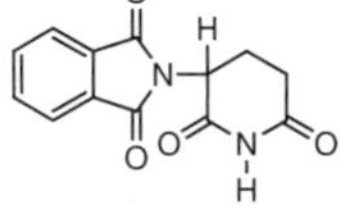

Thalidomide

Thalidomide (Thalomid)

The development of painful, tender, inflamed subcutaneous nodules which may last a week or two, but may reappear and last for long periods is seen in a number of disease. In the case of leprosy the condition is referred to as erythema nodosum leprosum (ENL). The condition appears to by a hypersensitivity reaction and while it may appear in non-treated patients it is commonly seen as a complication of the chemotherapy of leprosy. In addition to painful nodules the patient may experience fever, malaise, wasting, vasculitis and peripheral neuritis. This condition has been successfully treated with thalidomide. Recently, racemic thalidomide has been approved by the FDA for treatment of ENL and is considered the drug of choice (69,70). The mechanism whereby thalidomide produces relief is thought to be associated with the drug's ability to control inflammatory cytokines. Specifically, thalidomide inhibits the synthesis and release of tumor necrosis factor alpha (TNFα). TNFα is synthesized and released by blood mononuclear cells and appears in the serum during ENL while concentrations drop when the patient is treated with thalidomide. In addition to treatment of ENL, thalidomide has been reported to exhibit beneficial effects in the treatment of aphthous ulcers in HIV-positive patients, Behcet's disease, chronic graft-versus-host disease, rash due to systemic of cutaneous lupus erythematosus, and pyoderma gangrenosum.

Thalidomide is a very potent teratogenic agent with a history of an estimated 10,000 deformed infants born to mothers using the drug during pregnancy. While the drug can be used safely in post-menopausal women, strict controls are required for women of child bearing age. And while there is no evidence to suggest that men can trans-

Fig. 37.21. Human metabolic products of clofazimine.

mit the drug during sex, the use of condoms by male patients will be required.

Therapeutic Considerations

From its introduction into the chemotherapy of leprosy in 1947, dapsone has proved to be the single most effective agent. This drug was used as a monotherapeutic agent despite the recognition that resistant strains were beginning to emerge. The problems of primary and secondary drug resistance are not the only treatment complications experienced. Relapse can result from bacterial persistence. Nonmultiplying microorganisms unsusceptible to dapsone may emerge at a later date causing reinfection. Since 1977, monotherapy with dapsone is no longer recognized as an acceptable method for treatment of leprosy. Today, combination chemotherapy is the method of choice. The combination consists of rifampin (600 mg monthly), dapsone (100 mg, daily) and clofazimine (300 mg, monthly and 50 mg, daily). This regimen is used for treatment of multibacillary leprosy, including lepromatous and borderline cases. Therapy is usually continued for at least 2 years or as long as skin smears are positive. The patient is kept under supervision for 5 years following completion of chemotherapy. For paucibacillary leprosy, including tuberculoid and indeterminate cases only rifampin and dapsone are used with doses as indicated above. Treatment may continue for 6 months and the patient kept under observation for an additional 2 years (71). Other combinations which have been reported include rifampin plus ofloxacin and minocycline or ofloxacin plus minocycline. The new regimens allow a shortened treatment period and a reduced rate of relapse.

CASE STUDY

Victoria F. Roche and S. William Zito

CW is a 38-year-old hot-head who's currently doing a 7–10 year stretch at the Texas State Penitentiary for viciously assaulting his brother-in-law with a frozen tuna after an oil field development deal turned sour. CW has led a rough life, and was previously busted for using and dealing heroin. He is now on methadone maintenance therapy, but suffers from hepatic dysfunction as a result of a bad bout of hepatitis from his days of sharing needles with other junkies. His wife of eight years left him six months ago, taking their two children back to Montana. CW is undergoing psychotherapy and, after unsuccessful attempts to treat his depression with tricyclic antidepressants and SSRIs, he has been stabilized on the monoamine oxidase inhibitor isocarboxazide. He is of the slow acetylator phenotype. CW has now contracted multi-drug resistant tuberculosis in the crowded prison. At this time the infection is localized in CW's lungs. A routine screen for AIDS is negative. The therapeutic choices for the treatment of CW's latest health crisis are shown as structures 1–4.

1. *Identify the therapeutic problem(s) where the pharmacist's intervention may benefit the patient.*

2. *Identify and prioritize the patient specific factors that must be considered to achieve the desired therapeutic outcomes.*

3. *Conduct a thorough and mechanistically oriented structure-activity analysis of all therapeutic alternatives provided in the case.*

4. *Evaluate the SAR findings against the patient specific factors and desired therapeutic outcomes and make a therapeutic decision.*

5. *Counsel your patient.*

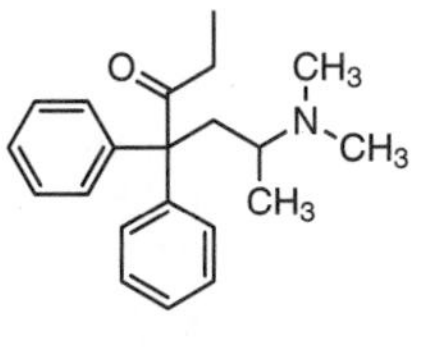

Methadone 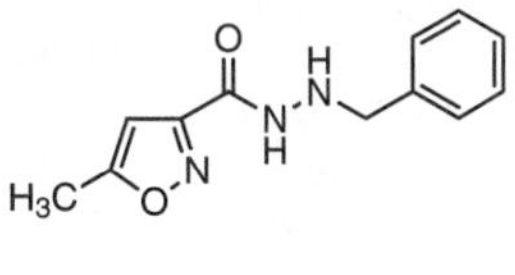   Isocarboxazide 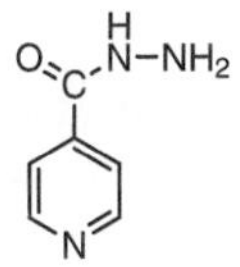   1

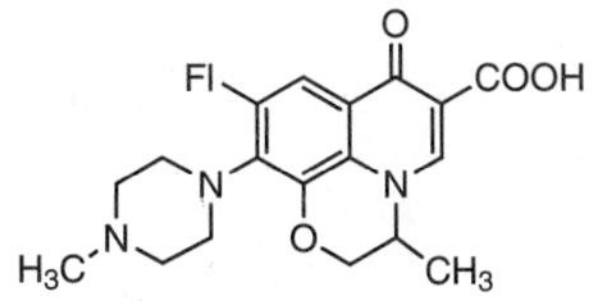

2 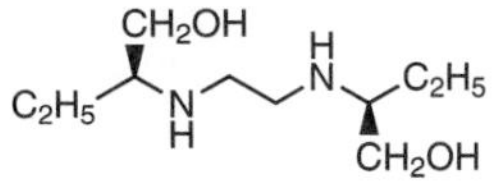   3 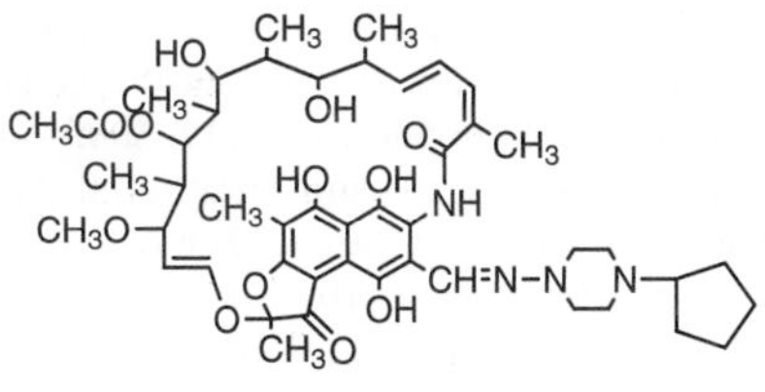   4

REFERENCES

1. Rastogi N. Structure and Functions of the Cell Envelope in Relation to Mycobacterial Virulence, Pathogenicity and Multiple Drug Resistance. 7th Form in Microbiology. Res Microbiol 1991; 142: 419–481.

2. Minnikin DE. Chemical Principles in the Organization of Lipid Components in the Mycobacterial Cell Envelope.Res Microbiol 1991; 142: 423–427.

3. McNeil MR, Brennan PJ. Structure, Function and Biogenesis of the Cell Envelope of Mycobacteria in Relation to Bacterial Physiology, Pathogenesis and Drug Resistance; Some thoughts and Possibilities Arising from Recent Structural Infromation. Res Microbiol 1991; 142: 451–463.

4. Marwick C. Do worldwide Outbreaks Mean Tuberculosis Again Becomes 'Captain of All thes Men of Death'?. JAMA 1992; 267: 1174–1175.

5. Daniel TM. Tuberculosis. In: Harrison's Principles of Internal Medicine, 12th ed. Jean D. Wilson, et.al., Ed., New York, McGraw-Hill, 1991.

6. Taylor HG. The Tuberculosis Epidemic and the Pharmacist's Role. Amer Pharm 1992; 32(7): 41–44.

7. Blanchard JS. Molecular Mechanisms of Drug Resistance in *Mycobacterium Tuberculosis*. Annu Rev Biochem 1996; 65, 215–239.

8. Zhang Y, Heym B, Allen B, et al. The catalase-peroxidase gene and isoniazid resistance of Mycobacterium tuberculosis. Nature 1992; 358: 591–593.

9. Johnsson K, Schultz PG. Mechanistic Studies of the Oxidation of Isoniazid by the Catalase Peroxidase from *Mycobacterium Tuberculosis*. J Am Chem Soc 1994; 116, 7425–7426.

10. Banerjee A, Dubnau E, Quemard A, et al. inhA, a Gene Encoding a Target for Isonaizid and Ethionamide in *Mycobacterium Tuberculosis*. Sci 1994; 263, 227–230.

11. Mdluli K, Sherman DR, Hickey MJ, et al. Biochemical and Genetic Data Suggest that inhA is not the Primary Target for Activated Isoniazid in *Mycobacterium tuberculosis*. J Infect Dis 1996; 174, 1085–1090.

12. Basso LA, Zheng R, Musser JM, et al. Mechanism of Isoniazide Resistance in *Mycobacterium Tuberculosis*: Enzymatic Characterization of Enoyl Reductase Mutants Identified in Isoniazid-Resistant Clinical Isolates. J Infect Dis 1998; 178: 769–775.

13. Quemard A, Sacchettini JC, Dessen A, et al. Enzymatic Characterization of the Target for Isoniazid in *Mycobacterium Tuberculosis*. Biochem 1995; 34: 8235–8241.

14. Johnsson K, King DS, Schultz PG. Studies on the Mechanism of Action of Isoniazid and Ethimamide in the Chemotherapy of Tuberculosis. J Am Chem Soc 1995; 117, 5009–5010.

15. Rozwarski DA, Grant GA, Barton DHR, et al. Modification of the NADH of the Isoniazid Target (Inha) from *Mycobacterium Tuberculosis*. Sci 1998; 279: 98–102.

16. Bavin EM, James B, Kay E, et al. Further Observations on the Antibacterial Activity to *Mycobacterium Tuberculosis* of a Derivative of Isoniazid, o-Hydroxybenzal Isonicotinylhydrazone (NUPASAL-213). J Pharm Pharmacol 1955; 7: 1032–1038.

17. Bavin EM, Drain DJ, Seiler M, et al. Some Further Studies on Tuberculostatic Compounds. J Pharm Pharmcol 1952: 4: 844–855.

18. Fox HH, Gibas JT. Synthetic Tuberculostats. IV. Pyridine Carboxylic Acid Hydrazides and Benzoic Acid Hydrazides. J Org Chem 1952; 17: 1653–1660.

19. Fox HH, Gibas JT. Synthetic Tuberculostats. VIII. Monoalkyl Derivatives of Isonicotinylhydrazine. J Org Chem 1953; 18: 994–1002.

20. Fox HH, Gibas JT. Synthetic Tuberculostats. IX. Dialkyl Derivatives of Isonicotinylhydrazine. J Org Chem 1955; 20: 60–69.

21. Fox HH, Gibas JT. Synthetic Tuberculostats. XI. Trialkyl and Other Derivatives of Isonicotinylhydrazine. J Org Chem 1956; 21: 356–361.

22. Weber WW, Hein DW. Clinical Pharmacokinetics of Isoniazid. Clin Pharmacokinetics 1979: 4: 401–422.

23. Holdiness MR. Clinical Pharmacokinetics of the Antituberculosis Drugs. Clin Pharmacokinetics 1984; 9: 511–544.

24. Timbrell JA, Mitchell JR, Snodgrass WR, et al. Isoniazid Hepatotoxicity: The Relationship between Covalent Binding and Metabolism *in vivo*. J Pharmacol Exper Therap 1980; 213: 364–369 .

25. Nolan CM, Goldberg SV, Buskin SE. Hepatotoxicity Associated with Isoniazid Preventing Therapy. J Am Med Assoc 1999; 281:1014–1018.

26. Lancini G. Ansamycins. In Pape H, Rehm H-J, ed. Biotechnology: Microbial Products II. vol 4. Deerfield Beach FL: VCH, 1986.

27. Arora SK. Correlation of Structure and Activity in Ansamycins: Structure, Conformation, and Interactions of Antibiotic Rifamycin S. J Med Chem 1985; 28: 1099–1102.

28. Levin ME, Hatfull GF. *Mycobacterium smegmatis* RNA polymerase: DNA supercoiling, Action of Rifampicin and Mechanism of Rifampicin Resistance. Mol Microbiol 1993; 8: 277–285.

29. Lancini G, Zanchelli W. Structure-Activity Relationship in Rifamycins. In Perlman D, ed. Structure-Activity Relationship Among the Semisynthetic Antibiotics. New York: Academic Press, 1977.

30. Jarvis B, Lamb HM. Rifapentine. Drugs 1998; 56: 607–616.

31. Reith K, Keung A, Toren PC, et al. Disposition and Metabolism of 14C-Rifapentine in Healthy Volunteers. Drug Met Disposition 1998; 26: 732–738.

32. Drugs for Tuberculosis. The Medical Letter, 37, The Medical Letter, Inc., New Rochelle, NY, August 4, 1995; 67–70.

33. Keung ACF, Eller MG, Weir SJ. Pharmacokinetics of Rifapentine in Patients with Varying Degrees of Hepatic Dysfunction. J Clin Pharmacol 1998; 38: 517–524.

34. Scorpio A, Zhang Y. Mutations in *pncA*, a Gene Encoding Pyrazinamidase/Nicotinamidase, Cause Resistance to the Antituberculous Drug Pyrazinamide in Tubercle Bacillus. Nature Med 1996; 2: 662–667.

35. Heifets LB, Flory MA, Lindholm-Levy PJ. Does Pyrazinoic Acid as an Active Moiety of Pyrazinamide Have Specific Activity Against *Mycobacterium tuberculosis?* Antimicrob Agents Chemo 1989; 33: 1252

36. Kushner S, Dalalian H, Sanjurjo JL, et al. Experimental Chemotherapy of Tuberculosis. II. The Synthesis of Pyrazinamides and Related Compounds. J Am Chem Soc 1952; 74: 3617–3621.

37. Bergmann KE, Cynamon MH, Welch JT. Quantitiative Structure-Activity Relationships for the *in Vitro* Antimycobacterial Activity of Pyrazinoic Acid Esters. J Med Chem 1996; 3394–3400.

38. Peloquin CA, Bulpitt AE, Jaresko GS, et al. Pharmacokinetics of Pyrazinamide under Fasting Conditions, with Food, and with Antacids. Pharmacother 1998; 18: 1205–1211.

39. Daffe M, Brennan PJ, McNeil MR. Predominant Structureal Features of the Cell Wall Arabinogalactan of *Mycobacterium tuberculosis* as Revealed through Characterization fo Oligoglycosyl Alditol Fragments by Gas Chromatography/Mass Spectrometry and by ^{1}H and ^{13}C NMR analysis. J Biol Chem 1990; 265: 6734–6743.

40. Wolucka BA, McNeil MR, de Hoffmann E, et al. Recognition of the Lipid Intermediate for Arabinoglactan/Arabinomannan Structure of Cell Wall of Mycobacterium: Biosynthesis and Its Relation to the Mode of Action of Ethambutol in Mycobacteria. J Biol Chem 1994; 269: 23328–23335.

41. Takayama K, Kilburn JO. Inhibition of synthesis of Arabinoglactan by Ethambutol in *Mycobacterium smegmatis*. Antimicrob Agents Chemother 1989; 33: 1493–1499.

42. Mikusova K, Slayden RAS, Besra GS, et al. Biogenesis of the Mycobacterial Cell Wall and the Site of Action of Ethambutol. Antimicrob Agents Chemo 1995; 39: 2484–2489.

43. Lee RE, Mikusova K, Brennan PJ, et al. "Synthesis of the Mycobacterial arabinose Donor β-D-Arabinofuranosyl-1-Monophosphoryldecaprenol, development of a basic Arabinosyl-transferase Assay, and identification of Ethambutol as an Arabinosyl transferase inhibitor." J Am Chem Soc 1995; 117: 11829–11832.

44. Khoo K-H, douglas E, Azadi P, et al. Truncated Structral Variants of Lopoarabinomannan in Ethambutol Drug-resistant Strains of *Mycobacterium smegmatis*. J Biol Chem 1996; 271: 28628–28690.

45. Belanger AE, Besra GS, Ford ME, et al. The *embAB* Genes of *Mycobacterium avium* Encode an Arabinosyl Transferase Involved in Cell Wall Arabinan Biosynthesis that is the Target for the Antimycobacterial Drug Ethambutol. Proc Natl Acad Sci 1996; 93: 11919–11924.

46. Kuehl FA, Peck RL, Hoffhine Jr. CE, et al. Streptomyces Antibiotics. XVIII. Structure of Streptomycin. J Amer Chem Soc 1945; 70: 2325–2329.

47. Finken M, Kirschner P, Meier A, et al. Molecular Basis of Streptomycin Resistance in *Mycobacterium tuberculosis*: Alterations of the 'Ribosomal Protein S12 Gene and Point Putations Within a Functional 16S Ribosomal RNA pseudoknot. Mol Microbiol 1993; 9: 1239–1246.

48. Bieder A, Brunel P, Mazeau L. Identification de Trois Nouveaux Metabolites de l'ethionamide: Chromatographie, Spectrophotometrie, Polarographie. Ann Pharmaceut Francais 1966; 24: 493–500.

49. Caceres NE, Harris NB, Wellehan JF, et al. Over Expression of the D-Alanine Racemase Gene Confers Resistance to D-Cycloserince in *Mycobacterium smegmatis*. J Bacteriol 1997; 179: 5046–5055.

50. Gale EF, Cundliffe E, Reynolds PE, Richmond MH, Waring MJ. In: The Molecular Basis of Antibiotic Action, 2nd Ed., London, Wiley & Son, 1981;500–502

51. Reinke CM, Albrant DH. An Old Scorge: Tuberculosis in the 1990s. U S Pharmacist Hospital Edition October, 1991; 16: 37–72.

52. Jacobs MR. Activity of Quinolones Against Mycobacteria. Drugs 1995; 49(Suppl.2): 67–75.

53. Renau TE, Sanchez JP, Gage JW, et al. Structure-activity Relationships of the Quinolone Antibacterials Against Mycobacteria: Effect of Structural Changes at N-1 and C-7. J Med Chem 1996; 39: 729–735.

54. Miyazaki E, Miyazaki M, Chen JM, et al. Moxifloxacin (BAY-12–8039), a New 8–Methoxyquinolone, Is active in Mouse Model of Tuberculosis. Antimicrob Agents Chemo 1999; 43: 85–89.

55. Zhao BY, Pine R, Domagala J, et al. Fluoroquinolone Action Against Clinical Isolates of *Mycobacterium tuberculosis*: Effects of a C-8 Methoxy Group on survival in Liquid Media and in Human Macrophages. Antimicrob Agents Chemo 1999; 43: 661–333.

56. Yew WW, Kwan SY, Ma WK, et al. In vitro Activity of Ofloxacin in *Mycobacterium tuberculosis* and its Clinical Efficacy in Mutiply Resistant Pulmonary Tuberculosis. J Antimicrob Chemo 1990; 26: 227–236.

57. Amsdenn GW, Peloquin CA, Berning SE. The Role of Advanced Generation Macrolides in the Prophylaxis and Treatment of *Mycobacterium avium* Complex (MAC) Infections. Drugs 1997; 54: 69–80.

58. Wright J. Current Strategies for the Prevention and Treatment of Disseminated *Mycobacterium avium* Complex Infection in Patients with AIDS. Pharmacotherapy 1998; 18: 738–747.

59. Faris MA, Raasch RH, Hopfer RL, et al. Treatment and Prophylaxis of Disseminated *Mycobacterium avium* Complex in HIV-Infected Individuals. Ann Pharmacotherapy 1998; 32: 561–573.

60. van Zyl JM, Basson K, Kriegler A, et al. Mechanisms by which Clofazimine and Dapsone Inhibit the Myeloperoxidase System. Biochem Pharmacol 1991; 42: 599–608.

61. Dhople AM. In vitro and in vivo Actitity of K-130, a Dihyrofolate Reductase Inhibitor, against *Mycobacterium leprae*. Arzneim-Forsch Drug Res 1999; 49: 267–271.

62. Ward KE, McCarthy MW. Dapsone-Induced Methemoglovinemia. Ann Pharmacotherapy 1998; 32: 549–552.

63. Savage JE, O'Sullivan JF, Zeis BM, et al. Investigation of the Structural Properties of Dihydrophenazines which Contribute to their Pro-oxidative Interaction with Human Phagocytes. J Antimicrob Chemo 1989; 23: 691–700.

64. Franzblau SG, White KE, O'Sullivan JF. Structure-Activity Relationships of Tetramethylpiperdine-Substituted Phenazines Against *Mycobacterium leprae* in vitro. Antimicrob Agenst Chemo 1989; 33: 2004–2005.

65. Arutla S, Arra GS, Prabhakar CM, et al. Pro- and Anti-oxidant Effects of Some Antileprotic drugs in vitro and Their Influence on Super Oxide Dismutase Actitivity. Arzneim— Forsch Drug Res 1998; 48: 1024–1027.

66. O'Sullivan JF, Conalty ML, Morrison NE. Clofazimine Analogues Active against a Clofazimine Resistant Orgnism. J Med Chem 1988; 31: 567–572.

67. Kapoor VK. Clofazimine. In: Analytical Profiles of Drug Substances, Vol 18, Florey K ed, San Diego, Academic Press, Inc., 1989.

68. Krishna DR, Mamidi RNVS, Hofmann U, et al. Characterization of Clofazimine Metabolites in Humans by HPLC-Electrospray Mass Spectrometry. Arzneim-Forsch Drug Res 1997; 47: 303–306.

69. Stirling D, Sherman M, Strauss S. Thalidomide A Surprising Recovery. J Am Pharm Assoc 1997; 37: 306–313.

70. Thalidomide. The Medical Letter, 40, The Medical Letter, Inc., New Rochelle, NY, October 23, 1998; 103–104.

71. Lambert HP, O'Grady FW. Antibiotic and Chemotherapy, 6th ed, Edinburgh, Churchill Livingstone, 1992.

38. Cancer and Cancer Chemotherapy

PAT CALLERY AND PETER GANNETT

INTRODUCTION
Historical

Among the first agents used to treat cancer were members of the mustards (Fig. 38.1). Originally, simple sulfur mustards were used as chemical warfare agents during World War I. A chance observation during an autopsy involving a case of mustard gas exposure revealed inhibition (aplasia) of bone marrow formation. This observation suggested the use of mustards in the treatment of leukemia. By the 1940s, nitrogen mustards had been extensively studied, especially in regard to their cytotoxic effects on lymphoid tissue. The first clinical trials with nitrogen mustards began in 1942, initiating the era of cancer chemotherapy.

During the next 20 years many cancer chemotherapeutic agents were synthesized and tested. In addition to the mustards, which are members of the alkylating cancer chemotherapeutic agents, additional classes of agents were discovered and developed including folic acid derivatives, pyrimidine and purine synthesis inhibitors, and the vinca alkaloids. A time-line for the introduction of some of the more significant cancer chemotherapeutic agents is shown in Table 38.1.

In the late 1950s, the National Cancer Institute (NCI) began to play a major role in the development of anticancer agents. NCI has since been involved in the development of drugs in a variety of ways including screening chemicals for antitumor activity, funding cancer related research at all levels, and conducting basic cancer research. In 1971, during the Nixon administration, the National Cancer Act was passed. The aim of this legislation was to "substantially reduce the overall death rates for most of the common carcinomas." In certain instances, significant strides toward this goal have been achieved. Examples include methotrexate in the treatment of choriocarcinoma in women; acute leukemia treatment with vincristine and doxorubicin; Wilm's tumor and Ewing's sarcoma treatment with dactinomycin and vincristine; rhabdomyosarcoma treatment with vincristine, dactinomycin and cyclophosphamide; retinoblastoma in children treatment with cyclophosphamide and vincristine; Hodgkin's disease treatment with a nitrogen mustard, vincristine, procarbazine and prednisone; Burkitt's lymphoma treated with chlorambucil; and testicular cancer treatment with cisplatin. Overall, however, only modest improvements have been made. For most cancers in the U.S., incidence rates are rising and mortality rates are flat or slightly declining (1).

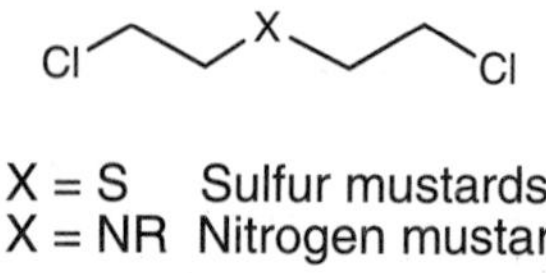

Definitions
Neoplasms

Selection of an appropriate agent to treat cancer depends on knowledge of the type of cancer, since many agents or classes of agents are only effective against certain types of cancer. There is no general classification system for cancer and some terminology that is used lacks precision. The term neoplasm is defined as a new and diseased form of tissue growth. Benign neoplasms are not cancerous while malignant neoplasms are. The key distinction between these two terms is that only malignant tumors metastasize. Benign tumors can typically be removed by surgery as easily as "shelling a pea from a pod" since they have well defined borders. In addition, any symptoms caused by them are usually a result of local effects that disappear subsequent to the removal of a benign neoplasm. In contrast, malignant neoplasms are invasive to the surrounding tissue and their complete removal is difficult, if not impossible. Furthermore, malignant tumors spread to sites discontinuous with the original tumor mass in a process termed metastasis.

Neoplasms have been named in a variety of ways. Many neoplasms have been named after their discoverer such as Wilm's tumor, Hodgkin's disease and Kaposi sarcoma. A second method for naming neoplasms is based on a histogenic classification of the tissue from which the neoplasm is derived (Table 38.2). The suffix -oma usually indicates a

X = S   Sulfur mustards
X = NR Nitrogen mustards

Fig. 38.1. Generalized chemical structure of the mustards.

Table 38.1. Time-line for the Introduction of Some Cancer Chemotherapeutic Agents

Agent or Class	Approximate Year of Introduction
Nitrogen Mustards	1949
Methotrexate	1948
Vinca Alkaloids	1958
Pyrimidine/Purine Synthesis Inhibitors	Early 1960s
Antitumor Antibiotics	Early 1960s
Hydroxyurea	1963
Hydrazines	1963
cis-Platin	Early 1970s
Epipodophyllotoxins	Late 1970s–early 1980s
Antiestrogens	1990s

Table 38.2. Histogenic Classification of Malignant Tumors

Normal Tissue	Malignant Neoplasm	Example
Bone Marrow	Leukemia	
Connective Tissue	Sarcoma	Chondrosarcoma (cartilage)
		Liposarcoma (fat)
		Osteosarcoma (bone)
Epithelium	Carcinoma	Hepatocellular carcinoma (liver) squamous carcinoma (squamos epithelium)
		Adenocarcinoma (glandular epithelium)
Atypical Names		
Lymphoid Tissue	Lymphoma	Hodgkin's disease
Myeloid stem cells	Myeloid Leukemia	
Endothelium	Kaposi's sarcoma	
Skin (melanocytes)	Malignant melanoma	

benign tumor such as adenoma (glandular epithelium), chondroma (cartilage) or osteoma (bone). Notable exceptions exist including the malignant tumors, myelomas and lymphomas. Both are examples of malignant neoplasms. Finally, some lesions ending in -oma, such as granulomas, are not tumors at all.

In the case of undifferentiated tumors, a distinction can be made between tumors of epithelial origin and those of connective tissue origin. The former are referred to as carcinomas while the latter are termed sarcomas. Finally, some tumor types are difficult to classify histogenically and include those of the neuroendocrine system comprising cells that store biogenic amines in granules. The suffix -blastoma is often used to classify these malignant neoplasms. Examples include neuroblastoma (sympathetic neurons), retinoblastoma (embryonal retina) and myoblastoma (muscle tissue).

Leukemia

Leukemia, a cancer of the cells in the blood, usually involves the over production of leukocytes by two to three orders of magnitude. There are two major classes of leukemia, acute and chronic. In acute leukemia, precursor white blood cells (blasts) do not mature and interfere with the production of normal, mature white blood cells. In contrast, chronic leukemia produces abnormal mature white blood cells that are unable to fulfill their role of preventing or resisting infection.

Metastases

Malignant tumors will eventually metastasize, if left untreated, while metastasis does not occur in the case of benign tumors. The result of this process is the formation of secondary tumors at locations different from that of the primary tumor. Malignant tumor cells can be shed from the primary tumor and distributed by the vascular or lymph systems. There are many barriers to this process that serve to protect against the spread of cancer. First, few cells survive transport in the blood. Second, the few cells that do survive transport must adhere themselves to and penetrate the underlying basement membrane. This re-

quires the concerted action of collagenases, plasminogen activators and cysteine proteases. Interestingly, metastasis does not appear to be mainly a random process. In part, this can be explained by a mechanism where tumor cells shed into the blood lodge in the first capillary network encountered. A third major factor affecting the formation of secondary tumors is whether or not a malignant cell is in a congenial environment. Also, the local production of either inhibitory or stimulatory growth factors has a significant influence.

Important Principles
Proliferation (2)

Two key aspects of cellular life are (1) DNA synthesis and mitosis to produce new cells and (2) cell differentiation which produces specialized cells. Normal cells, often referred to as nontransformed cells, have control mechanisms to modulate these two processes. The mechanisms may be regulated by chemical signals such as growth factors or growth inhibitors. Normal cells produce growth factors that stimulate growth. Simultaneously, many cells also have a negative feedback loop to counterbalance the effects of growth factors. If the organ is damaged, the amount of inhibitor produced is decreased and the rate of proliferation increases until the lost cells are replaced.

Growth factors and growth inhibitors exert their effects by binding to cell surface receptors (3,4). In cancer cells, these regulatory processes are aberrant. For example, cancer cells may over produce growth factors such as epidermal growth factor (EGF), under express growth inhibitors such as p53, or over express growth factor receptors. Regardless of mechanism, the aberrant activation of growth factors or decreased expression of growth inhibitors will lead to a loss of normal growth control resulting in abnormal and increased cell proliferation. The root causes of these aberrations, at the cellular level, have not been completely determined. However, the general belief is that proto-oncogenes, which control normal proliferation and differentiation, are transformed into oncogenes. In turn, oncogenes alter the cellular control mechanisms, stimulating processes that support cellular proliferation.

Cell Cycle and Regulation (5)

The cell cycle is pictorially represented in Figure 38.2. The cycle is divided into four main parts. The G_1 or Gap 1 phase is the period when a newly created cell is born. The period of time a cell remains in the G_1 phase depends on the tissue type and whether it is a normal cell or a tumor cell. If the cell is a proliferating cell, it will quickly move into the S or synthesis phase. It is during this period that nuclear DNA is replicated, and at the end of the S phase, two copies of DNA are present in the cell. The next phase is the G_2 or Gap 2 period and this phase is largely a time during which preparations are made for the final cell cycle phase, the M phase or mitosis. The time between mitoses is the cell cycle time, although this time can vary depending mainly on the duration of G_1 phase.

There are two major control points in the cell cycle. One of these is at G_1/S when cells commit to replicate. The second is at G_2/M when cells commit to divide. Of these two major points in the cell cycle, the G_1/S is of major importance in understanding cancer and cancer treatment.

During the G_1 phase a cell can take one of three routes. First, the cell may enter the S phase. Second, a cell in the G_1 phase may enter into a fifth phase called G_0, or Gap 0. Cells in G_0 are termed quiescent. Third, the cell may terminally differentiate and die. In normal cell populations cells may be proliferating, quiescent, or terminally differentiating such that there is no net change in the number of cells. However, in tumors, the fraction of cells proliferating increases at the expense of quiescent or terminally differentiating cells such that there is a net increase in the number of cells.

Cells can be born into a proliferative state or a nonproliferative state. In tumors, new cells that are produced in hypoxic regions, which typically are nearer the center of the tumor and poorly perfused, may be born into the nonproliferative state. These cells are not sensitive to drugs. Thus, after the tumor is exposed to a cancer chemotherapeutic agent and the outer most cells, which are mainly in the proliferative state, are susceptible to and destroyed by cancer chemotherapeutic agents, those cells that were in the nonproliferative state may then be recruited into a proliferative state. Thus, in order to eradicate a tumor it usually requires several rounds of the cancer chemotherapeutic agent.

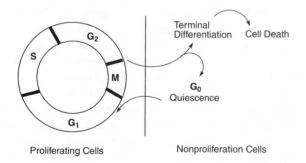

Fig. 38.2. The cell cycle.

Growth Factors and Growth Inhibitors (3,4)

The cell cycle key check points G_1/S and G_2/M appear to be controlled by water soluble proteins called growth factors that are secreted by cells and which bind to the membrane of other cells at a glycoprotein receptor. This binding then initiates a series of biochemical reactions that ultimately result in gene expression of growth factors. Growth factor concentrations are typically in the picomolar range. However, the response of the cell to growth factors appears to be limited by the number of cell receptors and not by growth factor concentration.

There are three main types of growth factors. Endocrine growth factors are hormones such as thyroxine or insulin. This type of growth factor is produced at one site and then distributed throughout the body. A second type of growth factor is the paracrine type which are produced at multiple locations but, due to short plasma half-life, only act on nearby cells. Finally, autocrine growth factors are produced by a cell and stimulate the same cell. In the latter case, a major role of the growth factor is to control the number of cells in either the proliferative or nonproliferative state and thus maintains homeostasis.

Many cancer cells produce excessive levels of growth factors. For example, epithelial growth factor receptor (EGFR) is often overexpressed in squamous carcinomas (breast, lung or bladder). The overexpression of autocrine growth factors by cancer cells offers a new approach to cancer therapy. In particular, antibodies can be prepared to target the autocrine growth factors. This approach has been shown to produce cell death in cultured tumor cells.

BIOCHEMICAL BASIS OF CANCER
Mutation (6)

There are two main types of mutations, germ-line and somatic mutations. Most mutations that result in cancer are of the latter type. In principle, only one mutation is necessary. However, because cells have many mechanisms for repairing damaged DNA, it is generally believed that multiple mutations are required as described by the multi-hit or multi-stage theory of cancer. This theory also claims that carcinogenesis requires both initiation (mutation) and then promotion. Thus, following (1) an initial mutation or mutations, (2) a promotion phase occurs during which time mutated cells proliferate aided by exposure to otherwise nongenotoxic compounds, (3) a small benign tumor forms or mild dysplasia occurs along with the development of the malignant phenotype, (4) the primary malignant tumor forms, and finally (5) cells break off, lodge at remote sites, and secondary tumors form (metastasis).

The distinction between initiators and promoters is an important one. Initiators, at least in low doses, do not produce cancer, though they usually produce mutations. Without a secondary stimulus, transformation to malignant cells is unlikely. However, if these cells are subsequently exposed to a promoter, emergence of the malignant phenotype occurs. Promoters, in the absence of

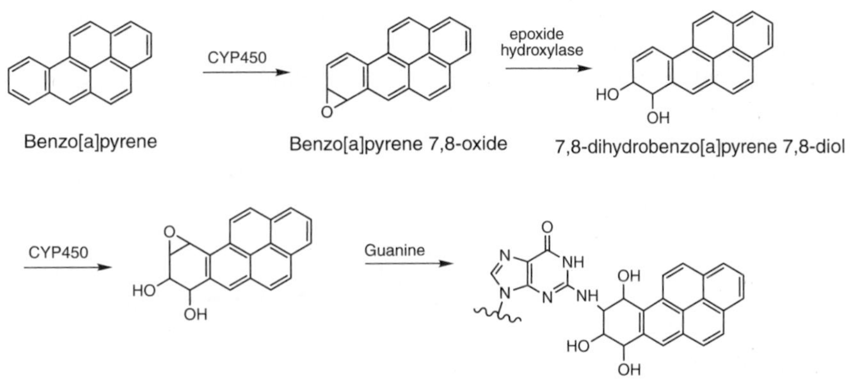

Fig. 38.3. Metabolic activation of benzo[a]pyrene.

initiators are generally not genotoxic or mutagenic. Some of the more important promoters include 12-O-tetrade-canoyl phorbol-13–acetate (TPA), organochlorine pesticides, and many hormones (e.g., estrogen).

Chemicals (7)

A key event in linking cancer to the exposure to chemicals occurred at the end of the 18th century when Sir Percival Pott, a surgeon in Britain noted the high incidence of cancer of the scrotum in chimney sweeps. Eventually, benzo[a]pyrene, a component of soot, was identified as the cause of the scrotal cancer. Subsequently, benzo[a]pyrene was shown to be metabolized to reactive intermediates by CYP450 enzymes. It is the current hypothesis that these reactive intermediates react with guanine and other bases in DNA and produce point (single) mutations (Fig. 38.3). These potentially cytotoxic mutations may be recognized and repaired, or may persist. In the latter case, mutations may be misread when DNA is replicated producing base transitions or transversions resulting in permanent mutations. Since the time that a link between exposure to a chemical and subsequent occurrence of cancer was first discovered, numerous other chemicals have been studied and established to be carcinogens. Some of these chemicals and the cancer they are associated with are shown in Table 38.3.

Table 38.3. Environmental Sources of Carcinogens

Carcinogen	Cancer Type	Environmental Source
β-Naphthylamine	Bladder	Dyes
Asbestos	Lung	Insulation
Ionizing Radiation	Lung, Bone	Uranium miners
Polyaromatic Hydrocarbons	Skin, Lung	Exposure to coal tar, combustion products
UV light	Skin	Sunbathers, outdoor workers
Aflatoxin	Liver	Contaminated foods
Tobacco smoke	Lung, Mouth	Smokers
Alkylating agents	Bone, Bladder	Cancer chemo-therapeutic agents

While many of the agents listed in Table 38.3 produce DNA adducts including β-naphthylamine, aflatoxins, and alkylating agents, other carcinogens such as asbestos or ionizing radiation produce DNA adducts indirectly by free radical mediated processes. In particular, the latter set of carcinogens produces reactive oxygen species (ROS), such as hydroxyl radical, that can react with DNA to produce adducts. ROS can also damage DNA in other ways such as producing single or double strand breaks.

Oncogenic Viruses (8)

There are several human cancers whose cause can be linked to a virus. There are fundamentally two types of viruses, DNA and RNA types. In either case, the virus inserts itself into the host genome. DNA viruses produce proteins that interact with growth regulatory proteins or tumor suppressor genes. In some cases, the viral genome may be integrated into cellular chromosomes, often near key regulatory genes. In addition, viral genes may produce other mutations.

RNA viruses, and in particular RNA retro viruses, may also cause tumors. RNA retro viruses produce a double stranded DNA provirus from RNA by the action of reverse transcriptase. The proviral DNA is then inserted into the host genome by the enzyme integrase. The insertion point is usually near a proto-oncogene and thus alterations in gene expression may occur and lead to tumors.

Altered Gene Expression

It is generally believed that most human malignancies result from incorrect proto-oncogene expression. The function of proto-oncogenes is to control cell growth. Abnormal expression of proto-oncogenes can take several forms; their protein product may be aberrant or is over or under expressed. Thus, two fundamentally different genetic mechanisms exist consisting of (1) enhanced or aberrant oncogene expression or (2) decreased activity of tumor suppressor (anti-oncogenes). Normal cells express these genes in such a fashion that the cell populations are maintained while tumor cells do not. The cause of altered gene expression may be a point mutation or a result of insertional mutagenesis.

A number of oncogenes are known and are grouped based on function. One group is associated with the ability to continuously produce growth factors such as the *hst* gene or the *int* gene. These two genes, when both are present, have been linked with breast cancer. Other categories include genes associated with growth factor receptors such as c-*erb*B-2, an epithelial growth factor receptor (EGFR) related proto-oncogene, and guanine nucleotide binding oncogenes such as *myc*.

Tumor suppressor genes have been identified and studied. Their original discovery was through the study of hereditary cancer, although this term does not signify that what is inherited is a predisposition to cancer. Their initial discovery was derived from research on a rare childhood tumor, retinoblastoma. Tumor formation is dependent on the presence of the retinoblastoma gene Rb. A second well-studied tumor suppressor gene is p53 which encodes a 53 KDa protein. This protein is involved in cell cycle regulation through its interaction with cyclins which act to slow cell proliferation. The study of p53 has led to the identification of other tumor suppressor genes including p21. Subsequent research has suggested that p21 and p53 work together to hold a cell in the G_1 phase. Mutation of p53, however, may allow proliferation of mutant cells.

CANCER THERAPY (9)
Overview

The specific approach used to treat cancer depends upon the specific type, location, and stage of the cancer. Regardless of the specific details, there are several fundamental techniques available to treat cancer including surgery, radiation therapy, immunologic treatment, and chemical based approaches. Each has its own merits. Generally, a combination of these methods is used, for example, surgery in combination with chemotherapy or radiation therapy with chemotherapy. In most therapeutic approaches to the treatment of cancer there will be a chemical component.

Surgery

Surgery is one of the oldest approaches to the treatment of cancer. In order for this approach to be effective, the cancer must still be in the primary tumor stage and there must be a high degree of confidence that the entire tumor can be excised. In addition, it should be possible to remove the tumor without causing significant damage to vital organs. Surgery can also be used for diagnostic purposes and in combination with other approaches.

Radiation Therapy

Radiation therapy is used to shrink or destroy tumors. It does so by causing damage to the DNA of the tumor cells so that they die. X-ray radiation is used by focusing an X-ray beam on the tumor. Radiation therapy is not painful and anesthetics are not required for the procedure. In addition, there are few after affects from the procedure unless the tumor is in the vicinity of the digestive tract. In which case, patients may experience nausea after treatment. Similar to surgery, the approach requires that the tumor be localized if the approach is to be successful.

Immunologic Therapy

This is a relatively new approach to the treatment of cancer. The approach attempts to utilize the immune system to eradicate the cancer. The methodology attempts to boost the levels of lymphocytes, specifically T-cell and B-cell lymphocytes. The major role of T-cells is to destroy foreign cells, including malignant and premalignant cells. B-cells, produced in the bone marrow and lymph nodes make antibodies in response to a foreign protein which may be expressed by cancer cells. Currently, therapy of this type primarily consists of the administration of highly purified interferons, especially interferon-2.

Chemotherapy

Cancer chemotherapeutic agents are used for a wide range of purposes. The intent of their administration may be to cure a specific cancer, reduce the size of a tumor prior to surgery, sensitize tumors to radiation therapy or to destroy microscopic metastases after tumors are surgically removed. Chemotherapeutic agents are complementary to either surgery or radiation therapy in that they are effective against metastasized tumors or residual tumor after surgery or radiation therapy. In other words, they are useful for eliminating tumors that are small in size. The reason they are less useful for larger tumors is that large tumors are not well perfused by blood and thus the inner reaches of a tumor are not accessible to cancer chemotherapeutic agents.

A second problem with cancer chemotherapy is the lack of selectivity of the agents for normal versus malignant cells. Chemotherapeutic agents are basically cytotoxic and they can kill both normal and malignant cell types. Their usefulness in the treatment of cancer relies on the assumption that malignant cells, which are rapidly proliferating cells, take up extracellular materials at a greater rate than normal cells. This is often the case although there are a few normal cell types that are rapidly proliferating including hair cells, bone marrow cells, and cells lining the gastrointestinal tract. A consequence of this is patients undergoing chemotherapy suffer hair loss, depression of their immune system, and nausea or diarrhea. These effects typically disappear once chemotherapy has been discontinued.

Cancer Chemotherapy Successes

The successful treatment of cancer has progressed over the past 40 years. The improvement, as measured by five-year survival rates, is attributed to a variety of factors including improved methods of detection and treatment. Early detection clearly has been a major player in improving the five-year survival rates since tumors are more likely to be small and secondary tumors are usually not present.

Several major success stories exist. For example, the treatment of testicular cancer with cisplatin has achieved partial or complete remission rates of 85% and five-year survival rates are better than 90%. Hodgkins disease is a second example. There is only a 5% spontaneous remission rate for Hodgkin's disease, but with treatment the complete remission rate is in excess of 80%.

However, other cancers have proven to be very difficult to successfully treat by chemotherapy or other methods. The five-year survival rates for lung cancer, the most prevalent form of cancer, is less than 15%. Likewise, cancers of the liver and pancreas have proven to be very difficult to treat and the five-year survival rates for these forms of cancer are less than 10%.

Summaries of the indications of drugs for specific cancer chemotherapy, as well as commonly used combination therapy, are included in the following sections. A useful source of drugs of choice is published periodically in *The Medical Letter*.

CLASSES OF ANTICANCER AGENTS—ALKYLATING AGENTS
Mechanism of Action

The alkylating agents are a structurally diverse class of chemicals that can be subdivided into three main classes. The first and perhaps the oldest class are the nitrogen mustards. Mechlorethamine was the first agent in this class and received FDA approval in 1949 (10). Several related compounds have since been developed including cyclophosphamide, ifosfamide, chlorambucil, estramustine phosphate, and melphalan. All of the agents in this class are considered to be classical alkylating agents that react with DNA through heterolytic mechanisms (11). Closely related to the mustards are thiotepa and busulfan and the nitrosoureas, carmustine and lomustine (12). These agents lack the mustard skeleton, although they behave as classical alkylating agents.

Regardless of which subgroup is considered, the alkylating agents act by alkylation of DNA. The most common site of alkylation is the N-7 position of guanine (Fig. 38.4). Other sites on the DNA bases (guanine, adenine, thymine or cytosine) or the phosphate oxygens of the DNA back-

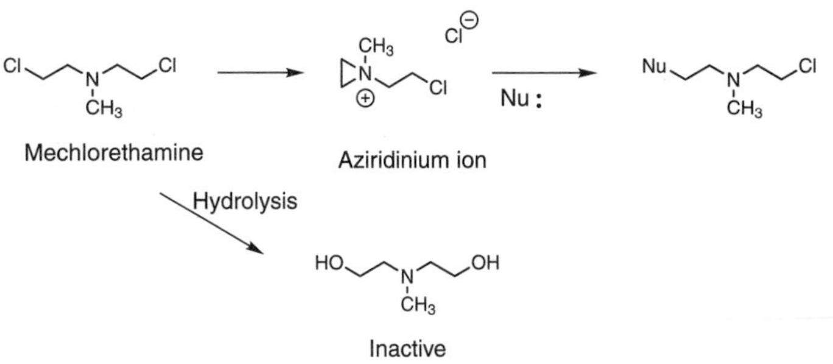

Fig. 38.5. Formation of aziridinium ion from nitrogen mustards. Nu: = a nucleophile such as the N-7 of guanine.

bone may also be alkylated. In the case of difunctional alkylating agents such as the mustards, two DNA sites may be alkylated by the same compound producing intra- or interstrand links. Once alkylation of DNA occurs, the alkylated sites become prone to cleavage resulting in the formation of single strand breaks of the nuclear DNA.

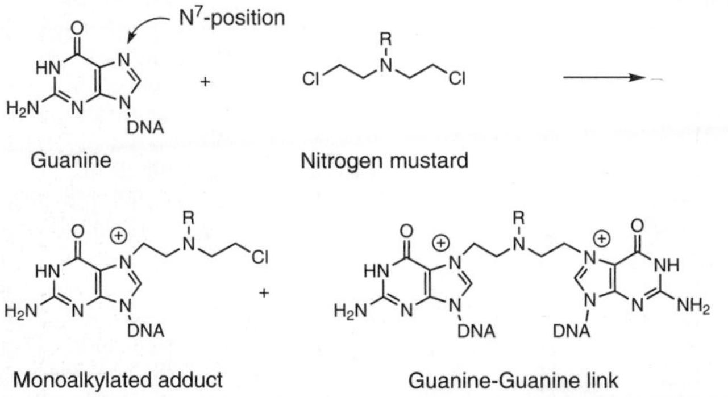

The consequences of DNA alkylation have been extensively studied. However, a mechanism for the cytotoxicity has yet to be established. Alkylating agents are known to react with DNA, RNA and proteins, although their reaction with DNA is believed to be the most important. Bifunctional alkylating agents can produce inter- and intrastrand cross-links. Inter-strand links, which form from mechlorethamine aziridinium ions (13), prevent DNA separation and are cytotoxic. Bifunctional alkylating agents do not necessarily produce inter-strand cross-links (14). Reaction with guanine at N-7 appears to occur to the greatest extent. Other sites on guanine, sites on other bases, and the phosphate oxygens also appear to be alkylated. Alkylation of the N-7 position of guanine can result in the formation of an apurinic site.

The alkylating agents appear to be the most effective in the G_1 or S phase. Repair can occur if DNA alkylation is discovered. When it is, an endonuclease cuts the damaged strand, an exonuclease excises the damaged piece and the region is then backfilled. Rapidly proliferating cells have insufficient time to repair damaged DNA, whereas cells in G_0 have considerable time to effect repair. Thus, alkylating agents should be most effective against rapidly proliferating cells, a prediction that is clinically observed.

Chloride, the leaving group present in the mustards, is not generally an easily replaced atom. However, in the case of mustards, the nitrogen atom activates the chloride by proceeding through an aziridinium ion intermediate as shown in Figure 38.5. The nitrogen mustards are, therefore, quite reactive agents and must be administered intravenously.

Specific Agents
Nitrogen Mustards

Mechlorethamine HCl. Mechlorethamine has the simplest chemical structure of a nitrogen mustard used as an antineoplastic agent (Fig. 38.5). Aqueous solutions of the

Fig. 38.4. Alkylation of guanine in DNA by an alkylating agent.

injectable formulation of mechlorethamine HCl triturated with NaCl at a concentration of 1 mg of mechlorethamine per ml are in a pH range of 3–5, as would be anticipated for a hydrochloride salt of a tertiary amine. Hydrolysis of mechlorethamine is rapid ($t_{1/2}$ = 15 min) *in vivo* and the drug is not present in an active form within a few minutes after administration. Dosage forms and pharmacologic indications are shown in Table 38.4.

Melphalan

Melphalan.   Melphalan, also known as L-phenylalanine mustard or L-PAM, is a nitrogen mustard chemically linked to a natural amino acid. An indication that the L-isomer is transported into cells preferentially, presumably with the assistance of an L-amino acid active transporter. This suggestion is supported by the observation that D-phenylalanine mustard requires a higher dose to reach the same cytotoxicity level against certain animal tumors than is the marketed enantiomer, L-phenylalanine mustard. Characteristic of a nitrogen mustard, approximately 30% of a dose of melphalan can be accounted for in a covalently bound form with plasma proteins. Dosage forms and pharmacologic indications are shown in Table 38.4.

Cyclophosphamide

Cyclophosphamide.   Although cyclophosphamide is chemically related to the nitrogen mustards, the nucleophilicity of the mustard nitrogen is substantially reduced through an amide-like phosphoramide linkage. As a result, cyclophosphamide is less likely to form an aziridinium ion than are the alkyl-substituted nitrogen mustards. In addition to being more stable chemically,

cyclophosphamide contains several polarizable functional groups that impart solubility in water. Cyclophosphamide is a classical example of a drug that requires metabolic activation (pro-drug). Bioactivation of cyclophosphamide by CYP450 enzyme mediated hydroxylation to an unstable carbinolamine intermediate is shown in Figure 38.6. This intermediate undergoes nonenzymatic fragmentation to acrolein and phosphoramide mustard. Whereas cyclophosphamide is thought to have little or no antineoplastic activity, phosphoramide mustard and its aziridinium derivative is an effective DNA-cross-linking agent associated with cytotoxic activity. Cyclophosphamide is well absorbed orally and is available as a tablet and as a lyophilized powder that can be prepared for parenteral use (Table 38.4).

Ifosfamide

Ifosphamide.   Ifosphamide is an analogue of cyclophosphamide that is also related in structure to the nitrogen mustards except that the two chloroethyl arms are not attached to the same nitrogen. Metabolic activation catalyzed by CYP450 enzymes is required for cytotoxic activity. Hydroxylation at C-4 produces the active, unstable carbinolamine metabolite, 4-hydroxyifosphamide, which degrades further to form additional cytotoxic metabolites. Mesna is a sulfhydryl-containing detoxifying agent used adjunctively to prevent hemorrhagic cystitis (see side bar p. 939).

Chlorambucil

Chlorambucil.   Chlorambucil is one of the original nitrogen mustards. An alternative approach to reducing

Table 38.4. Nitrogen Mustard Alkylating Agents

Generic Name	Trade Name	Indications@	Toxicity*	Dosage Form (mg/unit)**
Chlorambucil	Leukeran	CLL, Hodgkin's & non-Hodgkin's lymphoma	A	Tab (2.0)
Estramustine phosphate	Emcyt	Prostate carcinoma	C	Cap (140)
Mechlorethamine	Mustargen	Lung carcinoma, CLL, chronic myelocytic leukemia, Hodgkin's lymphoma lymphosarcoma	A	IV, Intracavitary (10/vial)
Melphalan	Alkeran	Ovarian carcinoma, multiple myeloma	A	Tab (2.0), IV (50/vial)
Cyclophosphamide	Cytoxan	Carcinoma of breast and ovaries, ALL, acute monocytic leukemia, AML, CLL chronic myelocytic leukemia, Hodgkin's & non-Hodgkin's lymphoma, multiple myeloma, neuroblastoma, retinoblastoma	A	Tab (25, 50), IV (100, 200, 500, 1000/vial)
Ifosphamide	Ifex	Testicular carcinoma	A,B	IV, Intracavitary (1000, 3000/vial)

@ALL = Acute lymphocytic leukemia; AML = acute myelogenous leukemia; CLL = chronic lymphocytic leukemia.
*A = Bone marrow depression; B = Hemorrhagic cystitis.
**IV = Intravenous; Cap = capsule; Tab = tablet; C = gynecomastia, nausea, and vomiting.

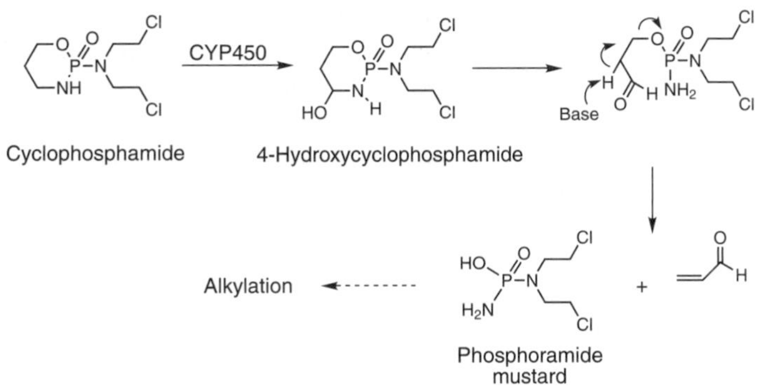

Fig. 38.6. Metabolic activation of cyclophosphamide.

the reactivity of alkyl nitrogen mustards is to attach an aromatic group to the nitrogen atom of the mustard, as in the drug chlorambucil. This decreases the basicity, and hence the nucleophilicity, of the mustard nitrogen. Chlorambucil is absorbed orally and undergoes metabolism in the liver to form phenylacetic acid mustard as the major metabolite (Fig. 38.7). This two-carbon loss from the butanoic acid side-chain is reminiscent of a fatty acid metabolism pathway. The metabolite retains the nitrogen mustard moiety and shows antineoplastic activity. Both chlorambucil and its metabolite follow the general rule that acidic compounds are highly protein bound. Pharmacologic indications and dosage forms are shown in Table 38.4.

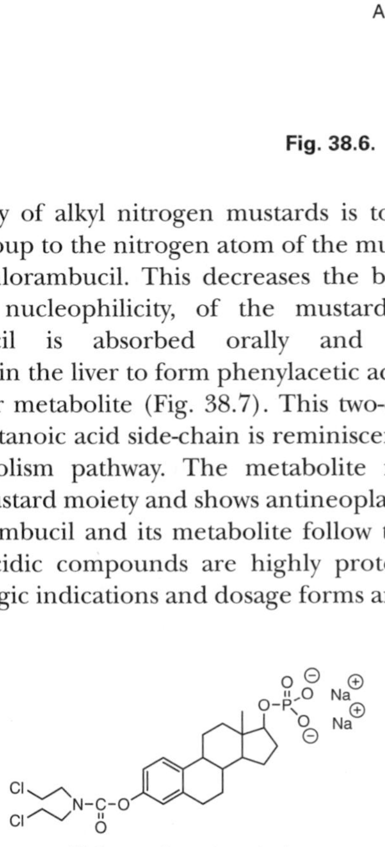

Estramustine phosphate

Estramustine. Estramustine phosphate sodium for oral administration is formulated from estramustine phosphate sodium as the disodium salt monohydrate equivalent on a molar basis to 140 mg of estramustine phosphate. The structure of estramustine consists of an estradiol molecule esterified at C-17 with phosphoric acid and carbamoylated with a nitrogen mustard analogue. The phosphate ester imparts the capacity to form a disodium salt and water solubility. The alkylating moiety is not a true mustard in that the nitrogen atom is acylated as part of the carbamate functionality. After oral administration, estramustine phosphate is rapidly dephosphorylated during absorption. The major metabolites in plasma are estramustine, an estrone analogue of estramustine, estradiol, and its oxidation product, estrone.

Other Alkylating Agents

Busulfan. The classical alkylating agents alkylate nucleophilic species as shown in Figure 38.4.

In the context of antineoplastic agents, the nucleophile is commonly an atom in DNA, which is usually either nitrogen or oxygen. The specific atom, and thus the site of alkylation, depends upon the relative nucleophilicity. As noted, one of the more nucleophilic sites in DNA is the N-7 atom of guanine. In the case of busulfan, Figure 38.8 shows the product of both monoalkylation and dialkylation. Busulfan is a sulfonic acid ester that is an electrophile with methane sulfonic acid acting as a leaving group. Although no unchanged drug is found in the urine of patients treated with busulfan, the bulk of sulfur-35 radiolabeled busulfan was recovered in urine as labeled methanesulfonic acid, suggesting that hydrolysis or alkylation reactions may account for the major metabolic pathway. Determination of 3-hydroxytetrahydrothiophene-1,1-dioxide as a major urinary metabolite in animals supports the suggested electrophilic reactivity of busulfan with sulfhydryl groups in the body. Busulfan is a neutral molecule with poor water solubility. It is commercially formulated as a tablet. Dosage forms and pharmacologic indications are presented in Table 38.5

Thiotepa. Less reactive agents have been developed. For example, thiotepa (Fig. 38.9) is an aziridine-containing

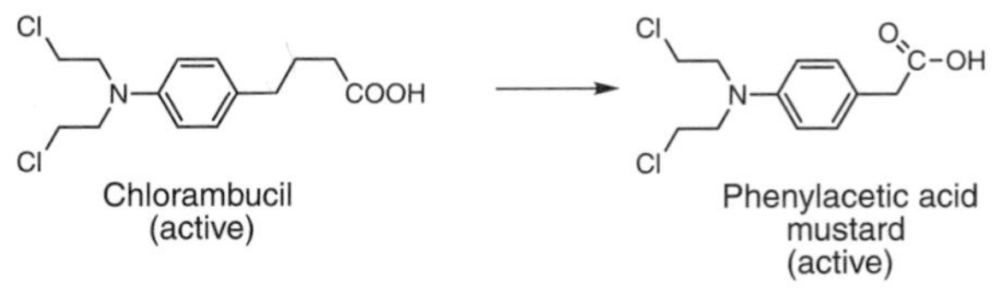

Fig. 38.7. Metabolism of chlorambucil.

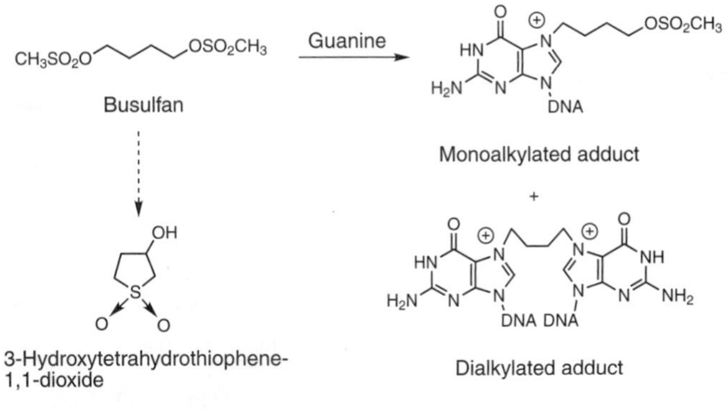

Fig. 38.8. Alkylation of DNA by busulfan.

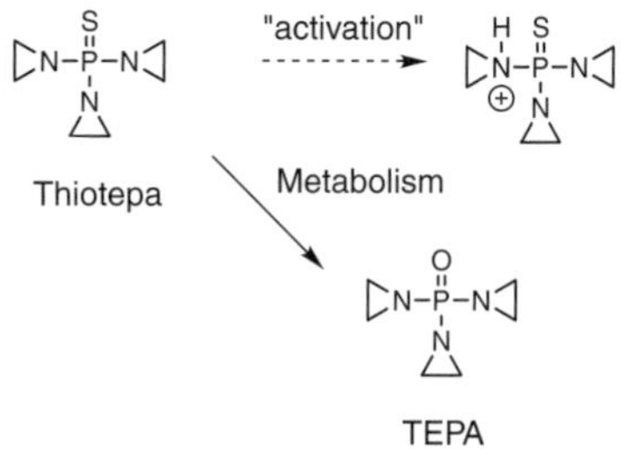

Fig. 38.9. Thiotepa and its metabolic product TEPA.

drug. Aziridine is a three-membered nitrogen heterocycle that reacts with nucleophiles in order to relieve ring strain. At acidic pH, the aziridine group is protonated to provide a reactive aziridinium ion that is known to alkylate DNA. At physiologic pH, aziridine with a pKa of approximately 6 is primarily in the free base form that is less reactive as an alkylating species. Metabolic desulfuration of thiotepa leads to a toxic metabolite, TEPA (triethylenephosphoramide).

Dosage forms and pharmacologic indications are shown in Table 38.5.

Procarbazine.   Alkylation of DNA can also occur by way of free radical intermediates. This may occur from substituted hydrazines, compounds known to produce radical intermediates *in vitro*. A case in point is procarbazine which is used to treat Hodgkin's disease. At physiologic pH and in the presence of oxygen, procarbazine decomposes by an auto-oxidation pathway with release of hydrogen peroxide. The azo derivative formed during oxidation undergoes hydrolysis to yield a benzaldehyde derivative and methylhydrazine (Figure 38.10). Methylhydrazine oxidation, which occurs both *in vitro* and *in vivo*, produces methyldiazene and then methyl radical. Methyl hydrazine has been shown to methylate RNA (15) and DNA (16). In DNA, methylation occurs on the C-8 position of guanine.

The benzaldehyde derivative is excreted in the urine as a further oxidation product, *N*-isopropylterephthalamic acid. Procarbazine inhibits enzymes involved in alcohol metabolism and catecholamine metabolism. Patients tak-

ing procarbazine may experience Antabuse (disulfuram)-like effects with ethyl alcohol intake. Monoamine oxidase is inhibited by procarbazine. Drug interactions with procarbazine and sympathomimetic drugs, tricyclic antidepressant agents, and other drugs and food high in tyramine content are possible.

Dosage forms and pharmacologic indications are shown in Table 38.5.

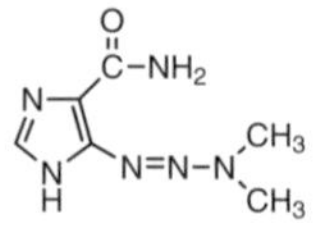

Dacarbazine

Dacarbazine (DTIC) and Temozolomide.   Dacarbazine is a dimethyl triazenyl imidiazole carboxamide (DTIC) which is thought to act as an alkylating agent. Although its anticancer mechanism of action is not fully understood, DTIC appears to be metabolically bioactivated through a series of reactions involving CYP450 (Fig. 38.11). Initial demethylation to MTIC is followed by formation of diazomethane a potent methylating agent. Diazomethane in turn is capable of methylating the N-7 position of guanine. Dacarbazine must be administered intravenously and has a large volume of distribution and is rapidly removed from the plasma. Supportive of the proposed mechanism of action is the isolation of the major metabolite in urine, 5-aminoimidazole-4-carboxamide.

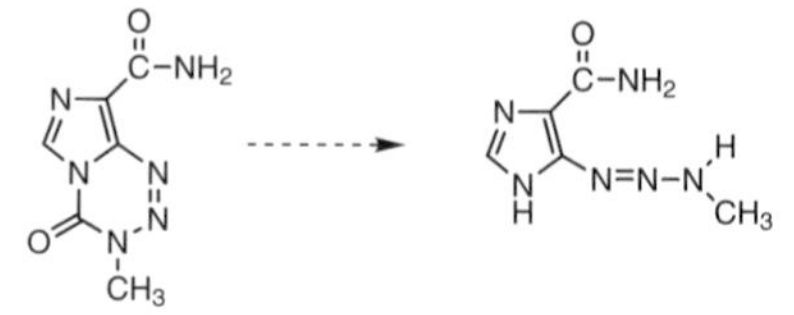

Temozolomide   MTIC

Temozolomide is a pro-drug which is nonenzymaticly converted into MTIC which then alkylates DNA in a manor similar to that of DTIC (Fig. 38.11). Recently, the FDA has approved this MTIC pro-drug for the treatment of brain tumors. A major advantage of temozolomide over DTIC is the fact this drug is administered orally and is rap-

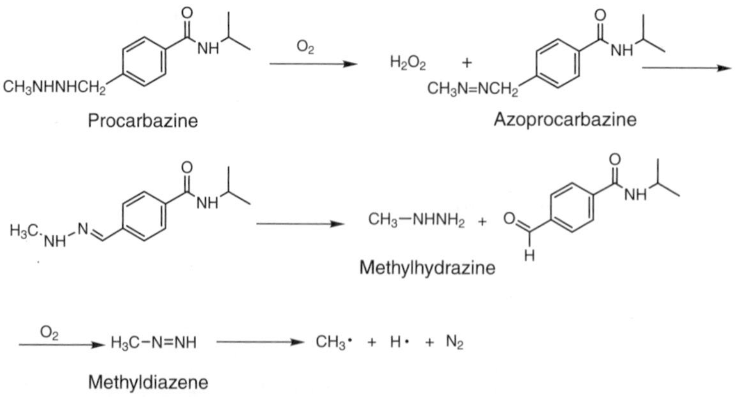

Fig. 38.10. Metabolic activation of procarbazine.

Table 38.5. Miscellaneous Alkylating Agents

Generic Name	Trade Name	Indications	Toxicity*	Dosage Form (mg/unit)**
Carmustine	BiCNU	Hodgkin's & nonHodgkin's lymphoma, multiple myeloma, primary brain tumor	A	IV (100/vial), IW (7.7)
Lomustine	CeeNU	Hodgkin's lymphoma, primary and metastatic brain tumor	A	Cap (10, 40, 100)
Streptozocin	Zanosar	Pancreatic carcinoma	C	IV (1000/vial)
Busulfan	Myleran	Chronic myelocytic leukemia	A,D	Tab (2.0)
Dacarbazine	DTIC-Dome	Hodgkin's lymphoma, metastatic maligant melanoma	A	IV, IM (200/vial)
Temozolomide	Temnodal	Brain tumor	A	Cap (5, 20, 100, 250)
Procarbazine	Matulane	Hodgkin's lymphoma	A	Cap (50)
Thiotepa	Thioplex	Carcinoma of breast, bladder, ovaries, Hodgkin's & nonHodgkin's lymphoma, malignant effusions, lymphosarcoma	A	IV, Intracavitary, Intravesical (15/vial)
Cisplatin	Platinol	Carcinoma of bladder, ovaries, testes	C	IV (1/ml [50, 100ml])
Carboplatin	Paraplatin	Carcinoma of ovaries	A	IV (50, 150, 450/vial)

*A = Bone marrow depression; C = Renal damage; D = Pneumonitis/pulmonary fibrosis.
**IV = Intravenous; IW = implant wafer; Cap = capsule; Tab = tablet; IM = intramuscular.

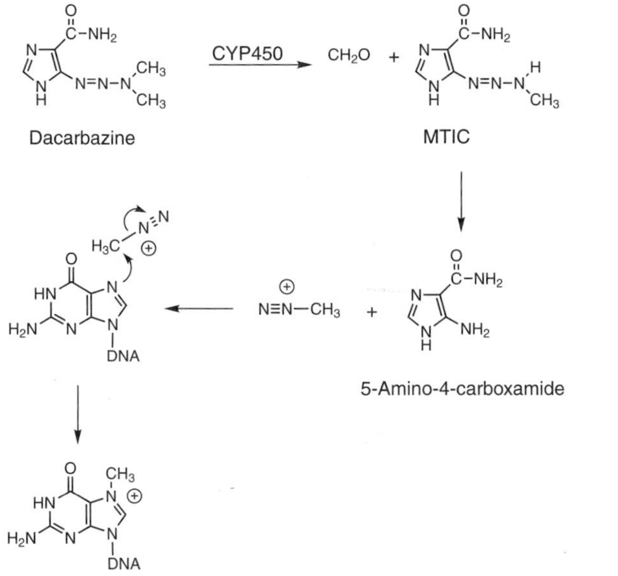

Fig. 38.11. Proposed metabolism and mechanism of action of DTIC.

idly absorbed via this route. The recommended initial dose is 150 mg/m² which will result in the patient taking a combination of capsules of different sizes and colors to make up the required dose. Reported common side effects include nausea, vomiting, constipation, headache, and fatigue.

Nitrosoureas

Mechanism of action. The nitrosoureas are examples of a third mechanism whereby an alkylating species is produced. These compounds are fairly reactive with water, similar to the reactivity of the mustards and decompose as shown in Figure 38.12. In water the urea NH is deprotonated and the negatively charged oxygen then displaces the chloride to give a cyclic oxazolidine. This intermediate then fragments to a vinyl diazohydroxide and 2-chloroethylisocyanate. The

former species is very reactive and loses nitrogen forming the even more reactive vinyl cation, the ultimate alkylating species. The isocyanate is also reactive and in water yields 2-chloroethylamine, an additional alkylating agent.

Carmustine. Carmustine is also known as BCNU, which is an acronym derived from the chemical name, 1,3-*bis*(chloroethyl)-1-nitrosourea (Fig. 38.12). As are the other nitrosourea antineoplastic agents, carmustine is a neutral molecule that is highly lipophilic and poorly soluble in water. These properties allow for efficient crossing of the blood-brain barrier providing higher CSF to plasma ratios of drug in comparison to other alkylating agents. Although carmustine administration is thought to lead to alkylation of DNA and RNA as a mechanism of antineoplastic activity, it is not cross resistant with nitrogen mustards and alternate mechanisms of action involving enzyme inhibition by carbamoylation of proteins have been suggested. Carmustine is rapidly metabolized after intravenous administration to form metabolites that have

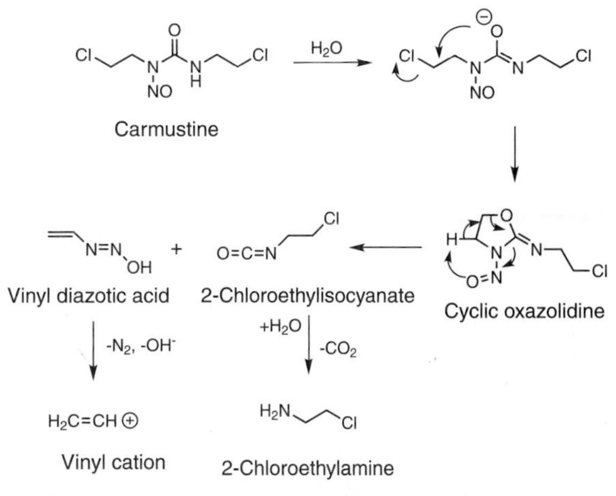

Fig. 38.12. Formation of a vinyl cation from carmustine.

antineoplastic activity. Carmustine is a low melting solid. As carmustine decomposes, the melting point drops such that partially degraded preparations may be in a liquid form at room temperature. Vials of carmustine that show an oily film indicate that the drug has decomposed and these vials should not be used. For intravenous use, lyophilized carmustine is dissolved in absolute ethanol and diluted with sterile water to make a 10% ethanol solution that can be diluted further. Dosage forms and pharmacologic indications are shown in Table 38.5.

Lomustine

Lomustine. Lomustine, also known as CCNU (1-(2-chloroethyl)-3-cyclohexyl-1-nitrosourea), is a nitrosourea antineoplastic agent with similar structure, solubility, and activity characteristics to carmustine.

Streptozocin

Streptozocin. Streptozocin is composed of a combination of a glucopyranose amino sugar and a nitrosourea. The sugar moiety, existing in both anomeric forms, imparts good water solubility as compared to the lipophilic nitrosourea antineoplastic agents. In addition to antineoplastic activity that is thought to be a result of inhibition of DNA synthesis or inhibition of cell proliferation, streptozocin has long been known to produce a diabetes-like syndrome in animals. This syndrome appears to be mediated by a lowering of beta cell concentrations of nicotinamide adenine dinucleotide (NAD).

cis-Dichlorodiammineplatinum (II)

Cisplatin. Cisplatin is a platinum complex containing two ammonia molecules and two chloride atoms in a *cis* configuration. Cisplatin has nominal solubility in water or saline at 1 mg/mL. Reactivity with cellular nucleophiles or water proceeds at a faster rate than drug metabolism reactions. The injectable formulation is at a concentration near its solubility in saline and should not be refrigerated. In pH 7.4, 0.1 M NaCl solutions, cisplatin is in equilibrium with monohydroxymonochloro *cis*-diammine platinum (II). After a dose of cisplatin, most of the platinum becomes tightly bound to plasma proteins including albumin, transferrin and gamma globulin. Because cisplatin is highly protein bound, hemodialysis as an antidote started four hours after overdosing has little effect. Platinum has been detected in tissues up to 180 days after the last dose. For administration of cisplatin intravenously, needles or intravenous sets containing aluminum parts should not be used because cisplatin reacts with aluminum resulting in a precipitate and a loss of potency. Dosage forms and pharmacologic indications are shown in Table 38.5.

The action of cisplatin, like other alkylating agents, appears to be associated with the ability of the drug to alkylate the N-7 position of guanine forming intrastrand and interstrand cross-links.

Carboplatin

Carboplatin. Carboplatin is similar in structure to cisplatin in containing *cis*-diammine groups and platinum (II). In place of the two chloride groups of cisplatin, carboplatin has two organometallic cyclobutaneplatinum groups. Carboplatin is sufficiently soluble in water (14 mg/mL) to make an injectable formulation, although it is virtually insoluble in organic solvents such as acetone or ethanol. Replacement of a chloride with water in carboplatin forms a monohydroxy derivative that is thought to retain anticancer activity. This aquation reaction occurs at a slower rate than it does in the case of cisplatin which may explain why carboplatin is less potent than cisplatin.

Antimetabolites and Nucleoside Analogs

Antimetabolites are compounds that prevent the biosynthesis of normal cellular metabolites. Usually, this suggests a close chemical similarity between the natural metabolite and the antimetabolite. Two well-known examples are the competitive inhibitor, methotrexate, and the suicide-substrate enzyme inhibitor, 5-fluorouracil.

Pyrimidine Antimetabolites

There are a large number of pyrimidine based antimetabolites. They are usually structurally related to the endogenous substrate that they antagonize. The structural modification may be on the pyrimidine ring or, if present, on the pendant sugar group. Their possible mechanisms of action are diverse and may involve: 1) inhibition of kinases, 2) inhibition of enzymes involved in pyrimidine biosynthesis, 3) incorporation into RNA or DNA and subsequently cause misreading, or 4) inhibition of DNA polymerase.

5-Fluorouracil. One of the early antimetabolites prepared was 5-fluorouracil (5-FU Fig. 38.14), a pyrimidine with ring modifications. It was designed by Heidelberger in 1957 (17). The development of this compound was based on the observation that some tumors preferentially use uracil rather than orotic acid for pyrimidine biosynthesis. Thymidine synthesis from uracil involves thymidylate synthetase and in this process a thiol group of a cysteine residue in the enzyme (E-SH) adds to the C-6 position of

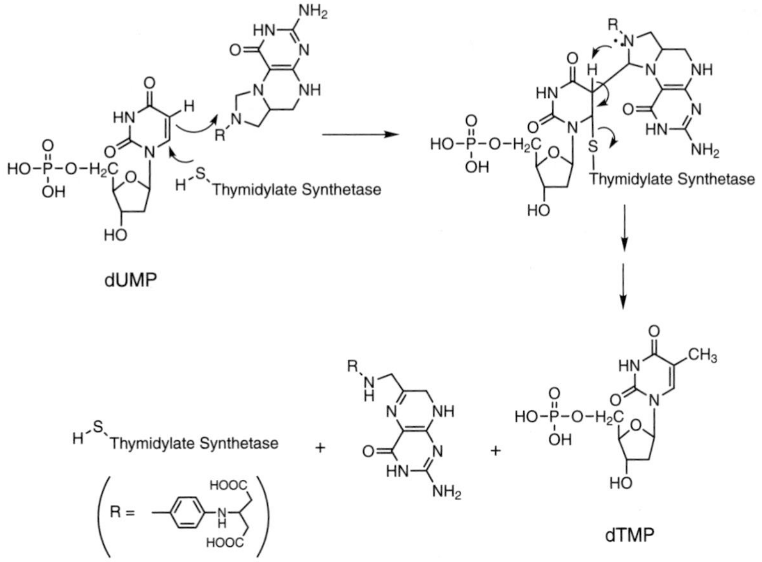

Fig. 38.13. Key intermediates in the synthesis of deoxythymidylic acid from deoxyuridylic acid.

deoxyuridylic acid and with subsequent addition of the C-5 carbon to the N^5,N^{10}-methylene of N^5,N^{10}-methylene-tetrahydrofolate (Fig. 38.13). The resulting intermediate transfers the C-5-hydrogen to the N^{10} position of the folate ultimately giving rise to deoxythymidylic acid, dihydrofolate, and the regenerated enzyme.

In vivo, 5-FU must first be activated by conversion to 5-fluoro-2′-deoxyuridylic acid (5-FdUMP). In general this occurs by conversion of 5-FU to 5-fluorouracil riboside which is then transformed directly into 5-FdUMP by ribonucleotide reductase (Fig. 38.14). The 5-FdUMP then binds to thymidylate synthetase to give an intermediate that resembles the intermediate formed with uridylic acid. However, the intermediate bears a fluorine at C-5 instead of a hydrogen and the latter is unable to transfer the fluorine. Thus, the intermediate cannot break down and the enzyme is inhibited. This, in turn, can lead to a deficiency of thymidine which is essential for the synthesis of DNA. Additional metabolic reactions are thought to lead to the formation of 5-FU intermediates which are incorporated into DNA and RNA and may contribute to the actions of the drug. 5-FU is also metabolized by dihydropyrimidine dehydrogenase leading to inactivated 5-fluoro-5,6-dihydroureal (Fig. 38.13). This enzyme can be inhibited by 5-ethynyluracil which improves the therapeutic index of 5-FU by 2- to 4-fold. An alternative form

of 5-FU is floxuridine (Sterile FUDR) which is a prodrug of 5-fluorouracil. Metabolically, the deoxysugar moiety of floxuridine is cleaved rapidly to provide 5-fluorouracil. In contrast to 5-fluorouracil, floxuridine is freely soluble in water. Pharmacologic indications and dosage forms are shown in Table 38.6.

Cytarabine. Cytarabine (ARA-C, Fig. 38.15) is an example of a pyrimidine antimetabolite in which the sugar has been modified. In this case, the sugar moiety is an arabinose as indicated by the 2′-OH group having a β-configuration rather than the normal α-configuration. Like 5-FU, ARA-C must be first converted into its monophosphate and then its triphosphate derivative (ARA-CTP) (Fig. 38.15). This subtle change in configuration of the 2′-carbon results in a

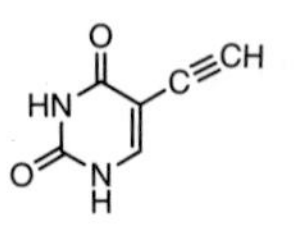

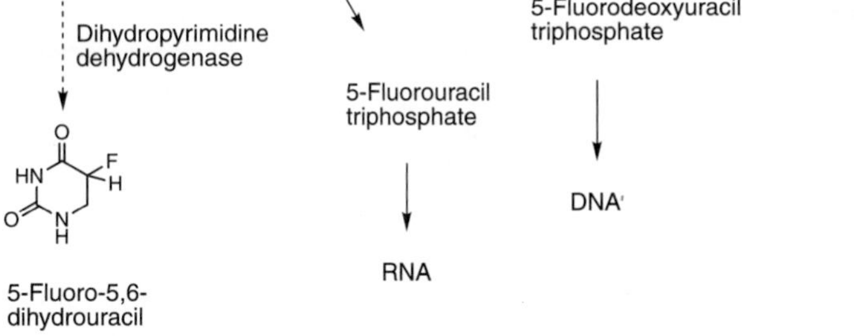

Fig. 38.14. Metabolism of 5-fluorouracil.

5-Ethynyluracil

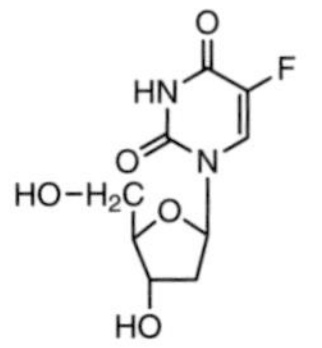

5-Fluorodeoxyuridine
(Floxuridine)

Table 38.6. Antimetabolites

Generic Name	Trade Name	Indications@	Toxicity*	Dosage Form (mg/unit)**
Cladribine	Leustatin	Hairy-cell leukemia	A	IV (10/10 ml vial)
Cytarabine	Cytosar-U	ALL, AML, chronic myelocytic leukemia, meningeal leukemia	A	IV, Intrathecal, SQ (20, 50, 100/ml)
Floxuridine	FUDR	Palliative manag. GI adenocarcinoma metastatic to liver	A,E	Intra-arterial (500/vial)
Fludarabine	Fludara	CLL	A	IV (50/vial)
Fluorouracil	Adrucil	Carcinoma of breast, colon, rectum, stomach, pancreas, carcinoma of the skin, actinic keratoses	A,E	Top (1, 2, 5%), IV (500/vial)
Gemcitabline	Gemzar	Locally advanced or metastatic adenocarcinoma of pancreas		IV (200, 1000/vial)
Mercaptopurine	Purinethol	ALL, AML, acute myelomonocytic leukemia	A	Tab (50)
Methotrexate	Folex	Trophoblasic neoplasms, acute leukemia, menigeal leukemia, carcinoma of breast, head, neck, lung, Burkitt's lymphoma, lymphosarcoma, nonmetastatic osteosarcoma	A,D,E	Tab (2.5), IV (20, 50, 100, 200, 250, 1000/vial)

@ALL = Acute lymphocytic leukemia; AML = acute myelogenous leukemia; CLL = chronic lymphocytic leukemia.
*A = Bone marrow depression; D = Pneumonitis/pulmonary fibrosis; E = Oral/GI ulceration.
**IV = Intravenous; Tab = tablet; IM = intramuscular.; Top = Topical; SQ = Subcutaneous.

compound that has multiple activities. First, ARA-CTP inhibits the conversion of cytidylic acid to 2'-deoxycytidylic acid (18). Second, ARA-CTP also inhibits DNA-dependent DNA polymerase (19). Finally, ARA-C causes miscoding after being incorporated into DNA or RNA (20). Cytarabine is available as a water-soluble sterile powder for intavenous, intrathecal, and subcutaneous use. Cytarabine is rapidly metabolized to an inactive product, arabinofuranosyluracil.

See Table 38.6 for pharmacologic indications and dosage forms.

Gemcitabine. Gemcitabine is a newer pyrimidine antimetabolite. This molecule bears two fluorines in place of the hydrogen and hydroxyl normally present on C-2' of the sugar group of cytosine. Unlike ARA-C, it shows excellent antitumor activity *in vivo* against a variety of murine solid tumors. Gemcitabine, like ARA-C, must first be phosphorylated to the active triphosphate analogue which can then be incorporated into DNA leading to cell death (Fig. 38.16). This has been shown to occur in several cell lines including CCRF-CEM, human T-lymphoblastoid, and human chronic myelogenous leukemia cell lines. More recently, the triphosphate analogue has been shown to be incorporated into RNA and to inhibit both DNA and RNA synthesis (21). Gemcitabine is extensively metabolized and its major urinary excretion product is the inactive uracil analogue metabolite, 2'-deoxy-2',2'-difluorouridine (dFdU).

Purine Antimetabolites
6-Mercaptopurine

Mechanism of Action. The purine antimetabolites, like the pyrimidine antimetabolites, have several potential modes of action. A well-studied example of a purine an-

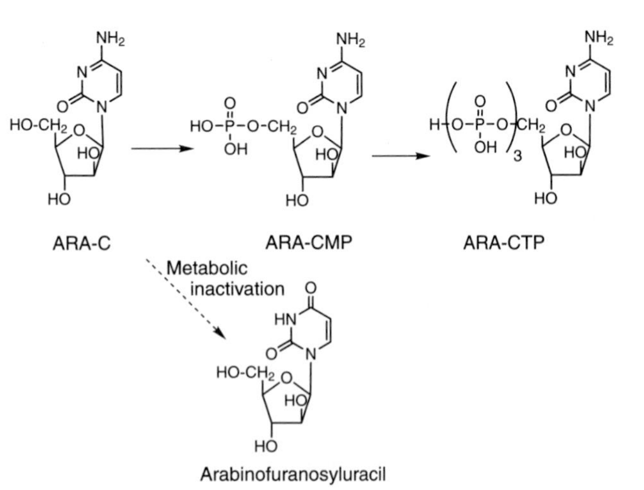

Fig. 38.15. Metabolic activation and inactivation of 1-β-D-arabinofuranosylcytosine (ARA-C).

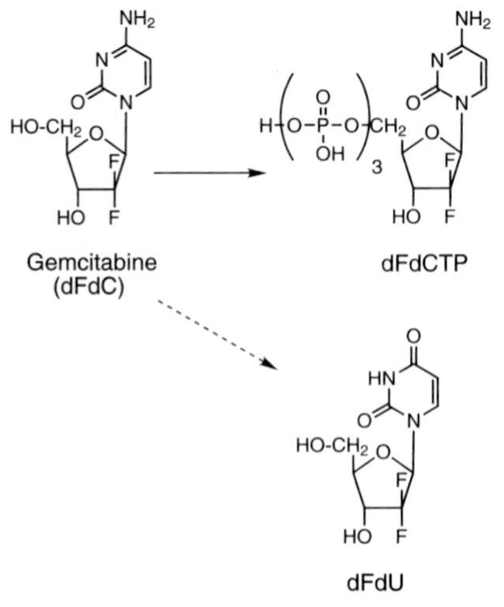

Fig. 38.16. Metabolic activation and inactivation of 2',2'-difluorocytosine (dFdC).

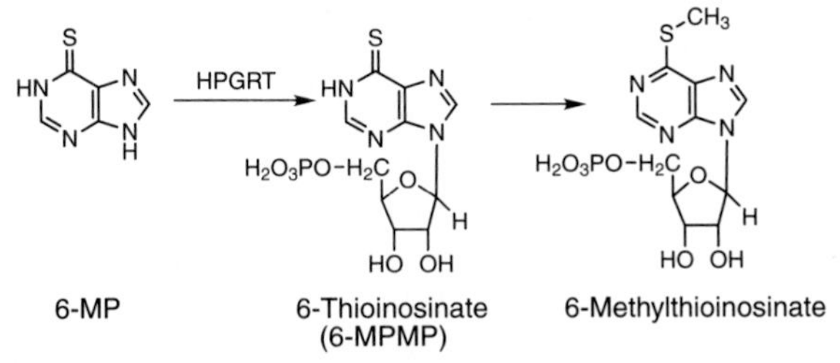

Fig. 38.17. Metabolic activation of 6-mercaptopurine (6-MP) to the corresponding ribose monophosphate (6-MPMP) and 6-Methylthioinosinate.

timetabolite is 6-mercaptopurine (6-MP). The drug is converted *in vivo* to the corresponding ribonucleotide, 6-thioinosinate, by the enzyme hypoxantine-guanine phosphoribosyltransferase (HGPRT) (Fig. 38.17). 6-Thioinosinate has been shown to be a powerful inhibitor of the conversion of 5-phosphoribosyl pyrophosphate into 5-phosphoribosylamine, involved in purine biosynthesis. In addition, 6-thioinosinate inhibits the conversion of inosinic acid to adenylic acid as well as the oxidation of inosinic acid to xanthylic acid (Fig. 38.18). Therefore, the overall action of 6-MP is inhibition of the *de novo* synthesis of purines (22).

The mechanism of action of 6-MP and its anabolite 6-thioinosinate is only part of the activity as 6-thioinosinate can be further transformed into its ribose diphosphate and triphosphate. Both of these species are enzyme inhibitors and the triphosphate can be used in DNA and RNA synthesis in place of guanine and, once incorporated, it inhibits chain elongation. Finally, 6-thioinosinate can be a substrate for 3-adenosylmethionine and is converted to 6-methylthioinosinate which is responsible for some of the antimetabolite properties of 6-MP (23).

Pharmacokinetic Properties. Mercaptopurine is orally available, although its oral absorption is incomplete and variable. Once absorbed, mercaptopurine has a large volume of distribution. Little unchanged drug is detected in urine and its metabolic fate, which includes the formation of cytotoxic metabolites, is complex. Urinary metabolites include thiouric acid, formed by xanthine oxidase, as well as a number of methylthiopurines. The concurrent administration of mercaptopurine with xanthine oxidase inhibitors, such as allopurinol, requires a dose reduction of mercaptopurine. Cross-resistance between the structurally related drugs, such as thioguanine, is likely. Pharmacologic indications and dosage forms are shown in Table 38.6.

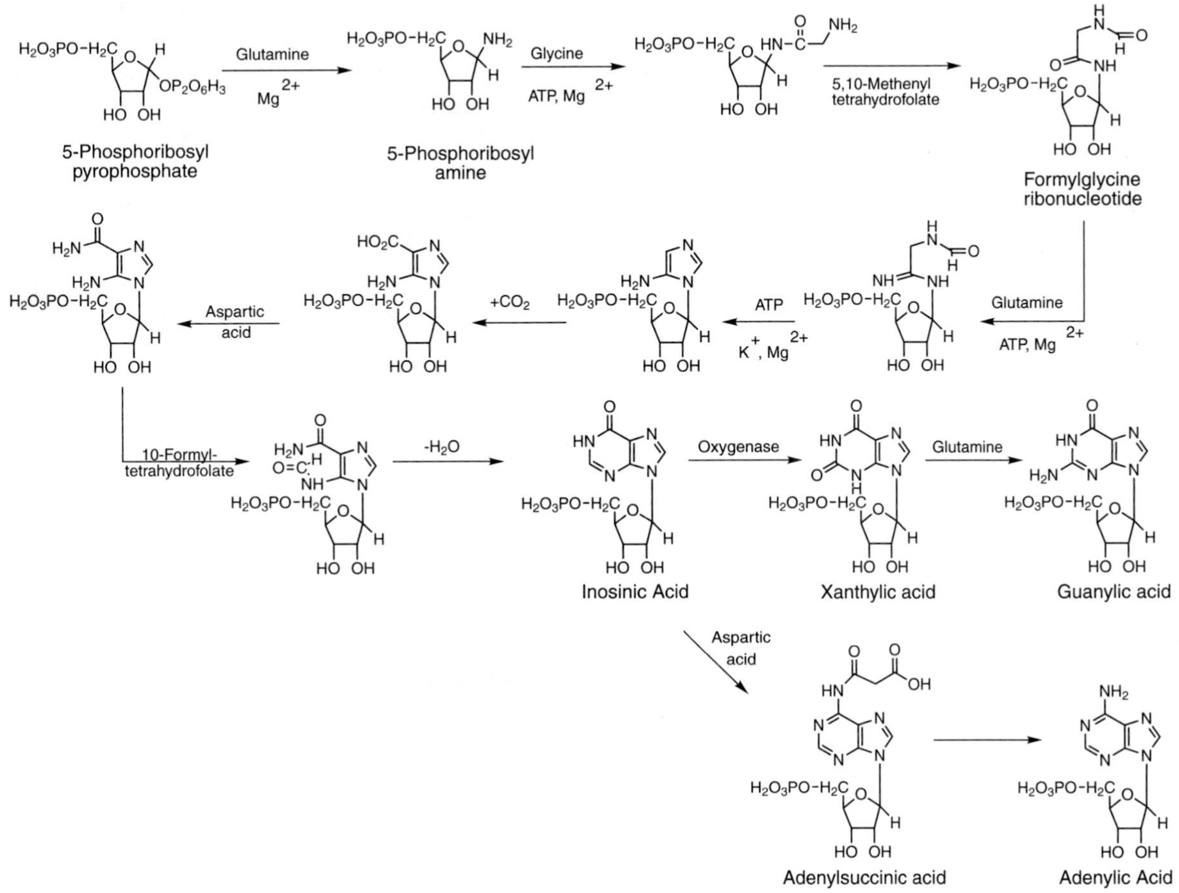

Fig. 38.18. Biosynthetic scheme for the synthesis of purines.

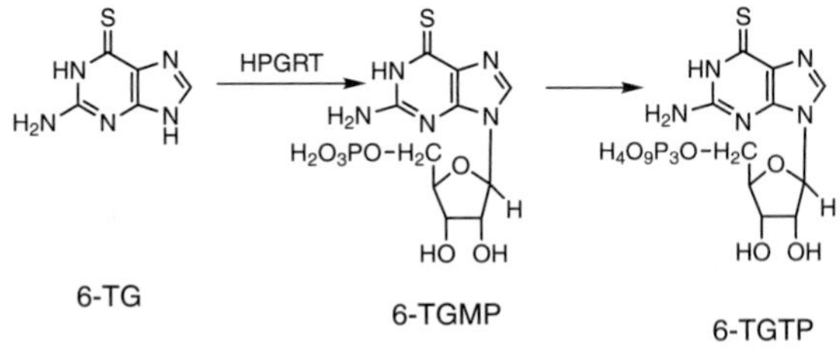

Fig. 38.19. Bioactivation of 6-thioguanine (6-TG) to the corresponding monophosphate (6-TGMP) and then the triphosphate (6-TGTP).

6-Thioguanine. An antimetabolite structurally related to 6-MP is 6-thioguanine (6-TG). Like 6-MP, 6-TG is first ribosylated to the monophosphate (6-TGMP) and is then converted into the diphosphate derivative (6-TGDP) and the triphosphate (6-TGTP) (Fig. 38.19). Each of these intermediate forms of 6-TG inhibit a range of enzymes and processes that generally parallels the activity previous noted for 6-MP. In addition, the ribosylated triphosphate of 6-TG can be incorporated into RNA or, after reduction to the 2′-deoxy derivative, into DNA. Subsequent to incorporation into DNA, 6-TG may inhibit DNA replication because of the inability of the replication enzymes to recognize 6-TG. Generally, 6-TG parallels the activity of 6-MP, although thioguanine deactivation is not dependent upon xanthine oxidase.

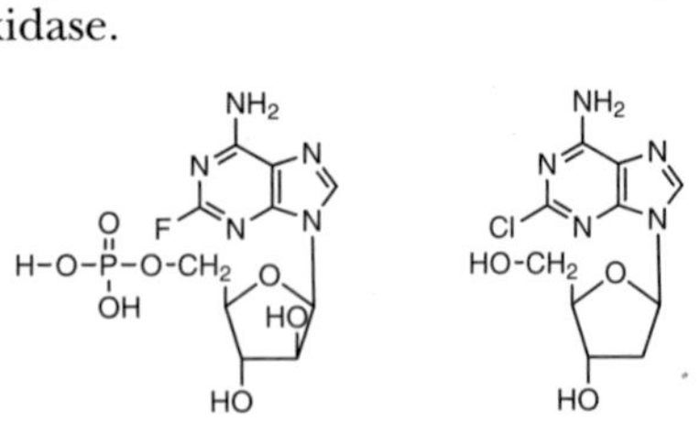

Fludarabine phosphate   Cladribine

Fludarabine Phosphate and Cladribine. Fludarabine phosphate is a purine antimetabolite that is structurally related to adenosine and embodies both purine ring and sugar modifications. Fludarabine is a derivative of vidarabine (ARA-A). Vidarabine is the 2′-β-anomer of adenosine (analogous to ARA-C) and has antimetabolite activity, although it is a good substrate for adenosine deaminase. In contrast, fludarabine is more effective than vidarabine because it is less susceptible to adenosine deaminase. *In vivo* it is converted to the 5′-triphosphate, an inhibitor of ribonucleotide reductase. In contrast, the activity of the 2-chloro analogue of fludarabine, cladribine, inhibits enzymes important for DNA repair.

Pharmacologic indications and dosage forms are shown in Table 38.6

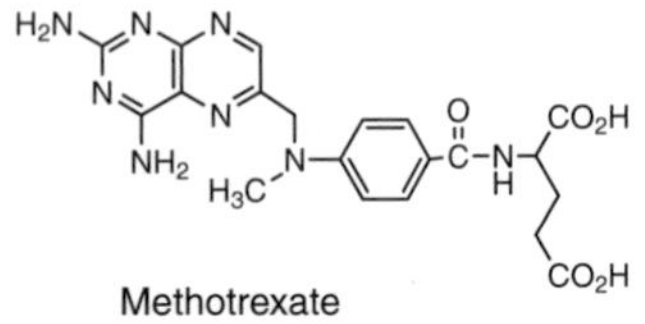

Methotrexate

Other Antimetabolites
Methotrexate

Mechanism of Action. Methotrexate (MTX) and its analogues are pteridines that compete with the normal substrates, folic acid and dihydrofolate, for the active site on the enzyme dihydrofolate reductase (DHFR). DHFR is involved in the reduction of folic acid, first to dihydrofolate and then to tetrahydrofolate (Fig. 38.20). MTX kills cells by inhibiting DNA synthesis in part due to inhibition of thymidine synthesis from uridylic acid. As indicated earlier and shown in Figure 38.20 tetrahydrofolic acid is converted into N^5,N^{10}-methylenetetrahydrofolic acid by transfer of a methylene group from serine. In turn, this methylene is transferred to the C-5 position of 2′-deoxyuridylic acid to give thymidylic acid and dihydrofolic acid which must be reduced by DHFR to tetrahydrofolate for the next round of uridylic to thymidylic acid biosynthesis (Fig. 38.13). Thus, by inhibiting DHFR, methotrexate prevents DNA synthesis and kills cells by depleting thymidylic acid.

The inhibition of DHFR by methotrexate can also inhibit purine synthesis. As part of the overall process for purine synthesis, N^5,N^{10}-methylenetetrahydrofolic acid is oxidized to N^5,N^{10}-methenyltetrahydrofolic acid and then, by hydrolysis of the latter compound to N^{10}-formyltetrahydrofolic acid, the compound which is the formyl donor to 5-aminoimidazole-4-carboxamide ribonucleotide in purine biosynthesis (Fig. 38.18). N^{10}-Formyltetrahydrofolic acid is derived from N^5-formyltetrahydrofolic acid by the action of an isomerase. N^5-formyltetrahydrofolic acid is also known as leucovorin and is utilized in "rescue" therapy with methotrexate as it prevents the lethal effects of methotrexate on normal cells. Interestingly, leucovorin also inhibits the active transport of methotrexate into cells.

Methotrexate is converted in the liver and intracellularly to polyglutamated forms which are enzymatically hydrolyzed back to methotrexate. Urinary metabolites are negligible in concentration and methotrexate is largely excreted unchanged. Pharmacologic indications and dosage forms are shown in Table 38.6

Antitumor Antibiotics

Several compounds that were originally evaluated for antibiotic activity have become clinically useful as anticancer or antitumor agents, Table 38.7. Many of these compounds have been known for a long time and were originally rejected as antibiotics because of toxicity. This property was subsequently turned into an asset with their application as anticancer agents. The source of most antitumor antibiotics is from microbial fermentations. Their preparation still typically depends on this source as many of these compounds are quite complex molecules that represent significant synthetic challenges. The clinically important antitumor antibiotics, will be considered.

Bleomycins

The bleomycins were first discovered in 1966. The current preparation, bleomycin sulfate isomers (bleomycin A_2

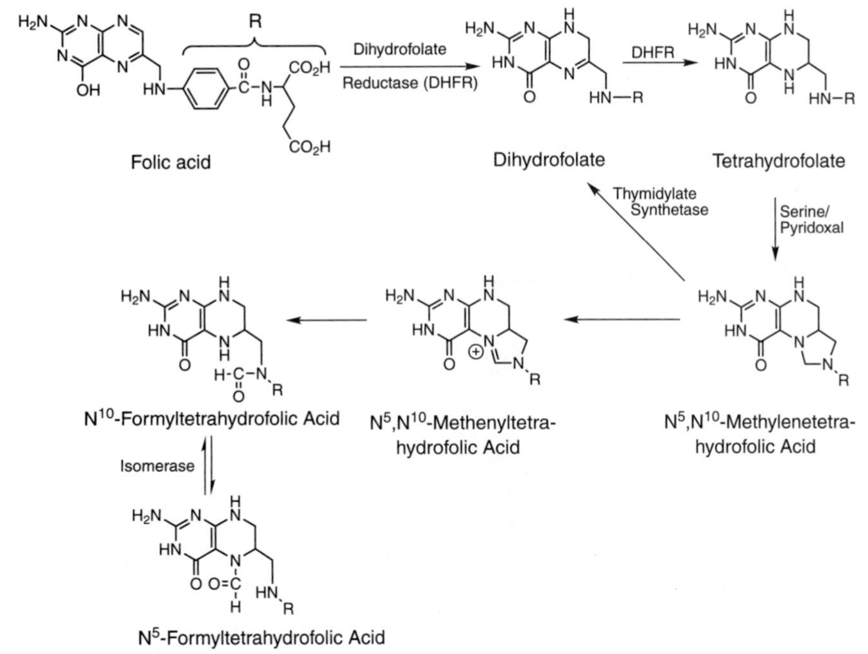

Fig. 38.20. Interconversion of folic acid derivatives important in the biosynthesis of thymidine and purines.

Table 38.7. Antitumor Antibiotics

Generic Name	Trade Name	Indications@	Toxicity*	Dosage Form (mg/unit)**
Bleomycin	Blenoxane	Carcinoma of cervix, head and neck, larynx, penis, skin, testes, Hodgkin's and nonHodgkin's lymphoma	D	IM, IV, SQ, Intrapleural (15, 30 unites/vial)
Dactinomycin	Cosmegen	Carcinoma of testes, ewing's sarcoma, trophoblasic tumors, Welm's tumor, rhabdomycosarcome, sarcoma botryoides	A,E,F	IV (0.5/vial)
Daunorubicin	Cerubidine	ALL, AML, acute monocytic leukemia	A,G	IV (20/vial)
Doxorubicin	Adriamycin	Acute lymphoblastic & myeloblastic leukemia, Welm's tumor, neuroblastoma, soft tissue and bone sarcomas, breast, ovarian, thyroid, gastric carcinoma, Hodgkin's disease, malignant lymphoma, bronchogenic carcinoma	A,G	IV (10, 20, 50, 100, 200/vial)
Idarubicin	Idamycin	ALL, AML	A	IV (5, 0, 20/vial)
Epirubicin	Ellence	Adjunct therapy in axillary node tumor in breast cancer		IV (2/ml)
Valrubicin	Valstar	BCG-refactory CIS of the urinary bladder		Intravesical (40/ml)
Mitomycin C	Mutamycin	Gastric and pancreatic carcinoma	A	IV (5, 20, 40/vial)
Mitoxantrone	Novantrone	Acute monocytic leukemia, AML, acute promyelocytic leukemia	A	IV (20, 25,3 0/vial)
Pentostatin	Nipent	Alpha interferon-refactory hairy-cell leukemia in adults	A	IV (10/vial)
Vincristine	Oncovin	ALL, Hodgkin's & and nonHodgkin's lymphoma, neuroblastoma, Wilm's tumor, rhabdomyosarcoma	H	IV (1, 2, 5/vial)
Vinblastine	Velban	Breast and testicular carcinoma, Hodgkin's & nonHodgkin's lymphoma, Kaposi sarcoma, mycosis fungoides	A	IV (10/vial)
Vinorelbine	Navelbine	Nonsmall cell lung cancer	A	IV (10, 50/vial)
Paclitaxel	Taxol	Refactory metastatic carcinoma of the ovary, metastatic breast cancer	A	IV (30/5 ml, 100/16.7 ml))
Docetaxel	Taxotere	Locally advanced or metastatic breast cancer, nonsmall cell lung cancer	A	IV (20, 80/vial)

@ALL = Acute lymphocytic leukemia; AML = acute myelogenous leukemia.
*A = Bone marrow depression; D = Pneumonitis/pulmonary fibrosis; E = Oral/GI ulceration; F = Stomatitis; G = Cardiotoxicity; H = Peripheral neuropathy.
**IV = Intravenous; Tab = tablet; SQ = Subcutaneous.

Anticancer Adjuncts

In various cancer chemotherapies a protective or rescue agent is administered in order to improve the drug regimen. Two such rescue/protective drugs are calcium leu-

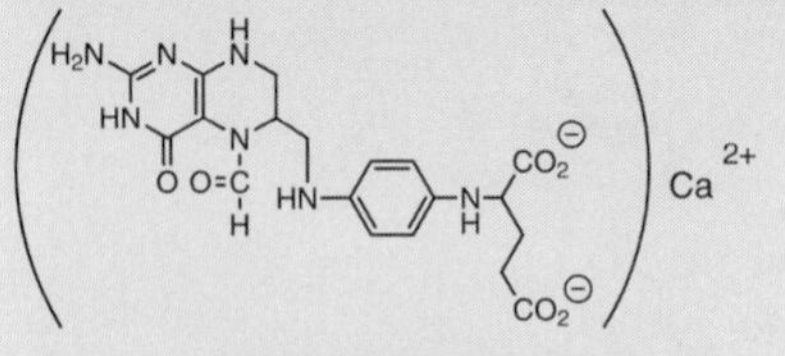

Calcium 5-Formyltetrahydrofolate
(Calcium leucovorin)

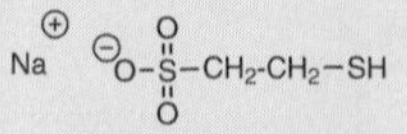

2-Mercaptoethanesulfonate
(MESNA [Mesnex])

covorin, the calcium salt of N^5- formyltetrahydrofolate and sodium 2-mercaptoethanesulfonate (MESNA). Calcium leucovorin is commonly used in combination with MTX. Toxicity of MTX is a function of the duration and dosage. Large doses of MTX are administered and the "leucovorin rescue" is then given intravenously to supply noncancer cells with tetrahydrofolate to diminish toxicity. Calcium leucovorin can also be combined with 5-FU to improve therapy. In this case by increasing the level of the complex formed between 5-FU, tetrahydrofolic acid, and thymidylate synthase. MESNA is co-administered with cyclophosphamide or ifosfamide to reduce the toxicity of acrolein metabolites of these drugs. Acrolein causes severe hemorrhagic cystitis leading to nephrotoxicity and urotoxicity. MESNA conjugates the toxic metabolite.

and bleomycin B_2) belongs to the bleomycin family of naturally occurring cytotoxic glycopeptide antibiotics isolated from *Streptomyces verticillus.*

Naturally, bleomycins occur as copper chelates with ligands provided by the pyrazine, imidazole, amide and amine functional groups. Although the copper is removed during processing, the tendency of the bleomycins to form metal chelates is key to antitumor activity. It is believed that in cells, bleomycin forms a chelate with iron (Fe^{2+}. Five of the six coordination positions are strongly coordi-

Bleomycin A_2 R =

Bleomycin B_2 R =

nated to bleomycin. The sixth is available for coordination to oxygen. The chelate also alters the redox potential of iron such that bound oxygen is reduced, converting the oxygen into a reactive radical species, the hydroxyl radical (•OH). The hydroxyl radical then reacts with nuclear DNA, degrading it in an ultimately cytotoxic event.

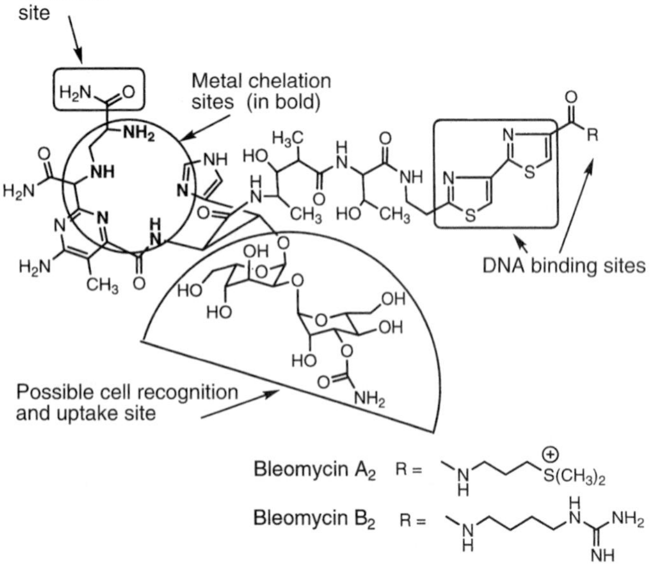

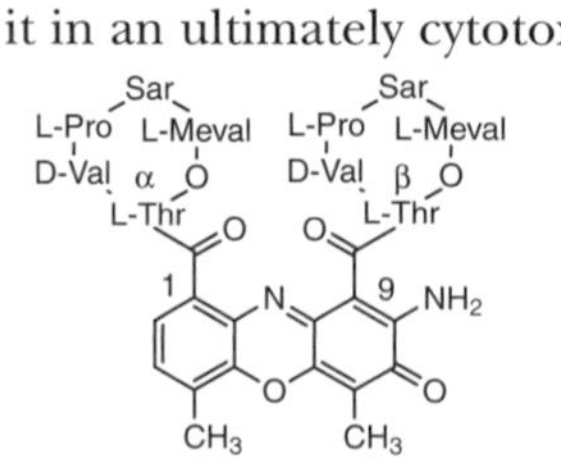

Dactinomycin

Dactinomycin or Actinomycin D

The actinomycins act by a fundamentally different mechanism relative to the bleomycins. All of the actinomycins contain the same root structure, a 3-phenoxazone-1,9-dicarboxylic acid (actinocin). This ring system is aromatic and planar and can intercalate or insert into DNA between base-pair steps. In the intercalation process, the helix must unwind some in order for there to be space for the actinocin moiety. Once inserted, the actinocin ring system is held in the DNA helix by π-π stacking interactions between the actinocin ring system and the DNA bases. The local distortion caused by the presence of the intercalating agent affects the action of topoisomerase II, which normally regulates unwinding of coiled double-stranded DNA. In turn, this interferes with DNA replication and transcription. Actinomycins may also cause DNA cleavage by nucleases. Intercalation of the actinomycins is ultimately lethal to cells. An example of an antineoplastic actinomycin is dactinomycin. Dactinomycin, which is the main antibiotic constituent of *Streptomyces parvullus,* consists of a tricyclic phenoxazone ring in the quinone oxidation state and two identical pentapeptide lactone appendages. The pentapeptides are made up of L-proline and L-threonine plus the nonessential amino acids, D-valine, sarcosine, and N-methylvaline. Dactinomycin undergoes minimal metabolism in humans and does not readily cross the blood-brain barrier. Crystals of actinomycin are dark red in color and dilute solutions are highly sensitive to degradation in light.

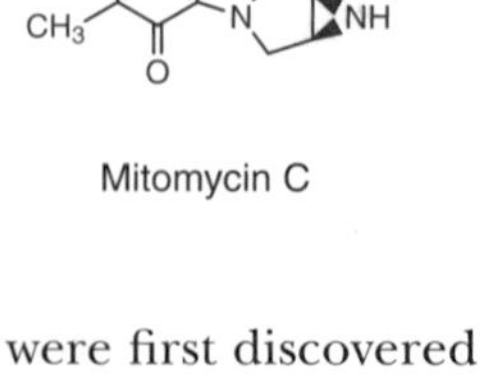

Mitomycin C

Mitomycin C

The mitomycins were first discovered in the 1950s but it was the mid-70s before they were approved for use as anticancer agents. Mitomycin C is an antitumor antibiotic isolated from *Streptomyces caespitosus.* Mitomycins are unique in that they possess several functional groups capable of anticancer activity. Of these, the quinone moiety,

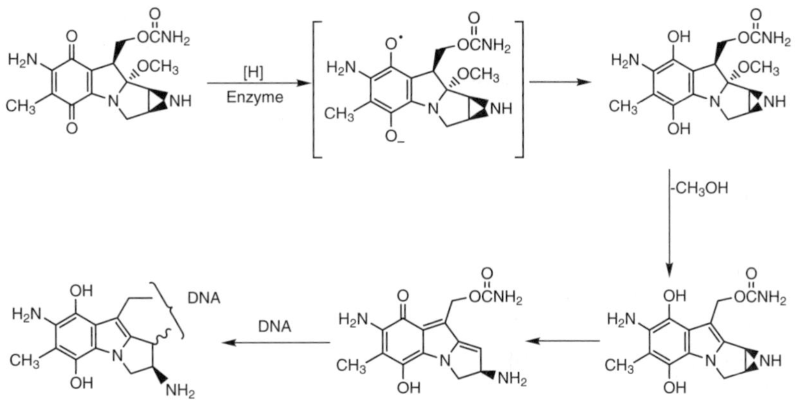

Fig. 38.21. Bio-reductive activation of mytomycin C and DNA alkylation.

the aziridine ring system, and the carbamate are thought to be intimately involved in the action of the drug. The drug is classified as a bio-reductive alkylating agent. After a bio-reductive activation, followed by the elimination of methanol, the compound is capable of reaction with nucleophiles in DNA leading to either mono- or dialkylation (cross-linking) products (Fig. 38.21). Alkylation appears to prefer CG rich regions of DNA with guanine alkylation at the 2-amino group of guanine having been demonstrated *in vitro*.

Mitomycin C is poorly absorbed via oral administration and must be administered IV (Table 38.7). Following administration mitomycin C is rapidly and extensively metabolized. The quinone moiety imparts a blue-violet color to mitomycin crystals. Mitomycin C is used primarily to treat pancreatic cancer.

Anthracyclines

The anthracycline antibiotics represent a major class of antineoplastic agents. This class of drugs is characterized as having a tetracyclic quinone containing ring nucleus to which is attached a unique daunosamine sugar. Because of the conjugated anthroquinone nucleus, the anthracyclines are reddish in color and impart a red color to the urine of the patient. First isolated from the fermentation broths of *Streptomyces peucetius*, literally hundreds of semisynthetic derivatives have been prepared in an attempt to reduce the cardiotoxicity common to this class of agents. Presently, four drugs are marketed and utilized for a diverse number of cancerous conditions. The drugs consist of daunorubicin, doxorubicin, idarubicin, and epirubicin.

Mechanism of Action. The mechanism of action of the anthracyclines has been attributed to a number of biologic actions that the anthracyclines produce. The flat topography of the anthroquinone nucleus results in the ability of the anthracyclines to intercalate with DNA perpendicular to its long axis. The amino sugar appears to confer added stability to this binding through its interaction with the sugar phosphate backbone of DNA. The result of intercalation can lead to single- and double-stranded DNA breaks. This may be the result of a repair process initiated by topoisomerase. In addition, because of the anthroquinone ring system, the anthracyclines are capable of generating reactive oxygen species such as hydroxyl radicals (•OH) and superoxide radical anions (•O-O$^{\ominus}$). These free radicals may produce destructive effects upon the cell which may include damage to the DNA. The generation of free radicals may also account for the cardiotoxicity demonstrated by the anthroquinone which results in the most troublesome side effect of the anthracyclines.

Specific Agents. Daunorubicin, Doxorubicin, Idarubicin, and Epirubicin.

Due to lack of oral activity all of the anthracyclines are administered intravenously. They are rapidly cleared from the plasma. Daunorubicin hydrochloride is isolated from fermentation broths of *Streptomyces peucetius*. Hydroxylation of daunorubicin to form daunorubinol yields an active metabolite. Other biotransformations include reductive cleavage of the glycosidic bond, O-demethylation, and conjugation with glucuronic acid and sulfate ester formation.

Doxorubicin hydrochloride is chemically similar to daunorubicin, differing by having an additional hydroxyl group on the 8–acetyl side chain. Doxorubicin hydrochloride liposome injection (Doxil) has different pharmacokinetic properties compared to doxorubicin hydrochloride displaying a smaller volume of distribution and slower clearance. The liposome encapsulated formulation is a translucent, red dispersion.

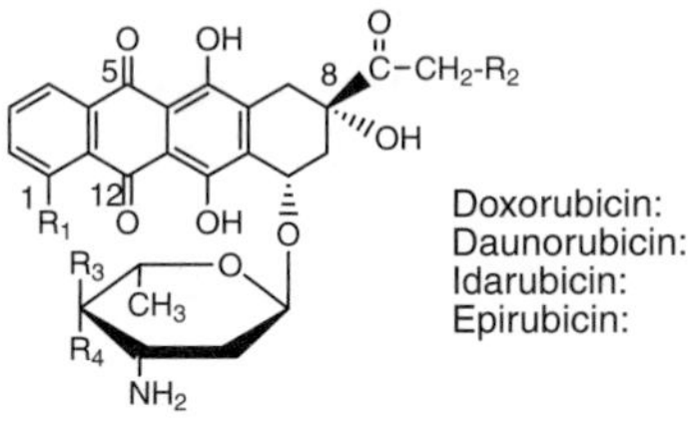

Doxorubicin: R$_1$ = CH$_3$O, R$_2$ = OH, R$_3$ = H, R$_4$ = OH
Daunorubicin: R$_1$ = CH$_3$O, R$_2$ = H, R$_3$ = H, R$_4$ = OH
Idarubicin: R$_1$ = R$_2$ = R$_3$ = H,   R$_4$ = OH
Epirubicin: R$_1$ = CH$_3$O, R$_2$ = OH, R$_3$ = OH, R$_4$ = H

Idarubicin is a synthetic analog of the natural occurring anthracyclines. The drug is claimed to have improved cellular uptake over previous agents which may be due to its high lipid solubility. The major metabolic product formed from idarubicin is the 13-hydroxyl derivative (idarubicinol) which retains biologic activity. Idarubicinol has a prolonged half-life (approximately 45 hours) as compared to idarubicin (approximately 22 hours). Because of the high lipophilicity of idarubicin the drug penetrates into cerebrospinal fluid.

Epirubicin differs in the stereochemistry of the alcohol present at the 4′-position of the daunosamine sugar. While not used as extensively as the other anthracyclines, epirubicin is indicated as a component of adjuvant therapy in patients with evidence of axillary node tumor involvement following resection of primary breast cancer.

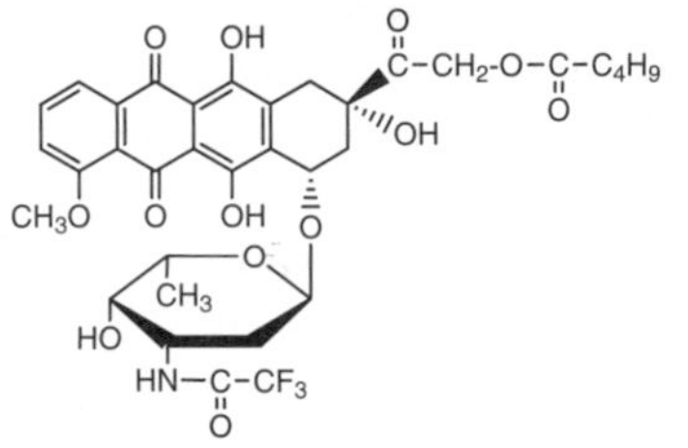

Valrubicin

Recently, the FDA has approved a new anthracycline under the orphan drug classification. The drug is valrubicin and it is specifically approved for use as intravesical therapy of BCG-refractory carcinoma in situ of the bladder (CIS) for which immediate cystectomy is not an option. The patient population for this condition is approximately 1000. Valrubicin is contraindicated in patients known to be hypersensitive to another anthracycline and valrubinicin has the same mechanism of action and physical chemical properties as other anthracyclines.

For dosage forms and indications of the anthracyclines see Table 38.7.

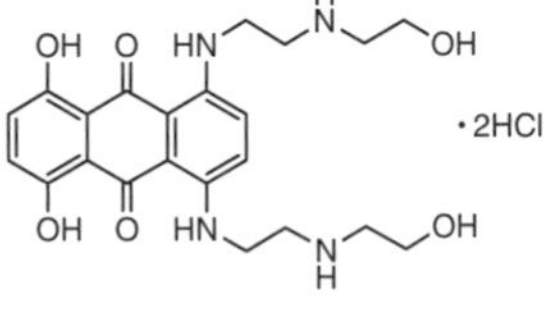

Mitoxantrone

Mitoxantrone

Mitoxantrone hydrochloride is an antineoplastic anthracenedione that is a cytostatic anthraquinone analogue. Because anthracenediones are highly conjugated quinones, aqueous solutions are colored dark blue. An acute effect of treatment with mitoxantrone is a blue-green pigment in urine and blue-green sclera. The mechanism of action of this drug is probably the same as that of the parent anthracylines. Parenteral formulations of mi-

toxantrone (pH 3.0–4.5) should not be mixed with heparin (pH 5.0–7.5) since a precipitate may form.

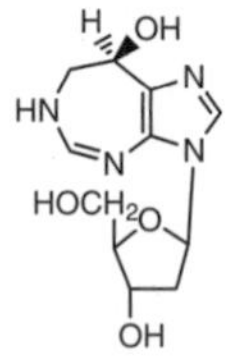

Pentostatin

Pentostatin

Pentostatin is an adenosine deaminase inhibitor that has been isolated from *Streptomyces antibioticus*. Related in structure to purines, pentostatin has an unusual 7-membered ring containing two nitrogens (a tetrahydrodiazepine). Also known as 2′-deoxycoformycin (DCF), pentostatin for injection is marketed as a lyophilized powder that is freely soluble in distilled water.

Antimitotic Agents

Mechanism of Action

Antimitotic agents, as the name suggests, prevent cellular mitosis, and in particular, interfere with the formation of the mitotic spindle. During mitosis, the protein tubulin undergoes polymerization ultimately to form the mitotic spindle. Antimitotic agents interfere with this process either by depolymerization of the microtubules or by causing structures other than the normal mitotic spindle to form, such as in ball or star shapes. In the absence of a properly formed mitotic spindle, the chromosomes cannot correctly segregate and this ultimately leads to cellular death.

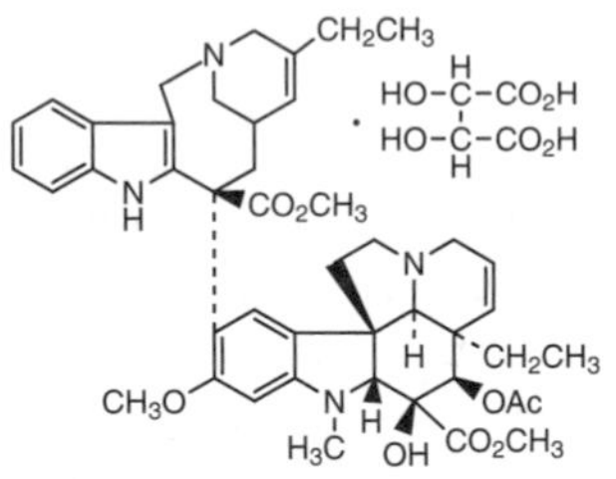

Vinorelbine

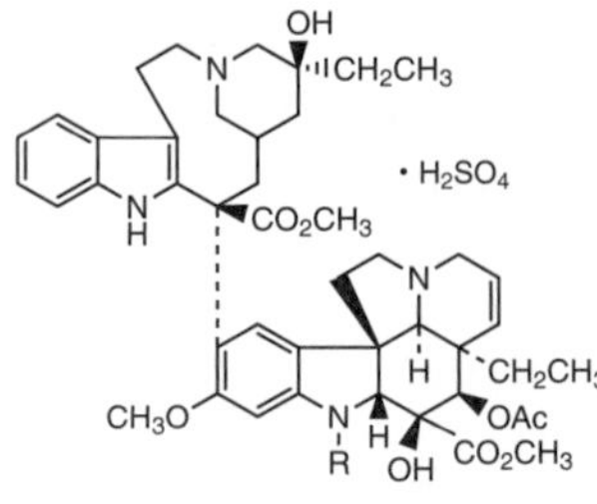

Vincristine: R = CHO
Vinblastine: R = CH₃

Specific Drugs

Vinca Alkaloids—Vincristine, Vinblastine, and Vinorelbine. The first antimitotic agents were the vinca alkaloids, vincristine sulfate, vinblastine sulfate, and the semi-synthetic derivative, vinorelbine tartrate, which are obtained from the periwinkle flower (*Vinca rosea*) (Table 38.7). They are composed of two multi-ringed units, vindoline and catharanthine. The vinca alkaloids contain tertiary amino groups that form salts freely soluble in water. The CYP3A isoform of CYP450 mediates the metabolism of these vinca alkaloids. Two of these alkaloids, vinblastine and vincristine, have become important clinical agents for the treatment of cancer. These two compounds block mitosis with metaphase arrest. It appears that both vinblastine and vincristine bind specifically with tubulin and cause its depolymerization. In fact, treatment of cells with vinblastine results in the formation of a 1-to-1 complex of vinblastine and tubulin.

Paclitaxel: $R_1 = C_6H_5$; $R_2 = Ac$
Docetaxel: $R_1 = (CH_3)_3C-O$; $R_2 = H$

Taxanes—Paclitaxel and Docetaxel. More recently, the antimitotic agent paclitaxel was discovered. This compound was isolated from the Pacific yew tree in the early 1960s, although its use as an anticancer agent for ovarian cancer was not approved until the mid-1990s (Table 38.7). Paclitaxel acts by binding to tubulin. However, unlike the vinca alkaloids, paclitaxel does not cause depolymerization. Paclitaxel causes microtubules to arrange themselves in a parallel array rather than the required arrangement of the mitotic spindle. Nevertheless, the ultimate effect is the same as the vinca alkaloids, and paclitaxel causes mitotic arrest. It is highly lipophilic, does not form stable salts with acids or bases, and is insoluble in water. For intravenous infusion, paclitaxel is prepared as a nonaqueous solution in polyoxyethylated castor oil and dehydrated alcohol. The primary metabolite of paclitaxel is 6-hydroxypaclitaxel formed by the action of CYP2C8. Two minor metabolites formed by CYP3A4 include 3'-p-hydroxypaclitaxel and 6,3'-p-dihydroxypaclitaxel.

Docetaxel is a taxoid differing in structure from paclitaxel in having one less acetate group and a tertiary butyl carbamate functionality in place of the benzamido group. The injectable formulation, consisting of docetaxel in polysorbate 80, must be diluted prior to use. The diluent consists of 13% ethanol in water for injection. Docetaxel is metabolized by CYP3A enzymes.

Miscellaneous Antineoplastics
Epipodophyllotoxins
Mechanism of action. The podophyllotoxins are obtained as extracts of the May Apple plant and were long used as a folk remedy by Native Americans and early settlers for their gastrointestinal effects (emetic and cathartic). Two compounds, etoposide and teniposide, are semi-synthetic derivatives and have been used to treat small-cell carcinomas of the lung and Hodgkins disease (Table 38.8). Etoposide and teniposide bind to tubulin. However, they bind to tubulin at sites different from the vinca alkaloids and do not appear to alter normal microtubular structure. Interestingly, etoposide and teniposide appear to exert their effects during G_2 phase and cause protein-DNA links and DNA strand breaks by inhibiting topoisomerase II. Etoposide has also been shown to stabilize the DNA-topoisomerase II complex.

Etoposide: $R_1 = CH_3$, $R_2 = H$
Etoposide phosphate: $R_1 = CH_3$, $R_2 = PO_3H_2$

Teniposide: $R_1 =$
$R_2 = H$

Etoposide, Etoposide phosphate and Teniposide. Etoposide and teniposide are podophyllotoxin analogues that have similar structural features. The significant difference between the structure of the originally isolated natural products and the semisynthetic antineoplastic drugs involves the stereochemical relationship between the substituents at the 1,4-position. The podophyllotoxins have a *cis* stereochemistry while the active drugs possess the *trans* configuration. A variety of functional groups are present in the structure of etoposide including lactone, phenol, aromatic ether, acetal, and glucopyranoside groups. Unfortunately, none of these functional groups form stable

Table 38.8. Miscellaneous Antineoplastic Agents

Generic Name	Trade Name	Indications	Toxicity*	Dosage Form (mg/unit)**
Etoposide	VePesid	Refractory testicular cancer, small cell lung cancer	A	IV (5, 7.5, 20, 25, 50/vial), Cap(50)
Teniposide	Vumon	Refractory childhood acute lymphoblastic leukemia	A	IV (50/5ml)
Irinotecan	Camptosar	Metastatic carcinoma of colon or rectum	I	IV (100/5ml)
Topotecan	Hycamtin	Metastatic ovarian carcinoma	A	IV (4/vial)
Hydroxyurea	Hydrea	Head and neck carcinoma, ovarian carcinoma, chronic myelocytic leukemia, malignant melanoma	A	Cap (500)
Mitotane	Lysodren	Adrenal cortex carcinoma	K	Tab (500)
Tretinoin	Vesanoid	Acute promyelocytic leukemia		
Alitretinoin	Panretin	Cutanious lesions in AIDS-related Kaposi's sarcoma		0.1% gel

*A = Bone marrow depression; I = Late diarrhea; K = CNS depression.
**IV = Intravenous; Cap = capsule; Tab = tablet.

salts that would be useful for solubilizing etoposide in aqueous solutions. The diluent for an injectable formulation of etoposide consists primarily of modified polysorbate 80/Tween 80, polyethylene glycol 300, and alcohol. Etoposide phosphate is a water soluble phosphate ester pro-drug of etoposide. Following intravenous infusion, etoposide phosphate is rapidly and completely hydrolyzed to etoposide. Teniposide is a cell cycle phase-specific semisynthetic podophyllotoxin analogue. Teniposide is highly lipophilic showing an octanol/water partition coefficient of approximately 100. The injectable formulation is a nonaqueous solution that is intended to be diluted prior to intravenous infusion. The nonaqueous solution in one commercial preparation consists of benzyl alcohol, N,N-dimethylacetamide, polyoxyethylated castor oil and dehydrated alcohol. When teniposide is diluted for intravenous infusion, precipitation may occur, especially in refrigerated solutions.

The major urinary metabolite of etoposide results from hydrolysis of the lactone moiety. In addition to glucuronidation and sulfate ester formation, etoposide is a substrate for CYP3A4 yielding catecholic metabolites by way of O-demethylation reactions. Teniposide is highly protein bound and extensively metabolized.

Hydroxyurea

Hydroxyurea

Hydroxyurea is a low molecular weight neutral molecule that is well absorbed orally and is excreted in the urine primarily as the parent compound. The mechanism of action appears to be inhibition of ribonucleotide diphosphate reductase. Thus, it causes decreased levels of deoxyribonucleotides required for DNA synthesis. Its mechanism of action may ultimately be due to chelation of an Fe^{2+} cofactor. The agent is cell-cycle specific for the S-phase and causes cells to arrest at the G_1-S interface. This is very useful for radiation therapy as cells in the G_1 phase are particularly sensitive to radiation. Other uses are shown in Table 38.8.

Mitotane

Mitotane

Mitotane known by its trivial name, o,p'-DDD is related in structure to the insecticide, DDT. Mitotane is an adrenal cytotoxic agent. After oral administration, only a small amount of mitotane and metabolites are excreted in urine or bile suggesting that most of the drug is stored in tissues.

The terminal plasma half-life after discontinuation of mitotane is long, ranging from 18–159 days. Mitotane is metabolized to a water-soluble phenylacetic acid metabolite, presumably through an acyl chloride intermediate. The drug is used in the treatment of adrenal cortex carcinoma (Table 38.8)

Tretinoin   Alitretinoin

Retinoids—Tretinoin, Alitretinoin

Tretinoin is a retinoid that induces the differentiation of acute promyelocytic leukemia cells. Tretinoin (all-*trans* retinoic acid) is similar in structure to vitamin A (retinol) and is a normal metabolite of vitamin A. Tretinoin is well absorbed orally and is highly protein bound by plasma proteins. Oxidative metabolism of tretinoin catalyzed by the CYP450 system includes formation of 4-oxo *trans* retinoic acid and its glucuronide and isomerization to 13-*cis* retinoic acid (isotretinoin) followed by oxidation to 4-oxo *cis* retinoic acid.

Alitretinoin, the 9-*cis*-retinoic acid, is a naturally occurring retinoid which functions by inhibiting the growth of Kaposi's sarcoma cells. The drug does this by activating intracellular retinoid receptors which when activated express genes which regulate cell growth, differentiation, and apoptosis. Alitretinoin is available for topical application for the treatment of cutaneous lesions in patients with AIDS-related Kaposi's sarcoma. The drug received priority review by the FDA and is designated as an orphan drug. Due to its topical use toxicities are expected to by minor. Clinical trials indicate that skin rash is the most common side effect. Studies are underway to determine the value of alitretinoin as a systemic agent for the treatment of a wide variety of systemic cancers as well as psoriasis.

Camptothecin: $R_1 = R_2 = R_3 = H$

Topotecan: $R_1 = H$, $R_2 = -CH_2-N(CH_3)_2$, $R_3 = OH$

Irinotecan: $R_1 = -C_2H_5$, $R_2 = H$, R =

Camptothecins—Topotecan and Irinotecan

Topotecan hydrochloride is a semisynthetic camptothecin. Modification of camptothecin by addition of the phenolic hydroxyl and dimethylaminomethyl groups improved water solubility and reduced the occurrence of unpredictable side effects without compromising its antitumor activity. The lactone form of topotecan is pharmacologically active, although the equilibrium between the lactone and hydrolysis product favors the ring-opened form at physiologic pH. Both camptothecin and topotecan are inhibitors of topoisomerase I and cause single-strand breaks in DNA. Either or both of these effects may be cytotoxic.

Irinotecan hydrochloride is a semisynthetic piperidine-containing analogue of the plant alkaloid, camptothecin. An active metabolite is formed by the action of hepatic carboxylesterases through the hydrolysis of the carbamate functional group. Although irinotecan is only slightly soluble in water, both irinotecan and its active metabolite exist in alkaline solutions in an equilibrium of lactone and ring-opened forms. For indications of the camptothecins see Table 38.8.

Porfimer

Porfimer sodium is a photosensitizing agent used in photodynamic therapy (PDT) of tumors. Porfimer is a mixture of oligomers made consisting of up to eight porphyrin units linked together by ester and ether linkages. It is dark red to reddish-brown in color. Clearance from tissues other than tumors, skin, and tissues of the reticuloendothelial system is rapid. Illumination of the tumor with a laser at 630 nm wavelength is performed after porfimer has accumulated in tumor tissue. The laser light promotes the porfimer polymer to an excited state which results in the initiation and propagation of radical reactions. Singlet oxygen ($\uparrow$O–O$\uparrow$) may be formed in the reaction by spin transfer from porfimer to molecular oxygen. Further reaction products include superoxide ($\bullet$O-O$^{\ominus}$) and hydroxyl radical ($\bullet$ OH). Patients experience photosensitivity for up to 30 days and are cautioned to avoid exposure of skin and eyes to direct sunlight or bright indoor light. UV sunscreens are of no value against porfimer photosensitivity because photoactivation is caused by visible light.

Hormonal Therapy

Hormonal manipulation in the treatment of hormone supportive cancers has become a common practice today and is most notably seen in the treatment of breast cancer with antiestrogens and prostate cancer with gonadotropin-releasing hormone (GnRH) agonists and with antiandrogens (Table 38.9).

Tamoxifen

Antiestrogens

The reader is referred to Chapter 44 for an in depth discussion of the history and present use of antiestrogens for the treatment of breast cancer. Tamoxifen has been a prototype structure for the development of antiestrogens, but while tamoxifen's antiestrogen action appears to play a significant role in its anticancer activity the complete action is more complex than simply estrogen antagonism. Added to the arsenal of estrogen antagonists is the drug toremifene.

An additional approach to the treatment of breast cancer has been the use of aromatase inhibitors. A key step in estrogen biosynthesis involves the conversion of androstenedione to estrone catalyzed by the enzyme aromatase. Blocking aromatase significantly lowers the level of circulating estradiol. Two aromatase inhibitors have been approved by the FDA for first-line treatment of postmenopausal women with hormone receptor-positive locally advanced or metastatic breast cancer. Anastrazole and letrozole are nonsteroidal inhibitors of aromatase which competitively inhibit aromatase by binding to the CYP450 subunit of the enzyme. Both drugs are well absorbed following oral administration. Metabolism and excretion of

Table 38.9. Hormonal Antineoplastic Agents

Generic Name	Trade Name	Indications	Toxicity*	Dosage Form (mg/unit)**
Tamoxifen	Novladex	Breast cancer	L	Tab (10, 20)
Toremifene	Fareston	Breast cancer	L	Tab (88.5)
Anastrazole	Arimidex	Advanced breast cancer	L	Tab (1.0)
Letrozole	Femara	Advanced breast cancer	L	Tab (2.5)
Leuprolide	Lupron	Prostatic carcinoma, endometriosis	G,L	IV (5/ml)
	Lupron Depot			IV (3.75, 7.5/vial)
Goserelin	Zoladex	Advanced prostatic carcinoma	G,L	IV (3.6/vial, 10.8/implant)
Flutamide	Eulexin	Prostatic carcinoma	G,L	Cap (125)
Bicalutamide	Casodex	Metastatic prostatic carcinoma	G,L	Tab (50)
Nilutamide	Nilandron	Metastatic prostatic carcinoma	L	Tab (50)

*G = Gynecomastia and impotence; L = Hot flashes, nausea and vomiting.
**IV = Intravenous; Cap = capsule; Tab = tablet.

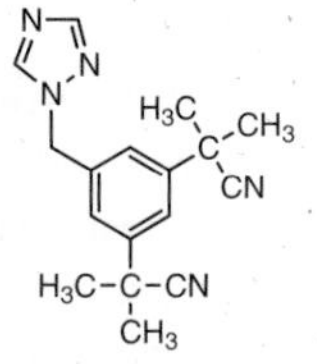

Fig. 38.22. Metabolism of flutamide.

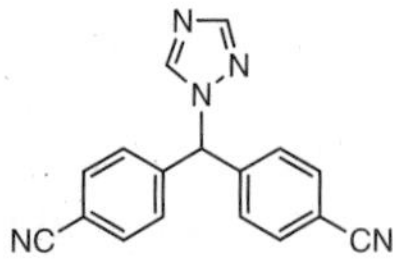

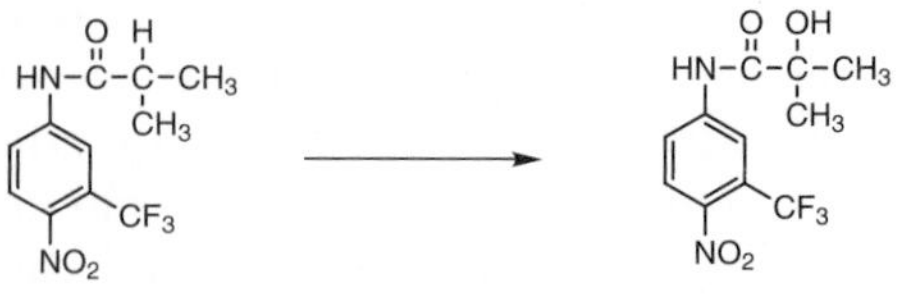

letrozole is slow in humans. In vitro, letrozole is a substrate of CYP3A4 and CYP2A6, and an inhibitor of CYP2A6 and CYP2C19. The latter isoform of CYP has been linked to the aramotase enzyme.

GnRH Agonists and Antiandrogens

Hormonal therapy is quite common for the treatment of metastatic prostate cancer. The goal of such therapy is to remove the stimulatory effects of male hormones (testosterone and dihydrotestosterone) on the prostate cancer cells. A variety of medical approaches can be taken in an attempt to control the levels of male hormones one of which is the use of drug therapy. The use of gonadotropin-releasing hormone (GnRH, also known as Luteinizing Hormone Releasing Hormone-LHRH) agonists is based upon the fact that while such agents initially increase the levels of testosterone, they later cause a decline in testosterone levels through downregulation (desensitization). This process takes approximately 4 weeks and leads to castrate levels of testosterone. Recognizing that GnRH agonists cause an initial increase in testosterone and in prostate growth, known as the flare phenomenon, explains the benefit of combination therapy utilizing an antiadrogen agent with the GnRH agonist.

The two most common GnRH agonists used today are leuprolide and goserelin. Both are nonapeptides differing at only two locations from the natural hormone

GnRH (see Chapter 6 for additional discussion of leuprolide and goserelin). Leuprolide acetate is administered by injection daily or as a depot injection monthly, every 3 or 4 months, as a palliative treatment in advanced prostatic carcinoma.

The use of antiandrogen drug in the treatment of prostate cancer is now common practice. Three antiandrogen drugs have been approved by the FDA and they are of flutamide, bicalutamide, and nilutamide. These drugs are classified as nonsteroidal antiandrogens which inhibit androgen receptor translocation to the nucleus in target tissue which in this case includes the hypothalamus and prostate. As a result these drugs block the action of testosterone and dihydrotestosterone. The first two drugs, flutamide and bicalutamide, are administered in combination with a GnRH agonist for prevention of the flare phenomenon in the treatment of metastatic prostate cancer. Both drugs are readily absorbed following oral administration. Flutamide is metabolized by oxidation to the α-hydroxylated derivative which also possess biologic activity (Fig. 38.22).

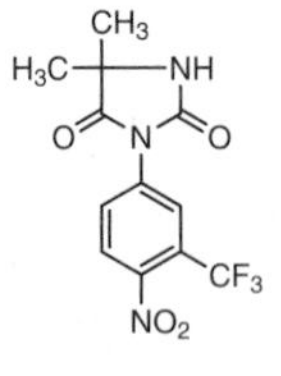

A third antiandrogen drug, nilutamide, is used as single drug therapy in combination with surgical castration to block the action of testosterone and dihydrotestosterone.

Finally, an additional approach to the treatment of prostate cancer is the development of GnRH antagonists. One such agent is the drug abarelix for which a new drug application has been submitted. This agent is a peptide drug which bears some similarity to the natural hormone GnRH.

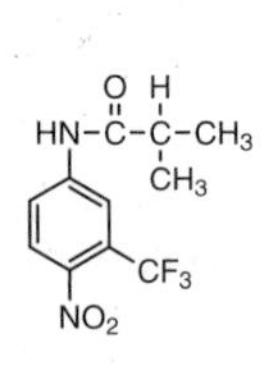

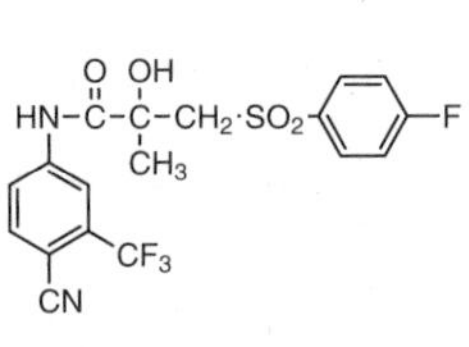

COMBINATION THERAPY

Combination drug therapy is a common and highly effective method of treating a wide variety of cancer conditions. The basic principles underlying combination therapy consist of using drugs which individually are effective

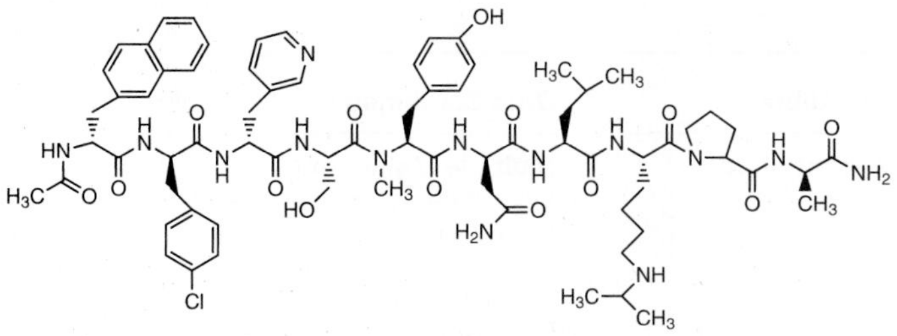

Abarelix

against a particular cancer and using the individual drug at a dose which in single drug therapy would be expected to be effective against the cancer. Each drug in the combination should have a unique mechanism of action and it would be beneficial if the drugs did not have overlapping toxicities. The intent of combination therapy is to totally destroy all of the abnormal cells. An exhaustive review of the large number of combinations used in cancer chemotherapy is beyond the scope of this chapter. A summary of some of the combinations is given in Table 38.10. The reader is referred to reference 24 and 25 for a more detailed listing of drug dosing. The reader is also referred to reference 26 for a listing of individual drugs, indications, chemical stability of reconstituted preparations, dosages, special precautions and instructions, as well as adverse reactions.

Table 38.10. Combination Cancer Chemotherapeutic Regimens (24)

Drug Combination	Abbrev.	Drug Combination	Abbrev.	Drug Combination	Abbrev.
Adenocarcinoma		**Gastric Cancer**		**Genitourinary Melignancy—Testicular—** *continued*	
Cisplatin	EP	Leucovorin			
Etoposide		Etoposide	ELF	Bleomycin	
Paclitaxel		Fluorouracil		Etoposide	BEP
Carboplatin		Methotrexate		Cisplatin	
Etoposide		Fluorouracil	FAMTX	Cisplatin	PVB
		Leucovorin		Vinblastine	
		Doxorubicin		Bleomycin	
Breast Cancer		Fluorouracil	FUP	Vinblastine or	
Cyclophosphamide	CAF	Cisplatin		Etoposide	
Doxorubicin	FAC			Ifosfamide	VIP
Fluorouracil		**Genitourinary Malignancy—Bladder**		Cisplatin	
Cyclophosphamide	CEF	Cyclophosphamide	CISCA	Mesna	
Epirubicin	FEC	Doxorubicin			
Fluorouracil		Cisplatin		**Gynecologic Malignancy—Cervical**	
Cyclophosphamide	CFM	Cisplatin		Cisplatin	
Fluorouracil	CNF	Docetaxel		Fluorouracil	
Mitoxantrone	FNC	Cisplatin	CMV	Cisplatin	
Cyclophosphamide		Methotrexate		Vinorelbine	
Methotrexate	CMF	Vinblastine			
Fluorouracil		Gemcitabine		**Gynecologic Malignancy—Endometrial**	
Mitoxantrone	NFL	Cisplatin		Doxorubicin	AP
Fluorouracil		Methotrexate		Cisplatin	
Leucovorin		Vinblastine			
Paclitacel		Doxorubicin	MVAC	**Gynecologic Malignancy—** **Ovarian/Epithelial**	
Vinorelbine		Cisplatin			
Doxorubicin	Sequential	Paclitaxel	PC	Carboplatin	CC
Cyclophosphamide	AC/Paclitacel	Carboplatin		Cyclophosphamide	
Paclitaxel				Cyclophosphamide	CP
Vinorelbine		**Genitourinary Malignancy—Prostate**		Cisplatin	
Doxorubicin	NA	Estramustine		Paclitaxel	CT
Doxorubicin	Sequential	Vinblastine		Cisplatin	
Cyclophosphamide	DOX-CMF	Flutamide	FL	Paclitaxel	Carbo-Tax
Methotrexate		Leuprolide		Carboplatin	
Fluorouracil		Flutamide	FZ		
Trastuzumab		Goserelin		**Head & Neck/Esophageal Malignancies**	
Paclitaxel		Mitoxantrone		Carboplatin	
		Prednisone		Fluorouracil	
		Paclitaxel	PE	Cisplatin	
Colon Cancer		Estramustine		Fluorouracil	
Leucovorin	Roswell Park				
Fluorouracil	Mayo regimen			**Leukemia—AML**	
Irinotecan	5-FU/LV/	**Genitourinary Melignancy—Testicular**		Cytarabine	
Fluorouracil	CPT-11	Etoposide	EP	Daunorubicin	7+3+7
Leucovorin	(Saltz regimen)	Cisplatin		Etoposide	

Continued

Table 38.10—continued

Drug Combination	Abbrev.
Leukemia-AML—continued	
Idarubicin	
Cytarabine	
Etoposide	
Cytarabine with	
Daunorubicin or	
Idarubicin or	7+3
Mitoxantrone	
Cytarabine with	
Daunorubicin or	5+2
Mitoxantrone	
Lung Cancer—Small Cell	
Cyclophosphamide	
Doxorubicin	CAE
Etoposide	
Cyclophosphamide	
Doxorubicin	CAV
Vincristine	
Cyclophosphamide	
Doxorubicin	CAV/
Vindristine	EP
Etoposide	
Cisplatin	
Etoposide	EP
Cisplatin	
Etoposide	VIP
Ifosfamide	
Cisplatin	
Mesna	
Lung Cancer—Non-Small Cell	
Gemcitabline	
Carboplatin	
Gemcitabline	
Cisplatin	
Gemcitabline	
Vinorelbine	
Paclitaxel	PC
Cisplatin	
Vinorelbine	
Cisplatin	
Lymphoma—Hodgkin's	
Doxorubicin	
Bleomycin	ABDV
Vinblastine	
Dacarbazine	
Chlorambucil	
Vinblastine	ChIVPP
Procarbazine	
Prednisone	

Drug Combination	Abbrev.
Lymphoma-Hodgkin's—continued	
Mechlorethamine	MOPP
Vincristine	
Procarbazine	
Prednisone	
Doxorubicin	Stanford V
Vinblastine	
Mechlorethamine	
Vincristine	
Bleomycin	
Etoposide	
Prednisone	
Lymphoma—Non-Hodgkin's	
Cyclophosphamide	
Doxorubicin	CHOP
Vincristine	
Prednisone	
Cyclophosphamide	
Mitoxantrone	
Vincristine	CNOP
Prednisone	
Cyclophosphamide	
Vincristine	COP
Prednisone	
Dexamethasone	
Cisplatin	DHAP
Cytarabine	
Etoposide	
Methylprednisolone	
Cytarabine	
Cisplatin	ESHAP
or	
Mesna	
Ifosfamide	
Metoxantrone	
Etoposide	
Melanoma	
Cisplatin	
Vinblastine	CVD
Dacarbazine	
Cisplatin	
Vinblastine	CVD+
Dacarbazine	IL-21
Interleukin-2	
Interferon alfa	
Cisplatin	
Dacarbazine	
Carmustine	

Drug Combination	Abbrev.
Multiple Melanoma	
Vincristine	
Carmustine	M2
Cyclophosphamide	
Melphalan	
Prednisone	
Melphalan	MP
Prednisone	
Vincristine	
Doxorubicin	VAD
Dexamethasone	
Vincristine	
Carmustine	
Melphalan	VBMCP
Cyclophosphamide	
Prednisone	
Pancreatic Cancer	
Streptozocin	
Mitomycin-C	SMF
Fluorouracil	
Sarcoma	
Doxorubicin	
Ifosfamide	DI
Mesna	
Doxorubicin	
Dacarbazine	AD
Mesna	
Doxorubicin	MAID
Ifosfamide	
Dacarbazine	
Pediatric Regimens—ALL	
Consolidation	
Methotrexate	
Mercaptopurine	IDMTX/
Leucovorin	6-MP
Pediatric Regimens—ALL	
Continuation	
Methotrexate	MTX/
Mercaptopurine	6-MP
Methotrexate	MTC/
Mercaptopurine	6-MP/VP
Vincristine	
Prednisone	
Induction	
Prednisone	
Vincristine	PVA
Asparaginase	

Table 38.10—*continued*

Drug Combination	Abbrev.
Pediatric Regimens-ALL—*continued*	
Prednisone	
Vincristine	PVDA
Daunorubicin	
Asparaginase	
Pediatric Regiments—AML	
Induction	
Cytarabine	CA
Asparaginase	
Daunorubicin	DA
Cytarabine	
Daunorubicin	
Cytarabine	DAT
Thioguanine	
Daunorubicin	
Cytarabine	DAV
Etoposide	
Daunorubicin	
Cytarabine	HI-
Etoposide	CDAZE
Azacitidine	
Pediatric Regimens—Brain Tumors	
Cisplatin	CDDP/
Etoposide	VP-16
Vincristine	
Cyclophosphamide	
Cycle A:	
Vincristine	COPE
Cyclophosphamide	Baby
Cycle B:	Brain I
Cisplatin	
Etoposide	
Methylprednisolone	
Vincristine Lomustine	
Procarbazine	"8 in 1"
Hydroxyurea	
Cisplatin	
Cytarabine	
Dacarbazine	
Also used: MOPP, POC	

Drug Combination	Abbrev.
Pediatric Regimens—Lymphoma	
Cyclophosphamide	
Vincristine	COMP
Methotrexate	
Prednisone	
Cyclophosphamide	
Vincristine	COPP
Procarbazine	
Prednisone	
Vincristine	
Prednisone	OPA
Doxorubicin	
Pediatric Regimens—Lymphoma	
Vincristine	
Procarbazine	
Prednisone	
Doxorubicin	
Also used: ABVD, CHOP, MOPP	
Pediatric Regimens—Neuroblastoma	
Cyclophosphamide	Cy/A
Doxorubicin	
Cisplatin	Pt/VM
Tenioside	
Pediatric Regimens—Osteosarcoma	
Ifosfamide	
Etoposide	IfoVP
Mesna	
Pediatric Regimens—Sarcomas	
Ifosfamide	
Carboplatin	ICE
Etoposide	
Cyclophosphamide	Tope/CTX
Topotecan	

Drug Combination	Abbrev.
Vincristine	
Cyclophosphamide	VAC/Adr
Doxorubicin	
Dactinomycin	
Vincristine	
Dactinomycin	VAC
Cyclophosphamide	

CASE STUDY

Victoria F. Roche and S. William Zito

GM is a 62-year-old architect who has been diagnosed with stage III ovarian cancer. She underwent surgical ovarian debulking and is now about to begin an aggressive chemotherapeutic regimen. GM's medical history reveals two previous myocardial infarctions, and she underwent double bypass surgery three years ago. She currently has mild congestive heart failure that is being treated with low dose furosemide (a loop diuretic). In addition to furosemide, her current medication regimen includes the HMG CoA reductase inhibitor lovastatin and estrogen replacement therapy with estradiol.

The physician has ordered compound 1 (cisplatin) and wants to add a second compound to the regimen. Your advice on an appropriate second agent for combination therapy is solicited.

1. Identify the therapeutic problem(s) where the pharmacist's intervention may benefit the patient.

2. Identify and prioritize the patient specific factors that must be considered to achieve the desired therapeutic outcomes.

3. Conduct a thorough and mechanistically oriented structure-activity analysis of all therapeutic alternatives provided in the case.

4. Evaluate the SAR findings against the patient specific factors and desired therapeutic outcomes and make a therapeutic decision.

5. Counsel your patient.

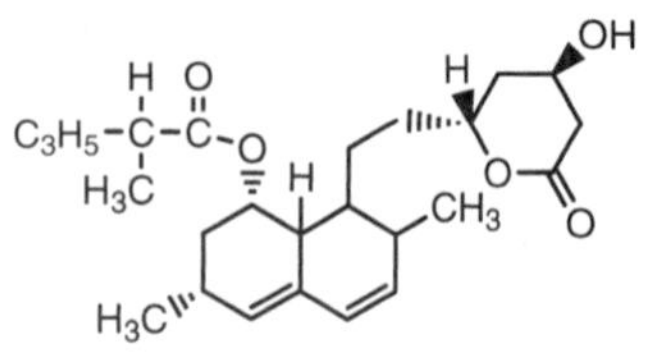

Lovastatin 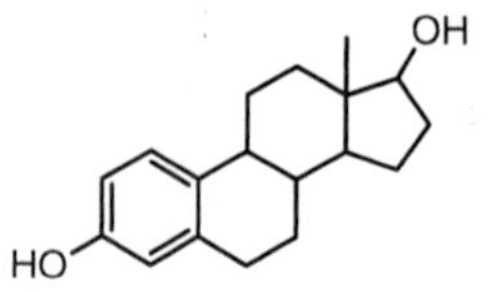   Estradiol 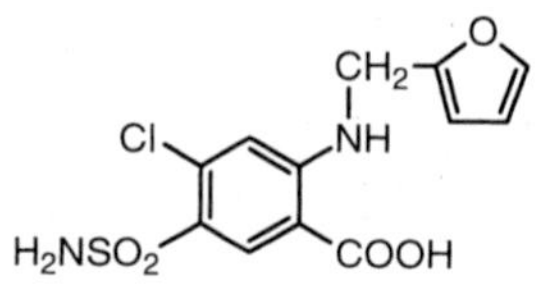   Furosemide

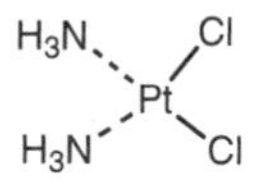

1 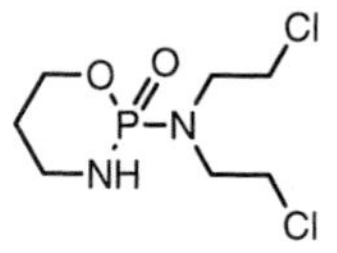   2 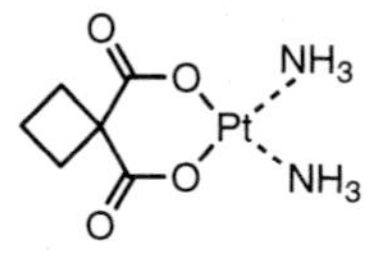   3

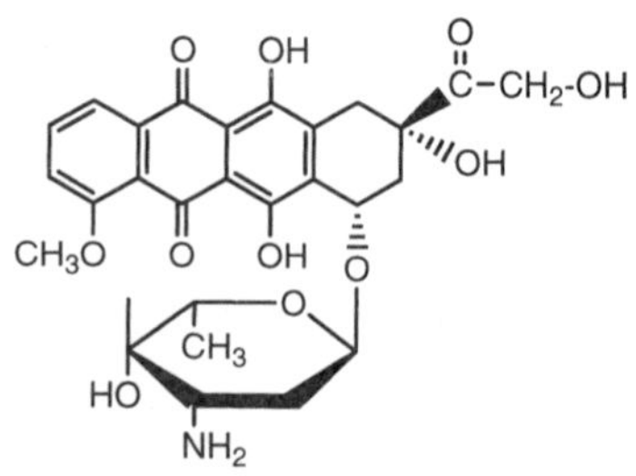

4 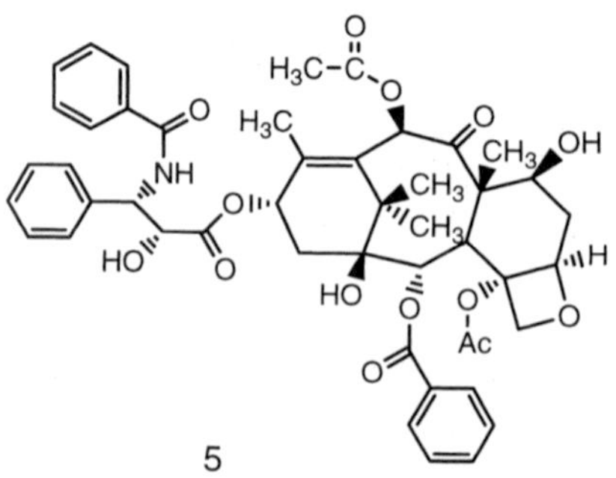   5

REFERENCES

1. "Cancer: Rates and Risks"; 4ᵗʰ ed.; Harras A, ed.; National Institutes of Health—National Cancer Instititue, 1996.
2. Bertino JR. Encyclopedia of Cancer, Vol 2. New York, NY: Academic Press, 1997, pp 760–782.
3. Aaronson SA. Growth factors and cancer. Science 1991; 254:1146–1153.
4. Weinberg RA. Tumor suppressor genes. Science 1991; 254:1138–1146.
5. Holland JF, Frei III E, Kufe DW, et al, eds. Cancer Medicine, 3ʳᵈ ed. Philadelphia: Williams & Williams, 1997.
6. Solomon E, Borrow J, Goddard AD. Chromosome aberrations and cancer. Science 1991; 254:1153–1160.
7. Band P, ed. Recent Results in Cancer Research, V. 120, Occupational Cancer Epidemiology. New York, NY:Springer-Verlag, 1990.
8. zur Hausen H. Viruses in human cancers. Science, 1991; 254:1167–1173.
9. Dollinger M, Rosenbaum EH, Cable G. Everyones Guide to Cancer Therapy. Kansas City, MO:Andrews McMeel, 1997.
10. Gilman A, Philips FS. The biological actions and therapeutic applications ofthe β-chloroethyl amines and sulfides. Science 1946; 103:409–415.
11. Conners TA. Mechanism of action of 2-chloroethylamine, derivatives, sulfur mustards, epoxides and aziridines. In Sartorelli AC and Johns DJ, eds. Handbook of Experimental Pharmacology. New York, NY:Springer-Verlag, 1975; 38(2):4.
12. Montgomery JA, James R, McCaleb GS, et al. The modes of decomposition of 1,3-bis(2-chloroethyl)-1-nitrosourea and related compounds. J Med Chem 1967; 10:668.
13. Brooks P and Lawley PD. The reaction of mono- and di-functional alkylating agents with nucleic acids Biochem J 1961; 80:496–503.
14. Kohn KW, Green, DM. Transforming activity of nitrogen mustard-linked DNA J Mol Biol 1966; 19:289–302.
15. Kreis W and Yen W. An antineoplastic C¹⁴-labeled methylhydrazine derivative in P815 mouse leukemia. A metabolic study. Experientia 1965; 21:284.
16. Augusto O, Cavalieri EL, Rogan EG, et al. Formation of 8-methylguanine as a result of DNA alkylation by methyl radicals generated during horseradish peroxidase-catalyzed oxidation of methylhydrazine. J Biol Chem 1990; 256:22093–22096.
17. Heidelberger, C. Fluorinated pyrimidines and their nucleosides. In Sartorelli, A.C., and Johns, D.J. (eds.). Handbook of Experimental Pharmacology, Vol. 38, part 2, p. 193. New York, Springer-Verlag, 1975
18. Chu MY and Fischer GA. A proposed mechanism of action of 1-β-D-arabinofuranosyl-cytosine as an inhibitor of the growth of leukemic cells. Biochem Pharmacol 1962; 11:423–430.
19. Creasey WA, DoConti RC, and Kaplan SR Biochemical studies with 1-β-D-arabinofuranosylcytosine in human leukemic leuko-cytes and normal bone marrow cells. Cancer Res. 1968; 28:1074–1081.
20. Borun TW, Scharff MD, and Robbins E. Rapidly labeled polyribosome-associated RNA having the properties of histone messenger. Proc Nat'l Acad Sci, USA 1967; 58:1977–1983.
21. Ruiz van haperen VWT, Veerman G, Vermorken JB, et al. "2′2-Difluoro-deoxycytidine (Gemcitabine) Incorporation into RNA and DNA of Tumour Cell Lines" iochem. Pharmacol. 46:762–766 (1993)
22. Lukens LN, and Herrington KA. Enzymic formation of 6-mercaptopurine ribotide. Biochem Biophys Acta 1957; 24:432–433.
23. Bennett LL, Jr., and Allan PW. Formation and significance of 6-methylthiopurine ribonucleotide as a metabolite of 6-mercaptopurine. Cancer Res. 1971; 31:152–158.
24. Valgus JM, Treish I, Shifflett SL, et al. 2001 Guide to Cancer Chemotherapeutic Regimens. Pharm Pract News Special Edition Nov 2000; 71–80.
25. Adams VR, Sheehin JB, Holdsworth MT. Guide to Cancer chemotherapy Regiments. Pharm Pract News. Oct 2001;25–35.
26. McFarland HM, Almuete V, Brisby J, et al. 2001 Guide for the Administration and Use of Cancer Chemotherapeutic Agents. Pharm Pract News Special Edition Nov 2000; 35–42.

SUGGESTED READINGS

AMA Council Report. Guidelines for Handling Parenteral Antineoplastics. J Amer Med Assoc 1985; 253:1590–1592.

American Society of Hospital Pharmacists Technical Assistance Bulletin on Handling Cytotoxic and Hazardous Drugs. Am J Hosp Pharm 1990; 47:1033–1049.

Clinical Oncological Society of Australia. Guidelines and Recommendations for Safe Handling of Antineoplastic Agents. Med J Australia 1983; 1:426–428.

Controlling occupational exposure to hazardous drugs. (OSHA Work-Practice Guidelines). Am J Health-Syst Pharm 1996; 53: 1669–1685.

Drugs of Choice for Cancer Chemotherapy, Medical Letter, 2000; 42:83–92. Recommendations for the Safe Handling of Parenteral Antineoplastic Drugs. NIH Publication No. 83–2621. For sale by the Superintendent of Documents, U.S. Government Printing Office, Washington, DC 20402.

Jones RB, et al.: Safe Handling of Chemotherapeutic Agents: A Report from the Mount Sinai Medical Center. CA-A Cancer Journal for Clinicians 1983; (Sept/Oct) 258–263.

National Study Commission on Cytotoxic Exposure-Recommendations for Handling Cytotoxic Agents. Available from Louis P Jeffrey, Chairman, National Study Commission on Cytotoxic Exposure. Massachusetts College of Pharmacy and Allied Health Sciences, 179 Longwood Avenue, Boston, Massachusetts 02115.

39. Antiviral Agents and Protease Inhibitors

MANOHAR L. SETHI

INTRODUCTION
Virus Structure
and Classification

Viruses are among the smallest microorganisms, varying in size from 0.02–0.40μm (1). They are filterable through porcelain filters and can be seen and identified with the help of an electron microscope. Viruses consist of a nucleic acid core that contains either deoxyribonucleic acid (DNA) or ribonucleic acid (RNA), which constitutes the genetic material and provides a basis for classification of viruses. A protein coat known as a capsid surrounds the nucleic acid core. The entire structure is called the nucleocapsid. On the basis of the structural characteristics of the nucleocapsid, most viruses are divided into two groups classified by their symmetry or shape. One group of viruses may show helical symmetry and the other icosahedral (20-sided) symmetry of the nucleocapsid. The nucleocapsid may or may not be covered by another protein coat called an envelope. The envelope is composed of glycoproteins that are important virus antigens. The arrangement of coat proteins defines the overall shape of the viruses. Spheres, rods, filaments, bullets, rectangles, triangles, and elongated tubes are some of the shapes of viruses. The complete infectious virus particle is called a virion.

Viruses have long been recognized as the cause of a wide variety of infections in animals and humans (2). The disease type and symptoms depend on the group and species of viruses. Fundamentally, viruses are classified into two main groups, DNA viruses and RNA viruses (retroviruses). Other methods of classification are based on traditional taxonomy, properties of the viruses (composition, structure, shapes, and relative sizes), induction and carriage of polymerases (DNA- or RNA-directed RNA), and presence or absence of a lipid-containing envelope.

The protein coats of the nucleocapsid and envelope and the absence or the presence of the envelope play an important role in the initial stages of viral infection. Reactive sites on the capsid or envelope (glycoprotein) become attached to the receptor sites (polypeptide) on the host cell. The penetration, uncoating, and release of the virions in the host cell depend on the structural coat proteins. This process influences the susceptibility of the virus to the actions of antiviral agents. The study of the structure of viral coat proteins and their properties are therefore important in the development of effective antiviral agents.

Viral Replication and Transformation of Cells (3,4)

Because viruses do not multiply without living cells, they depend solely on the host cell to carry out their metabolic activities. The enzyme system of the host cell is used for the synthesis of DNA and virus replication. The viruses (DNA and RNA) may replicate and or transform the cell simultaneously. When oncogenic or infectious viruses attack the host cell, they adsorb onto the host cell surface receptor by electrostatic interaction, penetrate the cell surface, and remove their viral coat, liberating the nucleic acid into the host cell. Viral nucleic acid is replicated within the host by viral enzymes catalyzing the synthesis of mRNAs for formation of viral structural and nonstructural proteins. The assembled viral particles are released from the cell by a budding process or after lysis. In the case of replication of DNA viruses (Fig. 39.1), the liberated DNA integrates into the host cell DNA. As a result, viral DNA becomes a permanent part of the host's genetic material. It may remain latent for years or duplicate into progeny viral DNA during cell division. Viral DNA transcribes into early and late mRNA, which is then translated into viral proteins under the direction of viral and host enzymes. In the case of oncogenic DNA viruses, synthesized viral proteins may act on the host cell to change the normal functions or morphologic characters of the cell. As a result, the infected cell behaves like a transformed or cancer cell. During the translation process, mRNA synthesizes the structural proteins of the viral capsid and envelope. The viral DNA in conjunction with the structural proteins assembles into progeny virions that escape from the host cell.

Replication of oncogenic RNA viruses is conceivably different from that of the DNA viruses. In 1970, Temin and Mizutani (5) and Baltimore (6) discovered an enzyme from RNA tumor viruses, reverse transcriptase (RT), which reverses the usual information flow (DNA→RNA) in a cell to opposite order which means that DNA is produced on an RNA template (RNA→DNA). RT (RNA-directed DNA polymerase) has been found in almost all oncogenic RNA viruses. In oncogenic virus replication and transformation (Fig. 39.2), RNA viruses must first form a DNA copy that is integrated into host cell chromosomes. Thus an oncogenic RNA virus after entry into the host cell forms a viral DNA from RNA with the help of reverse transcriptase. A double-stranded helix (RNA/DNA duplex) is formed in which one strand is the original RNA viral chromosome and the other is a new complementary DNA chain. The strand of viral RNA is then removed by another enzyme (RNase H), leav-

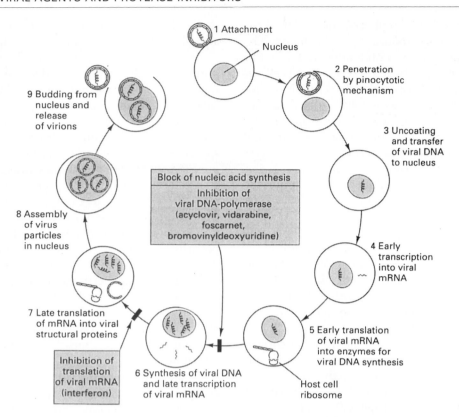

Fig. 39.1. Schematic diagram of replication of a DNA virus (e.g., herpes simplex) in a host cell with the probable sites of action of antiviral agents. In some viruses, assembly (stage 8) takes place in the host cell cytoplasm. Reproduced with permission from Churchill Livingstone, New York from the book "Pharmacology" 1995, page 745 by H. P. Rang, M. M. Dale, J. M. Ritter and P. Gardner.

ing a single-stranded DNA molecule. Replication of single-stranded viral DNA with the host's enzyme results in the duplex viral DNA that is then integrated into the host's DNA by integrase. The integrated DNA copy of viral RNA into the host DNA is called a "provirus," which is transmitted to the daughter cell in the same way as other cellular genes. The "provirus" contains the same genetic information that was present in the viral RNA chromosome.

Subsequently, the "provirus" is transcribed into viral mRNA, which is translated into viral proteins with the help of host enzymes. One or more of these viral proteins may alter cell behavior, resulting in the transformation of a cell into a cancer cell. Furthermore, viral mRNA synthesizes structural proteins for the viral capsid and envelope, which enclose viral nucleic acid. New RNA viral particles assembled by acquiring viral and envelope proteins escape from the host cell by budding process with the help of protease enzymes.

Infectious RNA viruses replicate in the cytoplasm via RNA polymerases. In some RNA viruses, for example poliomyelitis, the RNA of the infecting particles is capable of acting as mRNA. In other RNA viruses, such as influenza and measles, a complementary strand of mRNA is synthesized with the RNA of the infecting particles serving as a template. Translation of mRNA into viral proteins and the release of viral particles from the host cells are analogous to those described for oncogenic RNA viruses.

After the replication of DNA and RNA viruses, the release of viruses may occur after lysis of the host cell or by "budding" from the cell. The latter process is less harmful to the host cell. Released particles may infect adjacent cells immediately or be carried by tissue body fluids, lymph, or blood to distant cells, where the infectious cycle is repeated. By this sequence, a large number of infected cells are formed, leading to transformation of normal cells to cancer cells.

Virus Properties (7)

Viruses are microscopic organisms that can infect all living cells. They are parasitic in nature and multiply at the expense of the host's metabolic system. Viruses may start their infectious cycle immediately on attack or remain dormant in the cellular site of the host for extended periods until an etiologic agent triggers them to reproduce. Once the viral become active, they may produce cytotoxic effects or cause numerous diseases in animals and humans. The major routes of transmission of viral infections in humans are through the respiratory, gastrointestinal (GI) and genital tracts, skin, urine, blood, and placenta. Viral infections may occur through air, water, food, milk, or environmental sources. Whether the host survives the effects of the viral infection depends on the immune response of the host and also on the severity and type of infection. Immune response is obtained by the production of B lymphocytes derived from the bone marrow and T lymphocytes derived from the thymus with the help of macrophages. Specific immune response to viral diseases depends on antibodies formed by humoral (B cells), local (secretory IgA system), and cell-mediated (T cell) immunities. Discussion of immunizing biologics and virus-specific immunoglobulins that provide active and passive immunity is beyond the scope of this chapter. To understand the mechanisms of antiviral chemotherapy, however, some aspects of viral characteristics are reviewed, including viral replication and transformation of cells. Detailed information on the molecular biology of viruses is found in the suggested readings.

Viral Diseases (8,9)

Many diseases are produced by the different groups of DNA- and RNA-containing viruses (Table 39.1). The herpes group of viruses, namely herpes simplex virus (HSV), varicella-zoster virus (VZV), cytomegalovirus (CMV), and Epstein-Barr (EB) virus primarily cause ocular viral diseases. Herpetic keratoconjunctivitis, a serious infection of the eye caused by the HSV, is the leading cause of corneal blindness in the United States. Herpes zoster (shingles) is a severe skin infection affecting mostly the elderly. It is caused by the VZV that also causes chickenpox. Herpes zoster is the reactivated form of the VZV infection. The virus enters the sensory nerve endings in the skin and re-

mains dormant until reactivation. Varicella infection is also considered a minor form of smallpox (variola).

The herpes labialis (common cold sore) virus often lies dormant in early life, but may affect the mucous membrane, skin, eye, and genital tract in later life. CMV, HSV, and rubella virus produces chronic intrauterine and perinatal infections. Several viruses, such as EB virus, mumps, smallpox, CMV, HSV, viral hepatitis A and B, and togaviruses are responsible for systemic and viral infections of immunosuppressed patients. Herpes simplex virus types 1 (HSV-1) and 2 (HSV-2) are also involved in localized diseases of the skin.

Acute respiratory diseases are the most common manifestation of viral infections. Both DNA (adenovirus) and RNA viruses (influenza, parainfluenza, picornavirus, herpesvirus, and oncornavirus) are involved in respiratory diseases. Viruses are also associated with such diseases as viral rhinitis, pharyngitis, laryngitis, laryngotracheo-bronchitis, influenza, parainfluenza, and respiratory syncytial virus (RSV) pneumonia. Diseases of the nervous system include poliomyelitis, rabies, and meningoencephalitis associated with mumps, measles, vaccinia, and "slow" viral infections.

Viruses are also linked with various other diseases, such as rheumatoid arthritis, multiple sclerosis, diabetes mellitus, cancer of the cervix, certain heart diseases, hepatitis, and acquired immunodeficiency syndrome (AIDS). The

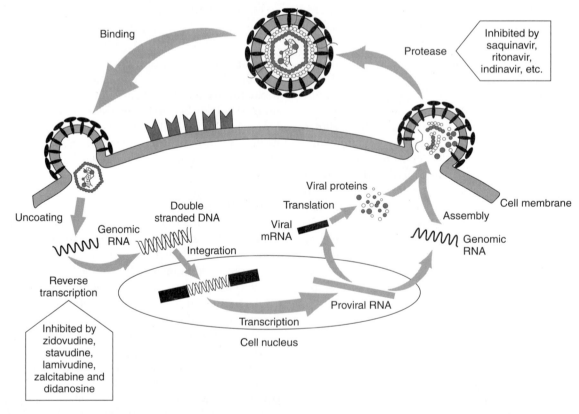

Fig. 39.2. The life cycle of HIV and the site of action of nelfinavir and other antiretroviral agents. PI = protease inhibitors (e.g., nelfinavir, indinavir, ritonavir, saquinavir); RTI = reverse transcriptase inhibitors (e.g., didanosine, lamivudine, stavudine, zalcitabine, zidovudine, efavirenz, delviradine, nevirapine). Reproduced with permission from Adis International Ltd., New Zealand from original article by M. Barry in Clinical Pharmacokinetics 1997, 32(3):194–209.

Table 39.1. Viruses Infecting Animals and Humans

Virus Group	Species	Disease
DNA-Containing Viruses		
Adenovirus*	Many types	Respiratory tract and eye infections (keratitis)
Herpesvirus	Herpes simplex virus types 1 and 2	Encephalitis, eye infections(keratoconjunctivitis), skin diseases, genital infections
	Varicella-zoster(Varicella)	Chickenpox (children)
	Herpes zoster	Shingles (adults)
	Cytomegalovirus	Cytomegalovirus diseases (mononucleosis), hepatitis (animals and humans), Marek's virus disease (avian leukemias)
	Epstein-Barr virus (EBV)	Epstein-Barr virus associated diseases (infectious mononucleosis, Burkitt's lymphoma, nasopharyngeal carcinoma), acute hepatitis as a complication
Papovavirus†	Human wart virus	Animal and human warts
	Polyoma virus	Salivary gland (parotid) infection, progressive
	SV 40	Multifocal leukoencephalopathy (PML) in human
Poxvirus	Variola	Smallpox (variola), cowpox (vaccinia), chickenpox,
	Vaccinia	infectious mononucleosis, eczema
RNA-Containing Viruses		
Arenavirus	Lymphocytic chorio-meningitis (LCM) virus	Lymphocytic choriomeningitis (LCM), Lassa fever, hemorrhagic fever
	Lassa fever virus	
Orthomyxovirus	Influenza A, B, and C viruses	Influenza A, B, and C
Paramyxovirus	Parainfluenza virus	Mumps, measles, parainfluenza (pneumonia, bronchiolitis)
	Respiratory syncytial virus	
	Measles (rubeola)	
Picornavirus	Rhinoviruses	Respiratory diseases, GI diseases, poliomyelitis, aseptic meningitis
	Enteroviruses (polio, coxsackie A, B,echovirus)	
Reovirus	Human reovirus (rotavirus)	Mild respiratory and GI symptoms
Retrovirus (Oncornavirus)	Human T-cell lymphotropic viruses (type C viruses)	Leukemia, lymphoma and sarcoma in animals (birds, cats, rodents, cows, gibbon apes etc.), mouse mammary tumor, human breast cancer, human T-cell leukemia, nasopharyngeal carcinoma
	B-type viruses	Mouse mammary tumor
	D-type viruses	Simian AIDS, monkey AIDS
	Human immuno deficiency virus type 1 (HIV-1, HTLV III/LAV) and type 2	Acquired immunodeficiency syndrome (AIDS) and AIDS-related complex (ARC)
Rhabdovirus	Rabies virus	Rabies, encephalitis
Togavirus	Encephalitis virus	Rubella (German measles), meningoencephalititis
	Rubella virus	encephalitis, hepatitis, yellow fever and sand fly fever
	Arbovirus	
Unclassified Hepatitis	Hepatitis A, B and C viruses	Hepatitis

*Adenoviruses were originally isolated from humans (children and throats of patients with respiratory diseases).
†Papovaviruses are derived from the names of papilloma, polyoma, and vacuolating viruses. Modified and adapted from G. J. Galasso, et al., eds., Antiviral agents and human viral diseases, New York, Raven Press, 1997, and W. L. Drew, ed., Viral infections, a clinical approach, Philadelphia, F. A. Davis, 1976.

latter usually has an associated opportunistic infection caused by bacteria, fungi and mycobacteria. However, the prime candidate involved in AIDS is the human T-cell lymphotropic virus (HTLV-III/LAV), currently known as human immunodeficiency virus (HIV) type 1 (HIV-1). Also, HIV type 2 (HIV-2) is involved in AIDS, which is spread by sexual contact, blood transfusion, blood-derived products, intravenous drug users or through intrauterine transmission (10). AIDS has become a significant health problem because of its fatal nature and lack of permanent cure.

Common to the HIV infections is the significant depletion of CD4 cells (helper, inducer) a subset of T-lympho-cytes. Monitoring CD4 cell counts is a measure of disease progression and success of drug therapy.

VIRAL DRUG THERAPY
General Approaches (11,12)

Because viruses are obligate intracellular parasites, their replication depends on the host's cellular processes. Ideally, a useful drug is considered most effective if it interferes with the viral replication without affecting normal cellular metabolic processes. Unfortunately, this objective has not been achieved with many antiviral compounds. Many of the early drugs have proven toxic to humans at therapeutic levels or had a limited spectrum of activity.

The lack of early success has been one reason why antiviral drugs have not been developed as rapidly as antibacterial, antiprotozoal, or antifungal agents. Despite much research on the molecular biology of viruses and understanding of the complexity of the virus-host interaction, few antiviral agents have been successful. Therefore, only licensed drugs are discussed in detail. In most viral infections, immunity of the specific host cell is not fully understood. Unfortunately, specific symptoms produced by viral infection may not appear until viral replication is complete or viral infection has already induced severe and sometimes irreversible changes in the infected cells. Because of this latent period, it may be difficult to determine the effectiveness of antiviral drugs. Administration of the antiviral agents may often be too late to inhibit a particular step of viral infection or to prevent host cells from performing abnormal functions. Perhaps because of these limitations and the life-long effects of viral vaccines, immunizing biologics rather than antiviral agents have been sought for the prevention of viral infections.

Because of the unique properties of viruses and the need for host cell metabolic activities, antiviral agents have been developed to act at various stages in the viral replication cycle, such as attachment, replication and release of virus. General approaches for treating viral infection by antiviral agents are:

1. Inhibition or interference of virus attachment to host cell receptor, virus penetration and uncoating.
2. Inhibition of virus-associated enzymes, such as DNA polymerases and others.
3. Inhibition of transcription processes.
4. Inhibition of translation processes.
5. Interference with viral regulatory proteins.
6. Interference with glucosylation, phosphorylation, sulfation etc.
7. Interference with assembly of viral proteins.
8. Interference with release of virus from cell surface membrane.

This chapter deals with antiviral agents that have been approved by the United States Food and Drug Administration (FDA) and are clinically effective in viral infections. Antiviral agents with specific activity against HIV are called anti-AIDS agents. They are discussed under antiretroviral (anti-HIV) agents and this includes protease inhibitors. Immunizing biologics and specific antineoplastic agents are not covered in this chapter. However, some important experimental antiviral agents are discussed under investigational antiviral agents. The medicinal agents that are used for viral infections are broadly grouped as virucidal (infection of intact viruses), antiviral (inhibition of viral replication at the cellular level) or immunomodulators (modification of the host's response to infection).

Antibiotics are used primarily in the treatment of bacterial infections, but some also inhibit viral replication. For example, rifamycin derivatives (rifampicin) were reported to inhibit the growth of poxviruses and aden-

oviruses, probably by blocking envelope formation or preventing release of infectious virions. Similarly, other antibiotics, such as bleomycin, adriamycin, and actinomycin D inhibited RNA tumor viruses and DNA and RNA-directed polymerases *in vitro*. Because these antibiotics do not interfere with the transcription or translation of viral mRNA, and because large concentrations of the drug were required to inhibit the growth of viruses, such antibiotics are not commonly used specifically for viral infections. Some natural and synthetic agents are inhibitors of RT activity but have limited use in the chemotherapy of viral infections due to cytotoxicity (13). The antibiotics are discussed in Chapter 38.

HIV RT and proteases play an important role in the HIV life cycle (14). These enzymes direct the infected cells to produce viral proteins and assembly of viral particles. HIV protease releases viral particles by a budding process from the infected cells. In order to treat HIV infection, drugs acting at different stages of HIV cell cycle are used. Basically, two types of anti-HIV drugs are used. One type belongs to RT inhibitors and the second is called protease inhibitors (PIs). The latter block the formation and release of viral particles from the infected cells. The drugs that inhibit HIV RT and proteases are shown in Figure 39.2. Although, each type of drug is used to treat AIDS, the combination of RT inhibitors and PIs are beneficial in decreasing the viral load to a negligible limit. A combination (cocktail) treatment consisting of triple anti-HIV drugs including one or two PIs has (have) an optimal antiretroviral effect(s). Such treatment has increased survival rate and awareness of compliance of drug therapy. However, it is suggested that an anti-HIV treatment should be started as early as possible. The measurements of viral load, tolerability and pharmacokinetics of drugs are some of the factors in the management of AIDS patients.

DRUG THERAPY (15,16)

Antiviral agents must be developed because viral vaccines, although successful in preventing some viral diseases, are not effective as curative measures. Because viruses direct the host cell to synthesize enzymes and proteins for their own growth and multiplication, inhibition of such processes and development of antiviral drugs with selective toxicity to viruses are important. An effective antiviral agent should have broad-spectrum antiviral activity and completely inhibit viral replication. It should also be able to reach the target organ without interfering with the immune system of the patient. In addition, it should have minimal toxicity to the host cells and be effective against resistant mutant viruses.

Anti-HIV drugs, as previously indicated, are mainly classified as RT inhibitors or PIs. Drugs arresting translation, glycosylation and immunomodulators for treatment of AIDS patients are under development. The antiviral agents are classified and used according to their mode of action and stage of infection. They act by preventing virus penetration and uncoating, inhibiting different stages of viral replication, interfering with viral nucleic acid replication or affecting ribosomal translation. Successful development of antiviral agents for clinical use must take into consideration factors such as underlying diseases and immunity of the host, age of the patient, severity of infection, dosage and pharmacokinetics of drug, toxicity and resistance of virus in order to be successful.

NH₂

Amantadine

Antiviral Agents (17,18)
Agents Inhibiting Virus Attachment, Penetration and Early Viral Replication
Amantadine

Mechanism of Action. Amantadine hydrochloride (1-adamantanamine hydrochloride) is a symmetric tricyclic primary amine that inhibits penetration of RNA virus particles into the host cell (19). It also inhibits the early stages of viral replication, blocking the uncoating of the viral genome and the transferring of nucleic acid into the host cell.

Clinical Application. Amantadine is effective clinically in preventing and treating all A strains of influenza, particularly A2 strains of Asian influenza virus, and to a lesser extent, German measles (rubella) or atoga virus. It also shows *in vitro* activity against influenza B, parainfluenza (paramyxovirus), RSV, and some RNA viruses (murine, Rous, and Esh sarcoma viruses). Many prototype influenza A viruses of different human subtypes (H1N1, Fort Dix, H2N2, Asian type and H3N2, Hongkong type) are also inhibited by amantadine hydrochloride *in vitro* and in animal model systems. If given within the first 48 hours of onset of symptoms, amantadine hydrochloride is effective in respiratory tract illness resulting from influenza A but not influenza B virus infection, adenoviruses and RSV.

Pharmacokinetics. Amantadine is well absorbed orally and the usual dosage for oral administration is 100 mg twice daily. The drug has been approved as capsule, tablet, and syrup for the treatment of HSV infection (keratoconjunctivitis) (Table 39.2). Amantadine hydrochloride oral solution should not be kept in a freezer. It should be stored in a tight container at 15–30°C. Capsules and tablets should be protected from moisture and light. A 100 mg oral dose produces blood serum levels of 0.3 μg/mL within 1–8 hours. Maximum tissue concentration is reached in 48 hours when a 100 mg dose is given every 12 hours. In healthy adults receiving 25, 100 or 150 mg dose of the drug twice daily, steady-state trough plasma concentrations were 110, 302 or 588 mg/mL, respectively. Usually, no neurotoxicity is observed if the plasma level of amantadine is no more than 1.00 μg/mL.

Amantadine crosses the blood-brain barrier and is distributed in saliva, nasal secretions, and breast milk (20). Approximately 90% of the drug is excreted unchanged by the kidney, primarily through glomerular filtration and tubular secretion and there are no reports of metabolic products. Acidification of urine increases the rate of amantadine excretion. The half-life of the drug is 15–20 hours in patients with normal renal function.

Side Effects. Generally, the drug has low toxicity at therapeutic levels but may cause severe central nervous system (CNS) symptoms such as nervousness, confusion, headache, drowsiness, insomnia, depression, and hallucinations. GI side effects include nausea, diarrhea, constipation and anorexia. Convulsions and coma occur with high doses and in patients with cerebral arteriosclerosis and convulsive disorders. Chronic toxicity with amantadine is unexpected since few side effects have been experienced when the drug has been used for long term therapy for Parkinson's disease. Some serious reactions, however, include depression, orthostatic hypotension, psychosis, urinary retention, and congestive heart failure. Amantadine hydrochloride should be used with caution in patients who have a history of epilepsy, severe arteriosclerosis, liver diseases and eczematoid dermatitis. Be-

Table 39.2. Antiviral Agents Interfering with Cellular Penetration and Early Replication

Generic Name	Trade Name	Spectrum of Activity	Dosage Form (mg/unit)
Amantadine	Symmetrel	Influenza A	Cap (100), Syrup (50/5 ml)
Rimantadine	Flumadine	Influenza A	Cap (100)
Interferon			
Interferon α-2a	Roferon A	Unlabeled use:	Inj (3,5,10,18,25,50
	Alferon	Chronic hepatitis, CMV,	million units/ml)
	Intron	HSV, Pappillomaviruses,	
	Wellferon	Rhinovirses, others	
Interferon α-2b	Interon A	Chronic hepatitis B	Inj (3,5,10,18,25,50
		and C, Unlabeled: many	million (units/ml)
		virus infections	
γ-Interferon	Actimmune		Inj (100 mcg/0.5ml)
Zanamivir	Relenza	Influenza A; Influenza B	Inhalation (5mg powder)
Oseltamivir	Tamiflu	Influenza A; Influenza B	Cap (75)

cause amantadine does not appear to interfere with the immunogenicity of inactivated influenza A virus vaccine, patients may continue the use of amantadine for 1 week after influenza A vaccination. A virus resistant to amantadine has been obtained in cell culture and from animals, but these reports are not confirmed in humans.

$$H_2N \quad CH_3$$

·HCl

Rimantadine

Rimantadine

Mechanism of Action. Rimantadine hydrochloride (α-methyl-1-adamantanemethylamine hydrochloride), is a synthetic adamatane derivative, which is structurally and pharmacologically related to amantadine (21). It appears more effective than amantadine hydrochloride against influenza A virus with fewer CNS side effects. Rimantadine hydrochloride appears to interfere with virus uncoating by inhibiting release of specific proteins. It may act by inhibiting RT or the synthesis of virus-specific RNA but does not inhibit virus adsorption or penetration. It appears to produce a virustatic effect early in the virus replication. It is used widely in Russia and Europe.

Clinical Application. Rimantadine hydrochloride has activity against most strains of influenza A including H1N1, H2N2 and H3N2 but has no activity against influenza B virus. It is used for prevention of infection caused by various human, animal, or avian strains of influenza A virus in adults and children. The side effects are nightmares, hallucinations, and vomiting. The most common side effects of rimantadine are associated with CNS and GI tract. Rimantadine is metabolized in the liver and about 20% is excreted unchanged as hydroxylated compound.

Pharmacokinetics. The half-life of rimantadine in adults ranges from 24–36 hours. Over 90% of rimantadine doses were absorbed in 3–6 hours. Steady-state plasma concentrations are from 0.10–2.60 μg/mL at doses of 3 mg/kg/d in infants to 100 mg twice daily in the elderly. Nasal fluid concentrations of rimantadine at steady state were 1.5 times higher than plasma concentration.

Interferon (22,23).

Isaacs and Lindenmann discovered interferon in 1957. When they infected cells with viruses, viral interference was observed. Interferon was isolated and found to protect the cells from further infection. When interferon was administered to other cells or animals, it displayed biologic properties such as inhibition of viral growth, cell multiplication, and immunomodulatory activities. The results led to the speculation that interferon may be a natural antiviral factor, possibly formed before antibody production, and may be involved in the normal mechanism of resistance displayed against viral infection. Some investiga-

tors relate interferon to the polypeptide hormones and suggest that interferon functions in cell-to-cell communication by transmitting specific messages. Recently, antitumor and anticancer properties of interferon have evoked worldwide interest in the possible use of this agent in therapy for viral diseases, cancer, and immunodeficiency disorders. Host cells in response to various inducers synthesize interferons.

Interferon Induction. Because viruses were found to induce release of interferon, the production or release of interferon in humans was attempted by the administration of chemical "inducers" (24). Various small molecules (substituted propanediamine) and large polymers (double-stranded polynucleotides) were used to induce interferons. Statolon, a natural double-stranded RNA produced in *Penicillium stoloniferum* culture, and a double-stranded complex of polyriboinosinic acid and polyribocytidylic acid (poly I:C) have been used as nonviral inducers for releasing preformed interferons. A modification of poly I:C stabilized with poly-L-lysine and carboxymethylcellulose (poly ICLC) has been used experimentally in humans. Clinically, it prevented coryza when used locally in the nose and conjunctival sacs. This substance was found to be a better interferon inducer than poly I:C. Another interferon inducer is ampligen, a polynucleotide derivative of poly I:C with spaced uridines. It has anti-HIV activity *in vitro* and is an immunomodulator.

Tilorone

Other chemical inducers, such as pyran copolymers, tilorone, diethylaminoethyl dextran, and heparin, have also been used. Tilorone is an effective inducer of interferon in mice but it is relatively ineffective in humans. Initial use of interferon and its inducers instilled intranasally after rhinovirus exposure was successful in the prevention of respiratory diseases. The clinical success of interferon and its inducers has not yet been established, although they may play a significant role in cell-mediated immunity to viral infections and cancer. Disadvantages of interferon use include unacceptable side effects, such as fever, headache, myalgias, leukopenia, nausea, vomiting, diarrhea, hypotension, alopecia, anorexia, and weight loss.

Interferon Structure. Interferon consists of a mixture of small proteins with molecular weights ranging from 20,000–160,000. They are glycoproteins that exhibit species-specific antiviral activity. Human interferons are classified into three types (25): alpha (α), beta (β), and gamma (γ). The α-type is secreted by human leukocytes (white blood cells, non-T-lymphocytes) and the β-type secreted by human fibroblasts. Lymphoid cells (T lymphocytes) secrete the alpha type of interferon, which either have been exposed to a presensitized antigen or have been stimulated to divide by mitogen. γ-Interferon is also called "immune" interferon. Interferons are active in extremely low concentrations.

Clinical Application. Interferon has been tested for use in chronic hepatitis B virus infection, herpetic keratitis, herpes genitalis, herpes zoster, varicella-zoster, chronic hepatitis, influenza, and common cold infections. Other uses of interferon are in the treatment of cancers, such as breast cancer, lung carcinoma, and multiple myeloma. Interferon has had some success when used as a prophylactic agent for CMV infection in renal transplant recipients. The scarcity of interferon and the difficulty in purifying it have limited clinical trials. Supplies have been augmented by recombinant DNA technology, which allows cloning of the interferon gene (26), although the high cost still hinders clinical application (Chapter 40). The FDA has approved recombinant interferon α-2a (Table 39.2), α-2b and γ-interferon for the treatment of hairy cell leukemia (a rare form of cancer), AIDS-related Kaposi's sarcoma, and genital warts (condyloma acuminatum). Subcutaneous injection of recombinant interferon α-2b has been approved for the treatment of chronic hepatitis C. Some foreign countries have approved α-interferon for the treatment of cancers such as multiple myeloma (cancer of plasma cells), malignant melanoma (skin cancer), and Kaposi's sarcoma (cancer associated with AIDS). Both β- and γ-interferons, and interleukin-2 may be commercial drugs of the future for the treatment of cancers and viral infections, including genital warts and the common cold.

Mechanism of Action. Although, interferons are mediators of immune response, different mechanisms for the antiviral action of interferon have been proposed. Alpha interferon possesses broad-spectrum antiviral activity, it acts on virus-infected cells by binding to the specific cell surface receptors. It inhibits the transcription and translation of mRNA into viral nucleic acid and protein. Studies in cell free systems have shown that the addition of adenosine triphosphate and double-stranded RNA to extracts of interferon-treated cells activates cellular RNA proteins and a cellular endonuclease. This activation causes the formation of translation inhibitory protein, which terminates production of viral enzyme, nucleic acid, and structural proteins (27). Interferon may also act by blocking synthesis of a cleaving enzyme required for viral release.

Pharmacokinetics. The pharmacokinetics of interferon is not well understood. Maximum levels in blood after intramuscular injection was obtained in 5–8 hours. Interferon does not penetrate well into cerebrospinal fluid (CSF). Oral administration of interferon does not indicate a detectable serum level thereby oral administration is not used clinically. After intramuscular or subcutaneous injection, drug concentration in plasma is dose related. Clinical use

of interferon is limited to topical administration (nasal sprays) for prophylaxis and treatment of rhinovirus infections. Adverse reactions and toxicity include influenza-like syndrome of fever, chills, headache, myalgias, nausea, vomiting, diarrhea, bone marrow suppression, mental confusion and behavioral changes. Intranasal administration produces mucosal friability, ulceration and dryness.

Neuraminidase Inhibitors (28). Influenza viruses are surrounded by a protein coat and a lipid envelop. Embedded in the lipid membrane are two surface glycoproteins: hemagglutinin (HA) an enzyme important for binding viruses to target cell receptors via a terminal sialic acid residue and neuraminidase (NA) an enzyme involved in various aspects of activation of influenza viruses. NA is found in both influenza A and B viruses and is thought to be involved in catalytically cleaving glycosidic bonds between a terminal sialic acid and an adjacent sugar. The cleavage of sialic acid bonds facilitates the spread of viruses and as a result increases the infectiveness or pathogenicity of the virus. In the absence of this cleavage, viral aggregation or binding to hemagglutinin will occur interfering with the spread of the infection. In addition, NA appears to be involved in preventing viral inactivation by respiratory mucus and induction of cytokine elaboration. When the new viruses are released from an infected cell (shed) the viruses are coated with sialic acid. The viruses are bound to the NA through the sialic acid and the NA cleaves the sialic acid moiety.

Mechanism of Action. Since NA plays such an important role in the activation of newly formed viruses, it is not surprising that the development of NA inhibitors has become an important potential means of inhibiting the spread of viral infections. X-ray crystalography of NA has shown that while the amino acid sequence in the NA from various viruses is considerably different, the sialic acid binding site is quite similar for type A and B influenza virus. In addition, it is believed that the hydrolysis of sialic acid proceeds through a oxonium cation stabilitized carbonium ion as shown in Figure 39.3. Mimicking the transition state with novel carbocyclic derivatives of sialic acid has led to the development of transition-state-based inhibitors (29). The first of such compounds, 2-deoxy-2,3-dehydro-N-acetylneuraminic acid (DANA, Fig. 39.4), was found to be an active neuraminidase inhibitor but lacked specificity for viral neuraminidase. Upon determination of the crystal structure of neuraminidase, more sophisticated measurements of the binding site for sialic acid lead to the development of zanamivir and later oseltamivir.

Zanamivir. Crystallographic studies of DANA bound to NA defined the receptor site to which the sialic acid portion of the virus binds. These studies suggested that substitution of the 4-hydroxy with an amino group or the larger guanidino group should increase binding of the inhibitor to NA. The 4-amino derivative was found to bind

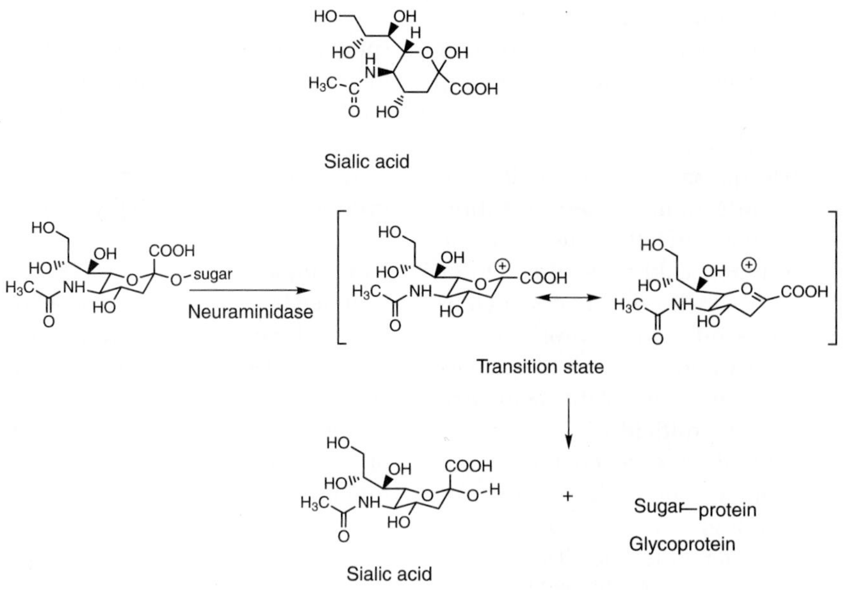

Fig. 39.3. Sialic acid hydrolysis catalyzed by neuraminidase.

to a glutamic acid (Glu 119) in the receptor through a salt bridge while the guanidino was able to form both a salt bridge to Glu 119 and a charge-charge interaction with a glutamic acid at position 227. The result of these substitutions was a dramatic increase in binding capacity of the amino and guanidino derivatives to NA leading to effective competitive inhibition of the enzyme. The result has been the development of zanamivir as an effective antiviral agent against influenza A and B virus.

Zanamirvir is effective when administered via the nasal, intraperitoneal, and intravenous routes, but is inactive when given orally (Table 39.2). Animal studies have shown 68% recovery of the drug in the urine following intraperitoneal administration, 43% urinary recovery following nasal administration and only 3% urinary recovery following oral administration. Human data gave similar results to those obtained in animal models. Human efficacy studies with nasal drops or sprays demonstrated that the drug was effective when administered before exposure and after exposure to influenza A or B virus. When given before viral inoculation, the drug reduced viral shedding, infection, and symptoms. When administered beginning at either 26 or 32 hours after inoculation there was a reduction in shedding, viral titre, and fibrile illness. Presently the drug is available as a dry powder for oral inhalation by adults and adolescents who have been symptomatic for no more than 2 days. Zanamirvir is able to more rapidly resolve influenza symptoms and improve recovery (from 7 days with placebo to 4 days with treatment). Additional studies have suggested the prophylactic benefit of zanamirvir when administered to family members after one member of the family developed flu-like symptoms. As a result, the manufacturer has submitted an application for the use of the drug for the prevention of influenza A and B.

Oseltamivir Phosphate. X-ray crystallographic studies further demonstrated that additional binding sites exist between NA and substrate involving the C-5 acetamido carbonyl and an arginine (Arg 152), the C-2 carboxyl and arginines as 118, 292, and 371, and the potential for hydrophobic binding to substituents at C-6 (with glutamic acid, alanine, arginine, and isoleucine) (Fig. 39.5). Structure-activity relationship studies showed that maximum binding occured to NA when C-6 was substituted with the 3-pentyloxy side chain as found in oseltamivir. In addition, esterification with ethanol gave rise to a compound which was orally effective. Oseltamivir was approved as the first orally administered NA inhibitor used against influenza A and B (Table 39.2). The drug is indicated for the treatment of uncomplicated acute illness due to influenza infection.

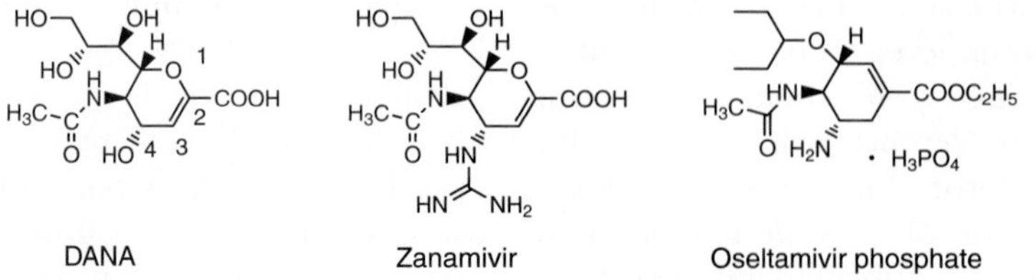

Fig. 39.4. Structural derivatives of sialic acid as neuraminidase inhibitors.

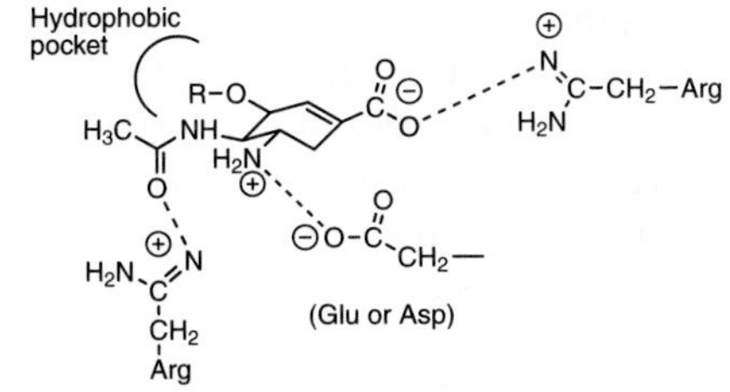

Fig. 39.5. Receptor binding for the transition-state-based carbocyclic sialic acid analogs.

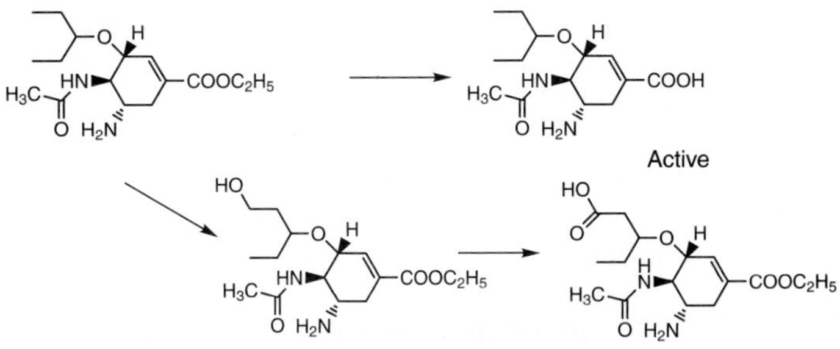

Fig. 39.6. Metabolism of oseltamivir.

Recently, the manufacturer has submitted a request for approval of the drug for prevention of influenza A and B for use in adults, adolescents, and children one year of age and older. The drug is effective in treating the flu if administered within 2 days after onset of symptoms. The recommended dose is 75mg twice daily for 5 days. The prophylactic dose is 75mg taken once daily for 7 days. Oseltamivir is readily absorbed from the GI tract following oral administration. Oseltamivir is a pro-drug which is extensively metabolized in the liver undergoing ester hydrolysis to the active carboxylic acid (Fig. 39.6). Two oxidative metabolites have also been isolated with the major oxidation product being the ω-carboxylic acid shown in Figure 39.6 (30).

Side effects with oseltamivir are minor and consist of nausea and vomiting and occur in the first two days of therapy.

Agents Interfering with Viral Nucleic Acid Replication (Table 39.3)

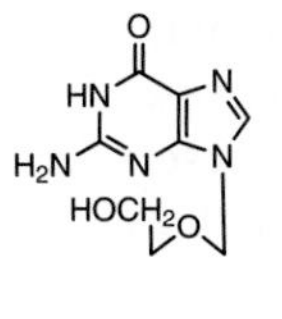

Acyclovir
(9-[(2-Hydroxyethoxy)methyl]guanine)

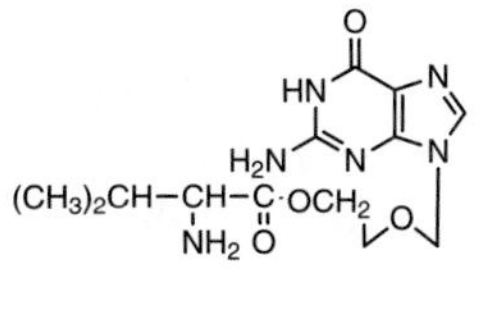

Valacyclovir

Acyclovir and Valacyclovir

Mechanism of Action. Acyclovir is a synthetic analogue of deoxyguanosine in which the carbohydrate moiety is acyclic (31). Because of this difference in structure as compared to other antiviral compounds (idoxuridine, vidarabine, and trifluridine), acyclovir possesses a unique mechanism of antiviral activity. The mode of action of acyclovir consists of three consecutive mechanisms (32) that are: (1) conversion to active acyclovir monophosphate within cells by viral thymidine kinase (Fig. 39.7). This phosphorylation reaction occurs faster by cells infected by herpesvirus than by normal cells because acyclovir is a poor substrate for the normal cell thymidine kinase. Acyclovir is further converted to di- and triphosphates by a normal cellular enzyme called guanosine monophosphate kinase. (2) Viral DNA polymerase is competitively inhibited by acyclovir triphosphate at lower concentrations than is cellular DNA polymerase. Acyclovir triphosphate is incorporated into the viral DNA chain during DNA synthesis. Because acyclovir triphosphate lacks the 3′-hydroxyl group of a cyclic sugar, it terminates further elongation of the DNA chain. (3) Preferential uptake of

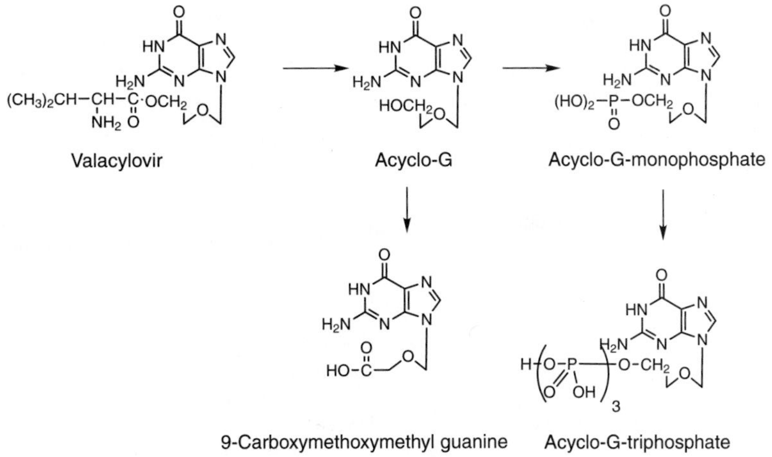

Valacylovir

Acyclo-G

Acyclo-G-monophosphate

9-Carboxymethoxymethyl guanine

Acyclo-G-triphosphate

Fig. 39.7. Metabolic reactions of valacyclovir and acyclovir (acyclo-G).

acyclovir by herpes-infected cells as compared to uninfected cells results in a higher concentration of acyclovir triphosphate, which leads to a high ratio of therapeutic value to toxicity ratio of herpes-infected cells to normal cells. Acyclovir is active against certain herpes virus infections. These viruses induce virus-specific thymidine kinase and DNA polymerase, which are inhibited by acyclovir. Thus, acyclovir significantly reduces DNA synthesis in virus-infected cells without disturbing the active replication of uninfected cells.

Clinical Application. Acyclovir has potent activity against several DNA viruses including HSV-1, the common cause of labial herpes (cold sore) and HSV-2, common cause of genital herpes (33). VZV and some isolates of EB viruses are affected to lesser extent by acyclovir. On the other hand, CMV is less sensitive to acyclovir, which has no activity against vaccinia virus, adenovirus, and parainfluenza infections.

An ointment containing 5% acyclovir has been used in a regimen of five times a day for up to 14 days for the treatment of herpetic keratitis and primary and recurrent infections of herpes genitalis; mild pain, transient burning, stinging, pruritus, rash, and vulvitis have been noted. The FDA has approved topical and intravenous (IV) acyclovir preparations for initial herpes genitalis and HSV-1 and HSV-2 infections in immunocompromised patients (34).

In these individuals, early use of acyclovir shortens the duration of viral shedding and lesion pain. Oral doses of 200 mg of acyclovir, taken five times a day for 5–10 days, have not proven successful because of the low bioavailability of current preparations. Oral doses of 800 mg of the drug given five times daily for 7–10 days have been approved by the FDA for treatment of herpes zoster infection. This treatment shortens the duration of viral shedding in chickenpox and shingles. The IV injection of the drug

(given 10 mg/kg three times daily for 10–12 days) has been approved for the treatment of herpes simplex encephalitis (35). Excessive and high doses of acyclovir have, however, caused viruses to develop resistance to the drug. This resistance results from reduction of virus-encoded thymidine kinase, which does not effectively activate the drug.

Acyclovir Pro-drug

6-Deoxyacyclovir is a pro-drug form of acyclovir which is rapidly metabolized to acyclovir by xanthine oxidase. This drug has the advantage of improved solubility.

6-Deoxyacyclovir

6-Deoxyacyclovir is used in the treatment of varicella-zoster infection.

Pharmacokinetics. Pharmacokinetic studies show that IV dose administration of 2.5 mg/kg, acyclovir results in peak plasma concentrations of 3.4–6.8 mg/mL (36,37). The bioavailability of acyclovir is 15–30%. It is metabolized to 9-carboxymethoxymethylguanine, which is inactive. Plasma protein binding averages 15%, and approximately 70% of acyclovir is excreted unchanged in the urine by both glomerular filtration and tubular secretion. The half-life of the drug is approximately 3 hours in patients with normal renal function. In an individual with renal diseases, the half-life of the drug is prolonged. Therefore, acyclovir dosage adjustment is necessary for patients with renal impairment. Because of its low molecular weight and protein binding, acyclovir is easily dialyzed. Thus, a full dose of the drug should be given after

Table 39.3. Antiviral Agents Interfering with Viral Nucleic Acid Replication

Generic Name	Common Name	Trade Name	Spectrum of Activity	Dosage Form (mg/unit)
Acyclovir	Acyclo-G	Zovirax	HSV-1; HSV-2; VZV; EB	5% Oint, Inj (5 mg/ml), Cap (200), Tab (400,800), Susp (200/5ml)
Valacyclovir		Valtrex	HSV-1; VZV; CMV;	Tab (500)
Cidofovir	HPMPC	Vistide	CMV; HSV-1; HSV-2; VZV; CMV; EBV	Inj (75/ml)
Cytarabine	Ara-C	Cytosar	Herpes Zoster	Inj (10,20,50,100/ml)
Famciclovir	FCV	Famvir	HSV; VZV; EB; Chronic HBV	Tab (125,250,500)
Fomivirsen		Vitravene	CMV retinitis;	Inj. (6.6/ml)
Foscarnet	PFA	Foscavir	CMV retinitis; HSV; VZV;	Inj (24/ml)
Ganciclovir	DHPG	Cytovene Vitrasert	CMV retinitis	Inj (50/ml), Cap (250,500) Insert (4.5/insert)
Idoxuridine	5-IUDR	Herplex	HSV keratitis	0.1% sol, 0.5% Oint.
Ribavirin		Virazole	RSV; Influenza A & B; HIV-1; Parainfluenza	Aerosol (20/ml)
Trifluoro-thymidine	TFT F3T	Viroptic	HSV-1	1% Sol.
Vidarabine	Ara-A	Vira A	HSV-1; HSV-2	3% Oint. (monohydrate)

hemodialysis. It should be infused slowly over at least 30 minutes to avoid acute transient and reversible renal failure. Acyclovir easily penetrates the lung, brain, muscle, spleen, uterus, vaginal mucosa, intestine, liver, and kidney. Acyclovir has relatively few side effects, except that IV injection causes reversible renal dysfunction and irritation, inflammation, and pain at the injection site. Infusion sites should therefore be inspected frequently and changed after every 72 hours. The drug is slightly toxic to bone marrow at higher doses. Less frequent side effects are nausea, vomiting, headache, skin rashes, hematuria, arthralgia, and insomnia.

Valacyclovir hydrochloride is an amino acid ester prodrug of acyclovir, which exhibits antiviral activity only after metabolism first in the intestine walls or liver to acyclovir and then conversion to the triphosphate as shown in Figure 39.7 (38). Structurally, it differs from acyclovir by the presence of the amino acid, valine, attached to the 5'-hydroxyl group of the nucleoside. Valacyclovir's benefit comes from an increased GI absorption resulting in a higher plasma concentrations of acyclovir, which is normally poorly absorbed from the GI tract. As with acyclovir, valacyclovir is active against HSV-1, VZV and CMV because of its affinity for the enzyme thymidine kinase encoded by the viruses. Oral valacyclovir is used for the treatment of acute, localized herpes zoster (shingles) in immunocompetent patients and may be given without meals. It is also used for the initial and recurrent episodes of genital herpes infections. The adverse effects are similar to acyclovir, which include nausea, headache, vomiting, constipation and anorexia. The binding of valacyclovir to human plasma proteins ranged between 13.5–17.9%. The plasma elimination half-life of acyclovir is 2.5–3.3 hours. The bioavailability of valacyclovir hydrochloride is 54% compared to approximately 20% for oral acyclovir. It is as effective as acyclovir in decreasing the duration of pain associated with post-therapeutic neuralgia and episodes of genital lesion healing.

Cidofovir
1-[(S)-3-hydroxy-2-(phosphonomethoxy)propyl]cytosine

Cidofovir

Mechanism of Action. Cidofovir is a synthetic acyclic purine nucleotide analog of cytosine (39). It is a phosphorylated nucleotide which is additionally phosphorylated by host cell enzymes to its active intracellular metabolite, cidofovir diphosphate. This reaction occurs without initial virus-dependent phosphorylation by viral nucleoside kinases. It has antiviral effects by interfering with DNA synthesis and inhibiting viral replication.

Pharmacokinetics. Topical cidofovir (0.2%) is as effective as trifluridine (1%) in reducing HSV-1 shedding and healing time in rabbits with dendritic keratitis. Cidofovir is administered IV, topically and by ocular implant (Table 39.3). Peak plasma concentration of 3.1–23.6 μg/mL is achieved with doses of 1.0–10.0 mg/kg, respectively. The terminal plasma half-life is 2.6 hours and 90% drug is excreted in the urine. It has a variable bioavailability (2–26%).

Clinical Application. Cidofovir is active against herpes viruses including, HSV-1 and HSV-2, VZV, CMV and EBV. It is effective against acyclovir resistant strains of HSV and ganciclovir-resistant strains of CMV. Cidofovir is a long acting drug for the treatment of CMV retinitis in AIDS patients given as IV infusion or intravitreal injection. It is not a curative drug and its benefit over foscarnet or ganciclovir is yet to be determined. The major adverse effect is nephrotoxicity, which appears to result in renal tubular damage. Concomitant administration of cidofovir with probenecid is contraindicated because of increased risk of nephrotoxicity.

Cytarabine
1-β'-Arabinofuranosylcytosine (ara-C)

Cytarabine

Mechanism of Action. Cytarabine is a pyrimidine nucleoside related to idoxuridine (40). It is used primarily as an anticancer rather than an antiviral agent. Cytarabine acts by blocking the utilization of deoxycytidine, thereby inhibiting the replication of viral DNA. The drug is first converted to mono-, di- and triphosphates, which interfere with DNA synthesis by inhibiting both DNA polymerase and the reductase that promotes the conversion of cytidine diphosphate into its deoxy derivatives.

Clinical Application. Cytarabine is used to treat Burkitt's lymphoma and both myeloid and lymphatic leukemias. Its antiviral use is in the treatment of herpes zoster (shingles) infection. It is also used to treat herpetic keratitis and viral infections resistant to idoxuridine. The drug is usually used topically, but it has been given by IV injection to individuals with serious herpes infection (Table 39.2) (41). Cytarabine is deaminated rapidly in the body to an inactive compound, arabinosyluracil, which is excreted in the urine. The half-life of the drug in plasma is 3–5 hours. The toxic effects of cytarabine are chiefly on bone marrow, the GI tract, and the kidney. The drug is not given in the early months of pregnancy because of its teratogenic and carcinogenic effects in animals.

Famciclovir   Penciclovir

Famciclovir

Mechanism of Action. Famciclovir is a synthetic purine nucleoside analogue related to guanine (42). It is the diacetyl 6-deoxy ester of penciclovir (PCV) which is structurally related to ganciclovir. Its pharmacologic and microbiologic activities are similar to acyclovir. Famciclovir is a pro-drug of penciclovir, which is formed *in vivo* by hydrolysis. Penciclovir and its metabolite, penciclovir triphosphate possesses antiviral activity resulting in inhibition of viral DNA polymerase.

Clinical Application. Famciclovir is active against recurrent HSV (genital herpes and cold sores), VZV and EB virus but less active against CMV (Table 39.3). It is used in the treatment of recurrent localized herpes zoster and genital herpes in immunocompetent adults. It is also promising for the treatment of chronic HBV reinfection after liver transplantation.

Pharmacokinetics. Famciclovir can be given with or without food. The most common adverse effects are headache and GI disturbances. Concomitant use of famciclovir with probenecid results in increased plasma concentrations of penciclovir. The recommended dose of famciclovir is 500 mg every 8 hours for 7 days. The absolute bioavailability of famciclovir is 77% and area under plasma-concentration-time curve (AUC) is 86 mcg/mL. Famciclovir with digoxin increased plasma concentration of digoxin to 19% as compared to digoxin given alone.

Fomivirsen. Fomivirsen sodium is used to treat CMV, which causes retinitis in patients with AIDS. Such patients respond to fomivirsen but not to other treatment for CMV retinitis, which leads to blindness (43). Fomivirsen is the first antisense oligonucleotide agent that has been approved as an alternative medicine for patients with CMV retinitis for whom other agents did not work. It works by inhibiting synthesis of proteins responsible for the regulation of viral gene expression that is involved in infection of CMV retinitis. Fomivirsen works only in the eye in which it is injected. It is not recommended if cidofovir is used within the last 2–4 weeks because of increased risk of eye inflammation. Fomivirsen is given in two induction doses followed by monthly maintenance doses, each 330 mcg administered by intravitreal injection. It causes increased pressure in the eye for which eye examination is necessary by the ophthalmologist.

Fomivirsen is also used in Crohn's disease and cancers. It causes eye inflammation, abnormal vision, cataract, eye pain and retinal problems. In addition, it has several other side effects, such as stomach pain, headache, fever, infection, rash, vomiting and liver dysfunction.

Foscarnet sodium

Foscarnet. Foscarnet sodium is a trisodium phosphoformate hexahydrate that inhibits DNA polymerase of herpes viruses including CMV and retroviral RT (44). It is not phosphorylated into an active form by viral host cell enzymes. Therefore, it has the advantage of not requiring an activation step before attacking the target viral enzyme.

Clinical Application. Foscarnet sodium was approved by the FDA for the treatment of CMV retinitis in AIDS patients. In combination with ganciclovir, the results have been promising, even in progressive disease with ganciclovir-resistant strains. Foscarnet sodium is also effective in the treatment of mucocutaneous diseases caused by acyclovir-resistant strains of HSV and VZV in AIDS patients. Foscarnet sodium is administered intravenously (60 mg/kg) three times a day for initial therapy and 90–120 mg/kg daily for maintenance therapy (Table 39.3). The plasma-half life is 3–6 hours. Foscarnet sodium penetrates CSF and the eye. The drug is neurotoxic and common adverse effects include phlebitis, anemia, nausea, vomiting, and seizures. Foscarnet sodium carries risk of severe hypocalcemia, especially with concurrent use of IV pentamidine. Foscarnet sodium used with zidovudine (ZDV) has an additive effect against CMV and acts synergistically against HIV.

Ganciclovir (DHPG)

Ganciclovir. Ganciclovir sodium is an acyclic deoxyguanosine analogue of acyclovir (45). Ganciclovir inhibits DNA polymerase. Its active form is ganciclovir triphosphate, which is an inhibitor of viral rather than cellular DNA polymerase. The phosphorylation of ganciclovir does not require a virus-specific thymidine kinase for its activity against CMV. The mechanism of action is similar to that of acyclovir; however, ganciclovir is more toxic to human cells than is acyclovir.

Ganciclovir has greater activity than acyclovir against CMV and EB virus infection in immunocompromised patients. It is also active against HSV infection and in some mutants resistant to acyclovir. In AIDS patients, ganciclovir stopped progressive hemorragic retinitis and symptomatic pneumonitis related to CMV infection.

Ganciclovir is absorbed and phosphorylated by infection-induced kinases of HSV and VZV infections. Common side effects are leukopenia, neutropenia, and thrombocytopenia. Ganciclovir with ZDV causes severe hematologic toxicity. Ganciclovir is available only as an IV infusion because oral bioavailability is poor (Table 39.3). It is given in doses of 5 mg/kg twice daily for 14–21 days. When ganciclovir is given by IV dose administration, concentrations of the drug in CSF and in the brain vary from 25–70% of the plasma concentration. After minimal metabolism, ganciclovir is excreted in the urine. In adults with normal renal function, the serum half-life of the drug is approximately 3 hours. Ganciclovir has been approved by the FDA for the treatment of CMV retinitis in immunocompromised and AIDS patients.

Idoxuridine

Idoxuridine

Mechanism of Action. Idoxuridine is a nucleoside containing a halogenated pyrimidine and is an analogue of thymidine (46). It acts as an antiviral agent against DNA viruses by interfering with their replication based on their similarity of structure. Idoxuridine is first phosphorylated by the host cell virus-encoded enzyme thymidine kinase to an active triphosphate form. The phosphorylated drug inhibits cellular DNA polymerase to a lesser extent than HSV DNA polymerase, which is necessary for the synthesis of viral DNA. The triphosphate form of the drug is then incorporated during viral nucleic acid synthesis by a false pairing system that replaces thymidine. On transcription, faulty viral proteins are formed, resulting in defective viral particles (47).

Clinical Application. Idoxuridine is available as ophthalmic drops (0.1%) and ointment (0.5%) for the treatment of HSV keratoconjunctivitis, the leading cause of blindness in the United States (Table 39.3). Because of its poor solubility, the drug is ineffective in labial or genital HSV or for cutaneous herpes zoster infection. Idoxuridine in dimethylsulfoxide (DMSO), however, has been used in mucocutaneous HSV infection of the mouth and nose. Because DMSO facilitates drug absorption and also has some therapeutic effect, a 40% solution of idoxuridine in DMSO is more effective than idoxuridine used without this vehicle. Therefore, the FDA approved idoxuridine only for topical treatment of herpes simplex keratitis, and is more effective in epithelial than in stromal infections. It is less effective for recurrent herpes keratitis, probably because of the development of drug-resistant virus strains.

Adverse reactions of idoxuridine include such local reactions as pain, pruritus, edema, burning, and hypersensitivity. Systemic administration of idoxuridine by IV injec-

Additional Hydrogenated Uridines

Fluorodeoxyuridine has *in vitro* antiviral activity but is not used in clinical practice.

Fluorodeoxyuridine (R = F, X = OH)
Bromodeoxyuridine (R = Br, X = OH)
5'-aminoidoxuridine (R = I, X = NH₂)

Bromodeoxyuridine is used in subacute sclerosing panencephalitis, a deadly virus-induced CNS disease. This agent appears to interfere with DNA synthesis in the same way as idoxuridine. The 5'-amino analogue of idoxuridine (5-iodo-5'-amino-2',5'-dideoxy-uridine) is a better antiviral agent than idoxuridine and it is less toxic. It is metabolized in herpesvirus-infected cells only by thymidine kinase to di- and triphosphoramidates. These metabolites inhibit HSV-specific late RNA transcription, causing reduction of less infective abnormal viral proteins. 5-Bromo-2'-deoxy-uridine has an action similar to that of other iodinated compounds.

tion may be given in an emergency but leads to bone marrow toxicities such as leukopenia, thrombocytopenia, and anemia. It may also induce stomatitis, nausea, vomiting, abnormalities of liver functions, and alopecia. Idoxuridine has a plasma half-life of 30 minutes and is rapidly metabolized in the blood to idoxuracil and uracil.

Ribavirin

Ribavirin

Mechanism of Action. Ribavirin, a guanosine analogue, has broad-spectrum antiviral activity against both DNA and RNA viruses (48,49). It is phosphorylated by adenosine kinase to the triphosphate resulting in inhibition of viral specific RNA polymerase, messenger RNA, and nucleic acid synthesis.

Clincial Application. Ribavirin is highly active against influenza A and B and the parainfluenza group of viruses, genital herpes, herpes zoster, measles, and acute hepatitis types A, B, and C. Aerosolized ribavirin has been approved by the FDA for the treatment of lower respiratory tract infections (bronchiolitis and pneumonia) serious RSV infection, but it can cause cardiopulmonary and immunologic disorders in children. Ribavirin inhibits *in vitro* replication of HIV-1, which is involved in AIDS. Clinically, ribavirin was shown to delay the onset of full-blown AIDS in patients with early symptoms of HIV infection. Some viruses are less susceptible, for example, poliovirus, herpes viruses excluding varicella, vaccinia, mumps, reovirus, and rotavirus. A randomized double-blind study of aerosolized ribavirin treatment of infants with RSV infections indicated significant improvement in the severity of infection with a decrease in viral shedding (50).

Pharmacokinetics. Oral or IV forms of ribavirin are useful in the prevention and treatment of Lassa fever. The oral bioavailability is approximately 45% and serum half-life is 9 hours. Peak plasma level after one hour is 1–3 µg/mL. IV administration of the drug has higher peak plasma levels. Aerosol preparation delivery of drug (0.8 mg/kg/hr) produced drug levels in respiratory secretions of 50–200 µg/mL (Table 39.3). The clinical benefits of this agent are yet to be confirmed. Its few side effects are generally limited to GI disturbances, such as nausea, vomiting, and diarrhea. The drug is contraindicated in asthma patients because of deterioration of pulmonary function. Viral strains susceptible to ribavirin have not been found to develop drug resistance, as is the case with other antiviral agents, such as acyclovir, idoxuridine, and bromovinyldeoxyuridine (BVDU).

Trifluorothymidine (TFT, F3T)

Trifluorothymidine

Mechanism of Action. Trifluorothymidine is a fluorinated pyridine nucleoside structurally related to idoxuridine (51).

It has been approved by the FDA and is a potent, specific inhibitor of replication of HSV-1 in vitro. Its mechanism of action is similar to that of idoxuridine. Like other antiherpes drugs, it is first phosphorylated by thymidine kinase to mono-, di- and triphosphate forms, which are then incorporated into viral DNA in place of thymidine to stop the formation of late virus mRNA and subsequent synthesis of the virion proteins.

Clinical Application. Trifluorothymidine, because of its greater solubility in water, is active against HSV-1 and 2. It is also useful in treating infections caused by human CMV and VZV infections. The advantage of use of this agent over idoxuridine is its high topical efficacy in the cure of primary keratoconjunctivitis and recurrent epithelial keratitis. It is also useful for difficult cases of herpetic iritis and established stromal keratitis.

Pharmacokinetics. Trifluorothymidine is available as a 1% ophthalmic solution, which is effective in dendritic ulcers (Table 39.3). Generally, a 1% eye solution of trifluorothymidine is well tolerated. Cross-hypersensitivity and cross-toxicity between trifluorothymidine, idoxuridine, and vidarabine are rare. The most frequent side ef-

fects are temporary burning, stinging, localized edema, and bone marrow toxicity. It is less toxic but more expensive than idoxuridine. Trifluorothymidine, given intravenously, shows a plasma half-life of 18 minutes and is excreted in urine unchanged or as the inactive metabolite 5-carboxyuracil.

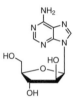

Vidarabine (ara-A)

Vidarabine

Mechanism of Action. Vidarabine is an adenosine nucleoside obtained from cultures of *Streptomyces antibioticus* (52). Cellular enzymes convert vidarabine to mono-, di- and triphosphate derivatives that interfere with viral nucleic acid replication, specifically inhibiting the early steps in DNA synthesis. This agent was used originally as an antineoplastic drug. Its antiviral effect is, in some cases, superior to that of idoxuridine or cytarabine.

Clinical Application. Vidarabine is used mainly in human HSV-1 and 2 encephalitis, decreasing the mortality rate from 70 to 30%. Whitley and co-workers reported that early vidarabine therapy is helpful in controlling complications of localized or disseminated herpes zoster in immunocompromised patients (53). Vidarabine is also useful in neonatal herpes labialis or genitalis, vaccinia virus, adenovirus, RNA viruses, papovavirus, CMV, and smallpox virus infections. Given the efficacy of vidarabine in certain viral infections, the FDA approved a 3% ointment for the treatment of herpes simplex keratoconjunctivitis and recurrent epithelial keratitis, and a 2% IV injection for the treatment of herpes simplex encephalitis and herpes zoster infections (Table 39.3). A topical ophthalmic preparation of vidarabine is useful in herpes simplex keratitis but shows little promise in herpes simplex labialis or genitalis. The monophosphate esters of vidarabine are more water-soluble and can be used in smaller volumes and even intramuscularly. These esters are under clinical investigation for the treatment of hepatitis B, systemic and cutaneous herpes simplex, and herpes zoster virus infections in immunocompromised patients.

Pharmacokinetics. Vidarabine is deaminated rapidly by adenine deaminase, which is present in serum and red blood cells. The enzyme converts vidarabine to its principal metabolite, arabinosyl hypoxanthine (ara-HX), which has weak antiviral activity (Fig. 39.8) (54). The half-life of vidarabine is approximately one hour, whereas ara-HX has a half-life of 3.5 hours. The drug is detected mostly in the kidney, liver, and spleen because 50% of it is recovered in

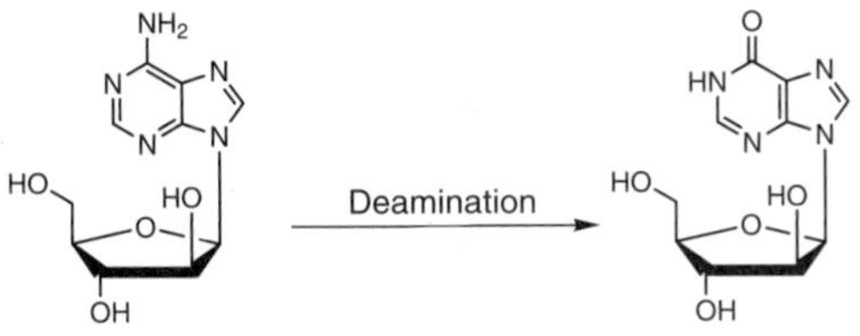

Fig. 39.8. Metabolism of vidarabine.

the urine as ara-HX. Levels of vidarabine in CSF fluid are 50% of those in the plasma.

Most side effects of vidarabine are GI disturbances, such as anorexia, nausea, vomiting, and diarrhea. CNS side effects include tremors, dizziness, pain syndromes, and seizures. Bone marrow suppression is reported at higher doses. Because vidarabine is reported to be mutagenic, carcinogenic, and teratogenic in animal studies, its use in pregnant women is to be avoided. Allopurinol and theophylline may interfere with the metabolism of vidarabine at higher doses because of the xanthine oxidase metabolism of vidarabine. Therefore, this agent should be avoided or given with caution to patients receiving these medications concurrently. Also, adjustment of the dose is necessary in patients with renal insufficiency.

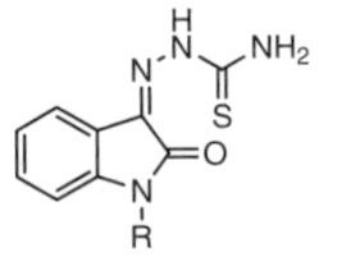

Methisazone, R = CH$_3$
(Marboran)

Agents Affecting Translation of Ribosomes—Methisazone (55)

Methisazone interferes with the translation of mRNA messages into protein synthesis on the cell ribosome. Ultimately, it produces a defect in protein incorporation into virus. Although viral DNA increases and host cells are damaged, an infectious virus is not produced.

Methisazone is active against poxviruses, including variola and vaccinia (56). Some RNA viruses, such as rhinoviruses, echoviruses, reoviruses, influenza, parainfluenza, and polioviruses are also inhibited. Therapeutically, methisazone is given in 1.5–3.0 g doses, twice daily by mouth. It has also been used as a prophylactic agent against smallpox. Historically, methisazone was one of the first antiviral compounds used in clinical practice. It is orally absorbed, with nausea and vomiting as the principal side effects. The drug is also used in vaccinia gangrenosa and disseminated vaccinia infections. This drug is not available in the United States, but it has been used in Europe for some time. Several analogs of methisazone (R = H, R = C$_2$H$_5$) possess activity against variola, neurovaccinia, smallpox in mice, Rous sarcoma virus, and vaccinia generalisata.

Antiretroviral (Anti-HIV) Agents Including Protease Inhibitors (57)

Although, billions of dollars have been spent on research and development of anti-AIDS drugs, the disease remains uncontrolled. Over 30 million people are infected worldwide with HIV and approximately 5 million cases are reported in the United States. Although a variety of drugs have been developed for treating AIDS patients none have proven successful in curing the disease. The basic difficulty experienced with this viral infections is the ability of virus to mutate leading to rapid drug resistance.

While there can be no permanent cure of AIDS without prevention or elimination of HIV infection, AIDS patients can prolong their life if early diagnosis and treatments are started. Initial HIV treatment requires specific drugs that inhibit RT and HIV protease. In an advanced HIV infection, AIDS is complicated by other infections called opportunistic infections, which are related to the loss of immunity in AIDS patients. Thus, such patients are treated symptomatically with a variety of drugs depending upon the opportunistic infections (58–60). Anti-HIV agents have side effects but patients can be managed by a careful monitoring of the drugs. Opportunistic diseases include infections by parasites, bacteria, fungi and viruses. Neoplasms include Kaposi's sarcoma and Burkitt's lymphoma may be common occurrences.

Anti-HIV agents are classified according to the mode of action. The drugs inhibiting RT interfere with replication of HIV and stop synthesis of infective viral particles. They are further classified into nucleoside and nonnucleoside RT inhibitors.

The drugs inhibiting HIV protease inactivate RT activity and block release of viral particles from the infected cells. The chemistry, pharmacokinetics, side effects, toxicity, and drug interactions of RT inhibitors and PIs are discussed below.

Nucleoside RT Inhibitors (NRTI) (61)

The synthesis of viral DNA under the direction of reverse transcriptase (RT) (Table 39.4) requires availability of purines and pyrimidine nucleosides and nucleotides. Therefore, it is not surprising that a variety of chemical modifications of natural nucleosides have been investigated. Two such modifications have resulted in active drugs. Removal of the 3'-hydroxyl group of the deoxynucleosides has given rise to dideoxy*adenosine* (didanosine is the pro-drug for this derivative) (62), dideoxy*cytodine* (63), and didehydrodideoxy*thymidine* (64). Replacement of the 3'-deoxy with an azido group has given 3'-azido*thymidine* (65–67) and 3'-azido*uridine* (no longer used as a drug) (68). All of these drugs have similar mechanisms of action in that their incorporation into the viral DNA will ultimately lead to chain terminating blockade due to the lack of a 3'-hydroxyl needed for the DNA propagation.

Table 39.4. HIV Reverse Transcriptase (RT) Inhibitors

Generic Name	Common Name	Trade Name	Dosage Form (mg/unit)
Nucleoside Reverse Transcriptase Inhibitors (NRTI)			
Zidovudine	AZT ZDV	Retrovir	Tab (300), Cap (100), Syrup (50/5ml), Inj (10/ml)
Didanosine (Dideoxyadenosine)	ddI (ddA)	Videx	Tab (25,50,100,150,200) Powder for po sol. (100,167,250)
Zalcitabine	ddC	Hivid	Tab (0.375)
Stavudine	D4T	Zerit	Cap (15,20,30,40) Powder for po sol. (1/ml)
Lamivudine	3TC	Epivir Epivir HBV	Tab (150), Sol. (10/ml) Tab (100), Sol. (5/ml)
Abacavir	ABC	Ziagen	Tab (300), Sol (20/ml)
Nonnucleoside Reverse Transcriptase Inhibitors (NNRTI)			
Nevirapine		Viramune	Tab (200)
Delavirdine		Rescriptor	Tab (100)
Efavirenz		Sustiva	Cap (50,100,200)

Zidovudine(AZT)

Zidovudine

Mechanism of Action. Zidovudine is an analogue of thymidine in which the azido group is substituted at the 3-carbon atom of the dideoxyribose moiety. It is active against RNA tumor viruses (retroviruses) that are the causative agents of AIDS and T cell leukemia. Retroviruses, by virtue of RT, direct the synthesis of a provirus (DNA copy of a viral RNA genome). Proviral DNA integrates into the normal cell DNA, leading to the HIV infection. ZDV is converted to 5'-mono- di- and triphosphates by the cellular thymidine kinase. These phosphates are then incorporated into proviral DNA, because RT uses ZDV- triphosphate as a substrate. This process prevents normal 5',3'-phosphodiester bonding, resulting in termination of DNA chain elongation owing to the presence of an azido group in ZDV. The multiplication of HIV is halted by selective inhibition of reverse transcriptase and thus viral DNA polymerase by ZDV-triphosphate at the required dose concentration. ZDV is a potent inhibitor of HIV-1 but also inhibits HIV-2 and EB virus.

Clinical Application. ZDV is used in AIDS and AIDS-related complex (ARC) to control opportunistic infections by raising absolute CD4+ lymphocyte counts. ZDV was first synthesized by Horwitz (1964), biologic activity was reported by Ostertag (1974), and in 1986 Yarchoan demonstrated application of ZDV in clinical trials of AIDS and related diseases (69). ZDV is recommended in the control of the disease in asymptomatic patients in whom absolute CD4+ lymphocyte counts are less than 200/mm³. It prolongs the life of patients affected with *Pneumocystis carinii* pneumonia (PCP) and improves the condition of patients with advanced ARC by reducing the severity and frequency of opportunistic infections. Substantial benefits are obtained when the drug is given after the CD4+ cell counts fall below 500/mm³. Therefore, ZDV is used in early and advanced symptomatic treatment of AIDS or ARC patients. ZDV with other RT inhibitors or in combination with PIs are more beneficial when resistance to ZDV occurs.

HIV attacks susceptible cells and interacts mainly with CD4+ cell surface proteins of helper T cells. The glycoprotein, gp 120 of virus coat, forms a complex with CD4 receptor on host cells and enters the cells by endocytosis. The sequence of events is shown in Fig. 39.2. Ultimately, the immune system of the host is altered and AIDS symptoms appear. AIDS patients have symptoms, such as high fever, weight loss, lymphadenopathy, chronic diarrhea, myalgias, fatigue, and night sweats. ZDV is given in such conditions. However, the drug is toxic to the bone marrow and causes macrocytic anemia, neutropenia, and granulocytopenia. Other adverse reactions include headache, insomnia, nausea, vomiting, seizures, myalgias, and confusion.

Pharmacokinetics. ZDV is available in 100-mg capsules for oral administration. For asymptomatic adults, the initial recommended dosage is 1200 mg daily (200 mg every 4 hours) reducing to 600 mg daily (100 mg every 4 hours) for patients with advanced disease. The maintenance dose is 600 mg daily in symptomatic patients. ZDV is sensitive to heat and light because of its azide group and should be stored in colored bottles at 15°–25° C.

ZDV is well absorbed through the GI tract. It concentrates in the body tissues and fluids, including CSF. The bioavailability of the drug was found to be approximately 65%. Its half-life is approximately 1 hour. IV doses of 2.5 mg/kg or oral doses of 5 mg/kg yielded peak plasma concentrations of 5 μg mol/L. Plasma protein binding was approximately 30%. Most of the drug is converted to its inactive glucuronide metabolite and is excreted unchanged through urine. ZDV also crosses the blood-brain barrier. Pentamidine, dapsone, amphotericin B, flucytosine, and doxorubicin may increase the toxic effects of ZDV. Probencid prolongs the plasma half-life of the drug.

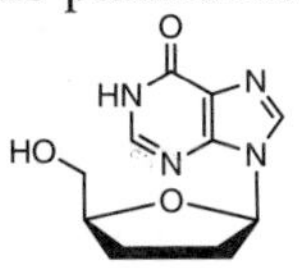

Didanosine(ddI)

Didanosine

Mechanism of Action. Didanosine is a purine dideoxynucleoside, which is an analogue of inosine. Chemically, it is 2,′ 3′-dideoxyinosine that differs from inosine by having hydrogen atoms in place of 2′- and 3′-hydroxyl groups on the ribose ring. Didanosine is a pro-drug which is bioactivated by metabolism to dideoxyadenosine treiphosphate (ddATP) (Fig. 39.9). ddATP is a competative inhibitor of viral reverse transcriptase and is incorporated into the developing viral DNA in place of deoxyladenosine triphosphate. As such this agent causes chain termination due to the absence of a 3′-hydroxyl group. Didanosine inhibits HIV RT and exerts a virustatic effect on the retroviruses. Combined with ZDV, antiretroviral activity of ddI is increased.

Pharmacokinetics. Didanosine has a plasma half-life of 1.5 hours and it is given in 200-mg dose twice daily. Oral bioavailability of the drug is approximately 25% at doses of 7 mg/kg or less. Didanosine decreased significantly p24 antigen level and increased CD4+ cell counts. Viral resistance to ddI occurred after treatment for one year. Didanosine is less toxic than ZDV. The CSF fluid/plasma ratio of ddI is 0.2. Didanosine is ultimately converted to hypoxanthine, xanthine and uric acid (Fig. 39.9). The latter is a nontoxic metabolic product.

Didanosine is given in advanced HIV infection, ZDV intolerance or significant clinical/immunologic deterioration. The major side effects of ddI are painful peripheral neuropathy and pancreatitis. Some of the minor side effects include abdominal pain, nausea and vomiting. The use of products, such as pentamidine, sulfonamides and cimetidine should be avoided with ddI. However, combination of ddI with ZDV is beneficial because of different toxicity profile.

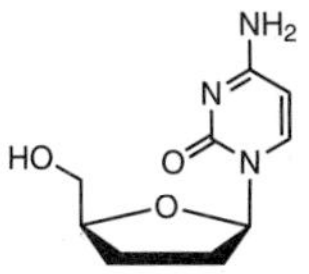

Zalcitabine
(2′,3′-Dideoxycytidine, ddC)

Zalcitabine. Zalcitabine is a useful alternate drug to ZDV. It is a synthetic pyrimidine nucleoside analogue. It differs from 2′-deoxycytidine in that the 3′-hydroxyl group of the 2′-deoxyribose moiety is replaced with a hydrogen atom. It is given in combination with zidovudine when CD4+ cell counts fall below 300 cells/mm³. Monotherapy with ddC was more active than ZDV. Its oral bioavailability is 87% and plasma half-life is approximately one hour. It has side effects, such as stomatitis, rash, fever, malaise, arthritis and arthralgia. In low doses (0.005 mg/kg every 4 hours), ddC produced sustained decrease in p24 antigen level and increase in CD4+ cell counts. The CSF fluid/plasma ratio of ddC is 0.2.

Following oral administration, bioavailability of ddC was less than 80%, which was further reduced with food. The mean maximum plasma concentration of the drug was also reduced from 25.2 ng/mL to 15.5 ng/mL when the drug was taken with food. Dideoxyuridine (ddU) is the major metabolite in urine and feces. The drug demonstrated penetration through blood-brain barrier. The major toxicity of ddC is peripheral neuropathy in which case, it should be discontinued. Pancreatitis occurs in some cases when given alone or in combination with ZDV.

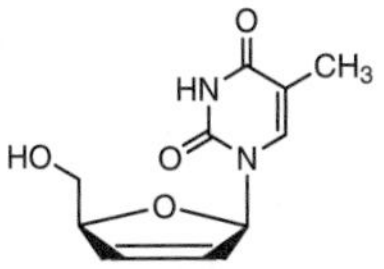

Stavudine
(2′,3′-Dideoxy-2′,3′-didehydrothymidine, D4T)

Stavudine. Stavudine is a pyrimidine nucleoside analogue, which has significant activity against HIV-1 after intracellular conversion of the drug to a D4T-triphosphate. It differs in structure from thymidine by the replacement of the 3′-hydroxyl group with a hydrogen atom and a double bond in the 2′ and 3′ positions on the deoxyribose ring. It decreased p24 antigen and raised CD4+ cell counts. D4T is beneficial for patients where CD4+ cell counts do not decrease below

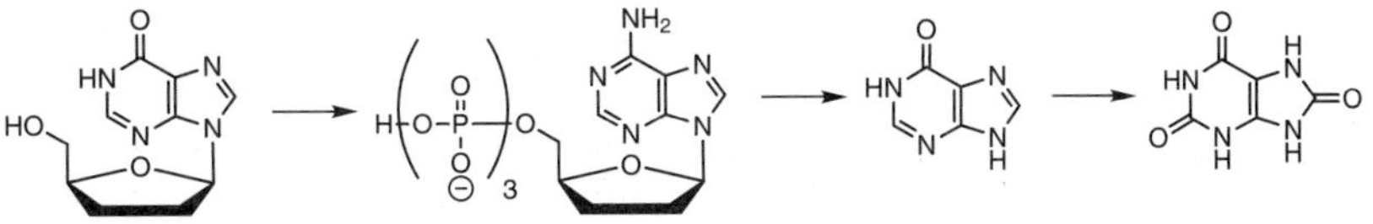

| ddI | ddATP | Hypoxanthine | Uric acid |

Fig. 39.9. Metabolism of didanosine.

300 cells/mm³ with ZDV and ddI. It was more effective than ZDV or ddC treated patients in delaying the progression of HIV infection. It is recommended for patients with advanced HIV infection.

D4T is rapidly absorbed and absolute bioavailability in adults is 85% at an oral dose of 4 mg/kg. A peak plasma concentration in dose dependent manner occurs within an hour. It can be taken with food. The apparent volume distribution after oral dose is 66 L. The plasma half-life of D4T is approximately 1.5 hours and intracellular half-life of D4T-triphosphate is 3.5 hours. It is less toxic to bone marrow but causes peripheral neuropathic toxicity. The side effects include pain, tingling and numbness in the hands and feet.

Lamivudine
(2'-Deoxy-3'-thiacytidine, 3TC)

Lamivudine. Lamivudine is an analogue of ddC in which 3'-methylene group is replaced with a sulfur (S) atom in the ribose ring (70). It exerts virustatic effect against retroviruses by competitively inhibiting HIV RT after intracellular conversion of the drug to its active 5'-3TC-triphosphate form. It is usually given with other antiretroviral agents, such as ZDV or D4T.

Pharmacokinetics. 3TC in 600 mg/day dose reduced HIV cells by 75% and in combination with ZDV, the reduction in viral load was 94%. 3TC are rapidly absorbed through the GI tract. Its bioavailability is approximately 86% and after oral administration of 2 mg/kg twice daily, peak serum 3TC concentration was approximately 2 mg/mL. 3TC binding to human plasma were approximately 36%. Mainly, it is converted to transsulfoxide metabolite and a majority of the drug is eliminated unchanged in urine.

The FDA approved 3TC in combination with ZDV for the treatment of disease progression caused by HIV infection. The combinations of 3TC with ddI, ddC or D4T also are used for advanced HIV infection. Such combinations have the ability to delay resistance to ZDV and restore ZDV sensitivity in AIDS patients. Recently, oral therapy in lower doses of 3TC (Table 39.4) has been approved by the FDA for treatment of chronic hepatitis B. Peripheral neuropathy and GI disturbances are the major side effects of 3TC. The minor side effects are nausea, vomiting and diarrhea.

Abacavir. Abacavir sulfate was approved in 1998 as a NRTI to be used in combination with other drugs for the treatment of HIV and AIDS. The drug is extensively metabolized via stepwise phosphorylation to 5'-mono-, di-, and triphosphate. Abacavir is well absorb (>75%) and penetrates the CNS. The drug can be taken without

Abacavir (ABC)

regard to meals. The drug does not show any clinically significant drug-drug interactions. The drug has been reported to produce life-threatening hypersensitivity reactions.

The major use of abacavir appears to be in combination with other NRTIs. A fixed combination product has recently been approved by the FDA under the trade name of Trizivir. This product contains 300mg of ABC, 150mg of 3TC, and 300mg of ZDV. The combination has been shown to be superior to other combinations in reducing viral load as well as showing improvement in CD4⁺cell count.

The most common adverse effects reported with abacavir include headache, nausea, vomiting, malaise, and diarrhea.

Nonnucleoside RT Inhibitors (NNRTI)

The FDA has recently approved several nonnucleosides that inhibit RT activity. They are used with nucleoside drugs to obtain synergistic activity in decreasing the viral load and increasing CD4⁺ cell counts. Mostly, these drugs are synthesized by protein structure-based drug design methodologies. Their use as monotherapy may be limited because of rapid onset of resistance and hypersensitivity reactions. However, interaction of nonnucleoside drugs with other protease inhibitors, such as saquinavir, indinavir and ritonavir is being investigated. Also, interaction of these drugs with clarithromycin, ketoconazole, rifabutin and rifampin are under study. Nonnucleosides that inhibit RT activity are discussed below:

Nevirapine

Nevirapine. Nevirapine and its analogues exhibit antiretroviral effect against AZT-resistant HIV strains (71). Nevirapine in combination with ZDV and ddI produced approximately 18% higher CD4⁺ cell counts and a decrease in viral load compared with patients who took ZDV and ddI. Nevirapine is recommended with nucleosides for HIV-1 infected patients who have experienced clinical or immunologic deterioration. The significant side effects of nevirapine are liver dysfunction and skin rashes.

Mechanism of Action. Nevirapine is a dipyridodiazepinone derivative, which binds directly to RT. Thus, it blocks RNA- and DNA-dependent polymerase activities by causing a disruption of the enzyme's catalytic site. The activity of nevirapine does not compete with template or nucleoside triphosphate. HIV-2 RT and human DNA polymerases are not inhibited by nevirapine. The 50% inhibitory concentration ranged within 10–100 nM against HIV-1.

Pharmacokinetics. Nevirapine is rapidly absorbed after oral administration and its bioavailability is approximately 95%. Peak plasma nevirapine concentrations of 2 ± 0.4 μg/mL (7.5 μM) are obtained in 4 hours following a single 200 mg dose (Table 39.4). Following multiple doses, nevirapine concentrations appear to increase linearly in the dose range of 200–400 mg/day. Nevirapine is about 60% bound to plasma proteins in the plasma concentration range of 1–10 μg/mL. It readily crossed the placenta and was found in breast milk.

Nevirapine is metabolized as glucuronide conjugates of hydroxylated metabolites, which are excreted in urine. *In vivo*, ketoconazole did not produce any significant inhibitory effect on nevirapine metabolism. The plasma concentrations of nevirapine were elevated or reduced in patients receiving cimetidine or rifabutin, respectively.

Delavirdine

Delavirdine. Delavirdine, a bisheteroarylpiperazine derivative, is a potent nonnucleoside RT inhibitor of activity specific for HIV-1 (72). The FDA has approved this drug in combination with other anti-HIV agents (Table 39.4). In phase I/II study trials, it demonstrated sustained improvements in CD4$^+$ cell counts, p24 antigen levels and RNA viral load. Promising results were obtained when the drug was used in two or three-drug combination with nucleoside drugs. Combination of delavirdine with ddI, ddC or ZDV demonstrated additive or synergistic effect. However, delavirdine with ZDV was more beneficial in early HIV infection. Combinations of nevirapine and delavirdine had an antagonistic effect on HIV-1 RT inhibition.

Mechanism of Action. Delavirdine directly inhibits RT and DNA-directed DNA polymerase activities of HIV-1 after the formation of the enzyme-substrate complexes thereby causing chain termination effects.

Pharmacokinetics. Delaviradine is rapidly absorbed by oral administration and peak plasma concentration was obtained in one hour. Following administration of delaviridine, 400 mg three times daily resulted in peak plasma concentration of 45 μM. The single dose

bioavailability of delaviridine tablets relative to oral solution was approximate 85%. The 50% inhibitory concentration for delavirdine against RT activity was 6.0 nM. Delaviridine is extensively bound to plasma protein (about 98%). Delavirdine is metabolized to its N-desisopropyl metabolite in liver and the pharmacokinetics is nonlinear. Clarithromycin, rifabutin or ergot alkaloid derivatives are predicted to increase plasma concentration of delaviridine. Skin rashes are the major side effect of delavirdine therapy. Cross-resistance between delavidine and PIs, such as indinavir, nelfinavir, ritonavir and saquinavir is unlikely because of action on different enzyme targets.

Efavirenz

Efavirenz. Efavirenz is a new nonnucleoside RT inhibitor that is recently approved by the FDA (Table 39.4) (73). It is a potent inhibitor of wild-type as well as resistant mutants HIV-1 that is inhibited up to 95% in efavirenz concentration of 1.5 mM. In combination with indinavir, a mean reduction in HIV-RNA of 1.68 log, and an increase in CD4$^+$ cell counts of 96 cells/mm^3 were reported. Coadministration of efavirenz with indinavir reduced indinavir concentration (AUC) by approximately 35%.

Efavirenz is administered once a day and can be used as a substitute for indinavir in combination therapy with standard drugs, such as ZDV and 3TC. Since, it is given once a day, it cuts down the number of pills that an AIDS patient has to swallow. In the current cocktail therapy of AIDS patients, efavirenz is a good option for reducing the many side effects of cocktail therapy. It is administered to both adults and children and may be less expensive than indinavir.

The side effects of efavirenz include dizziness, insomnia, impaired concentration, abnormal dreams and drowsiness. The most common adverse effect is a skin rash. Other side effects are diarrhea, headache and dizziness. Efavirenz is recommended to be taken at bedtime with or without food. Avoiding driving or operating machinery and intake of high fat meals are recommended. It should always be taken in combination with at least one other anti-HIV agent. Efavirenz is contraindicated with midazolam, triazolam or ergot derivatives.

HIV Protease Inhibitors (Table 39.5) (74)

HIV protease is an enzyme that is essential for viral growth. It is responsible for the post-translation modification of core proteins into structural proteins. The latter consists of p7, p9, p17, and p24, which play important roles in infectivity of HIV. These proteins are products of a *pol* gene. The HIV genome contains various sites (regions) designated as genes, such as *gag* and *gag-pol* genes

Table 39.5. HIV Protease Inhibitors

Generic Name	Trade Name	Dosage Form (mg/unit)
Saquinavir	Invirase	Cap (200)
	Fortovase	Cap (200)
Ritonavir	Norvir	Cap (100), Sol (80/ml)
Indinavir	Crixivan	Cap (200, 400)
Nelfinavir	Viracept	Tab (250), Powder (50/g)
Amprenavir	Agenerase	Cap (50, 150), Sol (15/ml)
Lopinavir/	Kaletra	Cap (133.3/33.3),
Ritonavir		Sol (80/20 per ml)

which are translated as polyproteins and form immature viral particles. The latter are precursor protein molecules that are cleaved by a viral *pol-encoded* aspartic proteinases to form the desired structural proteins of the mature viral particles. HIV protease activates RT and plays an important role in the release of infectious viral particles. Thus, an area of considerable interest has been the development of drugs that act as inhibitors of protease and *pol* gene. The inhibitors act on HIV protease and prevent post-translational processing and budding of immature viral particles from the infected cells. This group of drugs represents a major breakthrough in treatment of HIV when used in combination with RT inhibitors.

Mechanism of Action. HIV protease exists as a dimer in which each monomer contains one of two-conserved aspartic residues at the active sites. Drugs are designed as transition-state mimetics to align at the active site of HIV-1 protease, as defined by three-dimensional crystallographic analysis of this molecule (Chapter 40, Fig, 40.10). The best-fit compounds replace amino acids near the active site. A number of polypeptides have been synthesized to differentially inhibit viral and mammalian aspartic proteases with their target being HIV-1 protease. These agents may appear as either peptidomimetic and nonpeptide compounds. Their effectiveness is related to their ability to inhibit *gag-pol* gene, which process p24, p55 and p160. Consequently, infectivity of HIV-1 is diminished.

Although, some compounds exhibited *in vitro* and *in vivo* antiviral activities, optimization of their pharmacokinetics and pharmacodynamic properties have presented major problems. In view of the great demand for successful anti-AIDS drugs, the FDA has approved the following drugs as PIs under the accelerated approval process (Fig. 39.10).

Metabolism. The PIs have a high potential for drug interactions which is associated with the fact that these drugs are substrates for and inhibitors of the CYP3A4 enzyme system. As a result, concurrent use of PIs with other drugs metabolized by CYP3A4 (See Chapter 8) may be contraindicated and in some cases the drug interactions can be life-threatening. The most potent CYP450 inhibitor is ritonavir (used to advantage in combination with

lopinavir), followed by indinavir, nelfinavir and amprenavir as moderate inhibitors, and saquinavir as the least potent inhibitor. Drug interactions have been reported with bepridil, dihydroergotamine, and a number of benzodiazepines. Marked increase in activity of amiodarone, lidocaine (systemic), quinidine, the tricyclic antidepressants, and warfarin might be expected. Other interactions have been reported to include rifampin, rifabutin phenobarbital, phenytoin, dexamethasone or carbazepine.

Since the PIs are themselves metabolized by CYP450, the PIs action may be altered by other agents that induce or inhibit this system. With ketoconazole or the rifamycins, relative bioavailability of the PIs is increased and the dose of the PIs may need to be decreased.

Specific Drugs—Saquinavir. Saquinavir mesylate (Fig. 39.10) was the first protease inhibitor approved by the FDA in December 1995 (75). It is a carboxamide derivative that is specifically designed to inhibit HIV proteinase preventing post-translational formation of viral proteins. It contains an hydroxyethylamine moiety rather than the Phe-Pro scissle bond.

Clinical Application. Saquinavir is used in the treatment of advanced HIV infection in selected patients. Saquinavir is used concomitantly with either ZDV untreated patients or ddC patients previously treated with prolonged ZDV therapy. Although, combined therapy did not show slowing of progression of disease; CD4$^+$ cell counts were increased in patients infected with HIV in the United States and European countries. Triple therapy with saquinavir, ZDV and ddC has been more effective than double therapy with saquinavir plus ZDV or ddC. Thus, combination therapy slowed disease progression and mortality.

The 50% inhibitory concentration of saquinavir in both acutely and chronically infected cells was 1–30 nM. In combination with ZDV, ddC or ddI, the activity of saquinavir was increased without increased cytotoxicity. The resistance of HIV isolates to saquinavir was observed due to substitution mutations in the HIV protease at amino acid positions 48 (glycine to valine) and 90 (leucine to methionine).

Pharmacokinetics. The bioavailability of saquinavir in a single 600-mg dose following a high fat meal was shown to be about 4%. Approximately, 30% of a 600-mg dose of saquinavir reached the liver where it showed first-pass metabolism. The metabolites, mono- and dihydroxylated compounds, are not active. Approximately, 88% and 19% of a 600-mg oral dose was found in the feces and urine, respectively. The volume distribution following IV administration of a 12-mg dose of saquinavir was 700 L. The drug is bound 98% to the plasma protein and very low concentration of saquinavir was found in CSF. The steady-state AUC was 2.5 times higher than that observed after a single dose of 600 mg in HIV-infected patients after a meal as compared to multiple dosing. Saquinavir has a plasma half-life of approximately 1.8 hours. Although saquinavir hard-gel capsule in combination with other antiretroviral drugs reduced risk of disease progression or death, it has limited bioavailability. To overcome this limitation, the FDA has approved saquinavir soft-gel capsules.

Saquinavir is well tolerated with ZDV and or ddC with few side effects but GI disturbances were the most common adverse effects. Saquinavir has few side effects, such as headache, rhinitis, nausea and diarrhea.

Ritonavir (Fig. 39.10). Ritonavir is another HIV PI approved by the FDA in March 1996 (76). Ritonavir is a peptidomimetic inhibitor of both the HIV-1 and HIV-2 proteases. The 50% viral replication was obtained by 3.8 to 153 nM ritonavir concentration.

Pharmacokinetics. After a 600-mg dose of oral solution, peak concentrations of ritonavir were obtained in approximately 2 and 4 hours of fasting and nonfasting conditions, respectively. Under nonfasting conditions, peak ritonavir concentrations decreased 23% and the extent of absorption decreased 7% relative to fasting conditions. In two separate studies, the capsule and oral solution indicated AUC of 129.5 ± 47.1 and 129.0 ± 39.3 μg.h/mL, respectively when a 600 mg dose was given under nonfasting conditions.

Five ritonavir metabolites have been isolated from human urine and feces. The isopropylthiazole oxidation metabolite was the major active metabolite. As with saquinavir, ritonavir is metabolized by CYP3A4 and is an inhibitor of the CYP450 system. Ritonavir is contraindi-cated with several compounds, such as clarithromycin, desipramine, ethinyl estradiol, rifabutin, sulfamethoxazole and trimethoprim because of increased concentrations of these drugs in the plasma due their inhibited metabolism. Ritonavir alone or in combination with 3TC, ZDV, saquinavir or ddC increased CD4$^+$ cell counts and decreased HIV RNA particle levels. Cross-resistance between ritonavir and RT inhibitors is unlikely because of the different mode of action and enzyme involved.

The common adverse reactions, such as nausea, diarrhea, vomiting, anorexia, abdominal pain and neurologic disturbances were reported with the use of ritonavir alone or in combination with other nucleoside analogues. Ritonavir is used for the treatment of advanced HIV infection including opportunistic infections. In combination with nucleoside drugs, ritonavir reduced the risk of mortality and clinical progression.

Indinavir. Indinavir sulfate (Fig. 39.10), a pentanoic acid amide derivative, was approved by the FDA in March 1996 (77). The 95% inhibitory concentration against laboratory adapted HIV variants, primary clinical isolates and clinical resistant virus to indinavir analogues, is 25–100 nM in drug combination studies with ZDV and ddI. However, HIV has shown ritonavir resistance in some patients. This resistance is due to mutation of virus that is correlated with the expression of amino acid substitutions in the viral protease. Cross-resistance to indinavir is observed with other PIs but not with the RT inhibitor. For this reason, indinavir is beneficial with ZDV and other nucleoside drugs.

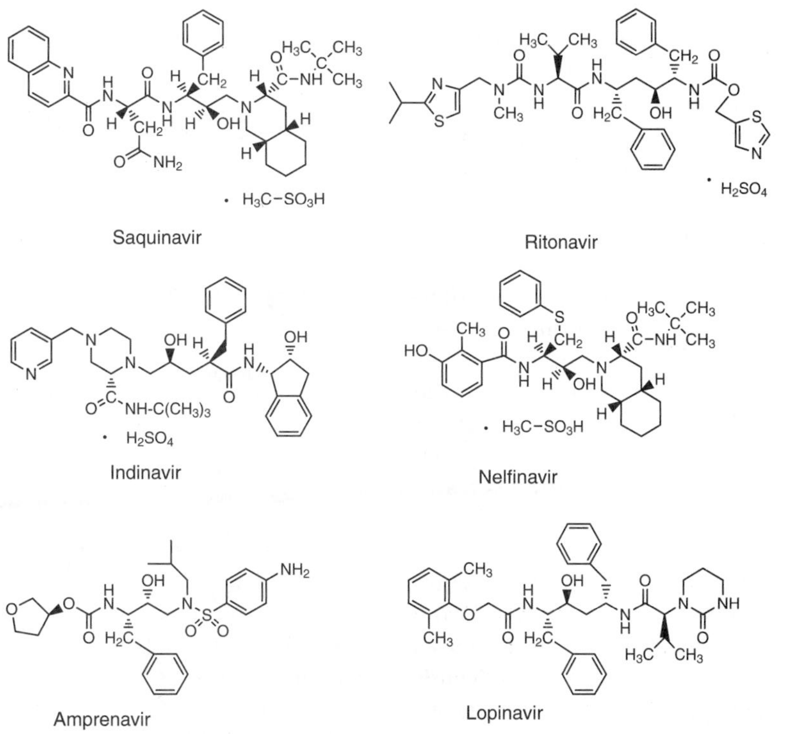

Fig. 39.10. Structures of FDA approved HIV protease inhibitors (PIs).

Pharmacokinetics. Indinavir is rapidly absorbed in the fasted patients and plasma peak concentration is observed in about one hour. At a dose of 800 mg every 8 hours, peak plasma concentration is approximately 300 nM. The drug is approximately 60% bound to human plasma proteins. Indinavir is metabolized via oxidation and glucuronide conjugation. These metabolites were recovered in feces and urine and with about 20% of the drug excreted in the urine. The half-life of indinavir is approximately 1.8 hours.

Because of indinavir's metabolism, a number of drug interactions are possible. Indinavir interacts with rifabutin or ketoconazole leading to increased or decreased indinavir concentration, respectively in the blood plasma. Administration of drug combinations of indinavir with antiviral nucleoside analogues, cimetidine, quinidine, trimethoprim/sulfamethoxazole, fluconazole or isoniazid resulted in an increased activity of indinavir. Indinavir is contraindicated in patients taking triazolam or midazolam because of inhibition of metabolism of these drugs may result in prolonged sedation, nephrolithiasis, asymptomatic hyperbilirubinemia and GI problems (anorexia, constipation, dyspepsia and gastritis).

The usual oral dose for indinavir alone or in combination with other antiviral agents is one 800-mg capsule every 8 hours. The drug is well absorbed if given on an empty stomach or 1 hour before or 2 hours after light meal with water. The dose is reduced to 600 mg every 8 hours if given concurrently with ketoconazole. Indinavir activity is increased when combined with RT inhibitors.

Nelfinavir. Nelfinavir mesylate (Fig. 39.10), is a peptidomimetic drug which is effective in HIV-1 and 2 and ZDV-resistant strains with 50% effective concentrations ranging from 9–60 nM (95% effective dose was 0.04 μg/mL)(78). After IV administration, the elimination half-life of nelfinavir was about an hour. In combination with D4T, nelfinavir reduced HIV viral load by about 98% after 4 weeks. It is well-tolerated when used with azole antifungals (ketoconazole, fluconazole, or itraconazole) or macrolide antibiotics (erythromycin, clarithromycin or azithromycin). However, it causes diarrhea and other side effects common to nonnucleoside drugs. Following oral administration, nelfinavir peak levels in plasma ranged from 0.34 μg/mL (10 mg/kg in the dog) to 1.7 μg/mL (50 mg/kg in the rat). Nelfinavir was slowly absorbed and bioavailability was 47% in the dog. The drug appeared to be metabolized in the liver and the major excretory route was in feces.

Amprenavir. Amprenavir (Fig. 39.10) is the fifth in a series of protease inhibitors to be approved for marketing in the U.S. While structurally unique from the previous agents, its pharmacologic profile does not appear to differ significantly from the previously marketed agents. Early studies suggest that a different resistance profile may exist and that the drug may be effective against some resistant strains of HIV.

Side effects appear to be more common than with other PIs and include nausea, vomiting, paresthesia, depression, and rash. Since amprenavir is a sulfonamide there is some concern for cross-sensitivity with antibacterial sulfonamides. Although this has not been reported, care should be taken if sensitivity to trimethoprim/sulfamethoxazole, used in PCP infections, is reported.

Amprenavir is rapidly absorbed following oral administration and may be taken with or without food. High-fat meals decrease the absorption of the drug and therefore should be avoided. The product is available in a capsule and liquid form. The recommended adult and adolescent dose of 1200mg twice daily requires the patient to take 8 capsules (150mg) twice daily. The liquid preparation is recommended for children between 4 and 12 years of age or for patients 13–16 years of age who weigh less than 50kg. The dose is 22.5mg/kg twice daily or 17mg/kg three times a day. Since this preparation contains the excipient propylene glycol it is not recommended for children less than 4 years of age and certain other individuals who are unable to metabolize this alcohol.

Lopinavir/Ritonavir. Recently, the FDA has approved the release of lopinavir/ritonavir (Fig. 39.10) combination in patients who have not responded to other regimens for treatment of HIV. The product is available in a soft gelatin capsule containing 133.3mg of lopinavir and 33.3mg of ritonavir as well as oral solutions containing 80mg of lopinavir and 20mg ritonavir/mL. The small amount of ritonavir is not expected to have antiretroviral activity, but

Investigational PIs

Several additional peptidomimetics are under investigation as potential PIs. These agents, tipranavir and palinavir, are presently under clinical investigation.

Tipranavir   Palinavir

DMP-850: R₁ = Benzyl, R₂ =
DMP-851: R₁ = n-Butyl, R₂ =

Tipranavir is a nonpeptidic PI which is in Phase II clinical studies. The latter compound, palinavir, is quite similar in structure to saquinavir. A number of cyclic ureas have shown promise as PIs (DMP-850 and DMP-851). While these compounds have excellent *in vitro* potency comparable to presently used PIs, they have had variable pharmacokinetic properties.

rather the ritonavir is meant to increase the plasma concentrations of lopinavir by inhibiting lopinavir's metabolism by CYP3A4. The drugs in combination with other antiretroviral agents have been approved for use in adults as well as patients between the ages of 6 months and 12 years. This is the first PI to be indicated for the very young.

Combination Drug Therapy (79,80). Combination drug therapy for viral infections is another approach under investigation. The synergistic antiviral effects of rimantadine with ribavirin and tiazofurin against influenza B virus and DHPG with foscarnet against HSV-1 and 2 are noteworthy. The synergistic action of either trifluorothymidine or acyclovir with leukocyte interferon has been used in the topical treatment of human herpetic keratitis.

During the past decade, combination antiretroviral therapy for AIDS patients has made remarkable progress. ZDV, the first approved drug for HIV-infected patients, produced bone marrow toxicity. To overcome toxic effects, combinations of ZDV with foscarnet, ddC or ddI have been used. Such combination therapy indicated improved efficacy and decreased side effects as compared to either drug used alone. The combination of ZDV with α-interferon has been used to treat patients with AIDS-related Kaposi's sarcoma. The combination drug therapy delayed emergence of ZDV-resistant HIV strains.

A combination of granulocyte-macrophage colony-stimulating factor with ZDV and α-interferon has been successful in managing treatment-related cytopenia in HIV-infected patients. The advantages of combination therapy include therapeutic antiviral effect, decreased toxicity, and low incidence of drug-resistant infection. In recent years, emergence of drug resistance has been demonstrated in patients receiving single antiviral agent therapy. Resistance to amantadine, acyclovir, ribavirin, ganciclovir, ZDV and other antiviral agents is noteworthy.

The combined antiretroviral drug therapy serves different purposes. It prolongs the life of AIDS patients; removes drug resistance and or reduce toxicity of drugs. With these objectives, successful combinations of ZDV have been reported with ddC, ddI, 3TC or D4T. Recently, combination of nucleosides drugs (ZDV, ddC, ddI, 3TC) are used with PIs (saquinavir, indinavir, ritonavir) for delaying HIV infection. Combined nucleoside drugs delay progression of HIV infection.

Antiretroviral therapy includes nucleosides or nonnucleoside RT inhibitors and PIs. These drugs inhibit HIV replication at different stage of viral infection. Nucleoside and nonnucleoside drugs inhibit RT by preventing RNA formation or viral protein synthesis. Nonnucleoside drugs inhibit RT by inactivating the catalytic site of the enzyme. PIs act after HIV provirus has integrated into the human genome. These drug inhibit protease, which is an enzyme responsible for cleaving viral precursor polypeptides into effective virions. Thus, PIs combined with RT inhibitors act by a synergistic mechanism to interupt HIV replication.

Two-drug combination, such as ZDV plus ddI or ddC; 3TC and ZDV; and D4T and ddI has been successful in raising CD4$^+$ cell counts and decreasing HIV RNA viral load. Triple drug therapy consisting of ZDV, 3TC and one of PIs (indinavir, ritonavir, nelfinavir) has been more effective than double drug therapy consisting of two nonnucleoside analogue combinations. Also fewer opportunistic infections were noted when patients took the three-drug combination.

ZDV is combined with immunomodulators to increase immunologic response in AIDS patients. ZDV has been combined with alpha interferon to obtain synergistic activity of the drug. An ideal approach of combined antiretroviral drug therapy would be drugs acting at different stages of HIV cell replication.

Investigational Antiviral Agents

New and advanced analytical techniques coupled with a good understanding of the multiplication cycle of viruses including HIV, has greatly improved the potential for the development of new antiviral agents. In the past decade, development of safe and effective antiviral therapies for the management of life-threatening infections with herpes viruses, respiratory viruses and HIV have been reported. However, future growth areas for antiviral therapy are required for virus infections of CNS, cardiovascular and emergence of new and mutant viruses. New approaches such as, antisense oligonucleotides synthesis, lyposome carrying antivirals, computer modeling, biotechnology, and gene therapy are future areas of development.

CASE STUDY

Victoria F. Roche and S. William Zito

Mrs. VG, an octogenarian widow who frequents the pharmacy where you intern, tells you that some of her neighbors have got the "grippe" and she's starting to feel a little achy herself. Last year she took the "flu shot" from her doctor and the pain in her skinny arm lasted for 5 days. She said it hurt so badly that it was almost impossible for her to lift the teakettle or make herself dinner. She was wondering if you could recommend any alternative. VG is relatively healthy for an 80-year-old and only takes Dyrenium (triamterene) once a day for mild hypertension. Evaluate antiviral structures 1–4 and make a recommendation.

1. *Identify the therapeutic problem(s) where the pharmacist's intervention may benefit the patient.*

2. *Identify and prioritize the patient specific factors that must be considered to achieve the desired therapeutic outcomes.*

3. *Conduct a thorough and mechanistically oriented structure-activity analysis of all therapeutic alternatives provided in the case.*

4. *Evaluate the SAR findings against the patient specific factors and desired therapeutic outcomes and make a therapeutic decision.*

5. *Counsel your patient.*

Triamterene   1   2   3   4

REFERENCES

1. Fraenkel-Conrat H, ed. The chemistry and biology of viruses. New York: Academic Press, 1969; 45–109.

2. Evans AS, Kaslow RA, ed. Viral infections of humans, epidemiology and control, 4th ed. New York: Plenum Medical Book Company, 1997.

3. Rothschild H, Allison F Jr, Howe C, et al, eds. Human diseases caused by viruses. New York: Oxford University Press, 1978; 61–258.

4. Drew WL, ed. Viral infections: a clinical approach. Philadelphia: F. A. Davis, 1976; 8–10.

5. Temin HM, Mizutani S. RNA-dependent DNA polymerase in virions of Rouse sarcoma viruss. Nature 1970; 226: 1211–1213.

6. Baltimore D. RNA dependent DNA polymerase in virions of RNA tumor viruses. Nature 1970; 226: 1209–1211.

7. Choppin PW. Basic virology. In: Rothschild H, Cohen JC, eds., Virology in medicine. New York: Oxford University, 1986; 3–45.

8. Galasso GJ, Whitley RJ, Merigan T, eds. Antiviral agents and viral diseases of man. New York: Raven Press, 1990;1–48.

9. Halsey NA. The epidemiology of viral diseases, In: Rothschild H, Cohen JC, eds. Virology in medicine. New York: Oxford University, 1986; 87–110.

10. Calio R, Nistico G, eds. Antiviral drugs, basic and therapeutic aspects. Rome-Milan: Pythagora Press, 1989; 1–9.

11. Mandell GL, Bennett SE, Dolin R, eds. Principles and practice of infectious diseases. New York: Churchill Livingstone, 1995.

12. Mills J, Corey L , eds. Antiviral chemotherapy: new directions for clinical application and research, Vol. 3, Englewood Cliffs, NJ: PTR Prentice Hall, 1993.

13. Sethi VS, Sethi ML. Inhibition of reverse transcriptase activity of RNA tumor viruses by fagaronine. Biochem Biophys Res Commun 1975; 63: 1070–1076; Sethi ML. Inhibition of reverse transcriptase activity by benzophenanthridine alkaloids. J Nat Prod 1979; 42:187–196; Sethi ML. Screening of benzophenanthridine alkaloids for their inhibition of reverse transcriptase activity and preliminary report on the structure-activity relationships. Can J Pharm Sci 1981; 16:29–34.

14. Rosenberg M, Debouck C. HIV protease: a molecular target for therapeutic intervention In: Mills J, Corey M, eds. Antiviral chemotherapy, vol 3, 1993;327–44.

15. Boyd JR, Editor-in-Chief, Drug Facts and comparison. St. Louis: J. B. Lippincott Company, 1997; 2346–2437.

16. Douglas RG. Jr. Antiviral drugs 1983, Med Clin North Amer 1983; 67: 1163–1172.

17. Keating MR. Antiviral agents. Mayo Clin. Proc. 1992; 67 (2): 160–178.

18. Hammer SM, Inouye RT. Antiviral agents In: Whitley RJ, Hayden FG, eds. Clinical virology New York: Churchill Livingstone, 1997.

19. Burlington DB, Meiklejohn G, Mostow SR. Antiinfluenza A virus activity of amantadine hydrochloride and rimantadine hydrochloride in ferret tracheal ciliated epithelium. Antimicrob Agents Chemother 1982; 21:794–799.

20. Hayden FG. Combinations of antiviral agents for treatment of influenza virus infection. J antimicrob chemother 1986; suppl B: 177–183.

21. Wingfield WL, Pollack D, Grunert RR. Therapeutic efficacy of an amantadine and rimantadine hydrochloride in naturally occurring influenza A2 respiratory illness inman. N Engl J Med 1969; 28: 579–584; Wintermeyer, SM, Nahata MC. Rimantadine: a clinical prospective. Ann Pharmacother 1995; 29:299–310.

22. Francis ML, Meltzer MS, Gendelman HE. Interferons in the persistence, pathogenesis, and treatment of HIV infection. AIDS Res. Human Retroviruses 1992, 8:199–207.

23. Hayden FG. In: Revel M, ed. Clinical aspects of interferons. Boston: Kluwer Academic Publishers, 1988.

24. Pollard RB. Interferons and interferon inducers: development of clinical usefulness and therapeutic promise. Drugs. 1982; 23: 37–55.

25. Streuli M, Nagata S, Weismann C. At least three human type α interferons: structure of α_2. Science 1980; 209: 1343–1347.

26. Taniguchi T, Guarente L, Roberts TM, et al. Expression of the human fibroblast interferon gene in Escherichia coli. Proc Nat. Acad Sci USA. 1980; 77: 5230–5233.

27. Baglioni C, Maroney PA. Mechanisms of action of human interferons, induction of 2,′5′-oligo (A) polymerase. J Biol Chem 1980; 255: 8390–8393.

28. Calfee DP, Hayden FG. New approaches to influenza chemotherapy: neuraminidase inhibitors. Drugs 1998: 56:537–553.

29. Kim CU, Lew W, Williams MA, et al. Influenza neuraminidase inhibitors possessing a novel hydrophobic interaction in the enzyme active site: design, synthesis, and structural analysis of carbocyclic sialic acid analogues with potent anti-influenza activity. J Amer Chem Soc 1997; 119: 681–690.

30. Sweeny DJ, Lynch G, Bidgood AM, et al. Metabolism of the influenza neuraminidase inhibitor prodrug oseltamivir in the rat. Drug Met Disp 2000: 28:737–741.

31. Field HJ. A perspective on resistance to acyclovir in herpes simplex virus. Antimicrob Chemother 1983; 12 (Suppl. B): 129–135.

32. Elion GB, Furman PA, Fyfe JA, et al. Selectivity of action of an antiherpetic agent, 9-(2-hydroxyethoxymethyl) guanine. Proc Natl Acad Sci USA 1977; 74: 5716–5720.

33. Whitley RJ, Alford CA. Antiviral agents: clinical status report. Hosp Pract 1981; 16:109–121.

34. Mitchell CD, Bean B, Gentry SR, et al. Acyclovir therapy for mucucutaneous herpes simplex infections in immunocompromised patients. Lancet 1981;1:1389–1392.

35. Whitley RJ, Alford CA, Hirsch MS, et al. Vidarabine versus acyclovir therapy in herpes simplex encephalitis. N Engl J Med 1986; 314: 144–149.

36. Brigden D, Bye A, Fowle AS, et al. Human pharmacokinetics of acyclovir (an antiviral agent) following rapid intravenous injection. J Antimicrob Chemother 1981, 7:399–404.

37. de Miranda P, Whitley RJ, Blum MR, et al. Acyclovir kinetics after intravenous infusion. Clin Pharmacol Ther 1979; 26: 718–728.

38. Perry CM, Faulds D. Valaciclovir, a review of its antiviral activity, pharmacokinetic properties and therapeutic efficacy in herpes virus infection. Drugs 1996; 52:754–772.

39. Martinez CM, Lucks-Golger DB. Cidofovir use in acyclovir-resistant herpes infection. Ann Pharmacother 1997; 31: 1519–1521

40. Ward RL, Stevens JG. Effect of cytosine arabinoside on viral-specific protein synthesis in cells infected with herpes simplex virus. J Virol 1975; 15: 71–80.

41. Nutter RL, Rapp F. The effect of cytosine arabinoside on virus production in various cells infected with herpes simplex virus types 1 and 2. Cancer Res 1973; 33: 166–170.

42. Schacker T, Hu HL, Koell DM, et al. Famciclovir for the suppression of symptomatic and asymptomatic herpes simplex virus reactivation in HIV-infected person. A double blind, placebo-control trial. Ann Intern Med 1998; 128 (1): 21–28.

43. Field AK. Viral targets for antisense oligonucleotides: a mini review. Antiviral Res 1998; 37:67–81.

44. Chrisp P, Clissold SP. Foscarnet: A review of its antiviral activity, pharmacokinetic properties and therapeutic use in immunocompromised patients with cytomegalovirus retinitis. Drugs 1991; 41: 104–129.

45. Fletcher CV, Balfour HH. Evaluation of ganciclovir for cytomagalovirus disease. Drug Intell Clin Pharm 1989; 23: 5–11.

46. Whitley RJ. The past as prelude to the future: history, status and future of antiviral drugs. Annals Pharmacotherapy 1996; 30: 967–971.

47. Farah A, eds. Handbook of experimental biology. Vol. 38/2, Berlin: Springer, 1975; 272–347.

48. Sidwell RW, Huffman JH, Khare GP, et al. Broas-spectrum antiviral activity of virazole: 1-beta-D-ribofuranosyl-1,2,4-triazole-3-carboxamide. Science 1972; 177: 705–706.

49. Hall CB, McBride JT. Vapors, viruses and views. Ribavirin and respiratory syncytial virus. Am J Dis Child 1986; 140: 331–332.

50. Fox CF, Robinson WS, eds. Virus research. New York: Academic Press 1973; 415–436.

51. Power WJ, Benedict SA, Hillery M, et al. Randomised double-blind trial of bromovinyldeoxyuridine (BUVD) and trifluorothymidine (TFT) in dendritic corneal ulceration. Br J Ophthalmology 1991; 75: 649–651.

52. Whitley RJ, Soong SJ, Dolin R, et al. Adenine arabinoside therapy of biopsy-proved herpes simplex encephalitis. National Institute of Allergy and Infectious diseases collaborative antiviral study. N Engl J Med 1977; 297: 289–294.

53. Whitley RJ, Soong SJ, Dolin R, et al. Early vidarabine therapy to control the complications of herpes zooster in immunocompromised patients. N Engl J Med 1982; 307: 971–975.

54. Chao DL, Kimblall AP. Determination of arabinosyladenine by adenosine deaminase and inhibition by arabinosyl-6-mercaptopurine. Cancer Res 1972; 32: 1721–1724.

55. Blair E, Darby G. eds. Antiviral Therapy. New York: BIOS Scientific Publishers, 1998.

56. Valle LA do, Melo PR de, Gomes LF de. Methisazone in prevention of variola minor among contacts. Lancet 1965; 2: 976–978.

57. Mohan P, Baba M, eds. Anti-AIDS drug development: challenges, strategies and prospects. Chur Switzerland: Harwood Academic, 1995; Sethi ML. Current concepts in HIV/AIDS pharmacotherapy. The Cosultant Pharmacists. 1998; 13:12241245.

58. Berger TG. Treatment of bacterial, fungal and parasitic infections in the HIV-infected host. Semin Dermatol 1993; 12: 296–300.

59. Sattler FR, Feinberg J. New developments in the treatment of Pneumocystis carinii pneumonia. Chest 1992; 101: 451–457.

60. Goa KL, Barradell LB. Fluconazole. An update of its pharmacodynamic and pharmacokinetic properties and therapeutic use in major superficial and systemic mycosis in immunocompromised patients. Drugs 1995; 50: 658–690.

61. Mitsuya H, ed. Anti-HIV nucleosides: past, present and future. New York: Chapman and Hall, 1997; Gorbach SL, Barlett JG, Blacklow NR, eds. Infectious diseases. Philadelphia: WB Saunders Company, 1998; 330–350, 1154–1168.

62. MacDonald L, Kazanjian P. Antiretroviral therapy in HIV-infection: an update. Formulary 1996; 31: 780–804; Faulds D, Brogden RN. Didanosine. A review of its antiviral activity, pharmacokinetic properties and therapeutic potential in human immunodeficiency virus infection. Drugs 1992; 44: 94–116.

63. Beach, JW. Chemotherapeutic agents for human immunodeficiency virus infection: mechanism of action, pharmacokinetics, metabolism and adverse reactions, Clin Ther 1998; 20: 2–25; Lipsky JJ. Zalcitabine and didanosine, Lancet 1993; 341:30–32; Shelton MH, O'Donnell AM, Morse GD. Zalcitabine. Ann Pharmacother 1993; 27: 480–489.

64. Neuzil KM. Pharmacologic therapy for HIV infection: a review. Am J Med Sci 1994; 307:368–373.

65. Fischl MA, Richmann DD, Greico MH, et al. The efficacy of the azothymidine (AZT) in the treatment of patients with AIDS and AIDS-related complex, a double-blinded, placebo controlled trial. N Engl J Med 1987; 317: 185–191.

66. Fischl MA, Richmann DD, Hansen N, et al. The safety and efficacy of zidovudine (AZT) in the treatment of subjects with mildly symptomatic human immunodeficiency virus type 1 (HIV) infection: a double-blind, placebo-controlled trial. Ann Intern Med 1990; 112: 727–737; Sethi ML. Zidovudine. In: Florey K, ed. Analytical profiles of drug substances. San Diego: Academic Press, 1991, Vol 20; 729–765.

67. Nasr M, Littest C, McGowan J. Computer-assisted structure-activity correlations of dideoxynucleoside analogs as potential anti-HIV drugs. Antiviral Res 1990; 14: 125–148.

68. Hoth DF, Myers MW, Stein, DS. Current status of HIV therapy I. Antiviral agents. Hospital Practice 1992;. 27: 145–156.

69. Horowitz JP, Chua J, Noel M. Nucleosides V. The monomesylates of 1-(2′-deoxy-β-D-lyxofuranosyl) thymine. J Org Chem 1964: 29:2076–2079: Ostertag W, Roesler G, Krieg CJ, et al. Induction of endogenous virus and of thymidine kinase by bromodeoxyuridine in cell cultures transformed by Friend virus. Proc Natl Acad Sci USA 1974: 71:4980–4985; Yarchoan R, Klecker RW, Weinhold KJ, Markham PD, et al. Administration of 3′-azido-3′′-deoxythymidine, an inhibitor of HTLV-III/LAV replication to patients with AIDS or AIDS-related complex. Lancet 1986: 1:575–580.

70. Perry CM, Faulds D. Lamivudine. A review of its antiviral activity, pharmacokineticproperties and therapeutic efficacy in the management of HIV infection. Drugs 1997; 53: 657–680.

71. Tan B, Ratner L. The use of new antiretroviral therapy in combination with chemotherapy. Curr Opin Oncol 1997; 9: 455–464.

72. Freimuth WW. Delaviridine mesylate, a potent non-nucleoside HIV-1 reverse transcriptase inhibitor. Adv Exp Med Biol 1996; 394:279–289.

73. Graul A, Rabasseda X, Castaner J. Efavirenz. Drugs of the Future 1998; 23:133–141.

74. Deeks SG, Volberding PA. HIV-1 protease inhibitors. AIDS Clin Rev, 1997–1998: 145–185.

75. Hoetelmans RM, Meenhorst PL, Mulder JW, et al. Clinical pharmacology of HIV protease inhibitors: focus on saquanivir, indinavir and ritonavir. Pharm World Sci 1997; 19: 159–175; Perry CM, Noble S. Saquinavir soft-gel capsule formulation. Drugs 1998; 56: 461–486.

76. Markowitz M, Saag M, Powderly WG, et al. A preliminary study of ritonavir, an inhibitor HIV-1 protease to treat HIV-1 infection. N Engl J Med 1995; 333:1534–1539.

77. Deeks SG, Smith M, Holodniy M, et al. HIV-1 protease inhibitor: a review for clinician. JAMA 1997; 277 (2):145–153.

78. Perry CM, Benfield P. Nelfinavir. Drugs 1997; 54:81–88.

79. Fischl MA, Stanley K, Collier AC, et al. Combination and monotherapy with zidovudine and zalcitabine in patients with advanced HIV disease. The NIAID AIDS clinical trial group. Ann Intern Med 1995; 122 (1):24–32.

80. Havlir DV, Lange JM. New antivirals and new combinations. AIDS 1998; 12 Suppl A:S 165–174.

SUGGESTED READINGS

Arrand JA, Harper DR, eds. Viruses and human cancer, Oxford: BIOS Scientific Publishers, 1998.

Blair ED, Darby G. In: Molecular biology of HIV/AIDS, Lever AM, ed. The Molecular Biology of HIV/AIDS, Chichester, New York: Wiley, 1996.

Collier LH, Oxford JS, eds. Developments in antiviral therapy. New York: Academic Press, 1980.

Collier LH, Oxford J, ed. Human virology: a text for students of medicine, dentistry, and microbiology. Oxford: Oxford University Press, 1993.

Fraenkel-Conrat H, ed. Molecular basis of virology. New York: Reinhold, 1968.

Fraenkel-Conrat H, Wagner RR, ed. Comprehensive virology, vol. 16, 19, New York: Plenum Press, 1980, 1997.

Galasso GJ, Whitley RJ, Mergan TC, eds. Antiviral agents and human viral diseases. 4th ed., Philadelphia: Lippencott-Raven Publishers, 1997.

Harper D, ed. Molecular virology New York, Oxford: BIOS Scientific Publishers 1998.

Knight CA, ed. Chemistry of viruses, 2nd ed. New York: Springer, 1975.

Levine AJ. ed, Viruses. New York: Scientific American Library, 1992.

Merigan TC. Antivirals with clinical potential introduction. J Infect Dis. 1976; 133: Suppl., A1–2.

Molla A, Granneman GR, Sun E, et al. Recent developments in HIV protease inhibitor therapy. Antiviral Res 1998; 39:1–23.

Rothschild H, Cohan JC, ed. Virology in medicine. New York: Oxford University Press, 1986.

Stuart-Harris CH, Oxford JS, eds. Problems of antiviral therapy. London: New York: Academic Press, 1983.

Wolff ME, ed. Burger's medicinal chemistry.and drug discovery. 5th ed. Vol 5, New York: Wiley, 1997.

PART III

Recent Advances
in Drug Discovery

40. Pharmaceutical Biotechnology

ROBERT D. SINDELAR, Ph.D.

INTRODUCTION

Pharmaceutical biotechnology is advancing with unprecedented methodology and achievements. The early 1980s saw the products of modern pharmaceutical biotechnology come to the marketplace as the Food and Drug Administration (FDA) approved recombinant DNA-produced insulin in 1982, and second-generation home pregnancy test kits containing monoclonal antibodies were developed. In an article entitled "Biotechnology: Are you ready for it?," appearing as the cover story in the May 1990 issue of *Drug Topics,* Conlan (1) suggested that "pharmacists will skillfully ride the coming biotechnology drug wave into the 21st century, where they'll reign as the unchallenged drug therapy experts, designing, dispensing, counseling, and monitoring medicines in the brave new world of genetic engineering." Although a decade later this vision has yet to be fulfilled in its entirety, this is certainly an attractive scenario and represents an exciting opportunity for pharmacists (2). Pharmaceutical biotechnology generates basic scientific knowledge, useful therapeutic and diagnostic products, and promising methodologies for future research and clinical applications. There is little doubt that the techniques of biotechnology have led to the development and marketing of new and novel therapies residing on pharmacists' shelves today; improved methods of manufacture of pharmaceuticals; and significant contributions to our better understanding of disease etiology, pathophysiology, and biochemistry. Obviously, advances in biotechnology are going to have an increasing impact on pharmacy practice in the first decade of the 21st century and

well into the future. Rapid advances in deciphering the code of life, the human genome, provides the potential for unparalleled therapeutic opportunities. The clinician of the future will have the tools to routinely screen for the genetic implications of new drugs, improving a patient's response to drug treatment and making therapeutics a true science. Although many of the first biotechnology-derived therapeutics were initially used in acutely ill hospital patients, products of today's pharmaceutical biotechnology increasingly have an impact on the chronic disease patient populations constituting much of ambulatory care practice.

Biotechnology, innovation harnessing nature's own biochemical tools, uses living organisms and their cellular, sub-cellular, and molecular components. In its broadest definition, Sumerian and Babylonian beer brewing around 6000 BC, the baking of leavened bread by the Egyptians (by 4000 BC), cheese making, and even Alexander Fleming's discovery of penicillin in 1928 are products of biotechnology. Therefore, biotechnology is an evolutionary technology, not a revolutionary one. What we may think of as modern biotechnology is enabled by a collection of techniques arising out of developments in molecular and cell biology, microbiology, genetics, biochemistry, protein chemistry, organic chemistry, and immunology in the 1970s and 1980s (Fig. 40.1). The FDA defines biotechnology as a technique that uses living organisms or a part of a living organism to produce or modify a product, to improve a plant or animal, or to develop a microorganism to be used for a specific purpose. Applications of biotech-

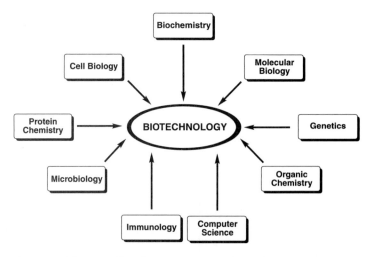

Fig. 40.1. Enabling technologies of biotechnology.

nology are found in medicine, pharmaceutical sciences, agriculture, environmental science, food science, forensics, and materials science. As applied to pharmaceuticals, the techniques of biotechnology discover, develop, and produce useful therapeutic agents and diagnostics. Pioneering strategies for exploring the causes of disease, new drug design, and therapeutic intervention tailored for the individual are products of today's modern pharmaceutical biotechnology.

Several textbooks on the pharmaceutical aspects of biotechnology are available (3–8). Additionally, encyclopedias and dictionaries of biotechnology (9–12) and other biotechnology texts (13–17) appeared in print. Most biochemistry and molecular biology textbooks are fine sources of biotechnology-related material.(18–21) Excellent chapters on biotechnology in medicinal chemistry (22–24)and numerous reviews of biotechnology for pharmacists(1–2,25–45) are also available. In addition, listings of biotechnology-produced pharmaceuticals in development(46) and a biotechnology reference resource catalog(47) have been published.

IMPACT OF BIOTECHNOLOGY ON PHARMACEUTICAL CARE

The biotechnology industry has grown explosively over the past 25 years, with estimated sales of human therapeutic and diagnostic products for fiscal 2000 reaching $14.2 billion (48). This is a doubling in 7 years. These sales are projected for an increase to $71.9 billion in the year 2025, escalating to $233 billion by the year 2050. Approximately 90% of the nearly $16 billion in total worldwide biotechnology sales expected in 2000 will come from biotechnology-produced pharmaceuticals. As reported in the 1998 survey of Biotechnology Medicines in Development, the Pharmaceutical Research and Manufacturers of America (PhRMA)found 350 new biotechnology-produced medicines in development and 140 pharmaceutical and biotechnology companies testing biotech products (46). The survey represents a significant increase over the past decade (Fig. 40.2). Of the 350 medicines, 151 products are for cancer or cancer-related conditions, 29 are in the development for human immunodeficiency virus (HIV) infection and acquired immunodeficiency syndrome (AIDS), 36 for other infectious diseases, 28 are for the treatment of heart disease, and 20 products are under development for respiratory disease. A further analysis of the survey data reveals that 77 of the 350 medicines in development are new vaccines. In addition, 74 are monoclonal antibody-based products and 38 are gene therapy approaches.

Improved manufacturing of pharmaceuticals was the first major contribution of biotechnology to pharmaceutical care in the 1980s. Biotechnology-produced human insulin, growth hormone, and erythropoietin, all replacements of highly specific, endogenous molecules, were major advances in therapy. Since the late 1980s, however, pharmaceutical biotechnology has also helped to identify

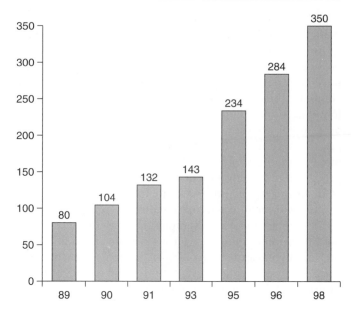

Fig. 40.2. Increasing number of biotechnology-produced medicines in development by year. (Data from Biotechnology Medicines in Development, 1998 Annual Survey. Washington, D.C.: Pharmaceutical Research and Manufacturers of America, 1998.)

new compounds with new mechanisms of action. Significant contributions to the understanding of the mechanism of disease at the molecular level continue to be made by biotechnology researchers and will translate into newer, better pharmaceuticals. The impact of biotechnology on pharmaceutical care is expected to exponentially increase as advances in technology continue to yield novel medicinal agents such as the colony-stimulating factors (CSFs), tissue-type plasminogen activator (tPA), new vaccines, DNase, fusion protein drugs (e.g., leukin diftitox), and specific monoclonal antibodies including trastuzumab. Products of biotechnology are playing a critical role in the discovery and design as well as the production of treatments for life-threatening diseases, such as cancer, AIDS, and cardiovascular disease.

Pharmaceutical care using biotechnology-derived products requires (43–44):

1. An understanding of how the handling and stability of biopharmaceuticals differs from other drugs pharmacists dispense.
2. A preparation of the product for patient use, including reconstitution or compounding, if required.
3. Patient education on their disease, benefits of the prescribed biopharmaceutical, potential side effects or drug interactions to be aware of, and the techniques to self-administer the biotechnology drug.
4. Patient counseling on the reimbursement issues involving an expensive product.
5. Monitoring of the patient for compliance.

A decade ago, it was predicted that by the turn of the century biotechnology-produced pharmaceuticals would overtake nonbiotech medicines in sales and approvals

(49). While this prediction has not happened, the biotechnology medicine evolution is gaining momentum. The techniques of pharmaceutical biotechnology will make it possible to: prevent, cure and treat more diseases than possible today; anticipate and prevent disease symptoms; eliminate the contamination risks of infectious pathogens found in human blood derived biopharmaceuticals; target drug therapy toward the underlying cause of diseases, not just the treatment of disease symptoms; produce replacement human proteins on large scale; and develop more precise and effective medicines with fewer side effects (46). Key areas of future growth for biotech in the 21st century will include pharmacogenomics/pharmacogenetics, recombinant-based therapies such as vaccines delivered by novel administrative routes, genetic modification of the patient, and the cloning of human tissues and organs (50). It will be interesting to view the impact of these future biotech advances on the practice of pharmacy.

TECHNIQUES OF BIOTECHNOLOGY
Overview

The techniques made available by advances in biotechnology that have provided new medicinal agents fall into several broad areas. First, recombinant DNA (rDNA) technology, the ability to manipulate the genetic information inherent within the nucleus of living cells, provides the ability to take identified gene sequences from one organism and place them functionally into another to permit the production of protein medicines. Second, hybridoma techniques permit the production of monoclonal antibodies (MAb). MAbs are ultrasensitive hybrid immune system-derived proteins designed to recognize specific antigens and are used as diagnostic agents for laboratory and home kits and site-directed therapeutics.

Additionally, the development of technologies to study DNA-DNA and DNA-RNA interactions has led to the formation of RNA and DNA probes (antisense technology) for a variety of research purposes with potential uses as diagnostics and therapeutics. Tools of modern pharmaceutical biotechnology also include polymerase chain reaction, genomics, proteomics, gene therapy, transgenics, glycobiology and a host of other evolving techniques (Table 40.1).

Table 40.1. Major Techniques of Biotechnology

Recombinant DNA technology (rDNA)
Hybridoma technology (monoclonal antibodies)
Antisense technology
Polymerase chain reaction (PCR)
Genomics (including DNA microarrays)
Proteomics
Gene therapy
Transgenics
Glycobiology
Proteomics
Cloning
Molecular modeling
Peptidomimetics

Recombinant DNA Technology

The revolution in biology and genetics that has occurred over the past 25 years, affecting both the basic research and its practical aspects, has been fueled by rDNA technology. Sometimes also referred to as genetic engineering, gene cloning, or *in vitro* genetic manipulation, rDNA technology provides the ability to introduce genetic material from any source into cells (bacterial, fungal, plant, or animal) or whole plants and animals (51). A general understanding of the technologies involved should readily help the pharmacist better gain insight into and comprehension of a biotechnology drug's use, stability, handling, side effects, and potential toxicity: in other words, how these agents differ from traditional drugs. Also, such an understanding should readily demonstrate the impact that rDNA technology is having on both current and future pharmacy practice.

Normal Process of Protein Synthesis by the Cell

To understand the impact of rDNA technology, a general understanding of the process of protein synthesis by a cell is essential. Sections on protein synthesis in any biochemistry or molecular biology textbook (18–21) furnish a detailed review. A general review of gene expression and the process of protein synthesis follows and is schematically represented in Figure 40.3.

The active working components of the cellular machinery are proteins, which constitute more than half the total dry weight of a cell. Proteins carry out most biologic activities of cells. A protein's particular function is determined by the exact linear order of amino acids composing that protein, its primary structure. Therefore, protein synthesis is critical to cell development, maintenance, and growth. The information or coding for protein synthesis and the chemical synthesis of the protein are the central dogma of molecular biology: DNA to RNA to protein (52–53).

The genetic information necessary for a cell to live and function, i.e., to encode for the synthesis of specific proteins, is stored in discrete genes within the linear molecules of 2'-deoxyribonucleic acid (DNA) making up the chromosomes in the cell nucleus. As a result of the efforts of the Human Genome Project and genomics, the number of functional genes is estimated to be 30,000–35,000. This number is nearly one-third previous predictions. The estimated genome size of several species is shown in Table 40.2.

The genes consist of double helical strands of DNA. The exact sequence of building blocks of the cell's DNA, the nucleic acid bases, contain the genetic code to synthesize a specific protein. A detailed discussion of the structure of DNA, the complementary binding between the two strands of DNA, and DNA replication can be found in Chapter 41. In addition, the reader is referred to Chapter 41 for details of the step-by-step processes shown in Figure 40.3 in which transcription from DNA to messenger RNA (mRNA) occurs through the intermediate pre-mRNA and the enzyme RNA polyerase.

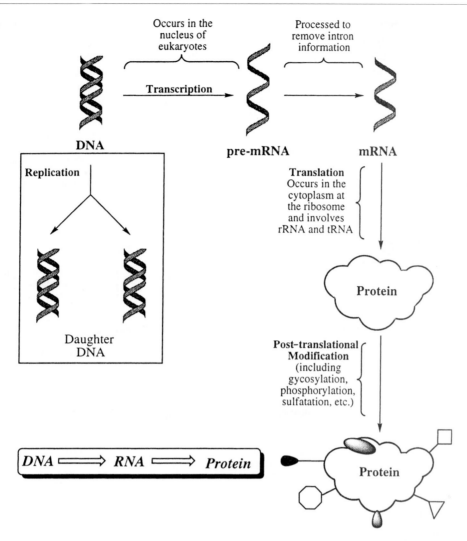

Fig. 40.3. Gene expression: the synthesis of proteins.

Table 40.2. Estimated Genome Size of Some Selected Organisms

Organism	Genome Size (in base pairs)
Amoeba	290,000,000,000
Cow	3,651,500,000
Frog	3,000,000,000
Gorilla	3,523,200,000
HIV-1	9,750
Housefly	900,000,000
Human	**3,400,000,000**
Mouse	3,454,200,000
Pig	3,108,700,000
Pine tree	68,000,000,000
Yeast	12,067,280

Israel RK, Lesney MS. SNPs and snails and genome tails. Mod Drug Discov. 1999;2:104.

The relay of genetic information from RNA into protein involving transfer RNA (tRNA) at the cytoplasmic ribosome is referred to as translation. The ribosome is composed of ribosomal RNA (rRNA) along with a set of proteins (Fig. 40.3). The tRNA bearing specific amino acids binds to a codon on the mRNA at the ribosome and under the influence of enzymes called aminoacyl tRNA synthetase begins the synthesis of a protein. As amino acid addition occurs, the newly synthesized protein begins to assume its characteristic three-dimensional shape (secondary and tertiary structure). In addition, post-translational modifications of the protein can commonly occur in the endoplasmic reticulum or Golgi apparatus after completion of the protein chain (Fig. 40.3). In most cases, these enzymatic chemical reactions alter the side chains of some of the amino acids in the protein. Some examples of post-translational modifications include O-glycosylation of threonine or tyrosine; N-glycosylation of asparagine; sulfate conjugation of thyrosine; hydroxylation of proline or lysine; and phosphorylation of tyrosine, serine, or threonine (54). Although the codon system is consistent among all organisms (thus allowing rDNA technology), it is important to note that many post-translational modifications occur only in higher organisms (not bacteria).

Protein Synthesis Through Recombinant DNA

Useful reviews detailing the process of recombinant DNA are available (4–8,13–16,52,55–56). Applicable sections in any biochemistry or molecular biology textbooks(18–21) provide more detailed reviews. Several reviews of rDNA technology have been written for practicing pharmacists.(26,30,33,35,43) In addition, a biotechnology resource catalog listing references of various aspects of rDNA has been published (46). A general summary of the typical rDNA production of a protein follows and is schematically presented in Figure 40.4.

In theory, one can produce any protein desired as long as a copy of the corresponding gene is made available. Reproducing the DNA involved is called cloning. There are two major methods to obtain the necessary gene. The first is genomic cloning, in which identification and isolation of the DNA coding for the protein is achieved by breaking up the entire genome into fragments and using DNA probes to screen the resulting genomic library for the desired gene. DNA probes are the standard method for identifying a DNA sequence within a mixture (57 and Chapter 41). The probes are labeled (radioactive or fluorescent) spe-

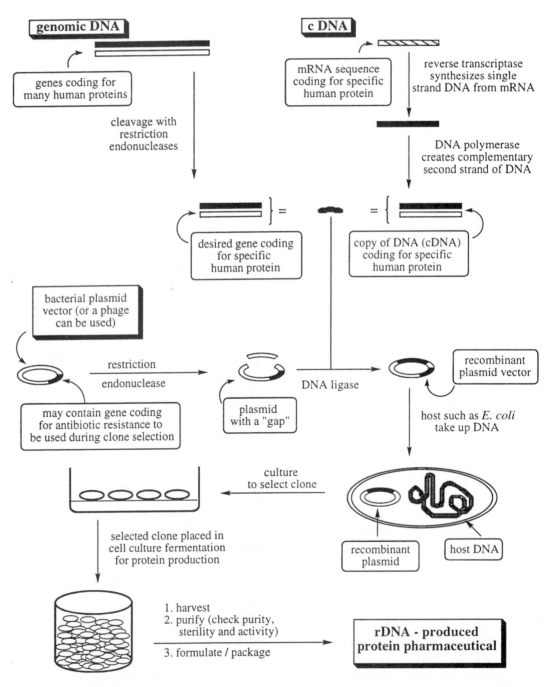

Fig. 40.4. Summary of typical rDNA production of a protein from either a) genomic DNA or b) cDNA.

cific nucleotide sequences that bind only to their complementary or copy DNA (cDNA) in the mixture of DNA fragments to form a double helix. The resulting double helix is detected using the label. Probes are the basis for DNA fingerprinting, the method of making a pattern of the DNA of an individual unique from any other individual.

The second method, cDNA cloning, involves the isolation of the mRNA that codes for the amino acid sequence of the protein and is achieved using the viral enzyme reverse transcriptase to "retro"-synthesize the cDNA. Reverse transcriptase, also called RNA-dependent DNA polymerase, is an enzyme capable of converting mRNA into complementary single-stranded DNA. The enzyme DNA polymerase synthesizes a complementary second strand of DNA on the created single strand of DNA.

An additional method to obtain DNA for use in rDNA technology is the automated synthesis of the gene through biochemical means, if the amino acid sequence of the protein is known so the codon sequence can be deduced. At present, however, this method is practical only for relatively small proteins.

Once the gene coding for the desired protein has been identified and isolated, the genetic material is introduced into cells using restriction endonucleases and a vector to enable DNA replication and to produce protein. The discovery of restriction endonuclease enzymes that recognize explicit sequences of bases in double-stranded DNA and precisely hydrolyzes the phosphodiester bonds of the nucleic acids at specific sites along the DNA strands offered a way of isolating predictable fragments of any DNA molecule. This family of "scissors-like" enzymes is used to provide the DNA fragment coding for the protein of interest by "cutting" or "clipping" the DNA (Fig. 40.5). The bacterial enzymes, numbering greater than 100 variations isolated (see Table 40.3 for representative examples), have led to the powerful techniques of DNA sequencing and rDNA technology. Most restriction endonucleases create two single-strand breaks, one in each strand generating a 5′-phospho*mono*ester and 3′-hydroxyl group from each cleavage. The breaks are not necessarily opposite one another as can be seen in Table 40.3 with examples ASU II, Bal I, and Eco RV. For instance, Eco RI causes breaks that are not opposite one another creating sticky (or cohesive or complementary) ends to the DNA strands. The DNA fragments can be isolated, purified, and identified.

A cloning vector is a carrier molecule, the vehicle that is used to insert foreign DNA into a host cell. Typically, vectors are genetic elements that can be replicated in a host cell separately from that cell's chromosomes. Bacterial plasmids, circular DNA of only a few thousand base pairs outside of the nucleus that replicate freely within the cell, are ideal to carry the gene into the host organism (see discussion of gene vectors in Chapter 41). In the first such rDNA experiments in early 1973, Cohen and associates(58) used the small *Escherichia coli* plasmid pSC101 containing only a single Eco RI recognition site as the vec-

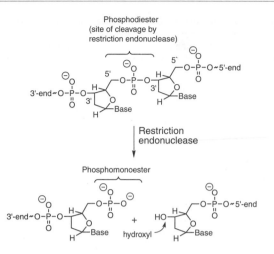

Fig. 40.5. Cleavage by restriction endonuclease.

tor to insert foreign plasmid DNA into *E. coli*. Other vectors include the constructed plasmids pBR322 and pUC18 and bacteriophages. Bacteriophages are bacterial viruses modified to accept large pieces (7–20 kilobases in length) of exogenous DNA without altering their ability to infect and replicate inside the bacteria (59). Large genomic libraries have been created by fragmenting all of the embryonic or sperm cell DNA of an organism, inserting them into bacteriophage lambda, and screening with DNA probes to identify the gene sequences.

The DNA fragments coding for the desired protein can be cloned from genomic DNA or cDNA as described previously. The piece of DNA coding for the protein of interest is then inserted into the vector that carries the code to synthesize the protein into the host. The plasmid or bacteriophage DNA is opened with a restriction enzyme, and the exogenous gene is pasted into it by an enzyme called DNA ligase with the assistance of special sections of DNA called linkers. DNA ligase seals the single-strand breaks in double-stranded DNA. Also, promoter or enhancer DNA sequences are added to increase plasmid replication and increase protein synthesis by the gene. A promoter is a short DNA sequence that amplifies the expression of protein by the adjacent target gene. An enhancer is a viral DNA sequence that dramatically increases the level of transcription of adjacent DNA. A gene providing antibiotic resistance (as a selection tool) may also be placed in a plasmid that is inserted into a bacterial host. This gene confers a particular antibiotic resistance on the clone and may be used in the clone selection later in the rDNA process. This vector is now a rDNA molecule consisting of the gene, linker, promoter/enhancer, and vector DNA.

The vector containing the code for the target protein is then inserted into the host. Host cells are typically bacteria (e.g., *E. coli*), eukaryotic yeast such as *Saccharomyces cerevisiae* (baker's yeast), or mammalian cell lines. Examples of mammalian cell lines include CHO (Chinese hamster ovary), VERO (African green monkey kidney), and BHK

Table 40.3. Some Representative Examples of Restriction Endonucleases (1)

Restriction Endonucleases	Source	Recognition Sequence*	Cleavage Products	
Alu I	*Arthrobacter*	5'- TT/CGAA -3'	-TT-	-CGAA-
	luteus	3'- AAGC/TT -5'	-AAGC-	-TT-
Asu II	*Ananaena*	5'- AG/CT -3'	-AG-	-CT-
	subcylindria	3'- TC/GA -5'	-TC-	-GA-
Bal I	*Brevibacterium*	5'- TGG/CCA -3'	-TGG-	-CCA-
	albidum	3'- ACC/GGT -5'	-ACC-	-GGT-
Eco RI	*Escherichia*	5'- G/AATTC -3'	-G-	-AATTCT-
	coli	3'- CTTAA/G -5'	-CTTAA-	-G-
Eco RV	*Escherichia*	5'- GAT/ATC -3'	-GAT-	-ATC-
	coli	3'- CTA/TAG -5'	-CTA-	-TAG-
Hha I	*Haemophilus*	5'- GCG/C -3'	-GCG-	-C-
	haemolyticus	3'- C/GCG -5'	-C-	-GCG-

* Illustrates the position where the DNA strands are cleaved.

(baby hamster kidney). The choice of host system is influenced primarily by the type of protein to be expressed and the key differences among the various host cells (60). Bacterial and yeast cells are more easily cultured in large fermentors. Overall protein yields are generally much lower in mammalian cells, but, in some cases, this may be the only system that produces some mammalian proteins. Another difference is that yeast and mammalian cells do not form toxins, whereas gram-negative bacteria produce endotoxins. Finally, an important distinction is that post-translational modification reactions such as glycosylation do not occur in bacteria.

The host cells containing the vector are grown in small-scale culture to select only for the correct clone containing the desired gene and able to express the best yields of the protein (61). The selected cloned cells (or cell bank cells) are used as inoculum first for a small-scale cell culture/fermentation, which is then followed by larger fermentations in bioreactors. The medium is carefully controlled to enhance cell reproduction and protein synthesis. The host cells divide, and the vectors within the hosts multiply. The host produces its natural proteins along with the desired protein, which may be secreted into the growth medium. The protein of interest can then be isolated from the fermentation, purified and formulated to give a potential rDNA-produced pharmaceutical.

Protein Isolation and Purification

The isolation and purification of the final protein product from the complex mixture of cells, cellular debris, medium nutrients, and other host metabolites is a challenging task (60–61). The structure, purity, potency, and stability of the recombinant protein must be assayed and taken into consideration in this process. Often, sophisticated filtrations, phase separations, precipitation, and complex multiple-column chromatographic procedures are required to obtain the desired protein. Although isolation of the recombinant protein, produced in culture in relatively large amounts, is generally easier than isolating

the native protein, ensuring the stability and retention of the bioactive three-dimensional structure (correct protein folding) of any biopharmaceutical is a more arduous task. In addition, recombinant proteins from bacterial hosts require removal of endotoxins, whereas viral particles may need to be removed from mammalian cell culture products (62). A discussion of these techniques is beyond the scope of this chapter, however. Useful reviews on the extraction and purification (60–61, 63), and analysis and chromatography(64–68) of biotechnology products are available as a resource for further information.

SOME GENERAL PROPERTIES OF BIOTECHNOLOGY-PRODUCED MEDICINAL AGENTS

Although a majority of traditional medicinal agents are relatively small organic molecules, rDNA and hybridoma technologies have made it possible to produce large quantities of highly pure, therapeutically useful proteins. Recombinant DNA-derived proteins and monoclonal antibodies are not dissimilar to the other protein pharmaceuticals or biopharmaceuticals that pharmacists have dispensed in the past. As polymers of amino acids joined by peptide bonds, properties of these proteins differ generally from small organic molecule pharmaceuticals. An overview of the general properties of biotechnology-produced medicinal agents is actually a review of the general physicochemical properties of proteins. Therefore, to study the stability, handling, storage, route of administration, and metabolism of biotechnology-produced pharmaceuticals, it is valuable to understand the chemical nature of proteins. Chapter 6 of this text and other publications(69–73) review the physical biochemistry of protein drugs. Related chapters in any biochemistry textbook also review this topic.

Stability of Biotech Pharmaceuticals

Several detailed reviews on the stability of proteins and protein pharmaceuticals written for pharmaceutical scientists are available (70,71,73,74–78). A brief overview of these resources follows and provides additional information. The instability of proteins, including protein pharmaceuticals, can be separated into two distinct classes. Chemical instability results from bond formation or cleavage yielding a modification of the protein and a new chemical entity. Physical instability involves a change to the secondary or higher-order structure of the protein rather than a covalent bond-breaking modification.

Chemical Instability

A variety of reactions give rise to the chemical instability of proteins, including hydrolysis, oxidation, racemization, β-elimination, and disulfide exchange (Fig. 40.6 a-c). Each of these changes may cause a loss of biologic activity. Proteolytic hydrolysis of peptide bonds results in fragmentation of the protein chain. It is well established that in dilute acids, aspartic acid (Asp) residues in proteins are hydrolyzed at a rate of at least 100 times faster than other peptide bonds owing to the mechanism of the reaction. An additional hydrolysis reaction is the deamidation of the neutral residue of asparagine (Asn) and glutamine (Gln) side-chain linkages forming the ionizable carboxylic acid residues aspartic acid (Asp) and glutamic acid (Glu) (Fig. 40.6a). This conversion may be considered primary sequence isomerization.

Oxidative degradative reactions can occur to the side chains of sulfur-containing methionine (Met) and cysteine (Cys) residues and the aromatic amino acid residues histidine (His), tryptophan (Trp), and tyrosine (Tyr) in proteins during their isolation and storage. The weakly nucleophilic thioether group of Met ($R-S-CH_3$) can be oxidized at low pH by hydrogen peroxide as well as by oxygen in the air to the sulfoxide ($R-SO-CH_3$) and the sulfone ($R-SO_2-CH_3$). The thiol (sulfhydryl, $R-SH$) group of Cys can be succes-

sively oxidized to the corresponding sulfenic acid ($R-SOH$), disulfide ($R-SS-R$), sulfinic acid ($R-SO_2H$), and, finally, sulfonic acid ($R-SO_3H$). A number of factors, including pH, influence the rate of this oxidation. Oxidation of His, Trp, and Tyr residues is believed to occur with a variety of oxidizing agents resulting in the cleavage of the aromatic rings.

Base-catalyzed racemization reactions may occur in any of the amino acids except achiral glycine (Gly) to yield residues in proteins with mixtures of L- and D-configurations. The α-methine hydrogen is removed to form a carbanion intermediate (Fig. 40.6b). The degree of stabilization of this intermediate controls the rate of this reaction. Racemization generally alters the proteins' physicochemical properties and biologic activity. Also, racemization generates nonmetabolizable D-configuration forms of the amino acids. Generally, most amino acid residues are relatively stable to racemization, with a notable exception. Aspartate residues in proteins racemize at 10^5-fold faster rate than when free, in contrast to the 2-fold to 4-fold increase for the other residues. The facilitated rate of racemization for Asp residues is believed to result from the formation of a stabilized cyclic imide.

Proteins containing cysteine (Cys), serine (Ser), threonine (Thr), phenylalanine (Phe), and lysine (Lys) are prone to β-elimination reactions under alkaline conditions (Fig. 40.6c). The reaction proceeds through the same carbanion intermediate as racemization. It is influenced by a number of additional factors, including temperature and the presence of metal ions.

The interrelationships of disulfide bonds and free sulfhydryl groups in proteins are important factors influencing the chemical and biologic properties of protein pharmaceuticals. Disulfide exchange can result in incor-

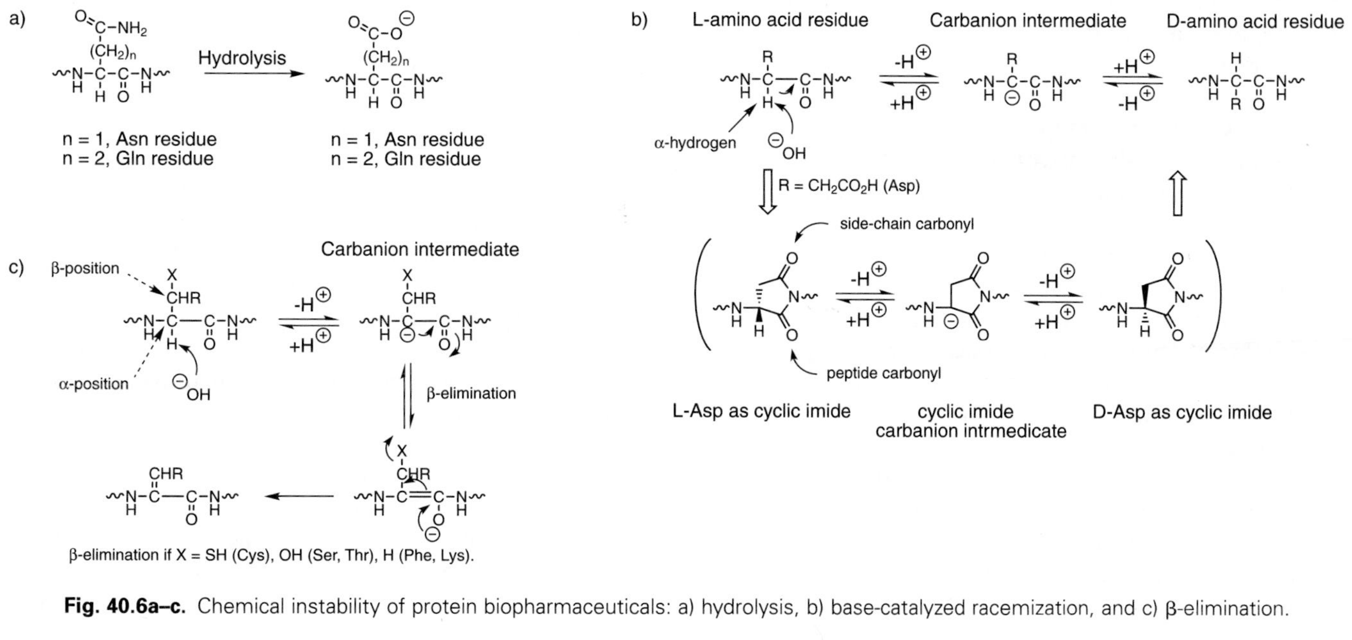

Fig. 40.6a–c. Chemical instability of protein biopharmaceuticals: a) hydrolysis, b) base-catalyzed racemization, and c) β-elimination.

rect pairings and major changes in the higher-order structure (secondary and above) of proteins. The exchange may occur in neutral, acidic, and alkaline media.

Physical Instability

Generally not encountered in most small organic molecules, physical instability is a consequence of the polymeric nature of proteins. Proteins adopt secondary, tertiary, and quaternary structures, which influence their three-dimensional shape and, therefore, their biologic activity. Any change to the higher-order structure of a protein may alter both. Physical instability includes denaturation, adsorption to surfaces, and noncovalent self-aggregation (soluble and precipitation). The most widely studied aspect of protein instability is denaturation. Noncovalent aggregation, however, is one of the primary mechanisms of protein degradation (70).

A protein, in principle, can be folded into a virtually infinite number of conformations. The combination of spatial arrangements and noncovalent intramolecular interactions of nearby amino acid residues providing the lowest energy conformation is the most stable secondary structure. Longer-distance interactions cause the globular nature of proteins (tertiary structure), including their ability to fold so that hydrophilic amino acid side chains are directed toward the exterior surface of the protein exposed to an aqueous environment. In general, all molecules of any protein species adopt the same conformation, or native state. Denaturation occurs by disrupting the weaker noncovalent interactions that hold a protein together in its secondary and tertiary structures. Temperature, pH, and the addition of organic solvents and solutes may cause denaturation. The process can be reversible or irreversible. In general, denaturation affects the protein by decreasing aqueous solubility, altering three-dimensional molecular shape, increasing susceptibility to enzymatic hydrolysis, and causing the loss of the native protein's biologic activity.

Handling and Storage of Biotechnology-Produced Products

The preparation and administration of drugs of recombinant or hybridoma origin are dissimilar to the other nonprotein pharmaceuticals that pharmacists have been dispensing in the past. Proteins generally have more limited shelf stability. The average shelf life for a biotechnology product is 12–18 months versus more than 36 months for a small molecule drug. Although each individual biotechnology drug may be different, several generalizations can be made.

Proper storage of the lyophilized and the reconstituted drug is essential. As most are expensive drugs, special care must be taken not to inactivate the therapeutic protein during storage and handling. The human proteins have limited chemical and physical stability, which is shortened

on reconstitution. Expiration dating ranges from 2 hours to 30 days. The self-association of either native state or misfolded protein subunits may readily occur under certain conditions. This can lead to aggregation and precipitation and results in a loss of biologic activity. Self-association mechanisms depend on the conditions of formulation and may occur as a result of hydrophobic interactions.

Many of the biotechnology-produced drugs are stored refrigerated, but not frozen, between 2–8°C. In general, temperature extremes must be avoided. One example is the rDNA-produced blood clot dissolving drug alteplase. A recombinant version of a naturally occurring human tissue plasminogen activator, lyophilized alteplase is stable at room temperature for several years if protected from light (79). Freezing or exposure to excessive heat decreases the physical stability of the protein. Anything that causes denaturation or self-aggregation, even though labile peptide bonds are not broken, may inactivate the protein. Some pharmacy facilities may need to increase cold storage capacity in order to accommodate biotech storage needs. If the patient must travel any distance home after receiving the medication, the pharmacist should help package the biotechnology product according to the manufacturer's directions. This may mean supplying a reusable cooler for the patient's use. Because the protein drug should not be frozen, the cooler should contain an ice pack rather than dry ice.

Some rDNA-derived pharmaceuticals, in particular, the cytokines (such as the interferons, interleukin-2, and colony-stimulating factors), require human serum albumin in their formulation to prevent adhesion of the protein drug to the glass surface of the vial, which results in loss of protein (80–81). The amount of human serum albumin added varies with the biotech product. The vials should not be shaken in order to prevent foaming of the albumin, which causes protein loss or inactivation of the biotechnology-derived proteins. Care must be exercised in reconstituting protein pharmaceuticals. The diluent used for reconstitution of biotechnology drugs varies with the product and is specified by the manufacturer. Diluents can include normal saline, bacteriostatic water, and 5% dextrose. Several reviews of biotechnology drugs written for pharmacists contain additional information on the subjects of handling and storage (32,34–35,43, 45,81–82).

Biotechnology Drug Delivery

Protein-based pharmaceuticals, whether produced by biotechnology or isolated from traditional sources, present challenges to drug delivery owing to the unique demands imposed by their physicochemical and biologic properties. Although a detailed discussion of this topic is beyond the scope of this chapter, a brief overview follows. Useful reviews are available for further information (78,83–87).

Delivery of large-molecular-weight, biotechnology-produced drugs into the body is difficult because of the poor

Light Catalyzed Instability in Biotech Products

It is important to be knowledgeable about the conditions for handling biotech products that may affect therapeutic action. For instance, some biotech drugs are sensitive to light. The chemical nature of their sidechains and various substituents make them susceptible to chemical reactions catalyzed by light. Thus, many products are distributed in light-protective containers. For instance, lyophilized alteplase is light sensitive and must be protected from light to retain its pharmacologic activity. It is not light sensitive when reconstituted into a solution, however (81).

absorption of these compounds, the acid lability of peptide bonds, and their rapid enzymatic degradation in the body. In addition, protein pharmaceuticals are susceptible to physical instability, complex feedback control mechanisms, and peculiar dose-response relationships.

Given the limitations of today's technology, the strongly acidic environment of the stomach, peptidases in the gastrointestinal tract, and the barrier to absorption presented by gastrointestinal mucosal cells preclude successful oral administration of most protein drugs. Therefore, administration of all of the biotechnology-produced protein drugs is currently parenteral (by intravenous, subcutaneous, or intramuscular injections) to provide a better therapeutic profile. Manufacturers supply most of these drugs as sterile solutions without a preservative. In such cases, it is recommended that only one dose be prepared from each vial to prevent bacterial contamination. Novel solutions to overcome delivery problems associated with biotechnology protein products are being explored. Oral drug delivery approaches in development for various biotechnology-derived drugs include conjugated systems (such as with polyethylene glycol [PEG]), liposomes, microspheres, erythrocytes as carriers, and viruses as drug carriers (73). Specialized delivery methods being examined are transdermal systems, pulmonary delivery, intranasal sprays, buccal administration, ocular delivery systems, rectal administration, iontophoresis, phonophoresis, metered pumps, protein prodrugs, lymphatic uptake, co-administration of peptidase inhibitors, and penetration enhancers.

Some Pharmacokinetic Considerations of Biotechnology-Produced Proteins

The processes of adsorption into the body, distribution within the body, metabolism by the body and excretion from the body (i.e., ADME) of biotechnology-produced pharmaceuticals are important factors affecting the time-course of their pharmacologic effect. To deliver quality pharmaceutical care with biotech products, a pharmacist must be able to apply pharmacokinetic principles to establish and maintain a nontoxic, therapeutic effect. The pharmacokinetics of these protein drugs differ in some

pharmacokinetic aspects from those of the small molecule organic agents for which we are most familiar. Although a lengthy discussion of this topic is beyond the scope of this chapter, a brief overview of metabolism follows. Useful reviews are available for further information (88–89).

The plasma half-life of most administered proteins is relatively short because they are susceptible to a wide variety of metabolic reactions. Rapid hydrolytic degradation of peptide bonds by both nonspecific enzymes and highly structurally selective aminopeptidases, carboxypeptidases, deamidases, and proteinases occurs at the site of administration, while crossing the vascular endothelia, at the site of action, in the liver, in the blood, in the kidney, and, in fact, in most tissues and fluids of the body. Overall, the metabolic products of most proteins are not considered to be a safety issue. They are generally broken down into amino acids and re-incorporated into new, endogenously biosynthesized proteins.

Metabolic oxidation reactions may occur to the side chains of sulfur-containing residues similar to that observed for in vitro chemical instability. Methionine can be oxidized to the sulfoxide, whereas metabolic oxidation of cysteine residues forms a disulfide. Metabolic reductive cleavage of disulfide bridges in proteins may occur yielding free sulfhydryl groups.

Adverse Effects
Overview

An important consideration in the pharmaceutical care of a patient being administered a biotechnology-produced medicinal agent is the potential for adverse reactions. Many of the protein agents are biotechnology-derived versions of endogenous human proteins normally present, on stimulus, in minute quantities near their specific site of action. Therefore, the same protein administered in much larger quantities may cause adverse effects not commonly observed at normal physiologic concentrations (29,88–89). Careful monitoring of patients administered biotechnology-produced drugs is critical for the health care team.

Immunogenicity

The immune system may respond to an antigen such as a protein pharmaceutical triggering the production of antibodies. Biotechnology-derived proteins may possess a different set of antigenic determinants (regions of a protein recognized by an antibody) owing to structural differences between the recombinant protein and the natural human protein (70,85,89). Factors that can contribute to this immunogenicity include incorrect or lack of glycosylation, amino acid modifications, and amino acid additions and deletions. A number of recombinant proteins produced with bacterial vectors contain an N-terminal methionine in addition to the natural human amino acid sequence. Bacterial vector-derived recombinant protein preparations may also contain small amounts of immunoreactive bacterial polypeptides as possible contaminants. Also, immunogenicity may result from proteins that are misfolded, denatured, or aggregated.

RECOMBINANT DNA-PRODUCED MEDICINAL AGENTS

Recombinant DNA technology provides a powerful tool for new pharmaceutical product development and production. Table 40.4 lists the rDNA-produced drugs and vaccines approved by the U.S. FDA through 2000. The biotech products include hormones, enzymes, cytokines, hematopoietic growth factors, other growth factors, blood clotting factors and anticoagulants, and vaccines.

Hormones

Insulin

Biotechnology has provided hormone replacement therapy with the introduction of human insulin,(90–92) the first FDA-approved rDNA drug in 1982, for the treatment of insulin-dependent diabetes. The human insulin molecule has the structural characteristics of a large protein yet is only the size of a polypeptide totaling 51 amino acid residues. Two disulfide bonds (cysteine [Cys] A7 to Cys B7 and Cys A20 to Cys B19) link two polypeptide chains, the A-chain consisting of 21 amino acids and the 30-residue B-chain. An additional disulfide loop is found in the A-chain between Cys A6 and Cys A11 (Fig. 6.14 and Fig. 27.2). Insulin formulation development focused on modifying the time-action profile (onset, peak plasma concentration, and duration of action) through the uses of various levels of zinc and protamine. Also, the chemical stability of insulin was improved by moving from acidic to neutral formulations. A more complete medicinal chemistry discussion of insulin may be found in Chapter 27.

Before the availability of rDNA-produced human insulin, porcine and bovine insulin were the most commonly used pharmaceutical preparations. Both porcine and bovine insulin differ in primary structure from human with alanine (Ala) replacing Thr at the C-terminal of the B-chain (B30). Bovine insulin also differs from human insulin by Ala replacing Thr at A8 and valine (Val) substituting for isoleucine (Ile) at A10. These subtle differences can result in immunologic responses to the nonhuman insulins requiring a modification of therapeutic regimen. The biotechnology solution has several advantages over insulin derived from animal sources: (1) it should have potentially fewer serious immune reactions; (2) it is pyrogen free; (3) it is not contaminated with other peptide hormones, such as glucagon, somatostatin, and proinsulin found in isolated products; and (4) it can be produced in larger amounts. The first successful attempts to tailor a protein hormone for therapy by rDNA techniques has yielded interesting insulin analogs (90–92).

Human insulin rDNA origin is available commercially as Humulin, Novolin, and as several analogs. The Humulin and Novolin products are produced using genetically modified strains of two different microorganisms. Humulin is prepared using recombinant *Escherichia coli* bacteria. The pharmaceutical preparation is reported to contain less than 4 ppm of immunoreactive bacterial polypeptides that act as possible contaminants. *Saccharomyces cerevisiae*, baker's yeast, serves as the recombinant organism for the production of Novolin. Before 1986, Humulin was produced by chemically joining together the separately rDNA-derived A-chain and B-chain. Today the product is prepared by enzymatically cleaving the connecting peptide in recombinant proinsulin. Humulin and Novolin are available in a variety of forms as indicated in Chapter 27 and shown in Table 27.4.

Studies in animals, healthy adults, and patients with type I diabetes mellitus have shown human insulin to have identical pharmacologic effects as purified porcine insulin. A comparable pharmacokinetic profile has also been shown. Human insulin, however, administered intramuscularly or intravenously may have a slightly faster onset and slightly shorter duration of action when compared with purified porcine insulin in patients with diabetes. The usual precautions concerning toxic potentials observed with insulin of animal origin should be followed with rDNA human insulin. As would be expected the recombinant product has been shown to be less immunogenic than animal insulins.

Insulin remains the only treatment option for type 1 diabetes and is still widely used to treat type 2 diabetes patients who do not respond adequately to other pharmacotherapies. Recombinant DNA technology has lead recently to the development of insulin analogs that have greater utility in certain situations and may more closely resemble the normal diurnal pattern of insulin secretion. The newly engineered analogs have specific amino acid sequence modifications that improve absorption properties and biologic profiles (93). Insulin lispro (Humalog) has a more rapid onset and shorter duration of action than regular human insulin. Unlike regular insulin that must be injected 30–60 minutes before a meal, recombinant insulin lispro is effective when injected 15 minutes before a meal. The analog differs from natural human insulin because the B-chain amino acids B28 proline and B29 lysine are exchanged. Insulin aspart (Novolog), homologous with human insulin except for the single amino acid substitution of aspartic acid for proline at B28, is effective when injected 5–10 minutes before a meal. Insulin glargine (Lantus) is the newest rDNA-derived human insulin analog. An ultra-long-acting agent, insulin glargine differs from human insulin in that the amino acid asparagine at residue A21 is replaced by glycine, and two arginines are added to the C-terminus of the β chain. When administered subcutaneously, insulin glargine has a duration of action up to 24–48 hours. This action profile change resulted from structural modifications that enhanced the products basicity, thus causing the product to precipitate at neutral

Table 40.4. Drugs and Vaccines of rDNA Origin Approved by the U.S. FDA

Class	Generic Name	Indication
Hormone	Insulin (human)	Insulin-dependent diabetes mellitus
Hormone	Insulin (human) lispro	Insulin-dependent diabetes mellitus
Hormone	Insulin (human) aspart	Insulin-dependent diabetes mellitus
Hormone	Insulin (human) glargine	Insulin-dependent diabetes mellitus
Hormone	Glucagon	Treatment of hypoglycemia, diagnostic aid
Hormone	Somatrem	hGH deficiency in children
Hormone	Somatropin	hGH deficiency in children
		Growth failure in children due to chronic renal insufficiency
		Turner's syndrome
		hGH deficiency in adults
		Children with Prader-Willi syndrome
Hormone	Follitropin alfa	Infertility
Hormone	Follitropin beta	Infertility
Hormone	Thyrotropin alfa	Delection and treatment of thyroid cancer
Enzyme	Alteplase	Acute myocardial infaction
		Acute myocardial embolism
		Ischemic stroke
Enzyme	Retavase	Acute myocardial Infaction
Enzyme	Tenecteplase	Acute myocardial infaction
Enzyme	Dornase alpha	Cystic fibrosis
Enzyme	Imiglucerase	Treatment of Gaucher's disease
Cytokine	Interferon alfa-2a	Hairy cell leukemia
		AIDS-related Kaposi's sarcoma
		Chronic myelogenous leukemia
		Hepatitis C
Cytokine	Interferon alfa-2b	Hairy cell leukemia
		Genital warts
		AIDS-related Kaposi's sarcoma
		Hepatitis B
		Hepatitis C
		Malignant melanoma
		Follicular lymphoma in conjuction with chemotherapy
Cytokine	Interferon alfacon-1	Treatment of chronic hepatitis C viral infection
Cytokine	Interferon beta-1a	Relapsing multiple sclerosis
Cytokine	Interferon beta-1b	Relapsing, remitting multiple sclerosis
Cytokine	Interferon gamma-1b	Management of chronic granulomatous disease
Cytokine	Aldesleukin	Renal cell carcinoma
		Metastatic melanoma
Cytokine	Denileukin diftitox	Persistant or recurrent cutaneous T-cell lymphoma
Cytokine	Oprrelvekin	Prevention of severe chemotherapy-induced thrombocytopenia
Cytokine	Etanercept	Moderate to severe active rheumatoid arthritis
Hematopoietic growth factor	Epoetin alpha	Anemia related to AZT therapy in HIV-infected patients
		Anemia associated with chronic renal failure
		Anemia caused by chemotherapy in patients with non-myeloid malignanacies
		Prevention of anemia associated with surgical blood loss
		Anemia in children—chronic renal failure undergoing dialysis
Hematopoietic growth factor	Filgrastim	Decrease incidence of infection—patients with non-myeloid malignancies receiving myelosuppressive drugs
		Autologous or allogeneic bone marrow transplantation
		Chronic severe neutropenia
Hematopoietic growth factor	Sargramostim	Myeloid recovery in patients after autologous bone marrow transplantation
		Neutropenia—result of chemo. in acute myelogenous leukemia
		Allogenic bone marrow transplantation
		Support for peripheral blood progenitor cell mobilization and transplantation
Other growth factors	Becaplermin	Lower extremity diabetic neuropathic ulcers
Blood clotting factor	Recombinant factor VIII	Hemophilia B
Blood clotting factor	Recombinant factor IX	Hemophilia A
Anticoagulant	Lepirudin	Heparin-inducer thrombocytopenia type II
Vaccine	Hepatitis B vaccine	Prevention of hepatitis B
Vaccine	Lyme disease vaccine	Prevention of Lyme disease

pH post-injection and therefore increasing its duration of action.

Insulin Toxicity

In a recent paper, Argo and co-workers quote statistics that suggest "medication errors cause at least one death every day and injure roughly 1.3 million people in the United States every year." In their opinion, they list insulin errors as among the 10 most common lethal medication errors based on literature review (94). Insulin is an extremely potent molecule. Pharmacists should always listen to and evaluate information provided by their patients and always double check large dose prescriptions. Remember that most biopharmaceuticals have their dose expressed in units rather than a weight as common for small molecule drugs. A 10 unit dose written as "10U" may be mistakenly read as a 100 unit dose.

Glucagon (Glucagen)

Like insulin, glucagon is a hormone normally biosynthesized as a high-molecular mass protein from which the mature peptide hormone is released by selective proteolytic cleavage. The single-chain 29 amino acid polypeptide has an overall catabolic effect that tends to oppose the actions of insulin. Interestingly, the amino acid sequence of human, bovine, and porcine glucagon are identical. Glucagon of rDNA origin is now available (95). Replacing the bovine product with the rDNA-derived drug would eliminate the risk of acquiring bovine spongiform encephalopathy from glucagon therapy.

Growth Hormones

The introduction of rDNA human growth hormone (hGH) (96–97), previously isolated from cadaver pituitaries, greatly improved the long-term treatment of children who have growth failure caused by a lack of adequate endogenous hGH. The major, circulating form of human pituitary hGH is a globular protein of 191 amino acids in a single polypeptide chain with a molecular weight of 22,000 daltons. Pituitary hGH is a roughly spherical protein with a hydrophobic interior. It is nonglycosylated. Degradation pathways of hGH include typical proteolysis reactions; deamidation of Asn and Gln residues; oxidation of Met, Trp, His, and Tyr residues; disulfide exchange; and aggregation.

Somatrem, first introduced in 1985, contains the identical 191-amino acid sequence found in the pituitary-derived hGH plus the addition of a methionine amino acid at the N-terminus of the peptide chain (resulting in a 192-amino acid protein; also known as Met-rhGH) (Table 40.5). Somatropin products contain the 191-amino acid sequence identical to that of hGH of pituitary origin. Marketed somatropin products are shown in Table 40.5. Actions of rDNA-derived hGHs include an increase in the linear growth of the patient, increased skeletal growth, increased protein synthesis, reduction in body fat stores,

and increased organ growth (Table 40.4). Clearance and bioavailability do not appear to be clinically or statistically significantly different for somatrem and somatropin. Although the direct clinical comparison of the efficacy of the two forms of hGH have yet to be performed, separate controlled studies of growth hormone-deficient patients were similar. Recombinant hGHs are safe and effective therapies with relatively few side effects. A long-acting dosage form of somatropin has recently received FDA approval for use in children with Prader-Willi syndrome (PWS), a rare genetic disorder. PWS, causes short stature; an involuntary, continuous urge to eat (that is life-long and may be life threatening); low muscle tone; and cognitive disorders. The new formulation was designed to reduce the frequency of injections to 1–2/month by encapsulating the agent in biodegradable microspheres.

Gonadotropins (FSH)—Follitropin Alpha (Gonal-F) and Follitropin Beta (Fillistim)

The gonadotropins are a family of protein hormones that include follicle-stimulating hormone (FSH) and primarily target their actions to the gonads. FSH is synthesized and released by the pituitary gland. The hormone enhances spermatogenesis in males and stimulates folicular growth in females. FSH is a 34 kDa glycoprotein (approximately 14% carbohydrate) containing two polypeptide subunits, an α- and a β-chain. Follitropin alpha and follitropin beta are human FSH preparations produced by recombinant DNA technology (98–99). Gonadotropin preparations are utilized for infertility treatments in men and women. The production of r-hFSH in a Chinese Hamster Ovary (CHO) cell line has proved particularly challenging. Follitropin alfa was the first heterodimeric glycoprotein to be produced by rDNA technology. Before the product of rDNA origin was available for infertility treatment, FSH was isolated from urine at less than 5% purity.

Thyrotropin (TSH)

Thyroid-stimulating hormone (TSH, thyrotropin) is a 28,000–30,000 molecular weight glycoprotein secreted by the anterior lobe of the pituitary gland that is necessary for the growth and function of the thyroid. A recombinant

Table 40.5. Commercially Available rDNA hGH

Generic Name	Trade Name	Chemical Nature
Somatrem	Protropin	hGH + methionine (192 amino acids)
Somatropin	GenoTropin	hGH (191 amino acids)
	Humatrope	hGH
	Norditropin	hGH
	Nutropin	hGH
	Nutropin Depot	hGH-long acting
	Saizen	hGH
	Serostim	hGh

thyrotropin alpha useful for the detection and treatment of cancer was approved in November, 1998 (46).

Enzymes

Tissue Plasminogen Activators

The fibrinolytic system is activated in response to the presence of an intracellular thrombus or clot. The process of clot dissolution is initiated by the conversion of plasminogen to plasmin. Plasminogen activation is catalyzed by two endogenous highly specific serine proteases, urokinase-type plasminogen activator (u-PA) and tissue-type plasminogen activator (t-PA) (100–105) (also see Chapter 26).

The mature human t-PA, is a glycoprotein consisting of a single chain of 527 amino acids. Its molecular weight is about 70,000 daltons. Human t-PA contains 35 cysteines assigned to 17 disulfide bonds. A serine protease domain of about 260 residues is located at the carboxy-terminal end of this protein. A fibronectin "finger" domain, two kringle domains, and an epidermal growth factor domain are also present. The tPA protease domain is approximately 35–40% homologous with typical serine protease, such as bovine trypsin and chymotrypsin.

Mammalian cells produce two t-PA variants of N-linked glycosylation, type 1 (at asparagines 117, 184, and 448) and type 2 (only as asparagines 117 and 448). The rate of fibrin-dependent plasminogen activation is 2–3 times faster for type 2 compared with type 1. The cDNA obtained from a human melanoma cell line was expressed in CHO cells to achieve glycosylation and a protein identical to the natural protein. Protein engineering studies have produced variant t-PA molecules with modified pharmacokinetics, affinity for fibrin, catalytic activity, and side effects.

There are three rDNA thrombolytic agents approved in the United States (100–105) (Table 40.6). The first is alteplase an enzyme equivalent to human t-PA. It is supplied as vials of a white to off-white lyophilized powder for injection. The powder should be stored at a room temperature of 15–30°C or refrigerated at 2–8°C. The expiration date is 2 years after manufacture. Reconstituted solutions (diluent supplied) contain no preservatives and should be stored at 2–30°C for no more than 8 hours.

Alteplase is indicated for the treatment of acute myocardial infarction (administered as a bolus), acute massive pulmonary embolism (administered by intravenous infusion), and ischemic stroke (Table 40.4). The mechanism of action of t-PA is unlike that of streptokinase and urokinase. It is the first fibrin-selective thrombolytic agent preferentially activating fibrinogen bound to fibrin. Thus, the thrombolytic effect is localized to a blood clot and avoids systemic activation of fibrinogen, preventing bleeding elsewhere in the body. Plasma t-PA concentrations are proportional to the rate of infusion. Alteplase is rapidly cleared from circulating plasma, with 50% cleared within 5 minutes after termination of infusion. The mechanisms for clearance of t-PA from the blood are poorly understood. Detectable levels of antibody against alteplase have been

Table 40.6. Commerically Available rDNA Tissue Plaminogen Activators

Generic Name	Trade Name	Chemical Nature
Alteplase	Activase	Human t-PA (527 amino acids)
Reteplase	Retavase	Modified human t-PA (355 amino acids)
Tenecteplase	TNKase, TNK-tPA	Modified human t-PA (527 amino acids)

found in patients receiving the drug, although 12 days to 10 months later antibody determinations were negative.

Reteplase recombinant is a nonglycosylated deletion mutation of human t-PA containing 355 of 527 amino acids of native t-PA. The drug is indicated for acute myocardial infarction and is given as a 10 Units + 10 Units double bolus. Searching for t-PA derivatives having a: prolonged half-life, allowing single bolus administration; a higher level of fibrin specificity, minimizing superficial and internal bleeding problems; and resistance to the endogenous t-PA inactivator, plasminogen activator inhibitor (PAI-1). The most recent addition to the marketed rDNA-derived t-PAs is tenecteplase. The recombinant protein contains three modifications from natural human t-PA. These are: in the kringle 1 domain of natural t-PA, threonine (T) 103 replaced by arginine (R); the kringle 1 domain asparagine (N) 117 replaced by glutamine (Q); and in the protease domain, four amino acids [lysine (K), histadine (H), and two arginines (R)] are replaced by four alanines (A). The drug is indicated for acute myocardial infarction. Bleeding at the injection site is similar to alteplase, but there is a reduction in the noncerebral bleeding complications. It is administered as a single 5 second bolus.

DNase—Dornase Alpha (Pulmozyme)

According to the Cystic Fibrosis Foundation, cystic fibrosis (CF) is the most common fatal genetic disorder, afflicting approximately 30,000 patients, most of whom die before the age of 30. They develop thick mucous secretions and suffer from severe, frequent lung infections. Studies during the 1950s and 1960s determined that CF-related secretions in the lungs contained large amounts of DNA. Mucus-thickening DNA release resulted from an inflammatory response and ensuing white blood cell death. The enzyme deoxyribonuclease I (DNase I) specifically cleaves extracellular DNA such as that found in the mucous secretion of CF patients and has no effect on the DNA of intact cells. The FDA has approved a recombinant human DNase (106–108).

DNase I is a glycoprotein containing 260 amino acids with an approximate molecular weight of 37,000 daltons. The recombinant protein is expressed by genetically engineered CHO cells encoding for the native enzyme, although DNase I was not purified or sequenced from human sources at the time. A degenerate sequence, based on the sequence of bovine DNase (263 amino acids), was used to synthesize probes and screen a human pancreatic DNA library. The primary amino acid sequence of rhD-Nase is identical to native human DNase I.

The only FDA-approved DNase product, dornase alpha (inhalation solution), has been developed as a therapeutic agent for the management of CF. The product is supplied in single-use ampules delivering 2.5 ml of a sterile, clear, colorless solution containing 1.0 mg/ml dornase alpha with no preservative. Administration is by nebulizer aerosol delivery systems.

Dornase alpha is indicated for daily administration in conjunction with standard CF therapies to reduce the frequency of respiratory infections requiring parental antibiotics to improve pulmonary function. The breakdown of DNA in infected sputum results in improved airflow in the lung and reduced risk of bacterial infection. The medicinal agent has been shown in clinical trials to have a positive effect on pulmonary function, which returned to baseline on stopping therapy. Although effective for the management of the respiratory symptoms of CF, dornase alpha is not a replacement for antibiotics, bronchodilators, and daily physical therapy. Two short-term studies have reported no adverse reactions. The agent is also in early clinical trials for the treatment of chronic bronchitis, a disease afflicting 400,000 patients in the United States alone.

Imiglucerase (Cerezyme)

Type 1 Gaucher disease, the most common form, is an inherited disorder. Fewer than 1 in 40,000 people in the general population have Gaucher disease. Patients with the disease lack the normal form of the enzyme glucocerebrosidase. They cannot break down glucocerebroside, causing a buildup of the compound within the lysosomes. This leads to the poor functioning of macrophages, and an accumulation of "Gaucher cells" in the spleen, liver and bone marrow. Some individuals experience few symptoms while others develop life-threatening conditions. Imiglucerase is an analog of glucocerebrosidase produced by recombinant DNA technology (109).

Cytokines

Cytokine is a generic term for the soluble protein molecules released by participating and interacting cells in the innate and adaptive immune systems. Cytokines communicate in a dynamic cellular network during an immune/inflammatory response to an antigen (110–112). Lymphokine and monokine are the terms used for a cytokine derived from lymphocytes and macrophages, respectively. Chemokines are a group of at least 25 structurally homologous, low molecular weight cytokines that stimulate leukocyte movement and regulate the migration of leukocytes from the blood to tissues. Cytokines, usually released and targeted to produce a localized effect, regu-

late the growth, differentiation, and activation of the hematopoietic cells responsible for the maintenance of the immune response. A wide array of glycoproteins, including interferons, interleukins, hematopoietic growth factors, and tumor necrosis factors, are cytokines. Cytokines can only act on target cells that express receptors for that cytokine. There are five families of cytokine receptor proteins: Class I cytokine receptors, Class II cytokine receptors, TNF receptors, Chemokine receptors, and immunoglobulin superfamily receptors (Table 40.7). Cytokine research has entered an exciting growth phase fueled by genomics, cancer research and a growing understanding of apoptosis. Over 100 human cytokines are being studied. Currently, the National Library of Medicine has well over 260,000 papers on the topic (113). Among the many reviews discussing the cytokines, several written for pharmacists or pharmaceutical scientists are excellent sources for a readable overview of the area (114–123).

Interferons

The interferons (120, 123) are a family of cytokines discovered in the late 1950s, with broad-spectrum antiviral and potential anticancer activity making them biologic response modifiers (BRM). Biotherapy (the therapeutic use of any substance of biologic origin) of cancer is different than standard chemotherapy. That is, biotherapy agents belong to a group of compounds that enhanced normal immune interactions (therefore, they are also immunomodulators) with cells in a specific or nonspecific fashion. Chemotherapeutics interact directly with the cancer cells themselves. Three types of naturally occurring interferons have been found present in small quantities: leukocyte interferon (interferon alpha, IFN-α), produced by lymphocytes and macrophages; fibroblast interferon (interferon beta, IFN-β) produced by fibroblasts, epithelial cells, and macrophages; and immune interferon (interferon gamma, IFN-γ) synthesized by CD4+, CD8+, and natural killer lymphocytes. IFN-α and IFN-β, also known as type I interferons, exhibit approximately 30% primary sequence homology but no structural similarity to IFN-γ, a type II interferon. All three are glycoproteins. Previously only available in low yields by chemical synthesis or isolation, several rDNA interferon pharmaceuticals now have been mar-

Table 40.7. The Five Families of Cytokine Receptors and Some Ligands

Receptor Families	Ligands
Class I Cytokine Receptors	IL-2 - IL-7, IL-9, IL-11 - IL-13, IL-15, CM-CSF, G-CSF
Class II Cytokine Receptors	INF-α, INF-β, INF-γ
TNF Receptors	TNF-α, TNF-β, CD30, CD40, FAS
Chemokine Receptors	IL-8, RANTES, MIP-1, PF-4, MCAF
Immunoglobin Superfamily Receptors	IL-1, M-CSF

Table 40.8. Commerically Available rDNA Cytokines

Generic Name	Trade Name	Chemical Nature
Interferon alpha-2a	Roferon-A	Human interferon-165 amino acids
Interferon alpha-2b	Intron A	Human interferon-165 amino acids
Interferon alfacon-1	Infergen, CIFN	Modified interferon-166 amino acids
Interferon beta-1ba	Avonex	Human interferon-165 amino acids
Interferon beta-1b	Betaseron	Modified interferon-165 amino acids
Interferon gamma-1b	Actimmune	Human interferon- 140 amino acids
Aldesleukin	Proleukin	Modified human IL-2 -132 amino acids
Denileuin diftitox	Ontak	Modified interleukin + modified diphtheria toxin
Oprelvekin	Neumega	Modified interleukin 11-177 amino acids
Etanercept	Enbrel	Modified TNF + human IgG1

keted in the United States including three interferon alpha products, two interferon beta agents and an interferon gamma drug (see Table 40.4).

Interferon Alpha. At least 24 different human genes producing 16 distinct mature IFN-α molecules with slight structural variations are known (120,123–126). Human IFN-α proteins generally are composed of either 165 or 166 amino acids. IFN-α-2a and IFN-α-2b, the two primary subtypes, both contain 165 amino acids differing only at position 23, with IFN-α-2a containing a lysine group and IFN-α-2b an arginine group at this position. They have molecular weights of approximately 19,000 daltons. Although cultures of genetically modified *E. coli* produce two recombinant FDA-approved interferon alphas, IFN-α-2a and IFN-α-2b, their method of purification differs. IFN-α-2a's purification includes affinity chromatography using a murine MAb, whereas IFN-α-2b's does not.

IFN-α-2a is commercially available as a sterile solution or a sterile white-to-beige lyophilized powder to reconstitute for subcutaneous or intramuscular injection (Table 40.8). IFN-α-2b is available as a sterile white-to-cream-colored lyophilized powder to reconstitute for subcutaneous or intramuscular injection and in combination with the antiviral ribavirin. Storage of the lyophilized powders or the reconstituted solutions should be at 2–8°C. IFN-α-2a and IFN-α-2b, as lyophilized powders, have expiration dates of 36 and 24 months after manufacture, respectively. Reconstituted solutions, if stored properly, are stable for up to 30 days. During the manufacture of the rDNA interferon alphas, human albumin is added to minimize adsorption to glass and plastic by these cytokines. Solutions, therefore, should not be shaken.

Interferon alpha possesses complex antiviral, antineoplastic, and immunomodulating activities. Approved indications are shown in Table 40.4. Although the precise mechanism of action of interferon alphas is not known, they are believed to interact with cell surface receptors to produce their biologic effects. The actions appear to result from a complex cascade of biologic modulation and pharmacologic effects that include the modulation of host immune responses; cellular antiproliferative effects; cell differentiation, transcription, and translation processes; and reduction of oncogene expression.

Interferon alpha is filtered through the glomeruli in the kidney and undergoes rapid proteolytic degradation during tubular reabsorption. Toxicity is generally dose and time dependent with fever, fatigue, myalgia, chills, and anorexia, all flu-like symptoms, generally occurring within 2–8 hours after administration of high doses.

Concensus Interferon. Hepatitis C infection results in a chronic disease state in 50–70% of cases and is now the most important known causes of chronic liver disease (127–128). Following the acute phase, as many as 80% of patients may progress to the chronic phase of the infectious disease. An estimated 20% of patients with a chronic form of the disease progress to cirrhosis. The only agents shown to be effective in the treatment of hepatitis C are the interferons. A unique recombinant molecule, a concensus interferon known as interferon alfacon-1 has been approved for the treatment of chronic hepatitis C infection. It contains 166 amino acids in a relationship in which each amino acid position in the molecule contains the most commonly occurring amino acid among all the natural interferon alpha subtypes. Interferon alfacon-1 exhibits 5–10 times higher biologic activity when compared to either IFN-α-2a or IFN-α-2b.

Interferon Beta. Normally produced by fibroblasts, human interferon beta (120, 123, 126, 129–130) (Table 40.8) was first cloned and expressed in 1980; however, its instability made it unsuitable for clinical use. The more stable recombinant interleukin beta-1b, a 165-amino acid analog of human interferon beta, differs from the native protein with a serine residue substituted for cysteine at position 17. The highly purified product of biotechnology has a molecular weight of 18,500 daltons. It is produced in a recombinant *E. coli*.

Approved in December 1993, IFN-β-1b is indicated for the treatment of patients with exacerbating-remitting multiple sclerosis (MS). The National Multiple Sclerosis Society says that 250,000–300,000 Americans have this disease, with greater than 60% of the patients falling into the exacerbating-remitting category. A vial of recombinant IFN-β-1b contains 0.3 mg of protein with dextrose and human albumin as stabilizers. The sterile white lyophilized powder is reconstituted without preservative for single-use subcutaneous injection every other day. Before and after reconstitution, the preparation should be refrigerated at 2–8°C. The refrigerated solution should be administered within 3 hours of reconstitution.

Results from a large double-blind, placebo-controlled study have found that 8 million IU subcutaneously (the low-dose treatment group) of interferon beta every other day brought the most promising results, with a one-third reduction in exacerbations and a decrease by half in the frequency of severe attacks. Cranial magnetic resonance imaging scans showed that treated patients did not develop new lesions in the central nervous system and had less active lesions than placebo patients. The exact mechanism of action of IFN-β-1b is not known. Its immunomodulating effects, however, may benefit MS patients by decreasing the levels of endogenous interferon gamma. Levels of IFN-gamma are believed to rise before and during acute attacks in MS patients.

As observed with other interferons, flu-like symptoms are common on administration. During clinical trials, a suicide and four attempted suicides were reported. Depression and suicide have previously also been reported with patients receiving interferon alfa.

While IFN-β-1b of rDNA origin was the first to the market, IFN-β-1a is also now available. IFN-β-1a is produced in mammalian cells and has the same amino acid sequence and carbohydrate side chain as natural IFN-β. Recombinant IFN-β-1a is administered to patients once weekly by intramuscular injection (30 mcg). This differs from the subcutaneous every other day administration of rDNA produced IFN-β-1b. Similar to pharmacotherapy with IFN-β-1b, the most common side effects of IFN-β-1 therapy include flu-like symptoms.

Interferon Gamma. Human interferon gamma (120, 123, 126, 131–132) is a single-chain glycoprotein with a molecular weight of approximately 15,500 daltons. The cytokine mainly exists as a noncovalent dimer of differentially glycosylated chains in solution in vivo. Glycosylation does not appear to be necessary for biologic activity. The 140-amino acid IFN-γ-1b is produced by fermentation of a recombinant *E. coli*. Approved in 1990 (Table 40.8), IFN-γ-1b is supplied as a sterile solution containing 100 mcg of the drug for subcutaneous injection. Vials must be placed in a refrigerator at 2–8°C and neither frozen nor shaken.

IFN-γ-1b possesses biologic activity identical to the natural human gamma interferon derived from lymphoid cells. Although all the interferons share certain biologic effects, gamma interferon differs distinctly from alpha and beta interferons by its potent capacity to activate phago-

cytes involved in host defense. These activating effects include the ability to enhance the production of toxic oxygen metabolites within phagocytes, resulting in a more efficient killing of various microorganisms. This activity is the basis for the use of IFN-γ-1b in the management of chronic granulomatous disease. Chronic granulomatous disease is a group of rare X-linked or autosomal genetic disorders of the phagocytic oxygen metabolite generating system leaving patients susceptible to severe infections. The drug extends the time patients spend without being hospitalized for infectious episodes. Investigational applications of gamma interferon include the treatment of renal cell carcinoma, small-cell lung cancer, infectious disease, trauma, atopic dermatitis, asthma, allergies, rheumatoid arthritis, and venereal warts. Adverse reactions are similar to those reported for interferon alpha.

Interleukins

Interleukins are cytokines involved in immune cell communication. Synthesized by monocytes, macrophages, and lymphocytes, interleukins serve as soluble messengers between leukocytes. Currently, at least 18 interleukins have been observed. One of the most studied cytokines is interleukin-2 (IL-2), originally called T cell growth factor owing to its ability to stimulate growth of T lymphocytes.

Interleukin-2. Human IL-2 is a 133-amino acid, 15,400-dalton protein O-glycosylated at a threonine in position 3. An intramolecular disulfide bond between cysteine 58 and cysteine 105 is essential for biologic activity. A recombinant version of IL-2 is marketed as aldesleukin (Table 40.8) (121, 126, 133–138). Aldesleukin differs from the native protein by the absence of glycosylation, a lack of the N-terminal alanine residue at position 1 (132 amino acids), and the replacement of cysteine with serine at position 125 of the primary sequence. Sequence changes were accomplished by site-directed mutagenesis to the IL-2 gene before cloning and expression. Aldesleukin exists as noncovalent microaggregates with an average size of 27 recombinant IL-2 molecules. The recombinant drug does possess the biologic activity of the native protein.

Aldesleukin is supplied as a lyophilized formulation of protein admixed with mannitol to provide bulk in the vial. Sodium dodecyl sulfate is present to ensure sufficient water solubility on reconstitution. The drug is administered as an intravenous infusion. Handling and storage considerations for aldesleukin are consistent with the other cytokines. Recombinant IL-2 should be administered within 48 hours after reconstitution.

Aldesleukin is used in cancer biotherapy (therapeutic use of any substance of biologic origin) as a biologic response modifier for the treatment of metastatic renal cell carcinoma and metastatic melanoma. Aldesleukin has recently been studied in the management of HIV infection. Although the exact mechanism of action is not established, IL-2 is known to bind to an IL-2 receptor that has been well studied. In vitro, IL-2 induces killer cell activity, enhances lymphocyte mitogenesis and cytotoxicity, and induces interferon gamma production. The extent of its antitumor effect is directly proportional to the amount of IL-2 administered. Side effects are the major dose-limiting factor because aldesleukin is an extremely toxic drug. The manufacturer's labeling should be consulted for full details. Careful patient selection and thorough patient monitoring are essential. The incidence of non-neutralizing anti-IL-2 antibodies in patients treated on an every-8-hour regimen is quite high (76% in one clinical study).

IL-2 Fusion Protein. Using ligation chemistry approaches during the preparation of recombinant proteins, researchers have created biologically active molecules that combine the activities of two individual proteins into "fusion molecules." These fusion technologies hold promise for developing custom molecules expressing a wide variety of dual activities. The FDA recently approved the fusion protein denileukin diftitox for the treatment of patients with persistent or recurrent cutaneous T-cell lymphoma whose malignant cells express the CD25 component of the interleukin-2 receptor (139–142). Cutaneous T-cell lymphoma (CTCL) is a general term for a group of low-grade nonHodgkin's lymphomas affecting approximately 1000 new patients/year. Malignant T cells manifest initially in the skin. Over time, there is systemic involvement. For many patients, CTCL is a persistent, disfiguring and debilitating disease that requires multiple treatments. Malignant CTCL cells express one or more of the components of the IL-2 receptor. Thus, the IL-2 receptor may be a homing device to attract a "killer drug."

Denileukin diftitox is a rDNA derived cytotoxic IL-2 "fusion" protein that contains the first 389 amino acids of diphtheria toxin fused to amino acid residues 2-133 of human IL-2 (the IL-2 residues replace the amino acids of the receptor binding domain of native diphtheria toxin). Thus, the biotech drug targets IL-2 receptors, and brings the diphtheria toxin directly to kill the CTCL target. Studies have shown that 30% of patients treated with the therapeutic fusion protein experience at least 50% reduction of tumor burden that is sustained for minimally 6 weeks.

Interleukin 11. IL-11 is a thrombopoietic growth factor that directly stimulates the proliferation of hematopoietic stem cells and the proliferation of megakaryocyte progenitor cells (143–144). This induces megakaryocyte maturation, resulting in increased platelet production. IL-11 is a 178 amino acid glycosylated cytokine produced by bone marrow stromal cells. Primary osteoblasts and mature osteoclasts express mRNAs for an IL-11 receptor (IL-11R alpha). Thus, bone-forming cells and bone-resorbing cells are potential targets of IL-11. In 1997, the FDA approved a rDNA-derived version of IL-11 produced

in *E. coli.* Oprelvekin (Table 40.8) contains only 177 amino acids, lacking the amino terminal proline of the native IL-11. Produced in *E. coli,* the cytokine analog is nonglycosylated. Oprelvekin has potent thrombopoietic activity in animal models of compromised hematopoiesis. It is indicated for the prevention of thrombocytopenia following myelosuppressive chemotherapy. Pharmacists should monitor for possible fluid retention and electrolyte states when used with chronic diuretic therapy.

Tumor Necrosis Factor

Tumor necrosis factors (TNFs), a family of cytokines produced mainly by activated mononuclear phagocytes, have both beneficial and potentially harmful effects, mediating cytotoxic and inflammatory reactions(121). TNFs are endogenous pyrogens capable of inducing chills, fever, and other flu-like symptoms. TNF-α, also called cachectin (and commonly referred to as TNF), and TNF-β, also called lymphotoxin, both bind to the same receptor and induce similar biologic activities. Biologic effects of TNF-α include selective toxicity against a range of tumor cells, mediation of septic shock, activation of elements of the immune system in response to Gram-negative bacteria and induction/regulation of inflammation. TNF-α of rDNA origin has been studies extensively, but has not been developed into a useful drug.

Etanercept is a rDNA-produced fusion protein that binds specifically to TNF and blocks its interaction with cell surface TNF receptors.(145–147) It is indicated for the treatment of moderate to severe active rheumatoid arthritis in adults and juvenile rheumatoid arthritis in patients who have had an inadequate response to one or more disease-modifying antirheumatic drugs (DMARDs). It is a genetically-engineered protein that includes two components. The extracellular, ligand-binding portion (p75) of the human TNF receptor (TNFR) is linked as a fusion protein to the Fc portion of the human IgG1 antibody. Each etanercept molecule binds specifically to two TNF molecules found in the synovial fluid of RA patients, blocking TNF's interaction with the TNFR. The drug inhibits both TNF-α and TNF-β. The Fc portion of the fusion protein helps to clear the etanercept-TNF complex from the body.

Hematopoietic Growth Factors

Hematopoiesis is the complex series of events involved in the formation, proliferation, differentiation, and activation of red blood cells, white blood cells, and platelets. Hematopoietic growth factors are cytokines that regulate these events.(122, 148–151) Investigators have identified and cloned at least 20 factors, including IL-3 (or multi-CSF), IL-4, IL-5, IL-6, IL-7, erythropoietin (EPO), granulocyte-macrophage colony-stimulating factor (GM-CSF), granulocyte colony-stimulating factor (G-CSF), macrophage colony-stimulating factor (M-CSF), and stem cell factor (SCF). Figure 40.7 summarizes the elaborate hematopoietic cascade. All blood cells originate within the bone marrow from a single class of pluripotent stem cells. In response to various external and internal stimuli, regulated by hematopoietic growth factors, stem cells give rise to additional new stem cells (self-renewal) and differentiate into mature specialized blood cells.

Erythropoietin—Epoetin Alpha (Epogen, Procrit)

Erythropoietin (EPO), (122, 149, 152–158) a 30,000–34,000 molecular weight glycoprotein produced by the kidney, stimulates the division and differentiation of erythroid progenitors in the bone marrow, increasing the production of red blood cells. Epoetin alpha (rHuEPO-α), a recombinant EPO prepared from cultures of genetically engineered mammalian CHO cells, consists of the identical 165-amino acid sequence of endogenous EPO. The molecular weight is approximately 30,400 daltons. The protein contains two disulfide bonds (linking cysteine 7 with 161 and 29 with 33) and four sites of glycosylation (one O-site and three N-sites); the disulfide bonds and glycosylation are necessary for the hormone's biologic activity. Deglycosylated natural EPO or bacterial-derived EPO (without glycosylation) have greatly de-

creased *in vivo* activity, although *in vitro* activity is largely conserved. The sugars may play a role in thermal stability or the prevention of aggregation *in vivo*.

The marketed products are formulated as a sterile, colorless, preservative-free liquid for intravenous or subcutaneous administration. The vial should not be shaken, or the glycoprotein may become denatured rendering it inactive. Epoetin alpha is indicated for the treatment of various anemias. Several of the conditions are listed in Table 40.4. Epoetin alpha represents a major scientific advance in the treatment of patients with chronic renal failure, serving as a replacement therapy for inadequate production of endogenous EPO by failing kidneys. Epoetin alpha may decrease the need for infusions in dialysis patients. By several mechanisms related to elevating the erythroid progenitor cell pool, epoetin alpha increases the production of red blood cells.

The manufacturer's full prescribing information should be consulted for dosing regimens because the dose is titrated individually to maintain the patient's target hematocrit. The circulating half-life is 4–13 hours in patients with chronic renal failure. Peak serum levels are achieved within 5–24 hours following subcutaneous administration.

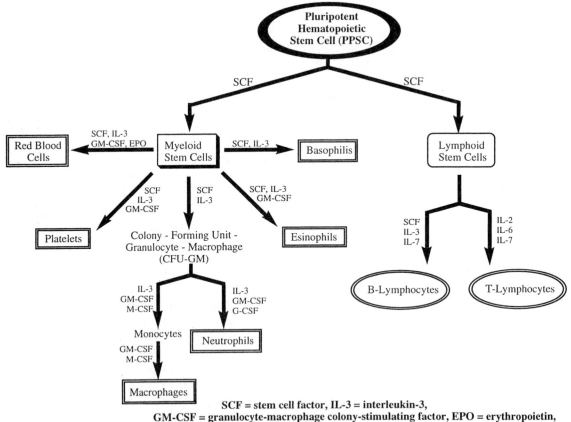

SCF = stem cell factor, IL-3 = interleukin-3,
GM-CSF = granulocyte-macrophage colony-stimulating factor, EPO = erythropoietin,
G-CSF = granulocyte colony-stimulating factor, M-CSF = macrophage
colony-stimulating factor. (adapted from reference 151)

Fig. 40.7. Schematic overview of hematopoiesis.

Colony-stimulating Factors

Colony-stimulating factors (CSFs) are glycoprotein cytokines that promote progenitor proliferation, differentiation, and some functional activation. The name colony-stimulating factor results from the fact that these proteins are often assayed by their ability to stimulate the formation of cell colonies in bone marrow cultures. The names added to CSF reflect the types of cell colonies that arise in these assays.

Granulocyte Colony-stimulating Factor—Filgration (Neuprogen). Recombinant DNA-derived G-CSF (122,149–149,159–166) or filgrastim, was approved in 1991 to decrease the incidence of infection in patients with nonmyeloid malignancies receiving myelosuppressive anticancer drugs. Additional indications are shown in Table 40.4. Filgrastim is a 175-amino acid, single-chain protein with a molecular weight of 18,800 daltons. Filgrastim, produced by a recombinant bacteria, differs from the endogenous human protein by the addition of a methionine at the N-terminus (recombinant methionyl G-CSF is sometimes called r-metHuG-CSF) and the lack of glycosylation. Glycosylation, however, does not appear to be necessary for the biologic activity.

Filgrastim injectable solution should be refrigerated at 2–8°C and is packaged with a patented indicator that turns red at temperatures below –4°C. The vials should never be shaken before the dose is withdrawn (contains human albumin). Administration is by intravenous infusion or by subcutaneous injection or infusion. The drug is rapidly absorbed with perk serum concentrations in 4–5 hours. Elimination half-life is approximately 3.5 hours.

Filgrastim is lineage selective for the neutrophil lineage type of white blood cells, whereas GM-CSF is multilineage stimulating progenitors of neutrophils, monocytes, basophils, and eosinophils. The drug reduces the period of neutropenia, the number of infections, and the number of days the patient is on antibiotics. Filgrastim is generally well tolerated, with medullary bone pain being the most frequently encountered side effect.

Granulocyte-Macrophage Colony-stimulating Factor—Sargramostim (Leukine). GM-CSF (122,149,159–163, 167–168) has been produced by rDNA technology in the yeast *S. cerevisiae*. Sargramostim is a glycoprotein of 127 amino acids differing from the endogenous human GM-CSF by substituting leucine at position 23. Also, the glycosylation pattern may differ from the native protein.

Sargramostim is supplied in vials of lyophilized powder (with mannitol) for intravenous infusion. Reconstituted with 1 ml of Sterile Water for Injection, USP (without preservative), the drug should be administered within 6 hours. Vials are intended for single use only. The powder, reconstituted solution, and diluted solution require refrigeration at 2-8°C without being frozen or shaken.

Sargramostim's indications are shown in Table 40.1. Cellular division, maturation, and activation are induced through GM-CSF's binding to specific receptors expressed on the surface of target cells. On 2-hour intravenous infusion, the alpha half-life is 12–17 minutes followed by a slower decrease (beta half-life) of 2 hours. The manufacturer's label should be consulted for precautions. Additional indications for GM-CSF under study are as an adjuvant to chemotherapy and an adjuvant to AIDS therapy.

Other Growth Factors—Becaplermin (Regranex)

Growth factors are cytokines responsible for regulating cell proliferation, differentiation, and function(169). They act as intercellular signals. Each cell type's response is specific for each particular growth factor and differs from growth factor to growth factor. Platelet-derived growth factor (PDGF) is an endogenous growth-promoting protein that is released from cells involved in the healing process. PDGF is evident at the cell proliferation stage of a healing open wound. A recombinant human PDGF B homodimer has been produced from genetically engineered *S. cerevisiae* cells (172–174). Becaplermin is the B-chain of the PDGF B protein. Thus, becaplermin is also referred to as rhPDGF-BB. The 25 kDa protein is formulated into a gel that mimics natural PDGF when applied to diabetic foot ulcers.

Clotting Factors VIII (Recombinate, KoGENate, Bioclate, Helixate), Factor IX (BeneFix) and Anticoagulants—Lepriudin (Refludan)

Antihemophiliac factor (AHF), or factor VIII, is required for the transformation of prothrombin (factor II) to thrombin by the intrinsic clotting pathway (102,104,171) (Chapter 26, Fig. 26.1). Hemophilia A, a life-long bleeding disorder, results from a deficiency of factor VIII. Conventional biotherapy for the treatment of hemophilia A includes protein concentrates from human plasma collected by transfusion services or commercial organizations. Therefore, the concentrates may possibly contain other native human proteins and microorganisms, such as viruses (e.g., HIV, hepatitis), derived from infected blood. Four versions of recombinant factor VIII (antihemophiliac factor), highly purified, microorganism-free proteins, are now available. All four therapeutic proteins are produced by the insertion of cDNA encoding for the entire factor VIII protein into mammalian cells. The mature, heavily glycosylated protein is composed of 2332 amino acids (1–2 million daltons) and contains sulfate groups. Stability of the large protein is a concern. The products have proved to be safe and effective in reducing bleeding time in patients. There is the possibility of induction of inhibitors in previously untreated patients. Hemophilia B results when a patient is deficient in specific clotting factor IX (106,175). It affects males primarily and makes up approximately 15% of all hemophilia cases. A recombinant human factor IX is now available.

Surgeons have used medicinal leeches (*Hirudo medicinalis*) for years to prevent thrombosis in fine vessels of reattached digits. Hirudin is the potent, specific thrombin inhibitor isolated from the leech. Lepirudin is a rDNA-derived (recombinant yeast) polypeptide that differs from the natural polypeptide with a terminal leucine instead of isoleucine and missing the sulfate group at Tyr 63 (174).

Vaccines

There are two types of immunization: active immunization and passive immunization. Active immunization is the induction of an immune response either through exposure to an infectious agent or by deliberate immunization with a vaccine (vaccination) made from the microorganism or its products to develop protective immunity. Passive immunization involves the transfer of products produced by an immune animal or human (preformed antibody or sensitized lymphoid cells) to a previously nonimmune recipient host, usually by injection. While sufficient active immunity may take days, several weeks or even months to induce (possibly including booster vaccinations), it is generally long-lasting (even life-long) through the clonal selection of genetically specific immunological memory B- and T-lymphocytes. Passive immunity, while often providing effective protection against some infection, is relatively brief, lasting only until the injected immunoglobulin or lymphoid cells have disappeared (a few weeks or months). Thus, vaccines enable the body to resist infection by diseases. In response to an injection of vaccine, the immune system makes antibodies, which recognize surface antigens found in the vaccine. If the subject is later exposed to a virulent form of the virus, the immune system is primed and ready to eliminate it. Many viral vaccines are produced from the antigens isolated from pooled human plasma of virus carriers. Vaccinations are among the most cost-effective and widely used public health interventions. Although generally safe, the minimal risk of vaccine-produced infections can be eliminated by administration of highly purified vaccine antigens of recombinant origin (175–178).

Two hepatitis B vaccines (175–179), Recombivax HB and Engerix-B were marketed in 1986 and 1989. Both are derived from a hepatitis B surface antigen and are produced in yeast cells. The primary difference between the two appears to be in exact dosing regimens. The immunization regimen consists of three injections: initial, at 1 month, and at 6 months. The immune response and clinical reactions for both intramuscular and subcutaneous administration are comparable. Vials containing the vaccine in solution should be stored at 2–8°C; freezing destroys potency.

There is also marketed a Lyme disease vaccine containing recombinant OspA (175–177,180). The vaccine is a sterile suspension of a noninfectious recombinant vaccine containing an immunodominant outer surface protein of *Borrelia burgdorferi* known as lipoprotein OspA. The antigen is adsorbed onto aluminum hydroxide as an adjuvant. Vaccine efficacy against definite Lyme disease was 78% after three doses.

VI. RECOMBINANT DNA-PRODUCED AGENTS IN DEVELOPMENT

According to the Pharmaceutical Research and Manufacturers Association 2000 survey of "Biotechnology Medicines in Development," companies are developing 369 biotechnology pharmaceuticals targeting more than 200 diseases. Nearly half of the medicines in the drug pipeline are for the treatment and detection of cancer. Table 40.9 lists some interesting examples of rDNA drugs in development.

Table 40.9. Some rDNA-derived Medicines in Development

Medicines	Status	Indications
HIV-1 immunogen	Phase III	HIV seropositive
AnervaX.RA	Phase II completed	Rheumatoid arthritis
Interleukin-1 receptor antagonist	Application accepted	Rheumatoid arthritis
Interleukin-10	Phase III	Rheumatoid arthritis
Gene-activated erythropoietin	Phase III	Anemia associated with renal disease
NESP	Application submitted	Stimulates production of RBCs
Abarelix	Phase III	Prostate cancer
Colon cancer vaccine	Phase I	Treat colon cancer
GeneVax	Phase I	Gene vaccine for various cancers
GVAX	Phase II	Cancer vaccine
Leridistim	Phase III	Myelorestoration with multicycle chemo
SomatoKine	Phase III	Growth factor for diabetes
TNF-binding protein 1	Phase II	Crohn's disease
Fibroblast growth factor	Phase II	Coronary artery disease
TP-10	Phase I	Heart attack
Malaria vaccine	Phase III	Malaria prevention
Brain-derived neurotropic factor	Phase III	Amyotrophic lateral sclerosis
Neutrophil inhibitory factor	Phase III	Stroke
Superoxide dismutase	Phase II	Asthma, displasia in premature infants
Recombinant osteogenic protein-1	Phase II/III	Fresh fractures, spinal fusion
Recombinant human albumin	Phase I	Excipient use

For example, IL-1, released in response to microbial challenge, interacts with receptors on lymphocytes, macrophages, and other cell types and is one of the most powerful cytokines driving inflammatory responses. Thus, blocking IL-1 synthesis or receptor interaction could be helpful in treating autoimmune diseases. Anakinra or IL-1 receptor antagonist is a recombinant derivative of a naturally occurring IL-1 receptor antagonist, currently undergoing clinical trials for the treatment of sepsis arthritis, ocular allergies, asthma, and inflammatory bowel disease.

Several rDNA-produced growth factors are now undergoing clinical trials. Epidermal growth factor (EGF) stimulates epidermal cell proliferation. Indications being explored include tissue repair in corneal and cataract surgeries, angiogenesis (new capillary formation), anti-angiogenesis (cancer treatment) and improvement in wound healing including burns and tendon repair. Because EGF assists in nerve regeneration, the potential may exist for the treatment of damaged spinal cords sometime in the future. Fibroblast growth factor (FGF), a member of a family of heparin-binding growth factors, is similar to EGF in its potential therapeutic uses. Platelet-derived growth factor (PDGF) is in early clinical trials for wound healing and ulcer repair. Other exciting growth factors being studied by the pharmaceutical industry include nerve factor, insulin-like growth factor, and stem cell growth factor.

Superoxide dismutase (SOD) is an enzyme that destroys oxygen free radicals. Recombinant SOD has the potential to be useful in the treatment of oxygen toxicity in premature infants, myocardial infarction, organ transplantation, and stroke.

Recombinant vaccines in human clinical trials are directed against HIV, melanoma, herpes simplex 2 virus, and malaria. Each of the vaccines uses a recombinant surface protein or protein fragment. The HIV proteins used in vaccine development include the gp120 envelope glycoprotein (gp), the entire gp 160 glycoprotein, and the p24 core protein. Advances in biotechnology and immunology have fueled efforts to create an engineered plant that possesses the antigen currently found in today's vaccines. Upon eating this recombinant DNA-produced plant (such as an apple or potato), the patient would ingest a subunit vaccine (such as the recombinant hepatitis B antigen now produced in yeast) genetically-engineered to be produced by the plant. The patient would then develop immunity to the antigen present in the subunit vaccine (i.e., an antigen found in measles, HIV, hepatitis B, etc.). Other vaccine strategies undergoing investigation include DNA vaccines and vector vaccines. There are at least two HIV DNA vaccines in clinical trials and a much-publicized vector vaccine using attenuated canarypox virus to deliver HIV genes to uninfected patients. Malaria vaccine development has continued to progress, despite the current lack of an effective vaccine. It appears that the multi-component DNA vaccines under development offer significant advantages over conventional vaccines. Several vaccines developed by various strategies have or are undergoing clinical trials.

VII. MONOCLONAL ANTIBODIES (MABS)

Introduction to Antibodies

The human immune system is composed of two major branches or arms: the cell-mediated immune system (which includes macrophages, lymphocytes, and granulocytes) and the humoral immune system (which includes the antibody-secreting B cells or plasma cells) (181–183). In contrast to the cell-mediated nature of the immune actions carried out by most lymphocytes, antibodies (Abs) or immunoglobulins (Igs) are soluble proteins that are produced in response to an antigenic stimulus. Antibodies are proteins. As part of the normal immune system, each B cell produces as many as a hundred million antibody proteins (polyclonal antibodies) directed against bacteria, viruses, and other foreign invaders. Antibodies act by binding to a particular antigen (Ag), thereby "tagging" it for removal or destruction by other immune system components.

The production of antigen "neutralizing" antibodies or immunoglobulins and the detection of a sufficient antibody titer are important concepts to an understanding of vaccinations and the exposure to antigens. The humoral response to an antigen involves the creation of memory B-cells and B-lymphocyte transformation into plasma cells that serve as factories for the production of secreted antibodies. Approximately four days after initial contact with an antigen (immunization), IgM antibodies (one of five types of immunoglobulin structure) appear and peak about four hours later. Approximately seven days after exposure, IgG, the major class of circulating immunoglobulin, appears. The antibodies bind to the antigen and effect additional immune system-mediated events, "neutralizing" the antigen and leading to its elimination. The concentration of an immunoglobulin specific for a given antigen at a given time is referred to as the antibody titer and may be a measure of the effectiveness of the initial antigen exposure/vaccination to illicit immunologic memory.

Antibody Structure

Antibodies are glycoproteins. The simplest structure of an immunoglobulin molecule consists of two identical long peptide chains (the heavy chains), and two identical short polypeptide chains (the light chains) interconnected by several disulfide bonds. The selectivity of any immunoglobulin for a particular antigen is determined by its structure and specifically by the variable or antigen-binding regions (Fig. 40.8). Enzymatic digestion of the antibody with papain yields the Fab fragment, which contains the antigen binding sites, and the Fc fragment, which specifies the other biologic activities of the molecule.

Hybridoma Technology

MAbs are ultrasensitive hybrid immune system-derived proteins designed to recognize specific antigens. Nobel, Laureates, Kohler, and Milstein first reported MAbs in 1975(184). MAbs have been used in laboratory diagnostics, site-directed drugs, and home test kits (177,185–189).

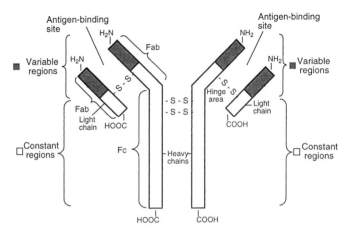

Fig. 40.8. Schematic model of an antibody molecule.

The B lymphocyte produces a wide range of structurally diverse antibody proteins with varying degrees of specificity in response to a single antigen stimulus. Because of their structural diversity, these antibodies would be called polyclonal antibodies. MAbs are homogeneous hybrid proteins produced by a selected single clone of an engineered B lymphocyte. They are designed to recognize specific sites or epitopes on antigens.

Hybridoma technology, the technology used to produce MAbs, consists of combining or fusing two different cell lines: a myeloma cell (generally from a mouse) and a plasma spleen cell (B lymphocyte) capable of producing an antibody that recognizes a specific antigen (Fig. 40.9). The resulting fused cell or hybridoma possesses some of the characteristics of both original cells: the myeloma cell's ability to survive and reproduce in culture (immortality) and the plasma spleen cell's ability to produce antibodies to a specific antigen.

Two myeloma variant cell lines with defects in nucleotide synthesis pathways are commonly used as fusion partners (185, 187, 189–191). One lacks the HGPRT gene coding for an essential enzyme in purine biosynthesis. The other lacks the Tk gene coding for a pyrimidine biosynthetic enzyme. Following fusion, the cells are cultured in a medium containing hypoxanthine, aminopterin, and thymidine (HAT medium). Correct hybridomas (1 myeloma plus 1 spleen cell), although missing the gene from the myeloma partner, possess the gene from its spleen cell partner. Fused myeloma hybrids do not survive because they lack the essential gene, and fused spleen cell hybrids do not grow in culture. Hybridomas can be grown in large quantities, and clones producing antibodies with the appropriate specificity for the original antigen can be isolated from culture. Various techniques have been developed to select the single hybridoma clone producing the desired antibody (thus MAb). Hybridomas are grown in *in vitro* cell culture or *in vivo* in mouse (murine) ascites to yield large amounts of MAbs (1–100 mcg/mL in culture and 1 mg/mL in ascites).

MAbs are more attractive than polyclonal antibodies for diagnostic and therapeutic applications because of their increased specificity of antigen recognition. Thus, they can serve as target-directed "homing devices" to find and attach to the targeted antigen. Developments in hybridoma technology have led to highly specific diagnostic agents for: home use in pregnancy testing and ovulation prediction kits; laboratory use in detection of colorectal cancer, ovarian cancer, and others; and the design of site-directed therapeutic agents such as trastuzumab to combat metastatic breast cancer and abciximab as an adjunct for the prevention of cardiac ischemic complications.

Monoclonal Antibody Immunogenicity

Nearly 25 years after Kohler and Milstein's pioneering work, monoclonal antibodies began to realize their therapeutic potential. Until recently, most monoclonal antibodies were murine proteins based on their production. Initial clinical trials of murine MAbs showed that these mouse proteins were highly immunogenic in patients after just a single dose (192–194). Human patients formed antibodies to combat the foreign MAb that was administered. The human anti-mouse antibody response is known as HAMA. Far from being the "magic bullets" that were proposed, im-

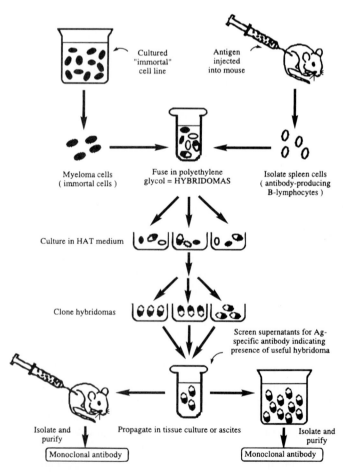

Fig. 40.9. Outline of hybridoma creation and MAb production.

Table 40.10. Some FDA-approved MAb Therapeutic Agents

Generic Name	Trade Name	MAb Type	Description	Indication
Trastuzumab	Herceptin	Humanized	Binds to extracellular domain of human epidermal growth factor receptor (HER2) mediating an antibody-dependent cellular toxicity in cells that over express HER protein	Refractory breast cancer
Muromonab-CD3	Orthoclone-OKT3	Murine	First FDA-approved MAb therapeutic	Reversal of transplant rejection
Infliximab	Remicade	Chimeric	An anti-tumor necrosis factor-alpha MAb	Crohn's disease
Abciximab	ReoPro	Chimeric	LgG-derived F(ab')2 fragment blocks GPIIb/IIIa receptor site on activated platelet	Adjunct to PTCA for prevention of acute cardia complications
Ritiximab	Rituxan	Chimeric	Binds to the CD20 antigen found on >90% of all B-cell lymphomas	Treatment od B-cell non-Hodgkin's lymphoma
Basiliximab	Simulect	Chimeric	Binds to subunit of high-affinity IL-2 receptor found on activated T-cells	Prevention of transplant rejection
Daclizumab	Zenapax	Humanized	Binds to subunit of high-affinity IL-2 receptor found on activated T-cells	Prevention of transplant rejection
Palivizumab	Synagis	Humanized	Binds to "F" protein on surface of virus preventing virus from infecting cells	Respiratory syncitial virus prophylaxis
Gemtuzumab Ozoganicin	Mylotarg	Fusion MAb	Composed of humanized anti-CD33 MAb conjugated with the cytotoxic antibiotic calicheamicin	Treatment of CD33 positive acute myeloid leukemia

munogenic murine MAbs were useless in chronic therapy. Thus, some approach was needed to eliminate the unwanted immune response (HAMA) in patients.

The variable regions of an immunoglobulin must be of a specific chemical structure with the ability to bind to the antigen they "recognize." The part within the variable region that forms the intermolecular interactions with the antigen is the complementarity determining region (CDR). The variable domains of antibody light and heavy chains each contain three CDRs.

It was determined that immune responses against the mouse-produced MAbs were directed against both the variable and the constant regions of the antibody. Human and murine antibodies are very homologous in chemical structure. Thus, a MAb should be engineered to decrease the immunogenicity of a MAb by replacing the mouse constant regions of an IgG with human constant regions, making the antibody less mouse-like (185, 195–199). In practice what generally occurs is the variable heavy and variable light chain domains (CDRs) of human immunoglobulins are replaced with those of a murine antibody which possesses the requisite antigen specificity. This "chimeric" MAb will retain its ability to recognize the antigen (a property of the murine MAb), retain the many effector functions of an immunoglobulin (both murine and human), while being much less immunogenic (a property of a human immunoglobulin). A chimeric MAb, containing approximately 70% human sequence, will have a longer half-life than its murine counterpart in a human patient. Therapeutic monoclonal antibodies that are chimeric include abciximab, ritiximab, infliximab, and basiliximab.

While the discovery that the conserved structure of antibodies, in particular IgGs, across many species suggested the possibility of chimeric antibodies, the realization that the homology extended to the antigen-binding site facilitated the engineering of humanized immunoglobulins. Advances in phage display technology and the production of transgenic animals has lead to the production of humanized or fully human MAbs (185, 195–199). Functional human antibody fragments (e.g., Fab fragments) can be displayed on the surface of bacteriophages. A bacteriophage, also called a phage, is a virus that infects bacteria. The expression of these human antibody fragments on the phage surface has facilitated efficient screening of large numbers of phage clones (phage display) for antigen-binding specificity (200). Once a fragmented with the requisite antigen specificity is selected, it can be isolated and engineered into a humanized MAb (replacing up to 95% of the murine protein sequence) or a fully human MAb (100% human sequence). Transgenic strains of mice have been genetically engineered to possess most and now all of the essential human antibody genes. Thus, upon immunization with a foreign antigen, the transgenic mice will develop humanized or fully human antibodies in response. Both of these techniques, while very complex and expensive, have yielded FDA-approved humanized antibody pharmaceuticals such as daclizumab, palivuzumab, and trastuzumab. The half-life of humanized antibodies are dramatically enhanced (from hours to weeks) and immunogenicity is drastically reduced.

Monoclonal Antibody Therapeutic Agents

Hybridoma technology and advanced antibody engineering has led to the design of an increasing number of site-directed therapeutic agents for the treatment and prevention of transplant rejection, therapy in rheumatoid arthritis, the treatment of nonHodgkin's lymphoma and other indications. These products (Table 40.10) are examples of murine, chimeric and humanized MAbs and represent significant advances in pharmacotherapy.

Monoclonal Antibody Diagnostic Agents

Several ultra-sensative diagnostic MAb-based products have enjoyed great success and include a variety of imaging agents for the detection of blood clots and cancer cells. A monoclonal Fab fragment, technetium-99m-arcitumomab (CEA-Scan), can detect the presence and indicate the location of recurrent and metastatic colorectal cancer. Colorectal cancer and ovarian cancer can be detected with satumomab pendetide (OncoScint CR/OV). Capromab pentetate (ProstaScint) is used for detection, staging and follow-up of prostate adenocarcinoma patients. Small-cell lung cancer can be detected with nofetumomab (Verluma). The first imaging MAb for myocardial infarction is imiciromab pentetate (MyoScint). PhRMA reports that 59 of the 369 biotechnology agents in testing are MAb-based products, most diagnostics (46).

Monoclonal Antibody-Based In-Home Diagnostic Kits

The strong trend toward self-care coupled with a heightened awareness by the public of available technology and an emphasis on preventive medicine has increased the use of in-home diagnostics (201–203). Sales of in-home diagnostics were predicted to exceed $1 billion by the mid-1990s. MAb specifically minimizes the possibilities of interference from other substances that might yield false-positive test results. The antigen being selectively detected by MAb-based pregnancy test kits is human chorionic gonadotropin (hCG), the hormone produced if fertilization occurs and that continues to increase in concentration during the pregnancy. Table 40.11 lists some examples of MAb-containing in-home pregnancy test kits. Luteinizing hormone present in the urine is the antigen detected by MAb ovulation prediction home test kits. These test kits can help determine when a woman is most fertile because ovulation occurs 20–48 hours after the luteinizing hormone surge. Table 40.11 also provides some examples of MAb-based in-home ovulation prediction kits.

INFLUENCE OF BIOTECHNOLOGY ON DRUG DISCOVERY

The search for novel, efficacious, and safer medicinal agents is an increasingly costly and complex process. R&D costs are climbing, the number of drug candidates in the pipeline are increasing, there is an information onslaught, and growing regulatory requirements. The past 25 years has brought recombinant DNA technology, hybridoma and advanced MAb production, genomics, and a host of other innovative technologies that are transforming drug discovery. While taking advantage of any opportunity or technique available to aid in the drug discovery process, the challenge for medicinal chemists remains lead identification. Traditionally, medicinal chemistry research programs aimed at discovering new therapeutic agents relied heavily on random screening followed by analog synthesis and lead optimization. In discovering a lead, medicinal chemists encounter a problem. What biologic property does one screen for that directly correlates with the desired therapeutic outcome?

Biotechnology's contribution to pharmaceutical care in the 1980s and 1990s was an improvement in the methods used to manufacture peptide-based and protein-based biopharmaceuticals, such as insulin and human

Table 40.11. Some MAb-based In-home Test Kits*

Product	Manufacturer/Distributor	End Point
Pregnancy		
Answer Plus	Carter Products	Plus in test window = +
Answer Quick & Simple	Carter Products	Plus in test window = +
Clear Blue Easy	Unipath	Blue line in large window = +
Clear Blue Easy One Min.	Unipath	Blue line in large window = +
Conceive	Quidel	Pink to purple test line = +
1 Step E.P.T.	Warner Lambert	Pink color in test and control = +
Fact Plus One Step	Advanced Care	Pink plus sign in window = +
Fact Plus	Advanced Care	Pink plus sign in window = +
First Response1 Step	Carter Products	Two pink lines in window = +
Fortel Plus	Biomerica	Purple stick line darker than reference = +
One Step Fortel Early	Biomerica	Purple stick line darker than reference = +
Q Test	Quidel	Blue control line and pink plus sign = +
Ovulation		
Answer Quick & Simple	Carter Products	Purple stick line darker than reference = +
Conceive 1 Step	Quidel	Pink to purple test line darker than reference = +
First Response1 Step	Carter Products	Purple test line darker than reference = +
ClearPlan Easy	Unipath	Blue test line in large window similar or darker than line in small window = +
Ovukit Self Test	Quidel	White to shades of blue compared to LH surge guide = +
OvuQuick	Quidel	Test spot appears darker than reference = +
Q Test	Quidel	Purple test line darker than reference = +

*Information from references 201–203.

growth hormone. Manufacturing shifted to highly controlled, well-characterized microbial fermentation or culture techniques from extraction, from blood, or other biologic materials. This improved the availability, safety, and, to some extent, the efficacy of widely used hormones and vaccines. Since the late 1980s, advances in biotechnology have not only affected manufacturing, but also have contributed to a greater understanding of the cause and progression of disease and have identified new therapeutic targets forming the basis of novel drug screens. The revolution in biotechnology, (including molecular and cellular biology, biochemistry, immunology, genetics, etc.) has generated new strategies for the identification of targets for therapeutic intervention. George Scangos, a biotech pharmaceutical company CEO, has stated that "For the first time, pharmaceutical researchers have the opportunity to identify optimal drug screening targets based on a logical, systematic program. By identifying targets that antagonize disease gene activity and then rationally choosing among those targets based on select criteria, researchers should, for the first time, be able to rationally choose drug targets, and therefore maximize chances for the safety and efficacy of the drugs against those targets" (204). These advances are changing the paradigm for drug discovery and have facilitated the design of new agents with novel mechanisms of action for diseases that were previously difficult or impossible to treat.(205–209) Having entered all areas of the drug discovery process, there is little doubt that biotechnology is playing a pivotal role in shaping the medicinal agents that pharmacists will dispense in the future.

With the evolution of biotechnology and, in particular, recombinant DNA techniques, detailed structural information about therapeutic targets is becoming increasingly available. The editor of the *Journal of Medicinal Chemistry* Phillip Portoghese has said that "as a graduate student in medicinal chemistry, it was inconceivable that we know as much about drug receptors as we do today. It is mind-boggling to think that in the relatively short span of two decades, the amino acid sequences of well over a thousand G protein-coupled receptors have been deposited in electronic data bases"(210). The application of the techniques of biotechnology (to the identification of proteins and other macromolecules as drug targets, and their production in meaningful quantities) as discovery tools thus can provide an answer to at least one of the persistent problems of lead detection. The number of different receptor classes as well as the number of genes encoding receptor subtypes within each class is continually growing and is far greater than previously expected. Detailed structural analysis of cloned receptors and receptor subtypes has provided insight into receptor function through comparisons of sequence and molecular modeling. Cloned and expressed receptors have proved helpful in highlighting the pharmacologic differences between humans and animals, in developing ligand binding assays for drug discovery, and in reevaluating the mechanism of action of known medicinal agents.

Receptor Structure Determination

Recombinant drug targets (receptors) can be crystallized and their three-dimensional structure determined by the well-established technique of X-ray crystallography (211–212). Macromolecules such as recombinant proteins require specialized procedures to obtain suitable crystals for X-ray analysis. At present, it is the only available technique that elucidates the complete three-dimensional structure of a molecule in high-resolution detail, including bond distances, angles, stereochemistry, and absolute configuration. X-ray crystallography can provide atomic resolution structures of protein receptor targets and protein-ligand interactions with other molecules, such as substrates, cofactors, or inhibitors. The structure of these complexes can be obtained by co-crystallizing the protein and the ligand or by soaking the ligand into an existing protein crystal.

Rational drug design (sometimes called mechanistic drug design or computer-assisted drug design) is an iterative process in which three-dimensional structure determination, analysis, design, synthesis, and bioassay form a dynamic feedback cycle. Rational drug design requires a structure for the target receptor, a demand satisfied by the availability of macromolecular crystal structures, including recombinant proteins. Drug design approaches can use crystal structures in a priori design (the terms de novo design or ab initio design have sometimes been used in the same context) and a posteriori analysis (205–206, 209). A priori design, a rational drug design approach, employs the crystal structure to create the initial, structurally novel lead compound with the aid of molecular graphics. A retrospective method, a posteriori analysis rationalizes existing structure-activity relationship data with X-ray structure and proposes design improvements.

HIV encodes for a protease (HIV-1 PR) required for viral replication. An example of the use of X-ray crystallography in drug design is the intensive study of inhibitors of HIV-1 PR as potential anti-AIDS drugs. Medicinal chemists have applied a priori design and a posteriori analysis to the problem. Crystallographic studies of both recombinant expressed and synthetic HIV-1 PR suggested a substrate binding site. In addition, the crystal structure of a complex of an inhibitor bound to HIV-1 PR was determined, resulting in a closest contact map detailing hydrogen bonding interactions that serves as an aid to future HIV-1 PR inhibitor design (Fig. 40.10) (213). Also, high-throughput enzyme inhibition assays based on recombinant HIV-1 PR have facilitated the drug design studies. There are six HIV protease inhibitors now on the market, all products of rational drug design; amprenavir, indinavir, nelfinavir, ritonavir, saquinavir, and lopinavir (See Chapter 39, Table 39.5).

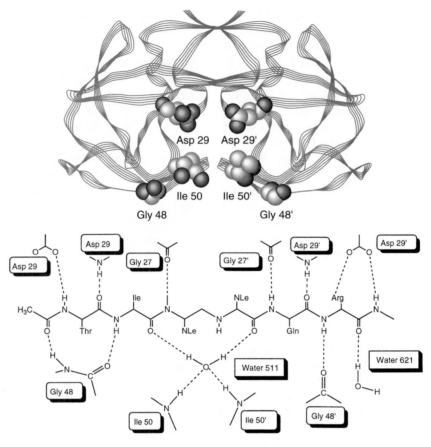

Fig. 40.10. Representation of H-bonding interactions of an inhibitor of HIV-1 PR as determined by X-ray analysis (Miller M, et al., Science 1989; 246:1149–1152).

Although X-ray crystallography may not reflect the three-dimensional molecular structure of a recombinant receptor protein under biologic conditions in solution, multidimensional nuclear magnetic resonance (NMR) spectroscopy may be the most powerful technique for such examinations. NMR can often provide structural information faster than X-ray crystallography and more easily study the dynamic interaction of ligand and receptor because the technique does not require crystals (214–216).

Genomics, Proteomics, Bioinformatics and Pharmacogenomics/genetics

It has been stated "No meaningful discussion of 21st-century healthcare can ignore the promise of genomics" (217). Research in genomics, proteomics, bioinformatics and pharmacogenomics are heralded as the next important supply source of innovative future drug design targets. With the Human Genome Project rapidly approaching closure, researchers are turning increasingly to the task of converting the DNA sequence data into information that will potentially improve, and perhaps even revolutionize, human medicine and healthcare. Pharmacists and pharmaceutical scientists are poised to take advantage of this scientific break-through by incorporating state-of-the-art genomics techniques into a new drug discovery

and development paradigm (218–222). Techniques that will be required to solve today's and tomorrows' drug discovery problems include genomics, proteomics, bioinformatics and pharmacogenomics/genetics.

Genomics and the Human Genome Project

Genomics is the study of genes and their functions. The Human Genome Project or Human Genome Initiative began in 1990 to map and sequence human DNA (223). Mapping the genome would require locating all genes and other markers as well as their relative positions on the chromosomes. The goal of the project was to learn not only what is contained in the genetic code, but also how to manipulate it to cure or help prevent the estimated 4000 genetic diseases afflicting humankind. In May 1999, 700 million base pairs of the humane genome were deposited in public archives. Fifteen months later, the figure had ballooned to more than 4 billion (224). A milestone in genomic science was reached on June 26, 2000, two years earlier then projected, when researchers at Celera Genomics and the international Genome Project jointly announced that they had completed sequencing 97–99% of the human genome. The journal *Science* ranks the mapping of the human genome as its breakthrough of the year in its December 22, 2000 issue. Sequencing the entire genome may be a reality, but the job of sorting through human and pathogen diversity factors and correlating them with genomic data to provide real benefits has barely begun. Solving this monumental problem will usher in an era of molecular medicine. The human genome consisting of 23 pairs of chromosomes and three billion base pair (bp) codes for approximately 100,000 functional genes (some recent estimates of 30,000–35,000 genes suggest that the previous estimates of 90,000–120,000 may be incorrect) is now being interpreted. Determining gene functionality in any organism opens the door for linking a disease to specific genes or proteins, which become targets for new drugs or ways to detect organisms.

Deciphering the biochemical pathways at the molecular level that provide the underlying basis of disease states will result in the identification of a vast array of proteins that will serve as candidates for therapeutic intervention. Medicinal chemists anticipate that many of the proteins will be entirely novel and have unknown functions offering a unique opportunity to identify previously unknown molecular targets and the ultrsensitive detection of organisms to address unmet therapeutic needs. Analyzing the data will be an enormous task

Proteomics

The study of proteomics seeks to define the function and expression profiles of all proteins encoded within a genome (225–228). To date, we are unable to identify valid drug targets and new detection methodology simply by examining gene sequence information. Often, multiple genes are involved in a single disease process. Since few proteins act alone, studying protein interactions will be paramount to a full understanding of functionality. There is a wide gap between genomics and drug discovery that reflects the fact that gene sequence rarely reveals protein function or disease relevance. Therefore, the real value of human genome sequence information will only be realized after a function has been assigned for each and every protein. Applying proteomics technologies will not only provide validated targets for drug discovery and disease detection, but will also increase the efficiency of the drug discovery process. Proteomics is far more challenging than genomics because there are so many more proteins then genes. Again, sifting through the enormous amount of proteomic data to select a group of drug targets from all proteins in the human body presents a Herculean task.

Bioinformatics and Microarrays

Scientists have applied information technology and innovative software to the research in genomics and molecular biology to give birth to the new field of bioinformatics (229–230). With bioinformatics, a researcher can now search the tremendous flood of Human Genome Project data looking for a drug discovery "needle" in that massive "haystack." Because of the mass of data that is generated, bioinformatics capabilities are required to conduct ge-

nomics and proteomics research including "microarray screening." Another goal of bioinformatics is to be able to study the molecules and processes discovered by genomics and proteomics research in silico. That is, to be able to product chemical and physical structure and properties by computer.

A DNA microarray, also called a biochip, is a surface collection of immobilized genes that can be simultaneously examined with specialized robotic equipment to conduct expression analysis (231–233). Microarray analysis has gained increasing importance as a direct result of the Human Genome Project. These miniature laboratories provide the medicinal chemist with the quick and easy capability to simultaneously analyze thousands of gene expression levels under specific conditions. Microarray technology is a platform for studying functional genomics since the data obtained may link expression to function. The biochips provide polymorphism detection and genotyping as well as hybridization-based expression monitoring. Microarrays of DNAs provide expression analysis for each gene represented on the microarray. Biochips may contain a particular set of gene sequences (i.e., sequences coding for all human cytochrome P450 isozymes) or may contain sequences representing all human genes. The potential to study key areas of molecular medicine are unlimited at this stage of the technology's development. For example, gene expression levels of thousands of mRNA species may be studied simultaneously in normal versus tumor cells each challenged with anticancer drug candidates.

Pharmacogenomics/Genetics

Advances in biotechnology have created a dramatic change in the way new pharmacotherapeutic agents are discovered and developed. Pharmaceutical care will experience similar significant changes as health care providers utilize the pharmacogenomic/genetic knowledge gained from genomics and proteomics to tailor drug therapy to meet the needs of their individual patients (234–238).

Pharmacogenetics is the field of study concerned with how genetic differences influence drug action including drug safety and efficacy. The field of pharmacogenetics is almost 50 years old, but is undergoing exponential growth at this time. A good example of pharmacogenetics is our understanding of the genetic variations among patients affecting liver enzymes such as the cytochrome P-450 class. For instance, some patients lack an enzymatically active form of CYP2D6 and will metabolize certain drugs differently than other patients expressing an active enzyme.

Pharmacogenomics, a form of genotyping, is a much newer term that correlates an individual patients genetic make-up with his or her response to pharmacotherapy using genomics or proteomics techniques. Molecular medicine utilizing pharmacogenomics would first perform a detailed genetic analysis of a patient assembling a comprehensive list of single nucleotide polymorphisms (SNPs) within the genome. Pharmacogenomic tests are

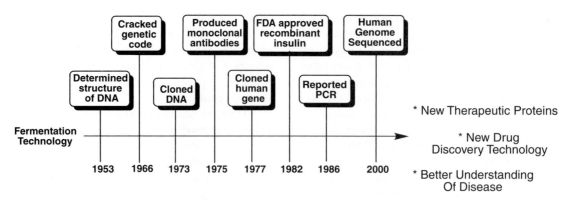

Fig. 40.11. Major advances in biotechnology.

performed to pre-identify patients who may respond to a specific agent. The relationship of the SNPs to a drug response is pharmacogenetics. The impact of the patient's SNPs on the use of new or existing drugs would be predicted and individualized drug therapy would be identified that assures maximal efficacy and minimal toxicity. The rational, individualize drug therapy based on the tests is pharmacogenomics. Identifying SNPs will help differentiate responders and nonresponders to drug therapy. The right drug to the right patient at the right time. Pharmaceutical care in the near-future will certainly be driven by pharmacogenetic and pharmacogenomic considerations.

CONCLUSION

Many advances have occurred in biotechnology since Watson and Crick determined the structure of DNA (Fig. 40.11). Pharmaceutical biotechnology and, in particular, recombinant DNA technology, hybridoma methodology and advanced MAb production techniques have provided improved pharmaceuticals, novel therapeutic agents, unique diagnostic products, and new drug design tools. Disease processes are being defined at the molecular level and new drug targets are being identified that will contribute to innovative drug discovery. Pharmacogenomics and pharmacogenetics will bring individualized pharmacotherapy into the provision of pharmaceutical care. Pharmacists and medicinal chemists are poised to be among the great beneficiaries of the advances made in the techniques and products of biotechnology, if they are prepared. Many other techniques of biotechnology exist and impact medicinal chemists, beyond those discussed in this chapter. Antisense technology and gene therapy are discussed in other chapters of this textbook. Additional important biotechnologies pharmacists and pharmaceutical scientists should be familiar with include PCR, site-directed mutagenesis, ribozymes, abzymes, transgenic animals, glycobiology, tissue engineering, and biosensors. Novel technologies or innovative extensions of existing biotechnologies are being developed with increasing frequencies. The suggested readings listed in this chapter serve as useful resources on each of these topics and the

internet has proven to be an excellent source of up-to-date biotech information. Some useful websites include: www.ornl.gov/hgmis/; www.hgsc.bcm.tmc.edu/; genomics.phrma.org/; snp.cshl.org; and www.ncbi.nlm.nih.gov/.

REFERENCES

1. Conlan MF. Drug Top 1990;134:34.
2. Wade DA, Levy RA. Biotechnology: A opportunity for pharmacists. Am Pharm 1992;NS32:33–37.
3. Crommelin, DJA, Sindelar RD eds. Pharmaceutical Biotechnology, An introduction for pharmacists and pharmaceutical scientists. Amsterdam, The Netherlands: Harwood Academic Publishers, 1997.
4. Zito SW, ed. Pharmaceutical Biotechnology, A Programmed Text. 2nd ed. Lancaster, PA:Technomic Publishing, 1997.
5. Walsh G. Biopharmaceutical: Biochemistry and Biotechnology. Chichester, England: John Wiley & Sons Ltd., 1998.
6. Pezzuto JM, Johnson ME, Manasse HR, eds. Biotechnology and Pharmacy. New York, NY: Chapman & Hall, 1993.
7. Klegerman ME, Groves MJ, eds. Pharmaceutical Biotechnology-Fundamentals and Essentials. Buffalo Grove, IL: Interpharm Press, 1992.
8. Wu-Pong S, Rojanasakul Y, eds. Bioharmaceutical Drug Design and Development. Totowa, NJ: Humana Press, 1999.
9. Creighton TE, ed., Encyclopedia of Molecular Biology, Volumes 1–4. New York, NY: John Wiley & Sons, 1999.
10. Bains W. Biotechnology from A to Z. 2nd ed. Oxford, England: Oxford University Press, 1998.
11. Coombs J. Dictionary of Biotechnology. 2nd ed. New York, NY: MacMillan Press, 1992.
12. Nill KR. Glossary of Biotechnology terms. 2nd ed. Lancaster, PA: Technomic Publishing, 1998.
13. Glick BR, Pasternak JJ, eds. Molecular Biotechnology: Principles & Applications of Recombinant DNA. 2nd ed. Washington, D.C.: ASM Press, 1998.
14. Franks F, ed., Protein Biotechnology. Totowa, NJ: Humana Press, 1993.
15. Moses V, Cape RE, eds. Biotechnology—The Science and the Business. Chur, Switzerland: Harwood Academic Publishers GmbH, 1991.
16. Walker JM, Gingold EB, eds. Molecular Biology and Biotechnology. 3rd ed. Cambridge, England: Royal Society of Chemistry, 1993.
17. Davies J, Reznikoff WS, eds. Milestones in Biotechnology: Classic Papers on Genetic Engineering. Stoneham, MA: Butterworth-Heinemann, 1992.

18. Alberts B, Bray D, Lewis J, et al, eds. Molecular Biology of the Cell. 3rd ed. New York, NY: Garland Publishing, 1994.

19. Lodish H, Baltimore D, Berk A, et al, eds. Molecular Cell Biology, 3rd ed. New York, NY: Scientific American Books, 1995.

20. Freifelder D, Malacinski GM, eds. Essentials of Molecular Biology. 2nd ed. Boston, MA: Jones & Bartlett Publishers, 1993.

21. Wolfe SL. An introduction to Cell and Molecular Biology. Belmont, CA: Wadsworth Publishing Co., 1995.

22. Regan JW. Biotechnology and drug discovery. In: Delgado JN, Remers WA, eds. Textbook of Organic Medicinal and Pharmaceutical Chemistry. 10th ed. Phildelphia, PA: Lippincott-Raven, 1998; 139–152.

23. Harris TJR. The current and future impact of molecular biology in drug discovery. In: Ganellin CR, Roberts SM, eds. Medicinal Chemistry, The Role of Organic Chemistry in Drug Research. 2nd ed. San Diego, CA: Academic Press, 1993; 103–128.

24. Drlica K. Genetic engineering: the gene. In: Hansch C, Sammes PG, Taylor JB eds. Comprehensive Medicinal Chemistry. Volume 1. New York, NY: Pergamon Press, 1990;361–408.

25. Brixner D. Biotechnology's impact on pharmacists. Pharm Times 1991; Nov:39–42.

26. Demuth JE, ed. An introduction to pharmaceutical biotechnology. Madison, WI: The Regents of the University of Wisconsin System, 1992.

27. Piascik MM. Research and development of drugs and biologic entities. Am J Hosp Pharm 1991;48(Suppl.1):S4–13.

28. Speedie MK. The impact of biotechnology upon pharmacy education. Am J Pharm Educ 1990;53,55–61.

29. Stewart CF, Fleming RA. Biotechnology products: new opportunities and responsibilities for the pharmacist. Am J Hosp Pharm 1989;46(Suppl. 2):S4–8.

30. Tami JA. Recombinant DNA technology and therapeutics. Am Pharm 1991;NS31(2):1–8.

31. Sindelar RD. Overview/preview of current and future recombinant DNA-produced pharmaceuticals. Drug Top 1992 (Suppl.):3–13.

32. Kane BJ, Kuhn JG. Biotechnology: new roles and challenges for the pharmacist in ambulatory care. Drug Top 1992 (Suppl.):3–13.

33. Hudson RA, Black CD. Biotechnology—The New Dimension in Pharmacy Practice: A Working Pharmacist's Guide. 2nd ed. Toledo,OH: Council of Ohio Colleges of Pharmacy, 1999.

34. Fields S. Dispensing biotechnology products. Am Pharm 1993; NS33:28–29.

35. Hall P. Pharmaceutical Biotechnology. New York, NY: Global Medical Communications, 1992.

36. Gore MJ. Pharmacy prepares for a new era. Consult Pharm 1992; 7:369–386.

37. Dasher T. Reimbursement for outpatient biotech drugs, Part 1. Am Pharm 1993;NS33:16–17.

38. Dasher T. Reimbursement for outpatient biotech drugs, Part 2. Am Pharm 1993;NS33:24–25.

39. Roth R. Specializing in biotechnology pharmaceuticals. Am Pharm 1994;NS34:31–33.

40. Allen LV. Compounding biotechnology drug products. Am Pharm 1994;NS34:18–21.

41. Roth R, Constantine LM. Biotech pharmacy addresses patient compliance. Am Pharm 1995;NS35:19–21.

42. Kennedy HG, Dong LG. Reimbursement and patient assistance programs for biotech drugs. Am Pharm 1997;NS37: 136–138.

43. Sindelar RD. The pharmacy of the future—biotechnology and your practice. Drug Top 1993;137:66–78.

44. McKinnon B. Disease management—biotechnology and managed care pharmacy. Drug Benefit Trends 1997; Dec:30–34.

45. Evens R, Louie SG, Sindelar R, et al. Biotech Rx: Biotechnology in Pharmacy Practice: Science, Clinical Applications and Pharmaceutical Care—Opportunities in Therapy Management. Washington, D.C.: American Pharmaceutical Association, 1997.

46. Biotechnology Medicines in Development, 2000 Annual Survey. Washington, D.C.: Pharmaceutical Research and Manufacturers of America, 2000.

47. Biotechnology Resource Catalog. Philadelphia, PA: Philadelphia College of Pharmacy and Science, 1993.

48. Shamel RE, Udis-Kessler AU. Biotechnology in the 21st century. Genetic Engin News 1999;19:19,75.

49. Dibner MD. Biotechnology and pharmaceuticals—10 years later. Biopharm 1997;11:24–30.

50. Dutton G. Key areas of growth for biotech. Genetic Engin News 1999;19:17,22.

51. Gingold EB. An introduction to recombinant DNA technology. In: JM, Gingold EB, eds. Molecular Biology and Biotechnology, 3rd ed. Cambridge, England: Royal Society of Chemistry, 1993, 23.

52. Watson JD, Gilman M, Witkowski J, et al. Recombinant DNA, 2nd ed. New York, NY: Scientific American Books, 1992, 13–32.

53. Lewin B. Genes VI. Oxford, England: Oxford University Press, 1997, 97–113.

54. Voet D., Voet JG, Pratt CW. Fundamentals of Biochemistry. New York, NY: John Wiley & Sons, Inc., 1999, 881–882.

55. Greene JJ, Rao VB, eds. Recombinant DNA Principles and Methodologies. New York, NY: Marcel Dekker, Inc., 1998.

56. Kreuzer H, Massey A. Recombinant DNA and Biotechnology. Washington, D.C.: ASM Press, 1996.

57. Hoekstra WPM, Smeekens SCM. Molecular biotechnology. In: Crommelin, DJA, Sindelar RD eds. Pharmaceutical Biotechnology, An introduction for pharmacists and pharmaceutical scientists. Amsterdam, The Netherlands: Harwood Academic Publishers, 1997, 1–25.

58. Cohen SN, Chang A, Boyer H, et al. Construction of biologically functional bacterial plasmids in vitro. Proc Natl Acad Sci U.S.A. 1973;70:3240–3244.

59. Davis LG. Background to recombinant DNA technology. In: Pezzuto JM, Johnson ME, Manasse HR, eds. Biotechnology and Pharmacy. New York, NY: Chapman & Hall, 1993, 3–38.

60. Walsh G. Biopharmaceutical: Biochemistry and Biotechnology. Chichester, England: John Wiley & Sons Ltd., 1998, 75–157.

61. Kadir F. Production of biotech compounds—Cultivation and downstream processing. In: Crommelin, DJA, Sindelar RD eds. Pharmaceutical Biotechnology, An introduction for pharmacists and pharmaceutical scientists. Amsterdam, The Netherlands: Harwood Academic Publishers, 1997, 53–70.

62. Crommelin DJA. Formulation of biotech products, including biopharmaceutical considerations. In: Crommelin, DJA, Sindelar RD eds. Pharmaceutical Biotechnology, An introduction for pharmacists and pharmaceutical scientists. Amsterdam, The Netherlands: Harwood Academic Publishers, 1997, 71–99.

63. Seetharam R, Sharma SK, eds. Purification and Analysis of Recombinant Proteins. New York, NY: Marcel Dekker, 1991.

64. Hancock W, Willis B. The future of analytical chemistry in the characterization of biopharmaceuticals. Am Lab 1996; June:31–34.

65. Briggs J. Panfili PR. Quantitation of DNA and protein impurities in biopharmaceuticals. Anal Chem 1991;63:850–859.

66. Prankerd RJ, Schulman SG. Analytical methods in biotechnology. In: Pezzuto JM, Johnson ME, Manasse HR, eds. Biotechnology and Pharmacy. New York, NY: Chapman & Hall, 1993, 71–96.

67. Dwyer JL. Analytical chromatography of amino acids, peptides, and proteins. In: Franks F, ed., Protein Biotechnology. Totowa, NJ: Humana Press, 1993, 49–90.

68. Horvath C, Ettre LS, eds. Chromatography in Biotechnology. Washington, D.C.: American Chemical Society, 1993.

69. Samanen JM. Physical biochemistry of peptide drugs: structure, properties, and stabilities of peptides compared with proteins. In: Lee VHL, ed. Peptide and Protein Drug Delivery. New York, NY: Marcel Dekker, 1991, 137–166.

70. Oeswein JQ, Shire SJ. Physical biochemistry of protein drugs. In: Lee VHL, ed. Peptide and Protein Drug Delivery. New York, NY: Marcel Dekker, 1991, 167–202.

71. Kenney WC, Arakawa T. Biophysical and biochemical analyses of recombinant proteins. In: Crommelin, DJA, Sindelar RD eds. Pharmaceutical Biotechnology, An introduction for pharmacists and pharmaceutical scientists. Amsterdam, The Netherlands: Harwood Academic Publishers, 1997, 27–51.

72. Franks F. Solution properties of proteins. In: Franks F, ed., Protein Biotechnology. Totowa, NJ: Humana Press, 1993, 133–189.

73. Wang YJ, Pearlman R, eds. Stability and Characterization of Protein and Peptide Drugs, Case Histories. New York, NY: Plenum Press, 1993.

74. Manning MC, Patel K, Borchardt RT. Stability of Protein Pharmaceuticals. Pharmaceut Res 1989;6:903–918.

75. Powell MF. Peptide Stability in Drug development: In vitro Peptide degradation in Plasma and Serum. Ann Reports Med Chem 1993;28:285–294.

76. Lemke TL. Review of Organic Functional Groups. 3rd Ed., Malvern, PA, Lea & Febiger, 1992.

77. Li S, Schoneich C, Borchardt RT. Chemical Instability of Proteins. Pharmaceut News 1995;2:12–16.

78. Burgess DJ. Drug Delivery Aspects of Biotechnology Products. In: Pezzuto JM, Johnson ME, Manasse HR, eds., Biotechnology and Pharmacy. New York: Chapman & Hall, 1993,116–151.

79. Genentech, Inc. Written information on storage, reconstitution, compatibility, stability, and administration on file. South San Francisco: 1995.

80. Koeller J, Fields S. Biologic Response Modifiers. Contemp Pharm Issues 1991; (April): 4.

81. Banga AK, Reddy IK. Biotechnology Drug: Pharmaceutical Issues. Pharm Times 1994; (March): 68–76.

82. Smith GH, Piascik P. Dispensing Biotechnology Products: Handling, Professional Education and Product Information. In: Crommelin, DJA, Sindelar RD eds. Pharmaceutical Biotechnology, An introduction for pharmacists and pharmaceutical scientists. Amsterdam, The Netherlands: Harwood Academic Publishers, 1997, 321–335.

83. Lee VHL, ed. Peptide and Protein Drug Delivery. New York, NY: Marcel Dekker, 1991.

84. Ansel HC, Popovich NG. Pharmaceutical Dosage Forms and Drug Delivery Systems. 5th ed. Malvern, PA: Lea & Febiger, 1990.

85. Reddy IK. Protein and Peptide Drug Delivery. In: Zito SW, ed. Pharmaceutical Biotechnology, A Programmed Text. 2nd ed. Lancaster, PA: Technomic Publishing, 1997, 159–182.

86. Bayley H. Protein therapy—delivery guaranteed. Nature Biotech 1999;17(11):1066–1067.

87. Bailon P, Berthold W. Polyethylene glycol—conjugated pharmaceutical proteins. PSTT 1998;1:352–356.

88. Reddy IK, Belmonte AA. Pharmacokinetics of Protein and Peptide Drugs. In: Zito SW, ed. Pharmaceutical Biotechnology, A Programmed Text. 2nd ed. Lancaster, PA: Technomic Publishing, 1997, 183–203.

89. Braeckman R. Pharmacokinetics and Pharmacodynamics of Peptide and Protein and Drugs. In: Crommelin, DJA, Sindelar RD eds. Pharmaceutical Biotechnology, An introduction for pharmacists and pharmaceutical scientists. Amsterdam, The Netherlands: Harwood Academic Publishers, 1997, 101–121.

90. Facts and Comparisons. St. Louis, MO: Facts and Comparisons, 2000, 287–290.

91. AHFS Drug Information. Bethesda, MD: American Society of Hospital Pharmacists, 1999, 2714–2728.

92. Beals JM, Kovach PM. Insulin. In: Crommelin, DJA, Sindelar RD eds. Pharmaceutical Biotechnology, An introduction for pharmacists and pharmaceutical scientists. Amsterdam, The Netherlands: Harwood Academic Publishers, 1997, 229–239.

93. Riley TN, DeRuiter J. How effective are the new insulin analogs in regulating glucose metabolism? U.S. Pharmacist 2000;25 (10):56–64.

94. Argo AL, Cox KK, Kelly WN. The Ten Most Common Lethal Medication Errors in Hospital Patients. Hosp Pharm 2000; 35 (5):470–474.

95. Facts and Comparisons. St. Louis, MO: Facts and Comparisons, 2000, 313–314.

96. Facts and Comparisons. St. Louis, MO: Facts and Comparisons, 2000, 344–346.

97. Marian M. Growth Hormones. In: Crommelin, DJA, Sindelar RD eds. Pharmaceutical Biotechnology, An introduction for pharmacists and pharmaceutical scientists. Amsterdam, The Netherlands: Harwood Academic Publishers, 1997, 241–253.

98. Facts and Comparisons. St. Louis, MO: Facts and Comparisons, 2000, 247–250.

99. Sam T, De Boer W. Follicle-Stimulating Hormone (FSH). In: Crommelin, DJA, Sindelar RD eds. Pharmaceutical Biotechnology, An introduction for pharmacists and pharmaceutical scientists. Amsterdam, The Netherlands: Harwood Academic Publishers, 1997, 315–320.

100. Facts and Comparisons. St. Louis, MO: Facts and Comparisons, 2000, 183–186b.

101. AHFS Drug Information. Bethesda, MD: American Society of Hospital Pharmacists, 1999, 1333–1343.

102. Modi NB. Recombinant Tissue-Type Plasminogen Activator and Factor VIII. In: Crommelin, DJA, Sindelar RD eds. Pharmaceutical Biotechnology, An introduction for pharmacists and pharmaceutical scientists. Amsterdam, The Netherlands: Harwood Academic Publishers, 1997, 297–306.

103. Higgins DL, Bennett WF. Tissue Plasminogen Activator: Biochemistry and Pharmacology of Variants Produced by Mutagenesis. Annu Rev Pharmacol Toxicol 1990;30:91–121.

104. Walsh G. Biopharmaceutical: Biochemistry and Biotechnology. Chichester, England: John Wiley & Sons Ltd., 1998, 293–336.

105. Brixner D. Biotechnology Products: An Overview. In: Pezzuto JM, Johnson ME, Manasse HR, eds., Biotechnology and Pharmacy. New York: Chapman & Hall, 1993,392–395.

106. Facts and Comparisons. St. Louis, MO: Facts and Comparisons, 2000, 679–680.

107. AHFS Drug Information. Bethesda, MD: American Society of Hospital Pharmacists, 1999, 2358–2360.

108. Marian M, Baughman S. Recombinant Human Deoxyribonuclease. In: Crommelin, DJA, Sindelar RD eds. Pharmaceutical Biotechnology, An introduction for pharmacists and pharmaceutical scientists. Amsterdam, The Netherlands: Harwood Academic Publishers, 1997, 307–314.

109. Facts and Comparisons. St. Louis, MO: Facts and Comparisons, 2000, 355.

110. Janeway CA, Travers P, Walport M, et al. Immunobiology, The Immune System in Health and Disease, 4th ed. New York: Elsevier Science Ltd/Garland Publishing, 1999, 288–292.

111. Abbas AK, Lichtman AH, Pober JS. Cellular and Molecular Immunology, 4th ed. Philadelphia, Pennsylvania: W.B. Saunders 2000, 235–269.

112. Roitt I, Brostoff J, Male D. Immunology, 5th ed. London, England: Mosby International, 1998, 121–125.

113. Wrotnowski C. Cytokines, Growth Factors and Chemokines. Genetic Eng News 2000; 20(12):8.

114. Mire-Sluis AR. Cytokines: from technology to therapeutics. TIBTECH 1999; 17:319–325.

115. Xing Z, Wang J. Consideration of Cytokines as Therapeutic Targets. Curr Pharmaceut Design 2000; 6:599–611.

116. Rodriguez FH, Nelson S, Kolls JK. Cytokine Therapeutics for Infectious Diseases. Curr Pharmaceut Design 2000; 6:665–680.

117. Arai K, Lee F, Miyajima A, et al. Cytokines: Coordinators of Immune and Inflammatory Responses. Annu Rev Biochem 1990; 59:783–836.

118. Louie SG, Jung B. Clinical effects of biological response modifiers. Am J Hosp Pharm 1993; 50(7, S3):S10–S18.

119. Urdal DL. Cytokine Receptors. Ann Rep Med Chem 1991; 26:221–228.

120. Walsh G. Biopharmaceutical: Biochemistry and Biotechnology. Chichester, England: John Wiley & Sons Ltd., 1998, 158–188.

121. Walsh G. Biopharmaceutical: Biochemistry and Biotechnology. Chichester, England: John Wiley & Sons Ltd., 1998, 189–215.

122. Walsh G. Biopharmaceutical: Biochemistry and Biotechnology. Chichester, England: John Wiley & Sons Ltd., 1998, 216–234.

123. Klegerman ME, Plotnikoff NP. Lymphokines and Monokines. In: Pezzuto JM, Johnson ME, Manasse HR, eds., Biotechnology and Pharmacy. New York: Chapman & Hall, 1993, 53–70.

124. Facts and Comparisons. St. Louis, MO: Facts and Comparisons, 2000, 1571d–1571l.

125. AHFS Drug Information. Bethesda, MD: American Society of Hospital Pharmacists, 1999, 897–927.

126. Tami J. Interleukins and Interferons. In: Crommelin, DJA, Sindelar RD eds. Pharmaceutical Biotechnology, An introduction for pharmacists and pharmaceutical scientists. Amsterdam, The Netherlands: Harwood Academic Publishers, 1997, 215–227.

127. Facts and Comparisons. St. Louis, MO: Facts and Comparisons, 2000, 1572–1573.

128. Ebert S, De Muth JE. Hepatitis C, From Pathogenesis to Prognosis. Thousand Oaks, California: Amgen, 1997.

129. Facts and Comparisons. St. Louis, MO: Facts and Comparisons, 2000, 1577–1580.

130. AHFS Drug Information. Bethesda, MD: American Society of Hospital Pharmacists, 1999, 3272–3273.

131. Facts and Comparisons. St. Louis, MO: Facts and Comparisons, 2000, 1575–1576.

132. Todd PA, Goa KL. Interferon Gamma-1b, A Review of its Pharmacology and Therapeutic Potential in Chronic Granulomatous Disease. Drugs 1992; 43(1), 111–122.

133. Facts and Comparisons. St. Louis, MO: Facts and Comparisons, 2000, 1946–1949.

134. AHFS Drug Information. Bethesda, MD: American Society of Hospital Pharmacists, 1999, 786–791.

135. Solimando, Jr. DA, Hanna WJ. Aldesleukin and Levamisole. Hosp Pharm 1998; 33(10), 1172–1177.

136. Romanelli F. Interleukin-2 for the Management of HIV Infection. J Am Pharmaceut Assoc 1999; 39:867–868.

137. Siegel JP, Puri RK. Interleukin-2 Toxicity. J Clin Oncol 1991; 9:694–704.

138. Rosenberg SA, Lotze MT, Mule JJ. New Approaches to the Immunotherapy of Cancer Using Interleukin-2. Ann Intern Med 1988; 108:853–864.

139. Facts and Comparisons. St. Louis, MO: Facts and Comparisons, 2000, 1951–1953.

140. Mancano MA. New Drugs 1999. Pharm Times 2000; Mar:67–91.

141. Hussan DA. New Drugs of 1999. J Am Pharmaceut Assoc 2000; 40:181–221.

142. Piascik P. FDA Approves Fusion Protein for Treatment of Lymphoma. J Am Pharmaceut Assoc 1999; 39:571–572.

143. Facts and Comparisons. St. Louis, MO: Facts and Comparisons, 2000, 144–146.

144. Vu K, Solimando, Jr. DA. Oprelvekin. Hosp Pharm 1998; 33:387–389.

145. Facts and Comparisons. St. Louis, MO: Facts and Comparisons, 2000, 1580–1581.

146. Newton RC, Decicco CP. Therapeutic Potential and Strategies for Inhibiting Tumor Necrosis Factor-a. J Med Chem 1999; 42:2295–2314.

147. Cada DJ, Baker DE. Etanercept. Hosp Pharm 1999; 34:462–481.

148. Huber SL, Yee G, Michau D. New Product Bulletin, Filgrastim. Washington, D.C.: American Pharmaceutical Association, 1993.

149. Flynn J, Rosman AW. Interleukins and Interferons. In: Crommelin, DJA, Sindelar RD eds. Pharmaceutical Biotechnology, An introduction for pharmacists and pharmaceutical scientists. Amsterdam, The Netherlands: Harwood Academic Publishers, 1997, 185–214.

150. Summerhayes M. Myeloid haematopoietic growth factors in clinical practice—a comparative review—Parts 1 and II. Eur Hosp Pharm 1995; 1, 30–36 and 67–74.

151. Kouides PA, DiPersio JF. The Hematopoietic Growth Factors. In: Haskell CM, ed., Cancer Treatment, 4th ed. Philadelphia, Pennsylvania: W.B. Saunders Company, 1995, 69–77.

152. Facts and Comparisons. St. Louis, MO: Facts and Comparisons, 2000, 135–138.

153. AHFS Drug Information. Bethesda, MD: American Society of Hospital Pharmacists, 1999, 1298–1310.

154. Faulds D, Sorkin EM. Epoetin (Recombinant Human Erythropoietin). Drugs 1989; 38:863–899.

155. Jensen JD, Madsen JK, Jensen LW, et al. Pharmacokinetics of Epoetin in Dialysis Patients Before and After Correction of the Anaemia. Drug Invest 1994; 8:278–287.

156. Graber SE, Krantz SB. Erythropoietin: Biology and Clinical Use Hematol/Oncol Clinics N Amer 1989; 3:369–400.

157. Johnson CA. Epoetin Alfa: A Therapeutic Achievement from Pharmaceutical B Biotechnology. U.S. Pharmacist, Hosp ed 1989; Nov:1–11.

158. Watson E, Bhide A. Carbohydrate Analysis of Recombinant-Derived Erythropoietin. LC-GC 1993; 11:216–220.

159. Louie S, Rho J. Pharmacotherapeutics of Biotechnology-Produced Drugs. In: Zito SW, ed. Pharmaceutical Biotechnology, A Programmed Text. 2nd ed. Lancaster, PA: Technomic Publishing, 1997, 224–231.

160. Lieschke GJ, Burgess AW. Granulocyte Colony-Stimulating Factor and Granulocyte-Macrophage Colony-Stimulating Factor. N Engl J. Med 1992; 327(July 2), 28–35.

161. Smith SP, Yee GC. Hematopoiesis. Pharmacotherapy 1992; 12(2, Pt 2), 11S–19S.

162. Blackwell S, Crawford J. Colony-Stimulating Factors: Clinical Applications. Pharmacotherapy 1992; 12(2, Pt 2), 20S–31S.

163. Petros WP. Pharmacokinetics and Administration of Colony-Stimulating Factors. Pharmacotherapy 1992; 12(2, Pt 2), 32S–38S.

164. Hollingshead LM, Goa KL. Recombinant Granulocyte Colony-Stimulating Factor Colony-Stimulating Factor (rG-CSF). Drugs 1991; 42:300–330.

165. Facts and Comparisons. St. Louis, MO: Facts and Comparisons, 2000, 139–141.

166. AHFS Drug Information. Bethesda, MD: American Society of Hospital Pharmacists, 1999, 1310–1319.

167. Facts and Comparisons. St. Louis, MO: Facts and Comparisons, 2000, 141–144.

168. AHFS Drug Information. Bethesda, MD: American Society of Hospital Pharmacists, 1999, 1319–1329.

169. Walsh G. Biopharmaceutical: Biochemistry and Biotechnology. Chichester, England: John Wiley & Sons Ltd., 1998, 235–255.

170. Facts and Comparisons. St. Louis, MO: Facts and Comparisons, 2000, 1703.

171. Piascik P. Use of Regranex Gel for Diabetic Foot Ulcers. J Am Pharmaceut Assoc 1998; 38:628–629.

172. Becaplermin. Drugs Fut 1999; 24(2):123–127.

173. Facts and Comparisons. St. Louis, MO: Facts and Comparisons, 2000, 192–194.

174. Facts and Comparisons. St. Louis, MO: Facts and Comparisons, 2000, 174–176.

175. Walsh G. Biopharmaceutical: Biochemistry and Biotechnology. Chichester, England: John Wiley & Sons Ltd., 1998, 337–386.

176. Jiskoot W, Kersten GFA, Beuvery EC. Vaccines. In: Crommelin, DJA, Sindelar RD eds. Pharmaceutical Biotechnology, An introduction for pharmacists and pharmaceutical scientists. Amsterdam, The Netherlands: Harwood Academic Publishers, 1997, 255–278.

177. Glick BR, Pasternak JJ, eds. Molecular Biotechnology: Principles & Applications of Recombinant DNA. Washington, D.C.: ASM Press, 1994, 207–233.

178. Hikal AH, Hikal EM. The ABCs of hepatitis Drug Topics 1998; 146,60–69.

179. Facts and Comparisons. St. Louis, MO: Facts and Comparisons, 2000, 1529–1531.

180. Facts and Comparisons. St. Louis, MO: Facts and Comparisons, 2000, 1505–1508.

181. Janeway CA, Travers P, Walport M, et al. Immunobiology, The Immune System in Health and Disease, 4th ed. New York: Elsevier Science Ltd/Garland Publishing, 1999, 79–113.

182. Abbas AK, Lichtman AH, Pober JS. Cellular and Molecular Immunology, 4th ed. Philadelphia, Pennsylvania: W.B. Saunders 2000, 41–62.

183. Roitt I, Brostoff J, Male D. Immunology, 5th ed. London, England: Mosby International, 1998, 71–82.

184. Kohler G, Milstein C. Continous cultures of fused cells secreting antibody of predefined specificity. Nature 1975; 256, 495–497.

185. Adair JR, Zivin RA, Guzman NA, et al. Monoclonal Antibody-Based Pharmaceuticals. In: Crommelin, DJA, Sindelar RD eds. Pharmaceutical Biotechnology, An introduction for pharmacists and pharmaceutical scientists. Amsterdam, The Netherlands: Harwood Academic Publishers, 1997, 279–290.

186. Chamow SM, Ashkenazi A. Overview. In: Chamow SM, Ashkenazi A, eds. Antibody Fusion Proteins. New York, New York: Wiley-Liss,1999, 1–12.

187. Adams VR, Karlix JL. Monoclonal Antibodies. In: American Society of Health-System Pharmacists' Production Office. Concepts in Immunology and Immunotherapeutics, 3rd ed. Bethesda, Maryland: American Society of Health-System Pharmacists,'1997, 269–299.

188. Shen W-C, Louie SG. Immunology for Pharmacy Students. Amsterdam, The Netherlands: Harwood Academic Publishers, 1999, 45–58.

189. Klegerman ME. Background to Monoclonal Antibodies. In: Pezzuto JM, Johnson ME, Manasse HR, eds., Biotechnology and Pharmacy. New York: Chapman & Hall, 1993,39–52.

190. Van Duijn G, Schram AW. Production and Application of Polyclonal and Monoclonal Antibodies. In: Franks F, ed. Protein Biotechnology, 3rd Ed. Totowa, New Jersey: Humana Press, 1993, 365–393.

191. Mayforth RD. Designing Antibodies. San Diego, California: Academic Press, 1993, 54–79.

192. Hakimi J, Mould D, Waldmann TA, et al. Development of Zenapax: A humanized anti-Tac antibody. In: Harris WJ, Adair JR, eds. Antibody Therapeutics. Boca Raton, Florida: CRC Press, 1997, 277–300.

193. Chatenoud L. Restriction of the Human In Vivo Immune Response Against the Mouse Monoclonal Antibody OKT3. J Immunol 1986; 137(3), 830–838.

194. Saleh MN. Phase I Trial of the Murine Monoclonal Anti-GD2 Antibody 14G2a in Metastic Melanoma. Cancer Res 1992; 52, 4342–4347.

195. Vaughan TJ, Osbourn JK, Tempest PR. Human antibodies by design. Nature Biotech 1998; 16, 535–539.

196. Holliger P, Hoogenboom H. Antibodies come back from the brink. Nature Biotech 1998; 16, 1015–1016.

197. Adair F. Immunogenicity: The Last Hurdle for Clinically Successful Therapeutic Antibodies. Pharmaceut Tech 2000; 24(10), 50–56.

198. Kling J. Restoring magic to the bullets. Mod Drug Dis 1999; 2(March/April), 33–45.

195. Glover D. Fully human monoclonal antibodies come to fruition. Scrip Mag 1999; May, 16–19.

200. Huse W. Combinatorial Antibody Expression Libraries in Filamentous Phage. In: Borrebaeck CAK, ed. Antibody Engineering—A Practical Guide. New York, New York: W.H. Freeman and Company 1992, 103–120.

201. Rosenthal WM, Briggs GC. Home Testing and Monitoring Devices. In: Allen Jr. LV, Berardi, RR, DeSimone II EM, et al. eds. Handbook of Nonprescription Drugs. Washington, DC: American Pharmaceutical Association 2000, 917–942.

202. Quattrocchi E, Hove I. Ovulation & Pregnancy Home Testing Products. U.S. Pharmacist 1998; 23(9), 54–63.

203. Pray WS. Nonprescription Product Therapeutics. Philadelphia, Pennsylvania: Lippincott Williams & Wilkins, 1999, 717–735.

204. Scangos G. Drug discovery in the postgenomic era. Nature Biotech 1997; 15, 1220–1221.

205. Setti EL, Micetich R. Modern drug Discovery and Lead Discovery: A Overview. Curr Med Chem 1996; 3, 317–324.

206. Dean PM, Jolles G, Newton CG. New Perspectives in Drug Design. San Diego, California: Academic Press, 1995.

207. Ashton MJ, Jaye M, Mason JS. New perspectives in lead generation I: Discovery of biological targets. DDT 1996; 1(1), 11–15.

208. Steinmetz M. Venturing into drug discovery. Nature Biotech 1998; 16 (suppl), 17.

209. Hobden AN. The Contribution of Molecular Biology to Drug Discovery. In: Wermuth CG, ed. The Practice of Medicinal Chemistry. San Diego, California: Academic Press 1996, 153–166.

210. Portoghese PS. Impact of Recombinant DNA Technology and Molecular Modeling on the Practice of Medicinal Chemistry: Structure-Activity Analysis of Opioid Ligands. Am J Pharmaceut Ed 1999, 63(Fall), 342–346.

211. Rondeau J-M, Schreuder H. The use of X-ray Structures of Receptors and Enzymes in drug Discovery. In: Wermuth CG, ed. The Practice of Medicinal Chemistry. San Diego, California: Academic Press 1996, 485–522.

212. Comello V. Protein Crystallography Pinpoints Drug Candidates. Mod Drug Dis 2000; 3(April), 26–28.

213. Miller M, Schneider J, Sathyanarayana BK, et al. Structure of Complex of Synthetic HIV-1 Protease with a Substrate-Based Inhibitor at 2.3 A Resolution. Science 1989, 246, 1149–1152.

214. Archer SJ, Domaille PJ, Laue ED. New NMR Methods for Structural Studies of Proteins to Aid in Drug Design. Ann Rep Med Chem 1996, 31, 299–307.

215. Clore GM, Gronenborn AM. Determining the structures of large proteins and protein complexes by NMR. TIBECH 1998, 16, 22–34.

216. Greer J, Erickson JW, Baldwin JJ, et al. Application of the Three-Dimensional Structures of Protein Target Molecules in Structure-Based Drug Design. J Med Chem 1994, 37(8), 1035–1054.

217. Rios M. An Interview with J. Craig Venter—Genomics and the Future of the Pharmaceutical Industry. Pharmaceut Tech 2001, 25(1), 34–40.

218. Nelson R. Genome Pharmacy. Hosp Pharm Rep 2000, 14(10), 22–24.

219. Ukens C. Prepare for genomics, expert advises pharmacists. Drug Top 2000, 144(23), 38.

220. Carrico JM. Human Genome Project and Pharmacogenomics—Implications for Pharmacy. J Am Pharmaceut Assoc 2000, 40(1), 115–116.

221. Beavers N. Genomics, A New Age in Therapy. Drug Top 1998, 142(20), 73–80.

222. R&D Staff. Beyond Genomics. R&D Direct 1999, 5(4), 40–44.

223. Cantor CR, Smith CL. Genomics—The Science and Technology Behind the Human Genome Project. New York, New York: John Wiley & Sons, Inc., 1999.

224. Pennisi E. Genomics Comes of Age. Science 2000, 290, 2220–2221.

225. Persidis A. Proteomics. Nature Biotech 1998; 16, 393–394.

226. Blackstock WP, Weir MP. Proteomics: quantitative and physical mapping of cellular proteins. TIBECH 1999, 17, 121–127.

227. Borman S. Proteomics: Taking Over Where Genomics Leaves Off. Chem Eng News 2000, 78(July 31), 31–37.

228. Edwards AM, Arrowsmith CH, Pallieres B. Proteomics: New tools for a new era. Mod Drug Dis 2000; 3(September), 34–44.

229. Felton MJ. Bioinformatics: The child of success. Mod Drug Dis 2001; 4(January), 25–28.

230. Emmett A. The State of Bioinformatics. The Scientist 2000, 14(23), 1, 10, 12, 19.

231. Ramsey G. DNA chips: State-of-the-art. Nature Biotech 1998, 16, 40–44.

232. Khan J, Bittner ML, Chen Y, Meltzer PS, et al. DNA microarray technology: the anticipated impact on the study of human disease. Biochim Biophys Acta 1999, 1423, M17-M28.

233. Schena M, Heller RA, Theriault TP, et al. Microarrays: biotechnology's discovery platform for functional genomics. TIBTECH 1998, 16, 301–306.

234. Evans WE, Relling MV. Pharmacogenomics: Translating functional genomics into rational therapies. Science 1999, 286, 487–491.

235. Lau KF, Sakul H. Pharmacogenomics. Ann Rep Med Chem 2000, 36, 261–269.

236. Pettipher R, Holford R. Pharmacogenetics Paves the Way. Crug Discov Develop 2000, (January/February), 53–54.

237. Persidis A. Pharmacogenomics and diagnostics. Nature Biotech 1998; 16, 791–792.

238. Ball S, Borman N. Pharmacogenomics and drug metabolism. Nature Biotech 1997; 15, 925–926.

SUGGESTED READINGS

Crommelin, DJA, Sindelar RD, eds. Pharmaceutical Biotechnology, An introduction for pharmacists and pharmaceutical scientists. Amsterdam, The Netherlands: Harwood Academic Publishers, 1997.

Glick BR, Pasternak JJ, eds. Molecular Biotechnology: Principles & Applications of Recombinant DNA. 2nd ed. Washington, D.C.: ASM Press, 1998.

Klegerman ME, Groves MJ, eds. Pharmaceutical Biotechnology—Fundamentals and Essentials. Buffalo Grove, IL: Interpharm Press, 1992.

Pezzuto JM, Johnson ME, Manasse HR, eds. Biotechnology and Pharmacy. New York, NY: Chapman & Hall, 1993.

Walsh G. Biopharmaceutical: Biochemistry and Biotechnology. Chichester, England: John Wiley & Sons Ltd., 1998.

Zito SW, ed. Pharmaceutical Biotechnology, A Programmed Text. 2nd ed. Lancaster, PA: Technomic Publishing, 1997.

41. Gene Therapy

RONALD E. REID

INTRODUCTION

The human species is a product of millions of years of evolution. The living organism that has evolved is supported by a complex chemical machinery that senses and responds to environmental signals, nourishes and protects the trillions of cells that are the basic unit of the living organism, determines and regulates cellular function, and finally assures that cellular multiplication and organism reproduction will occur. Disruptions of this chemical machinery are the sources of disease and disability and a detailed understanding of these mechanisms at the molecular level is critical to understanding disease pathology and developing an effective defense or aggressive therapy against disease and disability. Much information of the human condition to date arises from studies on simpler organisms like the bacteriophage and viruses, bacteria, yeasts, nematodes, fruit flies, and the more complex mouse. Through such studies we seek understanding to be able to detect the damage potential of a particular internal or external environment, repair damage that has already occurred, or sustain the body in the presence of damage.

Current dogma places biochemical information and its transfer as the basis of the function of a living organism regulating the nervous, immune, digestive, and reproductive systems. This information flow originates at the deoxyribonucleic acid (DNA) molecule, proceeds to ribonucleic acid (RNA) which is then translated into protein (1). Proteins are the main components of the functional organization of the cell and are critical to the relationship of the organism's DNA structure or genotype to the organism's functional organization or phenotype. Therefore, intervention in the regulatory system to detect or repair disease, or sustain the organism in the event of disease may occur at any level between the genotype and the phenotype. Genetic intervention has many levels from direct tinkering with the genes (the information source) to manipulating the many processes involved in the transcription and translation of the genetic information into proteins. Protein function may be altered through direct manipulation of proteins or through altering the many events occurring between protein production and the physical response noted by the organism. Regardless of the particular approach taken in any isolated instance, our understanding of the molecular mechanisms of the chemical mediated information transfer will be the basis for rationalizing any therapeutic initiative. It is highly likely that any approach to disease therapy will utilize a mixture of techniques, only a few of which will involve the direct manipulation of genes in the form of gene replacement therapy. Further development of the knowledge of molecular processes involved in this information transfer and how it is related to disease may help us make better use of the current therapeutic technologies and allow us to treat the individual patient rather than treating the disease symptoms (2).

The premise of gene therapy is that genes can be used as pharmaceutical products to cause *in vivo* production of therapeutic proteins. There is considerable confidence that gene therapy, as a therapeutic paradigm, will provide a number of novel pharmaceutical products, diagnostics, and therapeutic approaches in the next decade (3).

Historical Background

Gene therapy is broadly defined as the application of genetic principles to the treatment of human disease. This novel approach to disease therapy has emerged over the past 20 years as a result of major scientific advances in microbiology, genetics, and biochemistry that combined to produce the new science of molecular biology. However, a historical account of the development in science leading up to the present day gene therapy goes back even further in time and the events can be divided into three phases (Table 41.1).

Phase I consists of the early developments in understanding of the chemical composition of the genetic material and how the chemistry could be related to an understanding of the function of this material as the chemical basis of heredity. The father of modern genetics was the Franciscan monk Gregor Mendel whose experiments in the mid 19th century on the garden pea *Pisum savitum* and other plants led to the concept of a gene and the principles of inheritance that can be summarized as follows (4):

1. The heredity and variation of characters are controlled by factors, now called genes, which occur in pairs. Mendel called these factors *formbuildungellementen* (formbuilding elements)
2. Contrasting traits are specified by different forms of each gene (different alleles).
3. When two dissimilar alleles are present in the same individual (i.e., in a heterozygote), one trait displays dominance over the other: the phenotype associated with one allele (the dominant allele) is expressed at the expense of that of the other (the recessive allele).
4. Genes do not blend, but remain discrete (particulate) as they are transmitted.

Table 41.1. Historical Highlights of the Evolution of Gene Therapy

Phase I—Emergence and Acceptance of the Concept of a Gene

Date	Event
1866	Gregor Mendel publishes his studies on inherited traits and develops the concept of the factors (genes) as the units of heredity.
1871	Friedrich Miescher discovers that the nuclei of white blood cells release a white gummy substance upon treatment with pepsin. He calls the substance nuclein.
1897	Edward Büchner uses a cell free yeast extract to reproduce sugar fermentation *in vitro.*
1902	Sir Archibald Garrod suggests that alkaptonuria (black urine due to the presence of homogentisic acid) is caused by a defect in a gene.
1906	Thomas Hunt Morgan demonstrates that genes for specific physical characteristics could be located on specific chromosomes.
1935	W.M. Stanley crystallizes the tobacco mosaic virus.
1941	George Beadle and Edward Tatum demonstrate conclusively that the function of genes is to direct the production of enzymes and other proteins. This is the first demonstration of a link between genetics and biochemistry.
1944	Ostwald T. Avery identifies deoxyribonucleic acid as the chief chemical in the gene.
1946	Tatum and Lederberg demonstrate that *E. coli* bacteria fertilize one another to produce crossbreeds possessing the genetic qualities of both.
1949	Linus Pauling shows that sickle-cell anemia is linked to an abnormal structure of hemoglobin.
1952	Zinder and Lederberg recognize the capacity for viruses to transmit genes in *Salmonella.* Alfred Hershey and Martha Chase make the first use of radiolabeled proteins (^{35}S) and DNA (^{32}P) to demonstrate that bacteriophage DNA is fundamental for phage replication.
1953	James Watson and Francis Crick postulate the double helix structure of and explain the auto-replication of deoxyribonucleic acid.

Phase II—Technical Implementation

Date	Event
1955	Hoagland discovers tRNA by demonstrating that activated amino acids are linked to a soluble ribonucleic acid.
1956	Lederberg recognizes the bacteriophage as a potential "gene carrier" therapeutic agent. Ingram demonstrates that the mutation responsible for sickle-cell anemia is linked to a change in a single amino acid in a single protein.
1957	Crick and Orgel propose a triplet genetic code for DNA that is read in a "reading frame" to provide the correct protein amino acid sequence.
1958	Kornberg purifies and characterizes deoxyribonucleic acid polymerase.
1959	Jacob and Monod discover regulator genes and develop the concepts of gene induction and repression.
1960	Doty and Marmur demonstrate that the two strands of DNA after separation by heating, will re-anneal if slowly cooled.
1961	Matthaei and Nirenberg decipher the first word of the genetic code—UUU = Phe. Discovery of messenger ribonucleic acid.
1968	Discovery of enzymes that cleave DNA at specific base sequences—the restriction enzymes.
1969	Isolation and purification of the first bacterial gene—the *lac* operon.
1970	Total chemical synthesis of the gene for yeast alanine transfer RNA. Discovery of reverse transcriptase in RNA viruses.
1972	Discovery that the restriction enzyme EcoRI cleaved DNA leaving cohesive ends that could be re-annealed with other pieces of DNA that have been cleaved by the same enzyme.
1973	*In vitro* construction of biologically active bacterial plasmids containing resistance genes and DNA sequences from different species of bacteria.
1974	Demonstration that DNA from a toad introduced into a bacterium could be transcribed to RNA opening up the possibility of producing proteins from higher organism in bacteria. Techniques developed for producing a genomic library.
1975	Asilomar Conference addressing the risks and benefits of the new genetic manipulation technology. Isolation of the first mammalian gene as the DNA complementary to mRNA (i.e., cDNA)-β-globin from the rabbit.
1977	Discovery of split genes and gene splicing. Sanger and Gilbert independently introduce DNA sequencing techniques. Introduction of the solid phase synthesis technology for rapid synthesis of oligonucleotides. Bacterial synthesis of human somatostatin by expression of an artificially synthesized gene.
1978	Isolation of the β-globin gene from genomic DNA libraries using cDNA oligonucleotide probes. Smith introduces a technique for directed mutagenesis using synthetic oligonucleotides.
1980	Integration of DNA into plant cells for the first time. Production of the first transgenic mice.
1983	Mullis develops the polymerase chain reaction.

Phase III—Clinical Development

Date	Event
1975	Discovery of cancer genes—oncogenes. Unsuccessful attempt at gene therapy in arginase deficiency.
1976	First genetic diagnosis: Detection of the presence of the gene coding for α-thalassaemia.
1980	Martin Cline transfects bone marrow cells from thalassaemia patients *in vitro* with plasmids containing the human globin gene and re-infuses the transfected bone marrow cells into the patients. The clinical trial was criticized for procedural and scientific reasons and Cline is censured by his University (UCLA) and the NIH.
1988	Rosenberg uses tumor infiltrating lymphocytes as targets for gene therapy in the treatment of cancer.
9/14/1990	First clinical trial for gene therapy of adenosine deaminase deficiency.
1992	Clinical trials begin for the treatment of cystic fibrosis.
1993	Clinical trials begin for familial hypercholesterolemia.

5. During meiosis, pairs of alleles segregate equally so that equivalent numbers of gametes carrying each allele are formed.

6. The segregation of each pair of alleles is independent from that of any other pair.

Mendel's work remained obscure until the beginning of the 20th century. The search was on for the nature of Mendel's *formbuildungellementen* or genes as they were called by Wilhelm Johannsen in 1909. Phase I culminated in 1953 with the postulation by Watson and Crick that the genetic material, deoxyribonucleic acid (DNA) had a complementary double helical structure (5).

Phase II of developments in gene therapy concentrated on understanding the chemical nature of the genetic process based on the Watson and Crick model of DNA and how its chemical nature (genotype) could lead to the expression of physical features (phenotype). Soon after the publication of the Watson and Crick model, proof was obtained that DNA replication involves separation of the complementary strands. The enzymes DNA and RNA polymerase and DNA ligase were isolated and messenger RNA (mRNA) was demonstrated to carry information that placed the amino acids in the correct sequence in proteins. The techniques of isolating and sequencing genes led to the development of complementary and recombinant DNA (cDNA and rDNA, respectively) and the use of viruses, bacteriophage, and plasmids as vehicles for DNA transport. Relationships of DNA sequence to protein structure and biologic function resulted in an understanding of the relation of genetic mutation to disease.

Phase III involves the development of gene therapy in the clinic and has considerable temporal overlap with Phase II. There was recognition of the relevance of gene replacement therapy to a number of genetic diseases very early on in the development of modern molecular biology (6). However, recognition of the potential for gene therapy preceded the technology and the early attempts at treating arginase deficiency and thalassemia resulted in failure and, in the case of UCLA's Martin Cline, drastic consequences for the scientists involved (7–11). The first gene therapy clinical protocol involving gene marking with neomycin phosphotransferse was approved by the National Institutes of Health (NIH) in 1989. On September 6, 1990, the NIH approved two gene therapy trials. One involved the use of tumor infiltrating lymphocytes transduced with the gene coding for tumor necrosis factor and the other involved the treatment of severe combined immune deficiency due to adenosine deaminase deficiency (ADA) with autologus lymphocytes transduced with the human ADA gene. The ADA trial, which actually began on September 14, 1990, enrolled two young girls with adenosine deaminase deficiency and limited success was obtained (12–15). These initial trials were followed by NIH approval for clinical trials for a variety of gene therapy approaches to the treatment of a number of cancers as well as the treatment of cystic fibrosis (11, 16–18), familial hy-

percholesterolemia (19), AIDS, Gaucher's Disease (glucocerebrosidase deficiency), α-1-antitrypsin deficiency, rheumatoid arthritis, Fanconi's anemia, Hunter Syndrome (mucopolysaccharidosis type II), peripheral artery disease, chronic Granulomatous Disease, purine nucleoside phosphorylase deficiency, and restenosis.

Between 1989 and May 2000, more than 280 new gene transfer INDs were submitted to the FDA, with 55 submitted in 1999. As of May 1, 2000, 206 INDs were still active. For an update see the NIH web site (http://www.nih.gov/ and search for "protocol list").

Chemical Basis of Heredity

Gene therapy could be more fundamentally defined as nucleic acid therapeutics denoting manipulations of DNA, RNA, and their components (purine and pyrimidine bases, nucleosides, and nucleotides) (20). A fundamental understanding of gene therapy must therefore be based on a sound understanding of the molecular composition of the genetic material and the structure and functional nature of the gene.

DNA

The eukaryotic chromosome makes a brief appearance when the cell is actively dividing and can be seen as a pair

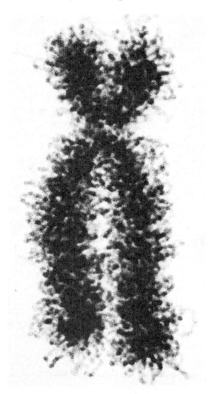

Fig. 41.1. Sister chromatids of a mitotic pair. The sister chromosomes are produced by the previous replication event and are still joined together at this stage of mitosis. Each of the chromosomes consists of a fiber with a diameter of approximately 30 nm. The DNA is 5–10 times more condensed in chromosomes than it is at interphase. Taken from Lewin B. Genes IV. 4th ed. by permission of Oxford University Press and Cell Press.

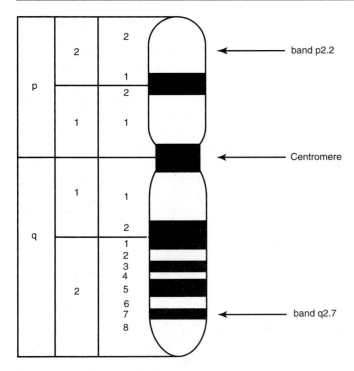

Fig. 41.2. The human X chromosome can be divided into distinct regions by its banding pattern. Taken from Lewin B. Genes IV. 4th ed. by permission of Oxford University Press and Cell Press.

of chromatids (daughter chromosomes produced during replication of DNA prior to mitosis) (Fig. 41.1). The individual chromosome can be divided along its length into many clear striations of dark bands and light interband regions (Fig. 41.2). The dark bands are dense clumps of protein and DNA while the interbands are regions of lower density of protein and DNA. The reasons for this highly regular banding are not known. Each of these bands and interbands of the chromosome is composed of a well defined mixture of protein and DNA called chromatin

The main protein component of chromatin is histones which are basic proteins associated with the DNA in the form of structures called nucleosomes (Fig. 41.3) (21). DNA can be stored in very small compact forms, condensed DNA, that is 10^4–10^6 times less volume than uncondensed DNA. The main force that must be overcome in the condensation process is charge repulsion due to the negatively charged phosphates in the polyanion. This repulsion may be overcome by DNA interaction with multivalent organic and inorganic cations. The histones, which are the major components of the nucleosome, are cationic organic proteins that interact with DNA in the compact nucleosome structure.

The nucleosome consists of a 200bp (200 base pairs) DNA strand making two left-handed coils around an octamer of histone proteins consisting of two copies each of histones H2A, H2B, H3, and H4 and a single copy of the histone H1 (Fig. 41.3).

Separation of the protein spools from chromatin leaves a very long string-like DNA molecule. DNA is composed of purine bases (adenine (A), and guanine (G), pyrimidine bases (cytosine (C), and thymine (T) or uracil (U) in the case or RNA), deoxyribose sugars (or ribose sugars in the case of RNA), and phosphates (Fig. 41.4). The bases combine with the 1′ position of the ribose sugar molecule to form a nucleoside (Fig. 41.4). The DNA structural unit, a nucleotide, is a 3′ or 5′-monophosphate ester of a nucleoside. Nucleotides are covalently linked through phosphate esters to form the DNA polymer chain. Each nucleotide is linked to one neighbor by a 5′, 3′-phosphodiester bond and to the other neighbor by a 3′,5′-phosphodiester bond (Fig. 41.5). All the 3′ and 5′ hydroxyl groups in the DNA molecule are involved in phosphodiester bonds except the first and last nucleotides in the chain. The first nucleotide in the chain has a 5′-phosphate nonbonded to a nucleotide and the last nucleotide in the chain has a free 3′-hydroxyl group

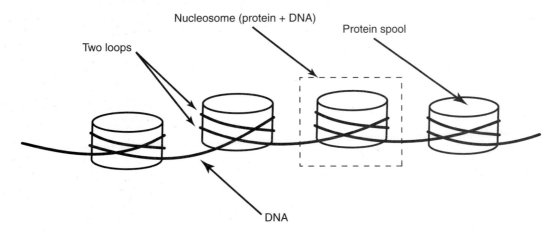

Fig. 41.3. A DNA thread making two left-handed coils around each of a series of protein spools. A single spool consists of an octamer of histone proteins, two each of H2A, H2B, H3 and H4. The ninth histone protein, H1, may be located in the linker region between spools immediately adjacent to the spool. The DNA and histones make up the nucleosome. Adapted from Calladine CR, Drew HR, Understanding DNA: The Molecule and How It Works. 2nd ed. New York: Academic Press with permission.

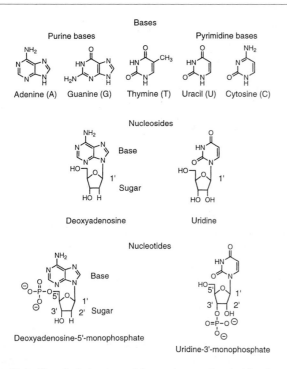

Fig. 41.4. Chemical structure of the purines and pyrimidine bases as well as representative nucleosides and nucleotides.

(Fig. 41.5). The DNA sugar-phosphate backbone chain has polarity, meaning it has a 5'-end and a 3'-end.

The structure of deoxyribonucleic acid was determined in 1953 by Watson and Crick to consist of two antiparallel strands of deoxyribonucleic acid coiled around a common axis in a "double helix" (Fig. 41.6). The purine and pyrimidine bases are on the inside of the helix, whereas the phosphate and deoxyribose units are on the outside. The planes of the bases are perpendicular to the helix axis. The planes of the sugars are at approximately 70° to those of the bases. The helix diameter is 20 angstroms; adjacent

bases are separated by 3.4 angstroms along the helix and related by a rotation of 36°. Hence, the helical structure repeats after 10 residues on each chain, that is, at intervals of 34 angstroms. The two chains are held together by hydrogen bonds between base pairs. Adenine is always paired with thymine and guanine is always paired with cytosine thus providing a specific interaction between the two DNA strands such that the nucleotide sequence of the strand can be exploited as a method of transmitting information, i.e., the amino acid sequence coded for by the nucleotide sequence in the nucleic acid.

The double helix stability is determined by a longitudinal interaction of neighboring bases, called base stacking, which is due to complex interactions of π-electron orbitals of the planar bases, dipole, dipole-induced dipole, London dispersion forces, and hydrophobic interactions. The stability of base stacking is of the order: purine-purine > purine-pyrimidine > pyrimidine-pyrimidine. Since G/C pairs are more stable than A/T pairs because they have three hydrogen bonds as opposed to two (Fig. 41.7), stacked dimers high in G/C content are energetically preferred to those rich in A/T content (22).

Nucleic acids are water soluble because of the polyanionic character of the molecule. It is possible to obtain viscous aqueous solutions of DNA up to 1% w/v. The long, thin DNA structure means that the molecule is very susceptible to cleavage by shearing or sonication in solution, which results in a reduction in solution viscosity. The nucleic acids are precipitated from aqueous solution by the addition of alcohol.

Strong acid at high temperatures will result in complete hydrolysis of nucleic acids into their constituent bases,

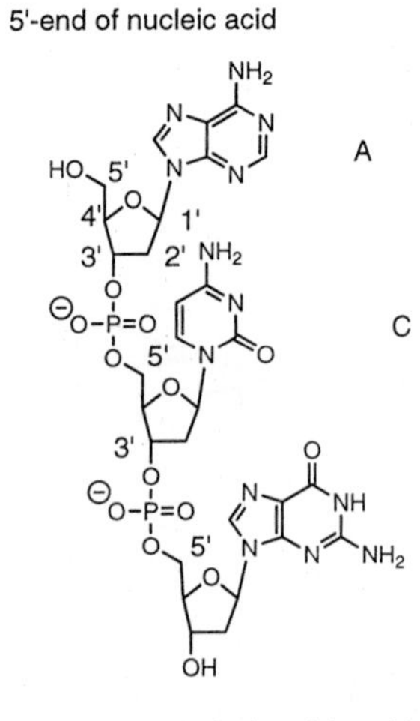

5'-end of nucleic acid

3'-end of nucleic acid

Fig. 41.5. Chemical structure of a DNA fragment ACG.

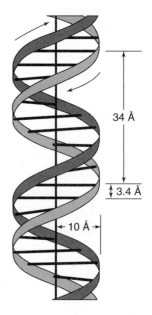

Fig. 41.6. Schematic representation of the Watson and Crick double helical model of DNA. The radius of the double helix is 10 angstroms, the vertical rise per base pair is 3.4 angstroms, and one complete turn of the double helix traverses 10 base pairs or 34 angstroms.

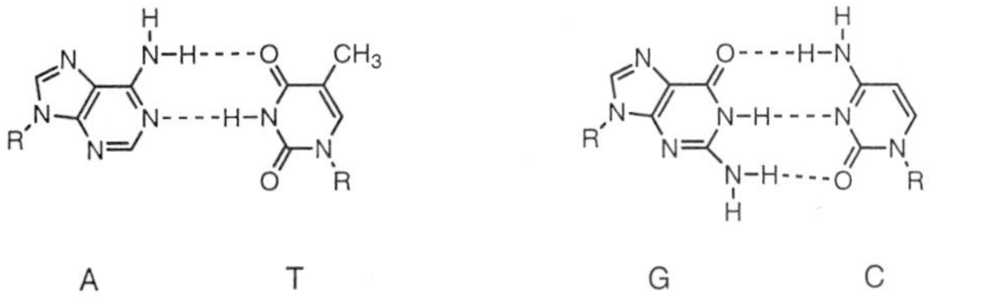

Fig. 41.7. Watson and Crick base pairing in double stranded DNA. The purine A pairs with the pyrimidine T and the purine G pairs with the pyrimidine C.

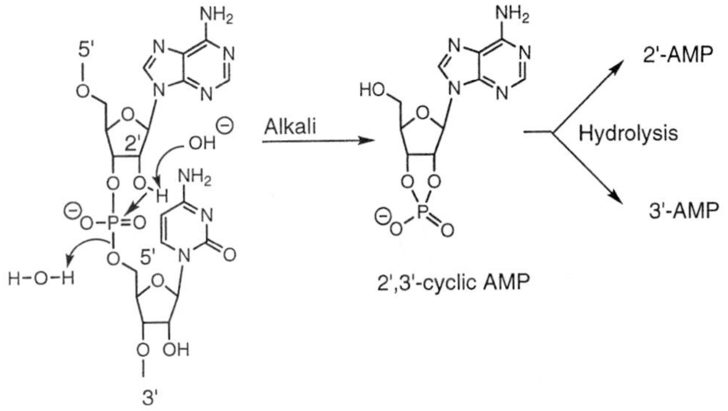

Fig. 41.9. Alkaline hydrolysis of RNA to produce the intermediate 2′,3′-cyclic nucleotide monophosphate which undergoes further hydrolysis to 2′ and 3′ nucleotide monophosphates.

sugars, and phosphate. Milder acidic conditions (pH 3–4) at 37° C will result in hydrolysis of the most susceptible bonds, those being the glycosyl bonds linking the purine bases, A and G, to the sugar molecules resulting in depurination of the nucleic acid. Depyrimidation is less frequently seen but may also occur.

Heterocyclic molecules containing nitrogen tautomerize to yield a mixture of molecular species in solution because the hydrogens attached to the nitrogens in the ring systems are able to migrate to other nitrogens or keto oxygens in the same molecule (Fig. 41.8).

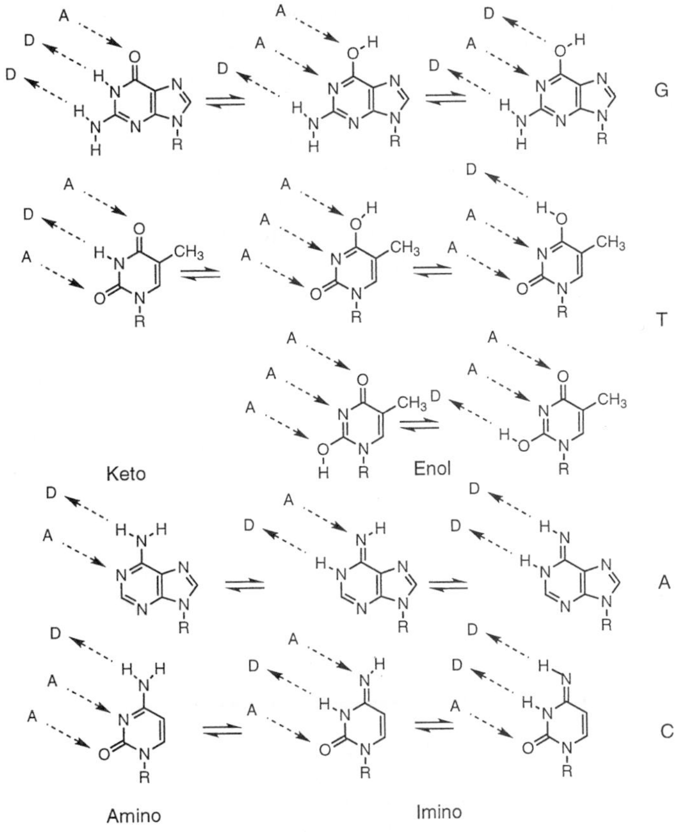

Fig. 41.8. Keto-enol and amino-imino tautomerism in nucleoside bases. Arrows denote A and D which symbolize acceptor and donor sites for hydrogen bond formation. Note that in the enol forms, G becomes equivalent to A, and U to C; in the imino forms, A is equivalent to U or G, and C to U. The situation changes if the imino or enol groups rotate, giving rise to a diversity of hydrogen-bonding possibilities.

Since correct base pairing is critical to information transfer in the replication, transcription and translation of DNA structure, base tautomerization could be a disaster for living systems. Fortunately, the keto and amino structures are the predominant tautomeric structures with less than 0.1% in the imino and enol tautomeric states. However, increasing pH of the nucleic acid environment will shift the keto/enol tautomeric equilibrium to the enol form due to ionization of the enolic hydroxyl group with the net result being disruption of the hydrogen bonding in DNA and denaturation of the double stranded molecule. The double helical structure of DNA can also be denatured through heat or relatively high concentrations of chemical agents such as urea and formamide that also disrupt the critical hydrogen bond system.

Helical regions of RNA are similarly denatured by alkali, however, hydrolysis of RNA is the predominant reaction occurring in alkali. The hydrolysis is assisted by the 2′-OH group on the sugar (Fig. 41.9). DNA is not as susceptible to the alkaline hydrolysis because the 2′-OH group is missing.

The spectroscopic properties of DNA provide a wealth of information concerning concentration, structure, stability, and purity of a particular DNA preparation. Nucleic acids absorb UV light at $\lambda_{max} = 260$ nm due to the conjugated/aromatic ring systems of the bases. The absorption intensity is greatest for single stranded DNA (ssDNA) and RNA and least for double stranded DNA (dsDNA) (Fig. 41.10). The hydrophobic environment of the stacked bases in dsDNA is responsible for the lower intensity of UV absorption of this molecule at 260 nm. ssDNA is said to be hyperchromic relative to dsDNA, thus dsDNA undergoes a hyperchromic shift during denaturation to ssDNA.

The extinction coefficient of a nucleic acid is not suitable for determination of the concentration of the nucleic acid because it is dependent upon the length of the molecule. The extinction coefficient is instead expressed in terms of concentration where a 1 mg/mL solution of dsDNA has an A_{260nm} of 20. Similar concentrations of ssDNA or RNA have

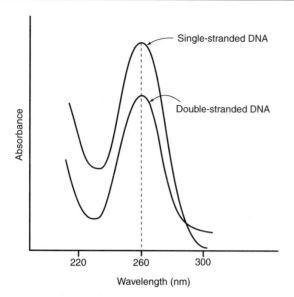

Fig. 41.10. Hyperchromic shift between double-stranded and single-stranded DNA. Single-stranded DNA has a higher ultraviolet absorbance at 260 nm than does double-stranded DNA.

A_{260nm} of approximately 25. This value is approximate for ss-DNA and RNA because the absorbance of purines is greater than pyrimidines at 260 nm and the ratio of purines to pyrimidines in ssDNA and RNA will vary whereas the same ratio is 1 in dsDNA. The A_{260nm} is also dependent upon base stacking which is also variable in ssDNA and RNA but constant in dsDNA.

The spectroscopic properties of a DNA solution can also be used to determine approximate purity of the preparation. Since the shape and λ_{max} of the UV absorption spectra will vary depending upon the environment of the bases, one can use the ratio of A_{260nm}/A_{280nm} to estimate the RNA and protein content of a dsDNA preparation. Pure dsDNA has a ratio of 1.8 and pure RNA has a ratio of 2.0. Since protein has a λ_{max} around 280 nm, the A_{260nm}/A_{280nm} of a protein solution will always be less than 1. Therefore a sample of dsDNA with a A_{260nm}/A_{280nm} greater than 1.8 suggests RNA contamination, while a ratio less than 1.8 suggests protein contamination.

The stability of dsDNA can be determined through a temperature denaturation study. Native dsDNA will denature to ssDNA as the temperature of the solution is increased. This is a reversible process and the ssDNA will anneal to dsDNA upon slowly cooling the denatured solution. This behavior can be followed spectroscopically (Fig. 41.11) by noting the increase in A_{260nm} with temperature indicating the hyperchromic shift as the dsDNA denatures to ssDNA. The midpoint of the sigmoid curve is termed the melting temperature of the dsDNA (T_m). Stability of different dsDNA molecules can be demonstrated by comparing the T_m values of the solutions (Fig. 41.11).

Replication. Replication of prokaryotic and eukaryotic DNA proceeds from the origin (single origins in

prokaryotes and multiple origins in eukaryotes) which is a region high in A and T residues that make opening of the double helix easier due to fewer base pairing hydrogen bonds between A/T compared to G/C. Since each strand of the DNA carries the same information, replication produces two daughter strands built from the parent strands acting as templates.

The process of replication takes place at the replication fork where the parent strands are unwound and the daughter strands are synthesized in the $5' \rightarrow 3'$ direction (reading the parent template in the $3' \rightarrow 5'$ direction) (Fig. 41.12). Both daughter strands are synthesized at the same time. One is synthesized as a continuous strand called the leading strand. The other, lagging strand, must be made in the reverse direction to the leading strand starting at the replicating fork and proceeding $5' \rightarrow 3'$ back to the origin resulting in the necessity of synthesizing blocks of nucleic acids (100–200 nucleotides (nts) in eukaryotes and 1000–2000 nts in prokaryotes) known as Okazaki fragments. These fragments are subsequently joined into a continuous daughter strand later by a DNA ligase. The DNA polymerase responsible for adding deoxynucleoside triphosphates to the growing strands requires short strands of nucleic acids as primers to start the synthetic process. These primer fragments are short RNA strands that are replaced with DNA by a proof reading exonuclease associated with the polymerase. The use of RNA primers assures the fidelity of DNA replication at the 5' end of the newly synthesized strands because the increased mobility of the "unanchored" base at the 5' end of a DNA strand can never appear as a "correct" residue and therefore cannot be proofread. However, a short RNA strand is recognized as low fidelity material and replaced

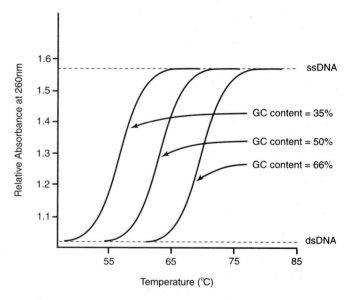

Fig. 41.11. Stability of dsDNA based upon the GC content of the nucleic acid. The melting temperature is detected by a hyperchromic shift that occurs during the temperature induced melting of dsDNA to ssDNA and is shown to increase as the GC content of dsDNA increases.

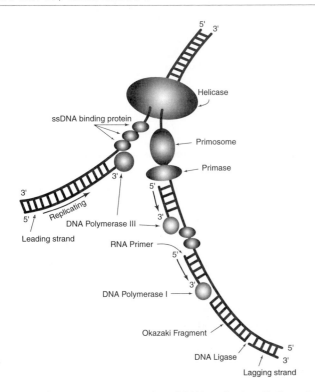

Fig. 41.12. Schematic representation of DNA replication. Helicase is responsible for unwinding the dsDNA and the ssDNA is stabilized by ssDNA binding proteins. The leading strand is synthesized continuously by DNA polymerase III. A primosome and primase are responsible for making the RNA primers that are used by DNA pol III to synthesize the initial fragments in the lagging strand, which are then elongated by DNA polymerase I to make the Okazaki fragments that are finally ligated by DNA ligase to complete the lagging strand.

with DNA. The polymerases responsible for DNA replication are different in prokaryotes and eukaryotes. DNA polymerase III (DNA pol III) synthesizes both the leading and lagging strands in prokaryotes but DNA pol I replaces the RNA primers in the lagging strand with DNA. Eukaryotic polymerases are more complex. DNA pol α starts both the lagging and leading strands in eukaryotes but is replaced by DNA pol δ on the leading strand and DNA pol ε on the lagging strand.

Transcription. It is impossible for DNA to act as a direct template in the ordering of amino acids in protein synthesis because almost all DNA is located in the nucleus and protein synthesis occurs in the cytoplasm. The genetic information in DNA is transcribed to the intermediate RNA molecule that moves to the cytoplasm where it directs the synthesis of the gene product on the ribosomes. RNA differs chemically from DNA in that the sugar molecule is ribose and thymine in DNA is replaced by uracil in RNA. Structurally, RNA is predominantly a single-stranded molecule with short double-helical regions providing some three-dimensional structure.

There are several types of RNA molecules in the cell, three of which play major roles in the message transcrip-

tion and protein synthesis. Messenger RNA (mRNA) is transcribed from a particular DNA sequence and carries the specific message from DNA in the nucleus to the cytoplasm. The molecule is very unstable with a relatively short half-life of only a few minutes. Transfer RNAs (tRNA) are relatively small molecules approximately 80 nucleotides in length. These molecules are covalently linked to specific amino acids and they carry the anticodon triplet that recognizes a particular complementary trinucleotide sequence of mRNA specific for the amino acid that it carries. tRNA is involved in protein synthesis and is metabolically unstable, being degraded once it has transferred it's amino acid to the growing protein chain. Ribosomal RNA (rRNA) is a metabolically stable complex of ribonucleic acids and proteins. rRNA provides the site of mRNA and tRNA interaction at which proteins are synthesized in the cytoplasm. While there are several differences in the mechanism of transcription between prokaryotes and eukaryotes, the more complex eukaryotic system will be described here.

Transcription is carried out by RNA polymerases (RNA pols) of which there are three types in the eukaryote. RNA pol I catalyzes the synthesis of rRNAs. RNA pol II is responsible for the synthesis of mRNA and RNA pol III synthesizes tRNA. All three polymerases are large enzymes containing 12 or more subunits.

Like prokaryotic RNA polymerase, each eukaryotic enzyme copies DNA from the 3' end thus catalyzing mRNA formation in the 5' ⇒ 3' direction and synthesizing RNA complementary to the antisense DNA template strand. The reaction requires the precursor nucleotides ATP, GTP, CTP, and UTP and does not require a primer for transcription initiation. Unlike the bacterial polymerases, the eukaryotic RNA polymerases require the presence of additional initiation proteins before they are able to bind to promoters and initiate transcription. The five stages of eukaryotic transcription include initiation, elongation and termination, capping, polyadenylation, and splicing.

Initiation. Eukaryotes have different RNA polymerase binding promoter sequences than prokaryotes. The TATA consensus sequence of the eukaryotic promoter region is located 25-35 bp upstream from the transcription start site (Fig. 41.13). The low activity of basal promoters is greatly increased by the presence of other elements located upstream from the promoter called upstream regulatory elements (UREs). These elements are located 40–200 bp upstream of the promoter sequence and include the SP1 box, the CCAAT box, and the hormone response elements. Transcription from many eukaryotic promoters can be stimulated by control elements called enhancers located many thousands of base pairs away from the transcription start site and they are usually 100–200 bp in length.

The length of DNA between the enhancer and the promoter region loops out to allow the transcription factors

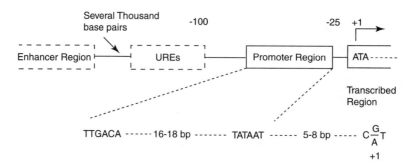

Fig. 41.13. Schematic representation of the eukaryotic transcription unit showing the relative relationship between the promoter, upstream regulatory elements and enhancer regions. Note that transcription usually starts with a purine base in the +1 position.

bound to the enhancer to interact with the general transcription factors, other regulatory proteins, or the RNA polymerase itself to bring about initiation of polymerization. RNA pol II requires a number of other proteins or protein complexes, called general transcription factors, to initiate transcription (Fig. 41.14). All these have the generic name of TFII (for transcription factor for RNA pol II). The first event in initiation is binding of TFIID to the TATA box. The key subunit of TFIID is TBP (TATA box-binding protein). After TFIID binding, TFIIA binds followed by TFIIB and then RNA pol II already complexed with TFIIF, followed in turn by TFII E, H, and J. This final complex contains at least 40 polypeptides and is called the transcription initiation complex.

Elongation and Termination. The RNA polymerase moves along the DNA template until a terminator sequence is reached. RNA pol II does not terminate at specific sites but stops at varying distances downstream of the gene. Eukaryotic termination of transcription is not as well understood as that of prokaryotic transcription. The RNA molecule made from a protein-coding gene by RNA pol II in eukaryotes is called pre-mRNA. The pre-mRNA from a eukaryotic protein coding gene is extensively processed *en route* to creating mRNA ready for translation.

Capping. At the end of polymerization, the 5′ end of the pre-mRNA molecule is modified by addition of a N-7 methyl guanine molecule (Fig. 41.15). The 5′ terminal phosphate is removed by a phosphatase and the resulting diphosphate 5′ end reacts with the α-phosphate of GTP to form an unusual 5′,5′-triphosphate link (Cap 0). The 5′-cap may also be methylated by S-adenosylmethionine on the 2′-OH of the ribose sugar of the adjacent nucleotide (Cap 1) or on both ribose sugars in the 2 and 3 positions (Cap 2) (Fig. 41.15). This cap structure protects the 5′ end of the primary transcript against attack by ribonucleases that have specificity for 3′,5′-phosphodiester bonds and so cannot hydrolyze the 5′,5′ bond in the cap structure. The cap structure also plays a role in the initiation step of protein synthesis in eukaryotes. Only RNA transcripts from eukaryotic protein-coding genes

become capped; prokaryotic mRNA and eukaryotic rRNA and tRNA are uncapped.

Polyadenylation. The 3′ end of the pre-mRNA is generated by cleavage by nucleases followed by the addition of a run, or tail, of 100–200 adenosine nucleotides resulting

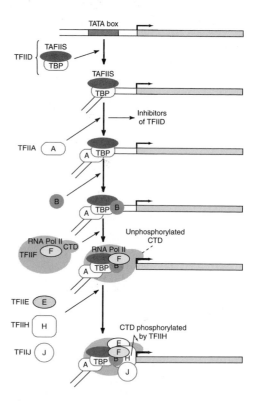

Fig. 41.14. Schematic representation of the assembly of the RNA pol II transcription initiation complex at a TATA box promoter. The transcription factors are labelled TFIIA, B, E, F, H, and J. TFIID is a complex of TATA binding protein (TBP) and multiple accessory factors called TBP-associated factors of TAFIIs. TFIID binds to the TATA box and this binding is enhanced by TFIIA, which appears to stop some inhibitory factors from binding to TFIID and preventing further assembly of the complex. TFIIB binds to the complex and acts as a bridge for binding the RNA polymerase which attaches itself to the complex along with TFIIF. When RNA pol II binding occurs, the transcription factors E, H and J, which are required for transcription, bind in a defined sequence. The carboxyl-terminal domain (CTD) of RNA pol II is phosphorylated by TFIIH thus allowing the polymerase to leave the promoter region.

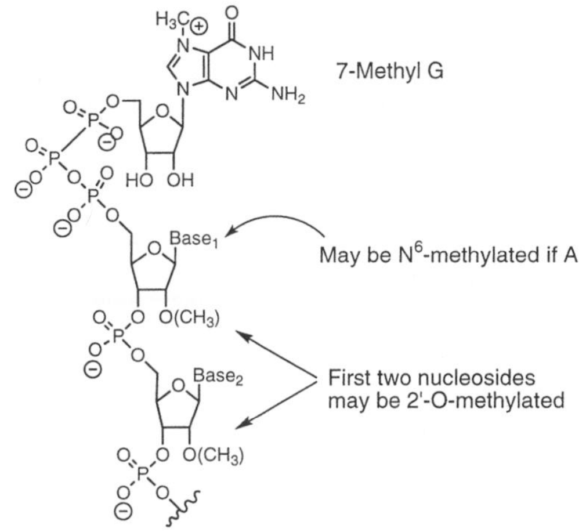

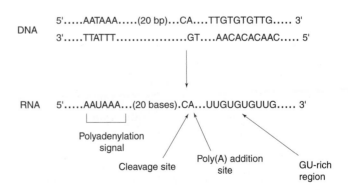

Fig. 41.15. Chemical structure of the 5'-cap of mRNA. Cap 0 consists of the 7-methylguanosine triphosphate attached to the 5' end of the mRNA. Cap 1 consists of the 7-methylguanosine and 2'-O-methylation of the 5'-base. Cap 2 consists of the 7-methylguanosine and the 2'-O-methylation of the first two bases in the sequence.

in what is called the poly(A) tail. Cleavage and polyadenylation requires specific sequences in the DNA and its pre-mRNA transcript that is part of the transcription termination signal (Fig. 41.16). A 5'-AAUAAA-3' sequence followed by a 5'-PyA-3' (Py = pyrimidine) within the next 11–20 nucleotides and a GU rich sequence further downstream collectively make up the requirements for a polyadenylation site. The poly(A) tail is thought to help stabilize the molecule since a poly(A)-binding protein interacts with the tail reducing the pre-mRNA's sensitivity to 3'-nuclease activity. In addition, the poly(A) tail may have a role to play in the translation of mature RNA in the cytoplasm.

Splicing. The next step in pre-mRNA processing is the precise cutting out of the intron sequences and joining the ends of neighboring exons to produce a functional mRNA molecule, a process termed RNA splicing. The exon-intron boundaries are marked by specific sequences. Introns are sequences that interrupt those sequences that will eventually become adjacent regions in mature RNA. Exons become the protein-coding regions of mRNA. The exon-intron boundary at the 5'-splice site always starts the intron with a GU sequence (Fig. 41.17a). The boundary at the 3' splice site always ends the intron with an AG sequence. Each sequence at the 5' and 3' splice sites lie within a larger consensus sequence. The intron also has a stretch of 10 pyrimidines near the 3'splice site and an internal branch site containing an important adenosine residue located about 20–50 nucleotides upstream of the 3' splice site. Splicing takes place in a two step reaction (Fig. 41.17b). First the bond in front of the G at the 5' splice site is attacked by the 2'-hydroxyl group of the A residue at the branch point sequence creating a tailed circular molecule called the lariat and a free exon. In the

second step, cleavage of the 3' splice site occurs after G of the AG sequence as the two exons are joined together.

Translation.   Protein synthesis occurs when the triplet genetic code carried by mRNA is translated into a protein sequence on the ribosome. As mentioned earlier, tRNA carries a specific amino acid attached to its 3' terminus based upon the anticodon present in its structure. The anticodon complements the triplet codon sequence in mRNA. A triplet is the minimum number of nucleotides necessary to provide a unique sequence for each of the 20 amino acids. With a triplet code, there is a possibility of 64 different combinations of which 61 actually code for amino acids (Table 41.2). The remaining three codons are nonsense or stop codons. Eighteen of the 20 common amino acids are coded for by more than one codon meaning the code is degenerate or redundant. Two amino acids, Met (AUG) and Trp (UGG) each have one unique codon. From a fixed start point on the mRNA (start codon–AUG) which establishes the reading frame, each group of three bases in the coding region of the mRNA represents a codon that is recognized by a complementary triplet on the end of a particular tRNA molecule. One triplet on an mRNA molecule is directly followed by the next one without any additional bases between them indicating that the code is commaless and nonoverlapping. Because each triplet is independent of any other and there are no gaps between codons, any reading frame can be divided up in three ways. Once the start codon is found, the reading frame is fixed and the protein sequence begins.

There are four stages in the protein synthesis in both prokaryotes and eukaryotes;

1. Initiation—assembly of the ribosome on an mRNA molecule.
2. Elongation—repeated cycles of amino acid addition.
3. Termination—recognition of the stop codon, release of the new protein chain, and breakdown of the synthetic complex.

```
         5'.....AATAAA.....(20 bp)...CA....TTGTGTGTTG..... 3'
DNA
         3'.....TTATTT.................GT....AACACACAAC..... 5'

                                    |
                                    |
                                    ↓

RNA      5'.....AAUAAA...(20 bases).CA...UUGUGUGUUG..... 3'
              └──────┘
         Polyadenylation
             signal
                          Cleavage site    Poly(A) addition    GU-rich
                                                site            region
```

Fig. 41.16. Sequence of a typical polyadenylation site showing the polyadenylation signal, cleavage site, and GU rich region (Turner PC, McLennan AG, Bates AD, White MRH. Notes in Molecular Biology. Oxford, New York: BIOS Scientific Publishers, 1997).

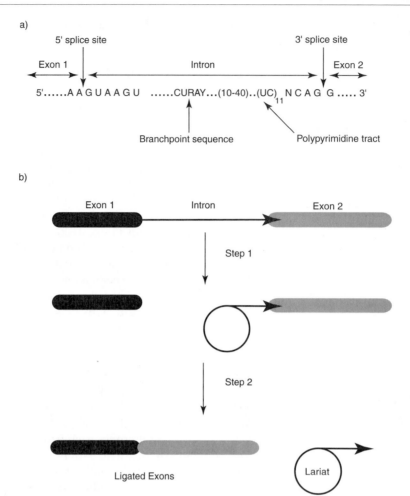

Fig. 41.17. a) Splice site concensus sequences showing the 5′ and 3′ splice sites; R = purine, Y = pyrimidine; b) Two steps in the splicing sequence showing formation of the lariat at the branchpoint sequence.

4. Post-translational modification—usually include protein cleavage by carboxy or amino peptidases, and chemical modification such as acetylation, sulfonylation, phosphorylation, hydroxylation, or addition of polysaccharides.

There are distinct differences in detail between the mechanism in prokaryotes and eukaryotes most of which occur in the initiation stage.

Genes

Manipulation of genes for therapeutic effect is the broad goal of gene therapy, so it is rather important to have an understanding of the tools used in gene manipulation. A gene is not equated with the gene product. We have seen how several changes may occur to the gene product during the production process and the final product seldom corresponds to a direct decoding of a linear nucleic acid chain. A gene is defined as the segment of DNA involved in producing a polypeptide chain; it includes regions preceding (the leader or 5′-untranslated region) and following (the trailer or 3′-untranslated region) the coding region as well as intervening sequences

(introns) between individual coding segments (exons) (23). The details of cell function that are attainable using the current tools of molecular biology will find exceptions to the above definition. Another concept critical to the understanding of gene therapy is the relationship between the genetic constitution of the organism (the genotype) and the appearance or other characteristics of the organism (phenotype). This relationship is critical since it is the objective of gene therapy to change phenotype by altering the genotype or more simply to alter gene function by changing gene structure. A direct, unalterable relationship between the structure and function of genes is known as genetic determinism and can be summed up by the statement; "He can't help it, it's in his genes."

An explanation of the relationship between the genotype and the phenotype will include a detailed description at the molecular level of the mechanism by which the genotype appears as a particular characteristic of the organism. In the majority of cases little is understood of this mechanistic relationship and we frequently compare the beginning and the end—genotype and phenotype—and if a correlation exists between the genetic makeup and a particular characteristic we say that he has a gene "for" the characteristic. However, a key player in this mechanistic description about which we have little or no information is the environment in which the organism is located and the effect that the environment will have on the genotype in producing a particular phenotype (2). A narrow concept of gene therapy ignores environmental factors and concentrates on finding the gene "for" a particular trait, characterizing a mutation of that gene that "causes" a malfunction of the trait, and correcting the mutation to correct the malfunction. The appearance of genetic determinism rises from a lack of understanding of the mechanism of genotype expression in phenotype that may be a complex mixture of several genes and the environment. An example of this complexity can be found in the attempts to relate emotions and personality to genetic composition. Genes for intelligence, aggression, or homosexuality are not likely to exist on their own. However, the implication of genes in a complex interaction between genetic and environmental factors to effect a phenotype like intelligence, aggression or homosexuality is a likely scenario. For what is evolution if not a product of interaction between genes and the environment. While the current

concept of gene therapy dwells on the narrow side, one cannot lose sight of the importance of environment and how it may be part of the gene therapy to include modifying the organism's environment to permit the continuation of a healthy life. Therefore, gene therapy will include genetic alteration to correct a defect or environment modification to fix some molecular condition that, if left untreated, would have a high probability of producing a genetic disease (2).

Cloning and the Preparation of DNA Libraries. Studies on the nature of DNA, genes and chromosomes ground to a near halt in the early 1960s due to the fact that DNA was just too large a molecule to work with and attempts to break it up into manageable pieces were thwarted by the inability to put the pieces back together in the correct order. The discovery in the early 1970s of bacterial enzymes capable of cleaving nucleic acids at specific, palindromic (symmetrical) base sequences was a major breakthrough in nucleic acid chemistry (Fig. 41.18). The second discovery in molecular biology that advanced genetic analysis was the use of bacterial plasmids as vehicles (vectors) to amplify gene fragments produced by restriction enzymes. Plasmids are small, circular, extrachromosomal nucleic acid molecules in bacteria that replicate independently within the bacterial cell. Restriction enzymes are used to produce relatively small DNA fragments that are inserted into bacterial plasmid vectors forming recombinant DNA molecules (rDNA). The rDNA vectors are inserted into bacterial hosts where the plasmid replicates with the bacteria producing a large number of identical rDNA molecules known as clones, completing the process known as DNA cloning.

There are two sources of DNA that are used to prepare fragments or libraries of DNA fragments. Genomic DNA isolated from the species of interest is digested with restriction enzymes and the fragments are inserted into plasmids to produce a genomic DNA (gDNA) library. Alternatively, one can use mRNA fragments from restriction enzyme digests of mRNA from a cell or tissue and prepare DNA copies of the mRNA fragments using reverse transcription. The DNA fragment copies are complementary to the mRNA and are called complementary DNA (cDNA) fragments thus producing a cDNA library. Different genetic information is provided by the two types of DNA libraries. The gDNA library would have the gene regulatory sequences along with the introns in the gene coding sequence while the cDNA would be missing these and other nontranscribed features of the gene sequence.

Finding a Gene in the Library. A well-prepared gene library has a high probability of containing a particular gene sequence. Library screening is the process through which one or more clones containing the gene of interest can be identified (24). If one wishes to screen for a particular gene, sufficient knowledge of that gene sequence

Table 41.2. The Genetic Code

First Position	Second Position				Third Position
	U	C	A	G	
U	Phe UUU	Ser UCU	Tyr UAU	Cys UGU	U
	Phe UUC	Ser UCC	Tyr UAC	Cys UGC	C
	Leu UUA	Ser UCA	Stop UAA	Stop UGA	A
	Leu UUG	Ser UCG	Stop UAG	Trp UGG	G
C	Leu CUU	Pro CCU	His CAU	Arg CGU	U
	Leu CUC	Pro CCC	His CAC	Arg CGC	C
	Leu CUA	Pro CCA	Gln CAA	Arg CGA	A
	Leu CUG	Pro CCG	Gln CAG	Arg CGG	G
A	Ile AUU	Thr ACU	Asn AAU	Ser AGU	U
	Ile AUC	Thr ACC	Asn AAC	Ser AGC	C
	Ile AUA	Thr ACA	Lys AAA	Arg AGA	A
	Met AUG	Thr ACG	Lys AAG	Arg AGG	G
G	Val GUU	Ala GCU	Asp GAU	Gly GGU	U
	Val GUC	Ala GCC	Asp GAC	Gly GGC	C
	Val GUA	Ala GCA	Glu GAA	Gly GGA	A
	Val GUG	Ala GCG	Glu GAG	Gly GGG	G

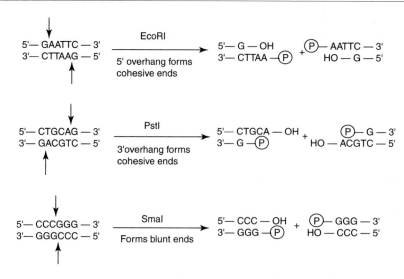

Fig. 41.18. Actions of restriction endonucleases EcoRI, PstI, and SmaI at their recognition sequences. Note: EcoRI and PstI enzymes produce "sticky ends," with overlapping sequences while SmaI produces "blunt ends" or nonoverlapping sequences.

must be available to allow synthesis of oligonucleotide fragments complementary to parts of the gene. These fragments can be radiolabeled and used as nucleic acid probes to screen the library by hybridization. Assuming the library was made by ligating the gene fragments to bacterial vectors and inserting the vectors into *E. coli*, the library is spread on several agar plates and the bacteria are allowed to grow to form colonies such that each colony rises from a single bacteria carrying a single vector with a single gene fragment (Fig. 41.19).

After the colonies have grown to a size visible to the naked eye, nitrocellulose filters are carefully laid onto the surface of the agar plates to make an exact replica of the agar plate by blotting up a small amount of each colony on the plate (Fig. 41.19). The bacteria on the filter are lysed by soaking in sodium dodecyl sulfate and a protease and the DNA is denatured using alkali (NaOH) then baking the filter to bond the ssDNA to the filter. The filter is then incubated in a solution of radiolabeled nucleic acid probe complementary to a portion of the gene of interest and allowed to hybridize to the ssDNA on the filter. The filters are carefully washed to remove the nonspecifically bound probe and the specifically bound probes are located on the filter by exposing the filter to X-ray film (autoradiography). The bacterial colony that specifically bound the probe likely contains a fragment of the gene in question and this colony will show up on the autoradiogram as a dark spot and its position on the original agar plate can be located by comparing the nitrocellulose filter to the agar plate. Once located, the colony can be picked off the original plate and grown in culture to provide a large sample of the bacteria carrying the vector with the gene fragment.

Characterizing the Cloned Gene Fragment

Restriction Mapping and Southern Blotting. The size of DNA fragments is generally determined by agarose gel electro-

phoresis. The dsDNA samples are placed in wells in the surface of the gel in separate lanes and when an electric current is applied to an agarose gel in the presence of a buffer that will conduct electricity, the dsDNA fragments will travel through the gel toward the cathode (positive electrode) at a rate dependent upon the size of the linear

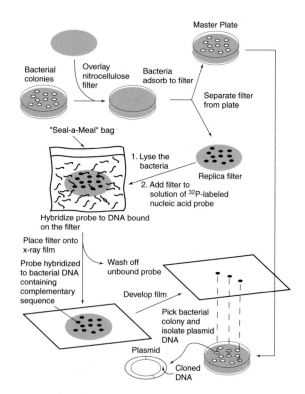

Fig. 41.19. Screening a library with a nucleic acid probe to find a clone of the pattern of bacterial colonies. Adapted from Watson JD, Gilman M, Witkowski J, Zoller M. Recombinant DNA. 2nd ed. New York: Scientific American Books, W.H. Freeman and Company; 1992 with permission.

molecule. Small fragments will travel faster than larger fragments separating the mixture of DNA fragments according to size. The fragments are generally viewed by staining the gel with ethidium bromide, a chemical that intercalates into dsDNA. The molecular weight of fragments may be roughly determined by running a standard sample of DNA fragments with known molecular weights in a lane on the same gel as the unknown fragments. A DNA fragment isolated by the cloning technique described above may be characterized further by restriction enzyme mapping. This procedure consists of isolating the DNA fragment from the cloning vector and digesting it with one or more restriction enzymes then separating the fragments on gel electrophoresis and staining them with ethidium bromide.

The number and size of the restriction fragments provide valuable information about the original DNA fragment. The individual restriction fragments may be extracted from the gels and the nucleotide sequence determined by Sanger's dideoxy method (see below) (25). When the nucleotide sequences of the restriction fragments are determined, overlapping fragments may be found and the fragments reassembled to determine the sequence of the original fragment. If examination of the sequence indicates the presence of a start and stop codon, an open reading frame exists in the sequence and it is possible that the sequence codes for an expressed gene. However, further studies are necessary to determine if the sequence is expressed in the cell from which the original DNA fragment was isolated.

It is also possible to analyze DNA fragments by hybridization with particular radiolabeled probes using a technique called Southern Blotting (Fig. 41.20). The DNA solutions that have been digested with restriction enzymes are placed in wells at the top of the gel and electrophoresis separates the fragments that are then denatured with alkali and blotted onto nitrocellulose paper to make an exact replica of the gel. This is done by placing the agarose gel on a sponge in a tray of buffer. The nitrocellulose filter is placed over the gel and covered with a large stack of paper towels that act as a wick pulling the buffer through the gel and filter. The DNA fragments are carried from the gel to the filter where they stick. The filter is removed and hybridized with a radioactively labeled probe that specifically tags the sequence of interest through hybridization. The stringency with which the hybridization and washing is carried out is critical and is determined by temperature and salt concentration in the hybridization buffer—high temperature and low salt being the most stringent conditions. If the conditions are not too stringent then the probe may bind to too many nonhomologus sequences to be useful. Unbound probe is removed by washing and the filter is placed on an X-ray film and the bound probe appears as a band on the film. A similar technique utilizing RNA fragments is called Northern Blotting.

Sequencing DNA Fragments. The two major methods of nucleic acid sequencing are the Maxam and Gilbert

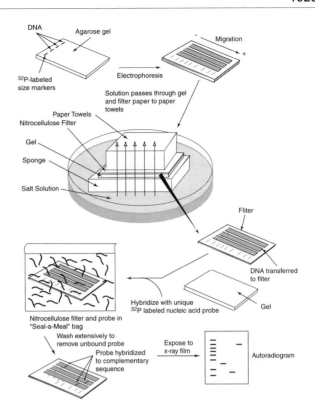

Fig. 41.20. Analyzing DNA by gel electrophoresis and Southern blotting. Adapted from Watson JD, Gilman M, Witkowski J, Zoller M. Recombinant DNA. 2nd ed. New York: Scientific American Books, W.H. Freeman and Company; 1992 with permission.

chemical method (26) and Sanger's dideoxy method (25). The dideoxy method of Sanger is largely the method of choice to sequence DNA fragments. The method capitalizes on the use of DNA polymerase to catalyze the synthesis of a copy of the DNA fragment that one wishes to sequence. The method relies on the fact that when 2′,3′-dideoxynucleotide triphosphates (ddNTPs) are incorporated into growing nucleic acid chains, the growth ceases because the dideoxynucleotide does not have a 3′-hydroxyl group on which to add the next nucleotide in the chain. The method consists of four reagent vials each containing the ssDNA template fragment to be sequenced, DNA polymerase, short radiolabeled oligonucleotide primer that hybridizes to the 3′ end of the template fragment, and the four nucleotide triphosphates (dATP, dGTP, dCTP, and dTTP). Each vial contains one of the four ddNTPs either ddATP, ddGTP, ddCTP, or ddTTP and the vial is labeled according to which ddNTP is present (Fig. 41.21). The ratio of the ddNTP to the normal dNTPs in the vial is carefully controlled such that the polymerase catalyzed synthesis of the fragment will go to completion but a small, yet detectable portion of the synthesis will be terminated each time a ddNTP is attached to the growing fragment. The reaction is initiated by the addition of the polymerase to the vials and when the synthesis is complete, a sample from each vial is applied to wells at the top of a polyacrylamide gel and the gel is developed to separate the DNA fragments

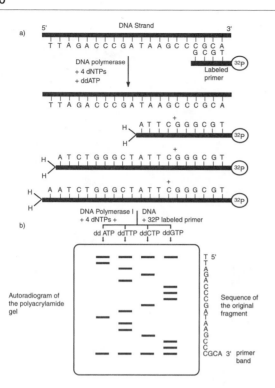

Fig. 41.21. The Sanger DNA-sequencing procedure; a) the Sanger dideoxy nucleotide sequencing reaction with 32P labeled primers; b) acrylamide gel separation of the labeled fragments. Taken from Watson JD, Gilman M, Witkowski J, Zoller M. Recombinant DNA. 2nd ed. New York: Scientific American Books, W.H. Freeman and Company; 1992 with permission.

in each vial by size (Fig. 41.21). All fragments that arise in each of the vials as a result of termination of the synthesis at the incorporation of a ddNTP can be visualized on the gel by autoradiography because the primer is radiolabeled (usually with a 32P phosphate at the 5'-end) and all fragments will contain the primer sequence. The nucleotide sequence of the **complementary** strand of the fragment that acted as template in the DNA polymerase catalyzed reaction can be read from the bottom of the gel starting with the sequence of the 5'-end primer and adding nucleotides based on the lane in which the next largest fragment occurs (Fig. 41.21). The smallest visible fragment will be the primer and the largest visible fragment will be the complete fragment, both of which will appear in all the vials. The intermediate fragment sizes will be different in each lane depending upon the sequence of the template and which ddNTP was present.

Synthesizing Oligonucleotides. The need for short oligonucleotides of known sequence has grown tremendously with the need for radiolabeled probes to isolate and characterize nucleic acids as well as the need for primers of the DNA polymerase catalyzed synthesis of nucleic acids. It is now possible to synthesize an entire gene by enzymatically linking chemically synthesized oligonucleoside fragments making up the gene sequence. The phosphite-triester (27)

and the phosphotriester methods (28) are convenient solid-phase automated techniques for the synthesis of oligonucleotides. The solid phase technique synthesizes the nucleic acid in the 3' to 5' direction by attaching the 3'-hydroxyl group of a 5'-O-dimethoxytrityl protected deoxyribonucleoside to an insoluble solid support that may be polystyrene resin, silica gel, glass beads, polyamide, or cellulose paper. The subsequent 5'-protected nucleosides are coupled as 3'-phospho or phosphite triesters to the 5'-deprotected nucleic acid attached to the solid support. The 6-amino group of adenine and the 4-amino group of cytosine are protected as benzoyl amides and the 2-amino group of guanine is protected by the isobutyryl amide.

The basic steps in the phosphite-triester method are as follows (Fig. 41.22) (27):

1. Removal of the 5'-O-dimethoxytrityl group from the deoxyribonucleoside attached to the solid support is carried out by treatment of the reaction mixture with 3% dichloroacetic acid in dichloromethane.
2. The free 5'-OH group is coupled with excess 5'-O-dimethoxytrityl deoxyribonucleoside-3'-phosphoramidite using tetrazole as an acid catalyst.
3. The new 3',5'-phosphite-triester linking the two nucleotides is converted to the more stable phosphotriester by iodine catalyzed oxidation.
4. Any 5'-OH groups that failed to react are capped by acetylation with acetic anhydride.
5. The 5'-O-dimethoxytrityl protecting group is removed by treatment of the reaction mixture with 3% dichloroacetic acid in dichloromethane.

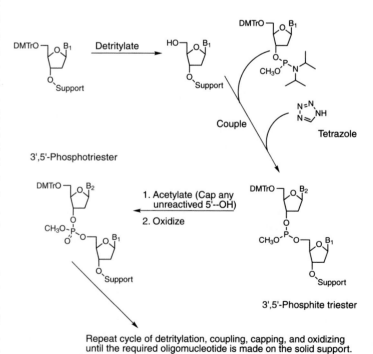

Fig. 41.22. Solid-phase phosphite-triester method of oligodeoxyribonucleotide synthesis.

6. The sequence of deprotection, coupling, oxidation, and capping is repeated until the oligodeoxyribonucleotide of desired length is obtained.

7. The final product is deprotected, removed from the solid support, and purified.

Polymerase Chain Reaction. The problem of working with small quantities of nucleic acids isolated from cell and tissue sources was solved to a certain extent with the development of cloning techniques that would amplify a DNA fragment as part of a replicating vector in bacteria. The polymerase chain reaction was the second development that tremendously increased the ease with which a fragment of DNA could be amplified without the need for the complications of cloning (29). Through this procedure there was no need to isolate the fragment to be amplified. The only requirement was for DNA polymerase oligonucleotide primers at the boundaries of the fragment to be amplified.

The dsDNA fragment is targeted for amplification by designing oligonucleotide primers that anneal to the 3′ ends of the double-stranded fragment (Fig. 41.23). A DNA polymerase uses the oligonucleotides as primers to synthesize the two strands from the 3′ ends producing two new dsDNA strands carrying the DNA fragment bounded by the two primers. A series of cycles of denaturation, annealing primers, and DNA polymerization results in greatly amplified quantities of the fragment of interest (Fig. 41.23). The original technique used a DNA polymerase from *E. coli* that was heat sensitive and hence had to be replaced at every cycle of the reaction. The finding that thermophilic bacteria made DNA polymerases were resistant to the high temperatures used in the denaturation step of the polymerase cycle provided a source for the polymerase enzyme that would not have to be replaced after each cycle and the reaction could be automated without interruption. The most common temperature resistant enzyme used is *Taq* polymerase isolated from *Thermus aquaticus*. This enzyme survives a 1–2 minute exposure to 95°C temperature but lacks a 3′–5′ proofreading exonuclease activity so it may introduce errors during DNA replication. Other enzymes with better features have been isolated and are being used in place of the *Taq* polymerase. The technique has many different applications in molecular biology and is really a corner stone in the research on genetic structure/function relationships.

MOLECULAR PATHOLOGY OF GENETIC DISORDERS

The hemoglobin diseases of sickle cell anemia and thalassemia have provided much of the early insight into genetic diseases (30,31). The demonstration that sickle cell anemia was due to a single mutation in the hemoglobin gene where the normal glutamic acid (GAG codon) in position 6 of the β chain is mutated to valine (GTG) by a single A → T base change provided direct support for the one gene one protein concept. Once technology developed sufficiently to allow the studies on the α and β chains

of the adult $\alpha_2\beta_2$ hemoglobin, it was found that the hemoglobin molecule was incredibly polymorphic. The hemolytic anemias, α and β thalassaemia, arise from a family of unstable hemoglobins involving single amino acid changes in the gene sequence for the α and β globins. It has been found that human proteins in general are widely polymorphic and some of the polymorphic variability results in defective function of the gene product (32). These mutations will produce disease in one of two ways:

1. The mutation alters the function or stability of the gene product.
2. The mutation causes a reduction or absence of the gene product.

Genetic polymorphisms are not the only determining factors of an individual's phenotype. As discussed earlier (Chemical Basis of Heredity) environmental factors may also impact the phenotypic expression of genotypic variation. The role of environment appears to become greater in the phenotype that arises from the interactions of multiple genes. These complex phenotypes are encountered in some of the major death producing diseases of western culture such as heart disease, stroke, hypertension, diabetes, and cancer as well as a number of severely debilitating psychiatric

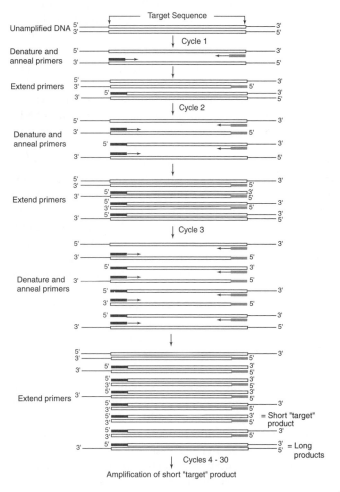

Fig. 41.23. The polymerase chain reaction.

disorders. The treatment of complex multigenic diseases will require consideration of both the patient's genotype and the environmental factors specific to that individual ("envirotype") that may impact on the patient's phenotype. The greater complexity of the molecular pathology of the multigenic disorders compared to monogenic disorders will also be reflected in the different approaches to therapy.

Mutation

Mutations are the result of heritable, permanent changes in the DNA base sequence. These usually come about by one of three mechanisms; substitution, addition, or deletion. The number of base pairs involved in a single gene mutation can vary from a single base pair change, called a point mutation, to a large number of gross changes in the gene structure involving insertion, deletion or rearrangements of a very large number of base pairs.

Point mutations may result in a variety of changes to the gene product. If the base change occurs within the reading frame of the gene product and produces a single change in one amino acid in the amino acid sequence of the gene product it is termed a **missense point mutation.** Some of these missense mutations result in a change in the gene product that has no effect on its function and is termed a silent mutation. Generally speaking, a point mutation in a gene that does not result in functional change of the gene product is called a polymorphism. Mutations are defined as base changes causing a change in function of the gene product. However, this distinction is not rigidly adhered to and many single base mutations causing changes in function of gene product are frequently called single nucleotide polymorphisms or SNPs. In fact, SNPs have been defined as single base mutations that occur in 1% or more of the population (33). Many of these SNPs may be responsible for the production of a malfunctioning gene product that in turn is responsible for a serious disease. The well used example here is the previously mentioned A → T mutation in the β globin gene where the GAG glutamic acid codon is changed to the GTG valine codon resulting in abnormal aggregation of the hemoglobin molecules and leading to sickle cell anemia.

Point mutations occurring in the reading frame that convert an amino acid codon to a stop codon (TAA, TAG, TGA) are termed **nonsense mutations** and result in the truncation of the gene product due to a premature stop in the translation process. These changes are very serious, and may lead to loss of a large sequence of the carboxy terminus of the gene product especially if they occur in the 5′ region of the gene. β-thalassemia is a result of mutation of a CAG glutamine codon to the TAG stop codon early in the DNA sequence resulting in premature termination of the translation process and total loss of the β subunit of the adult hemoglobin molecule.

A **frameshift mutation** occurs when, instead of changing a base pair, a base pair is inserted or deleted in the gene sequence. An insertion/deletion of more or less than three bases will result in a shift of the reading frame and a different set of codons will be read 3′ (downstream) of the mutation (Fig. 41.24). These mutations have very serious effects and frequently result in the total loss of the gene product.

Point mutations occurring in the boundaries between the exons and introns may result in the inability of the pre-mRNA to splice properly and are called **splice mutations.** These mutations may result in the loss of many amino acids in the gene product sequence or may cause a frameshift resulting in total loss of functional gene product. Mutations may also occur in introns with the resultant formation of splice sites that also cause the pre-mRNA to splice abnormally.

Point mutations in promoter regions known as **promoter mutations** occur frequently and are responsible for reducing or eliminating the expression of a gene.

One of the gross changes in gene structure involves an unusual form of gene mutation known as the trinucleotide repeat where a trinucleotide sequence undergoes a dramatic increase in the number of copies of the trinucleotide in a gene sequence. Fragile X Syndrome and Huntington's Disease are both the result of this unusual mutation.

Inheritance of Single Gene Mutations

Many inherited genetic disorders are the result of mutations in a single gene. These disorders include sickle cell anemia, immune deficiency disorders such as adenosine deaminase deficiency, hemophilias, hypercholesterolemia resulting from LDL receptor mutations, and cystic fibrosis. In many cases of monogenic disorders, the pathology indicates a direct relationship between the disease and the loss of the proper function of a gene product. Hemophilia and the loss of a proper functioning gene producing Factor VIII is an example. Delivery of a normal Factor VIII gene should cure the disease in the hemophiliac patient. A more indirect pathologic relationship between the mutated gene and the disease occurs in sickle cell anemia. In this case, the mutation stabilizes the hemoglobin molecules in the deoxy form causing the hemoglobin molecules to polymerize under low oxygen tension which in

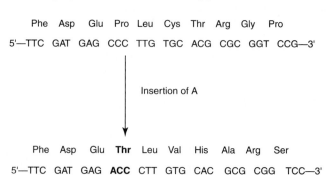

Fig. 41.24. An example of a frameshift point mutation. Adenosine is inserted between guanosine, the last nucleotide in the glutamic acid triplet, and cytosine, the first nucleic acid in the proline triplet. The reading frame is shifted to the left by one nucleic acid thereby changing the sequence of amino acids from glutamic acid onward.

turn causes the red blood cell to form a sickle shape. The sickled red blood cells are prematurely destroyed in the circulation and lead to blockage of small blood vessels and resulting tissue damage (34).

Single gene mutations are passed on from parents to children through these possible patterns of inheritance: autosomal dominant, autosomal recessive, and X linked. All human cells contain 22 pairs of homologous chromosomes or autosomes and a pair of sex chromosomes. One copy of each gene called an allele occurs on each of the autosomes.

Where a mutation is autosomal dominant such as Huntington's Disease, the inheritance of a single mutated allele is sufficient to cause the disease. Those individuals affected with the disease and having one normal and one mutated allele are known as heterozygotes. These individuals have a 50% chance of passing on the disease to their offspring.

An autosomal recessive mutation means that both mutant alleles must be inherited from the parents before the disease will be exhibited. The individuals with the disease are said to be homozygous for the mutant allele. Those individuals who inherit a single mutant allele do not exhibit the disease but are said to be carriers of the diseased gene. The carriers of the autosomal recessive allele will have a 25% chance of passing the disease on to their children if the other parent is also a carrier. In this case, there is a 25% chance that the offspring will be normal and a 50% chance that the offspring will be carriers of the disease. If one parent is a carrier and the other is homozygous for the normal allele then there is a 50% chance of having a normal child and a 50% chance that the offspring will be carriers.

The X-linked diseases are recessive and appear predominantly in males. Since males carry one X and one Y chromosome a mutated recessive allele on the X chromosome would automatically appear in males who are said to be hemizygous. Since females carry two X chromosomes the recessive allele on one chromosome is not likely to affect females. Females are carriers of X linked disorders and 50% of their male offspring are likely to display the disease while 50% of their female offspring will be carriers of the disease.

Inherited Polygenic Disorders

Many diseases of western civilizations are far more complicated than the monogenic disorders mentioned above. Heart disease, stroke, hypertension, diabetes, cancer, psychiatric illnesses, and rheumatoid arthritis are serious diseases with a strong genetic component. However, the genetic disorder cannot be traced through family histories in the same way that suggests a single gene disorder. Environmental complications, commonly called risk factors, also play a major role in the pathogenesis of these diseases. In these cases, one may identify a particular gene that may be an indicator of the possibility of developing one of these more complicated diseases. However, the probability

of developing the disease depends upon several other genetic and environmental factors coming into play all of which may be unknown at the time. This obviously leads to several dilemmas on the part of the health care worker in that the probability of the individual developing the disease may not be known with any accuracy and yet the probability is still there. This leads to a new approach to health care called the predict-and-manage paradigm (35). The ability to predict the course of any disease based on genetic and biochemical background, physiologic state, and disease history is combined with advanced therapies that include behavior modification.

These multigenic disorders are the major challenges facing gene therapy in the immediate future. Symptomatic management of these diseases will be replaced by an understanding of the biochemical basis of the underlying causes of the disease which in turn should lead to a better treatment if not cure of the disease. The replacement of one of the many genes involved in the disease may reverse or retard the disease processes at the cellular level (36).

GENERAL THERAPEUTIC APPLICATIONS
Approaches

There are four stages of study that a therapeutic agent of any sort must pass before government regulatory bodies will deem it acceptable for human use (Table 41.3).

As of May 1, 2000 the Human Gene Therapy Protocol List at the U.S. National Institutes of Health web site listed a total of 206 gene therapy protocols, the majority of which were Phase I protocols. Cancer and infectious diseases (AIDS is the only infectious disease being treated through gene therapy with 25 RAC approved trials currently underway) are the therapeutic areas most heavily represented as candidates for gene therapy. A wide variety of technological approaches are used in these gene therapy protocols but basically they include modification to the somatic cell performed either *in vivo* or *ex vivo*.

Choice of Cell Type (Germ Cell vs. Somatic Cell)

The choice of the cell type to be used in gene therapy will have a major impact on the extent to which the therapy will alter the gene pool. Somatic cell gene therapy is intended to alter the individual's genetic constitution without altering the genetic makeup of the children of

Table 41.3. Stages of Study Before a Drug is Marketed

Preclinical Studies	Animal testing of the therapeutic agent to determine a rationale for therapeutic use, toxicities, dose details, and risks involved.
Phase I	A small human trial generally involving dose escalation and focusing on safety and pharmacology of the therapeutic agent.
Phase II	An expanded human trial with the focus on efficacy in a particular patient population(s).
Phase III	A large human trial intended to establish a definitive role for a drug or biologic.

that individual. Presumably the alteration in the somatic cell genetic makeup would be for the lifetime of the individual, however, this is not always the case and depends upon whether or not the new gene is inserted into the genome or remains epichromosomal and whether or not the altered cells are replaced rapidly or in a more prolonged time frame. Naturally, if the gene is inserted into the cell genome, the new gene should be carried on from cell to cell as the old cells are replaced. However, if the new gene is inserted as epichromosomal material, then there is the possibility that it may be lost to one daughter cell during cell division.

Germ cell gene therapy is a more ethically problematic approach to gene therapy. This approach alters both the somatic cell and the germ cell lines of the individual and insures that the genetic alteration will be passed on to the individual's offspring. The ethical issues involved in this approach to gene therapy are currently prohibitive but provide a lively area for debate and discussion about the future of gene therapy (37).

In vivo vs. Ex vivo

The various approaches for implementing somatic cell gene therapy may be described under two categories—*in vivo* gene therapy and *ex vivo* gene therapy. The *ex vivo* approach involves the following steps:

i)   Collect and culture the cells to be manipulated.
ii) Transfer the gene to the cultured cells.
iii) Select for the cells that have been transformed and expand the cell numbers in culture.
iv) Infuse or transplant the cells into the patient.

The source of cells for genetic manipulation can either be autologus or from a compatible donor. The autologus source would naturally avoid the problems that may arise with adverse immune responses. Some cells that are currently used for *ex vivo* gene therapy are the totipotent embryonic blood stem cells from bone marrow, hepatocytes, vascular smooth muscle cells, and tumor infiltrating lymphocytes. The totipotent bone marrow cells are a popular choice for gene therapy because these will differentiate into a number of different cell types in mature blood including B and T lymphocytes, macrophages, red blood cells, platelets, and osteoclasts.

The *in vivo* approach involves the direct delivery of the gene to the cells of a particular tissue. A major difference between the *ex vivo* and *in vivo* techniques is that it is possible to screen the *ex vivo* modified cells for gene delivery and function prior to returning them to the patient but the *in vivo* technique does not allow this luxury. The *in vivo* delivery systems are discussed later and each have their particular advantages and disadvantages. In general the *in vivo* delivery should be efficient in that all targeted cells should receive the gene. The delivery should be tissue specific in that the delivery system should deliver the gene to the diseased tissue only. *In vivo* delivery should also place the gene in a predetermined position in the chromosome. This chromosomal targeting should avert the danger of disrupting other essential genes by inserting the gene into the coding region for another gene. It will also prevent activation of oncogenes through uncontrolled gene insertion into the chromosome. *In vivo* delivery obviously has some tough standards to live up to and the various approaches being used are discussed under Gene Delivery.

Strategies

In attempting to carry out gene therapy on somatic cells there are several requirements that must be met in order to have even a remote chance of success. The gene for the particular disorder should be isolated along with its regulatory sequences. There must also be an efficient way of targeting the gene to a particular set of cells either *in vivo* or *ex vivo*. In the case of the *ex vivo* approach, it must be possible to obtain a sufficient number of cells in which to insert the gene and return the cells to the patient. Last of all, it is important that the gene function in the cellular environment by producing the gene product in sufficient quantities over a reasonable length of time to have a therapeutic effect without significant side effects.

Genes may also be thought of a being either house keeping genes or tissue specific genes. The house keeping genes are not tightly regulated and are generally expressed in all tissues at all levels of development. Since regulation of gene expression is one of the difficult areas of gene therapy, the house keeping genes would be a simplified approach for gene therapy since regulation is not an important feature of the gene function. The tissue specific genes are generally tightly regulated and abnormal expression of these genes could lead to major disease problems. The thalassemias are good examples of this type of gene in that poorly regulated expression of the α and β subunits of hemoglobin results in disruptions in the structure of hemoglobin with the ultimate problem of poor oxygen binding to the molecule.

Diagnosis

Before any attempts can be made to a correct genetic disorder, one must first determine which gene is responsible for the disorder. In many cases nothing is known about the gene or the gene product and one must then begin by determining the chromosomal location of the gene. The approximate position of the gene can be determined through positional cloning. Positional cloning, once called reverse genetics, consists of first establishing a linkage between the gene and a genetic marker in the human genome then using linkage to locate the position of the gene. Markers are genes the genome location of which is known and linkage analysis follows the coinheritance of both the marker and the gene under study. If the gene is linked to a particular marker and can be located within approximately two megabases of the marker, then the region can be searched for coding sequences. A technique called chromosome walking uses DNA probes to find fragments of the region being searched and these fragments then produce new probes that are again used to find new fragments further along the DNA sequence. If a coding sequence is found, the entire gene can be sequenced, the amino acid sequence of the gene product deduced, the function postulated, and finally the relationship between the gene and the abnormality estimated by comparing the mutant with a wild type gene.

Variations in the DNA sequence that occurs in 1% or more of the population are called polymorphisms (See Mutations, p. 1032). Occasionally a polymorphism may be found in an enzyme restriction site that is unique to a particular gene of interest in a genetic disorder and this polymorphism is used to determine the presence of the gene by digesting the gene into fragments and analyzing the fragment sizes by Southern blotting. These types of polymorphisms are called restriction fragment length polymorphisms (RFLPs) and are very useful because they may be used as markers of the genes in which they arise. Once a gene is found that is related to a particular inherited disorder it is sometimes possible to use the RFLPs to identify the presence of that particular allele in an individual. If the RFLP allows identification of the presence of a mutant allele responsible for a particular genetic disorder then this RFLP may be used as a diagnostic test for the determination of the inheritance of a potentially dangerous genetic trait. The use of RFLPs in carrier or prenatal diagnosis entails three steps (34):

i) An appropriate RFLP marker is chosen that is either within or closely linked to the disease locus and for which an individual at risk of carrying the disease is heterozygous.
ii) Determine which of the marker alleles is on the chromosome carrying the disease allele.
iii) Using the markers the DNA samples (fetal or adult) are examined to see whether the individual has inherited the chromosome(s) carrying the abnormal phenotype.

The development of the polymerization chain reaction and the synthesis of oligonucleotide probes are two other techniques aside from restriction fragment length polymorphisms that have greatly facilitated the detection of carrier and prenatal genetic disorders. A particular polymorphic sequence can be recognized by amplification through the PCR and using a labeled synthetic oligonucleotide probe that anneals to the polymorphic sequence of interest to detect the sequence through Southern blot analysis (Fig. 41.25).

A number of genetic diagnostic tests are in the process of being developed and commercial diagnostic kits are becoming available for some tests. With the first phase of the Human Genome Project complete, more genes related to

disease are being sequenced by positional cloning and many more tests will become available for carrier and prenatal detection of monogenetic disorders. Multigenic disorders such as cardiovascular disease, diabetes, and cancer are far more complex than the monogenic disorders and subject to complications by environmental effects. However, the new DNA chips are capable of detecting all 6200 genes in the yeast genome reading frame through the use of 260,000 25bp of oligonucleotide probes. DNA chips should soon have the capacity of analyzing all 30,000–40,000 genes in the human genome (38–40).

Genetic polymorphisms in the CYP450 drug metabolizing enzymes are also being exploited using the above technologies to tailor drug therapies to genetic makeup (41, 42). Knowledge of CYP450 polymorphisms are becoming important in the prescribing of drug therapy since knowledge of a particular CYP450 polymorphism in a particular patient could prevent serious side effects or wasted, expensive, drug therapy.

Correcting Monogenic Disease

The monogenic disorders, where a defect in a single gene can be directly related to a particular disease, are the most readily amenable to gene therapy. The ideal situation would be to remove the defective gene and replace it with a normal gene returning the cell to its normal genotype with the concomitant correction of phenotype. Since it is not an easy task to locate and remove a gene from the human genome either *in vivo* or *ex vivo*, such a strategy for monogenic disease is not currently feasible. An alternative strategy would be to correct the genetic defect through site directed mutagenesis, bypassing the need to remove the defective gene. Again, this strategy is problematic since it is not an easy task to locate the gene defect in the human genome either *in vivo* or *ex vivo*.

The most technically feasible strategy currently used is gene augmentation. This consists of introducing the gene into cells such that it will produce sufficient gene product to compensate for the lack of expression of the correct gene product by the defective gene. Recessive monogenic disorders should respond well to this strategy, however, dominantly inherited disorders are not likely to be good candidates for gene augmentation therapy.

Cell and Tissue Engineering

Synthetic polymers have found extensive use in drug delivery and are now finding use in the engineering of cell and tissue substitutes (43,44). It is possible to coat synthetic polymer scaffolds such as polytetrafluoroethylene or natural polymers like collagen with genetically altered cells and implant the "neo-organoid" into the body to function as a source of the gene product for which the cells were altered (45,46). The large surface to volume ratio of the polymer scaffolds make them capable of supporting large numbers of cells and therefore they may play

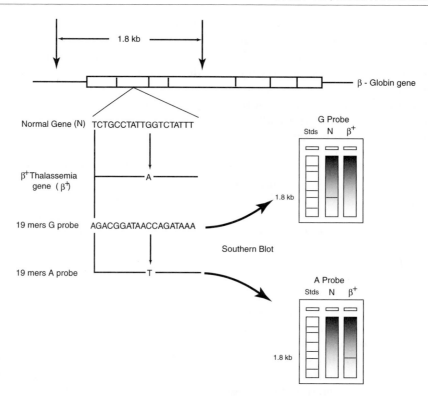

Fig. 41.25. Schematic representation of the use of oligonucleotide probes for prenatal diagnosis. The mutation that is being analyzed is the G → A change at position 110 in the first intervening sequence of the β globin gene which causes the common variety of β⁺ thalassaemia in Mediterranean populations. Two probes, each 19 nucleotides long, are made. One has the normal sequence (G probe); the other has the same sequence except for the G → A change (A probe). The region of DNA to be studied is part of a 1.8 kb restriction enzyme fragment, as indicated. The patient's DNA and normal DNA are digested with the appropriate enzyme and the mixture is separated and hybridized with both G and A probes. Under appropriate conditions the G probe hybridizes to the abnormal but not to the normal (β⁺) DNA; the A probe hybridizes to the abnormal but not to the normal DNA. Taken from Weatherall DJ. The New Genetics and Clinical Practice. 3rd ed., 1991 by permission of Oxford University Press.

a major role in implanting large numbers of genetically engineered cells into patients (47).

Controlled Delivery of Therapeutic Protein—Regulating Gene Expression

The concept of cell implants as a source of therapeutic proteins can be carried a step further by genetically engineering the cell to secrete the protein in response to an external stimulus. The external stimulus will be a molecule that interacts with the gene regulatory elements. The gene product may be secreted systemically, released locally, or remain attached to the cell surface (48). Regulation of gene function is a complex series of events. There are two classes of regulatory elements. The *cis*-acting elements are nucleic acid sequences that function as promoters of a gene and are found on the same chromosome as the regulated gene. As promoters, these nucleic acid sequences are found immediately upstream (5′) and parallel to the gene initiation sequence. However, they may also act as enhancers that are found up or downstream at considerable distance from the gene. The *trans*-acting elements are regulatory proteins that act on both pairs of homologous genes and are usually encoded on chromosomes other than the chromosome carrying the gene that is regulated by them. When insert-

ing a gene into a foreign cell it will likely be necessary to provide some of the *cis*-acting nucleic acid sequences while the *trans*-acting regulatory proteins will be provided by genes in the recipient cells (49).

Cancer

The monogenic and polygenic disorders discussed above are those genetic mutations that are passed on through parental germ cells. While a number of cancers can be related to germline mutations of particular genes, breast cancer being a particularly good example where, the majority of mutations causing cancer are somatic cell mutations. There are also possibilities that some cancers are a combination of somatic and germ cell mutations, where the cancer phenotype resulting from the germ cell genotype is not seen until a second somatic cell mutation occurs to allow expression of the cancer phenotype (34).

Mutations in protooncogenes and tumor suppressor genes are major causes of cancer. Oncogenes were first discovered in tumor cells but are also found in normal cells where they are termed protooncogenes. The protooncogene product functions as a regulator of cell growth and differentiation where it is involved in the transmission of external cellular environment growth stimuli to the cell apparatus inside the nucleus controlling cell growth. These protooncogene products are usually involved in phosphorylation/dephosphorylation mechanisms. Inappropriate activation or deregulation of the protooncogene results in an oncogene that produces inappropriate or uncontrolled cell growth (Table 41.4). The transformation of protooncogenes to oncogenes may occur *via* the following molecular mechanisms:

i) Point mutation of the protooncogene, altering the structure of the gene product such that it becomes a more efficient or unregulated protein.

ii) Juxtaposition of a promoter sequence adjacent to a protooncogene increasing its transcription.

iii) Amplification of the protooncogene through production of multiple independent single gene copies.

Obviously, in many cases, the oncogene and protooncogene products are identical but differ in the fact that the latter is regulated in its function while the former is not. Oncogenes produce uncontrolled growth through (50):

i) Excess production of growth factors.

ii) Enriched or aberrant growth factor receptors signaling growth stimulation even in the absence of growth factor.

iii) Protein kinases (phosphorylating enzymes) abnormally altering cell regulation proteins through phosphorylation.

iv) Abnormal cell regulation protein signaling growth.

v) Altered transcription factors stimulating cell replication.

Tumor suppressor genes (Table 41.5) are also normal components of cell regulation. Normally, the suppressor gene product will arrest replication of a cell with damaged DNA until the DNA is repaired. Failure to repair the DNA and resume normal function will result in programmed cell death (apoptosis). Therefore, the loss of suppressor genes may result in uncontrolled cell growth arising from cell transformation. Gene therapy can be carried out in which the tumor suppressor gene (p53 and RBI as examples) is inserted into tumor cell lines to stimulate apoptosis killing the tumor cells.

Gene therapy for cancers may take one or more of the following forms (36,51):

i) Insertion of a gene into the cancer cell to alter the malignant phenotype. Attempts to repair or replace oncogenes or mutated tumor suppressor genes would be examples.

ii) Cell surface expression of foreign proteins. The gene encoding the human leukocyte antigen B7 (HLA-B7) can be injected into unwanted cells. The expression of HLA-B7 on the surface of a cell stimulates a cytotoxic T-cell (CTL) response that destroys the cell.

iii) Secretion of cytokine proteins that immunopotentiate an antitumor response. The tumor cells can be removed and grown in tissue culture, transfected with the gene encoding such immune stimulating cytokines as the granulocyte-macrophage-colony stimulating factor, IL-1, IL-2, IL-4, IL-6, tumor necrosis factor (TNF), or gamma interferon (IFN). The cultured transformed tumor cells are then reimplanted into the patient and stimulate a strong immune response against the tumor cells. This approach not only destroys the tumor cells but has the potential to immunize against recurrence of the tumor. There are also tumor-infiltrating leukocytes that are transformed with the tumor necrosis factor (TNF-TILs) *ex vivo* and then reintroduced into the body. These transformed TILs will seek out tumors and stimulate an immune response through secretion of TNF.

iv) Enzyme conversion of a pro-drug to its toxic metabolite (51). Ganciclovir is a nucleoside analogue related to acyclovir that inhibits DNA polymerase. The drug is first monophosphorylated by thymidine kinase, followed by di- and triphosphorylation and the triphosphorylated form acts as a substrate for DNA polymerase and the en-

Table 41.4. Functional Classification of Selected Oncogenes and Associated Human Tumors*

Function	Oncogene	Associated Tumors
Growth factor	HST	Gastric cancer
	KS3	Kaposi sarcoma
Growth factor receptor	NEU/ERB-B2	Breast, ovary, gastric cancers
	ERB-B	Breast cancer, glioblastoma
	TRK	Papillary thyroid, colon cancers
Signal transducing (GTP-binding) proteins	Ha-RAS	Bladder cancer
	Ki-RAS	Lung, colon cancers
	N-RAS	Leukemias
	GSP	Pituitary tumors
Protein kinases	RAF	Gastric cancer
	MET	Osteosarcoma
	ABL	Leukemia/lymphoma
Nuclear transcription factor	MYC	Lymphomas, carcinomas
	N-MYC	Neuroblastoma
	L-MYC	Small cell lung cancer
Membrane proteins	BCL-2	Follicular, undifferentiated lymphoma
	MAS	Breast cancer
	RET	Papillary thyroid cancer

*Taken from reference 50.

Table 41.5. Tumor Suppressor Genes*

Gene	Gene Product	Tumor Associations
RBI (13q)**	110-kDa nuclear hypophosphorylated protein, negative cell cycle regulator	Retinoblastoma Osteosarcoma Small cell lung cancer Soft tissue sarcoma Breast cancer Bladder cancer
P53 (17p)	53-kDa sequence-specific DNA-binding protein and transcriptional activator	Li-Fraumeni syndrome Most common alteration in human cancer
DCC (18q)	1447 amino acid transmembrane protein with homology to known adhesion molecules, role in terminal cell differentiation	Colorectal cancer
APC (Sq21)	2843 amino acid protein which interacts with membrane-associated cadherin catenin complexes and with microtubules	Familial adenomatous polyposis Gardner's Syndrome
MTSI (9q21)	148 amino acid protein inhibitor of cyclin dependent kinase-4	Familial melanoma
BRCA1 (17q)	1863 amino acid protein with zinc finger-like domains suggesting functions as a transcriptional factor	Breast cancer Ovarian cancer
BRCA2 (13q)	Possibly BRUSH 1	Familial breast cancer
VHL (3p)	Protein with short homology to a glycan-anchored membrane protein to T. brucei, no function assigned	Pheochromocytoma Renal cell cancer Pancreatic cancer Hemangioblastomas of CNS and retina
WT-1 (11q)	50-kDa gene related to the early growth response gene, encodes four 46- to 49-kDa proteins that appear to function as DNA binding transcriptional repressors	Wilms' tumor
NF-1 (17q11.2)	Neurofibromin (about 2500 amino acids), probably negative regulator for p21 ras	Von Recklinghausen's neurofibromatosis
NF-2 (22q12)	Schwannomin (about 600 amino acids), regulator of cellular response to external environment	Neurofibromatosis type 2

*Taken from reference 50.
**Number in brackets indicates the chromosomal location.

zyme is subsequently inhibited. The herpes simplex virus thymidine kinase has a much higher selectivity for ganciclovir than does the mammalian cell thymidine kinase and is therefore much more efficient at phosphorylating the drug. The gene coding for herpes simplex virus thymidine kinase (HSV-tk) is introduced into tumor cells and ganciclovir is administered to the patient resulting in a selective inhibition of DNA polymerization in the tumor cells carrying HSV-tk. The technology does not permit transformation of the entire tumor mass with the HSV-tk gene but the treatment is designed to reduce the tumor burden. The "bystander effect" where the toxic metabolite of ganciclovir formed in transfected tumor cells is transferred to surrounding unmodified tumor cells, possibly through phagocytosis of the apoptotic vesicles, is thought to be responsible for instances where the HSV-tk/ganciclovir treatment has resulted in complete tumor elimination.

v) Delivery of genes to bone marrow cells providing resistance to conventional chemotherapeutic agents which are then used to reconstitute the bone marrow of patients before treatment with intensive, and otherwise lethal, chemotherapeutic regimens.

Infectious Disease

Infectious diseases such as hepatitis, herpes and HIV are chronic infectious diseases that may be suitable targets for gene therapy. Two general areas are the focus of current efforts in controlling infectious diseases (20,36,52). The first is the post-exposure vaccination that attempts to boost the host immune response to the infection. This polynucleotide vaccine approach delivers genes encoding viral or microbial antigens that are designed to trigger cytotoxic T cells (CTLs) to assist in the elimination of the infected cells.

Intracellular immunization is an alternative approach that attempts to express genes in target cells that render them incapable of being infected or of supporting viral replication. The ways in which intracellular immunization through gene therapy can be used to inhibit viral or microbial replication include:

i) Antisense RNA targeting specific viral or microbial mRNA sequences that interferes with the normal replication and expression of those sequences.

ii) Ribozymes are RNA molecules that act as catalysts and are designed to cleave microbial or viral RNA at specific unique sites.

iii) Decoy RNAs are short sequences of RNA that compete with important nucleic acid binding proteins that are required for viral replication.

iv) Genes that express single chain antibodies that are specifically designed to bind viral proteins.

Gene Delivery

A major problem in gene therapy is similar to the problem encountered in all forms of drug therapy that being the assurance of drug efficacy through efficient delivery of the therapeutic agent to its biologic target in a fully functional form (53). Gene delivery is unique in the sense that it is the product of gene function, the protein, not the gene itself that is the therapeutic agent. Hence, we must not only deliver the gene to its proper target but we must also assure that when the gene reaches its target it will arrive in a form that will produce the therapeutic agent in such a form that it too will be assured of reaching its specified target. What is most critical in gene delivery is the effective modulation of the production of the therapeutic protein. Constitutive expression of some proteins may occur without adversely affecting the therapeutic efficacy. However, constitutive expression of most genes is not desirable and can even be life threatening. For example, as seen above, many forms of cancer involve the constitutive expression of proteins involved in stimulation of cell division. The proper, controlled delivery of the protein necessitates the prior delivery of the gene to the cell nucleus and this special consideration for gene delivery compared to conventional drugs warrants the development of novel vehicles for the delivery of genes to the cell nucleus.

Most gene therapy protocols involve the use of viruses as gene carriers or vectors. However, there are also nonviral methods of gene delivery appearing in the NIH approved gene therapy protocols. In both cases, the steps involved in the delivery of the therapeutic agent include (Fig. 41.26) (54):

i) **Administration** or introduction of the nucleic acid (DNA) into the body which usually involves either *in vivo* or *in vitro (ex vivo)* techniques.

ii) **Delivery** of the nucleic acid from the site of administration to the nucleus which includes directing the bioavailability, uptake of the nucleic acid (DNA) into the cell, and translocation of the nucleic acid from the cytosol to the nucleus.

iii) **Expression** of the nucleic acid product including the normal steps in gene expression—transcription, translation, and post-translational modification. Expression is vital to the therapeutic efficacy of the gene in the sense that controlled expression of genes is important to proper biological function. With few exceptions delivery technologies result in continuous gene expression.

The viral and nonviral vectors approach the nucleic acid delivery problem from opposite directions. Viral vectors are reduced in complexity to make them less immunogenic yet maintain the efficient delivery properties while nonviral vectors are altered to increase the com-

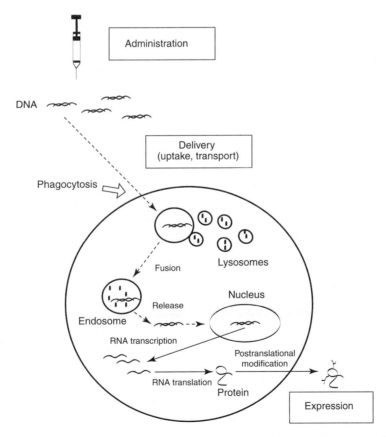

Fig. 41.26. Steps in gene therapy. Gene therapy involves the steps of administration, delivery and expression (Note: dashed arrow represents uptake and transport).

Table 41.6. Comparison of the Properties of Various Vector Systems*

Features	Retroviral	Adenoviral	AAV	Herpes
Maximum Insert Size	7–7.5 kb	~30 kb	3.5–4 kb	150 kb
Concentrations (Viral particles per ml)	$>10^8$	$>10^8$	$>10^{12}$	$>10^8$
Route of gene delivery	Ex vivo	Ex/in vivo	Ex/in vivo	Ex/in vivo
Integration	Yes	No	Yes/no	No
Duration of expression in vivo	Short	Short	Long	Long
Stability	Good	Good	Good	Good
Ease of preparation (scale up)	Pilot scale up, up to 20–50 liters	Easy to scale up	Difficult to purify, difficult to scale up	—
Immunologic problems	Few	Extensive	Not known	—
Pre-existing host immunity	Unlikely	Yes	Yes	—
Safety problems	Insertional mutagenesis	Inflammatory response, toxicity	Inflammatory response, toxicity	—

*Adapted from reference 55.

plexity of their delivery systems to improve the specificity and efficiency of nucleic acid delivery. It is likely that the ideal vector will be a composite of viral and nonviral delivery vehicles. Nonviral gene delivery systems are composed of synthetic or semisynthetic gene formulations. Some of the properties that might be features of the ideal delivery vector include:

i) No limit in the size of the gene that can be incorporated into the vector.
ii) Absence of immunogenicity.
iii) Ability to target specific tissue or cell populations.
iv) Incorporation of elements that limit the expression of delivered genes to specific cell types.
v) Ability to modulate the levels of gene expression in response to exogenous and endogenous signals.
vi) Stability and ease of productivity in large quantities at high concentrations.

Viral Vectors

Virus-based gene delivery arose from the attempt to exploit the highly evolved viral pathways for infection to achieve efficient delivery and expression of therapeutic genes in the body (3,55,56). Viral vectors are attenuated or defective viruses engineered to carry therapeutic genes. Several different viruses have been developed as vectors for gene therapy including the murine C-type oncovirus and human immunodeficiency virus (retroviruses), adenovirus, adeno-associated virus, and the herpes simplex virus (Table 41.6). Ultimately, the therapeutic gene vectors should target specific types of genetically damaged cells, insert into a specific position in the cell's genome, and produce large amounts of the corrective protein in a regulated fashion.

Retrovirus. The retroviruses (*Retroviridae*) have three subfamilies: the *Spumavirinae* (foamy viruses), the *Lentivirinae* and the *Oncovirinae* (57). The oncoviruses based on the murine C type oncovirus are the vector of choice for gene therapy protocols. The retrovirus enters the target cells where its RNA genome is converted to proviral DNA and transported to the nucleus. In the nucleus, the proviral DNA becomes integrated into the host chromosomal DNA thus ensuring long term persistence and stable transmission to all progeny of the transduced cell (Fig. 41.27).

The murine leukemia viruses (MLVs) have been the most widely used vectors for gene therapy. Human retroviral gene therapy requires replication defective vectors capable of delivering the therapeutic gene to the target cells without causing severe infection by further replication. The proviral genome has a complex sequence of essential components necessary for mRNA reverse transcription and integration of the viral RNA (57). These elements serve to carry out packaging to ensure encapsidation of: 1) vector RNA; 2) portions of the genome directing reverse transcription; 3) regions necessary for the integration of the vector DNA into the host cell chromosome in the ordered and reproducible manner characteristic of retroviruses. However, the protein coding sequences *gag, pol,* and *env* can be discarded and replaced with the therapeutic gene (Fig. 41.28).

The modified vector carrying the cDNA of the therapeutic gene is incapable of forming viral particles since the *gag, pol,* and *env* genes are missing. Therefore, a retroviral packaging cell line is required to provide the viral "helper" functions that have been deleted from the vector. The *gag, pol,* and *env* genes are stably expressed in the packaging cell from helper plasmids that lack the ψ packaging sequence and therefore the transcripts from the helper plasmid are not packaged in viral particles (Fig. 42.28). The *gag, pol,* and *env* proteins are produced and form the viral core as well as the envelop proteins. The vector transcript carrying the ψ packaging sequence and the therapeutic gene is recognized by the gag proteins and incorporated into the core particle which then buds off into a one-time-only infective particle delivering the therapeutic gene to the target cell. The *gag, pol,* and *env* genes are not packaged in a viral particle because the sequence carrying these genes is lacking the packaging signal (Fig. 41.28B).

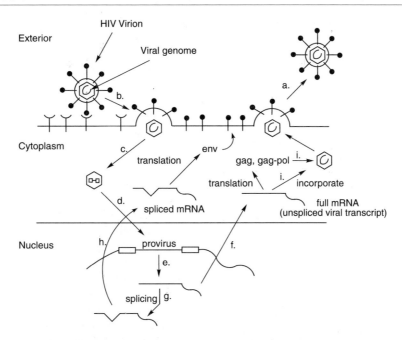

Fig. 41.27. Retroviral entry into target cells. The HIV virion is composed of a nucleotprotein core surrounded by an envelope. The core contains the viral genome, which consists of two identical positive single-stranded RNA molecules and viral proteins. a) The envelope is derived from the cell membrane when the virion buds from the cell; b) penetration into the cell is initiated by and dependent on specific interactions between the viral gp120 molecule, which is embedded in the viral envelope, and the cellular receptor, the CD4 molecule; c) after partial uncoating of the virus, viral RNA is reverse transcribed to form a linear double-stranded DNA molecule; d) this is then translocated into the nucleus as part of a pre-integration complex, where it integrates into the host genome; e) the integrated viral DNA, called a provirus, is the template for transcription, a process that is under the strict regulation of the viral *tat* gene; the initial viral transcript is; f) either transported to the cytoplasm without further processing to serve as genomic RNA, or; g) remains in the nucleus where it undergoes a series of splicing reactions regulated by the viral *rev* gene; h) which generates mRNAs for viral protein synthesis; i) the newly synthesized viral proteins (gag, and gag-pol) associate with unspliced viral transcripts to form viral cores; j) which bud through the cell membrane, acquiring the viral envelope.

Adenovirus (58). Adenoviruses (AV) are DNA viruses that belong to the *Adenoviridae* family of viruses. They are the most widely used DNA viruses for gene transfer vectors. The primary target for AV infection is the respiratory epithelial cells. The AVs are large viruses and hence can carry large DNA inserts up to 35kb (see Table 41.6). They can transduce nondividing cells and produce very high titers in culture. They are also human viruses and are able to transduce a large number of different human cell types at a very high efficiency. Unlike the retroviruses, the adenoviruses do not integrate into the host cell chromosome but remain in the nucleus as an extrachromosomal element or episome. Due to the extra-chromosomal nature of the double-stranded DNA insert, the therapeutic gene is eliminated over time.

The major problem with adenoviral vectors is immunotoxicity. Since the recombinant adenoviral vectors are attenuated (not defective) viruses, they express several viral proteins. The result is induction of cytopathic and immunogenic responses *in vivo*. Some of the attempts to improve the adenovirus as a therapeutic gene vector include (3):

1. Reduction of immunogenicity by further mutation of genome to reduce viral protein production.
2. Increasing the potency of the virus to reduce the immune challenge.

3. Co-administration of immunosuppressants with the vector therapy.

Adeno-associated Virus (58). The adeno-associated virus (AAV) is a nonpathogenic, single-stranded DNA virus belonging to the *Parvoviridae* family of viruses. This virus has two genes; the *cap* gene encodes for three viral coat proteins and the *rep* gene encodes for four proteins involved in viral replication and integration. This virus needs additional genes to replicate that are provided by the helper virus which is usually the adenovirus or herpes virus. Interest in this virus as a vector arose from the discovery that the *rep* gene product directs the virus to integrate the viral DNA preferentially into human chromosome 19. The AAV vector is produced by replacing the *rep* and *cap* genes with the therapeutic gene. Without a helper virus, the AAV will integrate into the host genome and remain as a provirus. Because of the toxic nature of the *rep* gene products, it is difficult to develop a packaging cell line in which all the protein can be stably produced and this is a major problem with the AAV as a therapeutic gene vector. Also, since the rep proteins are missing in the therapeutic gene vector, the site specific insertion in chromosome 19 is not observed. The AAV is a small vector that can only carry genes of ~4.8 kb and the defective vector does not efficiently integrate into the genome of nondividing cells.

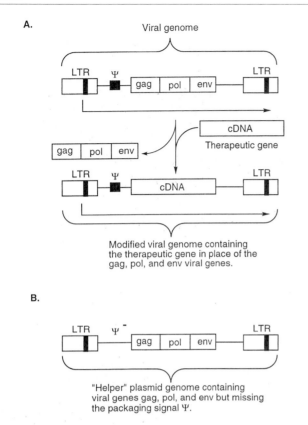

Fig. 41.28. A. Schematic representation of the preparation of a single gene retroviral construct. The therapeutic gene replaces the retroviral gag, pol, and env genes. Expression of the therapeutic gene is driven off the viral long terminal repeat (LTR) containing the retroviral packaging signal sequence (ψ); **B.** Schematic representation of a helper cell genome containing the retroviral gag, pol, and env genes but lacking the packaging signal sequence (ψ-).

Herpes Simplex. Herpes simplex virus (HSV) is a member of the alpha-herpes virus family that are nuclear DNA viruses with large genomes capable of carrying therapeutic genes up to 150 kb. These viruses are able to establish lifelong latent infections in which the viral genome exists as a stable episome in the host cell (59, 60). Genes delivered by the HSV vector can be maintained indefinitely as an episome in long-lived cells such as those of the nervous system. HSVs made replication deficienct by deleting the transcriptional regulator gene IE-3 are used as therapeutic gene vectors. Plasmids containing the HSV origin of replication and packaging signal are called "amplicons." The amplicon can also be used as a vector in the presence of a helper virus which is usually the IE-3 deficient HSV. In this case, the amplicon/helper virus requires a complementary cell line that provides the IE-3 gene product to assist in forming the replication deficient viral vectors. Long term expression is a major obstacle to routine use of this virus as a therapeutic vector.

Nonviral Vectors

Compared to the conventional small molecule drugs that are the mainstay of pharmaceutical care, the plasmids that are utilized to carry the therapeutic DNA (gene) in nonviral vectors are large, circular, hydrophilic macromolecules of bacterial origin with a hydrodynamic diameter between 100–200 nm approximating 3000 kDa in molecular weight (5–10 kbp) (see Fig. 41.29) (3). Plasmids carry a net negative charge, are susceptible to nucleases, and their potential as a class of pharmaceuticals is limited by their colloidal and surface properties. The size and charge density of these particles are problematic when it comes to their delivery as therapeutic agents and these properties depend upon the number of base pairs and the DNA conformation. Supercoiled DNA has higher negative charge density than linear, or nicked-circular DNA and therefore has a more negative zeta potential (electrophoretic mobility) than nicked-circular DNA that is slightly more negative than linear DNA (3). The zeta potential varies between -30 and -70 mV and effectively prevents the plasmid from crossing biologic membranes. Plasmids contain the therapeutic gene of mammalian origin and other DNA sequences to control the gene expression *in vivo*. The plasmid may also contain genetic elements controlling mRNA stability and the timing of protein production, cell specific promoters and enhancers to limit gene expression to specific sites in the body, as well as sequences to direct post translational processing and secretion of the gene product. Plasmids delivered by nonviral techniques do not integrate into the host genome at doses used but remain in the nucleus as extrachromosomal material called episomes. The plasmids will therefore persist in the target cells according to the biochemical half-life of the molecule that can be any where from several months to a few hours. Therefore, as the transfected cells replicate, the DNA is gradually lost over time. The nonviral techniques thus provide a finite period of expression of the therapeutic gene. The advantage is that the techniques may be applied to both chronic and acute diseases where the dose and frequency of administration is controlled by the clinician and the level of expression may be quickly adjusted or even terminated in response to a patient's changing clinical needs. Plasmids also contain nucleic acid sequences that allow them to be grown in bacteria including a prokaryotic origin of replication and selectable markers thus allowing the plasmids to be amplified through cloning in bacteria.

Some of the specific barriers to the *in vivo* delivery of DNA have been identified (3):

1. Rapid degradation of DNA within tissues or blood by nucleases.
2. Limited dispersion of DNA from the site of interstitial administration.
3. The inability of DNA to cross intact basement membranes of the endothelium or epithelium effectively.
4. The rapid clearance of DNA from the vascular compartment by cells of the reticuloendothelial system.
5. The need for effective interaction with the surface of the target cell to induce internalization.
6. Destruction of DNA in the endosomal/lysosomal compartments by nuclease, acid, and reducing agents.

7. The need to penetrate to the nucleus of cells across the perilasmic membrane and nuclear membrane.

The elements of a nonviral gene delivery system include a gene coding for the therapeutic gene, a plasmid-based expression system, and a synthetic delivery system.

Direct Injection (61). The microinjection of naked DNA in the form of circular plasmids is often used for introducing genes into embryos to engineer transgenic animals. Delivery is localized to the site of injection and unless the injection is made directly into the cell, the problem of uptake of naked DNA into the cell limits the efficiency of the technique. There has been some success in using this technique to deliver genes to skeletal and cardiac muscle tissue that has been attributed to the possibility that the sarcoplasmic reticulum and transverse tubules found in muscle tissue are favorable structures for DNA uptake. DNA uptake through the cavelolae in muscle via potocytosis involves invagination of the caveloae rich membranes. There is potential for using direct injection of naked DNA in DNA vaccinations where delivery need not be widespread since stimulation of the immune system is the goal of vaccination.

Electroporation. Electroporation is used in research for the transfection of a wide range of plant and animal cells many of which are not amenable to transfection by other methods such as calcium phosphate coprecipitation. Electroporation likely involves a physical interaction between the cell membrane and the applied electric field and as such may be relatively independent of cell type. The procedure involves charging a capacitor with a conventional power supply and then discharging the capacitor (2–10 kV/cm) through a cell suspension containing DNA over a very short time period (<5 μs). Mammalian cells have been transfected with a weaker pulse (0.53 kV/cm) and a longer duration (7000 μs) (62). The DNA enters when the cells are exposed to a pulsed electric field presumably disrupting the membrane lipids and creating pores in the cell membrane without damaging the membrane structure (63). DNA concentration and voltage are critical parameters for electroporation. There is a sharply defined voltage for efficient transfection depending upon the buffer and capacitance. The procedure should be applied over a range of voltages to determine the best voltage for the experimental conditions. The local potential difference across the cell is the driving force for membrane pore formation and is proportional to the product of the capacitor voltage and the cell diameter (64). Therefore, the voltage optimum for transfection will depend inversely on cell size (62).

Particle Bombardment. Particle bombardment involves the generation of a shockwave *via* an explosive device (65), compressed gas (66), or electrical discharge (67) to propel DNA coated gold or tungsten particles into the target tissue. The gold particles are usually 1–3μm in size while the tungsten particles are slightly larger (around 4μm). The particles are coated with DNA by precipitation through addition of calcium chloride and spermidine solutions to the plasmid DNA in the presence of a suspension of the gold or tungsten particles. The DNA coated particles are deposited on macrocarrier discs and a

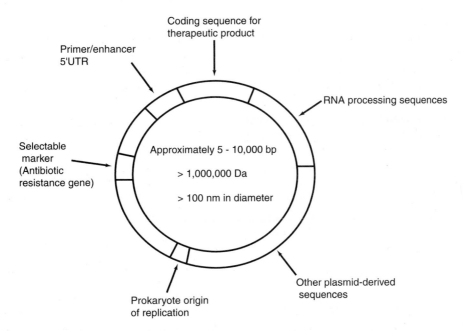

Fig. 41.29. Plasmid DNA constructed for gene delivery contains a therapeutic gene sequence, eukaryotic gene promoter regions, prokaryotic origins of replication, selectable markers, as well as RNA processing sequences and other plasmid derived sequences. Adapted from Ledley FD. Pharm Res 1996;13:1595–1614, with permission.

shockwave generated as described above accelerates the particles to a high velocity enabling efficient penetration of target organs, tissues, or single cells in their path. Some acceleration devices can be finely tuned to adjust the velocity and resulting distribution of particles in various target tissues by varying the discharge voltage or gas pressure, bead density, and bead size. This technique is not likely to be widely used for gene delivery because it is essentially a surgical procedure and the particles are only able to penetrate several millimeters into the target tissue, however, it may well have widespread use as a gene vaccine delivery vehicle (68).

Calcium Phosphate Precipitation. One of the early methods of facilitating the transport of DNA into cells was the coprecipitation of DNA with calcium phosphate or calcium chloride and applying the precipitate to a monolayer of cells (69). While the mechanism of uptake is not fully understood it is postulated that the particulate nature of the calcium phosphate/DNA complex adheres to the cell membrane and is taken up by endocytosis. The pH of the buffer during the formation of the precipitate, the gradual formation of the precipitate (overnight incubation of the DNA in the calcium phosphate 2X N,N-bis(2-hydroxyethyl)-2-aminoethane sulfonic acid buffered saline [2X BBS]), and the concentration of the DNA are critical factors in determining the efficiency of the procedure in delivering DNA to the cell (70, 71). pH of approximately 7.0 and DNA concentrations of 40 µg/ml result in the most efficient uptake of DNA by the mammalian cells. Calcium is an efficient facilitator of DNA uptake for a number of reasons. It increases the concentration of DNA on the cell surface through precipitation, it protects the DNA from digestion by serum and intracellular nucleases and calcium phosphate itself induces phagocytosis. The calcium phosphate precipitate may also neutralize the negative charge on the DNA molecule thus facilitating penetration of the lipid membrane and also reducing repulsion of the negatively charged DNA by the negatively charged cell membrane. Other cations including polyornithine, polylysine, polybrene, and diethylamnoethylamine have also been used as cationic facilitators for cellular uptake of DNA (72,73). The most efficient facilitated DNA uptake is observed in cells at the exponential stage of growth. However, this technique depends upon the phagocytosis of the DNA/Calcium Phosphate particle resulting in endosome formation and the exposure of the DNA to the intracellular endosome/lysosome degradation process.

Cationic Lipids

Cationic lipids, or "cytofectins" as they are sometimes called, are positively charged amphiphilic molecules that interact with the negatively charged phosphate backbone of DNA molecules neutralizing the charge and promoting the condensation of DNA into a more compact structure

(74–76). The chemical composition of the cationic lipids consists of (Fig. 41.30):

1. A hydrophobic lipid anchor that aids in the formation of cationic liposomes that are critical components of the complex with DNA.
2. A linker group that is located between the cationic head group of the molecule and the lipid tail. The linker determines the chemical stability and biodegradability of the cationic lipids. The most common link is the alkyl ether.
3. The cationic head group that is responsible for the complexation of the liposome with the negatively charged DNA. The cationic group is a singly or multiply charged primary, secondary, tertiary, or quaternary amine. The common counter ions found with the cationic lipids are the bromide, chloride, or trifluoroacetate anion.

The cationic lipids are most frequently used in a 0.5 molar ratio with a neutral, zwitterinic phospholipid (usually dioleoyloxyphophatidylethanolamine—DOPE) called the colipid. The cationic lipid and colipid form unilamellar (ULV) and multiamellar (MLV) liposomes that are approximately 100 nm and 300–700 nm in diameter, respectively. The role played by the cationic lipid in the cationic liposome is multifold and includes causing the condensation of DNA to form a particle with specific colloidal properties, controlling the distribution of DNA particles

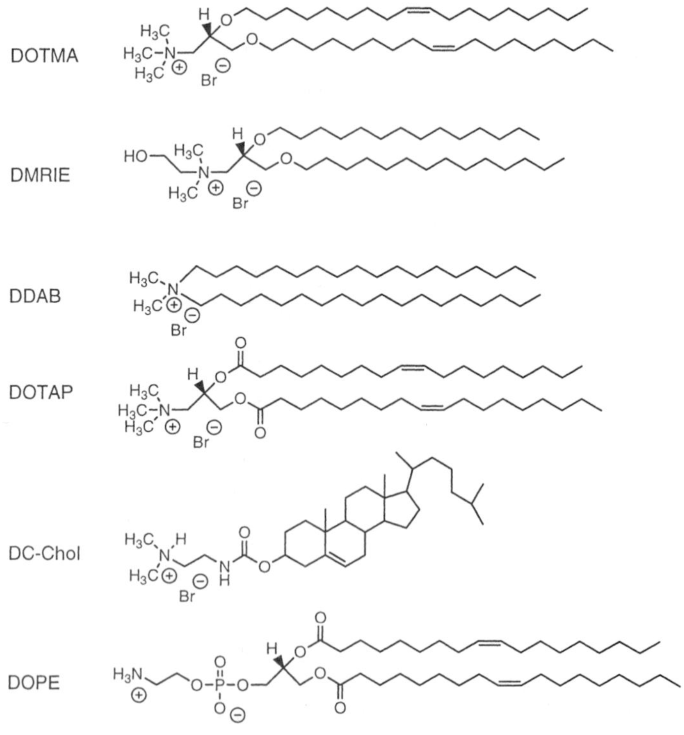

Fig. 41.30. Chemical structures of common cationic lipids: 1,2-dioleyl-oxypropyl-3-trimethylammonium bromide (DOTMA), 1,1-dimyristyl-oxypropyl-3,3-dimethyl-3(2-hydroxyethyl) ammonium bromide (DMRIE), N,N-dimethyl-N,N-dioctadecylammonium bromide (DDAB), 1,2-dioleoyloxy-propyl-3-trimethylammonium bromide (DOTAP), 3β-[N-(N,N-dimethylaminoethyl)carbamoyl]cholesterol hydrobromide (DC-Chol), 1,2-dioleoylpropyloxyphosphatidylethanolamine (DOPE).

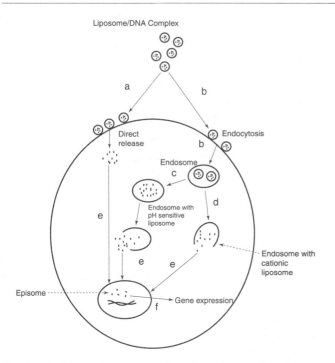

Liposome/DNA Complex

Fig. 41.31. Schematic representation of possible modes of interaction of liposomes with cells that lead to intracellular delivery. Liposomes can enter the cell by local destabilization of plasma membrane or fusion (a) or endocytosis (b). The release of DNA by fusion is still not clear (c or d). The released DNA or cationic liposome-DNA complexes reach into the nucleus (e) and gene expression occurs (f). Adapted from Singhal A, Huang L. Gene Transfer in Mamalian Cells Using Liposomes as Carriers. In: JA Wolff ed., Gene Therapeutics, p118, 1994, with permission.

in the body, causing the particles to interact with the target cell, and finally inducing cytosis to aid entry of the particle into the cell. The colipid may play an active role in the internalization of DNA into the cell through facilitating the fusion of the DNA/lipid complex with the cell membrane or endosome membrane releasing the DNA into the cytoplasm (Fig. 41.31).

The cationic liposomes are absorbed onto the surface of the negatively charged cyclic polynucleotide (plasmid) to form aggregates that gradually surround the larger segments of the DNA. At a critical lipid concentration, the processes of lipid fusion and DNA collapse are initiated. Subsequent increase in the lipid concentration causes the collapsed DNA structures to become coated in the lipid bilayers. The final product is like a "condensed nanoparticle" with the lipid bilayers providing an internal structure that looks like the ridges of a fingerprint (77). Generally, the complexes formed with the larger multilamellar vesicles are more active than those formed with the smaller unilamellar vesicles.

The plasmid/lipid complexes tend to aggregate over time and this aggregation is a function of a number of factors which may include: cationic lipid species, the DNA/cationic lipid ratio and concentrations, shearing force, temperature, solution viscosity, time, and salt and serum protein content. This instability necessitates that the plasmid/lipid complex be formed immediately prior to use and therefore limits the ability of the user to characterize and control the parameters of the formulations. The positive charge on the complex also results in an unfavorable interaction with negatively charged cellular proteins leading to aggregation of the complex and premature release of the DNA. Cationic lipids also interact with the complement system of the body and are therefore opsonized by the C3b/C4b components resulting in rapid clearance by macrophages in the reticuloendothelial systems. The particle size and the zeta potential of the plasmid/lipid complexes depends upon various factors including the cationic lipid species, the amount and type of colipid, the particle size and composition of the liposomes used in the preparation, the molecular weight, the form and type of plasmid, the stoichiometry of the cationic lipid and DNA, concentration of lipid and DNA in the final preparation, and the mixing procedure.

Interaction of the plasmid/lipid complex with the target cell membrane occurs when the cationic lipid preparation has a high positive charge that results in an ionic interaction with the negatively charged cell membrane. The mechanism of transfer of the plasmid to the nucleus is poorly understood. Two hypotheses currently describe the mechanism, neither of which is mutually exclusive of the other (Fig. 41.31). One hypothesis suggests that the plasmid/lipid complex fuses with the target cell membrane and expels the plasmid into the cytosol where it then makes its way to the nucleus where it is taken up and remains as extrachromosomal material (episome). The second hypothesis suggests that the nanoparticle plasmid/lipid complex interacts with the target cell membrane and is absorbed through endocytosis. The colipid then aids in the fusion of the plasmid/lipid complex with the endosomal membrane and the disintegration of the endosome prior to interaction with the lysosome and destruction of the plasmid.

The presence of cationic lipids in the preparation may enhance gene delivery in several ways as indicated in Table 41.7.

Similar delivery systems have been designed using other cationic polymers including lipopolyamines (78), amphipathic peptides (79), polylysine lipids (80), cholesterol (81), quaternary ammonium detergents (82), polyamidoamines

Table 41.7. Actions of Cationic Lipids Which Enhance Gene Delivery

- Protect the DNA against degradation by nucleases.
- Modify the size, charge, and surface characteristics of the DNA containing particulate to control its biodistribution within the body and access to the target cell.
- Improve the interaction of DNA with the surface of the target cell.
- Induce endocytosis.
- Improve release of DNA from the endosome.
- Improve the entry of DNA into the nucleus.

called dendrimers, polyethylenimines or chitosan, DEAE dextran, and polybrene.

Nonviral Targeted Gene Transfer.   Receptor mediated uptake of nucleic acids is approached through the complexation of the DNA with protein ligands specific for cellular receptors. This technique is carried out by covalently linking the protein ligand to a positively charged polylysine polymer and then complexing the ligand/polymer unit to DNA by ionic interaction with the negatively charged phosphate groups. The interaction of polylysine with DNA causes the condensation of DNA into a compact torus shaped (toroidal) protein/DNA structure that may be as small as 80 nm in diameter (83) and similar to that seen for the interaction of the cationic lipids with DNA. The protein retains its ability to interact with its receptor on the cell surface and the resulting complex causes internalization of the DNA through endocytosis of the protein/receptor complex. The procedure for preparation of the covalent polylysine/ligand complex is illustrated in Figure 41.32. The amino groups on the lysine side chains of polymers of lysine containing 90, 270, or 450 lysine monomers ($pLys_{90}$, $pLys_{270}$, or $pLys_{450}$) are derivatized with 3-(2-pyridyldithio)propionate (SPDP) to give a pyridyldithiopropionate (PDP) intermediate that is

then reduced with dithiothreitol to give the 3-mercaptopropionate-modified polylysine containing approximately one mercaptopropionate group per 50 lysine residues in the polymer. A PDP derivative of the ligand is also prepared and conjugated with the mercaptopropionate polylysine polymer through disulfide bond formation. This procedure generally results in approximately one ligand linked to every 50 residues of the polylysine polymer.

The ligand/polylysine covalent complex is subsequently mixed with DNA plasmids containing the therapeutic gene to be targeted to the cells carrying the ligand receptor to condense the DNA and form the ligand/polylysine/DNA complex (Fig. 41.32). The targeted cells are exposed to the complex either *in vitro* through exposure of a cell culture to the complex or *in vivo* through intravenous injection of the complex into the host. The following ligand/complexes have been used to deliver genes to specific cell targets:

- Transferrin/polylysine/DNA—hematopoietic cells, T-cells, pulmonary epithelial cells.
- Asialoorosomucoid/polylysine/DNA—liver cells.
- Insulin/polylysine/DNA—liver cells.
- Surfactant B/polylysine/DNA—epithelial airway cells.
- Antithromobmodulin/polylysine/DNA—epithelial airway cells.

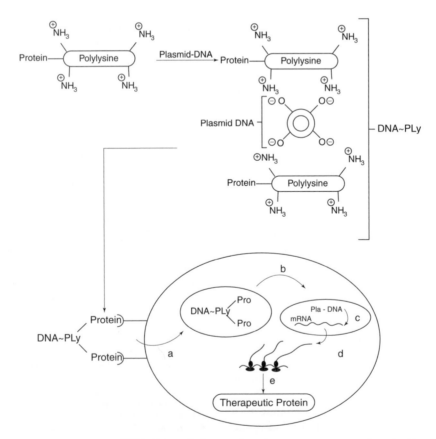

Fig. 41.32. Schematic representation of nonviral targeted gene transfer. The process involves complexation of a protein-polylysine component to plasmid-DNA (DNA~PLy) followed by protein assisted cellular absorption (a) into hepatocytes, transfer into the nucleus (b), transcription of the plasmid~DNA (Pla~DNA) into mRNA (c), and translation into therapeutic protein (e). Note that the protein is linked to the polylysine by a disulfide bond.

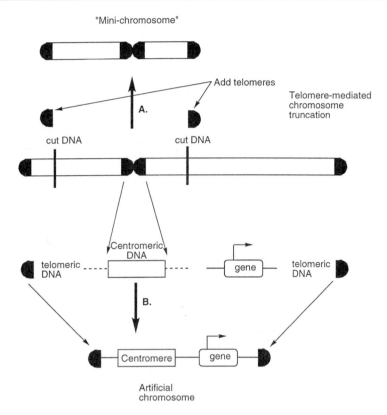

Fig. 41.33. Two approaches for manipulation of a human chromosome. **A)** Mini-chromosomes can be generated in cultured cells by chromosome truncation mediated by the integration of telomeric sequences into chromosome arms. **B)** Alternatively, artificial chromosomes might be constructed by combining the known functional elements of a human chromosome: telomeric DNA, centromeric DNA, and genomic DNA containing a human gene or selectable genetic marker.

Several small molecules including folate, galactose, lactose, and N-acetyl galactosamine have also been used to prepare polylysine/DNA complexes for delivery of DNA by receptor mediated endocytosis.

The major factors limiting the *in vivo* effectiveness of the protein/DNA complexes may be the poor bioavailability to many target cells and their colloidal instability in physiologic media. The endocytotic uptake of the recetor complex also limits the effectiveness of the delivery system since the DNA is quickly destroyed in the endosome/lysosome pathway.

Artificial Chromosomes—YACs, and HACs

A more recent development in gene delivery that has potential for developing into a therapeutic gene delivery system is the artificial chromosome. Genetic manipulation of the yeast genome has resulted in the development of yeast artificial chromosomes (YACs). These linear structures utilize the same basic functional elements as the normal linear mammalian and yeast chromosomes.

The capacity for YACs to carry very large fragments of foreign DNA permits the cloning of genes with all their natural genomic elements in correct spatial orientation. YACs have been used in the preparation of large DNA fragments for sequencing in the Human Genome Pro-

ject. They have also been very useful in the analysis of gene function and the creation of chromosome transgenic mice.

The potential of artificial chromosomes for gene therapy is currently being investigated (84–86). The development of a properly segregating, autonomously replicating "mini-chromosome" has the potential to eliminate the disadvantages of viral vectors such as genomic insertional position effects, gene size restrictions, and the lack of proper regulation of gene function.

The human chromosome is far larger and more complex than the yeast chromosome. In spite of numerous complications, the human artificial chromosome (HAC or MAC) is being developed and the potential applications to gene therapy investigated (87). Two approaches are currently being used to create the HAC (Fig. 41.33). Small human chromosomes called "mini-chromosomes" are being developed through truncation of the normal chromosome mediated by insertion of human telomeres (the specialized structure of the ends of the chromosome) into the chromosome arms creating shortened chromosomes 3.5–9 Mb in size (87). Alternatively, many steps have been taken toward creating an artificial chromosome through the assembly of the known functional elements of a human chromosome with genomic DNA containing a human gene (88).

Pharmacokinetics and Metabolism of DNA

Genes can be delivered using either *ex vivo* or *in vivo* strategy (see above). The *ex vivo* strategy encounters intracellular barriers presented by the cell that include the cell, endosome, and nuclear membranes (Fig. 41.34).

Depending upon the *ex vivo* vector used, the DNA can be delivered directly to the cell cytosol through fusion of the vector with the cell membrane of the DNA may enter the cell through endocytosis creating the endosomal membrane barrier. Endosomal DNA can be released from the endosome into the cytosol or the endosome may fuse with the lysosome resulting in degradation of the DNA by nucleases and the acidic environment of the lysosome. Cytosolic DNA is susceptible to a variety of nucleases found in cellular cytosol and that which reaches the nuclear membrane is taken up by an active transport mechanism possibly similar to that of protein uptake by the nuclear membrane (89). Once inside the nucleus, the transgene DNA is still susceptible to degradation by nucleases.

DNA delivery *in vivo* faces additional extracellular barriers posed by specific tissues and the immune system (Fig. 41.34). The blood-brain barrier, connective tissue, and epithelial cell linings are particular examples of cellular structures that may impede delivery of DNA to the target cells. Humoral and cellular immune responses also pose serious barriers to successful delivery of DNA to target cells.

DNA is rapidly eliminated from the compartment into which it is administered as a result of both degradation through endo- and exonucleases and distribution to other compartments. DNA is eliminated from the blood compartment by interaction with Kuppfer cells through a specific scavenger/receptor interaction (90). An IV administered asialo-orosomucoidpolylysine-DNA complex was cleared from the blood with an apparent half life of 2.5 min. (91). The DNA taken up by the liver was eliminated with a half life of 1–1.3 hours, gene transcripts were evident for 1–12 hours, and the gene product persisted for 6–24 hours.

Different tissues have been shown to display different DNA pharmacokinetics. Genes and gene products have been observed as long as 19 months after direct injection without indication of plasmid integration or replication (92). Direct injection of the chloramphenicol acetyltransferase gene into the thyroid resulted in elimination of DNA from the gland with a half-life of 10 hours. The enzyme activity was maximal for 24 hours and eliminated through first order kinetics with an apparent half-life of 40 hours (93). Similar results were recorded for synovial fluid intra-articular administration of plasmid DNA (94).

If the therapeutic gene is not incorporated into the host cell genome, the level of the therapeutic product can be controlled by adjusting the dose and administration schedule as for any conventional drug therapy. However, the for-

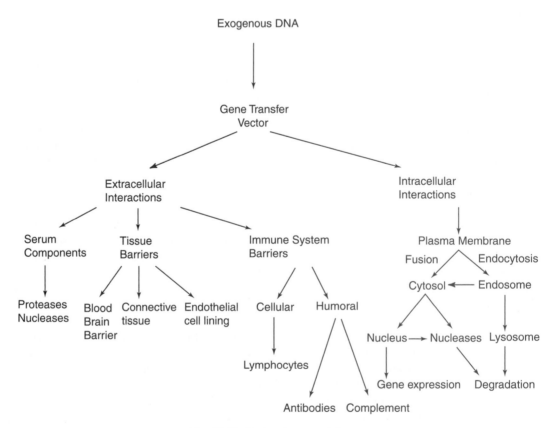

Fig. 41.34. Barriers to gene delivery.

mulation of the delivery vehicle and the design of the gene expression vector affects the duration and level of therapeutic activity. Gene therapy also provides unique pharmacokinetic issues in that the apparent kinetic properties of the therapeutic agent are a combination of the intrinsic kinetic properties of the DNA vector, the RNA transcript, and the translated protein product (95). The intrinsic kinetic parameters are described by a six component model of DNA pharmacokinetics (95). Flux between the compartments labeled Milieu, Endosome, Cell, RNA, protein, and Product will reflect the biologic process of uptake, endosomal transport into cells, transcription, translation, and secretion. DNA will also be subjected to degradation in each of the compartments. While this is a first approximation of the processes involved in using genes as medicines, a total description of DNA pharmacokinetics will likely include:

- Compartmental distribution and extracellular elimination of DNA after *in vivo* administration.
- Efficiency of DNA uptake into cells.
- Compartmentalization of DNA within the endosomal, cytoplasmic, and nuclear compartments of the cell.
- Rate of degradation of DNA within the cell.
- Rate of transcription of RNA from DNA.
- Stability of the mRNA.
- Rate of translation of the mRNA to create the new gene product.
- Rate of post-translational modification of the gene product.
- Intracellular compartmentalization or secretion of the gene product.
- Pharmacokinetics of the gene product in the body.

CONCLUSIONS

Genetic technology has evolved over the past 30 years to the stage where we are on the verge of determining the entire sequence of the 3 billion base pairs in the human genome. The impact that such a scientific advance will have on our lives has yet to be determined but the social, legal, ethical, and economic issues are certain to be extensive and complex. The Human Genome Project (HGP) is developing scientific technology for the manipulation and analysis of the human genome. This analysis will in turn provide valuable information on the relationship between genotype and potential for serious genetic disease. The HGP is already paying dividends in the analysis and therapy of monogeneic diseases such as cystic fibrosis. However, the greatest killers of western society such as cancer, diabetes, cardiovascular disease, and many others not only involve multiple genes but are also subject to environmental factors. As a result, many serious diseases will only be predicted with a certain potential and the possibility of preventative therapy that manipulates an individual's environment to reduce the potential will add another dimension to health care.

We are likely to be inundated with information on the genetic composition of individuals and populations. Information management will be a daunting task in the wake of the completion of the HGP. Already the relatively new science of Bioinformatics is developing methods for storing and retrieving the vast amounts of information that the HGP is generating (see National center for Biotechnology Information web page at www.ncbi.nlm.nih.gov). The social, legal, and ethical implications involved in the storage and release of information about the human individual must balance the individual's right to self determination and control of personal information against the interests of third parties and the public (2,37,96). One can see that the HGP is not only creating a revolution in the medical sciences but the social, legal, and economic sciences are also being challenged to reevaluate their vision of the social structure. The future will see an altered form of health care utilizing a genetic information infrastructure to contain costs and predict outcomes, create advanced personalized therapies, and develop a predict-and-manage paradigm of health care (35).

Acknowledgments: I am grateful to Scott Loucks for proofreading this chapter and providing many criticisms and suggestions. However, any errors or omissions remain my responsibility.

REFERENCES

1. Crick FH. On Protein Synthesis. Symposium of the Society for Experimental Biology 1957;12:138–163.
2. Kitcher P. The Lives To Come: The Genetic Relationship and Human Possibilities. 1st Touchstone ed: Simon and Schuster; 1997.
3. Ledley FD. Pharmaceutical approach to somatic gene therapy. Pharmaceutical Research 1996;13(11):1595–1614.
4. Twyman RM. Advanced Molecular Biology: A Concise Reference: Bios Scientific Publisher, Springer; 1998.
5. Watson JD, Crick FHC. Molecular structure of nucleic acid. Nature 1953:171:737–738.
6. Wolff JA, Lederberg J. An early history of gene transfer and therapy. Human Gene Therapy 1994;5(4):469–80.
7. Terheggen HG, Lowenthal A, Lavinha F, et al. Unsuccessful trial of gene replacement in arginase deficiency. Journal of Experimental Medicine 1975;119:1–3.
8. Wade N. UCLA gene therapy racked by friendly fire. Science 1980;210:509–511.
9. Wade N. Gene therapy pioneer draws Mikadoesque rap. Science 1981;212:1253.
10. Wade N. Gene therapy caught in more entanglements. Science 1981;212:24–25.
11. Crystal RG, McElvaney NG, Rosenfeld MA, et al. Administration of an adenovirus containing the human CFTR cDNA to the respiratory tract of individuals with cystic fibrosis [see comments]. Nature Genetics 1994;8(1):42–51.
12. Blaese RM, Culver KW. Gene therapy for primary immunodeficiency disease. Immunodeficiency Reviews 1992;3(4):329–349.
13. Bordignon C, Mavilio F, Ferrari G, et al. Transfer of the ADA gene into bone marrow cells and peripheral blood lymphocytes for the treatment of patients affected by ADA-deficient SCID. Human Gene Therapy 1993;4(4):513–520.
14. Bordignon C, Notarangelo LD, Nobili N, et al. Gene therapy in peripheral blood lymphocytes and bone marrow for ADA-immunodeficient patients. Science 1995;270(5235):470–475.

15. Kohn DB. Gene therapy for hematopoietic and immune disorders. Bone Marrow Transplant 1996;18 Suppl 3:S55–58.

16. Hay JG, McElvaney NG, Herena J, et al. Modification of nasal epithelial potential differences of individuals with cystic fibrosis consequent to local administration of a normal CFTR cDNA adenovirus gene transfer vector. Human Gene Therapy 1995;6(11):1487–1496.

17. Knowles MR. New therapies for cystic fibrosis. Introduction. Chest 1995;107(2 Suppl):59S–60S.

18. Zabner J, Couture LA, Gregory RJ, et al. Adenovirus-mediated gene transfer transiently corrects the chloride transport defect in nasal epithelia of patients with cystic fibrosis. Cell 1993;75(2):207–216.

19. Grossman M, Rader DJ, Muller DW, et al. A pilot study of ex vivo gene therapy for homozygous familial hypercholesterolaemia [see comments]. Nature Medicine 1995;1(11):1148–1154.

20. Hess P. Gene therapy: a brief review. Clinical Laboratory Medicine 1996;16(1):197–211.

21. Calladine CR, Drew HR, Understanding DNA: The Molecule and How it Works. 2nd ed. New York: Academic Press; 1997.

22. Saenger W. Principles of Nucleic Acid Structure. New York, Berlin, Heifdelberg. Tokyo: Springer-Verlag: 1994.

23. Lewin B. Genes IV. 4th ed. Oxford, England and Cambridge, Mass.: Oxford University Press and Cell Press; 1990.

24. Watson JD, Gilman M, Witkowski J, et al. Recombinant DNA. 2nd ed. New York: Scientific American Books, W.H. Freeman and Company; 1992.

25. Sanger F, Nicklen S, Coulson AR. DNA sequencing with chain-terminating inhibitors. Proc Nat Acad Sci USA 1977;74: 5463–5467.

26. Maxam AM, Gilbert W. A new method of sequencing DNA. Proc Nat Acad Sci USA 1977;74:560–564.

27. Atkinson A, Smith M. Solid-phase synthesis of oligodeoxyribonucleotides by the phosphitetriester method. In: Gait MJ, editor. Oligonucleotide Synthesis: A Practical Approach. Oxford, England: IRL Press Limited; 1984. p. 35–82.

28. Sproat BS, Gait MJ. Solid-phase synthesis of Oligodeoxyribonucleotides by the phosphotriester method. In: Gait MJ, editor. Oligonucleotide Synthesis: A Practical Approach. Oxford, England: IRL Press Limited; 1984. p. 83–115.

29. Newton CR, Graham A. PCR. 2nd ed. New York, NY.: Springer-Verlag: 1997.

30. Conley CL. Sickle Cell Anemia: The First Molecular Disease. In: Wintrobe MM, editor. Blood, Pure and Eloquent. New York: McGraw-Hill; 1980. p. 320–359.

31. Weatherall DJ. Towards an Understanding of the Molecular Biology of Some Common Inherited Anemias: The Story of Thalassemia. In: Wintrobe WW, editor. Blood, Pure and Eloquent. New York: McGraw-Hill; 1980. p. 373–407.

32. Weatherall DJ. Science and the Quiet Art: The Role of Medical Research in Health Care. New York and London: W.W. Norton and Company; 1995.

33. Wang DG, et al. Large-scale indentification, mapping, and genotyping of single-nucleotide polymorphisms in the human genome. Science 1998;208:1077–1082.

34. Weatherall DJ. The New Genetics and Clinical Practice. 3rd ed. Oxford, New York, Tokyo: Oxford University Press; 1991.

35. Bezold C, Halperin JA, Eng JL, editors. 20/20 Visions: Health Care Information Standards and Technologies. Rockville, Maryland: The United States Pharamacopeial Convention, Inc.; 1993.

36. Orkin SH, Motulsky AG. Report and Recommendations of the Panel to Assess the NIH Investment in Research on Gene Therapy. Washington D.C.: National Institutes of Health; 1995.

37. Harris J. Clones, Genes, and Immortality: Ethics and Genetic Revolution. Oxford: Oxford University Press; 1998.

38. Marshall A, Hodgson J. DNA chips: An array of possibilities. Nature Biotechnology 1998;16:27–31.

39. Davis B. Speed freaks. New Scientist 1998;160:47–50.

40. Ramsay G. DNA chips: State-of-the-art. Nature Biotechnology 1998;16:40–44.

41. Schmidt K. Just for you. New Scientist 1998;2160:32–36.

42. Nebert D. Polymorphisms in drug-metabolizing enzymes: What is their clinical relevance and why do they exist? The Am J Human Genetics 1991;60:265.

43. Langer R. New Methods of drug Delivery. Science 1990;249:1527–1533.

44. Langer R, Vacanti J. Tissue Engienering. Science 1993;260: 920–926.

45. Naffakh N, Henri A, Villeval JL, et al. Sustained delivery of erythropoietin in mice by genetically modified skin fibroblasts. Proc Nat Acad Sci USA 1995;92:3194–3198.

46. Moullier P, Bohl D, Heard J-M, et al. Correction of lysosomal storage in the liver and spleen of MPS VII mice by implantation of genetically modified skin fibroblasts. Nature Genetics 1993;4:154–159.

47. Langer R. Tissue Engineering: A New Field and Its Challenges. Pharmaceutical Reserach 1997;14:840–841.

48. Bohl D, Heard J-M. Modulation of erythropoietin delivery from engineered muscles in mice. Human Gene Therapy 1997;8:195–204.

49. Weatherall DJ. Scope and limitations of gene therapy. Brit Med Bull 1995;51:1–11.

50. Mastrangelo MJ, Berd D, Nathan FE, et al. Gene Therapy for Human Cancer: An Essay for Clinicians. Seminars in Oncology 1996;23:4–21.

51. Freeman SM, Wartenby KA, Freeman JL, et al. In Situ Use of Suicide Genes for Cancer Therapy. Seminars in Oncology 1996;23:31–45.

52. Gilboa E, Smith C. Gene therapy for infectious diseases: the AIDS model. Trends in Genetics 1994;10:139–144.

53. Blau HM, Springer ML. Molecular Medicine: Gene Therapy—A novel form of drug delivery. New Engl J Med 1995;333(18): 1204–1207.

54. Ledley FD. Nonviral gene therapy: The promise of genes as pharmaceutical products. Human Gene Therapy 1995;6: 1129–1144.

55. Verma IM, Somia N. Gene therapy—promises, problems and prospects. Nature 1997;389:239–242.

56. Anderson WF. Human gene therapy. Nature 1998;392 S25–30.

57. Vile RG, Russel SJ. Retroviruses as vectors. Brit Med Bull 1995;51:12–30.

58. Kremer EJ, Perricaudet M. Adenovirus and adeno-associated virus mediated gene transfer. Brit Med Bull 1995;51(1):31–44.

59. Efstathiou S, Minson AC. Herpes virus-based vectors. Brit Med Bull 1995;51(1):45–55.

60. Fink DJ, Glorioso JC. Engineering herpes simplex virus vectors for gene transfer to neurons. Nature Medicine 1997;3(3):357–359.

61. Davis HL, Whalen RG, Demeneix BA. Direct gene transfer into skeletal muscle in vivo: factors affecting efficiency of transfer and stability of expression. Human Gene Therapy 1993;4:151–159.

62. Chu G, Hayakawa H, Berg P. Electroporation for the efficient transfection of mammalian cells with DNA. Nucleic Acids Research 1987;15(3):1311–1326.

63. Kinosita K, Jr., Tsong TY. Voltage-induced pore formation and hemolysis of human erythrocytes. Biochimica et Biophysica Acta 1997;471:227–242.

64. Neumann E, Schaefer-Ridder M, Wang Y, et al. Gene transfer into mouse lyoma cells by electroporation in high electric fields. EMBO Journal. 1982;1:841–845.

65. Klein TM, Wolf ED, Wu R, et al. High-velocity microprojectiles for delivering nucleic acids into living cells. Nature 1987;327:70–73.

66. Williams RS, Johnston SA, Riedy M, et al. Introduction of foreign genes into tissues of living mice by DNA-coated microprojectiles. Proc Nat Acad Sci USA 1991;88:2726–2730.

67. Christou P, McCabew DE, Martinell BJ, et al. Soybean genetic engineering—commercial production of transgenic plants. Trends in Biotechnology 1990;8:145–151.

68. Tang D-C, DeVit M, Johnston SA. Genetic immunization is a simple method for eliciting an immune response. Nature 1993;356:152–154.

69. Graham FL, Van der Eb AJ. A new technique for the assay of infectivity of human adenovirus 5 DNA. Virology 1973;52:456–460.

70. Loyter A, Scangon GA, Ruddle FH. Mechanisms of DNA uptake by mammalian cells: Fate of exogenously added DNA monitored by the use of fluorescent dyes. Proc Nat Acad Sci USA 1982;79:422–426.

71. Chen C, Okayama H. High-efficiency transformation of mammalian cells by plasmid DNA. Mol Cell Biol 1987;7:2745–2752.

72. Kawai S, Nishizawa M. New procedure for DNA transfection with polycation and dimethyl sulfoxide. Mol Cell Biol 1984;4:1172–1174.

73. Farber FE, Melnick JL, Butel JS. Optimal conditions for uptake of exogenous DNA by chinese hamster lung cells deficient in hypoxanthine-guanine phosphoribosyltransferase. Biochemica et Biophysica Acta 1975;390:298–311.

74. Mahato RI, Rolland A, Thomlinson E. Cationic lipid-based gene delivery systems: Pharmaceutical perspectives. Pharmaceutical Research 1997;14:853–859.

75. Felgner JH, Kumar R, Sridhar CN, et al. Enhanced gene delivery and mechanism studies with a novel series of cationic lipid formulations. J Biol Chem 1994;269:2550–2561.

76. Felgner PL, Gadek TR, Holm M, et al. Lipofection: A highly efficient, lipid-mediated DNA-transfection procedure. Proc Nat Acad Sci USA 1987;84:7413–7417.

77. Tomlinson E, Rolland AP. Controllable gene therapy. Pharmceutics of non-vial gene delivery systems. Journal of Controlled Release 1996;39:357–372.

78. Behr J-P, Demeneix B, Loeffler J-P, et al. Efficient gene transfer into mammalian primary endocrine cells with lipopolyamine-coated DNA. Proc Nat Acad Sci USA 1989;86:6982–6986.

79. Legendre J-Y, Szoka FCJ. Cyclic amphiphathic peptide-DNA complexes mediate high-efficiency transfection of adherent mammalian cells. Proc Natl Acad Sci USA 1993;90:893–897.

80. Zhou X, Huang L. DNA transfection mediated by cationic liposomes containing lipopolylysine: characterization and mechanism of action. Biochimica et Biophysica Acta 1994;1189:195–203.

81. Li S, Gao X, Son K, et al. DC-Chol lipid system in gene transfer. Journal of Controlled Release 1996;39:373–381.

82. Pinnaduwage P, Schmit L, Huang L. Use of quaternary ammonium detergent in liposome mediated DNA transfection of mouse L-cells. Biochimica et Biophysica Acta 1989;985:33–37.

83. Wagner E, Cotton M, Foisner R, et al. Transferrin-polycation-DNA complexes: The effect of polycations on the structure of the complex DNA delivery to cells. Proc Nat Acad Sci USA 1991;88:4255–4259.

84. Huxley C. Mammalian artificial chromosomes: a new tool for gene therapy. Gene Therapy 1994;1:7–12.

85. Calos MP. The potential of extrachromosomal replicating vectors for gene therapy. Trends in Genetics 1996;12:463–466.

86. Vos J-MH. Mammalian artificial chromosomes as tools for gene therapy. Current Opinion in Genetics and Development 1998;8:351–359.

87. Willard HF. A systematic approach toward understanding human chromosome structure and function. Proc Natl Acad Sci USA 1996;93:6847–6850.

88. Willard HF. Human artificial chromosomes coming into focus. Nature Biotechnology 1998;16:415–416.

89. Melchior F, Gerace L. Mechanisms of nuclear protein import. Current Opinion in Cell Biology 1995;7:310–318.

90. Kawabata K, Takakura Y, Hashida M. The fate of plasmid DNA after intravenous injection in mice: involvement of scavenger receptors in its hepatic uptake. Pharmaceutical Research 1995;12:825–830.

91. Stankovics J, Crane AM, Andrevos E, et al. Over expression of human methylmalonyl CoA mutase in mice after in vivo gene transfer with asialoglycoprotein/polylysine/DNA complexes. Human Gene Therapy 1994;5:1095–1104.

92. Manthorpe M, Cornefort-Jensen F, Hartikka J, et al. Gene therapy by intramuscular injection of plasmid DNA: Studies on firefly luciferase gene expression in mice. Human Gene Therapy 1993;4:419–431.

93. Sikes M, O'Malley BWJ, Finegold MJ, et al. In vivo gene transfer into rabbit and thyroid follicular cells by direct DNA injection. Human Gene Therapy 1994;5:837–844.

94. Yovandich J, O'Malley BWJ, Sikes M, et al. Gene transfer to synovial cells by intraarticular administration of plasmid DNA. Human Gene Therapy 1995;6:603–610.

95. Ledley TS, Ledley FD. Multicompartment, numerical model of cellular events in the pharmacokinetics of gene therapies. Human Gene Therapy 1994;5:679–691.

96. Wood-Harper J, Harris J. Ethics of human genome analysis: some virtues and vices. In: Marteau T, Richards M, editors. The Troubled Helix. Cambridge: Cambridge University Press: 1996, p. 274–294.

42. Antisense Therapeutic Agents

MARILYN SPEEDIE

INTRODUCTION
Principles

Antisense therapeutic agents are based upon a simple and elegant concept as illustrated in Figure 42.1. As genes are expressed to produce specific proteins, the two complementary strands of DNA begin uncoiling within the nucleus. The "sense" strand carries nucleic acid bases in an order which specifies which amino acids should be assembled to produce the protein. The complementary strand or "antisense" strand is used as a template for assembling a complementary strand of messenger RNA (mRNA) in the process called transcription. The mRNA will have the same sequence as the "sense" strand of DNA, but is made up of ribose sugars instead of deoxyribose sugars in the nucleotide backbone (ribonucleotides versus deoxyribonucleotides). In eucaryotes, the mRNA is further processed in the nucleus by capping and splicing and is transported into the cytoplasm where ribosomes translate the mRNA into proteins. Antisense drugs are short stretches of deoxyribonucleotide analogs which bind to specific complementary areas of the mRNA (which have a "sense" sequence) by Watson-Crick base pairing. In doing so, they can induce a nuclease (RNase H) which cleaves the mRNA at the site of the binding or can physically block translation or other steps in mRNA processing and transport, thus stopping protein synthesis. Antisense drugs thus work at an early stage in the production of a disease-causing protein and theoretically can be applied to a number of diseases where the basic pathophysiology involves an overexpression or aberrant expression of a given protein molecule. Viral diseases, cancers, and inflammatory diseases are all examples of such diseases that potentially can be treated via antisense mechanisms.

History

The beginning of antisense technology may be traced to a report of sequence specific binding of a modified DNA to complementary mRNA in 1978 (1). However, the road from demonstration of the binding to an approved human therapeutic agent has been one filled with alternating optimism and pessimism. Development steps included identification of the optimum chemistry for getting antisense molecules into cells and preventing nuclease destruction of the molecules while optimizing binding to messenger. Design of antisense molecules to achieve selective binding to the target mRNA was essential if side effects were to be minimized. After several years of optimizing the parameters to improve efficacy *in vitro* (in tissue culture), scientists moved to testing antisense candidates in animal models. This did not prove to be an easy challenge and resulted in pessimism about the ultimate utility of the products. For a period medical researchers were skeptical about the efficacy of the approach. There were questions about the reproducibility of experiments and about whether the pharmacologic effects being observed in animal experiments were the result of sequence specific antisense activity. However, careful design of experiments to provide appropriate controls eventually reversed the skepticism and now scientists generally agree that antisense approaches can lead to useful medicinal agents (2,3).

Problems associated with the automated synthesis and cost of antisense molecules have been overcome. Initially, each compound could only be synthesized in small amounts and the costs of each synthesis would have limited their clinical use. However, improvements to the technology during scale-up have resulted in prices between $50 and $100 per gram, well within a useful range for pharmaceutical agents (2).

Many people believe that we are only beginning to exploit the full potential of antisense drug development. The first generation drugs are mostly of a single chemical design and several second generation products are under development. Only time will tell how useful this approach to drug design will be.

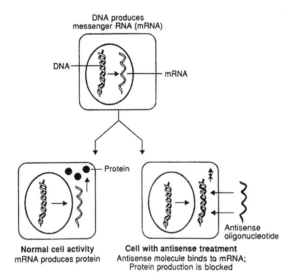

Fig. 42.1. Concept of antisense oligonucleotide inhibition of gene expression. The antisense oligonucleotide enters the cell and binds to specific complementary mRNA, causing it to be degraded or otherwise inhibiting synthesis of the corresponding protein.

**Steps in
gene expression**

**Outcome of
antisense
intervention**

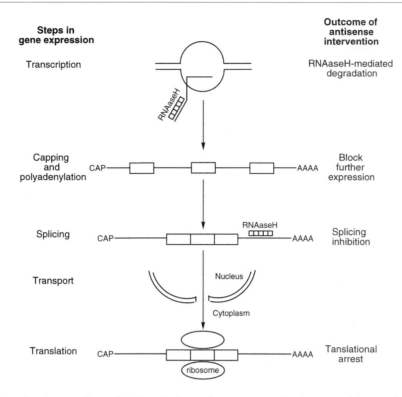

Transcription

RNAaseH-mediated
degradation

Capping
and
polyadenylation

Block
further
expression

Splicing

Splicing
inhibition

Transport

Translation

Tanslational
arrest

Fig. 42.2. Mechanism of action of antisense oligonucleotides. Each step in gene expression is a potential target for antisense oligonucleotide activity. Steps in gene expression are indicated on the left and the outcome of antisense binding is shown on the right. (Adapted from reference 7.)

DESIGN OF ANTISENSE AGENTS

While conceptually the design of an antisense strand is simple, designing an antisense therapeutic agent that will function in human disease is quite complicated. Many conditions must be satisfied for an antisense drug to function. It must be administered in a manner that delivers it to the site of action in the body without it being degraded by nucleases which are ubiquitous in human cells. It must get into the cell of the target tissue and it must colocalize with its target RNA at a sufficient concentration for a bimolecular reaction to occur. It must have a structure that favors association with the target RNA and must be designed to bind to a RNA region that is vulnerable to binding. Identification of the molecule with optimum binding is generally performed in tissue culture experiments for which 30 or 40 oligonucleotides, each about 30 nucleotides in length, are synthesized. These oligonucleotides are complementary to different portions of the target mRNA and are used to determine where the binding can be best achieved, as indicated by inhibition of synthesis of the target protein. This "brute force" effort is usually quite successful but limits initial drug discovery, in general, to industrial laboratories that have the capability to efficiently synthesis large numbers of antisense molecules. Getting to the target cell, binding to the target mRNA and inhibiting protein synthesis are necessary, but are still insufficient, to define successful antisense activity. In order for a target gene (and protein) to be suitable for

an antisense approach, there must be sufficient turnover of the resultant protein that inhibiting its synthesis will have the desired effect within a reasonable time period. This can be tested in tissue culture and in whole animals once the initial conditions are met.

Modifications in the base, sugar and phosphate moieties, as well as in the length of the polymer, have been reported in attempts to create molecules with enhanced affinity and more selective affinity for specific sites on the RNA, to enhance nuclease stability, to improve cellular uptake and distribution and to optimize distribution and clearance. There is much work remaining to define the medicinal chemistry of these molecules and to correlate the chemistry with the biologic effects. To date, the most detailed work has been done with phosphorothioate deoxyoligonucleotides, as described below, but even with this class of molecules, our knowledge is not yet at a state where optimal structures can be predicted and developed without screening multiple drug candidates.

We know that at some sites the binding of antisense oligonucleotides to mRNA creates a substrate for RNase H, leading to greater efficacy since the mRNA is actually cleaved. The antisense deoxyoligonucleotide is released and can bind to yet another mRNA molecule, thus amplifying its effect (4). Screens incorporating RNase H-mediated cleavage offer the potential to improve identification of the optimal antisense drug molecules, although these cell-free systems still leave many critical parameters undefined in

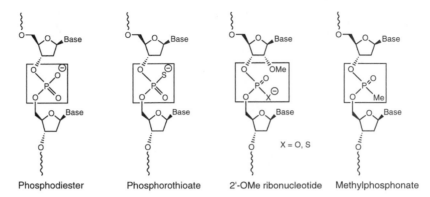

Phosphodiester   **Phosphorothioate**   **2'-OMe ribonucleotide**   **Methylphosphonate**

Fig. 42.3. Generalized structures of natural DNA (phosphodiester) and three antisense oligonucleotide derivatives tested as antisense drugs. (Adapted from reference 9.)

terms of achieving a drug that will be active *in vivo* (5). Phosphorothioate oligonucleotide complexes with mRNA can serve as substrates for Rnase H while many other oligonucleotides do not create Rnase H susceptible complexes. This appears to account, at least in part, for the efficacy of the phospohorothiates and second-generation molecules attempt to maintain the ability to be a RNase H substrate while improving other properties.

Although many studies focus on antisense drugs creating substrates for RNase H, it is important to realize that a number of other mechanisms have been identified, including inhibition of translation, inhibition of splicing and degradation of RNA via other mechanisms. Furthermore, studies, especially with antiviral antisense molecules, have shown antisense-sequence-independent effects, e.g., decreasing the adsorption of the virus, in addition to the antisense-sequence-dependent effects. Therefore, studies that attribute the effect of a given antisense molecule to an antisense mechanism must be carefully controlled to demonstrate dose-response effects, sequence specific effects, and measurement of the loss of the target RNA or protein or both (6). Figure 42.2 illustrates some of the possible sites of antisense oligonucleotide action in the transcription, processing and translation of a specific gene product. As shown in Figure 42.2, favorite targets have included RNA splice sites, 5'-capping, 3'-adenylation sites and translation start and termination sites (8). In reality, the choice of the portion of a mRNA to be a target for antisense drug action is quite empirical. Little is known about the shape of the mRNA molecules within cells and there is no common structure among the target sequences for a variety of successful antisense drugs. Therefore, there is no easy way to predict what portion of the mRNA molecule will be available for binding to the drug. Scientists make 30–40 oligonucleotides of appropriate length that complement different portions of the mRNA and use them to "march down the message" in tissue culture experiments to see where binding is best (2).

The generalized structures illustrating some of the first generation antisense oligonucleotides that were tested

are shown in Figure 42.3. Each was designed and tested with the goal of optimizing and balancing the affinity of binding for mRNA, nuclease resistance and uptake into the cells. As is seen in Figure 42.3, the first generation antisense oligonucleotide agents used methylphosphonate modifications, 2'-O-methylribonucleotides, and phosphorothioate linkages. The methylphosphonate backbone yields a molecule that is nonionic, has good nuclease resistance and forms a stable duplex with mRNA. The duplex formed is not a substrate for RNaase H. Uptake is via passive diffusion. Of the first-generation oligonucleotide antisense molecules, the class that has resulted in the broadest range of activities is the phosphorothioate class, in which one of the oxygen atoms in the phosphate group is replaced with a sulfur. The resulting compound is negatively charged, is chiral at each phosphorothioate, and is much more resistant to nuclease digestion than the parent phosphodiester compound. Compound length has been determined empirically. Molecules must have at least 7–8 complementary bases to bind to the target site and induce RNase H activity. Molecules with fewer than 13–15 bases have lower specificity with complementary mRNA and molecules longer than 20-mers result in more nonsequence specific interactions. Molecules in the range of approximately 15–20 bases (15- to 20-mers) are commonly synthesized with 18 or 20 bases generally considered optimum (3).

Although the phosphorothioate molecules (unbound to mRNA) are relatively resistant to nucleases, some nuclease degradation occurs, primarily by exonucleases (which cleave the terminal bases), and perhaps with a modest contribution by endonucleases (which cleave within the chain) as well. Phosphorothioates are taken up by a wide range of cells *in vitro* and it is thought that uptake is enhanced by the negative charge which allows binding to specific uptake proteins resulting in receptor-mediated endocytosis. Uptake is time and temperature dependent and is influenced by the cell-type, the specific sequence and length of the oligonucleotide. Cationic lipids have been used *in vitro* to enhance uptake of phosphorothioate oligonucleotides in cells that otherwise take up little of the compounds (10).

The negative charge also affects protein binding *in vivo*. The kD for albumin is approximately 150 micromolar which is similar to aspirin or penicillin (11). Phosphorothioates are rapidly and extensively absorbed after parenteral administration and are rapidly and extensively distributed to all peripheral tissues. There is no evidence of penetration of the blood-brain barrier. Clearance is primarily through metabolism by nucleases with the degraded compounds being eliminated through the urine. Oral bioavailability is less than 5%, but the limiting factor may be degradation in the gut rather than absorption *per se*. Studies with a more stable 2′-methoxyphosphorothioate oligonucleotide showed a significant increase in oral bioavailability that appeared to be associated with improved stabilty of the analogs (9).

Toxicologic studies with phosphorothioate oligonucleotides have been performed with mice, monkeys, and, to a lesser extent, with humans. The dose-limiting effect in mice is a reversible immune stimulation observed as lymphoid hyperplasia, splenomegaly and multiorgan monocellular infiltrate. These effects appear to be sequence independent and therefore are not related to the antisense mechanism. In monkeys, the dose-limiting effect is sporadic drops in blood pressure associated with bradycardia and, at higher doses, abnormalities in blood clotting, perhaps due to interactions with thrombin. In humans, systemic IV administration of ISIS 2302 (a phosphorothioate that inhibits intercellular adhesion molecule, ICAM-1) caused no significant toxicities, including no evidence of immune stimulation and no hypotension. A slight subclinical increase in activated partial thromboplastin time was observed at the highest dose (2 mg/kg) (12). Inflammation of the anterior chamber of the eye is the most common side effect of local administration of fomivirsen (see below) into the vitreous fluid (intravitreal injection) for CMV retinitis.

DRUG THERAPY

To re-emphasize, antisense drugs block the overexpression or aberrant expression of a given protein molecule linked to a disease.

Current Product—Fomivirsen

The first antisense therapeutic agent to reach the market is fomivirsen (ISIS 2922; sold as Vitravene (13). Fomivirsen is a 21-mer phosphorothioate oligodeoxynucleotide. Its structure is shown in Figure 42.4. It inhibits human cytomegalovirus, a ubiquitous herpes-virus that is the most common cause of viral retinitis in immunocompromised patients, especially those with HIV infection. Cytomegalovirus infection is characterized by the progressive destruction of retinal cells and, if untreated, leads to retinal detachment and blindness. Even with treatment, some degree of visual loss occurs in nearly all

patients with a diagnosis of CMV retinitis. It can affect one or both eyes.

Fomivirsen inhibits cytomegalovirus by at least two mechanisms. The first is a sequence-specific antisense binding to inhibit expression of immediate-early genes, thus preventing viral replication. The second is sequence-independent and involves inhibition of adsorption of cytomegalovirus to host cells, probably by direct binding to viral coat proteins (14,15). The reduction of immediate-early protein synthesis occurs in a dose-dependent manner. While it inhibits viral replication, fomivirsen does not eradicate the virus whose DNA, as for all herpes viruses, is integrated into the human genome. Therefore, treatment will have to continue for the life of the patient.

The series of clinical trials that led to FDA approval involved 430 eyes in 330 patients. Fomivirsen significantly delayed progression of cytomegalovirus retinitis in patients with AIDS, including those who had failed treatment with ganciclovir or foscarnet, the first-line therapies. Fomivirsen is administered by intravitreal injection at doses of 165 ug once weekly for three weeks of induction and then once every two weeks. It can also be administered in a dose of 330 ug on days 1, 15 and then once monthly. Mean maximum retinal concentrations of fomivirsen occur at 2 days and the elimination half-life after a single 115 ug dose in monkey retina was 78 hours. There are no systemic side effects. Ocular side effects include increased intraocular pressure and mild to moderate intraocular inflammation that can be reversed with topical steroid treatment. It is important that side effects be minor since treatment will be lifelong.

The FDA approved fomivirsen as second-line treatment of cytomegalovirus retinitis in patients with AIDS who are intolerant or unresponsive to previous treatment(s) for the disease (16). Alternative treatments include intravenous or oral ganciclovir, ganciclovir implant, cidofovir and foscarnet (17) (Chapter 39). All are virustatic and share a common mechanism, inhibition of DNA polymerase. The disadvantages of these agents include the need for an indwelling catheter for intravenous administration of ganciclovir or foscarnet and the high cost and repeated surgeries needed for the surgically implanted, controlled release ganciclovir pellets. However, in cell culture assays, fomivirsen showed additive antiviral activity with ganciclovir or foscarnet so further study may show some benefit to combination therapy in human patients who haven't yet failed with these agents.

The significance of fomivirsen goes beyond its efficacy for cytomegalovirus retinitis. The better control of AIDS that is currently being achieved fortunately is decreasing the incidence of cytomegalovirus retinitis. However, the impact of fomivirsen on the quality of life of patients with the disease is dramatic. The further significance lies in the fact that it is the first antisense therapeutic agent. This achievement indicates that the concept can be developed into efficacious and safe drug products, including solving

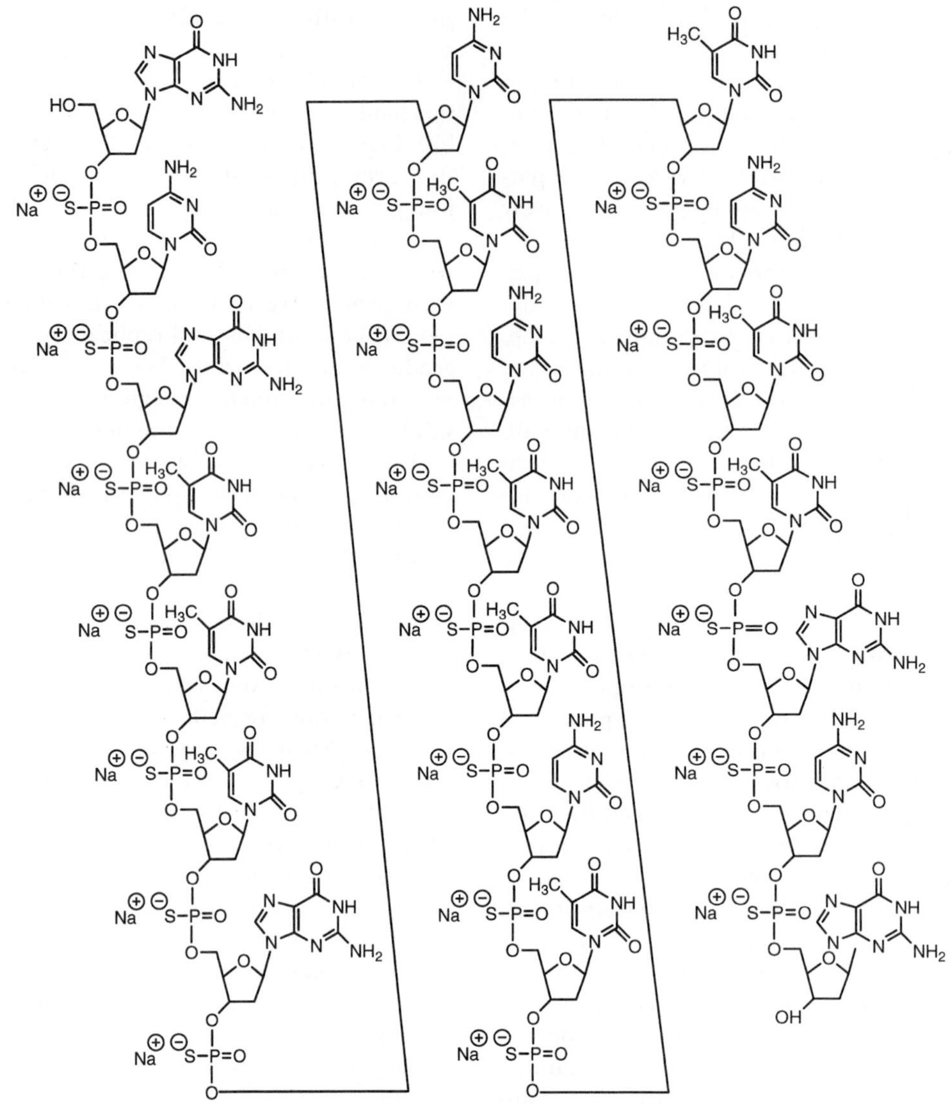

Fig. 42.4. Structure of fomivirsen, the first marketed antisense therapeutic agent. (Redrawn from reference 13.)

all the manufacturing, formulation, and analytical problems that process entails.

Products in Development

ISIS 2302 is a phosphorothioate oligodeoxynucleotide 20 bases in length with a sequence complementary to the 3'-untranslated region of the mRNA of human intercellular adhesion molecule I (ICAM-1) (18). Hybridization of ISIS 2302 to mRNA inhibits expression of the ICAM-1 protein in response to inflammatory stimuli. Initial tests of activity were performed in mice using a analogous antisense oligonucleotide that is active against the analogous mouse ICAM molecule. Studies with this oligonucleotide showed that it had anti-inflammatory activity in models of organ transplant rejection, ulcerative colitis and collagen-induced arthritis. Toxicities in the mouse model were sim-

ilar to those observed with other antisense oligonucleotides and were independent of the suppression of ICAM-1 expression. Immune stimulation, kidney changes, liver abnormalities, and increased clotting times were observed, but all toxicities were reversible and occurred at doses well above those required for pharmacologic activity. No genetic toxicity was observed (19). In a phase II human trial, 47% of patients with Crohn's disease treated intravenously with ISIS 2302, but none on placebo, were in remission after one month's treatment. No clinically significant complications were observed (18). Further clinical trials are underway.

Another potential antisense therapeutic agent for Crohn's disease is being developed in Europe. It targets nuclear-factor-kB (NF-kB) which is a transcription factor that regulates the expression of several proteins such as cytokines, adhesion molecules and acute-phase proteins, all involved in inflammation. Initial clinical trials of rectally-administered antisense DNA are underway (20). By blocking the protein synthesis of NF-kB and subsequently the molecules involved in the inflammatory response, the progression of Crohn's disease becomes limited and patient improvement is observed.

HIV is another target for antisense therapy. Trecovirsen is a 25-mer antisense phosphorothioate oligodeoxynucleotide targeted at the initiation site of mRNA from the *gag* gene of the HIV genome (21). It has a strong affinity for the complementary mRNA and produces potent, long-lasting HIV inhibitory effects in cultured HIV-infected cells. Phase I results in HIV-positive volunteers showed that it was well tolerated at single IV doses up to 2.5 mg/kg with the only significant adverse effect being a transitory increase in activated thromboplastin time at higher doses. This effect is attributed to the polyanion nature of the molecule and is independent of the antisense activity. Further clinical trials to study efficacy and safety are underway. A variety of other viral diseases are also being studied as targets for antisense pharmaceuticals (8).

FUTURE TARGETS AND DIRECTIONS

Antisense RNA produced intracellularly provides an alternative approach to regulating gene expression. In this approach one administers a synthetic gene as gene therapy that encodes an antisense RNA that can bind to the RNA transcript of the target gene and prevent that transcript from being further processed. If the gene can be administered and incorporated into the patient's genome, it can have a long-lived effect on the expression of the target gene, thus eliminating some of the delivery problems associated with more traditional antisense approach. It does however, then entail all of the problems of delivery and stability associated with gene therapy (Chapter 41). This approach has been successfully applied in plants in producing the Flavr-Savr tomato which contains an artificial gene which expresses an antisense transcript which prevents the expression and protein synthesis of polygalacturonase, thus slowing the ripening of the tomato to improve shipping characteristics (22). Its use for human therapy is still in its infancy (23).

Several alternative structures are being tested as second-generation antisense oligonucleotides. One of these involves a mixed backbone oligonucleotide (24). Studies have shown that the toxicity and immune stimulatory effects of phosphorothioates was correlated with the nuclease cleavage of a terminal CG dinucleotide. The toxicity could be minimized by the use of 2'-O-methylribonucleosides in place of four deoxynucleotides at both the 3'-end and 5'-end of the phosphorothioate oligonucleotide. It retained the RNase H substrate properties of the original phosphorothiate molecule (oligonucleotides made up

entirely of 2'-O-methylribonucleotides do not form RNase H susceptible duplexes) and had good duplex stability and better nuclease resistance. Upon intravenous administration the hybrid oligonucleotides had rapid uptake and longer elimination half-lives and analysis of tissues showed that mainly full-length oligonucleotides were present, consistent with the greater resistance to nuclease-mediated degradation compared to the nonhybrid phosphorothioate oligonucleotide. Excretion was primarily in the urine and, like phosphorothiates, these were mainly degraded products with only trace amounts of the intact molecule. Studies in rats suggest that the mixed backbone oligonucleotides may also be orally bioavailable (25–30% of the administered dose) which would present a major advantage in the utility of antisense therapeutic agents, especially for chronic diseases.

Mixed backbone hybrid oligonucleotides have also been made using methylphosphonate linkages at the ends. Methylphosphonates are nonionic, are resistant to nucleases, but do not lead to RNase H degradation. The reduced polyanionic nature of the mixed backbone oligonucleotide with methylphosphonate moieties has the potential to reduce the clotting abnormality associated with the use of phosphorothioate agents (9).

One goal for future development would be the design of orally available antisense products. Some attempts have included attaching a 2-methoxyethoxy group at the 2' site of ribose on the bases at both ends of the oligonucleotide, creating 2'-methoxyphosphorothioate analogs, and substituting aminopropoxy groups at the 2' ribose site (2). Work will continue to develop orally available compounds, particularly for chronic diseases. However, the oral availability must be balanced with penetration into target cells and tissues, binding to the mRNA, and RNase H induction.

Many additional disease targets are being studied with antisense drug candidates. Several anticancer drugs are under investigation, including drugs that target protein kinase A and c-raf kinase, a protein involved in signaling cell proliferation (2).

In summary, the concept of antisense technology has been proven, one first generation phosphorothioate oligonucleotide drug has reached the market, and second generation drugs with improved properties are under development. It seems likely that the list of marketed antisense drugs will continue to grow.

REFERENCES

1. Zamecnik PC, Stephenson ML. Inhibition of Rous sarcoma virus replication and cell transformation by a specific oligodeoxynucleotide. Proc Natl Acad Sci USA 1978; 75:280–284.
2. Rawls RL. Optimistic about antisense: Promising clinical results and chemical strategies for further improvements delight antisense drug researchers. Chem Engin News 1997; 75:35–38.
3. Stein CA. How to design an antisense oligonucleotide experiment: a consensus approach. Antisense Nucl Acid Drug Dev 1998; 8:129–132.

4. Lavrovsky Y, Chen S, Roy AK. Therapeutic potential and mechanism of action of oligonucleotides and ribozymes. Biochem Mol Medicine 1997;62:11–22.

5. Branch AD. Antisense drug discovery: can cell-free screens speed the process? Antisense Nucl Acid Drug Dev 1998; 8:249–254.

6. Crooke ST. An overview of progress in antisense therapeutics. Antisense Nucl Acid Drug Dev 1998;8:115–122.

7. Crooke ST. Molecular mechanisms of antisense drugs: RNase H. Antisense Nucl Acid Drug Dev 1998;8:133–134.

8. Field AK. Viral targets for antisense oligonucleotides: a mini review. Antiviral Res 1998;37:67–81.

9. Agrawal S, Iyer RP. Perspectives in antisense therapeutics. Pharmacol Ther 1997; 76: 151–160.

10. Juliano RL, Alahari S, Yoo H, et al. Antisense pharamcodynamics: Critical issue in the transport and delivery of antisense oligonucleotides. Pharmaceutical Res 1999; 16:494–502.

11. Crooke ST, Graham MJ, Zuckerman JE, et al. Pharmacokinetic properties of several novel oligonucleotide analogs in mice. J Pharmacol Exp Ther 1996;277:923–937.

12. Glover JM, Leeds JM, Mant TGK, et al. Phase I safety and pharmacokinetic profile of an intracellular adhesion molecule-1 antisense oligodeoxynucleotide (ISIS 2302). J Pharmacol Exp Ther 1997; 282:1173–1180.

13. Perry CM, Balfour JAB. Fomivirsen. Drugs 1999; 57(3): 375–380.

14. Azad RF, Driver VB, Tanaka K. Antiviral activity of a phosphorothioate oligonucleotide complementary to RNA of the human cytomegalovirus major immediate-early region. Antimicrob Agents Chemother 1993; 37:1945–1954.

15. Anderson KP, Fox MC, Brown-Driver V. Inhibition of human cytomegalovirus immediate-early gene expression by an oligonucleotide complementary to immediate early RNA. Antimicrob Agents Chemother 1996;40:2004–2011.

16. Crooke ST, Guest editorial: Vitravene®—Another piece in the mosaic. Antisense Nucl Acid Drug Dev 1998; 8:vii-viii.

17. Piascik P. Fomivirsen sodium approved to treat CMV retinitis. J Amer Pharm Assoc 1999; 39:84–85.

18. Yacyshyn BR, Bowen-Yacyshyn MB, Jewell L, et al. A placebo-controlled trial of ICAM-1 antisense oligonucleotide in the treatment of Crohn's disease. Gastroenterology 1998;114:1133–1142.

19. Henry SP, Templin MV, Gillett N, et al. Correlation of toxicity and pharmacokinetic properties of a phosphorothioate oligonucleotide designed to inhibit ICAM-1. Toxicol Pathol 1999; 27:95–100.

20. Bonn D. Tackling the real culprits in Crohn's disease. Lancet 1998;351:1710.

21. Sereni D, Tubiana R, Lascoux C, et al. Tolerability of intravenous trecovirsen (GEM 91), an antisense phosphorothioate oligonucleotide in HIV-positive subjects. J Clin Pharmacol 1999; 39:47–54.

22. Fray RG, Grierson D. Molecular genetics of tomato fruit ripening. Trends Genet 1993; 9:438.

23. Weiss B, Darikova G, Zhou LW. Antisense RNA gene therapy for studying and modulating biological processes. Cell Mol Life Sci 1999; 55(3):334–358.

24. Agrawal S, Zhou Q. Mixed backbone oligonucleotides:Improvement in oligonucleotide-induced toxicity in vivo. Antisense Nucl Acid Drug Dev 1998;8:135–139.

43. Selective Estrogen Receptor Modulators

V. CRAIG JORDAN

INTRODUCTION

Antiestrogenic drugs have many potential applications in medicine ranging from the regulation of fertility and the treatment of gynecologic conditions to the treatment of estrogen-responsive breast and endometrial cancers. However, the evolution of antiestrogens from failed contraceptives to the discovery that these drugs have the potential to modulate selectively the different estrogen target tissues in a woman's body is an important example of translational research that has created multifunctional drugs. The compounds block estrogen action in the breast and uterus but can maintain bone density and reduce circulating levels of cholesterol as estrogen-like molecules. The concept is known as selective estrogen receptor (ER) modulation and the drugs are collectively known as selective estrogen receptor modulators (SERMs) or designer estrogens (1).

The precise mechanism of SERM action is not well understood, but it is clear that the ER is a primary target, as a signal transduction pathway, to modulate drug action in different tissues. This chapter will describe the ER target, the pharmacologic structure-activity relationships of SERMs, and discuss their current clinical applications. However, it must be emphasized that it is the clinical success of antiestrogen therapy in breast cancer and the knowledge gained from the clinical use of tamoxifen which has opened the door to all of the other clinical applications of SERMs.

Treatment of Breast Cancer

Tamoxifen is the first antiestrogen to be used successfully for the treatment of all stages of breast cancer (33). Several laboratory principles, described 20 years ago, have been tested in clinical trials and become the standard treatment approach for women with breast cancer. After surgery only micrometastases remain, and there is no way to determine who will be cured or who will have a recurrence of their disease at a distant site. Adjuvant chemotherapy and tamoxifen treatment are designed to destroy micrometastases and increase patient survival. In the 1970s it was proposed that ER-positive patients would receive the most benefit from tamoxifen treatment (87), longer adjuvant therapy would be more beneficial than shorter therapy (88), and tamoxifen could reduce primary breast cancer incidence (89). Now, it is clear that each principle is correct and the adjuvant treatment of patients for 5 years with ER-positive primary tumors saves lives and reduces the incidence of second breast cancers by 50% (90).

HORMONE-DEPENDENT BREAST CANCER

Breast cancer is one of the most common cancers in women; one of nine women will have breast cancer in her lifetime.

In 1896, Beatson demonstrated that premenopausal women with advanced breast cancer could show improvement if their ovaries were removed (2). However, by 1900 it was clear (3) that only one in three women would receive benefit, but the reason for this clinical observation would remain obscure until the 1950s and the discovery of the ER and the description of the early events of estrogen action.

Tritium-labeled hexestrol (4) (the hydrogenated derivative of the synthetic estrogen diethylstilbestrol (5)) and estradiol (6) (the natural steroidal estrogen from the ovaries) (Fig. 43.1) bind to, and are retained by, the estrogen target tissues (uterus, vagina and pituitary gland) of laboratory animals. These findings led to the identification of an ER protein in estrogen target tissues (7) and the subsequent development of a subcellular ER model by Jensen (8) and Gorski (9) and their coworkers. The current simplified model proposes that the ER is a nuclear protein and that the steroid must diffuse into the nucleus to form a receptor complex to initiate estrogen action. Clearly, estrogen will control only those cells that contain the ER.

Jensen extrapolated the concept to preselect breast cancer patients who might respond to endocrine therapy (10). Different concentrations of ER are present in breast cancers, which can be explained by a heterogeneity of the tumor cell population. The more cells in the tumor that contain ERs, the higher the overall ER content in the tumor. Approximately 60% of ER-positive (receptor-rich) tumors are responsive to any form of additive or ablative en-

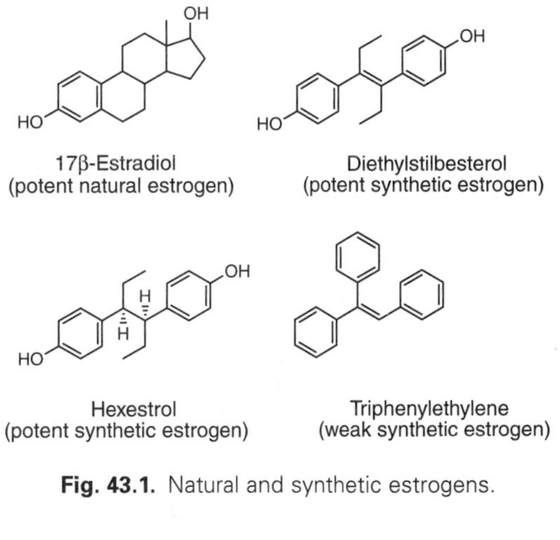

17β-Estradiol
(potent natural estrogen)

Diethylstilbesterol
(potent synthetic estrogen)

Hexestrol
(potent synthetic estrogen)

Triphenylethylene
(weak synthetic estrogen)

Fig. 43.1. Natural and synthetic estrogens.

docrine therapy, whereas only 10% of ER-negative (receptor-poor) tumors respond to endocrine therapy (11). It is now the standard of care to determine the ER status of the tumor of all patients with breast cancer.

Prevention of Breast Cancer

In 1936 Professor Antoine Lacassagne (91) suggested that if breast cancer occurred because of a specific hereditary sensitivity to estrogen then an antagonist could prevent the disease in high-risk women. Tamoxifen is the first drug that prevents breast cancer in high-risk women. However, the drug could not have been evaluated if it was not a SERM. Estrogen is essential to maintain bone density in women and to protect them from coronary heart disease. Clearly, the long-term use of an antiestrogen could have been catastrophic in well women. Breast cancer might have been prevented, but there would have been an increase in osteoporosis and heart attacks. The fact that tamoxifen has estrogen-like actions in bones (39,58) and on circulating cholesterol (59) created the appropriate drug to test as a breast cancer preventive.

In 1998 tamoxifen was found to reduce the incidence of breast cancer by 49% in high-risk women between the ages of 35 and 75 years (34). If the 20th century was the era of chemotherapy, the 21st century is marked as the era of chemoprevention.

SUBCELLULAR MECHANISM OF ESTROGEN ACTION
Overview

Two different ERs have been identified, ERα, the protein identified in estrogen target tissues (6–9), and ERβ, a new molecule cloned from a rat prostate cDNA library (12). Most knowledge about estrogen action has been derived from the study of ERα, and as a result, this model will be presented.

However, ERβ may have similar effects or modulate other aspects of estrogen action that have yet to be discovered.

A current subcellular model of estrogen action is illustrated in Figure 43.2. Estradiol diffuses into all cells but binds to the nuclear ER specifically located in estrogen target tissues (e.g., uterus, vagina, some breast cancers, etc) (13). The steroid receptor complex undergoes a conformational change and dimerizes before binding to an estrogen respose element (ERE) in the promoter region of an estrogen-responsive gene (14). A transcription unit is formed by interaction with coactivator (CoA) molecules to initiate RNA synthesis and, ultimately, the estrogen-specific cellular response (15). Corepressor (CoR) molecules are believed to prevent transcription by interacting with antiestrogen ER complexes (16). However, this aspect of antiestrogen pharmacology is not well understood.

The ER is divided into six regions (A-F) (17). The DNA-binding domain (C) is essential for the interaction of the ER with an ERE (18). The ligand-binding domain (E) is the site of E_2 binding and the site of competitive binding by antiestrogens. The AA351 is illustrated in the E region because it is the known site of interaction of the protein with the antiestrogenic side chain in raloxifene (19). The activating function (AF-1 and AF-2) regions are the areas of the ER that interact with coactivator molecules to form an effective transcription unit at an estrogen-responsive gene (20).

Based on this subcellular model of E_2 action at ERα, it is now possible to describe the action of antiestrogens and consider their molecular mechanisms of action.

Antiestrogens
Triphenylethylene Analogs

Lerner and coworkers (21) described the first non-steroidal antiestrogen, ethamoxytriphetol (MER25) (Fig.

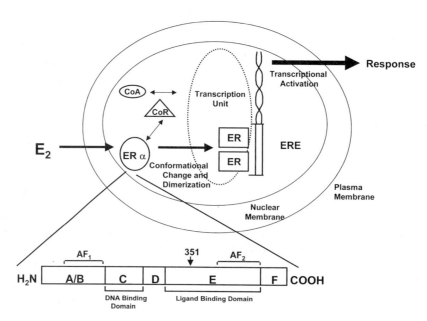

Fig. 43.2. A subcellular model of estradiol (E_2) action in a target tissue. The abbreviations used are described in the text.

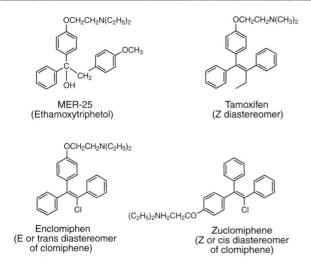

Fig. 43.3. Triphenylethylene antiestrogens.

43.3). This compound is an antiestrogen in all species tested and possesses no other hormonal or antihormonal properties. An interesting action of the compound, that sparked the interest of the pharmaceutical industry, was its ability to act as a "morning after" pill in laboratory animals (22). Unfortunately, the clinical trials of MER25 for reproductive and gynecologic applications showed that the drug had low potency and the high doses required caused central nervous system (CNS) toxicity (23). A search for more potent compounds related to the estrogen triphenylethylene showed that clomiphene (formerly MRL41) was also an effective postcoital contraceptive in laboratory animals (Fig. 43.3) (24). Clinical trials in humans, however, demonstrated that clomiphene induces ovulation (25) and does not prevent implantation. Clomiphene a mixture of E (*trans*) and Z (*cis*) geometric isomers, is used to induce ovulation in subfertile women (26). A related triphenylethylene, tamoxifen (formerly ICI46,474) (Fig. 43.3) was also discovered as part of a fertility control program (27). The drug is the separated Z diastereomer and it is also used in some countries to induce ovulation (28). However, tamoxifen, clomiphene, and a rigid analog of tamoxifen, nafoxidine (Fig. 43.4), were all found to inhibit the binding of [³H]estradiol to ER and, therefore, it was logical to test their efficacy as breast cancer treatments. Clomiphene and nafoxidine were not developed further after initial testing because of concerns about toxic side effects (29). Only tamoxifen was found to have a very low incidence of side effects compared to other endocrine therapies (30,31). Tamoxifen has now replaced endocrine ablative surgery in both pre- and postmenopausal patients with advanced breast cancer. Over the past 25 years tamoxifen has become the endocrine treatment of choice for all stages of breast cancer (32,33) and the first agent to reduce the incidence of breast cancer in high-risk pre- and postmenopausal women (34).

The pharmacologic activity of triphenylethylenes is dependent upon geometric isomerization. Clomiphene is a mixture of E and Z geometric isomers. The Z diastere-

omer (*cis*) (zuclomiphene) is an estrogen in rat uterine weight tests whereas the E diastereomer (*trans*) (enclomiphene) is a partial agonist with antiestrogenic properties (Fig. 43.3) (35). Tamoxifen, the Z diastereomer, is an antiestrogen in rat uterine weight tests but the E diastereomer (*cis*) (ICI, 47,699) is an estrogen (35). Numerous rigid analogs of the triphenylethylene structure using the 3,4-dihydronaphthalene and benzothiophene structures as building blocks, have now been tested and developed to avoid potential problems of geometric isomerization (Fig. 43.4). Nafoxidine (U-11, 100A) is antiestrogenic with antitumor properties but the drug is too toxic for human use (29). Trioxifene (LY 133314) deviates from nafoxidine by the introduction of a ketone bridging group that links the phenyl ring containing the pyrrolidinyl side chain with the rest of the molecule (36). The compound has been tested, but not developed, as a breast cancer drug. In contrast, raloxifene (formerly keoxifene, LY 156,758) has a high affinity for ER, low uterotropic activity (37) and antitumor properties in animals (38), but it was not developed as a breast cancer drug. Paradoxically, raloxifene was found to be a SERM because it maintained bone density in laboratory animals (39). The drug is available for the prevention of osteoporosis and is currently being tested in a Study of Tamoxifen And Raloxifene (STAR) for the prevention of breast cancer.

Molecular Mechanism of Antiestrogen Activity

The crystallization of the ligand-binding domain of the ER with estradiol, diethylstilbestrol, raloxifene (19) and 4-hydroxytamoxifen (40) has provided an important insight into the conformational changes that occur with agonist or antiagonist ER complexes. Figure 43.5A shows the crystal structure of estradiol or raloxifene receptor complexes (Fig. 43.5B). The most important difference is the position of helix 12 that is essential for the correct binding of coactivators to form a transcription complex at an estrogen responsive gene. Estradiol causes helix 12 to seal the ligand inside the hydrophobic pocket of the ligand-binding domain (19). It is

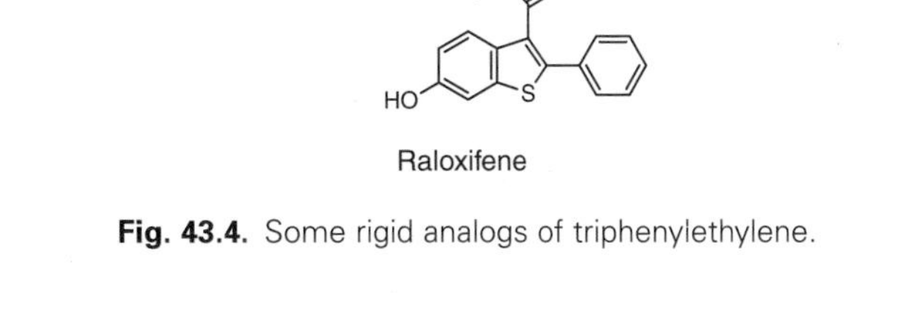

Fig. 43.4. Some rigid analogs of triphenylethylene.

A

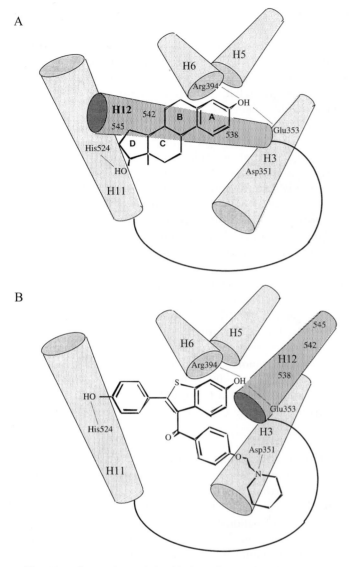

B

Fig. 43.5. Comparison of the binding of estradiol (diagram A) and raloxifene (diagram B) in the ligand binding domain of the human estrogen receptor (ER). The key event in estrogen action is the repositioning of helix 12 (H12) to seal the steroid into the hydrophobic pocket so that coactivators can bind at the key amino acids indicated on H12. This cannot happen in the raloxifene ER complex.

hypothesized that this conformation allows coactivator binding. By contrast, raloxifene prevents helix 12 from sealing the hydrophobic pocket and gene transcription is prevented because coactivators cannot bind (19). A similar model is proposed for the 4-hydroxytamoxifen ER complex, but it is clear from studies in vitro that the raloxifene and 4-hydroxytamoxifen receptor complexes have different efficacies (41). 4-Hydroxytamoxifen ER complexes are more promiscuous than raloxifene ER complexes (41,42).

Metabolism

Antiestrogens such as tamoxifen or raloxifene are metabolized extensively. Tamoxifen (Fig. 43.6) is hydroxylated mainly by CYP2D6, but also by CYP3A4 and CYP2C9 to

4-hydroxytamoxifen (43), which has a higher binding affinity for the ER (44) than the parent drug. As a rule hydroxylated metabolites have a shorter biologic half-life because of rapid phase II metabolism. Continuous administration of tamoxifen results in the accumulation of the drug to steady state within 4–6 weeks (28). Additionally, side chain demethylation by CYP3A4 to N-desmethyl tamoxifen is the principal metabolite in rats and women. Circulating levels at steady state are up to twice the level of the parent drug because the elimination half-life of N-desmethyl tamoxifen is 14 days vs. 7 days for tamoxifen (43). Obviously, drug levels are detectable in patients for many weeks after tamoxifen treatment is stopped. Tamoxifen and its metabolites, as conjugates, are primarily excreted via the bile duct into the feces. Enterohepatic recirculation of hydrolyzed conjugated metabolites has been observed in the rat (45).

The dimethylaminoethoxy side chain of tamoxifen is essential for antiestrogenic activity. Although, N-desmethyl tamoxifen and the deaminated metabolite Y are antiestrogens in laboratory tests, breaking the ether bond to form the phenolic metabolite, metabolite E, results in a change in pharmacology from an antiestrogen to an estrogen (46).

The oral bioavailability of raloxifene, a polyhydroxylated compound, is poor, with about 2% absolute bioavailability of the administered dose. Raloxifene suffers from severe first pass metabolism to the glucuronide conjugates, which are primarily excreted into the feces via enterohepatic cycling. The elimination half-life for raloxifene is 27–37 hours. There is no significant CYP450 metabolism for raloxifene. A new compound targeted for breast cancer treatment, LY 353385, is designed for better bioavailability by protecting one phenolic group through methylation (47). The same principle is used with the novel antiestrogen EM-800 that is metabolically activated by hydrolysis of the ester links to the active agent EM652 (48).

EM 800

EM 652

DISCOVERY OF SELECTIVE ER MODULATION
Overview

In the 1970s, antiestrogen action was correlated with antitumor activity. However, the finding that compounds expressed increased estrogenic properties in mice, i.e., vaginal cornification and increases in uterine weight

(49,50), raised questions about the reason for the species specificity. One obvious possibility was species-specific metabolism, i.e., the mouse converts antiestrogens to estrogens via novel metabolic pathways. However, no species-specific metabolic routes to known estrogens have been identified (51–53), but knowledge of the mouse model created a new dimension for study that ultimately led to the recognition of selective estrogen-receptor modulation or the target-site specificity of antiestrogen molecules.

ER-positive breast cancer cell lines can be heterotransplanted into immune-deficient athymic mice but the cells only grow into tumors with estrogen support. Paradoxically, tamoxifen, an estrogen in the mouse (49), does not support tumor growth (54) but stimulates mouse uterine growth with the same spectrum of metabolites present in both the uterus and the transplanted human breast tumor (55). To explain the selective actions of tamoxifen in different estrogen target tissues of the same host, it was suggested that the ER complex could be interpreted as a stimulatory signal at one site and an inhibitory signal at another site (55). The concept was consolidated with experimental evidence from two further models. First, tamoxifen and raloxifene maintain bone density in the ovariectomized rat (39), but both compounds significantly inhibit estradiol-stimulating increases in uterine weight (39) and, most importantly, prevent carcinogen-induced rat mammary tumorigenesis (38). Second, tamoxifen completely blocks estradiol-stimulated breast tumor growth in athymic mice but tamoxifen alone causes the partial growth of a human endometrial carcinoma transplanted into the same mouse (56). The range of tamoxifen metabolites in the breast and endometrial tumors was found to be the same, so the ER ligand complexes must be interpreted as antagonists or agonist signals in different target tissues.

These observations in the laboratory were translated to clinical medicine to develop SERMs to their full potential.

Clinical Demonstration of SERM Action

Tamoxifen exhibits estrogen-like activity in the postmenopausal woman. Gonadotropins are depressed, antithrombin III is depressed, and estrogen-regulated serum proteins are elevated (28). Tamoxifen causes partial cornification of vaginal epithelium, and there is a modest estrogen-like rise in endometrial cancer risk (57). Most importantly, tamoxifen causes an estrogen-like increase in bone density (58) and this translates into a small decrease in hip and wrist fractures in well women (34). Additionally, tamoxifen causes a drop in low-density lipoprotein (LDL) cholesterol but does not decrease high-density lipoprotein cholesterol (HDL) (59), which may result in a decrease in the incidence of coronary heart disease in high-risk individuals (60). In contrast, tamoxifen causes an antiestrogenic effect in the breast by preventing primary breast cancer (34). Raloxifene also causes a decrease in LDL cholesterol but HDL cholesterol remains the same (61). As a result of these findings, raloxifene is being tested as a preventive for coronary heart disease in high-risk women. Raloxifene maintains bone density in postmenopausal women (62). It is used for the prevention of osteoporosis and reduces spinal fractures. A beneficial side effect is a decrease in the incidence of breast cancer in women taking raloxifene to prevent osteoporosis (63) with no endometrial stimulation (64). The drug is being tested in the STAR trial as a preventive for breast cancer in high-risk postmenopausal women. Both tamoxifen and raloxifene cause an increase in the incidence of hot flashes (an antiestrogenic action), and cause an increased incidence of blood clots (an estrogenic action). The incidence of blood clots is the same as for hormone replacement therapy.

Mechanism of SERM Action

The antiestrogenic and some of the estrogen-like actions of SERMs can be explained by the different confor-

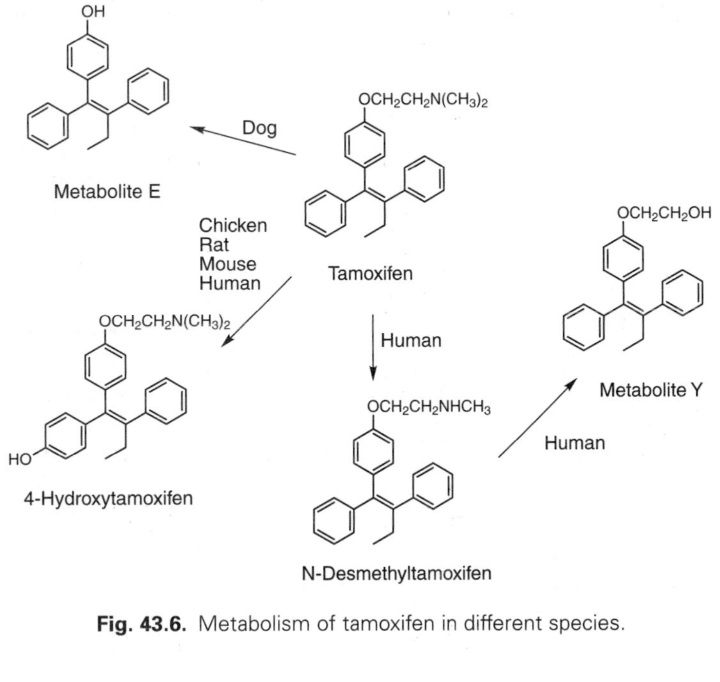

Fig. 43.6. Metabolism of tamoxifen in different species.

mations of the ERα complexes attracting novel coactivators or corepressors to modulate estrogen action at different sites. In this model, the receptor would be the same at each site but coactivators and corepressors would be distributed differently at different targets (65).

Alternatively, ERα could be modulated by different concentrations of ERβ at different sites. It has been suggested that ERβ could enhance estrogen-like gene activation through a protein-protein interaction at AP-1 (*fos* and *jun*) sites (66). At present, it is not precisely clear how SERM action is modulated at each target. Indeed, more than one mechanism may occur.

Tamoxifen Analogs

Knowledge of the structure-activity relationships of tamoxifen and its metabolites has resulted in the development of several analogs for clinical testing (Fig. 43.7). Toremifene (chlorotamoxifen) is available for the treatment of advanced breast cancer in postmenopausal women (67) but has estrogen-like effects to lower circulating cholesterol (68) and to maintain bone density (69). Droloxifene (3-hydroxytamoxifen) has been tested as a breast cancer therapy (70) but also maintains bone density in ovariectomized rats (71). The drug has been tested as an agent for the prevention of osteoporosis but no information is available. Idoxifene is metabolically blocked at the 4 position (72) and builds on the earlier structure-activity relationship studies with tamoxifen (73). The compounds are not metabolically activated to 4-hydroxy derivatives so it was reasoned that the resulting compound idoxifene would be less toxic. Idoxifene has been tested as a breast cancer treatment, but trials for the prevention of osteoporosis were terminated in 1999.

One toxicological concern with tamoxifen is the modest increase in the incidence of endometrial cancer observed in postmenopausal women (57). This estrogen-like effect of tamoxifen, which encourages the detection of

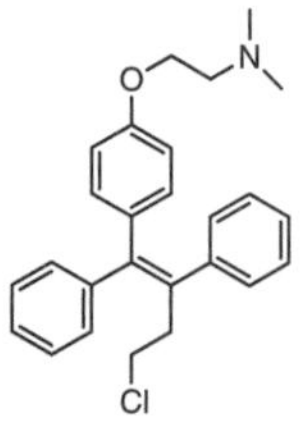

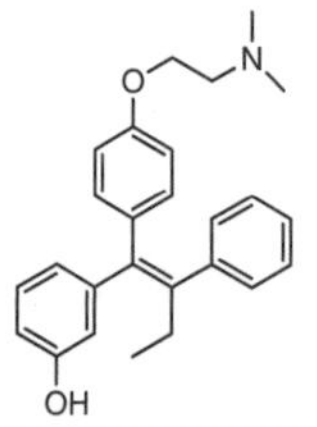

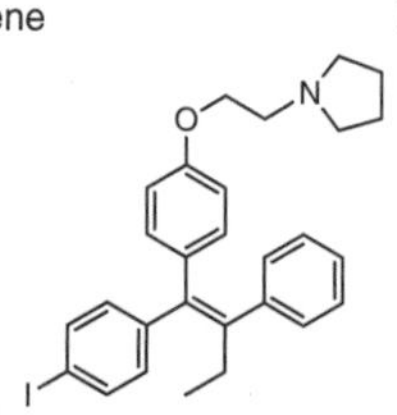

Fig. 43.7. SERM analogs of tamoxifen.

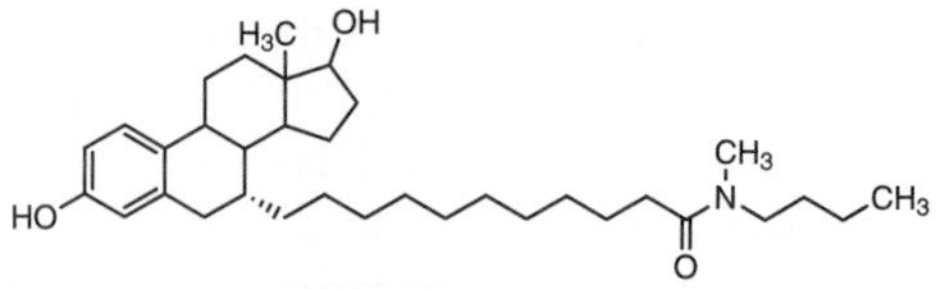

Fig. 43.8. Antiestrogen analogs of estradiol.

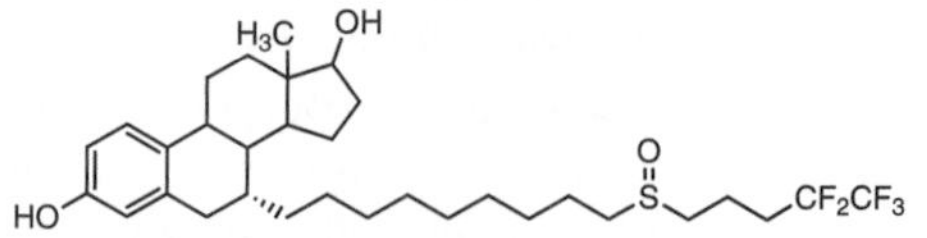

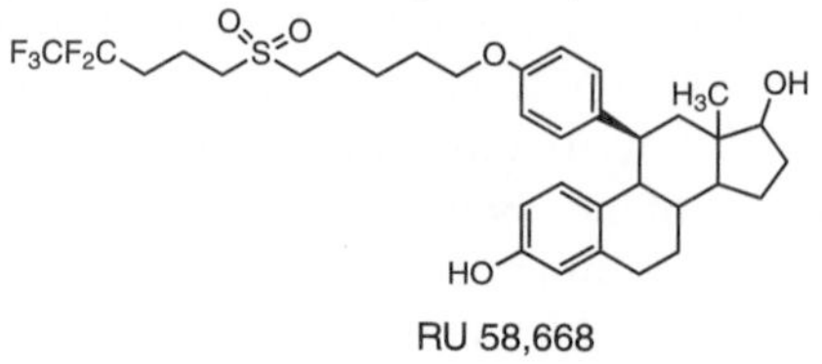

pre-existing disease, increases the normal incidence from 1 endometrial cancer per 1000 women per year to 4 endometrial cancers per 1000 women per year. There is no evidence that any of the SERMs that are tamoxifen analogs will decrease the incidence of endometrial cancer.

Pure Antiestrogens

These compounds do not possess any estrogen-like activity in any species or target tissue. As a result, they cannot be classified as SERMs. The first nonsteroidal antiestrogen, MER25, had virtually no estrogen-like activity in any species or target tissue (21), but it was not until the mid 1980s that the concept was revisited with the discovery of ICI 164,384 (Fig. 43.8) (74). The reason for the reexamination of pure antiestrogens was to outwit drug resistance to tamoxifen. The estrogen-like properties of tamoxifen eventually encouraged the selection of tamoxifen-stimulated clones of breast cancer cells (75) so pure antiestrogens were developed as a second-line endocrine therapy for breast cancer or a more effective first-line treatment for advanced breast cancer. The compound ICI 182,780 (Fig. 43.8) is effective both in the laboratory (76,77) and in clinical trial to prevent the growth of tamoxifen-resistant breast cancers (78). The drug is currently in large-scale clinical trials for the treatment of advanced breast cancer. Side effects appear to be minimal and there is no evidence of uterine stimulation clinically, or for the stimulation of endometrial carcinoma models in the laboratory (79). Faslodex is administered by intramuscular injection once a month. Oral bioavailability is poor, despite metabolic protection with a pentafluoro tip to the hydrophobic side chain, because the steroid is virtually insoluble.

Faslodex has the hydrophobic side chain in the 7α position of estradiol; however, the pure antiestrogen RU

58,688 has an analogous side chain oriented in the 11β position of estradiol (80). The compound is not orally active and has not yet been pursued for clinical applications.

The compound EM-800 is an orally active nonsteroidal drug that is a rigid analog of the triphenylethylene series of antiestrogens. It closely resembles raloxifene with a benzopyran ring substituting for the benzothiophene ring. As previously mentioned, EM-800 is metabolically activated by hydrolysis of the ester links to the active metabolite EM652 (48). However, the structure-activity relationship of the steroidal pure antiestrogens demonstrate that activity is lost if the long hydrophobic side chain is shortened (81). Additionally, the placing of only a dimethylaminoethoxy phenol side chain in the 11β position of estradiol does not result in a pure antiestrogen. The active metabolite EM-652 (48) binds to the ER in a similar manner (82). The drug EM-652, now renamed SC-5705, is being tested as a second-line therapy after tamoxifen treatment failure. However, it is possible that SC-5705 could be a SERM and enjoy a wider application.

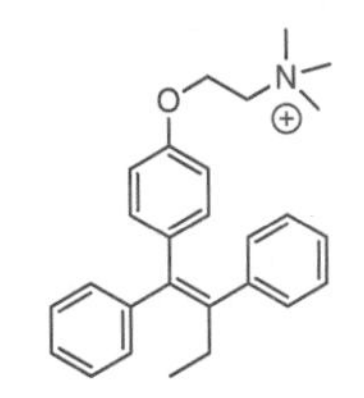

Trimethyltamoxifen 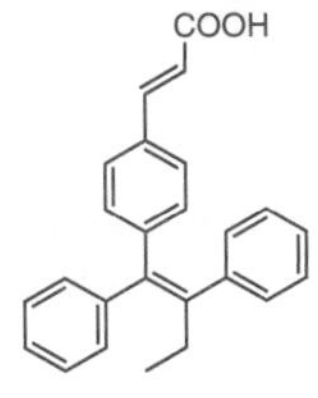   GW 5638

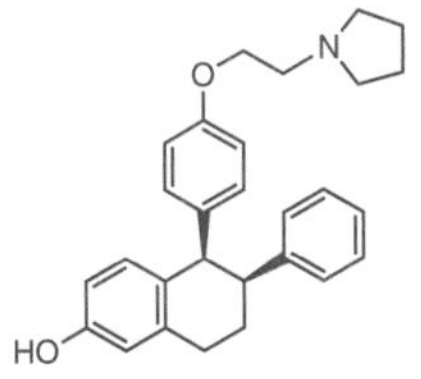

CP 336,156

Fig. 43.9. Novel SERMs.

Novel SERMs

One problem with administering SERMs is that they increase hot flashes and mimic menopausal symptoms, even in women who have passed menopause within the past decade. This effect is considered to be an antiestrogenic action of the drugs. The side effect is believed to be regulated in the brain, so one approach to drug design would be to prevent the compound from crossing the blood-brain barrier. Two drugs, trimethyltamoxifen and GW-5638, are charged molecules that could be peripherally specific (Fig. 43.9). Although trimethyltamoxifen has only been tested in animals (83), GW-5638 is being considered for clinical trials as a breast cancer drug. Laboratory studies show that GW-5638 has bone-sparing properties (84) but virtually no uterotropic activity (85). Clearly, women could take hormone replacement therapy to provide CNS benefit but have peripheral protection from breast and endometrial cancer. Finally, CP336,156, an hydrogenated derivative of a nafoxidine metabolite, has been reported to maintain bone density in rats (86), but there is no evidence of peripheral selectivity.

THE PERFECT SERM

The identification of selective ER modulation has opened the door to the discovery of new drugs and to refine the target site-specific effects of novel molecules. Clearly, an agent that could maintain bone density and protect against coronary heart disease, but at the same time prevent breast and endometrial cancer, is a possibility with the completion of the clinical testing of raloxifene. However, the main problem with administering drugs to well women is the issue of quality of life. SERMs produce an increase in hot flashes, and there is no information about the incidence of Alzheimer's disease with long-term therapy. The ideal agent would be an estrogen in the brain but with an enhanced estrogen-like effect on bones and risk factors for coronary heart disease. The challenge for medicinal chemists will be to retain absolute antiestrogenic action in the breast and uterus.

CASE STUDY

Victoria F. Roche and S. William Zito

LR is a 59-year-old librarian who was diagnosed with stage II invasive ductal adenocarcinoma of the breast eight months ago. She underwent a unilateral radical mastectomy and has just completed a six month course of adriamycin/ cyclophosphamide/fluorouracil chemotherapy. Her cancer was ER positive, and LR's oncologist wants to initiate a prolonged course of anti-estrogen therapy. Since she practices at a major hospital located on a large, research-intensive academic medical center, she has the option of enrolling LR in one of several clinical trials ongoing at the facility, and seeks your guidance.

LR's mother and grandmother suffered from severe osteoporosis and she is considered to be at risk. She is lactose-intolerant and had learned to avoid dairy products long before the availability of *lactobacillus* tablets, so her diet is calcium-poor. Her blood lipid profile had been normal up to menopause, but her LDL levels are now a bit above normal while her HDL levels are slightly below normal. Her cardiovascular health is considered good, but several male relatives have died from myocardial infarcts or strokes. Prior to her diagnosis,

LR was taking phytoestrogens in an attempt to treat the hot flashes she was experiencing with menopause, but has stopped all herbal drugs with the onset of the cancer. Her hot flashes have been troublesome, especially at night, but she considers them minor now that she has the cancer to worry about.

1. *Identify the therapeutic problem(s) where the pharmacist's intervention may benefit the patient.*

2. *Identify and prioritize the patient specific factors that must be considered to achieve the desired therapeutic outcomes.*

3. *Conduct a thorough and mechanistically oriented structure-activity analysis of all therapeutic alternatives provided in the case.*

4. *Evaluate the SAR findings against the patient specific factors and desired therapeutic outcomes and make a therapeutic decision.*

5. *Counsel your patient.*

REFERENCES

1. Jordan VC. Designer estrogens. Sci Am 1998;279: 60–67.
2. Beatson GT. On the treatment of inoperable cases of carcinoma of the mamma: suggestions for a new method of treatment with illustrative cases. Lancet 1896; 2: 104–107.
3. Boyd S. On oophorectomy in cancer of the breast. B M J 1900; ii: 1161–1167.
4. Glascock RF, Hoekstra WG. Selective accumulation of tritium labelled hexoestrol by the reproductive organs of immature female goats and sheep. Biochem J 1959; 72: 673–682.
5. Dodds EC, Lawson W, Noble RL. Biological effects of the synthetic oestrogenic substance 4:4'-dihydroxy-alpha:beta-diethyl-stilbene. Lancet 1938; 1: 1389–1391.
6. Jensen EV, Jacobson HI. Basic guides to the mechanism of estrogen action. Recent Prog Horm Res 1962; 18: 387–414.
7. Toft D, Gorski J. A receptor molecule for estrogens: isolation from the rat uterus and preliminary characterization. Proc Natl Acad Sci U S A 1966; 55: 1574–1581.
8. Jensen EV, Suzuki T, Kawashima T, et al. A two-step mechanism for the interaction of estradiol with rat uterus. Proc Natl Acad Sci U S A 1968; 59: 632–638.
9. Gorski J, Toft D, Shyamala G, et al. Hormone receptors: studies on the interaction of estrogen with the uterus. Recent Prog Horm Res 1968; 24: 45–80.
10. Jensen EV, Block GE, Smith S, et al. Estrogen receptors and breast cancer response to adrenalectomy. Natl Cancer Inst Monogr 1971; 34: 55–70.
11. McGuire WL, Carbone PP, Volliner EP. Estrogen receptors in human breast cancer; New York: Raven Press, 1975.
12. Kuiper GG, Enmark E, Pelto-Huikko M, et al. Cloning of a novel receptor expressed in rat prostate and ovary. Proc Natl Acad Sci U S A 1996; 93: 5925–5930.
13. Gorski J, Welshons W, Sakai D. Remodeling the estrogen receptor model. Mol Cell Endocrinol 1984; 36: 11–15.
14. Kumar V, Chambon P. The estrogen receptor binds tightly to its responsive element as a ligand-induced homodimer. Cell 1988; 55: 145–156.
15. Halachmi S, Marden E, Martin G, et al. Estrogen receptor-associated proteins: possible mediators of hormone- induced transcription. Science 1994; 264: 1455–1458.
16. Jenster G. Coactivators and corepressors as mediators of nuclear receptor function: an update. Mol Cell Endocrinol 1998; 143: 1–7.
17. Kumar V, Green S, Stack G, et al. Functional domains of the human estrogen receptor. Cell 1987; 51: 941–951.
18. Green S, Chambon P. Oestradiol induction of a glucocorticoid-responsive gene by a chimaeric receptor. Nature 1987; 325: 75–78.
19. Brzozowski AM, Pike AC, Dauter Z, et al. Molecular basis of agonism and antagonism in the oestrogen receptor. Nature 1997; 389: 753–758.
20. Kraus WL, McInerney EM, Katzenellenbogen BS. Ligand-dependent, transcriptionally productive association of the amino- and carboxyl-terminal regions of a steroid hormone nuclear receptor. Proc Natl Acad Sci U S A 1995; 92: 12314–12318.
21. Lerner LJ, Holthaus JF, Thompson CR. A non-steroidal estrogen antagonist 1-(p-2-diethylaminoethoxyphenyl)-1-phenyl-2-p-methoxyphenylethanol. Endocrinology 1958; 63: 295–318.
22. Segal JS, Nelson WO. An orally active compound with antifertility effects in rats. Proc Soc Exp Biol Med 1958; 98: 431–436.
23. Lerner LJ. The first non-steroidal antiestrogen-MER 25. Non-steroidal Antioestrogens: Molecular Pharmacology and Antitumour Activity; Sydney, Australia: Sydney Academic Press; 1981; pp 1–6.
24. Holtkamp DE, Greslin SC, Root CA, et al. Gonadotropin inhibiting and antifecundity effects of chloramiphene. Proc Soc Exp Biol Med 1960; 105: 197–201.
25. Greenblatt R, Roy S, Mahesh V. The induction of ovulation. Am J Obstet Gynecol 1962; 84: 900–912.
26. Huppert LC. Induction of ovulation with clomiphene citrate. Fertil Steril 1979; 31: 1–8.
27. Harper MJ, Walpole AL. A new derivative of triphenylethylene: effect on implantation and mode of action in rats. J Reprod Fertil 1967; 13: 101–119.
28. Furr BJ, Jordan VC. The pharmacology and clinical uses of tamoxifen. Pharmacol Ther 1984; 25: 127–205.
29. Legha SS, Carter SK. Antiestrogens in the treatment of breast cancer. Cancer Treat Rev 1976; 3: 205–216.
30. Cole MP, Jones CT, Todd ID. A new anti-oestrogenic agent in late breast cancer. An early clinical appraisal of ICI46474. Br J Cancer 1971; 25: 270–275.
31. Ward HW. Anti-oestrogen therapy for breast cancer: a trial of tamoxifen at two dose levels. Br Med J 1973; 1: 13–14.
32. Lerner LJ, Jordan V C. Development of antiestrogens and their use in breast cancer: Eighth Cain memorial award lecture. Cancer Res 1990; 50: 4177–4189.
33. Osborne CK. Tamoxifen in the treatment of breast cancer. N Engl J Med 1998; 339: 1609–1618.
34. Fisher B, Costantino JP, Wickerham DL, et al. Tamoxifen for prevention of breast cancer: report of the National Surgical Adjuvant Breast and Bowel Project P-1 Study. J Natl Cancer Inst 1998; 90: 1371–1388.
35. Jordan VC, Haldemann B, Allen KE. Geometric isomers of substituted triphenylethylenes and antiestrogen action. Endocrinology 1981; 108: 1353–1361.
36. Jones CD, Suarez T, Massey EH, et al. Synthesis and antiestrogenic activity of [3,4-dihydro-2-(4-methoxyphenyl)-1-naphthalenyl][4-[2-(1-pyrrolidinyl)ethoxy]-phenyl]methanone, methanesulfonic acid salt. J Med Chem 1979; 22: 962–966.
37. Black LJ, Jones CD, Falcone JF. Antagonism of estrogen action with a new benzothiophene derived antiestrogen. Life Sci 1983; 32: 1031–1036.
38. Gottardis MM, Jordan VC. Antitumor actions of keoxifene and tamoxifen in the N-nitrosomethylurea- induced rat mammary carcinoma model. Cancer Res 1987; 47: 4020–4024.
39. Jordan VC, Phelps E, Lindgren JU. Effects of anti-estrogens on bone in castrated and intact female rats. Breast Cancer Res Treat 1987; 10: 31–35.
40. Shiau AK, Barstad D, Loria PM, et al. The structural basis of estrogen receptor/coactivator recognition and the antagonism of this interaction by tamoxifen. Cell 1998; 95: 927–937.
41. Jordan VC. Antiestrogenic action of raloxifene and tamoxifen: today and tomorrow. J Natl Cancer Inst 1998; 90: 967–971.
42. Levenson AS, Jordan VC. The key to the antiestrogenic mechanism of raloxifene is amino acid 351 (aspartate) in the estrogen receptor. Cancer Res 1998; 58: 1872–1875.
43. Jordan VC. Biochemical pharmacology of antiestrogen action. Pharmacol Rev 1984; 36: 245–276.
44. Jordan VC, Collins MM, Rowsby L, et al. A monohydroxylated metabolite of tamoxifen with potent antioestrogenic activity. J Endocrinol 1977; 75: 305–316.
45. Fromson JM, Pearson S, Bramah S. The metabolism of tamoxifen (I.C.I. 46,474). I. In laboratory animals. Xenobiotica 1973; 3: 693–709.
46. Jordan VC, Bain RR, Brown RR, et al. Determination and pharmacology of a new hydroxylated metabolite of tamoxifen observed in patient sera during therapy for advanced breast cancer. Cancer Res 1983; 43: 1446–1450.

47. Munster PN, Buzdar A, Dhingra K, et al. Phase I study of a third-generation selective estrogen receptor modulator, LY353381.HCl, in metastatic breast cancer. J Clin Oncol 2001; 19:2002–2009.

48. Simard J, Sanchez R, Poirier D, et al. Blockade of the stimulatory effect of estrogens, OH-tamoxifen, OH- toremifene, droloxifene, and raloxifene on alkaline phosphatase activity by the antiestrogen EM-800 in human endometrial adenocarcinoma Ishikawa cells. Cancer Res 1997; 57: 3494–3497.

49. Harper MJ, Walpole AL. Contrasting endocrine activities of cis and trans isomers in a series of substituted triphenylethylenes. Nature 1966; 212: 87.

50. Terenius L. Structure-activity relationships of anti-oestrogens with regard to interaction with 17-beta-oestradiol in the mouse uterus and vagina. Acta Endocrinol (Copenh) 1971; 66: 431–447.

51. Lyman SD, Jordan VC. Metabolism of nonsteroidal antiestrogens. Estrogen/Antiestrogen Action and Breast Cancer Therapy; Madison: University of Wisconsin Press; 1986; pp 191–219.

52. Robinson SP, Langan-Fahey SM, Jordan VC. Implications of tamoxifen metabolism in the athymic mouse for the study of antitumor effects upon human breast cancer xenografts. Eur J Cancer Clin Oncol 1989; 25: 1769–1776.

53. Robinson SP, Langan-Fahey SM, Johnson DA, et al. Metabolites, pharmacodynamics, and pharmacokinetics of tamoxifen in rats and mice compared to the breast cancer patient. Drug Metab Dispos 1991; 19: 36–43.

54. Osborne CK, Hobbs K, Clark GM. Effect of estrogens and antiestrogens on growth of human breast cancer cells in athymic nude mice. Cancer Res 1985; 45: 584–590.

55. Jordan VC, Robinson SP. Species-specific pharmacology of antiestrogens: role of metabolism. Fed Proc 1987; 46: 1870–1874.

56. Gottardis MM, Robinson SP, Satyaswaroop PG, et al. Contrasting actions of tamoxifen on endometrial and breast tumor growth in the athymic mouse. Cancer Res 1988; 48: 812–815.

57. Assikis VJ, Neven P, Jordan VC, et al. A realistic clinical perspective of tamoxifen and endometrial carcinogenesis. Eur J Cancer 1996; 32A: 1464–1476.

58. Love RR, Mazess RB, Barden HS, et al. Effects of tamoxifen on bone mineral density in postmenopausal women with breast cancer. N Engl J Med 1992; 326: 852–856.

59. Love RR, Wiebe DA, Newcomb P, et al. Effects of tamoxifen on cardiovascular risk factors in postmenopausal women. Ann Intern Med 1991; 115: 860–864.

60. McDonald CC, Alexander FE, Whyte BW, et al. Cardiac and vascular morbidity in women receiving adjuvant tamoxifen for breast cancer in a randomised trial. The Scottish Cancer Trials Breast Group. BMJ 1995; 311: 977–980.

61. Walsh BW, Kuller LH, Wild RA, et al. Effects of raloxifene on serum lipids and coagulation factors in healthy postmenopausal women. JAMA 1998; 279: 1445–1451.

62. Delmas PD, Bjarnason NH, Mitlak BH, et al. Effects of raloxifene on bone mineral density, serum cholesterol concentrations, and uterine endometrium in postmenopausal women [see comments]. N Engl J Med 1997; 337: 1641–1647.

63. Cummings SR, Eckert S, Krueger KA, et al. The effect of raloxifene on risk of breast cancer in postmenopausal women: results from the MORE randomized trial. Multiple Outcomes of Raloxifene Evaluation. JAMA 1999; 281: 2189–2197.

64. Boss SM, Huster WJ, Neild JA, et al. Effects of raloxifene hydrochloride on the endometrium of postmenopausal women. Am J Obstet Gynecol 1997; 177: 1458–1464.

65. Wijayaratne AL, Nagel SC, Paige LA, et al. Comparative analyses of mechanistic differences among antiestrogens. Endocrinology 1999; 140: 5828–5840.

66. Paech K, Webb P, Kuiper GG, et al. Differential ligand activation of estrogen receptors ERalpha and ERbeta at AP1 sites. Science 1997; 277: 1508–1510.

67. Hayes DF, Van Zyl JA, Hacking A, et al. Randomized comparison of tamoxifen and two separate doses of toremifene in postmenopausal patients with metastatic breast cancer. J Clin Oncol 1995; 13: 2556–2566.

68. Gylling H, Pyrhonen S, Mantyla E, et al. Tamoxifen and toremifene lower serum cholesterol by inhibition of delta 8-cholesterol conversion to lathosterol in women with breast cancer [see comments]. J Clin Oncol 1995; 13: 2900–2905.

69. Saarto T, Blomqvist C, Valimaki M, et al. Clodronate improves bone mineral density in post-menopausal breast cancer patients treated with adjuvant antioestrogens. Br J Cancer 1997; 75: 602–605.

70. Rauschning W, Pritchard KI. Droloxifene, a new antiestrogen: its role in metastatic breast cancer. Breast Cancer Res Treat 1994; 31: 83–94.

71. Ke HZ, Simmons HA, Pirie CM, et al. Droloxifene a new estrogen antagonist/agonist, prevents bone loss in ovariectomized rats. Endocrinology 1995; 136: 2435–2441.

72. McCague R, Parr IB, Haynes BP. Metabolism of the 4-iodo derivative of tamoxifen by isolated rat hepatocytes. Demonstration that the iodine atom reduces metabolic conversion and identification of four metabolites. Biochem Pharmacol 1990; 40: 2277–2283.

73. Allen KE, Clark ER, Jordan VC. Evidence for the metabolic activation of non-steroidal antioestrogens: a study of structure-activity relationships. Br J Pharmacol 1980; 71: 83–91.

74. Wakeling AE, Bowler J. Steroidal pure antioestrogens. J Endocrinol 1987; 112: R7–10.

75. Gottardis MM, Jordan VC. Development of tamoxifen-stimulated growth of MCF-7 tumors in athymic mice after long-term antiestrogen administration. Cancer Res 1988; 48: 5183–5187.

76. Wakeling AE, Dukes M, Bowler J. A potent specific pure antiestrogen with clinical potential. Cancer Res 1991; 51: 3867–3873.

77. Osborne CK, Coronado-Heinsohn EB, Hilsenbeck SG, et al. Comparison of the effects of a pure steroidal antiestrogen with those of tamoxifen in a model of human breast cancer. J Natl Cancer Inst 1995; 87: 746–750.

78. Howell A, DeFriend DJ, Robertson JF, et al. Pharmacokinetics, pharmacological and anti-tumour effects of the specific antioestrogen ICI 182780 in women with advanced breast cancer. Br J Cancer 1996; 74: 300–308.

79. O'Regan RM, Cisneros A, England GM, et al. Effects of the antiestrogens tamoxifen, toremifene, and ICI 182,780 on endometrial cancer growth. J Natl Cancer Inst 1998; 90: 1552–1558.

80. Van de Velde P, Nique F, Planchon P, et al. RU 58668: further in vitro and in vivo pharmacological data related to its antitumoral activity. J Steroid Biochem Mol Biol 1996; 59: 449–457.

81. Bowler J, Lilley TJ, Pittam JD, et al. Novel steroidal pure antiestrogens. Steroids 1989; 54: 71–99.

82. MacGregor-Schafer JI, Liu H, Tonetti DA, et al. The interaction of raloxifene and the active metabolite of the antiestrogen EM-800 (SC 5705) with the human estrogen receptor. Cancer Res 1999; 59: 4308–4313.

83. Biegon A, Brewster M, Degani H, et al. A permanently charged tamoxifen derivative displays anticancer activity and improved tissue selectivity in rodents. Cancer Res 1996; 56: 4328–4331.

84. Willson TM, Henke BR, Momtahen TM, et al. 3-[4-(1,2-Diphenylbut-1-enyl)phenyl]acrylic acid: a non-steroidal estrogen with functional selectivity for bone over uterus in rats. J Med Chem 1994; 37: 1550–1552.

85. Willson TM, Norris JD, Wagner BL, et al. Dissection of the molecular mechanism of action of GW5638, a novel estrogen receptor ligand, provides insights into the role of estrogen receptor in bone. Endocrinology 1997; 138, 3901–3911.

86. Ke HZ, Paralkar VM, Grasser WA, et al. Effects of CP-336,156, a new, nonsteroidal estrogen agonist/antagonist, on bone, serum cholesterol, uterus and body composition in rat models. Endocrinology 1998; 139: 2068–2076.

87. Jordan VC, Jaspan T. Tamoxifen as an antitumour agent: oestrogen binding as a predictive test for tumour response. J Endocrinol 1976; 68: 453–460.

88. Jordan VC, Allen K, Dix CJ. Pharmacology of tamoxifen in laboratory animals. Cancer Treat Rep 1980; 64: 745–759.

89. Jordan VC. Effect of tamoxifen (ICI 46,474) on initiation and growth of DMBA-induced rat mammary carcinomata. Eur J Cancer 1976; 12: 419–424.

90. EBCTCG Tamoxifen for early breast cancer: an overview of the randomised trials. Lancet 1998; 351: 1451–1467.

91. Lacassagne A. Hormonal pathogenesis of adenocarcinoma of the breast. Am J Cancer 1936; 27: 217–225.

pKa Values for Some Drugs and Miscellaneous Organic Acids and Bases
pH Values for Tissue Fluids

DAVID A. WILLIAMS

Table A–1. pKa Values for Some Drugs and Miscellaneous Organic Acids and Bases

| Drug | pKa Values | | Reference |
	HA	HB+	
Acebutolol		9.2	1
Acenocoumarol	4.7		1
Acetaminophen	9.7		1
Acetanilide		0.5	1
Acetazolamide	7.4, 9.1		3
Acetohydroxamic acid	9.4		1
α-Acetylmethadol		8.6	1
Acetysalicylic acid	3.5		1
Acyclovir	9.3	2.3	1
Adriamycin		8.2	1
Ajamaline		8.2	1
Albuterol	10.3	9.3	9
Alclofenac	4.3		1
Alfentanil		6.5	1
Allobarbital	7.8		1
Allopurinol	9.4		1,4
Alphaprodine		8.7	1
Alprenolol		9.7	1,5
Altretamine		10.3	1
Amantadine		9.0	1
Amidinocillin	3.4	8.9	1
Amiloride		8.7	1
Aminoacrine		10.0	1
p-Aminobenzoic acid	4.9	2.5	1
Aminocaproic acid	4.4	10.8	1
Aminohippuric acid	3.8		1
Aminopterin	5.5		1
Aminopyrine		5.0	1
p-Aminosalicylic acid	3.6	1.8	1
Aminothiadiazole		3.2	1
Amiodarone		6.6	1
Amitriptyline		9.4	15
Amobarbital	7.8		1
Amoxapine		7.6	1,4
Amoxicillin	2.4	9.6	12
Amphetamine		10.0	1
Amphotericin B	5.5	10.0	11
Ampicillin	2.5	7.2	16
Anileridine		3.7, 7.5	1
Antazoline		2.5, 10.1	1
Antipyrine		1.5	1
Apomorphine	8.9	7.0	1
Aprobarbital	8.0		1
Ascorbic acid	4.2, 11.6		1
Atenolol		9.6	6
Atropine		9.8	1
Azatadine		9.3	1
Azathioprine	8.0		9
Azlocillin	2.8		1
Aztrenam	0.7, 2.9	3.9	1
Bacampicillin		6.8	1
Baclofen	5.4	9.5	1
Barbital	7.9		1
Bendroflumethiazide	8.5		5

Table A–1. *Continued*

Drug	pK_a Values		Reference
	HA	**HB⁺**	
Benzocaine		2.5	1
Benzphetamine		6.6	1
Benzquinamide		5.9	1
Benztropine		10.0	1
Betahistine		3.5, 9.8	1
Betaprodine		8.7	1
Bethanidine		10.6	1
Bromazepam	11.0	2.9	1
Bromocriptine[a]		9.8	1
Bromodiphenhydramine		4.9	7
Brompheniramine		3.6, 9.8	1
Brucine		8.2, 2.5	1
Bufuralol		8.9	1
Bumetanide	5.2, 10.0		1
Bunolol		9.3	1
Bupivacaine		8.1	1
Bupropion		7.0	8
Burimamide		7.5	1
Butabarbital	7.9		1
Butacaine		9.0	1
Butaclamol		7.2	1
Butamben		5.4	1
Butorphanol		8.6	1
Butylated hydroxytoluene	7.5		1
Butylparaben	8.5		3
Caffeine	>14.0	0.6	1
Camptothecin		10.8	1
Captopril	3.7, 9.8		4
Carbachol		4.8	1
Carbenicillin	2.7		1
Carbenoxolone	6.7, 7.1		1
Carbinoxamine		8.1	1
Carisoprodol		4.2	4
Carpindolol		8.8	1
Cefaclor	1.5	7.2	8
Cefamandole	2.7		9
Cefazolin	2.1		1
Cefoperazone	2.6		4
Cefotaxime	3.4		4
Cefoxitin	2.2		10
Ceftazidime	1.8, 2.7	4.1	11
Ceftizoxime	2.7	2.1	4
Ceftriaxone	3.2, 4.1	3.2	1
Cefuroxime			4
Cephacetrile			3
Cephalexin[b]	3.2		1
L-Cephaloglycin	4.6	7.1	1
Cephaloridine	3.4		1
Cephalothin	2.5		1
Cephapirin			4
Cephradine			4
Chenodiol	4.3		1,4
Chloral hydrate	10.0		16
Chlorambucil	5.8		4
Chlorcyclizine		2.1, 8.2	1
Chlordiazepoxide		4.8	1
Chlorhexidine		10.8	1
Chlorocresol	9.6		1
Chloroquin		8.1, 9.9	1
8-Chlorotheophylline	8.2		1
Chlorothiazide	6.8, 9.5		1
Chlorpheniramine		9.0	1
Chlorphentermine		9.6	1
Chlorpromazine		9.3	1
Chlorpropamide	4.9		1

Continued

Table A–1. *Continued*

Drug	pK$_a$ Values HA	HB$^+$	Reference
Chlorprothixene		8.8, 7.6	16
Chlortetracycline[c]	3.3, 7.4	9.3	1
Chlorthalidone	9.4	1	
Chlorzoxazone	8.3		1
Cimetidine		6.8	1
Cinchonine		4.3, 8.4	1
Ciprofloxacin	6.0	8.8	1
Clindamycin		7.5	9
Clofibrate	3.5		1
Clonazepam	10.5	1.5	1
Clonidine		8.3	1
Clopenthixol		6.7, 7.6	1
Clotrimazole		4.7	10
Cloxacillin	2.8		1
Clozapine		8.0	1
Cocaine		8.7	1
Codeine		8.2	1
Colchicine		1.9	1
Cromolyn	1.1, 1.9		1
Cyanocobalamin		3.4	9
Cyclacillin	2.7	7.5	4
Cyclazocine		9.4	1
Cyclizine		8.0, 2.5	1
Cyclobarbital	8.6		1
Cyclobenzapine		8.5	1
Cyclopentamine		11.5	1
Cyclopentolate		7.9	1
Cycloserine		4.5, 7.4	1
Cyclothiazide[c]	9.1, 10.5		1
Cyproheptadine		8.9	4
Cytarabine		4.3	1
Dacarbazine		4.4	1
Dantrolene	7.5		1
Dapsone		1.3, 2.5	1
Daunorubicin		8.4	1,4
Debrisoquin		11.9	1
Dehydrocholic acid	5.12		1
Demeclocycline	3.3, 7.2	9.4	1
Demoxepam		4.5, 10.6	1
Deserpidine[d]		6.7	1
Desipramine		10.4	1
Dextroamphetamine		9.9	1
Dextrobrompheniramine		9.3	1
Dextrochlorpheniramine		9.2	1
Dextrofenfluramine		9.1	1
Dextroindoprofen	4.6		1
Dextromethorphan		8.3	1
Dextromoramide		7.0	1
Diacetylmorphine (heroin)		7.8	1
Diatrizoic acid	3.4		1
Diazepam		3.4	1
Diazoxide	8.5		1
Dibenzepin		8.3	8
Dibucaine		8.9	1
Dichlorphenamide	7.4, 8.6		1
Diclofenac	4.5		1
Dicloxacillin	2.8		1
Dicoumarol	4.4, 8.0		1
Dicyclomine		9.0	1
Diethazine		9.1	1
Diethylcarbamazepine		7.7	1
Diflunisal	3.0		1
Dihydroergocriptine		6.9	1
Dihydroergocristine		6.9	1
Dihydroergotamine		6.9	1

Table A–1. *Continued*

Drug	pK$_a$ Values		Reference
	HA	HB$^+$	
Dihydrostreptomycin		7.8	1
Dilevolol		9.5	1
Diltiazem		7.7	1
Dimethadione	6.1		1
Dimethisoquin		6.3	1
Dinoprost[e]	4.9		1
Dinoprostone	4.6		1
Diperodon		8.4	11
Diphenhydramine		9.1	1
Diphenoxylate		7.1	1
Diphenylpyraline		8.9	1
Dipipanone		8.5	1
Dipyridamole		6.4	1
Disopyramide	10.2	8.4	1
Dobutamine		9.5	1,4
Dopamine	10.6	8.9	1
Doxepin		9.0	1
Doxorubicin		8.2, 10.2	1
Doxycycline	3.4, 7.7	9.5	1
Doxylamine		4.4, 9.2	1
Droperidol		7.6	1
Emetine		8.2, 7.4	1
Enalapril	3.0	5.5	1
Enalaprilat	2.3, 3.4	8.0	1
Ephedrine		9.6	1
Epinephrine	8.9	10.0	1
Ergometrine		7.3	1
Ergonovine		6.8	1
Ergotamine		6.4	1
Erythromycin		8.8	1
Estrone[f]	10.8		13
Ethacrynic acid	3.50		1
Ethambutol		6.3, 9.5	1
Ethoheptazine		8.5	1
Ethopropazine		9.6	1
Ethosuximide	9.5		1
Ethoxazolamide	8.1		1
Ethyl biscoumacetate	7.5		1
Ethylmorphine		8.2	1
Ethylnorepinephrine		8.4	1
Etidocaine		7.9	1
Etileprine	9.0	10.2	1
Etomidate		4.2	1
Eugenol	9.8		1
Fenclofenac	4.5		1
Fenfluramine		9.1	1
Fenoterol	10.0	8.6	1
Fenprofen	4.5		1
Fentanyl		8.4	14
Floxuridine	7.4		1
Flubiprofen	4.3		1
Flucloxacillin	2.7		1
Flucytosine	10.7	2.9	1
Flufenamic acid	3.9		10
Flumizole	10.7		1
Flunitrazepam		1.8	1
Fluorouracil	8.0, 13.0		1
Flupenthixol		7.8	1
Fluphenazine enanthate		3.5, 8.2	1
Fluphenazine		3.9, 8.1	1
Flupromazine		9.2	1
Flurazepam	8.2	1.9	1
Furosemide	3.9		1
Fusidic acid	5.4		1
Gentamicin[b]		8.2	1

Continued

Table A–1. *Continued*

Drug	pK$_a$ Values		Reference
	HA	HB$^+$	
Glibenclamide	5.3		9
Glipizide	5.9		1
Glutethimide	9.2		1
Glyburide	5.3		1
Glycyclamine		5.5	1
Guanethidine		8.3, 11.9	1
Guanoxan		12.3	1
Haloperidol		8.3	1
Hexetidine		8.3	12
Hexobarbital	8.2		1
Hexylcaine		9.1	1
Hexylresorcinol	9.5		1
Hippuric acid	3.6		1
Histamine		5.9, 9.8	1
Homatropine		9.7	1
Hycanthone		3.4	1
Hydralazine		0.5, 7.1	1
Hydrochlorothiazide	7.0, 9.2		1
Hydrocodone		8.9	1
Hydrocortisone sodium succinate	5.1		1
Hydroflumethiazide	8.9, 10.7		1
Hydromorphone		8.2	1
Hydroquinone	10.0, 12.0		1
Hydroxyamphetamine		9.3	1
Hydroxyzine		2.0, 7.1	1
Hyoscyamine		9.7	1
Ibuprofen	5.2		1
Idoxuridine	8.3		1
Imipramine		9.5	1
Indapamide	8.8		5
Indomethacin	4.5		1
Indoprofen	5.8		1
Indoramin		7.7	1
Iocetamic acid[g]	4.1 or 4.3		4
Iodipamide	3.5		1
Iodoquinol	8.0		1
Iopanoic acid	4.8		4
Iprindole	8.2		1
Ipronidazole		2.7	1
Isocarboxazid		10.4	1
Isoniazid		2.0, 3.5, 10.8	1
Isoproterenol	10.1, 12.1	8.6	1
Isoxsuprine	9.8	8.0	1
Kanamycin		7.2	1
Ketamine		7.5	1,11
Ketobemidone		8.7	1
Ketoconazole		2.9, 6.5	1,4
Ketoprofen[h]	4.8		1,9
Labetalol	8.7	7.4	1
Leucovorin	3.1, 8.1, 10.4		1
Levallorphan tartrate	4.5	6.9	1
Levobunolol		9.2	1
Levodopa	2.3, 9.7, 13.4	8.7	1
Levomethorphan		8.3	1
Levomoramide		7.0	1
Levonordefrin	9.8	8.6	1
Levopropoxyphene		6.3	1
Levorphanol		9.2	1
Levothyroxine	2.2, 6.7	10.1	1
Lidocaine		7.8	1
Lincomycin		7.5	1
Liothyronine	8.4		1
Lisinopril	1.7, 3.3, 11.1	7.0	1
Loperamide		8.6	1

Table A–1. *Continued*

Drug	pK_a Values		Reference
	HA	HB⁺	
Lorazepam	11.5	1.3	1
Loxapine		6.6	1
Lysergide		7.5	1
Maprotiline		10.2	4
Mazindol		8.6	1
Mecamylamine		11.2	1
Mechlorethamine		6.4	1
Meclizine		3.1, 6.2	1
Meclofenamic acid	4.0		4
Medazepam		6.2	1
Mefenamic acid	4.2		1
Mepazine		9.3	1
Meperidine		8.7	1
Mephentermine		10.4	1
Mephobarbital	7.7		1
Mepindolol		8.9	1
Mepivacaine		7.7	1
Mercaptomerin	3.7, 5.1		1
Mercaptopurine	7.8	11.0	1
Mesalamine	2.7	5.8	1
Mesna	9.1		1
Metaproterenol	11.8	8.8	1
Metaraminol		8.6	1
Methacycline	3.5, 7.6	9.5	1
Methadone		8.3	1
Methamphetamine		10.0	1
Methapyrilene		3.7, 8.9	1
Methaqualone		2.5	1
Metharbital	8.2		1
Methazolamide	7.3		1
Methdilazine		7.5	1
Methenamine		4.8	4
Methicillin	3.0		1
Methohexital	8.3		1
Methotrexate	3.8, 4.8	5.6	1
Methotrimeprazine		9.2	1
Methoxamine		9.2	1
Methoxyphenamine		10.1	1
Methyclothiazide	9.4		1
Methyl nicotinate		3.1	1
Methyl paraben	8.4		1
Methyl salicylate	9.9		1
Methyldopa	2.3, 10.4, 12.6	9.2	1
Methylergonovine		6.6	1
Methylphenidate		8.8	1
Methylthiouracil	8.2		1
Methyprylon	12.0		1
Methysergide		6.62	1
Metoclopramide		0.6, 9.3	1
Metolazone	9.7		1
Metopon		8.1	1
Metoprolol		9.7	1
Metronidazole		2.6	4
Metyrosine	2.7, 10.1		1
Mexiletine		9.1	1
Mezlocillin	2.7		1
Miconazole		6.7	1
Midazolam		6.2	1
Minocycline	2.8, 5.0, 7.8	9.5	1
Minoxidil		4.6	4
Mitomycin		10.9	1
Molindone		6.9	1
Morphine	9.9	8.0	1
Moxalactam	2.5, 7.7, 10.2		4

Continued

Table A–1. *Continued*

Drug	pK_a Values HA	pK_a Values HB⁺	Reference
Nabilone[b]	13.5		9
Nadolol		9.4	5
Nafcillin	2.7		1
Nalbuphine	10.0	8.7	4
Nalidixic acid	6.0		1
Nalorphine		7.8	1
Naloxone		7.9	1
Naphazoline		10.9	1
Naproxen	4.2		1
Natamycin	4.6	8.4	8
Neostigmine		12.0	1
Niacin	2.0	4.8	1
Nicotinamide		0.5, 3.4	1
Nicotine		3.1, 8.0	1
Nikethamide		3.5	1
Nitrazepam	10.8	3.2	1
Nitrofurantoin	7.1		1
Norcodeine		5.7	1
Nordefrin	9.8	8.5	1
Norepinephrine	9.8, 12.0	8.6	1,2
Norfenephrine		8.7	1
Normorphine		9.8	1
Nortriptyline		9.7	1
Noscapine		6.2	1
Novobiocin	4.3, 9.1		1
Nystatin[i]	8.9	5.1	11
Octopamine	9.5	8.9	1
Orphenadrine		8.4	1
Oxacillin	2.7		1
Oxazepam	11.6	1.8	
Oxprenolol		9.5	5
Oxybutynin		7.0	4
Oxycodone		8.9	1
Oxymorphone	9.3	8.5	1
Oxyphenbutazone	4.7		1
Oxypurinol	7.7		1
Oxytetracycline[c]	3.3, 7.3	9.1	1
Pamaquine		1.3, 3.5, 10.0	1
Papaverine		6.4	1
Pargyline		6.9	1
Pemoline		10.5	1,2
Penbutolol[c]		9.3	1
Penicillamine	1.8, 10.5	7.9	1
Penicillin G	2.8		1
Penicillin V	2.7		1
Pentamidine		11.4	4
Pentazocine	10.0	8.5	2,9
Pentobarbital	8.1		1
Pentoxiphylline		0.3	1
Perphenazine		3.7, 7.8	1
Phenacetin		2.2	1
Phenazocine		8.5	1
Phencyclidine		8.5	2
Phendimetrazine		7.6	1
Phenethicillin	2.8		1
Phenformin		2.7, 11.8	1
Phenindamine		8.3	1
Phenindione	4.1		1
Pheniramine		4.2, 9.3	1
Phenmetrazine		8.5	1
Phenobarbital	7.4		1
Phenolphthalein	9.7		1
Phenolsulfonphthalein	8.1		1
Phenothiazine		2.5	1
Phenoxybenzamine		4.4	4

Table A–1. *Continued*

Drug	pK$_a$ Values		Reference
	HA	HB$^+$	
Phenoxypropazine		6.9	1
Phentermine		10.1	1
Phentolamine		7.7	1
Phenylbutazone	4.5		1
Phenylephrine	10.1	8.8	1
Phenylpropanolamine		9.4	1
Phenyltoloxamine		9.1	1
Phenyramidol		5.9	1
Phenytoin	8.3		1
Physostigmine		2.0, 8.2	1
Pilocarpine		1.6, 7.1	1
Pimozide		7.3, 8.6	1
Pindolol		8.8	1
Piperazine		5.6, 9.8	1
Pipradrol		9.7	1
Pirbuterol		3.0, 7.0, 10.3	1
Piroxicam	4.6		1
Pivampicillin		7.0	1
Polymyxin		8.9	1
Polythiazide	9.8		1
Practolol		9.5	1
Pralidoxime		7.9	1
Pramoxine		6.2	1
Prazepam		2.9	1
Prazosin		6.5	1
Prenalterol	10.0	9.5	1
Prilocaine		7.9	1
Probenecid	3.4		1
Procainamide		9.2	1
Procaine		8.8	1
Procarbazine		6.8	1
Prochlorperazine		3.7, 8.1	1
Promazine		9.4	1
Promethazine		9.1	1
Proparacaine		3.2	11
Propiomazine		9.1	1
Propoxycaine		8.6	1
Propoxyphene		6.3	1
Propranolol		9.5	1
Propylhexedrine		10.4	1
Propylthiouracil	7.8		1
Pseudoephedrine		9.5	1
Pyrathiazine		8.9	1
Pyrazinamide		0.5	1
Pyridoxine	8.96	5.0	1
Pyrilamine		4.0, 8.9	1
Pyrimethamine		7.3	1
Pyrrobutamine		8.8	1
Quinacrine		8.2, 10.2	1
Quinethazone	9.3, 10.7		1
Quinidine		4.2, 7.9	1
Quinine		4.2, 8.5	1
Ranitidine		2.3, 8.2	4
Rescinnamine		6.4	4
Reserpine		6.6	1
Rifampin	1.7	7.9	1
Rimoterol	10.3	8.7	1
Ritodrine		9.0	1
Rolitetracycline	7.4		1
Rotoxamine		8.1	1
Saccharin	1.6		1
Salicylamide	8.2		3
Salicylic acid	3.0, 13.4		1
Salsalate	3.5, 9.8		1,2
Scopolamine		7.6	1

Continued

Table A–1. *Continued*

Drug	pK$_a$ Values		Reference
	HA	HB$^+$	
Secobarbital	7.9, 12.6		1
Serotonin	9.8	4.9, 9.1	1
Sotalol	8.5	9.8	1
Sparteine		4.8, 12.0	1
Spiperone		8.3, 9.1	1
Streptozocin		1.3	4
Strychnine		2.3, 8.0	1
Succinylsulfathiazole	4.5		1
Sufentanil		8.0	4
Sulfacetamide	5.4	1.8	1
Sulfadiazine	6.5	2.0	1
Sulfadimethoxine	6.7	2.0	1
Sulfaguanidine	12.1	2.8	1
Sulfamerazine	7.1	2.3	1
Sulfamethazine	7.4	2.4	1
Sulfamethizole	5.5	2.0	1
Sulfamethoxazole	5.6		1
Sulfaphenazole	6.5	1.9	1
Sulfapyridine	8.43	2.6	1
Sulfasalazine	2.4, 9.7, 11.8		1
Sulfathiazole	7.1	2.4	1
Sulfinpyrazone	2.8		1
Sulfisoxazole	5.0		1
Sulindac	4.5		1
Sulpiride		9.1	1
Sulthiame	10.0		1
p-Synephrine	10.2	9.3	1
Talbutal	7.8		1
Tamoxifen		8.9	4
Temazepam		1.6	1
Terbutaline	10.1, 11.2	8.8	1
Tetracaine		8.4	1
Tetracycline	3.3, 7.7	9.7	1
Tetrahydrocannabinol (THC)	10.6		2
Tetrahydrozoline		10.5	1
Thenyldiamine		3.9, 8.9	1
Theobromine	10.1	0.1	1
Theophylline	8.6	3.5	1
Thiazbendazole		4.7	4
Thiamine		4.8, 9.0	1
Thiamylal	7.5		1
Thioguanine	8.2		3
Thiopental	7.5		1
Thiopropazate		3.2, 7.2	1
Thioridazine		9.5	1
Thiothixene		7.7, 7.9	1
Thiouracil	7.5		1
Thonzylamine		2.2, 9.0	1
L-Thyroxine	2.2, 6.7	10.1	1
Ticarcillin	2.6, 3.4		1
Ticrynafen	2.7		1
Timolol		8.8	1
Timoprazole		3.1, 8.8	1
Tiotidine		6.8	1
Tiprofenic acid	30.		1
Tobramycin		6.7, 8.3, 9.9	2
Tocainide		7.5	1
Tolamolol		7.9	5
Tolazamide	3.1	5.7	1
Tolazoline		10.3	1
Tolbutamide	5.4		1
Tolmetin	3.5		1
Tramzoline		10.7	1
Tranylcypromine		8.2	1
Trazodone		6.7	1

Table A–1. *Continued*

Drug	pK_a Values HA	HB+	Reference
Triamterene		6.2	1
Trichlormethiazide	8.6		1
Trifluperazine		3.9, 8.1	1,3
Triflupromazine		9.2	1
Trimeprazine		9.0	1
Trimethobenzamide		8.3	1
Trimethoprim		6.6	3
Trimipramine		8.0	4
Tripelennamine		4.2, 8.7	1
Triprolidine		6.5	1
Troleandomycin		6.6	1
Tromethamine		8.1	1
Tropicamide		5.3	1
Tuaminoheptane		10.5	1
Tubocurarine		8.1, 9.1	1
Tyramine	10.9	9.3	1
Valproic acid	4.8		1,3
Verapamil		8.9	1
Vidarabine		3.5, 12.5	1
Viloxazine		8.1	1
Vinbarbital	8.0		1
Vinblastine		5.4, 7.4	1
Vincristine[j]		5.0, 7.4	1
Vindesine		6.0, 7.7	1
Warfarin	5.1		1
Xylometazoline		10.2	1
Zimeldine		3.8, 8.74	1

Miscellaneous Organic Acids and Bases

Drug	pK_a Values HA	HB+	Reference
Acetic acid	4.8		
Allylamine		10.7	
6-Aminopenicillanic acid	2.3	4.9	
Ammonia		9.3	
Aniline		4.6	
Benzoic acid	4.2		
Benzyl alcohol	18.0		
Benzylamine		9.3	
Butyric acid	4.8		
Carbonic acid	6.4, 10.4		
Citric acid	3.1, 4.8, 5.4		
Diethanolamine		8.9	
Diethylamine		11.0	
Dimethylamine		10.7	
p-Dimethylaminobenzoic acid	5.1		
Ethanol	15.6		
Ethanolamine		9.5	
Ethylamine		10.7	
Ethylenediamine		7.2, 10.0	
Fumaric acid	3.0, 4.4		
Gluconic acid	3.6		
Glucuronic acid	3.2		
Guanidine		13.6	
Imidazole		7.0	
Isopropylamine		10.6	
Lactic acid	3.9		
Maleic acid	1.9		
Mandelic acid	3.4		
Monochloroacetic acid	2.9		
N-propylamine		10.6	
Nitromethane	11.0		
Phenol	9.9		
Phthalic acid	2.9		
Resorcinol	9.2, 11.3		

Continued

Table A–1. *Continued*

Miscellaneous Organic Acids and Bases	HA	HB+
Sorbic acid	4.8	
Succinimide	9.6	
Tartaric acid	3.0, 4.4	
p-Toluidine		5.3
Trichloroacetic acid	0.9	
Triethanolamine		7.8
Triethylamine		10.7
Tropic acid	4.1	
Tropine		10.4
Uric acid	5.4	

[a] Determined in methyl cellosolve-water, 8:2 w/w mixture.
[b] Determined in 66% dimethylformamide.
[c] Determined in 25–30% ethanol.
[d] Determined in 40% methanol.
[e] Prostaglandin $F_{2\alpha}$.
[f] Spectrophotometric determination.
[g] The pK_a values are 4.1 for two and 4.25 for two of the four optical isomers.
[h] Determined in methanol-water, 3:1 mixture.
[i] Determined in dimethylformamide-water, 1:1 mixture.
[j] Determined in 33% dimethylformamide.

Table A.2. pH Values for Tissue Fluids

Fluid	pH
Aqueous humor	7.2
Blood, arterial	7.4
Blood, venous	7.4
Blood, maternal umbilical	7.3
Cerebrospinal fluid	7.4
Colon[a]	
fasting	5–8
fed	5–8
Duodenum[a]	
fasting	4.4–6.6
fed	5.2–6.2
Feces[b]	7.1 (4.6–8.8)
Ileum[a]	
fasting	6.8–8.6
fed	6.8–8.0
Intestine, microsurface	5.3
Lacrimal fluid (tears)	7.4
Milk, breast	7.0
Muscle, skeletal[c]	6.0
Nasal secretions	6.0
Prostatic fluid	6.5
Saliva	6.4
Semen	7.2
Stomach[a]	
fasting	1.4–2.1
fed	3–7
Sweat	5.4
Urine	5.8 (5.5–7.0)
Vaginal secretions, premenopause	4.5
Vaginal secretions, postmenopause	7.0

[a] Dressman JB, Amidon GL, Reppas C, Shah UP. Dissolution testing as a prognostic tool for oral drug absorption. Pharm, Res, 1998; 15:11–22.
[b] Value for normal soft, formed stools; hard stools tend to be more alkaline, whereas watery, unformed stools are acidic.
[c] Studies conducted intracellularly on the rat.

REFERENCES

1. C. Hansch, et al., *Comprehensive Medicinal Chemistry*, Vol. 6, New York, Pergamon Press, 1990.
2. A. Albert and EP Serjeant, *The Determination of Ionization Constants*, 3rd ed., New York, Chapman and Hall, 1984.
3. Merck Index, 11th ed., Rahway, N.J., Merck and Co., 1989.
4. G.K. McEvoy, Ed., *American Hospital Formulary Service: Drug Information 2000*, Bethesda, American Society of Hospital Pharamcists, 2000.
5. P.H. Welling, et al., *J. Pharmacokinet. Biopharm., 12*, 263 (1984).
6. K. Florey, Ed., *Analytical Profiles of Drug Substances*, Vol. 13, New York, Academic Press, 1984.
7. Ibid., Vol. 8, 1979.
8. Ibid., Vol. 9, 1980.
9. Ibid., Vol. 10, 1981.
10. Ibid., Vol. 11, 1982.
11. Ibid., Vol. 6, 1977.
12. Ibid., Vol. 7, 1978.
13. Ibid., Vol. 12, 1983.
14. Ibid., Vol. 5, 1976.
15. Ibid., Vol. 3, 1974.
16. Ibid., Vol. 2, 1973.

SUGGESTED READINGS

A. Albert and E.P. Serjeant, *The Determination of Ionization Constants*, 3rd ed., New York, Chapman and Hall, 1984.

A. Martin, *Physical Pharmacy*, 4th ed., Philadelphia, Lea & Febiger, 1993.

Drug Index

Page numbers followed by "f" indicate illustrations and chemical structures; those followed by "t" indicate tables. Drugs are listed under the generic name.

Subject Index